2007 Product Alert

Ingenix Has You Covered!

April ICD-9-CM Updates
With semi-annual ICD-9-CM changes effective April 1 and October 1, it is more important than ever to have up-to-date ICD-9-CM coding information in order to stay in compliance with HIPAA regulations. Ingenix is committed to providing you and your staff with the ICD-9-CM code update information you need to code accurately and efficiently. We are offering several ways to make sure you are always up-to-date.

- **Updateable *Expert* ICD-9-CM code books.**
  The February update will have any new April 1 codes.

- **Annual *Expert* and *Professional ICD-9-CM* editions.**
  Just visit *Ingenix Online* and look for the ICD-9, CPT® and HCPCS Alerts link under the Quick Access Resources menu.

  No extra charges for code changes. No additional cost for updated books. No hassle for you or your staff.

Revised Coding Guidelines
Revised official ICD-9-CM guidelines have been released and became effective December 1, 2005. Significant revisions were made to chapter-specific guidelines, the V code table and the use of terminology.

Only this set of guidelines, approved by the Cooperating Parties, is official. Adherence to these guidelines when assigning ICD-9-CM diagnosis and procedure codes is required under the Health Insurance Portability and Accountability Act (HIPAA).

Medicare Code Edits Notice
Not all Medicare edits for the new 2007 ICD-9-CM codes were released in time to be published in this edition. Once these edits are released we will post them on our Web site. Please visit www.ingenixonline.com and click on the ICD-9, CPT® and HCPCS Alerts link under the Quick Access Resources menu to view these edits.

Online Quick Access Resources
Ingenix is committed to providing you with current coding information. Ingenix hopes to assist you in correct application of coding conventions and guidelines in order to support your coding practices, training processes and ongoing quality and compliance initiatives. Included in these free resources are informative articles, regulatory updates and clinical coding scenarios that you can use to keep your facility, practice and staff informed on the latest changes.

Visit *Ingenix Online,* look for the Quick Access Resources menu and click on the Code This! and Ingenix Insights: Free eAlerts links to take advantage of the following free informative resources.

Code This!: Practical clinical coding scenarios demonstrate accurate classification of codes based on interpretation of documentation in compliance with official coding guidelines and conventions. These scenarios often reflect correct application of new codes and changes or updates of official coding guidelines in a clinical format. This feature is updated monthy.

Ingenix Insights: Free eAlerts: Access coding, billing and reimbursement analysis and breaking news that matters to you. These articles include regulatory, policy and other timely topics. Visit often for late-breaking news.

CPT is a registered trademark of the American Medical Association.

2007 Web Products — INGENIX

SAVE 5% when you order online—use source code FOBW7.

SAVE MORE and qualify for REWARDS when you order at IngenixOnline.com.

HERE ARE THE TOP THREE REASONS TO PLACE YOUR ORDER ONLINE:

1. Save an additional 5% when you order online*—use source **FOBW7**.
2. Get rewards for every $500 you spend at Ingenix Online with our eSmart program.**
3. Experience a quick, hassle-free purchase process with streamlined checkout options.

ingenix online frequent buyer program

Get rewards when you order online.

Ingenix eSmart is a program designed to reward our best Ingenix Online customers. If you are a registered online customer and qualify to participate**, all you have to do is use the returning customer checkout option for your web purchases every time you shop online. We keep track of your purchases. Once you reach $500, we send you a FREE product—it's that easy!

If you are not yet registered, go to IngenixOnline.com and register right away so we can get you started with the Ingenix eSmart program.

Are you part of our Medallion program?

Ingenix Online has enhanced options for you, for a hassle-free, streamlined purchase and account management experience!

To view your enhanced online account options, simply register with us at IngenixOnline.com. You will then be able to easily place orders from your Price List, get access to your purchase history, track shipments, change your profile, manage your address book and much more.

Could you benefit from an easy, quick way to consolidate orders for your company?

The Ingenix web-based consolidation tool is designed to streamline the purchasing process and enhance your productivity. For more information log into your account or visit www.ingenixonline.com/orderconsolidation.

(*) Additional 5% savings offer valid online, cannot be combined with any other offer and is not applicable to Partner accounts. Bookstore products, package items, eLearning products, Academy Credential Study Guides, online exams, Worker's Compensation items and conferences not included. For Medallion accounts, we compare the Price List discounts against the offer discounts and honor the better of the two.

(**) eSmart program valid for Ingenix customers who are NOT part of Medallion or Partner Accounts programs. You must be registered at Ingenix Online to have your online purchases tracked for rewards purposes. Shipping charges and taxes still apply and cannot be used for rewards. eSmart reward offers valid online only.

100% Money Back Guarantee

If our merchandise* ever fails to meet your expectations, please contact our Customer Service Department toll-free at 1.800.INGENIX (464.3649), option 1, for an immediate response. *Software and Data File: Credit will be granted for unopened packages only.

SAVE 5% when you order at www.ingenixonline.com (reference source code FOBW7)

or call toll-free 1.800.INGENIX (464.3649), option 1.

Also available from your medical bookstore or distributor.

FOBA7

2007 Web Products   **INGENIX**®

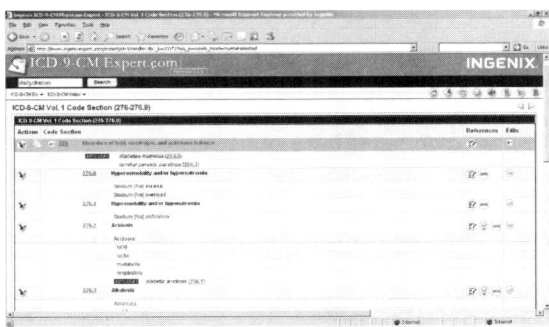

Fast Code Look Up and Access to Real-Time Updates All Year.

ICD-9-CM Expert.com for Physicians
Item No.: 1402 $79.95*
Available: Now   *Call for multi-user pricing.

ICD-9-CM Expert.com for Hospitals
Item No.: 1403 $89.95*
Available: Now   *Call for multi-user pricing.

CPT® Expert.com
Item No.: 1400 $74.95*
Available: Now   *Call for multi-user pricing.

HCPCS Expert.com
Item No.: 1401 $69.95*
Available: Now   *Call for multi-user pricing.

The *Expert.com* applications allow you to reference the same codes, edits, tables and indexes that appear in our *Expert* code books. Affordable and convenient, these online solutions deliver every code description, guideline and instruction you need.

- **Look up codes faster than ever.** Locate the code you need with a term search, or scroll through the index to access sections from the code book.

- **Get user-friendly guidance from Ingenix and Medicare with color code edits, guidelines and instructions.** Spend less time searching for information; avoid having to thumb through multiple pages or various books.

- **Up-to-date code descriptions and clinical information.** Code more confidently by accessing always up-to-date information, extensive appendices, commonly miscoded procedures, Medicare requirements and glossaries with a click of the mouse.

- **Anatomical illustrations.** Large display of anatomical illustrations on your screen will help you to better understand procedures and anatomy, so you can make the best possible coding selection.

CPT is a registered trademark of the American Medical Association.

CPT® Expert.com is not a replacement for the American Medical Associations' CPT® 2007 Standard or Professional code books.

100% Money Back Guarantee
If our merchandise* ever fails to meet your expectations, please contact our Customer Service Department toll-free at 1.800.INGENIX (464.3649), option 1, for an immediate response. *Software: Credit will be granted for unopened packages only.

SAVE 5% when you order at www.ingenixonline.com (reference source code FOBW7)
or call toll-free 1.800.INGENIX (464.3649), option 1.
Also available from your medical bookstore or distributor.

FOBA7

2007 Web Products — INGENIX

Online Code Lookup Across ICD-9-CM, CPT® and HCPCS Level II Code Sets.

EncoderPro.com (Single User)
Item No.: 1137 — $249.95*
*Call for multi-user pricing.
Available: Now

EncoderPro.com Professional (Single User)
Item No.: 1221 — $499.95*
*Call for multi-user pricing.
Available: Now

EncoderPro.com Expert (Single User)
Item No.: 1127 — $899.95*
*Call for multi-user pricing.
Available: Now

EncoderPro.com is the coder's essential CPT®, ICD-9-CM and HCPCS online code lookup software, providing users with fast search capabilities across all three code sets in real time.

- **Ingenix Edge — Ingenix CodeLogic™ search engine.** Search all three code sets simultaneously using lay terms, acronyms, abbreviations and even misspelled words.

- **Ingenix Edge — Receive *Coders' Desk Reference* lay descriptions for thousands of ICD-9-CM, CPT® and HCPCS codes.** Enhance your understanding of diagnoses, procedures, supplies and services with easy-to-understand descriptions.

- **Ingenix Edge — Real-time application service.** Rest assured you are always using accurate codes. You can code confidently throughout the year with free code updates.

- **All new color-coded edits.** Understand whether a code carries an age or sex edit, is covered by Medicare or contains bundled procedures.

EncoderPro.com Professional and *Expert* also contain the following features:

- **Access local coverage determinations (LCDs) and Medicare's Pub 100.** Check procedures for Medicare coverage instructions and medical necessity edits.

- **Modifier crosswalk.** Guides you to the correct modifiers when billing payers.

- **Medicare CCI edits.** Check your selected procedure for unbundling against four quarters of CCI edits.

EncoderPro.com Expert also contains the following features:

- **Compliance editor.** Check for coding accuracy and review your code selections for CCI unbundle edits, ICD-9-CM specificity, age, medical necessity and gender.

- **View entire LCD and NCD policies.** Reference comprehensive guidelines in every active policy, updated monthly.

- **Fee calculator.** Helps you calculate the Medicare reimbursement rate for your area.

CPT is a registered trademark of the American Medical Association.

100% Money Back Guarantee
If our merchandise* ever fails to meet your expectations, please contact our Customer Service Department toll-free at 1.800.INGENIX (464.3649), option 1, for an immediate response. *Software: Credit will be granted for unopened packages only.

SAVE 5% when you order at www.ingenixonline.com (reference source code FOBW7)
or call toll-free 1.800.INGENIX (464.3649), option 1.
Also available from your medical bookstore or distributor.

2007 Publications

INGENIX.

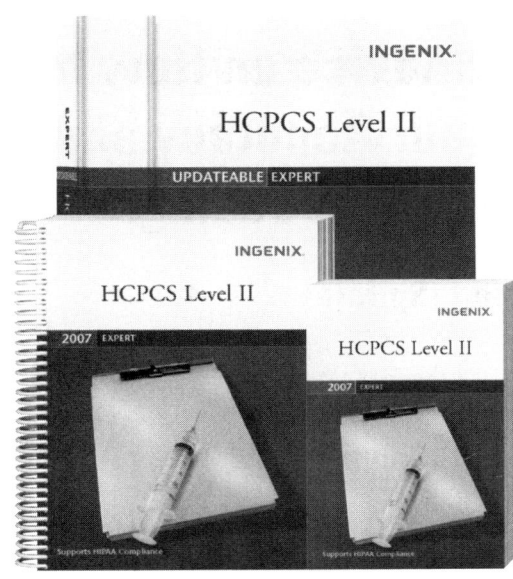

The Expert is on Your Side.

2007 HCPCS Level II Expert (Spiral)
Item No.: 4693 $94.95
Available: December 2006   ISBN: 978-156337-850-8

2007 HCPCS Level II Expert (Compact)
Item No.: 4695 $79.95
Available: December 2006   ISBN: 978-1-56337-852-2

HCPCS Level II Expert (Updateable)
Item No.: 4524 $139.95
Available: Now

Rest assured that you will be getting the most current and complete collection of HCPCS Level II codes — the **HCPCS Level II Expert** pulls codes from all of the sources that generate HCPCS codes, including CMS, OPPS addendum B, the physician fee schedule and other official sources. Not only does this book have an expanded table of drugs and an expanded index, but Ingenix is the only publisher to put the drug names right under the code descriptions to make it easier for you to find the code you're looking for.

- **Ingenix Edge — Includes all 2007 HCPCS Level II codes and modifiers from CMS.** Know you have the most complete, up-to-date HCPCS codes available to submit accurate claims.

- **Ingenix Edge — Enhanced table of drugs with generic and brand drug names and their corresponding codes.** This comprehensive table also includes the amount and route of administration.

- **Ingenix Edge — ASP status indicators.** Easily determine which codes are payable under OPPS.

- **Ingenix Edge — DMEPOS icon distinguishes codes paid under that fee schedule.** Improve efficiency when coding for supplies that should be submitted under the DMEPOS to your durable medical payer.

- **Ingenix Edge — Age and sex edits indicated by icons.** Improve coding accuracy by knowing for what specific ages and sex a code is meant.

- **Ingenix Edge — In-depth illustrations.** Makes coding various supplies and services easier and more accurate.

- **Ingenix Edge — AHA *Coding Clinic for HCPCS* references.** These references help users find advice about difficult-to-code HCPCS Level II codes or sections.

- **Ingenix Edge — Email alerts inform you of the latest changes to HCPCS Level II from CMS.** Keep current with late-breaking news through special reports and code using the most up-to-date codes and regulations.

- **Ingenix Edge — National Medicare and commercial fees for most HCPCS Level II codes.** This information helps identify reimbursement based on Medicare and private payer fee data for HCPCS Level II codes.

100% Money Back Guarantee
If our merchandise* ever fails to meet your expectations, please contact our Customer Service Department toll-free at 1.800.INGENIX (464.3649), option 1, for an immediate response. *Software: Credit will be granted for unopened packages only.

SAVE 5% when you order at www.ingenixonline.com (reference source code FOBW7)
or call toll-free 1.800.INGENIX (464.3649), option 1.
Also available from your medical bookstore or distributor.

2007 Publications

INGENIX

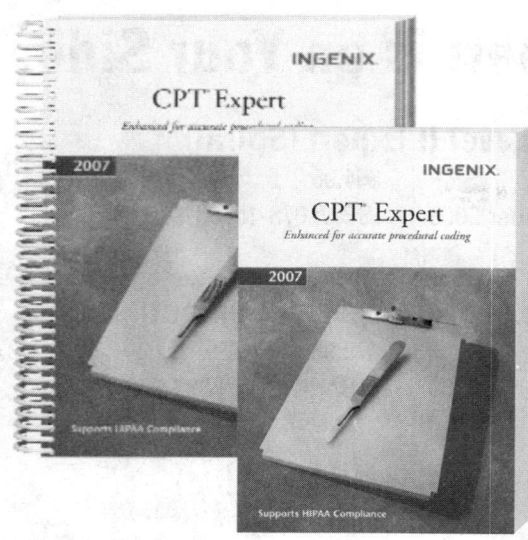

Get Expert Advice on How to Increase Your Accuracy and Understand CPT® Coding.

2007 CPT® Expert (Spiral)

Item No.: 4575 $97.95
Available: December 2006   ISBN: 978-1-56337-846-1

2007 CPT® Expert (Compact)

Item No.: 4770 $82.95
Available: December 2006   ISBN: 978-156337-847-8

A one-of-a-kind resource, the *CPT® Expert* includes all of the CPT® codes, plus detailed guidance on how to improve coding accuracy, increase coding efficiency and expedite claim submission by clarifying annual CPT® code changes and detailing the implications of the changes.

- **Ingenix Edge—All 2007 CPT® codes with official, full descriptions.** Access a complete, comprehensive listing of CPT® codes.

- **Ingenix Edge—Coding instruction sections at the beginning of each chapter.** Simple, short introductions to each chapter describe how best to ensure accuracy and speed claims.

- **Ingenix Edge—Edit symbols distinguish codes meant for specific populations.** Prevent denials due to restrictions based on age or sex.

- **Ingenix Edge—Information from the AMA, CMS, National Coverage Manual and Ingenix experts.** Better understand the rules and regulations and improve the precision of CPT® code selection.

- **Ingenix Edge—Illustrations.** Better understand procedures so that you can select the right codes the first time.

- **Ingenix Edge—Alerts sent via email provide valuable code change information.** Keep current with corrections to CPT® codes and other late-breaking news.

- **Ingenix Edge—National Coverage Manual references (formerly MCM and CIM).** This feature helps you understand federal regulations.

- **CPT® Assistant references.** Provides guidance and practical advice so you know exactly how to apply a CPT® code.

- **Deleted codes for 2007 and their complete descriptions.** Complete unfinished claims requiring deleted CPT® codes.

- **APC and ASC edits help you determine payment.** Start off on the right foot by knowing what status or group your service falls under.

- **Extensive index.** An easy-to-use index helps you save time locating the information you need to submit accurate claims.

- **Glossary.** Terms found in the nomenclature are defined in an easy-to-understand glossary.

CPT is a registered trademark of the American Medical Association.

CPT® Expert is not a replacement for the American Medical Association's CPT® Standard or Professional code books.

100% Money Back Guarantee

If our merchandise* ever fails to meet your expectations, please contact our Customer Service Department toll-free at 1.800.INGENIX (464.3649), option 1, for an immediate response. *Software: Credit will be granted for unopened packages only.

SAVE 5% when you order at www.ingenixonline.com (reference source code FOBW7)

or call toll-free **1.800.INGENIX (464.3649), option 1.**

Also available from your medical bookstore or distributor.

2007 Publications

INGENIX.

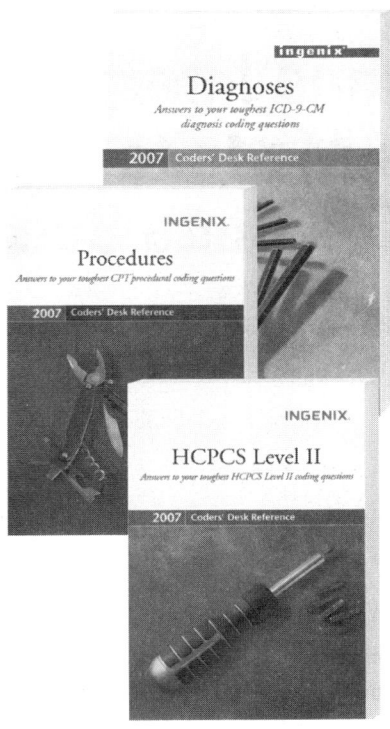

Get answers to your toughest coding questions from the experts.

2007 Coders' Desk Reference for Procedures

Item No.: 5700 $129.95
Available: December 2006 ISBN: 978-1-56337-848-5

2007 Coders' Desk Reference for Diagnoses

Item No.: 4995 $129.95
Available: September 2006 ISBN: 978-1-56337-921-5

2007 Coders' Desk Reference for HCPCS Level II

Item No.: 1083 $129.95
Available: December 2006 ISBN: 978-1-56337-849-2

With the nationwide shortage of coders continuing, new coders are expected to be proficient right away...while experienced coders are under pressure to be more productive than ever before. That's why Ingenix has created a comprehensive *Coders' Desk Reference* suite for all three code sets, creating an essential power suite for every health care professional.

- **Decrease coding time with comprehensive lay descriptions.** Clinical explanations clarify procedures in *Coders' Desk Reference for Procedures,* indicate the disease processes and causes of conditions in *Coders' Desk Reference for Diagnoses* and simplify HCPCS Level II codes by describing supplies and services in *Coders' Desk Reference for HCPCS Level II.*

- **Reduce costly claim delays and denials by always using the latest code sets.** All *Coders' Desk References* conform to standard code book organization and use updated codes for 2007.

- **New coders: Master the intricacies of coding, documentation and billing.** Veteran health care professionals: Code faster and more efficiently. The suite offers advice to avoid common coding errors and includes anatomical charts, eponyms, acronyms and medical abbreviations.

100% Money Back Guarantee

If our merchandise* ever fails to meet your expectations, please contact our Customer Service Department toll-free at 1.800.INGENIX (464.3649), option 1, for an immediate response. *Software: Credit will be granted for unopened packages only.

SAVE 5% when you order at www.ingenixonline.com (reference source code FOBW7)

or call toll-free 1.800.INGENIX (464.3649), option 1.

Also available from your medical bookstore or distributor.

FOBA7

2007 Publications

INGENIX.

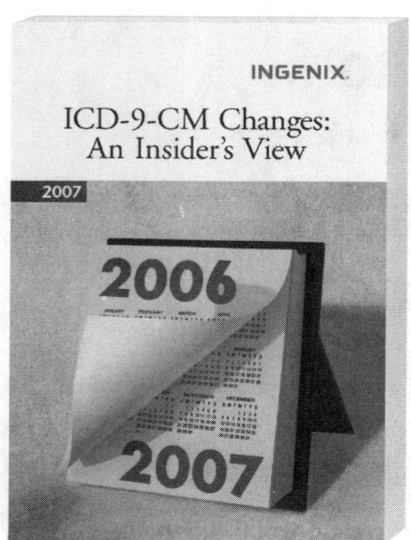

Understand and Interpret the Changes Made to the 2007 ICD-9-CM Code Set.

2007 ICD-9-CM Changes: An Insider's View

Item No.: 1077 $59.95
Available: September 2006   ISBN: 978-1-56337-920-8

A must-have resource for ICD-9-CM users! *ICD-9-CM Changes: An Insider's View* is a reference for understanding each of the code changes for 2007.

- **Ingenix Edge — Rationale for new and revised codes for 2007.** Knowing the reasons behind every new or revised code change is critical to adapting coding practices.

- **Ingenix Edge — Explanation of changes to indexes, conventions and instructional notes.** Understand what other changes will affect coding practices.

- **Ingenix Edge — Clinical presentation and treatment.** Coders must understand the clinical presentation of a condition or the intricacies of a procedure to code correctly to prevent "undercoding" or "overcoding."

- **Ingenix Edge — Clinical definitions of diagnoses and procedures.** Recognize terms in the medical records that pertain to new codes, ensuring correct application of the code changes.

- **Coding history and changes.** Understanding how the condition was coded in the past and how the change will impact coding practices.

- **Coding scenarios.** Examples of coding scenarios clarify application of the new codes.

- **Organized by chapter of ICD-9-CM.** Organizing the code changes in the context of their relationship to other codes provides insight into the rationale of the changes.

- **Detailed illustrations.** Illustrations are worth a thousand words and clarify some of the complex issues surrounding many of the code changes.

- **Annotated official addenda.** View the official addenda that contain all the changes with annotations to the three volumes of ICD-9-CM, including text deletions.

100% Money Back Guarantee

If our merchandise* ever fails to meet your expectations, please contact our Customer Service Department toll-free at 1.800.INGENIX (464.3649), option 1, for an immediate response. *Software: Credit will be granted for unopened packages only.

SAVE 5% when you order at www.ingenixonline.com (reference source code FOBW7)

or call toll-free 1.800.INGENIX (464.3649), option 1.

Also available from your medical bookstore or distributor.

FOBA7

2007 Publications

INGENIX

Essential links from CPT® codes to ICD-9-CM and HCPCS Level II codes.

2007 Cross Coders

Radiology Cross Coder
Item No.: 4960 $174.95
Available: December 2006 ISBN: 978-1-56337-893-5

Surgical Cross Coder
Item No.: 4962 $174.95
Available: December 2006 ISBN: 978-1-56337-894-2

Medical Services Cross Coder
Item No.: 4958 $134.95
Available: December 2006 ISBN: 978-1-56337-891-1

Anesthesia Cross Coder
Item No.: 4956 $174.95
Available: December 2006 ISBN: 978-1-56337-889-8

Speed and simplify code selection for various services billed to Medicare and third-party payers with the 2007 *Cross Coders*. Providing essential links from CPT® codes to the appropriate ICD-9-CM and HCPCS Level II codes, these guides are sure to help you code it right — the first time!

- **Quickly locate the necessary code information.** Procedure and diagnosis code information for your specialty is organized by CPT® code.

- **Spend less time correcting erroneous claims.** Prior to claim submission, consult complete CPT®, ICD-9-CM and HCPCS Level II code descriptions providing clear code explanations and guidance.

- **Identify anatomical sites and procedure specifics.** Intricate, detailed illustrations are included.

- **Recognize when primary/secondary codes are required.** ICD-9-CM code icons indicate when additional codes are needed and if the code selected is appropriate for the sex of the patient.

- **Ideal for quick reference.** Solve problematic coding concerns with the help of the glossary or appendix.

- **Earn CEUs from the American Academy of Professional Coders.**

CPT is a registered trademark of the American Medical Association.

100% Money Back Guarantee

If our merchandise* ever fails to meet your expectations, please contact our Customer Service Department toll-free at 1.800.INGENIX (464.3649), option 1, for an immediate response. *Software and Data File: Credit will be granted for unopened packages only.

SAVE 5% when you order at www.ingenixonline.com (reference source code FOBW7)

or call toll-free 1.800.INGENIX (464.3649), option 1.

Also available from your medical bookstore or distributor.

INGENIX.

Four simple ways to place an order.

Call
1.800.ingenix (464.3649), option 1. Mention source code FOBA7 when ordering.

Mail
PO Box 27116
Salt Lake City, UT 84127-0116
With payment and/or purchase order.

Fax
801.982.4033
With credit card information and/or purchase order.

Click
www.ingenixonline.com
Save 5% when you order online today—use source code FOBW7.

ingenix esmart
ingenix online frequent buyer program

GET REWARDS FOR SHOPPING ONLINE!
To find out more, visit IngenixOnline.com

eSmart program available only to Ingenix customers who are not part of Medallion, Gold Medallion or Partner Accounts programs. You must be registered at Ingenix Online to have your online purchases tracked for rewards purposes. Shipping charges and taxes still apply and cannot be used for rewards. Offer valid online only.

100% Money Back Guarantee

If our merchandise* ever fails to meet your expectations, please contact our Customer Service Department toll-free at 1.800.ingenix (464.3649), option 1 for an immediate response.

*Software: Credit will be granted for unopened packages only.

Customer Service Hours
7:00 am - 5:00 pm Mountain Time
9:00 am - 7:00 pm Eastern Time

Shipping and Handling

no. of items	fee
1	$10.95
2-4	$12.95
5-7	$14.95
8-10	$19.95
11+	Call

Order Form

Information.

Customer No. _____ Contact No. _____
Source Code _____
Contact Name _____
Title _____ Specialty _____
Company _____
Street Address _____
City _____ NO PO BOXES, PLEASE State _____ Zip _____
Telephone (   ) _____ Fax (   ) _____
                IN CASE WE HAVE QUESTIONS ABOUT YOUR ORDER
E-mail _____ @ _____
REQUIRED FOR ORDER CONFIRMATION AND SELECT PRODUCT DELIVERY.

Ingenix respects your right to privacy. We will not sell or rent your e-mail address or fax number to anyone outside Ingenix and its business partners. If you would like to remove your name from Ingenix promotion, please call 1.800.ingenix (464.3649), option 1.

Product

Item No.	Qty	Description	Price	Total

Subtotal _____
UT & VA residents, please add applicable Sales tax _____
(See chart on the left) Shipping & handling charges _____
All foreign orders, please call for shipping costs
Total _____

Payment

○ Please bill my credit card ○ MasterCard ○ VISA ○ Amex ○ Discover

Card No. | | | | | | | | | | | | | | | | | Expires _____
                                                                              MONTH   YEAR
Signature _____

○ Check enclosed, made payable to: Ingenix, Inc. ○ Please bill my office

Purchase Order No. _____
ATTACH COPY OF PURCHASE ORDER

©2006 Ingenix, Inc. All prices subject to change without notice.

FOBA7

2007

INGENIX®

ICD-9-CM Expert

*for Physicians
Volumes 1 & 2*

*International Classification of Diseases
9th Revision
Clinical Modification*

Seventh Edition

*Edited by:
Anita C. Hart, RHIA, CCS, CCS-P
Beth Ford, RHIT, CCS*

Ingenix is committed to providing you with the ICD-9-CM code update information you need to code accurately and to be in compliance with HIPAA regulations. In the case of adoption of additional ICD-9-CM code changes effective April 1, 2007, Ingenix will provide these code changes to you at no additional cost! Just check back at http://www.IngenixOnline.com and look for the ICD-9, CPT® and HCPCS Alerts link under the Quick Access Resources Menu to review the latest information concerning any new code changes.

Codes Valid October 1, 2006, through September 30, 2007

© 2006 Ingenix

All Rights Reserved

First Printing — August 2005

Made in the USA

This book, or parts hereof, may not be reproduced in any form without permission.

Additional copies may be ordered from:

Your local bookstore
or
1-800-INGENIX (464-3649)

IPES ISBN 978-1-56337-911-6

PUBLISHER'S NOTICE

All the codes, indexes and other material in the ICD-9-CM are compiled from official ICD-9-CM codes and instructions as well as the Medicare regulations and manuals issued or authorized by the Centers for Medicare and Medicaid Services. The code book is designed to provide accurate and authoritative information in regard to the subject covered, and every reasonable effort has been made to ensure the accuracy of the information within these pages. However, the ultimate responsibility for correct coding lies with the provider of services.

Ingenix, its employees, agents and staff make no representation, warranty or guarantee that this compilation of codes and narratives is error-free or that the use of this code book will prevent differences of opinion or disputes with Medicare or other third-party payers as to the codes that are accepted or the amounts that will be paid to providers of services, and will bear no responsibility or liability for the results or consequences of the use of this code book.

CONTINUING EDUCATION UNITS FOR CERTIFIED MEMBERS OF THE AMERICAN ACADEMY OF PROFESSIONAL CODERS

This publication has prior approval by the American Academy of Professional Coders for continuing education units (CEUs). Granting of prior approval in no way constitutes endorsement by the Academy of the publication content nor the publisher. Instructions to submit CEUs are available within the "Preapproved CEU Vendor List" file at www.aapc.com/education/CEUs/ceus.html.

OUR COMMITMENT TO ACCURACY

Ingenix is committed to producing accurate and reliable materials. To report corrections, please visit www.ingenixonline.com/accuracy or email accuracy@ingenix.com. You can also reach customer service by calling 1.800.INGENIX (464.3649), option 1.

SPECIAL REPORTS AND ANNOUNCEMENTS

Purchase of this publication entitles you to Special Reports and announcements via e-mail. Please call customer service at 800 INGENIX (464-3649) or contact your bookstore to take advantage of this exciting free service that will keep you abreast of important code changes and regulatory developments.

Review, download, and print the Special Reports in .pdf format. Log on to http://www.ingenixonline.com/content/2007I9Expert

Preface

ICD-9-CM for Physicians has been designed with the physician office coder in mind. The most recent official government versions of volumes 1 and 2 have been combined to provide physicians and their office staff with an ICD-9-CM book that is easy to use.

In addition, our technical experts have drawn upon their extensive hands-on experience to enhance the government's official version with valuable features essential to correct coding and reimbursement. With these enhancements, physician office health information professionals will increase the efficiency and timeliness of claim submission for both Medicare and other third-party payers.

As you review the content, you'll find the following:

- All the official ICD-9-CM codes, indexes, notes, footnotes and symbols
- Complete official coding guidelines
- Our exclusive color coding, symbols, and footnotes that alert coders to coding and reimbursement issues. Medicare outpatient code edits, such as invalid fourth or fifth digit for diagnosis codes are identified.
- Illustrations and clinically oriented definitions to aid in correct code assignment
- Symbols identifying new codes and text revisions; pages are dated to indicate when the changes were made
- Exclusive QuickFlip Color Tabs for quick, easy location of terms and codes in the index and Tabular List

USE OF OFFICIAL SOURCES

This *ICD-9-CM for Physicians* contains the official U.S. Department of Health and Human Services, ICD-9-CM codes, effective for the current year.

The color coding, footnotes and symbols, which identify coding and reimbursement issues, are derived from official federal government sources, including the Medicare Outpatient Code Editor as well as the knowledge of our technical experts.

The American Hospital Association's (AHA) *Coding Clinic for ICD-9-CM* references are used with permission of the AHA.

IMPORTANT INFORMATION ABOUT YOUR SUBSCRIPTION SERVICE

If you have purchased the updateable *ICD-9-CM for Physicians*, your subscription includes an updating service throughout the year to keep the code book current and accurate. Whenever CMS issues changes or corrections to the ICD-9-CM codes, We will issue an update to the book. In July you will receive a list of all new, revised, and invalid codes for the upcoming year.

TECHNICAL EDITORS

Anita C. Hart, RHIA, CCS, CCS-P
Product Manager, Ingenix
Ms. Hart's experience includes 15 years conducting and publishing research in clinical medicine and human genetics for Yale University, Massachusetts General Hospital, and Massachusetts Institute of Technology. In addition, Ms. Hart has supervised medical records management, health information management, coding and reimbursement, and worker's compensation issues as the office manager for a physical therapy rehabilitation clinic. Ms. Hart is an expert in physician and facility coding, reimbursement systems, and compliance issues. Ms. Hart developed the *ICD-9-CM Changes: An Insider View*, and has served as technical consultant for numerous other publications for hospital and physician practices. Currrently, Ms. Hart is the Product Manager and Technical Editor for the ICD-9-CM and ICD-10-CM/PCS product lines.

Beth Ford, RHIT, CCS
Clinical/Technical Editor, Ingenix
Ms. Ford is a clinical/technical editor for Ingenix. She has extensive background in both the professional and technical components of CPT/HCPCS and ICD-9-CM coding. Ms. Ford has served as a coding supervisor and coding consultant, as well as a health information management director. She is an active member of the American Heath Information Management Association (AHIMA).

In addition to the editors, the following people have contributed to this book:

Michael E. Desposito, *Product Director & Client Relationships*
Lynn Speirs, *Senior Director, Editorial/Desktop Publishing*
Stacy Perry, *Manager, Desktop Publishing*
Tracy Betzler, *Desktop Publishing Specialist*
Irene Day, *Desktop Publishing Specialist*
Hope Dunn, *Desktop Publishing Specialist*
Kerrie Hornsby, *Desktop Publishing Specialist*
Kate Holden, *Editor*

WHAT TO DO IF YOU HAVE QUESTIONS

If you have any questions call our customer service department toll-free at 800-INGENIX (464-3649), option 1.

If you have comments on the content of this book, please e-mail them to customerservice@ingenix.com or fax to 801-982-4033.

ADDITIONAL COPIES

Contact the customer service order department toll-free at 800-INGENIX (464-3649), option 1.

Introduction

HISTORY AND FUTURE OF ICD-9

The *International Classification of Diseases, Ninth Revision, Clinical Modification* (ICD-9-CM) is based on the official version of the World Health Organization's Ninth Revision, International Classification of Diseases (ICD-9). ICD-9-CM classifies morbidity and mortality information for statistical purposes, indexing of hospital records by disease and operations, data storage, and retrieval.

This modification of ICD-9 supplants the Eighth Revision International Classification of Diseases, Adapted for Use in the United States (ICDA-8) and the Hospital Adaptation of ICDA (H-ICDA).

The concept of extending the *International Classification of Diseases* for use in hospital indexing was originally developed in response to a need for a more efficient basis for storage and retrieval of diagnostic data. In 1950, the U.S. Public Health Service and the Veterans Administration began independent tests of the International Classification of Diseases for hospital indexing purposes. The following year, the Columbia Presbyterian Medical Center in New York City adopted the International Classification of Diseases, Sixth Revision, with some modifications for use in its medical record department. A few years later, the Commission on Professional and Hospital Activities (CPHA) in Ann Arbor, Mich., adopted the International Classification of Diseases with similar modifications for use in hospitals participating in the Professional Activity Study.

The problem of adapting ICD for indexing hospital records was addressed by the U.S. National Committee on Vital and Health Statistics through its subcommittee on hospital statistics. The subcommittee reviewed the modifications made by the various users of ICD and proposed that uniform changes be made. This was done by a small working party.

In view of the growing interest in the use of the International Classification of Diseases for hospital indexing, a study was undertaken in 1956 by the American Hospital Association and the American Medical Record Association (then the American Association of Medical Record Librarians) of the relative efficiencies of coding systems for diagnostic indexing. This study indicated the International Classification of Diseases provided a suitable and efficient framework for indexing hospital records. The major users of the International Classification of Diseases for hospital indexing purposes then consolidated their experiences, and an adaptation was first published in December 1959. A revision was issued in 1962 and the first "Classification of Operations and Treatments" was included.

In 1966, the international conference for revising the International Classification of Diseases noted the eighth revision of ICD had been constructed with hospital indexing in mind and considered the revised classification suitable, in itself, for hospital use in some countries. However, it was recognized that the basic classification might provide inadequate detail for diagnostic indexing in other countries. A group of consultants was asked to study the eighth revision of ICD (ICD-8) for applicability to various users in the United States. This group recommended that further detail be provided for coding of hospital and morbidity data. The American Hospital Association was requested to develop the needed adaptation proposals. This was done by an advisory committee (the Advisory Committee to the Central Office on ICDA). In 1968 the United States Public Health Service published the product, Eighth Revision International Classification of Diseases, Adapted for Use in the United States. This became commonly known as ICDA-8, and beginning in 1968 it served as the basis for coding diagnostic data for both official morbidity and mortality statistics in the United States.

In 1968, the CPHA published the Hospital Adaptation of ICDA (H-ICDA) based on both the original ICD-8 and ICDA-8. In 1973, CPHA published a revision of H-ICDA, referred to as H-ICDA-2. Hospitals throughout the United States were divided in their use of these classifications until January 1979, when ICD-9-CM was made the single classification intended primarily for use in the United States, replacing these earlier related, but somewhat dissimilar, classifications.

Physicians have been required by law to submit diagnosis codes for Medicare reimbursement since the passage of the Medicare Catastrophic Coverage Act of 1988. This act requires physician offices to include the appropriate diagnosis codes when billing for services provided to Medicare beneficiaries on or after April 1, 1989. The Centers for Medicare and Medicaid Services (CMS) designated ICD-9-CM as the coding system physicians must use.

In 1993 the World Health Organization published the newest version of International Classification of Diseases, Tenth Revision, ICD-10. This version contains the greatest number of changes in the history of ICD. There are more codes (5,500 more than ICD-9) to allow more specific reporting of diseases and newly recognized conditions. ICD-10 consists of three volumes; Tabular List (volume I), instructions (volume 2) and the Alphabetic Index (volume 3). It contains 21 chapters including two supplementary ones. The codes are alphanumeric (A00–T98, V01–Y98 and Z00–Z99). Currently ICD-10 is being used in some European countries with implementation expected after the year 2009 in the United States.

ICD-9-CM BACKGROUND

In February 1977, a steering committee was convened by the National Center for Health Statistics to provide advice and counsel in developing a clinical modification of ICD-9. The organizations represented on the steering committee included the following:

- American Association of Health Data Systems
- American Hospital Association
- American Medical Record Association
- Association for Health Records
- Council on Clinical Classifications
- Centers for Medicare and Medicaid Services, Department of Health and Human Services
- WHO Center for Classification of Diseases for North America, sponsored by the National Center for Health Statistics, Department of Health and Human Services

The Council on Clinical Classifications was sponsored by the following:

- American Academy of Pediatrics
- American College of Obstetricians and Gynecologists
- American College of Physicians
- American College of Surgeons
- American Psychiatric Association
- Commission on Professional and Hospital Activities

The steering committee met periodically in 1977. Clinical guidance and technical input were provided by task forces on classification from the Council on Clinical Classification's sponsoring organizations.

ICD-9-CM is a clinical modification of the World Health Organization's ICD-9. The term "clinical" is used to emphasize the modification's intent: to serve as a useful tool to classify morbidity data for indexing medical records, medical care review, and ambulatory and other medical care programs, as well as for basic health statistics. To describe the clinical picture of the patient, the codes must be more precise than those needed only for statistical groupings and trend analysis.

CHARACTERISTICS OF ICD-9-CM

ICD-9-CM far exceeds its predecessors in the number of codes provided. The disease classification has been expanded to include health-related conditions and to provide greater specificity at the fifth-digit level of detail. These fifth digits are not optional; they are intended for use in recording the information substantiated in the clinical record.

Volume I (Tabular List) of ICD-9-CM contains four appendices:

Appendix A:	Morphology of Neoplasms
Appendix B:	Deleted effective October 1, 2004
Appendix C:	Classification of Drugs by American Hospital Formulary Service List Number and Their ICD-9-CM Equivalents

Appendix D:	Classification of Industrial Accidents According to Agency
Appendix E:	List of Three-Digit Categories

These appendices are included as a reference to provide further information about the patient's clinical picture, to further define a diagnostic statement, to aid in classifying new drugs or to reference three-digit categories.

Volume 2 (Alphabetic Index) of ICD-9-CM contains many diagnostic terms that do not appear in volume I since the index includes most diagnostic terms currently in use.

THE DISEASE CLASSIFICATION

ICD-9-CM is totally compatible with its parent system, ICD-9, thus meeting the need for comparability of morbidity and mortality statistics at the international level. A few fourth-digit codes were created in existing three-digit rubrics only when the necessary detail could not be accommodated by the use of a fifth-digit subclassification. To ensure that each rubric of ICD-9-CM collapses back to its ICD-9 counterpart the following specifications governed the ICD-9-CM disease classification:

Specifications for the Tabular List:

1. Three-digit rubrics and their contents are unchanged from ICD-9.
2. The sequence of three-digit rubrics is unchanged from ICD-9.
3. Three-digit rubrics are not added to the main body of the classification.
4. Unsubdivided three-digit rubrics are subdivided where necessary to
   - add clinical detail
   - isolate terms for clinical accuracy
5. The modification in ICD-9-CM is accomplished by adding a fifth digit to existing ICD-9 rubrics, except as noted under #7 below.
6. The optional dual classification in ICD-9 is modified.
   - Duplicate rubrics are deleted:
     - four-digit manifestation categories duplicating etiology entries
     - manifestation inclusion terms duplicating etiology entries
   - Manifestations of disease are identified, to the extent possible, by creating five-digit codes in the etiology rubrics.
   - When the manifestation of a disease cannot be included in the etiology rubrics, provision for its identification is made by retaining the ICD-9 rubrics used for classifying manifestations of disease.
7. The format of ICD-9-CM is revised from that used in ICD-9.
   - American spelling of medical terms is used.
   - Inclusion terms are indented beneath the titles of codes.
   - Codes not to be used for primary tabulation of disease are printed in italics with the notation, "*code first underlying disease.*"

Specifications for the Alphabetic Index:

1. The format of the Alphabetic Index follows that of ICD-9.
2. When two codes are required to indicate etiology and manifestation, the manifestation code appears in brackets (e.g., diabetic cataract 250.5 *[366.41]*).

THE ICD-9-CM COORDINATION AND MAINTENANCE COMMITTEE

The four cooperating parties involved in maintaining the ICD-9-CM classification system include representatives of the American Hospital Association (AHA), the Centers for Medicare and Medicaid Services (CMS), the National Center for Health Statistics (NCHS), and the American Health Information Management Association (AHIMA).

Proposals for changes to the ICD-9-CM classification system are submitted and discussed in two open forum meetings held in April and October of each year at the Headquarters of the Centers for Medicare and Medicaid Services, Baltimore, Maryland. Comments received during and after the meetings are then discussed by the Committee. A notice of the new codes and code revisions approved by the Committee are published in the *Federal Register* as part of the proposed and final rule for the changes to the inpatient prospective payment system. The complete official document of changes to the classification system is released as the Addenda for the *International Classification of Diseases, Ninth Revision, Clinical Modification, Sixth Edition, Volumes 1, 2 and 3*.

How to Use the ICD-9-CM for Physicians (Volumes 1 & 2)

This *ICD-9-CM for Physicians* is based on the official version of the International Classification of Diseases, Ninth Revision, Clinical Modification, Sixth Edition, issued by the U.S. Department of Health and Human Services. Annual code changes are implemented by the government and are effective Oct. 1 and valid through Sept. 30 of the following year.

To accommodate the coder's approach to coding, the Alphabetic Index (Volume 2) has been placed before the Tabular List (Volume 1). This allows the user to locate the term in the index, then confirm the accuracy of the code in the Tabular List.

10 STEPS TO CORRECT CODING

To code accurately, it is necessary to have a working knowledge of medical terminology and to understand the characteristics, terminology and conventions of ICD-9-CM. Transforming descriptions of diseases, injuries, conditions and procedures into numerical designations (coding) is a complex activity and should not be undertaken without proper training.

Originally, coding allowed retrieval of medical information by diagnoses and operations for medical research, education and administration. Coding today is used to describe the medical necessity of a procedure and facilitate payment of health services, to evaluate utilization patterns and to study the appropriateness of health care costs. Coding provides the basis for epidemiological studies and research into the quality of health care. Incorrect or inaccurate coding can lead to investigations of fraud and abuse. Therefore, coding must be performed correctly and consistently to produce meaningful statistics to aid in planning for the health needs of the nation.

Follow the steps below to code correctly:

Step 1: Identify the reason for the visit (e.g., sign, symptom, diagnosis, condition to be coded).

Physicians describe the patient's condition using terminology that includes specific diagnoses as well as symptoms, problems or reasons for the encounter. If symptoms are present but a definitive diagnosis has not yet been determined, code the symptoms. Do not code conditions that are referred to as "rule out," "suspected," "probable" or "questionable."

Step 2: Always consult the Alphabetic Index, Volume 2, before turning to the Tabular List.

The most critical rule is to begin a code search in the index. Never turn first to the Tabular List (Volume 1), as this will lead to coding errors and less specificity in code assignments. To prevent coding errors, use both the Alphabetic Index and the Tabular List when locating and assigning a code.

Step 3: Locate the main entry term.

The Alphabetic Index is arranged by condition. Conditions may be expressed as nouns, adjectives and eponyms. Some conditions have multiple entries under their synonyms. Main terms are identified using boldface type.

Step 4: Read and interpret any notes listed with the main term

Notes are identified using italicized type.

Step 5: Review entries for modifiers

Nonessential modifiers are in parentheses. These parenthetical terms are supplementary words or explanatory information that may either be present or absent in the diagnostic statement and do not affect code assignment.

Step 6: Interpret abbreviations, cross-references, symbols and brackets

Cross-references used are "*see*," "*see* category" or "*see also*." The abbreviation NEC may follow main terms or subterms. NEC (not elsewhere classified) indicates that there is no specific code for the condition even though the medical documentation may be very specific. The ☑ box indicates the code requires an additional digit. If the appropriate digits are not found in the index, in a box beneath the main term, you MUST refer to the Tabular List. Italicized brackets [ ], are used to enclose a second code number that must be used with the code immediately preceding it and in that sequence.

Step 7: Choose a tentative code and locate it in the Tabular List.

Be guided by any inclusion or exclusion terms, notes or other instructions, such as "*code first*" and "use additional code," that would direct the use of a different or additional code from that selected in the index for a particular diagnosis, condition or disease.

Step 8: Determine whether the code is at the highest level of specificity.

Assign three-digit codes (category codes) if there are no four-digit codes within the code category. Assign four-digit codes (subcategory codes) if there are no five-digit codes for that category. Assign five-digit codes (fifth-digit subclassification codes) for those categories where they are available.

Step 9: Consult the color coding and reimbursement prompts, including the age, sex and Medicare as secondary payer edits.

Consult the official ICD-9-CM guidelines for coding and reporting, and refer to the AHA's *Coding Clinic for ICD-9-CM* for coding guidelines governing the use of specific codes.

Step 10: Assign the code.

ORGANIZATION

Introduction
The introductory material in this book includes the history and future of ICD-9-CM as well as an overview of the classification system

Official ICD-9-CM Conventions
This section provides a full explanation of all the official footnotes, symbols, instructional notes, and conventions found in the official government version

Additional Conventions
Exclusive color-coding, symbols, and notations have been included in the *ICD-9-CM for Physicians, Volumes 1 and 2* to alert coders to important coding and reimbursement issues. This section provides a full explanation of the additional conventions used throughout this book.

Summary of Code Changes
This section includes a complete listing of all code changes for the current year.

Summary of AHA's *Coding Clinic for ICD-9-CM* Topics
This is a brief summary of the official advice concerning coding topics covered in the latest issues of *AHA's Coding Clinic for ICD-9-CM* and is found ONLY in the *ICD-9-CM Expert for Physicians* updateable edition.

Coding Guidelines
Included in this book are the official ICD-9-CM coding guidelines as approved by the four cooperating parties of the ICD-9-CM Coordination and Maintenance Committee. Failure to comply with these official coding guidelines may result in denied or delayed claims.

Disease Classification: Alphabetic Index to Diseases

The Alphabetic Index to Diseases is separated by tabs labeled with the letters of the alphabet, contains diagnostic terms for illnesses, injuries and reasons for encounters with health care professionals. Both the Table of Drugs and Chemicals and the Alphabetic Index to External Causes of Injury and Poisoning are easily located with the tabs in this section.

The warning statement at the bottom of every page of the index, Subterms under main terms may continue to next column or page, is a reminder to always check for additional subterms before making final selection.

Disease Classification: Tabular List of Diseases

The Tabular List of Diseases arranges the ICD-9-CM codes and descriptors numerically. Tabs divide this section into chapters, identified by the code range on the tab.

The Tabular List includes two supplementary classifications:

- V Codes—Supplementary Classification of Factors Influencing Health Status and Contact with Health Services (V01–V86)
- E Codes—Supplementary Classification of External Causes of Injury and Poisoning (E800–E999)

ICD-9-CM includes four official appendixes.

- Appendix A   Morphology of Neoplasms
- Appendix B   Deleted effective October 1, 2004
- Appendix C   Classification of Drugs by AHFS List
- Appendix D   Classification of Industrial Accidents According to Agency
- Appendix E   List of Three-digit Categories

These appendices are included as a reference to provide further information about the patient's circumstances, help further define a diagnostic statement, maintain a tumor registry and aid in classifying new drugs.

Resources

Listed below are the exclusive resources found ONLY in the *ICD-9-CM Expert for Physicians, Volumes 1 & 2*.

Valid Three-digit Code Table

ICD-9-CM is composed of codes with either 3, 4, or 5 digits. A code is invalid if it has not been coded to the full number of digits required for that code. There are a certain number codes that are valid for reporting as three digit codes. A list of these valid three-digit code is included as a convenient reference when auditing claims.

Code Tables

Exclusive coding tables covering abortion, burns, complications, diabetes, hernia, pregnancy, and others are provided to simplify those complex coding issues.

ICD-9-CM Official Conventions

ICD-9-CM FOOTNOTES, SYMBOLS, INSTRUCTIONAL NOTES AND CONVENTIONS

This *ICD-9-CM for Physicians* preserves all the footnotes, symbols, instructional notes and conventions found in the government's official version. Accurate coding depends upon understanding the meaning of these elements.

The following appear in the disease Tabular List, unless otherwise noted.

OFFICIAL GOVERNMENT SYMBOLS

§   The section mark preceding a code denotes a footnote on the page. This symbol is used only in the Tabular List of Diseases.

ICD-9-CM CONVENTIONS USED IN THE TABULAR LIST

In addition to the symbols and footnotes above, the ICD-9-CM disease tabular has certain abbreviations, punctuation, symbols and other conventions. Our *ICD-9-CM for Physicians* preserves these conventions. Proper use of the conventions will lead to efficient and accurate coding.

Abbreviations

NEC   Not elsewhere classifiable

This abbreviation is used when the ICD-9-CM system does not provide a code specific for the patient's condition.

NOS   Not otherwise specified

This abbreviation is the equivalent of 'unspecified' and is used only when the coder lacks the information necessary to code to a more specific four-digit subcategory.

[ ]   Brackets enclose synonyms, alternative terminology or explanatory phrases:

482.2   Pneumonia due to Hemophilus influenzae [H. influenzae]

Brackets that appear beneath a code indicate the fifth digits that are considered valid fifth digits for the code. This convention is applied for those instances in ICD-9-CM where not all common fifth digits are considered valid for each subcategory within a category.

715.0   Osteoarthrosis, generalized
[0,4,9]

Generalized arthrosis can only be assigned in cases for which the degenerative joint disease involves multiple joints. Therefore, this code is considered for arthrosis in the sites described as unspecified, hand (which consists of multiple joints), or multiple sites. Therefore, only fifth digits 0, 4, and 9 are valid with subcategory 715.0.

[ ]   Slanted brackets that appear in the Alphabetic Index indicates mandatory multiple coding. Both codes must be assigned to fully describe the condition and are sequenced in the order listed.

Tachycardia
    ventricular (paroxysmal)
      psychogenic 316 *[427.1]*

Psychogenic paroxysmal tachycardia is reported using both 316, Psychogenic factors associated with diseases classified elsewhere, and 427.1, Paroxysmal ventricular tachydcardia.

( )   Parentheses enclose supplementary words, called nonessential modifiers, that may be present in the narrative description of a disease without affecting the code assignment:

198.4   Other parts of nervous system
     Meninges (cerebral) (spinal)

:   Colons are used in the Tabular List after an incomplete term that needs one or more of the modifiers that follow in order to make it assignable to a given category:

021.1   Enteric tularemia
    Tularemia:
      cryptogenic
      intestinal
      typhoidal

}   Braces enclose a series of terms, each of which is modified by the statement appearing to the right of the brace:

560.2   Volvulus
    Knotting
    Strangulation   } of intestine, bowel, or colon
    Torsion
    Twist

OTHER CONVENTIONS

Boldface   Boldface type is used for all codes and titles in the Tabular List.

Italicized   Italicized type is used for all exclusion notes and to identify codes that should not be used for describing the primary diagnosis.

INSTRUCTIONAL NOTES

These notes appear only in the Tabular List of Diseases:

Includes   An includes note further defines or clarifies the content of the chapter, subchapter, category, subcategory or subclassification. The includes note in the example below applies only to category 461.

Excludes   Terms following the word "*Excludes*" are not classified to the chapter, subchapter, category, subcategory or specific subclassification code under which it is found. The note also may provide the location of the excluded diagnosis. Excludes notes are italicized.

461   Acute sinusitis
    INCLUDES   abscess
                    empyema   acute, of sinus
                    infection   (accessory)
                    inflammation   (nasal)
                    suppuration

    EXCLUDES   *chronic or unspecified sinusitis (473.0-473.9)*

Use additional code:

This instruction signals the coder that an additional code should be used if the information is available to provide a more complete picture of that diagnosis.

362.13   Changes in vascular appearance
    Vascular sheathing of retina
    Use additional code for any associated
       atherosclerosis (440.8)

There are coding circumstances outside of the etiology/manifestation convention when multiple coding for a single condition is required. The 'Use additional code' note will be found under the associated condition code in the tabular. In the index, the multiple coding requirement is indicated by the use of the slanted bracket. The two codes are to be sequenced as listed in the index. For example, retinal arteriosclerosis must be coded using two codes sequenced as listed in the index.

Arteriosclerosis, arteriosclerotic
    retinal (vascular) 440.8 *[362.13]*

Code first underlying disease:

The *Code first underlying disease* instructional note found under certain codes is a sequencing rule. Most often this sequencing rule applies to the etiology/manifestation convention and is found under the manifestation code. The manifestation code may never be used alone or as a primary diagnosis (i.e., sequenced first). The instructional note, the code and its descriptor appear in italics in the Tabular List.

> *590.81 Pyelitis or pyelonephritis in diseases classified elsewhere*
>> *Code first underlying disease as:*
>>> *tuberculosis (016.0)*

Not all codes with a 'Code first underlying disease' instructional note are part of the etiology/manifestation convention. The 'Code first' note will appear, but the title of the code and the instructional note are not in italics. These codes may be reported alone or as the secondary diagnosis. For example, disseminated chorioretinitis may be reported as a principal diagnosis. However, if the underlying condition that caused disseminated chorioretinitis is known, such as tuberculous disseminated chorioretinitis, two codes are required and sequenced as listed in the index.

> **363.13 Disseminated choroiditis and chorioretinitis, generalized**
>> Code first underlying disease as:
>>> tuberculosis (017.3)

Code, if applicable, any causal condition first:

A code with this note indicates that this code may be assigned as a principal diagnosis when the causal condition is unknown or not applicable. If a causal condition is known, then the code for that condition should be sequenced as the principal or first-listed diagnosis.

> **590.0 Chronic pyelonephritis**
>> Chronic pyelitis
>> Chronic pyonephrosis
>> Code, if applicable, any causal condition first

Omit code:

"*Omit code*" is used to instruct the coder that no code is to be assigned. When this instruction is found in the Alphabetic Index to Diseases the medical term should not be coded as a diagnosis.

> **Metaplasia**
>> cervix — *omit code*

See Condition:

The "*see* condition' note found in the Alphabetic Index to Disease instructs the coder to refer to a main term for the condition. This note will follow index terms that are nouns for anatomical sites or adjectival forms of disease term. In the example below, the index terms 'Cervix' and 'Diffuse' are followed by the — see condition. Coders should search the index using a condition term such as atrophy or prolapse.

> **Cervix** — *see* condition
> **Diffuse** — *see* condition

Morphology Codes:

For each neoplastic disease listed in the index, a morphology code is provided that identifies histological type and behavior.

> **Myelolipoma** (M8870/0) — *see* Neoplasm, by site, benign

The histology is identified by the first four digits and the behavior is identified by the digit following the slash. Appendix A of Volume 1 contains a listing of morphology codes. This appendix is helpful when the pathology report identifies the neoplasm by using an M code. The coder may refer to Appendix A to determine the nomenclature of the neoplasm that will be the main term to search in the Index. The behavior classification is as follows:

0	Benign
1	Uncertain behavior
2	Carcinoma in situ
3	Malignant, primary site
6	Malignant, secondary site.

Additional Conventions

SYMBOLS AND NOTATIONS

New and Revised Text Symbols
- ●   A bullet at a code or line of text indicates that that the entry is new.
- ▲   A triangle in the Tabular List indicates that the code title is revised. In the Alphabetic Index the triangle indicates that a code has changed.
- ▶◀   These symbols appear at the beginning and at the end of a section of new or revised text.

When these symbols appear on a page there will be a date on the lower outside corner of the page indicating the date of the change, (e.g., October 2006).

Additional Digits Required
- ✓4th   This symbol indicates that the code requires a fourth digit.
- ✓5th   This symbol indicates that a code requires a fifth digit.
- ✓   This symbol found only in the Alphabetic Index sections and the Table of Drugs and Chemicals indicates that an additional digit is required. Referring to the tabular section is essential to locate the appropriate additional digit.

AHA's Coding Clinic for ICD-9-CM References
The four cooperating parties have designated the AHA's *Coding Clinic for ICD-9-CM* as the official publication for coding guidelines. The references are identified by the notation **AHA:** followed by the issue, year and page number.

In the example below, AHA's *Coding Clinic for ICD-9-CM*, third quarter 1991, page 15, contains a discussion on code assignment for vitreous hemorrhage:

    379.23   **Vitreous hemorrhage**
                    AHA: 3Q, '91, 15

The table below explains the abbreviations in the *Coding Clinic* references:

J-F	January/February
M-A	March/April
M-J	May/June
J-A	July/August
S-O	September/October
N-D	November/December
1Q	First quarter
2Q	Second quarter
3Q	Third quarter
4Q	Fourth quarter

Age and Sex Edit Symbols
The age edits below address OCE edits and are used to detect inconsistencies between the patient's age and diagnosis. They appear in the Tabular List of Diseases to the right of the code description.

Newborn Age: 0
These diagnoses are intended for newborns and neonates and the patient's age must be 0 years.

Pediatric Age: 0-17
These diagnoses are intended for children and the patient's age must be between 0 and 17 years.

Maternity Age: 12-55
These diagnoses are intended for the patients between the age of 12 and 55 years.

Adult Age 15-124
These diagnoses are intended for the patients between the age of 15 and 124 years.

The sex symbols below address OCE edits and are used to detect inconsistencies between the patient's sex and diagnosis. They appear in the Tabular List of Diseases to the right of the code description:

♂   **Male diagnosis only**
This symbol appears to the right of the code description. This reference appears in the disease Tabular List.

♀   **Female diagnosis only**
This symbol appears to the right of the code description. This reference appears in the disease Tabular List.

COLOR CODING
To alert the coder to Medicare outpatient code edits and other important reimbursement issues, color bars have been added over the code descriptors in the Tabular List. Some codes carry more than one color.

Carriers use the Medicare Outpatient Code Editor (OCE) to examine claims for coding and billing accuracy and completeness. Color codes in this book signify Medicare code edits for manifestation codes not to be reported as a primary diagnosis, and when a more specific diagnosis code should be used.

Manifestation Code
These codes will appear in italic type as well as with a blue color bar over the code title. A manifestation code is not allowed to be reported as a primary diagnosis because each describes a manifestation of some other underlying disease, not the disease itself. This is referred to as mandatory multiple coding of etiology and manifestation. Code the underlying disease first. A *Code first underlying disease* instructional note will appear with underlying disease codes identified. In the Alphabetic Index these codes are listed as the secondary code in slanted brackets with the code for the underlying disease listed first.

Other Specified Code
These codes will appear with a gray color bar over the code title. Use these codes when the documentation indicates a specified diagnosis, but the ICD-9-CM system does not have a specific code that describes the diagnosis. These codes are may be stated as "Other" or "Not elsewhere classified (NEC)."

Unspecified Code
These codes will have a yellow color bar over the code title. Use these codes when the neither the diagnostic statement nor the documentation provides enough information to assign a more specified diagnosis code. These codes may be stated as "Unspecified" or "Not otherwise specified (NOS)." Note: Do not assign these codes when a more specific diagnosis has been determined.

OTHER NOTATIONS
DEF: This symbol indicates a definition of disease term. The definition will appear in blue type in the Disease Tabular Lists.

PDx   This symbol identifies a V code that can only be used as a primary diagnosis.

SDx   This symbol identifies a V code that can only be used as a secondary diagnosis.

    Note: A V code without a symbol may be used as either a primary or secondary diagnosis

Medicare as Secondary Payer (MSP)
    Note: The Medicare as Secondary Payer (MSP) alert identified trauma diagnoses that may be covered under automobile insurance, no-fault insurance, workmen's compensation or other types of liability insurance for which Medicare should be a secondary payer. Providers must verify MSP information prior to submitting the claim to Medicare. Therefore, this edit is no longer included in the official Medicare Code Editor (MCE).

Alphabetic Indexes
▽ Subterms under main terms may continue to next column or page.

This warning statement is a reminder to always check for additional subterms and information that may continue on to the next page or column before making a final selection.

Summary of Code Changes

DISEASE TABULAR LIST (VOLUME 1)

- ● 052.2 Postvaricella myelitis
  Includes note added
- ● 053.14 Herpes zoster myelitis
- ● 054.74 Herpes simplex myelitis
- 136.3 Includes term added
- 151 Excludes note added
- 152 Excludes note added
- 171 Includes term added
  Excludes term revised
- 174 Use additional code note added
- 175 Use additional code note added
- 202.1 Includes term deleted
- 211 Excludes note added
- 215.5 Includes term added
- 233.1 Includes term added
  Excludes term revised
- 235 Excludes note added
- 238.1 Includes term added
- 238.7 Includes note deleted
  Excludes terms added
  Excludes term revised
- ● 238.71 Essential thrombocythemia
  Includes note added
- ● 238.72 Low grade myelodysplastic syndrome lesions
  Includes note added
- ● 238.73 High grade myelodysplastic syndrome lesions
  Includes note added
- ● 238.74 Myelodysplastic syndrome with 5q deletion
  Includes note added
  Excludes note added
- ● 238.75 Myelodysplastic syndrome, unspecified
- ● 238.76 Myelofibrosis with myeloid metaplasia
  Includes note added
  Excludes note added
- ● 238.79 Other lymphatic and hematopoietic tissues
  Includes note added
- ▲ 255.10 Primary Aldosteronism ▶Hyperaldosteronism, unspecified◀
  Includes note added
  Includes term deleted
- 277.3 Includes note deleted
- ● 277.30 Amyloidosis, unspecified
  Includes note added
- ● 277.31 Familial Mediterranean fever
  Includes note added
- ● 277.39 Other amyloidosis
  Includes note added
- 278.0 Use additional code note revised
- ▲ 284 Aplastic anemia and ▶other bone marrow failure syndromes◀
- 284.0 Includes note deleted
- ● 284.01 Constitutional red blood cell aplasia
  Includes note added
- ● 284.09 Other constitutional aplastic anemia
  Includes note added
- ● 284.1 Pancytopenia
  Excludes note added
- ● 284.2 Myelophthisis
  Includes note added
  Code first note added
- 284.8 Includes term deleted
  Excludes term deleted
- 284.9 Excludes term revised
- 285.0 Excludes term revised
- ▲ 285.2 Anemia in ▶of◀ other chronic illness ▶disease◀
  Includes note added
- ▲ 285.29 Anemia of other chronic illness ▶disease◀
  Includes note added
- 285.8 Includes term deleted
- 287 Excludes term revised

- ▲ 288.0 Agranulocytosis ▶Neutropenia◀
  Includes term added
  Includes terms deleted
  Use additional code note deleted
  Use additional code note added
  Excludes term added
- ● 288.00 Neutropenia, unspecified
- ● 288.01 Congenital neutropenia
  Includes note added
- ● 288.02 Cyclic neutropenia
- ● 288.03 Drug induced neutropenia
  Use additional code note added
- ● 288.04 Neutropenia due to infection
- ● 288.09 Other neutropenia
  Includes note added
- ● 288.4 Hemophagocytic syndromes
  Includes note added
- ● 288.5 Decreased white blood cell count
  Excludes note added
- ● 288.50 Leukocytopenia, unspecified
  Includes note added
- ● 288.51 Lymphocytopenia
  Includes note added
- ● 288.59 Other decreased white blood cell count
  Includes note added
- ● 288.6 Elevated white blood cell count
  Excludes note added
- ● 288.60 Leukocytosis, unspecified
  Includes note added
- ● 288.61 Lymphocytosis (symptomatic)
  Includes note added
- ● 288.62 Leukemoid reaction
  Includes note added
- ● 288.63 Monocytosis (symptomatic)
  Excludes note added
- ● 288.64 Plasmacytosis
- ● 288.65 Basophilia
- ● 288.69 Other elevated white blood cell count
- 288.8 Includes note deleted
  Excludes terms added
- 289.4 Excludes term revised
- ● 289.53 Neutropenic splenomegaly
- ● 289.83 Myelofibrosis
  Includes note added
  Code first note added
  Excludes note added
- 289.89 Includes term deleted
- 305.1 Excludes terms added
- 307.89 Code first note revised
- 309.81 Includes terms added
- 323 Includes terms revised
  Excludes terms added
- ▲ 323.0 Encephalitis, ▶myelitis, and encephalomyelitis◀ in viral diseases classified elsewhere
  Excludes note deleted
- ● 323.01 Encephalitis and encephalomyelitis in viral diseases classified elsewhere
  Excludes note added
- ● 323.02 Myelitis in viral diseases classified elsewhere
  Excludes note added
- ▲ 323.1 Encephalitis ▶, myelitis, and encephalomyelitis◀ in rickettsial diseases classified elsewhere
- ▲ 323.2 Encephalitis ▶, myelitis, and encephalomyelitis◀ in protozoal diseases classified elsewhere
- ▲ 323.4 Other encephalitis ▶, myelitis, and encephalomyelitis◀ due to infection classified elsewhere
  Excludes note deleted
- ● 323.41 Other encephalitis and encephalomyelitis due to infection classified elsewhere
  Excludes note added
- ● 323.42 Other myelitis due to infection classified elsewhere
  Excludes note added

- ▲ 323.5 Encephalitis ▶, myelitis, and encephalomyelitis◀ following immunization procedures
  Includes note deleted
- ● 323.51 Encephalitis and encephalomyelitis following immunization procedures
  Includes note added
- ● 323.52 Myelitis following immunization procedures
  Includes note added
- ▲ 323.6 Postinfectious encephalitis▶, myelitis, and encephalomyelitis◀
  Includes note deleted
  Excludes note deleted
- ● 323.61 Infectious acute disseminated encephalomyelitis [ADEM]
  Includes note added
  Excludes note added
- ● 323.62 Other postinfectious encephalitis and encephalomyelitis
  Excludes note added
- ● 323.63 Postinfectious myelitis
  Excludes note added
- ▲ 323.7 Toxic encephalitis▶, myelitis, and encephalomyelitis◀
- ● 323.71 Toxic encephalitis and encephalomyelitis
- ● 323.72 Toxic myelitis
- ▲ 323.8 Other causes of encephalitis ▶, myelitis, and encephalomyelitis◀
  Excludes note deleted
- ● 323.81 Other causes of encephalitis and encephalomyelitis
  Includes note added
- ● 323.82 Other causes of myelitis
  Includes note added
- ▲ 323.9 Unspecified causes of encephalitis ▶, myelitis, and encephalomyelitis◀
- 326 Instructional note revised
- 327 Section title added
- 327.5 Excludes term revised
- ● 331.83 Mild cognitive impairment, so stated
  Excludes note added
- ▲ 333.6 Idiopathic ▶Genetic◀ torsion dystonia
- ▲ 333.7 Symptomatic ▶Acquired◀torsion dystonia
  Includes note deleted
  Use additional code note deleted
- ● 333.71 Athetoid cerebral palsy
  Includes note added
  Excludes note added
- ● 333.72 Acute dystonia due to drugs
  Includes note added
  Use additional code note added
  Excludes note added
- ● 333.79 Other acquired torsion dystonia
- 333.81 Excludes note added
- 333.82 Includes term deleted
  Excludes note added
- ● 333.85 Subacute dyskinesia due to drugs
  Includes note added
  Use additional code note added
  Excludes note added
- 333.92 Excludes note added
- ● 333.94 Restless legs syndrome [RLS]
- 333.99 Excludes term deleted
- 336.9 Excludes term revised
- 337.1 Code first note revised
- 338 Section title added
- ● 338 Pain, not elsewhere classified
  Use additional code note added
  Excludes note added
- ● 338.0 Central pain syndrome
  Includes note added
- ● 338.1 Acute pain
- ● 338.11 Acute pain due to trauma
- ● 338.12 Acute post-thoracotomy pain
  Includes note added
- ● 338.18 Other acute postoperative pain
  Includes note added

▶◀ Revised Text ● New Code ▲ Revised Code Title

2007 ICD·9·CM ix

● 338.19	Other acute pain	● 389.16	Sensorineural hearing loss, asymmetrical	▲ 404.90	Hypertensive heart and ▶chronic◀ kidney disease, unspecified, without heart failure or ▶and with◀ chronic kidney disease ▶stage I through stage IV, or unspecified◀
	Excludes note added	▲ 389.18	Sensorineural hearing loss of combined types, ▶bilateral◀		
● 338.2	Chronic pain	▲ 403	Hypertensive ▶chronic◀ kidney disease		
	Excludes note added		Use additional code note deleted		
● 338.21	Chronic pain due to trauma	▲ 403.0	Hypertensive ▶chronic◀ kidney disease, malignant		Use additional code note added
● 338.22	Chronic post-thoracotomy pain			▲ 404.91	Hypertensive heart and ▶chronic◀ kidney disease, unspecified, with heart failure ▶and with◀ chronic kidney disease stage I through stage IV, or unspecified◀
● 338.28	Other chronic postoperative pain	▲ 403.00	Hypertensive ▶chronic◀ kidney disease, malignant, ~~without~~ ▶with◀ chronic kidney disease ▶stage I through stage IV, or unspecified◀		
● 338.29	Other chronic pain				
● 338.3	Neoplasm related pain (acute) (chronic)				Use additional code note added
	Includes note added		Use additional code note added	▲ 404.92	Hypertensive heart and ▶chronic◀ kidney disease, unspecified ,▶ without heart failure and◀ with chronic kidney disease ▶stage V or end stage renal disease◀
● 338.4	Chronic pain syndrome	▲ 403.01	Hypertensive ▶chronic◀ kidney disease, malignant, with chronic kidney disease ▶stage V or end stage renal disease◀		
	Includes note added				
● 341.2	Acute (transverse) myelitis				
	Excludes note added		Use additional code note added		Use additional code note added
● 341.20	Acute (transverse) myelitis NOS	▲ 403.10	Hypertensive ▶chronic◀ kidney disease, benign, ~~without~~ ▶with◀ chronic kidney disease ▶stage I through stage IV, or unspecified◀	▲ 404.93	Hypertensive heart and ▶chronic◀ kidney disease, unspecified, with heart failure or ▶and with◀ chronic kidney disease ▶stage V or end stage renal disease◀
● 341.21	Acute (transverse) myelitis in conditions classified elsewhere				
	Code first note added				
● 341.22	Idiopathic transverse myelitis		Use additional code note added		Use additional code note added
343	Excludes terms added	▲ 403.11	Hypertensive ▶chronic◀ kidney disease, benign, with chronic kidney disease ▶stage V or end stage renal disease◀	420.0	Code first note revised
	Excludes term revised			425.7	Code first note revised
▲ 345	Epilepsy ▶and recurrent seizures◀			● 429.83	Takotsubo syndrome
345.1	Excludes terms revised		Use additional code note added		Includes note added
▲ 345.4	~~Partial epilepsy, with impairment of consciousness~~ ▶Localization-related (focal) (partial) epilepsy and epileptic syndromes with complex partial seizures◀	▲ 403.90	Hypertensive▶chronic◀ kidney disease, unspecified, ~~without~~ ▶with◀ chronic kidney disease ▶stage I through stage IV, or unspecified◀	440.24	Use additional code note added
				445.81	Use additional code note revised
				478.1	Includes note deleted
				● 478.11	Nasal mucositis (ulcerative)
	Includes terms added		Use additional code note added		Use additional code note added
▲ 345.40	~~Partial epilepsy, with impairment of consciousness~~ ▶Localization-related (focal) (partial) epilepsy and epileptic syndromes with complex partial seizures◀, without mention of intractable epilepsy	▲ 403.91	Hypertensive ▶chronic◀ kidney disease, unspecified, with chronic kidney disease ▶stage I through stage IV, or unspecified◀	● 478.19	Other disease of nasal cavity and sinuses
					Includes note added
				496	Excludes term added
				514	Excludes term added
				517.8	Code first note revised
			Use additional code note added	● 518.7	Transfusion related acute lung injury [TRALI]
▲ 345.41	~~Partial epilepsy, with impairment of consciousness~~ ▶Localization-related (focal) (partial) epilepsy and epileptic syndromes with complex partial seizures◀, with intractable epilepsy	▲ 404	Hypertensive heart and ▶chronic◀ kidney disease		
				519.1	Includes note deleted
			Use additional code note deleted	● 519.11	Acute bronchospasm
		▲ 404.0	Hypertensive heart and ▶chronic◀ kidney disease, malignant		Includes note added
					Excludes note added
▲ 345.5	~~Partial epilepsy, without impairment of consciousness~~ ▶Localization-related (focal) (partial) epilepsy and epileptic syndromes with simple partial seizures◀	▲ 404.00	Hypertensive heart and ▶chronic◀ kidney disease, malignant, without heart failure or ▶and with◀ chronic kidney disease ▶stage I through stage IV, or unspecified◀	● 519.19	Other diseases of trachea and bronchus
					Includes note added
				520.6	Includes terms added
				521.06	Includes note added
	Includes terms added			521.97	Includes note added
▲ 345.50	~~Partial epilepsy, without impairment of consciousness~~ ▶Localization-related (focal) (partial) epilepsy and epileptic syndromes with simple partial seizures◀, without mention of intractable epilepsy		Use additional code note added	521.08	Includes note added
		▲ 404.01	Hypertensive heart and ▶chronic◀ kidney disease, malignant, with heart failure ▶and with chronic kidney disease stage I through stage IV, or unspecified◀	521.8	Includes note deleted
				● 521.81	Cracked tooth
					Excludes note added
				● 521.89	Other specific diseases of hard tissues of teeth
			Use additional code note added		Includes note added
▲ 345.51	~~Partial epilepsy, without impairment of consciousness~~ ▶Localization-related (focal) (partial) epilepsy and epileptic syndromes with simple partial seizures◀, with intractable epilepsy	▲ 404.02	Hypertensive heart and ▶chronic◀ kidney disease, malignant,▶ without heart failure and◀ with chronic kidney disease ▶stage V or end stage renal disease◀	● 523.00	Acute gingivitis, plaque induced
					Includes note added
				● 523.01	Acute gingivitis, non-plaque induced
				523.1	Includes terms deleted
▲ 345.8	Other forms of epilepsy ▶and recurrent seizures◀,		Use additional code note added	● 523.10	Chronic gingivitis, plaque induced
		▲ 404.03	Hypertensive heart and ▶chronic◀ kidney disease, malignant, with heart failure or ▶and with◀ chronic kidney disease ▶stage V or end stage renal disease◀		Includes note added
▲ 345.80	Other forms of epilepsy ▶and recurrent seizures◀, without mention of intractable epilepsy			● 523.11	Chronic gingivitis, non-plaque induced
				▲ 523.3	▶Aggressive and◀ Aacute periodontitis
					Excludes terms deleted
			Use additional code note added	● 523.30	Aggressive periodontitis, unspecified
▲ 345.81	Other forms of epilepsy ▶and recurrent seizures◀, with intractable epilepsy	▲ 404.1	Hypertensive heart and ▶chronic◀ kidney disease, benign	● 523.31	Aggressive periodontitis, localized
					Includes note added
345.9	Includes terms added	▲ 404.10	Hypertensive heart and ▶chronic◀ kidney disease, benign, without heart failure or ▶and with◀ chronic kidney disease ▶stage I through stage IV, or unspecified◀	● 523.32	Aggressive periodontitis, generalized
	Excludes terms added			● 523.33	Acute periodontitis
	Excludes term revised			523.4	Excludes term deleted
348.31	Excludes note added			● 523.40	Chronic periodontitis, unspecified
349.82	Includes note added			● 523.41	Chronic periodontitis, localized
357.4	Code first note added		Use additional code note added	● 523.42	Chronic periodontitis, generalized
	Code first note revised	▲ 404.11	Hypertensive heart and ▶chronic◀ kidney disease, benign, with heart failure ▶and with chronic kidney disease stage I through stage IV, or unspecified◀	524.07	Includes note added
359.6	Code first note revised			524.2	Includes note added
360.0	Excludes note added			▲ 524.21	▶Malocclusion,◀ Angle's class I
360.1	Excludes note added			▲ 524.22	▶Malocclusion,◀ Angle's class II
● 377.43	Optic nerve hypoplasia			▲ 524.23	▶Malocclusion,◀ Angle's class III
● 379.6	Inflammation (infection) of postprocedural bleb		Use additional code note added	524.24	Includes note added
		▲ 404.12	Hypertensive heart and ▶chronic◀ kidney disease, benign,▶ without heart failure and◀ with chronic kidney disease ▶stage V or end stage renal disease◀	524.25	Includes note added
	Includes note added			524.26	Includes note added
● 379.60	Inflammation (infection) of postprocedural bleb, unspecified			524.27	Includes term added
				524.28	Includes term added
● 379.61	Inflammation (infection) of postprocedural bleb, stage 1			524.29	Includes note added
		▲ 404.13	Hypertensive heart and ▶chronic◀ kidney disease, benign, with heart failure or ▶and with◀ chronic kidney disease ▶stage V or end stage renal disease◀	524.33	Includes note added
● 379.62	Inflammation (infection) of postprocedural bleb, stage 2			524.34	Includes term added
				▲ 524.35	Rotation of ▶tooth/◀teeth
● 379.63	Inflammation (infection) of postprocedural bleb, stage 3			524.36	Includes note added
			Use additional code note added	524.37	Includes term added
	Includes note added	▲ 404.9	Hypertensive heart and ▶chronic◀ kidney disease, unspecified		
▲ 389.11	Sensory hearing loss, ▶bilateral◀				
▲ 389.12	Neural hearing loss, ▶bilateral◀				
▲ 389.14	Central hearing loss, ▶bilateral◀				
● 389.15	Sensorineural hearing loss, unilateral				

▶◀ Revised Text   ● New Code   ▲ Revised Code Title

524.54	Includes note added	
524.55	Includes note added	
524.56	Includes note added	
● 525.6	Unsatisfactory restoration of tooth	
	Includes note added	
	Excludes note added	
● 525.60	Unspecified unsatisfactory restoration of tooth	
	Includes note added	
● 525.61	Open restoration margins	
	Includes note added	
● 525.62	Unrepairable overhanging of dental restorative materials	
	Includes note added	
● 525.63	Fractured dental restorative material without loss of material	
	Excludes note added	
● 525.64	Fractured dental restorative material with loss of material	
	Excludes note added	
● 525.65	Contour of existing restoration of tooth biologically incompatible with oral health	
	Includes note added	
● 525.66	Allergy to existing dental restorative material	
	Use additional code note added	
● 525.67	Poor aesthetics of existing restoration	
	Includes note added	
● 525.69	Other unsatisfactory restoration of existing tooth	
● 526.6	Periradicular pathology associated with previous endodontic treatment	
● 526.61	Perforation of root canal space	
● 526.62	Endodontic overfill	
● 526.63	Endodontic underfill	
● 526.69	Other periradicular pathology associated with previous endodontic treatment	
▲ 528.0	Stomatitis ▶and mucositis (ulcerative)◀	
	Includes note deleted	
	Excludes terms added	
● 528.00	Stomatitis and mucositis, unspecified	
	Includes note added	
● 528.01	Mucositis (ulcerative) due to antineoplastic therapy	
	Use additional code note added	
● 528.02	Mucositis (ulcerative) due to other drugs	
	Use additional code note added	
● 528.09	Other stomatitis and mucositis (ulcerative)	
528.3	Excludes term revised	
528.71	Includes note added	
528.72	Includes note added	
528.79	Includes term added	
530-538	Section title revised	
536.8	Includes term added	
● 538	Gastrointestinal mucositis (ulcerative)	
	Use additional code note added	
	Excludes note added	
567	Excludes terms revised	
567.23	Excludes note added	
573	Excludes term revised	
580-589	Section title revised	
581.81	Code first note revised	
582.81	Code first note revised	
583.81	Code first note revised	
585	Excludes note deleted	
	Code first note added	
585.5	Excludes note added	
585.6	Includes note added	
599.6	Excludes term deleted	
599.69	Code first note added	
600	Includes note added	
	Use additional code note deleted	
▲ 600.00	Hypertrophy (benign) of prostate without urinary obstruction ▶and other lower urinary tract symptoms [LUTS]◀	
▲ 600.01	Hypertrophy (benign) of prostate with urinary obstruction ▶and other lower urinary tract symptoms [LUTS]◀	
	Use additional code note added	
▲ 600.20	Benign localized hyperplasia of prostate without urinary obstruction ▶and other lower urinary tract symptoms [LUTS]◀	
▲ 600.21	Benign localized hyperplasia of prostate with urinary obstruction ▶and other lower urinary tract symptoms [LUTS]◀	
	Use additional code note added	
▲ 600.90	Hyperplasia of prostate, unspecified, without urinary obstruction ▶and other lower urinary tract symptoms [LUTS]◀	
▲ 600.91	Hyperplasia of prostate, unspecified, with urinary obstruction ▶and other lower urinary tract symptoms [LUTS]◀	
	Use additional code note added	
608.2	Includes note deleted	
● 608.20	Torsion of testis, unspecified	
● 608.21	Extravaginal torsion of spermatic cord	
● 608.22	Intravaginal torsion of spermatic cord	
● 608.23	Torsion of appendix testis	
● 608.24	Torsion of appendix epididymis	
616.8	Includes note deleted	
● 616.81	Mucositis (ulcerative) of cervix, vagina, and vulva	
	Use additional code note added	
● 616.89	Other inflammatory disease of cervix, vagina and vulva	
● 618.84	Cervical stump prolapse	
629.2	Includes term added	
629.20	Includes term added	
629.21	Includes term added	
629.22	Includes term added	
629.23	Includes term added	
● 629.29	Other female genital mutilation status	
	Includes note added	
● 629.81	Habitual aborter without current pregnancy	
	Excludes note added	
● 629.89	Other specified disorders of female genital organs	
629.9	Includes note deleted	
640-649	Section title revised	
	Instructional note revised [5th digit box]	
641.3	Excludes note added	
642.2	Includes terms revised	
646.8	Includes term deleted	
648.4	Instructional note revised	
● 649	Other conditions or status of the mother complicating pregnancy, childbirth, or puerperium	
● 649.0	Tobacco use disorder complicating pregnancy, childbirth, or puerperium	
	Includes note added	
● 649.00	Tobacco use disorder complicating pregnancy, childbirth, or the puerperium, unspecified as to episode of care or not applicable	
● 649.01	Tobacco use disorder complicating pregnancy, childbirth, or the puerperium, delivered, with or without mention of antepartum condition	
● 649.02	Tobacco use disorder complicating pregnancy, childbirth, or the puerperium, delivered, with mention of postpartum complication	
● 649.03	Tobacco use disorder complicating pregnancy, childbirth, or the puerperium, antepartum condition or complication	
● 649.04	Tobacco use disorder complicating pregnancy, childbirth, or the puerperium, postpartum condition or complication	
● 649.1	Obesity complicating pregnancy, childbirth, or puerperium	
	Use additional code note added	
● 649.10	Obesity complicating pregnancy, childbirth, or the puerperium, unspecified as to episode of care or not applicable	
● 649.11	Obesity complicating pregnancy, childbirth, or the puerperium, delivered, with or without mention of antepartum condition	
● 649.12	Obesity complicating pregnancy, childbirth, or the puerperium, delivered, with mention of postpartum complication	
● 649.13	Obesity complicating pregnancy, childbirth, or the puerperium, antepartum condition or complication	
● 649.14	Obesity complicating pregnancy, childbirth, or the puerperium, postpartum condition or complication	
● 649.2	Bariatric surgery status complicating pregnancy, childbirth, or puerperium	
	Includes note added	
● 649.20	Bariatric surgery status complicating pregnancy, childbirth, or the puerperium, unspecified as to episode of care or not applicable	
● 649.21	Bariatric surgery status complicating pregnancy, childbirth, or the puerperium, delivered, with or without mention of antepartum condition	
● 649.22	Bariatric surgery status complicating pregnancy, childbirth, or the puerperium, delivered, with mention of postpartum complication	
● 649.23	Bariatric surgery status complicating pregnancy, childbirth, or the puerperium, antepartum condition or complication	
● 649.24	Bariatric surgery status complicating pregnancy, childbirth, or the puerperium, postpartum condition or complication	
● 649.3	Coagulation defects complicating pregnancy, childbirth, or puerperium	
	Use additional code note added	
	Excludes note added	
● 649.30	Coagulation defects complicating pregnancy, childbirth, or the puerperium, unspecified as to episode of care or not applicable	
● 649.31	Coagulation defects complicating pregnancy, childbirth, or the puerperium, delivered, with or without mention of antepartum condition	
● 649.32	Coagulation defects complicating pregnancy, childbirth, or the puerperium, delivered, with mention of postpartum complication	
● 649.33	Coagulation defects complicating pregnancy, childbirth, or the puerperium, antepartum condition or complication	
● 649.34	Coagulation defects complicating pregnancy, childbirth, or the puerperium, postpartum condition or complication	
● 649.4	Epilepsy complicating pregnancy, childbirth, or puerperium	
	Use additional code note added	
	Excludes note added	
● 649.40	Epilepsy complicating pregnancy, childbirth, or the puerperium, unspecified as to episode of care or not applicable	
● 649.41	Epilepsy complicating pregnancy, childbirth, or the puerperium, delivered, with or without mention of antepartum condition	
● 649.42	Epilepsy complicating pregnancy, childbirth, or the puerperium, delivered, with mention of postpartum complication	
● 649.43	Epilepsy complicating pregnancy, childbirth, or the puerperium, antepartum condition or complication	
● 649.44	Epilepsy complicating pregnancy, childbirth, or the puerperium, postpartum condition or complication	
● 649.5	Spotting complicating pregnancy, childbirth, or puerperium	
	Excludes note added	
● 649.50	Spotting complicating pregnancy, unspecified as to episode of care or not applicable	
● 649.51	Spotting complicating pregnancy, delivered, with or without mention of antepartum condition	
● 649.53	Spotting complicating pregnancy, antepartum condition or complication	
● 649.6	Uterine size date discrepancy complicating pregnancy, childbirth, or puerperium	
● 649.60	Uterine size date discrepancy, unspecified as to episode of care or not applicable	
● 649.61	Uterine size date discrepancy, delivered, with or without mention of antepartum condition	
● 649.62	Uterine size date discrepancy, delivered, with mention of postpartum complication	
● 649.63	Uterine size date discrepancy, antepartum condition or complication	
● 649.64	Uterine size date discrepancy, postpartum condition or complication	
666.1	Includes term revised	
692.3	Excludes term revised	
693	Excludes term revised	

▶◀ Revised Text ● New Code ▲ Revised Code Title

713.7	Code first note revised
● 729.7	Nontraumatic compartment syndrome Excludes note added
● 729.71	Nontraumatic compartment syndrome of upper extremity Includes note added
● 729.72	Nontraumatic compartment syndrome of lower extremity Includes note added
● 729.73	Nontraumatic compartment syndrome of abdomen
● 729.79	Nontraumatic compartment syndrome of other sites
730.0	Use additional code note added
730.1	Use additional code note added
730.2	Use additional code note added
● 731.3	Major osseous defects Code first note added
733.0	Use additional code note added
733.4	Use additional code note added
743.8	Excludes term added
768	Excludes note added
▲ 768.3	Fetal distress first noted during labor ▶and delivery,◀ in liveborn infant Includes term revised
768.5	Excludes note added
768.6	Excludes note added
● 768.7	Hypoxic-ischemic encephalopathy [HIE]
768.9	Excludes term deleted
770.8	Excludes note added
● 770.87	Respiratory arrest of newborn
● 770.88	Hypoxemia of newborn Includes note added
▲ 775.8	Other transitory neonatal endocrine and metabolic disturbances Excludes term deleted
● 775.81	Other acidosis of newborn Includes note added
● 775.89	Other neonatal endocrine and metabolic disturbances Includes note added
776.7	Excludes term revised
779.2	Includes term added Excludes note added
● 779.85	Cardiac arrest of newborn
▲ 780.31	Febrile convulsions ▶(simple), unspecified◀ Includes term revised
● 780.32	Complex febrile convulsions Includes note added Excludes note added
780.39	Excludes term added
780.58	Excludes term revised
780.6	Code first note added
▲ 780.95	Excessive crying ▶of child, adolescent, or adult◀
● 780.96	Generalized pain Includes note added
● 780.97	Altered mental status Includes note added Excludes note added
780.99	Excludes terms deleted
783.2	Use additional code note revised
784.3	Excludes term added
784.9	Includes note deleted
● 784.91	Postnasal drip
● 784.99	Other symptoms involving head and neck Includes note added
785.52	Code first note deleted
788	Excludes term added
788.2	Excludes note deleted Code first note added
788.3	Code first note added
788.4	Code first note added
788.6	Code first note added
● 788.64	Urinary hesitancy
● 788.65	Straining on urination
790	Excludes term revised
790.29	Includes note added
790.6	Includes term added Excludes terms added
793.81	Excludes note added
793.89	Includes note added
793.9	Includes note deleted
● 793.91	Image test inconclusive due to excess body fat Use additional code note added
● 793.99	Other nonspecific abnormal findings on radiological and other examinations of body structure Includes note added
795.04	Includes note deleted
● 795.06	Papanicolaou smear of cervix with cytologic evidence of malignancy
795.7	Excludes terms added
795.8	Abnormal tumor markers Includes note added Excludes note added
● 795.81	Elevated carcinoembryonic antigen [CEA]
● 795.82	Elevated cancer antigen 125 [CA 125]
● 795.89	Other abnormal tumor markers
799.4	Code first note added Excludes note deleted
▲ 873.63	Tooth (broken) ▶(fractured) (due to trauma)◀ [Category 873.6 Internal structures of mouth, without mention of complications] Excludes note added
▲ 873.73	Tooth (broken) ▶(fractured) (due to trauma)◀ [Category 873.7 Internal structures of mouth, complicated] Excludes note added
● 958.9	Traumatic compartment syndrome Excludes note added
● 958.90	Compartment syndrome, unspecified
● 958.91	Traumatic compartment syndrome of upper extremity Includes note added
● 958.92	Traumatic compartment syndrome of lower extremity Includes note added
● 958.93	Traumatic compartment syndrome of abdomen
● 958.99	Traumatic compartment syndrome of other sites
960-979	Section Excludes note revised
▲ 995.2	▶Other and◀ uUnspecified adverse effect of drug, medicinal and biological substance
● 995.20	Unspecified adverse effect of unspecified drug, medicinal and biological substance
● 995.21	Arthus phenomenon Includes note added
● 995.22	Unspecified adverse effect of anesthesia
● 995.23	Unspecified adverse effect of insulin
● 995.27	Other drug allergy Includes note added
● 995.29	Unspecified adverse effect of other drug, medicinal and biological substance
995.3	Excludes term added Excludes term revised
995.4	Excludes term revised
995.9	Code first note deleted
▲ 995.91	Systemic inflammatory response syndrome, unspecified ▶Sepsis◀ Includes term added Includes term deleted Code first note added Excludes note added
▲ 995.92	Systemic inflammatory response syndrome due to infectious process without organ dysfunction ▶Severe sepsis◀ Includes terms added Includes term deleted Code first note added Use additional code note revised Use additional code note added
▲ 995.93	Systemic inflammatory response syndrome due to noninfectious process without ▶acute◀ organ dysfunction Code first note added Excludes note added
▲ 995.94	Systemic inflammatory response syndrome due to noninfectious process with ▶acute◀ organ dysfunction Code first note added Use additional code note added Use additional code note deleted Excludes note added
996.45	Use additional code note added
996.7	Use additional code note added
997.3	Excludes terms added
998.5	Excludes terms added
999	Excludes terms revised
999.8	Excludes terms added
V01-V86	Section title revised
V07.39	Excludes terms revised
● V18.51	Colonic polyps Excludes note added
● V18.59	Other digestive disorders
V20.2	Includes term added
V26.21	Excludes term revised
V26.3	Excludes term added
▲ V26.31	Testing ▶of female◀ for genetic disease carrier status
▲ V26.32	Other genetic testing ▶of female◀ Use additional code note added
● V26.34	Testing of male for genetic disease carrier status
● V26.35	Encounter for testing of male partner of habitual aborter
● V26.39	Other genetic testing of male
▲ V28	▶Encounter for◀ Aantenatal screening ▶of mother◀
V45.3	Excludes note added
V45.77	Excludes term revised
● V45.86	Bariatric surgery status Includes note added Excludes note added
V54.1	Excludes note added
▲ V58.3	Attention to surgical dressings and sutures Includes terms deleted Includes term added Excludes note added
● V58.30	Encounter for change or removal of nonsurgical wound dressing Includes note added
● V58.31	Encounter for change or removal of surgical wound dressing
● V58.32	Encounter for removal of sutures
V58.41	Excludes term added
V58.49	Includes note added
V65.3	Use additional code note added
V65.4	Excludes terms revised
V70-V82	Section title revised
V72.11	Encounter for hearing examination following failed hearing screening
● V72.19	Other examination of ears and hearing
● V82.7	Genetic screening Excludes note added
● V82.71	Screening for genetic disease carrier status
● V82.79	Other genetic screening
V83-V84	Section title added
V85	Section title added
▲ V85	Body Mass Index ▶[BMI]◀
V85.5	Body Mass Index, pediatric Instructional note added
● V85.51	Body Mass Index, pediatric, less than 5th percentile for age
● V85.52	Body Mass Index, pediatric, 5th percentile to less than 85th percentile for age
● V85.53	Body Mass Index, pediatric, 85th percentile to less than 95th percentile for age
● V85.54	Body Mass Index, pediatric, greater than or equal to 95th percentile for age
V86	Section title added
● V86	Estrogen receptor status Code first note added
● V86.0	Estrogen receptor positive status [ER+]
● V86.1	Estrogen receptor negative status [ER-]

▶◀ Revised Text   ● New Code   ▲ Revised Code Title

Coding Guidelines

ICD-9-CM OFFICIAL GUIDELINES FOR CODING AND REPORTING
Effective December 1, 2005
Narrative changes appear in bold text
The guidelines have been updated to include the V Code Table.

The Centers for Medicare and Medicaid Services (CMS) and the National Center for Health Statistics (NCHS), two departments within the U.S. Federal Government's Department of Health and Human Services (DHHS) provide the following guidelines for coding and reporting using the International Classification of Diseases, 9th Revision, Clinical Modification (ICD-9-CM). These guidelines should be used as a companion document to the official version of the ICD-9-CM as published on CD-ROM by the U.S. Government Printing Office (GPO).

These guidelines have been approved by the four organizations that make up the Cooperating Parties for the ICD-9-CM: the American Hospital Association (AHA), the American Health Information Management Association (AHIMA), CMS, and NCHS. These guidelines are included in the official government version of the ICD-9-CM and also appear in *Coding Clinic for ICD-9-CM*, published by the AHA.

These guidelines are a set of rules that have been developed to accompany and complement the official conventions and instructions provided within the ICD-9-CM itself. These guidelines are based on the coding and sequencing instructions in Volumes 1, 2, and 3 of ICD-9-CM, but provide additional instruction. Adherence to these guidelines when assigning ICD-9-CM diagnosis and procedure codes is required under the Health Insurance Portability and Accountability Act (HIPAA). The diagnosis codes (Volumes 1-2) have been adopted under HIPAA for all health care settings. Volume 3 procedure codes have been adopted for inpatient procedures reported by hospitals. A joint effort between the health care provider and the coder is essential to achieve complete and accurate documentation, code assignment, and reporting of diagnoses and procedures. These guidelines have been developed to assist both the health care provider and the coder in identifying those diagnoses and procedures that are to be reported. The importance of consistent, complete documentation in the medical record cannot be overemphasized. Without such documentation accurate coding cannot be achieved. The entire record should be reviewed to determine the specific reason for the encounter and the conditions treated.

The term "encounter" is used for all settings, including hospital admissions. In the context of these guidelines, the term "provider" is used throughout the guidelines to mean physician or any qualified health care practitioner who is legally accountable for establishing the patient's diagnosis. Only this set of guidelines, approved by the cooperating parties, is official.

The guidelines are organized into sections. Section I includes the structure and conventions of the classification and general guidelines that apply to the entire classification, and chapter-specific guidelines that correspond to the chapters as they are arranged in the classification. Section II includes guidelines for selection of principal diagnosis for non-outpatient settings. Section III includes guidelines for reporting additional diagnoses in non-outpatient settings. Section IV is for outpatient coding and reporting.

Section I. Conventions, general coding guidelines and chapter-specific guidelines
A. Conventions for the ICD-9-CM
1. Format
2. Abbreviations
   a. Index abbreviations
   b. Tabular abbreviations
3. Punctuation
4. Includes and excludes notes and inclusion terms
5. Other and Unspecified codes
   a. "Other" codes
   b. "Unspecified" codes
6. Etiology/manifestation convention ("code first," "use additional code," and "in diseases classified elsewhere" notes)
7. "And"
8. "With"
9. "See" and "see also"
B. General coding guidelines
1. Use of both Alphabetic Index and Tabular List
2. Locate each term in the Alphabetic Index
3. Level of detail in coding
4. Code or codes from 001.0 through V86.1
5. Selection of codes 001.0 through 999.9
6. Signs and symptoms
7. Conditions that are an integral part of a disease process
8. Conditions that are not an integral part of a disease process
9. Multiple coding for a single condition
10. Acute and chronic conditions
11. Combination code
12. Late effects
13. Impending or threatened condition
C. Chapter-specific coding guidelines
1. Chapter 1: Infectious and Parasitic Diseases (001–139)
   a. Human immunodeficiency virus (HIV) infections
   b. Septicemia, systemic inflammatory response syndrome . . . (SIRS), sepsis, severe sepsis, and septic shock
2. Chapter 2: Neoplasms (140–239)
   a. Treatment directed at the malignancy
   b. Treatment of secondary site
   c. Coding and sequencing of complications
   d. Primary malignancy previously excised
   e. Admissions/encounters involving chemotherapy and radiation therapy
   f. Admission/encounter to determine extent of malignancy
   g. Symptoms, signs, and ill-defined conditions listed in chapter 16
   h. Encounter for prophylactic organ removal
3. Chapter 3: Endocrine, Nutritional, and Metabolic Diseases and Immunity Disorders (240–279)
   a. Diabetes mellitus
4. Chapter 4: Diseases of Blood and Blood-Forming Organs (280–289)
   a. Anemia of chronic disease
5. Chapter 5: Mental Disorders (290–319)
   Reserved for future guideline expansion
6. Chapter 6: Diseases of Nervous System and Sense Organs (320–389)
   Reserved for future guideline expansion
7. Chapter 7: Diseases of Circulatory System (390–459)
   a. Hypertension
   b. Cerebral infarction/stroke/cerebrovascular accident (CVA)
   c. Postoperative cerebrovascular accident
   d. Late effects of cerebrovascular disease
   e. Acute myocardial infarction (AMI)
8. Chapter 8: Diseases of Respiratory System (460–519)
   a. Chronic obstructive pulmonary disease [COPD] and asthma
   b. Chronic obstructive pulmonary disease [COPD] and bronchitis
9. Chapter 9: Diseases of Digestive System (520–579)
   Reserved for future guideline expansion
10. Chapter 10: Diseases of Genitourinary System (580–629)
    a. Chronic kidney disease
11. Chapter 11: Complications of Pregnancy, Childbirth, and the Puerperium (630–677)
    a. General rules for obstetric cases
    b. Selection of OB principal or first-listed diagnosis
    c. Fetal conditions affecting the management of the mother
    d. HIV infection in pregnancy, childbirth and the puerperium
    e. Current conditions complicating pregnancy
    f. Diabetes mellitus in pregnancy
    g. Gestational diabetes
    h. Normal delivery, code 650
    i. The postpartum and peripartum eriods
    j. Code 677 Late effect of complication of pregnancy
    k. Abortions
12. Chapter 12: Diseases Skin and Subcutaneous Tissue (680–709)
    Reserved for future guideline expansion
13. Chapter 13: Diseases of Musculoskeletal and Connective Tissue (710–739)
    Reserved for future guideline expansion

14. Chapter 14: Congenital Anomalies (740–759)
    a. Codes in categories 740-759, Congenital anomalies
15. Chapter 15: Newborn (Perinatal) Guidelines (760-779)
    a. General perinatal rules
    b. Use of codes V30-V39
    c. Newborn transfers
    d. Use of category V29
    e. Use of other V codes on perinatal records
    f. Maternal causes of perinatal morbidity
    g. Congenital anomalies in newborns
    h. Coding additional perinatal diagnoses
    i. Prematurity and fetal growth retardation
    j. Newborn sepsis
16. Chapter 16: Signs, Symptoms and Ill-Defined Conditions (780–799)
17. Chapter 17: Injury and Poisoning (800-999)
    a. Coding of injuries
    b. Coding of fractures
    c. Coding of burns
    d. Coding of debridement of wound, infection, or burn
    e. Adverse effects, poisoning and toxic effects
    f. Complications of care
18. Classification of Factors Influencing Health Status and Contact with Health Service (Supplemental V01-V86)
    a. Introduction
    b. V codes use in any health care setting
    c. V codes indicate a reason for an encounter
    d. Categories of V codes
    e. V Code Table
19. Supplemental Classification of External Causes of Injury and Poisoning (E codes, E800–E999)
    a. General E code coding guideline
    b. Place of occurrence guideline
    c. Adverse effects of drugs, medicinal and biological substances guidelines
    d. Multiple cause E code coding guidelines
    e. Child and adult abuse guideline
    f. Unknown or suspected intent guideline
    g. Undetermined cause
    h. Late effects of external cause guidelines
    i. Misadventures and complications of care guidelines
    j. Terrorism guidelines

Section II. Selection of Principal Diagnosis
A. Codes for symptoms, signs, and ill-defined conditions
B. Two or more interrelated conditions, each potentially meeting the definition for principal diagnosis
C. Two or more diagnoses that equally meet the definition for principal diagnosis
D. Two or more comparative or contrasting conditions
E. A symptom(s) followed by contrasting/comparative diagnoses
F. Original treatment plan not carried out
G. Complications of surgery and other medical care
H. Uncertain diagnosis
I. Admission from observation unit
   1. Admission following medical observation
   2. Admission following post-operative observation
J. Admission from outpatient surgery

Section III. Reporting Additional Diagnoses
A. Previous conditions
B. Abnormal findings
C. Uncertain diagnosis

Section IV. Diagnostic Coding and Reporting Guidelines for Outpatient Services
A. Selection of first-listed condition
B. Codes from 001.0 through V86.1
C. Accurate reporting of ICD-9-CM diagnosis codes
D. Selection of codes 001.0 through 999.9
E. Codes that describe symptoms and signs
F. Encounters for circumstances other than a disease or injury
G. Level of detail in coding
   1. ICD-9-CM codes with three, four, or five digits
   2. Use of full number of digits required for a code
H. ICD-9-CM code for the diagnosis, condition, problem, or other reason for encounter/visit

I. "Probable," "suspected," "questionable," "rule out," or "working diagnosis"
J. Chronic diseases
K. Code all documented conditions that coexist
L. Patients receiving diagnostic services only
M. Patients receiving therapeutic services only
N. Patients receiving preoperative evaluations only
O. Ambulatory surgery
P. Routine outpatient prenatal visits

Section I. Conventions, general coding guidelines and chapter-specific guidelines
The conventions, general guidelines, and chapter-specific guidelines are applicable to all health care settings unless otherwise indicated.

A. Conventions for the ICD-9-CM
The conventions for the ICD-9-CM are the general rules for use of the classification independent of the guidelines. These conventions are incorporated within the index and tabular of the ICD-9-CM as instructional notes. The conventions are as follows:

1. **Format:**
   The ICD-9-CM uses an indented format for ease in reference

2. **Abbreviations**
   a. Index abbreviations
   NEC "Not elsewhere classifiable"—This abbreviation in the index represents "other specified." When a specific code is not available for a condition, the index directs the coder to the "other specified" code in the tabular.

   b. Tabular abbreviations
   NEC "Not elsewhere classifiable"—This abbreviation in the tabular represents "other specified." When a specific code is not available for a condition, the tabular includes an NEC entry under a code to identify the code as the "other specified" code (See section I.A.5.a.,"Other" codes).

   NOS "Not otherwise specified"—This abbreviation is the equivalent of unspecified. (See section I.A.5.b., "Unspecified" codes)

3. **Punctuation**
   [ ] Brackets are used in the Tabular List to enclose synonyms, alternative wording, or explanatory phrases. Brackets are used in the index to identify manifestation codes. (See section I.A.6., Etiology/manifestations)

   ( ) Parentheses are used in both the index and tabular to enclose supplementary words that may be present or absent in the statement of a disease or procedure without affecting the code number to which it is assigned. The terms within the parentheses are referred to as nonessential modifiers.

   : Colons are used in the Tabular List after an incomplete term needs one or more of the modifiers following the colon to make it assignable to a given category.

4. **Includes and excludes notes and inclusion terms**
   Includes: This note appears immediately under a three-digit code title to further define, or give examples of, the content of the category.

   Excludes: An excludes note under a code indicates that the terms excluded from the code are to be coded elsewhere. In some cases the codes for the excluded terms should not be used in conjunction with the code from which they are excluded. An example of this is a congenital condition excluded from an acquired form of the same condition. The congenital and acquired codes should not be used together. In other cases, the excluded terms may be used together with an excluded code. An example of this is when fractures of different bones are coded to different codes. Both codes may be used together if both types of fractures are present.

   Inclusion terms: List of terms included under certain four- and five-digit codes. These terms are the conditions for which that code number is to be used. The terms may be synonyms of the code title, or, in the case of "other specified" codes, the terms are a list of the various conditions assigned to that code. The inclusion terms are not necessarily exhaustive. Additional terms found only in the index may also be assigned to a code.

5. **Other and unspecified codes**
   a."Other" codes—Codes titled "other" or "other specified" (usually a code with a fourth digit of 8 or fifth digit of 9 for diagnosis codes) are for use when the information in the medical record provides detail for which a specific code does not exist. Index entries with NEC in the line designate "other" codes in the tabular. These index entries

represent specific disease entities for which no specific code exists so the term is included within an "other" code.

    b. **"Unspecified" codes**—Codes (usually a code with a fourth digit of 9 or fifth of 0 for diagnosis codes) titled "unspecified" are for use when the information in the medical record is insufficient to assign a more specific code.

6. **Etiology/manifestation convention ("code first," "use additional code," and "in diseases classified elsewhere" notes)**—Certain conditions have both an underlying etiology and multiple body system manifestations due to the underlying etiology. For such conditions, the ICD-9-CM has a coding convention that requires the underlying condition to be sequenced first followed by the manifestation. Wherever such a combination exists, there is a "use additional code" note at the etiology code, and a "code first" note at the manifestation code. These instructional notes indicate the proper sequencing order of the codes, etiology followed by manifestation.

   In most cases the manifestation codes will have in the code title, "in diseases classified elsewhere." Codes with this title are a component of the etiology/manifestation convention. The code title indicates that it is a manifestation code. "In diseases classified elsewhere," codes are never permitted to be used as first listed or principal diagnosis codes. They must be used in conjunction with an underlying condition code, and they must be listed following the underlying condition.

   There are manifestation codes that do not have "in diseases classified elsewhere" in the title. For such codes a "use additional code" note will still be present and the rules for sequencing apply.

   In addition to the notes in the tabular, these conditions also have a specific index entry structure. In the index both conditions are listed together with the etiology code first followed by the manifestation codes in brackets. The code in brackets is always to be sequenced second.

   The most commonly used etiology/manifestation combinations are the codes for diabetes mellitus, category 250. For each code under category 250 there is a use additional code note for the manifestation that is specific for that particular diabetic manifestation. Should a patient have more than one manifestation of diabetes, more than one code from category 250 may be used with as many manifestation codes as are needed to fully describe the patient's complete diabetic condition. The category 250 diabetes codes should be sequenced first, followed by the manifestation codes.

   "Code first" and "use additional code" notes are also used as sequencing rules in the classification for certain codes that are not part of an etiology/manifestation combination. See section I.B.9., "Multiple coding for a single condition."

7. **"And"**
   The word "and" should be interpreted to mean either "and" or "or" when it appears in a title.

8. **"With"**
   The word "with" in the Alphabetic Index is sequenced immediately following the main term, not in alphabetical order.

9. **"See" and "see also"**
   The "see" instruction following a main term in the index indicates that another term should be referenced. It is necessary to go to the main term referenced with the "see" note to locate the correct code.

   A "see also" instruction following a main term in the index instructs that there is another main term that may also be referenced that may provide additional index entries that may be useful. It is not necessary to follow the "see also" note when the original main term provides the necessary code.

B. General coding guidelines

1. **Use of both Alphabetic Index and Tabular List**—Use both the Alphabetic Index and the Tabular List when locating and assigning a code. Reliance on only the Alphabetic Index or the Tabular List leads to errors in code assignments and less specificity in code selection.

2. **Locate each term in the alphabetic index**—Locate each term in the Alphabetic Index and verify the code selected in the Tabular List. Read and be guided by instructional notations that appear in both the Alphabetic Index and the Tabular List.

3. **Level of detail in coding**—Diagnosis and procedure codes are to be used at their highest number of digits available.

   ICD-9-CM diagnosis codes are composed of codes with either three, four, or five digits. Codes with three digits are included in ICD-9-CM as the heading of a category of codes that may be further subdivided by the use of four and/or fifth digits, which provide greater detail.

   A three-digit code is to be used only if it is not further subdivided. Where fourth-digit subcategories and/or fifth-digit subclassifications are provided, they must be assigned. A code is invalid if it has not been coded to the full number of digits required for that code. For example, acute myocardial infarction, code 410, has fourth digits that describe the location of the infarction (e.g., 410.2 Of inferolateral wall), and fifth digits that identify the episode of care. It would be incorrect to report a code in category 410 without a fourth and fifth digit.

   ICD-9-CM Volume 3 procedure codes are composed of codes with either three or four digits. Codes with two digits are included in ICD-9-CM as the heading of a category of codes that may be further subdivided by the use of third and/or fourth digits, which provide greater detail.

4. **Code or codes from 001.0 through V86.1**—The appropriate code or codes from 001.0 through V86.1 must be used to identify diagnoses, symptoms, conditions, problems, complaints, or other reason(s) for the encounter/visit.

5. **Selection of codes 001.0 through 999.9**—The selection of codes 001.0 through 999.9 will frequently be used to describe the reason for the admission/encounter. These codes are from the section of ICD-9-CM for the classification of diseases and injuries (e.g., infectious and parasitic diseases; neoplasms; symptoms, signs, and ill-defined conditions, etc.).

6. **Signs and symptoms**—Codes that describe symptoms and signs, as opposed to diagnoses, are acceptable for reporting purposes when a related definitive diagnosis has not been established (confirmed) by the provider. Chapter 16 of ICD-9-CM, "Symptoms, Signs, and Ill-defined Conditions" (codes 780.0-799.9) contain many, but not all, codes for symptoms.

7. **Conditions that are an integral part of a disease process**—Signs and symptoms that are integral to the disease process should not be assigned as additional codes.

8. **Conditions that are not an integral part of a disease process**—Additional signs and symptoms that may not be associated routinely with a disease process should be coded when present.

9. **Multiple coding for a single condition**—In addition to the etiology/manifestation convention that requires two codes to fully describe a single condition that affects multiple body systems, there are other single conditions that also require more than one code. "Use additional code" notes are found in the tabular at codes that are not part of an etiology/manifestation pair where a secondary code is useful to fully describe a condition. The sequencing rule is the same as the etiology/manifestation pair where a secondary code is useful to fully describe a condition. The sequencing rule is the same; "use additional code" indicates that a secondary code should be added.

   For example, for infections that are not included in chapter 1, a secondary code from category 041 Bacterial infection in conditions classified elsewhere and of unspecified site, may be required to identify the bacterial organism causing the infection. A "use additional code" note will normally be found at the infectious disease code, indicating a need for the organism code to be added as a secondary code.

   "Code first" notes are also under certain codes that are not specifically manifestation codes but may be due to an underlying cause. When a "code first" note is present and an underlying condition is present, the underlying condition should be sequenced first.

   "Code, if applicable, any causal condition first" notes indicate that this code may be assigned as a principal diagnosis when the causal condition is unknown or not applicable. If a causal condition is known, then the code for that condition should be sequenced as the principal or first-listed diagnosis.

   Multiple codes may be needed for late effects, complication codes, and obstetric codes to more fully describe a condition. See the specific guidelines for these conditions for further instruction.

10. **Acute and chronic conditions**—If the same condition is described as both acute (subacute) and chronic, and separate subentries exist in the Alphabetic Index at the same indentation level, code both and sequence the acute (subacute) code first.

11. **Combination code**—A combination code is a single code used to classify:
    - Two diagnoses
    - A diagnosis with an associated secondary process (manifestation)
    - A diagnosis with an associated complication

    Combination codes are identified by referring to subterm entries in the Alphabetic Index and by reading the inclusion and exclusion notes in the Tabular List.

    Assign only the combination code when that code fully identifies the diagnostic conditions involved or when the Alphabetic Index so directs. Multiple coding should not be used when the classification provides a combination code that clearly identifies all of the elements documented in the diagnosis. When the combination code lacks necessary specificity in describing the manifestation or complication, an additional code should be used as a secondary code.

12. **Late effects**—A late effect is the residual effect (condition produced) after the acute phase of an illness or injury has terminated. There is no time limit on when a late effect code can be used. The residual may be apparent early, such as in cerebrovascular accident cases, or it may occur months or years later, such as that due to a previous injury. Coding of late effects generally requires two codes sequenced in the following order: The condition or nature of the late effect is sequenced first... The late effect code is sequenced second.

    An exception to the above guidelines are those instances where the code for late effect is followed by a manifestation code identified in the Tabular List and title, or the late effect code has been expanded (at the fourth- and fifth-digit levels) to include the manifestation(s). The code for the acute phase of an illness or injury that led to the late effect is never used with a code for the late effect.

13. **Impending or threatened condition**—Code any condition described at the time of discharge as "impending" or "threatened" as follows:

    If it did occur, code as confirmed diagnosis. If it did not occur, reference the Alphabetic Index to determine if the condition has a subentry term for "impending" or "threatened" and also reference main term entries for "Impending" and for "Threatened." If the subterms are listed, assign the given code. If the subterms are not listed, code the existing underlying condition(s) and not the condition described as impending or threatened.

C. Chapter-specific coding guidelines

In addition to general coding guidelines, there are guidelines for specific diagnoses and/or conditions in the classification. Unless otherwise indicated, these guidelines apply to all health care settings. Please refer to section II for guidelines on the selection of principal diagnosis.

1. **Chapter 1: Infectious and Parasitic Diseases (001-139)**
    a. **Human immunodeficiency virus (HIV) infections**
       1) **Code only confirmed cases**—Code only confirmed cases of HIV infection/illness. This is an exception to the hospital inpatient guideline section II, H.

          In this context, "confirmation" does not require documentation of positive serology or culture for HIV; the provider's diagnostic statement that the patient is HIV positive or has an HIV-related illness is sufficient.

       2) **Selection and sequencing of HIV codes**
          (a) Patient admitted for HIV-related condition—If a patient is admitted for an HIV-related condition, the principal diagnosis should be 042, followed by additional diagnosis codes for all reported HIV-related conditions.

          (b) Patient with HIV disease admitted for unrelated condition—If a patient with HIV disease is admitted for an unrelated condition (such as a traumatic injury), the code for the unrelated condition (e.g., the nature of injury code) should be the principal diagnosis. Other diagnoses would be 042 followed by additional diagnosis codes for all reported HIV-related conditions.

          (c) Whether the patient is newly diagnosed—Whether the patient is newly diagnosed or has had previous admissions/encounters for HIV conditions is irrelevant to the sequencing decision.

          (d) Asymptomatic human immunodeficiency virus—V08 Asymptomatic human immunodeficiency virus [HIV] infection, is to be applied when the patient without any documentation of symptoms is listed as being "HIV positive," "known HIV," "HIV test positive," or similar terminology. Do not use this code if the term "AIDS" is used or if the patient is treated for any HIV-related illness or is described as having any condition(s) resulting from his/her HIV positive status; use 042 in these cases.

          (e) Patients with inconclusive HIV serology—Patients with inconclusive HIV serology, but no definitive diagnosis or manifestations of the illness, may be assigned code 795.71 Inconclusive serologic test for human immunodeficiency virus [HIV].

          (f) Previously diagnosed HIV-related illness—Patients with any known prior diagnosis of an HIV-related illness should be coded to 042. Once a patient has developed an HIV-related illness, the patient should always be assigned code 042 on every subsequent admission/encounter. Patients previously diagnosed with any HIV illness (042) should never be assigned to 795.71 or V08.

          (g) HIV infection in pregnancy, childbirth and the puerperium—During pregnancy, childbirth, or the puerperium, a patient admitted (or presenting for a health care encounter) because of an HIV-related illness should receive a principal diagnosis code of 647.6x Other specified infectious and parasitic diseases in the mother classifiable elsewhere but complicating the pregnancy, childbirth or the puerperium, followed by 042 and the code(s) for the HIV-related illness(es). Codes from chapter 15 always take sequencing priority. Patients with asymptomatic HIV infection status admitted (or presenting for a health care encounter) during pregnancy, childbirth, or the puerperium should receive codes of 647.6x and V08.

          (h) Encounters for testing for HIV—If a patient is being seen to determine his/her HIV status, use code V73.89 Screening for other specified viral disease. Use code V69.8 Other problems related to lifestyle, as a secondary code if an asymptomatic patient is in a known high risk group for HIV. Should a patient with signs or symptoms or illness, or a confirmed HIV related diagnosis be tested for HIV, code the signs and symptoms or the diagnosis. An additional counseling code V65.44 may be used if counseling is provided during the encounter for the test.

          When a patient returns to be informed of his/her HIV test results, use code V65.44 HIV counseling, if the results of the test are negative.

          If the results are positive but the patient is asymptomatic, use code V08 Asymptomatic HIV infection. If the results are positive and the patient is symptomatic, use code 042 HIV infection, with codes for the HIV-related symptoms or diagnosis. The HIV counseling code may also be used if counseling is provided for patients with positive test results.

    b. **Septicemia, systemic inflammatory response syndrome (SIRS), sepsis, severe sepsis, and septic shock**
       1) **Sepsis as principal diagnosis or secondary diagnosis**
          (a) **Sepsis as principal diagnosis**—If sepsis is present on admission and meets the definition of principal diagnosis, the underlying systemic infection code (e.g., 038.xx, 112.5, etc.) should be assigned as the principal diagnosis, followed by code 995.91 Systemic inflammatory response syndrome due to infectious process without organ dysfunction, as required by the sequencing rules in the Tabular List. Codes from subcategory 995.9 can never be assigned as a principal diagnosis.

          (b) **Sepsis as secondary diagnoses**—When sepsis develops during the encounter (it was not present on admission), the sepsis codes may be assigned as secondary diagnoses, following the sequencing rules provided in the Tabular List.

          (c) **Documentation unclear as to whether sepsis present on admission**—If the documentation is not clear whether the sepsis was present on admission, the provider should be queried. After provider query, if sepsis is determined at that point to have met the definition of principal diagnosis, the underlying systemic infection (038.xx, 112.5, etc.) may be used as the principal diagnosis along with code 995.91 Systemic inflammatory response syndrome due to infectious process without organ dysfunction.

       2) **Septicemia/sepsis**—In most cases, it will be a code from category 038 Septicemia, that will be used in conjunction with a code from subcategory 995.9 such as the following:

          (a) Streptococcal sepsis—If the documentation in the record states streptococcal sepsis, codes 038.0 and code 995.91 should be used, in that sequence.

          (b) Streptococcal septicemia—If the documentation states streptococcal septicemia, only code 038.0 should be assigned; however, the provider should be queried whether the patient has sepsis, an infection with SIRS.

          (c) Sepsis or SIRS must be documented—Either the term sepsis or SIRS must be documented to assign a code from subcategory 995.9.

       3) **Terms "sepsis," " severe sepsis," or "SIRS"**—If the terms sepsis, severe sepsis, or SIRS are used with an underlying infection other than septicemia, such as pneumonia, cellulitis, or a nonspecified urinary tract infection, a code from category 038 should be assigned first, then code 995.91, followed by the code for the initial infection. The use of the terms sepsis or SIRS indicates that the patient's infection has advanced to the point of a systemic infection so the systemic infection should be sequenced before the localized infection. The instructional note under subcategory 995.9 instructs to assign the underlying systemic infection first.

          Note: The term "urosepsis" is a nonspecific term. If that is the only term documented then only code 599.0 should be assigned based on the default for the term in the ICD-9-CM index, in addition to the code for the causal organism if known.

       4) **Severe sepsis**—For patients with severe sepsis, the code for the systemic infection (e.g., 038.xx, 112.5, etc) or trauma should be sequenced first, followed by either code 995.92 Systemic inflammatory response syndrome due to infectious process with organ dysfunction, or code 995.94 Systemic inflammatory response syndrome due to noninfectious process with organ dysfunction. Codes for the specific organ dysfunctions should also be assigned.

5) **Septic shock**
   (a) Sequencing of septic shock—Septic shock is a form of organ dysfunction associated with severe sepsis. A code for the initiating underlying systemic infection followed by a code for SIRS (code 995.92) must be assigned before the code for septic shock. As noted in the sequencing instructions in the Tabular List, the code for septic shock cannot be assigned as a principal diagnosis.
   (b) Septic shock without documentation of severe sepsis—Septic shock cannot occur in the absence of severe sepsis. A code from subcategory 995.9 must be sequenced before the code for septic shock. The use additional code notes and the code first note provide sequencing instructions.

6) **Sepsis and septic shock associated with abortion**—Sepsis and septic shock associated with abortion, ectopic pregnancy, and molar pregnancy are classified to category codes in chapter 11 (630-639).

7) **Negative or inconclusive blood cultures**—Negative or inconclusive blood cultures do not preclude a diagnosis of septicemia or sepsis in patients with clinical evidence of the condition; however, the provider should be queried.

8) **Newborn sepsis**—See section I.C.15.j for information on the coding of newborn sepsis.

9) **Sepsis due to a postprocedural infection**—Sepsis resulting from a postprocedural infection is a complication of care. For such cases code 998.59 Other postoperative infections, should be coded first followed by the appropriate codes for the sepsis. The other guidelines for coding sepsis should then be followed for the assignment of additional codes.

10) External cause of injury codes with SIRS—An external cause code is not needed with codes 995.91 Systemic inflammatory response syndrome due to infectious process without organ dysfunction, or 995.92 Systemic inflammatory response syndrome due to infectious process with organ dysfunction.

Refer to section I.C.19.a.7 for instruction on the use of external cause of injury codes with codes for SIRS resulting from trauma.

2. Chapter 2: Neoplasms (140-239)
General guidelines

Chapter 2 of the ICD-9-CM contains the codes for most benign and all malignant neoplasms. Certain benign neoplasms, such as prostatic adenomas, may be found in the specific body system chapters. To properly code a neoplasm it is necessary to determine from the record if the neoplasm is benign, in situ, malignant, or of uncertain histologic behavior. If malignant, any secondary (metastatic) sites should also be determined.

The neoplasm table in the Alphabetic Index should be referenced first. However, if the histological term is documented, that term should be referenced first, rather than going immediately to the neoplasm table, in order to determine which column in the neoplasm table is appropriate. For example, if the documentation indicates "adenoma," refer to the term in the Alphabetic Index to review the entries under this term and the instructional note to "see also neoplasm, by site, benign." The table provides the proper code based on the type of neoplasm and the site. It is important to select the proper column in the table that corresponds to the type of neoplasm. The tabular should then be referenced to verify that the correct code has been selected from the table and that a more specific site code does not exist.

See section I. C. 18.d.4. for information regarding V codes for genetic susceptibility to cancer.

a. **Treatment directed at the malignancy**—If the treatment is directed at the malignancy, designate the malignancy as the principal diagnosis.

b. **Treatment of secondary site**—When a patient is admitted because of a primary neoplasm with metastasis and treatment is directed toward the secondary site only, the secondary neoplasm is designated as the principal diagnosis even though the primary malignancy is still present.

c. **Coding and sequencing of complications**—Coding and sequencing of complications associated with the malignancies or with the therapy thereof are subject to the following guidelines:

   1) **Anemia associated with malignancy**—When admission/encounter is for management of an anemia associated with the malignancy, and the treatment is only for anemia, **the appropriate anemia code (such as code 285.22 Anemia in neoplastic disease)** is designated as the principal diagnosis and is followed by the appropriate code(s) for the malignancy.

   Code 285.22 may also be used as a secondary code if the patient suffers from anemia and is being treated for the malignancy.

   2) **Anemia associated with chemotherapy, immunotherapy and radiation therapy**—When the admission/encounter is for management of an anemia associated with chemotherapy, **immunotherapy,** or radiotherapy and the only treatment is for the anemia, the anemia is sequenced first followed by **code E933.1. The appropriate neoplasm code should be assigned as an additional code.**

   3) **Management of dehydration due to the malignancy**—When the admission/encounter is for management of dehydration due to the malignancy or the therapy, or a combination of both, and only the dehydration is being treated (intravenous rehydration), the dehydration is sequenced first, followed by the code(s) for the malignancy.

   4) **Treatment of a complication resulting from a surgical procedure**—When the admission/encounter is for treatment of a complication resulting from a surgical procedure, designate the complication as the principal or first-listed diagnosis if treatment is directed at resolving the complication.

d. **Primary malignancy previously excised**—When a primary malignancy has been previously excised or eradicated from its site and there is no further treatment directed to that site and there is no evidence of any existing primary malignancy, a code from category V10 Personal history of malignant neoplasm, should be used to indicate the former site of the malignancy. Any mention of extension, invasion, or metastasis to another site is coded as a secondary malignant neoplasm to that site. The secondary site may be the principal or first-listed with the V10 code used as a secondary code.

e. **Admissions/encounters involving chemotherapy, immunotherapy, and radiation therapy**

   1) **Episode of care involves surgical removal of neoplasm**—When an episode of care involves the surgical removal of a neoplasm, primary or secondary site, followed by adjunct chemotherapy or radiation treatment **during the same episode of care,** the neoplasm code should be assigned as principal or first-listed diagnosis, using codes in the 140-198 series or where appropriate in the 200-203 series.

   2) **Patient admission/encounter solely for administration of chemotherapy, immunotherapy, and radiation therapy**—If a patient admission/encounter is solely for the administration of chemotherapy, **immunotherapy** or radiation therapy, assign code V58.0 Encounter for radiation therapy, **V58.11 Encounter for antineoplastic chemotherapy, or V58.12 Encounter for antineoplastic immunotherapy as** the first-listed or principal diagnosis. If a patient receives **more than one of these therapies during the same admission, more than one of these codes may be assigned, in any sequence.**

   3) **Patient admitted for radiotherapy/chemotherapy and immunotherapy and develops complications**—When a patient is admitted for the purpose of radiotherapy, **immunotherapy,** or chemotherapy and develops complications such as uncontrolled nausea and vomiting or dehydration, the principal or first-listed diagnosis is V58.0 Encounter for radiotherapy, **V58.11 Encounter for antineoplastic chemotherapy, or V58.12 Encounter for antineoplastic immunotherapy** followed by any codes for the complications.

   See section I.C.18.d.8. for additional information regarding aftercare V codes.

f. **Admission/encounter to determine extent of malignancy**—When the reason for admission/encounter is to determine the extent of the malignancy, or for a procedure such as paracentesis or thoracentesis, the primary malignancy or appropriate metastatic site is designated as the principal or first-listed diagnosis, even though chemotherapy or radiotherapy is administered.

g. **Symptoms, signs, and ill-defined conditions listed in chapter 16**—Symptoms, signs, and ill-defined conditions listed in chapter 16 characteristic of, or associated with, an existing primary or secondary site malignancy cannot be used to replace the malignancy as principal or first-listed diagnosis, regardless of the number of admissions or encounters for treatment and care of the neoplasm.

h. See section I.C.18.d.14, Encounter for prophylactic organ removal

3. Chapter 3: Endocrine, Nutritional, and Metabolic Diseases and Immunity Disorders (240-279)

a. **Diabetes mellitus**—Codes under category 250 Diabetes mellitus, identify complications/manifestations associated with diabetes mellitus. A fifth-digit is required for all category 250 codes to identify the type of diabetes mellitus and whether the diabetes is controlled or uncontrolled.

1) **Fifth digits for category 250:** The following are the fifth digits for the codes under category 250:
   0 type II or unspecified type, not stated as uncontrolled
   1 type I, [juvenile type], not stated as uncontrolled
   2 type II or unspecified type, uncontrolled
   3 type I, [juvenile type], uncontrolled

   The age of a patient is not the sole determining factor, though most type I diabetics develop the condition before reaching puberty. For this reason type I diabetes mellitus is also referred to as juvenile diabetes.

2) **Type of diabetes mellitus not documented**—If the type of diabetes mellitus is not documented in the medical record the default is type II.

3) **Diabetes mellitus and the use of insulin**—All type I diabetics must use insulin to replace what their bodies do not produce. However, the use of insulin does not mean that a patient is a type I diabetic. Some patients with type II diabetes mellitus are unable to control their blood sugar through diet and oral medication alone and do require insulin. If the documentation in a medical record does not indicate the type of diabetes but does indicate that the patient uses insulin, the appropriate fifth digit for type II must be used. For type II patients who routinely use insulin, code V58.67 Long-term (current) use of insulin, should also be assigned to indicate that the patient uses insulin. Code V58.67 should not be assigned if insulin is given temporarily to bring a type II patient's blood sugar under control during an encounter.

4) **Assigning and sequencing diabetes codes and associated conditions**—When assigning codes for diabetes and its associated conditions, the code(s) from category 250 must be sequenced before the codes for the associated conditions. The diabetes codes and the secondary codes that correspond to them are paired codes that follow the etiology/manifestation convention of the classification (See section I.A.6., Etiology/manifestation convention). Assign as many codes from category 250 as needed to identify all of the associated conditions that the patient has. The corresponding secondary codes are listed under each of the diabetes codes.

   (a) **Diabetic retinopathy/diabetic macular edema—Diabetic macular edema, code 362.07, is only present with diabetic retinopathy. Another code from subcategory 362.0 Diabetic retinopathy, must be used with code 362.07. Codes under subcategory 362.0 are diabetes manifestation codes, so they must be used following the appropriate diabetes code.**

5) **Diabetes mellitus in pregnancy and gestational diabetes**
   (a) For diabetes mellitus complicating pregnancy, see aection I.C.11.f., Diabetes mellitus in pregnancy.
   (b) For gestational diabetes, see section I.C.11, g., Gestational diabetes.

6) **Insulin pump malfunction**
   (a) Underdose of insulin due to insulin pump failure—An underdose of insulin due to an insulin pump failure should be assigned 996.57 Mechanical complication due to insulin pump, as the principal or first listed code, followed by the appropriate diabetes mellitus code based on documentation.
   (b) Overdose of insulin due to insulin pump failure—The principal or first-listed code for an encounter due to an insulin pump malfunction resulting in an overdose of insulin should also be 996.57 Mechanical complication due to insulin pump, followed by code 962.3 Poisoning by insulins and antidiabetic agents, and the appropriate diabetes mellitus code based on documentation.

4. **Chapter 4: Diseases of Blood and Blood Forming Organs (280-289)**

   a. **Anemia of chronic disease**—Subcategory 285.2 Anemia in chronic illness, has codes for anemia in chronic kidney disease, code 285.21; anemia in neoplastic disease, code 285.22; and anemia in other chronic illness, code 285.29. These codes can be used as the principal/first-listed code if the reason for the encounter is to treat the anemia. They may also be used as secondary codes if treatment of the anemia is a component of an encounter but not the primary reason for the encounter. When using a code from subcategory 285 it is also necessary to use the code for the chronic condition causing the anemia.

   1) **Anemia in chronic kidney disease**—When assigning code 285.21 Anemia in chronic kidney disease. It is also necessary to assign a code from category 585 Chronic kidney disease to indicate the stage of chronic kidney disease. See I.C.10.a., Chronic kidney disease (CKD).

   2) **Anemia in neoplastic disease**—When assigning code 285.22 Anemia in neoplastic disease, it is also necessary to assign the neoplasm code that is responsible for the anemia. Code 285.22 is for use for anemia that is due to the malignancy, not for anemia due to antineoplastic chemotherapy drugs, which is an adverse effect.

   See I.C.2.c.1., Anemia associated with malignancy.
   See I.C.2.c.2., Anemia associated with chemotherapy, immunotherapy and radiation therapy.
   See I.C.17.e.1., Adverse effects.

5. **Chapter 5: Mental Disorders (290-319)**
   Reserved for future guideline expansion

6. **Chapter 6: Diseases of Nervous System and Sense Organs (320-389)**
   Reserved for future guideline expansion

7. **Chapter 7: Diseases of Circulatory System (390-459)**
   a. **Hypertension**

   <u>Hypertension Table</u>

   The hypertension table, found under the main term, "Hypertension," in the Alphabetic Index, contains a complete listing of all conditions due to or associated with hypertension and classifies them according to malignant, benign, and unspecified.

   1) **Hypertension, essential, or NOS**—Assign hypertension (arterial) (essential) (primary) (systemic) (NOS) to category code 401 with the appropriate fourth digit to indicate malignant (.0), benign (.1), or unspecified (.9). Do not use either .0 malignant or .1 benign unless medical record documentation supports such a designation.

   2) **Hypertension with heart disease**—Heart conditions (425.8, 429.0–429.3, 429.8, 429.9) are assigned to a code from category 402 when a causal relationship is stated (due to hypertension) or implied (hypertensive). Use an additional code from category 428 to identify the type of heart failure in those patients with heart failure. More than one code from category 428 may be assigned if the patient has systolic or diastolic failure and congestive heart failure.

   The same heart conditions (425.8, 429.0–429.3, 429.8, 429.9) with hypertension, but without a stated casual relationship, are coded separately. Sequence according to the circumstances of the admission/encounter.

   3) **Hypertensive kidney disease with chronic renal failure**—Assign codes from category 403, Hypertensive **kidney** disease, when conditions classified to categories 585-587 are present. Unlike hypertension with heart disease, ICD-9-CM presumes a cause-and-effect relationship and classifies renal failure with hypertension as hypertensive renal disease.

   4) **Hypertensive heart and kidney disease**—Assign codes from combination category 404, Hypertensive heart and **kidney** disease, when both hypertensive **kidney** disease and hypertensive heart disease are stated in the diagnosis. Assume a relationship between the hypertension and the **kidney** disease, whether or not the condition is so designated. Assign an additional code from category 428 to identify the type of heart failure. More than one code from category 428 may be assigned if the patient has systolic or diastolic failure and congestive heart failure.

   5) **Hypertensive cerebrovascular disease**—First assign codes from 430-438 Cerebrovascular disease, then the appropriate hypertension code from categories 401–405.

   6) **Hypertensive retinopathy**—Two codes are necessary to identify the condition. First assign the code from subcategory 362.11 Hypertensive retinopathy, then the appropriate code from categories 401–405 to indicate the type of hypertension.

   7) **Hypertension, secondary**—Two codes are required: one to identify the underlying etiology and one from category 405 to identify the hypertension. Sequencing of codes is determined by the reason for admission/encounter.

   8) **Hypertension, transient**—Assign code 796.2 Elevated blood pressure reading without diagnosis of hypertension, unless patient has an established diagnosis of hypertension. Assign code 642.3x for transient hypertension of pregnancy.

   9) **Hypertension, controlled**—Assign appropriate code from categories 401–405. This diagnostic statement usually refers to an existing state of hypertension under control by therapy.

10) **Hypertension, uncontrolled**—Uncontrolled hypertension may refer to untreated hypertension or hypertension not responding to current therapeutic regimen. In either case, assign the appropriate code from categories 401-405 to designate the stage and type of hypertension. Code to the type of hypertension.

11) **Elevated blood pressure**—For a statement of elevated blood pressure without further specificity, assign code 796.2, Elevated blood pressure reading without diagnosis of hypertension, rather than a code from category 401.

b. **Cerebral infarction/stroke/cerebrovascular accident (CVA)**—The terms stroke and CVA are often used interchangeably to refer to a cerebral infarction. The terms stroke, CVA, and cerebral infarction NOS are all indexed to the default code 434.91, Cerebral artery occlusion, unspecified, with infarction. Code 436, Acute, but ill-defined, cerebrovascular disease, should not be used when the documentation states stroke or CVA.

c. **Postoperative cerebrovascular accident**—A cerebrovascular hemorrhage or infarction that occurs as a result of medical intervention is coded to 997.02, Iatrogenic cerebrovascular infarction or hemorrhage. Medical record documentation should clearly specify the cause- and-effect relationship between the medical intervention and the cerebrovascular accident in order to assign this code. A secondary code from the code range 430-432 or from a code from subcategories 433 or 434 with a fifth digit of "1" should also be used to identify the type of hemorrhage or infarct.

This guideline conforms to the use additional code note instruction at category 997. Code 436, Acute, but ill-defined, cerebrovascular disease, should not be used as a secondary code with code 997.02.

d. **Late effects of cerebrovascular disease**

1) **Category 438, late effects of cerebrovascular disease**—Category 438 is used to indicate conditions classifiable to categories 430–437 as the causes of late effects (neurologic deficits), themselves classified elsewhere. These "late effects" include neurologic deficits that persist after initial onset of conditions classifiable to 430–437. The neurologic deficits caused by cerebrovascular disease may be present from the onset or may arise at any time after the onset of the condition classifiable to 430-437.

2) **Codes from category 438 with codes from 430–437**—Codes from category 438 may be assigned on a health care record with codes from 430–437, if the patient has a current cerebrovascular accident (CVA) and deficits from an old CVA.

3) **Code V12.59**—Assign code V12.59 (and not a code from category 438) as an additional code for history of cerebrovascular disease when no neurologic deficits are present.

e. **Acute myocardial infarction (AMI)**

1) **ST elevation myocardial infarction (STEMI) and non-ST elevation myocardial infarction (NSTEMI)**—The ICD-9-CM codes for acute myocardial infarction (AMI) identify the site, such as anterolateral wall or true posterior wall. Subcategories 410.0-410.6 and 410.8 are used for ST elevation myocardial infarction (STEMI). Subcategory 410.7 Subendocardial infarction, is used for non-ST elevation myocardial infarction (NSTEMI) and nontransmural MIs.

2) **Acute myocardial infarction, unspecified**—Subcategory 410.9 is the default for the unspecified term acute myocardial infarction. If only STEMI or transmural MI without the site is documented, query the provider as to the site or assign a code from subcategory 410.9.

3) **AMI documented as nontransmural or subendocardial, but site provided**—If an AMI is documented as nontransmural or subendocardial but the site is provided, it is still coded as a subendocardial AMI. If NSTEMI evolves to STEMI, assign the STEMI code. If STEMI converts to NSTEMI due to thrombolytic therapy, it is still coded as STEMI.

8. **Chapter 8: Diseases of Respiratory System (460-519)**

a. **Chronic obstructive pulmonary disease [COPD] and asthma**

1) **Conditions that comprise COPD and asthma**—The conditions that comprise COPD are obstructive chronic bronchitis, subcategory 491.2, and emphysema, category 492. All asthma codes are under category 493 Asthma. Code 496 Chronic airway obstruction, not elsewhere classified, is a nonspecific code that should be used only when the documentation in a medical record does not specify the type of COPD being treated.

2) **Acute exacerbation of chronic obstructive bronchitis and asthma**—The codes for chronic obstructive bronchitis and asthma distinguish between uncomplicated cases and those in acute exacerbation. An acute exacerbation is a worsening or a decompensation of a chronic condition. An acute exacerbation is not equivalent to an infection superimposed on a chronic condition, though an exacerbation may be triggered by an infection.

3) **Overlapping nature of the conditions that comprise COPD and asthma**—Due to the overlapping nature of the conditions that make up COPD and asthma, there are many variations in the way these conditions are documented. Code selection must be based on the terms as documented. When selecting the correct code for the documented type of COPD and asthma, it is essential to first review the index and then verify the code in the Tabular List. There are many instructional notes under the different COPD subcategories and codes. It is important that all such notes be reviewed to ensure correct code assignment.

4) **Acute exacerbation of asthma and status asthmaticus**—An acute exacerbation of asthma is an increased severity of the asthma symptoms, such as wheezing and shortness of breath. Status asthmaticus refers to a patient's failure to respond to therapy administered during an asthmatic episode and is a life-threatening complication that requires emergency care. If status asthmaticus is documented by the provider with any type of COPD or with acute bronchitis, the status asthmaticus should be sequenced first. It supersedes any type of COPD, including that with acute exacerbation or acute bronchitis. It is inappropriate to assign an asthma code with fifth-digit 2, with acute exacerbation, together with an asthma code with fifth-digit 1, with status asthmaticus. Only the fifth-digit 1 should be assigned.

b. **Chronic obstructive pulmonary disease [COPD] and bronchitis**

1) **Acute bronchitis with COPD**—Acute bronchitis, code 466.0, is due to an infectious organism. When acute bronchitis is documented with COPD, code 491.22 Obstructive chronic bronchitis with acute bronchitis, should be assigned. It is not necessary to also assign code 466.0. If a medical record documents acute bronchitis with COPD with acute exacerbation, only code 491.22 should be assigned. The acute bronchitis included in code 491.22 supersedes the acute exacerbation. If a medical record documents COPD with acute exacerbation without mention of acute bronchitis, only code 491.21 should be assigned.

9. **Chapter 9: Diseases of Digestive System (520-579)**
Reserved for future guideline expansion

10. **Chapter 10: Diseases of Genitourinary System (580-629)**

a. **Chronic kidney disease**

1) **Stages of chronic kidney disease (CKD)**—The ICD-9-CM classifies CKD based on severity. The severity of CKD is designated by stages I-V. Stage II, code 585.2, equates to mild CKD; stage III, code 585.3, equates to moderate CKD; and stage IV, code 585.4, equates to severe CKD. Code 585.6 End-stage renal disease (ESRD), is assigned when the provider has documented end-stage renal disease (ESRD). If both a stage of CKD and ESRD are documented, assign code 585.6 only.

2) **Chronic kidney disease and kidney transplant status**—Patients who have undergone kidney transplant may still have some form of CKD because the kidney transplant may not fully restore kidney function. Code V42.0 may be assigned with the appropriate CKD code for patients who are status post kidney transplant, based on the patient's post-transplant stage. The use additional code note under category 585 provides this instruction.

Use of a 585 code with V42.0 does not necessarily indicate transplant rejection or failure. Patients with mild or moderate CKD following a transplant should not be coded as having transplant failure unless it is documented in the medical record. For patients with severe CKD or ESRD it is appropriate to assign code 996.81 Complications of transplanted organ, kidney transplant, when kidney transplant failure is documented. If a post kidney transplant patient has CKD and it is unclear from the documentation whether there is transplant failure or rejection, it is necessary to query the provider.

3) **Chronic kidney disease with other conditions**—Patients with CKD may also suffer from other serious conditions, most commonly diabetes mellitus and hypertension. The sequencing of the CKD code in relationship to codes for other contributing conditions is based on the conventions in the tabular list. See I.C.3.a.4. for sequencing instructions for diabetes.

See I.C.4.a.1. for anemia in CKD.

See I.C.7.a.3. for hypertensive kidney disease.

See I.C.17.f.1.b. Transplant complications, for instructions on coding of documented rejection or failure.

11. **Chapter 11: Complications of Pregnancy, Childbirth, and the Puerperium (630-677)**
    a. **General rules for obstetric cases**
       1) **Codes from chapter 11 and sequencing priority**—Obstetric cases require codes from chapter 11, codes in the range 630-677 Complications of pregnancy, childbirth, and the puerperium. Chapter 11 codes have sequencing priority over codes from other chapters. Additional codes from other chapters may be used in conjunction with chapter 11 codes to further specify conditions. Should the provider document that the pregnancy is incidental to the encounter, then code V22.2 should be used in place of any chapter 11 codes. It is the provider's responsibility to state that the condition being treated is not affecting the pregnancy.
       2) **Chapter 11 codes used only on the maternal record**—Chapter 11 codes are to be used only on the maternal record, never on the record of the newborn.
       3) **Chapter 11 fifth digits**—Categories 640-648, 651-676 have required fifth-digits, which indicate whether the encounter is antepartum, postpartum and whether a delivery has also occurred.
       4) **Fifth digits, appropriate for each code**—The fifth digits, which are appropriate for each code number, are listed in brackets under each code. The fifth digits on each code should all be consistent with each other. That is, should a delivery occur all of the fifth digits should indicate the delivery.
    b. **Selection of OB principal or first-listed diagnosis**
       1) **Routine outpatient prenatal visits**—For routine outpatient prenatal visits when no complications are present, codes V22.0 Supervision of normal first pregnancy, and V22.1 Supervision of other normal pregnancy, should be used as the first-listed diagnoses. These codes should not be used in conjunction with chapter 11 codes.
       2) **Prenatal outpatient visits for high-risk patients**—For prenatal outpatient visits for patients with high-risk pregnancies, a code from category V23 Supervision of high-risk pregnancy, should be used as the principal or first-listed diagnosis. Secondary chapter 11 codes may be used in conjunction with these codes if appropriate.
       3) **Episodes when no delivery occurs**—In episodes when no delivery occurs, the principal diagnosis should correspond to the principal complication of the pregnancy, which necessitated the encounter. Should more than one complication exist, all of which are treated or monitored, any of the complication codes may be sequenced first.
       4) **When a delivery occurs**—When a delivery occurs, the principal diagnosis should correspond to the main circumstances or complication of the delivery. In cases of cesarean delivery, the selection of the principal diagnosis should correspond to the reason the cesarean delivery was performed unless the reason for admission/encounter was unrelated to the condition resulting in the cesarean delivery.
       5) **Outcome of delivery**—An outcome of delivery code, V27.0-V27.9, should be included on every maternal record when a delivery has occurred. These codes are not to be used on subsequent records or on the newborn record.
    c. **Fetal conditions affecting the management of the mother**
       1) **Fetal condition responsible for modifying the management of the mother**—Codes from category 655 Known or suspected fetal abnormality affecting management of the mother, and category 656 Other fetal and placental problems affecting the management of the mother, are assigned only when the fetal condition is actually responsible for modifying the management of the mother, i.e., by requiring diagnostic studies, additional observation, special care, or termination of pregnancy. The fact that the fetal condition exists does not justify assigning a code from this series to the mother's record.
       2) **In utero surgery**—In cases when surgery is performed on the fetus, a diagnosis code from category 655 Known or suspected fetal abnormalities affecting management of the mother, should be assigned identifying the fetal condition. Procedure code 75.36 Correction of fetal defect, should be assigned on the hospital inpatient record.

No code from chapter 15, the perinatal codes, should be used on the mother's record to identify fetal conditions. Surgery performed in utero on a fetus is still to be coded as an obstetric encounter.

   d. **HIV infection in pregnancy, childbirth and the puerperium**
      During pregnancy, childbirth, or the puerperium, a patient admitted because of an HIV-related illness should receive a principal diagnosis of 647.6X Other specified infectious and parasitic diseases in the mother classifiable elsewhere, but complicating the pregnancy, childbirth, or the puerperium, followed by 042 and the code(s) for the HIV-related illness(es).

      Patients with asymptomatic HIV infection status admitted during pregnancy, childbirth, or the puerperium should receive codes of 647.6X and V08.
   e. **Current conditions complicating pregnancy**—Assign a code from subcategory 648.x for patients that have current conditions when the condition affects the management of the pregnancy, childbirth, or the puerperium. Use additional secondary codes from other chapters to identify the conditions, as appropriate.
   f. **Diabetes mellitus in pregnancy**—Diabetes mellitus is a significant complicating factor in pregnancy. Pregnant women who are diabetic should be assigned code 648.0x Diabetes mellitus complicating pregnancy, and a secondary code from category 250 Diabetes mellitus, to identify the type of diabetes.

      Code V58.67 Long-term (current) use of insulin, should also be assigned if the diabetes mellitus is being treated with insulin.
   g. **Gestational diabetes**—Gestational diabetes can occur during the second and third trimester of pregnancy in women who were not diabetic prior to pregnancy. Gestational diabetes can cause complications in the pregnancy similar to those of pre-existing diabetes mellitus. It also puts the woman at greater risk of developing diabetes after the pregnancy. Gestational diabetes is coded to 648.8x Abnormal glucose tolerance. Codes 648.0x and 648.8x should never be used together on the same record.

      Code V58.67 Long-term (current) use of insulin, should also be assigned if the gestational diabetes is being treated with insulin.
   h. **Normal delivery, code 650**
      1) **Normal delivery**—Code 650 is for use in cases when a woman is admitted for a full-term normal delivery and delivers a single, healthy infant without any complications antepartum, during the delivery, or postpartum during the delivery episode. Code 650 is always a principal diagnosis. It is not to be used if any other code from chapter 11 is needed to describe a current complication of the antenatal, delivery, or perinatal period. Additional codes from other chapters may be used with code 650 if they are not related to or are in any way complicating the pregnancy.
      2) **Normal delivery with resolved antepartum complication**—Code 650 may be used if the patient had a complication at some point during her pregnancy, but the complication is not present at the time of the admission for delivery.
      3) **V27.0 Single liveborn, outcome of delivery**—V27.0 Single liveborn, is the only outcome of the delivery code appropriate for use with 650.
   i. **The postpartum and peripartum periods**
      1) **Postpartum and peripartum periods**—The postpartum period begins immediately after delivery and continues for six weeks following delivery. The peripartum period is defined as the last month of pregnancy to five months postpartum.
      2) **Postpartum complication**—A postpartum complication is any complication occurring within the six-week period.
      3) **Pregnancy-related complications after six-week period**—Chapter 11 codes may also be used to describe pregnancy-related complications after the six-week period should the provider document that a condition is pregnancy related.
      4) **Postpartum complications occurring during the same admission as delivery**—Postpartum complications that occur during the same admission as the delivery are identified with a fifth digit of 2. Subsequent admissions/encounters for postpartum complications should be identified with a fifth digit of 4.
      5) **Admission for routine postpartum care following delivery outside hospital**—When the mother delivers outside the hospital prior to admission and is admitted for routine postpartum care and no complications are noted, code V24.0 Postpartum care and examination immediately after delivery, should be assigned as the principal diagnosis.

6) **Admission following delivery outside hospital with postpartum conditions**—A delivery diagnosis code should not be used for a woman who has delivered prior to admission to the hospital. Any postpartum conditions and/or postpartum procedures should be coded.

j. **Code 677 Late effect of complication of pregnancy**

1) **Code 677**—Code 677 Late effect of complication of pregnancy, childbirth, and the puerperium is for use in those cases when an initial complication of a pregnancy develops a sequelae requiring care or treatment at a future date.

2) **After the initial postpartum period**—This code may be used at any time after the initial postpartum period.

3) **Sequencing of code 677**—This code, like all late effect codes, is to be sequenced following the code describing the sequelae of the complication.

k. **Abortions**

1) **Fifth digits required for abortion categories**—Fifth digits are required for abortion categories 634-637. Fifth-digit 1, incomplete, indicates that all of the products of conception have not been expelled from the uterus. Fifth-digit 2, complete, indicates that all products of conception have been expelled from the uterus prior to the episode of care.

2) **Code from categories 640-648 and 651-659**—A code from categories 640-648 and 651-659 may be used as additional codes with an abortion code to indicate the complication leading to the abortion.

Fifth-digit 3 is assigned with codes from these categories when used with an abortion code because the other fifth digits will not apply. Codes from the 660-669 series are not to be used for complications of abortion.

3) **Code 639 for complications**—Code 639 is to be used for all complications following abortion. Code 639 cannot be assigned with codes from categories 634-638.

4) **Abortion with liveborn fetus**—When an attempted termination of pregnancy results in a liveborn fetus assign code 644.21 Early onset of delivery, with an appropriate code from category V27 Outcome of delivery. The procedure code for the attempted termination of pregnancy should also be assigned.

5) **Retained products of conception following an abortion**—Subsequent admissions for retained products of conception following a spontaneous or legally induced abortion are assigned the appropriate code from category 634 Spontaneous abortion, or 635 Legally induced abortion, with a fifth digit of 1 (incomplete). This advice is appropriate even when the patient was discharged previously with a discharge diagnosis of complete abortion.

12. **Chapter 12: Diseases of Skin and Subcutaneous Tissue (680-709)**
Reserved for future guideline expansion

13. **Chapter 13: Diseases of Musculoskeletal and Connective Tissue (710-739)**
Reserved for future guideline expansion

14. **Chapter 14: Congenital Anomalies (740-759)**

a. **Codes in categories 740-759 Congenital anomalies**—Assign an appropriate code(s) from categories 740-759, Congenital anomalies, when an anomaly is documented. A congenital anomaly may be the principal/first-listed diagnosis on a record or a secondary diagnosis. **When a congenital anomaly does not have a unique code assignment, assign additional code(s) for any manifestations that may be present.**

When the code assignment specifically identifies the congenital anomaly, manifestations that are an inherent component of the anomaly should not be coded separately. Additional codes should be assigned for manifestations that are not an inherent component.

Codes from Chapter 14 may be used throughout the life of the patient. If a congenital anomaly has been corrected, a personal history code should be used to identify the history of the anomaly. **Although present at birth, a congenital anomaly may not be identified until later in life. Whenever the condition is diagnosed by the physician, it is appropriate to assign a code from codes 740-759.**

For the birth admission, the appropriate code from category V30 Liveborn infants, according to type of birth should be sequenced as the principal diagnosis, followed by any congenital anomaly codes, 740-759.

15. **Chapter 15: Newborn (Perinatal) Guidelines (760-779)**
For coding and reporting purposes the perinatal period is defined as birth through the 28th day following birth. The following guidelines are provided for reporting purposes. Hospitals may record other diagnoses as needed for internal data use.

a. **General perinatal rules**

1) **Chapter 15 codes**—They are never for use on the maternal record. Codes from chapter 11, the obstetric chapter, are never permitted on the newborn record. Chapter 15 code may be used throughout the life of the patient if the condition is still present.

2) **Sequencing of perinatal codes**—Generally, codes from chapter 15 should be sequenced as the principal/first-listed diagnosis on the newborn record, with the exception of the appropriate V30 code for the birth episode, followed by codes from any other chapter that provide additional detail. The "use additional code" note at the beginning of the chapter supports this guideline. If the index does not provide a specific code for a perinatal condition, assign code 779.89 Other specified conditions originating in the perinatal period, followed by the code from another chapter that specifies the condition. Codes for signs and symptoms may be assigned when a definitive diagnosis has not been established.

3) **Birth process or community acquired conditions**—If a newborn has a condition that may be either due to the birth process or community acquired and the documentation does not indicate which it is, the default is due to the birth process and the code from chapter 15 should be used. If the condition is community acquired, a code from chapter 15 should not be assigned.

4) **Code all clinically significant conditions**—All clinically significant conditions noted on routine newborn examination should be coded. A condition is clinically significant if it requires:

- Clinical evaluation; or
- Therapeutic treatment; or
- Diagnostic procedures; or
- Extended length of hospital stay; or
- Increased nursing care and/or monitoring; or
- Has implications for future health care needs

Note: The perinatal guidelines listed above are the same as the general coding guidelines for "additional diagnoses," except for the final point regarding implications for future health care needs. Codes should be assigned for conditions that have been specified by the provider as having implications for future health care needs. Codes from the perinatal chapter should not be assigned unless the provider has established a definitive diagnosis.

b. **Use of codes V30-V39**—When coding the birth of an infant, assign a code from categories V30-V39, according to the type of birth. A code from this series is assigned as a principal diagnosis and assigned only once to a newborn at the time of birth.

c. **Newborn transfers**—If the newborn is transferred to another institution, the V30 series is not used at the receiving hospital.

d. **Use of category V29**

1) **Assigning a code from category V29**—Assign a code from category V29 Observation and evaluation of newborns and infants for suspected conditions not found, to identify those instances when a healthy newborn is evaluated for a suspected condition that is determined after study not to be present. Do not use a code from category V29 when the patient has identified signs or symptoms of a suspected problem; in such cases, code the sign or symptom.

A code from category V29 may also be assigned as a principal diagnosis for readmissions or encounters when the V30 code no longer applies. Codes from category V29 are for use only for healthy newborns and infants for which no condition after study is found to be present.

2) **V29 code on a birth record**—A V29 code is to be used as a secondary code after the V30 Outcome of delivery, code.

e. **Use of other V codes on perinatal records**—V codes other than V30 and V29 may be assigned on a perinatal or newborn record code. The codes may be used as a principal or first-listed diagnosis for specific types of encounters or for readmissions or encounters when the V30 code no longer applies.

See section I.C.18 for information regarding the assignment of V codes.

f. **Maternal causes of perinatal morbidity**—Codes from categories 760-763 Maternal causes of perinatal morbidity and mortality, are assigned only when the maternal condition has actually affected the fetus or newborn. The fact that the mother has an associated medical condition or experiences some complication of pregnancy, labor, or delivery does not justify the routine assignment of codes from these categories to the newborn record.

g. **Congenital anomalies in newborns**—For the birth admission, the appropriate code from category V30 Liveborn infants according to type of birth, should be used, followed by any congenital anomaly codes, categories 740-759. Use additional secondary codes from other chapters to specify conditions associated with the anomaly, if applicable.

Also, see section I.C.14 for information on the coding of congenital anomalies.

h. **Coding additional perinatal diagnoses**

1) **Assigning codes for conditions that require treatment**—Assign codes for conditions that require treatment or further investigation, prolong the length of stay, or require resource utilization.

2) **Codes for conditions specified as having implications for future health care needs**—Assign codes for conditions that have been specified by the provider as having implications for future health care needs.

Note: This guideline should not be used for adult patients.

3) **Codes for newborn conditions originating in the perinatal period**—Assign a code for newborn conditions originating in the perinatal period (categories 760-779), as well as complications arising during the current episode of care classified in other chapters, only if the diagnoses have been documented by the responsible provider at the time of transfer or discharge as having affected the fetus or newborn.

i. **Prematurity and fetal growth retardation**—Providers utilize different criteria in determining prematurity. A code for prematurity should not be assigned unless it is documented. The fift-digit assignment for codes from category 764 and subcategories 765.0 and 765.1 should be based on the recorded birth weight and estimated gestational age.

A code from subcategory 765.2 Weeks of gestation, should be assigned as an additional code with category 764 and codes from 765.0 and 765.1 to specify weeks of gestation as documented by the provider in the record.

j. **Newborn sepsis**—Code 771.81 Septicemia [sepsis] of newborn, should be assigned with a secondary code from category 041 Bacterial infections in conditions classified elsewhere and of unspecified site, to identify the organism. It is not necessary to use a code from subcategory 995.9 Systemic inflammatory response syndrome (SIRS), on a newborn record. A code from category 038 Septicemia, should not be used on a newborn record. Code 771.81 describes the sepsis.

16. **Chapter 16: Signs, Symptoms and Ill-Defined Conditions (780-799)**
Reserved for future guideline expansion

17. **Chapter 17: Injury and Poisoning (800-999)**
a. **Coding of injuries**—When coding injuries, assign separate codes for each injury unless a combination code is provided, in which case the combination code is assigned. Multiple injury codes are provided in ICD-9-CM but should not be assigned unless information for a more specific code is not available. These codes are not to be used for normal, healing surgical wounds or to identify complications of surgical wounds.

The code for the most serious injury, as determined by the provider and the focus of treatment, is sequenced first.

1) **Superficial injuries**—Superficial injuries such as abrasions or contusions are not coded when associated with more severe injuries of the same site.

2) **Primary injury with damage to nerves/blood vessels**—When a primary injury results in minor damage to peripheral nerves or blood vessels, the primary injury is sequenced first with additional code(s) from categories 950-957 Injury to nerves and spinal cord, and/or 900-904 Injury to blood vessels. When the primary injury is to the blood vessels or nerves, that injury should be sequenced first.

b. **Coding of fractures**—The principles of multiple coding of injuries should be followed in coding fractures. Fractures of specified sites are coded individually by site in accordance with both the provisions within categories 800-829 and the level of detail furnished by medical record content. Combination categories for multiple fractures are provided for use when there is insufficient detail in the medical record (such as trauma cases transferred to another hospital), when the reporting form limits the number of codes that can be used in reporting pertinent clinical data, or when there is insufficient specificity at the fourth-digit or fifth-digit level. More specific guidelines are as follows:

1) **Multiple fractures of same limb**—Multiple fractures of same limb classifiable to the same three-digit or four-digit category are coded to that category.

2) **Multiple unilateral or bilateral fractures of same bone**—Multiple unilateral or bilateral fractures of same bone(s) but classified to different fourth-digit subdivisions (bone part) within the same three-digit category are coded individually by site.

3) **Multiple fracture categories 819 and 828**—Multiple fracture categories 819 and 828 classify bilateral fractures of both upper limbs (819) and both lower limbs (828), but without any detail at the fourth-digit level other than open and closed type of fractures.

4) **Multiple fractures sequencing**—Multiple fractures are sequenced in accordance with the severity of the fracture. The provider should be asked to list the fracture diagnoses in the order of severity.

c. **Coding of burns**—Current burns (940-948) are classified by depth, extent, and by agent (E code). Burns are classified by depth as first degree (erythema), second degree (blistering), and third degree (full-thickness involvement).

1) **Sequencing of burn codes and related condition**—Sequence first the code that reflects the highest degree of burn when more than one burn is present.

(a) **When the reason for the admission or encounter is for treatment of external multiple burns, sequence first the code that reflects the burn of the highest degree.**

(b) **When a patient has both internal and external burns, the circumstances of admission govern the selection of the principal diagnosis or first-listed diagnosis.**

(c) **When a patient is admitted for burn injuries and other related conditions such as smoke inhalation and/or respiratory failure, the circumstances of admission govern the selection of the principal or first-listed diagnosis.**

2) **Burns of the same local site**—Classify burns of the same local site (three-digit category level, 940-947) but of different degrees to the subcategory identifying the highest degree recorded in the diagnosis.

3) **Non-healing burns**—Non-healing burns are coded as acute burns. Necrosis of burned skin should be coded as a non-healed burn.

4) **Code 958.3 Posttraumatic wound infection**—Assign code 958.3 Posttraumatic wound infection, not elsewhere classified, as an additional code for any documented infected burn site.

5) **Assign separate codes for each burn site**—When coding burns, assign separate codes for each burn site. Category 946 Burns of multiple specified sites, should only be used if the locations of the burns are not documented. Category 949 Burn, unspecified, is extremely vague and should rarely be used.

6) **Burns classified according to extent of body surface involved**—Assign codes from category 948 Burns, when the site of the burn is not specified or when there is a need for additional data. It is advisable to use category 948 as additional coding when needed to provide data for evaluating burn mortality, such as that needed by burn units. It is also advisable to use category 948 as an additional code for reporting purposes when there is mention of a third-degree burn involving 20 percent or more of the body surface.

In assigning a code from category 948:

- Fourth-digit codes are used to identify the percentage of total body surface involved in a burn (all degree).
- Fifth digits are assigned to identify the percentage of body surface involved in third-degree burn.
- Fifth-digit zero (0) is assigned when less than 10 percent or when no body surface is involved in a third-degree burn.
- Category 948 is based on the classic "rule of nines" in estimating body surface involved: head and neck are assigned 9 percent, each arm 9 percent, each leg 18 percent, the anterior trunk 18 percent, posterior trunk 18 percent, and genitalia 1 percent. Providers may change these percentage assignments where necessary to accommodate infants and children who have proportionately larger heads than adults and patients who have large buttocks, thighs, or abdomen that involve burns.

7) **Encounters for treatment of late effects of burns**—Encounters for the treatment of the late effects of burns (i.e., scars or joint contractures) should be coded to the residual condition (sequelae) followed by the appropriate late effect code (906.5-906.9). A late effect E code may also be used, if desired.

8) **Sequelae with a late effect code and current burn**—When appropriate, both a sequelae with a late effect code, and a current burn code may be assigned on the same record (when both a current burn and sequelae of an old burn exist).

d. **Coding of debridement of wound, infection, or burn**—Excisional debridement involves an excisional debridement (surgical removal or cutting away), as opposed to a mechanical (brushing, scrubbing, washing) debridement.

For coding purposes, excisional debridement is assigned to code 86.22.

Nonexcisional debridement is assigned to code 86.28.

e. **Adverse effects, poisoning and toxic effects**—The properties of certain drugs, medicinal and biological substances, or combinations of such substances, may cause toxic reactions. The occurrence of drug toxicity is classified in ICD-9-CM as follows:

1) **Adverse effect**—When the drug was correctly prescribed and properly administered, code the reaction plus the appropriate code from the E930-E949 series. Codes from the E930-E949 series must be used to identify the causative substance for an adverse effect of drug, medicinal and biological substances, correctly prescribed and properly administered. The effect, such as tachycardia, delirium, gastrointestinal hemorrhaging, vomiting, hypokalemia, hepatitis, renal failure, or respiratory failure, is coded and followed by the appropriate code from the E930-E949 series.

Adverse effects of therapeutic substances correctly prescribed and properly administered (toxicity, synergistic reaction, side effect, and idiosyncratic reaction) may be due to (1) differences among patients, such as age, sex, disease, and genetic factors, and (2) drug-related factors, such as type of drug, route of administration, duration of therapy, dosage, and bioavailability.

2) **Poisoning**

(a) **Error was made in drug prescription**—Errors made in drug prescription or in the administration of the drug by provider, nurse, patient, or other person, use the appropriate poisoning code from the 960-979 series.

(b) **Overdose of a drug intentionally taken**—If an overdose of a drug was intentionally taken or administered and resulted in drug toxicity, it would be coded as a poisoning (960-979 series).

(c) **Nonprescribed drug taken with correctly prescribed and properly administered drug**—If a nonprescribed drug or medicinal agent was taken in combination with a correctly prescribed and properly administered drug, any drug toxicity or other reaction resulting from the interaction of the two drugs would be classified as a poisoning.

(d) **Sequencing of poisoning**—When coding a poisoning or reaction to the improper use of a medication (e.g., wrong dose, wrong substance, wrong route of administration) the poisoning code is sequenced first, followed by a code for the manifestation. If there is also a diagnosis of drug abuse or dependence to the substance, the abuse or dependence is coded as an additional code.

See section I.C.3.a.6.b. if poisoning is the result of insulin pump malfunctions and section I.C.19 for general use of E codes.

3) **Toxic effects**

(a) **Toxic effect codes**—When a harmful substance is ingested or comes in contact with a person, this is classified as a toxic effect. The toxic effect codes are in categories 980-989.

(b) **Sequencing toxic effect codes**—A toxic effect code should be sequenced first, followed by the codes that identify the result of the toxic effect.

(c) **External cause codes for toxic effects**—An external cause code from categories E860-E869 for accidental exposure, code E950.6 or E950.7 for intentional self-harm, category E962 for assault, or categories E980-E982 for undetermined, should also be assigned to indicate intent.

f. **Complications of care**

1) **Transplant complications**

(a) **Transplant complications other than kidney—Codes under subcategory 996.8 Complications of transplanted organ, are for use for both complications and rejection of transplanted organs. A transplant complication code is only assigned if the complication affects the function of the transplanted organ. Two codes are required to fully describe a transplant complication, the appropriate code from subcategory 996.8 and a secondary code that identifies the complication.**

Pre-existing conditions or conditions that develop after the transplant are not coded as complications unless they affect the function of the transplanted organs.

Post-transplant surgical complications that do not relate to the function of the transplanted organ are classified to the specific complication. For example, a surgical wound dehiscence would be coded as a wound dehiscence, not as a transplant complication.

Post-transplant patients who are seen for treatment unrelated to the transplanted organ should be assigned a code from category V42 Organ or tissue replaced by transplant, to identify the transplant status of the patient. A code from category V42 should never be used with a code from subcategory 996.8.

(b) **Kidney transplant and chronic kidney disease—Patients with chronic kidney disease (CKD) following a transplant should not be assumed to have transplant failure or rejection unless it is documented by the provider. If documentation supports the presence of failure or rejection, then it is appropriate to assign code 996.81 Complications of transplanted organs, kidney, followed by the appropriate CKD code.**

18. **Classification of Factors Influencing Health Status and Contact with Health Service (Supplemental V01-V86)**

Note: The chapter-specific guidelines provide additional information about the use of V codes for specified encounters.

a. **Introduction**—ICD-9-CM provides codes to deal with encounters for circumstances other than a disease or injury. The Supplementary Classification of Factors Influencing Health Status and Contact with Health Services (V01-V86) is provided to deal with occasions when circumstances other than a disease or injury (codes 001-999) are recorded as a diagnosis or problem.

There are four primary circumstances for the use of V codes:

1) A person who is not currently sick encounters the health services for some specific reason, such as to act as an organ donor, to receive prophylactic care, such as inoculations or health screenings, or to receive counseling on health related issues.

2) A person with a resolving disease or injury, or a chronic, long-term condition requiring continuous care, encounters the health care system for specific aftercare of that disease or injury (e.g., dialysis for renal disease; chemotherapy for malignancy; cast change). A diagnosis/symptom code should be used whenever a current, acute diagnosis is being treated or a sign or symptom is being studied.

3) Circumstances or problems influence a person's health status but are not in themselves a current illness or injury.

4) Newborns, to indicate birth status

b. **V codes use in any health care setting**—V codes are for use in any healthcare setting. V codes may be used as either a first-listed (principal diagnosis code in the inpatient setting) or secondary code, depending on the circumstances of the encounter. Certain V codes may only be used as first listed, others only as secondary codes. See section I.C.18.e, V code table.

c. **V codes indicate a reason for an encounter**—They are not procedure codes. A corresponding procedure code must accompany a V code to describe the procedure performed.

d. **Categories of V codes**

1) **Contact/exposure**—Category V01 indicates contact with or exposure to communicable diseases. These codes are for patients who do not show any sign or symptom of a disease but have been exposed to it by close personal contact with an infected individual or are in an area where a disease is epidemic. These codes may be used as a first-listed code to explain an encounter for testing, or, more commonly, as a secondary code to identify a potential risk.

2) **Inoculations and vaccinations**—Categories V03-V06 are for encounters for inoculations and vaccinations. They indicate that a patient is being seen to receive a prophylactic inoculation against a disease. The injection itself must be represented by the appropriate procedure code. A code from V03-V06 may be used as a secondary code if the inoculation is given as a routine part of preventive health care, such as a well-baby visit.

3) **Status**—Status codes indicate that a patient is either a carrier of a disease or has the sequelae or residual of a past disease or condition. This includes such things as the presence of prosthetic or mechanical devices resulting from past treatment.

A status code is informative, because the status may affect the course of treatment and its outcome. A status code is distinct from a history code. The history code indicates that the patient no longer has the condition.

A status code should not be used with a diagnosis code from one of the body system chapters, if the diagnosis code includes the information provided by the status code. For example, code V42.1 Heart transplant status, should not be used with code 996.83 Complications of transplanted heart. The status code does not provide additional information. The complication code indicates that the patient is a heart transplant patient.

The status V codes/categories are:

V02 Carrier or suspected carrier of infectious diseases—Carrier status indicates that a person harbors the specific organisms of a disease without manifest symptoms and is capable of transmitting the infection.

V08 Asymptomatic HIV infection status—This code indicates that a patient has tested positive for HIV but has manifested no signs or symptoms of the disease.

V09 Infection with drug-resistant microorganisms—This category indicates that a patient has an infection that is resistant to drug treatment. Sequence the infection code first.

V21 Constitutional states in development

V22.2 Pregnant state, incidental—This code is a secondary code only for use when the pregnancy is in no way complicating the reason for visit. Otherwise, a code from the obstetric chapter is required.

V26.5x Sterilization status

V42 Organ or tissue replaced by transplant

V43 Organ or tissue replaced by other means

V44 Artificial opening status

V45 Other postsurgical states

V46 Other dependence on machines

V49.6 Upper limb amputation status

V49.7 Lower limb amputation status

V49.81 Postmenopausal status

V49.82 Dental sealant status

V49.83 Awaiting organ transplant status

V58.6 Long-term (current) drug use—This subcategory indicates a patient's continuous use of a prescribed drug (including such things as aspirin therapy) for the long-term treatment of a condition or for prophylactic use. It is not for use for patients who have addictions to drugs.

Assign a code from subcategory V58.6 Long-term (current) drug use, if the patient is receiving a medication for an extended period as a prophylactic measure (such as for the prevention of deep vein thrombosis) or as treatment of a chronic condition (such as arthritis) or a disease requiring a lengthy course of treatment (such as cancer). Do not assign a code from subcategory V58.6 for medication being administered for a brief period of time to treat an acute illness or injury (such as a course of antibiotics to treat acute bronchitis).

V83 Genetic carrier status—Genetic carrier status indicates that a person carries a gene, associated with a particular disease, which may be passed to offspring who may develop that disease. The person does not have the disease and is not at risk of developing the disease.

V84 Genetic susceptibility status—Genetic susceptibility indicates that a person has a gene that increases the risk of that person developing the disease.

Codes from category V84 Genetic susceptibility to disease, should not be used as principal or first-listed codes. If the patient has the condition to which he/she is susceptible and that condition is the reason for the encounter, the code for the current condition should be sequenced first. If the patient is being seen for follow-up after completed treatment for this condition and the condition no longer exists, a follow-up code should be sequenced first, followed by the appropriate personal history and genetic susceptibility codes. If the purpose of the encounter is genetic counseling associated with procreative management, a code from subcategory V26.3 Genetic counseling and testing, should be assigned as the first-listed code, followed by a code from category V84.

Additional codes should be assigned for any applicable family or personal history. See Section I.C.18.d.14. for information on prophylactic organ removal due to a genetic susceptibility.

Note: Categories V42-V46, and subcategories V49.6, V49.7 are for use only if there are no complications or malfunctions of the organ or tissue replaced, the amputation site, or the equipment on which the patient is dependent.

4) **History (of)**—There are two types of history V codes, personal and family. Personal history codes explain a patient's past medical condition that no longer exists and is not receiving any treatment but that has the potential for recurrence, and therefore may require continued monitoring. The exceptions to this general rule are category V14 Personal history of allergy to medicinal agents, and subcategory V15.0 Allergy, other than to medicinal agents. A person who has had an allergic episode to a substance or food in the past should always be considered allergic to the substance.

Family history codes are for use when a patient has a family member(s) who has had a particular disease that causes the patient to be at higher risk of also contracting the disease.

Personal history codes may be used in conjunction with follow-up codes and family history codes may be used in conjunction with screening codes to explain the need for a test or procedure. History codes are also acceptable on any medical record regardless of the reason for visit. A history of an illness, even if no longer present, is important information that may alter the type of treatment ordered.

The history V code categories are:

V10 Personal history of malignant neoplasm

V12 Personal history of certain other diseases

V13 Personal history of other diseases

Except: V13.4 Personal history of arthritis, and V13.6 Personal history of congenital malformations. These conditions are life-long so are not true history codes.

V14 Personal history of allergy to medicinal agents

V15 Other personal history presenting hazards to health
Except: V15.7 Personal history of contraception

V16 Family history of malignant neoplasm

V17 Family history of certain chronic disabling diseases

V18 Family history of certain other specific diseases

V19 Family history of other conditions

5) **Screening**—Screening is the testing for disease or disease precursors in seemingly well individuals so that early detection and treatment can be provided for those who test positive for the disease. Screenings that are recommended for many subgroups in a population include routine mammograms for women over 40, a fecal occult blood test for everyone over 50, an amniocentesis to rule out a fetal anomaly for pregnant women over 35, because the incidence of breast cancer and colon cancer in these subgroups is higher than in the general population, as is the incidence of Down's syndrome in older mothers.

The testing of a person to rule out or confirm a suspected diagnosis because the patient has some sign or symptom is a diagnostic examination, not a screening. In these cases, the sign or symptom is used to explain the reason for the test.

A screening code may be a first-listed code if the reason for the visit is specifically the screening exam. It may also be used as an additional code if the screening is done during an office visit for other health problems. A screening code is not necessary if the screening is inherent to a routine examination, such as a Pap smear done during a routine pelvic examination.

Should a condition be discovered during the screening then the code for the condition may be assigned as an additional diagnosis.

The V code indicates that a screening exam is planned. A procedure code is required to confirm that the screening was performed.

The screening V code categories:

V28 Antenatal screening

V73-V82 Special screening examinations

6) **Observation**—There are two observation V code categories. They are for use in very limited circumstances when a person is being observed for a suspected condition that is ruled out. The observation codes are not for use if an injury or illness or any signs or symptoms related to the suspected condition are present. In such cases the diagnosis/symptom code is used with the corresponding E code to identify any external cause.

The observation codes are to be used as principal diagnosis only. The only exception to this is when the principal diagnosis is required to be a code from the V30 Live born infant, category. Then the V29 observation code is sequenced after the V30 code. Additional codes may be used in addition to the observation code but only if they are unrelated to the suspected condition being observed.

The observation V code categories:

V29 Observation and evaluation of newborns for suspected condition not found
For the birth encounter, a code from category V30 should be sequenced before the V29 code.

V71 Observation and evaluation for suspected condition not found

7) Aftercare—Aftercare visit codes cover situations when the initial treatment of a disease or injury has been performed and the patient requires continued care during the healing or recovery phase, or for the long-term consequences of the disease. The aftercare V code should not be used if treatment is directed at a current, acute disease or injury, the diagnosis code is to be used in these cases. Exceptions to this rule are codes V58.0 Radiotherapy, and **codes from subcategory V58.1 Encounter for chemotherapy and immunotherapy for neoplastic conditions**. These codes are to be first listed, followed by the diagnosis code when a patient's encounter is solely to receive radiation therapy or chemotherapy for the treatment of a neoplasm. Should a patient receive both chemotherapy and radiation therapy during the same encounter, codes V58.0 and V58.1 may be used together on a record with either one being sequenced first.

The aftercare codes are generally first listed to explain the specific reason for the encounter. An aftercare code may be used as an additional code when some type of aftercare is provided in addition to the reason for admission and no diagnosis code is applicable. An example of this would be the closure of a colostomy during an encounter for treatment of another condition.

Certain aftercare V code categories need a secondary diagnosis code to describe the resolving condition or sequelae, for others, the condition is inherent in the code title.

Additional V code aftercare category terms include fitting and adjustment, and attention to artificial openings.

Status V codes may be used with aftercare V codes to indicate the nature of the aftercare. For example code V45.81 Aortocoronary bypass status, may be used with code V58.73 Aftercare following surgery of the circulatory system, NEC, to indicate the surgery for which the aftercare is being performed. Also, a transplant status code may be used following code V58.44 Aftercare following organ transplant, to identify the organ transplanted. A status code should not be used when the aftercare code indicates the type of status, such as using V55.0 Attention to tracheostomy with V44.0 Tracheostomy status.

The aftercare V category/codes:

V52 Fitting and adjustment of prosthetic device and implant
V53 Fitting and adjustment of other device
V54 Other orthopedic aftercare
V55 Attention to artificial openings
V56 Encounter for dialysis and dialysis catheter care
V57 Care involving the use of rehabilitation procedures
V58.0 Radiotherapy
V58.11 Encounter for antineoplastic chemotherapy
V58.12 Encounter for antineoplastic immunotherapy
V58.3 Attention to surgical dressings and sutures
V58.41 Encounter for planned post-operative wound closure
V58.42 Aftercare, surgery, neoplasm
V58.43 Aftercare, surgery, trauma
V58.44 Aftercare involving organ transplant
V58.49 Other specified aftercare following surgery
V58.7x Aftercare following surgery
V58.81 Fitting and adjustment of vascular catheter
V58.82 Fitting and adjustment of non-vascular catheter
V58.83 Monitoring therapeutic drug
V58.89 Other specified aftercare

8) Follow-up—The follow-up codes are used to explain continuing surveillance following completed treatment of a disease, condition, or injury. They imply that the condition has been fully treated and no longer exists. They should not be confused with aftercare codes that explain current treatment for a healing condition or its sequelae. Follow-up codes may be used in conjunction with history codes to provide the full picture of the healed condition and its treatment. The follow-up code is sequenced first, followed by the history code.

A follow-up code may be used to explain repeated visits. Should a condition be found to have recurred on the follow-up visit, then the diagnosis code should be used in place of the follow-up code.

The follow-up V code categories:

V24 Postpartum care and evaluation
V67 Follow-up examination

9) Donor—Category V59 is the donor codes. They are used for living individuals who are donating blood or other body tissue. These codes are only for individuals donating for others, not for self-donations. They are not for use to identify cadaveric donations.

10) Counseling—Counseling V codes are used when a patient or family member receives assistance in the aftermath of an illness or injury, or when support is required in coping with family or social problems. They are not necessary for use in conjunction with a diagnosis code when the counseling component of care is considered integral to standard treatment.

The counseling V categories/codes:

V25.0 General counseling and advice for contraceptive management
V26.3 Genetic counseling
V26.4 General counseling and advice for procreative management
V61 Other family circumstances
V65.1 Person consulted on behalf of another person
V65.3 Dietary surveillance and counseling
V65.4 Other counseling, not elsewhere classified

11) Obstetrics and related conditions—See section I.C.11., the obstetrics guidelines for further instruction on the use of these codes.

V codes for pregnancy are for use in those circumstances when none of the problems or complications included in the codes from the obstetrics chapter exist (a routine prenatal visit or postpartum care). Codes V22.0 Supervision of normal first pregnancy, and V22.1 Supervision of other normal pregnancy, are always first listed and are not to be used with any other code from the OB chapter.

The outcome of delivery, category V27, should be included on all maternal delivery records. It is always a secondary code.

V codes for family planning (contraceptive) or procreative management and counseling should be included on an obstetric record either during the pregnancy or the postpartum stage, if applicable.

Obstetrics and related conditions V code categories:

V22 Normal pregnancy
V23 Supervision of high-risk pregnancy
Except: V23.2 Pregnancy with history of abortion. Code 646.3 Habitual aborter, from the OB chapter is required to indicate a history of abortion during a pregnancy.
V24 Postpartum care and evaluation
V25 Encounter for contraceptive management
Except V25.0x (See section I.C.18.d.11, Counseling)
V26 Procreative management
Except V26.5x Sterilization status, V26.3 and V26.4 (See section I.C.18.d.11., Counseling)
V27 Outcome of delivery
V28 Antenatal screening (See section I.C.18.d.6., Screening)

12) Newborn, infant and child—See section I.C.15, the newborn guidelines, for further instruction on the use of these codes.

Newborn V code categories:

V20 Health supervision of infant or child
V29 Observation and evaluation of newborns for suspected condition not found (See section I.C.18.d.7, Observation).
V30-V39 Liveborn infant according to type of birth

13) Routine and administrative examinations—The V codes allow for the description of encounters for routine examinations, such as a general check-up or, examinations for administrative purposes, such as a pre-employment physical. The codes are for use as first-listed codes only, and are not to be used if the examination is for diagnosis of a suspected condition or for treatment purposes. In such cases the diagnosis code is used. During a routine exam, should a diagnosis or condition be discovered, it should be coded as an additional code. Pre-existing and chronic conditions and history codes may also be included as additional codes as long as the examination is for administrative purposes and not focused on any particular condition.

Preoperative examination V codes are for use only in those situations when a patient is being cleared for surgery and no treatment is given.

The V code categories/code for routine and administrative examinations:

- V20.2 Routine infant or child health check Any injections given should have a corresponding procedure code.
- V70 General medical examination
- V72 Special investigations and examinations
  Except V72.5 and V72.6

14) Miscellaneous V codes—The miscellaneous V codes capture a number of other health care encounters that do not fall into one of the other categories. Certain of these codes identify the reason for the encounter, others are for use as additional codes that provide useful information on circumstances that may affect a patient's care and treatment.

Prophylactic Organ Removal

For encounters specifically for prophylactic removal of breasts, ovaries, or another organ due to a genetic susceptibility to cancer or a family history of cancer, the principal or first-listed code should be a code from subcategory V50.4 Prophylactic organ removal, followed by the appropriate genetic susceptibility code and the appropriate family history code.

If the patient has a malignancy of one site and is having prophylactic removal at another site to prevent either a new primary malignancy or metastatic disease, a code for the malignancy should also be assigned in addition to a code from subcategory V50.4. A V50.4 code should not be assigned if the patient is having organ removal for treatment of a malignancy, such as the removal of the testes for the treatment of prostate cancer.

Miscellaneous V code categories/codes:

- V07 Need for isolation and other prophylactic measures
- V50 Elective surgery for purposes other than remedying health states
- V58.5 Orthodontics
- V60 Housing, household, and economic circumstances
- V62 Other psychosocial circumstances
- V63 Unavailability of other medical facilities for care
- V64 Persons encountering health services for specific procedures, not carried out
- V66 Convalescence and palliative care
- V68 Encounters for administrative purposes
- V69 Problems related to lifestyle

15) Nonspecific V codes—Certain V codes are so nonspecific, or potentially redundant with other codes in the classification, that there can be little justification for their use in the inpatient setting. Their use in the outpatient setting should be limited to those instances when there is no further documentation to permit more precise coding. Otherwise, any sign or symptom or any other reason for a visit that is captured in another code should be used.

Nonspecific V code categories/codes:

- V11 Personal history of mental disorder—A code from the mental disorders chapter, with an in remission fifth digit, should be used.
- V13.4 Personal history of arthritis
- V13.6 Personal history of congenital malformations
- V15.7 Personal history of contraception
- V23.2 Pregnancy with history of abortion
- V40 Mental and behavioral problems
- V41 Problems with special senses and other special functions
- V47 Other problems with internal organs
- V48 Problems with head, neck, and trunk
- V49 Problems with limbs and other problems
  Exceptions:
  - V49.6 Upper limb amputation status
  - V49.7 Lower limb amputation status
  - V49.81 Postmenopausal status
  - V49.82 Dental sealant status
- V49.83 Awaiting organ transplant status
- V51 Aftercare involving the use of plastic surgery
- V58.2 Blood transfusion, without reported diagnosis
- V58.9 Unspecified aftercare

- V72.5 Radiological examination, NEC
- V72.6 Laboratory examination
  Codes V72.5 and V72.6 are not to be used if any sign or symptoms, or reason for a test is documented. See section IV.K. and section IV.L. of the outpatient guidelines.

V Code Table

Items in bold indicate a change from the April 2005 table. Items underlined have been moved within the table since April 2005.

FIRST LISTED: V codes/categories/subcategories which are only acceptable as principal/first listed.

Codes:

- V22.0 Supervision of normal first pregnancy
- V22.1 Supervision of other normal pregnancy
- V46.12 Encounter for respirator dependence during power failure
- **V46.13 Encounter for weaning from respirator [ventilator]**
- V56.0 Extracorporeal dialysis
- V58.0 Radiotherapy
  V58.0 and **V58.1** may be used together on a record with either one being sequenced first, when a patient receives both chemotherapy and radiation therapy during the same encounter.
- **V58.11 Encounter for antineoplastic chemotherapy**
  V58.0 and V58.11 may be used together on a record, with either one being sequenced first, when a patient receives both chemotherapy and radiation therapy during the same encounter.
- **V58.12 Encounter for antineoplastic immunotherapy**

Categories/Subcategories:

- V20 Health supervision of infant or child
- V24 Postpartum care and examination
- V29 Observation and evaluation of newborns for suspected condition not found
  Exception: A code from the V30-V39 may be sequenced before the V29 if it is the newborn record.
- V30-V39 Liveborn infants according to type of birth
- <u>V57</u> <u>Care involving use of rehabilitation procedures</u>
- V59 Donors
- V66 Convalescence and palliative care
  Exception: V66.7 Palliative care
- V68 Encounters for administrative purposes
- V70 General medical examination
  Exception: V70.7 Examination of participant in clinical trial
- V71 Observation and evaluation for suspected conditions not found
- V72 Special investigations and examinations
  Exceptions:
  V72.4 Pregnancy examination or test
  V72.5 Radiological examination, NEC
  V72.6 Laboratory examination
  V72.86 Encounter for blood typing

FIRST OR ADDITIONAL: V code categories/subcategories which may be either principal/first-listed, or additional codes.

Codes:

- **V15.88 History of fall**
- V43.22 Fully implantable artificial heart status
- **V46.14 Mechanical complication of respirator [ventilator]**
- V49.81 Asymptomatic postmenopausal status (age-related) (natural)
- V49.84 Bed confinement status
- <u>V49.89</u> <u>Other specified conditions influencing health status</u>
- V70.7 Examination of participant in clinical trial
- <u>V72.5</u> <u>Radiological examination, NEC</u>
- <u>V72.6</u> <u>Laboratory examination</u>
- **V72.86 Encounter for blood typing**

Categories/Subcategories:

- V01 Contact with or exposure to communicable diseases
- V02 Carrier or suspected carrier of infectious diseases
- V03-V06 Need for prophylactic vaccination and inoculations
- V07 Need for isolation and other prophylactic measures
- V08 Asymptomatic HIV infection status
- V10 Personal history of malignant neoplasm
- V12 Personal history of certain other diseases
- V13 Personal history of other diseases
  Exception:
  V13.4 Personal history of arthritis
  V13.69 Personal history of other congenital malformations

V16-V19	Family history of disease		V13.69	Personal history of congenital malformations
V23	Supervision of high-risk pregnancy		V15.7	Personal history of contraception
V25	Encounter for contraceptive management		V40	Mental and behavioral problems
V26	Procreative management		V41	Problems with special senses and other special functions
	Exception: V26.5 Sterilization status		V47	Other problems with internal organs
V28	Antenatal screening		V48	Problems with head, neck, and trunk
V45.7	Acquired absence of organ		**V49.0**	**Deficiencies of limbs**
V49.6x	**Upper limb amputation status**		**V49.1**	**Mechanical problems with limbs**
V49.7x	**Lower limb amputation status**		**V49.2**	**Motor problems with limbs**
V50	Elective surgery for purposes other than remedying health states		**V49.3**	**Sensory problems with limbs**
V52	Fitting and adjustment of prosthetic device and implant		**V49.4**	**Disfigurements in limbs**
V53	Fitting and adjustment of other device		**V49.5**	**Other problems with limbs**
V54	Other orthopedic aftercare		**V49.9**	**Unspecified condition influencing health status**
V55	Attention to artificial openings		V51	Aftercare involving the use of plastic surgery
V56	Encounter for dialysis and dialysis catheter care		V58.2	Blood transfusion, without reported diagnosis
	Exception: V56.0 Extracorporeal dialysis		V58.5	Orthodontics
V58.3	Attention to surgical dressings and sutures		V58.9	Unspecified aftercare
V58.4	Other aftercare following surgery		V72.5	Radiological examination, NEC
V58.7	Aftercare following surgery to specified body systems, not elsewhere classified		V72.6	Laboratory examination
V58.8	Other specified procedures and aftercare			
V61	Other family circumstances			
V63	Unavailability of other medical facilities for care			
V65	Other persons seeking consultation without complaint or sickness			
V67	Follow-up examination			
V69	Problems related to lifestyle			
V72.4	**Pregnancy examination or test**			
V73-V82	Special screening examinations			
V83	Genetic carrier status			

ADDITIONAL ONLY: V code categories/subcategories which may only be used as additional codes, not principal/first listed.

Codes:
V13.61	Personal history of hypospadias
V22.2	Pregnancy state, incidental
V46.11	**Dependence on respirator, status**
V49.82	Dental sealant status
V49.83	Awaiting organ transplant status
V66.7	Palliative care
V85	Body mass index

Categories/Subcategories:
V09	Infection with drug-resistant microorganisms
V14	Personal history of allergy to medicinal agents
V15	Other personal history presenting hazards to health
	Exception: V15.7 Personal history of contraception
V15.88	**History of fall**
V21	Constitutional states in development
V26.5	Sterilization status
V27	Outcome of delivery
V42	Organ or tissue replaced by transplant
V43	Organ or tissue replaced by other means
	Exception: V43.22 Fully implantable artificial heart status
V44	Artificial opening status
V45	Other postsurgical states
	Exception: Subcategory V45.7 Acquired absence of organ
V46	Other dependence on machines
	Exception: V46.12 Encounter for respirator dependence during power failure
V46.13	**Encounter for weaning from respirator [ventilator]**
~~V49.6x~~	~~Upper limb amputation status~~
~~V49.7x~~	~~Lower limb amputation status~~
V58.6	**Long-term current drug use**
V60	Housing, household, and economic circumstances
V62	Other psychosocial circumstances
V64	Persons encountering health services for specified procedure, not carried out
V84	Genetic susceptibility to disease
V85	**Body Mass Index**

NONSPECIFIC CODES AND CATEGORIES:
V11	Personal history of mental disorder
V13.4	Personal history of arthritis

19. Supplemental Classification of External Causes of Injury and Poisoning (E-codes, E800-E999)

Introduction: These guidelines are provided for those who are currently collecting E codes in order that there will be standardization in the process. If your institution plans to begin collecting E codes, these guidelines are to be applied. The use of E codes is supplemental to the application of ICD-9-CM diagnosis codes. E codes are never to be recorded as principal diagnoses (first-listed in non-inpatient setting) and are not required for reporting to CMS.

External causes of injury and poisoning codes (E codes) are intended to provide data for injury research and evaluation of injury prevention strategies. E codes capture how the injury or poisoning happened (cause), the intent (unintentional or accidental; or intentional, such as suicide or assault), and the place where the event occurred.

Some major categories of E codes include:
- Transport accidents
- Poisoning and adverse effects of drugs, medicinal substances and biologicals
- Accidental falls
- Accidents caused by fire and flames
- Accidents due to natural and environmental factors
- Late effects of accidents, assaults or self injury
- Assaults or purposely inflicted injury
- Suicide or self inflicted injury

These guidelines apply to the coding and collection of E codes from records in hospitals, outpatient clinics, emergency departments, other ambulatory care settings and provider offices, and nonacute care settings, except when other specific guidelines apply.

a. **General E code coding guidelines**

1) **Used with any code in the range of 001-V86.1**—An E code may be used with any code in the range of 001-V86.1, which indicates an injury, poisoning, or adverse effect due to an external cause.

2) **Assign the appropriate E code for all initial treatments**—Assign the appropriate E code for the initial encounter of an injury, poisoning, or adverse effect of drugs, not for subsequent treatment.

3) **Use the full range of E codes**—Use the full range of E codes to completely describe the cause, the intent and the place of occurrence, if applicable, for all injuries, poisonings, and adverse effects of drugs.

4) **Assign as many E codes as necessary**
Assign as many E codes as necessary to fully explain each cause. If only one E code can be recorded, assign the E code most related to the principal diagnosis.

5) **The selection of the appropriate E code**—The selection of the appropriate E code is guided by the Index to External Causes, which is located after the Alphabetical Index to Diseases and by inclusion and exclusion notes in the Tabular List.

6) **E code can never be a principal diagnosis**—An E code can never be a principal (first-listed) diagnosis.

7) **External cause code(s) with systemic inflammatory response syndrome (SIRS)**—An external cause code(s) may be used with codes 995.93 Systemic inflammatory response syndrome due to noninfectious process without organ dysfunction, and 995.94 Systemic inflammatory response syndrome due to noninfectious process with organ dysfunction, if trauma was the initiating insult that precipitated the

SIRS. The external cause(s) code should correspond to the most serious injury resulting from the trauma. The external cause code(s) should only be assigned if the trauma necessitated the admission in which the patient also developed SIRS. If a patient is admitted with SIRS but the trauma has been treated previously, the external cause codes should not be used.

b. **Place of occurrence guideline**—Use an additional code from category E849 to indicate the place of occurrence for injuries and poisonings. The place of occurrence describes the place where the event occurred and not the patient's activity at the time of the event.

Do not use E849.9 if the place of occurrence is not stated.

c. **Adverse effects of drugs, medicinal and biological substances guidelines**

1) **Do not code directly from the Table of Drugs**—Do not code directly from the Table of Drugs and Chemicals. Always refer back to the Tabular List.

2) **Use as many codes as necessary to describe**—Use as many codes as necessary to describe completely all drugs, medicinal or biological substances.

3) **If the same E code would describe the causative agent**—If the same E code would describe the causative agent for more than one adverse reaction, assign the code only once.

4) **If two or more drugs, medicinal or biological substances**—If two or more drugs, medicinal or biological substances are reported, code each individually unless the combination code is listed in the Table of Drugs and Chemicals. In that case, assign the E code for the combination.

5) **When a reaction results from the interaction of a drug(s)**—When a reaction results from the interaction of a drug(s) and alcohol, use poisoning codes and E codes for both.

6) **If the reporting format limits the number of E codes**—If the reporting format limits the number of E codes that can be used in reporting clinical data, code the one most related to the principal diagnosis. Include at least one from each category (cause, intent, place) if possible.

If there are different fourth-digit codes in the same three-digit category, use the code for "other specified" of that category. If there is no "other specified" code in that category, use the appropriate "unspecified" code in that category.

If the codes are in different three-digit categories, assign the appropriate E code for other multiple drugs and medicinal substances.

7) **Codes from the E930-E949 series**—Codes from the E930-E949 series must be used to identify the causative substance for an adverse effect of drug, medicinal and biological substances, correctly prescribed and properly administered. The effect, such as tachycardia, delirium, gastrointestinal hemorrhaging, vomiting, hypokalemia, hepatitis, renal failure, or respiratory failure, is coded and followed by the appropriate code from the E930-E949 series.

d. **Multiple cause E code coding guidelines**—If two or more events cause separate injuries, an E code should be assigned for each cause. The first listed E code will be selected in the following order:

E codes for child and adult abuse take priority over all other E codes. See section I.C.19.e., Child and adult abuse guidelines.

E codes for terrorism events take priority over all other E codes except child and adult abuse.

E codes for cataclysmic events take priority over all other E codes except child and adult abuse and terrorism.

E codes for transport accidents take priority over all other E codes except cataclysmic events and child and adult abuse and terrorism.

The first-listed E code should correspond to the cause of the most serious diagnosis due to an assault, accident, or self-harm, following the order of hierarchy listed above.

e. **Child and adult abuse guideline**

1) **Intentional injury**—When the cause of an injury or neglect is intentional child or adult abuse, the first-listed E code should be assigned from categories E960-E968 Homicide and injury purposely inflicted by other persons, (except category E967). An E code from category E967 Child and adult battering and other maltreatment, should be added as an additional code to identify the perpetrator, if known.

2) **Accidental intent**—In cases of neglect when the intent is determined to be accidental E code E904.0 Abandonment or neglect of infant and helpless person, should be the first-listed E code.

f. **Unknown or suspected intent guideline**

1) **If the intent (accident, self-harm, assault) of the cause of an injury or poisoning is unknown**—If the intent (accident, self-harm, assault) of the cause of an injury or poisoning is unknown or unspecified, code the intent as undetermined, E980-E989.

2) **If the intent (accident, self-harm, assault) of the cause of an injury or poisoning is questionable**—If the intent (accident, self-harm, assault) of the cause of an injury or poisoning is questionable, probable or suspected, code the intent as undetermined, E980-E989.

g. **Undetermined cause**—When the intent of an injury or poisoning is known, but the cause is unknown, use codes E928.9 Unspecified accident, E958.9 Suicide and self-inflicted injury by unspecified means, and E968.9 Assault by unspecified means.

These E codes should rarely be used, as the documentation in the medical record, in both the inpatient outpatient and other settings, should normally provide sufficient detail to determine the cause of the injury.

h. **Late effects of external cause guidelines**

1) **Late effect E codes**—Late effect E codes exist for injuries and poisonings but not for adverse effects of drugs, misadventures, and surgical complications.

2) **Late effect E codes (E929, E959, E969, E977, E989, or E999.1)**—A late effect E code (E929, E959, E969, E977, E989, or E999.1) should be used with any report of a late effect or sequela resulting from a previous injury or poisoning (905-909).

3) **Late effect E code with a related current injury**—A late effect E code should never be used with a related current nature of injury code.

4) **Use of late effect E codes for subsequent visits**—Use a late effect E code for subsequent visits when a late effect of the initial injury or poisoning is being treated. There is no late effect E code for adverse effects of drugs. Do not use a late effect E code for subsequent visits for follow-up care (e.g., to assess healing, to receive rehabilitative therapy) of the injury or poisoning when no late effect of the injury has been documented.

i. **Misadventures and complications of care guidelines**

1) **Code range E870-E876**—Assign a code in the range of E870-E876 if misadventures are stated by the provider.

2) **Code range E878-E879**—Assign a code in the range of E878-E879 if the provider attributes an abnormal reaction or later complication to a surgical or medical procedure, but does not mention misadventure at the time of the procedure as the cause of the reaction.

j. **Terrorism guidelines**

1) **Cause of injury identified by the federal government (FBI) as terrorism**—When the cause of an injury is identified by the federal government (FBI) as terrorism, the first-listed E code should be a code from category E979 Terrorism. The definition of terrorism employed by the FBI is found at the inclusion note at E979. The terrorism E code is the only E code that should be assigned. Additional E codes from the assault categories should not be assigned.

2) **Cause of an injury is suspected to be the result of terrorism**—When the cause of an injury is suspected to be the result of terrorism a code from category E979 should not be assigned. Assign a code in the range of E codes based on the documentation of intent and mechanism.

3) **Code E979.9 Terrorism, secondary effects**—Assign code E979.9 Terrorism, secondary effects, for conditions occurring subsequent to the terrorist event. This code should not be assigned for conditions that are due to the initial terrorist act.

4) **Statistical tabulation of terrorism codes**—For statistical purposes these codes will be tabulated within the category for assault, expanding the current category from E960-E969 to include E979 and E999.1.

Section II. Selection of Principal Diagnosis

The circumstances of inpatient admission always govern the selection of principal diagnosis. The principal diagnosis is defined in the Uniform Hospital Discharge Data Set (UHDDS) as "that condition established after study to be chiefly responsible for occasioning the admission of the patient to the hospital for care."

The UHDDS definitions are used by hospitals to report inpatient data elements in a standardized manner. These data elements and their definitions can be found in the July 31, 1985, *Federal Register* (vol. 50, no. 147), pp. 31038-40.

Since that time the application of the UHDDS definitions has been expanded to include all non-outpatient settings (acute care, short-term, long-term care and psychiatric hospitals; home health agencies; rehab facilities; nursing homes, etc.).

In determining principal diagnosis the coding conventions in the ICD-9-CM, Volumes 1 and 2 take precedence over these official coding guidelines. (See section I.A., Conventions, for the ICD-9-CM).

The importance of consistent, complete documentation in the medical record cannot be overemphasized. Without such documentation the application of all coding guidelines is a difficult, if not impossible, task.

A. Codes for symptoms, signs, and ill-defined conditions
Codes for symptoms, signs, and ill-defined conditions from chapter 16 are not to be used as principal diagnosis when a related definitive diagnosis has been established.

B. Two or more interrelated conditions, each potentially meeting the definition for principal diagnosis.
When there are two or more interrelated conditions (such as diseases in the same ICD-9-CM chapter or manifestations characteristically associated with a certain disease) potentially meeting the definition of principal diagnosis, either condition may be sequenced first, unless the circumstances of the admission, the therapy provided, the Tabular List, or the Alphabetic Index indicate otherwise.

C. Two or more diagnoses that equally meet the definition for principal diagnosis
In the unusual instance when two or more diagnoses equally meet the criteria for principal diagnosis as determined by the circumstances of admission, diagnostic workup and/or therapy provided, and the Alphabetic Index, Tabular List, or another coding guidelines do not provide sequencing direction, any one of the diagnoses may be sequenced first.

D. Two or more comparative or contrasting conditions.
In those rare instances when two or more contrasting or comparative diagnoses are documented as "either/or" (or similar terminology), they are coded as if the diagnoses were confirmed and the diagnoses are sequenced according to the circumstances of the admission. If no further determination can be made as to which diagnosis should be principal, either diagnosis may be sequenced first.

E. A symptom(s) followed by contrasting/comparative diagnoses
When a symptom(s) is followed by contrasting/comparative diagnoses, the symptom code is sequenced first. All the contrasting/comparative diagnoses should be coded as additional diagnoses.

F. Original treatment plan not carried out
Sequence as the principal diagnosis the condition, which after study occasioned the admission to the hospital, even though treatment may not have been carried out due to unforeseen circumstances.

G. Complications of surgery and other medical care
When the admission is for treatment of a complication resulting from surgery or other medical care, the complication code is sequenced as the principal diagnosis. If the complication is classified to the 996-999 series and the code lacks the necessary specificity in describing the complication, an additional code for the specific complication should be assigned.

H. Uncertain diagnosis
If the diagnosis documented at the time of discharge is qualified as "probable," "suspected," "likely," "questionable," "possible," or "still to be ruled out," code the condition as if it existed or was established. The bases for these guidelines are the diagnostic workup, arrangements for further workup or observation, and initial therapeutic approach that correspond most closely with the established diagnosis.

Note: This guideline is applicable only to short-term, acute, long-term care and psychiatric hospitals.

I. Admission from observation unit

1. Admission following medical observation—When a patient is admitted to an observation unit for a medical condition that either worsens or does not improve, and is subsequently admitted as an inpatient of the same hospital for this same medical condition, the principal diagnosis would be the medical condition that led to the hospital admission.
2. Admission following post-operative observation—When a patient is admitted to an observation unit to monitor a condition (or complication) that develops following outpatient surgery and then is subsequently admitted as an inpatient of the same hospital, hospitals should apply the Uniform Hospital Discharge Data Set (UHDDS) definition of principal diagnosis as "that condition established after study to be chiefly responsible for occasioning the admission of the patient to the hospital for care."

J. Admission from outpatient surgery
When a patient receives surgery in the hospital's outpatient surgery department and is subsequently admitted for continuing inpatient care at the same hospital, the following guidelines should be followed in selecting the principal diagnosis for the inpatient admission:

- **If the reason for the inpatient admission is a complication, assign the complication as the principal diagnosis.**
- **If no complication, or other condition, is documented as the reason for the inpatient admission, assign the reason for the outpatient surgery as the principal diagnosis.**
- **If the reason for the inpatient admission is another condition unrelated to the surgery, assign the unrelated condition as the principal diagnosis.**

Section III. Reporting Additional Diagnoses
GENERAL RULES FOR OTHER (ADDITIONAL) DIAGNOSES

For reporting purposes the definition for "other diagnoses" is interpreted as additional conditions that affect patient care in terms of requiring:

- Clinical evaluation; or
- Therapeutic treatment; or
- Diagnostic procedures; or
- Extended length of hospital stay; or
- Increased nursing care and/or monitoring.

The UHDDS item #11-b defines other diagnoses as "all conditions that coexist at the time of admission, that develop subsequently, or that affect the treatment received and/or the length of stay. Diagnoses that relate to an earlier episode which have no bearing on the current hospital stay are to be excluded." UHDDS definitions apply to inpatients in acute care, short-term, long-term care and psychiatric hospital settings. The UHDDS definitions are used by acute care short-term hospitals to report inpatient data elements in a standardized manner. These data elements and their definitions can be found in the July 31, 1985, *Federal Register* (vol. 50, no. 147), pp. 31038-40.

Since that time the application of the UHDDS definitions has been expanded to include all non-outpatient settings (acute care, short-term, long-term care and psychiatric hospitals; home health agencies; rehab facilities; nursing homes, etc.).

The following guidelines are to be applied in designating other diagnoses when neither the Alphabetic Index nor the Tabular List in ICD-9-CM provides direction. The listing of the diagnoses in the patient record is the responsibility of the attending provider.

A. Previous conditions
If the provider has included a diagnosis in the final diagnostic statement, such as the discharge summary or the face sheet, it should ordinarily be coded. Some providers include in the diagnostic statement resolved conditions or diagnoses and status-post procedures from previous admission that have no bearing on the current stay. Such conditions are not to be reported and are coded only if required by hospital policy.

However, history codes (V10-V19) may be used as secondary codes if the historical condition or family history has an impact on current care or influences treatment.

B. Abnormal findings
Abnormal findings (laboratory, x-ray, pathologic, and other diagnostic results) are not coded and reported unless the provider indicates their clinical significance. If the findings are outside the normal range and the attending provider has ordered other tests to evaluate the condition or prescribed treatment, it is appropriate to ask the provider whether the abnormal finding should be added.

Please note: This differs from the coding practices in the outpatient setting for coding encounters for diagnostic tests that have been interpreted by a provider.

C. Uncertain Diagnosis
If the diagnosis documented at the time of discharge is qualified as "probable," "suspected," "likely," "questionable," "possible," or "still to be ruled out," code the condition as if it existed or was established. The bases for these guidelines are the diagnostic workup, arrangements for further workup or observation, and initial therapeutic approach that correspond most closely with the established diagnosis.

Note: This guideline is applicable only to short-term, acute, long-term care and psychiatric hospitals.

Section IV. Diagnostic Coding and Reporting Guidelines for Outpatient Services
These coding guidelines for outpatient diagnoses have been approved for use by hospitals/providers in coding and reporting hospital-based outpatient services and provider-based office visits.

Coding Guidelines

Information about the use of certain abbreviations, punctuation, symbols, and other conventions used in the ICD-9-CM Tabular List (code numbers and titles), can be found in section IA of these guidelines, under "Conventions for the ICD-9-CM." Information about the correct sequence to use in finding a code is also described in section I.

The terms "encounter" and "visit" are often used interchangeably in describing outpatient service contacts and, therefore, appear together in these guidelines without distinguishing one from the other.

Though the conventions and general guidelines apply to all settings, coding guidelines for outpatient and provider reporting of diagnoses will vary in a number of instances from those for inpatient diagnoses, recognizing that:

- The Uniform Hospital Discharge Data Set (UHDDS) definition of principal diagnosis applies only to inpatients in acute, short-term, long-term care and psychiatric hospitals.
- Coding guidelines for inconclusive diagnoses (probable, suspected, rule out, etc.) were developed for inpatient reporting and do not apply to outpatients.

A. Selection of first-listed condition

In the outpatient setting, the term "first-listed diagnosis" is used in lieu of principal diagnosis.

In determining the first-listed diagnosis the coding conventions of ICD-9-CM, as well as the general and disease-specific guidelines take precedence over the outpatient guidelines.

Diagnoses often are not established at the time of the initial encounter/visit. It may take two or more visits before the diagnosis is confirmed.

The most critical rule involves beginning the search for the correct code assignment through the Alphabetic Index. Never begin searching initially in the Tabular List as this will lead to coding errors.

1. **Outpatient surgery—When a patient presents for outpatient surgery, code the reason for the surgery as the first-listed diagnosis (reason for the encounter), even if the surgery is not performed due to a contraindication.**
2. **Observation stay—When a patient is admitted for observation for a medical condition, assign a code for the medical condition as the first-listed diagnosis. When a patient presents for outpatient surgery and develops complications requiring admission to observation, code the reason for the surgery as the first reported diagnosis (reason for the encounter), followed by codes for the complications as secondary diagnoses.**

B. Codes from 001.0 through V86.1

The appropriate code or codes from 001.0 through V86.1 must be used to identify diagnoses, symptoms, conditions, problems, complaints, or other reason(s) for the encounter/visit.

C. Accurate reporting of ICD-9-CM diagnosis codes

For accurate reporting of ICD-9-CM diagnosis codes, the documentation should describe the patient's condition, using terminology which includes specific diagnoses as well as symptoms, problems, or reasons for the encounter. There are ICD-9-CM codes to describe all of these.

D. Selection of codes 001.0 through 999.9

The selection of codes 001.0 through 999.9 will frequently be used to describe the reason for the encounter. These codes are from the section of ICD-9-CM for the classification of diseases and injuries (e.g. infectious and parasitic diseases; neoplasms; symptoms, signs, and ill-defined conditions, etc.).

E. Codes that describe symptoms and signs

Codes that describe symptoms and signs, as opposed to diagnoses, are acceptable for reporting purposes when a diagnosis has not been established (confirmed) by the provider. Chapter 16 of ICD-9-CM, Symptoms, Signs, and Ill-defined Conditions (codes 780.0-799.9) contain many, but not all, codes for symptoms.

F. Encounters for circumstances other than a disease or injury

ICD-9-CM provides codes to deal with encounters for circumstances other than a disease or injury. The Supplementary Classification of Factors Influencing Health Status and Contact with Health Services (V01.0-V84.8) is provided to deal with occasions when circumstances other than a disease or injury are recorded as diagnosis or problems.

G. Level of Detail in Coding

1. **ICD-9-CM codes with three, four, or five digits**—ICD-9-CM is composed of codes with either three, four, or five digits. Codes with three digits are included in ICD-9-CM as the heading of a category of codes that may be further subdivided by the use of fourth and/or fifth digits, which provide greater specificity.

2. **Use of full number of digits required for a code**—A three-digit code is to be used only if it is not further subdivided. Where fourth-digit subcategories and/or fifth-digit subclassifications are provided, they must be assigned. A code is invalid if it has not been coded to the full number of digits required for that code. See also discussion under section I.b.3., General coding guidelines, Level of detail in coding.

H. ICD-9-CM code for the diagnosis, condition, problem, or other reason for encounter/visit

List first the ICD-9-CM code for the diagnosis, condition, problem, or other reason for encounter/visit shown in the medical record to be chiefly responsible for the services provided. List additional codes that describe any coexisting conditions. In some cases the first-listed diagnosis may be a symptom when a diagnosis has not been established (confirmed) by the physician.

I. "Probable," "suspected," "questionable," "rule out," or "working diagnosis"

Do not code diagnoses documented as "probable," "suspected," "questionable," "rule out," or "working diagnosis." Rather, code the condition(s) to the highest degree of certainty for that encounter/visit, such as symptoms, signs, abnormal test results, or other reason for the visit.

Please note: This differs from the coding practices used by short-term, acute care, long-term care, and psychiatric hospitals.

J. Chronic diseases

Chronic diseases treated on an ongoing basis may be coded and reported as many times as the patient receives treatment and care for the condition(s).

K. Code all documented conditions that coexist

Code all documented conditions that coexist at the time of the encounter/visit, and require or affect patient care treatment or management. Do not code conditions that were previously treated and no longer exist. However, history codes (V10-V19) may be used as secondary codes if the historical condition or family history has an impact on current care or influences treatment.

L. Patients receiving diagnostic services only

For patients receiving diagnostic services only during an encounter/visit, sequence first the diagnosis, condition, problem, or other reason for encounter/visit shown in the medical record to be chiefly responsible for the outpatient services provided during the encounter/visit. Codes for other diagnoses (e.g., chronic conditions) may be sequenced as additional diagnoses.

For outpatient encounters for diagnostic tests that have been interpreted by a physician and the final report is available at the time of coding, code any confirmed or definitive diagnosis(es) documented in the interpretation. Do not code related signs and symptoms as additional diagnoses.

Please note: This differs from the coding practice in the hospital inpatient setting regarding abnormal findings on test results.

M. Patients receiving therapeutic services only

For patients receiving therapeutic services only during an encounter/visit, sequence first the diagnosis, condition, problem, or other reason for encounter/visit shown in the medical record to be chiefly responsible for the outpatient services provided during the encounter/visit. Codes for other diagnoses (e.g., chronic conditions) may be sequenced as additional diagnoses.

The only exception to this rule is that when the primary reason for the admission/encounter is chemotherapy, radiation therapy, or rehabilitation, the appropriate V code for the service is listed first, and the diagnosis or problem for which the service is being performed is listed second.

N. Patients receiving preoperative evaluations only

For patients receiving preoperative evaluations only, sequence first a code from category V72.8 Other specified examinations, to describe the pre-op consultations. Assign a code for the condition to describe the reason for the surgery as an additional diagnosis. Code also any findings related to the pre-op evaluation.

O. Ambulatory surgery

For ambulatory surgery, code the diagnosis for which the surgery was performed. If the postoperative diagnosis is known to be different from the preoperative diagnosis at the time the diagnosis is confirmed, select the postoperative diagnosis for coding, since it is the most definitive.

P. Routine outpatient prenatal visits

For routine outpatient prenatal visits when no complications are present, code V22.0 Supervision of normal first pregnancy, or V22.1 Supervision of other normal pregnancy, should be used as the principal diagnosis. These codes should not be used in conjunction with chapter 11 codes.

Index to Diseases

A

AAT (alpha-1 antitrypsin) deficiency 273.4
AAV (disease) (illness) (infection) — see Human immunodeficiency virus (disease) (illness) (infection)
Abactio — see Abortion, induced
Abactus venter — see Abortion, induced
Abarognosis 781.99
Abasia (-astasia) 307.9
  atactica 781.3
  choreic 781.3
  hysterical 300.11
  paroxysmal trepidant 781.3
  spastic 781.3
  trembling 781.3
  trepidans 781.3
Abderhalden-Kaufmann-Lignac syndrome (cystinosis) 270.0
Abdomen, abdominal — see also condition
  accordion 306.4
  acute 789.0 ☑
  angina 557.1
  burst 868.00
  convulsive equivalent (see also Epilepsy) 345.5 ☑
  heart 746.87
  muscle deficiency syndrome 756.79
  obstipum 756.79
Abdominalgia 789.0 ☑
  periodic 277.31 ▲
Abduction contracture, hip or other joint — see Contraction, joint
Abercrombie's syndrome (amyloid degeneration) 277.39 ▲
Aberrant (congenital) — see also Malposition, congenital
  adrenal gland 759.1
  blood vessel NEC 747.60
    arteriovenous NEC 747.60
    cerebrovascular 747.81
    gastrointestinal 747.61
    lower limb 747.64
    renal 747.62
    spinal 747.82
    upper limb 747.63
  breast 757.6
  endocrine gland NEC 759.2
  gastrointestinal vessel (peripheral) 747.61
  hepatic duct 751.69
  lower limb vessel (peripheral) 747.64
  pancreas 751.7
  parathyroid gland 759.2
  peripheral vascular vessel NEC 747.60
  pituitary gland (pharyngeal) 759.2
  renal blood vessel 747.62
  sebaceous glands, mucous membrane, mouth 750.26
  spinal vessel 747.82
  spleen 759.0
  testis (descent) 752.51
  thymus gland 759.2
  thyroid gland 759.2
  upper limb vessel (peripheral) 747.63
Aberratio
  lactis 757.6
  testis 752.51
Aberration — see also Anomaly
  chromosome — see Anomaly, chromosome(s)
  distantial 368.9
  mental (see also Disorder, mental, nonpsychotic) 300.9
Abetalipoproteinemia 272.5
Abionarce 780.79
Abiotrophy 799.89
Ablatio
  placentae — see Placenta, ablatio
  retinae (see also Detachment, retina) 361.9
Ablation
  pituitary (gland) (with hypofunction) 253.7

Ablation — continued
  placenta — see Placenta, ablatio
  uterus 621.8
Ablepharia, ablepharon, ablephary 743.62
Ablepsia — see Blindness
Ablepsy — see Blindness
Ablutomania 300.3
Abnormal, abnormality, abnormalities
  — see also Anomaly
  acid-base balance 276.4
    fetus or newborn — see Distress, fetal
  adaptation curve, dark 368.63
  alveolar ridge 525.9
  amnion 658.9 ☑
    affecting fetus or newborn 762.9
  anatomical relationship NEC 759.9
  apertures, congenital, diaphragm 756.6
  auditory perception NEC 388.40
  autosomes NEC 758.5
    13 758.1
    18 758.2
    21 or 22 758.0
    D_1 758.1
    E_3 758.2
    G 758.0
  ballistocardiogram 794.39
  basal metabolic rate (BMR) 794.7
  biosynthesis, testicular androgen 257.2
  blood level (of)
    cobalt 790.6
    copper 790.6
    iron 790.6
    lead 790.6 ●
    lithium 790.6
    magnesium 790.6
    mineral 790.6
    zinc 790.6
  blood pressure
    elevated (without diagnosis of hypertension) 796.2
    low (see also Hypotension) 458.9
      reading (incidental) (isolated) (nonspecific) 796.3
  bowel sounds 787.5
  breathing behavior — see Respiration
  caloric test 794.19
  cervix (acquired) NEC 622.9
    congenital 752.40
    in pregnancy or childbirth 654.6 ☑
      causing obstructed labor 660.2 ☑
      affecting fetus or newborn 763.1
  chemistry, blood NEC 790.6
  chest sounds 786.7
  chorion 658.9 ☑
    affecting fetus or newborn 762.9
  chromosomal NEC 758.89
    analysis, nonspecific result 795.2
    autosomes (see also Abnormal, autosomes NEC) 758.5
    fetal, (suspected) affecting management of pregnancy 655.1 ☑
    sex 758.81
  clinical findings NEC 796.4
  communication — see Fistula
  configuration of pupils 379.49
  coronary
    artery 746.85
    vein 746.9
  cortisol-binding globulin 255.8
  course, Eustachian tube 744.24
  dentofacial NEC 524.9
    functional 524.50
    specified type NEC 524.89
  development, developmental NEC 759.9
    bone 756.9
    central nervous system 742.9
  direction, teeth 524.30
  Dynia (see also Defect, coagulation) 286.9

Abnormal, abnormality, abnormalities
  — see also Anomaly — continued
  Ebstein 746.2
  echocardiogram 793.2
  echoencephalogram 794.01
  echogram NEC — see Findings, abnormal, structure
  electrocardiogram (ECG) (EKG) 794.31
  electroencephalogram (EEG) 794.02
  electromyogram (EMG) 794.17
    ocular 794.14
  electro-oculogram (EOG) 794.12
  electroretinogram (ERG) 794.11
  erythrocytes 289.9
    congenital, with perinatal jaundice 282.9 [774.0]
  Eustachian valve 746.9
  excitability under minor stress 301.9
  fat distribution 782.9
  feces 787.7
  fetal heart rate — see Distress, fetal
  fetus NEC
    affecting management of pregnancy — see Pregnancy, management affected by, fetal
    causing disproportion 653.7 ☑
      affecting fetus or newborn 763.1
      causing obstructed labor 660.1 ☑
        affecting fetus or newborn 763.1
    findings without manifest disease — see Findings, abnormal
  fluid
    amniotic 792.3
    cerebrospinal 792.0
    peritoneal 792.9
    pleural 792.9
    synovial 792.9
    vaginal 792.9
  forces of labor NEC 661.9 ☑
    affecting fetus or newborn 763.7
  form, teeth 520.2
  function studies
    auditory 794.15
    bladder 794.9
    brain 794.00
    cardiovascular 794.30
    endocrine NEC 794.6
    kidney 794.4
    liver 794.8
    nervous system
      central 794.00
      peripheral 794.19
    oculomotor 794.14
    pancreas 794.9
    placenta 794.9
    pulmonary 794.2
    retina 794.11
    special senses 794.19
    spleen 794.9
    thyroid 794.5
    vestibular 794.16
  gait 781.2
    hysterical 300.11
  gastrin secretion 251.5
  globulin
    cortisol-binding 255.8
    thyroid-binding 246.8
  glucagon secretion 251.4
  glucose 790.29
    in pregnancy, childbirth, or puerperium 648.8 ☑
    fetus or newborn 775.0
    non-fasting 790.29
  gravitational (G) forces or states 994.9
  hair NEC 704.2
  hard tissue formation in pulp 522.3
  head movement 781.0
  heart
    rate
      fetus, affecting liveborn infant
        before the onset of labor 763.81
        during labor 763.82

Abnormal, abnormality, abnormalities
  — see also Anomaly — continued
  heart — continued
    rate — continued
      fetus, affecting liveborn infant — continued
        unspecified as to time of onset 763.83
      intrauterine
        before the onset of labor 763.81
        during labor 763.82
        unspecified as to time of onset 763.83
      newborn
        before the onset of labor 763.81
        during labor 763.82
        unspecified as to time of onset 763.83
    shadow 793.2
    sounds NEC 785.3
  hemoglobin (see also Disease, hemoglobin) 282.7
    trait — see Trait, hemoglobin, abnormal
  hemorrhage, uterus — see Hemorrhage, uterus
  histology NEC 795.4
  increase
    in
      appetite 783.6
      development 783.9
  involuntary movement 781.0
  jaw closure 524.51
  karyotype 795.2
  knee jerk 796.1
  labor NEC 661.9 ☑
    affecting fetus or newborn 763.7
  laboratory findings — see Findings, abnormal
  length, organ or site, congenital — see Distortion
  loss of height 781.91
  loss of weight 783.21
  lung shadow 793.1
  mammogram 793.80
    calcification 793.89 ●
    calculus 793.89 ●
    microcalcification 793.81
  Mantoux test 795.5
  membranes (fetal)
    affecting fetus or newborn 762.9
    complicating pregnancy 658.8 ☑
  menstruation — see Menstruation
  metabolism (see also condition) 783.9
  movement 781.0
    disorder NEC 333.90
      sleep related, unspecified 780.58
      specified NEC 333.99
    head 781.0
    involuntary 781.0
    specified type NEC 333.99
  muscle contraction, localized 728.85
  myoglobin (Aberdeen) (Annapolis) 289.9
  narrowness, eyelid 743.62
  optokinetic response 379.57
  organs or tissues of pelvis NEC
    in pregnancy or childbirth 654.9 ☑
      affecting fetus or newborn 763.89
      causing obstructed labor 660.2 ☑
        affecting fetus or newborn 763.1
  origin — see Malposition, congenital
  palmar creases 757.2
  Papanicolaou (smear)
    cervix 795.00

Abnormal, abnormality, abnormalities

Abnormal, abnormality, abnormalities
— see also Anomaly —
continued
  Papanicolaou — continued
    cervix — continued
      with
        atypical squamous cells
          cannot exclude high grade squamous intraepithelial lesion (ASC-H) 795.02
          of undetermined significance (ASC-US) 795.01
        cytologic evidence of malignancy 795.06
        high grade squamous intraepithelial lesion (HGSIL) 795.04
        low grade squamous intraepithelial lesion (LGSIL) 795.03
        nonspecific finding NEC 795.09
      other site 795.1
  parturition
    affecting fetus or newborn 763.9
    mother — see Delivery, complicated
  pelvis (bony) — see Deformity, pelvis
  percussion, chest 786.7
  periods (grossly) (see also Menstruation) 626.9
  phonocardiogram 794.39
  placenta — see Placenta, abnormal
  plantar reflex 796.1
  plasma protein — see Deficiency, plasma, protein
  pleural folds 748.8
  position (see also Malposition)
    gravid uterus 654.4
      causing obstructed labor 660.2
        affecting fetus or newborn 763.1
  posture NEC 781.92
  presentation (fetus) — see Presentation, fetus, abnormal
  product of conception NEC 631
  puberty — see Puberty
  pulmonary
    artery 747.3
    function, newborn 770.89
    test results 794.2
    ventilation, newborn 770.89
      hyperventilation 786.01
  pulsations in neck 785.1
  pupil reflexes 379.40
  quality of milk 676.8
  radiological examination 793.99
    abdomen NEC 793.6
    biliary tract 793.3
    breast 793.89
      mammogram NOS 793.80
      mammographic
        calcification 793.89
        calculus 793.89
        microcalcification 793.81
    gastrointestinal tract 793.4
    genitourinary organs 793.5
    head 793.0
    image test inconclusive due to excess body fat 793.91
    intrathoracic organ NEC 793.2
    lung (field) 793.1
    musculoskeletal system 793.7
    retroperitoneum 793.6
    skin and subcutaneous tissue 793.99
    skull 793.0
  red blood cells 790.09
    morphology 790.09
    volume 790.09
  reflex NEC 796.1
  renal function test 794.4
  respiration signs — see Respiration
  response to nerve stimulation 794.10

Abnormal, abnormality, abnormalities
— see also Anomaly —
continued
  retinal correspondence 368.34
  rhythm, heart (see also Arrhythmia)
    fetus — see Distress, fetal
  saliva 792.4
  scan
    brain 794.09
    kidney 794.4
    liver 794.8
    lung 794.2
    thyroid 794.5
  secretion
    gastrin 251.5
    glucagon 251.4
  semen 792.2
  serum level (of)
    acid phosphatase 790.5
    alkaline phosphatase 790.5
    amylase 790.5
    enzymes NEC 790.5
    lipase 790.5
  shape
    cornea 743.41
    gallbladder 751.69
    gravid uterus 654.4
      affecting fetus or newborn 763.89
      causing obstructed labor 660.2
        affecting fetus or newborn 763.1
    head (see also Anomaly, skull) 756.0
    organ or site, congenital NEC — see Distortion
  sinus venosus 747.40
  size
    fetus, complicating delivery 653.5
      causing obstructed labor 660.1
    gallbladder 751.69
    head (see also Anomaly, skull) 756.0
    organ or site, congenital NEC — see Distortion
    teeth 520.2
  skin and appendages, congenital NEC 757.9
  soft parts of pelvis — see Abnormal, organs or tissues of pelvis
  spermatozoa 792.2
  sputum (amount) (color) (excessive) (odor) (purulent) 786.4
  stool NEC 787.7
    bloody 578.1
      occult 792.1
    bulky 787.7
    color (dark) (light) 792.1
    content (fat) (mucus) (pus) 792.1
    occult blood 792.1
  synchondrosis 756.9
  test results without manifest disease — see Findings, abnormal
  thebesian valve 746.9
  thermography — see Findings, abnormal, structure
  threshold, cones or rods (eye) 368.63
  thyroid-binding globulin 246.8
  thyroid product 246.8
  toxicology (findings) NEC 796.0
  tracheal cartilage (congenital) 748.3
  transport protein 273.8
  ultrasound results — see Findings, abnormal, structure
  umbilical cord
    affecting fetus or newborn 762.6
    complicating delivery 663.9
    specified NEC 663.8
  union
    cricoid cartilage and thyroid cartilage 748.3
    larynx and trachea 748.3

Abnormal, abnormality, abnormalities
— see also Anomaly —
continued
  union — continued
    thyroid cartilage and hyoid bone 748.3
  urination NEC 788.69
    psychogenic 306.53
    stream
      intermittent 788.61
      slowing 788.62
      splitting 788.61
      weak 788.62
    urgency 788.63
  urine (constituents) NEC 791.9
  uterine hemorrhage (see also Hemorrhage, uterus) 626.9
    climacteric 627.0
    postmenopausal 627.1
  vagina (acquired) (congenital)
    in pregnancy or childbirth 654.7
      affecting fetus or newborn 763.89
      causing obstructed labor 660.2
        affecting fetus or newborn 763.1
  vascular sounds 785.9
  vectorcardiogram 794.39
  visually evoked potential (VEP) 794.13
  vulva (acquired) (congenital)
    in pregnancy or childbirth 654.8
      affecting fetus or newborn 763.89
      causing obstructed labor 660.2
        affecting fetus or newborn 763.1
  weight
    gain 783.1
      of pregnancy 646.1
        with hypertension — see Toxemia, of pregnancy
    loss 783.21
  x-ray examination — see Abnormal, radiological examination
Abnormally formed uterus — see Anomaly, uterus
Abnormity (any organ or part) — see Anomaly
ABO
  hemolytic disease 773.1
  incompatibility reaction 999.6
Abocclusion 524.20
Abolition, language 784.69
Aborter, habitual or recurrent NEC
  without current pregnancy 629.81
  current abortion (see also Abortion, spontaneous) 634.9
    affecting fetus or newborn 761.8
  observation in current pregnancy 646.3
Abortion (complete) (incomplete) (inevitable) (with retained products of conception) 637.9

Note — Use the following fifth-digit subclassification with categories 634–637:
  0 unspecified
  1 incomplete
  2 complete

  with
    complication(s) (any) following previous abortion — see category 639
    damage to pelvic organ (laceration) (rupture) (tear) 637.2
    embolism (air) (amniotic fluid) (blood clot) (pulmonary) (pyemic) (septic) (soap) 637.6
    genital tract and pelvic infection 637.0

Abortion — continued
  with — continued
    hemorrhage, delayed or excessive 637.1
    metabolic disorder 637.4
    renal failure (acute) 637.3
    sepsis (genital tract) (pelvic organ) 637.0
    urinary tract 637.7
    shock (postoperative) (septic) 637.5
    specified complication NEC 637.7
    toxemia 637.3
    unspecified complication(s) 637.8
    urinary tract infection 637.7
  accidental — see Abortion, spontaneous
  artificial — see Abortion, induced
  attempted (failed) — see Abortion, failed
  criminal — see Abortion, illegal
  early — see Abortion, spontaneous
  elective — see Abortion, legal
  failed (legal) 638.9
    with
      damage to pelvic organ (laceration) (rupture) (tear) 638.2
      embolism (air) (amniotic fluid) (blood clot) (pulmonary) (pyemic) (septic) (soap) 638.6
      genital tract and pelvic infection 638.0
      hemorrhage, delayed or excessive 638.1
      metabolic disorder 638.4
      renal failure (acute) 638.3
      sepsis (genital tract) (pelvic organ) 638.0
      urinary tract 638.7
      shock (postoperative) (septic) 638.5
      specified complication NEC 638.7
      toxemia 638.3
      unspecified complication(s) 638.8
      urinary tract infection 638.7
  fetal indication — see Abortion, legal
  fetus 779.6
  following threatened abortion — see Abortion, by type
  habitual or recurrent (care during pregnancy) 646.3
    with current abortion (see also Abortion, spontaneous) 634.9
      affecting fetus or newborn 761.8
    without current pregnancy 629.81
  homicidal — see Abortion, illegal
  illegal 636.9
    with
      damage to pelvic organ (laceration) (rupture) (tear) 636.2
      embolism (air) (amniotic fluid) (blood clot) (pulmonary) (pyemic) (septic) (soap) 636.6
      genital tract and pelvic infection 636.0
      hemorrhage, delayed or excessive 636.1
      metabolic disorder 636.4
      renal failure 636.3
      sepsis (genital tract) (pelvic organ) 636.0
      urinary tract 636.7
      shock (postoperative) (septic) 636.5
      specified complication NEC 636.7
      toxemia 636.3

Abortion — *continued*
  illegal — *continued*
    with — *continued*
      unspecified complication(s) 636.8 ☑
      urinary tract infection 636.7 ☑
    fetus 779.6
  induced 637.9 ☑
    illegal — *see* Abortion, illegal
    legal indications — *see* Abortion, legal
    medical indications — *see* Abortion, legal
    therapeutic — *see* Abortion, legal
  late — *see* Abortion, spontaneous
  legal (legal indication) (medical indication) (under medical supervision) 635.9 ☑
    with
      damage to pelvic organ (laceration) (rupture) (tear) 635.2 ☑
      embolism (air) (amniotic fluid) (blood clot) (pulmonary) (pyemic) (septic) (soap) 635.6 ☑
      genital tract and pelvic infection 635.0 ☑
      hemorrhage, delayed or excessive 635.1 ☑
      metabolic disorder 635.4 ☑
      renal failure (acute) 635.3 ☑
      sepsis (genital tract) (pelvic organ) 635.0 ☑
      urinary tract 635.7 ☑
      shock (postoperative) (septic) 635.5 ☑
      specified complication NEC 635.7 ☑
      toxemia 635.3 ☑
      unspecified complication(s) 635.8 ☑
      urinary tract infection 635.7 ☑
    fetus 779.6
  medical indication — *see* Abortion, legal
  mental hygiene problem — *see* Abortion, legal
  missed 632
  operative — *see* Abortion, legal
  psychiatric indication — *see* Abortion, legal
  recurrent — *see* Abortion, spontaneous
  self-induced — *see* Abortion, illegal
  septic — *see* Abortion, by type, with sepsis
  spontaneous 634.9 ☑
    with
      damage to pelvic organ (laceration) (rupture) (tear) 634.2 ☑
      embolism (air) (amniotic fluid) (blood clot) (pulmonary) (pyemic) (septic) (soap) 634.6 ☑
      genital tract and pelvic infection 634.0 ☑
      hemorrhage, delayed or excessive 634.1 ☑
      metabolic disorder 634.4 ☑
      renal failure 634.3 ☑
      sepsis (genital tract) (pelvic organ) 634.0 ☑
      urinary tract 634.7 ☑
      shock (postoperative) (septic) 634.5 ☑
      specified complication NEC 634.7 ☑
      toxemia 634.3 ☑
      unspecified complication(s) 634.8 ☑
      urinary tract infection 634.7 ☑
    fetus 761.8
    threatened 640.0 ☑

Abortion — *continued*
  spontaneous — *continued*
    threatened — *continued*
      affecting fetus or newborn 762.1
  surgical — *see* Abortion, legal
  therapeutic — *see* Abortion, legal
  threatened 640.0 ☑
    affecting fetus or newborn 762.1
  tubal — *see* Pregnancy, tubal
  voluntary — *see* Abortion, legal
Abortus fever 023.9
Aboulomania 301.6
Abrachia 755.20
Abrachiatism 755.20
Abrachiocephalia 759.89
Abrachiocephalus 759.89
Abrami's disease (acquired hemolytic jaundice) 283.9
Abramov-Fiedler myocarditis (acute isolated myocarditis) 422.91
Abrasion — *see also* Injury, superficial, by site
  cornea 918.1
  dental 521.20
    extending into
      dentine 521.22
      pulp 521.23
    generalized 521.25
    limited to enamel 521.21
    localized 521.24
  teeth, tooth (dentifrice) (habitual) (hard tissues) (occupational) (ritual) (traditional) (wedge defect) (*see also* Abrasion, dental) 521.20
Abrikossov's tumor (M9580/0) — *see also* Neoplasm, connective tissue, benign
  malignant (M9580/3) — *see* Neoplasm, connective tissue, malignant
Abrism 988.8
Abruption, placenta — *see* Placenta, abruptio
Abruptio placentae — *see* Placenta, abruptio
Abscess (acute) (chronic) (infectional) (lymphangitic) (metastatic) (multiple) (pyogenic) (septic) (with lymphangitis) — *see also* Cellulitis 682.9
  abdomen, abdominal
    cavity 567.22
    wall 682.2
  abdominopelvic 567.22
  accessory sinus (chronic) (*see also* Sinusitis) 473.9
  adrenal (capsule) (gland) 255.8
  alveolar 522.5
    with sinus 522.7
  amebic 006.3
    bladder 006.8
    brain (with liver or lung abscess) 006.5
    liver (without mention of brain or lung abscess) 006.3
      with
        brain abscess (and lung abscess) 006.5
        lung abscess 006.4
    lung (with liver abscess) 006.4
      with brain abscess 006.5
    seminal vesicle 006.8
    specified site NEC 006.8
    spleen 006.8
  anaerobic 040.0
  ankle 682.6
  anorectal 566
  antecubital space 682.3
  antrum (chronic) (Highmore) (*see also* Sinusitis, maxillary) 473.0
  anus 566
  apical (tooth) 522.5
    with sinus (alveolar) 522.7
  appendix 540.1

Abscess — *see also* Cellulitis — *continued*
  areola (acute) (chronic) (nonpuerperal) 611.0
    puerperal, postpartum 675.1 ☑
  arm (any part, above wrist) 682.3
  artery (wall) 447.2
  atheromatous 447.2
  auditory canal (external) 380.10
  auricle (ear) (staphylococcal) (streptococcal) 380.10
  axilla, axillary (region) 682.3
    lymph gland or node 683
  back (any part) 682.2
  Bartholin's gland 616.3
    with
      abortion — *see* Abortion, by type, with sepsis
      ectopic pregnancy (*see also* categories 633.0–633.9) 639.0
      molar pregnancy (*see also* categories 630–632) 639.0
      complicating pregnancy or puerperium 646.6 ☑
    following
      abortion 639.0
      ectopic or molar pregnancy 639.0
  bartholinian 616.3
  Bezold's 383.01
  bile, biliary, duct or tract (*see also* Cholecystitis) 576.8
  bilharziasis 120.1
  bladder (wall) 595.89
    amebic 006.8
  bone (subperiosteal) (*see also* Osteomyelitis) 730.0
    accessory sinus (chronic) (*see also* Sinusitis) 473.9
    acute 730.0
    chronic or old 730.1 ☑
    jaw (lower) (upper) 526.4
    mastoid — *see* Mastoiditis, acute
    petrous (*see also* Petrositis) 383.20
    spinal (tuberculous) (*see also* Tuberculosis) 015.0 ☑ [730.88]
    nontuberculous 730.08
  bowel 569.5
  brain (any part) 324.0
    amebic (with liver or lung abscess) 006.5
    cystic 324.0
    late effect — *see* category 326
    otogenic 324.0
    tuberculous (*see also* Tuberculosis) 013.3 ☑
  breast (acute) (chronic) (nonpuerperal) 611.0
    newborn 771.5
    puerperal, postpartum 675.1 ☑
    tuberculous (*see also* Tuberculosis) 017.9 ☑
  broad ligament (chronic) (*see also* Disease, pelvis, inflammatory) 614.4
    acute 614.3
  Brodie's (chronic) (localized) (*see also* Osteomyelitis) 730.1 ☑
  bronchus 519.19 ▲
  buccal cavity 528.3
  bulbourethral gland 597.0
  bursa 727.89
    pharyngeal 478.29
  buttock 682.5
  canaliculus, breast 611.0
  canthus 372.20
  cartilage 733.99
  cecum 569.5
    with appendicitis 540.1
  cerebellum, cerebellar 324.0
    late effect — *see* category 326
  cerebral (embolic) 324.0
    late effect — *see* category 326
  cervical (neck region) 682.1
    lymph gland or node 683

Abscess — *see also* Cellulitis — *continued*
  cervical — *continued*
    stump (*see also* Cervicitis) 616.0
  cervix (stump) (uteri) (*see also* Cervicitis) 616.0
  cheek, external 682.0
    inner 528.3
  chest 510.9
    with fistula 510.0
    wall 682.2
  chin 682.0
  choroid 363.00
  ciliary body 364.3
  circumtonsillar 475
  cold (tuberculous) (*see also* Tuberculosis, abscess)
    articular — *see* Tuberculosis, joint
  colon (wall) 569.5
  colostomy or enterostomy 569.61
  conjunctiva 372.00
  connective tissue NEC 682.9
  cornea 370.55
    with ulcer 370.00
  corpus
    cavernosum 607.2
    luteum (*see also* Salpingo-oophoritis) 614.2
  Cowper's gland 597.0
  cranium 324.0
  cul-de-sac (Douglas') (posterior) (*see also* Disease, pelvis, inflammatory) 614.4
    acute 614.3
  dental 522.5
    with sinus (alveolar) 522.7
  dentoalveolar 522.5
    with sinus (alveolar) 522.7
  diaphragm, diaphragmatic 567.22
  digit NEC 681.9
  Douglas' cul-de-sac or pouch (*see also* Disease, pelvis, inflammatory) 614.4
    acute 614.3
  Dubois' 090.5
  ductless gland 259.8
  ear
    acute 382.00
    external 380.10
    inner 386.30
    middle — *see* Otitis media
  elbow 682.3
  endamebic — *see* Abscess, amebic
  entamebic — *see* Abscess, amebic
  enterostomy 569.61
  epididymis 604.0
  epidural 324.9
    brain 324.0
    late effect — *see* category 326
    spinal cord 324.1
  epiglottis 478.79
  epiploon, epiploic 567.22
  erysipelatous (*see also* Erysipelas) 035
  esophagostomy 530.86
  esophagus 530.19
  ethmoid (bone) (chronic) (sinus) (*see also* Sinusitis, ethmoidal) 473.2
  external auditory canal 380.10
  extradural 324.9
    brain 324.0
    late effect — *see* category 326
    spinal cord 324.1
  extraperitoneal — *see* Abscess, peritoneum
  eye 360.00
  eyelid 373.13
  face (any part, except eye) 682.0
  fallopian tube (*see also* Salpingo-oophoritis) 614.2
  fascia 728.89
  fauces 478.29
  fecal 569.5
  femoral (region) 682.6
  filaria, filarial (*see also* Infestation, filarial) 125.9

Abscess

Abscess — see also Cellulitis — continued
- finger (any) (intrathecal) (periosteal) (subcutaneous) (subcuticular) 681.00
- fistulous NEC 682.9
- flank 682.2
- foot (except toe) 682.7
- forearm 682.3
- forehead 682.0
- frontal (sinus) (chronic) (see also Sinusitis, frontal) 473.1
- gallbladder (see also Cholecystitis, acute) 575.0
- gastric 535.0 ☑
- genital organ or tract NEC
  - female 616.9
    - with
      - abortion — see Abortion, by type, with sepsis
      - ectopic pregnancy (see also categories 633.0–633.9) 639.0
      - molar pregnancy (see also categories 630–632) 639.0
    - following
      - abortion 639.0
      - ectopic or molar pregnancy 639.0
    - puerperal, postpartum, childbirth 670.0 ☑
  - male 608.4
- genitourinary system, tuberculous (see also Tuberculosis) 016.9 ☑
- gingival 523.30 ▲
- gland, glandular (lymph) (acute) NEC 683
- glottis 478.79
- gluteal (region) 682.5
- gonorrheal NEC (see also Gonococcus) 098.0
- groin 682.2
- gum 523.30 ▲
- hand (except finger or thumb) 682.4
- head (except face) 682.8
- heart 429.89
- heel 682.7
- helminthic (see also Infestation, by specific parasite) 128.9
- hepatic 572.0
  - amebic (see also Abscess, liver, amebic) 006.3
  - duct 576.8
- hip 682.6
  - tuberculous (active) (see also Tuberculosis) 015.1 ☑
- ileocecal 540.1
- ileostomy (bud) 569.61
- iliac (region) 682.2
  - fossa 540.1
- iliopsoas 567.31
  - nontuberculous 728.89
  - tuberculous (see also Tuberculosis) 015.0 ☑ [730.88]
- infraclavicular (fossa) 682.3
- inguinal (region) 682.2
  - lymph gland or node 683
- intersphincteric (anus) 566
- intestine, intestinal 569.5
  - rectal 566
- intra-abdominal (see also Abscess, peritoneum) 567.22
  - postoperative 998.59
- intracranial 324.0
  - late effect — see category 326
- intramammary — see Abscess, breast
- intramastoid (see also Mastoiditis, acute) 383.00
- intraorbital 376.01
- intraperitoneal 567.22
- intraspinal 324.1
  - late effect — see category 326
- intratonsillar 475
- iris 364.3
- ischiorectal 566

Abscess — see also Cellulitis — continued
- jaw (bone) (lower) (upper) 526.4
  - skin 682.0
- joint (see also Arthritis, pyogenic) 711.0 ☑
  - vertebral (tuberculous) (see also Tuberculosis) 015.0 ☑ [730.88]
  - nontuberculous 724.8
- kidney 590.2
  - with
    - abortion — see Abortion, by type, with urinary tract infection
    - calculus 592.0
    - ectopic pregnancy (see also categories 633.0–633.9) 639.8
    - molar pregnancy (see also categories 630–632) 639.8
    - complicating pregnancy or puerperium 646.6 ☑
      - affecting fetus or newborn 760.1
    - following
      - abortion 639.8
      - ectopic or molar pregnancy 639.8
- knee 682.6
  - joint 711.06
  - tuberculous (active) (see also Tuberculosis) 015.2 ☑
- labium (majus) (minus) 616.4
  - complicating pregnancy, childbirth, or puerperium 646.6 ☑
- lacrimal (passages) (sac) (see also Dacryocystitis) 375.30
  - caruncle 375.30
  - gland (see also Dacryoadenitis) 375.00
- lacunar 597.0
- larynx 478.79
- lateral (alveolar) 522.5
  - with sinus 522.7
- leg, except foot 682.6
- lens 360.00
- lid 373.13
- lingual 529.0
  - tonsil 475
- lip 528.5
- Littre's gland 597.0
- liver 572.0
  - amebic 006.3
    - with
      - brain abscess (and lung abscess) 006.5
      - lung abscess 006.4
    - due to Entamoeba histolytica 006.3
  - dysenteric (see also Abscess, liver, amebic) 006.3
  - pyogenic 572.0
  - tropical (see also Abscess, liver, amebic) 006.3
- loin (region) 682.2
- lumbar (tuberculous) (see also Tuberculosis) 015.0 ☑ [730.88]
  - nontuberculous 682.2
- lung (miliary) (putrid) 513.0
  - amebic (with liver abscess) 006.4
    - with brain abscess 006.5
- lymphangitic, acute — see Cellulitis
- lymph, lymphatic, gland or node (acute) 683
  - any site, except mesenteric 683
  - mesentery 289.2
- malar 526.4
- mammary gland — see Abscess, breast
- marginal (anus) 566
- mastoid (process) (see also Mastoiditis, acute) 383.00
  - subperiosteal 383.01
- maxilla, maxillary 526.4
  - molar (tooth) 522.5
    - with sinus 522.7
  - premolar 522.5

Abscess — see also Cellulitis — continued
- maxilla, maxillary — continued
  - sinus (chronic) (see also Sinusitis, maxillary) 473.0
- mediastinum 513.1
- meibomian gland 373.12
- meninges (see also Meningitis) 320.9
- mesentery, mesenteric 567.22
- mesosalpinx (see also Salpingo-oophoritis) 614.2
- milk 675.1 ☑
- Monro's (psoriasis) 696.1
- mons pubis 682.2
- mouth (floor) 528.3
- multiple sites NEC 682.9
- mural 682.2
- muscle 728.89
  - psoas 567.31
- myocardium 422.92
- nabothian (follicle) (see also Cervicitis) 616.0
- nail (chronic) (with lymphangitis) 681.9
  - finger 681.02
  - toe 681.11
- nasal (fossa) (septum) 478.19 ▲
  - sinus (chronic) (see also Sinusitis) 473.9
- nasopharyngeal 478.29
- nates 682.5
- navel 682.2
  - newborn NEC 771.4
- neck (region) 682.1
  - lymph gland or node 683
- nephritic (see also Abscess, kidney) 590.2
- nipple 611.0
  - puerperal, postpartum 675.0 ☑
- nose (septum) 478.19 ▲
  - external 682.0
- omentum 567.22
- operative wound 998.59
- orbit, orbital 376.01
- ossifluent — see Abscess, bone
- ovary, ovarian (corpus luteum) (see also Salpingo-oophoritis) 614.2
- oviduct (see also Salpingo-oophoritis) 614.2
- palate (soft) 528.3
  - hard 526.4
- palmar (space) 682.4
- pancreas (duct) 577.0
- paradontal 523.30 ▲
- parafrenal 607.2
- parametric, parametrium (chronic) (see also Disease, pelvis, inflammatory) 614.4
  - acute 614.3
- paranephric 590.2
- parapancreatic 577.0
- parapharyngeal 478.22
- pararectal 566
- parasinus (see also Sinusitis) 473.9
- parauterine (see also Disease, pelvis, inflammatory) 614.4
  - acute 614.3
- paravaginal (see also Vaginitis) 616.10
- parietal region 682.8
- parodontal 523.30 ▲
- parotid (duct) (gland) 527.3
  - region 528.3
- parumbilical 682.2
  - newborn 771.4
- pectoral (region) 682.2
- pelvirectal 567.22
- pelvis, pelvic
  - female (chronic) (see also Disease, pelvis, inflammatory) 614.4
    - acute 614.3
  - male, peritoneal (cellular tissue) — see Abscess, peritoneum
  - tuberculous (see also Tuberculosis) 016.9 ☑
- penis 607.2
  - gonococcal (acute) 098.0

Abscess — see also Cellulitis — continued
- penis — continued
  - gonococcal — continued
    - chronic or duration of 2 months or over 098.2
- perianal 566
- periapical 522.5
  - with sinus (alveolar) 522.7
- periappendiceal 540.1
- pericardial 420.99
- pericecal 540.1
- pericemental 523.30 ▲
- pericholecystic (see also Cholecystitis, acute) 575.0
- pericoronal 523.30 ▲
- peridental 523.30 ▲
- perigastric 535.0 ☑
- perimetric (see also Disease, pelvis, inflammatory) 614.4
  - acute 614.3
- perinephric, perinephritic (see also Abscess, kidney) 590.2
- perineum, perineal (superficial) 682.2
  - deep (with urethral involvement) 597.0
  - urethra 597.0
- periodontal (parietal) 523.31 ▲
  - apical 522.5
- periosteum, periosteal (see also Periostitis) 730.3 ☑
  - with osteomyelitis (see also Osteomyelitis) 730.2 ☑
    - acute or subacute 730.0 ☑
    - chronic or old 730.1 ☑
- peripleuritic 510.9
  - with fistula 510.0
- periproctic 566
- periprostatic 601.2
- perirectal (staphylococcal) 566
- perirenal (tissue) (see also Abscess, kidney) 590.2
- perisinuous (nose) (see also Sinusitis) 473.9
- peritoneum, peritoneal (perforated) (ruptured) 567.22
  - with
    - abortion — see Abortion, by type, with sepsis
    - appendicitis 540.1
    - ectopic pregnancy (see also categories 633.0–633.9) 639.0
    - molar pregnancy (see also categories 630–632) 639.0
  - following
    - abortion 639.0
    - ectopic or molar pregnancy 639.0
  - pelvic, female (see also Disease, pelvis, inflammatory) 614.4
    - acute 614.3
  - postoperative 998.59
  - puerperal, postpartum, childbirth 670.0 ☑
  - tuberculous (see also Tuberculosis) 014.0 ☑
- peritonsillar 475
- perityphlic 540.1
- periureteral 593.89
- periurethral 597.0
  - gonococcal (acute) 098.0
    - chronic or duration of 2 months or over 098.2
- periuterine (see also Disease, pelvis, inflammatory) 614.4
  - acute 614.3
- perivesical 595.89
- pernicious NEC 682.9
- petrous bone — see Petrositis
- phagedenic NEC 682.9
  - chancroid 099.0
- pharynx, pharyngeal (lateral) 478.29
- phlegmonous NEC 682.9
- pilonidal 685.0
- pituitary (gland) 253.8

Index to Diseases

Abscess

Abscess — see also Cellulitis — continued
pleura 510.9
  with fistula 510.0
popliteal 682.6
postanal 566
postcecal 540.1
postlaryngeal 478.79
postnasal 478.19
postpharyngeal 478.24
posttonsillar 475
posttyphoid 002.0
Pott's (see also Tuberculosis) 015.0 ☑ [730.88]
pouch of Douglas (chronic) (see also Disease, pelvis, inflammatory) 614.4
premammary — see Abscess, breast
prepatellar 682.6
prostate (see also Prostatitis) 601.2
  gonococcal (acute) 098.12
    chronic or duration of 2 months or over 098.32
psoas 567.31
  nontuberculous 728.89
  tuberculous (see also Tuberculosis) 015.0 ☑ [730.88]
pterygopalatine fossa 682.8
pubis 682.2
puerperal — see Puerperal, abscess, by site
pulmonary — see Abscess, lung
pulp, pulpal (dental) 522.0
  finger 681.01
  toe 681.10
pyemic — see Septicemia
pyloric valve 535.0 ☑
rectovaginal septum 569.5
rectovesical 595.89
rectum 566
regional NEC 682.9
renal (see also Abscess, kidney) 590.2
retina 363.00
retrobulbar 376.01
retrocecal 567.22
retrolaryngeal 478.79
retromammary — see Abscess, breast
retroperineal 682.2
retroperitoneal 567.38
  postprocedural 998.59 ●
retropharyngeal 478.24
  tuberculous (see also Tuberculosis) 012.8 ☑
retrorectal 566
retrouterine (see also Disease, pelvis, inflammatory) 614.4
  acute 614.3
retrovesical 595.89
root, tooth 522.5
  with sinus (alveolar) 522.7
round ligament (see also Disease, pelvis, inflammatory) 614.4
  acute 614.3
rupture (spontaneous) NEC 682.9
sacrum (tuberculous) (see also Tuberculosis) 015.0 ☑ [730.88]
  nontuberculous 730.08
salivary duct or gland 527.3
scalp (any part) 682.8
scapular 730.01
sclera 379.09
scrofulous (see also Tuberculosis) 017.2 ☑
scrotum 608.4
seminal vesicle 608.0
  amebic 006.8
septal, dental 522.5
  with sinus (alveolar) 522.7
septum (nasal) 478.19 ▲
serous (see also Periostitis) 730.3 ☑
shoulder 682.3
side 682.2
sigmoid 569.5
sinus (accessory) (chronic) (nasal) (see also Sinusitis) 473.9
  intracranial venous (any) 324.0

Abscess — see also Cellulitis — continued
sinus (see also Sinusitis) — continued
  intracranial venous — continued
    late effect — see category 326
Skene's duct or gland 597.0
skin NEC 682.9
  tuberculous (primary) (see also Tuberculosis) 017.0 ☑
sloughing NEC 682.9
specified site NEC 682.8
  amebic 006.8
spermatic cord 608.4
sphenoidal (sinus) (see also Sinusitis, sphenoidal) 473.3
spinal
  cord (any part) (staphylococcal) 324.1
    tuberculous (see also Tuberculosis) 013.5 ☑
  epidural 324.1
spine (column) (tuberculous) (see also Tuberculosis) 015.0 ☑ [730.88]
  nontuberculous 730.08
spleen 289.59
  amebic 006.8
staphylococcal NEC 682.9
stitch 998.59
stomach (wall) 535.0 ☑
strumous (tuberculous) (see also Tuberculosis) 017.2 ☑
subarachnoid 324.9
  brain 324.0
  cerebral 324.0
  late effect — see category 326
  spinal cord 324.1
subareolar (see also Abscess, breast)
  puerperal, postpartum 675.1 ☑
subcecal 540.1
subcutaneous NEC 682.9
subdiaphragmatic 567.22
subdorsal 682.2
subdural 324.9
  brain 324.0
  late effect — see category 326
  spinal cord 324.1
subgaleal 682.8
subhepatic 567.22
sublingual 528.3
  gland 527.3
submammary — see Abscess, breast
submandibular (region) (space) (triangle) 682.0
  gland 527.3
submaxillary (region) 682.0
  gland 527.3
submental (pyogenic) 682.0
  gland 527.3
subpectoral 682.2
subperiosteal — see Abscess, bone
subperitoneal 567.22
subphrenic (see also Abscess, peritoneum) 567.22
  postoperative 998.59
subscapular 682.2
subungual 681.9
suburethral 597.0
sudoriparous 705.89
suppurative NEC 682.9
supraclavicular (fossa) 682.3
suprahepatic 567.22
suprapelvic (see also Disease, pelvis, inflammatory) 614.4
  acute 614.3
suprapubic 682.2
suprarenal (capsule) (gland) 255.8
sweat gland 705.89
syphilitic 095.8
teeth, tooth (root) 522.5
  with sinus (alveolar) 522.7
  supporting structures NEC 523.30 ▲
temple 682.0
temporal region 682.0

Abscess — see also Cellulitis — continued
temporosphenoidal 324.0
  late effect — see category 326
tendon (sheath) 727.89
testicle — see Orchitis
thecal 728.89
thigh (acquired) 682.6
thorax 510.9
  with fistula 510.0
throat 478.29
thumb (intrathecal) (periosteal) (subcutaneous) (subcuticular) 681.00
thymus (gland) 254.1
thyroid (gland) 245.0
toe (any) (intrathecal) (periosteal) (subcutaneous) (subcuticular) 681.10
tongue (staphylococcal) 529.0
tonsil(s) (lingual) 475
tonsillopharyngeal 475
tooth, teeth (root) 522.5
  with sinus (alveolar) 522.7
  supporting structure NEC 523.30 ▲
trachea 478.9
trunk 682.2
tubal (see also Salpingo-oophoritis) 614.2
tuberculous — see Tuberculosis, abscess
tubo-ovarian (see also Salpingo-oophoritis) 614.2
tunica vaginalis 608.4
umbilicus NEC 682.2
  newborn 771.4
upper arm 682.3
upper respiratory 478.9
urachus 682.2
urethra (gland) 597.0
urinary 597.0
uterus, uterine (wall) (see also Endometritis) 615.9
  ligament (see also Disease, pelvis, inflammatory) 614.4
    acute 614.3
  neck (see also Cervicitis) 616.0
uvula 528.3
vagina (wall) (see also Vaginitis) 616.10
vaginorectal (see also Vaginitis) 616.10
vas deferens 608.4
vermiform appendix 540.1
vertebra (column) (tuberculous) (see also Tuberculosis) 015.0 ☑ [730.88]
  nontuberculous 730.0 ☑
vesical 595.89
vesicouterine pouch (see also Disease, pelvis, inflammatory) 614.4
vitreous (humor) (pneumococcal) 360.04
vocal cord 478.5
von Bezold's 383.01
vulva 616.4
  complicating pregnancy, childbirth, or puerperium 646.6 ☑
vulvovaginal gland (see also Vaginitis) 616.3
web-space 682.4
wrist 682.4
Absence (organ or part) (complete or partial)
acoustic nerve 742.8
adrenal (gland) (congenital) 759.1
  acquired V45.79
albumin (blood) 273.8
alimentary tract (complete) (congenital) (partial) 751.8
  lower 751.5
  upper 750.8
alpha-fucosidase 271.8
alveolar process (acquired) 525.8
  congenital 750.26

Absence — continued
anus, anal (canal) (congenital) 751.2
aorta (congenital) 747.22
aortic valve (congenital) 746.89
appendix, congenital 751.2
arm (acquired) V49.60
  above elbow V49.66
  below elbow V49.65
  congenital (see also Deformity, reduction, upper limb) 755.20
    lower — see Absence, forearm, congenital
    upper (complete) (partial) (with absence of distal elements, incomplete) 755.24
      with
        complete absence of distal elements 755.21
        forearm (incomplete) 755.23
artery (congenital) (peripheral) NEC (see also Anomaly, peripheral vascular system) 747.60
  brain 747.81
  cerebral 747.81
  coronary 746.85
  pulmonary 747.3
  umbilical 747.5
atrial septum 745.69
auditory canal (congenital) (external) 744.01
auricle (ear) (with stenosis or atresia of auditory canal), congenital 744.01
bile, biliary duct (common) or passage (congenital) 751.61
bladder (acquired) V45.74
  congenital 753.8
bone (congenital) NEC 756.9
  marrow 284.9
    acquired (secondary) 284.8
    congenital 284.09 ▲
    hereditary 284.09 ▲
    idiopathic 284.9
  skull 756.0
bowel sounds 787.5
brain 740.0
  specified part 742.2
breast(s) (acquired) V45.71
  congenital 757.6
broad ligament (congenital) 752.19
bronchus (congenital) 748.3
calvarium, calvaria (skull) 756.0
canaliculus lacrimalis, congenital 743.65
carpal(s) (congenital) (complete) (partial) (with absence of distal elements, incomplete) (see also Deformity, reduction, upper limb) 755.28
  with complete absence of distal elements 755.21
cartilage 756.9
caudal spine 756.13
cecum (acquired) (postoperative) (posttraumatic) V45.72
  congenital 751.2
cementum 520.4
cerebellum (congenital) (vermis) 742.2
cervix (acquired) (uteri) V45.77
  congenital 752.49
chin, congenital 744.89
cilia (congenital) 743.63
  acquired 374.89
circulatory system, part NEC 747.89
clavicle 755.51
clitoris (congenital) 752.49
coccyx, congenital 756.13
cold sense (see also Disturbance, sensation) 782.0
colon (acquired) (postoperative) V45.72
  congenital 751.2
congenital
  lumen — see Atresia

Absence

Absence — *continued*
  congenital — *continued*
    organ or site NEC — *see* Agenesis
    septum — *see* Imperfect, closure
  corpus callosum (congenital) 742.2
  cricoid cartilage 748.3
  diaphragm (congenital) (with hernia) 756.6
    with obstruction 756.6
  digestive organ(s) or tract, congenital (complete) (partial) 751.8
    acquired V45.79
    lower 751.5
    upper 750.8
  ductus arteriosus 747.89
  duodenum (acquired) (postoperative) V45.72
    congenital 751.1
  ear, congenital 744.09
    acquired V45.79
    auricle 744.01
    external 744.01
    inner 744.05
    lobe, lobule 744.21
    middle, except ossicles 744.03
      ossicles 744.04
    ossicles 744.04
  ejaculatory duct (congenital) 752.89
  endocrine gland NEC (congenital) 759.2
  epididymis (congenital) 752.89
    acquired V45.77
  epiglottis, congenital 748.3
  epileptic (atonic) (typical) (*see also* Epilepsy) 345.0 ☑
  erythrocyte 284.9
  erythropoiesis 284.9
    congenital 284.01 ▲
  esophagus (congenital) 750.3
  Eustachian tube (congenital) 744.24
  extremity (acquired)
    congenital (*see also* Deformity, reduction) 755.4
    lower V49.70
    upper V49.60
  extrinsic muscle, eye 743.69
  eye (acquired) V45.78
    adnexa (congenital) 743.69
    congenital 743.00
    muscle (congenital) 743.69
  eyelid (fold), congenital 743.62
    acquired 374.89
  face
    bones NEC 756.0
    specified part NEC 744.89
  fallopian tube(s) (acquired) V45.77
    congenital 752.19
  femur, congenital (complete) (partial) (with absence of distal elements, incomplete) (*see also* Deformity, reduction, lower limb) 755.34
    with
      complete absence of distal elements 755.31
      tibia and fibula (incomplete) 755.33
  fibrin 790.92
  fibrinogen (congenital) 286.3
    acquired 286.6
  fibula, congenital (complete) (partial) (with absence of distal elements, incomplete) (*see also* Deformity, reduction, lower limb) 755.37
    with
      complete absence of distal elements 755.31
      tibia 755.35
        with
          complete absence of distal elements 755.31
          femur (incomplete) 755.33
            with complete absence of distal elements 755.31
  finger (acquired) V49.62

Absence — *continued*
  finger — *continued*
    congenital (complete) (partial) (*see also* Deformity, reduction, upper limb) 755.29
      meaning all fingers (complete) (partial) 755.21
      transverse 755.21
  fissures of lungs (congenital) 748.5
  foot (acquired) V49.73
    congenital (complete) 755.31
  forearm (acquired) V49.65
    congenital (complete) (partial) (with absence of distal elements, incomplete) (*see also* Deformity, reduction, upper limb) 755.25
    with
      complete absence of distal elements (hand and fingers) 755.21
      humerus (incomplete) 755.23
  fovea centralis 743.55
  fucosidase 271.8
  gallbladder (acquired) V45.79
    congenital 751.69
  gamma globulin (blood) 279.00
  genital organs
    acquired V45.77
    congenital
      female 752.89
        external 752.49
        internal NEC 752.89
      male 752.89
        penis 752.69
  genitourinary organs, congenital NEC 752.89
  glottis 748.3
  gonadal, congenital NEC 758.6
  hair (congenital) 757.4
    acquired — *see* Alopecia
  hand (acquired) V49.63
    congenital (complete) (*see also* Deformity, reduction, upper limb) 755.21
  heart (congenital) 759.89
    acquired — *see* Status, organ replacement
  heat sense (*see also* Disturbance, sensation) 782.0
  humerus, congenital (complete) (partial) (with absence of distal elements, incomplete) (*see also* Deformity, reduction, upper limb) 755.24
    with
      complete absence of distal elements 755.21
      radius and ulna (incomplete) 755.23
  hymen (congenital) 752.49
  ileum (acquired) (postoperative) (posttraumatic) V45.72
    congenital 751.1
  immunoglobulin, isolated NEC 279.03
    IgA 279.01
    IgG 279.03
    IgM 279.02
  incus (acquired) 385.24
    congenital 744.04
  internal ear (congenital) 744.05
  intestine (acquired) (small) V45.72
    congenital 751.1
      large 751.2
    large V45.72
      congenital 751.2
  iris (congenital) 743.45
  jaw — *see* Absence, mandible
  jejunum (acquired) V45.72
    congenital 751.1
  joint, congenital NEC 755.8
  kidney(s) (acquired) V45.73
    congenital 753.0
  labium (congenital) (majus) (minus) 752.49
  labyrinth, membranous 744.05

Absence — *continued*
  lacrimal apparatus (congenital) 743.65
  larynx (congenital) 748.3
  leg (acquired) V49.70
    above knee V49.76
    below knee V49.75
    congenital (partial) (unilateral) (*see also* Deformity, reduction, lower limb) 755.31
      lower (complete) (partial) (with absence of distal elements, incomplete) 755.35
        with
          complete absence of distal elements (foot and toes) 755.31
        thigh (incomplete) 755.33
          with complete absence of distal elements 755.31
      upper — *see* Absence, femur
  lens (congenital) 743.35
    acquired 379.31
  ligament, broad (congenital) 752.19
  limb (acquired)
    congenital (complete) (partial) (*see also* Deformity, reduction) 755.4
    lower 755.30
      complete 755.31
      incomplete 755.32
      longitudinal — *see* Deficiency, lower limb, longitudinal
      transverse 755.31
    upper 755.20
      complete 755.21
      incomplete 755.22
      longitudinal — *see* Deficiency, upper limb, longitudinal
      transverse 755.21
    lower NEC V49.70
    upper NEC V49.60
  lip 750.26
  liver (congenital) (lobe) 751.69
  lumbar (congenital) (vertebra) 756.13
    isthmus 756.11
    pars articularis 756.11
  lumen — *see* Atresia
  lung (bilateral) (congenital) (fissure) (lobe) (unilateral) 748.5
    acquired (any part) V45.76
  mandible (congenital) 524.09
  maxilla (congenital) 524.09
  menstruation 626.0
  metacarpal(s), congenital (complete) (partial) (with absence of distal elements, incomplete) (*see also* Deformity, reduction, upper limb) 755.28
    with all fingers, complete 755.21
  metatarsal(s), congenital (complete) (partial) (with absence of distal elements, incomplete) (*see also* Deformity, reduction, lower limb) 755.38
    with complete absence of distal elements 755.31
  muscle (congenital) (pectoral) 756.81
    ocular 743.69
  musculoskeletal system (congenital) NEC 756.9
  nail(s) (congenital) 757.5
  neck, part 744.89
  nerve 742.8
  nervous system, part NEC 742.8
  neutrophil 288.00 ▲
  nipple (congenital) 757.6
  nose (congenital) 748.1
    acquired 738.0
  nuclear 742.8
  ocular muscle (congenital) 743.69
  organ
    of Corti (congenital) 744.05

Absence — *continued*
  organ — *continued*
    or site
      acquired V45.79
      congenital NEC 759.89
  osseous meatus (ear) 744.03
  ovary (acquired) V45.77
    congenital 752.0
  oviduct (acquired) V45.77
    congenital 752.19
  pancreas (congenital) 751.7
    acquired (postoperative) (posttraumatic) V45.79
  parathyroid gland (congenital) 759.2
  parotid gland(s) (congenital) 750.21
  patella, congenital 755.64
  pelvic girdle (congenital) 755.69
  penis (congenital) 752.69
    acquired V45.77
  pericardium (congenital) 746.89
  perineal body (congenital) 756.81
  phalange(s), congenital 755.4
    lower limb (complete) (intercalary) (partial) (terminal) (*see also* Deformity, reduction, lower limb) 755.39
      meaning all toes (complete) (partial) 755.31
      transverse 755.31
    upper limb (complete) (intercalary) (partial) (terminal) (*see also* Deformity, reduction, upper limb) 755.29
      meaning all digits (complete) (partial) 755.21
      transverse 755.21
  pituitary gland (congenital) 759.2
  postoperative — *see* Absence, by site, acquired
  prostate (congenital) 752.89
    acquired V45.77
  pulmonary
    artery 747.3
    trunk 747.3
    valve (congenital) 746.01
    vein 747.49
  punctum lacrimale (congenital) 743.65
  radius, congenital (complete) (partial) (with absence of distal elements, incomplete) 755.26
    with
      complete absence of distal elements 755.21
      ulna 755.25
        with
          complete absence of distal elements 755.21
          humerus (incomplete) 755.23
  ray, congenital 755.4
    lower limb (complete) (partial) (*see also* Deformity, reduction, lower limb) 755.38
      meaning all rays 755.31
      transverse 755.31
    upper limb (complete) (partial) (*see also* Deformity, reduction, upper limb) 755.28
      meaning all rays 755.21
      transverse 755.21
  rectum (congenital) 751.2
    acquired V45.79
  red cell 284.9
    acquired (secondary) 284.8
    congenital 284.01 ▲
    hereditary 284.01 ▲
    idiopathic 284.9
  respiratory organ (congenital) NEC 748.9
  rib (acquired) 738.3
    congenital 756.3
  roof of orbit (congenital) 742.0
  round ligament (congenital) 752.89
  sacrum, congenital 756.13
  salivary gland(s) (congenital) 750.21
  scapula 755.59

Absence — *continued*
   scrotum, congenital 752.89
   seminal tract or duct (congenital) 752.89
      acquired V45.77
   septum (congenital) (*see also* Imperfect, closure, septum)
      atrial 745.69
         and ventricular 745.7
      between aorta and pulmonary artery 745.0
      ventricular 745.3
         and atrial 745.7
   sex chromosomes 758.81
   shoulder girdle, congenital (complete) (partial) 755.59
   skin (congenital) 757.39
   skull bone 756.0
      with
         anencephalus 740.0
         encephalocele 742.0
         hydrocephalus 742.3
            with spina bifida (*see also* Spina bifida) 741.0 ☑
         microcephalus 742.1
   spermatic cord (congenital) 752.89
   spinal cord 742.59
   spine, congenital 756.13
   spleen (congenital) 759.0
      acquired V45.79
   sternum, congenital 756.3
   stomach (acquired) (partial) (postoperative) V45.75
      with postgastric surgery syndrome 564.2
      congenital 750.7
   submaxillary gland(s) (congenital) 750.21
   superior vena cava (congenital) 747.49
   tarsal(s), congenital (complete) (partial) (with absence of distal elements, incomplete) (*see also* Deformity, reduction, lower limb) 755.38
   teeth, tooth (congenital) 520.0
      with abnormal spacing 524.30
      acquired 525.10
         with malocclusion 524.30
         due to
            caries 525.13
            extraction 525.10
            periodontal disease 525.12
            trauma 525.11
   tendon (congenital) 756.81
   testis (congenital) 752.89
      acquired V45.77
   thigh (acquired) 736.89
   thumb (acquired) V49.61
      congenital 755.29
   thymus gland (congenital) 759.2
   thyroid (gland) (surgical) 246.8
      with hypothyroidism 244.0
      cartilage, congenital 748.3
      congenital 243
   tibia, congenital (complete) (partial) (with absence of distal elements, incomplete) (*see also* Deformity, reduction, lower limb) 755.36
      with
         complete absence of distal elements 755.31
         fibula 755.35
            with
               complete absence of distal elements 755.31
            femur (incomplete) 755.33
               with complete absence of distal elements 755.31
   toe (acquired) V49.72
      congenital (complete) (partial) 755.39
         meaning all toes 755.31
         transverse 755.31
      great V49.71
   tongue (congenital) 750.11
   tooth, teeth (congenital) 520.0

Absence — *continued*
   tooth, teeth — *continued*
      with abnormal spacing 524.30
      acquired 525.10
         with malocclusion 524.30
         due to
            caries 525.13
            extraction 525.10
            periodontal disease 525.12
            trauma 525.11
   trachea (cartilage) (congenital) (rings) 748.3
   transverse aortic arch (congenital) 747.21
   tricuspid valve 746.1
   ulna, congenital (complete) (partial) (with absence of distal elements, incomplete) (*see also* Deformity, reduction, upper limb) 755.27
      with
         complete absence of distal elements 755.21
         radius 755.25
            with
               complete absence of distal elements 755.21
               humerus (incomplete) 755.23
   umbilical artery (congenital) 747.5
   ureter (congenital) 753.4
      acquired V45.74
   urethra, congenital 753.8
      acquired V45.74
   urinary system, part NEC, congenital 753.8
      acquired V45.74
   uterus (acquired) V45.77
      congenital 752.3
   uvula (congenital) 750.26
   vagina, congenital 752.49
      acquired V45.77
   vas deferens (congenital) 752.89
      acquired V45.77
   vein (congenital) (peripheral) NEC (*see also* Anomaly, peripheral vascular system) 747.60
      brain 747.81
      great 747.49
      portal 747.49
      pulmonary 747.49
   vena cava (congenital) (inferior) (superior) 747.49
   ventral horn cell 742.59
   ventricular septum 745.3
   vermis of cerebellum 742.2
   vertebra, congenital 756.13
   vulva, congenital 752.49
Absentia epileptica — *see also* Epilepsy 345.0 ☑
Absinthemia — *see also* Dependence 304.6 ☑
Absinthism — *see also* Dependence 304.6 ☑
Absorbent system disease 459.89
Absorption
   alcohol, through placenta or breast milk 760.71
   antibiotics, through placenta or breast milk 760.74
   anticonvulsants, through placenta or breast milk 760.77
   antifungals, through placenta or breast milk 760.74
   anti-infective, through placenta or breast milk 760.74
   antimetabolics, through placenta or breast milk 760.78
   chemical NEC 989.9
      specified chemical or substance — *see* Table of Drugs and Chemicals
      through placenta or breast milk (fetus or newborn) 760.70
         alcohol 760.71
         anticonvulsants 760.77
         antifungals 760.74

Absorption — *continued*
   chemical — *continued*
      through placenta or breast milk — *continued*
         anti-infective agents 760.74
         antimetabolics 760.78
         cocaine 760.75
         "crack" 760.75
         diethylstilbestrol [DES] 760.76
         hallucinogenic agents 760.73
         medicinal agents NEC 760.79
         narcotics 760.72
         obstetric anesthetic or analgesic drug 763.5
         specified agent NEC 760.79
         suspected, affecting management of pregnancy 655.5 ☑
   cocaine, through placenta or breast milk 760.75
   drug NEC (*see also* Reaction, drug)
      through placenta or breast milk (fetus or newborn) 760.70
         alcohol 760.71
         anticonvulsants 760.77
         antifungals 760.74
         anti-infective agents 760.74
         antimetabolics 760.78
         cocaine 760.75
         "crack" 760.75
         diethylstilbestrol [DES] 760.76
         hallucinogenic agents 760.73
         medicinal agents NEC 760.79
         narcotics 760.72
         obstetric anesthetic or analgesic drug 763.5
         specified agent NEC 760.79
         suspected, affecting management of pregnancy 655.5 ☑
   fat, disturbance 579.8
   hallucinogenic agents, through placenta or breast milk 760.73
   immune sera, through placenta or breast milk 760.79
   lactose defect 271.3
   medicinal agents NEC, through placenta or breast milk 760.79
   narcotics, through placenta or breast milk 760.72
   noxious substance — *see* Absorption, chemical
   protein, disturbance 579.8
   pus or septic, general — *see* Septicemia
   quinine, through placenta or breast milk 760.74
   toxic substance — *see* Absorption, chemical
   uremic — *see* Uremia
Abstinence symptoms or syndrome
   alcohol 291.81
   drug 292.0
Abt-Letterer-Siwe syndrome (acute histiocytosis X) (M9722/3) 202.5 ☑
Abulia 799.89
Abulomania 301.6
Abuse
   adult 995.80
      emotional 995.82
      multiple forms 995.85
      neglect (nutritional) 995.84
      physical 995.81
      psychological 995.82
      sexual 995.83
   alcohol — *see also* Alcoholism 305.0 ☑
      dependent 303.9 ☑
      non-dependent 305.0 ☑
   child 995.50
      counseling
         perpetrator
            non-parent V62.83
            parent V61.22
         victim V61.21
      emotional 995.51

Abuse — *continued*
   child — *continued*
      multiple forms 995.59
      neglect (nutritional) 995.52
      physical 995.54
         shaken infant syndrome 995.55
      psychological 995.51
      sexual 995.53
   drugs, nondependent 305.9 ☑

> Note — Use the following fifth-digit subclassification with the following codes: 305.0, 305.2–305.9:
> 0   unspecified
> 1   continuous
> 2   episodic
> 3   in remission

   amphetamine type 305.7 ☑
   antidepressants 305.8 ☑
   anxiolytic 305.4 ☑
   barbiturates 305.4 ☑
   caffeine 305.9 ☑
   cannabis 305.2 ☑
   cocaine type 305.6 ☑
   hallucinogens 305.3 ☑
   hashish 305.2 ☑
   hypnotic 305.4 ☑
   inhalant 305.9 ☑
   LSD 305.3 ☑
   marijuana 305.2 ☑
   mixed 305.9 ☑
   morphine type 305.5 ☑
   opioid type 305.5 ☑
   phencyclidine (PCP) 305.9 ☑
   sedative 305.4 ☑
   specified NEC 305.9 ☑
   tranquilizers 305.4 ☑
   spouse 995.80
   tobacco 305.1
Acalcerosis 275.40
Acalcicosis 275.40
Acalculia 784.69
   developmental 315.1
Acanthocheilonemiasis 125.4
Acanthocytosis 272.5
Acanthokeratodermia 701.1
Acantholysis 701.8
   bullosa 757.39
Acanthoma (benign) (M8070/0) — *see also* Neoplasm, by site, benign
   malignant (M8070/3) — *see* Neoplasm, by site, malignant
Acanthosis (acquired) (nigricans) 701.2
   adult 701.2
   benign (congenital) 757.39
   congenital 757.39
   glycogenic
      esophagus 530.89
   juvenile 701.2
   tongue 529.8
Acanthrocytosis 272.5
Acapnia 276.3
Acarbia 276.2
Acardia 759.89
Acardiacus amorphus 759.89
Acardiotrophia 429.1
Acardius 759.89
Acariasis 133.9
   sarcoptic 133.0
Acaridiasis 133.9
Acarinosis 133.9
Acariosis 133.9
Acarodermatitis 133.9
   urticarioides 133.9
Acarophobia 300.29
Acatalasemia 277.89
Acatalasia 277.89
Acatamathesia 784.69
Acataphasia 784.5
Acathisia 781.0
   due to drugs 333.99
Acceleration, accelerated
   atrioventricular conduction 426.7
   idioventricular rhythm 427.89

Accessory

Index to Diseases

Accessory (congenital)
  adrenal gland 759.1
  anus 751.5
  appendix 751.5
  atrioventricular conduction 426.7
  auditory ossicles 744.04
  auricle (ear) 744.1
  autosome(s) NEC 758.5
    21 or 22 758.0
  biliary duct or passage 751.69
  bladder 753.8
  blood vessels (peripheral) (congenital)
    NEC (see also Anomaly, peripheral vascular system) 747.60
    cerebral 747.81
    coronary 746.85
  bone NEC 756.9
    foot 755.67
  breast tissue, axilla 757.6
  carpal bones 755.56
  cecum 751.5
  cervix 752.49
  chromosome(s) NEC 758.5
    13-15 758.1
    16-18 758.2
    21 or 22 758.0
    autosome(s) NEC 758.5
    D$_1$ 758.1
    E$_3$ 758.2
    G 758.0
    sex 758.81
  coronary artery 746.85
  cusp(s), heart valve NEC 746.89
    pulmonary 746.09
  cystic duct 751.69
  digits 755.00
  ear (auricle) (lobe) 744.1
  endocrine gland NEC 759.2
  external os 752.49
  eyelid 743.62
  eye muscle 743.69
  face bone(s) 756.0
  fallopian tube (fimbria) (ostium)
    752.19
  fingers 755.01
  foreskin 605
  frontonasal process 756.0
  gallbladder 751.69
  genital organ(s)
    female 752.89
      external 752.49
      internal NEC 752.89
    male NEC 752.89
      penis 752.69
  genitourinary organs NEC 752.89
  heart 746.89
    valve NEC 746.89
      pulmonary 746.09
  hepatic ducts 751.69
  hymen 752.49
  intestine (large) (small) 751.5
  kidney 753.3
  lacrimal canal 743.65
  leaflet, heart valve NEC 746.89
    pulmonary 746.09
  ligament, broad 752.19
  liver (duct) 751.69
  lobule (ear) 744.1
  lung (lobe) 748.69
  muscle 756.82
  navicular of carpus 755.56
  nervous system, part NEC 742.8
  nipple 757.6
  nose 748.1
  organ or site NEC — see Anomaly,
    specified type NEC
  ovary 752.0
  oviduct 752.19
  pancreas 751.7
  parathyroid gland 759.2
  parotid gland (and duct) 750.22
  pituitary gland 759.2
  placental lobe — see Placenta, abnormal
  preauricular appendage 744.1
  prepuce 605

Accessory — continued
  renal arteries (multiple) 747.62
  rib 756.3
    cervical 756.2
  roots (teeth) 520.2
  salivary gland 750.22
  sesamoids 755.8
  sinus — see condition
  skin tags 757.39
  spleen 759.0
  sternum 756.3
  submaxillary gland 750.22
  tarsal bones 755.67
  teeth, tooth 520.1
    causing crowding 524.31
  tendon 756.89
  thumb 755.01
  thymus gland 759.2
  thyroid gland 759.2
  toes 755.02
  tongue 750.13
  tragus 744.1
  ureter 753.4
  urethra 753.8
  urinary organ or tract NEC 753.8
  uterus 752.2
  vagina 752.49
  valve, heart NEC 746.89
    pulmonary 746.09
  vertebra 756.19
  vocal cords 748.3
  vulva 752.49
Accident, accidental — see also condition
  birth NEC 767.9
  cardiovascular (see also Disease, cardiovascular) 429.2
  cerebral (see also Disease, cerebrovascular, acute) 434.91
  cerebrovascular (current) (CVA) (see also Disease, cerebrovascular, acute) 434.91
    embolic 434.11
    healed or old V12.59
    hemorrhagic — see Hemorrhage, brain
    impending 435.9
    ischemic 434.91
    late effect — see Late effect(s) (of) cerebrovascular disease
    postoperative 997.02
    thrombotic 434.01
  coronary (see also Infarct, myocardium) 410.9 ☑
  craniovascular (see also Disease, cerebrovascular, acute) 436
  during pregnancy, to mother, affecting fetus or newborn 760.5
  heart, cardiac (see also Infarct, myocardium) 410.9 ☑
  intrauterine 779.89
  vascular — see Disease, cerebrovascular, acute
Accommodation
  disorder of 367.51
    drug-induced 367.89
    toxic 367.89
  insufficiency of 367.4
  paralysis of 367.51
    hysterical 300.11
  spasm of 367.53
Accouchement — see Delivery
Accreta placenta (without hemorrhage) 667.0 ☑
  with hemorrhage 666.0 ☑
Accretio cordis (nonrheumatic) 423.1
Accretions on teeth 523.6
Accumulation secretion, prostate 602.8
Acephalia, acephalism, acephaly 740.0
Acephalic 740.0
Acephalobrachia 759.89
Acephalocardia 759.89
Acephalocardius 759.89
Acephalochiria 759.89
Acephalochirus 759.89
Acephalogaster 759.89

Acephalostomus 759.89
Acephalothorax 759.89
Acephalus 740.0
Acetonemia 790.6
  diabetic 250.1 ☑
Acetonglycosuria 982.8
Acetonuria 791.6
Achalasia 530.0
  cardia 530.0
  digestive organs congenital NEC 751.8
  esophagus 530.0
  pelvirectal 751.3
  psychogenic 306.4
  pylorus 750.5
  sphincteral NEC 564.89
Achard-Thiers syndrome (adrenogenital) 255.2
Ache(s) — see Pain
Acheilia 750.26
Acheiria 755.21
Achillobursitis 726.71
Achillodynia 726.71
Achlorhydria, achlorhydric 536.0
  anemia 280.9
  diarrhea 536.0
  neurogenic 536.0
  postvagotomy 564.2
  psychogenic 306.4
  secondary to vagotomy 564.2
Achloroblepsia 368.52
Achloropsia 368.52
Acholia 575.8
Acholuric jaundice (familial) (splenomegalic) — see also Spherocytosis 282.0
  acquired 283.9
Achondroplasia 756.4
Achrestic anemia 281.8
Achroacytosis, lacrimal gland 375.00
  tuberculous (see also Tuberculosis) 017.3 ☑
Achroma, cutis 709.00
Achromate (congenital) 368.54
Achromatopia 368.54
Achromatopsia (congenital) 368.54
Achromia
  congenital 270.2
  parasitica 111.0
  unguium 703.8
Achylia
  gastrica 536.8
    neurogenic 536.3
    psychogenic 306.4
  pancreatica 577.1
Achylosis 536.8
Acid
  burn (see also Burn, by site)
    from swallowing acid — see Burn, internal organs
  deficiency
    amide nicotinic 265.2
    amino 270.9
    ascorbic 267
    folic 266.2
    nicotinic (amide) 265.2
    pantothenic 266.2
  intoxication 276.2
  peptic disease 536.8
  stomach 536.8
  psychogenic 306.4
Acidemia 276.2
  arginosuccinic 270.6
  fetal
    affecting management of pregnancy 656.3 ☑
    before onset of labor, in liveborn infant 768.2
    during labor ▶and delivery◀ in liveborn infant 768.3
    intrauterine 656.3 ☑
    unspecified as to time of onset, in liveborn infant 768.4
  newborn 775.81 ●
  pipecolic 270.7
Acidity, gastric (high) (low) 536.8
  psychogenic 306.4

Acidocytopenia 288.59 ▲
Acidocytosis 288.3
Acidopenia 288.59 ▲
Acidosis 276.2
  diabetic 250.1 ☑
  fetal, affecting management of pregnancy 775.81 ▲
  fetal, affecting newborn 775.81 ▲
  kidney tubular 588.89
    newborn 775.81 ●
  lactic 276.2
  metabolic NEC 276.2
    with respiratory acidosis 276.4
      of newborn 775.81 ●
    late, of newborn 775.7
  newborn 775.81 ●
  renal
    hyperchloremic 588.89
    tubular (distal) (proximal) 588.89
  respiratory 276.2
    complicated by
      metabolic acidosis 276.4
        of newborn 775.81 ●
      metabolic alkalosis 276.4
Aciduria 791.9
  arginosuccinic 270.6
  beta-aminoisobutyric (BAIB) 277.2
  glutaric
    type I 270.7
    type II (type IIA, IIB, IIC) 277.85
    type III 277.86
  glycolic 271.8
  methylmalonic 270.3
    with glycinemia 270.7
  organic 270.9
  orotic (congenital) (hereditary) (pyrimidine deficiency) 281.4
Acladiosis 111.8
  skin 111.8
Aclasis
  diaphyseal 756.4
  tarsoepiphyseal 756.59
Acleistocardia 745.5
Aclusion 524.4
Acmesthesia 782.0
Acne (pustular) (vulgaris) 706.1
  agminata (see also Tuberculosis) 017.0 ☑
  artificialis 706.1
  atrophica 706.0
  cachecticorum (Hebra) 706.1
  conglobata 706.1
  conjunctiva 706.1
  cystic 706.1
  decalvans 704.09
  erythematosa 695.3
  eyelid 706.1
  frontalis 706.0
  indurata 706.1
  keloid 706.1
  lupoid 706.0
  necrotic, necrotica 706.0
    miliaris 704.8
  neonatal 706.1
  nodular 706.1
  occupational 706.1
  papulosa 706.1
  rodens 706.0
  rosacea 695.3
  scorbutica 267
  scrofulosorum (Bazin) (see also Tuberculosis) 017.0 ☑
  summer 692.72
  tropical 706.1
  varioliformis 706.0
Acneiform drug eruptions 692.3
Acnitis (primary) — see also Tuberculosis 017.0 ☑
Acomia 704.00
Acontractile bladder 344.61
Aconuresis — see also Incontinence 788.30
Acosta's disease 993.2
Acousma 780.1
Acoustic — see condition
Acousticophobia 300.29

Index to Diseases

Acquired — see condition
Acquired immune deficiency syndrome — see Human immunodeficiency virus (disease) (illness) (infection)
Acquired immunodeficiency syndrome — see Human immunodeficiency virus (disease) (illness) (infection)
Acragnosis 781.99
Acrania 740.0
Acroagnosis 781.99
Acroasphyxia, chronic 443.89
Acrobrachycephaly 756.0
Acrobystiolith 608.89
Acrobystitis 607.2
Acrocephalopolysyndactyly 755.55
Acrocephalosyndactyly 755.55
Acrocephaly 756.0
Acrochondrohyperplasia 759.82
Acrocyanosis 443.89
  newborn 770.83
    meaning transient blue hands and feet — omit code
Acrodermatitis 686.8
  atrophicans (chronica) 701.8
  continua (Hallopeau) 696.1
  enteropathica 686.8
  Hallopeau's 696.1
  perstans 696.1
  pustulosa continua 696.1
  recalcitrant pustular 696.1
Acrodynia 985.0
Acrodysplasia 755.55
Acrohyperhidrosis — see also Hyperhidrosis 780.8
Acrokeratosis verruciformis 757.39
Acromastitis 611.0
Acromegaly, acromegalia (skin) 253.0
Acromelalgia 443.82
Acromicria, acromikria 756.59
Acronyx 703.0
Acropachyderma 757.39
Acropachy, thyroid — see also Thyrotoxicosis 242.9 ✓
Acroparesthesia 443.89
  simple (Schultz's type) 443.89
  vasomotor (Nothnagel's type) 443.89
Acropathy thyroid — see also Thyrotoxicosis 242.9 ✓
Acrophobia 300.29
Acroposthitis 607.2
Acroscleriasis — see also Scleroderma 710.1
Acroscleroderma — see also Scleroderma 710.1
Acrosclerosis — see also Scleroderma 710.1
Acrosphacelus 785.4
Acrosphenosyndactylia 755.55
Acrospiroma, eccrine (M8402/0) — see Neoplasm, skin, benign
Acrostealgia 732.9
Acrosyndactyly — see also Syndactylism 755.10
Acrotrophodynia 991.4
Actinic — see also condition
  cheilitis (due to sun) 692.72
    chronic NEC 692.74
    due to radiation, except from sun 692.82
  conjunctivitis 370.24
  dermatitis (due to sun) (see also Dermatitis, actinic) 692.70
    due to
      roentgen rays or radioactive substance 692.82
      ultraviolet radiation, except from sun 692.82
    sun NEC 692.70
  elastosis solare 692.74
  granuloma 692.73
  keratitis 370.24
  ophthalmia 370.24
  reticuloid 692.73
Actinobacillosis, general 027.8
Actinobacillus
  lignieresii 027.8

Actinobacillus — continued
  mallei 024
  muris 026.1
Actinocutitis NEC — see also Dermatitis, actinic 692.70
Actinodermatitis NEC — see also Dermatitis, actinic 692.70
Actinomyces
  israelii (infection) — see Actinomycosis
  muris-ratti (infection) 026.1
Actinomycosis, actinomycotic 039.9
  with
    pneumonia 039.1
  abdominal 039.2
  cervicofacial 039.3
  cutaneous 039.0
  pulmonary 039.1
  specified site NEC 039.8
  thoracic 039.1
Actinoneuritis 357.89
Action, heart
  disorder 427.9
    postoperative 997.1
  irregular 427.9
    postoperative 997.1
    psychogenic 306.2
Active — see condition
Activity decrease, functional 780.99
Acute — see also condition
  abdomen NEC 789.0 ✓
  gallbladder (see also Cholecystitis, acute) 575.0
Acyanoblepsia 368.53
Acyanopsia 368.53
Acystia 753.8
Acystinervia — see Neurogenic, bladder
Acystineuria — see Neurogenic, bladder
Adactylia, adactyly (congenital) 755.4
  lower limb (complete) (intercalary) (partial) (terminal) (see also Deformity, reduction, lower limb) 755.39
    meaning all digits (complete) (partial) 755.31
    transverse (complete) (partial) 755.31
  upper limb (complete) (intercalary) (partial) (terminal) (see also Deformity, reduction, upper limb) 755.29
    meaning all digits (complete) (partial) 755.21
    transverse (complete) (partial) 755.21
Adair-Dighton syndrome (brittle bones and blue sclera, deafness) 756.51
Adamantinoblastoma (M9310/0) — see Ameloblastoma
Adamantinoma (M9310/0) — see Ameloblastoma
Adamantoblastoma (M9310/0) — see Ameloblastoma
Adams-Stokes (-Morgagni) disease or syndrome (syncope with heart block) 426.9
Adaptation reaction — see also Reaction, adjustment 309.9
Addiction — see also Dependence
  absinthe 304.6 ✓
  alcoholic (ethyl) (methyl) (wood) 303.9 ✓
    complicating pregnancy, childbirth, or puerperium 648.4 ✓
      affecting fetus or newborn 760.71
    suspected damage to fetus affecting management of pregnancy 655.4 ✓
  drug (see also Dependence) 304.9 ✓
  ethyl alcohol 303.9 ✓
  heroin 304.0 ✓
  hospital 301.51
  methyl alcohol 303.9 ✓
  methylated spirit 303.9 ✓
  morphine (-like substances) 304.0 ✓
  nicotine 305.1

Addiction — see also Dependence — continued
  opium 304.0 ✓
  tobacco 305.1
  wine 303.9 ✓
Addison's
  anemia (pernicious) 281.0
  disease (bronze) (primary adrenal insufficiency) 255.4
    tuberculous (see also Tuberculosis) 017.6 ✓
  keloid (morphea) 701.0
  melanoderma (adrenal cortical hypofunction) 255.4
Addison-Biermer anemia (pernicious) 281.0
Addison-Gull disease — see Xanthoma
Addisonian crisis or melanosis (acute adrenocortical insufficiency) 255.4
Additional — see also Accessory
  chromosome(s) 758.5
    13-15 758.1
    16-18 758.2
    21 758.0
    autosome(s) NEC 758.5
    sex 758.81
Adduction contracture, hip or other joint — see Contraction, joint
ADEM (acute disseminated encephalomyelitis) (postinfectious) 136.9 [323.61] ▲
  infectious 136.9 [323.61] ▲
  noninfectious 323.81 ▲
Adenasthenia gastrica 536.0
Aden fever 061
Adenitis — see also Lymphadenitis 289.3
  acute, unspecified site 683
    epidemic infectious 075
  axillary 289.3
    acute 683
    chronic or subacute 289.1
  Bartholin's gland 616.89 ▲
  bulbourethral gland (see also Urethritis) 597.89
  cervical 289.3
    acute 683
    chronic or subacute 289.1
  chancroid (Ducrey's bacillus) 099.0
  chronic (any lymph node, except mesenteric) 289.1
    mesenteric 289.2
  Cowper's gland (see also Urethritis) 597.89
  epidemic, acute 075
  gangrenous 683
  gonorrheal NEC 098.89
  groin 289.3
    acute 683
    chronic or subacute 289.1
  infectious 075
  inguinal (region) 289.3
    acute 683
    chronic or subacute 289.1
  lymph gland or node, except mesenteric 289.3
    acute 683
    chronic or subacute 289.1
    mesenteric (acute) (chronic) (nonspecific) (subacute) 289.2
  mesenteric (acute) (chronic) (nonspecific) (subacute) 289.2
    due to Pasteurella multocida (P. septica) 027.2
  parotid gland (suppurative) 527.2
  phlegmonous 683
  salivary duct or gland (any) (recurring) (suppurative) 527.2
  scrofulous (see also Tuberculosis) 017.2 ✓
  septic 289.3
  Skene's duct or gland (see also Urethritis) 597.89
  strumous, tuberculous (see also Tuberculosis) 017.2 ✓
  subacute, unspecified site 289.1

Adenitis — see also Lymphadenitis — continued
  sublingual gland (suppurative) 527.2
  submandibular gland (suppurative) 527.2
  submaxillary gland (suppurative) 527.2
  suppurative 683
  tuberculous — see Tuberculosis, lymph gland
  urethral gland (see also Urethritis) 597.89
  venereal NEC 099.8
  Wharton's duct (suppurative) 527.2
Adenoacanthoma (M8570/3) — see Neoplasm, by site, malignant
Adenoameloblastoma (M9300/0) 213.1
  upper jaw (bone) 213.0
Adenocarcinoma (M8140/3) — see also Neoplasm, by site, malignant

> Note — The list of adjectival modifiers below is not exhaustive. A description of adenocarcinoma that does not appear in this list should be coded in the same manner as carcinoma with that description. Thus, "mixed acidophil-basophil adenocarcinoma," should be coded in the same manner as "mixed acidophil-basophil carcinoma," which appears in the list under "Carcinoma."
>
> Except where otherwise indicated, the morphological varieties of adenocarcinoma in the list below should be coded by site as for "Neoplasm, malignant."

  with
    apocrine metaplasia (M8573/3)
    cartilaginous (and osseous) metaplasia (M8571/3)
    osseous (and cartilaginous) metaplasia (M8571/3)
    spindle cell metaplasia (M8572/3)
    squamous metaplasia (M8570/3)
  acidophil (M8280/3)
    specified site — see Neoplasm, by site, malignant
    unspecified site 194.3
  acinar (M8550/3)
  acinic cell (M8550/3)
  adrenal cortical (M8370/3) 194.0
  alveolar (M8251/3)
    and
      epidermoid carcinoma, mixed (M8560/3)
      squamous cell carcinoma, mixed (M8560/3)
  apocrine (M8401/3)
    breast — see Neoplasm, breast, malignant
    specified site NEC — see Neoplasm, skin, malignant
    unspecified site 173.9
  basophil (M8300/3)
    specified site — see Neoplasm, by site, malignant
    unspecified site 194.3
  bile duct type (M8160/3)
    liver 155.1
    specified site NEC — see Neoplasm, by site, malignant
    unspecified site 155.1
  bronchiolar (M8250/3) — see Neoplasm, lung, malignant
  ceruminous (M8420/3) 173.2
  chromophobe (M8270/3)
    specified site — see Neoplasm, by site, malignant
    unspecified site 194.3
  clear cell (mesonephroid type) (M8310/3)
  colloid (M8480/3)
  cylindroid type (M8200/3)
  diffuse type (M8145/3)
    specified site — see Neoplasm, by site, malignant
    unspecified site 151.9

Adenocarcinoma

Adenocarcinoma — see also Neoplasm, by site, malignant — *continued*
  duct (infiltrating) (M8500/3)
    with Paget's disease (M8541/3) — see Neoplasm, breast, malignant
    specified site — see Neoplasm, by site, malignant
    unspecified site 174.9
  embryonal (M9070/3)
  endometrioid (M8380/3) — see Neoplasm, by site, malignant
  eosinophil (M8280/3)
    specified site — see Neoplasm, by site, malignant
    unspecified site 194.3
  follicular (M8330/3)
    and papillary (M8340/3) 193
    moderately differentiated type (M8332/3) 193
    pure follicle type (M8331/3) 193
    specified site — see Neoplasm, by site, malignant
    trabecular type (M8332/3) 193
    unspecified type 193
    well differentiated type (M8331/3) 193
  gelatinous (M8480/3)
  granular cell (M8320/3)
  Hürthle cell (M8290/3) 193
  in
    adenomatous
      polyp (M8210/3)
      polyposis coli (M8220/3) 153.9
    polypoid adenoma (M8210/3)
    tubular adenoma (M8210/3)
    villous adenoma (M8261/3)
  infiltrating duct (M8500/3)
    with Paget's disease (M8541/3) — see Neoplasm, breast, malignant
    specified site — see Neoplasm, by site, malignant
    unspecified site 174.9
  inflammatory (M8530/3)
    specified site — see Neoplasm, by site, malignant
    unspecified site 174.9
  in situ (M8140/2) — see Neoplasm, by site, in situ
  intestinal type (M8144/3)
    specified site — see Neoplasm, by site, malignant
    unspecified site 151.9
  intraductal (noninfiltrating) (M8500/2)
    papillary (M8503/2)
      specified site — see Neoplasm, by site, in situ
      unspecified site 233.0
    specified site — see Neoplasm, by site, in situ
    unspecified site 233.0
  islet cell (M8150/3)
    and exocrine, mixed (M8154/3)
    specified site — see Neoplasm, by site, malignant
    unspecified site 157.9
    pancreas 157.4
    specified site NEC — see Neoplasm, by site, malignant
    unspecified site 157.4
  lobular (M8520/3)
    specified site — see Neoplasm, by site, malignant
    unspecified site 174.9
  medullary (M8510/3)
  mesonephric (M9110/3)
  mixed cell (M8323/3)
  mucinous (M8480/3)
  mucin-producing (M8481/3)
  mucoid (M8480/3) (see also Neoplasm, by site, malignant)
    cell (M8300/3)
      specified site — see Neoplasm, by site, malignant
      unspecified site 194.3

Adenocarcinoma — see also Neoplasm, by site, malignant — *continued*
  nonencapsulated sclerosing (M8350/3) 193
  oncocytic (M8290/3)
  oxyphilic (M8290/3)
  papillary (M8260/3)
    and follicular (M8340/3) 193
    intraductal (noninfiltrating) (M8503/2)
      specified site — see Neoplasm, by site, in situ
      unspecified site 233.0
    serous (M8460/3)
      specified site — see Neoplasm, by site, malignant
      unspecified site 183.0
  papillocystic (M8450/3)
    specified site — see Neoplasm, by site, malignant
    unspecified site 183.0
  pseudomucinous (M8470/3)
    specified site — see Neoplasm, by site, malignant
    unspecified site 183.0
  renal cell (M8312/3) 189.0
  sebaceous (M8410/3)
  serous (M8441/3) (see also Neoplasm, by site, malignant)
    papillary
      specified site — see Neoplasm, by site, malignant
      unspecified site 183.0
  signet ring cell (M8490/3)
  superficial spreading (M8143/3)
  sweat gland (M8400/3) — see Neoplasm, skin, malignant
  trabecular (M8190/3)
  tubular (M8211/3)
  villous (M8262/3)
  water-clear cell (M8322/3) 194.1

Adenofibroma (M9013/0)
  clear cell (M8313/0) — see Neoplasm, by site, benign
  endometrioid (M8381/0) 220
    borderline malignancy (M8381/1) 236.2
    malignant (M8381/3) 183.0
  mucinous (M9015/0)
    specified site — see Neoplasm, by site, benign
    unspecified site 220
  prostate 600.20
    with ●
      other lower urinary tract ●
        symptoms (LUTS) ●
          600.21 ●
      urinary ●
        obstruction 600.21 ●
        retention 600.21 ●
  serous (M9014/0)
    specified site — see Neoplasm, by site, benign
    unspecified site 220
  specified site — see Neoplasm, by site, benign
  unspecified site 220

Adenofibrosis
  breast 610.2
  endometrioid 617.0

Adenoiditis 474.01
  acute 463
  chronic 474.01
    with chronic tonsillitis 474.02

Adenoids (congenital) (of nasal fossa) 474.9
  hypertrophy 474.12
  vegetations 474.2

Adenolipomatosis (symmetrical) 272.8

Adenolymphoma (M8561/0)
  specified site — see Neoplasm, by site, benign
  unspecified 210.2

Adenomatosis (M8220/0)
  endocrine (multiple) (M8360/1)
    single specified site — see Neoplasm, by site, uncertain behavior
    two or more specified sites 237.4
    unspecified site 237.4
  erosive of nipple (M8506/0) 217
  pluriendocrine — see Adenomatosis, endocrine
  pulmonary (M8250/1) 235.7
    malignant (M8250/3) — see Neoplasm, lung, malignant
  specified site — see Neoplasm, by site, benign
  unspecified site 211.3

Adenomatous
  cyst, thyroid (gland) — see Goiter, nodular
  goiter (nontoxic) (see also Goiter, nodular) 241.9
    toxic or with hyperthyroidism 242.3 ☑

Adenoma (sessile) (M8140/0) — see also Neoplasm, by site, benign

> *Note — Except where otherwise indicated, the morphological varieties of adenoma in the list below should be coded by site as for "Neoplasm, benign."*

  acidophil (M8280/0)
    specified site — see Neoplasm, by site, benign
    unspecified site 227.3
  acinar (cell) (M8550/0)
  acinic cell (M8550/0)
  adrenal (cortex) (cortical) (functioning) (M8370/0) 227.0
    clear cell type (M8373/0) 227.0
    compact cell type (M8371/0) 227.0
    glomerulosa cell type (M8374/0) 227.0
    heavily pigmented variant (M8372/0) 227.0
    mixed cell type (M8375/0) 227.0
  alpha cell (M8152/0)
    pancreas 211.7
    specified site NEC — see Neoplasm, by site, benign
    unspecified site 211.7
  alveolar (M8251/0)
  apocrine (M8401/0)
    breast 217
    specified site NEC — see Neoplasm, skin, benign
    unspecified site 216.9
  basal cell (M8147/0)
  basophil (M8300/0)
    specified site — see Neoplasm, by site, benign
    unspecified site 227.3
  beta cell (M8151/0)
    pancreas 211.7
    specified site NEC — see Neoplasm, by site, benign
    unspecified site 211.7
  bile duct (M8160/0) 211.5
  black (M8372/0) 227.0
  bronchial (M8140/1) 235.7
    carcinoid type (M8240/3) — see Neoplasm, lung, malignant
    cylindroid type (M8200/3) — see Neoplasm, lung, malignant
  ceruminous (M8420/0) 216.2
  chief cell (M8321/0) 227.1
  chromophobe (M8270/0)
    specified site — see Neoplasm, by site, benign
    unspecified site 227.3
  clear cell (M8310/0)
  colloid (M8334/0)
    specified site — see Neoplasm, by site, benign
    unspecified site 226
  cylindroid type, bronchus (M8200/3) — see Neoplasm, lung, malignant

Adenoma — see also Neoplasm, by site, benign — *continued*
  duct (M8503/0)
  embryonal (M8191/0)
  endocrine, multiple (M8360/1)
    single specified site — see Neoplasm, by site, uncertain behavior
    two or more specified sites 237.4
    unspecified site 237.4
  endometrioid (M8380/0) (see also Neoplasm, by site, benign)
    borderline malignancy (M8380/1) — see Neoplasm, by site, uncertain behavior
  eosinophil (M8280/0)
    specified site — see Neoplasm, by site, benign
    unspecified site 227.3
  fetal (M8333/0)
    specified site — see Neoplasm, by site, benign
    unspecified site 226
  follicular (M8330/0)
    specified site — see Neoplasm, by site, benign
    unspecified site 226
  hepatocellular (M8170/0) 211.5
  Hürthle cell (M8290/0) 226
  intracystic papillary (M8504/0)
  islet cell (functioning) (M8150/0)
    pancreas 211.7
    specified site NEC — see Neoplasm, by site, benign
    unspecified site 211.7
  liver cell (M8170/0) 211.5
  macrofollicular (M8334/0)
    specified site NEC — see Neoplasm, by site, benign
    unspecified site 226
  malignant, malignum (M8140/3) — see Neoplasm, by site, malignant
  mesonephric (M9110/0)
  microfollicular (M8333/0)
    specified site — see Neoplasm, by site, benign
    unspecified site 226
  mixed cell (M8323/0)
  monomorphic (M8146/0)
  mucinous (M8480/0)
  mucoid cell (M8300/0)
    specified site — see Neoplasm, by site, benign
    unspecified site 227.3
  multiple endocrine (M8360/1)
    single specified site — see Neoplasm, by site, uncertain behavior
    two or more specified sites 237.4
    unspecified site 237.4
  nipple (M8506/0) 217
  oncocytic (M8290/0)
  oxyphilic (M8290/0)
  papillary (M8260/0) (see also Neoplasm, by site, benign)
    intracystic (M8504/0)
  papillotubular (M8263/0)
  Pick's tubular (M8640/0)
    specified site — see Neoplasm, by site, benign
    unspecified site
      female 220
      male 222.0
  pleomorphic (M8940/0)
  polypoid (M8210/0)
  prostate (benign) 600.20
    with ●
      other lower urinary tract ●
        symptoms (LUTS) ●
          600.21 ●
      urinary ●
        obstruction 600.21 ●
        retention 600.21 ●
  rete cell 222.0

Adenoma — see also Neoplasm, by site, benign — continued
- sebaceous, sebaceum (gland) (senile) (M8410/0) (see also Neoplasm, skin, benign)
  - disseminata 759.5
- Sertoli cell (M8640/0)
  - specified site — see Neoplasm, by site, benign
  - unspecified site
    - female 220
    - male 222.0
- skin appendage (M8390/0) — see Neoplasm, skin, benign
- sudoriferous gland (M8400/0) — see Neoplasm, skin, benign
- sweat gland or duct (M8400/0) — see Neoplasm, skin, benign
- testicular (M8640/0)
  - specified site — see Neoplasm, by site, benign
  - unspecified site
    - female 220
    - male 222.0
- thyroid 226
- trabecular (M8190/0)
- tubular (M8211/0) (see also Neoplasm, by site, benign)
  - papillary (M8460/3)
  - Pick's (M8640/0)
    - specified site — see Neoplasm, by site, benign
    - unspecified site
      - female 220
      - male 222.0
- tubulovillous (M8263/0)
- villoglandular (M8263/0)
- villous (M8261/1) — see Neoplasm, by site, uncertain behavior
- water-clear cell (M8322/0) 227.1
- wolffian duct (M9110/0)

Adenomyoma (M8932/0) — see also Neoplasm, by site, benign
- prostate 600.20
  - with
    - other lower urinary tract symptoms (LUTS) 600.21
    - urinary
      - obstruction 600.21
      - retention 600.21

Adenomyometritis 617.0
Adenomyosis (uterus) (internal) 617.0
Adenopathy (lymph gland) 785.6
- inguinal 785.6
- mediastinal 785.6
- mesentery 785.6
- syphilitic (secondary) 091.4
- tracheobronchial 785.6
  - tuberculous (see also Tuberculosis) 012.1 ☑
    - primary, progressive 010.8 ☑
  - tuberculous (see also Tuberculosis, lymph gland) 017.2 ☑
    - tracheobronchial 012.1 ☑
      - primary, progressive 010.8 ☑

Adenopharyngitis 462
Adenophlegmon 683
Adenosalpingitis 614.1
Adenosarcoma (M8960/3) 189.0
Adenosclerosis 289.3
Adenosis
- breast (sclerosing) 610.2
- vagina, congenital 752.49

Adentia (complete) (partial) — see also Absence, teeth 520.0

Adherent
- labium (minus) 624.4
- pericardium (nonrheumatic) 423.1
  - rheumatic 393
- placenta 667.0 ☑
  - with hemorrhage 666.0 ☑
- prepuce 605
- scar (skin) NEC 709.2
- tendon in scar 709.2

Adhesion(s), adhesive (postinfectional) (postoperative)
- abdominal (wall) (see also Adhesions, peritoneum) 568.0
- amnion to fetus 658.8 ☑
  - affecting fetus or newborn 762.8
- appendix 543.9
- arachnoiditis — see Meningitis
- auditory tube (Eustachian) 381.89
- bands (see also Adhesions, peritoneum)
  - cervix 622.3
  - uterus 621.5
- bile duct (any) 576.8
- bladder (sphincter) 596.8
- bowel (see also Adhesions, peritoneum) 568.0
- cardiac 423.1
  - rheumatic 398.99
- cecum (see also Adhesions, peritoneum) 568.0
- cervicovaginal 622.3
  - congenital 752.49
  - postpartal 674.8 ☑
  - old 622.3
- cervix 622.3
- clitoris 624.4
- colon (see also Adhesions, peritoneum) 568.0
- common duct 576.8
- congenital (see also Anomaly, specified type NEC)
  - fingers (see also Syndactylism, fingers) 755.11
  - labium (majus) (minus) 752.49
  - omental, anomalous 751.4
  - ovary 752.0
  - peritoneal 751.4
  - toes (see also Syndactylism, toes) 755.13
  - tongue (to gum or roof of mouth) 750.12
- conjunctiva (acquired) (localized) 372.62
  - congenital 743.63
  - extensive 372.63
- cornea — see Opacity, cornea
- cystic duct 575.8
- diaphragm (see also Adhesions, peritoneum) 568.0
- due to foreign body — see Foreign body
- duodenum (see also Adhesions, peritoneum) 568.0
  - with obstruction 537.3
- ear, middle — see Adhesions, middle ear
- epididymis 608.89
- epidural — see Adhesions, meninges
- epiglottis 478.79
- Eustachian tube 381.89
- eyelid 374.46
  - postoperative 997.99
    - surgically created V45.69
- gallbladder (see also Disease, gallbladder) 575.8
- globe 360.89
- heart 423.1
  - rheumatic 398.99
- ileocecal (coil) (see also Adhesions, peritoneum) 568.0
- ileum (see also Adhesions, peritoneum) 568.0
- intestine (postoperative) (see also Adhesions, peritoneum) 568.0
  - with obstruction 560.81
    - with hernia (see also Hernia, by site, with obstruction)
    - gangrenous — see Hernia, by site, with gangrene
- intra-abdominal (see also Adhesions, peritoneum) 568.0
- iris 364.70
  - to corneal graft 996.79
- joint (see also Ankylosis) 718.5 ☑
- kidney 593.89

Adhesion(s), adhesive — continued
- labium (majus) (minus), congenital 752.49
- liver 572.8
- lung 511.0
- mediastinum 519.3
- meninges 349.2
  - cerebral (any) 349.2
    - congenital 742.4
  - congenital 742.8
  - spinal (any) 349.2
    - congenital 742.59
  - tuberculous (cerebral) (spinal) (see also Tuberculosis, meninges) 013.0 ☑
- mesenteric (see also Adhesions, peritoneum) 568.0
- middle ear (fibrous) 385.10
  - drum head 385.19
    - to
      - incus 385.11
      - promontorium 385.13
      - stapes 385.12
  - specified NEC 385.19
- nasal (septum) (to turbinates) 478.19 ▲
- nerve NEC 355.9
  - spinal 355.9
  - root 724.9
    - cervical NEC 723.4
    - lumbar NEC 724.4
    - lumbosacral 724.4
    - thoracic 724.4
- ocular muscle 378.60
- omentum (see also Adhesions, peritoneum) 568.0
- organ or site, congenital NEC — see Anomaly, specified type NEC
- ovary 614.6
  - congenital (to cecum, kidney, or omentum) 752.0
- parauterine 614.6
- parovarian 614.6
- pelvic (peritoneal)
  - female (postoperative) (postinfection) 614.6
  - male (postoperative) (postinfection) (see also Adhesions, peritoneum) 568.0
  - postpartal (old) 614.6
  - tuberculous (see also Tuberculosis) 016.9 ☑
- penis to scrotum (congenital) 752.69
- periappendiceal (see also Adhesions, peritoneum) 568.0
- pericardium (nonrheumatic) 423.1
  - rheumatic 393
  - tuberculous (see also Tuberculosis) 017.9 ☑ [420.0]
- pericholecystic 575.8
- perigastric (see also Adhesions, peritoneum) 568.0
- periovarian 614.6
- periprostatic 602.8
- perirectal (see also Adhesions, peritoneum) 568.0
- perirenal 593.89
- peritoneum, peritoneal (fibrous) (postoperative) 568.0
  - with obstruction (intestinal) 560.81
    - with hernia (see also Hernia, by site, with obstruction)
    - gangrenous — see Hernia, by site, with gangrene
  - duodenum 537.3
  - congenital 751.4
  - female (postoperative) (postinfective) 614.6
  - pelvic, female 614.6
  - pelvic, male 568.0
  - postpartal, pelvic 614.6
  - to uterus 614.6
- peritubal 614.6
- periureteral 593.89
- periuterine 621.5
- perivesical 596.8

Adhesion(s), adhesive — continued
- perivesicular (seminal vesicle) 608.89
- pleura, pleuritic 511.0
  - tuberculous (see also Tuberculosis, pleura) 012.0 ☑
- pleuropericardial 511.0
- postoperative (gastrointestinal tract) (see also Adhesions, peritoneum) 568.0
  - eyelid 997.99
    - surgically created V45.69
  - pelvic female 614.9
  - pelvic male 568.0
  - urethra 598.2
- postpartal, old 624.4
- preputial, prepuce 605
- pulmonary 511.0
- pylorus (see also Adhesions, peritoneum) 568.0
- Rosenmüller's fossa 478.29
- sciatic nerve 355.0
- seminal vesicle 608.89
- shoulder (joint) 726.0
- sigmoid flexure (see also Adhesions, peritoneum) 568.0
- spermatic cord (acquired) 608.89
  - congenital 752.89
- spinal canal 349.2
  - nerve 355.9
    - root 724.9
      - cervical NEC 723.4
      - lumbar NEC 724.4
      - lumbosacral 724.4
      - thoracic 724.4
- stomach (see also Adhesions, peritoneum) 568.0
- subscapular 726.2
- tendonitis 726.90
  - shoulder 726.0
- testicle 608.89
- tongue (congenital) (to gum or roof of mouth) 750.12
  - acquired 529.8
- trachea 519.19 ▲
- tubo-ovarian 614.6
- tunica vaginalis 608.89
- ureter 593.89
- uterus 621.5
  - to abdominal wall 614.6
  - in pregnancy or childbirth 654.4 ☑
    - affecting fetus or newborn 763.89
- vagina (chronic) (postoperative) (postradiation) 623.2
- vaginitis (congenital) 752.49
- vesical 596.8
- vitreous 379.29

Adie (-Holmes) syndrome (tonic pupillary reaction) 379.46
Adiponecrosis neonatorum 778.1
Adiposa dolorosa 272.8
Adiposalgia 272.8
Adiposis
- cerebralis 253.8
- dolorosa 272.8
- tuberosa simplex 272.8

Adiposity 278.02
- heart (see also Degeneration, myocardial) 429.1
- localized 278.1

Adiposogenital dystrophy 253.8
Adjustment
- prosthesis or other device — see Fitting of
- reaction — see Reaction, adjustment

Administration, prophylactic
- antibiotics V07.39
- antitoxin, any V07.2
- antivenin V07.2
- chemotherapeutic agent NEC V07.39
- chemotherapy NEC V07.39
- diphtheria antitoxin V07.2
- fluoride V07.31
- gamma globulin V07.2
- immune sera (gamma globulin) V07.2

Administration, prophylactic

Administration, prophylactic — *continued*
- passive immunization agent V07.2
- RhoGAM V07.2

Admission (encounter)
- as organ donor — *see* Donor
- by mistake V68.9
- for
  - adequacy testing (for)
    - hemodialysis V56.31
    - peritoneal dialysis V56.32
  - adjustment (of)
    - artificial
      - arm (complete) (partial) V52.0
      - eye V52.2
      - leg (complete) (partial) V52.1
    - brain neuropacemaker V53.02
    - breast
      - implant V52.4
      - prosthesis V52.4
    - cardiac device V53.39
      - defibrillator, automatic implantable V53.32
      - pacemaker V53.31
        - carotid sinus V53.39
    - catheter
      - non-vascular V58.82
      - vascular V58.81
    - cerebral ventricle (communicating) shunt V53.01
    - colostomy belt V55.3
    - contact lenses V53.1
    - cystostomy device V53.6
    - dental prosthesis V52.3
    - device, unspecified type V53.90
      - abdominal V53.5
      - cardiac V53.39
        - defibrillator, automatic implantable V53.32
        - pacemaker V53.31
        - carotid sinus V53.39
      - cerebral ventricle (communicating) shunt V53.01
      - insulin pump V53.91
      - intrauterine contraceptive V25.1
      - nervous system V53.09
      - orthodontic V53.4
      - other device V53.99
      - prosthetic V52.9
        - breast V52.4
        - dental V52.3
        - eye V52.2
        - specified type NEC V52.8
      - special senses V53.09
      - substitution
        - auditory V53.09
        - nervous system V53.09
        - visual V53.09
      - urinary V53.6
    - dialysis catheter
      - extracorporeal V56.1
      - peritoneal V56.2
    - diaphragm (contraceptive) V25.02
    - growth rod V54.02
    - hearing aid V53.2
    - ileostomy device V55.2
    - intestinal appliance or device NEC V53.5
    - intrauterine contraceptive device V25.1
    - neuropacemaker (brain) (peripheral nerve) (spinal cord) V53.02
    - orthodontic device V53.4
    - orthopedic (device) V53.7
      - brace V53.7
      - cast V53.7
      - shoes V53.7
    - pacemaker
      - brain V53.02
      - cardiac V53.31
      - carotid sinus V53.39
      - peripheral nerve V53.02

Admission — *continued*
- for — *continued*
  - adjustment — *continued*
    - pacemaker — *continued*
      - spinal cord V53.02
    - prosthesis V52.9
      - arm (complete) (partial) V52.0
      - breast V52.4
      - dental V52.3
      - eye V52.2
      - leg (complete) (partial) V52.1
      - specified type NEC V52.8
    - spectacles V53.1
    - wheelchair V53.8
  - adoption referral or proceedings V68.89
  - aftercare (*see also* Aftercare) V58.9
    - cardiac pacemaker V53.31
    - chemotherapy V58.11
    - dialysis
      - extracorporeal (renal) V56.0
      - peritoneal V56.8
      - renal V56.0
    - fracture (*see also* Aftercare, fracture) V54.9
    - medical NEC V58.89
    - organ transplant V58.44
    - orthopedic V54.9
      - specified care NEC V54.89
    - pacemaker device
      - brain V53.02
      - cardiac V53.31
      - carotid sinus V53.39
      - nervous system V53.02
      - spinal cord V53.02
    - postoperative NEC V58.49
      - wound closure, planned V58.41
    - postpartum
      - immediately after delivery V24.0
      - routine follow-up V24.2
    - postradiation V58.0
    - radiation therapy V58.0
    - removal of
      - non-vascular catheter V58.82
      - vascular catheter V58.81
    - specified NEC V58.89
    - surgical NEC V58.49
      - wound closure, planned V58.41
  - antineoplastic
    - chemotherapy V58.11
    - immunotherapy V58.12
  - artificial insemination V26.1
  - attention to artificial opening (of) V55.9
    - artificial vagina V55.7
    - colostomy V55.3
    - cystostomy V55.5
    - enterostomy V55.4
    - gastrostomy V55.1
    - ileostomy V55.2
    - jejunostomy V55.4
    - nephrostomy V55.6
    - specified site NEC V55.8
      - intestinal tract V55.4
      - urinary tract V55.6
    - tracheostomy V55.0
    - ureterostomy V55.6
    - urethrostomy V55.6
  - battery replacement
    - cardiac pacemaker V53.31
  - blood typing V72.86
    - Rh typing V72.86 ●
  - boarding V65.0
  - breast
    - augmentation or reduction V50.1
    - removal, prophylactic V50.41
  - change of
    - cardiac pacemaker (battery) V53.31
    - carotid sinus pacemaker V53.39

Admission — *continued*
- for — *continued*
  - change of — *continued*
    - catheter in artificial opening — *see* Attention to, artificial, opening
    - drains V58.49 ●
    - dressing
      - wound V58.30 ●
        - nonsurgical V58.30 ●
        - surgical V58.31 ●
    - fixation device
      - external V54.89
      - internal V54.01
    - Kirschner wire V54.89
    - neuropacemaker device (brain) (peripheral nerve) (spinal cord) V53.02
    - nonsurgical wound dressing ● V58.30 ●
    - pacemaker device
      - brain V53.02
      - cardiac V53.31
      - carotid sinus V53.39
      - nervous system V53.02
    - plaster cast V54.89
    - splint, external V54.89
    - Steinmann pin V54.89
    - surgical ▶wound◀ dressing V58.31 ▲
    - traction device V54.89
    - wound packing V58.30 ●
      - nonsurgical V58.30 ●
      - surgical V58.31 ●
  - checkup only V70.0
  - chemotherapy, antineoplastic V58.11
  - circumcision, ritual or routine (in absence of medical indication) V50.2
  - clinical research investigation (control) (normal comparison) (participant) V70.7
  - closure of artificial opening — *see* Attention to, artificial, opening
  - contraceptive
    - counseling V25.09
      - emergency V25.03
      - postcoital V25.03
    - management V25.9
      - specified type NEC V25.8
  - convalescence following V66.9
    - chemotherapy V66.2
    - psychotherapy V66.3
    - radiotherapy V66.1
    - surgery V66.0
    - treatment (for) V66.5
      - combined V66.6
      - fracture V66.4
      - mental disorder NEC V66.3
      - specified condition NEC V66.5
  - cosmetic surgery NEC V50.1
    - following healed injury or operation V51
  - counseling (*see also* Counseling) V65.40
    - without complaint or sickness V65.49
    - contraceptive management V25.09
      - emergency V25.03
      - postcoital V25.03
    - dietary V65.3
    - exercise V65.41
    - for
      - nonattending third party V65.19
      - pediatric pre-birth visit for expectant mother V65.11
    - victim of abuse
      - child V61.21
      - partner or spouse V61.11
    - genetic V26.33

Admission — *continued*
- for — *continued*
  - counseling (*see also* Counseling) — *continued*
    - gonorrhea V65.45
    - HIV V65.44
    - human immunodeficiency virus V65.44
    - injury prevention V65.43
    - insulin pump training V65.46
    - procreative management V26.4
    - sexually transmitted disease NEC V65.45
      - HIV V65.44
    - specified reason NEC V65.49
    - substance use and abuse V65.42
    - syphilis V65.45
    - victim of abuse
      - child V61.21
      - partner or spouse V61.11
  - desensitization to allergens V07.1
  - dialysis V56.0
    - catheter
      - fitting and adjustment
        - extracorporeal V56.1
        - peritoneal V56.2
      - removal or replacement
        - extracorporeal V56.1
        - peritoneal V56.2
    - extracorporeal (renal) V56.0
    - peritoneal V56.8
    - renal V56.0
  - dietary surveillance and counseling V65.3
  - drug monitoring, therapeutic V58.83
  - ear piercing V50.3
  - elective surgery V50.9
    - breast
      - augmentation or reduction V50.1
      - removal, prophylactic V50.41
    - circumcision, ritual or routine (in absence of medical indication) V50.2
    - cosmetic NEC V50.1
      - following healed injury or operation V51
    - ear piercing V50.3
    - face-lift V50.1
    - hair transplant V50.0
    - plastic
      - cosmetic NEC V50.1
      - following healed injury or operation V51
    - prophylactic organ removal V50.49
      - breast V50.41
      - ovary V50.42
    - repair of scarred tissue (following healed injury or operation) V51
    - specified type NEC V50.8
  - end-of-life care V66.7
  - examination (*see also* Examination) V70.9
    - administrative purpose NEC V70.3
    - adoption V70.3
    - allergy V72.7
    - at health care facility V70.0
    - athletic team V70.3
    - camp V70.3
    - cardiovascular, preoperative V72.81
    - clinical research investigation (control) (participant) V70.7
    - dental V72.2
    - developmental testing (child) (infant) V20.2
    - donor (potential) V70.8
    - driver's license V70.3
    - ear V72.19 ▲
    - employment V70.5

Index to Diseases

Admission

Admission — *continued*
- for — *continued*
  - examination (*see also* Examination) — *continued*
    - eye V72.0
    - follow-up (routine) — *see* Examination, follow-up
    - for admission to
      - old age home V70.3
      - school V70.3
    - general V70.9
      - specified reason NEC V70.8
    - gynecological V72.31
    - health supervision (child) (infant) V20.2
    - hearing V72.19
      - following failed hearing screening V72.11
    - immigration V70.3
    - infant, routine V20.2
    - insurance certification V70.3
    - laboratory V72.6
    - marriage license V70.3
    - medical (general) (*see also* Examination, medical) V70.9
    - medicolegal reasons V70.4
    - naturalization V70.3
    - pelvic (annual) (periodic) V72.31
    - postpartum checkup V24.2
    - pregnancy (possible) (unconfirmed) V72.40
      - negative result V72.41
      - positive result V72.42
    - preoperative V72.84
      - cardiovascular V72.81
      - respiratory V72.82
      - specified NEC V72.83
    - preprocedural V72.84
      - cardiovascular V72.81
      - general physical V72.83
      - respiratory V72.82
      - specified NEC V72.83
    - prison V70.3
    - psychiatric (general) V70.2
      - requested by authority V70.1
    - radiological NEC V72.5
    - respiratory, preoperative V72.82
    - school V70.3
    - screening — *see* Screening
    - skin hypersensitivity V72.7
    - specified type NEC V72.85
    - sport competition V70.3
    - vision V72.0
    - well baby and child care V20.2
  - exercise therapy V57.1
  - face-lift, cosmetic reason V50.1
  - fitting (of)
    - artificial
      - arm (complete) (partial) V52.0
      - eye V52.2
      - leg (complete) (partial) V52.1
    - biliary drainage tube V58.82
    - brain neuropacemaker V53.02
    - breast V52.4
      - implant V52.4
      - prosthesis V52.4
    - cardiac pacemaker V53.31
    - catheter
      - non-vascular V58.82
      - vascular V58.81
    - cerebral ventricle (communicating) shunt V53.01
    - chest tube V58.82
    - colostomy belt V55.2
    - contact lenses V53.1
    - cystostomy device V53.6
    - dental prosthesis V52.3
    - device, unspecified type V53.90
      - abdominal V53.5
      - cerebral ventricle (communicating) shunt V53.01
      - insulin pump V53.91
      - intrauterine contraceptive V25.1
      - nervous system V53.09

Admission — *continued*
- for — *continued*
  - fitting — *continued*
    - device, unspecified type — *continued*
      - orthodontic V53.4
      - other device V53.99
      - prosthetic V52.9
        - breast V52.4
        - dental V52.3
        - eye V52.2
        - special senses V53.09
      - substitution
        - auditory V53.09
        - nervous system V53.09
        - visual V53.09
    - diaphragm (contraceptive) V25.02
    - fistula (sinus tract) drainage tube V58.82
    - growth rod V54.02
    - hearing aid V53.2
    - ileostomy device V55.2
    - intestinal appliance or device NEC V53.5
    - intrauterine contraceptive device V25.1
    - neuropacemaker (brain) (peripheral nerve) (spinal cord) V53.02
    - orthodontic device V53.4
    - orthopedic (device) V53.7
      - brace V53.7
      - cast V53.7
      - shoes V53.7
    - pacemaker
      - brain V53.02
      - cardiac V53.31
      - carotid sinus V53.39
      - spinal cord V53.02
    - pleural drainage tube V58.82
    - prosthesis V52.9
      - arm (complete) (partial) V52.0
      - breast V52.4
      - dental V52.3
      - eye V52.2
      - leg (complete) (partial) V52.1
      - specified type NEC V52.8
    - spectacles V53.1
    - wheelchair V53.8
  - follow-up examination (routine) (following) V67.9
    - cancer chemotherapy V67.2
    - chemotherapy V67.2
    - high-risk medication NEC V67.51
    - injury NEC V67.59
    - psychiatric V67.3
    - psychotherapy V67.3
    - radiotherapy V67.1
    - specified surgery NEC V67.09
    - surgery V67.00
      - vaginal pap smear V67.01
    - treatment (for) V67.9
      - combined V67.6
      - fracture V67.4
      - involving high-risk medication NEC V67.51
      - mental disorder V67.3
      - specified NEC V67.59
  - hair transplant, for cosmetic reason V50.0
  - health advice, education, or instruction V65.4 ☑
  - hormone replacement therapy (postmenopausal) V07.4
  - hospice care V66.7
  - immunotherapy, antineoplastic V58.12
  - insertion (of)
    - subdermal implantable contraceptive V25.5
  - insulin pump titration V53.91
  - insulin pump training V65.46

Admission — *continued*
- for — *continued*
  - intrauterine device
    - insertion V25.1
    - management V25.42
  - investigation to determine further disposition V63.8
  - isolation V07.0
  - issue of
    - medical certificate NEC V68.0
    - repeat prescription NEC V68.1
      - contraceptive device NEC V25.49
  - kidney dialysis V56.0
  - lengthening of growth rod V54.02
  - mental health evaluation V70.2
    - requested by authority V70.1
  - nonmedical reason NEC V68.89
  - nursing care evaluation V63.8
  - observation (without need for further medical care) (*see also* Observation) V71.9
    - accident V71.4
    - alleged rape or seduction V71.5
    - criminal assault V71.6
    - following accident V71.4
      - at work V71.3
    - foreign body ingestion V71.89
    - growth and development variations, childhood V21.0
    - inflicted injury NEC V71.6
    - ingestion of deleterious agent or foreign body V71.89
    - injury V71.6
    - malignant neoplasm V71.1
    - mental disorder V71.09
    - newborn — *see* Observation, suspected, condition, newborn
    - rape V71.5
    - specified NEC V71.89
    - suspected disorder V71.9
      - abuse V71.81
      - accident V71.4
        - at work V71.3
      - benign neoplasm V71.89
      - cardiovascular V71.7
      - exposure
        - anthrax V71.82
        - biological agent NEC V71.83
        - SARS V71.83
      - heart V71.7
      - inflicted injury NEC V71.6
      - malignant neoplasm V71.1
      - mental NEC V71.09
      - neglect V71.81
      - specified condition NEC V71.89
      - tuberculosis V71.2
    - tuberculosis V71.2
  - occupational therapy V57.21
  - organ transplant, donor — *see* Donor
  - ovary, ovarian removal, prophylactic V50.42
  - palliative care V66.7
  - Papanicolaou smear
    - cervix V76.2
      - for suspected malignant neoplasm V76.2
      - no disease found V71.1
      - routine, as part of gynecological examination V72.31
      - to confirm findings of recent normal smear following initial abnormal smear V72.32
    - vaginal V76.47
      - following hysterectomy for malignant condition V67.01
  - passage of sounds or bougie in artificial opening — *see* Attention to, artificial, opening

Admission — *continued*
- for — *continued*
  - paternity testing V70.4
  - peritoneal dialysis V56.32
  - physical therapy NEC V57.1
  - plastic surgery
    - cosmetic NEC V50.1
    - following healed injury or operation V51
  - postmenopausal hormone replacement therapy V07.4
  - postpartum observation
    - immediately after delivery V24.0
    - routine follow-up V24.2
  - poststerilization (for restoration) V26.0
  - procreative management V26.9
    - specified type NEC V26.8
  - prophylactic
    - administration of
      - antibiotics V07.39
      - antitoxin, any V07.2
      - antivenin V07.2
      - chemotherapeutic agent NEC V07.39
      - chemotherapy NEC V07.39
      - diphtheria antitoxin V07.2
      - fluoride V07.31
      - gamma globulin V07.2
      - immune sera (gamma globulin) V07.2
      - RhoGAM V07.2
      - tetanus antitoxin V07.2
    - breathing exercises V57.0
    - chemotherapy NEC V07.39
    - fluoride V07.31
    - measure V07.9
      - specified type NEC V07.8
    - organ removal V50.49
      - breast V50.41
      - ovary V50.42
    - psychiatric examination (general) V70.2
      - requested by authority V70.1
  - radiation management V58.0
  - radiotherapy V58.0
  - reforming of artificial opening — *see* Attention to, artificial, opening
  - rehabilitation V57.9
    - multiple types V57.89
    - occupational V57.21
    - orthoptic V57.4
    - orthotic V57.81
    - physical NEC V57.1
    - specified type NEC V57.89
    - speech V57.3
    - vocational V57.22
  - removal of
    - cardiac pacemaker V53.31
    - cast (plaster) V54.89
    - catheter from artificial opening — *see* Attention to, artificial, opening
    - cerebral ventricle (communicating) shunt V53.01
    - cystostomy catheter V55.5
    - device
      - cerebral ventricle (communicating) shunt V53.01
      - fixation
        - external V54.89
        - internal V54.01
      - intrauterine contraceptive V25.42
      - traction, external V54.89
    - drains V58.49
    - dressing
      - wound V58.30
        - nonsurgical V58.30
        - surgical V58.31
    - fixation device
      - external V54.89
      - internal V54.01
    - intrauterine contraceptive device V25.42

Admission

Admission — *continued*
  for — *continued*
    removal of — *continued*
      Kirschner wire V54.89
      neuropacemaker (brain) (peripheral nerve) (spinal cord) V53.02
      nonsurgical wound dressing V58.30 ●
      orthopedic fixation device
        external V54.89
        internal V54.01
      pacemaker device
        brain V53.02
        cardiac V53.31
        carotid sinus V53.39
        nervous system V53.02
      plaster cast V54.89
      plate (fracture) V54.01
      rod V54.01
      screw (fracture) V54.01
      splint, traction V54.89
      staples V58.32 ●
      Steinmann pin V54.89
      subdermal implantable contraceptive V25.43
      surgical ▶wound◀ dressing V58.31 ▲
      sutures V58.32 ●
      traction device, external V54.89
      ureteral stent V53.6
      wound packing V58.30 ●
        nonsurgical V58.30 ●
        surgical V58.31 ●
    repair of scarred tissue (following healed injury or operation) V51
    reprogramming of cardiac pacemaker V53.31
    respirator [ventilator] dependence during
      mechanical failure V46.14
      power failure V46.12
      for weaning V46.13
    restoration of organ continuity (poststerilization) (tuboplasty) (vasoplasty) V26.0
    Rh typing V72.86 ●
    sensitivity test (*see also* Test, skin)
      allergy NEC V72.7
      bacterial disease NEC V74.9
      Dick V74.8
      Kveim V82.89
      Mantoux V74.1
      mycotic infection NEC V75.4
      parasitic disease NEC V75.8
      Schick V74.3
      Schultz-Charlton V74.8
    social service (agency) referral or evaluation V63.8
    speech therapy V57.3
    sterilization V25.2
    suspected disorder (ruled out) (without need for further care) — *see* Observation
    terminal care V66.7
    tests only — *see* Test
    therapeutic drug monitoring V58.83
    therapy
      blood transfusion, without reported diagnosis V58.2
      breathing exercises V57.0
      chemotherapy, antineoplastic V58.11
        prophylactic NEC V07.39
          fluoride V07.31
      dialysis (intermittent) (treatment)
        extracorporeal V56.0
        peritoneal V56.8
        renal V56.0
        specified type NEC V56.8
      exercise (remedial) NEC V57.1
        breathing V57.0

Admission — *continued*
  for — *continued*
    therapy — *continued*
      immunotherapy, antineoplastic V58.12
      long-term (current) drug use NEC V58.69
        antibiotics V58.62
        anticoagulants V58.61
        anti-inflammatories, non-steroidal (NSAID) V58.64
        antiplatelets V58.63
        antithrombotics V58.63
        aspirin V58.66
        insulin V58.67
        steroids V58.65
      occupational V57.21
      orthoptic V57.4
      physical NEC V57.1
      radiation V58.0
      speech V57.3
      vocational V57.22
    toilet or cleaning
      of artificial opening — *see* Attention to, artificial, opening
      of non-vascular catheter V58.82
      of vascular catheter V58.81
    tubal ligation V25.2
    tuboplasty for previous sterilization V26.0
    vaccination, prophylactic (against)
      arthropod-borne virus, viral NEC V05.1
        disease NEC V05.1
        encephalitis V05.0
      Bacille Calmette Guérin (BCG) V03.2
      BCG V03.2
      chickenpox V05.4
      cholera alone V03.0
        with typhoid-paratyphoid (cholera + TAB) V06.0
      common cold V04.7
      dengue V05.1
      diphtheria alone V03.5
      diphtheria-tetanus-pertussis (DTP) (DTaP) V06.1
        with
          poliomyelitis (DTP + polio) V06.3
          typhoid-paratyphoid (DTP + TAB) V06.2
      diphtheria-tetanus [Td] [DT] without pertussis V06.5
      disease (single) NEC V05.9
        bacterial NEC V03.9
          specified type NEC V03.89
        combinations NEC V06.9
          specified type NEC V06.8
        specified type NEC V05.8
        viral NEC V04.89
      encephalitis, viral, arthropod-borne V05.0
      Hemophilus influenzae, type B [Hib] V03.81
      hepatitis, viral V05.3
      immune sera (gamma globulin) V07.2
      influenza V04.81
        with
          Streptococcus pneumoniae [pneumococcus] V06.6
      Leishmaniasis V05.2
      measles alone V04.2
      measles-mumps-rubella (MMR) V06.4
      mumps alone V04.6
        with measles and rubella (MMR) V06.4
      not done because of contraindication V64.09
      pertussis alone V03.6
      plague V03.3
      pneumonia V03.82

Admission — *continued*
  for — *continued*
    vaccination, prophylactic — *continued*
      poliomyelitis V04.0
        with diphtheria-tetanus-pertussis (DTP+ polio) V06.3
      rabies V04.5
      respiratory syncytial virus (RSV) V04.82
      rubella alone V04.3
        with measles and mumps (MMR) V06.4
      smallpox V04.1
      specified type NEC V05.8
      Streptococcus pneumoniae [pneumococcus] V03.82
        with
          influenza V06.6
      tetanus toxoid alone V03.7
        with diphtheria [Td] [DT] V06.5
          and pertussis (DTP) (DTaP) V06.1
      tuberculosis (BCG) V03.2
      tularemia V03.4
      typhoid alone V03.1
        with diphtheria-tetanus-pertussis (TAB + DTP) V06.2
      typhoid-paratyphoid alone (TAB) V03.1
      typhus V05.8
      varicella (chicken pox) V05.4
      viral encephalitis, arthropod-borne V05.0
      viral hepatitis V05.3
      yellow fever V04.4
    vasectomy V25.2
    vasoplasty for previous sterilization V26.0
    vision examination V72.0
    vocational therapy V57.22
    waiting period for admission to other facility V63.2
      undergoing social agency investigation V63.8
    well baby and child care V20.2
    x-ray of chest
      for suspected tuberculosis V71.2
      routine V72.5

Adnexitis (suppurative) — *see also* Salpingo-oophoritis 614.2
Adolescence NEC V21.2
Adoption
  agency referral V68.89
  examination V70.3
  held for V68.89
Adrenal gland — *see* condition
Adrenalism 255.9
  tuberculous (*see also* Tuberculosis) 017.6 ☑
Adrenalitis, adrenitis 255.8
  meningococcal hemorrhagic 036.3
Adrenarche, precocious 259.1
Adrenocortical syndrome 255.2
Adrenogenital syndrome (acquired) (congenital) 255.2
  iatrogenic, fetus or newborn 760.79
Adrenoleukodystrophy 277.86
  neonatal 277.86
  x-linked 277.86
Adrenomyeloneuropathy 277.86
Adventitious bursa — *see* Bursitis
Adynamia (episodica) (hereditary) (periodic) 359.3
Adynamic
  ileus or intestine (*see also* Ileus) 560.1
  ureter 753.22
Aeration lung, imperfect, newborn 770.5
Aerobullosis 993.3
Aerocele — *see* Embolism, air

Aerodermectasia
  subcutaneous (traumatic) 958.7
    surgical 998.81
  surgical 998.81
Aerodontalgia 993.2
Aeroembolism 993.3
Aerogenes capsulatus infection — *see also* Gangrene, gas 040.0
Aero-otitis media 993.0
Aerophagy, aerophagia 306.4
  psychogenic 306.4
Aerosinusitis 993.1
Aerotitis 993.0
Affection, affections — *see also* Disease
  sacroiliac (joint), old 724.6
  shoulder region NEC 726.2
Afibrinogenemia 286.3
  acquired 286.6
  congenital 286.3
  postpartum 666.3 ☑
African
  sleeping sickness 086.5
  tick fever 087.1
  trypanosomiasis 086.5
    Gambian 086.3
    Rhodesian 086.4
Aftercare V58.9
  amputation stump V54.89 ●
  artificial openings — *see* Attention to, artificial, opening
  blood transfusion without reported diagnosis V58.2
  breathing exercise V57.0
  cardiac device V53.39
    defibrillator, automatic implantable V53.32
    pacemaker V53.31
      carotid sinus V53.39
  carotid sinus pacemaker V53.39
  cerebral ventricle (communicating) shunt V53.01
  chemotherapy session (adjunctive) (maintenance) V58.11
  defibrillator, automatic implantable cardiac V53.32
  exercise (remedial) (therapeutic) V57.1
    breathing V57.0
  extracorporeal dialysis (intermittent) (treatment) V56.0
  following surgery NEC V58.49
    for
      injury V58.43
      neoplasm V58.42
      organ transplant V58.44
      trauma V58.43
    joint replacement V54.81
    of
      circulatory system V58.73
      digestive system V58.75
      genital organs V58.76
      genitourinary system V58.76
      musculoskeletal system V58.78
      nervous system V58.72
      oral cavity V58.75
      respiratory system V58.74
      sense organs V58.71
      skin V58.77
      subcutaneous tissue V58.77
      teeth V58.75
      urinary system V58.76
    wound closure, planned V58.41
  fracture V54.9
    healing V54.89
      pathologic
        ankle V54.29
        arm V54.20
          lower V54.22
          upper V54.21
        finger V54.29
        foot V54.29
        hand V54.29
        hip V54.23
        leg V54.24
          lower V54.26
          upper V54.25
        pelvis V54.29

Index to Diseases

Aftercare — continued
  fracture — continued
    healing — continued
      pathologic — continued
        specified site NEC V54.29
        toe(s) V54.29
        vertebrae V54.27
        wrist V54.29
      traumatic
        ankle V54.19
        arm V54.10
          lower V54.12
          upper V54.11
        finger V54.19
        foot V54.19
        hand V54.19
        hip V54.13
        leg V54.14
          lower V54.16
          upper V54.15
        pelvis V54.19
        specified site NEC V54.19
        toe(s) V54.19
        vertebrae V54.17
        wrist V54.19
      removal of
        external fixation device V54.89
        internal fixation device V54.01
      specified care NEC V54.89
  gait training V57.1
    for use of artificial limb(s) V57.81
  internal fixation device V54.09
  involving
    dialysis (intermittent) (treatment)
      extracorporeal V56.0
      peritoneal V56.8
      renal V56.0
    gait training V57.1
      for use of artificial limb(s) V57.81
    growth rod
      adjustment V54.02
      lengthening V54.02
    internal fixation device V54.09
    orthoptic training V57.4
    orthotic training V57.81
    radiotherapy session V58.0
    removal of
      drains V58.49
      dressings
        wound V58.30
          nonsurgical V58.30
          surgical V58.31
      fixation device
        external V54.89
        internal V54.01
      fracture plate V54.01
      nonsurgical wound dressing V58.30
      pins V54.01
      plaster cast V54.89
      rods V54.01
      screws V58.32 ▲
      staples V58.32
      surgical ▶wound◀ dressings V58.31 ▲
      sutures V58.32
      traction device, external V54.89
      wound packing V58.30
        nonsurgical V58.30
        surgical V58.31
  neuropacemaker (brain) (peripheral nerve) (spinal cord) V53.02
  occupational therapy V57.21
  orthodontic V58.5
  orthopedic V54.9
    change of external fixation or traction device V54.89
    following joint replacement V54.81
    internal fixation device V54.09
    removal of fixation device
      external V54.89
      internal V54.01
    specified care NEC V54.89
  orthoptic training V57.4
  orthotic training V57.81

Aftercare — continued
  pacemaker
    brain V53.02
    cardiac V53.31
    carotid sinus V53.39
    peripheral nerve V53.02
    spinal cord V53.02
  peritoneal dialysis (intermittent) (treatment) V56.8
  physical therapy NEC V57.1
    breathing exercises V57.0
  radiotherapy session V58.0
  rehabilitation procedure V57.9
    breathing exercises V57.0
    multiple types V57.89
    occupational V57.21
    orthoptic V57.4
    orthotic V57.81
    physical therapy NEC V57.1
    remedial exercises V57.1
    specified type NEC V57.89
    speech V57.3
    therapeutic exercises V57.1
    vocational V57.22
  renal dialysis (intermittent) (treatment) V56.0
  specified type NEC V58.89
    removal of non-vascular catheter V58.82
    removal of vascular catheter V58.81
  speech therapy V57.3
  stump, amputation V54.89 ●
  vocational rehabilitation V57.22

After-cataract 366.50
  obscuring vision 366.53
  specified type, not obscuring vision 366.52

Agalactia 676.4 ☑

Agammaglobulinemia 279.00
  with lymphopenia 279.2
  acquired (primary) (secondary) 279.06
  Bruton's X-linked 279.04
  infantile sex-linked (Bruton's) (congenital) 279.04
  Swiss-type 279.2

Aganglionosis (bowel) (colon) 751.3

Age (old) — see also Senile 797

Agenesis — see also Absence, by site, congenital
  acoustic nerve 742.8
  adrenal (gland) 759.1
  alimentary tract (complete) (partial) NEC 751.8
    lower 751.2
    upper 750.8
  anus, anal (canal) 751.2
  aorta 747.22
  appendix 751.2
  arm (complete) (partial) (see also Deformity, reduction, upper limb) 755.20
  artery (peripheral) NEC (see also Anomaly, peripheral vascular system) 747.60
    brain 747.81
    coronary 746.85
    pulmonary 747.3
    umbilical 747.5
  auditory (canal) (external) 744.01
  auricle (ear) 744.01
  bile, biliary duct or passage 751.61
  bone NEC 756.9
  brain 740.0
    specified part 742.2
  breast 757.6
  bronchus 748.3
  canaliculus lacrimalis 743.65
  carpus NEC (see also Deformity, reduction, upper limb) 755.28
  cartilage 756.9
  cecum 751.2
  cerebellum 742.2
  cervix 752.49
  chin 744.89
  cilia 743.63

Agenesis — see also Absence, by site, congenital — continued
  circulatory system, part NEC 747.89
  clavicle 755.51
  clitoris 752.49
  coccyx 756.13
  colon 751.2
  corpus callosum 742.2
  cricoid cartilage 748.3
  diaphragm (with hernia) 756.6
  digestive organ(s) or tract (complete) (partial) NEC 751.8
    lower 751.2
    upper 750.8
  ductus arteriosus 747.89
  duodenum 751.1
  ear NEC 744.09
    auricle 744.01
    lobe 744.21
  ejaculatory duct 752.89
  endocrine (gland) NEC 759.2
  epiglottis 748.3
  esophagus 750.3
  Eustachian tube 744.24
  extrinsic muscle, eye 743.69
  eye 743.00
    adnexa 743.69
  eyelid (fold) 743.62
  face
    bones NEC 756.0
    specified part NEC 744.89
  fallopian tube 752.19
  femur NEC (see also Absence, femur, congenital) 755.34
  fibula NEC (see also Absence, fibula, congenital) 755.37
  finger NEC (see also Absence, finger, congenital) 755.29
  foot (complete) (see also Deformity, reduction, lower limb) 755.31
  gallbladder 751.69
  gastric 750.8
  genitalia, genital (organ)
    female 752.89
      external 752.49
      internal NEC 752.89
    male 752.89
      penis 752.69
  glottis 748.3
  gonadal 758.6
  hair 757.4
  hand (complete) (see also Deformity, reduction, upper limb) 755.21
  heart 746.89
    valve NEC 746.89
      aortic 746.89
      mitral 746.89
      pulmonary 746.01
  hepatic 751.69
  humerus NEC (see also Absence, humerus, congenital) 755.24
  hymen 752.49
  ileum 751.1
  incus 744.04
  intestine (small) 751.1
    large 751.2
  iris (dilator fibers) 743.45
  jaw 524.09
  jejunum 751.1
  kidney(s) (partial) (unilateral) 753.0
  labium (majus) (minus) 752.49
  labyrinth, membranous 744.05
  lacrimal apparatus (congenital) 743.65
  larynx 748.3
  leg NEC (see also Deformity, reduction, lower limb) 755.30
  lens 743.35
  limb (complete) (partial) (see also Deformity, reduction) 755.4
    lower NEC 755.30
    upper 755.20
  lip 750.26
  liver 751.69
  lung (bilateral) (fissures) (lobe) (unilateral) 748.5
  mandible 524.09

Agenesis — see also Absence, by site, congenital — continued
  maxilla 524.09
  metacarpus NEC 755.28
  metatarsus NEC 755.38
  muscle (any) 756.81
  musculoskeletal system NEC 756.9
  nail(s) 757.5
  neck, part 744.89
  nerve 742.8
  nervous system, part NEC 742.8
  nipple 757.6
  nose 748.1
  nuclear 742.8
  organ
    of Corti 744.05
    or site not listed — see Anomaly, specified type NEC
  osseous meatus (ear) 744.03
  ovary 752.0
  oviduct 752.19
  pancreas 751.7
  parathyroid (gland) 759.2
  patella 755.64
  pelvic girdle (complete) (partial) 755.69
  penis 752.69
  pericardium 746.89
  perineal body 756.81
  pituitary (gland) 759.2
  prostate 752.89
  pulmonary
    artery 747.3
    trunk 747.3
    vein 747.49
  punctum lacrimale 743.65
  radioulnar NEC (see also Absence, forearm, congenital) 755.25
  radius NEC (see also Absence, radius, congenital) 755.26
  rectum 751.2
  renal 753.0
  respiratory organ NEC 748.9
  rib 756.3
  roof of orbit 742.0
  round ligament 752.89
  sacrum 756.13
  salivary gland 750.21
  scapula 755.59
  scrotum 752.89
  seminal duct or tract 752.89
  septum
    atrial 745.69
    between aorta and pulmonary artery 745.0
    ventricular 745.3
  shoulder girdle (complete) (partial) 755.59
  skull (bone) 756.0
    with
      anencephalus 740.0
      encephalocele 742.0
      hydrocephalus 742.3
        with spina bifida (see also Spina bifida) 741.0 ☑
      microcephalus 742.1
  spermatic cord 752.89
  spinal cord 742.59
  spine 756.13
    lumbar 756.13
      isthmus 756.11
      pars articularis 756.11
  spleen 759.0
  sternum 756.3
  stomach 750.7
  tarsus NEC 755.38
  tendon 756.81
  testicular 752.89
  testis 752.89
  thymus (gland) 759.2
  thyroid (gland) 243
    cartilage 748.3
  tibia NEC (see also Absence, tibia, congenital) 755.36
  tibiofibular NEC 755.35
  toe (complete) (partial) (see also Absence, toe, congenital) 755.39

☑ Additional Digit Required — Refer to the Tabular List for Digit Selection
▶◀ Revised Text ● New Line ▲ Revised Code
Subterms under main terms may continue to next column or page

Agenesis

Agenesis — *see also* Absence, by site, congenital — *continued*
   tongue 750.11
   trachea (cartilage) 748.3
   ulna NEC (*see also* Absence, ulna, congenital) 755.27
   ureter 753.4
   urethra 753.8
   urinary tract NEC 753.8
   uterus 752.3
   uvula 750.26
   vagina 752.49
   vas deferens 752.89
   vein(s) (peripheral) NEC (*see also* Anomaly, peripheral vascular system) 747.60
      brain 747.81
      great 747.49
      portal 747.49
      pulmonary 747.49
      vena cava (inferior) (superior) 747.49
   vermis of cerebellum 742.2
   vertebra 756.13
      lumbar 756.13
         isthmus 756.11
         pars articularis 756.11
   vulva 752.49
Ageusia — *see also* Disturbance, sensation 781.1
Aggressiveness 301.3
Aggressive outburst — *see also* Disturbance, conduct 312.0
   in children or adolescents 313.9
Aging skin 701.8
Agitated — *see* condition
Agitation 307.9
   catatonic (*see also* Schizophrenia) 295.2
Aglossia (congenital) 750.11
Aglycogenosis 271.0
Agnail (finger) (with lymphangitis) 681.02
Agnosia (body image) (tactile) 784.69
   verbal 784.69
      auditory 784.69
         secondary to organic lesion 784.69
      developmental 315.8
      secondary to organic lesion 784.69
      visual 784.69
         developmental 315.8
         secondary to organic lesion 784.69
   visual 368.16
      developmental 315.31
Agoraphobia 300.22
   with panic disorder 300.21
Agrammatism 784.69
Agranulocytopenia ▶ — *see also* Agranulocytosis◀ 288.09
Agranulocytosis (angina) 288.09
   chronic 288.09
   cyclical 288.02
   genetic 288.01
   infantile 288.01
   periodic 288.02
   pernicious 288.09
Agraphia (absolute) 784.69
   with alexia 784.61
   developmental 315.39
Agrypnia — *see also* Insomnia 780.52
Ague — *see also* Malaria 084.6
   brass-founders' 985.8
   dumb 084.6
   tertian 084.1
Agyria 742.2
Ahumada-del Castillo syndrome (nonpuerperal galactorrhea and amenorrhea) 253.1
AIDS 042
AIDS-associated retrovirus (disease) (illness) 042
   infection — *see* Human immunodeficiency virus, infection
AIDS-associated virus (disease) (illness) 042

AIDS-associated virus — *continued*
   infection — *see* Human immunodeficiency virus, infection
AIDS-like disease (illness) (syndrome) 042
AIDS-related complex 042
AIDS-related conditions 042
AIDS-related virus (disease) (illness) 042
   infection — *see* Human immunodeficiency virus, infection
AIDS virus (disease) (illness) 042
   infection — *see* Human immunodeficiency virus, infection
Ailment, heart — *see* Disease, heart
Ailurophobia 300.29
Ainhum (disease) 136.0
Air
   anterior mediastinum 518.1
   compressed, disease 993.3
   embolism (any site) (artery) (cerebral) 958.0
      with
         abortion — *see* Abortion, by type, with embolism
         ectopic pregnancy (*see also* categories 633.0–633.9) 639.6
         molar pregnancy (*see also* categories 630–632) 639.6
      due to implanted device — *see* Complications, due to (presence of) any device, implant, or graft classified to 996.0–996.5 NEC
      following
         abortion 639.6
         ectopic or molar pregnancy 639.6
         infusion, perfusion, or transfusion 999.1
      in pregnancy, childbirth, or puerperium 673.0
      traumatic 958.0
   hunger 786.09
      psychogenic 306.1
   leak (lung) (pulmonary) (thorax) 512.8
      iatrogenic 512.1
      postoperative 512.1
   rarefied, effects of — *see* Effect, adverse, high altitude
   sickness 994.6
Airplane sickness 994.6
Akathisia, acathisia 781.0
   due to drugs 333.99
   neuroleptic-induced acute 333.99
Akinesia algeria 352.6
Akiyami 100.89
Akureyri disease (epidemic neuromyasthenia) 049.8
Alacrima (congenital) 743.65
Alactasia (hereditary) 271.3
Alagille syndrome 759.89
Alalia 784.3
   developmental 315.31
      receptive-expressive 315.32
   secondary to organic lesion 784.3
Alaninemia 270.8
Alastrim 050.1
Albarrán's disease (colibacilluria) 791.9
Albers-Schönberg's disease (marble bones) 756.52
Albert's disease 726.71
Albinism, albino (choroid) (cutaneous) (eye) (generalized) (isolated) (ocular) (oculocutaneous) (partial) 270.2
Albinismus 270.2
Albright (-Martin) (-Bantam) disease (pseudohypoparathyroidism) 275.49
Albright (-McCune) (-Sternberg) syndrome (osteitis fibrosa disseminata) 756.59
Albuminous — *see* condition
Albuminuria, albuminuric (acute) (chronic) (subacute) 791.0
   Bence-Jones 791.0

Albuminuria, albuminuric — *continued*
   cardiac 785.9
   complicating pregnancy, childbirth, or puerperium 646.2
      with hypertension — *see* Toxemia, of pregnancy
      affecting fetus or newborn 760.1
   cyclic 593.6
   gestational 646.2
   gravidarum 646.2
      with hypertension — *see* Toxemia, of pregnancy
      affecting fetus or newborn 760.1
   heart 785.9
   idiopathic 593.6
   orthostatic 593.6
   postural 593.6
   pre-eclamptic (mild) 642.4
      affecting fetus or newborn 760.0
      severe 642.5
         affecting fetus or newborn 760.0
   recurrent physiologic 593.6
   scarlatinal 034.1
Albumosuria 791.0
   Bence-Jones 791.0
   myelopathic (M9730/3) 203.0
Alcaptonuria 270.2
Alcohol, alcoholic
   abstinence 291.81
   acute intoxication 305.0
      with dependence 303.0
   addiction (*see also* Alcoholism) 303.9
      maternal
         with suspected fetal damage affecting management of pregnancy 655.4
         affecting fetus or newborn 760.71
   amnestic disorder, persisting 291.1
   anxiety 291.89
   brain syndrome, chronic 291.2
   cardiopathy 425.5
   chronic (*see also* Alcoholism) 303.9
   cirrhosis (liver) 571.2
   delirium 291.0
      acute 291.0
      chronic 291.1
      tremens 291.0
      withdrawal 291.0
   dementia NEC 291.2
   deterioration 291.2
   drunkenness (simple) 305.0
   hallucinosis (acute) 291.3
   induced
      circadian rhythm sleep disorder 291.82
      hypersomnia 291.82
      insomnia 291.82
      mental disorder 291.9
         anxiety 291.89
         mood 291.89
         sexual 291.89
         sleep 291.82
         specified type 291.89
      parasomnia 291.82
      persisting
         amnestic disorder 291.1
         dementia 291.2
      psychotic disorder
         with
            delusions 291.5
            hallucinations 291.3
      sleep disorder 291.82
   insanity 291.9
   intoxication (acute) 305.0
      with dependence 303.0
      pathological 291.4
   jealousy 291.5
   Korsakoff's, Korsakov's, Korsakow's 291.1
   liver NEC 571.3
      acute 571.1
      chronic 571.2
   mania (acute) (chronic) 291.9

Alcohol, alcoholic — *continued*
   mood 291.89
   paranoia 291.5
   paranoid (type) psychosis 291.5
   pellagra 265.2
   poisoning, accidental (acute) NEC 980.9
      specified type of alcohol — *see* Table of Drugs and Chemicals
   psychosis (*see also* Psychosis, alcoholic) 291.9
   Korsakoff's, Korsakov's, Korsakow's 291.1
   polyneuritic 291.1
      with
         delusions 291.5
         hallucinations 291.3
   related disorder 291.9
   withdrawal symptoms, syndrome NEC 291.81
      delirium 291.0
      hallucinosis 291.3
Alcoholism 303.9

> Note — Use the following fifth-digit subclassification with category 303:
> 0 unspecified
> 1 continuous
> 2 episodic
> 3 in remission

   with psychosis (*see also* Psychosis, alcoholic) 291.9
   acute 303.0
   chronic 303.9
      with psychosis 291.9
   complicating pregnancy, childbirth, or puerperium 648.4
      affecting fetus or newborn 760.71
   history V11.3
   Korsakoff's, Korsakov's, Korsakow's 291.1
   suspected damage to fetus affecting management of pregnancy 655.4
Alder's anomaly or syndrome (leukocyte granulation anomaly) 288.2
Alder-Reilly anomaly (leukocyte granulation) 288.2
Aldosteronism (primary) 255.10
   congenital 255.10
   familial type I 255.11
   glucocorticoid-remediable 255.11
   secondary 255.14
Aldosteronoma (M8370/1) 237.2
Aldrich (-Wiskott) syndrome (eczema-thrombocytopenia) 279.12
Aleppo boil 085.1
Aleukemic — *see* condition
Aleukia
   congenital 288.09
   hemorrhagica 284.9
      acquired (secondary) 284.8
      congenital 284.09
      idiopathic 284.9
   splenica 289.4
Alexia (congenital) (developmental) 315.01
   secondary to organic lesion 784.61
Algoneurodystrophy 733.7
Algophobia 300.29
Alibert-Bazin disease (M9700/3) 202.1
Alibert's disease (mycosis fungoides) (M9700/3) 202.1
Alice in Wonderland syndrome 293.89
Alienation, mental — *see also* Psychosis 298.9
Alkalemia 276.3
Alkalosis 276.3
   metabolic 276.3
      with respiratory acidosis 276.4
   respiratory 276.3
Alkaptonuria 270.2
Allen-Masters syndrome 620.6

Index to Diseases

Allergic bronchopulmonary aspergillosis 518.6
Allergy, allergic (reaction) 995.3
  air-borne substance — *see also* Fever, hay 477.9
    specified allergen NEC 477.8
  alveolitis (extrinsic) 495.9
    due to
      Aspergillus clavatus 495.4
      cryptostroma corticale 495.6
      organisms (fungal, thermophilic actinomycete, other)
        growing in ventilation (air conditioning systems) 495.7
    specified type NEC 495.8
  anaphylactic shock 999.4
    due to food — *see* Anaphylactic shock, due to, food
  angioneurotic edema 995.1
  animal (cat) (dog) (epidermal) 477.8
    dander 477.2
    hair 477.2
  arthritis (*see also* Arthritis, allergic) 716.2 ☑
  asthma — *see* Asthma
  bee sting (anaphylactic shock) 989.5
  biological — *see* Allergy, drug
  bronchial asthma — *see* Asthma
  conjunctivitis (eczematous) 372.14
  dander, animal (cat) (dog) 477.2
  dandruff 477.8
  dermatitis (venenata) — *see* Dermatitis
  diathesis V15.09
  drug, medicinal substance, and biological (any) (correct medicinal substance properly administered) (external) (internal) 995.27 ▲
    wrong substance given or taken NEC 977.9
      specified drug or substance — *see* Table of Drugs and Chemicals
  dust (house) (stock) 477.8
  eczema — *see* Eczema
  endophthalmitis 360.19
  epidermal (animal) 477.8
  existing dental restorative maerial 525.66 ●
  feathers 477.8
  food (any) (ingested) 693.1
    atopic 691.8
    in contact with skin 692.5
  gastritis 535.4 ☑
  gastroenteritis 558.3
  gastrointestinal 558.3
  grain 477.0
  grass (pollen) 477.0
    asthma (*see also* Asthma) 493.0 ☑
    hay fever 477.0
  hair, animal (cat) (dog) 477.2
  hay fever (grass) (pollen) (ragweed) (tree) (*see also* Fever, hay) 477.9
  history (of) V15.09
    to
      eggs V15.03
      food additives V15.05
      insect bite V15.06
      latex V15.07
      milk products V15.02
      nuts V15.05
        peanuts V15.01
      radiographic dye V15.08
      seafood V15.04
      specified food NEC V15.05
      spider bite V15.06
  horse serum — *see* Allergy, serum
  inhalant 477.9
    dust 477.8
    pollen 477.0
    specified allergen other than pollen 477.8
  kapok 477.8
  medicine — *see* Allergy, drug

Allergy, allergic — *continued*
  migraine 346.2 ☑
  milk protein 558.3
  pannus 370.62
  pneumonia 518.3
  pollen (any) (hay fever) 477.0
    asthma (*see also* Asthma) 493.0 ☑
  primrose 477.0
  primula 477.0
  purpura 287.0
  ragweed (pollen) (Senecio jacobae) 477.0
    asthma (*see also* Asthma) 493.0 ☑
    hay fever 477.0
  respiratory (*see also* Allergy, inhalant) 477.9
    due to
      drug — *see* Allergy, drug
      food — *see* Allergy, food
  rhinitis (*see also* Fever, hay) 477.9
    due to food 477.1
  rose 477.0
  Senecio jacobae 477.0
  serum (prophylactic) (therapeutic) 999.5
    anaphylactic shock 999.4
  shock (anaphylactic) (due to adverse effect of correct medicinal substance properly administered) 995.0
    food — *see* Anaphylactic shock, due to, food
    from serum or immunization 999.5
      anaphylactic 999.4
  sinusitis (*see also* Fever, hay) 477.9
  skin reaction 692.9
    specified substance — *see* Dermatitis, due to
  tree (any) (hay fever) (pollen) 477.0
    asthma (*see also* Asthma) 493.0 ☑
  upper respiratory (*see also* Fever, hay) 477.9
  urethritis 597.89
  urticaria 708.0
  vaccine — *see* Allergy, serum
Allescheriosis 117.6
Alligator skin disease (ichthyosis congenita) 757.1
  acquired 701.1
Allocheiria, allochiria — *see also* Disturbance, sensation 782.0
Almeida's disease (Brazilian blastomycosis) 116.1
Alopecia (atrophicans) (pregnancy) (premature) (senile) 704.00
  adnata 757.4
  areata 704.01
  celsi 704.01
  cicatrisata 704.09
  circumscripta 704.01
  congenital, congenitalis 757.4
  disseminata 704.01
  effluvium (telogen) 704.02
  febrile 704.09
  generalisata 704.09
  hereditaria 704.09
  marginalis 704.01
  mucinosa 704.09
  postinfectional 704.09
  seborrheica 704.09
  specific 091.82
  syphilitic (secondary) 091.82
  telogen effluvium 704.02
  totalis 704.09
  toxica 704.09
  universalis 704.09
  x-ray 704.09
Alpers' disease 330.8
Alpha-lipoproteinemia 272.4
Alpha thalassemia 282.49
Alphos 696.1
Alpine sickness 993.2
Alport's syndrome (hereditary hematuria-nephropathy-deafness) 759.89
Alteration (of), altered
  awareness 780.09

Alteration, altered — *continued*
  awareness — *continued*
    transient 780.02
    consciousness 780.09
      persistent vegetative state 780.03
      transient 780.02
    mental status 780.97 ▲
      amnesia (retrograde) 780.93
      memory loss 780.93
Alternaria (infection) 118
Alternating — *see* condition
Altitude, high (effects) — *see* Effect, adverse, high altitude
Aluminosis (of lung) 503
Alvarez syndrome (transient cerebral ischemia) 435.9
Alveolar capillary block syndrome 516.3
Alveolitis
  allergic (extrinsic) 495.9
    due to organisms (fungal, thermophilic actinomycete, other)
      growing in ventilation (air conditioning systems) 495.7
    specified type NEC 495.8
  due to
    Aspergillus clavatus 495.4
    Cryptostroma corticale 495.6
  fibrosing (chronic) (cryptogenic) (lung) 516.3
    idiopathic 516.3
    rheumatoid 714.81
  jaw 526.5
  sicca dolorosa 526.5
Alveolus, alveolar — *see* condition
Alymphocytosis (pure) 279.2
Alymphoplasia, thymic 279.2
Alzheimer's
  dementia (senile)
    with behavioral disturbance 331.0 [294.11]
    without behavioral disturbance 331.0 [294.10]
  disease or sclerosis 331.0
    with dementia — *see* Alzheimer's, dementia
Amastia — *see also* Absence, breast 611.8
Amaurosis (acquired) (congenital) — *see also* Blindness 369.00
  fugax 362.34
  hysterical 300.11
  Leber's (congenital) 362.76
  tobacco 377.34
  uremic — *see* Uremia
Amaurotic familial idiocy (infantile) (juvenile) (late) 330.1
Ambisexual 752.7
Amblyopia (acquired) (congenital) (partial) 368.00
  color 368.59
    acquired 368.55
  deprivation 368.02
  ex anopsia 368.00
  hysterical 300.11
  nocturnal 368.60
    vitamin A deficiency 264.5
  refractive 368.03
  strabismic 368.01
  suppression 368.01
  tobacco 377.34
  toxic NEC 377.34
  uremic — *see* Uremia
Ameba, amebic (histolytica) — *see also* Amebiasis
  abscess 006.3
    bladder 006.8
    brain (with liver and lung abscess) 006.5
    liver 006.3
      with
        brain abscess (and lung abscess) 006.5
        lung abscess 006.4
    lung (with liver abscess) 006.4
      with brain abscess 006.5

Ameba, amebic — *see also* Amebiasis — *continued*
  abscess — *continued*
    seminal vesicle 006.8
    spleen 006.8
  carrier (suspected of) V02.2
  meningoencephalitis
    due to Naegleria (gruberi) 136.2
    primary 136.2
Amebiasis NEC 006.9
  with
    brain abscess (with liver or lung abscess) 006.5
    liver abscess (without mention of brain or lung abscess) 006.3
    lung abscess (with liver abscess) 006.4
      with brain abscess 006.5
  acute 006.0
  bladder 006.8
  chronic 006.1
  cutaneous 006.6
  cutis 006.6
  due to organism other than Entamoeba histolytica 007.8
  hepatic (*see also* Abscess, liver, amebic) 006.3
  nondysenteric 006.2
  seminal vesicle 006.8
  specified
    organism NEC 007.8
    site NEC 006.8
Ameboma 006.8
Amelia 755.4
  lower limb 755.31
  upper limb 755.21
Ameloblastoma (M9310/0) 213.1
  jaw (bone) (lower) 213.1
    upper 213.0
  long bones (M9261/3) — *see* Neoplasm, bone, malignant
  malignant (M9310/3) 170.1
    jaw (bone) (lower) 170.1
      upper 170.0
  mandible 213.1
  tibial (M9261/3) 170.7
Amelogenesis imperfecta 520.5
  nonhereditaria (segmentalis) 520.4
Amenorrhea (primary) (secondary) 626.0
  due to ovarian dysfunction 256.8
  hyperhormonal 256.8
Amentia — *see also* Retardation, mental 319
  Meynert's (nonalcoholic) 294.0
    alcoholic 291.1
  nevoid 759.6
American
  leishmaniasis 085.5
  mountain tick fever 066.1
  trypanosomiasis — *see* Trypanosomiasis, American
Ametropia — *see also* Disorder, accommodation 367.9
Amianthosis 501
Amimia 784.69
Amino acid
  deficiency 270.9
    anemia 281.4
  metabolic disorder (*see also* Disorder, amino acid) 270.9
Aminoaciduria 270.9
  imidazole 270.5
Amnesia (retrograde) 780.93
  auditory 784.69
    developmental 315.31
    secondary to organic lesion 784.69
  dissociative 300.12
  hysterical or dissociative type 300.12
  psychogenic 300.12
  transient global 437.7
Amnestic (confabulatory) **syndrome** 294.0
  alcohol-induced persisting 291.1
  drug-induced persisting 292.83
  posttraumatic 294.0
Amniocentesis screening (for) V28.2

Amniocentesis screening

Amniocentesis screening — continued
  alphafetoprotein level, raised V28.1
  chromosomal anomalies V28.0
Amnion, amniotic — see also condition
  nodosum 658.8 ☑
Amnionitis (complicating pregnancy) 658.4 ☑
  affecting fetus or newborn 762.7
Amoral trends 301.7
Amotio retinae — see also Detachment, retina 361.9
Ampulla
  lower esophagus 530.89
  phrenic 530.89
Amputation
  any part of fetus, to facilitate delivery 763.89
  cervix (supravaginal) (uteri) 622.8
    in pregnancy or childbirth 654.6 ☑
      affecting fetus or newborn 763.89
  clitoris — see Wound, open, clitoris
  congenital
    lower limb 755.31
    upper limb 755.21
  neuroma (traumatic) (see also Injury, nerve, by site)
  surgical complication (late) 997.61
  penis — see Amputation, traumatic, penis
  status (without complication) — see Absence, by site, acquired
  stump (surgical) (posttraumatic)
    abnormal, painful, or with complication (late) 997.60
    healed or old NEC (see also Absence, by site, acquired)
      lower V49.70
      upper V49.60
  traumatic (complete) (partial)

Note — "Complicated" includes traumatic amputation with delayed healing, delayed treatment, foreign body, or infection.

    arm 887.4
      at or above elbow 887.2
        complicated 887.3
      below elbow 887.0
        complicated 887.1
      both (bilateral) (any level(s)) 887.6
        complicated 887.7
      complicated 887.5
    finger(s) (one or both hands) 886.0
      with thumb(s) 885.0
        complicated 885.1
      complicated 886.1
    foot (except toe(s) only) 896.0
      and other leg 897.6
        complicated 897.7
      both (bilateral) 896.2
        complicated 896.3
      complicated 896.1
      toe(s) only (one or both feet) 895.0
        complicated 895.1
    genital organ(s) (external) NEC 878.8
      complicated 878.9
    hand (except finger(s) only) 887.0
      and other arm 887.6
        complicated 887.7
      both (bilateral) 887.6
        complicated 887.7
      complicated 887.1
      finger(s) (one or both hands) 886.0
        with thumb(s) 885.0
          complicated 885.1
        complicated 886.1
      thumb(s) (with fingers of either hand) 885.0
        complicated 885.1
    head 874.9

Amputation — continued
  traumatic — continued
    late effect — see Late, effects (of), amputation
    leg 897.4
      and other foot 897.6
        complicated 897.7
      at or above knee 897.2
        complicated 897.3
      below knee 897.0
        complicated 897.1
      both (bilateral) 897.6
        complicated 897.7
      complicated 897.5
    lower limb(s) except toe(s) — see Amputation, traumatic, leg
    nose — see Wound, open, nose
    penis 878.0
      complicated 878.1
    sites other than limbs — see Wound, open, by site
    thumb(s) (with finger(s) of either hand) 885.0
      complicated 885.1
    toe(s) (one or both feet) 895.0
      complicated 895.1
    upper limb(s) — see Amputation, traumatic, arm
Amputee (bilateral) (old) — see also Absence, by site, acquired V49.70
Amusia 784.69
  developmental 315.39
  secondary to organic lesion 784.69
Amyelencephalus 740.0
Amyelia 742.59
Amygdalitis — see Tonsillitis
Amygdalolith 474.8
Amyloid disease or degeneration 277.30
  heart 277.39 [425.7] ▲
Amyloidosis (familial) (general) (generalized) (genetic) (primary) 277.39 ▲
  with lung involvement 277.39 [517.8] ▲
  cardiac, hereditary 277.39 ●
  heart 277.39 [425.7] ▲
  nephropathic 277.39 [583.81] ▲
  neuropathic (Portuguese) (Swiss) 277.39 [357.4] ▲
  pulmonary 277.39 [517.8] ▲
  secondary 277.39 ●
  systemic, inherited 277.39 ▲
Amylopectinosis (brancher enzyme deficiency) 271.0
Amylophagia 307.52
Amyoplasia, congenita 756.89
Amyotonia 728.2
  congenita 358.8
Amyotrophia, amyotrophy, amyotrophic 728.2
  congenita 756.89
  diabetic 250.6 ☑ [358.1]
  lateral sclerosis (syndrome) 335.20
  neuralgic 353.5
  sclerosis (lateral) 335.20
  spinal progressive 335.21
Anacidity, gastric 536.0
  psychogenic 306.4
Anaerosis of newborn 770.88 ▲
Analbuminemia 273.8
Analgesia — see also Anesthesia 782.0
Analphalipoproteinemia 272.5
Anaphylactic shock or reaction (correct substance properly administered) 995.0
  due to
    food 995.60
      additives 995.66
      crustaceans 995.62
      eggs 995.68
      fish 995.65
      fruits 995.63
      milk products 995.67
      nuts (tree) 995.64
      peanuts 995.61

Anaphylactic shock or reaction — continued
  due to — continued
    food — continued
      seeds 995.64
      specified NEC 995.69
      tree nuts 995.64
      vegetables 995.63
    immunization 999.4
    overdose or wrong substance given or taken 977.9
      specified drug — see Table of Drugs and Chemicals
    serum 999.4
  following sting(s) 989.5
  purpura 287.0
  serum 999.4
Anaphylactoid shock or reaction — see Anaphylactic shock
Anaphylaxis — see Anaphylactic shock
Anaplasia, cervix 622.10
Anarthria 784.5
Anarthritic rheumatoid disease 446.5
Anasarca 782.3
  cardiac (see also Failure, heart) 428.0
  fetus or newborn 778.0
  lung 514
  nutritional 262
  pulmonary 514
  renal (see also Nephrosis) 581.9
Anaspadias 752.62
Anastomosis
  aneurysmal — see Aneurysm
  arteriovenous, congenital NEC (see also Anomaly, arteriovenous) 747.60
    ruptured, of brain (see also Hemorrhage, subarachnoid) 430
  intestinal 569.89
    complicated NEC 997.4
      involving urinary tract 997.5
  retinal and choroidal vessels 743.58
    acquired 362.17
Anatomical narrow angle (glaucoma) 365.02
Ancylostoma (infection) (infestation) 126.9
  americanus 126.1
  braziliense 126.2
  caninum 126.8
  ceylanicum 126.3
  duodenale 126.0
  Necator americanus 126.1
Ancylostomiasis (intestinal) 126.9
  ancylostoma
    americanus 126.1
    caninum 126.8
    ceylanicum 126.3
    duodenale 126.0
    braziliense 126.2
    Necator americanus 126.1
Anders' disease or syndrome (adiposis tuberosa simplex) 272.8
Andersen's glycogen storage disease 271.0
Anderson's disease 272.7
Andes disease 993.2
Andrews' disease (bacterid) 686.8
Androblastoma (M8630/1)
  benign (M8630/0)
    specified site — see Neoplasm, by site, benign
    unspecified site
      female 220
      male 222.0
  malignant (M8630/3)
    specified site — see Neoplasm, by site, malignant
    unspecified site
      female 183.0
      male 186.9
  specified site — see Neoplasm, by site, uncertain behavior

Androblastoma — continued
  tubular (M8640/0)
    with lipid storage (M8641/0)
      specified site — see Neoplasm, by site, benign
      unspecified site
        female 220
        male 222.0
    specified site — see Neoplasm, by site, benign
    unspecified site
      female 220
      male 222.0
  unspecified site
    female 236.2
    male 236.4
Android pelvis 755.69
  with disproportion (fetopelvic) 653.3 ☑
    affecting fetus or newborn 763.1
  causing obstructed labor 660.1 ☑
    affecting fetus or newborn 763.1
Anectasis, pulmonary (newborn or fetus) 770.5
Anemia 285.9
  with
    disorder of
      anaerobic glycolysis 282.3
      pentose phosphate pathway 282.2
    koilonychia 280.9
  6-phosphogluconic dehydrogenase deficiency 282.2
  achlorhydric 280.9
  achrestic 281.8
  Addison's (pernicious) 281.0
  Addison-Biermer (pernicious) 281.0
  agranulocytic 288.09 ▲
  amino acid deficiency 281.4
  aplastic 284.9
    acquired (secondary) 284.8
    congenital 284.01 ▲
    constitutional 284.01 ▲
    due to
      chronic systemic disease 284.8
      drugs 284.8
      infection 284.8
      radiation 284.8
    idiopathic 284.9
    myxedema 244.9
    of or complicating pregnancy 648.2 ☑
    red cell (acquired) (with thymoma) 284.8
      congenital 284.01 ▲
      pure 284.01 ●
    specified type NEC 284.8
    toxic (paralytic) 284.8
  aregenerative 284.9
    congenital 284.01 ▲
  asiderotic 280.9
  atypical (primary) 285.9
  autohemolysis of Selwyn and Dacie (type I) 282.2
  autoimmune hemolytic 283.0
  Baghdad Spring 282.2
  Balantidium coli 007.0
  Biermer's (pernicious) 281.0
  blood loss (chronic) 280.0
    acute 285.1
  bothriocephalus 123.4
  brickmakers' (see also Ancylostomiasis) 126.9
  cerebral 437.8
  childhood 282.9
  chlorotic 280.9
  chronica congenita aregenerativa 284.01 ▲
  chronic simple 281.9
  combined system disease NEC 281.0 [336.2]
    due to dietary deficiency 281.1 [336.2]
  complicating pregnancy or childbirth 648.2 ☑
  congenital (following fetal blood loss) 776.5

Index to Diseases — Anemia

Anemia — *continued*
- congenital — *continued*
  - aplastic 284.01 ▲
  - due to isoimmunization NEC 773.2
  - Heinz-body 282.7
  - hereditary hemolytic NEC 282.9
  - nonspherocytic
    - Type I 282.2
    - Type II 282.3
  - pernicious 281.0
  - spherocytic (*see also* Spherocytosis) 282.0
- Cooley's (erythroblastic) 282.49
- crescent — *see* Disease, sickle-cell
- cytogenic 281.0
- Dacie's (nonspherocytic)
  - type I 282.2
  - type II 282.3
- Davidson's (refractory) 284.9
- deficiency 281.9
  - 2, 3 diphosphoglycurate mutase 282.3
  - 2, 3 PG 282.3
  - 6-PGD 282.2
  - 6-phosphogluronic dehydrogenase 282.2
  - amino acid 281.4
  - combined B_{12} and folate 281.3
  - enzyme, drug-induced (hemolytic) 282.2
  - erythrocytic glutathione 282.2
  - folate 281.2
    - dietary 281.2
    - drug-induced 281.2
  - folic acid 281.2
    - dietary 281.2
    - drug-induced 281.2
  - G-6-PD 282.2
  - GGS-R 282.2
  - glucose-6-phosphate dehydrogenase (G-6-PD) 282.2
  - glucose-phosphate isomerase 282.3
  - glutathione peroxidase 282.2
  - glutathione reductase 282.2
  - glyceraldehyde phosphate dehydrogenase 282.3
  - GPI 282.3
  - G SH 282.2
  - hexokinase 282.3
  - iron (Fe) 280.9
    - specified NEC 280.8
  - nutritional 281.9
    - with
      - poor iron absorption 280.9
      - specified deficiency NEC 281.8
    - due to inadequate dietary iron intake 280.1
    - specified type NEC 281.8
  - of or complicating pregnancy 648.2 ☑
  - pentose phosphate pathway 282.2
  - PFK 282.3
  - phosphofructo-aldolase 282.3
  - phosphofructokinase 282.3
  - phosphoglycerate kinase 282.3
  - PK 282.3
  - protein 281.4
  - pyruvate kinase (PK) 282.3
  - TPI 282.3
  - triosephosphate isomerase 282.3
  - vitamin B_{12} NEC 281.1
    - dietary 281.1
    - pernicious 281.0
- Diamond-Blackfan (congenital hypoplastic) 284.01 ▲
- dibothriocephalus 123.4
- dimorphic 281.9
- diphasic 281.8
- diphtheritic 032.89
- Diphyllobothrium 123.4
- drepanocytic (*see also* Disease, sickle-cell) 282.60
- due to
  - blood loss (chronic) 280.0
    - acute 285.1

Anemia — *continued*
- due to — *continued*
  - defect of Embden-Meyerhof pathway glycolysis 282.3
  - disorder of glutathione metabolism 282.2
  - fetal blood loss 776.5
  - fish tapeworm (D. latum) infestation 123.4
  - glutathione metabolism disorder 282.2
  - hemorrhage (chronic) 280.0
    - acute 285.1
  - hexose monophosphate (HMP) shunt deficiency 282.2
  - impaired absorption 280.9
  - loss of blood (chronic) 280.0
    - acute 285.1
  - myxedema 244.9
  - Necator americanus 126.1
  - prematurity 776.6
  - selective vitamin B_{12} malabsorption with proteinuria 281.1
- Dyke-Young type (secondary) (symptomatic) 283.9
- dyserythropoietic (congenital) (types I, II, III) 285.8
- dyshemopoietic (congenital) 285.8
- Egypt (*see also* Ancylostomiasis) 126.9
- elliptocytosis (*see also* Elliptocytosis) 282.1
- enzyme deficiency, drug-induced 282.2
- epidemic (*see also* Ancylostomiasis) 126.9
- EPO resistant 285.21
- erythroblastic
  - familial 282.49
  - fetus or newborn (*see also* Disease, hemolytic) 773.2
  - late 773.5
- erythrocytic glutathione deficiency 282.2
- erythropoietin-resistant (EPO resistant anemia) 285.21
- essential 285.9
- Faber's (achlorhydric anemia) 280.9
- factitious (self-induced blood letting) 280.0
- familial erythroblastic (microcytic) 282.49
- Fanconi's (congenital pancytopenia) 284.09 ▲
- favism 282.2
- fetal, following blood loss 776.5
- fetus or newborn
  - due to
    - ABO
      - antibodies 773.1
      - incompatibility, maternal/fetal 773.1
      - isoimmunization 773.1
    - Rh
      - antibodies 773.0
      - incompatibility, maternal/fetal 773.0
      - isoimmunization 773.0
    - following fetal blood loss 776.5
  - fish tapeworm (D. latum) infestation 123.4
- folate (folic acid) deficiency 281.2
  - dietary 281.2
  - drug-induced 281.2
- folate malabsorption, congenital 281.2
- folic acid deficiency 281.2
  - dietary 281.2
  - drug-induced 281.2
- G-6-PD 282.2
- general 285.9
- glucose-6-phosphate dehydrogenase deficiency 282.2
- glutathione-reductase deficiency 282.2
- goat's milk 281.2
- granulocytic 288.09 ▲
- Heinz-body, congenital 282.7
- hemoglobin deficiency 285.9

Anemia — *continued*
- hemolytic 283.9
  - acquired 283.9
    - with hemoglobinuria NEC 283.2
    - autoimmune (cold type) (idiopathic) (primary) (secondary) (symptomatic) (warm type) 283.0
    - due to
      - cold reactive antibodies 283.0
      - drug exposure 283.0
      - warm reactive antibodies 283.0
    - fragmentation 283.19
    - idiopathic (chronic) 283.9
    - infectious 283.19
      - autoimmune 283.0
    - non-autoimmune 283.10
    - toxic 283.19
    - traumatic cardiac 283.19
  - acute 283.9
    - due to enzyme deficiency NEC 282.3
    - fetus or newborn (*see also* Disease, hemolytic) 773.2
      - late 773.5
    - Lederer's (acquired infectious hemolytic anemia) 283.19
  - autoimmune (acquired) 283.0
  - chronic 282.9
    - idiopathic 283.9
  - cold type (secondary) (symptomatic) 283.0
  - congenital (spherocytic) (*see also* Spherocytosis) 282.0
    - nonspherocytic — *see* Anemia, hemolytic, nonspherocytic, congenital
  - drug-induced 283.0
    - enzyme deficiency 282.2
    - due to
      - cardiac conditions 283.19
      - drugs 283.0
      - enzyme deficiency NEC 282.3
        - drug-induced 282.2
      - presence of shunt or other internal prosthetic device 283.19
      - thrombotic thrombocytopenic purpura 446.6
  - elliptocytotic (*see also* Elliptocytosis) 282.1
  - familial 282.9
  - hereditary 282.9
    - due to enzyme deficiency NEC 282.3
    - specified NEC 282.8
  - idiopathic (chronic) 283.9
  - infectious (acquired) 283.19
  - mechanical 283.19
  - microangiopathic 283.19
  - non-autoimmune NEC 283.10
  - nonspherocytic
    - congenital or hereditary NEC 282.3
      - glucose-6-phosphate dehydrogenase deficiency 282.2
      - pyruvate kinase (PK) deficiency 282.3
      - type I 282.2
      - type II 282.3
    - type I 282.2
    - type II 282.3
  - of or complicating pregnancy 648.2 ☑
  - resulting from presence of shunt or other internal prosthetic device 283.19
  - secondary 283.19
    - autoimmune 283.0
  - sickle-cell — *see* Disease, sickle-cell

Anemia — *continued*
- hemolytic — *continued*
  - Stransky-Regala type (Hb-E) (*see also* Disease, hemoglobin) 282.7
  - symptomatic 283.19
    - autoimmune 283.0
  - toxic (acquired) 283.19
  - uremic (adult) (child) 283.11
  - warm type (secondary) (symptomatic) 283.0
- hemorrhagic (chronic) 280.0
  - acute 285.1
- HEMPAS 285.8
- hereditary erythroblast multinuclearity-positive acidified serum test 285.8
- Herrick's (hemoglobin S disease) 282.61
- hexokinase deficiency 282.3
- high A_2 282.49
- hookworm (*see also* Ancylostomiasis) 126.9
- hypochromic (idiopathic) (microcytic) (normoblastic) 280.9
  - with iron loading 285.0
  - due to blood loss (chronic) 280.0
    - acute 285.1
  - familial sex linked 285.0
  - pyridoxine-responsive 285.0
- hypoplasia, red blood cells 284.8
  - congenital or familial 284.01 ▲
- hypoplastic (idiopathic) 284.9
  - congenital 284.01 ▲
  - familial 284.01 ▲
  - of childhood 284.09 ▲
- idiopathic 285.9
  - hemolytic, chronic 283.9
- in
  - chronic illness NEC 285.29
  - chronic kidney disease 285.21
  - end-stage renal disease 285.21
  - neoplastic disease 285.22
- infantile 285.9
- infective, infectional 285.9
- intertropical (*see also* Ancylostomiasis) 126.9
- iron (Fe) deficiency 280.9
  - due to blood loss (chronic) 280.0
    - acute 285.1
  - of or complicating pregnancy 648.2 ☑
  - specified NEC 280.8
- Jaksch's (pseudoleukemia infantum) 285.8
- Joseph-Diamond-Blackfan (congenital hypoplastic) 284.01 ▲
- labyrinth 386.50
- Lederer's (acquired infectious hemolytic anemia) 283.19
- leptocytosis (hereditary) 282.49
- leukoerythroblastic 284.2 ▲
- macrocytic 281.9
  - nutritional 281.2
  - of or complicating pregnancy 648.2 ☑
  - tropical 281.2
- malabsorption (familial), selective B_{12} with proteinuria 281.1
- malarial (*see also* Malaria) 084.6
- malignant (progressive) 281.0
- malnutrition 281.9
- marsh (*see also* Malaria) 084.6
- Mediterranean (with hemoglobinopathy) 282.49
- megaloblastic 281.9
  - combined B_{12} and folate deficiency 281.3
  - nutritional (of infancy) 281.2
  - of infancy 281.2
  - of or complicating pregnancy 648.2 ☑
  - refractory 281.3
  - specified NEC 281.3
- megalocytic 281.9
- microangiopathic hemolytic 283.19

Anemia

Anemia — *continued*
  microcytic (hypochromic) 280.9
    due to blood loss (chronic) 280.0
      acute 285.1
    familial 282.49
    hypochromic 280.9
  microdrepanocytosis 282.49
  miners' (*see also* Ancylostomiasis) 126.9
  myelopathic 285.8
  myelophthisic (normocytic) 284.2 ▲
  newborn (*see also* Disease, hemolytic) 773.2
    due to isoimmunization (*see also* Disease, hemolytic) 773.2
    late, due to isoimmunization 773.5
    posthemorrhagic 776.5
  nonregenerative 284.9
  nonspherocytic hemolytic — *see* Anemia, hemolytic, nonspherocytic
  normocytic (infectional) (not due to blood loss) 285.9
    due to blood loss (chronic) 280.0
      acute 285.1
    myelophthisic 284.2 ▲
  nutritional (deficiency) 281.9
    with
      poor iron absorption 280.9
      specified deficiency NEC 281.8
    due to inadequate dietary iron intake 280.1
    megaloblastic (of infancy) 281.2
  of childhood 282.9
  of chronic •
    disease NEC 285.29 •
    illness NEC 285.29 •
  of or complicating pregnancy 648.2 ☑
    affecting fetus or newborn 760.8
  of prematurity 776.6
  orotic aciduric (congenital) (hereditary) 281.4
  osteosclerotic 289.89
  ovalocytosis (hereditary) (*see also* Elliptocytosis) 282.1
  paludal (*see also* Malaria) 084.6
  pentose phosphate pathway deficiency 282.2
  pernicious (combined system disease) (congenital) (dorsolateral spinal degeneration) (juvenile) (myelopathy) (neuropathy) (posterior sclerosis) (primary) (progressive) (spleen) 281.0
    of or complicating pregnancy 648.2 ☑
  pleochromic 285.9
    of sprue 281.8
  portal 285.8
  posthemorrhagic (chronic) 280.0
    acute 285.1
    newborn 776.5
  postoperative
    due to blood loss 285.1
    other 285.9
  postpartum 648.2 ☑
  pressure 285.9
  primary 285.9
  profound 285.9
  progressive 285.9
    malignant 281.0
    pernicious 281.0
  protein-deficiency 281.4
  pseudoleukemica infantum 285.8
  puerperal 648.2 ☑
  pure red cell 284.8
    congenital 284.01 ▲
  pyridoxine-responsive (hypochromic) 285.0
  pyruvate kinase (PK) deficiency 282.3
  refractoria sideroblastica 238.72 ▲
  refractory (primary) 238.72 ▲
    with
      excess •
        blasts-1 (RAEB-1) 238.73 •
        blasts-2 (RAEB-2) 238.73 •
      hemochromatosis 238.72 •

Anemia — *continued*
  refractory — *continued*
    with — *continued*
      ringed sideroblasts (RARS) • 238.72 •
      megaloblastic 281.3
      sideroblastic 238.72
      sideropenic 280.9
    Rietti-Greppi-Micheli (thalassemia minor) 282.49
  scorbutic 281.8
  secondary (to) 285.9
    blood loss (chronic) 280.0
      acute 285.1
    hemorrhage 280.0
      acute 285.1
    inadequate dietary iron intake 280.1
  semiplastic 284.9
  septic 285.9
  sickle-cell (*see also* Disease, sickle-cell) 282.60
  sideroachrestic 285.0
  sideroblastic (acquired) (any type) (congenital) (drug-induced) (due to disease) (hereditary) (primary) (secondary) (sex-linked hypochromic) (vitamin B_6 responsive) 285.0
    refractory 238.72 ▲
  sideropenic (refractory) 280.9
    due to blood loss (chronic) 280.0
      acute 285.1
  simple chronic 281.9
  specified type NEC 285.8
  spherocytic (hereditary) (*see also* Spherocytosis) 282.0
  splenic 285.8
    familial (Gaucher's) 272.7
  splenomegalic 285.8
  stomatocytosis 282.8
  syphilitic 095.8
  target cell (oval) 282.49
  thalassemia 282.49
  thrombocytopenic (*see also* Thrombocytopenia) 287.5
  toxic 284.8
  triosephosphate isomerase deficiency 282.3
  tropical, macrocytic 281.2
  tuberculous (*see also* Tuberculosis) 017.9 ☑
  vegan's 281.1
  vitamin
    B_6-responsive 285.0
    B_{12} deficiency (dietary) 281.1
      pernicious 281.0
  von Jaksch's (pseudoleukemia infantum) 285.8
  Witts' (achlorhydric anemia) 280.9
  Zuelzer (-Ogden) (nutritional megaloblastic anemia) 281.2
Anencephalus, anencephaly 740.0
  fetal, affecting management of pregnancy 655.0 ☑
Anergasia — *see also* Psychosis, organic 294.9
  senile 290.0
Anesthesia, anesthetic 782.0
  complication or reaction NEC 995.22 ▲
    due to
      correct substance properly administered 995.22 ▲
      overdose or wrong substance given 968.4
      specified anesthetic — *see* Table of Drugs and Chemicals
  cornea 371.81
  death from
    correct substance properly administered 995.4
    during delivery 668.9 ☑
    overdose or wrong substance given 968.4

Anesthesia, anesthetic — *continued*
  death from — *continued*
    specified anesthetic — *see* Table of Drugs and Chemicals
  eye 371.81
  functional 300.11
  hyperesthetic, thalamic 338.0 ▲
  hysterical 300.11
  local skin lesion 782.0
  olfactory 781.1
  sexual (psychogenic) 302.72
  shock
    due to
      correct substance properly administered 995.4
      overdose or wrong substance given 968.4
      specified anesthetic — *see* Table of Drugs and Chemicals
  skin 782.0
  tactile 782.0
  testicular 608.9
  thermal 782.0
Anetoderma (maculosum) 701.3
Aneuploidy NEC 758.5
Aneurin deficiency 265.1
Aneurysm (anastomotic) (artery) (cirsoid) (diffuse) (false) (fusiform) (multiple) (ruptured) (saccular) (varicose) 442.9
  abdominal (aorta) 441.4
    ruptured 441.3
    syphilitic 093.0
  aorta, aortic (nonsyphilitic) 441.9
    abdominal 441.4
      dissecting 441.02
      ruptured 441.3
      syphilitic 093.0
    arch 441.2
      ruptured 441.1
    arteriosclerotic NEC 441.9
      ruptured 441.5
    ascending 441.2
      ruptured 441.1
    congenital 747.29
    descending 441.9
      abdominal 441.4
        ruptured 441.3
      ruptured 441.5
      thoracic 441.2
        ruptured 441.1
    dissecting 441.00
      abdominal 441.02
      thoracic 441.01
      thoracoabdominal 441.03
    due to coarctation (aorta) 747.10
    ruptured 441.5
    sinus, right 747.29
    syphilitic 093.0
    thoracoabdominal 441.7
      ruptured 441.6
    thorax, thoracic (arch) (non-syphilitic) 441.2
      dissecting 441.01
      ruptured 441.1
      syphilitic 093.0
    transverse 441.2
      ruptured 441.1
    valve (heart) (*see also* Endocarditis, aortic) 424.1
  arteriosclerotic NEC 442.9
    cerebral 437.3
      ruptured (*see also* Hemorrhage, subarachnoid) 430
    arteriovenous (congenital) (peripheral) NEC (*see also* Anomaly, arteriovenous) 747.60
      acquired NEC 447.0
      brain 437.3
        ruptured (*see also* Hemorrhage, subarachnoid) 430
      coronary 414.11
      pulmonary 417.0
    brain (cerebral) 747.81

Aneurysm — *continued*
  arteriovenous (*see also* Anomaly, arteriovenous) — *continued*
    brain — *continued*
      ruptured (*see also* Hemorrhage, subarachnoid) 430
    coronary 746.85
    pulmonary 747.3
    retina 743.58
    specified site NEC 747.89
      acquired 447.0
    traumatic (*see also* Injury, blood vessel, by site) 904.9
  basal — *see* Aneurysm, brain
  berry (congenital) (ruptured) (*see also* Hemorrhage, subarachnoid) 430
  brain 437.3
    arteriosclerotic 437.3
      ruptured (*see also* Hemorrhage, subarachnoid) 430
    arteriovenous 747.81
      acquired 437.3
        ruptured (*see also* Hemorrhage, subarachnoid) 430
      ruptured (*see also* Hemorrhage, subarachnoid) 430
    berry (congenital) (ruptured) (*see also* Hemorrhage, subarachnoid) 430
    congenital 747.81
      ruptured (*see also* Hemorrhage, subarachnoid) 430
    meninges 437.3
      ruptured (*see also* Hemorrhage, subarachnoid) 430
    miliary (congenital) (ruptured) (*see also* Hemorrhage, subarachnoid) 430
    mycotic 421.0
      ruptured (*see also* Hemorrhage, subarachnoid) 430
    nonruptured 437.3
      ruptured (*see also* Hemorrhage, subarachnoid) 430
    syphilitic 094.87
    syphilitic (hemorrhage) 094.87
    traumatic — *see* Injury, intracranial
  cardiac (false) (*see also* Aneurysm, heart) 414.10
  carotid artery (common) (external) 442.81
    internal (intracranial portion) 437.3
      extracranial portion 442.81
      ruptured into brain (*see also* Hemorrhage, subarachnoid) 430
    syphilitic 093.89
      intracranial 094.87
  cavernous sinus (*see also* Aneurysm, brain) 437.3
    arteriovenous 747.81
      ruptured (*see also* Hemorrhage, subarachnoid) 430
    congenital 747.81
      ruptured (*see also* Hemorrhage, subarachnoid) 430
  celiac 442.84
  central nervous system, syphilitic 094.89
  cerebral — *see* Aneurysm, brain
  chest — *see* Aneurysm, thorax
  circle of Willis (*see also* Aneurysm, brain) 437.3
    congenital 747.81
      ruptured (*see also* Hemorrhage, subarachnoid) 430
    ruptured (*see also* Hemorrhage, subarachnoid) 430
  common iliac artery 442.2
  congenital (peripheral) NEC 747.60
    brain 747.81
      ruptured (*see also* Hemorrhage, subarachnoid) 430

Aneurysm — continued
- congenital — continued
  - cerebral — see Aneurysm, brain, congenital
  - coronary 746.85
  - gastrointestinal 747.61
  - lower limb 747.64
  - pulmonary 747.3
  - renal 747.62
  - retina 743.58
  - specified site NEC 747.89
  - spinal 747.82
  - upper limb 747.63
- conjunctiva 372.74
- conus arteriosus (see also Aneurysm, heart) 414.10
- coronary (arteriosclerotic) (artery) (vein) (see also Aneurysm, heart) 414.11
  - arteriovenous 746.85
  - congenital 746.85
  - syphilitic 093.89
- cylindrical 441.9
  - ruptured 441.5
  - syphilitic 093.9
- dissecting 442.9
  - aorta 441.00
    - abdominal 441.02
    - thoracic 441.01
    - thoracoabdominal 441.03
  - syphilitic 093.9
- ductus arteriosus 747.0
- embolic — see Embolism, artery
- endocardial, infective (any valve) 421.0
- femoral 442.3
- gastroduodenal 442.84
- gastroepiploic 442.84
- heart (chronic or with a stated duration of over 8 weeks) (infectional) (wall) 414.10
  - acute or with a stated duration of 8 weeks or less (see also Infarct, myocardium) 410.9 ✓
  - congenital 746.89
  - valve — see Endocarditis
- hepatic 442.84
- iliac (common) 442.2
- infective (any valve) 421.0
- innominate (nonsyphilitic) 442.89
  - syphilitic 093.89
- interauricular septum (see also Aneurysm, heart) 414.10
- interventricular septum (see also Aneurysm, heart) 414.10
- intracranial — see Aneurysm, brain
- intrathoracic (nonsyphilitic) 441.2
  - ruptured 441.1
  - syphilitic 093.0
- jugular vein 453.8
- lower extremity 442.3
- lung (pulmonary artery) 417.1
- malignant 093.9
- mediastinal (nonsyphilitic) 442.89
  - syphilitic 093.89
- miliary (congenital) (ruptured) (see also Hemorrhage, subarachnoid) 430
- mitral (heart) (valve) 424.0
- mural (arteriovenous) (heart) (see also Aneurysm, heart) 414.10
- mycotic, any site 421.0
  - without endocarditis — see Aneurysm by site ●
  - ruptured, brain (see also Hemorrhage, subarachnoid) 430
- myocardium (see also Aneurysm, heart) 414.10
- neck 442.81
- pancreaticoduodenal 442.84
- patent ductus arteriosus 747.0
- peripheral NEC 442.89
  - congenital NEC (see also Aneurysm, congenital) 747.60
- popliteal 442.3
- pulmonary 417.1

Aneurysm — continued
- pulmonary — continued
  - arteriovenous 747.3
    - acquired 417.0
  - syphilitic 093.89
  - valve (heart) (see also Endocarditis, pulmonary) 424.3
- racemose 442.9
  - congenital (peripheral) NEC 747.60
- radial 442.0
- Rasmussen's (see also Tuberculosis) 011.2 ✓
- renal 442.1
- retinal (acquired) 362.17
  - congenital 743.58
  - diabetic 250.5 ✓ [362.01]
- sinus, aortic (of Valsalva) 747.29
- specified site NEC 442.89
- spinal (cord) 442.89
  - congenital 747.82
  - syphilitic (hemorrhage) 094.89
- spleen, splenic 442.83
- subclavian 442.82
  - syphilitic 093.89
- superior mesenteric 442.84
- syphilitic 093.9
  - aorta 093.0
  - central nervous system 094.89
  - congenital 090.5
  - spine, spinal 094.89
- thoracoabdominal 441.7
  - ruptured 441.6
- thorax, thoracic (arch) (nonsyphilitic) 441.2
  - dissecting 441.01
  - ruptured 441.1
  - syphilitic 093.0
- traumatic (complication) (early) — see Injury, blood vessel, by site
- tricuspid (heart) (valve) — see Endocarditis, tricuspid
- ulnar 442.0
- upper extremity 442.0
- valve, valvular — see Endocarditis
- venous 456.8
  - congenital NEC (see also Aneurysm, congenital) 747.60
- ventricle (arteriovenous) (see also Aneurysm, heart) 414.10
- visceral artery NEC 442.84

Angiectasis 459.89
Angiectopia 459.9
Angiitis 447.6
- allergic granulomatous 446.4
- hypersensitivity 446.20
  - Goodpasture's syndrome 446.21
  - specified NEC 446.29
- necrotizing 446.0
- Wegener's (necrotizing respiratory granulomatosis) 446.4

Angina (attack) (cardiac) (chest) (effort) (heart) (pectoris) (syndrome) (vasomotor) 413.9
- abdominal 557.1
- accelerated 411.1
- agranulocytic 288.03 ▲
- aphthous 074.0
- catarrhal 462
- crescendo 411.1
- croupous 464.4
- cruris 443.9
  - due to atherosclerosis NEC (see also Arteriosclerosis, extremities) 440.20
- decubitus 413.0
- diphtheritic (membranous) 032.0
- erysipelatous 034.0
- erythematous 462
- exudative, chronic 476.0
- faucium 478.29
- gangrenous 462
  - diphtheritic 032.0
- infectious 462
- initial 411.1
- intestinal 557.1

Angina — continued
- ludovici 528.3
- Ludwig's 528.3
- malignant 462
  - diphtheritic 032.0
- membranous 464.4
  - diphtheritic 032.0
- mesenteric 557.1
- monocytic 075
- nocturnal 413.0
- phlegmonous 475
  - diphtheritic 032.0
- preinfarctional 411.1
- Prinzmetal's 413.1
- progressive 411.1
- pseudomembranous 101
- psychogenic 306.2
- pultaceous, diphtheritic 032.0
- scarlatinal 034.1
- septic 034.0
- simple 462
- stable NEC 413.9
- staphylococcal 462
- streptococcal 034.0
- stridulous, diphtheritic 032.3
- syphilitic 093.9
  - congenital 090.5
- tonsil 475
- trachealis 464.4
- unstable 411.1
- variant 413.1
- Vincent's 101

Angioblastoma (M9161/1) — see Neoplasm, connective tissue, uncertain behavior
Angiocholecystitis — see also Cholecystitis, acute 575.0
Angiocholitis — see also Cholecystitis, acute 576.1
Angiodysgenesis spinalis 336.1
Angiodysplasia (intestinalis) (intestine) 569.84
- with hemorrhage 569.85
- duodenum 537.82
  - with hemorrhage 537.83
- stomach 537.82
  - with hemorrhage 537.83

Angioedema (allergic) (any site) (with urticaria) 995.1
- hereditary 277.6

Angioendothelioma (M9130/1) — see also Neoplasm, by site, uncertain behavior
- benign (M9130/0) (see also Hemangioma, by site) 228.00
- bone (M9260/3) — see Neoplasm, bone, malignant
- Ewing's (M9260/3) — see Neoplasm, bone, malignant
- nervous system (M9130/0) 228.09

Angiofibroma (M9160/0) — see also Neoplasm, by site, benign
- juvenile (M9160/0) 210.7
- specified site — see Neoplasm, by site, benign
- unspecified site 210.7

Angiohemophilia (A) (B) 286.4
Angioid streaks (choroid) (retina) 363.43
Angiokeratoma (M9141/0) — see also Neoplasm, skin, benign
- corporis diffusum 272.7

Angiokeratosis
- diffuse 272.7

Angioleiomyoma (M8894/0) — see Neoplasm, connective tissue, benign
Angioleucitis 683
Angiolipoma (M8861/0) — see also Lipoma, by site 214.9
- infiltrating (M8861/1) — see Neoplasm, connective tissue, uncertain behavior

Angioma (M9120/0) — see also Hemangioma, by site 228.00
- capillary 448.1
- hemorrhagicum hereditaria 448.0

Angioma — see also Hemangioma, by site — continued
- malignant (M9120/3) — see Neoplasm, connective tissue, malignant
- pigmentosum et atrophicum 757.33
- placenta — see Placenta, abnormal
- plexiform (M9131/0) — see Hemangioma, by site
- senile 448.1
- serpiginosum 709.1
- spider 448.1
- stellate 448.1

Angiomatosis 757.32
- bacillary 083.8
- corporis diffusum universale 272.7
- cutaneocerebral 759.6
- encephalocutanea 759.6
- encephalofacial 759.6
- encephalotrigeminal 759.6
- hemorrhagic familial 448.0
- hereditary familial 448.0
- heredofamilial 448.0
- meningo-oculofacial 759.6
- multiple sites 228.09
- neuro-oculocutaneous 759.6
- retina (Hippel's disease) 759.6
- retinocerebellosa 759.6
- retinocerebral 759.6
- systemic 228.09

Angiomyolipoma (M8860/0)
- specified site — see Neoplasm, connective tissue, benign
- unspecified site 223.0

Angiomyoliposarcoma (M8860/3) — see Neoplasm, connective tissue, malignant
Angiomyoma (M8894/0) — see Neoplasm, connective tissue, benign
Angiomyosarcoma (M8894/3) — see Neoplasm, connective tissue, malignant
Angioneurosis 306.2
Angioneurotic edema (allergic) (any site) (with urticaria) 995.1
- hereditary 277.6

Angiopathia, angiopathy 459.9
- diabetic (peripheral) 250.7 ✓ [443.81]
- peripheral 443.9
  - diabetic 250.7 ✓ [443.81]
  - specified type NEC 443.89
- retinae syphilitica 093.89
- retinalis (juvenilis) 362.18
  - background 362.10
  - diabetic 250.5 ✓ [362.01]
  - proliferative 362.29
  - tuberculous (see also Tuberculosis) 017.3 ✓ [362.18]

Angiosarcoma (M9120/3) — see Neoplasm, connective tissue, malignant
Angiosclerosis — see Arteriosclerosis
Angioscotoma, enlarged 368.42
Angiospasm 443.9
- brachial plexus 353.0
- cerebral 435.9
- cervical plexus 353.2
- nerve
  - arm 354.9
    - axillary 353.0
    - median 354.1
    - ulnar 354.2
  - autonomic (see also Neuropathy, peripheral, autonomic) 337.9
  - axillary 353.0
  - leg 355.8
    - plantar 355.6
  - lower extremity — see Angiospasm, nerve, leg
  - median 354.1
  - peripheral NEC 355.9
  - spinal NEC 355.9
  - sympathetic (see also Neuropathy, peripheral, autonomic) 337.9
  - ulnar 354.2

Angiospasm — continued
   nerve — continued
      upper extremity — see Angiospasm, nerve, arm
     peripheral NEC 443.9
     traumatic 443.9
       foot 443.9
       leg 443.9
       vessel 443.9
Angiospastic disease or edema 443.9
Angle's
   class I 524.21
   class II 524.22
   class III 524.23
Anguillulosis 127.2
Angulation
   cecum (see also Obstruction, intestine) 560.9
   coccyx (acquired) 738.6
     congenital 756.19
   femur (acquired) 736.39
     congenital 755.69
   intestine (large) (small) (see also Obstruction, intestine) 560.9
   sacrum (acquired) 738.5
     congenital 756.19
   sigmoid (flexure) (see also Obstruction, intestine) 560.9
   spine (see also Curvature, spine) 737.9
   tibia (acquired) 736.89
     congenital 755.69
   ureter 593.3
   wrist (acquired) 736.09
     congenital 755.59
Angulus infectiosus 686.8
Anhedonia 302.72
Anhidrosis (lid) (neurogenic) (thermogenic) 705.0
Anhydration 276.51
   with
     hypernatremia 276.0
     hyponatremia 276.1
Anhydremia 276.52
   with
     hypernatremia 276.0
     hyponatremia 276.1
Anidrosis 705.0
Aniridia (congenital) 743.45
Anisakiasis (infection) (infestation) 127.1
Anisakis larva infestation 127.1
Aniseikonia 367.32
Anisocoria (pupil) 379.41
   congenital 743.46
Anisocytosis 790.09
Anisometropia (congenital) 367.31
Ankle — see condition
Ankyloblepharon (acquired) (eyelid) 374.46
   filiforme (adnatum) (congenital) 743.62
   total 743.62
Ankylodactly — see also Syndactylism 755.10
Ankyloglossia 750.0
Ankylosis (fibrous) (osseous) 718.50
   ankle 718.57
   any joint, produced by surgical fusion V45.4
   cricoarytenoid (cartilage) (joint) (larynx) 478.79
   dental 521.6
   ear ossicle NEC 385.22
     malleus 385.21
   elbow 718.52
   finger 718.54
   hip 718.55
   incostapedial joint (infectional) 385.22
   joint, produced by surgical fusion NEC V45.4
   knee 718.56
   lumbosacral (joint) 724.6
   malleus 385.21
   multiple sites 718.59
   postoperative (status) V45.4
   sacroiliac (joint) 724.6

Ankylosis — continued
   shoulder 718.51
   specified site NEC 718.58
   spine NEC 724.9
   surgical V45.4
   teeth, tooth (hard tissues) 521.6
   temporomandibular joint 524.61
   wrist 718.53
Ankylostoma — see Ancylostoma
Ankylostomiasis (intestinal) — see Ancylostomiasis
Ankylurethria — see also Stricture, urethra 598.9
Annular — see also condition
   detachment, cervix 622.8
   organ or site, congenital NEC — see Distortion
   pancreas (congenital) 751.7
Anodontia (complete) (partial) (vera) 520.0
   with abnormal spacing 524.30
   acquired 525.10
     causing malocclusion 524.30
     due to
       caries 525.13
       extraction 525.10
       periodontal disease 525.12
       trauma 525.11
Anomaly, anomalous (congenital) (unspecified type) 759.9
   abdomen 759.9
   abdominal wall 756.70
   acoustic nerve 742.9
   adrenal (gland) 759.1
   Alder (-Reilly) (leukocyte granulation) 288.2
   alimentary tract 751.9
     lower 751.5
     specified type NEC 751.8
     upper (any part, except tongue) 750.9
       tongue 750.10
       specified type NEC 750.19
   alveolar 524.70
     ridge (process) 525.8
     specified NEC 524.79
   ankle (joint) 755.69
   anus, anal (canal) 751.5
   aorta, aortic 747.20
     arch 747.21
     coarctation (postductal) (preductal) 747.10
     cusp or valve NEC 746.9
     septum 745.0
     specified type NEC 747.29
   aorticopulmonary septum 745.0
   apertures, diaphragm 756.6
   appendix 751.5
   aqueduct of Sylvius 742.3
     with spina bifida (see also Spina bifida) 741.0 ☑
   arm 755.50
     reduction (see also Deformity, reduction, upper limb) 755.20
   arteriovenous (congenital) (peripheral) NEC 747.60
     brain 747.81
     cerebral 747.81
     coronary 746.85
     gastrointestinal 747.61
       acquired — see Angiodysplasia
     lower limb 747.64
     renal 747.62
     specified site NEC 747.69
     spinal 747.82
     upper limb 747.63
   artery (see also Anomaly, peripheral vascular system) NEC 747.60
     brain 747.81
     cerebral 747.81
     coronary 746.85
     eye 743.9
     pulmonary 747.3
     renal 747.62
     retina 743.9
     umbilical 747.5

Anomaly, anomalous — continued
   arytenoepiglottic folds 748.3
   atrial
     bands 746.9
     folds 746.9
     septa 745.5
   atrioventricular
     canal 745.69
     common 745.69
     conduction 426.7
     excitation 426.7
     septum 745.4
   atrium — see Anomaly, atrial
   auditory canal 744.3
     specified type NEC 744.29
       with hearing impairment 744.02
   auricle
     ear 744.3
       causing impairment of hearing 744.02
     heart 746.9
     septum 745.5
   autosomes, autosomal NEC 758.5
   Axenfeld's 743.44
   back 759.9
   band
     atrial 746.9
     heart 746.9
     ventricular 746.9
   Bartholin's duct 750.9
   biliary duct or passage 751.60
     atresia 751.61
   bladder (neck) (sphincter) (trigone) 753.9
     specified type NEC 753.8
   blood vessel 747.9
     artery — see Anomaly, artery
     peripheral vascular — see Anomaly, peripheral vascular system
     vein — see Anomaly, vein
   bone NEC 756.9
     ankle 755.69
     arm 755.50
     chest 756.3
     cranium 756.0
     face 756.0
     finger 755.50
     foot 755.67
     forearm 755.50
     frontal 756.0
     head 756.0
     hip 755.63
     leg 755.60
     lumbosacral 756.10
     nose 748.1
     pelvic girdle 755.60
     rachitic 756.4
     rib 756.3
     shoulder girdle 755.50
     skull 756.0
       with
         anencephalus 740.0
         encephalocele 742.0
         hydrocephalus 742.3
           with spina bifida (see also Spina bifida) 741.0 ☑
         microcephalus 742.1
     toe 755.66
   brain 742.9
     multiple 742.4
     reduction 742.2
     specified type NEC 742.4
     vessel 747.81
   branchial cleft NEC 744.49
     cyst 744.42
     fistula 744.41
     persistent 744.41
     sinus (external) (internal) 744.41
   breast 757.9
   broad ligament 752.10
     specified type NEC 752.19
   bronchus 748.3
   bulbar septum 745.0
   bulbus cordis 745.9

Anomaly, anomalous — continued
   bulbus cordis — continued
     persistent (in left ventricle) 745.8
   bursa 756.9
   canal of Nuck 752.9
   canthus 743.9
   capillary NEC (see also Anomaly, peripheral vascular system) 747.60
   cardiac 746.9
     septal closure 745.9
       acquired 429.71
     valve NEC 746.9
       pulmonary 746.00
       specified type NEC 746.89
   cardiovascular system 746.9
     complicating pregnancy, childbirth, or puerperium 648.5 ☑
   carpus 755.50
   cartilage, trachea 748.3
   cartilaginous 756.9
   caruncle, lacrimal, lachrymal 743.9
   cascade stomach 750.7
   cauda equina 742.59
   cecum 751.5
   cerebral (see also Anomaly, brain vessels) 747.81
   cerebrovascular system 747.81
   cervix (uterus) 752.40
     with doubling of vagina and uterus 752.2
     in pregnancy or childbirth 654.6 ☑
       affecting fetus or newborn 763.89
       causing obstructed labor 660.2 ☑
         affecting fetus or newborn 763.1
   Chédiak-Higashi (-Steinbrinck) (congenital gigantism of peroxidase granules) 288.2
   cheek 744.9
   chest (wall) 756.3
   chin 744.9
     specified type NEC 744.89
   chordae tendineae 746.9
   choroid 743.9
     plexus 742.9
   chromosomes, chromosomal 758.9
     13 (13-15) 758.1
     18 (16-18) 758.2
     21 or 22 758.0
     autosomes NEC (see also Abnormal, autosomes) 758.5
     deletion 758.39
     Christchurch 758.39
     D_1 758.1
     E_3 758.2
     G 758.0
     mitochondrial 758.9
     mosaics 758.89
     sex 758.81
       complement, XO 758.6
       complement, XXX 758.81
       complement, XXY 758.7
       complement, XYY 758.81
       gonadal dysgenesis 758.6
       Klinefelter's 758.7
       Turner's 758.6
     trisomy 21 758.0
   cilia 743.9
   circulatory system 747.9
     specified type NEC 747.89
   clavicle 755.51
   clitoris 752.40
   coccyx 756.10
   colon 751.5
   common duct 751.60
   communication
     coronary artery 746.85
     left ventricle with right atrium 745.4
   concha (ear) 744.3
   connection
     renal vessels with kidney 747.62
     total pulmonary venous 747.41

Index to Diseases

Anomaly, anomalous

Anomaly, anomalous — *continued*
  connective tissue 756.9
    specified type NEC 756.89
  cornea 743.9
    shape 743.41
    size 743.41
    specified type NEC 743.49
  coronary
    artery 746.85
    vein 746.89
  cranium — *see* Anomaly, skull
  cricoid cartilage 748.3
  cushion, endocardial 745.60
    specified type NEC 745.69
  cystic duct 751.60
  dental arch 524.20
    specified NEC 524.29
  dental arch relationship 524.20
    angle's class I 524.21
    angle's class II 524.22
    angle's class III 524.23
    articulation
      anterior 524.27
      posterior 524.27
      reverse 524.27
    disto-occlusion 524.22
      division I 524.22
      division II 524.22
    excessive horizontal overlap 524.26
    interarch distance (excessive) (inadequate) 524.28
    mesio-occlusion 524.23
    neutro-occlusion 524.21
    open
      anterior occlusal relationship 524.24
      posterior occlusal relationship 524.25
    specified NEC 524.29
  dentition 520.6
  dentofacial NEC 524.9
    functional 524.50
    specified type NEC 524.89
  dermatoglyphic 757.2
  Descemet's membrane 743.9
    specified type NEC 743.49
  development
    cervix 752.40
    vagina 752.40
    vulva 752.40
  diaphragm, diaphragmatic (apertures) NEC 756.6
  digestive organ(s) or system 751.9
    lower 751.5
    specified type NEC 751.8
    upper 750.9
  distribution, coronary artery 746.85
  ductus
    arteriosus 747.0
    Botalli 747.0
  duodenum 751.5
  dura 742.9
    brain 742.4
    spinal cord 742.59
  ear 744.3
    causing impairment of hearing 744.00
      specified type NEC 744.09
    external 744.3
      causing impairment of hearing 744.02
      specified type NEC 744.29
    inner (causing impairment of hearing) 744.05
    middle, except ossicles (causing impairment of hearing) 744.03
      ossicles 744.04
    ossicles 744.04
    prominent auricle 744.29
    specified type NEC 744.29
      with hearing impairment 744.09
  Ebstein's (heart) 746.2
    tricuspid valve 746.2
  ectodermal 757.9
  Eisenmenger's (ventricular septal defect) 745.4
  ejaculatory duct 752.9
    specified type NEC 752.89
  elbow (joint) 755.50
  endocardial cushion 745.60
    specified type NEC 745.69
  endocrine gland NEC 759.2
  epididymis 752.9
  epiglottis 748.3
  esophagus 750.9
    specified type NEC 750.4
  Eustachian tube 744.3
    specified type NEC 744.24
  eye (any part) 743.9
    adnexa 743.9
      specified type NEC 743.69
    anophthalmos 743.00
    anterior
      chamber and related structures 743.9
        angle 743.9
          specified type NEC 743.44
        specified type NEC 743.44
      segment 743.9
        combined 743.48
        multiple 743.48
        specified type NEC 743.49
    cataract (*see also* Cataract) 743.30
    glaucoma (*see also* Buphthalmia) 743.20
    lid 743.9
      specified type NEC 743.63
    microphthalmos (*see also* Microphthalmos) 743.10
    posterior segment 743.9
      specified type NEC 743.59
      vascular 743.58
      vitreous 743.9
        specified type NEC 743.51
    ptosis (eyelid) 743.61
    retina 743.9
      specified type NEC 743.59
    sclera 743.9
      specified type NEC 743.47
    specified type NEC 743.8
  eyebrow 744.89
  eyelid 743.9
    specified type NEC 743.63
  face (any part) 744.9
    bone(s) 756.0
    specified type NEC 744.89
  fallopian tube 752.10
    specified type NEC 752.19
  fascia 756.9
    specified type NEC 756.89
  femur 755.60
  fibula 755.60
  finger 755.50
    supernumerary 755.01
    webbed (*see also* Syndactylism, fingers) 755.11
  fixation, intestine 751.4
  flexion (joint) 755.9
    hip or thigh (*see also* Dislocation, hip, congenital) 754.30
  folds, heart 746.9
  foot 755.67
  foramen
    Botalli 745.5
    ovale 745.5
  forearm 755.50
  forehead (*see also* Anomaly, skull) 756.0
  form, teeth 520.2
  fovea centralis 743.9
  frontal bone (*see also* Anomaly, skull) 756.0
  gallbladder 751.60
  Gartner's duct 752.41
  gastrointestinal tract 751.9
    specified type NEC 751.8
    vessel 747.61
  genitalia, genital organ(s) or system
    female 752.9
      external 752.40
        specified type NEC 752.49
      internal NEC 752.9
    male (external and internal) 752.9
      epispadias 752.62
      hidden penis 752.65
      hydrocele, congenital 778.6
      hypospadias 752.61
      micropenis 752.64
      testis, undescended 752.51
        retractile 752.52
      specified type NEC 752.89
  genitourinary NEC 752.9
  Gerbode 745.4
  globe (eye) 743.9
  glottis 748.3
  granulation or granulocyte, genetic 288.2
    constitutional 288.2
    leukocyte 288.2
  gum 750.9
  gyri 742.9
  hair 757.9
    specified type NEC 757.4
  hand 755.50
  hard tissue formation in pulp 522.3
  head (*see also* Anomaly, skull) 756.0
  heart 746.9
    auricle 746.9
    bands 746.9
    fibroelastosis cordis 425.3
    folds 746.9
    malposition 746.87
    maternal, affecting fetus or newborn 760.3
    obstructive NEC 746.84
    patent ductus arteriosus (Botalli) 747.0
    septum 745.9
      acquired 429.71
      aortic 745.0
      aorticopulmonary 745.0
      atrial 745.5
      auricular 745.5
      between aorta and pulmonary artery 745.0
      endocardial cushion type 745.60
        specified type NEC 745.69
      interatrial 745.5
      interventricular 745.4
        with pulmonary stenosis or atresia, dextraposition of aorta, and hypertrophy of right ventricle 745.2
        acquired 429.71
      specified type NEC 745.8
      ventricular 745.4
        with pulmonary stenosis or atresia, dextraposition of aorta, and hypertrophy of right ventricle 745.2
        acquired 429.71
    specified type NEC 746.89
    tetralogy of Fallot 745.2
    valve NEC 746.9
      aortic 746.9
        atresia 746.89
        bicuspid valve 746.4
        insufficiency 746.4
        specified type NEC 746.89
        stenosis 746.3
          subaortic 746.81
          supravalvular 747.22
      mitral 746.9
        atresia 746.89
        insufficiency 746.6
        specified type NEC 746.89
        stenosis 746.5
      pulmonary 746.00
        atresia 746.01
        insufficiency 746.09
        stenosis 746.02
          infundibular 746.83
          subvalvular 746.83
      tricuspid 746.9
        atresia 746.1
        stenosis 746.1
    ventricle 746.9
  heel 755.67
  Hegglin's 288.2
  hemianencephaly 740.0
  hemicephaly 740.0
  hemicrania 740.0
  hepatic duct 751.60
  hip (joint) 755.63
  hourglass
    bladder 753.8
    gallbladder 751.69
    stomach 750.7
  humerus 755.50
  hymen 752.40
  hypersegmentation of neutrophils, hereditary 288.2
  hypophyseal 759.2
  ileocecal (coil) (valve) 751.5
  ileum (intestine) 751.5
  ilium 755.60
  integument 757.9
    specified type NEC 757.8
  interarch distance (excessive) (inadequate) 524.28
  intervertebral cartilage or disc 756.10
  intestine (large) (small) 751.5
    fixational type 751.4
  iris 743.9
    specified type NEC 743.46
  ischium 755.60
  jaw NEC 524.9
    closure 524.51
    size (major) NEC 524.00
    specified type NEC 524.89
  jaw-cranial base relationship 524.10
    specified NEC 524.19
  jejunum 751.5
  joint 755.9
    hip
      dislocation (*see also* Dislocation, hip, congenital) 754.30
      predislocation (*see also* Subluxation, congenital, hip) 754.32
      preluxation (*see also* Subluxation, congenital, hip) 754.32
      subluxation (*see also* Subluxation, congenital, hip) 754.32
    lumbosacral 756.10
      spondylolisthesis 756.12
      spondylosis 756.11
    multiple arthrogryposis 754.89
    sacroiliac 755.69
  Jordan's 288.2
  kidney(s) (calyx) (pelvis) 753.9
    vessel 747.62
  Klippel-Feil (brevicollis) 756.16
  knee (joint) 755.64
  labium (majus) (minus) 752.40
  labyrinth, membranous (causing impairment of hearing) 744.05
  lacrimal
    apparatus, duct or passage 743.9
      specified type NEC 743.65
    gland 743.9
      specified type NEC 743.64
  Langdon Down (mongolism) 758.0
  larynx, laryngeal (muscle) 748.3
    web, webbed 748.2
  leg (lower) (upper) 755.60
    reduction NEC (*see also* Deformity, reduction, lower limb) 755.30

Anomaly, anomalous

Anomaly, anomalous — *continued*
  lens 743.9
    shape 743.36
    specified type NEC 743.39
  leukocytes, genetic 288.2
    granulation (constitutional) 288.2
  lid (fold) 743.9
  ligament 756.9
    broad 752.10
    round 752.9
  limb, except reduction deformity 755.9
    lower 755.60
      reduction deformity (*see also* Deformity, reduction, lower limb) 755.30
      specified type NEC 755.69
    upper 755.50
      reduction deformity (*see also* Deformity, reduction, upper limb) 755.20
      specified type NEC 755.59
  lip 750.9
    harelip (*see also* Cleft, lip) 749.10
    specified type NEC 750.26
  liver (duct) 751.60
    atresia 751.69
  lower extremity 755.60
    vessel 747.64
  lumbosacral (joint) (region) 756.10
  lung (fissure) (lobe) NEC 748.60
    agenesis 748.5
    specified type NEC 748.69
  lymphatic system 759.9
  Madelung's (radius) 755.54
  mandible 524.9
    size NEC 524.00
  maxilla 524.9
    size NEC 524.00
  May (-Hegglin) 288.2
  meatus urinarius 753.9
    specified type NEC 753.8
  meningeal bands or folds, constriction of 742.8
  meninges 742.9
    brain 742.4
    spinal 742.59
  meningocele (*see also* Spina bifida) 741.9 ☑
    acquired 349.2
  mesentery 751.9
  metacarpus 755.50
  metatarsus 755.67
  middle ear, except ossicles (causing impairment of hearing) 744.03
    ossicles 744.04
  mitral (leaflets) (valve) 746.9
    atresia 746.89
    insufficiency 746.6
    specified type NEC 746.89
    stenosis 746.5
  mouth 750.9
    specified type NEC 750.26
  multiple NEC 759.7
    specified type NEC 759.89
  muscle 756.9
    eye 743.9
      specified type NEC 743.69
    specified type NEC 756.89
  musculoskeletal system, except limbs 756.9
    specified type NEC 756.9
  nail 757.9
    specified type NEC 757.5
  narrowness, eyelid 743.62
  nasal sinus or septum 748.1
  neck (any part) 744.9
    specified type NEC 744.89
  nerve 742.9
    acoustic 742.9
      specified type NEC 742.8
    optic 742.9
      specified type NEC 742.8
    specified type NEC 742.8
  nervous system NEC 742.9
    brain 742.9
      specified type NEC 742.4

Anomaly, anomalous — *continued*
  nervous system — *continued*
    specified type NEC 742.8
  neurological 742.9
  nipple 757.6
  nonteratogenic NEC 754.89
  nose, nasal (bone) (cartilage) (septum) (sinus) 748.1
  ocular muscle 743.9
  omphalomesenteric duct 751.0
  opening, pulmonary veins 747.49
  optic
    disc 743.9
      specified type NEC 743.57
    nerve 742.9
  opticociliary vessels 743.9
  orbit (eye) 743.9
    specified type NEC 743.66
  organ
    of Corti (causing impairment of hearing) 744.05
    or site 759.9
      specified type NEC 759.89
  origin
    both great arteries from same ventricle 745.11
    coronary artery 746.85
    innominate artery 747.69
    left coronary artery from pulmonary artery 746.85
    pulmonary artery 747.3
    renal vessels 747.62
    subclavian artery (left) (right) 747.21
  osseous meatus (ear) 744.03
  ovary 752.0
  oviduct 752.10
  palate (hard) (soft) 750.9
    cleft (*see also* Cleft, palate) 749.00
  pancreas (duct) 751.7
  papillary muscles 746.9
  parathyroid gland 759.2
  paraurethral ducts 753.9
  parotid (gland) 750.9
  patella 755.64
  Pelger-Huët (hereditary hyposegmentation) 288.2
  pelvic girdle 755.60
    specified type NEC 755.69
  pelvis (bony) 755.60
    complicating delivery 653.0 ☑
    rachitic 268.1
      fetal 756.4
  penis (glans) 752.69
  pericardium 746.89
  peripheral vascular system NEC 747.60
    gastrointestinal 747.61
    lower limb 747.64
    renal 747.62
    specified site NEC 747.69
    spinal 747.82
    upper limb 747.63
  Peter's 743.44
  pharynx 750.9
    branchial cleft 744.41
    specified type NEC 750.29
  Pierre Robin 756.0
  pigmentation 709.00
    congenital 757.33
    specified NEC 709.09
  pituitary (gland) 759.2
  pleural folds 748.8
  portal vein 747.40
  position tooth, teeth 524.30
    crowding 524.31
    displacement 524.30
      horizontal 524.33
      vertical 524.34
    distance
      interocclusal
        excessive 524.37
        insufficient 524.36
    excessive spacing 524.32
    rotation 524.35
    specified NEC 524.39

Anomaly, anomalous — *continued*
  preauricular sinus 744.46
  prepuce 752.9
  prostate 752.9
  pulmonary 748.60
    artery 747.3
    circulation 747.3
    specified type NEC 748.69
    valve 746.00
      atresia 746.01
      insufficiency 746.09
      specified type NEC 746.09
      stenosis 746.02
        infundibular 746.83
        subvalvular 746.83
    vein 747.40
    venous
      connection 747.49
        partial 747.42
        total 747.41
      return 747.49
        partial 747.42
        total (TAPVR) (complete) (subdiaphragmatic) (supradiaphragmatic) 747.41
  pupil 743.9
  pylorus 750.9
    hypertrophy 750.5
    stenosis 750.5
  rachitic, fetal 756.4
  radius 755.50
  rectovaginal (septum) 752.40
  rectum 751.5
  refraction 367.9
  renal 753.9
    vessel 747.62
  respiratory system 748.9
    specified type NEC 748.8
  rib 756.3
    cervical 756.2
  Rieger's 743.44
  rings, trachea 748.3
  rotation (*see also* Malrotation)
    hip or thigh (*see also* Subluxation, congenital, hip) 754.32
  round ligament 752.9
  sacroiliac (joint) 755.69
  sacrum 756.10
  saddle
    back 754.2
    nose 754.0
      syphilitic 090.5
  salivary gland or duct 750.9
    specified type NEC 750.26
  scapula 755.50
  sclera 743.9
    specified type NEC 743.47
  scrotum 752.9
  sebaceous gland 757.9
  seminal duct or tract 752.9
  sense organs 742.9
    specified type NEC 742.8
  septum
    heart — *see* Anomaly, heart, septum
    nasal 748.1
  sex chromosomes NEC (*see also* Anomaly, chromosomes) 758.81
  shoulder (girdle) (joint) 755.50
    specified type NEC 755.59
  sigmoid (flexure) 751.5
  sinus of Valsalva 747.29
  site NEC 759.9
  skeleton generalized NEC 756.50
  skin (appendage) 757.9
    specified type NEC 757.39
  skull (bone) 756.0
    with
      anencephalus 740.0
      encephalocele 742.0
      hydrocephalus 742.3
        with spina bifida (*see also* Spina bifida) 741.0 ☑
      microcephalus 742.1

Anomaly, anomalous — *continued*
  specified type NEC
    adrenal (gland) 759.1
    alimentary tract (complete) (partial) 751.8
      lower 751.5
      upper 750.8
    ankle 755.69
    anus, anal (canal) 751.5
    aorta, aortic 747.29
      arch 747.21
    appendix 751.5
    arm 755.59
    artery (peripheral) NEC (*see also* Anomaly, peripheral vascular system) 747.60
      brain 747.81
      coronary 746.85
      eye 743.58
      pulmonary 747.3
      retinal 743.58
      umbilical 747.5
    auditory canal 744.29
      causing impairment of hearing 744.02
    bile duct or passage 751.69
    bladder 753.8
      neck 753.8
    bone(s) 756.9
      arm 755.59
      face 756.0
      leg 755.69
      pelvic girdle 755.69
      shoulder girdle 755.59
      skull 756.0
        with
          anencephalus 740.0
          encephalocele 742.0
          hydrocephalus 742.3
            with spina bifida (*see also* Spina bifida) 741.0 ☑
          microcephalus 742.1
    brain 742.4
    breast 757.6
    broad ligament 752.19
    bronchus 748.3
    canal of Nuck 752.89
    cardiac septal closure 745.8
    carpus 755.59
    cartilaginous 756.9
    cecum 751.5
    cervix 752.49
    chest (wall) 756.3
    chin 744.89
    ciliary body 743.46
    circulatory system 747.89
    clavicle 755.51
    clitoris 752.49
    coccyx 756.19
    colon 751.5
    common duct 751.69
    connective tissue 756.89
    cricoid cartilage 748.3
    cystic duct 751.69
    diaphragm 756.6
    digestive organ(s) or tract 751.8
      lower 751.5
      upper 750.8
    duodenum 751.5
    ear 744.29
      auricle 744.29
        causing impairment of hearing 744.02
      causing impairment of hearing 744.09
      inner (causing impairment of hearing) 744.05
      middle, except ossicles 744.03
        ossicles 744.04
    ejaculatory duct 752.89
    endocrine 759.2
    epiglottis 748.3
    esophagus 750.4
    Eustachian tube 744.24
    eye 743.8

Anomaly, anomalous — *continued*
  specified type — *continued*
    eye — *continued*
      lid 743.63
      muscle 743.69
    face 744.89
      bone(s) 756.0
    fallopian tube 752.19
    fascia 756.89
    femur 755.69
    fibula 755.69
    finger 755.59
    foot 755.67
    fovea centralis 743.55
    gallbladder 751.69
    Gartner's duct 752.89
    gastrointestinal tract 751.8
    genitalia, genital organ(s)
      female 752.89
        external 752.49
        internal NEC 752.89
      male 752.89
        penis 752.69
        scrotal transposition 752.81
    genitourinary tract NEC 752.89
    glottis 748.3
    hair 757.4
    hand 755.59
    heart 746.89
      valve NEC 746.89
        pulmonary 746.09
    hepatic duct 751.69
    hydatid of Morgagni 752.89
    hymen 752.49
    integument 757.8
    intestine (large) (small) 751.5
      fixational type 751.4
    iris 743.46
    jejunum 751.5
    joint 755.8
    kidney 753.3
    knee 755.64
    labium (majus) (minus) 752.49
    labyrinth, membranous 744.05
    larynx 748.3
    leg 755.69
    lens 743.39
    limb, except reduction deformity 755.8
      lower 755.69
        reduction deformity (*see also* Deformity, reduction, lower limb) 755.30
      upper 755.59
        reduction deformity (*see also* Deformity, reduction, upper limb) 755.20
    lip 750.26
    liver 751.69
    lung (fissure) (lobe) 748.69
    meatus urinarius 753.8
    metacarpus 755.59
    mouth 750.26
    muscle 756.89
      eye 743.69
    musculoskeletal system, except limbs 756.9
    nail 757.5
    neck 744.89
    nerve 742.8
      acoustic 742.8
      optic 742.8
    nervous system 742.8
    nipple 757.6
    nose 748.1
    organ NEC 759.89
      of Corti 744.05
    osseous meatus (ear) 744.03
    ovary 752.0
    oviduct 752.19
    pancreas 751.7
    parathyroid 759.2
    patella 755.64
    pelvic girdle 755.69
    penis 752.69
    pericardium 746.89

Anomaly, anomalous — *continued*
  specified type — *continued*
    peripheral vascular system NEC (*see also* Anomaly, peripheral vascular system) 747.60
    pharynx 750.29
    pituitary 759.2
    prostate 752.89
    radius 755.59
    rectum 751.5
    respiratory system 748.8
    rib 756.3
    round ligament 752.89
    sacrum 756.19
    salivary duct or gland 750.26
    scapula 755.59
    sclera 743.47
    scrotum 752.89
      transposition 752.81
    seminal duct or tract 752.89
    shoulder girdle 755.59
    site NEC 759.89
    skin 757.39
    skull (bone(s)) 756.0
      with
        anencephalus 740.0
        encephalocele 742.0
        hydrocephalus 742.3
          with spina bifida (*see also* Spina bifida) 741.0 ☑
        microcephalus 742.1
    specified organ or site NEC 759.89
    spermatic cord 752.89
    spinal cord 742.59
    spine 756.19
    spleen 759.0
    sternum 756.3
    stomach 750.7
    tarsus 755.67
    tendon 756.89
    testis 752.89
    thorax (wall) 756.3
    thymus 759.2
    thyroid (gland) 759.2
      cartilage 748.3
    tibia 755.69
    toe 755.66
    tongue 750.19
    trachea (cartilage) 748.3
    ulna 755.59
    urachus 753.7
    ureter 753.4
      obstructive 753.29
    urethra 753.8
      obstructive 753.6
    urinary tract 753.8
    uterus 752.3
    uvula 750.26
    vagina 752.49
    vascular NEC (*see also* Anomaly, peripheral vascular system) 747.60
      brain 747.81
    vas deferens 752.89
    vein(s) (peripheral) NEC (*see also* Anomaly, peripheral vascular system) 747.60
      brain 747.81
      great 747.49
      portal 747.49
      pulmonary 747.49
      vena cava (inferior) (superior) 747.49
    vertebra 756.19
    vulva 752.49
  spermatic cord 752.9
  spine, spinal 756.10
    column 756.10
    cord 742.9
      meningocele (*see also* Spina bifida) 741.9 ☑
      specified type NEC 742.59
      spina bifida (*see also* Spina bifida) 741.9 ☑
      vessel 747.82

Anomaly, anomalous — *continued*
  spine, spinal — *continued*
    meninges 742.59
    nerve root 742.9
  spleen 759.0
  Sprengel's 755.52
  sternum 756.3
  stomach 750.9
    specified type NEC 750.7
  submaxillary gland 750.9
  superior vena cava 747.40
  talipes — *see* Talipes
  tarsus 755.67
    with complete absence of distal elements 755.31
  teeth, tooth NEC 520.9
    position 524.30
      crowding 524.31
      displacement 524.30
        horizontal 524.33
        vertical 524.34
      distance
        interocclusal
          excessive 524.37
          insufficient 524.36
      excessive spacing 524.32
      rotation 524.35
      specified NEC 524.39
      spacing 524.30
  tendon 756.9
    specified type NEC 756.89
  termination
    coronary artery 746.85
  testis 752.9
  thebesian valve 746.9
  thigh 755.60
    flexion (*see also* Subluxation, congenital, hip) 754.32
  thorax (wall) 756.3
  throat 750.9
  thumb 755.50
    supernumerary 755.01
  thymus gland 759.2
  thyroid (gland) 759.2
    cartilage 748.3
  tibia 755.60
    saber 090.5
  toe 755.66
    supernumerary 755.02
    webbed (*see also* Syndactylism, toes) 755.13
  tongue 750.10
    specified type NEC 750.19
  trachea, tracheal 748.3
    cartilage 748.3
    rings 748.3
  tragus 744.3
  transverse aortic arch 747.21
  trichromata 368.59
  trichromatopsia 368.59
  tricuspid (leaflet) (valve) 746.9
    atresia 746.1
    Ebstein's 746.2
    specified type NEC 746.89
    stenosis 746.1
  trunk 759.9
  Uhl's (hypoplasia of myocardium, right ventricle) 746.84
  ulna 755.50
  umbilicus 759.9
    artery 747.5
  union, trachea with larynx 748.3
  unspecified site 759.9
  upper extremity 755.50
    vessel 747.63
  urachus 753.7
    specified type NEC 753.7
  ureter 753.9
    obstructive 753.20
    specified type NEC 753.4
      obstructive 753.29
  urethra (valve) 753.9
    obstructive 753.6
    specified type NEC 753.8
  urinary tract or system (any part, except urachus) 753.9

Anomaly, anomalous — *continued*
  urinary tract or system — *continued*
    specified type NEC 753.8
    urachus 753.7
  uterus 752.3
    with only one functioning horn 752.3
    in pregnancy or childbirth 654.0 ☑
      affecting fetus or newborn 763.89
      causing obstructed labor 660.2 ☑
        affecting fetus or newborn 763.1
  uvula 750.9
  vagina 752.40
  valleculae 748.3
  valve (heart) NEC 746.9
    formation, ureter 753.29
    pulmonary 746.00
    specified type NEC 746.89
  vascular NEC (*see also* Anomaly, peripheral vascular system) 747.60
    ring 747.21
  vas deferens 752.9
  vein(s) (peripheral) NEC (*see also* Anomaly, peripheral vascular system) 747.60
    brain 747.81
    cerebral 747.81
    coronary 746.89
    great 747.40
      specified type NEC 747.49
    portal 747.40
    pulmonary 747.40
    retina 743.9
  vena cava (inferior) (superior) 747.40
  venous return (pulmonary) 747.49
    partial 747.42
    total 747.41
  ventricle, ventricular (heart) 746.9
    bands 746.9
    folds 746.9
    septa 745.4
  vertebra 756.10
  vesicourethral orifice 753.9
  vessels NEC (*see also* Anomaly, peripheral vascular system) 747.60
    optic papilla 743.9
  vitelline duct 751.0
  vitreous humor 743.9
    specified type NEC 743.51
  vulva 752.40
  wrist (joint) 755.50
Anomia 784.69
Anonychia 757.5
  acquired 703.8
Anophthalmos, anophthalmus (clinical) (congenital) (globe) 743.00
  acquired V45.78
Anopsia (altitudinal) (quadrant) 368.46
Anorchia 752.89
Anorchism, anorchidism 752.89
Anorexia 783.0
  hysterical 300.11
  nervosa 307.1
Anosmia — *see also* Disturbance, sensation 781.1
  hysterical 300.11
  postinfectional 478.9
  psychogenic 306.7
  traumatic 951.8
Anosognosia 780.99
Anosphrasia 781.1
Anosteoplasia 756.50
Anotia 744.09
Anovulatory cycle 628.0
Anoxemia 799.02
  newborn 770.88
Anoxia 799.02
  altitude 993.2
  cerebral 348.1

Anoxia — continued
cerebral — continued
with
abortion — see Abortion, by type, with specified complication NEC
ectopic pregnancy (see also categories 633.0–633.9) 639.8
molar pregnancy (see also categories 630–632) 639.8
complicating
delivery (cesarean) (instrumental) 669.4 ☑
ectopic or molar pregnancy 639.8
obstetric anesthesia or sedation 668.2 ☑
during or resulting from a procedure 997.01
following
abortion 639.8
ectopic or molar pregnancy 639.8
newborn (see also Distress, fetal, liveborn infant) 770.88 ▲
due to drowning 994.1
fetal, affecting newborn 770.88 ▲
heart — see Insufficiency, coronary
high altitude 993.2
intrauterine
fetal death (before onset of labor) 768.0
during labor 768.1
liveborn infant — see Distress, fetal, liveborn infant
myocardial — see Insufficiency, coronary
newborn 768.9
mild or moderate 768.6
severe 768.5
pathological 799.02
Anteflexion — see Anteversion
Antenatal
care, normal pregnancy V22.1
first V22.0
screening of mother (for) V28.9
based on amniocentesis NEC V28.2
chromosomal anomalies V28.0
raised alphafetoprotein levels V28.1
chromosomal anomalies V28.0
fetal growth retardation using ulatrasonics V28.4
isoimmunization V28.5
malformations using ulatrasonics V28.3
raised alphafetoprotein levels in amniotic fluid V28.1
specified condition NEC V28.8
Streptococcus B V28.6
Antepartum — see condition
Anterior — see also condition
spinal artery compression syndrome 721.1
Antero-occlusion 524.24
Anteversion
cervix — ▶see◀ Anteversion, uterus
femur (neck), congenital 755.63
uterus, uterine (cervix) (postinfectional) (postpartal, old) 621.6
congenital 752.3
in pregnancy or childbirth 654.4 ☑
affecting fetus or newborn 763.89
causing obstructed labor 660.2 ☑
affecting fetus or newborn 763.1
Anthracosilicosis (occupational) 500
Anthracosis (lung) (occupational) 500
lingua 529.3
Anthrax 022.9
with pneumonia 022.1 [484.5]
colitis 022.2
cutaneous 022.0

Anthrax — continued
gastrointestinal 022.2
intestinal 022.2
pulmonary 022.1
respiratory 022.1
septicemia 022.3
specified manifestation NEC 022.8
Anthropoid pelvis 755.69
with disproportion (fetopelvic) 653.2 ☑
affecting fetus or newborn 763.1
causing obstructed labor 660.1 ☑
affecting fetus or newborn 763.1
Anthropophobia 300.29
Antibioma, breast 611.0
Antibodies
maternal (blood group) (see also Incompatibility) 656.2 ☑
anti-D, cord blood 656.1 ☑
fetus or newborn 773.0
Antibody deficiency syndrome
agammaglobulinemic 279.00
congenital 279.04
hypogammaglobulinemic 279.00
Anticoagulant, circulating — see also Circulating anticoagulants 286.5
Antimongolism syndrome 758.39
Antimonial cholera 985.4
Antisocial personality 301.7
Antithrombinemia — see also Circulating anticoagulants 286.5
Antithromboplastinemia — see also Circulating anticoagulants 286.5
Antithromboplastinogenemia — see also Circulating anticoagulants 286.5
Antitoxin complication or reaction — see Complications, vaccination
Anton (-Babinski) syndrome (hemiasomatognosia) 307.9
Antritis (chronic) 473.0
maxilla 473.1
acute 461.0
stomach 535.4 ☑
Antrum, antral — see condition
Anuria 788.5
with
abortion — see Abortion, by type, with renal failure
ectopic pregnancy (see also categories 633.0–633.9) 639.3
molar pregnancy (see also categories 630–632) 639.3
calculus (impacted) (recurrent) 592.9
kidney 592.0
ureter 592.1
congenital 753.3
due to a procedure 997.5
following
abortion 639.8
ectopic or molar pregnancy 639.3
newborn 753.3
postrenal 593.4
puerperal, postpartum, childbirth 669.3 ☑
specified as due to a procedure 997.5
sulfonamide
correct substance properly administered 788.5
overdose or wrong substance given or taken 961.0
traumatic (following crushing) 958.5
Anus, anal — see condition
Anusitis 569.49
Anxiety (neurosis) (reaction) (state) 300.00
alcohol-induced 291.89
depression 300.4
drug-induced 292.89
due to or associated with physical condition 293.84
generalized 300.02
hysteria 300.20
in
acute stress reaction 308.0
transient adjustment reaction 309.24

Anxiety — continued
panic type 300.01
separation, abnormal 309.21
syndrome (organic) (transient) 293.84
Aorta, aortic — see condition
Aortectasia 441.9
Aortitis (nonsyphilitic) 447.6
arteriosclerotic 440.0
calcific 447.6
Döhle-Heller 093.1
luetic 093.1
rheumatic (see also Endocarditis, acute, rheumatic) 391.1
rheumatoid — see Arthritis, rheumatoid
specific 093.1
syphilitic 093.1
congenital 090.5
Apathetic thyroid storm — see also Thyrotoxicosis 242.9 ☑
Apepsia 536.8
achlorhydric 536.0
psychogenic 306.4
Aperistalsis, esophagus 530.0
Apert-Gallais syndrome (adrenogenital) 255.2
Apertognathia 524.20
Apert's syndrome (acrocephalosyndactyly) 755.55
Aphagia 787.2
psychogenic 307.1
Aphakia (acquired) (bilateral) (postoperative) (unilateral) 379.31
congenital 743.35
Aphalangia (congenital) 755.4
lower limb (complete) (intercalary) (partial) (terminal) 755.39
meaning all digits (complete) (partial) 755.31
transverse 755.31
upper limb (complete) (intercalary) (partial) (terminal) 755.29
meaning all digits (complete) (partial) 755.21
transverse 755.21
Aphasia (amnestic) (ataxic) (auditory) (Broca's) (choreatic) (classic) (expressive) (global) (ideational) (ideokinetic) (ideomotor) (jargon) (motor) (nominal) (receptive) (semantic) (sensory) (syntactic) (verbal) (visual) (Wernicke's) 784.3
developmental 315.31
syphilis, tertiary 094.89
uremic — see Uremia
Aphemia 784.3
uremic — see Uremia
Aphonia 784.41
clericorum 784.49
hysterical 300.11
organic 784.41
psychogenic 306.1
Aphthae, aphthous — see also condition
Bednar's 528.2
cachectic 529.0
epizootic 078.4
fever 078.4
oral 528.2
stomatitis 528.2
thrush 112.0
ulcer (oral) (recurrent) 528.2
genital organ(s) NEC
female 629.89 ▲
male 608.89
larynx 478.79
Apical — see condition
Apical ballooning syndrome 429.83 ▲
Aplasia — see also Agenesis
alveolar process (acquired) 525.8
congenital 750.26
aorta (congenital) 747.22
aortic valve (congenital) 746.89
axialis extracorticalis (congenital) 330.0
bone marrow (myeloid) 284.9

Aplasia — see also Agenesis — continued
bone marrow — continued
acquired (secondary) 284.8
congenital 284.01 ▲
idiopathic 284.9
brain 740.0
specified part 742.2
breast 757.6
bronchus 748.3
cementum 520.4
cerebellar 742.2
congenital ▶(pure)◀ red cell 284.01 ▲
corpus callosum 742.2
erythrocyte 284.8
congenital 284.01 ▲
extracortical axial 330.0
eye (congenital) 743.00
fovea centralis (congenital) 743.55
germinal (cell) 606.0
iris 743.45
labyrinth, membranous 744.05
limb (congenital) 755.4
lower NEC 755.30
upper NEC 755.20
lung (bilateral) (congenital) (unilateral) 748.5
nervous system NEC 742.8
nuclear 742.8
ovary 752.0
Pelizaeus-Merzbacher 330.0
prostate (congenital) 752.89
red cell (with thymoma) 284.8
acquired (secondary) 284.8
congenital 284.01 ▲
hereditary 284.01 ▲
of infants 284.01 ▲
primary 284.01 ●
pure 284.01 ●
round ligament (congenital) 752.89
salivary gland 750.21
skin (congenital) 757.39
spinal cord 742.59
spleen 759.0
testis (congenital) 752.89
thymic, with immunodeficiency 279.2
thyroid 243
uterus 752.3
ventral horn cell 742.59
Apleuria 756.3
Apnea, apneic (spells) 786.03
newborn, neonatorum 770.81
essential 770.81
obstructive 770.82
primary 770.81
sleep 770.81
specified NEC 770.82
psychogenic 306.1
sleep, unspecified 780.57
with
hypersomnia, unspecified 780.53
hyposomnia, unspecified 780.51
insomnia, unspecified 780.51
sleep disturbance 780.57
central, in conditions classified elsewhere 327.27
obstructive (adult) (pediatric) 327.23
organic 327.20
other 327.29
primary central 327.21
Apneumatosis newborn 770.4
Apodia 755.31
Aponeurosis 726.90
Apophysitis (bone) — see also Osteochondrosis 732.9
calcaneus 732.5
juvenile 732.6
Apoplectiform convulsions — see also Disease, cerebrovascular, acute 436
Apoplexia, apoplexy, apoplectic — see also Disease, cerebrovascular, acute 436

Index to Diseases — Arteriosclerosis, arteriosclerotic

Apoplexia, apoplexy, apoplectic — see also Disease, cerebrovascular, acute — continued
- abdominal 569.89
- adrenal 036.3
- attack 436
- basilar (see also Disease, cerebrovascular, acute) 436
- brain (see also Disease, cerebrovascular, acute) 436
- bulbar (see also Disease, cerebrovascular, acute) 436
- capillary (see also Disease, cerebrovascular, acute) 436
- cardiac (see also Infarct, myocardium) 410.9 ☑
- cerebral (see also Disease, cerebrovascular, acute) 436
- chorea (see also Disease, cerebrovascular, acute) 436
- congestive (see also Disease, cerebrovascular, acute) 436
  - newborn 767.4
- embolic (see also Embolism, brain) 434.1 ☑
- fetus 767.0
- fit (see also Disease, cerebrovascular, acute) 436
- healed or old V12.59
- heart (auricle) (ventricle) (see also Infarct, myocardium) 410.9 ☑
- heat 992.0
- hemiplegia (see also Disease, cerebrovascular, acute) 436
- hemorrhagic (stroke) (see also Hemorrhage, brain) 432.9
- ingravescent (see also Disease, cerebrovascular, acute) 436
- late effect — see Late effect(s) (of) cerebrovascular disease
- lung — see Embolism, pulmonary
- meninges, hemorrhagic (see also Hemorrhage, subarachnoid) 430
- neonatorum 767.0
- newborn 767.0
- pancreatitis 577.0
- placenta 641.2 ☑
- progressive (see also Disease, cerebrovascular, acute) 436
- pulmonary (artery) (vein) — see Embolism, pulmonary
- sanguineous (see also Disease, cerebrovascular, acute) 436
- seizure (see also Disease, cerebrovascular, acute) 436
- serous (see also Disease, cerebrovascular, acute) 436
- spleen 289.59
- stroke (see also Disease, cerebrovascular, acute) 436
- thrombotic (see also Thrombosis, brain) 434.0 ☑
- uremic — see Uremia
- uteroplacental 641.2 ☑

Appendage
- fallopian tube (cyst of Morgagni) 752.11
- intestine (epiploic) 751.5
- preauricular 744.1
- testicular (organ of Morgagni) 752.89

Appendicitis 541
- with
  - perforation, peritonitis (generalized), or rupture 540.0
    - with peritoneal abscess 540.1
  - peritoneal abscess 540.1
- acute (catarrhal) (fulminating) (gangrenous) (inflammatory) (obstructive) (retrocecal) (suppurative) 540.9
  - with
    - perforation, peritonitis, or rupture 540.0
      - with peritoneal abscess 540.1
    - peritoneal abscess 540.1

Appendicitis — continued
- amebic 006.8
- chronic (recurrent) 542
- exacerbation — see Appendicitis, acute
- fulminating — see Appendicitis, acute
- gangrenous — see Appendicitis, acute
- healed (obliterative) 542
- interval 542
- neurogenic 542
- obstructive 542
- pneumococcal 541
- recurrent 542
- relapsing 542
- retrocecal 541
- subacute (adhesive) 542
- subsiding 542
- suppurative — see Appendicitis, acute
- tuberculous (see also Tuberculosis) 014.8 ☑

Appendiclausis 543.9
Appendicolithiasis 543.9
Appendicopathia oxyurica 127.4
Appendix, appendicular — see also condition
- Morgagni (male) 752.89
  - fallopian tube 752.11

Appetite
- depraved 307.52
- excessive 783.6
  - psychogenic 307.51
- lack or loss (see also Anorexia) 783.0
  - nonorganic origin 307.59
- perverted 307.52
  - hysterical 300.11

Apprehension, apprehensiveness (abnormal) (state) 300.00
- specified type NEC 300.09

Approximal wear 521.10
Apraxia (classic) (ideational) (ideokinetic) (ideomotor) (motor) 784.69
- oculomotor, congenital 379.51
- verbal 784.69

Aptyalism 527.7
Aqueous misdirection 365.83
Arabicum elephantiasis — see also Infestation, filarial 125.9
Arachnidism 989.5
Arachnitis — see Meningitis
Arachnodactyly 759.82
Arachnoidism 989.5
Arachnoiditis (acute) (adhesive) (basic) (brain) (cerebrospinal) (chiasmal) (chronic) (spinal) — see also Meningitis 322.9
- meningococcal (chronic) 036.0
- syphilitic 094.2
- tuberculous (see also Tuberculosis, meninges) 013.0 ☑

Araneism 989.5
Arboencephalitis, Australian 062.4
Arborization block (heart) 426.6
Arbor virus, arbovirus (infection) NEC 066.9
ARC 042
Arches — see condition
Arcuatus uterus 752.3
Arcus (cornea)
- juvenilis 743.43
  - interfering with vision 743.42
- senilis 371.41

Arc-welders' lung 503
Arc-welders' syndrome (photokeratitis) 370.24
Areflexia 796.1
Areola — see condition
Argentaffinoma (M8241/1) — see also Neoplasm, by site, uncertain behavior
- benign (M8241/0) — see Neoplasm, by site, benign
- malignant (M8241/3) — see Neoplasm, by site, malignant
- syndrome 259.2

Argentinian hemorrhagic fever 078.7
Arginosuccinicaciduria 270.6

Argonz-Del Castillo syndrome (nonpuerperal galactorrhea and amenorrhea) 253.1
Argyll-Robertson phenomenon, pupil, or syndrome (syphilitic) 094.89
- atypical 379.45
- nonluetic 379.45
- nonsyphilitic 379.45
- reversed 379.45

Argyria, argyriasis NEC 985.8
- conjunctiva 372.55
- cornea 371.16
- from drug or medicinal agent
  - correct substance properly administered 709.09
  - overdose or wrong substance given or taken 961.2

Arhinencephaly 742.2
Arias-Stella phenomenon 621.30
Ariboflavinosis 266.0
Arizona enteritis 008.1
Arm — see condition
Armenian disease 277.31 ▲
Arnold-Chiari obstruction or syndrome — see also Spina bifida 741.0 ☑
- type I 348.4
- type II (see also Spina bifida) 741.0 ☑
- type III 742.0
- type IV 742.2

Arousals
- confusional 327.41

Arrest, arrested
- active phase of labor 661.1 ☑
  - affecting fetus or newborn 763.7
- any plane in pelvis
  - complicating delivery 660.1 ☑
    - affecting fetus or newborn 763.1
- bone marrow (see also Anemia, aplastic) 284.9
- cardiac 427.5
  - with
    - abortion — see Abortion, by type, with specified complication NEC
    - ectopic pregnancy (see also categories 633.0–633.9) 639.8
    - molar pregnancy (see also categories 630–632) 639.8
  - complicating
    - anesthesia
      - correct substance properly administered 427.5
      - obstetric 668.1 ☑
      - overdose or wrong substance given 968.4
        - specified anesthetic — see Table of Drugs and Chemicals
    - delivery (cesarean) (instrumental) 669.4 ☑
    - ectopic or molar pregnancy 639.8
    - surgery (nontherapeutic) (therapeutic) 997.1
  - fetus or newborn 779.85 ▲
  - following
    - abortion 639.8
    - ectopic or molar pregnancy 639.8
  - postoperative (immediate) 997.1
  - long-term effect of cardiac surgery 429.4
- cardiorespiratory (see also Arrest, cardiac) 427.5
- deep transverse 660.3 ☑
  - affecting fetus or newborn 763.1
- development or growth
  - bone 733.91
  - child 783.40
  - fetus 764.9 ☑
    - affecting management of pregnancy 656.5 ☑
  - tracheal rings 748.3
- epiphyseal 733.91
- granulopoiesis 288.09 ▲

Arrest, arrested — continued
- heart — see Arrest, cardiac
- respiratory 799.1
  - newborn 770.87 ▲
- sinus 426.6
- transverse (deep) 660.3 ☑
  - affecting fetus or newborn 763.1

Arrhenoblastoma (M8630/1)
- benign (M8630/0)
  - specified site — see Neoplasm, by site, benign
  - unspecified site
    - female 220
    - male 222.0
- malignant (M8630/3)
  - specified site — see Neoplasm, by site, malignant
  - unspecified site
    - female 183.0
    - male 186.9
- specified site — see Neoplasm, by site, uncertain behavior
- unspecified site
  - female 236.2
  - male 236.4

Arrhinencephaly 742.2
- due to
  - trisomy 13 (13-15) 758.1
  - trisomy 18 (16-18) 758.2

Arrhythmia (auricle) (cardiac) (cordis) (gallop rhythm) (juvenile) (nodal) (reflex) (sinus) (supraventricular) (transitory) (ventricle) 427.9
- bigeminal rhythm 427.89
- block 426.9
- bradycardia 427.89
- contractions, premature 427.60
- coronary sinus 427.89
- ectopic 427.89
- extrasystolic 427.60
- postoperative 997.1
- psychogenic 306.2
- vagal 780.2

Arrillaga-Ayerza syndrome (pulmonary artery sclerosis with pulmonary hypertension) 416.0

Arsenical
- dermatitis 692.4
- keratosis 692.4
- pigmentation 985.1
  - from drug or medicinal agent
    - correct substance properly administered 709.09
    - overdose or wrong substance given or taken 961.1

Arsenism 985.1
- from drug or medicinal agent
  - correct substance properly administered 692.4
  - overdose or wrong substance given or taken 961.1

Arterial — see condition
Arteriectasis 447.8
Arteriofibrosis — see Arteriosclerosis
Arteriolar sclerosis — see Arteriosclerosis
Arteriolith — see Arteriosclerosis
Arteriolitis 447.6
- necrotizing, kidney 447.5
- renal — see Hypertension, kidney

Arteriolosclerosis — see Arteriosclerosis
Arterionephrosclerosis — see also Hypertension, kidney 403.90
Arteriopathy 447.9
Arteriosclerosis, arteriosclerotic (artery) (deformans) (diffuse) (disease) (endarteritis) (general) (obliterans) (obliterative) (occlusive) (senile) (with calcification) 440.9
- with
  - gangrene 440.24
  - psychosis (see also Psychosis, arteriosclerotic) 290.40
  - ulceration 440.23
- aorta 440.0

Arteriosclerosis, arteriosclerotic

Arteriosclerosis, arteriosclerotic — *continued*
- arteries of extremities — *see* Arteriosclerosis, extremities
- basilar (artery) (*see also* Occlusion, artery, basilar) 433.0 ☑
- brain 437.0
- bypass graft
  - coronary artery 414.05
    - autologous artery (gastroepiploic) (internal mammary) 414.04
    - autologous vein 414.02
    - nonautologous biological 414.03
    - of transplanted heart 414.07
  - extremity 440.30
    - autologous vein 440.31
    - nonautologous biological 440.32
- cardiac — *see* Arteriosclerosis, coronary
- cardiopathy — *see* Arteriosclerosis, coronary
- cardiorenal (*see also* Hypertension, cardiorenal) 404.90
- cardiovascular (*see also* Disease, cardiovascular) 429.2
- carotid (artery) (common) (internal) (*see also* Occlusion, artery, carotid) 433.1 ☑
- central nervous system 437.0
- cerebral 437.0
  - late effect — *see* Late effect(s) (of) cerebrovascular disease
- cerebrospinal 437.0
- cerebrovascular 437.0
- coronary (artery) 414.00
  - graft — *see* Arteriosclerosis, bypass graft
  - native artery 414.01
  - of transplanted heart 414.06
- extremities (native artery) NEC 440.20
  - bypass graft 440.30
    - autologous vein 440.31
    - nonautologous biological 440.32
  - claudication (intermittent) 440.21
  - and
    - gangrene 440.24
    - rest pain 440.22
      - and
        - gangrene 440.24
        - ulceration 440.23
          - and gangrene 440.24
    - ulceration 440.23
      - and gangrene 440.24
  - gangrene 440.24
  - rest pain 440.22
    - and
      - gangrene 440.24
      - ulceration 440.23
        - and gangrene 440.24
  - specified site NEC 440.29
  - ulceration 440.23
    - and gangrene 440.24
- heart (disease) (*see also* Arteriosclerosis, coronary)
  - valve 424.99
    - aortic 424.1
    - mitral 424.0
    - pulmonary 424.3
    - tricuspid 424.2
- kidney (*see also* Hypertension, kidney) 403.90
- labyrinth, labyrinthine 388.00
- medial NEC (*see also* Arteriosclerosis, extremities) 440.20
- mesentery (artery) 557.1
- Mönckeberg's (*see also* Arteriosclerosis, extremities) 440.20
- myocarditis 429.0
- nephrosclerosis (*see also* Hypertension, kidney) 403.90
- peripheral (of extremities) — *see* Arteriosclerosis, extremities
- precerebral 433.9
  - specified artery NEC 433.8 ☑

Arteriosclerosis, arteriosclerotic — *continued*
- pulmonary (idiopathic) 416.0
- renal (*see also* Hypertension, kidney) 403.90
  - arterioles (*see also* Hypertension, kidney) 403.90
  - artery 440.1
- retinal (vascular) 440.8 *[362.13]*
- specified artery NEC 440.8
  - with gangrene 440.8 *[785.4]*
- spinal (cord) 437.0
- vertebral (artery) (*see also* Occlusion, artery, vertebral) 433.2 ☑

Arteriospasm 443.9

Arteriovenous — *see* condition

Arteritis 447.6
- allergic (*see also* Angiitis, hypersensitivity) 446.20
- aorta (nonsyphilitic) 447.6
  - syphilitic 093.1
- aortic arch 446.7
- brachiocephalica 446.7
- brain 437.4
  - syphilitic 094.89
- branchial 446.7
- cerebral 437.4
  - late effect — *see* Late effect(s) (of) cerebrovascular disease
  - syphilitic 094.89
- coronary (artery) (*see also* Arteriosclerosis, coronary)
  - rheumatic 391.9
    - chronic 398.99
  - syphilitic 093.89
- cranial (left) (right) 446.5
- deformans — *see* Arteriosclerosis
- giant cell 446.5
- necrosing or necrotizing 446.0
- nodosa 446.0
- obliterans (*see also* Arteriosclerosis)
  - subclaviocarotica 446.7
- pulmonary 417.8
- retina 362.18
- rheumatic — *see* Fever, rheumatic
- senile — *see* Arteriosclerosis
- suppurative 447.2
- syphilitic (general) 093.89
  - brain 094.89
  - coronary 093.89
  - spinal 094.89
- temporal 446.5
- young female, syndrome 446.7

Artery, arterial — *see* condition

Arthralgia — *see also* Pain, joint 719.4 ☑
- allergic (*see also* Pain, joint) 719.4 ☑
- in caisson disease 993.3
- psychogenic 307.89
- rubella 056.71
- Salmonella 003.23
- temporomandibular joint 524.62

Arthritis, arthritic (acute) (chronic) (subacute) 716.9 ☑
- meaning Osteoarthritis — *see* Osteoarthrosis

Note — Use the following fifth-digit subclassification with categories 711–712, 715–716:

0 site unspecified
1 shoulder region
2 upper arm
3 forearm
4 hand
5 pelvic region and thigh
6 lower leg
7 ankle and foot
8 other specified sites
9 multiple sites

- allergic 716.2 ☑
- ankylosing (crippling) (spine) 720.0
  - sites other than spine 716.9 ☑

Arthritis, arthritic — *continued*
- atrophic 714.0
  - spine 720.9
- back (*see also* Arthritis, spine) 721.90
- Bechterew's (ankylosing spondylitis) 720.0
- blennorrhagic 098.50
- cervical, cervicodorsal (*see also* Spondylosis, cervical) 721.0
- Charcôt's 094.0 *[713.5]*
  - diabetic 250.6 ☑ *[713.5]*
  - syringomyelic 336.0 *[713.5]*
  - tabetic 094.0 *[713.5]*
- chylous (*see also* Filariasis) 125.9 *[711.7]* ☑
- climacteric NEC 716.3 ☑
- coccyx 721.8
- cricoarytenoid 478.79
- crystal (-induced) — *see* Arthritis, due to crystals
- deformans (*see also* Osteoarthrosis) 715.9 ☑
  - spine 721.90
    - with myelopathy 721.91
- degenerative (*see also* Osteoarthrosis) 715.9 ☑
  - idiopathic 715.09
  - polyarticular 715.09
  - spine 721.90
    - with myelopathy 721.91
- dermatoarthritis, lipoid 272.8 *[713.0]*
- due to or associated with
  - acromegaly 253.0 *[713.0]*
  - actinomycosis 039.8 *[711.4]* ☑
  - amyloidosis 277.39 *[713.7]* ▲
  - bacterial disease NEC 040.89 *[711.4]* ☑
  - Behçet's syndrome 136.1 *[711.2]* ☑
  - blastomycosis 116.0 *[711.6]* ☑
  - brucellosis (*see also* Brucellosis) 023.9 *[711.4]* ☑
  - caisson disease 993.3
  - coccidioidomycosis 114.3 *[711.6]* ☑
  - coliform (Escherichia coli) 711.0 ☑
  - colitis, ulcerative (*see also* Colitis, ulcerative) 556.9 *[713.1]*
  - cowpox 051.0 *[711.5]* ☑
  - crystals (*see also* Gout)
    - dicalcium phosphate 275.49 *[712.1]* ☑
    - pyrophosphate 275.49 *[712.2]* ☑
    - specified NEC 275.49 *[712.8]* ☑
  - dermatoarthritis, lipoid 272.8 *[713.0]*
  - dermatological disorder NEC 709.9 *[713.3]*
  - diabetes 250.6 ☑ *[713.5]*
  - diphtheria 032.89 *[711.4]* ☑
  - dracontiasis 125.7 *[711.7]* ☑
  - dysentery 009.0 *[711.3]* ☑
  - endocrine disorder NEC 259.9 *[713.0]*
  - enteritis NEC 009.1 *[711.3]* ☑
    - infectious (*see also* Enteritis, infectious) 009.0 *[711.3]* ☑
    - specified organism NEC 008.8 *[711.3]* ☑
    - regional (*see also* Enteritis, regional) 555.9 *[713.1]*
    - specified organism NEC 008.8 *[711.3]* ☑
  - epiphyseal slip, nontraumatic (old) 716.8 ☑
  - erysipelas 035 *[711.4]* ☑
  - erythema
    - epidemic 026.1
    - multiforme 695.1 *[713.3]*
    - nodosum 695.2 *[713.3]*
  - Escherichia coli 711.0 ☑
  - filariasis NEC 125.9 *[711.7]* ☑
  - gastrointestinal condition NEC 569.9 *[713.1]*
  - glanders 024 *[711.4]* ☑
  - Gonococcus 098.50

Arthritis, arthritic — *continued*
- due to or associated with — *continued*
  - gout 274.0
  - helminthiasis NEC 128.9 *[711.7]* ☑
  - hematological disorder NEC 289.9 *[713.2]*
  - hemochromatosis 275.0 *[713.0]*
  - hemoglobinopathy NEC (*see also* Disease, hemoglobin) 282.7 *[713.2]*
  - hemophilia (*see also* Hemophilia) 286.0 *[713.2]*
  - Hemophilus influenzae (H. influenzae) 711.0 ☑
  - Henoch (-Schönlein) purpura 287.0 *[713.6]*
  - H. influenzae 711.0 ☑
  - histoplasmosis NEC (*see also* Histoplasmosis) 115.99 *[711.6]* ☑
  - hyperparathyroidism 252.00 *[713.0]*
  - hypersensitivity reaction NEC 995.3 *[713.6]*
  - hypogammaglobulinemia (*see also* Hypogamma-globulinemia) 279.00 *[713.0]*
  - hypothyroidism NEC 244.9 *[713.0]*
  - infection (*see also* Arthritis, infectious) 711.9 ☑
  - infectious disease NEC 136.9 *[711.8]* ☑
  - leprosy (*see also* Leprosy) 030.9 *[711.4]* ☑
  - leukemia NEC (M9800/3) 208.9 *[713.2]*
  - lipoid dermatoarthritis 272.8 *[713.0]*
  - Lyme disease 088.81 *[711.8]* ☑
  - Mediterranean fever, familial 277.31 *[713.7]* ▲
  - meningococcal infection 036.82
  - metabolic disorder NEC 277.9 *[713.0]*
  - multiple myelomatosis (M9730/3) 203.0 *[713.2]*
  - mumps 072.79 *[711.5]* ☑
  - mycobacteria 031.8 *[711.4]* ☑
  - mycosis NEC 117.9 *[711.6]* ☑
  - neurological disorder NEC 349.9 *[713.5]*
  - ochronosis 270.2 *[713.0]*
  - O'Nyong Nyong 066.3 *[711.5]* ☑
  - parasitic disease NEC 136.9 *[711.8]* ☑
  - paratyphoid fever (*see also* Fever, paratyphoid) 002.9 *[711.3]* ☑
  - Pneumococcus 711.0 ☑
  - poliomyelitis (*see also* Poliomyelitis) 045.9 ☑ *[711.5]* ☑
  - Pseudomonas 711.0 ☑
  - psoriasis 696.0
  - pyogenic organism (E. coli) (H. influenzae) (Pseudomonas) (Streptococcus) 711.0 ☑
  - rat-bite fever 026.1 *[711.4]* ☑
  - regional enteritis (*see also* Enteritis, regional) 555.9 *[713.1]*
  - Reiter's disease 099.3 *[711.1]* ☑
  - respiratory disorder NEC 519.9 *[713.4]*
  - reticulosis, malignant (M9720/3) 202.3 *[713.2]*
  - rubella 056.71
  - salmonellosis 003.23
  - sarcoidosis 135 *[713.7]*
  - serum sickness 999.5 *[713.6]*
  - Staphylococcus 711.0 ☑
  - Streptococcus 711.0 ☑
  - syphilis (*see also* Syphilis) 094.0 *[711.4]* ☑
  - syringomyelia 336.0 *[713.5]*
  - thalassemia 282.49 *[713.2]*
  - tuberculosis (*see also* Tuberculosis, arthritis) 015.9 ☑ *[711.4]* ☑

Index to Diseases

Arthritis, arthritic — *continued*
  due to or associated with — *continued*
    typhoid fever 002.0 *[711.3]* ☑
    ulcerative colitis (*see also* Colitis, ulcerative) 556.9 *[713.1]*
    urethritis
      nongonococcal (*see also* Urethritis, nongonococcal) 099.40 *[711.1]* ☑
      nonspecific (*see also* Urethritis, nongonococcal) 099.40 *[711.1]* ☑
      Reiter's 099.3
    viral disease NEC 079.99 *[711.5]* ☑
  erythema epidemic 026.1
  gonococcal 098.50
  gouty (acute) 274.0
  hypertrophic (*see also* Osteoarthrosis) 715.9 ☑
    spine 721.90
      with myelopathy 721.91
  idiopathic, blennorrheal 099.3
  in caisson disease 993.3 *[713.8]*
  infectious or infective (acute) (chronic) (subacute) NEC 711.9 ☑
    nonpyogenic 711.9
    spine 720.9
  inflammatory NEC 714.9
  juvenile rheumatoid (chronic) (polyarticular) 714.30
    acute 714.31
    monoarticular 714.33
    pauciarticular 714.32
  lumbar (*see also* Spondylosis, lumbar) 721.3
  meningococcal 036.82
  menopausal NEC 716.3 ☑
  migratory — *see* Fever, rheumatic
  neuropathic (Charcôt's) 094.0 *[713.5]*
    diabetic 250.6 *[713.5]*
    nonsyphilitic NEC 349.9 *[713.5]*
    syringomyelic 336.0 *[713.5]*
    tabetic 094.0 *[713.5]*
  nodosa (*see also* Osteoarthrosis) 715.9 ☑
    spine 721.90
      with myelopathy 721.91
  nonpyogenic NEC 716.9 ☑
    spine 721.90
      with myelopathy 721.91
  ochronotic 270.2 *[713.0]*
  palindromic (see also Rheumatism, palindromic) 719.3 ☑
  pneumococcal 711.0 ☑
  postdysenteric 009.0 *[711.3]*
  postrheumatic, chronic (Jaccoud's) 714.4
  primary progressive 714.0
    spine 720.9
  proliferative 714.0
    spine 720.0
  psoriatic 696.0
  purulent 711.0 ☑
  pyogenic or pyemic 711.0 ☑
  rheumatic 714.0
    acute or subacute — *see* Fever, rheumatic
    chronic 714.0
    spine 720.9
  rheumatoid (nodular) 714.0
    with
      splenoadenomegaly and leukopenia 714.1
      visceral or systemic involvement 714.2
    aortitis 714.89
    carditis 714.2
    heart disease 714.2
    juvenile (chronic) (polyarticular) 714.30
      acute 714.31
      monoarticular 714.33
      pauciarticular 714.32
    spine 720.0
  rubella 056.71

Arthritis, arthritic — *continued*
  sacral, sacroiliac, sacrococcygeal (*see also* Spondylosis, sacral) 721.3
  scorbutic 267
  senile or senescent (*see also* Osteoarthrosis) 715.9 ☑
    spine 721.90
      with myelopathy 721.91
  septic 711.0 ☑
  serum (nontherapeutic) (therapeutic) 999.5 *[713.6]*
  specified form NEC 716.8 ☑
  spine 721.90
    with myelopathy 721.91
    atrophic 720.9
    degenerative 721.90
      with myelopathy 721.91
    hypertrophic (with deformity) 721.90
      with myelopathy 721.91
    infectious or infective NEC 720.9
    Marie-Strümpell 720.0
    nonpyogenic 721.90
      with myelopathy 721.91
    pyogenic 720.9
    rheumatoid 720.0
    traumatic (old) 721.7
    tuberculous (*see also* Tuberculosis) 015.0 *[720.81]*
  staphylococcal 711.0 ☑
  streptococcal 711.0 ☑
  suppurative 711.0 ☑
  syphilitic 094.0 *[713.5]*
    congenital 090.49 *[713.5]*
  syphilitica deformans (Charcôt) 094.0 *[713.5]*
  temporomandibular joint 524.69
  thoracic (*see also* Spondylosis, thoracic) 721.2
  toxic of menopause 716.3 ☑
  transient 716.4 ☑
  traumatic (chronic) (old) (post) 716.1 ☑
    current injury — *see* nature of injury
  tuberculous (*see also* Tuberculosis, arthritis) 015.9 ☑ *[711.4]* ☑
  urethritica 099.3 *[711.1]* ☑
  urica, uratic 274.0
  venereal 099.3 *[711.1]* ☑
  vertebral (*see also* Arthritis, spine) 721.90
  villous 716.8 ☑
  von Bechterew's 720.0
Arthrocele — *see also* Effusion, joint 719.0
Arthrochondritis — *see* Arthritis
Arthrodesis status V45.4
Arthrodynia — *see also* Pain, joint 719.4 ☑
  psychogenic 307.89
Arthrodysplasia 755.9
Arthrofibrosis joint — *see also* Ankylosis 718.5 ☑
Arthrogryposis 728.3
  multiplex, congenita 754.89
Arthrokatadysis 715.35
Arthrolithiasis 274.0
Arthro-onychodysplasia 756.89
Arthro-osteo-onychodysplasia 756.89

Arthropathy — *see also* Arthritis 716.9 ☑

> Note — Use the following fifth-digit subclassification with categories 711–712, 716:
> 0   site unspecified
> 1   shoulder region
> 2   upper arm
> 3   forearm
> 4   hand
> 5   pelvic region and thigh
> 6   lower leg
> 7   ankle and foot
> 8   other specified sites
> 9   multiple sites

  Behçet's 136.1 *[711.2]* ☑
  Charcôt's 094.0 *[713.5]*
    diabetic 250.6 ☑ *[713.5]*
    syringomyelic 336.0 *[713.5]*
    tabetic 094.0 *[713.5]*
  crystal (-induced) — *see* Arthritis, due to crystals
  gouty 274.0
  neurogenic, neuropathic (Charcôt's) (tabetic) 094.0 *[713.5]*
    diabetic 250.6 ☑ *[713.5]*
    nonsyphilitic NEC 349.9 *[713.5]*
    syringomyelic 336.0 *[713.5]*
  postdysenteric NEC 009.0 *[711.3]* ☑
  postrheumatic, chronic (Jaccoud's) 714.4
  psoriatic 696.0
  pulmonary 731.2
  specified NEC 716.8 ☑
  syringomyelia 336.0 *[713.5]*
  tabes dorsalis 094.0 *[713.5]*
  tabetic 094.0 *[713.5]*
  transient 716.4 ☑
  traumatic 716.1 ☑
  uric acid 274.0
Arthrophyte — *see also* Loose, body, joint 718.1 ☑
Arthrophytis 719.80
  ankle 719.87
  elbow 719.82
  foot 719.87
  hand 719.84
  hip 719.85
  knee 719.86
  multiple sites 719.89
  pelvic region 719.85
  shoulder (region) 719.81
  specified site NEC 719.88
  wrist 719.83
Arthropyosis — *see also* Arthritis, pyogenic 711.0 ☑
Arthroscopic surgical procedure converted to open procedure V64.43
Arthrosis (deformans) (degenerative) — *see also* Osteoarthrosis 715.9 ☑
  Charcôt's 094.0 *[713.5]*
  polyarticular 715.09
  spine (*see also* Spondylosis) 721.90
Arthus phenomenon 995.21 ▲
  due to
    correct substance properly administered 995.21 ▲
    overdose or wrong substance given or taken 977.9
      specified drug — *see* Table of Drugs and Chemicals
    serum 999.5
Articular — *see also* condition
  disc disorder (reducing or non-reducing) 524.63
  spondylolisthesis 756.12
Articulation
  anterior 524.27
  posterior 524.27
  reverse 524.27

Artificial
  device (prosthetic) — *see* Fitting, device
  insemination V26.1
  menopause (states) (symptoms) (syndrome) 627.4
  opening status (functioning) (without complication) V44.9
    anus (colostomy) V44.3
    colostomy V44.3
    cystostomy V44.50
      appendico-vesicostomy V44.52
      cutaneous-vesicostomy V44.51
      specified type NEC V44.59
    enterostomy V44.4
    gastrostomy V44.1
    ileostomy V44.2
    intestinal tract NEC V44.4
    jejunostomy V44.4
    nephrostomy V44.6
    specified site NEC V44.8
    tracheostomy V44.0
    ureterostomy V44.6
    urethrostomy V44.6
    urinary tract NEC V44.6
    vagina V44.7
  vagina status V44.7
ARV (disease) (illness) (infection) — *see* Human immunodeficiency virus (disease) (illness) (infection)
Arytenoid — *see* condition
Asbestosis (occupational) 501
Asboe-Hansen's disease (incontinentia pigmenti) 757.33
Ascariasis (intestinal) (lung) 127.0
Ascaridiasis 127.0
Ascaridosis 127.0
Ascaris 127.0
  lumbricoides (infestation) 127.0
  pneumonia 127.0
Ascending — *see* condition
ASC-H (atypical squamous cells cannot exclude high grade squamous intraepithelial lesion) 795.02
Aschoff's bodies — *see also* Myocarditis, rheumatic 398.0
Ascites 789.5
  abdominal NEC 789.5
  cancerous (M8000/6) 197.6
  cardiac 428.0
  chylous (nonfilarial) 457.8
    filarial (*see also* Infestation, filarial) 125.9
  congenital 778.0
  due to S. japonicum 120.2
  fetal, causing fetopelvic disproportion 653.7 ☑
  heart 428.0
  joint (*see also* Effusion, joint) 719.0 ☑
  malignant (M8000/6) 197.6
  pseudochylous 789.5
  syphilitic 095.2
  tuberculous (*see also* Tuberculosis) 014.0 ☑
Ascorbic acid (vitamin C) **deficiency** (scurvy) 267
ASC-US (atypical squamous cells of undetermined significance) 795.01
ASCVD (arteriosclerotic cardiovascular disease) 429.2
Aseptic — *see* condition
Asherman's syndrome 621.5
Asialia 527.7
Asiatic cholera — *see also* Cholera 001.9
Asocial personality or trends 301.7
Asomatognosia 781.8
Aspergillosis 117.3
  with pneumonia 117.3 *[484.6]*
  allergic bronchopulmonary 518.6
  nonsyphilitic NEC 117.3
Aspergillus (flavus) (fumigatus) (infection) (terreus) 117.3
Aspermatogenesis 606.0
Aspermia (testis) 606.0
Asphyxia, asphyxiation (by) 799.01
  antenatal — *see* Distress, fetal

Asphyxia, asphyxiation

Asphyxia, asphyxiation — *continued*
  bedclothes 994.7
  birth (*see also* Asphyxia, newborn) 768.9
  bunny bag 994.7
  carbon monoxide 986
  caul (*see also* Asphyxia, newborn) 768.9
  cave-in 994.7
    crushing — *see* Injury, internal, intrathoracic organs
  constriction 994.7
  crushing — *see* Injury, internal, intrathoracic organs
  drowning 994.1
  fetal, affecting newborn 768.9
  food or foreign body (in larynx) 933.1
    bronchioles 934.8
    bronchus (main) 934.1
    lung 934.8
    nasopharynx 933.0
    nose, nasal passages 932
    pharynx 933.0
    respiratory tract 934.9
      specified part NEC 934.8
    throat 933.0
    trachea 934.0
  gas, fumes, or vapor NEC 987.9
    specified — *see* Table of Drugs and Chemicals
  gravitational changes 994.7
  hanging 994.7
  inhalation — *see* Inhalation
  intrauterine
    fetal death (before onset of labor) 768.0
    during labor 768.1
    liveborn infant — *see* Distress, fetal, liveborn infant
  local 443.0
  mechanical 994.7
    during birth (*see also* Distress, fetal) 768.9
  mucus 933.1
    bronchus (main) 934.1
    larynx 933.1
    lung 934.8
    nasal passages 932
    newborn 770.18
    pharynx 933.0
    respiratory tract 934.9
      specified part NEC 934.8
    throat 933.0
    trachea 934.0
    vaginal (fetus or newborn) 770.18
  newborn 768.9
    with neurologic involvement 768.5
    blue 768.6
    livida 768.6
    mild or moderate 768.6
    pallida 768.5
    severe 768.5
    white 768.5
  pathological 799.01
  plastic bag 994.7
  postnatal (*see also* Asphyxia, newborn) 768.9
    mechanical 994.7
  pressure 994.7
  reticularis 782.61
  strangulation 994.7
  submersion 994.1
  traumatic NEC — *see* Injury, internal, intrathoracic organs
  vomiting, vomitus — *see* Asphyxia, food or foreign body

Aspiration
  acid pulmonary (syndrome) 997.3
    obstetric 668.0 ☑
  amniotic fluid 770.13
    with respiratory symptoms 770.14
  bronchitis 507.0
  clear amniotic fluid 770.13
    with
      pneumonia 770.14
      pneumonitis 770.14

Aspiration — *continued*
  clear amniotic fluid — *continued*
    with — *continued*
      respiratory symptoms 770.14
  contents of birth canal 770.17
    with respiratory symptoms 770.18
  fetal 770.10
    blood 770.15
      with
        pneumonia 770.16
        pneumonitis 770.16
      pneumonitis 770.18
  food, foreign body, or gasoline (with asphyxiation) — *see* Asphyxia, food or foreign body
  meconium 770.11
    with
      pneumonia 770.12
      pneumonitis 770.12
      respiratory symptoms 770.12
    below vocal cords 770.11
      with respiratory symptoms 770.12
  mucus 933.1
    into
      bronchus (main) 934.1
      lung 934.8
      respiratory tract 934.9
        specified part NEC 934.8
      trachea 934.0
    newborn 770.17
    vaginal (fetus or newborn) 770.17
  newborn 770.10
    with respiratory symptoms 770.18
    blood 770.15
      with
        pneumonia 770.16
        pneumonitis 770.16
        respiratory symptoms 770.16
  pneumonia 507.0
    fetus or newborn 770.18
    meconium 770.12
  pneumonitis 507.0
    fetus or newborn 770.18
    meconium 770.12
    obstetric 668.0 ☑
  postnatal stomach contents 770.85
    with
      pneumonia 770.86
      pneumonitis 770.86
      respiratory symptoms 770.86
  syndrome of newborn (massive) 770.18
    meconium 770.12
  vernix caseosa 770.12

Asplenia 759.0
  with mesocardia 746.87

Assam fever 085.0

Assimilation, pelvis
  with disproportion 653.2 ☑
    affecting fetus or newborn 763.1
    causing obstructed labor 660.1 ☑
      affecting fetus or newborn 763.1

Assmann's focus — *see also* Tuberculosis 011.0 ☑

Astasia (-abasia) 307.9
  hysterical 300.11

Asteatosis 706.8
  cutis 706.8

Astereognosis 780.99

Asterixis 781.3
  in liver disease 572.8

Asteroid hyalitis 379.22

Asthenia, asthenic 780.79
  cardiac (*see also* Failure, heart) 428.9
    psychogenic 306.2
  cardiovascular (*see also* Failure, heart) 428.9
    psychogenic 306.2
  heart (*see also* Failure, heart) 428.9
    psychogenic 306.2
    hysterical 300.11
  myocardial (*see also* Failure, heart) 428.9
    psychogenic 306.2
  nervous 300.5

Asthenia, asthenic — *continued*
  neurocirculatory 306.2
  neurotic 300.5
  psychogenic 300.5
  psychoneurotic 300.5
  psychophysiologic 300.5
  reaction, psychoneurotic 300.5
  senile 797
  Stiller's 780.79
  tropical anhidrotic 705.1

Asthenopia 368.13
  accommodative 367.4
  hysterical (muscular) 300.11
  psychogenic 306.7

Asthenospermia 792.2

Asthma, asthmatic (bronchial) (catarrh) (spasmodic) 493.9 ☑

Note — Use the following fifth-digit subclassification with category 493:
  0 *without mention of status asthmaticus or acute exacerbation or unspecified*
  1 *with status asthmaticus*
  2 *with acute exacerbation*

  with
    chronic obstructive pulmonary disease (COPD) 493.2 ☑
    hay fever 493.0 ☑
    rhinitis, allergic 493.0 ☑
  allergic 493.9 ☑
    stated cause (external allergen) 493.0 ☑
  atopic 493.0 ☑
  cardiac (*see also* Failure, ventricular, left) 428.1
  cardiobronchial (*see also* Failure, ventricular, left) 428.1
  cardiorenal (*see also* Hypertension, cardiorenal) 404.90
  childhood 493.0 ☑
  Colliers' 500
  cough variant 493.82
  croup 493.9 ☑
  detergent 507.8
  due to
    detergent 507.8
    inhalation of fumes 506.3
    internal immunological process 493.0 ☑
  endogenous (intrinsic) 493.1 ☑
  eosinophilic 518.3
  exercise induced bronchospasm 493.81
  exogenous (cosmetics) (dander or dust) (drugs) (dust) (feathers) (food) (hay) (platinum) (pollen) 493.0 ☑
  extrinsic 493.0 ☑
  grinders' 502
  hay 493.0 ☑
  heart (*see also* Failure, ventricular, left) 428.1
  IgE 493.0 ☑
  infective 493.1 ☑
  intrinsic 493.1 ☑
  Kopp's 254.8
  late-onset 493.1 ☑
  meat-wrappers' 506.9
  Millar's (laryngismus stridulus) 478.75
  millstone makers' 502
  miners' 500
  Monday morning 504
  New Orleans (epidemic) 493.0 ☑
  platinum 493.0 ☑
  pneumoconiotic (occupational) NEC 505
  potters' 502
  psychogenic 316 [493.9] ☑
  pulmonary eosinophilic 518.3
  red cedar 495.8
  Rostan's (*see also* Failure, ventricular, left) 428.1

Asthma, asthmatic — *continued*
  sandblasters' 502
  sequoiosis 495.8
  stonemasons' 502
  thymic 254.8
  tuberculous (*see also* Tuberculosis, pulmonary) 011.9 ☑
  Wichmann's (laryngismus stridulus) 478.75
  wood 495.8

Astigmatism (compound) (congenital) 367.20
  irregular 367.22
  regular 367.21

Astroblastoma (M9430/3)
  nose 748.1
  specified site — *see* Neoplasm, by site, malignant
  unspecified site 191.9

Astrocytoma (cystic) (M9400/3)
  anaplastic type (M9401/3)
    specified site — *see* Neoplasm, by site, malignant
    unspecified site 191.9
  fibrillary (M9420/3)
    specified site — *see* Neoplasm, by site, malignant
    unspecified site 191.9
  fibrous (M9420/3)
    specified site — *see* Neoplasm, by site, malignant
    unspecified site 191.9
  gemistocytic (M9411/3)
    specified site — *see* Neoplasm, by site, malignant
    unspecified site 191.9
  juvenile (M9421/3)
    specified site — *see* Neoplasm, by site, malignant
    unspecified site 191.9
  nose 748.1
  pilocytic (M9421/3)
    specified site — *see* Neoplasm, by site, malignant
    unspecified site 191.9
  piloid (M9421/3)
    specified site — *see* Neoplasm, by site, malignant
    unspecified site 191.9
  protoplasmic (M9410/3)
    specified site — *see* Neoplasm, by site, malignant
    unspecified site 191.9
  specified site — *see* Neoplasm, by site, malignant
  subependymal (M9383/1) 237.5
    giant cell (M9384/1) 237.5
  unspecified site 191.9

Astroglioma (M9400/3)
  nose 748.1
  specified site — *see* Neoplasm, by site, malignant
  unspecified site 191.9

Asymbolia 784.60

Asymmetrical breathing 786.09

Asymmetry — *see also* Distortion
  chest 786.9
  face 754.0
  jaw NEC 524.12
    maxillary 524.11
  pelvis with disproportion 653.0 ☑
    affecting fetus or newborn 763.1
    causing obstructed labor 660.1 ☑
      affecting fetus or newborn 763.1

Asynergia 781.3

Asynergy 781.3
  ventricular 429.89

Asystole (heart) — *see also* Arrest, cardiac 427.5

Ataxia, ataxy, ataxic 781.3
  acute 781.3
  brain 331.89
  cerebellar 334.3
    hereditary (Marie's) 334.2
  in
    alcoholism 303.9 ☑ [334.4]

Ataxia, ataxy, ataxic — *continued*
  cerebellar — *continued*
    in — *continued*
      myxedema (*see also* Myxedema) 244.9 [334.4]
      neoplastic disease NEC 239.9 [334.4]
  cerebral 331.89
  family, familial 334.2
    cerebral (Marie's) 334.2
    spinal (Friedreich's) 334.0
  Friedreich's (heredofamilial) (spinal) 334.0
  frontal lobe 781.3
  gait 781.2
    hysterical 300.11
  general 781.3
  hereditary NEC 334.2
    cerebellar 334.2
    spastic 334.1
    spinal 334.0
  heredofamilial (Marie's) 334.2
  hysterical 300.11
  locomotor (progressive) 094.0
    diabetic 250.6 ☑ [337.1]
  Marie's (cerebellar) (heredofamilial) 334.2
  nonorganic origin 307.9
  partial 094.0
  postchickenpox 052.7
  progressive locomotor 094.0
  psychogenic 307.9
  Sanger-Brown's 334.2
  spastic 094.0
    hereditary 334.1
    syphilitic 094.0
  spinal
    hereditary 334.0
    progressive locomotor 094.0
  telangiectasia 334.8
Ataxia-telangiectasia 334.8
Atelectasis (absorption collapse) (complete) (compression) (massive) (partial) (postinfective) (pressure collapse) (pulmonary) (relaxation) 518.0
  newborn (congenital) (partial) 770.5
    primary 770.4
  primary 770.4
  tuberculous (*see also* Tuberculosis, pulmonary) 011.9 ☑
Ateleiosis, ateliosis 253.3
Atelia — *see* Distortion
Ateliosis 253.3
Atelocardia 746.9
Atelomyelia 742.59
Athelia 757.6
Atheroembolism
  extremity
    lower 445.02
    upper 445.01
  kidney 445.81
  specified site NEC 445.89
Atheroma, atheromatous — *see also* Arteriosclerosis 440.9
  aorta, aortic 440.0
    valve (*see also* Endocarditis, aortic) 424.1
  artery — *see* Arteriosclerosis
  basilar (artery) (*see also* Occlusion, artery, basilar) 433.0 ☑
  carotid (artery) (common) (internal) (*see also* Occlusion, artery, carotid) 433.1 ☑
  cerebral (arteries) 437.0
  coronary (artery) — *see* Arteriosclerosis, coronary
  degeneration — *see* Arteriosclerosis
  heart, cardiac — *see* Arteriosclerosis, coronary
  mitral (valve) 424.0
  myocardium, myocardial — *see* Arteriosclerosis, coronary
  pulmonary valve (heart) (*see also* Endocarditis, pulmonary) 424.3
  skin 706.2

Atheroma, atheromatous — *see also* Arteriosclerosis — *continued*
  tricuspid (heart) (valve) 424.2
  valve, valvular — *see* Endocarditis
  vertebral (artery) (*see also* Occlusion, artery, vertebral) 433.2 ☑
Atheromatosis — *see also* Arteriosclerosis
  arterial, congenital 272.8
Atherosclerosis — *see* Arteriosclerosis
Athetosis (acquired) 781.0
  bilateral 333.79 ▲
  congenital (bilateral) 333.6 ▲
  double 333.71 ▲
  unilateral 781.0
Athlete's
  foot 110.4
  heart 429.3
Athletic team examination V70.3
Athrepsia 261
Athyrea (acquired) — *see also* Hypothyroidism 244.9
  congenital 243
Athyreosis (congenital) 243
  acquired — *see* Hypothyroidism
Athyroidism (acquired) — *see also* Hypothyroidism 244.9
  congenital 243
Atmospheric pyrexia 992.0
Atonia, atony, atonic
  abdominal wall 728.2
  bladder (sphincter) 596.4
    neurogenic NEC 596.54
      with cauda equina syndrome 344.61
  capillary 448.9
  cecum 564.89
    psychogenic 306.4
  colon 564.89
    psychogenic 306.4
  congenital 779.89
  dyspepsia 536.3
    psychogenic 306.4
  intestine 564.89
    psychogenic 306.4
  stomach 536.3
    neurotic or psychogenic 306.4
    psychogenic 306.4
  uterus
    with hemorrhage 666.1 ☑ ●
    without hemorrhage 669.8 ☑ ●
  vesical 596.4
Atopy NEC V15.09
Atransferrinemia, congenital 273.8
Atresia, atretic (congenital) 759.89
  alimentary organ or tract NEC 751.8
    lower 751.2
    upper 750.8
  ani, anus, anal (canal) 751.2
  aorta 747.22
    with hypoplasia of ascending aorta and defective development of left ventricle (with mitral valve atresia) 746.7
    arch 747.11
    ring 747.21
  aortic (orifice) (valve) 746.89
    arch 747.11
  aqueduct of Sylvius 742.3
    with spina bifida (*see also* Spina bifida) 741.0 ☑
  artery NEC (*see also* Atresia, blood vessel) 747.60
    cerebral 747.81
    coronary 746.85
    eye 743.58
    pulmonary 747.3
    umbilical 747.5
  auditory canal (external) 744.02
  bile, biliary duct (common) or passage 751.61
    acquired (*see also* Obstruction, biliary) 576.2
  bladder (neck) 753.6
  blood vessel (peripheral) NEC 747.60
    cerebral 747.81

Atresia, atretic — *continued*
  blood vessel — *continued*
    gastrointestinal 747.61
    lower limb 747.64
    pulmonary artery 747.3
    renal 747.62
    spinal 747.82
    upper limb 747.63
  bronchus 748.3
  canal, ear 744.02
  cardiac
    valve 746.89
      aortic 746.89
      mitral 746.89
      pulmonary 746.01
      tricuspid 746.1
  cecum 751.2
  cervix (acquired) 622.4
    congenital 752.49
    in pregnancy or childbirth 654.6 ☑
      affecting fetus or newborn 763.89
      causing obstructed labor 660.2 ☑
        affecting fetus or newborn 763.1
  choana 748.0
  colon 751.2
  cystic duct 751.61
    acquired 575.8
      with obstruction (*see also* Obstruction, gallbladder) 575.2
  digestive organs NEC 751.8
  duodenum 751.1
  ear canal 744.02
  ejaculatory duct 752.89
  epiglottis 748.3
  esophagus 750.3
  Eustachian tube 744.24
  fallopian tube (acquired) 628.2
    congenital 752.19
  follicular cyst 620.0
  foramen of
    Luschka 742.3
      with spina bifida (*see also* Spina bifida) 741.0 ☑
    Magendie 742.3
      with spina bifida (*see also* Spina bifida) 741.0 ☑
  gallbladder 751.69
  genital organ
    external
      female 752.49
      male NEC 752.89
        penis 752.69
    internal
      female 752.89
      male 752.89
  glottis 748.3
  gullet 750.3
  heart
    valve NEC 746.89
      aortic 746.89
      mitral 746.89
      pulmonary 746.01
      tricuspid 746.1
  hymen 752.42
    acquired 623.3
    postinfective 623.3
  ileum 751.1
  intestine (small) 751.1
    large 751.2
  iris, filtration angle (*see also* Buphthalmia) 743.20
  jejunum 751.1
  kidney 753.3
  lacrimal, apparatus 743.65
    acquired — *see* Stenosis, lacrimal
  larynx 748.3
  ligament, broad 752.19
  lung 748.5
  meatus urinarius 753.6
  mitral valve 746.89

Atresia, atretic — *continued*
  mitral valve — *continued*
    with atresia or hypoplasia of aortic orifice or valve, with hypoplasia of ascending aorta and defective development of left ventricle 746.7
  nares (anterior) (posterior) 748.0
  nasolacrimal duct 743.65
  nasopharynx 748.8
  nose, nostril 748.0
    acquired 738.0
  organ or site NEC — *see* Anomaly, specified type NEC
  osseous meatus (ear) 744.03
  oviduct (acquired) 628.2
    congenital 752.19
  parotid duct 750.23
    acquired 527.8
  pulmonary (artery) 747.3
    valve 746.01
    vein 747.49
  pulmonic 746.01
  pupil 743.46
  rectum 751.2
  salivary duct or gland 750.23
    acquired 527.8
  sublingual duct 750.23
    acquired 527.8
  submaxillary duct or gland 750.23
    acquired 527.8
  trachea 748.3
  tricuspid valve 746.1
  ureter 753.29
  ureteropelvic junction 753.21
  ureterovesical orifice 753.22
  urethra (valvular) 753.6
  urinary tract NEC 753.29
  uterus 752.3
    acquired 621.8
  vagina (acquired) 623.2
    congenital 752.49
    postgonococcal (old) 098.2
    postinfectional 623.2
    senile 623.2
  vascular NEC (*see also* Atresia, blood vessel) 747.60
    cerebral 747.81
  vas deferens 752.89
  vein NEC (*see also* Atresia, blood vessel) 747.60
    cardiac 746.89
    great 747.49
    portal 747.49
    pulmonary 747.49
    vena cava (inferior) (superior) 747.49
  vesicourethral orifice 753.6
  vulva 752.49
    acquired 624.8
Atrichia, atrichosis 704.00
  congenital (universal) 757.4
Atrioventricularis commune 745.69
At risk for falling V15.88
Atrophia — *see also* Atrophy
  alba 709.09
  cutis 701.8
    idiopathica progressiva 701.8
    senilis 701.8
  dermatological, diffuse (idiopathic) 701.8
  flava hepatis (acuta) (subacuta) (*see also* Necrosis, liver) 570
  gyrata of choroid and retina (central) 363.54
    generalized 363.57
  senilis 797
    dermatological 701.8
  unguium 703.8
    congenita 757.5
Atrophoderma, atrophodermia 701.9
  diffusum (idiopathic) 701.8
  maculatum 701.3
    et striatum 701.3
      due to syphilis 095.8
    syphilitic 091.3
  neuriticum 701.8

Atrophoderma, atrophodermia — continued
- pigmentosum 757.33
- reticulatum symmetricum faciei 701.8
- senile 701.8
- symmetrical 701.8
- vermiculata 701.8

Atrophy, atrophic
- adrenal (autoimmune) (capsule) (cortex) (gland) 255.4
  - with hypofunction 255.4
- alveolar process or ridge (edentulous) 525.20
  - mandible 525.20
    - minimal 525.21
    - moderate 525.22
    - severe 525.23
  - maxilla 525.20
    - minimal 525.24
    - moderate 525.25
    - severe 525.26
- appendix 543.9
- Aran-Duchenne muscular 335.21
- arm 728.2
- arteriosclerotic — see Arteriosclerosis
- arthritis 714.0
  - spine 720.9
- bile duct (any) 576.8
- bladder 596.8
- blanche (of Milian) 701.3
- bone (senile) 733.99
  - due to
    - disuse 733.7
    - infection 733.99
    - tabes dorsalis (neurogenic) 094.0
  - posttraumatic 733.99
- brain (cortex) (progressive) 331.9
  - with dementia 290.10
  - Alzheimer's 331.0
    - with dementia — see Alzheimer's, dementia
  - circumscribed (Pick's) 331.11
    - with dementia
      - with behavioral disturbance 331.11 [294.11]
      - without behavioral disturbance 331.11 [294.10]
  - congenital 742.4
  - hereditary 331.9
  - senile 331.2
- breast 611.4
  - puerperal, postpartum 676.3 ☑
- buccal cavity 528.9
- cardiac (brown) (senile) (see also Degeneration, myocardial) 429.1
- cartilage (infectional) (joint) 733.99
- cast, plaster of Paris 728.2
- cerebellar — see Atrophy, brain
- cerebral — see Atrophy, brain
- cervix (endometrium) (mucosa) (myometrium) (senile) (uteri) 622.8
  - menopausal 627.8
- Charcôt-Marie-Tooth 356.1
- choroid 363.40
  - diffuse secondary 363.42
  - hereditary (see also Dystrophy, choroid) 363.50
    - gyrate
      - central 363.54
      - diffuse 363.57
      - generalized 363.57
  - senile 363.41
- ciliary body 364.57
- colloid, degenerative 701.3
- conjunctiva (senile) 372.89
- corpus cavernosum 607.89
- cortical (see also Atrophy, brain) 331.9
- Cruveilhier's 335.21
- cystic duct 576.8
- dacryosialadenopathy 710.2
- degenerative
  - colloid 701.3
  - senile 701.3
- Déjérine-Thomas 333.0

Atrophy, atrophic — continued
- diffuse idiopathic, dermatological 701.8
- disuse
  - bone 733.7
  - muscle 728.2
  - pelvic muscles and anal sphincter 618.83
- Duchenne-Aran 335.21
- ear 388.9
- edentulous alveolar ridge 525.20
  - mandible 525.20
    - minimal 525.21
    - moderate 525.22
    - severe 525.23
  - maxilla 525.20
    - minimal 525.24
    - moderate 525.25
    - severe 525.26
- emphysema, lung 492.8
- endometrium (senile) 621.8
  - cervix 622.8
- enteric 569.89
- epididymis 608.3
- eyeball, cause unknown 360.41
- eyelid (senile) 374.50
- facial (skin) 701.9
- facioscapulohumeral (Landouzy-Déjérine) 359.1
- fallopian tube (senile), acquired 620.3
- fatty, thymus (gland) 254.8
- gallbladder 575.8
- gastric 537.89
- gastritis (chronic) 535.1 ☑
- gastrointestinal 569.89
- genital organ, male 608.89
- glandular 289.3
- globe (phthisis bulbi) 360.41
- gum (see also Recession, gingival) 523.20
- hair 704.2
- heart (brown) (senile) (see also Degeneration, myocardial) 429.1
- hemifacial 754.0
  - Romberg 349.89
- hydronephrosis 591
- infantile 261
  - paralysis, acute (see also Poliomyelitis, with paralysis) 045.1 ☑
- intestine 569.89
- iris (generalized) (postinfectional) (sector shaped) 364.59
  - essential 364.51
  - progressive 364.51
  - sphincter 364.54
- kidney (senile) (see also Sclerosis, renal) 587
  - with hypertension (see also Hypertension, kidney) 403.90
  - congenital 753.0
  - hydronephrotic 591
  - infantile 753.0
- lacrimal apparatus (primary) 375.13
  - secondary 375.14
- Landouzy-Déjérine 359.1
- laryngitis, infection 476.0
- larynx 478.79
- Leber's optic 377.16
- lip 528.5
- liver (acute) (subacute) (see also Necrosis, liver) 570
  - chronic (yellow) 571.8
  - yellow (congenital) 570
    - with
      - abortion — see Abortion, by type, with specified complication NEC
      - ectopic pregnancy (see also categories 633.0–633.9) 639.8
      - molar pregnancy (see also categories 630–632) 639.8
    - chronic 571.8
    - complicating pregnancy 646.7 ☑

Atrophy, atrophic — continued
- liver (see also Necrosis, liver) — continued
  - yellow — continued
    - following
      - abortion 639.8
      - ectopic or molar pregnancy 639.8
    - from injection, inoculation or transfusion (onset within 8 months after administration) — see Hepatitis, viral
    - healed 571.5
    - obstetric 646.7 ☑
    - postabortal 639.8
    - postimmunization — see Hepatitis, viral
    - posttransfusion — see Hepatitis, viral
    - puerperal, postpartum 674.8 ☑
- lung (senile) 518.89
  - congenital 748.69
- macular (dermatological) 701.3
  - syphilitic, skin 091.3
  - striated 095.8
- muscle, muscular 728.2
  - disuse 728.2
  - Duchenne-Aran 335.21
  - extremity (lower) (upper) 728.2
  - familial spinal 335.11
  - general 728.2
  - idiopathic 728.2
  - infantile spinal 335.0
  - myelopathic (progressive) 335.10
  - myotonic 359.2
  - neuritic 356.1
  - neuropathic (peroneal) (progressive) 356.1
  - peroneal 356.1
  - primary (idiopathic) 728.2
  - progressive (familial) (hereditary) (pure) 335.21
    - adult (spinal) 335.19
    - infantile (spinal) 335.0
    - juvenile (spinal) 335.11
    - spinal 335.10
      - adult 335.19
      - hereditary or familial 335.11
      - infantile 335.0
  - pseudohypertrophic 359.1
  - spinal (progressive) 335.10
    - adult 335.19
    - Aran-Duchenne 335.21
    - familial 335.11
    - hereditary 335.11
    - infantile 335.0
    - juvenile 335.11
  - syphilitic 095.6
- myocardium (see also Degeneration, myocardial) 429.1
- myometrium (senile) 621.8
  - cervix 622.8
- myotatic 728.2
- myotonia 359.2
- nail 703.8
  - congenital 757.5
- nasopharynx 472.2
- nerve (see also Disorder, nerve)
  - abducens 378.54
  - accessory 352.4
  - acoustic or auditory 388.5
  - cranial 352.9
    - first (olfactory) 352.0
    - second (optic) (see also Atrophy, optic nerve) 377.10
    - third (oculomotor) (partial) 378.51
      - total 378.52
    - fourth (trochlear) 378.53
    - fifth (trigeminal) 350.8
    - sixth (abducens) 378.54
    - seventh (facial) 351.8
    - eighth (auditory) 388.5
    - ninth (glossopharyngeal) 352.2
    - tenth (pneumogastric) (vagus) 352.3

Atrophy, atrophic — continued
- nerve (see also Disorder, nerve) — continued
  - cranial — continued
    - eleventh (accessory) 352.4
    - twelfth (hypoglossal) 352.5
  - facial 351.8
  - glossopharyngeal 352.2
  - hypoglossal 352.5
  - oculomotor (partial) 378.51
    - total 378.52
  - olfactory 352.0
  - peripheral 355.9
  - pneumogastric 352.3
  - trigeminal 350.8
  - trochlear 378.53
  - vagus (pneumogastric) 352.3
- nervous system, congenital 742.8
- neuritic (see also Disorder, nerve) 355.9
- neurogenic NEC 355.9
  - bone
    - tabetic 094.0
- nutritional 261
- old age 797
- olivopontocerebellar 333.0
- optic nerve (ascending) (descending) (infectional) (nonfamilial) (papillomacular bundle) (postretinal) (secondary NEC) (simple) 377.10
  - associated with retinal dystrophy 377.13
  - dominant hereditary 377.16
  - glaucomatous 377.14
  - hereditary (dominant) (Leber's) 377.16
  - Leber's (hereditary) 377.16
  - partial 377.15
  - postinflammatory 377.12
  - primary 377.11
  - syphilitic 094.84
    - congenital 090.49
    - tabes dorsalis 094.0
- orbit 376.45
- ovary (senile), acquired 620.3
- oviduct (senile), acquired 620.3
- palsy, diffuse 335.20
- pancreas (duct) (senile) 577.8
- papillary muscle 429.81
- paralysis 355.9
- parotid gland 527.0
- patches skin 701.3
  - senile 701.8
- penis 607.89
- pharyngitis 472.1
- pharynx 478.29
- pluriglandular 258.8
- polyarthritis 714.0
- prostate 602.2
- pseudohypertrophic 359.1
- renal (see also Sclerosis, renal) 587
- reticulata 701.8
- retina (see also Degeneration, retina) 362.60
  - hereditary (see also Dystrophy, retina) 362.70
- rhinitis 472.0
- salivary duct or gland 527.0
- scar NEC 709.2
- sclerosis, lobar (of brain) 331.0
  - with dementia
    - with behavioral disturbance 331.0 [294.11]
    - without behavioral disturbance 331.0 [294.10]
- scrotum 608.89
- seminal vesicle 608.89
- senile 797
  - degenerative, of skin 701.3
  - skin (patches) (senile) 701.8
- spermatic cord 608.89
- spinal (cord) 336.8
  - acute 336.8
  - muscular (chronic) 335.10
    - adult 335.19
    - familial 335.11

Index to Diseases

Atrophy, atrophic — *continued*
  spinal — *continued*
    muscular — *continued*
      juvenile 335.10
      paralysis 335.10
        acute (*see also* Poliomyelitis, with paralysis) 045.1 ☑
  spine (column) 733.99
  spleen (senile) 289.59
  spots (skin) 701.3
    senile 701.8
  stomach 537.89
  striate and macular 701.3
    syphilitic 095.8
  subcutaneous 701.9
    due to injection 999.9
  sublingual gland 527.0
  submaxillary gland 527.0
  Sudeck's 733.7
  suprarenal (autoimmune) (capsule) (gland) 255.4
    with hypofunction 255.4
  tarso-orbital fascia, congenital 743.66
  testis 608.3
  thenar, partial 354.0
  throat 478.29
  thymus (fat) 254.8
  thyroid (gland) 246.8
    with
      cretinism 243
      myxedema 244.9
    congenital 243
  tongue (senile) 529.8
    papillae 529.4
    smooth 529.4
  trachea 519.19
  tunica vaginalis 608.89
  turbinate 733.99
  tympanic membrane (nonflaccid) 384.82
    flaccid 384.81
  ulcer (*see also* Ulcer, skin) 707.9
  upper respiratory tract 478.9
  uterus, uterine (acquired) (senile) 621.8
    cervix 622.8
    due to radiation (intended effect) 621.8
  vagina (senile) 627.3
  vascular 459.89
  vas deferens 608.89
  vertebra (senile) 733.99
  vulva (primary) (senile) 624.1
  Werdnig-Hoffmann 335.0
  yellow (acute) (congenital) (liver) (subacute) (*see also* Necrosis, liver) 570
    chronic 571.8
    resulting from administration of blood, plasma, serum, or other biological substance (within 8 months of administration) — *see* Hepatitis, viral

Attack
  akinetic (*see also* Epilepsy) 345.0 ☑
  angina — *see* Angina
  apoplectic (*see also* Disease, cerebrovascular, acute) 436
  benign shuddering 333.93
  bilious — *see* Vomiting
  cataleptic 300.11
  cerebral (*see also* Disease, cerebrovascular, acute) 436
  coronary (*see also* Infarct, myocardium) 410.9 ☑
  cyanotic, newborn 770.83
  epileptic (*see also* Epilepsy) 345.9 ☑
  epileptiform 780.39
  heart (*see also* Infarct, myocardium) 410.9 ☑
  hemiplegia (*see also* Disease, cerebrovascular, acute) 436
  hysterical 300.11
  jacksonian (*see also* Epilepsy) 345.5 ☑
  myocardium, myocardial (*see also* Infarct, myocardium) 410.9 ☑

Attack — *continued*
  myoclonic (*see also* Epilepsy) 345.1 ☑
  panic 300.01
  paralysis (*see also* Disease, cerebrovascular, acute) 436
  paroxysmal 780.39
  psychomotor (*see also* Epilepsy) 345.4 ☑
  salaam (*see also* Epilepsy) 345.6 ☑
  schizophreniform (*see also* Schizophrenia) 295.4 ☑
  sensory and motor 780.39
  syncope 780.2
  toxic, cerebral 780.39
  transient ischemic (TIA) 435.9
  unconsciousness 780.2
    hysterical 300.11
  vasomotor 780.2
  vasovagal (idiopathic) (paroxysmal) 780.2

Attention to
  artificial opening (of) V55.9
    digestive tract NEC V55.4
    specified site NEC V55.8
    urinary tract NEC V55.6
    vagina V55.7
  colostomy V55.3
  cystostomy V55.5
  dressing
    wound V58.30
      nonsurgical V58.30
      surgical V58.31
  gastrostomy V55.1
  ileostomy V55.2
  jejunostomy V55.4
  nephrostomy V55.6
  surgical dressings V58.31
  sutures V58.32
  tracheostomy V55.0
  ureterostomy V55.6
  urethrostomy V55.6

Attrition
  gum (*see also* Recession, gingival) 523.20
  teeth (hard tissues) 521.10
    excessive 521.10
      extending into
        dentine 521.12
        pulp 521.13
      generalized 521.15
      limited to enamel 521.11
      localized 521.14

Atypical — *see also* condition
  cells
    endocervical 795.00
    endometrial 795.00
    glandular 795.00
  distribution, vessel (congenital) (peripheral) NEC 747.60
  endometrium 621.9
  kidney 593.89

Atypism, cervix 622.10

Audible tinnitus — *see also* Tinnitus 388.30

Auditory — *see* condition

Audry's syndrome (acropachyderma) 757.39

Aujeszky's disease 078.89

Aura, jacksonian — *see also* Epilepsy 345.5 ☑

Aurantiasis, cutis 278.3

Auricle, auricular — *see* condition

Auriculotemporal syndrome 350.8

Australian
  Q fever 083.0
  X disease 062.4

Autism, autistic (child) (infantile) 299.0 ☑

Autodigestion 799.89

Autoerythrocyte sensitization 287.2

Autographism 708.3

Autoimmune
  cold sensitivity 283.0
  disease NEC 279.4
  hemolytic anemia 283.0
  thyroiditis 245.2

Autoinfection, septic — *see* Septicemia

Autointoxication 799.89

Automatism 348.8
  epileptic (*see also* Epilepsy) 345.4 ☑
  paroxysmal, idiopathic (*see also* Epilepsy) 345.4 ☑

Autonomic, autonomous
  bladder 596.54
    neurogenic 596.54
      with cauda equina 344.61
  dysreflexia 337.3
  faciocephalalgia (*see also* Neuropathy, peripheral, autonomic) 337.9
  hysterical seizure 300.11
  imbalance (*see also* Neuropathy, peripheral, autonomic) 337.9

Autophony 388.40

Autosensitivity, erythrocyte 287.2

Autotopagnosia 780.99

Autotoxemia 799.89

Autumn — *see* condition

Avellis' syndrome 344.89

Aviators
  disease or sickness (*see also* Effect, adverse, high altitude) 993.2
    ear 993.0
  effort syndrome 306.2

Avitaminosis (multiple NEC) — *see also* Deficiency, vitamin 269.2
  A 264.9
  B 266.9
    with
      beriberi 265.0
      pellagra 265.2
  B_1 265.1
  B_2 266.0
  B_6 266.1
  B_{12} 266.2
  C (with scurvy) 267
  D 268.9
    with
      osteomalacia 268.2
      rickets 268.0
  E 269.1
  G 266.0
  H 269.1
  K 269.0
  multiple 269.2
  nicotinic acid 265.2
  P 269.1

Avulsion (traumatic) 879.8
  blood vessel — *see* Injury, blood vessel, by site
  cartilage (*see also* Dislocation, by site)
    knee, current (*see also* Tear, meniscus) 836.2
    symphyseal (inner), complicating delivery 665.6 ☑
  complicated 879.9
  diaphragm — *see* Injury, internal, diaphragm
  ear — *see* Wound, open, ear
  epiphysis of bone — *see* Fracture, by site
  external site other than limb — *see* Wound, open, by site
  eye 871.3
  fingernail — *see* Wound, open, finger
  fracture — *see* Fracture, by site
  genital organs, external — *see* Wound, open, genital organs
  head (intracranial) NEC (*see also* Injury, intracranial, with open intracranial wound)
    complete 874.9
    external site NEC 873.8
    complicated 873.9
  internal organ or site — *see* Injury, internal, by site
  joint (*see also* Dislocation, by site)
    capsule — *see* Sprain, by site
  ligament — *see* Sprain, by site
  limb (*see also* Amputation, traumatic, by site)

Avulsion — *continued*
  limb (*see also* Amputation, traumatic, by site) — *continued*
    skin and subcutaneous tissue — *see* Wound, open, by site
  muscle — *see* Sprain, by site
  nerve (root) — *see* Injury, nerve, by site
  scalp — *see* Wound, open, scalp
  skin and subcutaneous tissue — *see* Wound, open, by site
  symphyseal cartilage (inner), complicating delivery 665.6 ☑
  tendon (*see also* Sprain, by site)
    with open wound — *see* Wound, open, by site
  toenail — *see* Wound, open, toe(s)
  tooth 873.63
    complicated 873.73

Awaiting organ transplant status V49.83

Awareness of heart beat 785.1

Axe grinders' disease 502

Axenfeld's anomaly or syndrome 743.44

Axilla, axillary — *see also* condition
  breast 757.6

Axonotmesis — *see* Injury, nerve, by site

Ayala's disease 756.89

Ayerza's disease or syndrome (pulmonary artery sclerosis with pulmonary hypertension) 416.0

Azoospermia 606.0

Azorean disease (of the nervous system) 334.8

Azotemia 790.6
  meaning uremia (*see also* Uremia) 586

Aztec ear 744.29

Azygos lobe, lung (fissure) 748.69

B

Baader's syndrome (erythema multiforme exudativum) 695.1

Baastrup's syndrome 721.5

Babesiasis 088.82

Babesiosis 088.82

Babington's disease (familial hemorrhagic telangiectasia) 448.0

Babinski-Fröhlich syndrome (adiposogenital dystrophy) 253.8

Babinski-Nageotte syndrome 344.89

Babinski's syndrome (cardiovascular syphilis) 093.89

Bacillary — *see* condition

Bacilluria 791.9
  asymptomatic, in pregnancy or puerperium 646.5 ☑
  tuberculous (*see also* Tuberculosis) 016.9 ☑

Bacillus — *see also* Infection, bacillus
  abortus infection 023.1
  anthracis infection 022.9
  coli
    infection 041.4
      generalized 038.42
      intestinal 008.00
    pyemia 038.42
    septicemia 038.42
  Flexner's 004.1
  fusiformis infestation 101
  mallei infection 024
  Shiga's 004.0
  suipestifer infection (*see also* Infection, Salmonella) 003.9

Back — *see* condition

Backache (postural) 724.5
  psychogenic 307.89
  sacroiliac 724.6

Backflow (pyelovenous) — *see also* Disease, renal 593.9

Backknee — *see* Genu, recurvatum 736.5

Bacteremia 790.7
  newborn 771.83

Bacteria
  in blood (*see also* Bacteremia) 790.7

Bacteria

Bacteria — *continued*
  in urine (*see also* Bacteriuria) 599.0
Bacterial — *see* condition
Bactericholia — *see also* Cholecystitis, acute 575.0
Bacterid, bacteride (Andrews' pustular) 686.8
Bacteriuria, bacteruria 791.9
  with
    urinary tract infection 599.0
  asymptomatic 791.9
    in pregnancy or puerperium 646.5 ☑
      affecting fetus or newborn 760.1
Bad
  breath 784.99 ▲
  heart — *see* Disease, heart
  trip (*see also* Abuse, drugs, nondependent) 305.3 ☑
Baehr-Schiffrin disease (thrombotic thrombocytopenic purpura) 446.6
Baelz's disease (cheilitis glandularis apostematosa) 528.5
Baerensprung's disease (eczema marginatum) 110.3
Bagassosis (occupational) 495.1
Baghdad boil 085.1
Bagratuni's syndrome (temporal arteritis) 446.5
Baker's
  cyst (knee) 727.51
    tuberculous (*see also* Tuberculosis) 015.2 ☑
  itch 692.89
Bakwin-Krida syndrome (craniometaphyseal dysplasia) 756.89
Balanitis (circinata) (gangraenosa) (infectious) (vulgaris) 607.1
  amebic 006.8
  candidal 112.2
  chlamydial 099.53
  due to Ducrey's bacillus 099.0
  erosiva circinata et gangraenosa 607.1
  gangrenous 607.1
  gonococcal (acute) 098.0
    chronic or duration of 2 months or over 098.2
  nongonococcal 607.1
  phagedenic 607.1
  venereal NEC 099.8
  xerotica obliterans 607.81
Balanoposthitis 607.1
  chlamydial 099.53
  gonococcal (acute) 098.0
    chronic or duration of 2 months or over 098.2
  ulcerative NEC 099.8
Balanorrhagia — *see* Balanitis
Balantidiasis 007.0
Balantidiosis 007.0
Balbuties, balbutio 307.0
Bald
  patches on scalp 704.00
  tongue 529.4
Baldness — *see also* Alopecia 704.00
Balfour's disease (chloroma) 205.3 ☑
Balint's syndrome (psychic paralysis of visual fixation) 368.16
Balkan grippe 083.0
Ball
  food 938
  hair 938
Ballantyne (-Runge) syndrome (postmaturity) 766.22
Balloon disease — *see also* Effect, adverse, high altitude 993.2
Ballooning posterior leaflet syndrome 424.0
Baló's disease or concentric sclerosis 341.1
Bamberger's disease (hypertrophic pulmonary osteoarthropathy) 731.2
Bamberger-Marie disease (hypertrophic pulmonary osteoarthropathy) 731.2
Bamboo spine 720.0
Bancroft's filariasis 125.0

Band(s)
  adhesive (*see also* Adhesions, peritoneum) 568.0
  amniotic 658.8 ☑
    affecting fetus or newborn 762.8
  anomalous or congenital (*see also* Anomaly, specified type NEC)
    atrial 746.9
    heart 746.9
    intestine 751.4
    omentum 751.4
    ventricular 746.9
  cervix 622.3
  gallbladder (congenital) 751.69
  intestinal (adhesive) (*see also* Adhesions, peritoneum) 568.0
    congenital 751.4
    obstructive (*see also* Obstruction, intestine) 560.81
  periappendiceal (congenital) 751.4
  peritoneal (adhesive) (*see also* Adhesions, peritoneum) 568.0
    with intestinal obstruction 560.81
    congenital 751.4
  uterus 621.5
  vagina 623.2
Bandl's ring (contraction)
  complicating delivery 661.4 ☑
    affecting fetus or newborn 763.7
Bang's disease (Brucella abortus) 023.1
Bangkok hemorrhagic fever 065.4
Bannister's disease 995.1
Bantam-Albright-Martin disease (pseudohypoparathyroidism) 275.49
Banti's disease or syndrome (with cirrhosis) (with portal hypertension) — *see* Cirrhosis, liver
Bar
  calcaneocuboid 755.67
  calcaneonavicular 755.67
  cubonavicular 755.67
  prostate 600.90
    with
      other lower urinary tract symptoms (LUTS) 600.91 ●
      urinary
        obstruction 600.91 ●
        retention 600.91 ●
  talocalcaneal 755.67
Baragnosis 780.99
Barasheh, barashek 266.2
Barcoo disease or rot — *see also* Ulcer, skin 707.9
Bard-Pic syndrome (carcinoma, head of pancreas) 157.0
Bärensprung's disease (eczema marginatum) 110.3
Baritosis 503
Barium lung disease 503
Barlow (-Möller) disease or syndrome (meaning infantile scurvy) 267
Barlow's syndrome (meaning mitral valve prolapse) 424.0
Barodontalgia 993.2
Baron Münchausen syndrome 301.51
Barosinusitis 993.1
Barotitis 993.0
Barotrauma 993.2
  odontalgia 993.2
  otitic 993.0
  sinus 993.1
Barraquer's disease or syndrome (progressive lipodystrophy) 272.6
Barré-Guillain syndrome 357.0
Barrel chest 738.3
Barré-Liéou syndrome (posterior cervical sympathetic) 723.2
Barrett's esophagus 530.85
Barrett's syndrome or ulcer (chronic peptic ulcer of esophagus) 530.85
Bársony-Polgár syndrome (corkscrew esophagus) 530.5
Bársony-Teschendorf syndrome (corkscrew esophagus) 530.5

Bartholin's
  adenitis (*see also* Bartholinitis) 616.89 ▲
  gland — *see* condition
Bartholinitis (suppurating) 616.89 ▲
  gonococcal (acute) 098.0
    chronic or duration of 2 months or over 098.2
Barth syndrome 759.89
Bartonellosis 088.0
Bartter's syndrome (secondary hyperaldosteronism with juxtaglomerular hyperplasia) 255.13
Basal — *see* condition
Basan's (hidrotic) **ectodermal dysplasia** 757.31
Baseball finger 842.13
Basedow's disease or syndrome (exophthalmic goiter) 242.0 ☑
Basic — *see* condition
Basilar — *see* condition
Bason's (hidrotic) **ectodermal dysplasia** 757.31
Basopenia 288.59 ▲
Basophilia 288.65 ▲
Basophilism (corticoadrenal) (Cushing's) (pituitary) (thymic) 255.0
Bassen-Kornzweig syndrome (abetalipoproteinemia) 272.5
Bat ear 744.29
Bateman's
  disease 078.0
  purpura (senile) 287.2
Bathing cramp 994.1
Bathophobia 300.23
Batten's disease, retina 330.1 [362.71]
Batten-Mayou disease 330.1 [362.71]
Batten-Steinert syndrome 359.2
Battered
  adult (syndrome) 995.81
  baby or child (syndrome) 995.54
  spouse (syndrome) 995.81
Battey mycobacterium infection 031.0
Battledore placenta — *see* Placenta, abnormal
Battle exhaustion — *see also* Reaction, stress, acute 308.9
Baumgarten-Cruveilhier (cirrhosis) **disease, or syndrome** 571.5
Bauxite
  fibrosis (of lung) 503
  workers' disease 503
Bayle's disease (dementia paralytica) 094.1
Bazin's disease (primary) — *see also* Tuberculosis 017.1 ☑
Beach ear 380.12
Beaded hair (congenital) 757.4
Beals syndrome 759.82
Beard's disease (neurasthenia) 300.5
Bearn-Kunkel (-Slater) syndrome (lupoid hepatitis) 571.49
Beat
  elbow 727.2
  hand 727.2
  knee 727.2
Beats
  ectopic 427.60
  escaped, heart 427.60
    postoperative 997.1
  premature (nodal) 427.60
    atrial 427.61
    auricular 427.61
    postoperative 997.1
    specified type NEC 427.69
    supraventricular 427.61
    ventricular 427.69
Beau's
  disease or syndrome (*see also* Degeneration, myocardial) 429.1
  lines (transverse furrows on fingernails) 703.8
Bechterew's disease (ankylosing spondylitis) 720.0
Bechterew-Strümpell-Marie syndrome (ankylosing spondylitis) 720.0

Becker's
  disease (idiopathic mural endomyocardial disease) 425.2
  dystrophy 359.1
Beck's syndrome (anterior spinal artery occlusion) 433.8 ☑
Beckwith (-Wiedemann) syndrome 759.89
Bedclothes, asphyxiation or suffocation by 994.7
Bed confinement status V49.84
Bednar's aphthae 528.2
Bedsore 707.00
  with gangrene 707.00 [785.4]
Bedwetting — *see also* Enuresis 788.36
Beer-drinkers' heart (disease) 425.5
Bee sting (with allergic or anaphylactic shock) 989.5
Begbie's disease (exophthalmic goiter) 242.0 ☑
Behavior disorder, disturbance — *see also* Disturbance, conduct
  antisocial, without manifest psychiatric disorder
    adolescent V71.02
    adult V71.01
    child V71.02
  dyssocial, without manifest psychiatric disorder
    adolescent V71.02
    adult V71.01
    child V71.02
  high risk — *see* Problem
Behçet's syndrome 136.1
Behr's disease 362.50
Beigel's disease or morbus (white piedra) 111.2
Bejel 104.0
Bekhterev's disease (ankylosing spondylitis) 720.0
Bekhterev-Strümpell-Marie syndrome (ankylosing spondylitis) 720.0
Belching — *see also* Eructation 787.3
Bell's
  disease (*see also* Psychosis, affective) 296.0 ☑
  mania (*see also* Psychosis, affective) 296.0 ☑
  palsy, paralysis 351.0
    infant 767.5
    newborn 767.5
    syphilitic 094.89
  spasm 351.0
Bence-Jones albuminuria, albuminosuria, or proteinuria 791.0
Bends 993.3
Benedikt's syndrome (paralysis) 344.89
Benign — *see also* condition
  cellular changes, cervix 795.09
  prostate
    with
      other lower urinary tract symptoms (LUTS) 600.21 ●
      urinary
        obstruction 600.21 ●
        retention 600.21 ●
    hyperplasia 600.20
    neoplasm 222.2
Bennett's
  disease (leukemia) 208.9 ☑
  fracture (closed) 815.01
    open 815.11
Benson's disease 379.22
Bent
  back (hysterical) 300.11
  nose 738.0
    congenital 754.0
Bereavement V62.82
  as adjustment reaction 309.0
Bergeron's disease (hysteroepilepsy) 300.11
Berger's paresthesia (lower limb) 782.0
Beriberi (acute) (atrophic) (chronic) (dry) (subacute) (wet) 265.0
  with polyneuropathy 265.0 [357.4]

Beriberi — continued
  heart (disease) 265.0 [425.7]
  leprosy 030.1
  neuritis 265.0 [357.4]
Berlin's disease or edema (traumatic) 921.3
Berloque dermatitis 692.72
Bernard-Horner syndrome — see also Neuropathy, peripheral, autonomic 337.9
Bernard-Sergent syndrome (acute adrenocortical insufficiency) 255.4
Bernard-Soulier disease or thrombopathy 287.1
Bernhardt's disease or paresthesia 355.1
Bernhardt-Roth disease or syndrome (paresthesia) 355.1
Bernheim's syndrome — see also Failure, heart 428.0
Bertielliasis 123.8
Bertolotti's syndrome (sacralization of fifth lumbar vertebra) 756.15
Berylliosis (acute) (chronic) (lung) (occupational) 503
Besnier's
  lupus pernio 135
  prurigo (atopic dermatitis) (infantile eczema) 691.8
Besnier-Boeck disease or sarcoid 135
Besnier-Boeck-Schaumann disease (sarcoidosis) 135
Best's disease 362.76
Bestiality 302.1
Beta-adrenergic hyperdynamic circulatory state 429.82
Beta-aminoisobutyric aciduria 277.2
Beta-mercaptolactate-cysteine disulfiduria 270.0
Beta thalassemia (major) (minor) (mixed) 282.49
Beurmann's disease (sporotrichosis) 117.1
Bezoar 938
  intestine 936
  stomach 935.2
Bezold's abscess — see also Mastoiditis 383.01
Bianchi's syndrome (aphasia-apraxia-alexia) 784.69
Bicornuate or bicornis uterus 752.3
  in pregnancy or childbirth 654.0 ☑
    with obstructed labor 660.2 ☑
      affecting fetus or newborn 763.1
  affecting fetus or newborn 763.89
Bicuspid aortic valve 746.4
Biedl-Bardet syndrome 759.89
Bielschowsky's disease 330.1
Bielschowsky-Jansky
  amaurotic familial idiocy 330.1
  disease 330.1
Biemond's syndrome (obesity, polydactyly, and mental retardation) 759.89
Biermer's anemia or disease (pernicious anemia) 281.0
Biett's disease 695.4
Bifid (congenital) — see also Imperfect, closure
  apex, heart 746.89
  clitoris 752.49
  epiglottis 748.3
  kidney 753.3
  nose 748.1
  patella 755.64
  scrotum 752.89
  toe 755.66
  tongue 750.13
  ureter 753.4
  uterus 752.3
  uvula 749.02
    with cleft lip (see also Cleft, palate, with cleft lip) 749.20
Biforis uterus (supraplex) 752.3
Bifurcation (congenital) — see also Imperfect, closure
  gallbladder 751.69

Bifurcation — see also Imperfect, closure — continued
  kidney pelvis 753.3
  renal pelvis 753.3
  rib 756.3
  tongue 750.13
  trachea 748.3
  ureter 753.4
  urethra 753.8
  uvula 749.02
    with cleft lip (see also Cleft, palate, with cleft lip) 749.20
  vertebra 756.19
Bigeminal pulse 427.89
Bigeminy 427.89
Big spleen syndrome 289.4
Bilateral — see condition
Bile duct — see condition
Bile pigments in urine 791.4
Bilharziasis — see also Schistosomiasis 120.9
  chyluria 120.0
  cutaneous 120.3
  galacturia 120.0
  hematochyluria 120.0
  intestinal 120.1
  lipemia 120.9
  lipuria 120.0
  Oriental 120.2
  piarhemia 120.9
  pulmonary 120.2
  tropical hematuria 120.0
  vesical 120.0
Biliary — see condition
Bilious (attack) — see also Vomiting
  fever, hemoglobinuric 084.8
Bilirubinuria 791.4
Biliuria 791.4
Billroth's disease
  meningocele (see also Spina bifida) 741.9 ☑
Bilobate placenta — see Placenta, abnormal
Bilocular
  heart 745.7
  stomach 536.8
Bing-Horton syndrome (histamine cephalgia) 346.2 ☑
Binswanger's disease or dementia 290.12
Biörck (-Thorson) syndrome (malignant carcinoid) 259.2
Biparta, bipartite — see also Imperfect, closure
  carpal scaphoid 755.59
  patella 755.64
  placenta — see Placenta, abnormal
  vagina 752.49
Bird
  face 756.0
  fanciers' lung or disease 495.2
Bird's disease (oxaluria) 271.8
Birth
  abnormal fetus or newborn 763.9
  accident, fetus or newborn — see Birth, injury
  complications in mother — see Delivery, complicated
  compression during NEC 767.9
  defect — see Anomaly
  delayed, fetus 763.9
  difficult NEC, affecting fetus or newborn 763.9
  dry, affecting fetus or newborn 761.1
  forced, NEC, affecting fetus or newborn 763.89
  forceps, affecting fetus or newborn 763.2
  hematoma of sternomastoid 767.8
  immature 765.1 ☑
    extremely 765.0 ☑
  inattention, after or at 995.52
  induced, affecting fetus or newborn 763.89
  infant — see Newborn
  injury NEC 767.9

Birth — continued
  injury — continued
    adrenal gland 767.8
    basal ganglia 767.0
    brachial plexus (paralysis) 767.6
    brain (compression) (pressure) 767.0
      cerebellum 767.0
      cerebral hemorrhage 767.0
    conjunctiva 767.8
    eye 767.8
    fracture
      bone, any except clavicle or spine 767.3
      clavicle 767.2
      femur 767.3
      humerus 767.3
      long bone 767.3
      radius and ulna 767.3
      skeleton NEC 767.3
      skull 767.3
      spine 767.4
      tibia and fibula 767.3
    hematoma 767.8
      liver (subcapsular) 767.8
      mastoid 767.8
      skull 767.19
      sternomastoid 767.8
      testes 767.8
      vulva 767.8
    intracranial (edema) 767.0
    laceration
      brain 767.0
      by scalpel 767.8
      peripheral nerve 767.7
    liver 767.8
    meninges
      brain 767.0
      spinal cord 767.4
    nerves (cranial, peripheral) 767.7
      brachial plexus 767.6
      facial 767.5
    paralysis 767.7
      brachial plexus 767.6
      Erb (-Duchenne) 767.6
      facial nerve 767.5
      Klumpke (-Déjerine) 767.6
      radial nerve 767.6
      spinal (cord) (hemorrhage) (laceration) (rupture) 767.4
    rupture
      intracranial 767.0
      liver 767.8
      spinal cord 767.4
      spleen 767.8
      viscera 767.8
    scalp 767.19
    scalpel wound 767.8
    skeleton NEC 767.3
    specified NEC 767.8
    spinal cord 767.4
    spleen 767.8
    subdural hemorrhage 767.0
    tentorial, tear 767.0
    testes 767.8
    vulva 767.8
  instrumental, NEC, affecting fetus or newborn 763.2
  lack of care, after or at 995.52
  multiple
    affected by maternal complications of pregnancy 761.5
    healthy liveborn — see Newborn, multiple
  neglect, after or at 995.52
  newborn — see Newborn
  palsy or paralysis NEC 767.7
  precipitate, fetus or newborn 763.6
  premature (infant) 765.1 ☑
  prolonged, affecting fetus or newborn 763.9
  retarded, fetus or newborn 763.9
  shock, newborn 779.89
  strangulation or suffocation
    due to aspiration of clear amniotic fluid 770.13

Birth — continued
  strangulation or suffocation — continued
    due to aspiration of clear amniotic fluid — continued
      with respiratory symptoms 770.14
    mechanical 767.8
    trauma NEC 767.9
  triplet
    affected by maternal complications of pregnancy 761.5
    healthy liveborn — see Newborn, multiple
  twin
    affected by maternal complications of pregnancy 761.5
    healthy liveborn — see Newborn, twin
  ventouse, affecting fetus or newborn 763.3
Birthmark 757.32
Bisalbuminemia 273.8
Biskra button 085.1
Bite(s)
  with intact skin surface — see Contusion
  animal — see Wound, open, by site
    intact skin surface — see Contusion
  centipede 989.5
  chigger 133.8
  fire ant 989.5
  flea — see Injury, superficial, by site
  human (open wound) (see also Wound, open, by site)
    intact skin surface — see Contusion
  insect
    nonvenomous — see Injury, superficial, by site
    venomous 989.5
  mad dog (death from) 071
  open
    anterior 524.24
    posterior 524.25
  poisonous 989.5
  red bug 133.8
  reptile 989.5
    nonvenomous — see Wound, open, by site
  snake 989.5
    nonvenomous — see Wound, open, by site
  spider (venomous) 989.5
    nonvenomous — see Injury, superficial, by site
  venomous 989.5
Biting
  cheek or lip 528.9
  nail 307.9
Black
  death 020.9
  eye NEC 921.0
  hairy tongue 529.3
  heel 924.20
  lung disease 500
  palm 923.20
Blackfan-Diamond anemia or syndrome (congenital hypoplastic anemia) 284.01
Blackhead 706.1
Blackout 780.2
Blackwater fever 084.8
Bladder — see condition
Blast
  blindness 921.3
  concussion — see Blast, injury
  injury 869.0
    with open wound into cavity 869.1
    abdomen or thorax — see Injury, internal, by site
    brain (see also Concussion, brain) 850.9
      with skull fracture — see Fracture, skull

Blast

Blast — *continued*
  injury — *continued*
    ear (acoustic nerve trauma) 951.5
      with perforation, tympanic
        membrane — *see* Wound,
        open, ear, drum
    lung (*see also* Injury, internal,
      lung) 861.20
    otitic (explosive) 388.11
Blastomycosis, blastomycotic (chronic)
  (cutaneous) (disseminated) (lung)
  (pulmonary) (systemic) 116.0
  Brazilian 116.1
  European 117.5
  keloidal 116.2
  North American 116.0
  primary pulmonary 116.0
  South American 116.1
Bleb(s) 709.8
  emphysematous (bullous) (diffuse)
    (lung) (ruptured) (solitary) 492.0
  filtering, eye (postglaucoma) (status)
    V45.69
    with complication 997.99
      postcataract extraction (complica-
        tion) 997.99
  lung (ruptured) 492.0
    congenital 770.5
  subpleural (emphysematous) 492.0
Bleeder (familial) (hereditary) — *see also*
  Defect, coagulation 286.9
  nonfamilial 286.9
Bleeding — *see also* Hemorrhage 459.0
  anal 569.3
  anovulatory 628.0
  atonic, following delivery 666.1 ☑
  capillary 448.9
  due to subinvolution 621.1
    puerperal 666.2 ☑
  ear 388.69
  excessive, associated with menopausal
    onset 627.0
  familial (*see also* Defect, coagulation)
    286.9
  following intercourse 626.7
  gastrointestinal 578.9
  gums 523.8
  hemorrhoids — *see* Hemorrhoids,
    bleeding
  intermenstrual
    irregular 626.6
    regular 626.5
  intraoperative 998.11
  irregular NEC 626.4
  menopausal 627.0
  mouth 528.9
  nipple 611.79
  nose 784.7
  ovulation 626.5
  postclimacteric 627.1
  postcoital 626.7
  postmenopausal 627.1
    following induced menopause
      627.4
  postoperative 998.11
  preclimacteric 627.0
  puberty 626.3
    excessive, with onset of menstrual
      periods 626.3
  rectum, rectal 569.3
  tendencies (*see also* Defect, coagula-
    tion) 286.9
  throat 784.8
  umbilical stump 772.3
  umbilicus 789.9
  unrelated to menstrual cycle 626.6
  uterus, uterine 626.9
    climacteric 627.0
    dysfunctional 626.8
    functional 626.8
    unrelated to menstrual cycle 626.6
  vagina, vaginal 623.8
    functional 626.8
  vicarious 625.8
Blennorrhagia, blennorrhagic — *see*
  Blennorrhea

Blennorrhea (acute) 098.0
  adultorum 098.40
  alveolaris 523.40 ▲
  chronic or duration of 2 months or
    over 098.2
  gonococcal (neonatorum) 098.40
  inclusion (neonatal) (newborn) 771.6
  neonatorum 098.40
Blepharelosis — *see also* Entropion
  374.00
Blepharitis (eyelid) 373.00
  angularis 373.01
  ciliaris 373.00
    with ulcer 373.01
  marginal 373.00
    with ulcer 373.01
  scrofulous (*see also* Tuberculosis)
    017.3 ☑ [373.00]
  squamous 373.02
  ulcerative 373.01
Blepharochalasis 374.34
  congenital 743.62
Blepharoclonus 333.81
Blepharoconjunctivitis — *see also*
  Conjunctivitis 372.20
  angular 372.21
  contact 372.22
Blepharophimosis (eyelid) 374.46
  congenital 743.62
Blepharoplegia 374.89
Blepharoptosis 374.30
  congenital 743.61
Blepharopyorrhea 098.49
Blepharospasm 333.81
  due to drugs 333.85 ●
Blessig's cyst 362.62
Blighted ovum 631
Blind
  bronchus (congenital) 748.3
  eye (*see also* Blindness)
    hypertensive 360.42
    hypotensive 360.41
  loop syndrome (postoperative) 579.2
  sac, fallopian tube (congenital) 752.19
  spot, enlarged 368.42
  tract or tube (congenital) NEC — *see*
    Atresia
Blindness (acquired) (congenital) (both
  eyes) 369.00
  blast 921.3
    with nerve injury — *see* Injury,
      nerve, optic
  Bright's — *see* Uremia
  color (congenital) 368.59
    acquired 368.55
    blue 368.53
    green 368.52
    red 368.51
    total 368.54
  concussion 950.9
  cortical 377.75
  day 368.10
    acquired 368.10
    congenital 368.10
    hereditary 368.10
    specified type NEC 368.10
  due to
    injury NEC 950.9
    refractive error — *see* Error, refrac-
      tive
  eclipse (total) 363.31
  emotional 300.11
  hysterical 300.11
  legal (both eyes) (USA definition) 369.4
    with impairment of better (less im-
      paired) eye
      near-total 369.02
        with
          lesser eye impairment
            369.02
          near-total 369.04
          total 369.03
      profound 369.05
        with
          lesser eye impairment
            369.05

Blindness — *continued*
  legal — *continued*
    with impairment of better eye —
      continued
      profound — *continued*
        with — *continued*
          lesser eye impairment —
            continued
            near-total 369.07
            profound 369.08
            total 369.06
      severe 369.21
        with
          lesser eye impairment
            369.21
          blind 369.11
          near-total 369.13
          profound 369.14
          severe 369.22
          total 369.12
      total
        with lesser eye impairment
          total 369.01
  mind 784.69
  moderate
    both eyes 369.25
      with impairment of lesser eye
        (specified as)
        blind, not further specified
          369.15
        low vision, not further speci-
          fied 369.23
        near-total 369.17
        profound 369.18
        severe 369.24
        total 369.16
    one eye 369.74
      with vision of other eye (speci-
        fied as)
        near-normal 369.75
        normal 369.76
  near-total
    both eyes 369.04
      with impairment of lesser eye
        (specified as)
        blind, not further specified
          369.02
        total 369.03
    one eye 369.64
      with vision of other eye (speci-
        fied as)
        near-normal 369.65
        normal 369.66
  night 368.60
    acquired 368.62
    congenital (Japanese) 368.61
    hereditary 368.61
    specified type NEC 368.69
    vitamin A deficiency 264.5
  nocturnal — *see* Blindness, night
  one eye 369.60
    with low vision of other eye 369.10
  profound
    both eyes 369.08
      with impairment of lesser eye
        (specified as)
        blind, not further specified
          369.05
        near-total 369.07
        total 369.06
    one eye 369.67
      with vision of other eye (speci-
        fied as)
        near-normal 369.68
        normal 369.69
  psychic 784.69
  severe
    both eyes 369.22
      with impairment of lesser eye
        (specified as)
        blind, not further specified
          369.11
        low vision, not further speci-
          fied 369.21
        near-total 369.13
        profound 369.14

Blindness — *continued*
  severe — *continued*
    both eyes — *continued*
      with impairment of lesser eye —
        continued
        total 369.12
    one eye 369.71
      with vision of other eye (speci-
        fied as)
        near-normal 369.72
        normal 369.73
  snow 370.24
  sun 363.31
  temporary 368.12
  total
    both eyes 369.01
    one eye 369.61
      with vision of other eye (speci-
        fied as)
        near-normal 369.62
        normal 369.63
  transient 368.12
  traumatic NEC 950.9
  word (developmental) 315.01
    acquired 784.61
    secondary to organic lesion 784.61
Blister — *see also* Injury, superficial, by
  site
  beetle dermatitis 692.89
  due to burn — *see* Burn, by site, sec-
    ond degree
  fever 054.9
  multiple, skin, nontraumatic 709.8
Bloating 787.3
Bloch-Siemens syndrome (incontinentia
  pigmenti) 757.33
Bloch-Stauffer dyshormonal dermato-
  sis 757.33
Bloch-Sulzberger disease or syndrome
  (incontinentia pigmenti)
  (melanoblastosis) 757.33
Block
  alveolar capillary 516.3
  arborization (heart) 426.6
  arrhythmic 426.9
  atrioventricular (AV) (incomplete)
    (partial) 426.10
    with
      2:1 atrioventricular response
        block 426.13
      atrioventricular dissociation
        426.0
    first degree (incomplete) 426.11
    second degree (Mobitz type I)
      426.13
      Mobitz (type) II 426.12
    third degree 426.0
    complete 426.0
      congenital 746.86
    congenital 746.86
    Mobitz (incomplete)
      type I (Wenckebach's) 426.13
      type II 426.12
    partial 426.13
  auriculoventricular (*see also* Block,
    atrioventricular) 426.10
    complete 426.0
      congenital 746.86
    congenital 746.86
  bifascicular (cardiac) 426.53
  bundle branch (complete) (false) (in-
    complete) 426.50
    bilateral 426.53
    left (complete) (main stem) 426.3
      with right bundle branch block
        426.53
      anterior fascicular 426.2
        with
          posterior fascicular block
            426.3
          right bundle branch block
            426.52
      hemiblock 426.2
      incomplete 426.2
        with right bundle branch
          block 426.53

Index to Diseases

Block — *continued*
  bundle branch — *continued*
    left — *continued*
      posterior fascicular 426.2
        with
          anterior fascicular block 426.3
          right bundle branch block 426.51
    right 426.4
      with
        left bundle branch block (incomplete) (main stem) 426.53
        left fascicular block 426.53
          anterior 426.52
          posterior 426.51
    Wilson's type 426.4
  cardiac 426.9
  conduction 426.9
    complete 426.0
  Eustachian tube (*see also* Obstruction, Eustachian tube) 381.60
  fascicular (left anterior) (left posterior) 426.2
  foramen Magendie (acquired) 331.3
    congenital 742.3
      with spina bifida (*see also* Spina bifida) 741.0 ☑
  heart 426.9
    first degree (atrioventricular) 426.11
    second degree (atrioventricular) 426.13
    third degree (atrioventricular) 426.0
    bundle branch (complete) (false) (incomplete) 426.50
      bilateral 426.53
      left (*see also* Block, bundle branch, left) 426.3
      right (*see also* Block, bundle branch, right) 426.4
    complete (atrioventricular) 426.0
    congenital 746.86
    incomplete 426.13
    intra-atrial 426.6
    intraventricular NEC 426.6
    sinoatrial 426.6
    specified type NEC 426.6
  hepatic vein 453.0
  intraventricular (diffuse) (myofibrillar) 426.6
    bundle branch (complete) (false) (incomplete) 426.50
      bilateral 426.53
      left (*see also* Block, bundle branch, left) 426.3
      right (*see also* Block, bundle branch, right) 426.4
  kidney (*see also* Disease, renal) 593.9
    postcystoscopic 997.5
  myocardial (*see also* Block, heart) 426.9
  nodal 426.10
  optic nerve 377.49
  organ or site (congenital) NEC — *see* Atresia
  parietal 426.6
  peri-infarction 426.6
  portal (vein) 452
  sinoatrial 426.6
  sinoauricular 426.6
  spinal cord 336.9
  trifascicular 426.54
  tubal 628.2
  vein NEC 453.9
Blocq's disease or syndrome (astasia-abasia) 307.9
Blood
  constituents, abnormal NEC 790.6
  disease 289.9
    specified NEC 289.89
  donor V59.01
    other blood components V59.09
    stem cells V59.02

Blood — *continued*
  donor — *continued*
    whole blood V59.01
  dyscrasia 289.9
    with
      abortion — *see* Abortion, by type, with hemorrhage, delayed or excessive
      ectopic pregnancy (*see also* categories 633.0–633.9) 639.1
      molar pregnancy (*see also* categories 630–632) 639.1
    fetus or newborn NEC 776.9
    following
      abortion 639.1
      ectopic or molar pregnancy 639.1
    puerperal, postpartum 666.3 ☑
  flukes NEC (*see also* Infestation, Schistosoma) 120.9
  in
    feces (*see also* Melena) 578.1
      occult 792.1
    urine (*see also* Hematuria) 599.7
  mole 631
  occult 792.1
  poisoning (*see also* Septicemia) 038.9
  pressure
    decreased, due to shock following injury 958.4
    fluctuating 796.4
    high (*see also* Hypertension) 401.9
      incidental reading (isolated) (nonspecific), without diagnosis of hypertension 796.2
    low (*see also* Hypotension) 458.9
      incidental reading (isolated) (nonspecific), without diagnosis of hypotension 796.3
  spitting (*see also* Hemoptysis) 786.3
  staining cornea 371.12
  transfusion
    without reported diagnosis V58.2
    donor V59.01
      stem cells V59.02
    reaction or complication — *see* Complications, transfusion
  tumor — *see* Hematoma
  vessel rupture — *see* Hemorrhage
  vomiting (*see also* Hematemesis) 578.0
Blood-forming organ disease 289.9
Bloodgood's disease 610.1
Bloodshot eye 379.93
Bloom (-Machacek) (-Torre) syndrome 757.39
Blotch, palpebral 372.55
Blount-Barber syndrome (tibia vara) 732.4
Blount's disease (tibia vara) 732.4
Blue
  baby 746.9
  bloater 491.20
    with
      acute bronchitis 491.22
      exacerbation (acute) 491.21
  diaper syndrome 270.0
  disease 746.9
  dome cyst 610.0
  drum syndrome 381.02
  sclera 743.47
    with fragility of bone and deafness 756.51
  toe syndrome 445.02
Blueness — *see also* Cyanosis 782.5
Blurring, visual 368.8
Blushing (abnormal) (excessive) 782.62
BMI (body mass index)
  adult
    25.0-25.9 V85.21
    26.0-26.9 V85.22
    27.0-27.9 V85.23
    28.0-28.9 V85.24
    29.0-29.9 V85.25

BMI — *continued*
  adult — *continued*
    30.0-30.9 V85.30
    31.0-31.9 V85.31
    32.0-32.9 V85.32
    33.0-33.9 V85.33
    34.0-34.9 V85.34
    35.0-35.9 V85.35
    36.0-36.9 V85.36
    37.0-37.9 V85.37
    38.0-38.9 V85.38
    39.0-39.9 V85.39
    40 and over V85.4
    between 19-24 V85.1
    less than 19 V85.0
  pediatric
    5th percentile to less than 85th percentile for age V85.52
    85th percentile to less than 95th percentile for age V85.53
    greater than or equal to 95th percentile for age V85.54
    less than 5th percentile for age V85.51
Boarder, hospital V65.0
  infant V65.0
Bockhart's impetigo (superficial folliculitis) 704.8
Bodechtel-Guttmann disease (subacute sclerosing panencephalitis) 046.2
Boder-Sedgwick syndrome (ataxia-telangiectasia) 334.8
Body, bodies
  Aschoff (*see also* Myocarditis, rheumatic) 398.0
  asteroid, vitreous 379.22
  choroid, colloid (degenerative) 362.57
    hereditary 362.77
  cytoid (retina) 362.82
  drusen (retina) (*see also* Drusen) 362.57
    optic disc 377.21
  fibrin, pleura 511.0
  foreign — *see* Foreign body
  Hassall-Henle 371.41
  loose
    joint (*see also* Loose, body, joint) 718.1 ☑
      knee 717.6
    knee 717.6
    sheath, tendon 727.82
  Mallory's 034.1
  mass index (BMI)
    adult
      25.0-25.9 V85.21
      26.0-26.9 V85.22
      27.0-27.9 V85.23
      28.0-28.9 V85.24
      29.0-29.9 V85.25
      30.0-30.9 V85.30
      31.0-31.9 V85.31
      32.0-32.9 V85.32
      33.0-33.9 V85.33
      34.0-34.9 V85.34
      36.0-36.9 V85.36
      37.0-37.9 V85.37
      38.0-38.9 V85.38
      39.0-39.9 V85.39
      40 and over V85.4
      between 19-24 V85.1
      less than 19 V85.0
    pediatric
      5th percentile to less than 85th percentile for age V85.52
      85th percentile to less than 95th percentile for age V85.53
      greater than or equal to 95th percentile for age V85.54
      less than 5th percentile for age V85.51
  Mooser 081.0
  Negri 071

Body, bodies — *continued*
  rice (joint) (*see also* Loose, body, joint) 718.1 ☑
    knee 717.6
  rocking 307.3
Boeck's
  disease (sarcoidosis) 135
  lupoid (miliary) 135
  sarcoid 135
Boerhaave's syndrome (spontaneous esophageal rupture) 530.4
Boggy
  cervix 622.8
  uterus 621.8
Boil — *see also* Carbuncle 680.9
  abdominal wall 680.2
  Aleppo 085.1
  ankle 680.6
  anus 680.5
  arm (any part, above wrist) 680.3
  auditory canal, external 680.0
  axilla 680.3
  back (any part) 680.2
  Baghdad 085.1
  breast 680.2
  buttock 680.5
  chest wall 680.2
  corpus cavernosum 607.2
  Delhi 085.1
  ear (any part) 680.0
  eyelid 373.13
  face (any part, except eye) 680.0
  finger (any) 680.4
  flank 680.2
  foot (any part) 680.7
  forearm 680.3
  Gafsa 085.1
  genital organ, male 608.4
  gluteal (region) 680.5
  groin 680.2
  hand (any part) 680.4
  head (any part, except face) 680.8
  heel 680.7
  hip 680.6
  knee 680.6
  labia 616.4
  lacrimal (*see also* Dacryocystitis) 375.30
    gland (*see also* Dacryoadenitis) 375.00
    passages (duct) (sac) (*see also* Dacryocystitis) 375.30
  leg, any part, except foot 680.6
  multiple sites 680.9
  natal 085.1
  neck 680.1
  nose (external) (septum) 680.0
  orbit, orbital 376.01
  partes posteriores 680.5
  pectoral region 680.2
  penis 607.2
  perineum 680.2
  pinna 680.0
  scalp (any part) 680.8
  scrotum 608.4
  seminal vesicle 608.0
  shoulder 680.3
  skin NEC 680.9
  specified site NEC 680.8
  spermatic cord 608.4
  temple (region) 680.0
  testis 608.4
  thigh 680.6
  thumb 680.4
  toe (any) 680.7
  tropical 085.1
  trunk 680.2
  tunica vaginalis 608.4
  umbilicus 680.2
  upper arm 680.3
  vas deferens 608.4
  vulva 616.4
  wrist 680.4
Bold hives — *see also* Urticaria 708.9
Bolivian hemorrhagic fever 078.7
Bombé, iris 364.74

Bomford-Rhoads anemia (refractory) 238.72 ▲
Bone — see condition
Bonnevie-Ullrich syndrome 758.6
Bonnier's syndrome 386.19
Bonvale Dam fever 780.79
Bony block of joint 718.80
　ankle 718.87
　elbow 718.82
　foot 718.87
　hand 718.84
　hip 718.85
　knee 718.86
　multiple sites 718.89
　pelvic region 718.85
　shoulder (region) 718.81
　specified site NEC 718.88
　wrist 718.83
Borderline
　intellectual functioning V62.89
　pelvis 653.1 ☑
　　with obstruction during labor 660.1 ☑
　　　affecting fetus or newborn 763.1
　psychosis (see also Schizophrenia) 295.5 ☑
　　of childhood (see also Psychosis, childhood) 299.8 ☑
　schizophrenia (see also Schizophrenia) 295.5 ☑
Borna disease 062.9
Bornholm disease (epidemic pleurodynia) 074.1
Borrelia vincentii (mouth) (pharynx) (tonsils) 101
Bostock's catarrh — see also Fever, hay 477.9
Boston exanthem 048
Botalli, ductus (patent) (persistent) 747.0
Bothriocephalus latus infestation 123.4
Botulism 005.1
　wound — see Wound, open, by site, complicated ●
Bouba — see also Yaws 102.9
Bouffée délirante 298.3
Bouillaud's disease or syndrome (rheumatic heart disease) 391.9
Bourneville's disease (tuberous sclerosis) 759.5
Boutonneuse fever 082.1
Boutonniere
　deformity (finger) 736.21
　hand (intrinsic) 736.21
Bouveret (-Hoffmann) disease or syndrome (paroxysmal tachycardia) 427.2
Bovine heart — see Hypertrophy, cardiac
Bowel — see condition
Bowen's
　dermatosis (precancerous) (M8081/2) — see Neoplasm, skin, in situ
　disease (M8081/2) — see Neoplasm, skin, in situ
　epithelioma (M8081/2) — see Neoplasm, skin, in situ
　type
　　epidermoid carcinoma in situ (M8081/2) — see Neoplasm, skin, in situ
　　intraepidermal squamous cell carcinoma (M8081/2) — see Neoplasm, skin, in situ
Bowing
　femur 736.89
　　congenital 754.42
　fibula 736.89
　　congenital 754.43
　forearm 736.09
　　away from midline (cubitus valgus) 736.01
　　toward midline (cubitus varus) 736.02
　leg(s), long bones, congenital 754.44
　radius 736.09

Bowing — continued
　radius — continued
　　away from midline (cubitus valgus) 736.01
　　toward midline (cubitus varus) 736.02
　tibia 736.89
　　congenital 754.43
Bowleg(s) 736.42
　congenital 754.44
　rachitic 268.1
Boyd's dysentery 004.2
Brachial — see condition
Brachman-de Lange syndrome (Amsterdam dwarf, mental retardation, and brachycephaly) 759.89
Brachycardia 427.89
Brachycephaly 756.0
Brachymorphism and ectopia lentis 759.89
Bradley's disease (epidemic vomiting) 078.82
Bradycardia 427.89
　chronic (sinus) 427.81
　newborn 779.81
　nodal 427.89
　postoperative 997.1
　reflex 337.0
　sinoatrial 427.89
　　with paroxysmal tachyarrhythmia or tachycardia 427.81
　　chronic 427.81
　sinus 427.89
　　with paroxysmal tachyarrhythmia or tachycardia 427.81
　　chronic 427.81
　　persistent 427.81
　　severe 427.81
　tachycardia syndrome 427.81
　vagal 427.89
Bradypnea 786.09
Brailsford's disease 732.3
　radial head 732.3
　tarsal scaphoid 732.5
Brailsford-Morquio disease or syndrome (mucopolysaccharidosis IV) 277.5
Brain — see also condition
　death 348.8
　syndrome (acute) (chronic) (nonpsychotic) (organic) (with neurotic reaction) (with behavioral reaction) (see also Syndrome, brain) 310.9
　with
　　presenile brain disease 290.10
　　psychosis, psychotic reaction (see also Psychosis, organic) 294.9
　congenital (see also Retardation, mental) 319
Branched-chain amino-acid disease 270.3
Branchial — see condition
Brandt's syndrome (acrodermatitis enteropathica) 686.8
Brash (water) 787.1
Brass-founders' ague 985.8
Bravais-Jacksonian epilepsy — see also Epilepsy 345.5 ☑
Braxton Hicks contractions 644.1 ☑
Braziers' disease 985.8
Brazilian
　blastomycosis 116.1
　leishmaniasis 085.5
BRBPR (bright red blood per rectum) 569.3
Break
　cardiorenal — see Hypertension, cardiorenal
　retina (see also Defect, retina) 361.30
Breakbone fever 061
Breakdown
　device, implant, or graft — see Complications, mechanical

Breakdown — continued
　nervous (see also Disorder, mental, nonpsychotic) 300.9
　perineum 674.2 ☑
Breast — see condition
Breast feeding difficulties 676.8 ☑
Breath
　foul 784.99 ▲
　holder, child 312.81
　holding spells 786.9
　shortness 786.05
Breathing
　asymmetrical 786.09
　bronchial 786.09
　exercises V57.0
　labored 786.09
　mouth 784.99 ▲
　　causing malocclusion 524.59
　periodic 786.09
　　high altitude 327.22
　tic 307.20
Breathlessness 786.09
Breda's disease — see also Yaws 102.9
Breech
　delivery, affecting fetus or newborn 763.0
　extraction, affecting fetus or newborn 763.0
　presentation (buttocks) (complete) (frank) 652.2 ☑
　　with successful version 652.1 ☑
　　before labor, affecting fetus or newborn 761.7
　　during labor, affecting fetus or newborn 763.0
Breisky's disease (kraurosis vulvae) 624.0
Brennemann's syndrome (acute mesenteric lymphadenitis) 289.2
Brenner's
　tumor (benign) (M9000/0) 220
　　borderline malignancy (M9000/1) 236.2
　　malignant (M9000/3) 183.0
　　proliferating (M9000/1) 236.2
Bretonneau's disease (diphtheritic malignant angina) 032.0
Breus' mole 631
Brevicollis 756.16
Bricklayers' itch 692.89
Brickmakers' anemia 126.9
Bridge
　myocardial 746.85
Bright's
　blindness — see Uremia
　disease (see also Nephritis) 583.9
　　arteriosclerotic (see also Hypertension, kidney) 403.90
Bright red blood per rectum (BRBPR) 569.3
Brill's disease (recrudescent typhus) 081.1
　flea-borne 081.0
　louse-borne 081.1
Brill-Symmers disease (follicular lymphoma) (M9690/3) 202.0 ☑
Brill-Zinsser disease (recrudescent typhus) 081.1
Brinton's disease (linitis plastica) (M8142/3) 151.9
Brion-Kayser disease — see also Fever, paratyphoid 002.9
Briquet's disorder or syndrome 300.81
Brissaud's
　infantilism (infantile myxedema) 244.9
　motor-verbal tic 307.23
Brissaud-Meige syndrome (infantile myxedema) 244.9
Brittle
　bones (congenital) 756.51
　nails 703.8
　　congenital 757.5
Broad — see also condition
　beta disease 272.2
　ligament laceration syndrome 620.6

Brock's syndrome (atelectasis due to enlarged lymph nodes) 518.0
Brocq's disease 691.8
　atopic (diffuse) neurodermatitis 691.8
　lichen simplex chronicus 698.3
　parakeratosis psoriasiformis 696.2
　parapsoriasis 696.2
Brocq-Duhring disease (dermatitis herpetiformis) 694.0
Brodie's
　abscess (localized) (chronic) (see also Osteomyelitis) 730.1 ☑
　disease (joint) (see also Osteomyelitis) 730.1 ☑
Broken
　arches 734
　　congenital 755.67
　back — see Fracture, vertebra, by site
　bone — see Fracture, by site
　compensation — see Disease, heart
　heart syndrome 429.83 ●
　implant or internal device — see listing under Complications, mechanical
　neck — see Fracture, vertebra, cervical
　nose 802.0
　open 802.1
　tooth, teeth 873.63
　　complicated 873.73
Bromhidrosis 705.89
Bromidism, bromism
　acute 967.3
　　correct substance properly administered 349.82
　　overdose or wrong substance given or taken 967.3
　chronic (see also Dependence) 304.1 ☑
Bromidrosiphobia 300.23
Bromidrosis 705.89
Bronchi, bronchial — see condition
Bronchiectasis (cylindrical) (diffuse) (fusiform) (localized) (moniliform) (postinfectious) (recurrent) (saccular) 494.0
　with acute exacerbation 494.1
　congenital 748.61
　tuberculosis (see also Tuberculosis) 011.5 ☑
Bronchiolectasis — see Bronchiectasis
Bronchiolitis (acute) (infectious) (subacute) 466.19
　with
　　bronchospasm or obstruction 466.19
　　influenza, flu, or grippe 487.1
　catarrhal (acute) (subacute) 466.19
　chemical 506.0
　chronic 506.4
　chronic (obliterative) 491.8
　due to external agent — see Bronchitis, acute, due to
　fibrosa obliterans 491.8
　influenzal 487.1
　obliterans 491.8
　　with organizing pneumonia (B.O.O.P.) 516.8
　status post lung transplant 996.84
　obliterative (chronic) (diffuse) (subacute) 491.8
　due to fumes or vapors 506.4
　respiratory syncytial virus 466.11
　vesicular — see Pneumonia, broncho-
Bronchitis (diffuse) (hypostatic) (infectious) (inflammatory) (simple) 490
　with
　　emphysema — see Emphysema
　　influenza, flu, or grippe 487.1
　　obstruction airway, chronic 491.20
　　　with
　　　　acute bronchitis 491.22
　　　　exacerbation (acute) 491.21
　　tracheitis 490
　　　acute or subacute 466.0

Index to Diseases

Bronchitis — *continued*
  with — *continued*
    tracheitis — *continued*
      acute or subacute — *continued*
        with bronchospasm or obstruction 466.0
      chronic 491.8
  acute or subacute 466.0
    with
      bronchospasm 466.0
      obstruction 466.0
      tracheitis 466.0
    chemical (due to fumes or vapors) 506.0
    due to
      fumes or vapors 506.0
      radiation 508.8
  allergic (acute) (*see also* Asthma) 493.9 ☑
  arachidic 934.1
  aspiration 507.0
    due to fumes or vapors 506.0
  asthmatic (acute) 493.90
    with
      acute exacerbation 493.92
      status asthmaticus 493.91
    chronic 493.2 ☑
  capillary 466.19
    with bronchospasm or obstruction 466.19
    chronic 491.8
  caseous (*see also* Tuberculosis) 011.3 ☑
  Castellani's 104.8
  catarrhal 490
    acute — *see* Bronchitis, acute
    chronic 491.0
  chemical (acute) (subacute) 506.0
    chronic 506.4
    due to fumes or vapors (acute) (subacute) 506.0
      chronic 506.4
  chronic 491.9
    with
      tracheitis (chronic) 491.8
    asthmatic 493.2 ☑
    catarrhal 491.0
    chemical (due to fumes and vapors) 506.4
    due to
      fumes or vapors (chemical) (inhalation) 506.4
      radiation 508.8
      tobacco smoking 491.0
    mucopurulent 491.1
    obstructive 491.20
      with
        acute bronchitis 491.22
        exacerbation (acute) 491.21
    purulent 491.1
    simple 491.0
    specified type NEC 491.8
  croupous 466.0
    with bronchospasm or obstruction 466.0
    due to fumes or vapors 506.0
  emphysematous 491.20
    with
      acute bronchitis 491.22
      exacerbation (acute) 491.21
  exudative 466.0
  fetid (chronic) (recurrent) 491.1
  fibrinous, acute or subacute 466.0
    with bronchospasm or obstruction 466.0
  grippal 487.1
  influenzal 487.1
  membranous, acute or subacute 466.0
    with bronchospasm or obstruction 466.0
  moulders' 502
  mucopurulent (chronic) (recurrent) 491.1
    acute or subacute 466.0

Bronchitis — *continued*
  obliterans 491.8
  obstructive (chronic) 491.20
    with
      acute bronchitis 491.22
      exacerbation (acute) 491.21
  pituitous 491.1
  plastic (inflammatory) 466.0
  pneumococcal, acute or subacute 466.0
    with bronchospasm or obstruction 466.0
  pseudomembranous 466.0
  purulent (chronic) (recurrent) 491.1
    acute or subacute 466.0
      with bronchospasm or obstruction 466.0
  putrid 491.1
  scrofulous (*see also* Tuberculosis) 011.3 ☑
  senile 491.9
  septic, acute or subacute 466.0
    with bronchospasm or obstruction 466.0
  smokers' 491.0
  spirochetal 104.8
  suffocative, acute or subacute 466.0
  summer (*see also* Asthma) 493.9 ☑
  suppurative (chronic) 491.1
    acute or subacute 466.0
  tuberculous (*see also* Tuberculosis) 011.3 ☑
  ulcerative 491.8
    Vincent's 101
  Vincent's 101
  viral, acute or subacute 466.0
Bronchoalveolitis 485
Bronchoaspergillosis 117.3
Bronchocele
  meaning
    dilatation of bronchus 519.19 ▲
    goiter 240.9
Bronchogenic carcinoma 162.9
Bronchohemisporosis 117.9
Broncholithiasis 518.89
  tuberculous (*see also* Tuberculosis) 011.3 ☑
Bronchomalacia 748.3
Bronchomoniliasis 112.89
Bronchomycosis 112.89
Bronchonocardiosis 039.1
Bronchopleuropneumonia — *see* Pneumonia, broncho-
Bronchopneumonia — *see* Pneumonia, broncho-
Bronchopneumonitis — *see* Pneumonia, broncho-
Bronchopulmonary — *see* condition
Bronchopulmonitis — *see* Pneumonia, broncho-
Bronchorrhagia 786.3
  newborn 770.3
  tuberculous (*see also* Tuberculosis) 011.3 ☑
Bronchorrhea (chronic) (purulent) 491.0
  acute 466.0
Bronchospasm 519.11 ▲
  with
    asthma — *see* Asthma
    bronchiolitis, acute 466.19
      due to respiratory syncytial virus 466.11
    bronchitis — *see* Bronchitis
    chronic obstructive pulmonary disease (COPD) 496
    emphysema — *see* Emphysema
    due to external agent — *see* Condition, respiratory, acute, due to
  acute 519.11 ●
  exercise induced 493.81
Bronchospirochetosis 104.8
Bronchostenosis 519.19 ▲
Bronchus — *see* condition
Bronze, bronzed
  diabetes 275.0

Bronze, bronzed — *continued*
  disease (Addison's) (skin) 255.4
    tuberculous (*see also* Tuberculosis) 017.6 ☑
Brooke's disease or tumor (M8100/0) — *see* Neoplasm, skin, benign
Brown enamel of teeth (hereditary) 520.5
Brown-Séquard's paralysis (syndrome) 344.89
Brown's tendon sheath syndrome 378.61
Brow presentation complicating delivery 652.4 ☑
Brucella, brucellosis (infection) 023.9
  abortus 023.1
  canis 023.3
  dermatitis, skin 023.9
  melitensis 023.0
  mixed 023.8
  suis 023.2
Bruck-de Lange disease or syndrome (Amsterdam dwarf, mental retardation, and brachycephaly) 759.89
Bruck's disease 733.99
Brugada syndrome 746.89
Brug's filariasis 125.1
Brugsch's syndrome (acropachyderma) 757.39
Bruhl's disease (splenic anemia with fever) 285.8
Bruise (skin surface intact) — *see also* Contusion
  with
    fracture — *see* Fracture, by site
    open wound — *see* Wound, open, by site
    internal organ (abdomen, chest, or pelvis) — *see* Injury, internal, by site
  umbilical cord 663.6 ☑
    affecting fetus or newborn 762.6
Bruit 785.9
  arterial (abdominal) (carotid) 785.9
  supraclavicular 785.9
Brushburn — *see* Injury, superficial, by site
Bruton's X-linked agammaglobulinemia 279.04
Bruxism 306.8
  sleep related 327.53
Bubbly lung syndrome 770.7
Bubo 289.3
  blennorrhagic 098.89
  chancroidal 099.0
  climatic 099.1
  due to Hemophilus ducreyi 099.0
  gonococcal 098.89
  indolent NEC 099.8
  inguinal NEC 099.8
    chancroidal 099.0
    climatic 099.1
    due to H. ducreyi 099.0
  scrofulous (*see also* Tuberculosis) 017.2 ☑
  soft chancre 099.0
  suppurating 683
  syphilitic 091.0
    congenital 090.0
  tropical 099.1
  venereal NEC 099.8
  virulent 099.0
Bubonic plague 020.0
Bubonocele — *see* Hernia, inguinal
Buccal — *see* condition
Buchanan's disease (juvenile osteochondrosis of iliac crest) 732.1
Buchem's syndrome (hyperostosis corticalis) 733.3
Buchman's disease (osteochondrosis, juvenile) 732.1
Bucket handle fracture (semilunar cartilage) — *see also* Tear, meniscus 836.2
Budd-Chiari syndrome (hepatic vein thrombosis) 453.0

Budgerigar-fanciers' disease or lung 495.2
Büdinger-Ludloff-Läwen disease 717.89
Buerger's disease (thromboangiitis obliterans) 443.1
Bulbar — *see* condition
Bulbus cordis 745.9
  persistent (in left ventricle) 745.8
Bulging fontanels (congenital) 756.0
Bulimia 783.6
  nervosa 307.51
  nonorganic origin 307.51
Bulky uterus 621.2
Bulla(e) 709.8
  lung (emphysematous) (solitary) 492.0
Bullet wound — *see also* Wound, open, by site
  fracture — *see* Fracture, by site, open
  internal organ (abdomen, chest, or pelvis) — *see* Injury, internal, by site, with open wound
  intracranial — *see* Laceration, brain, with open wound
Bullis fever 082.8
Bullying — *see also* Disturbance, conduct 312.0 ☑
Bundle
  branch block (complete) (false) (incomplete) 426.50
    bilateral 426.53
    left (*see also* Block, bundle branch, left) 426.3
      hemiblock 426.2
    right (*see also* Block, bundle branch, right) 426.4
  of His — *see* condition
  of Kent syndrome (anomalous atrioventricular excitation) 426.7
Bungpagga 040.81
Bunion 727.1
Bunionette 727.1
Bunyamwera fever 066.3
Buphthalmia, buphthalmos (congenital) 743.20
  associated with
    keratoglobus, congenital 743.22
    megalocornea 743.22
    ocular anomalies NEC 743.22
  isolated 743.21
  simple 743.21
Bürger-Grütz disease or syndrome (essential familial hyperlipemia) 272.3
Buried roots 525.3
Burke's syndrome 577.8
Burkitt's
  tumor (M9750/3) 200.2 ☑
  type malignant, lymphoma, lymphoblastic, or undifferentiated (M9750/3) 200.2 ☑

Burn

Burn (acid) (cathode ray) (caustic) (chemical) (electric heating appliance) (electricity) (fire) (flame) (hot liquid or object) (irradiation) (lime) (radiation) (steam) (thermal) (x-ray) 949.0

Note — *Use the following fifth-digit subclassification with category 948 to indicate the percent of body surface with third degree burn:*

0	Less than 10% or unspecified
1	10–19%
2	20–29%
3	30–39%
4	40–49%
5	50–59%
6	60–69%
7	70–79%
8	80–89%
9	90% or more of body surface

with
- blisters — *see* Burn, by site, second degree
- erythema — *see* Burn, by site, first degree
- skin loss (epidermal) (*see also* Burn, by site, second degree)
- full thickness (*see also* Burn, by site, third degree)
  - with necrosis of underlying tissues — *see* Burn, by site, third degree, deep
- first degree — *see* Burn, by site, first degree
- second degree — *see* Burn, by site, second degree
- third degree — *see* Burn, by site, third degree
- deep — *see* Burn, by site, third degree, deep

abdomen, abdominal (muscle) (wall) 942.03
  with
    trunk — *see* Burn, trunk, multiple sites
  first degree 942.13
  second degree 942.23
  third degree 942.33
    deep 942.43
      with loss of body part 942.53
ankle 945.03
  with
    lower limb(s) — *see* Burn, leg, multiple sites
  first degree 945.13
  second degree 945.23
  third degree 945.33
    deep 945.43
      with loss of body part 945.53
anus — *see* Burn, trunk, specified site NEC
arm(s) 943.00
  first degree 943.10
  second degree 943.20
  third degree 943.30
    deep 943.40
      with loss of body part 943.50
  lower — *see* Burn, forearm(s)
  multiple sites, except hand(s) or wrist(s) 943.09
    first degree 943.19
    second degree 943.29
    third degree 943.39
      deep 943.49
        with loss of body part 943.59
  upper 943.03
    first degree 943.13
    second degree 943.23
    third degree 943.33
      deep 943.43

Burn — *continued*
arm(s) — *continued*
  upper — *continued*
    third degree — *continued*
      deep — *continued*
        with loss of body part 943.53
auditory canal (external) — *see* Burn, ear
auricle (ear) — *see* Burn, ear
axilla 943.04
  with
    upper limb(s), except hand(s) or wrist(s) — *see* Burn, arm(s), multiple sites
  first degree 943.14
  second degree 943.24
  third degree 943.34
    deep 943.44
      with loss of body part 943.54
back 942.04
  with
    trunk — *see* Burn, trunk, multiple sites
  first degree 942.14
  second degree 942.24
  third degree 942.34
    deep 942.44
      with loss of body part 942.54
biceps
  brachii — *see* Burn, arm(s), upper
  femoris — *see* Burn, thigh
breast(s) 942.01
  with
    trunk — *see* Burn, trunk, multiple sites
  first degree 942.11
  second degree 942.21
  third degree 942.31
    deep 942.41
      with loss of body part 942.51
brow — *see* Burn, forehead
buttock(s) — *see* Burn, back
canthus (eye) 940.1
  chemical 940.0
cervix (uteri) 947.4
cheek (cutaneous) 941.07
  with
    face or head — *see* Burn, head, multiple sites
  first degree 941.17
  second degree 941.27
  third degree 941.37
    deep 941.47
      with loss of body part 941.57
chest wall (anterior) 942.02
  with
    trunk — *see* Burn, trunk, multiple sites
  first degree 942.12
  second degree 942.22
  third degree 942.32
    deep 942.42
      with loss of body part 942.52
chin 941.04
  with
    face or head — *see* Burn, head, multiple sites
  first degree 941.14
  second degree 941.24
  third degree 941.34
    deep 941.44
      with loss of body part 941.54
clitoris — *see* Burn, genitourinary organs, external
colon 947.3
conjunctiva (and cornea) 940.4
  chemical
    acid 940.3
    alkaline 940.2
cornea (and conjunctiva) 940.4
  chemical
    acid 940.3
    alkaline 940.2
costal region — *see* Burn, chest wall

Burn — *continued*
due to ingested chemical agent — *see* Burn, internal organs
ear (auricle) (canal) (drum) (external) 941.01
  with
    face or head — *see* Burn, head, multiple sites
  first degree 941.11
  second degree 941.21
  third degree 941.31
    deep 941.41
      with loss of a body part 941.51
elbow 943.02
  with
    hand(s) and wrist(s) — *see* Burn, multiple specified sites
    upper limb(s), except hand(s) or wrist(s) (*see also* Burn, arm(s), multiple sites)
  first degree 943.12
  second degree 943.22
  third degree 943.32
    deep 943.42
      with loss of body part 943.52
electricity, electric current — *see* Burn, by site
entire body — *see* Burn, multiple, specified sites
epididymis — *see* Burn, genitourinary organs, external
epigastric region — *see* Burn, abdomen
epiglottis 947.1
esophagus 947.2
extent (percent of body surface)
  less than 10 percent 948.0 ☑
  10-19 percent 948.1 ☑
  20-29 percent 948.2 ☑
  30-39 percent 948.3 ☑
  40-49 percent 948.4 ☑
  50-59 percent 948.5 ☑
  60-69 percent 948.6 ☑
  70-79 percent 948.7 ☑
  80-89 percent 948.8 ☑
  90 percent or more 948.9 ☑
extremity
  lower — *see* Burn, leg
  upper — *see* Burn, arm(s)
eye(s) (and adnexa) (only) 940.9
  with
    face, head, or neck 941.02
      first degree 941.12
      second degree 941.22
      third degree 941.32
        deep 941.42
          with loss of body part 941.52
  other sites (classifiable to more than one category in 940–945) — *see* Burn, multiple, specified sites
  resulting rupture and destruction of eyeball 940.5
  specified part — *see* Burn, by site
eyeball (*see also* Burn, eye)
  with resulting rupture and destruction of eyeball 940.5
eyelid(s) 940.1
  chemical 940.0
face — *see* Burn, head
finger (nail) (subungual) 944.01
  with
    hand(s) — *see* Burn, hand(s), multiple sites
    other sites — *see* Burn, multiple, specified sites
  thumb 944.04
    first degree 944.14
    second degree 944.24
    third degree 944.34
      deep 944.44
        with loss of body part 944.54

Burn — *continued*
finger — *continued*
  first degree 944.11
  second degree 944.21
  third degree 944.31
    deep 944.41
      with loss of body part 944.51
  multiple (digits) 944.03
    with thumb — *see* Burn, finger, with thumb
    first degree 944.13
    second degree 944.23
    third degree 944.33
      deep 944.43
        with loss of body part 944.53
flank — *see* Burn, abdomen
foot 945.02
  with
    lower limb(s) — *see* Burn, leg, multiple sites
  first degree 945.12
  second degree 945.22
  third degree 945.32
    deep 945.42
      with loss of body part 945.52
forearm(s) 943.01
  with
    upper limb(s), except hand(s) or wrist(s) — *see* Burn, arm(s), multiple sites
  first degree 943.11
  second degree 943.21
  third degree 943.31
    deep 943.41
      with loss of body part 943.51
forehead 941.07
  with
    face or head — *see* Burn, head, multiple sites
  first degree 941.17
  second degree 941.27
  third degree 941.37
    deep 941.47
      with loss of body part 941.57
fourth degree — *see* Burn, by site, third degree, deep
friction — *see* Injury, superficial, by site
from swallowing caustic or corrosive substance NEC — *see* Burn, internal organs
full thickness — *see* Burn, by site, third degree
gastrointestinal tract 947.3
genitourinary organs
  external 942.05
    with
      trunk — *see* Burn, trunk, multiple sites
    first degree 942.15
    second degree 942.25
    third degree 942.35
      deep 942.45
        with loss of body part 942.55
  internal 947.8
globe (eye) — *see* Burn, eyeball
groin — *see* Burn, abdomen
gum 947.0
hand(s) (phalanges) (and wrist) 944.00
  first degree 944.10
  second degree 944.20
  third degree 944.30
    deep 944.40
      with loss of body part 944.50
  back (dorsal surface) 944.06
    first degree 944.16
    second degree 944.26
    third degree 944.36
      deep 944.46
        with loss of body part 944.56
  multiple sites 944.08
    first degree 944.18
    second degree 944.28

Burn — continued
    hand(s) — continued
        multiple sites — continued
            third degree 944.38
                deep 944.48
                    with loss of body part 944.58
    head (and face) 941.00
        first degree 941.10
        second degree 941.20
        third degree 941.30
            deep 941.40
                with loss of body part 941.50
        eye(s) only 940.9
        specified part — see Burn, by site
        multiple sites 941.09
            with eyes — see Burn, eyes, with face, head, or neck
            first degree 941.19
            second degree 941.29
            third degree 941.39
                deep 941.49
                    with loss of body part 941.59
    heel — see Burn, foot
    hip — see Burn, trunk, specified site NEC
    iliac region — see Burn, trunk, specified site NEC
    infected 958.3
    inhalation (see also Burn, internal organs) 947.9
    internal organs 947.9
        from caustic or corrosive substance (swallowing) NEC 947.9
        specified NEC (see also Burn, by site) 947.8
    interscapular region — see Burn, back
    intestine (large) (small) 947.3
    iris — see Burn, eyeball
    knee 945.05
        with
            lower limb(s) — see Burn, leg, multiple sites
        first degree 945.15
        second degree 945.25
        third degree 945.35
            deep 945.45
                with loss of body part 945.55
    labium (majus) (minus) — see Burn, genitourinary organs, external
    lacrimal apparatus, duct, gland, or sac 940.1
        chemical 940.0
    larynx 947.1
    late effect — see Late, effects (of), burn
    leg 945.00
        first degree 945.10
        second degree 945.20
        third degree 945.30
            deep 945.40
                with loss of body part 945.50
        lower 945.04
            with other part(s) of lower limb(s) — see Burn, leg, multiple sites
            first degree 945.14
            second degree 945.24
            third degree 945.34
                deep 945.44
                    with loss of body part 945.54
        multiple sites 945.09
            first degree 945.19
            second degree 945.29
            third degree 945.39
                deep 945.49
                    with loss of body part 945.59
        upper — see Burn, thigh
    lightning — see Burn, by site
    limb(s)
        lower (including foot or toe(s)) — see Burn, leg

Burn — continued
    limb(s) — continued
        upper (except wrist and hand) — see Burn, arm(s)
    lip(s) 941.03
        with
            face or head — see Burn, head, multiple sites
        first degree 941.13
        second degree 941.23
        third degree 941.33
            deep 941.43
                with loss of body part 941.53
    lumbar region — see Burn, back
    lung 947.1
    malar region — see Burn, cheek
    mastoid region — see Burn, scalp
    membrane, tympanic — see Burn, ear
    midthoracic region — see Burn, chest wall
    mouth 947.0
    multiple (see also Burn, unspecified) 949.0
        specified sites classifiable to more than one category in 940-945 ☑, 946.0
            first degree 946.1
            second degree 946.2
            third degree 946.3
                deep 946.4
                    with loss of body part 946.5
    muscle, abdominal — see Burn, abdomen
    nasal (septum) — see Burn, nose
    neck 941.08
        with
            face or head — see Burn, head, multiple sites
        first degree 941.18
        second degree 941.28
        third degree 941.38
            deep 941.48
                with loss of body part 941.58
    nose (septum) 941.05
        with
            face or head — see Burn, head, multiple sites
        first degree 941.15
        second degree 941.25
        third degree 941.35
            deep 941.45
                with loss of body part 941.55
    occipital region — see Burn, scalp
    orbit region 940.1
        chemical 940.0
    oronasopharynx 947.0
    palate 947.0
    palm(s) 944.05
        with
            hand(s) and wrist(s) — see Burn, hand(s), multiple sites
        first degree 944.15
        second degree 944.25
        third degree 944.35
            deep 944.45
                with loss of a body part 944.55
    parietal region — see Burn, scalp
    penis — see Burn, genitourinary organs, external
    perineum — see Burn, genitourinary organs, external
    periocular area 940.1
        chemical 940.0
    pharynx 947.0
    pleura 947.1
    popliteal space — see Burn, knee
    prepuce — see Burn, genitourinary organs, external
    pubic region — see Burn, genitourinary organs, external
    pudenda — see Burn, genitourinary organs, external
    rectum 947.3

Burn — continued
    sac, lacrimal 940.1
        chemical 940.0
    sacral region — see Burn, back
    salivary (ducts) (glands) 947.0
    scalp 941.06
        with
            face or neck — see Burn, head, multiple sites
        first degree 941.16
        second degree 941.26
        third degree 941.36
            deep 941.46
                with loss of body part 941.56
    scapular region 943.06
        with
            upper limb(s), except hand(s) or wrist(s) — see Burn, arm(s), multiple sites
        first degree 943.16
        second degree 943.26
        third degree 943.36
            deep 943.46
                with loss of body part 943.56
    sclera — see Burn, eyeball
    scrotum — see Burn, genitourinary organs, external
    septum, nasal — see Burn, nose
    shoulder(s) 943.05
        with
            hand(s) and wrist(s) — see Burn, multiple, specified sites
            upper limb(s), except hand(s) or wrist(s) — see Burn, arm(s), multiple sites
        first degree 943.15
        second degree 943.25
        third degree 943.35
            deep 943.45
                with loss of body part 943.55
    skin NEC (see also Burn, unspecified) 949.0
    skull — see Burn, head
    small intestine 947.3
    sternal region — see Burn, chest wall
    stomach 947.3
    subconjunctival — see Burn, conjunctiva
    subcutaneous — see Burn, by site, third degree
    submaxillary region — see Burn, head
    submental region — see Burn, chin
    sun — see Sunburn
    supraclavicular fossa — see Burn, neck
    supraorbital — see Burn, forehead
    temple — see Burn, scalp
    temporal region — see Burn, scalp
    testicle — see Burn, genitourinary organs, external
    testis — see Burn, genitourinary organs, external
    thigh 945.06
        with
            lower limb(s) — see Burn, leg, multiple sites
        first degree 945.16
        second degree 945.26
        third degree 945.36
            deep 945.46
                with loss of body part 945.56
    thorax (external) — see Burn, chest wall
    throat 947.0
    thumb(s) (nail) (subungual) 944.02
        with
            finger(s) — see Burn, finger, with other sites, thumb
            hand(s) and wrist(s) — see Burn, hand(s), multiple sites
        first degree 944.12
        second degree 944.22
        third degree 944.32
            deep 944.42

Burn — continued
    thumb(s) — continued
        third degree — continued
            deep — continued
                with loss of body part 944.52
    toe (nail) (subungual) 945.01
        with
            lower limb(s) — see Burn, leg, multiple sites
        first degree 945.11
        second degree 945.21
        third degree 945.31
            deep 945.41
                with loss of body part 945.51
    tongue 947.0
    tonsil 947.0
    trachea 947.1
    trunk 942.00
        first degree 942.10
        second degree 942.20
        third degree 942.30
            deep 942.40
                with loss of body part 942.50
        multiple sites 942.09
            first degree 942.19
            second degree 942.29
            third degree 942.39
                deep 942.49
                    with loss of body part 942.59
        specified site NEC 942.09
            first degree 942.19
            second degree 942.29
            third degree 942.39
                deep 942.49
                    with loss of body part 942.59
    tunica vaginalis — see Burn, genitourinary organs, external
    tympanic membrane — see Burn, ear
    tympanum — see Burn, ear
    ultraviolet 692.82
    unspecified site (multiple) 949.0
        with extent of body surface involved specified
            less than 10 percent 948.0 ☑
            10-19 percent 948.1 ☑
            20-29 percent 948.2 ☑
            30-39 percent 948.3 ☑
            40-49 percent 948.4 ☑
            50-59 percent 948.5 ☑
            60-69 percent 948.6 ☑
            70-79 percent 948.7 ☑
            80-89 percent 948.8 ☑
            90 percent or more 948.9 ☑
        first degree 949.1
        second degree 949.2
        third degree 949.3
            deep 949.4
                with loss of body part 949.5
    uterus 947.4
    uvula 947.0
    vagina 947.4
    vulva — see Burn, genitourinary organs, external
    wrist(s) 944.07
        with
            hand(s) — see Burn, hand(s), multiple sites
        first degree 944.17
        second degree 944.27
        third degree 944.37
            deep 944.47
                with loss of body part 944.57
Burnett's syndrome (milk-alkali) 275.42
Burnier's syndrome (hypophyseal dwarfism) 253.3
Burning
    feet syndrome 266.2
    sensation (see also Disturbance, sensation) 782.0
    tongue 529.6
Burns' disease (osteochondrosis, lower ulna) 732.3
Bursa — see also condition
    pharynx 478.29

Bursitis

Bursitis NEC 727.3
- Achilles tendon 726.71
- adhesive 726.90
  - shoulder 726.0
- ankle 726.79
- buttock 726.5
- calcaneal 726.79
- collateral ligament
  - fibular 726.63
  - tibial 726.62
- Duplay's 726.2
- elbow 726.33
- finger 726.8
- foot 726.79
- gonococcal 098.52
- hand 726.4
- hip 726.5
- infrapatellar 726.69
- ischiogluteal 726.5
- knee 726.60
- occupational NEC 727.2
- olecranon 726.33
- pes anserinus 726.61
- pharyngeal 478.29
- popliteal 727.51
- prepatellar 726.65
- radiohumeral 727.3
- scapulohumeral 726.19
  - adhesive 726.0
- shoulder 726.10
  - adhesive 726.0
- subacromial 726.19
  - adhesive 726.0
- subcoracoid 726.19
- subdeltoid 726.19
  - adhesive 726.0
- subpatellar 726.69
- syphilitic 095.7
- Thornwaldt's, Tornwaldt's (pharyngeal) 478.29
- toe 726.79
- trochanteric area 726.5
- wrist 726.4

Burst stitches or sutures (complication of surgery) (external) 998.32
- internal 998.31

Buruli ulcer 031.1

Bury's disease (erythema elevatum diutinum) 695.89

Buschke's disease or scleredema (adultorum) 710.1

Busquet's disease (osteoperiostitis) — see also Osteomyelitis 730.1 ☑

Busse-Buschke disease (cryptococcosis) 117.5

Buttock — see condition

Button
- Biskra 085.1
- Delhi 085.1
- oriental 085.1

Buttonhole hand (intrinsic) 736.21

Bwamba fever (encephalitis) 066.3

Byssinosis (occupational) 504

Bywaters' syndrome 958.5

C

Cacergasia 300.9

Cachexia 799.4
- cancerous ▶(see also Neoplasm, by site, malignant)◀ 799.4 ▲
- cardiac — see Disease, heart
- dehydration 276.51
  - with
    - hypernatremia 276.0
    - hyponatremia 276.1
- due to malnutrition 799.4 ▲
- exophthalmic 242.0 ☑
- heart — see Disease, heart
- hypophyseal 253.2
- hypopituitary 253.2
- lead 984.9
  - specified type of lead — see Table of Drugs and Chemicals
- malaria 084.9
- malignant ▶(see also Neoplasm, by site, malignant)◀ 799.4 ▲

Cachexia — continued
- marsh 084.9
- nervous 300.5
- old age 797
- pachydermic — see Hypothyroidism
- paludal 084.9
- pituitary (postpartum) 253.2
- renal (see also Disease, renal) 593.9
- saturnine 984.9
  - specified type of lead — see Table of Drugs and Chemicals
- senile 797
- Simmonds' (pituitary cachexia) 253.2
- splenica 289.59
- strumipriva (see also Hypothyroidism) 244.9
- tuberculous NEC (see also Tuberculosis) 011.9 ☑

Café au lait spots 709.09

Caffey's disease or syndrome (infantile cortical hyperostosis) 756.59

Caisson disease 993.3

Caked breast (puerperal, postpartum) 676.2 ☑

Cake kidney 753.3

Calabar swelling 125.2

Calcaneal spur 726.73

Calcaneoapophysitis 732.5

Calcaneonavicular bar 755.67

Calcareous — see condition

Calcicosis (occupational) 502

Calciferol (vitamin D) **deficiency** 268.9
- with
  - osteomalacia 268.2
  - rickets (see also Rickets) 268.0

Calcification
- adrenal (capsule) (gland) 255.4
  - tuberculous (see also Tuberculosis) 017.6 ☑
- aorta 440.0
- artery (annular) — see Arteriosclerosis
- auricle (ear) 380.89
- bladder 596.8
  - due to S. hematobium 120.0
- brain (cortex) — see Calcification, cerebral
- bronchus 519.19 ▲
- bursa 727.82
- cardiac (see also Degeneration, myocardial) 429.1
- cartilage (postinfectional) 733.99
- cerebral (cortex) 348.8
  - artery 437.0
- cervix (uteri) 622.8
- choroid plexus 349.2
- conjunctiva 372.54
- corpora cavernosa (penis) 607.89
- cortex (brain) — see Calcification, cerebral
- dental pulp (nodular) 522.2
- dentinal papilla 520.4
- disc, intervertebral 722.90
  - cervical, cervicothoracic 722.91
  - lumbar, lumbosacral 722.93
  - thoracic, thoracolumbar 722.92
- fallopian tube 620.8
- falx cerebri — see Calcification, cerebral
- fascia 728.89
- gallbladder 575.8
- general 275.40
- heart (see also Degeneration, myocardial) 429.1
  - valve — see Endocarditis
- intervertebral cartilage or disc (postinfectional) 722.90
  - cervical, cervicothoracic 722.91
  - lumbar, lumbosacral 722.93
  - thoracic, thoracolumbar 722.92
- intracranial — see Calcification, cerebral
- intraspinal ligament 728.89
- joint 719.80
  - ankle 719.87
  - elbow 719.82
  - foot 719.87

Calcification — continued
- joint — continued
  - hand 719.84
  - hip 719.85
  - knee 719.86
  - multiple sites 719.89
  - pelvic region 719.85
  - shoulder (region) 719.81
  - specified site NEC 719.88
  - wrist 719.83
- kidney 593.89
  - tuberculous (see also Tuberculosis) 016.0 ☑
- larynx (senile) 478.79
- lens 366.8
- ligament 728.89
  - intraspinal 728.89
  - knee (medial collateral) 717.89
- lung 518.89
  - active 518.89
  - postinfectional 518.89
  - tuberculous (see also Tuberculosis, pulmonary) 011.9 ☑
- lymph gland or node (postinfectional) 289.3
  - tuberculous (see also Tuberculosis, lymph gland) 017.2 ☑
- mammographic 793.89 ●
- massive (paraplegic) 728.10
- medial NEC (see also Arteriosclerosis, extremities) 440.20
- meninges (cerebral) 349.2
- metastatic 275.40
- Mönckeberg's — see Arteriosclerosis
- muscle 728.10
  - heterotopic, postoperative 728.13
- myocardium, myocardial (see also Degeneration, myocardial) 429.1
- ovary 620.8
- pancreas 577.8
- penis 607.89
- periarticular 728.89
- pericardium (see also Pericarditis) 423.8
- pineal gland 259.8
- pleura 511.0
  - postinfectional 518.89
  - tuberculous (see also Tuberculosis, pleura) 012.0 ☑
- pulp (dental) (nodular) 522.2
- renal 593.89
- Rider's bone 733.99
- sclera 379.16
- semilunar cartilage 717.89
- spleen 289.59
- subcutaneous 709.3
- suprarenal (capsule) (gland) 255.4
- tendon (sheath) 727.82
  - with bursitis, synovitis or tenosynovitis 727.82
- trachea 519.19 ▲
- ureter 593.89
- uterus 621.8
- vitreous 379.29

Calcified — see also Calcification
- hematoma NEC 959.9

Calcinosis (generalized) (interstitial) (tumoral) (universalis) 275.49
- circumscripta 709.3
- cutis 709.3
- intervertebralis 275.49 [722.90]
- Raynaud's phenomenonsclerodactylytelangiectasis (CRST) 710.1

Calciphylaxis — see also Calcification, by site 275.49 ●

Calcium
- blood
  - high (see also Hypercalcemia) 275.42
  - low (see also Hypocalcemia) 275.41
- deposits (see also Calcification, by site)
  - in bursa 727.82
  - in tendon (sheath) 727.82
    - with bursitis, synovitis or tenosynovitis 727.82

Calcium — continued
- salts or soaps in vitreous 379.22

Calciuria 791.9

Calculi — see Calculus

Calculosis, intrahepatic — see Choledocholithiasis

Calculus, calculi, calculous 592.9
- ampulla of Vater — see Choledocholithiasis
- anuria (impacted) (recurrent) 592.0
- appendix 543.9
- bile duct (any) — see Choledocholithiasis
- biliary — see Cholelithiasis
- bilirubin, multiple — see Cholelithiasis
- bladder (encysted) (impacted) (urinary) 594.1
  - diverticulum 594.0
- bronchus 518.89
- calyx (kidney) (renal) 592.0
  - congenital 753.3
- cholesterol (pure) (solitary) — see Cholelithiasis
- common duct (bile) — see Choledocholithiasis
- conjunctiva 372.54
- cystic 594.1
  - duct — see Cholelithiasis
- dental 523.6
  - subgingival 523.6
  - supragingival 523.6
- epididymis 608.89
- gallbladder (see also Cholelithiasis)
  - congenital 751.69
- hepatic (duct) — see Choledocholithiasis
- intestine (impaction) (obstruction) 560.39
- kidney (impacted) (multiple) (pelvis) (recurrent) (staghorn) 592.0
  - congenital 753.3
- lacrimal (passages) 375.57
- liver (impacted) — see Choledocholithiasis
- lung 518.89
- mammographic 793.89 ●
- nephritic (impacted) (recurrent) 592.0
- nose 478.19 ▲
- pancreas (duct) 577.8
- parotid gland 527.5
- pelvis, encysted 592.0
- prostate 602.0
- pulmonary 518.89
- renal (impacted) (recurrent) 592.0
  - congenital 753.3
- salivary (duct) (gland) 527.5
- seminal vesicle 608.89
- staghorn 592.0
- Stensen's duct 527.5
- sublingual duct or gland 527.5
  - congenital 750.26
- submaxillary duct, gland, or region 527.5
- suburethral 594.8
- tonsil 474.8
- tooth, teeth 523.6
- tunica vaginalis 608.89
- ureter (impacted) (recurrent) 592.1
- urethra (impacted) 594.2
- urinary (duct) (impacted) (passage) (tract) 592.9
  - lower tract NEC 594.9
  - specified site 594.8
- vagina 623.8
- vesical (impacted) 594.1
- Wharton's duct 527.5

Caliectasis 593.89

California
- disease 114.0
- encephalitis 062.5

Caligo cornea 371.03

Callositas, callosity (infected) 700

Callus (infected) 700
- bone 726.91

Index to Diseases

Callus

Callus — *continued*
  excessive, following fracture (*see also* Late, effect (of), fracture)
Calvé (-Perthes) disease (osteochondrosis, femoral capital) 732.1
Calvities — *see also* Alopecia 704.00
Cameroon fever — *see also* Malaria 084.6
Camptocormia 300.11
Camptodactyly (congenital) 755.59
Camurati-Engelmann disease (diaphyseal sclerosis) 756.59
Canal — *see* condition
Canaliculitis (lacrimal) (acute) 375.31
  Actinomyces 039.8
  chronic 375.41
Canavan's disease 330.0
Cancer (M8000/3) — *see also* Neoplasm, by site, malignant

> *Note* — The term "cancer" when modified by an adjective or adjectival phrase indicating a morphological type should be coded in the same manner as "carcinoma" with that adjective or phrase. Thus, "squamous-cell cancer" should be coded in the same manner as "squamous-cell carcinoma," which appears in the list under "Carcinoma."

  bile duct type (M8160/3), liver 155.1
  hepatocellular (M8170/3) 155.0
Cancerous (M8000/3) — *see* Neoplasm, by site, malignant
Cancerphobia 300.29
Cancrum oris 528.1
Candidiasis, candidal 112.9
  with pneumonia 112.4
  balanitis 112.2
  congenital 771.7
  disseminated 112.5
  endocarditis 112.81
  esophagus 112.84
  intertrigo 112.3
  intestine 112.85
  lung 112.4
  meningitis 112.83
  mouth 112.0
  nails 112.3
  neonatal 771.7
  onychia 112.3
  otitis externa 112.82
  otomycosis 112.82
  paronychia 112.3
  perionyxis 112.3
  pneumonia 112.4
  pneumonitis 112.4
  skin 112.3
  specified site NEC 112.89
  systemic 112.5
  urogenital site NEC 112.2
  vagina 112.1
  vulva 112.1
  vulvovaginitis 112.1
Candidiosis — *see* Candidiasis
Candiru infection or infestation 136.8
Canities (premature) 704.3
  congenital 757.4
Canker (mouth) (sore) 528.2
  rash 034.1
Cannabinosis 504
Canton fever 081.9
Cap
  cradle 690.11
Capillariasis 127.5
Capillary — *see* condition
Caplan-Colinet syndrome 714.81
Caplan's syndrome 714.81
Capsule — *see* condition
Capsulitis (joint) 726.90
  adhesive (shoulder) 726.0
  hip 726.5
  knee 726.60
  labyrinthine 387.8
  thyroid 245.9
  wrist 726.4
Caput
  crepitus 756.0

Caput — *continued*
  medusae 456.8
  succedaneum 767.19
Carapata disease 087.1
Carate — *see* Pinta
Carbohydrate-deficient glycoprotein syndrome (CGDS) 271.8
Carboxyhemoglobinemia 986
Carbuncle 680.9
  abdominal wall 680.2
  ankle 680.6
  anus 680.5
  arm (any part, above wrist) 680.3
  auditory canal, external 680.0
  axilla 680.3
  back (any part) 680.2
  breast 680.2
  buttock 680.5
  chest wall 680.2
  corpus cavernosum 607.2
  ear (any part) (external) 680.0
  eyelid 373.13
  face (any part, except eye) 680.0
  finger (any) 680.4
  flank 680.2
  foot (any part) 680.7
  forearm 680.3
  genital organ (male) 608.4
  gluteal (region) 680.5
  groin 680.2
  hand (any part) 680.4
  head (any part, except face) 680.8
  heel 680.7
  hip 680.6
  kidney (*see also* Abscess, kidney) 590.2
  knee 680.6
  labia 616.4
  lacrimal
    gland (*see also* Dacryoadenitis) 375.00
    passages (duct) (sac) (*see also* Dacryocystitis) 375.30
  leg, any part except foot 680.6
  lower extremity, any part except foot 680.6
  malignant 022.0
  multiple sites 680.9
  neck 680.1
  nose (external) (septum) 680.0
  orbit, orbital 376.01
  partes posteriores 680.5
  pectoral region 680.2
  penis 607.2
  perineum 680.2
  pinna 680.0
  scalp (any part) 680.8
  scrotum 608.4
  seminal vesicle 608.0
  shoulder 680.3
  skin NEC 680.9
  specified site NEC 680.8
  spermatic cord 608.4
  temple (region) 680.0
  testis 608.4
  thigh 680.6
  thumb 680.4
  toe (any) 680.7
  trunk 680.2
  tunica vaginalis 608.4
  umbilicus 680.2
  upper arm 680.3
  urethra 597.0
  vas deferens 608.4
  vulva 616.4
  wrist 680.4
Carbunculus — *see also* Carbuncle 680.9
Carcinoid (tumor) (M8240/1) — *see also* Neoplasm, by site, uncertain behavior
  and struma ovarii (M9091/1) 236.2
  argentaffin (M8241/1) — *see* Neoplasm, by site, uncertain behavior
    malignant (M8241/3) — *see* Neoplasm, by site, malignant

Carcinoid — *see also* Neoplasm, by site, uncertain behavior — *continued*
  benign (M9091/0) 220
  composite (M8244/3) — *see* Neoplasm, by site, malignant
  goblet cell (M8243/3) — *see* Neoplasm, by site, malignant
  malignant (M8240/3) — *see* Neoplasm, by site, malignant
  nonargentaffin (M8242/1) (*see also* Neoplasm, by site, uncertain behavior)
    malignant (M8242/3) — *see* Neoplasm, by site, malignant
  strumal (M9091/1) 236.2
  syndrome (intestinal) (metastatic) 259.2
  type bronchial adenoma (M8240/3) — *see* Neoplasm, lung, malignant
Carcinoidosis 259.2
Carcinomaphobia 300.29
Carcinomatosis
  peritonei (M8010/6) 197.6
  specified site NEC (M8010/3) — *see* Neoplasm, by site, malignant
  unspecified site (M8010/6) 199.0
Carcinoma (M8010/3) — *see also* Neoplasm, by site, malignant

> *Note* — Except where otherwise indicated, the morphological varieties of carcinoma in the list below should be coded by site as for "Neoplasm, malignant."

  with
    apocrine metaplasia (M8573/3)
    cartilaginous (and osseous) metaplasia (M8571/3)
    osseous (and cartilaginous) metaplasia (M8571/3)
    productive fibrosis (M8141/3)
    spindle cell metaplasia (M8572/3)
    squamous metaplasia (M8570/3)
  acidophil (M8280/3)
    specified site — *see* Neoplasm, by site, malignant
    unspecified site 194.3
  acidophil-basophil, mixed (M8281/3)
    specified site — *see* Neoplasm, by site, malignant
    unspecified site 194.3
  acinar (cell) (M8550/3)
  acinic cell (M8550/3)
  adenocystic (M8200/3)
  adenoid
    cystic (M8200/3)
    squamous cell (M8075/3)
  adenosquamous (M8560/3)
  adnexal (skin) (M8390/3) — *see* Neoplasm, skin, malignant
  adrenal cortical (M8370/3) 194.0
  alveolar (M8251/3)
    cell (M8250/3) — *see* Neoplasm, lung, malignant
  anaplastic type (M8021/3)
  apocrine (M8401/3)
    breast — *see* Neoplasm, breast, malignant
    specified site NEC — *see* Neoplasm, skin, malignant
    unspecified site 173.9
  basal cell (pigmented) (M8090/3) (*see also* Neoplasm, skin, malignant)
    fibro-epithelial type (M8093/3) — *see* Neoplasm, skin, malignant
    morphea type (M8092/3) — *see* Neoplasm, skin, malignant
    multicentric (M8091/3) — *see* Neoplasm, skin, malignant
  basaloid (M8123/3)
  basal-squamous cell, mixed (M8094/3) — *see* Neoplasm, skin, malignant
  basophil (M8300/3)
    specified site — *see* Neoplasm, by site, malignant

Carcinoma

Carcinoma — *see also* Neoplasm, by site, malignant — *continued*
  basophil — *continued*
    unspecified site 194.3
  basophil-acidophil, mixed (M8281/3)
    specified site — *see* Neoplasm, by site, malignant
    unspecified site 194.3
  basosquamous (M8094/3) — *see* Neoplasm, skin, malignant
  bile duct type (M8160/3)
    and hepatocellular, mixed (M8180/3) 155.0
    liver 155.1
    specified site NEC — *see* Neoplasm, by site, malignant
    unspecified site 155.1
  branchial or branchiogenic 146.8
  bronchial or bronchogenic — *see* Neoplasm, lung, malignant
  bronchiolar (terminal) (M8250/3) — *see* Neoplasm, lung, malignant
  bronchiolo-alveolar (M8250/3) — *see* Neoplasm, lung, malignant
  bronchogenic (epidermoid) 162.9
  C cell (M8510/3)
    specified site — *see* Neoplasm, by site, malignant
    unspecified site 193
  ceruminous (M8420/3) 173.2
  chorionic (M9100/3)
    specified site — *see* Neoplasm, by site, malignant
    unspecified site
      female 181
      male 186.9
  chromophobe (M8270/3)
    specified site — *see* Neoplasm, by site, malignant
    unspecified site 194.3
  clear cell (mesonephroid type) (M8310/3)
  cloacogenic (M8124/3)
    specified site — *see* Neoplasm, by site, malignant
    unspecified site 154.8
  colloid (M8480/3)
  cribriform (M8201/3)
  cylindroid type (M8200/3)
  diffuse type (M8145/3)
    specified site — *see* Neoplasm, by site, malignant
    unspecified site 151.9
  duct (cell) (M8500/3)
    with Paget's disease (M8541/3) — *see* Neoplasm, breast, malignant
    infiltrating (M8500/3)
      specified site — *see* Neoplasm, by site, malignant
      unspecified site 174.9
  ductal (M8500/3)
  ductular, infiltrating (M8521/3)
  embryonal (M9070/3)
    and teratoma, mixed (M9081/3)
    combined with choriocarcinoma (M9101/3) — *see* Neoplasm, by site, malignant
    infantile type (M9071/3)
    liver 155.0
    polyembryonal type (M9072/3)
  endometrioid (M8380/3)
  eosinophil (M8280/3)
    specified site — *see* Neoplasm, by site, malignant
    unspecified site 194.3
  epidermoid (M8070/3) (*see also* Carcinoma, squamous cell)
    and adenocarcinoma, mixed (M8560/3)
    in situ, Bowen's type (M8081/2) — *see* Neoplasm, skin, in situ
    intradermal — *see* Neoplasm, skin, in situ

Carcinoma

Carcinoma — *see also* Neoplasm, by site, malignant — *continued*
- fibroepithelial type basal cell (M8093/3) — *see* Neoplasm, skin, malignant
- follicular (M8330/3)
  - and papillary (mixed) (M8340/3) 193
  - moderately differentiated type (M8332/3) 193
  - pure follicle type (M8331/3) 193
  - specified site — *see* Neoplasm, by site, malignant
  - trabecular type (M8332/3) 193
  - unspecified site 193
  - well differentiated type (M8331/3) 193
- gelatinous (M8480/3)
- giant cell (M8031/3)
  - and spindle cell (M8030/3)
- granular cell (M8320/3)
- granulosa cell (M8620/3) 183.0
- hepatic cell (M8170/3) 155.0
- hepatocellular (M8170/3) 155.0
  - and bile duct, mixed (M8180/3) 155.0
- hepatocholangiolitic (M8180/3) 155.0
- Hürthle cell (thyroid) 193
- hypernephroid (M8311/3)
- in
  - adenomatous
    - polyp (M8210/3)
    - polyposis coli (M8220/3) 153.9
  - pleomorphic adenoma (M8940/3)
  - polypoid adenoma (M8210/3)
  - situ (M8010/3) — *see* Carcinoma, in situ
  - tubular adenoma (M8210/3)
  - villous adenoma (M8261/3)
- infiltrating duct (M8500/3)
  - with Paget's disease (M8541/3) — *see* Neoplasm, breast, malignant
  - specified site — *see* Neoplasm, by site, malignant
  - unspecified site 174.9
- inflammatory (M8530/3)
  - specified site — *see* Neoplasm, by site, malignant
  - unspecified site 174.9
- in situ (M8010/2) (*see also* Neoplasm, by site, in situ)
  - epidermoid (M8070/2) (*see also* Neoplasm, by site, in situ)
    - with questionable stromal invasion (M8076/2)
    - specified site — *see* Neoplasm, by site, in situ
    - unspecified site 233.1
    - Bowen's type (M8081/2) — *see* Neoplasm, skin, in situ
  - intraductal (M8500/2)
    - specified site — *see* Neoplasm, by site, in situ
    - unspecified site 233.0
  - lobular (M8520/2)
    - specified site — *see* Neoplasm, by site, in situ
    - unspecified site 233.0
  - papillary (M8050/2) — *see* Neoplasm, by site, in situ
  - squamous cell (M8070/2) (*see also* Neoplasm, by site, in situ)
    - with questionable stromal invasion (M8076/2)
    - specified site — *see* Neoplasm, by site, in situ
    - unspecified site 233.1
  - transitional cell (M8120/2) — *see* Neoplasm, by site, in situ
- intestinal type (M8144/3)
  - specified site — *see* Neoplasm, by site, malignant
  - unspecified site 151.9
- intraductal (noninfiltrating) (M8500/2)
  - papillary (M8503/2)
    - specified site — *see* Neoplasm, by site, in situ
    - unspecified site 233.0
    - specified site — *see* Neoplasm, by site, in situ
    - unspecified site 233.0
- intraepidermal (M8070/2) (*see also* Neoplasm, skin, in situ)
  - squamous cell, Bowen's type (M8081/2) — *see* Neoplasm, skin, in situ
- intraepithelial (M8010/2) (*see also* Neoplasm, by site, in situ)
  - squamous cell (M8072/2) — *see* Neoplasm, by site, in situ
- intraosseous (M9270/3) 170.1
  - upper jaw (bone) 170.0
- islet (M8150/3)
  - and exocrine, mixed (M8154/3)
    - specified site — *see* Neoplasm, by site, malignant
    - unspecified site 157.9
  - pancreas 157.4
  - specified site NEC — *see* Neoplasm, by site, malignant
  - unspecified site 157.4
- juvenile, breast (M8502/3) — *see* Neoplasm, breast, malignant
- Kulchitsky's cell (carcinoid tumor of intestine) 259.2
- large cell (M8012/3)
  - squamous cell, non-keratinizing type (M8072/3)
- Leydig cell (testis) (M8650/3)
  - specified site — *see* Neoplasm, by site, malignant
  - unspecified site 186.9
  - female 183.0
  - male 186.9
- liver cell (M8170/3) 155.0
- lobular (infiltrating) (M8520/3)
  - non-infiltrating (M8520/3)
    - specified site — *see* Neoplasm, by site, in situ
    - unspecified site 233.0
  - specified site — *see* Neoplasm, by site, malignant
  - unspecified site 174.9
- lymphoepithelial (M8082/3)
- medullary (M8510/3)
  - with
    - amyloid stroma (M8511/3)
      - specified site — *see* Neoplasm, by site, malignant
      - unspecified site 193
    - lymphoid stroma (M8512/3)
      - specified site — *see* Neoplasm, by site, malignant
      - unspecified site 174.9
- mesometanephric (M9110/3)
- mesonephric (M9110/3)
- metastatic (M8010/6) — *see* Metastasis, cancer
- metatypical (M8095/3) — *see* Neoplasm, skin, malignant
- morphea type basal cell (M8092/3) — *see* Neoplasm, skin, malignant
- mucinous (M8480/3)
- mucin-producing (M8481/3)
- mucin-secreting (M8481/3)
- mucoepidermoid (M8430/3)
- mucoid (M8480/3)
  - cell (M8300/3)
    - specified site — *see* Neoplasm, by site, malignant
    - unspecified site 194.3
- mucous (M8480/3)
- nonencapsulated sclerosing (M8350/3) 193
- noninfiltrating
  - intracystic (M8504/2) — *see* Neoplasm, by site, in situ
  - intraductal (M8500/2)
    - papillary (M8503/2)
      - specified site — *see* Neoplasm, by site, in situ
      - unspecified site 233.0
    - specified site — *see* Neoplasm, by site, in situ
    - unspecified site 233.0
  - lobular (M8520/2)
    - specified site — *see* Neoplasm, by site, in situ
    - unspecified site 233.0
- oat cell (M8042/3)
  - specified site — *see* Neoplasm, by site, malignant
  - unspecified site 162.9
- odontogenic (M9270/3) 170.1
  - upper jaw (bone) 170.0
- onocytic (M8290/3)
- oxyphilic (M8290/3)
- papillary (M8050/3)
  - and follicular (mixed) (M8340/3) 193
  - epidermoid (M8052/3)
  - intraductal (noninfiltrating) (M8503/2)
    - specified site — *see* Neoplasm, by site, in situ
    - unspecified site 233.0
  - serous (M8460/3)
    - specified site — *see* Neoplasm, by site, malignant
    - unspecified site 183.0
    - surface (M8461/3)
      - specified site — *see* Neoplasm, by site, malignant
      - unspecified site 183.0
  - squamous cell (M8052/3)
  - transitional cell (M8130/3)
- papillocystic (M8450/3)
  - specified site — *see* Neoplasm, by site, malignant
  - unspecified site 183.0
- parafollicular cell (M8510/3)
  - specified site — *see* Neoplasm, by site, malignant
  - unspecified site 193
- pleomorphic (M8022/3)
- polygonal cell (M8034/3)
- prickle cell (M8070/3)
- pseudoglandular, squamous cell (M8075/3)
- pseudomucinous (M8470/3)
  - specified site — *see* Neoplasm, by site, malignant
  - unspecified site 183.0
- pseudosarcomatous (M8033/3)
- regaud type (M8082/3) — *see* Neoplasm, nasopharynx, malignant
- renal cell (M8312/3) 189.0
- reserve cell (M8041/3)
- round cell (M8041/3)
- Schmincke (M8082/3) — *see* Neoplasm, nasopharynx, malignant
- Schneiderian (M8121/3)
  - specified site — *see* Neoplasm, by site, malignant
  - unspecified site 160.0
- scirrhous (M8141/3)
- sebaceous (M8410/3) — *see* Neoplasm, skin, malignant
- secondary (M8010/6) — *see* Neoplasm, by site, malignant, secondary
- secretory, breast (M8502/3) — *see* Neoplasm, breast, malignant
- serous (M8441/3)
  - papillary (M8460/3)
    - specified site — *see* Neoplasm, by site, malignant
- serous — *continued*
  - papillary — *continued*
    - unspecified site 183.0
  - surface, papillary (M8461/3)
    - specified site — *see* Neoplasm, by site, malignant
    - unspecified site 183.0
- Sertoli cell (M8640/3)
  - specified site — *see* Neoplasm, by site, malignant
  - unspecified site 186.9
- signet ring cell (M8490/3)
  - metastatic (M8490/6) — *see* Neoplasm, by site, secondary
- simplex (M8231/3)
- skin appendage (M8390/3) — *see* Neoplasm, skin, malignant
- small cell (M8041/3)
  - fusiform cell type (M8043/3)
  - squamous cell, non-keratinizing type (M8073/3)
- solid (M8230/3)
  - with amyloid stroma (M8511/3)
    - specified site — *see* Neoplasm, by site, malignant
    - unspecified site 193
- spheroidal cell (M8035/3)
- spindle cell (M8032/3)
  - and giant cell (M8030/3)
- spinous cell (M8070/3)
- squamous (cell) (M8070/3)
  - adenoid type (M8075/3)
  - and adenocarcinoma, mixed (M8560/3)
  - intraepidermal, Bowen's type — *see* Neoplasm, skin, in situ
  - keratinizing type (large cell) (M8071/3)
  - large cell, non-keratinizing type (M8072/3)
  - microinvasive (M8076/3)
    - specified site — *see* Neoplasm, by site, malignant
    - unspecified site 180.9
  - non-keratinizing type (M8072/3)
  - papillary (M8052/3)
  - pseudoglandular (M8075/3)
  - small cell, non-keratinizing type (M8073/3)
  - spindle cell type (M8074/3)
  - verrucous (M8051/3)
- superficial spreading (M8143/3)
- sweat gland (M8400/3) — *see* Neoplasm, skin, malignant
- theca cell (M8600/3) 183.0
- thymic (M8580/3) 164.0
- trabecular (M8190/3)
- transitional (cell) (M8120/3)
  - papillary (M8130/3)
  - spindle cell type (M8122/3)
- tubular (M8211/3)
- undifferentiated type (M8020/3)
- urothelial (M8120/3)
- ventriculi 151.9
- verrucous (epidermoid) (squamous cell) (M8051/3)
- villous (M8262/3)
- water-clear cell (M8322/3) 194.1
- wolffian duct (M9110/3)

Carcinosarcoma (M8980/3) — *see also* Neoplasm, by site, malignant
- embryonal type (M8981/3) — *see* Neoplasm, by site, malignant

Cardiac — *see also* condition
- death — *see* Disease, heart
- device
  - defibrillator, automatic implantable V45.02
  - in situ NEC V45.00
  - pacemaker
    - cardiac
      - fitting or adjustment V53.31
      - in situ V45.01

Cardiac — see also condition — continued
  device — continued
    pacemaker — continued
      carotid sinus
        fitting or adjustment V53.39
        in situ V45.09
    pacemaker — see Cardiac, device, pacemaker
    tamponade 423.9
Cardia, cardial — see condition
Cardialgia — see also Pain, precordial 786.51
Cardiectasis — see Hypertrophy, cardiac
Cardiochalasia 530.81
Cardiomalacia — see also Degeneration, myocardial 429.1
Cardiomegalia glycogenica diffusa 271.0
Cardiomegaly — see also Hypertrophy, cardiac 429.3
  congenital 746.89
  glycogen 271.0
  hypertensive (see also Hypertension, heart) 402.90
  idiopathic 429.3
Cardiomyoliposis — see also Degeneration, myocardial 429.1
Cardiomyopathy (congestive) (constrictive) (familial) (infiltrative) (obstructive) (restrictive) (sporadic) 425.4
  alcoholic 425.5
  amyloid 277.39 [425.7] ▲
  beriberi 265.0 [425.7]
  cobalt-beer 425.5
  congenital 425.3
  due to
    amyloidosis 277.39 [425.7] ▲
    beriberi 265.0 [425.7]
    cardiac glycogenosis 271.0 [425.7]
    Chagas' disease 086.0
    Friedreich's ataxia 334.0 [425.8]
    hypertension — see Hypertension, with, heart involvement
    mucopolysaccharidosis 277.5 [425.7]
    myotonia atrophica 359.2 [425.8]
    progressive muscular dystrophy 359.1 [425.8]
    sarcoidosis 135 [425.8]
  glycogen storage 271.0 [425.7]
  hypertensive — see Hypertension, with, heart involvement
  hypertrophic
    nonobstructive 425.4
    obstructive 425.1
      congenital 746.84
  idiopathic (concentric) 425.4
  in
    Chagas' disease 086.0
    sarcoidosis 135 [425.8]
  ischemic 414.8
  metabolic NEC 277.9 [425.7]
    amyloid 277.39 [425.7] ▲
    thyrotoxic (see also Thyrotoxicosis) 242.9 ☑ [425.7]
    thyrotoxicosis (see also Thyrotoxicosis) 242.9 ☑ [425.7]
  newborn 425.4
    congenital 425.3
  nutritional 269.9 [425.7]
    beriberi 265.0 [425.7]
  obscure of Africa 425.2
  peripartum 674.5 ☑
  postpartum 674.5 ☑
  primary 425.4
  secondary 425.9
  stress inuced 429.83 ●
  takotsubo 429.83 ▲
  thyrotoxic (see also Thyrotoxicosis) 242.9 ☑ [425.7]
  toxic NEC 425.9
  tuberculous (see also Tuberculosis) 017.9 ☑ [425.8]
Cardionephritis — see Hypertension, cardiorenal

Cardionephropathy — see Hypertension, cardiorenal
Cardionephrosis — see Hypertension, cardiorenal
Cardioneurosis 306.2
Cardiopathia nigra 416.0
Cardiopathy — see also Disease, heart 429.9
  hypertensive (see also Hypertension, heart) 402.90
  idiopathic 425.4
  mucopolysaccharidosis 277.5 [425.7]
Cardiopericarditis — see also Pericarditis 423.9
Cardiophobia 300.29
Cardioptosis 746.87
Cardiorenal — see condition
Cardiorrhexis — see also Infarct, myocardium 410.9 ☑
Cardiosclerosis — see Arteriosclerosis, coronary
Cardiosis — see Disease, heart
Cardiospasm (esophagus) (reflex) (stomach) 530.0
  congenital 750.7
Cardiostenosis — see Disease, heart
Cardiosymphysis 423.1
Cardiothyrotoxicosis — see Hyperthyroidism
Cardiovascular — see condition
Carditis (acute) (bacterial) (chronic) (subacute) 429.89
  Coxsackie 074.20
  hypertensive (see also Hypertension, heart) 402.90
  meningococcal 036.40
  rheumatic — see Disease, heart, rheumatic
  rheumatoid 714.2
Care (of)
  child (routine) V20.1
  convalescent following V66.9
    chemotherapy V66.2
    medical NEC V66.5
    psychotherapy V66.3
    radiotherapy V66.1
    surgery V66.0
    surgical NEC V66.0
    treatment (for) V66.5
      combined V66.6
      fracture V66.4
      mental disorder NEC V66.3
      specified type NEC V66.5
  end-of-life V66.7
  family member (handicapped) (sick)
    creating problem for family V61.49
    provided away from home for holiday relief V60.5
    unavailable, due to
      absence (person rendering care) (sufferer) V60.4
      inability (any reason) of person rendering care V60.4
  holiday relief V60.5
  hospice V66.7
  lack of (at or after birth) (infant) (child) 995.52
    adult 995.84
  lactation of mother V24.1
  palliative V66.7
  postpartum
    immediately after delivery V24.0
    routine follow-up V24.2
  prenatal V22.1
    first pregnancy V22.0
    high-risk pregnancy V23.9
      specified problem NEC V23.89
  terminal V66.7
  unavailable, due to
    absence of person rendering care V60.4
    inability (any reason) of person rendering care V60.4
  well baby V20.1
Caries (bone) — see also Tuberculosis, bone 015.9 ☑ [730.8]

Caries — see also Tuberculosis, bone — continued
  arrested 521.04
  cementum 521.03
  cerebrospinal (tuberculous) 015.0 ☑ [730.88]
  dental (acute) (chronic) (incipient) (infected) 521.00
    with pulp exposure 521.03
    extending to
      dentine 521.02
      pulp 521.03
    other specified NEC 521.09
    pit and fissure 521.06
    primary ●
      pit and fissure origin 521.06 ●
      root surface 521.08 ●
      smooth surface origin 521.07 ●
    root surface 521.08
    smooth surface 521.07
  dentin (acute) (chronic) 521.02
  enamel (acute) (chronic) (incipient) 521.01
  external meatus 380.89
  hip (see also Tuberculosis) 015.1 ☑ [730.85]
  initial 521.01
  knee 015.2 ☑ [730.86]
  labyrinth 386.8
  limb NEC 015.7 ☑ [730.88]
  mastoid (chronic) (process) 383.1
  middle ear 385.89
  nose 015.7 ☑ [730.88]
  orbit 015.7 ☑ [730.88]
  ossicle 385.24
  petrous bone 383.20
  sacrum (tuberculous) 015.0 ☑ [730.88]
  spine, spinal (column) (tuberculous) 015.0 ☑ [730.88]
  syphilitic 095.5
    congenital 090.0 [730.8] ☑
  teeth (internal) 521.00
    initial 521.01
  vertebra (column) (tuberculous) 015.0 ☑ [730.88]
Carini's syndrome (ichthyosis congenita) 757.1
Carious teeth 521.00
Carneous mole 631
Carnosinemia 270.5
Carotid body or sinus syndrome 337.0
Carotidynia 337.0
Carotinemia (dietary) 278.3
Carotinosis (cutis) (skin) 278.3
Carpal tunnel syndrome 354.0
Carpenter's syndrome 759.89
Carpopedal spasm — see also Tetany 781.7
Carpoptosis 736.05
Carrier (suspected) of
  amebiasis V02.2
  bacterial disease (meningococcal, staphylococcal) NEC V02.59
  cholera V02.0
  cystic fibrosis gene V83.81
  defective gene V83.89
  diphtheria V02.4
  dysentery (bacillary) V02.3
    amebic V02.2
  Endamoeba histolytica V02.2
  gastrointestinal pathogens NEC V02.3
  genetic defect V83.89
  gonorrhea V02.7
  group B streptococcus V02.51
  HAA (hepatitis Australian-antigen) V02.61
  hemophilia A (asymptomatic) V83.01
    symptomatic V83.02
  hepatitis V02.60
    Australian-antigen (HAA) V02.61
    B V02.61
    C V02.62
    serum V02.61
    specified type NEC V02.69
    viral V02.60

Carrier (suspected) of — continued
  infective organism NEC V02.9
  malaria V02.9
  paratyphoid V02.3
  Salmonella V02.3
    typhosa V02.1
  serum hepatitis V02.61
  Shigella V02.3
  Staphylococcus NEC V02.59
  Streptococcus NEC V02.52
    group B V02.51
  typhoid V02.1
  venereal disease NEC V02.8
Carrión's disease (Bartonellosis) 088.0
Car sickness 994.6
Carter's
  relapsing fever (Asiatic) 087.0
Cartilage — see condition
Caruncle (inflamed)
  abscess, lacrimal (see also Dacryocystitis) 375.30
  conjunctiva 372.00
    acute 372.00
  eyelid 373.00
  labium (majus) (minus) 616.89 ▲
  lacrimal 375.30
  urethra (benign) 599.3
  vagina (wall) 616.89 ▲
Cascade stomach 537.6
Caseation lymphatic gland — see also Tuberculosis 017.2 ☑
Caseous
  bronchitis — see Tuberculosis, pulmonary
  meningitis 013.0 ☑
  pneumonia — see Tuberculosis, pulmonary
Cassidy (-Scholte) syndrome (malignant carcinoid) 259.2
Castellani's bronchitis 104.8
Castleman's tumor or lymphoma (mediastinal lymph node hyperplasia) 785.6
Castration, traumatic 878.2
  complicated 878.3
Casts in urine 791.7
Catalepsy 300.11
  catatonic (acute) (see also Schizophrenia) 295.2 ☑
  hysterical 300.11
  schizophrenic (see also Schizophrenia) 295.2 ☑
Cataphasia 307.0
Cataplexy (idiopathic) — see Narcolepsy
Cataract (anterior cortical) (anterior polar) (black) (capsular) (central) (cortical) (hypermature) (immature) (incipient) (mature) 366.9
  anterior
    and posterior axial embryonal 743.33
    pyramidal 743.31
    subcapsular polar
      infantile, juvenile, or presenile 366.01
      senile 366.13
  associated with
    calcinosis 275.40 [366.42]
    craniofacial dysostosis 756.0 [366.44]
    galactosemia 271.1 [366.44]
    hypoparathyroidism 252.1 [366.42]
    myotonic disorders 359.2 [366.43]
    neovascularization 366.33
  blue dot 743.39
  cerulean 743.39
  complicated NEC 366.30
  congenital 743.30
    capsular or subcapsular 743.31
    cortical 743.32
    nuclear 743.33
    specified type NEC 743.39
    total or subtotal 743.34
    zonular 743.32
  coronary (congenital) 743.39
    acquired 366.12

Cataract — *continued*
  cupuliform 366.14
  diabetic 250.5 ☑ *[366.41]*
  drug-induced 366.45
  due to
    chalcosis 360.24 *[366.34]*
    chronic choroiditis (*see also*
      Choroiditis) 363.20 *[366.32]*
    degenerative myopia
      360.21 *[366.34]*
    glaucoma (*see also* Glaucoma)
      365.9 *[366.31]*
    infection, intraocular NEC 366.32
    inflammatory ocular disorder NEC
      366.32
    iridocyclitis, chronic
      364.10 *[366.33]*
    pigmentary retinal dystrophy
      362.74 *[366.34]*
    radiation 366.46
  electric 366.46
  glassblowers' 366.46
  heat ray 366.46
  heterochromic 366.33
  in eye disease NEC 366.30
  infantile (*see also* Cataract, juvenile)
    366.00
  intumescent 366.12
  irradiational 366.46
  juvenile 366.00
    anterior subcapsular polar 366.01
    combined forms 366.09
    cortical 366.03
    lamellar 366.03
    nuclear 366.04
    posterior subcapsular polar 366.02
    specified NEC 366.09
    zonular 366.03
  lamellar 743.32
    infantile, juvenile, or presenile
      366.03
  morgagnian 366.18
  myotonic 359.2 *[366.43]*
  myxedema 244.9 *[366.44]*
  nuclear 366.16
  posterior, polar (capsular) 743.31
    infantile, juvenile, or presenile
      366.02
    senile 366.14
  presenile (*see also* Cataract, juvenile)
    366.00
  punctate
    acquired 366.12
    congenital 743.39
  secondary (membrane) 366.50
    obscuring vision 366.53
    specified type, not obscuring vision
      366.52
  senile 366.10
    anterior subcapsular polar 366.13
    combined forms 366.19
    cortical 366.15
    hypermature 366.18
    immature 366.12
    incipient 366.12
    mature 366.17
    nuclear 366.16
    posterior subcapsular polar 366.14
    specified NEC 366.19
    total or subtotal 366.17
  snowflake 250.5 ☑ *[366.41]*
  specified NEC 366.8
  subtotal (senile) 366.17
    congenital 743.34
  sunflower 360.24 *[366.34]*
  tetanic NEC 252.1 *[366.42]*
  total (mature) (senile) 366.17
    congenital 743.34
    localized 366.21
    traumatic 366.22
  toxic 366.45
  traumatic 366.20
    partially resolved 366.23
    total 366.22
  zonular (perinuclear) 743.32

Cataract — *continued*
  zonular — *continued*
    infantile, juvenile, or presenile
      366.03
Cataracta 366.10
  brunescens 366.16
  cerulea 743.39
  complicata 366.30
  congenita 743.30
  coralliformis 743.39
  coronaria (congenital) 743.39
    acquired 366.12
  diabetic 250.5 ☑ *[366.41]*
  floriformis 360.24 *[366.34]*
  membranacea
    accreta 366.50
    congenita 743.39
  nigra 366.16
Catarrh, catarrhal (inflammation) — *see also* condition 460
  acute 460
  asthma, asthmatic (*see also* Asthma)
    493.9 ☑
  Bostock's (*see also* Fever, hay) 477.9
  bowel — *see* Enteritis
  bronchial 490
    acute 466.0
    chronic 491.0
    subacute 466.0
  cervix, cervical (canal) (uteri) — *see*
    Cervicitis
  chest (*see also* Bronchitis) 490
  chronic 472.0
  congestion 472.0
  conjunctivitis 372.03
  due to syphilis 095.9
    congenital 090.0
  enteric — *see* Enteritis
  epidemic 487.1
  Eustachian 381.50
  eye (acute) (vernal) 372.03
  fauces (*see also* Pharyngitis) 462
  febrile 460
  fibrinous acute 466.0
  gastroenteric — *see* Enteritis
  gastrointestinal — *see* Enteritis
  gingivitis 523.00 ▲
  hay (*see also* Fever, hay) 477.9
  infectious 460
  intestinal — *see* Enteritis
  larynx (*see also* Laryngitis, chronic)
    476.0
  liver 070.1
    with hepatic coma 070.0
  lung (*see also* Bronchitis) 490
    acute 466.0
    chronic 491.0
  middle ear (chronic) — *see* Otitis media, chronic
  mouth 528.00 ▲
  nasal (chronic) (*see also* Rhinitis)
    472.0
    acute 460
  nasobronchial 472.2
  nasopharyngeal (chronic) 472.2
    acute 460
  nose — *see* Catarrh, nasal
  ophthalmia 372.03
  pneumococcal, acute 466.0
  pulmonary (*see also* Bronchitis) 490
    acute 466.0
    chronic 491.0
  spring (eye) 372.13
  suffocating (*see also* Asthma) 493.9 ☑
  summer (hay) (*see also* Fever, hay)
    477.9
  throat 472.1
  tracheitis 464.10
    with obstruction 464.11
  tubotympanal 381.4
    acute (*see also* Otitis media, acute, nonsuppurative) 381.00
    chronic 381.10
  vasomotor (*see also* Fever, hay) 477.9
  vesical (bladder) — *see* Cystitis

Catarrhus aestivus — *see also* Fever, hay 477.9
Catastrophe, cerebral — *see also* Disease, cerebrovascular, acute 436
Catatonia, catatonic (acute) 781.99
  with
    affective psychosis — *see* Psychosis, affective
    agitation 295.2 ☑
    dementia (praecox) 295.2 ☑
    due to or associated with physical condition 293.89
    excitation 295.2 ☑
    excited type 295.2 ☑
    in conditions classified elsewhere
      293.89
    schizophrenia 295.2 ☑
    stupor 295.2 ☑
Cat's ear 744.29
Cat-scratch — *see also* Injury, superficial
  disease or fever 078.3
Cauda equina — *see also* condition
  syndrome 344.60
Cauliflower ear 738.7
Caul over face 768.9
Causalgia 355.9
  lower limb 355.71
  upper limb 354.4
Cause
  external, general effects NEC 994.9
  not stated 799.9
  unknown 799.9
Caustic burn — *see also* Burn, by site
  from swallowing caustic or corrosive substance — *see* Burn, internal organs
Cavare's disease (familial periodic paralysis) 359.3
Cave-in, injury
  crushing (severe) (*see also* Crush, by site) 869.1
  suffocation 994.7
Cavernitis (penis) 607.2
  lymph vessel — *see* Lymphangioma
Cavernositis 607.2
Cavernous — *see* condition
Cavitation of lung — *see also* Tuberculosis 011.2 ☑
  nontuberculous 518.89
  primary, progressive 010.8 ☑
Cavity
  lung — *see* Cavitation of lung
  optic papilla 743.57
  pulmonary — *see* Cavitation of lung
  teeth 521.00
  vitreous (humor) 379.21
Cavovarus foot, congenital 754.59
Cavus foot (congenital) 754.71
  acquired 736.73
Cazenave's
  disease (pemphigus) NEC 694.4
  lupus (erythematosus) 695.4
CDGS (carbohydrate-deficient glycoprotein syndrome) 271.8
Cecitis — *see* Appendicitis
Cecocele — *see* Hernia
Cecum — *see* condition
Celiac
  artery compression syndrome 447.4
  disease 579.0
  infantilism 579.0
Cell, cellular — *see also* condition
  anterior chamber (eye) (positive aqueous ray) 364.04
Cellulitis (diffuse) (with lymphangitis) —
  see also Abscess 682.9
  abdominal wall 682.2
  anaerobic (*see also* Gas gangrene)
    040.0
  ankle 682.6
  anus 566
  areola 611.0
  arm (any part, above wrist) 682.3
  auditory canal (external) 380.10
  axilla 682.3

Cellulitis — *see also* Abscess — *continued*
  back (any part) 682.2
  breast 611.0
    postpartum 675.1 ☑
  broad ligament (*see also* Disease, pelvis, inflammatory) 614.4
    acute 614.3
  buttock 682.5
  cervical (neck region) 682.1
  cervix (uteri) (*see also* Cervicitis) 616.0
  cheek, external 682.0
    internal 528.3
  chest wall 682.2
  chronic NEC 682.9
  colostomy 569.61
  corpus cavernosum 607.2
  digit 681.9
  Douglas' cul-de-sac or pouch (chronic)
    (*see also* Disease, pelvis, inflammatory) 614.4
    acute 614.3
  drainage site (following operation)
    998.59
  ear, external 380.10
  enterostomy 569.61
  erysipelar (*see also* Erysipelas) 035
  esophagostomy 530.86
  eyelid 373.13
  face (any part, except eye) 682.0
  finger (intrathecal) (periosteal) (subcutaneous) (subcuticular) 681.00
  flank 682.2
  foot (except toe) 682.7
  forearm 682.3
  gangrenous (*see also* Gangrene) 785.4
  genital organ NEC
    female — *see* Abscess, genital organ, female
    male 608.4
  glottis 478.71
  gluteal (region) 682.5
  gonococcal NEC 098.0
  groin 682.2
  hand (except finger or thumb) 682.4
  head (except face) NEC 682.8
  heel 682.7
  hip 682.6
  jaw (region) 682.0
  knee 682.6
  labium (majus) (minus) (*see also* Vulvitis) 616.10
  larynx 478.71
  leg, except foot 682.6
  lip 528.5
  mammary gland 611.0
  mouth (floor) 528.3
  multiple sites NEC 682.9
  nasopharynx 478.21
  navel 682.2
    newborn NEC 771.4
  neck (region) 682.1
  nipple 611.0
  nose 478.19 ▲
    external 682.0
  orbit, orbital 376.01
  palate (soft) 528.3
  pectoral (region) 682.2
  pelvis, pelvic
    with
      abortion — *see* Abortion, by type, with sepsis
      ectopic pregnancy (*see also* categories 633.0–633.9)
        639.0
      molar pregnancy (*see also* categories 630–632) 639.0
    female (*see also* Disease, pelvis, inflammatory) 614.4
      acute 614.3
    following
      abortion 639.0
      ectopic or molar pregnancy
        639.0
    male 567.21

Index to Diseases

Cellulitis — see also Abscess — continued
pelvis, pelvic — continued
- puerperal, postpartum, childbirth 670.0 ☑
- penis 607.2
- perineal, perineum 682.2
- perirectal 566
- peritonsillar 475
- periurethral 597.0
- periuterine (see also Disease, pelvis, inflammatory) 614.4
  - acute 614.3
- pharynx 478.21
- phlegmonous NEC 682.9
- rectum 566
- retromammary 611.0
- retroperitoneal (see also Peritonitis) 567.38
- round ligament (see also Disease, pelvis, inflammatory) 614.4
  - acute 614.3
- scalp (any part) 682.8
  - dissecting 704.8
- scrotum 608.4
- seminal vesicle 608.0
- septic NEC 682.9
- shoulder 682.3
- specified sites NEC 682.8
- spermatic cord 608.4
- submandibular (region) (space) (triangle) 682.0
  - gland 527.3
- submaxillary 528.3
  - gland 527.3
- submental (pyogenic) 682.0
  - gland 527.3
- suppurative NEC 682.9
- testis 608.4
- thigh 682.6
- thumb (intrathecal) (periosteal) (subcutaneous) (subcuticular) 681.00
- toe (intrathecal) (periosteal) (subcutaneous) (subcuticular) 681.10
- tonsil 475
- trunk 682.2
- tuberculous (primary) (see also Tuberculosis) 017.0 ☑
- tunica vaginalis 608.4
- umbilical 682.2
  - newborn NEC 771.4
- vaccinal 999.3
- vagina — see Vaginitis
- vas deferens 608.4
- vocal cords 478.5
- vulva (see also Vulvitis) 616.10
- wrist 682.4

Cementoblastoma, benign (M9273/0) 213.1
- upper jaw (bone) 213.0

Cementoma (M9273/0) 213.1
- gigantiform (M9276/0) 213.1
  - upper jaw (bone) 213.0
- upper jaw (bone) 213.0

Cementoperiostitis 523.40 ▲

Cephalgia, cephalagia — see also Headache 784.0
- histamine 346.2 ☑
- nonorganic origin 307.81
- psychogenic 307.81
- tension 307.81

Cephalhematocele, cephalematocele
- due to birth injury 767.19
- fetus or newborn 767.19
- traumatic (see also Contusion, head) 920

Cephalhematoma, cephalematoma (calcified)
- due to birth injury 767.19
- fetus or newborn 767.19
- traumatic (see also Contusion, head) 920

Cephalic — see condition
Cephalitis — see Encephalitis
Cephalocele 742.0

Cephaloma — see Neoplasm, by site, malignant
Cephalomenia 625.8
Cephalopelvic — see condition
Cercomoniasis 007.3
Cerebellitis — see Encephalitis
Cerebellum (cerebellar) — see condition
Cerebral — see condition
Cerebritis — see Encephalitis
Cerebrohepatorenal syndrome 759.89
Cerebromacular degeneration 330.1
Cerebromalacia — see also Softening, brain 434.9 ☑
Cerebrosidosis 272.7
Cerebrospasticity — see Palsy, cerebral
Cerebrospinal — see condition
Cerebrum — see condition
Ceroid storage disease 272.7
Cerumen (accumulation) (impacted) 380.4
Cervical — see also condition
- auricle 744.43
- high risk human papillomavirus (HPV) DNA test positive 795.05
- intraepithelial glandular neoplasia ● 233.1
- low risk human papillomavirus (HPV) DNA test positive 795.09
- rib 756.2

Cervicalgia 723.1
Cervicitis (acute) (chronic) (nonvenereal) (subacute) (with erosion or ectropion) 616.0
- with
  - abortion — see Abortion, by type, with sepsis
  - ectopic pregnancy (see also categories 633.0–633.9) 639.0
  - molar pregnancy (see also categories 630–632) 639.0
  - ulceration 616.0
- chlamydial 099.53
- complicating pregnancy or puerperium 646.6 ☑
  - affecting fetus or newborn 760.8
- following
  - abortion 639.0
  - ectopic or molar pregnancy 639.0
- gonococcal (acute) 098.15
  - chronic or duration of 2 months or more 098.35
- senile (atrophic) 616.0
- syphilitic 095.8
- trichomonal 131.09
- tuberculous (see also Tuberculosis) 016.7 ☑

Cervicoaural fistula 744.49
Cervicocolpitis (emphysematosa) — see also Cervicitis 616.0
Cervix — see condition
Cesarean delivery, operation or section NEC 669.7 ☑
- affecting fetus or newborn 763.4
- post mortem, affecting fetus or newborn 761.6
- previous, affecting management of pregnancy 654.2 ☑

Céstan-Chenais paralysis 344.89
Céstan-Raymond syndrome 433.8 ☑
Céstan's syndrome 344.89
Cestode infestation NEC 123.9
- specified type NEC 123.8

Cestodiasis 123.9
CGF (congenital generalized fibromatosis) 759.89 ●
Chabert's disease 022.9
Chacaleh 266.2
Chafing 709.8
Chagas' disease — see also Trypanosomiasis, American 086.2
- with heart involvement 086.0

Chagres fever 084.0
Chalasia (cardiac sphincter) 530.81
Chalazion 373.2
Chalazoderma 757.39
Chalcosis 360.24

Chalcosis — continued
- cornea 371.15
- crystalline lens 360.24 [366.34]
- retina 360.24

Chalicosis (occupational) (pulmonum) 502
Chancre (any genital site) (hard) (indurated) (infecting) (primary) (recurrent) 091.0
- congenital 090.0
- conjunctiva 091.2
- Ducrey's 099.0
- extragenital 091.2
- eyelid 091.2
- Hunterian 091.0
- lip (syphilis) 091.2
- mixed 099.8
- nipple 091.2
- Nisbet's 099.0
- of
  - carate 103.0
  - pinta 103.0
  - yaws 102.0
- palate, soft 091.2
- phagedenic 099.0
- Ricord's 091.0
- Rollet's (syphilitic) 091.0
- seronegative 091.0
- seropositive 091.0
- simple 099.0
- soft 099.0
  - bubo 099.0
  - urethra 091.0
  - yaws 102.0

Chancriform syndrome 114.1
Chancroid 099.0
- anus 099.0
- penis (Ducrey's bacillus) 099.0
- perineum 099.0
- rectum 099.0
- scrotum 099.0
- urethra 099.0
- vulva 099.0

Chandipura fever 066.8
Chandler's disease (osteochondritis dissecans, hip) 732.7
Change(s) (of) — see also Removal of
- arteriosclerotic — see Arteriosclerosis
- battery
  - cardiac pacemaker V53.31
- bone 733.90
  - diabetic 250.8 ☑ [731.8]
  - in disease, unknown cause 733.90
- bowel habits 787.99
- cardiac (vascular) (see also Hypertension, cardiorenal) 404.90
- cardiovascular — see Disease, cardiovascular
- circulatory 459.9
- cognitive or personality change of other type, nonpsychotic 310.1
- color, teeth, tooth
  - during formation 520.8
  - extrinsic 523.6
  - intrinsic posteruptive 521.7
- contraceptive device V25.42
- cornea, corneal
  - degenerative NEC 371.40
  - membrane NEC 371.30
  - senile 371.41
- coronary (see also Ischemia, heart) 414.9
- degenerative
  - chamber angle (anterior) (iris) 364.56
  - ciliary body 364.57
  - spine or vertebra (see also Spondylosis) 721.90
- dental pulp, regressive 522.2
- drains V58.49
- dressing
  - wound V58.30
    - nonsurgical V58.30
    - surgical V58.31
- fixation device V54.89
  - external V54.89

Change(s) — see also Removal of — continued
- fixation device — continued
  - internal V54.01
- heart (see also Disease, heart)
- hip joint 718.95
- hyperplastic larynx 478.79
- hypertrophic
  - nasal sinus (see also Sinusitis) 473.9
  - turbinate, nasal 478.0
  - upper respiratory tract 478.9
- inflammatory — see Inflammation
- joint (see also Derangement, joint) 718.90
  - sacroiliac 724.6
- Kirschner wire V54.89
- knee 717.9
- macular, congenital 743.55
- malignant (M— —/3) (see also Neoplasm, by site, malignant)

> Note — for malignant change occurring in a neoplasm, use the appropriate M code with behavior digit /3 e.g., malignant change in uterine fibroid — M8890/3. For malignant change occurring in a nonneoplastic condition (e.g., gastric ulcer) use the M code M8000/3.

- mental (status) NEC 780.97 ▲
  - due to or associated with physical condition — see Syndrome, brain
- myocardium, myocardial — see Degeneration, myocardial
- of life (see also Menopause) 627.2
- pacemaker battery (cardiac) V53.31
- peripheral nerve 355.9
- personality (nonpsychotic) NEC 310.1
- plaster cast V54.89
- refractive, transient 367.81
- regressive, dental pulp 522.2
- retina 362.9
  - myopic (degenerative) (malignant) 360.21
  - vascular appearance 362.13
- sacroiliac joint 724.6
- scleral 379.19
  - degenerative 379.16
- senile (see also Senility) 797
- sensory (see also Disturbance, sensation) 782.0
- skin texture 782.8
- spinal cord 336.9
- splint, external V54.89
- subdermal implantable contraceptive V25.5
- suture V58.32 ▲
- traction device V54.89
- trophic 355.9
  - arm NEC 354.9
  - leg NEC 355.8
  - lower extremity NEC 355.8
  - upper extremity NEC 354.9
- vascular 459.9
- vasomotor 443.9
- voice 784.49
  - psychogenic 306.1
- wound packing V58.30 ●
  - nonsurgical V58.30 ●
  - surgical V58.31 ●

Changing sleep-work schedule, affecting sleep 327.36
Changuinola fever 066.0
Chapping skin 709.8
Character
- depressive 301.12

Charcôt's
- arthropathy 094.0 [713.5]
- cirrhosis — see Cirrhosis, biliary
- disease 094.0
  - spinal cord 094.0
- fever (biliary) (hepatic) (intermittent) — see Choledocholithiasis
- joint (disease) 094.0 [713.5]
  - diabetic 250.6 ☑ [713.5]
  - syringomyelic 336.0 [713.5]

Charcôt's — Chondritis — Index to Diseases

Charcôt's — *continued*
  syndrome (intermittent claudication) 443.9
    due to atherosclerosis 440.21
Charcôt-Marie-Tooth disease, paralysis, or syndrome 356.1
CHARGE association (syndrome) 759.89
Charleyhorse (quadriceps) 843.8
  muscle, except quadriceps — *see* Sprain, by site
Charlouis' disease — *see also* Yaws 102.9
Chauffeur's fracture — *see* Fracture, ulna, lower end
Cheadle (-Möller) (-Barlow) disease or syndrome (infantile scurvy) 267
Checking (of)
  contraceptive device (intrauterine) V25.42
  device
    fixation V54.89
      external V54.89
      internal V54.09
      traction V54.89
    Kirschner wire V54.89
    plaster cast V54.89
    splint, external V54.89
Checkup
  following treatment — *see* Examination
  health V70.0
  infant (not sick) V20.2
    newborn, routine
      initial V20.2
      subsequent V20.2
  pregnancy (normal) V22.1
    first V22.0
    high-risk pregnancy V23.9
      specified problem NEC V23.89
Chédiak-Higashi (-Steinbrinck) anomaly, disease, or syndrome (congenital gigantism of peroxidase granules) 288.2
Cheek — *see also* condition
  biting 528.9
Cheese itch 133.8
Cheese washers' lung 495.8
Cheilitis 528.5
  actinic (due to sun) 692.72
    chronic NEC 692.74
      due to radiation, except from sun 692.82
    due to radiation, except from sun 692.82
  acute 528.5
  angular 528.5
  catarrhal 528.5
  chronic 528.5
  exfoliative 528.5
  gangrenous 528.5
  glandularis apostematosa 528.5
  granulomatosa 351.8
  infectional 528.5
  membranous 528.5
  Miescher's 351.8
  suppurative 528.5
  ulcerative 528.5
  vesicular 528.5
Cheilodynia 528.5
Cheilopalatoschisis — *see also* Cleft, palate, with cleft lip 749.20
Cheilophagia 528.9
Cheiloschisis — *see also* Cleft, lip 749.10
Cheilosis 528.5
  with pellagra 265.2
  angular 528.5
  due to
    dietary deficiency 266.0
    vitamin deficiency 266.0
Cheiromegaly 729.89
Cheiropompholyx 705.81
Cheloid — *see also* Keloid 701.4
Chemical burn — *see also* Burn, by site
  from swallowing chemical — *see* Burn, internal organs

Chemodectoma (M8693/1) — *see* Paraganglioma, nonchromaffin
Chemoprophylaxis NEC V07.39
Chemosis, conjunctiva 372.73
Chemotherapy
  convalescence V66.2
  encounter (for) V58.11
  maintenance V58.11
  prophylactic NEC V07.39
    fluoride V07.31
Cherubism 526.89
Chest — *see* condition
Cheyne-Stokes respiration (periodic) 786.04
Chiari's
  disease or syndrome (hepatic vein thrombosis) 453.0
  malformation
    type I 348.4
    type II (*see also* Spina bifida) 741.0
    type III 742.0
    type IV 742.2
    network 746.89
Chiari-Frommel syndrome 676.6
Chicago disease (North American blastomycosis) 116.0
Chickenpox — *see also* Varicella 052.9
  exposure to V01.71
  vaccination and inoculation (prophylactic) V05.4
Chiclero ulcer 085.4
Chiggers 133.8
Chignon 111.2
  fetus or newborn (from vacuum extraction) 767.19
Chigoe disease 134.1
Chikungunya fever 066.3
Chilaiditi's syndrome (subphrenic displacement, colon) 751.4
Chilblains 991.5
  lupus 991.5
Child
  behavior causing concern V61.20
Childbed fever 670.0
Childbirth — *see also* Delivery
  puerperal complications — *see* Puerperal
Childhood, period of rapid growth V21.0
Chill(s) 780.99
  with fever 780.6
  congestive 780.99
    in malarial regions 084.6
  septic — *see* Septicemia
  urethral 599.84
Chilomastigiasis 007.8
Chin — *see* condition
Chinese dysentery 004.9
Chiropractic dislocation — *see also* Lesion, nonallopathic, by site 739.9
Chitral fever 066.0
Chlamydia, chlamydial — *see* condition
Chloasma 709.09
  cachecticorum 709.09
  eyelid 374.52
    congenital 757.33
    hyperthyroid 242.0
  gravidarum 646.8
  idiopathic 709.09
  skin 709.09
  symptomatic 709.09
Chloroma (M9930/3) 205.3
Chlorosis 280.9
  Egyptian (*see also* Ancylostomiasis) 126.9
  miners' (*see also* Ancylostomiasis) 126.9
Chlorotic anemia 280.9
Chocolate cyst (ovary) 617.1
Choked
  disk or disc — *see* Papilledema
  on food, phlegm, or vomitus NEC (*see also* Asphyxia, food) 933.1
  phlegm 933.1

Choked — *continued*
  while vomiting NEC (*see also* Asphyxia, food) 933.1
Chokes (resulting from bends) 993.3
Choking sensation 784.99 ▲
Cholangiectasis — *see also* Disease, gallbladder 575.8
Cholangiocarcinoma (M8160/3)
  and hepatocellular carcinoma, combined (M8180/3) 155.0
  liver 155.1
  specified site NEC — *see* Neoplasm, by site, malignant
  unspecified site 155.1
Cholangiohepatitis 575.8
  due to fluke infestation 121.1
Cholangiohepatoma (M8180/3) 155.0
Cholangiolitis (acute) (chronic) (extrahepatic) (gangrenous) 576.1
  intrahepatic 575.8
  paratyphoidal (*see also* Fever, paratyphoid) 002.9
  typhoidal 002.0
Cholangioma (M8160/0) 211.5
  malignant — *see* Cholangiocarcinoma
Cholangitis (acute) (ascending) (catarrhal) (chronic) (infective) (malignant) (primary) (recurrent) (sclerosing) (secondary) (stenosing) (suppurative) 576.1
  chronic nonsuppurative destructive 571.6
  nonsuppurative destructive (chronic) 571.6
Cholecystdocholithiasis — *see* Choledocholithiasis
Cholecystitis 575.10
  with
    calculus, stones in
      bile duct (common) (hepatic) — *see* Choledocholithiasis
      gallbladder — *see* Cholelithiasis
  acute 575.0
  acute and chronic 575.12
  chronic 575.11
  emphysematous (acute) (*see also* Cholecystitis, acute) 575.0
  gangrenous (*see also* Cholecystitis, acute) 575.0
  paratyphoidal, current (*see also* Fever, paratyphoid) 002.9
  suppurative (*see also* Cholecystitis, acute) 575.0
  typhoidal 002.0
Choledochitis (suppurative) 576.1
Choledocholith — *see* Choledocholithiasis
Choledocholithiasis 574.5

> Note — Use the following fifth-digit subclassification with category 574:
> 0   without mention of obstruction
> 1   with obstruction

  with
    cholecystitis 574.4
      acute 574.3
      chronic 574.4
    cholelithiasis 574.9
      with
        cholecystitis 574.7
          acute 574.6
          and chronic 574.8
          chronic 574.7
Cholelithiasis (impacted) (multiple) 574.2

> Note — Use the following fifth-digit subclassification with category 574:
> 0   without mention of obstruction
> 1   with obstruction

  with
    cholecystitis 574.1
      acute 574.0
      chronic 574.1

Cholelithiasis — *continued*
  with — *continued*
    choledocholithiasis 574.9
      with
        cholecystitis 574.7
          acute 574.6
          and chronic 574.8
        chronic cholecystitis 574.7
Cholemia — *see also* Jaundice 782.4
  familial 277.4
  Gilbert's (familial nonhemolytic) 277.4
Cholemic gallstone — *see* Cholelithiasis
Choleperitoneum, choleperitonitis — *see also* Disease, gallbladder 567.81
Cholera (algid) (Asiatic) (asphyctic) (epidemic) (gravis) (Indian) (malignant) (morbus) (pestilential) (spasmodic) 001.9
  antimonial 985.4
  carrier (suspected) of V02.0
  classical 001.0
  contact V01.0
  due to
    Vibrio
      cholerae (Inaba, Ogawa, Hikojima serotypes) 001.0
      El Tor 001.1
  El Tor 001.1
  exposure to V01.0
  vaccination, prophylactic (against) V03.0
Cholerine — *see also* Cholera 001.9
Cholestasis 576.8
  due to total parenteral nutrition (TPN) 573.8
Cholesteatoma (ear) 385.30
  attic (primary) 385.31
  diffuse 385.35
  external ear (canal) 380.21
  marginal (middle ear) 385.32
    with involvement of mastoid cavity 385.33
    secondary (with middle ear involvement) 385.33
  mastoid cavity 385.30
  middle ear (secondary) 385.32
    with involvement of mastoid cavity 385.33
  postmastoidectomy cavity (recurrent) 383.32
  primary 385.31
  recurrent, postmastoidectomy cavity 383.32
  secondary (middle ear) 385.32
    with involvement of mastoid cavity 385.33
Cholesteatosis (middle ear) — *see also* Cholesteatoma 385.30
  diffuse 385.35
Cholesteremia 272.0
Cholesterin
  granuloma, middle ear 385.82
  in vitreous 379.22
Cholesterol
  deposit
    retina 362.82
    vitreous 379.22
  imbibition of gallbladder (*see also* Disease, gallbladder) 575.6
Cholesterolemia 272.0
  essential 272.0
  familial 272.0
  hereditary 272.0
Cholesterosis, cholesterolosis (gallbladder) 575.6
  with
    cholecystitis — *see* Cholecystitis
    cholelithiasis — *see* Cholelithiasis
  middle ear (*see also* Cholesteatoma) 385.30
Cholocolic fistula — *see also* Fistula, gallbladder 575.5
Choluria 791.4
Chondritis (purulent) 733.99

Index to Diseases

Chondritis — *continued*
- auricle 380.03
- costal 733.6
  - Tietze's 733.6
- patella, posttraumatic 717.7
- pinna 380.03
- posttraumatica patellae 717.7
- tuberculous (active) (*see also* Tuberculosis) 015.9 ☑
  - intervertebral 015.0 ☑ *[730.88]*

Chondroangiopathia calcarea seu punctate 756.59

Chondroblastoma (M9230/0) — *see also* Neoplasm, bone, benign
- malignant (M9230/3) — *see* Neoplasm, bone, malignant

Chondrocalcinosis (articular) (crystal deposition) (dihydrate) — *see also* Arthritis, due to, crystals 275.49 *[712.3]* ☑
- due to
  - calcium pyrophosphate 275.49 *[712.2]* ☑
  - dicalcium phosphate crystals 275.49 *[712.1]* ☑
  - pyrophosphate crystals 275.49 *[712.2]* ☑

Chondrodermatitis nodularis helicis 380.00

Chondrodysplasia 756.4
- angiomatose 756.4
- calcificans congenita 756.59
- epiphysialis punctata 756.59
- hereditary deforming 756.4
- rhizomelic punctata 277.86

Chondrodystrophia (fetalis) 756.4
- calcarea 756.4
- calcificans congenita 756.59
- fetalis hypoplastica 756.59
- hypoplastica calcinosa 756.59
- punctata 756.59
- tarda 277.5

Chondrodystrophy (familial) (hypoplastic) 756.4

Chondroectodermal dysplasia 756.55

Chondrolysis 733.99

Chondroma (M9220/0) — *see also* Neoplasm cartilage, benign
- juxtacortical (M9221/0) — *see* Neoplasm, bone, benign
- periosteal (M9221/0) — *see* Neoplasm, bone, benign

Chondromalacia 733.92
- epiglottis (congenital) 748.3
- generalized 733.92
- knee 717.7
- larynx (congenital) 748.3
- localized, except patella 733.92
- patella, patellae 717.7
- systemic 733.92
- tibial plateau 733.92
- trachea (congenital) 748.3

Chondromatosis (M9220/1) — *see* Neoplasm, cartilage, uncertain behavior

Chondromyxosarcoma (M9220/3) — *see* Neoplasm, cartilage, malignant

Chondro-osteodysplasia (Morquio-Brailsford type) 277.5

Chondro-osteodystrophy 277.5

Chondro-osteoma (M9210/0) — *see* Neoplasm, bone, benign

Chondropathia tuberosa 733.6

Chondrosarcoma (M9220/3) — *see also* Neoplasm, cartilage, malignant
- juxtacortical (M9221/3) — *see* Neoplasm, bone, malignant
- mesenchymal (M9240/3) — *see* Neoplasm, connective tissue, malignant

Chordae tendineae rupture (chronic) 429.5

Chordee (nonvenereal) 607.89
- congenital 752.63
- gonococcal 098.2

Chorditis (fibrinous) (nodosa) (tuberosa) 478.5

Chordoma (M9370/3) — *see* Neoplasm, by site, malignant

Chorea (gravis) (minor) (spasmodic) 333.5
- with
  - heart involvement — *see* Chorea with rheumatic heart disease
  - rheumatic heart disease (chronic, inactive, or quiescent) (conditions classifiable to 393–398) (*see* rheumatic heart condition involved)
    - active or acute (conditions classifiable to 391) 392.0
- acute — *see* Chorea, Sydenham's
- apoplectic (*see also* Disease, cerebrovascular, acute) 436
- chronic 333.4
- electric 049.8
- gravidarum — *see* Eclampsia, pregnancy
- habit 307.22
- hereditary 333.4
- Huntington's 333.4
- posthemiplegic 344.89
- pregnancy — *see* Eclampsia, pregnancy
- progressive 333.4
  - chronic 333.4
  - hereditary 333.4
- rheumatic (chronic) 392.9
  - with heart disease or involvement — *see* Chorea, with rheumatic heart disease
- senile 333.5
- Sydenham's 392.9
  - with heart involvement — *see* Chorea, with rheumatic heart disease
  - nonrheumatic 333.5
- variabilis 307.23

Choreoathetosis (paroxysmal) 333.5

Chorioadenoma (destruens) (M9100/1) 236.1

Chorioamnionitis 658.4 ☑
- affecting fetus or newborn 762.7

Chorioangioma (M9120/0) 219.8

Choriocarcinoma (M9100/3)
- combined with
  - embryonal carcinoma (M9101/3) — *see* Neoplasm, by site, malignant
  - teratoma (M9101/3) — *see* Neoplasm, by site, malignant
- specified site — *see* Neoplasm, by site, malignant
- unspecified site
  - female 181
  - male 186.9

Chorioencephalitis, lymphocytic (acute) (serous) 049.0

Chorioepithelioma (M9100/3) — *see* Choriocarcinoma

Choriomeningitis (acute) (benign) (lymphocytic) (serous) 049.0

Chorionepithelioma (M9100/3) — *see* Choriocarcinoma

Chorionitis — *see also* Scleroderma 710.1

Chorioretinitis 363.20
- disseminated 363.10
  - generalized 363.13
  - in
    - neurosyphilis 094.83
    - secondary syphilis 091.51
  - peripheral 363.12
  - posterior pole 363.11
  - tuberculous (*see also* Tuberculosis) 017.3 ☑ *[363.13]*
- due to
  - histoplasmosis (*see also* Histoplasmosis) 115.92
  - toxoplasmosis (acquired) 130.2
    - congenital (active) 771.2
- focal 363.00

Chorioretinitis — *continued*
- focal — *continued*
  - juxtapapillary 363.01
  - peripheral 363.04
  - posterior pole NEC 363.03
- juxtapapillaris, juxtapapillary 363.01
- progressive myopia (degeneration) 360.21
- syphilitic (secondary) 091.51
  - congenital (early) 090.0 *[363.13]*
  - late 090.5 *[363.13]*
  - late 095.8 *[363.13]*
- tuberculous (*see also* Tuberculosis) 017.3 ☑ *[363.13]*

Choristoma — *see* Neoplasm, by site, benign

Choroid — *see* condition

Choroideremia, choroidermia (initial stage) (late stage) (partial or total atrophy) 363.55

Choroiditis — *see also* Chorioretinitis 363.20
- leprous 030.9 *[363.13]*
- senile guttate 363.41
- sympathetic 360.11
- syphilitic (secondary) 091.51
  - congenital (early) 090.0 *[363.13]*
  - late 090.5 *[363.13]*
  - late 095.8 *[363.13]*
- Tay's 363.41
- tuberculous (*see also* Tuberculosis) 017.3 ☑ *[363.13]*

Choroidopathy NEC 363.9
- degenerative (*see also* Degeneration, choroid) 363.40
- hereditary (*see also* Dystrophy, choroid) 363.50
- specified type NEC 363.8

Choroidoretinitis — *see* Chorioretinitis

Choroidosis, central serous 362.41

Choroidretinopathy, serous 362.41

Christian's syndrome (chronic histiocytosis X) 277.89

Christian-Weber disease (nodular nonsuppurative panniculitis) 729.30

Christmas disease 286.1

Chromaffinoma (M8700/0) — *see also* Neoplasm, by site, benign
- malignant (M8700/3) — *see* Neoplasm, by site, malignant

Chromatopsia 368.59

Chromhidrosis, chromidrosis 705.89

Chromoblastomycosis 117.2

Chromomycosis 117.2

Chromophytosis 111.0

Chromotrichomycosis 111.8

Chronic — *see* condition

Churg-Strauss syndrome 446.4

Chyle cyst, mesentery 457.8

Chylocele (nonfilarial) 457.8
- filarial (*see also* Infestation, filarial) 125.9
- tunica vaginalis (nonfilarial) 608.84
  - filarial (*see also* Infestation, filarial) 125.9

Chylomicronemia (fasting) (with hyperprebetalipoproteinemia) 272.3

Chylopericardium (acute) 420.90

Chylothorax (nonfilarial) 457.8
- filarial (*see also* Infestation, filarial) 125.9

Chylous
- ascites 457.8
- cyst of peritoneum 457.8
- hydrocele 603.9
- hydrothorax (nonfilarial) 457.8
  - filarial (*see also* Infestation, filarial) 125.9

Chyluria 791.1
- bilharziasis 120.0
- due to
  - Brugia (malayi) 125.1
  - Wuchereria (bancrofti) 125.0
  - malayi 125.1
- filarial (*see also* Infestation, filarial) 125.9

Chyluria — *continued*
- filariasis (*see also* Infestation, filarial) 125.9
- nonfilarial 791.1

Cicatricial (deformity) — *see* Cicatrix

Cicatrix (adherent) (contracted) (painful) (vicious) 709.2
- adenoid 474.8
- alveolar process 525.8
- anus 569.49
- auricle 380.89
- bile duct (*see also* Disease, biliary) 576.8
- bladder 596.8
- bone 733.99
- brain 348.8
- cervix (postoperative) (postpartal) 622.3
  - in pregnancy or childbirth 654.6 ☑
    - causing obstructed labor 660.2 ☑
- chorioretinal 363.30
  - disseminated 363.35
  - macular 363.32
  - peripheral 363.34
  - posterior pole NEC 363.33
- choroid — *see* Cicatrix, chorioretinal
- common duct (*see also* Disease, biliary) 576.8
- congenital 757.39
- conjunctiva 372.64
- cornea 371.00
  - tuberculous (*see also* Tuberculosis) 017.3 ☑ *[371.05]*
- duodenum (bulb) 537.3
- esophagus 530.3
- eyelid 374.46
  - with
    - ectropion — *see* Ectropion
    - entropion — *see* Entropion
- hypopharynx 478.29
- knee, semilunar cartilage 717.5
- lacrimal
  - canaliculi 375.53
  - duct
    - acquired 375.56
    - neonatal 375.55
  - punctum 375.52
  - sac 375.54
- larynx 478.79
- limbus (cystoid) 372.64
- lung 518.89
- macular 363.32
  - disseminated 363.35
  - peripheral 363.34
- middle ear 385.89
- mouth 528.9
- muscle 728.89
- nasolacrimal duct
  - acquired 375.56
  - neonatal 375.55
- nasopharynx 478.29
- palate (soft) 528.9
- penis 607.89
- prostate 602.8
- rectum 569.49
- retina 363.30
  - disseminated 363.35
  - macular 363.32
  - peripheral 363.34
  - posterior pole NEC 363.33
- semilunar cartilage — *see* Derangement, meniscus
- seminal vesicle 608.89
- skin 709.2
  - infected 686.8
  - postinfectional 709.2
  - tuberculous (*see also* Tuberculosis) 017.0 ☑
- specified site NEC 709.8
- throat 478.29
- tongue 529.8
- tonsil (and adenoid) 474.8
- trachea 478.9
- tuberculous NEC (*see also* Tuberculosis) 011.9 ☑

Cicatrix

Cicatrix — *continued*
  ureter 593.89
  urethra 599.84
  uterus 621.8
  vagina 623.4
    in pregnancy or childbirth 654.7 ☑
      causing obstructed labor 660.2 ☑
  vocal cord 478.5
  wrist, constricting (annular) 709.2
CIN I [cervical intraepithelial neoplasia I] 622.11
CIN II [cervical intraepithelial neoplasia II] 622.12
CIN III [cervical intraepithelial neoplasia III] 233.1
Cinchonism
  correct substance properly administered 386.9
  overdose or wrong substance given or taken 961.4
Circine herpes 110.5
Circle of Willis — *see* condition
Circular — *see also* condition
  hymen 752.49
Circulating anticoagulants 286.5
  following childbirth 666.3 ☑
  postpartum 666.3 ☑
Circulation
  collateral (venous), any site 459.89
  defective 459.9
    congenital 747.9
    lower extremity 459.89
  embryonic 747.9
  failure 799.89
    fetus or newborn 779.89
    peripheral 785.59
  fetal, persistent 747.83
  heart, incomplete 747.9
Circulatory system — *see* condition
Circulus senilis 371.41
Circumcision
  in absence of medical indication V50.2
  ritual V50.2
  routine V50.2
  status (post), female 629.20
Circumscribed — *see* condition
Circumvallata placenta — *see* Placenta, abnormal
Cirrhosis, cirrhotic 571.5
  with alcoholism 571.2
  alcoholic (liver) 571.2
  atrophic (of liver) — *see* Cirrhosis, portal
  Baumgarten-Cruveilhier 571.5
  biliary (cholangiolitic) (cholangitic) (cholestatic) (extrahepatic) (hypertrophic) (intrahepatic) (nonobstructive) (obstructive) (pericholangiolitic) (posthepatic) (primary) (secondary) (xanthomatous) 571.6
    due to
      clonorchiasis 121.1
      flukes 121.3
  brain 331.9
  capsular — *see* Cirrhosis, portal
  cardiac 571.5
    alcoholic 571.2
  central (liver) — *see* Cirrhosis, liver
  Charcôt's 571.6
  cholangiolitic — *see* Cirrhosis, biliary
  cholangitic — *see* Cirrhosis, biliary
  cholestatic — *see* Cirrhosis, biliary
  clitoris (hypertrophic) 624.2
  coarsely nodular 571.5
  congestive (liver) — *see* Cirrhosis, cardiac
  Cruveilhier-Baumgarten 571.5
  cryptogenic (of liver) 571.5
  dietary (*see also* Cirrhosis, portal) 571.5
  due to
    bronzed diabetes 275.0

Cirrhosis, cirrhotic — *continued*
  due to — *continued*
    congestive hepatomegaly — *see* Cirrhosis, cardiac
    cystic fibrosis 277.00
    hemochromatosis 275.0
    hepatolenticular degeneration 275.1
    passive congestion (chronic) — *see* Cirrhosis, cardiac
    Wilson's disease 275.1
    xanthomatosis 272.2
  extrahepatic (obstructive) — *see* Cirrhosis, biliary
  fatty 571.8
    alcoholic 571.0
  florid 571.2
  Glisson's — *see* Cirrhosis, portal
  Hanot's (hypertrophic) — *see* Cirrhosis, biliary
  hepatic — *see* Cirrhosis, liver
  hepatolienal — *see* Cirrhosis, liver
  hobnail — *see* Cirrhosis, portal
  hypertrophic (*see also* Cirrhosis, liver)
    biliary — *see* Cirrhosis, biliary
    Hanot's — *see* Cirrhosis, biliary
  infectious NEC — *see* Cirrhosis, portal
  insular — *see* Cirrhosis, portal
  intrahepatic (obstructive) (primary) (secondary) — *see* Cirrhosis, biliary
  juvenile (*see also* Cirrhosis, portal) 571.5
  kidney (*see also* Sclerosis, renal) 587
  Laennec's (of liver) 571.2
    nonalcoholic 571.5
  liver (chronic) (hepatolienal) (hypertrophic) (nodular) (splenomegalic) (unilobar) 571.5
    with alcoholism 571.2
    alcoholic 571.2
    congenital (due to failure of obliteration of umbilical vein) 777.8
    cryptogenic 571.5
      alcoholic 571.2
    fatty 571.8
      alcoholic 571.0
    macronodular 571.5
      alcoholic 571.2
    micronodular 571.5
      alcoholic 571.2
    nodular, diffuse 571.5
      alcoholic 571.2
    pigmentary 275.0
    portal 571.5
      alcoholic 571.2
    postnecrotic 571.5
      alcoholic 571.2
    syphilitic 095.3
  lung (chronic) (*see also* Fibrosis, lung) 515
  macronodular (of liver) 571.5
    alcoholic 571.2
  malarial 084.9
  metabolic NEC 571.5
  micronodular (of liver) 571.5
    alcoholic 571.2
  monolobular — *see* Cirrhosis, portal
  multilobular — *see* Cirrhosis, portal
  nephritis (*see also* Sclerosis, renal) 587
  nodular — *see* Cirrhosis, liver
  nutritional (fatty) 571.5
  obstructive (biliary) (extrahepatic) (intrahepatic) — *see* Cirrhosis, biliary
  ovarian 620.8
  paludal 084.9
  pancreas (duct) 577.8
  pericholangiolitic — *see* Cirrhosis, biliary
  periportal — *see* Cirrhosis, portal
  pigment, pigmentary (of liver) 275.0
  portal (of liver) 571.5
    alcoholic 571.2

Cirrhosis, cirrhotic — *continued*
  posthepatitic (*see also* Cirrhosis, postnecrotic) 571.5
  postnecrotic (of liver) 571.5
    alcoholic 571.2
  primary (intrahepatic) — *see* Cirrhosis, biliary
  pulmonary (*see also* Fibrosis, lung) 515
  renal (*see also* Sclerosis, renal) 587
  septal (*see also* Cirrhosis, postnecrotic) 571.5
  spleen 289.51
  splenomegalic (of liver) — *see* Cirrhosis, liver
  stasis (liver) — *see* Cirrhosis, liver
  stomach 535.4 ☑
  Todd's (*see also* Cirrhosis, biliary) 571.6
  toxic (nodular) — *see* Cirrhosis, postnecrotic
  trabecular — *see* Cirrhosis, postnecrotic
  unilobar — *see* Cirrhosis, liver
  vascular (of liver) — *see* Cirrhosis, liver
  xanthomatous (biliary) (*see also* Cirrhosis, biliary) 571.6
    due to xanthomatosis (familial) (metabolic) (primary) 272.2
Cistern, subarachnoid 793.0
Citrullinemia 270.6
Citrullinuria 270.6
Ciuffini-Pancoast tumor (M8010/3) (carcinoma, pulmonary apex) 162.3
Civatte's disease or poikiloderma 709.09
Clam diggers' itch 120.3
Clap — *see* Gonorrhea
Clarke-Hadfield syndrome (pancreatic infantilism) 577.8
Clark's paralysis 343.9
Clastothrix 704.2
Claude Bernard-Horner syndrome — *see also* Neuropathy, peripheral, autonomic 337.9
Claude's syndrome 352.6
Claudication, intermittent 443.9
  cerebral (artery) (*see also* Ischemia, cerebral, transient) 435.9
  due to atherosclerosis 440.21
  spinal cord (arteriosclerotic) 435.1
    syphilitic 094.89
  spinalis 435.1
  venous (axillary) 453.8
Claudicatio venosa intermittens 453.8
Claustrophobia 300.29
Clavus (infected) 700
Clawfoot (congenital) 754.71
  acquired 736.74
Clawhand (acquired) 736.06
  congenital 755.59
Clawtoe (congenital) 754.71
  acquired 735.5
Clay eating 307.52
Clay shovelers' fracture — *see* Fracture, vertebra, cervical
Cleansing of artificial opening — *see also* Attention to artificial opening V55.9
Cleft (congenital) — *see also* Imperfect, closure
  alveolar process 525.8
  branchial (persistent) 744.41
    cyst 744.42
  clitoris 752.49
  cricoid cartilage, posterior 748.3
  facial (*see also* Cleft, lip) 749.10
  lip 749.10
    with cleft palate 749.20
      bilateral (lip and palate) 749.24
        with unilateral lip or palate 749.25
        complete 749.23
        incomplete 749.24

Cleft — *see also* Imperfect, closure — *continued*
  lip — *continued*
    with cleft palate — *continued*
      unilateral (lip and palate) 749.22
        with bilateral lip or palate 749.25
        complete 749.21
        incomplete 749.22
      bilateral 749.14
        with cleft palate, unilateral 749.25
        complete 749.13
        incomplete 749.14
      unilateral 749.12
        with cleft palate, bilateral 749.25
        complete 749.11
        incomplete 749.12
  nose 748.1
  palate 749.00
    with cleft lip 749.20
      bilateral (lip and palate) 749.24
        with unilateral lip or palate 749.25
        complete 749.23
        incomplete 749.24
      unilateral (lip and palate) 749.22
        with bilateral lip or palate 749.25
        complete 749.21
        incomplete 749.22
    bilateral 749.04
      with cleft lip, unilateral 749.25
      complete 749.03
      incomplete 749.04
    unilateral 749.02
      with cleft lip, bilateral 749.25
      complete 749.01
      incomplete 749.02
  penis 752.69
  posterior, cricoid cartilage 748.3
  scrotum 752.89
  sternum (congenital) 756.3
  thyroid cartilage (congenital) 748.3
  tongue 750.13
  uvula 749.02
    with cleft lip (*see also* Cleft, lip, with cleft palate) 749.20
  water 366.12
Cleft hand (congenital) 755.58
Cleidocranial dysostosis 755.59
Cleidotomy, fetal 763.89
Cleptomania 312.32
Clérambault's syndrome 297.8
  erotomania 302.89
Clergyman's sore throat 784.49
Click, clicking
  systolic syndrome 785.2
Clifford's syndrome (postmaturity) 766.22
Climacteric — *see also* Menopause 627.2
  arthritis NEC (*see also* Arthritis, climacteric) 716.3
  depression (*see also* Psychosis, affective) 296.2 ☑
  disease 627.2
    recurrent episode 296.3 ☑
    single episode 296.2 ☑
  female (symptoms) 627.2
  male (symptoms) (syndrome) 608.89
  melancholia (*see also* Psychosis, affective) 296.2 ☑
    recurrent episode 296.3 ☑
    single episode 296.2 ☑
  paranoid state 297.2
  paraphrenia 297.2
  polyarthritis NEC 716.39
  male 608.89
  symptoms (female) 627.2
Clinical research investigation (control) (participant) V70.7
Clinodactyly 755.59

Index to Diseases

Clitoris — see condition
Cloaca, persistent 751.5
Clonorchiasis 121.1
Clonorchiosis 121.1
Clonorchis infection, liver 121.1
Clonus 781.0
Closed bite 524.20
Closed surgical procedure converted to open procedure
    arthroscopic V64.43
    laparoscopic V64.41
    thoracoscopic V64.42
Closure
    artificial opening (see also Attention to artificial opening) V55.9
    congenital, nose 748.0
    cranial sutures, premature 756.0
    defective or imperfect NEC — see Imperfect, closure
    fistula, delayed — see Fistula
    fontanelle, delayed 756.0
    foramen ovale, imperfect 745.5
    hymen 623.3
    interauricular septum, defective 745.5
    interventricular septum, defective 745.4
    lacrimal duct 375.56
        congenital 743.65
        neonatal 375.55
    nose (congenital) 748.0
        acquired 738.0
    vagina 623.2
    valve — see Endocarditis
    vulva 624.8
Clot (blood)
    artery (obstruction) (occlusion) (see also Embolism) 444.9
    atrial appendage 429.89 ●
    bladder 596.7
    brain (extradural or intradural) (see also Thrombosis, brain) 434.0 ☑
        late effect — see Late effect(s) (of) cerebrovascular disease
    circulation 444.9
    heart (see also Infarct, myocardium) 410.9 ☑
        without myocardial infarction 429.89 ●
    vein (see also Thrombosis) 453.9
Clotting defect NEC — see also Defect, coagulation 286.9
Clouded state 780.09
    epileptic (see also Epilepsy) 345.9 ☑
    paroxysmal (idiopathic) (see also Epilepsy) 345.9 ☑
Clouding
    corneal graft 996.51
Cloudy
    antrum, antra 473.0
    dialysis effluent 792.5
Clouston's (hidrotic) ectodermal dysplasia 757.31
Clubbing of fingers 781.5
Clubfinger 736.29
    acquired 736.29
    congenital 754.89
Clubfoot (congenital) 754.70
    acquired 736.71
    equinovarus 754.51
    paralytic 736.71
Club hand (congenital) 754.89
    acquired 736.07
Clubnail (acquired) 703.8
    congenital 757.5
Clump kidney 753.3
Clumsiness 781.3
    syndrome 315.4
Cluttering 307.0
Clutton's joints 090.5
Coagulation, intravascular (diffuse) (disseminated) — see also Fibrinolysis 286.6
    newborn 776.2
Coagulopathy — see also Defect, coagulation 286.9
    consumption 286.6

Coagulopathy — see also Defect, coagulation — continued
    intravascular (disseminated) NEC 286.6
    newborn 776.2
Coalition
    calcaneoscaphoid 755.67
    calcaneus 755.67
    tarsal 755.67
Coal miners'
    elbow 727.2
    lung 500
Coal workers' lung or pneumoconiosis 500
Coarctation
    aorta (postductal) (preductal) 747.10
    pulmonary artery 747.3
Coated tongue 529.3
Coats' disease 362.12
Cocainism — see also Dependence 304.2 ☑
Coccidioidal granuloma 114.3
Coccidioidomycosis 114.9
    with pneumonia 114.0
    cutaneous (primary) 114.1
    disseminated 114.3
    extrapulmonary (primary) 114.1
    lung 114.5
        acute 114.0
        chronic 114.4
        primary 114.0
    meninges 114.2
    primary (pulmonary) 114.0
        acute 114.0
    prostate 114.3
    pulmonary 114.5
        acute 114.0
        chronic 114.4
        primary 114.0
    specified site NEC 114.3
Coccidioidosis 114.9
    lung 114.5
        acute 114.0
        chronic 114.4
        primary 114.0
    meninges 114.2
Coccidiosis (colitis) (diarrhea) (dysentery) 007.2
Cocciuria 791.9
Coccus in urine 791.9
Coccydynia 724.79
Coccygodynia 724.79
Coccyx — see condition
Cochin-China
    diarrhea 579.1
        anguilluliasis 127.2
    ulcer 085.1
Cockayne's disease or syndrome (microcephaly and dwarfism) 759.89
Cockayne-Weber syndrome (epidermolysis bullosa) 757.39
Cocked-up toe 735.2
Cock's peculiar tumor 706.2
Codman's tumor (benign chondroblastoma) (M9230/0) — see Neoplasm, bone, benign
Coenurosis 123.8
Coffee workers' lung 495.8
Cogan's syndrome 370.52
    congenital oculomotor apraxia 379.51
    nonsyphilitic interstitial keratitis 370.52
Coiling, umbilical cord — see Complications, umbilical cord
Coitus, painful (female) 625.0
    male 608.89
    psychogenic 302.76
Cold 460
    with influenza, flu, or grippe 487.1
    abscess (see also Tuberculosis, abscess)
    articular — see Tuberculosis, joint
    agglutinin
        disease (chronic) or syndrome 283.0
        hemoglobinuria 283.0

Cold — continued
    agglutinin — continued
        hemoglobinuria — continued
            paroxysmal (cold) (nocturnal) 283.2
    allergic (see also Fever, hay) 477.9
    bronchus or chest — see Bronchitis
        with grippe or influenza 487.1
    common (head) 460
        vaccination, prophylactic (against) V04.7
    deep 464.10
    effects of 991.9
        specified effect NEC 991.8
    excessive 991.9
        specified effect NEC 991.8
    exhaustion from 991.8
    exposure to 991.9
        specified effect NEC 991.8
    grippy 487.1
    head 460
    injury syndrome (newborn) 778.2
    intolerance 780.99
    on lung — see Bronchitis
    rose 477.0
    sensitivity, autoimmune 283.0
    virus 460
Coldsore — see also Herpes, simplex 054.9
Colibacillosis 041.4
    generalized 038.42
Colibacilluria 791.9
Colic (recurrent) 789.0 ☑
    abdomen 789.0 ☑
        psychogenic 307.89
    appendicular 543.9
    appendix 543.9
    bile duct — see Choledocholithiasis
    biliary — see Cholelithiasis
    bilious — see Cholelithiasis
    common duct — see Choledocholithiasis
    Devonshire NEC 984.9
        specified type of lead — see Table of Drugs and Chemicals
    flatulent 787.3
    gallbladder or gallstone — see Cholelithiasis
    gastric 536.8
    hepatic (duct) — see Choledocholithiasis
    hysterical 300.11
    infantile 789.0 ☑
    intestinal 789.0 ☑
    kidney 788.0
    lead NEC 984.9
        specified type of lead — see Table of Drugs and Chemicals
    liver (duct) — see Choledocholithiasis
    mucous 564.9
        psychogenic 316 [564.9]
    nephritic 788.0
    painter's NEC 984.9
    pancreas 577.8
    psychogenic 306.4
    renal 788.0
    saturnine NEC 984.9
        specified type of lead — see Table of Drugs and Chemicals
    spasmodic 789.0 ☑
    ureter 788.0
    urethral 788.0
        due to calculus 594.2
    uterus 625.8
        menstrual 625.3
    vermicular 543.9
    virus 460
    worm NEC 128.9
Colicystitis — see also Cystitis 595.9
Colitis (acute) (catarrhal) (croupous) (cystica superficialis) (exudative) (hemorrhagic) (noninfectious) (phlegmonous) (presumed noninfectious) 558.9
    adaptive 564.9
    allergic 558.3

Colitis — continued
    amebic (see also Amebiasis) 006.9
        nondysenteric 006.2
    anthrax 022.2
    bacillary (see also Infection, Shigella) 004.9
    balantidial 007.0
    chronic 558.9
        ulcerative (see also Colitis, ulcerative) 556.9
    coccidial 007.2
    dietetic 558.9
    due to radiation 558.1
    functional 558.9
    gangrenous 009.0
    giardial 007.1
    granulomatous 555.1
    gravis (see also Colitis, ulcerative) 556.9
    infectious (see also Enteritis, due to, specific organism) 009.0
        presumed 009.1
    ischemic 557.9
        acute 557.0
        chronic 557.1
        due to mesenteric artery insufficiency 557.1
    membranous 564.9
        psychogenic 316 [564.9]
    mucous 564.9
        psychogenic 316 [564.9]
    necrotic 009.0
    polyposa (see also Colitis, ulcerative) 556.9
    protozoal NEC 007.9
    pseudomembranous 008.45
    pseudomucinous 564.9
    regional 555.1
    segmental 555.1
    septic (see also Enteritis, due to, specific organism) 009.0
    spastic 564.9
        psychogenic 316 [564.9]
    Staphylococcus 008.41
        food 005.0
    thromboulcerative 557.0
    toxic 558.2
    transmural 555.1
    trichomonal 007.3
    tuberculous (ulcerative) 014.8 ☑
    ulcerative (chronic) (idiopathic) (nonspecific) 556.9
        entero- 556.0
        fulminant 557.0
        ileo- 556.1
        left-sided 556.5
        procto- 556.2
        proctosigmoid 556.3
        psychogenic 316 [556] ☑
        specified NEC 556.8
        universal 556.6
Collagen disease NEC 710.9
    nonvascular 710.9
    vascular (allergic) (see also Angiitis, hypersensitivity) 446.20
Collagenosis — see also Collagen disease 710.9
    cardiovascular 425.4
    mediastinal 519.3
Collapse 780.2
    adrenal 255.8
    cardiorenal (see also Hypertension, cardiorenal) 404.90
    cardiorespiratory 785.51
        fetus or newborn 779.85 ▲
    cardiovascular (see also Disease, heart) 785.51
        fetus or newborn 779.85 ▲
    circulatory (peripheral) 785.59
        with
            abortion — see Abortion, by type, with shock
            ectopic pregnancy (see also categories 633.0–633.9) 639.5

Collapse — Index to Diseases

Collapse — *continued*
  circulatory — *continued*
    with — *continued*
      molar pregnancy (*see also* categories 630–632) 639.5
      during or after labor and delivery 669.1
      fetus or newborn 779.85 ▲
      following
        abortion 639.5
        ectopic or molar pregnancy 639.5
      during or after labor and delivery 669.1
      fetus or newborn 779.89
  external ear canal 380.50
    secondary to
      inflammation 380.53
      surgery 380.52
      trauma 380.51
    general 780.2
  heart — *see* Disease, heart
  heat 992.1
  hysterical 300.11
  labyrinth, membranous (congenital) 744.05
  lung (massive) (*see also* Atelectasis) 518.0
    pressure, during labor 668.0
  myocardial — *see* Disease, heart
  nervous (*see also* Disorder, mental, nonpsychotic) 300.9
  neurocirculatory 306.2
  nose 738.0
  postoperative (cardiovascular) 998.0
  pulmonary (*see also* Atelectasis) 518.0
    fetus or newborn 770.5
      partial 770.5
      primary 770.4
  thorax 512.8
    iatrogenic 512.1
    postoperative 512.1
  trachea 519.19 ▲
  valvular — *see* Endocarditis
  vascular (peripheral) 785.59
    with
      abortion — *see* Abortion, by type, with shock
      ectopic pregnancy (*see also* categories 633.0–633.9) 639.5
      molar pregnancy (*see also* categories 630–632) 639.5
    cerebral (*see also* Disease, cerebrovascular, acute) 436
    during or after labor and delivery 669.1
    fetus or newborn 779.89
    following
      abortion 639.5
      ectopic or molar pregnancy 639.5
  vasomotor 785.59
  vertebra 733.13
Collateral — *see also* condition
  circulation (venous) 459.89
  dilation, veins 459.89
Colles' fracture (closed) (reversed) (separation) 813.41
  open 813.51
Collet-Sicard syndrome 352.6
Collet's syndrome 352.6
Colliculitis urethralis — *see also* Urethritis 597.89
Colliers'
  asthma 500
  lung 500
  phthisis (*see also* Tuberculosis) 011.4
Collodion baby (ichthyosis congenita) 757.1
Colloid milium 709.3
Coloboma NEC 743.49
  choroid 743.59
  fundus 743.52
  iris 743.46

Coloboma — *continued*
  lens 743.36
  lids 743.62
  optic disc (congenital) 743.57
    acquired 377.23
  retina 743.56
  sclera 743.47
Coloenteritis — *see* Enteritis
Colon — *see* condition
Coloptosis 569.89
Color
  amblyopia NEC 368.59
    acquired 368.55
  blindness NEC (congenital) 368.59
    acquired 368.55
Colostomy
  attention to V55.3
  fitting or adjustment V55.3
  malfunctioning 569.62
  status V44.3
Colpitis — *see also* Vaginitis 616.10
Colpocele 618.6
Colpocystitis — *see also* Vaginitis 616.10
Colporrhexis 665.4
Colpospasm 625.1
Column, spinal, vertebral — *see* condition
Coma 780.01
  apoplectic (*see also* Disease, cerebrovascular, acute) 436
  diabetic (with ketoacidosis) 250.3
    hyperosmolar 250.2
  eclamptic (*see also* Eclampsia) 780.39
  epileptic 345.3
  hepatic 572.2
  hyperglycemic 250.2
  hyperosmolar (diabetic) (nonketotic) 250.2
  hypoglycemic 251.0
    diabetic 250.3
  insulin 250.3
    hyperosmolar 250.2
    non-diabetic 251.0
  organic hyperinsulinism 251.0
  Kussmaul's (diabetic) 250.3
  liver 572.2
  newborn 779.2
  prediabetic 250.2
  uremic — *see* Uremia
Combat fatigue — *see also* Reaction, stress, acute 308.9
Combined — *see* condition
Comedo 706.1
Comedocarcinoma (M8501/3) — *see also* Neoplasm, breast, malignant
  noninfiltrating (M8501/2)
    specified site — *see* Neoplasm, by site, in situ
    unspecified site 233.0
Comedomastitis 610.4
Comedones 706.1
  lanugo 757.4
Comma bacillus, carrier (suspected) of V02.3
Comminuted fracture — *see* Fracture, by site
Common
  aortopulmonary trunk 745.0
  atrioventricular canal (defect) 745.69
  atrium 745.69
  cold (head) 460
    vaccination, prophylactic (against) V04.7
  truncus (arteriosus) 745.0
  ventricle 745.3
Commotio (current)
  cerebri (*see also* Concussion, brain) 850.9
    with skull fracture — *see* Fracture, skull, by site
  retinae 921.3
  spinalis — *see* Injury, spinal, by site
Commotion (current)
  brain (without skull fracture) (*see also* Concussion, brain) 850.9

Commotion — *continued*
  brain (*see also* Concussion, brain) — *continued*
    with skull fracture — *see* Fracture, skull, by site
  spinal cord — *see* Injury, spinal, by site
Communication
  abnormal (*see also* Fistula)
    between
      base of aorta and pulmonary artery 745.0
      left ventricle and right atrium 745.4
      pericardial sac and pleural sac 748.8
      pulmonary artery and pulmonary vein 747.3
      congenital, between uterus and anterior abdominal wall 752.3
      bladder 752.3
      intestine 752.3
      rectum 752.3
    left ventricular — right atrial 745.4
    pulmonary artery — pulmonary vein 747.3
Compartment syndrome — *see* Syndrome, compartment ●
Compensation
  broken — *see* Failure, heart
  failure — *see* Failure, heart
  neurosis, psychoneurosis 300.11
Complaint — *see also* Disease
  bowel, functional 564.9
    psychogenic 306.4
  intestine, functional 564.9
    psychogenic 306.4
  kidney (*see also* Disease, renal) 593.9
  liver 573.9
  miners' 500
Complete — *see* condition
Complex
  cardiorenal (*see also* Hypertension, cardiorenal) 404.90
  castration 300.9
  Costen's 524.60
  ego-dystonic homosexuality 302.0
  Eisenmenger's (ventricular septal defect) 745.4
  homosexual, ego-dystonic 302.0
  hypersexual 302.89
  inferiority 301.9
  jumped process
    spine — *see* Dislocation, vertebra
  primary, tuberculosis (*see also* Tuberculosis) 010.0
  Taussig-Bing (transposition, aorta and overriding pulmonary artery) 745.11
Complications
  abortion NEC — *see* categories 634-639
  accidental puncture or laceration during a procedure 998.2
  amputation stump (late) (surgical) 997.60
    traumatic — *see* Amputation, traumatic
  anastomosis (and bypass) (*see also* Complications, due to (presence of) any device, implant, or graft classified to 996.0–996.5 NEC)
    hemorrhage NEC 998.11
    intestinal (internal) NEC 997.4
      involving urinary tract 997.5
    mechanical — *see* Complications, mechanical, graft
    urinary tract (involving intestinal tract) 997.5
  anesthesia, anesthetic NEC (*see also* Anesthesia, complication) 995.22 ▲
    in labor and delivery 668.9
      affecting fetus or newborn 763.5
      cardiac 668.1

Complications — *continued*
  anesthesia, anesthetic (*see also* Anesthesia, complication) — *continued*
    in labor and delivery — *continued*
      central nervous system 668.2
      pulmonary 668.0
      specified type NEC 668.8
  aortocoronary (bypass) graft 996.03
    atherosclerosis — *see* Arteriosclerosis, coronary
    embolism 996.72
    occlusion NEC 996.72
    thrombus 996.72
  arthroplasty (*see also* Complications, prosthetic joint) 996.49
  artificial opening
    cecostomy 569.60
    colostomy 569.60
    cystostomy 997.5
    enterostomy 569.60
    esophagostomy 530.87
      infection 530.86
      mechanical 530.87
    gastrostomy 536.40
    ileostomy 569.60
    jejunostomy 569.60
    nephrostomy 997.5
    tracheostomy 519.00
    ureterostomy 997.5
    urethrostomy 997.5
  bariatric surgery 997.4
  bile duct implant (prosthetic) NEC 996.79
    infection or inflammation 996.69
    mechanical 996.59
  bleeding (intraoperative) (postoperative) 998.11
  blood vessel graft 996.1
    aortocoronary 996.03
      atherosclerosis — *see* Arteriosclerosis, coronary
      embolism 996.72
      occlusion NEC 996.72
      thrombus 996.72
    atherosclerosis — *see* Arteriosclerosis, extremities
    embolism 996.74
    occlusion NEC 996.74
    thrombus 996.74
  bone growth stimulator NEC 996.78
    infection or inflammation 996.67
  bone marrow transplant 996.85
  breast implant (prosthetic) NEC 996.79
    infection or inflammation 996.69
    mechanical 996.54
  bypass (*see also* Complications, anastomosis)
    aortocoronary 996.03
      atherosclerosis — *see* Arteriosclerosis, coronary
      embolism 996.72
      occlusion NEC 996.72
      thrombus 996.72
    carotid artery 996.1
      atherosclerosis — *see* Arteriosclerosis, extremities
      embolism 996.74
      occlusion NEC 996.74
      thrombus 996.74
  cardiac (*see also* Disease, heart) 429.9
    device, implant, or graft NEC 996.72
      infection or inflammation 996.61
      long-term effect 429.4
      mechanical (*see also* Complications, mechanical, by type) 996.00
        valve prosthesis 996.71
          infection or inflammation 996.61
    postoperative NEC 997.1
      long-term effect 429.4

Index to Diseases — Complications

Complications — *continued*
- cardiorenal (*see also* Hypertension, cardiorenal) 404.90
- carotid artery bypass graft 996.1
  - atherosclerosis — *see* Arteriosclerosis, extremities
  - embolism 996.74
  - occlusion NEC 996.74
  - thrombus 996.74
- cataract fragments in eye 998.82
- catheter device NEC (*see also* Complications, due to (presence of) any device, implant, or graft classified to 996.0–996.5 NEC)
  - mechanical — *see* Complications, mechanical, catheter
- cecostomy 569.60
- cesarean section wound 674.3 ☑
- chin implant (prosthetic) NEC 996.79
  - infection or inflammation 996.69
  - mechanical 996.59
- colostomy (enterostomy) 569.60
  - specified type NEC 569.69
- contraceptive device, intrauterine NEC 996.76
  - infection 996.65
  - inflammation 996.65
  - mechanical 996.32
- cord (umbilical) — *see* Complications, umbilical cord
- cornea
  - due to
    - contact lens 371.82
- coronary (artery) bypass (graft) NEC 996.03
  - atherosclerosis — *see* Arteriosclerosis, coronary
  - embolism 996.72
  - infection or inflammation 996.61
  - mechanical 996.03
  - occlusion NEC 996.72
  - specified type NEC 996.72
  - thrombus 996.72
- cystostomy 997.5
- delivery 669.9 ☑
  - procedure (instrumental) (manual) (surgical) 669.4 ☑
  - specified type NEC 669.8 ☑
- dialysis (hemodialysis) (peritoneal) (renal) NEC 999.9
  - catheter NEC (*see also* Complications, due to (presence of) any device, implant, or graft classified to 996.0–996.5 NEC)
    - infection or inflammation 996.62
      - peritoneal 996.68
    - mechanical 996.1
      - peritoneal 996.56
- due to (presence of) any device, implant, or graft classified to 996.0–996.5 NEC 996.70
  - with infection or inflammation — *see* Complications, infection or inflammation, due to (presence of) any device, implant, or graft classified to 996.0–996.5 NEC
  - arterial NEC 996.74
    - coronary NEC 996.03
      - atherosclerosis — *see* Arteriosclerosis, coronary
      - embolism 996.72
      - occlusion NEC 996.72
      - specified type NEC 996.72
      - thrombus 996.72
    - renal dialysis 996.73
    - arteriovenous fistula or shunt NEC 996.74
    - bone growth stimulator 996.78
    - breast NEC 996.79
    - cardiac NEC 996.72
      - defibrillator 996.72
      - pacemaker 996.72
      - valve prosthesis 996.71

Complications — *continued*
- due to any device, implant, or graft classified to 996.0–996.5 — *continued*
  - catheter NEC 996.79
    - spinal 996.75
    - urinary, indwelling 996.76
    - vascular NEC 996.74
      - renal dialysis 996.73
    - ventricular shunt 996.75
  - coronary (artery) bypass (graft) NEC 996.03
    - atherosclerosis — *see* Arteriosclerosis, coronary
    - embolism 996.72
    - occlusion NEC 996.72
    - thrombus 996.72
  - electrodes
    - brain 996.75
    - heart 996.72
  - esophagostomy 530.87
  - gastrointestinal NEC 996.79
  - genitourinary NEC 996.76
  - heart valve prosthesis NEC 996.71
  - infusion pump 996.74
  - insulin pump 996.57
  - internal
    - joint prosthesis 996.77
    - orthopedic NEC 996.78
    - specified type NEC 996.79
  - intrauterine contraceptive device NEC 996.76
  - joint prosthesis, internal NEC 996.77
  - mechanical — *see* Complications, mechanical
  - nervous system NEC 996.75
  - ocular lens NEC 996.79
  - orbital NEC 996.79
  - orthopedic NEC 996.78
    - joint, internal 996.77
  - renal dialysis 996.73
  - specified type NEC 996.79
  - urinary catheter, indwelling 996.76
  - vascular NEC 996.74
  - ventricular shunt 996.75
- during dialysis NEC 999.9
- ectopic or molar pregnancy NEC 639.9
- electroshock therapy NEC 999.9
- enterostomy 569.60
  - specified type NEC 569.69
- esophagostomy 530.87
  - infection 530.86
  - mechanical 530.87
- external (fixation) device with internal component(s) NEC 996.78
  - infection or inflammation 996.67
  - mechanical 996.49
- extracorporeal circulation NEC 999.9
- eye implant (prosthetic) NEC 996.79
  - infection or inflammation 996.69
  - mechanical
    - ocular lens 996.53
    - orbital globe 996.59
- gastrointestinal, postoperative NEC (*see also* Complications, surgical procedures) 997.4
- gastrostomy 536.40
  - specified type NEC 536.49
- genitourinary device, implant or graft NEC 996.76
  - infection or inflammation 996.65
    - urinary catheter, indwelling 996.64
  - mechanical (*see also* Complications, mechanical, by type) 996.30
    - specified NEC 996.39
- graft (bypass) (patch) (*see also* Complications, due to (presence of) any device, implant, or graft classified to 996.0–996.5 NEC)
  - bone marrow 996.85
  - corneal NEC 996.79
    - infection or inflammation 996.69

Complications — *continued*
- graft (*see also* Complications, due to any device, implant, or graft classified to 996.0–996.5) — *continued*
  - corneal — *continued*
    - rejection or reaction 996.51
  - mechanical — *see* Complications, mechanical, graft
  - organ (immune or nonimmune cause) (partial) (total) 996.80
    - bone marrow 996.85
    - heart 996.83
    - intestines 996.87
    - kidney 996.81
    - liver 996.82
    - lung 996.84
    - pancreas 996.86
    - specified NEC 996.89
  - skin NEC 996.79
    - infection or inflammation 996.69
    - rejection 996.52
      - artificial 996.55
      - decellularized allodermis 996.55
- heart (*see also* Disease, heart transplant (immune or nonimmune cause)) 996.83
- hematoma (intraoperative) (postoperative) 998.12
- hemorrhage (intraoperative) (postoperative) 998.11
- hyperalimentation therapy NEC 999.9
- immunization (procedure) — *see* Complications, vaccination
- implant (*see also* Complications, due to (presence of) any device, implant, or graft classified to 996.0–996.5 NEC)
  - mechanical — *see* Complications, mechanical, implant
- infection and inflammation
  - due to (presence of) any device, implant or graft classified to 996.0–996.5 NEC 996.60
    - arterial NEC 996.62
      - coronary 996.61
      - renal dialysis 996.62
    - arteriovenous fistula or shunt 996.62
    - artificial heart 996.61
    - bone growth stimulator 996.67
    - breast 996.69
    - cardiac 996.61
    - catheter NEC 996.69
      - peritoneal 996.68
      - spinal 996.63
      - urinary, indwelling 996.64
      - vascular NEC 996.62
      - ventricular shunt 996.63
    - coronary artery bypass 996.61
    - electrodes
      - brain 996.63
      - heart 996.61
    - gastrointestinal NEC 996.69
    - genitourinary NEC 996.65
      - indwelling urinary catheter 996.64
    - heart assist device 996.61
    - heart valve 996.61
    - infusion pump 996.62
    - insulin pump 996.69
    - intrauterine contraceptive device 996.65
    - joint prosthesis, internal 996.66
    - ocular lens 996.69
    - orbital (implant) 996.69
    - orthopedic NEC 996.67
      - joint, internal 996.66
    - specified type NEC 996.69
    - urinary catheter, indwelling 996.64
    - ventricular shunt 996.63
- infusion (procedure) 999.9

Complications — *continued*
- infusion — *continued*
  - blood — *see* Complications, transfusion
  - infection NEC 999.3
  - sepsis NEC 999.3
- inhalation therapy NEC 999.9
- injection (procedure) 999.9
  - drug reaction (*see also* Reaction, drug) 995.27 ▲
  - infection NEC 999.3
  - sepsis NEC 999.3
  - serum (prophylactic) (therapeutic) — *see* Complications, vaccination
  - vaccine (any) — *see* Complications, vaccination
- inoculation (any) — *see* Complications, vaccination
- insulin pump 996.57
- internal device (catheter) (electronic) (fixation) (prosthetic) (*see also* Complications, due to (presence of) any device, implant, or graft classified to 996.0–996.5 NEC)
  - mechanical — *see* Complications, mechanical
- intestinal transplant (immune or nonimmune cause) 996.87
- intraoperative bleeding or hemorrhage 998.11
- intrauterine contraceptive device (*see also* Complications, contraceptive device) 996.76
  - with fetal damage affecting management of pregnancy 655.8 ☑
  - infection or inflammation 996.65
- jejunostomy 569.60
- kidney transplant (immune or nonimmune cause) 996.81
- labor 669.9 ☑
  - specified condition NEC 669.8 ☑
- liver transplant (immune or nonimmune cause) 996.82
- lumbar puncture 349.0
- mechanical
  - anastomosis — *see* Complications, mechanical, graft
  - artificial heart 996.09
  - bypass — *see* Complications, mechanical, graft
  - catheter NEC 996.59
    - cardiac 996.09
    - cystostomy 996.39
    - dialysis (hemodialysis) 996.1
      - peritoneal 996.56
    - during a procedure 998.2
    - urethral, indwelling 996.31
  - colostomy 569.62
  - device NEC 996.59
    - balloon (counterpulsation), intra-aortic 996.1
    - cardiac 996.00
      - automatic implantable defibrillator 996.04
      - long-term effect 429.4
      - specified NEC 996.09
    - contraceptive, intrauterine 996.32
    - counterpulsation, intra-aortic 996.1
    - fixation, external, with internal components 996.49
    - fixation, internal (nail, rod, plate) 996.40
    - genitourinary 996.30
      - specified NEC 996.39
    - insulin pump 996.57
    - nervous system 996.2
    - orthopedic, internal 996.40
      - prosthetic joint (*see also* Complications, mechanical, device, orthopedic, prosthetic, joint) 996.47
    - prosthetic NEC 996.59

Complications

Complications — *continued*
 mechanical — *continued*
  device — *continued*
   prosthetic — *continued*
    joint (*see also* Complications, prosthetic joint) 996.47
     articular bearing surface wear 996.46
     aseptic loosening 996.41
     breakage 996.43
     dislocation 996.42
     failure 996.43
     fracture 996.43
      around prosthetic 996.44
      peri-prosthetic 996.44
     instability 996.42
     loosening 996.41
     peri-prosthetic osteolysis 996.45
     subluxation 996.42
     wear 996.46
    umbrella, vena cava 996.1
    vascular 996.1
  dorsal column stimulator 996.2
  electrode NEC 996.59
   brain 996.2
   cardiac 996.01
   spinal column 996.2
  enterostomy 569.62
  esophagostomy 530.87
  fistula, arteriovenous, surgically created 996.1
  gastrostomy 536.42
  graft NEC 996.52
   aortic (bifurcation) 996.1
   aortocoronary bypass 996.03
   blood vessel NEC 996.1
   bone 996.49
   cardiac 996.00
   carotid artery bypass 996.1
   cartilage 996.49
   corneal 996.51
   coronary bypass 996.03
   decellularized allodermis 996.55
   genitourinary 996.30
    specified NEC 996.39
   muscle 996.49
   nervous system 996.2
   organ (immune or nonimmune cause) 996.80
    heart 996.83
    intestines 996.87
    kidney 996.81
    liver 996.82
    lung 996.84
    pancreas 996.86
    specified NEC 996.89
   orthopedic, internal 996.49
   peripheral nerve 996.2
   prosthetic NEC 996.59
   skin 996.52
    artificial 996.55
   specified NEC 996.59
   tendon 996.49
   tissue NEC 996.52
   tooth 996.59
   ureter, without mention of resection 996.39
   vascular 996.1
  heart valve prosthesis 996.02
   long-term effect 429.4
  implant NEC 996.59
   cardiac 996.00
    automatic implantable defibrillator 996.04
    long-term effect 429.4
    specified NEC 996.09
   electrode NEC 996.59
    brain 996.2
    cardiac 996.01
    spinal column 996.2
   genitourinary 996.30
   nervous system 996.2
   orthopedic, internal 996.49
   prosthetic NEC 996.59

Complications — *continued*
 mechanical — *continued*
  implant — *continued*
   prosthetic — *continued*
    in
     bile duct 996.59
     breast 996.54
     chin 996.59
     eye
      ocular lens 996.53
      orbital globe 996.59
    vascular 996.1
  insulin pump 996.57
  nonabsorbable surgical material 996.59
  pacemaker NEC 996.59
   brain 996.2
   cardiac 996.01
   nerve (phrenic) 996.2
  patch — *see* Complications, mechanical, graft
  prosthesis NEC 996.59
   bile duct 996.59
   breast 996.54
   chin 996.59
   ocular lens 996.53
   reconstruction, vas deferens 996.39
  reimplant NEC 996.59
   extremity (*see also* Complications, reattached, extremity) 996.90
   organ (*see also* Complications, transplant, organ, by site) 996.80
  repair — *see* Complications, mechanical, graft
  respirator [ventilator] V46.14
  shunt NEC 996.59
   arteriovenous, surgically created 996.1
   ventricular (communicating) 996.2
  stent NEC 996.59
  tracheostomy 519.02
  vas deferens reconstruction 996.39
  ventilator [respirator] V46.14
 medical care NEC 999.9
  cardiac NEC 997.1
  gastrointestinal NEC 997.4
  nervous system NEC 997.00
  peripheral vascular NEC 997.2
  respiratory NEC 997.3
  urinary NEC 997.5
  vascular
   mesenteric artery 997.71
   other vessels 997.79
   peripheral vessels 997.2
   renal artery 997.72
 nephrostomy 997.5
 nervous system
  device, implant, or graft NEC 349.1
   mechanical 996.2
  postoperative NEC 997.00
 obstetric 669.9
  procedure (instrumental) (manual) (surgical) 669.4
  specified NEC 669.8
  surgical wound 674.3
 ocular lens implant NEC 996.79
  infection or inflammation 996.69
  mechanical 996.53
 organ transplant — *see* Complications, transplant, organ, by site
 orthopedic device, implant, or graft
  internal (fixation) (nail) (plate) (rod) NEC 996.78
   infection or inflammation 996.67
   joint prosthesis 996.77
    infection or inflammation 996.66
   mechanical 996.40
 pacemaker (cardiac) 996.72
  infection or inflammation 996.61
  mechanical 996.01

Complications — *continued*
 pancreas transplant (immune or non-immune cause) 996.86
 perfusion NEC 999.9
 perineal repair (obstetrical) 674.3
  disruption 674.2
 pessary (uterus) (vagina) — *see* Complications, contraceptive device
 phototherapy 990
 postcystoscopic 997.5
 postmastoidectomy NEC 383.30
 postoperative — *see* Complications, surgical procedures
 pregnancy NEC 646.9
  affecting fetus or newborn 761.9
 prosthetic device, internal (*see also* Complications, due to (presence of) any device, implant or graft classified to 996.0–996.5 NEC)
  mechanical NEC (*see also* Complications, mechanical) 996.59
 puerperium NEC (*see also* Puerperal) 674.9
 puncture, spinal 349.0
 pyelogram 997.5
 radiation 990
 radiotherapy 990
 reattached
  body part, except extremity 996.99
  extremity (infection) (rejection) 996.90
   arm(s) 996.94
   digit(s) (hand) 996.93
    foot 996.95
   finger(s) 996.93
   foot 996.95
   forearm 996.91
   hand 996.92
   leg 996.96
   lower NEC 996.96
   toe(s) 996.95
   upper NEC 996.94
 reimplant NEC (*see also* Complications, due to (presence of) any device, implant, or graft classified to 996.0–996.5 NEC)
  bone marrow 996.85
  extremity (*see also* Complications, reattached, extremity) 996.90
   due to infection 996.90
  mechanical — *see* Complications, mechanical, reimplant
  organ (immune or nonimmune cause) (partial) (total) (*see also* Complications, transplant, organ, by site) 996.80
 renal allograft 996.81
 renal dialysis — *see* Complications, dialysis
 respirator [ventilator], mechanical V46.14
 respiratory 519.9
  device, implant or graft NEC 996.79
   infection or inflammation 996.69
   mechanical 996.59
  distress syndrome, adult, following trauma or surgery 518.5
  insufficiency, acute, postoperative 518.5
  postoperative NEC 997.3
  therapy NEC 999.9
 sedation during labor and delivery 668.9
  affecting fetus or newborn 763.5
  cardiac 668.1
  central nervous system 668.2
  pulmonary 668.0
  specified type NEC 668.8
 seroma (intraoperative) (postoperative) (noninfected) 998.13
  infected 998.51

Complications — *continued*
 shunt (*see also* Complications, due to (presence of) any device, implant, or graft classified to 996.0–996.5 NEC)
  mechanical — *see* Complications, mechanical, shunt
 specified body system NEC
  device, implant, or graft — *see* Complications, due to (presence of) any device, implant, or graft classified to 996.0–996.5 NEC
  postoperative NEC 997.99
 spinal puncture or tap 349.0
 stomach banding 997.4
 stomach stapling 997.4
 stoma, external
  gastrointestinal tract
   colostomy 569.60
   enterostomy 569.60
   esophagostomy 530.87
    infection 530.86
    mechanical 530.87
   gastrostomy 536.40
  urinary tract 997.5
 surgical procedures 998.9
  accidental puncture or laceration 998.2
  amputation stump (late) 997.60
  anastomosis — *see* Complications, anastomosis
  burst stitches or sutures (external) 998.32
   internal 998.31
  cardiac 997.1
   long-term effect following cardiac surgery 429.4
  cataract fragments in eye 998.82
  catheter device — *see* Complications, catheter device
  cecostomy malfunction 569.62
  colostomy malfunction 569.62
  cystostomy malfunction 997.5
  dehiscence (of incision) (external) 998.32
   internal 998.31
  dialysis NEC (*see also* Complications, dialysis) 999.9
  disruption
   anastomosis (internal) — *see* Complications, mechanical, graft
   internal suture (line) 998.31
   wound (external) 998.32
    internal 998.31
  dumping syndrome (postgastrectomy) 564.2
  elephantiasis or lymphedema 997.99
   postmastectomy 457.0
  emphysema (surgical) 998.81
  enterostomy malfunction 569.62
  esophagostomy malfunction 530.87
  evisceration 998.32
  fistula (persistent postoperative) 998.6
  foreign body inadvertently left in wound (sponge) (suture) (swab) 998.4
   from nonabsorbable surgical material (Dacron) (mesh) (permanent suture) (reinforcing) (Teflon) — *see* Complications, due to (presence of) any device, implant, or graft classified to 996.0–996.5 NEC
  gastrointestinal NEC 997.4
  gastrostomy malfunction 536.42
  hematoma 998.12
  hemorrhage 998.11
  ileostomy malfunction 569.62
  internal prosthetic device NEC (*see also* Complications, internal device) 996.70
   hemolytic anemia 283.19

Index to Diseases

Complications — continued
surgical procedures — continued
- internal prosthetic device (see also Complications, internal device) — continued
  - infection or inflammation 996.60
  - malfunction — see Complications, mechanical
  - mechanical complication — see Complications, mechanical
  - thrombus 996.70
- jejunostomy malfunction 569.62
- nervous system NEC 997.00
- obstruction, internal anastomosis — see Complications, mechanical, graft
- other body system NEC 997.99
- peripheral vascular NEC 997.2
- postcardiotomy syndrome 429.4
- postcholecystectomy syndrome 576.0
- postcommissurotomy syndrome 429.4
- postgastrectomy dumping syndrome 564.2
- postmastectomy lymphedema syndrome 457.0
- postmastoidectomy 383.30
  - cholesteatoma, recurrent 383.32
  - cyst, mucosal 383.31
  - granulation 383.33
  - inflammation, chronic 383.33
- postvagotomy syndrome 564.2
- postvalvulotomy syndrome 429.4
- reattached extremity (infection) (rejection) (see also Complications, reattached, extremity) 996.90
- respiratory NEC 997.3
- seroma 998.13
- shock (endotoxic) (hypovolemic) (septic) 998.0
- shunt, prosthetic (thrombus) (see also Complications, due to (presence of) any device, implant, or graft classified to 996.0–996.5 NEC)
  - hemolytic anemia 283.19
- specified complication NEC 998.89
- stitch abscess 998.59
- transplant — see Complications, graft
- ureterostomy malfunction 997.5
- urethrostomy malfunction 997.5
- urinary NEC 997.5
- vascular
  - mesenteric artery 997.71
  - other vessels 997.79
  - peripheral vessels 997.2
  - renal artery 997.72
- wound infection 998.59
- therapeutic misadventure NEC 999.9
- surgical treatment 998.9
- tracheostomy 519.00
- transfusion (blood) (lymphocytes) (plasma) NEC 999.8
  - acute lung injury (TRALI) 518.7 ●
  - atrophy, liver, yellow, subacute (within 8 months of administration) — see Hepatitis, viral
  - bone marrow 996.85
  - embolism
    - air 999.1
    - thrombus 999.2
  - hemolysis NEC 999.8
    - bone marrow 996.85
  - hepatitis (serum) (type B) (within 8 months after administration) — see Hepatitis, viral
  - incompatibility reaction (ABO) (blood group) 999.6
    - Rh (factor) 999.7
  - infection 999.3

Complications — continued
transfusion — continued
- jaundice (serum) (within 8 months after administration) — see Hepatitis, viral
- sepsis 999.3
- shock or reaction NEC 999.8
  - bone marrow 996.85
- subacute yellow atrophy of liver (within 8 months after administration) — see Hepatitis, viral
- thromboembolism 999.2
- transplant NEC (see also Complications, due to (presence of) any device, implant, or graft classified to 996.0–996.5 NEC)
  - bone marrow 996.85
  - organ (immune or nonimmune cause) (partial) (total) 996.80
    - bone marrow 996.85
    - heart 996.83
    - intestines 996.87
    - kidney 996.81
    - liver 996.82
    - lung 996.84
    - pancreas 996.86
    - specified NEC 996.89
- trauma NEC (early) 958.8
- ultrasound therapy NEC 999.9
- umbilical cord
  - affecting fetus or newborn 762.6
  - complicating delivery 663.9 ☑
    - affecting fetus or newborn 762.6
  - specified type NEC 663.8 ☑
- urethral catheter NEC 996.76
  - infection or inflammation 996.64
  - mechanical 996.31
- urinary, postoperative NEC 997.5
- vaccination 999.9
  - anaphylaxis NEC 999.4
  - cellulitis 999.3
  - encephalitis or encephalomyelitis 323.51 ▲
  - hepatitis (serum) (type B) (within 8 months after administration) — see Hepatitis, viral
  - infection (general) (local) NEC 999.3
  - jaundice (serum) (within 8 months after administration) — see Hepatitis, viral
  - meningitis 997.09 [321.8]
  - myelitis 323.52 ▲
  - protein sickness 999.5
  - reaction (allergic) 999.5
    - Herxheimer's 995.0
    - serum 999.5
  - sepsis 999.3
  - serum intoxication, sickness, rash, or other serum reaction NEC 999.5
  - shock (allergic) (anaphylactic) 999.4
  - subacute yellow atrophy of liver (within 8 months after administration) — see Hepatitis, viral
  - vaccinia (generalized) 999.0
    - localized 999.3
- vascular
  - device, implant, or graft NEC 996.74
    - infection or inflammation 996.62
    - mechanical NEC 996.1
      - cardiac (see also Complications, mechanical, by type) 996.00
  - following infusion, perfusion, or transfusion 999.2
  - postoperative NEC 997.2
    - mesenteric artery 997.71
    - other vessels 997.79
    - peripheral vessels 997.2
    - renal artery 997.72

Complications — continued
- ventilation therapy NEC 999.9
- ventilator [respirator], mechanical V46.14

Compound presentation, complicating delivery 652.8 ☑
- causing obstructed labor 660.0 ☑

Compressed air disease 993.3

Compression
- with injury — see specific injury
- arm NEC 354.9
- artery 447.1
  - celiac, syndrome 447.4
- brachial plexus 353.0
- brain (stem) 348.4
  - due to
    - contusion, brain — see Contusion, brain
    - injury NEC (see also Hemorrhage, brain, traumatic)
      - birth — see Birth, injury, brain
      - laceration, brain — see Laceration, brain
    - osteopathic 739.0
- bronchus 519.19 ▲
- by cicatrix — see Cicatrix
- cardiac 423.9
- cauda equina 344.60
  - with neurogenic bladder 344.61
- celiac (artery) (axis) 447.4
- cerebral — see Compression, brain
- cervical plexus 353.2
- cord (umbilical) — see Compression, umbilical cord
- cranial nerve 352.9
  - second 377.49
  - third (partial) 378.51
    - total 378.52
  - fourth 378.53
  - fifth 350.8
  - sixth 378.54
  - seventh 351.8
- divers' squeeze 993.3
- duodenum (external) (see also Obstruction, duodenum) 537.3
- during birth 767.9
- esophagus 530.3
  - congenital, external 750.3
- Eustachian tube 381.63
- facies (congenital) 754.0
- fracture — see Fracture, by site
- heart — see Disease, heart
- intestine (see also Obstruction, intestine) 560.9
  - with hernia — see Hernia, by site, with obstruction
- laryngeal nerve, recurrent 478.79
- leg NEC 355.8
- lower extremity NEC 355.8
- lumbosacral plexus 353.1
- lung 518.89
- lymphatic vessel 457.1
- medulla — see Compression, brain
- nerve NEC (see also Disorder, nerve)
  - arm NEC 354.9
  - autonomic nervous system (see also Neuropathy, peripheral, autonomic) 337.9
  - axillary 353.0
  - cranial NEC 352.9
  - due to displacement of intervertebral disc 722.2
    - with myelopathy 722.70
    - cervical 722.0
      - with myelopathy 722.71
    - lumbar, lumbosacral 722.10
      - with myelopathy 722.73
    - thoracic, thoracolumbar 722.11
      - with myelopathy 722.72
  - iliohypogastric 355.79
  - ilioinguinal 355.79
  - leg NEC 355.8
  - lower extremity NEC 355.8
  - median (in carpal tunnel) 354.0
  - obturator 355.79

Compression — continued
nerve (see also Disorder, nerve) — continued
- optic 377.49
- plantar 355.6
- posterior tibial (in tarsal tunnel) 355.5
- root (by scar tissue) NEC 724.9
  - cervical NEC 723.4
  - lumbar NEC 724.4
  - lumbosacral 724.4
  - thoracic 724.4
- saphenous 355.79
- sciatic (acute) 355.0
- sympathetic 337.9
- traumatic — see Injury, nerve
- ulnar 354.2
- upper extremity NEC 354.9
- peripheral — see Compression, nerve
- spinal (cord) (old or nontraumatic) 336.9
  - by displacement of intervertebral disc — see Displacement, intervertebral disc
  - nerve
    - root NEC 724.9
      - postoperative 722.80
        - cervical region 722.81
        - lumbar region 722.83
        - thoracic region 722.82
      - traumatic — see Injury, nerve, spinal
    - traumatic — see Injury, nerve, spinal
  - spondylogenic 721.91
    - cervical 721.1
    - lumbar, lumbosacral 721.42
    - thoracic 721.41
    - traumatic (see also Injury, spinal, by site)
      - with fracture, vertebra — see Fracture, vertebra, by site, with spinal cord injury
  - spondylogenic — see Compression, spinal cord, spondylogenic
- subcostal nerve (syndrome) 354.8
- sympathetic nerve NEC 337.9
- syndrome 958.5
- thorax 512.8
  - iatrogenic 512.1
  - postoperative 512.1
- trachea 519.19 ▲
  - congenital 748.3
- ulnar nerve (by scar tissue) 354.2
- umbilical cord
  - affecting fetus or newborn 762.5
    - cord prolapsed 762.4
  - complicating delivery 663.2 ☑
    - cord around neck 663.1 ☑
    - cord prolapsed 663.0 ☑
- upper extremity NEC 354.9
- ureter 593.3
- urethra — see Stricture, urethra
- vein 459.2
- vena cava (inferior) (superior) 459.2
- vertebral NEC — see Compression, spinal (cord)

Compulsion, compulsive
- eating 307.51
- neurosis (obsessive) 300.3
- personality 301.4
- states (mixed) 300.3
- swearing 300.3
  - in Gilles de la Tourette's syndrome 307.23
- tics and spasms 307.22
- water drinking NEC (syndrome) 307.9

Concato's disease (pericardial polyserositis) 423.2
- peritoneal 568.82
- pleural — see Pleurisy

Concavity, chest wall 738.3

Concealed
- hemorrhage NEC 459.0
- penis 752.65

Concentric fading

Concentric fading 368.12
Concern (normal) **about sick person in family** V61.49
Concrescence (teeth) 520.2
Concretio cordis 423.1
   rheumatic 393
Concretion — *see also* Calculus
   appendicular 543.9
   canaliculus 375.57
   clitoris 624.8
   conjunctiva 372.54
   eyelid 374.56
   intestine (impaction) (obstruction) 560.39
   lacrimal (passages) 375.57
   prepuce (male) 605
     female (clitoris) 624.8
   salivary gland (any) 527.5
   seminal vesicle 608.89
   stomach 537.89
   tonsil 474.8
Concussion (current) 850.9
   with
     loss of consciousness 850.5
       brief (less than one hour)
         30 minutes or less 850.11
         31-59 minutes 850.12
       moderate (1-24 hours) 850.2
       prolonged (more than 24 hours) (with complete recovery) (with return to pre-existing conscious level) 850.3
       without return to pre-existing conscious level 850.4
     mental confusion or disorientation (without loss of consciousness) 850.0
       with loss of consciousness — *see* Concussion, with, loss of consciousness
     without loss of consciousness 850.0
   blast (air) (hydraulic) (immersion) (underwater) 869.0
     with open wound into cavity 869.1
     abdomen or thorax — *see* Injury, internal, by site
     brain — *see* Concussion, brain
     ear (acoustic nerve trauma) 951.5
       with perforation, tympanic membrane — *see* Wound, open, ear drum
     thorax — *see* Injury, internal, intrathoracic organs NEC
   brain or cerebral (without skull fracture) 850.9
     with
       loss of consciousness 850.5
         brief (less than one hour)
           30 minutes or less 850.11
           31-59 minutes 850.12
         moderate (1-24 hours) 850.2
         prolonged (more than 24 hours) (with complete recovery) (with return to pre-existing conscious level) 850.3
         without return to pre-existing conscious level 850.4
       mental confusion or disorientation (without loss of consciousness) 850.0
         with loss of consciousness — *see* Concussion, brain, with, loss of consciousness
       skull fracture — *see* Fracture, skull, by site
     without loss of consciousness 850.0
   cauda equina 952.4
   cerebral — *see* Concussion, brain
   conus medullaris (spine) 952.4
   hydraulic — *see* Concussion, blast

Concussion — *continued*
   internal organs — *see* Injury, internal, by site
   labyrinth — *see* Injury, intracranial
   ocular 921.3
   osseous labyrinth — *see* Injury, intracranial
   spinal (cord) (*see also* Injury, spinal, by site)
     due to
       broken
         back — *see* Fracture, vertebra, by site, with spinal cord injury
         neck — *see* Fracture, vertebra, cervical, with spinal cord injury
       fracture, fracture dislocation, or compression fracture of spine or vertebra — *see* Fracture, vertebra, by site, with spinal cord injury
   syndrome 310.2
   underwater blast — *see* Concussion, blast
Condition — *see also* Disease
   psychiatric 298.9
   respiratory NEC 519.9
     acute or subacute NEC 519.9
       due to
         external agent 508.9
           specified type NEC 508.8
         fumes or vapors (chemical) (inhalation) 506.3
         radiation 508.0
     chronic NEC 519.9
       due to
         external agent 508.9
           specified type NEC 508.8
         fumes or vapors (chemical) (inhalation) 506.4
         radiation 508.1
       due to
         external agent 508.9
           specified type NEC 508.8
         fumes or vapors (chemical) (inhalation) 506.9
Conduct disturbance — *see also* Disturbance, conduct 312.9
   adjustment reaction 309.3
   hyperkinetic 314.2
Condyloma NEC 078.10
   acuminatum 078.11
   gonorrheal 098.0
   latum 091.3
   syphilitic 091.3
     congenital 090.0
   venereal, syphilitic 091.3
Confinement — *see* Delivery
Conflagration — *see also* Burn, by site
   asphyxia (by inhalation of smoke, gases, fumes, or vapors) 987.9
   specified agent — *see* Table of Drugs and Chemicals
Conflict
   family V61.9
     specified circumstance NEC V61.8
   interpersonal NEC V62.81
   marital V61.10
     involving divorce or estrangement V61.0
   parent-child V61.20
   partner V61.10
Confluent — *see* condition
Confusional arousals 327.41
Confusion, confused (mental) (state) — *see also* State, confusional 298.9
   acute 293.0
   epileptic 293.0
   postoperative 293.9
   psychogenic 298.2
   reactive (from emotional stress, psychological trauma) 298.2
   subacute 293.1
Congelation 991.9

Congenital — *see also* condition
   aortic septum 747.29
   generalized fibromatosis (CGF) 759.89
   intrinsic factor deficiency 281.0
   malformation — *see* Anomaly
Congestion, congestive (chronic) (passive)
   asphyxia, newborn 768.9
   bladder 596.8
   bowel 569.89
   brain (*see also* Disease, cerebrovascular NEC) 437.8
     malarial 084.9
   breast 611.79
   bronchi 519.19 ▲
   bronchial tube 519.19 ▲
   catarrhal 472.0
   cerebral — *see* Congestion, brain
   cerebrospinal — *see* Congestion, brain
   chest 514
   chill 780.99
     malarial (*see also* Malaria) 084.6
   circulatory NEC 459.9
   conjunctiva 372.71
   due to disturbance of circulation 459.9
   duodenum 537.3
   enteritis — *see* Enteritis
   eye 372.71
   fibrosis syndrome (pelvic) 625.5
   gastroenteritis — *see* Enteritis
   general 799.89
   glottis 476.0
   heart (*see also* Failure, heart) 428.0
   hepatic 573.0
   hypostatic (lung) 514
   intestine 569.89
   intracranial — *see* Congestion, brain
   kidney 593.89
   labyrinth 386.50
   larynx 476.0
   liver 573.0
   lung 514
     active or acute (*see also* Pneumonia) 486
       congenital 770.0
     chronic 514
     hypostatic 514
     idiopathic, acute 518.5
     passive 514
   malaria, malarial (brain) (fever) (*see also* Malaria) 084.6
   medulla — *see* Congestion, brain
   nasal 478.19 ▲
   orbit, orbital 376.33
     inflammatory (chronic) 376.10
       acute 376.00
   ovary 620.8
   pancreas 577.8
   pelvic, female 625.5
   pleural 511.0
   prostate (active) 602.1
   pulmonary — *see* Congestion, lung
   renal 593.89
   retina 362.89
   seminal vesicle 608.89
   spinal cord 336.1
   spleen 289.51
     chronic 289.51
   stomach 537.89
   trachea 464.11
   urethra 599.84
   uterus 625.5
     with subinvolution 621.1
   viscera 799.89
Congestive — *see* Congestion
Conical
   cervix 622.6
   cornea 371.60
   teeth 520.2
Conjoined twins 759.4
   causing disproportion (fetopelvic) 653.7 ☑
Conjugal maladjustment V61.10

Conjugal maladjustment — *continued*
   involving divorce or estrangement V61.0
Conjunctiva — *see* condition
Conjunctivitis (exposure) (infectious) (nondiphtheritic) (pneumococcal) (pustular) (staphylococcal) (streptococcal) NEC 372.30
   actinic 370.24
   acute 372.00
     atopic 372.05
     contagious 372.03
     follicular 372.02
     hemorrhagic (viral) 077.4
   adenoviral (acute) 077.3
   allergic (chronic) 372.14
     with hay fever 372.05
   anaphylactic 372.05
   angular 372.03
   Apollo (viral) 077.4
   atopic 372.05
   blennorrhagic (neonatorum) 098.40
   catarrhal 372.03
   chemical 372.01
     allergic 372.05
     meaning corrosion — *see* Burn, conjunctiva
   chlamydial 077.98
     due to
       Chlamydia trachomatis — *see* Trachoma
       paratrachoma 077.0
   chronic 372.10
     allergic 372.14
     follicular 372.12
     simple 372.11
     specified type NEC 372.14
     vernal 372.13
   diphtheritic 032.81
   due to
     dust 372.05
     enterovirus type 70 077.4
     erythema multiforme 695.1 [372.33]
     filariasis (*see also* Filariasis) 125.9 [372.15]
     mucocutaneous
       disease NEC 372.33
       leishmaniasis 085.5 [372.15]
     Reiter's disease 099.3 [372.33]
     syphilis 095.8 [372.10]
     toxoplasmosis (acquired) 130.1
       congenital (active) 771.2
     trachoma — *see* Trachoma
   dust 372.05
   eczematous 370.31
   epidemic 077.1
     hemorrhagic 077.4
   follicular (acute) 372.02
     adenoviral (acute) 077.3
     chronic 372.12
   glare 370.24
   gonococcal (neonatorum) 098.40
   granular (trachomatous) 076.1
     late effect 139.1
   hemorrhagic (acute) (epidemic) 077.4
   herpetic (simplex) 054.43
     zoster 053.21
   inclusion 077.0
   infantile 771.6
   influenzal 372.03
   Koch-Weeks 372.03
   light 372.05
   medicamentosa 372.05
   membranous 372.04
   meningococcic 036.89
   Morax-Axenfeld 372.02
   mucopurulent NEC 372.03
   neonatal 771.6
     gonococcal 098.40
   Newcastle's 077.8
   nodosa 360.14
   of Beal 077.3
   parasitic 372.15

Index to Diseases

Conjunctivitis — continued
  parasitic — continued
    filariasis (see also Filariasis) 125.9 [372.15]
    mucocutaneous leishmaniasis 085.5 [372.15]
  Parinaud's 372.02
  petrificans 372.39
  phlyctenular 370.31
  pseudomembranous 372.04
    diphtheritic 032.81
  purulent 372.03
  Reiter's 099.3 [372.33]
  rosacea 695.3 [372.31]
  serous 372.01
    viral 077.99
  simple chronic 372.11
  specified NEC 372.39
  sunlamp 372.04
  swimming pool 077.0
  trachomatous (follicular) 076.1
    acute 076.0
    late effect 139.1
  traumatic NEC 372.39
  tuberculous (see also Tuberculosis) 017.3 ☑ [370.31]
  tularemic 021.3
  tularensis 021.3
  vernal 372.13
    limbar 372.13 [370.32]
  viral 077.99
    acute hemorrhagic 077.4
    specified NEC 077.8
Conjunctivochalasis 372.81
Conjunctoblepharitis — see Conjunctivitis
Connective tissue — see condition
Conn (-Louis) syndrome (primary aldosteronism) 255.12
Conradi (-Hünermann) syndrome or disease (chondrodysplasia calcificans congenita) 756.59
Consanguinity V19.7
Consecutive — see condition
Consolidated lung (base) — see Pneumonia, lobar
Constipation 564.00
  atonic 564.09
  drug induced
    correct substance properly administered 564.09
    overdose or wrong substance given or taken 977.9
      specified drug — see Table of Drugs and Chemicals
  neurogenic 564.09
  other specified NEC 564.09
  outlet dysfunction 564.02
  psychogenic 306.4
  simple 564.00
  slow transit 564.01
  spastic 564.09
Constitutional — see also condition
  arterial hypotension (see also Hypotension) 458.9
  obesity 278.00
    morbid 278.01
  psychopathic state 301.9
  short stature in childhood 783.43
  state, developmental V21.9
    specified development NEC V21.8
  substandard 301.6
Constitutionally substandard 301.6
Constriction
  anomalous, meningeal bands or folds 742.8
  aortic arch (congenital) 747.10
  asphyxiation or suffocation by 994.7
  bronchus 519.19 ▲
  canal, ear (see also Stricture, ear canal, acquired) 380.50
  duodenum 537.3
  gallbladder (see also Obstruction, gallbladder) 575.2
    congenital 751.69

Constriction — continued
  intestine (see also Obstruction, intestine) 560.9
  larynx 478.74
    congenital 748.3
  meningeal bands or folds, anomalous 742.8
  organ or site, congenital NEC — see Atresia
  prepuce (congenital) 605
  pylorus 537.0
    adult hypertrophic 537.0
    congenital or infantile 750.5
    newborn 750.5
  ring (uterus) 661.4 ☑
    affecting fetus or newborn 763.7
  spastic (see also Spasm)
    ureter 593.3
    urethra — see Stricture, urethra
  stomach 537.89
  ureter 593.3
  urethra — see Stricture, urethra
  visual field (functional) (peripheral) 368.45
Constrictive — see condition
Consultation
  without complaint or sickness V65.9
    feared complaint unfounded V65.5
    specified reason NEC V65.8
  medical (see also Counseling, medical)
    specified reason NEC V65.8
Consumption — see Tuberculosis
Contact
  with
    AIDS virus V01.79
    anthrax V01.81
    cholera V01.0
    communicable disease V01.9
      specified type NEC V01.89
      viral NEC V01.79
    Escherichia coli (E. coli) V01.83
    German measles V01.4
    gonorrhea V01.6
    HIV V01.79
    human immunodeficiency virus V01.79
    meningococcus V01.84
    parasitic disease NEC V01.89
    poliomyelitis V01.2
    rabies V01.5
    rubella V01.4
    SARS-associated coronavirus V01.82
    smallpox V01.3
    syphilis V01.6
    tuberculosis V01.1
    varicella V01.71
    venereal disease V01.6
    viral disease NEC V01.79
  dermatitis — see Dermatitis
Contamination, food — see also Poisoning, food 005.9
Contraception, contraceptive
  advice NEC V25.09
    family planning V25.09
    fitting of diaphragm V25.02
    prescribing or use of
      oral contraceptive agent V25.01
      specified agent NEC V25.02
  counseling NEC V25.09
    emergency V25.03
    family planning V25.09
    fitting of diaphragm V25.02
    prescribing or use of
      oral contraceptive agent V25.01
      emergency V25.03
      postcoital V25.03
      specified agent NEC V25.02
  device (in situ) V45.59
    causing menorrhagia 996.76
    checking V25.42
    complications 996.32
    insertion V25.1
    intrauterine V45.51
    reinsertion V25.42
    removal V25.42

Contraception, contraceptive — continued
  device — continued
    subdermal V45.52
  fitting of diaphragm V25.02
  insertion
    intrauterine contraceptive device V25.1
    subdermal implantable V25.5
  maintenance V25.40
    examination V25.40
      oral contraceptive V25.41
      specified method NEC V25.49
      subdermal implantable V25.43
      intrauterine device V25.42
    intrauterine device V25.42
    oral contraceptive V25.41
    specified method NEC V25.49
    subdermal implantable V25.43
  management NEC V25.49
  prescription
    oral contraceptive agent V25.01
      emergency V25.03
      postcoital V25.03
      repeat V25.41
    specified agent NEC V25.02
      repeat V25.49
  sterilization V25.2
  surveillance V25.40
    intrauterine device V25.42
    oral contraceptive agent V25.41
    subdermal implantable V25.43
    specified method NEC V25.49
Contraction, contracture, contracted
  Achilles tendon (see also Short, tendon, Achilles) 727.81
  anus 564.89
  axilla 729.9
  bile duct (see also Disease, biliary) 576.8
  bladder 596.8
    neck or sphincter 596.0
  bowel (see also Obstruction, intestine) 560.9
  Braxton Hicks 644.1 ☑
  bronchus 519.19 ▲
  burn (old) — see Cicatrix
  cecum (see also Obstruction, intestine) 560.9
  cervix (see also Stricture, cervix) 622.4
    congenital 752.49
  cicatricial — see Cicatrix
  colon (see also Obstruction, intestine) 560.9
  conjunctiva trachomatous, active 076.1
    late effect 139.1
  Dupuytren's 728.6
  eyelid 374.41
  eye socket (after enucleation) 372.64
  face 729.9
  fascia (lata) (postural) 728.89
    Dupuytren's 728.6
    palmar 728.6
    plantar 728.71
  finger NEC 736.29
    congenital 755.59
    joint (see also Contraction, joint) 718.44
  flaccid, paralytic
    joint (see also Contraction, joint) 718.4 ☑
    muscle 728.85
    ocular 378.50
  gallbladder (see also Obstruction, gallbladder) 575.2
  hamstring 728.89
    tendon 727.81
  heart valve — see Endocarditis
  Hicks' 644.1 ☑
  hip (see also Contraction, joint) 718.4 ☑
  hourglass
    bladder 596.8
      congenital 753.8

Contraction, contracture, contracted — continued
  hourglass — continued
    gallbladder (see also Obstruction, gallbladder) 575.2
      congenital 751.69
    stomach 536.8
      congenital 750.7
      psychogenic 306.4
    uterus 661.4 ☑
      affecting fetus or newborn 763.7
  hysterical 300.11
  infantile (see also Epilepsy) 345.6 ☑
  internal os (see also Stricture, cervix) 622.4
  intestine (see also Obstruction, intestine) 560.9
  joint (abduction) (acquired) (adduction) (flexion) (rotation) 718.40
    ankle 718.47
    congenital NEC 755.8
      generalized or multiple 754.89
      lower limb joints 754.89
      hip (see also Subluxation, congenital, hip) 754.32
      lower limb (including pelvic girdle) not involving hip 754.89
      upper limb (including shoulder girdle) 755.59
    elbow 718.42
    foot 718.47
    hand 718.44
    hip 718.45
    hysterical 300.11
    knee 718.46
    multiple sites 718.49
    pelvic region 718.45
    shoulder (region) 718.41
    specified site NEC 718.48
    wrist 718.43
  kidney (granular) (secondary) (see also Sclerosis, renal) 587
    congenital 753.3
    hydronephritic 591
    pyelonephritic (see also Pyelitis, chronic) 590.00
    tuberculous (see also Tuberculosis) 016.0 ☑
  ligament 728.89
    congenital 756.89
  liver — see Cirrhosis, liver
  muscle (postinfectional) (postural) NEC 728.85
    congenital 756.89
      sternocleidomastoid 754.1
    extraocular 378.60
    eye (extrinsic) (see also Strabismus) 378.9
      paralytic (see also Strabismus, paralytic) 378.50
    flaccid 728.85
    hysterical 300.11
    ischemic (Volkmann's) 958.6
    paralytic 728.85
    posttraumatic 958.6
    psychogenic 306.0
      specified as conversion reaction 300.11
  myotonic 728.85
  neck (see also Torticollis) 723.5
    congenital 754.1
    psychogenic 306.0
  ocular muscle (see also Strabismus) 378.9
    paralytic (see also Strabismus, paralytic) 378.50
  organ or site, congenital NEC — see Atresia
  outlet (pelvis) — see Contraction, pelvis
  palmar fascia 728.6
  paralytic
    joint (see also Contraction, joint) 718.4 ☑
    muscle 728.85

Contraction, contracture, contracted

Contraction, contracture, contracted — continued
- paralytic — continued
  - muscle — continued
    - ocular (see also Strabismus, paralytic) 378.50
- pelvis (acquired) (general) 738.6
  - affecting fetus or newborn 763.1
  - complicating delivery 653.1 ☑
    - causing obstructed labor 660.1 ☑
  - generally contracted 653.1 ☑
    - causing obstructed labor 660.1 ☑
  - inlet 653.2 ☑
    - causing obstructed labor 660.1 ☑
  - midpelvic 653.8 ☑
    - causing obstructed labor 660.1 ☑
  - midplane 653.8 ☑
    - causing obstructed labor 660.1 ☑
  - outlet 653.3 ☑
    - causing obstructed labor 660.1 ☑
- plantar fascia 728.71
- premature
  - atrial 427.61
  - auricular 427.61
  - auriculoventricular 427.61
  - heart (junctional) (nodal) 427.60
  - supraventricular 427.61
  - ventricular 427.69
- prostate 602.8
- pylorus (see also Pylorospasm) 537.81
- rectosigmoid (see also Obstruction, intestine) 560.9
- rectum, rectal (sphincter) 564.89
  - psychogenic 306.4
- ring (Bandl's) 661.4 ☑
  - affecting fetus or newborn 763.7
- scar — see Cicatrix
- sigmoid (see also Obstruction, intestine) 560.9
- socket, eye 372.64
- spine (see also Curvature, spine) 737.9
- stomach 536.8
  - hourglass 536.8
    - congenital 750.7
  - psychogenic 306.4
- tendon (sheath) (see also Short, tendon) 727.81
- toe 735.8
- ureterovesical orifice (postinfectional) 593.3
- urethra 599.84
- uterus 621.8
  - abnormal 661.9 ☑
    - affecting fetus or newborn 763.7
  - clonic, hourglass or tetanic 661.4 ☑
    - affecting fetus or newborn 763.7
  - dyscoordinate 661.4 ☑
    - affecting fetus or newborn 763.7
  - hourglass 661.4 ☑
    - affecting fetus or newborn 763.7
  - hypotonic NEC 661.2 ☑
    - affecting fetus or newborn 763.7
  - incoordinate 661.4 ☑
    - affecting fetus or newborn 763.7
  - inefficient or poor 661.2 ☑
    - affecting fetus or newborn 763.7
  - irregular 661.2 ☑
    - affecting fetus or newborn 763.7
  - tetanic 661.4 ☑
    - affecting fetus or newborn 763.7
- vagina (outlet) 623.2
- vesical 596.8
  - neck or urethral orifice 596.0
- visual field, generalized 368.45
- Volkmann's (ischemic) 958.6

Contusion (skin surface intact) 924.9
- with
  - crush injury — see Crush

Contusion — continued
- with — continued
  - dislocation — see Dislocation, by site
  - fracture — see Fracture, by site
  - internal injury (see also Injury, internal, by site)
    - heart — see Contusion, cardiac
    - kidney — see Contusion, kidney
    - liver — see Contusion, liver
    - lung — see Contusion, lung
    - spleen — see Contusion, spleen
  - intracranial injury — see Injury, intracranial
  - nerve injury — see Injury, nerve
  - open wound — see Wound, open, by site
- abdomen, abdominal (muscle) (wall) 922.2
  - organ(s) NEC 868.00
- adnexa, eye NEC 921.9
- ankle 924.21
  - with other parts of foot 924.20
- arm 923.9
  - lower (with elbow) 923.10
  - upper 923.03
    - with shoulder or axillary region 923.09
- auditory canal (external) (meatus) (and other part(s) of neck, scalp, or face, except eye) 920
- auricle, ear (and other part(s) of neck, scalp, or face except eye) 920
- axilla 923.02
  - with shoulder or upper arm 923.09
- back 922.31
- bone NEC 924.9
- brain (cerebral) (membrane) (with hemorrhage) 851.8 ☑

Note — Use the following fifth-digit subclassification with categories 851-854:

0 unspecified state of consciousness
1 with no loss of consciousness
2 with brief [less than one hour] loss of consciousness
3 with moderate [1-24 hours] loss of consciousness
4 with prolonged [more than 24 hours] loss of consciousness and return to pre-existing conscious level
5 with prolonged [more than 24 hours] loss of consciousness, without return to pre-existing conscious level

Use fifth-digit 5 to designate when a patient is unconscious and dies before regaining consciousness, regardless of the duration of the loss of consciousness

6 with loss of consciousness of unspecified duration
9 with concussion, unspecified

- with
  - open intracranial wound 851.9 ☑
  - skull fracture — see Fracture, skull, by site
- cerebellum 851.4 ☑
  - with open intracranial wound 851.5 ☑
- cortex 851.0 ☑
  - with open intracranial wound 851.1 ☑
- occipital lobe 851.4 ☑
  - with open intracranial wound 851.5 ☑
- stem 851.4 ☑
  - with open intracranial wound 851.5 ☑

Contusion — continued
- breast 922.0
- brow (and other part(s) of neck, scalp, or face, except eye) 920
- buttock 922.32
- canthus 921.1
- cardiac 861.01
  - with open wound into thorax 861.11
- cauda equina (spine) 952.4
- cerebellum — see Contusion, brain, cerebellum
- cerebral — see Contusion, brain
- cheek(s) (and other part(s) of neck, scalp, or face, except eye) 920
- chest (wall) 922.1
- chin (and other part(s) of neck, scalp, or face, except eye) 920
- clitoris 922.4
- conjunctiva 921.1
- conus medullaris (spine) 952.4
- cornea 921.3
- corpus cavernosum 922.4
- cortex (brain) (cerebral) — see Contusion, brain, cortex
- costal region 922.1
- ear (and other part(s) of neck, scalp, or face except eye) 920
- elbow 923.11
  - with forearm 923.10
- epididymis 922.4
- epigastric region 922.2
- eye NEC 921.9
- eyeball 921.3
- eyelid(s) (and periocular area) 921.1
- face (and neck, or scalp, any part, except eye) 920
- femoral triangle 922.2
- fetus or newborn 772.6
- finger(s) (nail) (subungual) 923.3
- flank 922.2
- foot (with ankle) (excluding toe(s)) 924.20
- forearm (and elbow) 923.10
- forehead (and other part(s) of neck, scalp, or face, except eye) 920
- genital organs, external 922.4
- globe (eye) 921.3
- groin 922.2
- gum(s) (and other part(s) of neck, scalp, or face, except eye) 920
- hand(s) (except fingers alone) 923.20
- head (any part, except eye) (and face) (and neck) 920
- heart — see Contusion, cardiac
- heel 924.20
- hip 924.01
  - with thigh 924.00
- iliac region 922.2
- inguinal region 922.2
- internal organs (abdomen, chest, or pelvis) NEC — see Injury, internal, by site
- interscapular region 922.33
- iris (eye) 921.3
- kidney 866.01
  - with open wound into cavity 866.11
- knee 924.11
  - with lower leg 924.10
- labium (majus) (minus) 922.4
- lacrimal apparatus, gland, or sac 921.1
- larynx (and other part(s) of neck, scalp, or face, except eye) 920
- late effect — see Late, effects (of), contusion
- leg 924.5
  - lower (with knee) 924.10
- lens 921.3
- lingual (and other part(s) of neck, scalp, or face, except eye) 920
- lip(s) (and other part(s) of neck, scalp, or face, except eye) 920
- liver 864.01

Contusion — continued
- liver — continued
  - with
    - laceration — see Laceration, liver
    - open wound into cavity 864.11
- lower extremity 924.5
  - multiple sites 924.4
- lumbar region 922.31
- lung 861.21
  - with open wound into thorax 861.31
- malar region (and other part(s) of neck, scalp, or face, except eye) 920
- mandibular joint (and other part(s) of neck, scalp, or face, except eye) 920
- mastoid region (and other part(s) of neck, scalp, or face, except eye) 920
- membrane, brain — see Contusion, brain
- midthoracic region 922.1
- mouth (and other part(s) of neck, scalp, or face, except eye) 920
- multiple sites (not classifiable to same three-digit category) 924.8
  - lower limb 924.4
  - trunk 922.8
  - upper limb 923.8
- muscle NEC 924.9
- myocardium — see Contusion, cardiac
- nasal (septum) (and other part(s) of neck, scalp, or face, except eye) 920
- neck (and scalp or face, any part, except eye) 920
- nerve — see Injury, nerve, by site
- nose (and other part(s) of neck, scalp, or face, except eye) 920
- occipital region (scalp) (and neck or face, except eye) 920
  - lobe — see Contusion, brain, occipital lobe
- orbit (region) (tissues) 921.2
- palate (soft) (and other part(s) of neck, scalp, or face, except eye) 920
- parietal region (scalp) (and neck, or face, except eye) 920
  - lobe — see Contusion, brain
- penis 922.4
- pericardium — see Contusion, cardiac
- perineum 922.4
- periocular area 921.1
- pharynx (and other part(s) of neck, scalp, or face, except eye) 920
- popliteal space (see also Contusion, knee) 924.11
- prepuce 922.4
- pubic region 922.4
- pudenda 922.4
- pulmonary — see Contusion, lung
- quadriceps femoralis 924.00
- rib cage 922.1
- sacral region 922.32
- salivary ducts or glands (and other part(s) of neck, scalp, or face, except eye) 920
- scalp (and neck, or face any part, except eye) 920
- scapular region 923.01
  - with shoulder or upper arm 923.09
- sclera (eye) 921.3
- scrotum 922.4
- shoulder 923.00
  - with upper arm or axillar regions 923.09
- skin NEC 924.9
- skull 920
- spermatic cord 922.4
- spinal cord (see also Injury, spinal, by site)
  - cauda equina 952.4
  - conus medullaris 952.4
- spleen 865.01

Index to Diseases

Contusion — *continued*
spleen — *continued*
with open wound into cavity 865.11
sternal region 922.1
stomach — *see* Injury, internal, stomach
subconjunctival 921.1
subcutaneous NEC 924.9
submaxillary region (and other part(s) of neck, scalp, or face, except eye) 920
submental region (and other part(s) of neck, scalp, or face, except eye) 920
subperiosteal NEC 924.9
supraclavicular fossa (and other part(s) of neck, scalp, or face, except eye) 920
supraorbital (and other part(s) of neck, scalp, or face, except eye) 920
temple (region) (and other part(s) of neck, scalp, or face, except eye) 920
testis 922.4
thigh (and hip) 924.00
thorax 922.1
organ — *see* Injury, internal, intrathoracic
throat (and other part(s) of neck, scalp, or face, except eye) 920
thumb(s) (nail) (subungual) 923.3
toe(s) (nail) (subungual) 924.3
tongue (and other part(s) of neck, scalp, or face, except eye) 920
trunk 922.9
multiple sites 922.8
specified site — *see* Contusion, by site
tunica vaginalis 922.4
tympanum (membrane) (and other part(s) of neck, scalp, or face, except eye) 920
upper extremity 923.9
multiple sites 923.8
uvula (and other part(s) of neck, scalp, or face, except eye) 920
vagina 922.4
vocal cord(s) (and other part(s) of neck, scalp, or face, except eye) 920
vulva 922.4
wrist 923.21
with hand(s), except finger(s) alone 923.20
Conus (any type) (congenital) 743.57
acquired 371.60
medullaris syndrome 336.8
Convalescence (following) V66.9
chemotherapy V66.2
medical NEC V66.5
psychotherapy V66.3
radiotherapy V66.1
surgery NEC V66.0
treatment (for) NEC V66.5
combined V66.6
fracture V66.4
mental disorder NEC V66.3
specified disorder NEC V66.5
Conversion
closed surgical procedure to open procedure
arthroscopic V64.43
laparoscopic V64.41
thoracoscopic V64.42
hysteria, hysterical, any type 300.11
neurosis, any 300.11
reaction, any 300.11
Converter, tuberculosis (test reaction) 795.5
Convulsions (idiopathic) 780.39
apoplectiform (*see also* Disease, cerebrovascular, acute) 436
brain 780.39
cerebral 780.39
cerebrospinal 780.39

Convulsions — *continued*
due to trauma NEC — *see* Injury, intracranial
eclamptic (*see also* Eclampsia) 780.39
epileptic (*see also* Epilepsy) 345.9 ☑
epileptiform (*see also* Seizure, epileptiform) 780.39
epileptoid (*see also* Seizure, epileptiform) 780.39
ether
anesthetic
correct substance properly administered 780.39
overdose or wrong substance given 968.2
other specified type — *see* Table of Drugs and Chemicals
febrile ►(simple)◄ 780.31
complex 780.32 ●
generalized 780.39
hysterical 300.11
infantile 780.39
epilepsy — *see* Epilepsy
internal 780.39
jacksonian (*see also* Epilepsy) 345.5 ☑
myoclonic 333.2
newborn 779.0
paretic 094.1
pregnancy (nephritic) (uremic) — *see* Eclampsia, pregnancy
psychomotor (*see also* Epilepsy) 345.4 ☑
puerperal, postpartum — *see* Eclampsia, pregnancy
recurrent 780.39
epileptic — *see* Epilepsy
reflex 781.0
repetitive 780.39
epileptic — *see* Epilepsy
salaam (*see also* Epilepsy) 345.6 ☑
scarlatinal 034.1
spasmodic 780.39
tetanus, tetanic (*see also* Tetanus) 037
thymic 254.8
uncinate 780.39
uremic 586
Convulsive — *see also* Convulsions
disorder or state 780.39
epileptic — *see* Epilepsy
equivalent, abdominal (*see also* Epilepsy) 345.5 ☑
Cooke-Apert-Gallais syndrome (adrenogenital) 255.2
Cooley's anemia (erythroblastic) 282.49
Coolie itch 126.9
Cooper's
disease 610.1
hernia — *see* Hernia, Cooper's
Coordination disturbance 781.3
Copper wire arteries, retina 362.13
Copra itch 133.8
Coprolith 560.39
Coprophilia 302.89
Coproporphyria, hereditary 277.1
Coprostasis 560.39
with hernia (*see also* Hernia, by site, with obstruction)
gangrenous — *see* Hernia, by site, with gangrene
Cor
biloculare 745.7
bovinum — *see* Hypertrophy, cardiac
bovis (*see also* Hypertrophy, cardiac)
pulmonale (chronic) 416.9
acute 415.0
triatriatum, triatrium 746.82
triloculare 745.8
biatriatum 745.3
biventriculare 745.69
Corbus' disease 607.1
Cord — *see also* condition
around neck (tightly) (with compression)
affecting fetus or newborn 762.5
complicating delivery 663.1 ☑
without compression 663.3 ☑

Cord — *see also* condition — *continued*
around neck — *continued*
complicating delivery — *continued*
without compression — *continued*
affecting fetus or newborn 762.6
bladder NEC 344.61
tabetic 094.0
prolapse
affecting fetus or newborn 762.4
complicating delivery 663.0 ☑
Cord's angiopathy — *see also* Tuberculosis 017.3 ☑ [362.18]
Cordis ectopia 746.87
Corditis (spermatic) 608.4
Corectopia 743.46
Cori type glycogen storage disease — *see* Disease, glycogen storage
Cork-handlers' disease or lung 495.3
Corkscrew esophagus 530.5
Corlett's pyosis (impetigo) 684
Corn (infected) 700
Cornea — *see also* condition
donor V59.5
guttata (dystrophy) 371.57
plana 743.41
Cornelia de Lange's syndrome (Amsterdam dwarf, mental retardation, and brachycephaly) 759.89
Cornual gestation or pregnancy — *see* Pregnancy, cornual
Cornu cutaneum 702.8
Coronary (artery) — *see also* condition
arising from aorta or pulmonary trunk 746.85
Corpora — *see also* condition
amylacea (prostate) 602.8
cavernosa — *see* condition
Corpulence — *see* Obesity
Corpus — *see* condition
Corrigan's disease — *see* Insufficiency, aortic
Corrosive burn — *see* Burn, by site
Corsican fever — *see also* Malaria 084.6
Cortical — *see also* condition
blindness 377.75
necrosis, kidney (bilateral) 583.6
Corticoadrenal — *see also* condition
Corticosexual syndrome 255.2
Coryza (acute) 460
with grippe or influenza 487.1
syphilitic 095.8
congenital (chronic) 090.0
Costen's syndrome or complex 524.60
Costiveness — *see also* Constipation 564.00
Costochondritis 733.6
Cotard's syndrome (paranoia) 297.1
Cot death 798.0
Cotugno's disease 724.3
Cough 786.2
with hemorrhage (*see also* Hemoptysis) 786.3
affected 786.2
bronchial 786.2
with grippe or influenza 487.1
chronic 786.2
epidemic 786.2
functional 306.1
hemorrhagic 786.3
hysterical 300.11
laryngeal, spasmodic 786.2
nervous 786.2
psychogenic 306.1
smokers' 491.0
tea tasters' 112.89
Counseling NEC V65.40
without complaint or sickness V65.49
abuse victim NEC V62.89
child V61.21
partner V61.11
spouse V61.11

Counseling — *continued*
child abuse, maltreatment, or neglect V61.21
contraceptive NEC V25.09
device (intrauterine) V25.02
maintenance V25.40
intrauterine contraceptive device V25.42
oral contraceptive (pill) V25.41
specified type NEC V25.49
subdermal implantable V25.43
management NEC V25.9
oral contraceptive (pill) V25.01
emergency V25.03
postcoital V25.03
prescription NEC V25.02
oral contraceptive (pill) V25.01
emergency V25.03
postcoital V25.03
repeat prescription V25.41
repeat prescription V25.40
subdermal implantable V25.43
surveillance NEC V25.40
dietary V65.3
exercise V65.41
expectant mother, pediatric pre-birth visit V65.11
explanation of
investigation finding NEC V65.49
medication NEC V65.49
family planning V25.09
for nonattending third party V65.19
genetic V26.33
gonorrhea V65.45
health (advice) (education) (instruction) NEC V65.49
HIV V65.44
human immunodeficiency virus V65.44
injury prevention V65.43
insulin pump training V65.46
marital V61.10
medical (for) V65.9
boarding school resident V60.6
condition not demonstrated V65.5
feared complaint and no disease found V65.5
institutional resident V60.6
on behalf of another V65.19
person living alone V60.3
parent-child conflict V61.20
specified problem NEC V61.29
partner abuse
perpetrator V61.12
victim V61.11
pediatric pre-birth visit for expectant mother V65.11
perpetrator of
child abuse V62.83
parental V61.22
partner abuse V61.12
spouse abuse V61.12
procreative V65.49
sex NEC V65.49
transmitted disease NEC V65.45
HIV V65.44
specified reason NEC V65.49
spousal abuse
perpetrator V61.12
victim V61.11
substance use and abuse V65.42
syphilis V65.45
victim (of)
abuse NEC V62.89
child abuse V61.21
partner abuse V61.11
spousal abuse V61.11
Coupled rhythm 427.89
Couvelaire uterus (complicating delivery) — *see* Placenta, separation
Cowper's gland — *see* condition
Cowperitis — *see also* Urethritis 597.89
gonorrheal (acute) 098.0
chronic or duration of 2 months or over 098.2
Cowpox (abortive) 051.0

Index to Diseases

Cowpox — *continued*
  due to vaccination 999.0
    eyelid 051.0 *[373.5]*
      postvaccination 999.0 *[373.5]*
Coxa
  plana 732.1
  valga (acquired) 736.31
    congenital 755.61
    late effect of rickets 268.1
  vara (acquired) 736.32
    congenital 755.62
    late effect of rickets 268.1
Coxae malum senilis 715.25
Coxalgia (nontuberculous) 719.45
  tuberculous (*see also* Tuberculosis) 015.1 ☑ *[730.85]*
Coxalgic pelvis 736.30
Coxitis 716.65
Coxsackie (infection) (virus) 079.2
  central nervous system NEC 048
  endocarditis 074.22
  enteritis 008.67
  meningitis (aseptic) 047.0
  myocarditis 074.23
  pericarditis 074.21
  pharyngitis 074.0
  pleurodynia 074.1
  specific disease NEC 074.8
Crabs, meaning pubic lice 132.2
Crack baby 760.75
Cracked
  nipple 611.2
    puerperal, postpartum 676.1 ☑
  tooth 521.81
Cradle cap 690.11
Craft neurosis 300.89
Craigiasis 007.8
Cramp(s) 729.82
  abdominal 789.0 ☑
  bathing 994.1
  colic 789.0 ☑
    psychogenic 306.4
  due to immersion 994.1
  extremity (lower) (upper) NEC 729.82
  fireman 992.2
  heat 992.2
  hysterical 300.11
  immersion 994.1
  intestinal 789.0 ☑
    psychogenic 306.4
  linotypist's 300.89
    organic 333.84
  muscle (extremity) (general) 729.82
    due to immersion 994.1
    hysterical 300.11
  occupational (hand) 300.89
    organic 333.84
  psychogenic 307.89
  salt depletion 276.1
  sleep related leg 327.52
  stoker 992.2
  stomach 789.0 ☑
  telegraphers' 300.89
    organic 333.84
  typists' 300.89
    organic 333.84
  uterus 625.8
    menstrual 625.3
  writers' 333.84
    organic 333.84
    psychogenic 300.89
Cranial — *see* condition
Cranioclasis, fetal 763.89
Craniocleidodysostosis 755.59
Craniofenestria (skull) 756.0
Craniolacunia (skull) 756.0
Craniopagus 759.4
Craniopathy, metabolic 733.3
Craniopharyngeal — *see* condition
Craniopharyngioma (M9350/1) 237.0
Craniorachischisis (totalis) 740.1
Cranioschisis 756.0
Craniostenosis 756.0
Craniosynostosis 756.0
Craniotabes (cause unknown) 733.3
  rachitic 268.1

Craniotabes — *continued*
  syphilitic 090.5
Craniotomy, fetal 763.89
Cranium — *see* condition
Craw-craw 125.3
Creaking joint 719.60
  ankle 719.67
  elbow 719.62
  foot 719.67
  hand 719.64
  hip 719.65
  knee 719.66
  multiple sites 719.69
  pelvic region 719.65
  shoulder (region) 719.61
  specified site NEC 719.68
  wrist 719.63
Creeping
  eruption 126.9
  palsy 335.21
  paralysis 335.21
Crenated tongue 529.8
Creotoxism 005.9
Crepitus
  caput 756.0
  joint 719.60
    ankle 719.67
    elbow 719.62
    foot 719.67
    hand 719.64
    hip 719.65
    knee 719.66
    multiple sites 719.69
    pelvic region 719.65
    shoulder (region) 719.61
    specified site NEC 719.68
    wrist 719.63
Crescent or conus choroid, congenital 743.57
Cretin, cretinism (athyrotic) (congenital) (endemic) (metabolic) (nongoitrous) (sporadic) 243
  goitrous (sporadic) 246.1
  pelvis (dwarf type) (male type) 243
    with disproportion (fetopelvic) 653.1 ☑
      affecting fetus or newborn 763.1
      causing obstructed labor 660.1 ☑
        affecting fetus or newborn 763.1
  pituitary 253.3
Cretinoid degeneration 243
Creutzfeldt-Jakob disease (syndrome) (new variant) 046.1
  with dementia
    with behavioral disturbance 046.1 *[294.11]*
    without behavioral disturbance 046.1 *[294.10]*
Crib death 798.0
Cribriform hymen 752.49
Cri-du-chat syndrome 758.31
Crigler-Najjar disease or syndrome (congenital hyperbilirubinemia) 277.4
Crimean hemorrhagic fever 065.0
Criminalism 301.7
Crisis
  abdomen 789.0 ☑
  addisonian (acute adrenocortical insufficiency) 255.4
  adrenal (cortical) 255.4
  asthmatic — *see* Asthma
  brain, cerebral (*see also* Disease, cerebrovascular, acute) 436
  celiac 579.0
  Dietl's 593.4
  emotional NEC 309.29
    acute reaction to stress 308.0
    adjustment reaction 309.9
    specific to childhood or adolescence 313.9
  gastric (tabetic) 094.0
  glaucomatocyclitic 364.22
  heart (*see also* Failure, heart) 428.9

Crisis — *continued*
  hypertensive — *see* Hypertension
  nitritoid
    correct substance properly administered 458.29
    overdose or wrong substance given or taken 961.1
  oculogyric 378.87
    psychogenic 306.7
  Pel's 094.0
  psychosexual identity 302.6
  rectum 094.0
  renal 593.81
  sickle cell 282.62
  stomach (tabetic) 094.0
  tabetic 094.0
  thyroid (*see also* Thyrotoxicosis) 242.9 ☑
  thyrotoxic (*see also* Thyrotoxicosis) 242.9 ☑
  vascular — *see* Disease, cerebrovascular, acute
Crocq's disease (acrocyanosis) 443.89
Crohn's disease — *see also* Enteritis, regional 555.9
Cronkhite-Canada syndrome 211.3
Crooked septum, nasal 470
Cross
  birth (of fetus) complicating delivery 652.3 ☑
    with successful version 652.1 ☑
    causing obstructed labor 660.0 ☑
  bite, anterior or posterior 524.27 ▲
  eye (*see also* Esotropia) 378.00
Crossed ectopia of kidney 753.3
Crossfoot 754.50
Croup, croupous (acute) (angina) (catarrhal) (infective) (inflammatory) (laryngeal) (membranous) (nondiphtheritic) (pseudomembranous) 464.4
  asthmatic (*see also* Asthma) 493.9 ☑
  bronchial 466.0
  diphtheritic (membranous) 032.3
  false 478.75
  spasmodic 478.75
    diphtheritic 032.3
  stridulous 478.75
    diphtheritic 032.3
Crouzon's disease (craniofacial dysostosis) 756.0
Crowding, teeth 524.31
CRST syndrome (cutaneous systemic sclerosis) 710.1
Cruchet's disease (encephalitis lethargica) 049.8
Cruelty in children — *see also* Disturbance, conduct 312.9
Crural ulcer — *see also* Ulcer, lower extremity 707.10
Crush, crushed, crushing (injury) 929.9
  with
    fracture — *see* Fracture, by site
  abdomen 926.19
    internal — *see* Injury, internal, abdomen
  ankle 928.21
    with other parts of foot 928.20
  arm 927.9
    lower (and elbow) 927.10
    upper 927.03
      with shoulder or axillary region 927.09
  axilla 927.02
    with shoulder or upper arm 927.09
  back 926.11
  breast 926.19
  buttock 926.12
  cheek 925.1
  chest — *see* Injury, internal, chest
  ear 925.1
  elbow 927.11
    with forearm 927.10
  face 925.1
  finger(s) 927.3
    with hand(s) 927.20

Crush, crushed, crushing — *continued*
  finger(s) — *continued*
    with hand(s) — *continued*
      and wrist(s) 927.21
  flank 926.19
  foot, excluding toe(s) alone (with ankle) 928.20
  forearm (and elbow) 927.10
  genitalia, external (female) (male) 926.0
    internal — *see* Injury, internal, genital organ NEC
  hand, except finger(s) alone (and wrist) 927.20
  head — *see* Fracture, skull, by site
  heel 928.20
  hip 928.01
    with thigh 928.00
  internal organ (abdomen, chest, or pelvis) — *see* Injury, internal, by site
  knee 928.11
    with leg, lower 928.10
  labium (majus) (minus) 926.0
  larynx 925.2
  late effect — *see* Late, effects (of), crushing
  leg 928.9
    lower 928.10
      and knee 928.11
    upper 928.00
  limb
    lower 928.9
      multiple sites 928.8
    upper 927.9
      multiple sites 927.8
  multiple sites NEC 929.0
  neck 925.2
  nerve — *see* Injury, nerve, by site
  nose 802.0
    open 802.1
  penis 926.0
  pharynx 925.2
  scalp 925.1
  scapular region 927.01
    with shoulder or upper arm 927.09
  scrotum 926.0
  shoulder 927.00
    with upper arm or axillary region 927.09
  skull or cranium — *see* Fracture, skull, by site
  spinal cord — *see* Injury, spinal, by site
  syndrome (complication of trauma) 958.5
  testis 926.0
  thigh (with hip) 928.00
  throat 925.2
  thumb(s) (and fingers) 927.3
  toe(s) 928.3
    with foot 928.20
      and ankle 928.21
  tonsil 925.2
  trunk 926.9
    chest — *see* Injury, internal, intrathoracic organs NEC
    internal organ — *see* Injury, internal, by site
    multiple sites 926.8
    specified site NEC 926.19
  vulva 926.0
  wrist 927.21
    with hand(s), except fingers alone 927.20
Crusta lactea 690.11
Crusts 782.8
Crutch paralysis 953.4
Cruveilhier-Baumgarten cirrhosis, disease, or syndrome 571.5
Cruveilhier's disease 335.21
Cruz-Chagas disease — *see also* Trypanosomiasis 086.2

Index to Diseases

Cyst

Crying
  constant, continuous
    adolescent 780.95
    adult 780.95
    baby 780.92
    child 780.95
    infant 780.92
    newborn 780.92
  excessive
    adolescent 780.95
    adult 780.95
    baby 780.92
    child 780.95
    infant 780.92
    newborn 780.92
Cryoglobulinemia (mixed) 273.2
Crypt (anal) (rectal) 569.49
Cryptitis (anal) (rectal) 569.49
Cryptococcosis (European) (pulmonary) (systemic) 117.5
Cryptococcus 117.5
  epidermicus 117.5
  neoformans, infection by 117.5
Cryptopapillitis (anus) 569.49
Cryptophthalmos (eyelid) 743.06
Cryptorchid, cryptorchism, cryptorchidism 752.51
Cryptosporidiosis 007.4
Cryptotia 744.29
Crystallopathy
  calcium pyrophosphate (see also Arthritis) 275.49 [712.2] ☑
  dicalcium phosphate (see also Arthritis) 275.49 [712.1] ☑
  gouty 274.0
  pyrophosphate NEC (see also Arthritis) 275.49 [712.2] ☑
  uric acid 274.0
Crystalluria 791.9
Csillag's disease (lichen sclerosis et atrophicus) 701.0
Cuban itch 050.1
Cubitus
  valgus (acquired) 736.01
    congenital 755.59
    late effect of rickets 268.1
  varus (acquired) 736.02
    congenital 755.59
    late effect of rickets 268.1
Cultural deprivation V62.4
Cupping of optic disc 377.14
Curling esophagus 530.5
Curling's ulcer — see Ulcer, duodenum
Curschmann (-Batten) (-Steinert) disease or syndrome 359.2
Curvature
  organ or site, congenital NEC — see Distortion
  penis (lateral) 752.69
  Pott's (spinal) (see also Tuberculosis) 015.0 ☑ [737.43]
  radius, idiopathic, progressive (congenital) 755.54
  spine (acquired) (angular) (incorrect) (postural) 737.9
    congenital 754.2
    due to or associated with
      Charcôt-Marie-Tooth disease 356.1 [737.40]
      mucopolysaccharidosis 277.5 [737.40]
      neurofibromatosis 237.71 [737.40]
      osteitis
        deformans 731.0 [737.40]
        fibrosa cystica 252.01 [737.40]
      osteoporosis (see also Osteoporosis) 733.00 [737.40]
      poliomyelitis (see also Poliomyelitis) 138 [737.40]
      tuberculosis (Pott's curvature) (see also Tuberculosis) 015.0 ☑ [737.43]
    kyphoscoliotic (see also Kyphoscoliosis) 737.30
    kyphotic (see also Kyphosis) 737.10
    late effect of rickets 268.1 [737.40]
    Pott's 015.0 ☑ [737.40]
    scoliotic (see also Scoliosis) 737.30
    specified NEC 737.8
    tuberculous 015.0 ☑ [737.40]
Cushing's
  basophilism, disease, or syndrome (iatrogenic) (idiopathic) (pituitary basophilism) (pituitary dependent) 255.0
  ulcer — see Ulcer, peptic
Cushingoid due to steroid therapy
  correct substance properly administered 255.0
  overdose or wrong substance given or taken 962.0
Cut (external) — see Wound, open, by site
Cutaneous — see also condition
  hemorrhage 782.7
  horn (cheek) (eyelid) (mouth) 702.8
  larva migrans 126.9
Cutis — see also condition
  hyperelastic 756.83
    acquired 701.8
  laxa 756.83
    senilis 701.8
  marmorata 782.61
  osteosis 709.3
  pendula 756.83
    acquired 701.8
  rhomboidalis nuchae 701.8
  verticis gyrata 757.39
    acquired 701.8
Cyanopathy, newborn 770.83
Cyanosis 782.5
  autotoxic 289.7
  common atrioventricular canal 745.69
  congenital 770.83
  conjunctiva 372.71
  due to
    endocardial cushion defect 745.60
    nonclosure, foramen botalli 745.5
    patent foramen botalli 745.5
    persistent foramen ovale 745.5
  enterogenous 289.7
  fetus or newborn 770.83
  ostium primum defect 745.61
  paroxysmal digital 443.0
  retina, retinal 362.10
Cycle
  anovulatory 628.0
  menstrual, irregular 626.4
Cyclencephaly 759.89
Cyclical vomiting 536.2
  psychogenic 306.4
Cyclitic membrane 364.74
Cyclitis — see also Iridocyclitis 364.3
  acute 364.00
    primary 364.01
    recurrent 364.02
  chronic 364.10
    in
      sarcoidosis 135 [364.11]
      tuberculosis (see also Tuberculosis) 017.3 ☑ [364.11]
  Fuchs' heterochromic 364.21
  granulomatous 364.10
  lens induced 364.23
  nongranulomatous 364.00
  posterior 363.21
  primary 364.01
  recurrent 364.02
  secondary (noninfectious) 364.04
    infectious 364.03
  subacute 364.00
    primary 364.01
    recurrent 364.02
Cyclokeratitis — see Keratitis
Cyclophoria 378.44
Cyclopia, cyclops 759.89
Cycloplegia 367.51
Cyclospasm 367.53
Cyclosporiasis 007.5
Cyclothymia 301.13
Cyclothymic personality 301.13
Cyclotropia 378.33
Cyesis — see Pregnancy
Cylindroma (M8200/3) — see also Neoplasm, by site, malignant
  eccrine dermal (M8200/0) — see Neoplasm, skin, benign
  skin (M8200/0) — see Neoplasm, skin, benign
Cylindruria 791.7
Cyllosoma 759.89
Cynanche
  diphtheritic 032.3
  tonsillaris 475
Cynorexia 783.6
Cyphosis — see Kyphosis
Cyprus fever — see also Brucellosis 023.9
Cyriax's syndrome (slipping rib) 733.99
Cyst (mucus) (retention) (serous) (simple)

> Note — In general, cysts are not neoplastic and are classified to the appropriate category for disease of the specified anatomical site. This generalization does not apply to certain types of cysts which are neoplastic in nature, for example, dermoid, nor does it apply to cysts of certain structures, for example, branchial cleft, which are classified as developmental anomalies.
>
> The following listing includes some of the most frequently reported sites of cysts as well as qualifiers which indicate the type of cyst. The latter qualifiers usually are not repeated under the anatomical sites. Since the code assignment for a given site may vary depending upon the type of cyst, the coder should refer to the listings under the specified type of cyst before consideration is given to the site.

  accessory, fallopian tube 752.11
  adenoid (infected) 474.8
  adrenal gland 255.8
    congenital 759.1
  air, lung 518.89
  allantoic 753.7
  alveolar process (jaw bone) 526.2
  amnion, amniotic 658.8 ☑
  anterior chamber (eye) 364.60
    exudative 364.62
    implantation (surgical) (traumatic) 364.61
    parasitic 360.13
  anterior nasopalatine 526.1
  antrum 478.19
  anus 569.49
  apical (periodontal) (tooth) 522.8
  appendix 543.9
  arachnoid, brain 348.0
  arytenoid 478.79
  auricle 706.2
  Baker's (knee) 727.51
    tuberculous (see also Tuberculosis) 015.2 ☑
  Bartholin's gland or duct 616.2
  bile duct (see also Disease, biliary) 576.8
  bladder (multiple) (trigone) 596.8
  Blessig's 362.62
  blood, endocardial (see also Endocarditis) 424.90
  blue dome 610.0
  bone (local) 733.20
    aneurysmal 733.22
    jaw 526.2
      developmental (odontogenic) 526.0
      fissural 526.1
      latent 526.89
    solitary 733.21
    unicameral 733.21

Cyst — continued
  brain 348.0
    congenital 742.4
    hydatid (see also Echinococcus) 122.9
    third ventricle (colloid) 742.4
  branchial (cleft) 744.42
  branchiogenic 744.42
  breast (benign) (blue dome) (pedunculated) (solitary) (traumatic) 610.0
    involution 610.4
    sebaceous 610.8
  broad ligament (benign) 620.8
    embryonic 752.11
  bronchogenic (mediastinal) (sequestration) 518.89
    congenital 748.4
  buccal 528.4
  bulbourethral gland (Cowper's) 599.89
  bursa, bursal 727.49
    pharyngeal 478.26
  calcifying odontogenic (M9301/0) 213.1
    upper jaw (bone) 213.0
  canal of Nuck (acquired) (serous) 629.1
    congenital 752.41
  canthus 372.75
  carcinomatous (M8010/3) — see Neoplasm, by site, malignant
  cartilage (joint) — see Derangement, joint
  cauda equina 336.8
  cavum septi pellucidi NEC 348.0
  celomic (pericardium) 746.89
  cerebellopontine (angle) — see Cyst, brain
  cerebellum — see Cyst, brain
  cerebral — see Cyst, brain
  cervical lateral 744.42
  cervix 622.8
    embryonal 752.41
    nabothian (gland) 616.0
  chamber, anterior (eye) 364.60
    exudative 364.62
    implantation (surgical) (traumatic) 364.61
    parasitic 360.13
  chiasmal, optic NEC (see also Lesion, chiasmal) 377.54
  chocolate (ovary) 617.1
  choledochal (congenital) 751.69
    acquired 576.8
  choledochus 751.69
  chorion 658.8 ☑
  choroid plexus 348.0
  chyle, mesentery 457.8
  ciliary body 364.60
    exudative 364.64
    implantation 364.61
    primary 364.63
  clitoris 624.8
  coccyx (see also Cyst, bone) 733.20
  colloid
    third ventricle (brain) 742.4
    thyroid gland — see Goiter
  colon 569.89
  common (bile) duct (see also Disease, biliary) 576.8
  congenital NEC 759.89
    adrenal glands 759.1
    epiglottis 748.3
    esophagus 750.4
    fallopian tube 752.11
    kidney 753.10
      multiple 753.19
      single 753.11
    larynx 748.3
    liver 751.62
    lung 748.4
    mediastinum 748.8
    ovary 752.0
    oviduct 752.11
    pancreas 751.7
    periurethral (tissue) 753.8

Cyst

Cyst — *continued*
  congenital — *continued*
    prepuce NEC 752.69
      penis 752.69
    sublingual 750.26
    submaxillary gland 750.26
    thymus (gland) 759.2
    tongue 750.19
    ureterovesical orifice 753.4
    vulva 752.41
  conjunctiva 372.75
  cornea 371.23
  corpora quadrigemina 348.0
  corpus
    albicans (ovary) 620.2
    luteum (ruptured) 620.1
  Cowper's gland (benign) (infected) 599.89
  cranial meninges 348.0
  craniobuccal pouch 253.8
  craniopharyngeal pouch 253.8
  cystic duct (*see also* Disease, gallbladder) 575.8
  Cysticercus (any site) 123.1
  Dandy-Walker 742.3
    with spina bifida (*see also* Spina bifida) 741.0 ☑
  dental 522.8
    developmental 526.0
    eruption 526.0
    lateral periodontal 526.0
    primordial (keratocyst) 526.0
    root 522.8
  dentigerous 526.0
    mandible 526.0
    maxilla 526.0
  dermoid (M9084/0) (*see also* Neoplasm, by site, benign)
    with malignant transformation (M9084/3) 183.0
    implantation
      external area or site (skin) NEC 709.8
      iris 364.61
      skin 709.8
      vagina 623.8
      vulva 624.8
    mouth 528.4
    oral soft tissue 528.4
    sacrococcygeal 685.1
      with abscess 685.0
  developmental of ovary, ovarian 752.0
  dura (cerebral) 348.0
    spinal 349.2
  ear (external) 706.2
  echinococcal (*see also* Echinococcus) 122.9
  embryonal
    cervix uteri 752.41
    genitalia, female external 752.41
    uterus 752.3
    vagina 752.41
  endometrial 621.8
    ectopic 617.9
  endometrium (uterus) 621.8
    ectopic — *see* Endometriosis
  enteric 751.5
  enterogenous 751.5
  epidermal (inclusion) (*see also* Cyst, skin) 706.2
  epidermoid (inclusion) (*see also* Cyst, skin) 706.2
    mouth 528.4
    not of skin — *see* Cyst, by site
    oral soft tissue 528.4
  epididymis 608.89
  epiglottis 478.79
  epiphysis cerebri 259.8
  epithelial (inclusion) (*see also* Cyst, skin) 706.2
  epoophoron 752.11
  eruption 526.0
  esophagus 530.89
  ethmoid sinus 478.19 ▲
  eye (retention) 379.8
    congenital 743.03

Cyst — *continued*
  eye — *continued*
    posterior segment, congenital 743.54
  eyebrow 706.2
  eyelid (sebaceous) 374.84
    infected 373.13
    sweat glands or ducts 374.84
  falciform ligament (inflammatory) 573.8
  fallopian tube 620.8
  female genital organs NEC 629.89 ▲
  fimbrial (congenital) 752.11
  fissural (oral region) 526.1
  follicle (atretic) (graafian) (ovarian) 620.0
    nabothian (gland) 616.0
  follicular (atretic) (ovarian) 620.0
    dentigerous 526.0
  frontal sinus 478.19 ▲
  gallbladder or duct 575.8
  ganglion 727.43
  Gartner's duct 752.41
  gas, of mesentery 568.89
  gingiva 523.8
  gland of moll 374.84
  globulomaxillary 526.1
  graafian follicle 620.0
  granulosal lutein 620.2
  hemangiomatous (M9121/0) (*see also* Hemangioma) 228.00
  hydatid (*see also* Echinococcus) 122.9
    fallopian tube (Morgagni) 752.11
    liver NEC 122.8
    lung NEC 122.9
    Morgagni 752.89
      fallopian tube 752.11
    specified site NEC 122.9
  hymen 623.8
    embryonal 752.41
  hypopharynx 478.26
  hypophysis, hypophyseal (duct) (recurrent) 253.8
    cerebri 253.8
  implantation (dermoid)
    anterior chamber (eye) 364.61
    external area or site (skin) NEC 709.8
    iris 364.61
    vagina 623.8
    vulva 624.8
  incisor, incisive canal 526.1
  inclusion (epidermal) (epithelial) (epidermoid) (mucous) (squamous) (*see also* Cyst, skin) 706.2
    not of skin — *see* Neoplasm, by site, benign
  intestine (large) (small) 569.89
  intracranial — *see* Cyst, brain
  intraligamentous 728.89
    knee 717.89
  intrasellar 253.8
  iris (idiopathic) 364.60
    exudative 364.62
    implantation (surgical) (traumatic) 364.61
    miotic pupillary 364.55
    parasitic 360.13
  Iwanoff's 362.62
  jaw (bone) (aneurysmal) (extravasation) (hemorrhagic) (traumatic) 526.2
    developmental (odontogenic) 526.0
    fissural 526.1
  keratin 706.2
  kidney (congenital) 753.10
    acquired 593.2
    calyceal (*see also* Hydronephrosis) 591
    multiple 753.19
    pyelogenic (*see also* Hydronephrosis) 591
    simple 593.2
    single 753.11
    solitary (not congenital) 593.2

Cyst — *continued*
  labium (majus) (minus) 624.8
    sebaceous 624.8
  lacrimal
    apparatus 375.43
    gland or sac 375.12
  larynx 478.79
  lens 379.39
    congenital 743.39
  lip (gland) 528.5
  liver 573.8
    congenital 751.62
    hydatid (*see also* Echinococcus) 122.8
      granulosus 122.0
      multilocularis 122.5
  lung 518.89
    congenital 748.4
    giant bullous 492.0
  lutein 620.1
  lymphangiomatous (M9173/0) 228.1
  lymphoepithelial
    mouth 528.4
    oral soft tissue 528.4
  macula 362.54
  malignant (M8000/3) — *see* Neoplasm, by site, malignant
  mammary gland (sweat gland) (*see also* Cyst, breast) 610.0
  mandible 526.2
    dentigerous 526.0
    radicular 522.8
  maxilla 526.2
    dentigerous 526.0
    radicular 522.8
  median
    anterior maxillary 526.1
    palatal 526.1
  mediastinum (congenital) 748.8
  meibomian (gland) (retention) 373.2
    infected 373.12
  membrane, brain 348.0
  meninges (cerebral) 348.0
    spinal 349.2
  meniscus knee 717.5
  mesentery, mesenteric (gas) 568.89
    chyle 457.8
    gas 568.89
  mesonephric duct 752.89
  mesothelial
    peritoneum 568.89
    pleura (peritoneal) 568.89
  milk 611.5
  miotic pupillary (iris) 364.55
  Morgagni (hydatid) 752.89
    fallopian tube 752.11
  mouth 528.4
  mullerian duct 752.89
  multilocular (ovary) (M8000/1) 239.5
  myometrium 621.8
  nabothian (follicle) (ruptured) 616.0
  nasal sinus 478.19 ▲
  nasoalveolar 528.4
  nasolabial 528.4
  nasopalatine (duct) 526.1
    anterior 526.1
  nasopharynx 478.26
  neoplastic (M8000/1) (*see also* Neoplasm, by site, unspecified nature)
    benign (M8000/0) — *see* Neoplasm, by site, benign
    uterus 621.8
  nervous system — *see* Cyst, brain
  neuroenteric 742.59
  neuroepithelial ventricle 348.0
  nipple 610.0
  nose 478.19 ▲
    skin of 706.2
  odontogenic, developmental 526.0
  omentum (lesser) 568.89
    congenital 751.8
  oral soft tissue (dermoid) (epidermoid) (lymphoepithelial) 528.4
  ora serrata 361.19
  orbit 376.81

Cyst — *continued*
  ovary, ovarian (twisted) 620.2
    adherent 620.2
    chocolate 617.1
    corpus
      albicans 620.2
      luteum 620.1
    dermoid (M9084/0) 220
    developmental 752.0
    due to failure of involution NEC 620.2
    endometrial 617.1
    follicular (atretic) (graafian) (hemorrhagic) 620.0
    hemorrhagic 620.2
    in pregnancy or childbirth 654.4 ☑
      affecting fetus or newborn 763.89
      causing obstructed labor 660.2 ☑
        affecting fetus or newborn 763.1
    multilocular (M8000/1) 239.5
    pseudomucinous (M8470/0) 220
    retention 620.2
    serous 620.2
    theca lutein 620.2
    tuberculous (*see also* Tuberculosis) 016.6 ☑
    unspecified 620.2
  oviduct 620.8
  palatal papilla (jaw) 526.1
  palate 526.1
    fissural 526.1
    median (fissural) 526.1
  palatine, of papilla 526.1
  pancreas, pancreatic 577.2
    congenital 751.7
    false 577.2
    hemorrhagic 577.2
    true 577.2
  paranephric 593.2
  para ovarian 752.11
  paraphysis, cerebri 742.4
  parasitic NEC 136.9
  parathyroid (gland) 252.8
  paratubal (fallopian) 620.8
  paraurethral duct 599.89
  paroophoron 752.11
  parotid gland 527.6
    mucous extravasation or retention 527.6
  parovarian 752.11
  pars planus 364.60
    exudative 364.64
    primary 364.63
  pelvis, female
    in pregnancy or childbirth 654.4 ☑
      affecting fetus or newborn 763.89
      causing obstructed labor 660.2 ☑
        affecting fetus or newborn 763.1
  penis (sebaceous) 607.89
  periapical 522.8
  pericardial (congenital) 746.89
    acquired (secondary) 423.8
  pericoronal 526.0
  perineural (Tarlov's) 355.9
  periodontal 522.8
    lateral 526.0
  peripancreatic 577.2
  peripelvic (lymphatic) 593.2
  peritoneum 568.89
    chylous 457.8
  pharynx (wall) 478.26
  pilonidal (infected) (rectum) 685.1
    with abscess 685.0
    malignant (M9084/3) 173.5
  pituitary (duct) (gland) 253.8
  placenta (amniotic) — *see* Placenta, abnormal
  pleura 519.8
  popliteal 727.51
  porencephalic 742.4

Index to Diseases

Cyst — *continued*
- porencephalic — *continued*
  - acquired 348.0
- postanal (infected) 685.1
  - with abscess 685.0
- posterior segment of eye, congenital 743.54
- postmastoidectomy cavity 383.31
- preauricular 744.47
- prepuce 607.89
  - congenital 752.69
- primordial (jaw) 526.0
- prostate 600.3
- pseudomucinous (ovary) (M8470/0) 220
- pudenda (sweat glands) 624.8
- pupillary, miotic 364.55
- sebaceous 624.8
- radicular (residual) 522.8
- radiculodental 522.8
- ranular 527.6
- Rathke's pouch 253.8
- rectum (epithelium) (mucous) 569.49
- renal — *see* Cyst, kidney
- residual (radicular) 522.8
- retention (ovary) 620.2
- retina 361.19
  - macular 362.54
  - parasitic 360.13
  - primary 361.13
  - secondary 361.14
- retroperitoneal 568.89
- sacrococcygeal (dermoid) 685.1
  - with abscess 685.0
- salivary gland or duct 527.6
  - mucous extravasation or retention 527.6
- Sampson's 617.1
- sclera 379.19
- scrotum (sebaceous) 706.2
  - sweat glands 706.2
- sebaceous (duct) (gland) 706.2
  - breast 610.8
  - eyelid 374.84
  - genital organ NEC
    - female 629.89 ▲
    - male 608.89
  - scrotum 706.2
- semilunar cartilage (knee) (multiple) 717.5
- seminal vesicle 608.89
- serous (ovary) 620.2
- sinus (antral) (ethmoidal) (frontal) (maxillary) (nasal) (sphenoidal) 478.19 ▲
- Skene's gland 599.89
- skin (epidermal) (epidermoid, inclusion) (epithelial) (inclusion) (retention) (sebaceous) 706.2
  - breast 610.8
  - eyelid 374.84
  - genital organ NEC
    - female 629.89 ▲
    - male 608.89
  - neoplastic 216.3
  - scrotum 706.2
  - sweat gland or duct 705.89
- solitary
  - bone 733.21
  - kidney 593.2
- spermatic cord 608.89
- sphenoid sinus 478.19 ▲
- spinal meninges 349.2
- spine (*see also* Cyst, bone) 733.20
- spleen NEC 289.59
  - congenital 759.0
  - hydatid (*see also* Echinococcus) 122.9
- spring water (pericardium) 746.89
- subarachnoid 348.0
  - intrasellar 793.0
- subdural (cerebral) 348.0
  - spinal cord 349.2
- sublingual gland 527.6
  - mucous extravasation or retention 527.6

Cyst — *continued*
- submaxillary gland 527.6
  - mucous extravasation or retention 527.6
- suburethral 599.89
- suprarenal gland 255.8
- suprasellar — *see* Cyst, brain
- sweat gland or duct 705.89
- sympathetic nervous system 337.9
- synovial 727.40
  - popliteal space 727.51
- Tarlov's 355.9
- tarsal 373.2
- tendon (sheath) 727.42
- testis 608.89
- theca-lutein (ovary) 620.2
- Thornwaldt's, Tornwaldt's 478.26
- thymus (gland) 254.8
- thyroglossal (duct) (infected) (persistent) 759.2
- thyroid (gland) 246.2
  - adenomatous — *see* Goiter, nodular
  - colloid (*see also* Goiter) 240.9
- thyrolingual duct (infected) (persistent) 759.2
- tongue (mucous) 529.8
- tonsil 474.8
- tooth (dental root) 522.8
- tubo-ovarian 620.8
  - inflammatory 614.1
- tunica vaginalis 608.89
- turbinate (nose) (*see also* Cyst, bone) 733.99
- Tyson's gland (benign) (infected) 607.89
- umbilicus 759.89
- urachus 753.7
- ureter 593.89
- ureterovesical orifice 593.89
  - congenital 753.4
- urethra 599.84
- urethral gland (Cowper's) 599.89
- uterine
  - ligament 620.8
    - embryonic 752.11
  - tube 620.8
- utricle (ear) 386.8
  - prostatic 599.89
- utriculus masculinus 599.89
- vagina, vaginal (squamous cell) (wall) 623.8
  - embryonal 752.41
  - implantation 623.8
  - inclusion 623.8
- vallecula, vallecular 478.79
- ventricle, neuroepithelial 348.0
- verumontanum 599.89
- vesical (orifice) 596.8
- vitreous humor 379.29
- vulva (sweat glands) 624.8
  - congenital 752.41
  - implantation 624.8
  - inclusion 624.8
  - sebaceous gland 624.8
- vulvovaginal gland 624.8
- wolffian 752.89

Cystadenocarcinoma (M8440/3) — *see also* Neoplasm, by site, malignant
- bile duct type (M8161/3) 155.1
- endometrioid (M8380/3) — *see* Neoplasm, by site, malignant
- mucinous (M8470/3)
  - papillary (M8471/3)
    - specified site — *see* Neoplasm, by site, malignant
    - unspecified site 183.0
  - specified site — *see* Neoplasm, by site, malignant
  - unspecified site 183.0

Cystadenocarcinoma — *see also* Neoplasm, by site, malignant — *continued*
- papillary (M8450/3)
  - mucinous (M8471/3)
    - specified site — *see* Neoplasm, by site, malignant
    - unspecified site 183.0
  - pseudomucinous (M8471/3)
    - specified site — *see* Neoplasm, by site, malignant
    - unspecified site 183.0
  - serous (M8460/3)
    - specified site — *see* Neoplasm, by site, malignant
    - unspecified site 183.0
  - specified site — *see* Neoplasm, by site, malignant
  - unspecified site 183.0
- pseudomucinous (M8470/3)
  - papillary (M8471/3)
    - specified site — *see* Neoplasm, by site, malignant
    - unspecified site 183.0
  - specified site — *see* Neoplasm, by site, malignant
  - unspecified site 183.0
- serous (M8441/3)
  - papillary (M8460/3)
    - specified site — *see* Neoplasm, by site, malignant
    - unspecified site 183.0
  - specified site — *see* Neoplasm, by site, malignant
  - unspecified site 183.0

Cystadenofibroma (M9013/0)
- clear cell (M8313/0) — *see* Neoplasm, by site, benign
- endometrioid (M8381/0) 220
  - borderline malignancy (M8381/1) 236.2
  - malignant (M8381/3) 183.0
- mucinous (M9015/0)
  - specified site — *see* Neoplasm, by site, benign
  - unspecified site 220
- serous (M9014/0)
  - specified site — *see* Neoplasm, by site, benign
  - unspecified site 220
- specified site — *see* Neoplasm, by site, benign
- unspecified site 220

Cystadenoma (M8440/0) — *see also* Neoplasm, by site, benign
- bile duct (M8161/0) 211.5
- endometrioid (M8380/0) (*see also* Neoplasm, by site, benign)
  - borderline malignancy (M8380/1) — *see* Neoplasm, by site, uncertain behavior
- malignant (M8440/3) — *see* Neoplasm, by site, malignant
- mucinous (M8470/0)
  - borderline malignancy (M8470/1)
    - specified site — *see* Neoplasm, uncertain behavior
    - unspecified site 236.2
  - papillary (M8471/0)
    - borderline malignancy (M8471/1)
      - specified site — *see* Neoplasm, by site, uncertain behavior
      - unspecified site 236.2
    - specified site — *see* Neoplasm, by site, benign
    - unspecified site 220
  - specified site — *see* Neoplasm, by site, benign
  - unspecified site 220
- papillary (M8450/0)
  - borderline malignancy (M8450/1)
    - specified site — *see* Neoplasm, by site, uncertain behavior

Cystadenoma — *see also* Neoplasm, by site, benign — *continued*
- papillary — *continued*
  - borderline malignancy — *continued*
    - unspecified site 236.2
  - lymphomatosum (M8561/0) 210.2
  - mucinous (M8471/0)
    - borderline malignancy (M8471/1)
      - specified site — *see* Neoplasm, by site, uncertain behavior
      - unspecified site 236.2
    - specified site — *see* Neoplasm, by site, benign
    - unspecified site 220
  - pseudomucinous (M8471/0)
    - borderline malignancy (M8471/1)
      - specified site — *see* Neoplasm, by site, uncertain behavior
      - unspecified site 236.2
    - specified site — *see* Neoplasm, by site, benign
    - unspecified site 220
  - serous (M8460/0)
    - borderline malignancy (M8460/1)
      - specified site — *see* Neoplasm, by site, uncertain behavior
      - unspecified site 236.2
    - specified site — *see* Neoplasm, by site, benign
    - unspecified site 220
  - specified site — *see* Neoplasm, by site, benign
  - unspecified site 220
- pseudomucinous (M8470/0)
  - borderline malignancy (M8470/1)
    - specified site — *see* Neoplasm, by site, uncertain behavior
    - unspecified site 236.2
  - papillary (M8471/0)
    - borderline malignancy (M8471/1)
      - specified site — *see* Neoplasm, by site, uncertain behavior
      - unspecified site 236.2
    - specified site — *see* Neoplasm, by site, benign
    - unspecified site 220
  - specified site — *see* Neoplasm, by site, benign
  - unspecified site 220
- serous (M8441/0)
  - borderline malignancy (M8441/1)
    - specified site — *see* Neoplasm, by site, uncertain behavior
    - unspecified site 236.2
  - papillary (M8460/0)
    - borderline malignancy (M8460/1)
      - specified site — *see* Neoplasm, by site, uncertain behavior
      - unspecified site 236.2
    - specified site — *see* Neoplasm, by site, benign
    - unspecified site 220
  - specified site — *see* Neoplasm, by site, benign
  - unspecified site 220
- thyroid 226

Cystathioninemia 270.4
Cystathioninuria 270.4
Cystic — *see also* condition
- breast, chronic 610.1
- corpora lutea 620.1
- degeneration, congenital
  - brain 742.4

Cystic

Cystic — see also condition — continued
  degeneration, congenital — continued
    kidney (see also Cystic, disease, kidney) 753.10
  disease
    breast, chronic 610.1
    kidney, congenital 753.10
      medullary 753.16
      multiple 753.19
      polycystic — see Polycystic, kidney
      single 753.11
      specified NEC 753.19
    liver, congenital 751.62
    lung 518.89
      congenital 748.4
    pancreas, congenital 751.7
    semilunar cartilage 717.5
  duct — see condition
  eyeball, congenital 743.03
  fibrosis (pancreas) 277.00
    with
      manifestations
        gastrointestinal 277.03
        pulmonary 277.02
        specified NEC 277.09
      meconium ileus 277.01
      pulmonary exacerbation 277.02
  hygroma (M9173/0) 228.1
  kidney, congenital 753.10
    medullary 753.16
    multiple 753.19
    polycystic — see Polycystic, kidney
    single 753.11
    specified NEC 753.19
  liver, congenital 751.62
  lung 518.89
    congenital 748.4
  mass — see Cyst
  mastitis, chronic 610.1
  ovary 620.2
  pancreas, congenital 751.7
Cysticerciasis 123.1
Cysticercosis (mammary) (subretinal) 123.1

Cysticercus 123.1
  cellulosae infestation 123.1
Cystinosis (malignant) 270.0
Cystinuria 270.0
Cystitis (bacillary) (colli) (diffuse) (exudative) (hemorrhagic) (purulent) (recurrent) (septic) (suppurative) (ulcerative) 595.9
  with
    abortion — see Abortion, by type, with urinary tract infection
    ectopic pregnancy (see also categories 633.0–633.9) 639.8
    fibrosis 595.1
    leukoplakia 595.1
    malakoplakia 595.1
    metaplasia 595.1
    molar pregnancy (see also categories 630–632) 639.8
  actinomycotic 039.8 [595.4]
  acute 595.0
    of trigone 595.3
  allergic 595.89
  amebic 006.8 [595.4]
  bilharzial 120.9 [595.4]
  blennorrhagic (acute) 098.11
    chronic or duration of 2 months or more 098.31
  bullous 595.89
  calculous 594.1
    chlamydial 099.53
  chronic 595.2
    interstitial 595.1
    of trigone 595.3
  complicating pregnancy, childbirth, or puerperium 646.6 ✓
    affecting fetus or newborn 760.1
  cystic(a) 595.81
  diphtheritic 032.84
  echinococcal
    granulosus 122.3 [595.4]
    multilocularis 122.6 [595.4]
  emphysematous 595.89
  encysted 595.81
  follicular 595.3
  following
    abortion 639.8

Cystitis — continued
  following — continued
    ectopic or molar pregnancy 639.8
  gangrenous 595.89
  glandularis 595.89
  gonococcal (acute) 098.11
    chronic or duration of 2 months or more 098.31
  incrusted 595.89
  interstitial 595.1
  irradiation 595.82
  irritation 595.89
  malignant 595.89
  monilial 112.2
  of trigone 595.3
  panmural 595.1
  polyposa 595.89
  prostatic 601.3
  radiation 595.82
  Reiter's (abacterial) 099.3
  specified NEC 595.89
  subacute 595.2
  submucous 595.1
  syphilitic 095.8
  trichomoniasis 131.09
  tuberculous (see also Tuberculosis) 016.1 ✓
  ulcerative 595.1
Cystocele (-rectocele)
  female (without uterine prolapse) 618.01
    with uterine prolapse 618.4
      complete 618.3
      incomplete 618.2
    lateral 618.02
    midline 618.01
    paravaginal 618.02
    in pregnancy or childbirth 654.4 ✓
      affecting fetus or newborn 763.89
      causing obstructed labor 660.2 ✓
        affecting fetus or newborn 763.1
  male 596.8
Cystoid
  cicatrix limbus 372.64
  degeneration macula 362.53
Cystolithiasis 594.1

Cystoma (M8440/0) — see also Neoplasm, by site, benign
  endometrial, ovary 617.1
  mucinous (M8470/0)
    specified site — see Neoplasm, by site, benign
    unspecified site 220
  serous (M8441/0)
    specified site — see Neoplasm, by site, benign
    unspecified site 220
  simple (ovary) 620.2
Cystoplegia 596.53
Cystoptosis 596.8
Cystopyelitis — see also Pyelitis 590.80
Cystorrhagia 596.8
Cystosarcoma phyllodes (M9020/1) 238.3
  benign (M9020/0) 217
  malignant (M9020/3) — see Neoplasm, breast, malignant
Cystostomy status V44.50
  with complication 997.5
  appendico-vesicostomy V44.52
  cutaneous-vesicostomy V44.51
  specified type NEC V44.59
Cystourethritis — see also Urethritis 597.89
Cystourethrocele — see also Cystocele
  female (without uterine prolapse) 618.09
    with uterine prolapse 618.4
      complete 618.3
      incomplete 618.2
  male 596.8
Cytomegalic inclusion disease 078.5
  congenital 771.1
Cytomycosis, reticuloendothelial — see also Histoplasmosis, American 115.00
Cytopenia 289.9
  refractory
    with
      multilineage dysplasia (RCMD) 238.72
      and ringed sideroblasts (RCMD-RS) 238.72

Index to Diseases

D

Daae (-Finsen) disease (epidemic pleurodynia) 074.1
Dabney's grip 074.1
Da Costa's syndrome (neurocirculatory asthenia) 306.2
Dacryoadenitis, dacryadenitis 375.00
  acute 375.01
  chronic 375.02
Dacryocystitis 375.30
  acute 375.32
  chronic 375.42
  neonatal 771.6
  phlegmonous 375.33
  syphilitic 095.8
    congenital 090.0
  trachomatous, active 076.1
    late effect 139.1
  tuberculous (see also Tuberculosis) 017.3
Dacryocystoblenorrhea 375.42
Dacryocystocele 375.43
Dacryolith, dacryolithiasis 375.57
Dacryoma 375.43
Dacryopericystitis (acute) (subacute) 375.32
  chronic 375.42
Dacryops 375.11
Dacryosialadenopathy, atrophic 710.2
Dacryostenosis 375.56
  congenital 743.65
Dactylitis
  bone (see also Osteomyelitis) 730.2
  sickle-cell 282.62
    Hb-C 282.64
    Hb-SS 282.62
    specified NEC 282.69
  syphilitic 095.5
  tuberculous (see also Tuberculosis) 015.5
Dactylolysis spontanea 136.0
Dactylosymphysis — see also Syndactylism 755.10
Damage
  arteriosclerotic — see Arteriosclerosis
  brain 348.9
    anoxic, hypoxic 348.1
      during or resulting from a procedure 997.01
      ischemic, in newborn 768.7
    child NEC 343.9
    due to birth injury 767.0
    minimal (child) (see also Hyperkinesia) 314.9
    newborn 767.0
  cardiac (see also Disease, heart)
  cardiorenal (vascular) (see also Hypertension, cardiorenal) 404.90
  central nervous system — see Damage, brain
  cerebral NEC — see Damage, brain
  coccyx, complicating delivery 665.6
  coronary (see also Ischemia, heart) 414.9
  eye, birth injury 767.8
  heart (see also Disease, heart)
    valve — see Endocarditis
  hypothalamus NEC 348.9
  liver 571.9
    alcoholic 571.3
  myocardium (see also Degeneration, myocardial) 429.1
  pelvic
    joint or ligament, during delivery 665.6
    organ NEC
      with
        abortion — see Abortion, by type, with damage to pelvic organs
        ectopic pregnancy (see also categories 633.0–633.9) 639.2

Damage — continued
  pelvic — continued
    organ — continued
      with — continued
        molar pregnancy (see also categories 630–632) 639.2
      during delivery 665.5
      following
        abortion 639.2
        ectopic or molar pregnancy 639.2
  renal (see also Disease, renal) 593.9
  skin, solar 692.79
    acute 692.72
    chronic 692.74
  subendocardium, subendocardial (see also Degeneration, myocardial) 429.1
  vascular 459.9
Dameshek's syndrome (erythroblastic anemia) 282.49
Dana-Putnam syndrome (subacute combined sclerosis with pernicious anemia) 281.0 [336.2]
Danbolt (-Closs) syndrome (acrodermatitis enteropathica) 686.8
Dandruff 690.18
Dandy fever 061
Dandy-Walker deformity or syndrome (atresia, foramen of Magendie) 742.3
  with spina bifida (see also Spina bifida) 741.0
Dangle foot 736.79
Danielssen's disease (anesthetic leprosy) 030.1
Danlos' syndrome 756.83
Darier's disease (congenital) (keratosis follicularis) 757.39
  due to vitamin A deficiency 264.8
  meaning erythema annulare centrifugum 695.0
Darier-Roussy sarcoid 135
Darling's
  disease (see also Histoplasmosis, American) 115.00
  histoplasmosis (see also Histoplasmosis, American) 115.00
Dartre 054.9
Darwin's tubercle 744.29
Davidson's anemia (refractory) 284.9
Davies-Colley syndrome (slipping rib) 733.99
Davies' disease 425.0
Dawson's encephalitis 046.2
Day blindness — see also Blindness, day 368.60
Dead
  fetus
    retained (in utero) 656.4
      early pregnancy (death before 22 completed weeks gestation) 632
      late (death after 22 completed weeks gestation) 656.4
    syndrome 641.3
  labyrinth 386.50
  ovum, retained 631
Deaf and dumb NEC 389.7
Deaf mutism (acquired) (congenital) NEC 389.7
  endemic 243
  hysterical 300.11
  syphilitic, congenital 090.0
Deafness (acquired) (complete) (congenital) (hereditary) (middle ear) (partial) 389.9
  with blue sclera and fragility of bone 756.51
  auditory fatigue 389.9
  aviation 993.0
  nerve injury 951.5
  boilermakers' 951.5
  central, ▶bilateral◀ 389.14
    with conductive hearing loss 389.2

Deafness — continued
  conductive (air) 389.00
    with sensorineural hearing loss 389.2
    combined types 389.08
    external ear 389.01
    inner ear 389.04
    middle ear 389.03
    multiple types 389.08
    tympanic membrane 389.02
  emotional (complete) 300.11
  functional (complete) 300.11
  high frequency 389.8
  hysterical (complete) 300.11
  injury 951.5
  low frequency 389.8
  mental 784.69
  mixed conductive and sensorineural 389.2
  nerve, ▶bilateral◀ 389.12
    with conductive hearing loss 389.2
  neural, ▶bilateral◀ 389.12
    with conductive hearing loss 389.2
  noise-induced 388.12
    nerve injury 951.5
  nonspeaking 389.7
  perceptive 389.10
    with conductive hearing loss 389.2
    central, ▶bilateral◀ 389.14
    combined types, ▶bilateral◀ 389.18
    multiple types, ▶bilateral◀ 389.18
    neural, ▶bilateral◀ 389.12
    sensorineural 389.10
      asymmetrical 389.16
      bilateral 389.18
      unilateral 389.15
    sensory, ▶bilateral◀ 389.11
  psychogenic (complete) 306.7
  sensorineural (see also Deafness, perceptive) 389.10
    asymmetrical 389.16
    bilateral 389.18
    unilateral 389.15
  sensory, ▶bilateral◀ 389.11
    with conductive hearing loss 389.2
  specified type NEC 389.8
  sudden NEC 388.2
  syphilitic 094.89
  transient ischemic 388.02
  transmission — see Deafness, conductive
  traumatic 951.5
  word (secondary to organic lesion) 784.69
    developmental 315.31
Death
  after delivery (cause not stated) (sudden) 674.9
  anesthetic
    due to
      correct substance properly administered 995.4
      overdose or wrong substance given 968.4
      specified anesthetic — see Table of Drugs and Chemicals
    during delivery 668.9
  brain 348.8
  cardiac — see Disease, heart
  cause unknown 798.2
  cot (infant) 798.0
  crib (infant) 798.0
  fetus, fetal (cause not stated) (intrauterine) 779.9
    early, with retention (before 22 completed weeks gestation) 632
    from asphyxia or anoxia (before labor) 768.0
      during labor 768.1
    late, affecting management of pregnancy (after 22 completed weeks gestation) 656.4
  from pregnancy NEC 646.9

Death — continued
  instantaneous 798.1
  intrauterine (see also Death, fetus) 779.9
    complicating pregnancy 656.4
  maternal, affecting fetus or newborn 761.6
  neonatal NEC 779.9
  sudden (cause unknown) 798.1
    during delivery 669.9
      under anesthesia NEC 668.9
    infant, syndrome (SIDS) 798.0
    puerperal, during puerperium 674.9
  unattended (cause unknown) 798.9
  under anesthesia NEC
    due to
      correct substance properly administered 995.4
      overdose or wrong substance given 968.4
      specified anesthetic — see Table of Drugs and Chemicals
    during delivery 668.9
  violent 798.1
de Beurmann-Gougerot disease (sporotrichosis) 117.1
Debility (general) (infantile) (postinfectional) 799.3
  with nutritional difficulty 269.9
  congenital or neonatal NEC 779.9
  nervous 300.5
  old age 797
  senile 797
Débove's disease (splenomegaly) 789.2
Decalcification
  bone (see also Osteoporosis) 733.00
  teeth 521.89
Decapitation 874.9
  fetal (to facilitate delivery) 763.89
Decapsulation, kidney 593.89
Decay
  dental 521.00
  senile 797
  tooth, teeth 521.00
Decensus, uterus — see Prolapse, uterus
Deciduitis (acute)
  with
    abortion — see Abortion, by type, with sepsis
    ectopic pregnancy (see also categories 633.0–633.9) 639.0
    molar pregnancy (see also categories 630–632) 639.0
  affecting fetus or newborn 760.8
  following
    abortion 639.0
    ectopic or molar pregnancy 639.0
  in pregnancy 646.6
  puerperal, postpartum 670.0
Deciduoma malignum (M9100/3) 181
Deciduous tooth (retained) 520.6
Decline (general) — see also Debility 799.3
Decompensation
  cardiac (acute) (chronic) (see also Disease, heart) 429.9
    failure — see Failure, heart
  cardiorenal (see also Hypertension, cardiorenal) 404.90
  cardiovascular (see also Disease, cardiovascular) 429.2
  heart (see also Disease, heart) 429.9
    failure — see Failure, heart
  hepatic 572.2
  myocardial (acute) (chronic) (see also Disease, heart) 429.9
    failure — see Failure, heart
  respiratory 519.9
Decompression sickness 993.3
Decrease, decreased
  blood
    platelets (see also Thrombocytopenia) 287.5
    pressure 796.3

Decrease, decreased — *continued*
  blood — *continued*
    pressure — *continued*
      due to shock following
        injury 958.4
        operation 998.0
    white cell count 288.50
      specified NEC 288.59
  cardiac reserve — see Disease, heart
  estrogen 256.39
    postablative 256.2
  fetal movements 655.7 ☑
  fragility of erythrocytes 289.89
  function
    adrenal (cortex) 255.4
      medulla 255.5
    ovary in hypopituitarism 253.4
    parenchyma of pancreas 577.8
    pituitary (gland) (lobe) (anterior) 253.2
      posterior (lobe) 253.8
  functional activity 780.99
  glucose 790.29
  haptoglobin (serum) NEC 273.8
  leukocytes 288.50
  libido 799.81
  lymphocytes 288.51
  platelets (*see also* Thrombocytopenia) 287.5
  pulse pressure 785.9
  respiration due to shock following injury 958.4
  sexual desire 799.81
  tear secretion NEC 375.15
  tolerance
    fat 579.8
    salt and water 276.9
  vision NEC 369.9
  white blood cell count 288.50
Decubital gangrene 707.00 [785.4]
Decubiti — *see also* Decubitus 707.00
Decubitus (ulcer) 707.00
  with gangrene 707.00 [785.4]
  ankle 707.06
  back
    lower 707.03
    upper 707.02
  buttock 707.05
  elbow 707.01
  head 707.09
  heel 707.07
  hip 707.04
  other site 707.09
  sacrum 707.03
  shoulder blades 707.02
Deepening acetabulum 718.85
Defect, defective 759.9
  3-beta-hydroxysteroid dehydrogenase 255.2
  11-hydroxylase 255.2
  21-hydroxylase 255.2
  abdominal wall, congenital 756.70
  aorticopulmonary septum 745.0
  aortic septal 745.0
  atrial septal (ostium secundum type) 745.5
    acquired 429.71
    ostium primum type 745.61
    sinus venosus 745.8
  atrioventricular
    canal 745.69
    septum 745.4
      acquired 429.71
  atrium secundum 745.5
    acquired 429.71
  auricular septal 745.5
    acquired 429.71
  bilirubin excretion 277.4
  biosynthesis, testicular androgen 257.2
  bridge 525.60
  bulbar septum 745.0
  butanol-insoluble iodide 246.1
  chromosome — *see* Anomaly, chromosome
  circulation (acquired) 459.9

Defect, defective — *continued*
  circulation — *continued*
    congenital 747.9
    newborn 747.9
  clotting NEC (*see also* Defect, coagulation) 286.9
  coagulation (factor) (*see also* Deficiency, coagulation factor) 286.9
    with
      abortion — *see* Abortion, by type, with hemorrhage
      ectopic pregnancy (*see also* categories 634–638) 639.1
      molar pregnancy (*see also* categories 630–632) 639.1
    acquired (any) 286.7
    antepartum or intrapartum 641.3 ☑
      affecting fetus or newborn 762.1
    causing hemorrhage of pregnancy or delivery 641.3 ☑
    complicating pregnancy, childbirth, or puerperium 649.3 ☑
    due to
      liver disease 286.7
      vitamin K deficiency 286.7
    newborn, transient 776.3
    postpartum 666.3 ☑
    specified type NEC 286.3
  conduction (heart) 426.9
    bone (*see also* Deafness, conductive) 389.00
  congenital, organ or site NEC (*see also* Anomaly)
    circulation 747.9
    Descemet's membrane 743.9
      specified type NEC 743.49
    diaphragm 756.6
    ectodermal 757.9
    esophagus 750.9
    pulmonic cusps — *see* Anomaly, heart valve
    respiratory system 748.9
      specified type NEC 748.8
  crown 525.60
  cushion endocardial 745.60
  dental restoration 525.60
  dentin (hereditary) 520.5
  Descemet's membrane (congenital) 743.9
    acquired 371.30
    specific type NEC 743.49
  deutan 368.52
  developmental (*see also* Anomaly, by site)
    cauda equina 742.59
    left ventricle 746.9
      with atresia or hypoplasia of aortic orifice or valve, with hypoplasia of ascending aorta 746.7
      in hypoplastic left heart syndrome 746.7
    testis 752.9
    vessel 747.9
  diaphragm
    with elevation, eventration, or hernia — *see* Hernia, diaphragm
    congenital 756.6
      with elevation, eventration, or hernia 756.6
      gross (with elevation, eventration, or hernia) 756.6
  ectodermal, congenital 757.9
  Eisenmenger's (ventricular septal defect) 745.4
  endocardial cushion 745.60
    specified type NEC 745.69
  esophagus, congenital 750.9
  extensor retinaculum 728.9
  fibrin polymerization (*see also* Defect, coagulation) 286.3
  filling
    biliary tract 793.3
    bladder 793.5

Defect, defective — *continued*
  filling — *continued*
    dental 525.60
    gallbladder 793.3
    kidney 793.5
    stomach 793.4
    ureter 793.5
  fossa ovalis 745.5
  gene, carrier (suspected) of V83.89
  Gerbode 745.4
  glaucomatous, without elevated tension 365.89
  Hageman (factor) (*see also* Defect, coagulation) 286.3
  hearing (*see also* Deafness) 389.9
  high grade 317
  homogentisic acid 270.2
  interatrial septal 745.5
    acquired 429.71
  interauricular septal 745.5
    acquired 429.71
  interventricular septal 745.4
    with pulmonary stenosis or atresia, dextraposition of aorta, and hypertrophy of right ventricle 745.2
    acquired 429.71
    in tetralogy of Fallot 745.2
  iodide trapping 246.1
  iodotyrosine dehalogenase 246.1
  kynureninase 270.2
  learning, specific 315.2
  major osseous 731.3
  mental (*see also* Retardation, mental) 319
  osseous, major 731.3
  osteochondral NEC 738.8
  ostium
    primum 745.61
    secundum 745.5
  pericardium 746.89
  peroxidase-binding 246.1
  placental blood supply — *see* Placenta, insufficiency
  platelet (qualitative) 287.1
    constitutional 286.4
  postural, spine 737.9
  protan 368.51
  pulmonic cusps, congenital 746.00
  renal pelvis 753.9
    obstructive 753.29
    specified type NEC 753.3
  respiratory system, congenital 748.9
    specified type NEC 748.8
  retina, retinal 361.30
    with detachment (*see also* Detachment, retina, with retinal defect) 361.00
    multiple 361.33
      with detachment 361.02
    nerve fiber bundle 362.85
    single 361.30
      with detachment 361.01
  septal (closure) (heart) NEC 745.9
    acquired 429.71
    atrial 745.5
    specified type NEC 745.8
  speech NEC 784.5
    developmental 315.39
    secondary to organic lesion 784.5
  Taussig-Bing (transposition, aorta and overriding pulmonary artery) 745.11
  teeth, wedge 521.20
  thyroid hormone synthesis 246.1
  tritan 368.53
  ureter 753.9
    obstructive 753.29
  vascular (acquired) (local) 459.9
    congenital (peripheral) NEC 747.60
      gastrointestinal 747.61
      lower limb 747.64
      renal 747.62
      specified NEC 747.69
      spinal 747.82
      upper limb 747.63

Defect, defective — *continued*
  ventricular septal 745.4
    with pulmonary stenosis or atresia, dextraposition of aorta, and hypertrophy of right ventricle 745.2
    acquired 429.71
    atrioventricular canal type 745.69
    between infundibulum and anterior portion 745.4
    in tetralogy of Fallot 745.2
    isolated anterior 745.4
  vision NEC 369.9
  visual field 368.40
    arcuate 368.43
    heteronymous, bilateral 368.47
    homonymous, bilateral 368.46
    localized NEC 368.44
    nasal step 368.44
    peripheral 368.44
    sector 368.43
  voice 784.40
  wedge, teeth (abrasion) 521.20
Defeminization syndrome 255.2
Deferentitis 608.4
  gonorrheal (acute) 098.14
    chronic or duration of 2 months or over 098.34
Defibrination syndrome — *see also* Fibrinolysis 286.6
Deficiency, deficient
  3-beta-hydroxysteroid dehydrogenase 255.2
  6-phosphogluconic dehydrogenase (anemia) 282.2
  11-beta-hydroxylase 255.2
  17-alpha-hydroxylase 255.2
  18-hydroxysteroid dehydrogenase 255.2
  20-alpha-hydroxylase 255.2
  21-hydroxylase 255.2
  AAT (alpha-1 antitrypsin) 273.4
  abdominal muscle syndrome 756.79
  accelerator globulin (Ac G) (blood) (*see also* Defect, coagulation) 286.3
  AC globulin (congenital) (*see also* Defect, coagulation) 286.3
    acquired 286.7
  activating factor (blood) (*see also* Defect, coagulation) 286.3
  adenohypophyseal 253.2
  adenosine deaminase 277.2
  aldolase (hereditary) 271.2
  alpha-1-antitrypsin 273.4
  alpha-1-trypsin inhibitor 273.4
  alpha-fucosidase 271.8
  alpha-lipoprotein 272.5
  alpha-mannosidase 271.8
  amino acid 270.9
  anemia — *see* Anemia, deficiency
  aneurin 265.1
    with beriberi 265.0
  antibody NEC 279.00
  antidiuretic hormone 253.5
  antihemophilic
    factor (A) 286.0
    B 286.1
    C 286.2
    globulin (AHG) NEC 286.0
  antithrombin III 289.81
  antitrypsin 273.4
  argininosuccinate synthetase or lyase 270.6
  ascorbic acid (with scurvy) 267
  autoprothrombin
    I (*see also* Defect, coagulation) 286.3
    II 286.1
    C (*see also* Defect, coagulation) 286.3
  bile salt 579.8
  biotin 266.2
  biotinidase 277.6
  bradykinase-1 277.6
  brancher enzyme (amylopectinosis) 271.0

Index to Diseases

Deficiency, deficient

Deficiency, deficient — *continued*
- calciferol 268.9
  - with
    - osteomalacia 268.2
    - rickets (*see also* Rickets) 268.0
- calcium 275.40
  - dietary 269.3
- calorie, severe 261
- carbamyl phosphate synthetase 270.6
- cardiac (*see also* Insufficiency, myocardial) 428.0
- carnitine 277.81
  - due to
    - hemodialysis 277.83
    - inborn errors of metabolism 277.82
    - valproic acid therapy 277.83
  - iatrogenic 277.83
  - palmitoyltransferase (CPT1, CPT2) 277.85
  - palmityl transferase (CPT1, CPT2) 277.85
  - primary 277.81
  - secondary 277.84
- carotene 264.9
- Carr factor (*see also* Defect, coagulation) 286.9
- central nervous system 349.9
- ceruloplasmin 275.1
- cevitamic acid (with scurvy) 267
- choline 266.2
- Christmas factor 286.1
- chromium 269.3
- citrin 269.1
- clotting (blood) (*see also* Defect, coagulation) 286.9
- coagulation factor NEC 286.9
  - with
    - abortion — *see* Abortion, by type, with hemorrhage
    - ectopic pregnancy (*see also* categories 634–638) 639.1
    - molar pregnancy (*see also* categories 630–632) 639.1
  - acquired (any) 286.7
  - antepartum or intrapartum 641.3 ☑
    - affecting fetus or newborn 762.1
  - complicating pregnancy, childbirth, or puerperium 649.3 ☑
  - due to
    - liver disease 286.7
    - vitamin K deficiency 286.7
  - newborn, transient 776.3
  - postpartum 666.3 ☑
  - specified type NEC 286.3
- color vision (congenital) 368.59
  - acquired 368.55
- combined, two or more coagulation factors (*see also* Defect, coagulation) 286.9
- complement factor NEC 279.8
- contact factor (*see also* Defect, coagulation) 286.3
- copper NEC 275.1
- corticoadrenal 255.4
- craniofacial axis 756.0
- cyanocobalamin (vitamin B_{12}) 266.2
- debrancher enzyme (limit dextrinosis) 271.0
- desmolase 255.2
- diet 269.9
- dihydrofolate reductase 281.2
- dihydropteridine reductase 270.1
- disaccharidase (intestinal) 271.3
- disease NEC 269.9
- ear(s) V48.8
- edema 262
- endocrine 259.9
- enzymes, circulating NEC (*see also* Deficiency, by specific enzyme) 277.6
- ergosterol 268.9
  - with
    - osteomalacia 268.2

Deficiency, deficient — *continued*
- ergosterol — *continued*
  - with — *continued*
    - rickets (*see also* Rickets) 268.0
- erythrocytic glutathione (anemia) 282.2
- eyelid(s) V48.8
- factor (*see also* Defect, coagulation) 286.9
  - I (congenital) (fibrinogen) 286.3
    - antepartum or intrapartum 641.3 ☑
      - affecting fetus or newborn 762.1
    - newborn, transient 776.3
    - postpartum 666.3 ☑
  - II (congenital) (prothrombin) 286.3
  - V (congenital) (labile) 286.3
  - VII (congenital) (stable) 286.3
  - VIII (congenital) (functional) 286.0
    - with
      - functional defect 286.0
      - vascular defect 286.4
  - IX (Christmas) (congenital) (functional) 286.1
  - X (congenital) (Stuart-Prower) 286.3
  - XI (congenital) (plasma thromboplastin antecedent) 286.2
  - XII (congenital) (Hageman) 286.3
  - XIII (congenital) (fibrin stabilizing) 286.3
  - Hageman 286.3
  - multiple (congenital) 286.9
    - acquired 286.7
- fibrinase (*see also* Defect, coagulation) 286.3
- fibrinogen (congenital) (*see also* Defect, coagulation) 286.3
  - acquired 286.6
- fibrin-stabilizing factor (congenital) (*see also* Defect, coagulation) 286.3
- finger — *see* Absence, finger
- fletcher factor (*see also* Defect, coagulation) 286.9
- fluorine 269.3
- folate, anemia 281.2
- folic acid (vitamin B_c) 266.2
  - anemia 281.2
- follicle-stimulating hormone (FSH) 253.4
- fructokinase 271.2
- fructose-1, 6-diphosphate 271.2
- fructose-1-phosphate aldolase 271.2
- FSH (follicle-stimulating hormone) 253.4
- fucosidase 271.8
- galactokinase 271.1
- galactose-1-phosphate uridyl transferase 271.1
- gamma globulin in blood 279.00
- glass factor (*see also* Defect, coagulation) 286.3
- glucocorticoid 255.4
- glucose-6-phosphatase 271.0
- glucose-6-phosphate dehydrogenase anemia 282.2
- glucuronyl transferase 277.4
- glutathione-reductase (anemia) 282.2
- glycogen synthetase 271.0
- growth hormone 253.3
- Hageman factor (congenital) (*see also* Defect, coagulation) 286.3
- head V48.0
- hemoglobin (*see also* Anemia) 285.9
- hepatophosphorylase 271.0
- hexose monophosphate (HMP) shunt 282.2
- HGH (human growth hormone) 253.3
- HG-PRT 277.2
- homogentisic acid oxidase 270.2
- hormone (*see also* Deficiency, by specific hormone)
  - anterior pituitary (isolated) (partial) NEC 253.4

Deficiency, deficient — *continued*
- hormone (*see also* Deficiency, by specific hormone) — *continued*
  - anterior pituitary — *continued*
    - growth (human) 253.3
    - follicle-stimulating 253.4
    - growth (human) (isolated) 253.3
    - human growth 253.3
    - interstitial cell-stimulating 253.4
    - luteinizing 253.4
    - melanocyte-stimulating 253.4
    - testicular 257.2
- human growth hormone 253.3
- humoral 279.00
  - with
    - hyper-IgM 279.05
      - autosomal recessive 279.05
      - X-linked 279.05
    - increased IgM 279.05
    - congenital hypogammaglobulinemia 279.04
    - non-sex-linked 279.06
  - selective immunoglobulin NEC 279.03
    - IgA 279.01
    - IgG 279.03
    - IgM 279.02
      - increased 279.05
  - specified NEC 279.09
- hydroxylase 255.2
- hypoxanthine-guanine phosphoribosyltransferase (HG-PRT) 277.2
- ICSH (interstitial cell-stimulating hormone) 253.4
- immunity NEC 279.3
  - cell-mediated 279.10
    - with
      - hyperimmunoglobulinemia 279.2
      - thrombocytopenia and eczema 279.12
    - specified NEC 279.19
  - combined (severe) 279.2
    - syndrome 279.2
  - common variable 279.06
  - humoral NEC 279.00
  - IgA (secretory) 279.01
  - IgG 279.03
  - IgM 279.02
- immunoglobulin, selective NEC 279.03
  - IgA 279.01
  - IgG 279.03
  - IgM 279.02
- inositol (B complex) 266.2
- interferon 279.4
- internal organ V47.0
- interstitial cell-stimulating hormone (ICSH) 253.4
- intrinsic factor (Castle's) (congenital) 281.0
- intrinsic (urethral) sphincter (ISD) 599.82
- invertase 271.3
- iodine 269.3
- iron, anemia 280.9
- labile factor (congenital) (*see also* Defect, coagulation) 286.3
  - acquired 286.7
- lacrimal fluid (acquired) 375.15
  - congenital 743.64
- lactase 271.3
- Laki-Lorand factor (*see also* Defect, coagulation) 286.3
- lecithin-cholesterol acyltranferase 272.5
- LH (luteinizing hormone) 253.4
- limb V49.0
  - lower V49.0
    - congenital (*see also* Deficiency, lower limb, congenital) 755.30
  - upper V49.0
    - congenital (*see also* Deficiency, upper limb, congenital) 755.20

Deficiency, deficient — *continued*
- lipocaic 577.8
- lipoid (high-density) 272.5
- lipoprotein (familial) (high density) 272.5
- liver phosphorylase 271.0
- long chain 3-hydroxyacyl CoA dehydrogenase (LCHAD) 277.85
- long chain/very long chain acyl CoA dehydrogenase (LCAD, VLCAD) 277.85
- lower limb V49.0
  - congenital 755.30
    - with complete absence of distal elements 755.31
    - longitudinal (complete) (partial) (with distal deficiencies, incomplete) 755.32
      - with complete absence of distal elements 755.31
      - combined femoral, tibial, fibular (incomplete) 755.33
      - femoral 755.34
      - fibular 755.37
      - metatarsal(s) 755.38
      - phalange(s) 755.39
        - meaning all digits 755.31
      - tarsal(s) 755.38
      - tibia 755.36
      - tibiofibular 755.35
    - transverse 755.31
- luteinizing hormone (LH) 253.4
- lysosomal alpha-1, 4 glucosidase 271.0
- magnesium 275.2
- mannosidase 271.8
- medium chain acyl CoA dehydrogenase (MCAD) 277.85
- melanocyte-stimulating hormone (MSH) 253.4
- menadione (vitamin K) 269.0
  - newborn 776.0
- mental (familial) (hereditary) (*see also* Retardation, mental) 319
- mineral NEC 269.3
- molybdenum 269.3
- moral 301.7
- multiple, syndrome 260
- myocardial (*see also* Insufficiency, myocardial) 428.0
- myophosphorylase 271.0
- NADH-diaphorase or reductase (congenital) 289.7
- NADH (DPNH)-methemoglobin-reductase (congenital) 289.7
- neck V48.1
- niacin (amide) (-tryptophan) 265.2
- nicotinamide 265.2
- nicotinic acid (amide) 265.2
- nose V48.8
- number of teeth (*see also* Anodontia) 520.0
- nutrition, nutritional 269.9
  - specified NEC 269.8
- ornithine transcarbamylase 270.6
- ovarian 256.39
- oxygen (*see also* Anoxia) 799.02
- pantothenic acid 266.2
- parathyroid (gland) 252.1
- phenylalanine hydroxylase 270.1
- phosphoenolpyruvate carboxykinase 271.8
- phosphofructokinase 271.2
- phosphoglucomutase 271.0
- phosphohexosisomerase 271.0
- phosphomannomutase 271.8
- phosphomannose isomerase 271.8
- phosphomannosyl mutase 271.8
- phosphorylase kinase, liver 271.0
- pituitary (anterior) 253.2
  - posterior 253.5
- placenta — *see* Placenta, insufficiency
- plasma
  - cell 279.00

Deficiency, deficient — continued
  plasma — continued
    protein (paraproteinemia) (pyroglobulinemia) 273.8
      gamma globulin 279.00
    thromboplastin
      antecedent (PTA) 286.2
      component (PTC) 286.1
  platelet NEC 287.1
    constitutional 286.4
  polyglandular 258.9
  potassium (K) 276.8
  proaccelerin (congenital) (see also Defect, coagulation) 286.3
    acquired 286.7
  proconvertin factor (congenital) (see also Defect, coagulation) 286.3
    acquired 286.7
  prolactin 253.4
  protein 260
    anemia 281.4
    C 289.81
    plasma — see Deficiency, plasma, protein
    S 289.81
  prothrombin (congenital) (see also Defect, coagulation) 286.3
    acquired 286.7
  Prower factor (see also Defect, coagulation) 286.3
  PRT 277.2
  pseudocholinesterase 289.89
  psychobiological 301.6
  PTA 286.2
  PTC 286.1
  purine nucleoside phosphorylase 277.2
  pyracin (alpha) (beta) 266.1
  pyridoxal 266.1
  pyridoxamine 266.1
  pyridoxine (derivatives) 266.1
  pyruvate carboxylase 271.8
  pyruvate dehydrogenase 271.8
  pyruvate kinase (PK) 282.3
  riboflavin (vitamin B_2) 266.0
  saccadic eye movements 379.57
  salivation 527.7
  salt 276.1
  secretion
    ovary 256.39
    salivary gland (any) 527.7
    urine 788.5
  selenium 269.3
  serum
    antitrypsin, familial 273.4
    protein (congenital) 273.8
  short chain acyl CoA dehydrogenase (SCAD) 277.85
  smooth pursuit movements (eye) 379.58
  sodium (Na) 276.1
  SPCA (see also Defect, coagulation) 286.3
  specified NEC 269.8
  stable factor (congenital) (see also Defect, coagulation) 286.3
    acquired 286.7
  Stuart (-Prower) factor (see also Defect, coagulation) 286.3
  sucrase 271.3
  sucrase-isomaltase 271.3
  sulfite oxidase 270.0
  syndrome, multiple 260
  thiamine, thiaminic (chloride) 265.1
  thrombokinase (see also Defect, coagulation) 286.3
    newborn 776.0
  thrombopoieten 287.39
  thymolymphatic 279.2
  thyroid (gland) 244.9
  tocopherol 269.1
  toe — see Absence, toe
  tooth bud (see also Anodontia) 520.0
  trunk V48.1
  UDPG-glycogen transferase 271.0
  upper limb V49.0

Deficiency, deficient — continued
  upper limb — continued
    congenital 755.20
      with complete absence of distal elements 755.21
      longitudinal (complete) (partial) (with distal deficiencies, incomplete) 755.22
        carpal(s) 755.28
        combined humeral, radial, ulnar (incomplete) 755.23
        humeral 755.24
        metacarpal(s) 755.28
        phalange(s) 755.29
          meaning all digits 755.21
        radial 755.26
        radioulnar 755.25
        ulnar 755.27
      transverse (complete) (partial) 755.21
  vascular 459.9
  vasopressin 253.5
  viosterol (see also Deficiency, calciferol) 268.9
  vitamin (multiple) NEC 269.2
    A 264.9
      with
        Bitôt's spot 264.1
          corneal 264.2
            with corneal ulceration 264.3
        keratomalacia 264.4
        keratosis, follicular 264.8
        night blindness 264.5
        scar of cornea, xerophthalmic 264.6
        specified manifestation NEC 264.8
        ocular 264.7
        xeroderma 264.8
        xerophthalmia 264.7
        xerosis
          conjunctival 264.0
            with Bitôt's spot 264.1
          corneal 264.2
            with corneal ulceration 264.3
    B (complex) NEC 266.9
      with
        beriberi 265.0
        pellagra 265.2
      specified type NEC 266.2
    B_1 NEC 265.1
      beriberi 265.0
    B_2 266.0
    B_6 266.1
    B_{12} 266.2
    B_c (folic acid) 266.2
    C (ascorbic acid) (with scurvy) 267
    D (calciferol) (ergosterol) 268.9
      with
        osteomalacia 268.2
        rickets (see also Rickets) 268.0
    E 269.1
    folic acid 266.2
    G 266.0
    H 266.2
    K 269.0
      of newborn 776.0
    nicotinic acid 265.2
    P 269.1
    PP 265.2
    specified NEC 269.1
  zinc 269.3
Deficient — see also Deficiency
  blink reflex 374.45
  craniofacial axis 756.0
  number of teeth (see also Anodontia) 520.0
  secretion of urine 788.5
Deficit
  neurologic NEC 781.99

Deficit — continued
  neurologic — continued
    due to
      cerebrovascular lesion (see also Disease, cerebrovascular, acute) 436
        late effect — see Late effect(s) (of) cerebrovascular disease
      transient ischemic attack 435.9
  oxygen 799.02
Deflection
  radius 736.09
  septum (acquired) (nasal) (nose) 470
  spine — see Curvature, spine
  turbinate (nose) 470
Defluvium
  capillorum (see also Alopecia) 704.00
  ciliorum 374.55
  unguium 703.8
Deformity 738.9
  abdomen, congenital 759.9
  abdominal wall
    acquired 738.8
    congenital 756.70
    muscle deficiency syndrome 756.79
  acquired (unspecified site) 738.9
    specified site NEC 738.8
  adrenal gland (congenital) 759.1
  alimentary tract, congenital 751.9
    lower 751.5
      specified type NEC 751.8
    upper (any part, except tongue) 750.9
      specified type NEC 750.8
      tongue 750.10
        specified type NEC 750.19
  ankle (joint) (acquired) 736.70
    abduction 718.47
    congenital 755.69
    contraction 718.47
    specified NEC 736.79
  anus (congenital) 751.5
    acquired 569.49
  aorta (congenital) 747.20
    acquired 447.8
    arch 747.21
      acquired 447.8
    coarctation 747.10
  aortic
    arch 747.21
      acquired 447.8
    cusp or valve (congenital) 746.9
      acquired (see also Endocarditis, aortic) 424.1
    ring 747.21
  appendix 751.5
  arm (acquired) 736.89
    congenital 755.50
  arteriovenous (congenital) (peripheral) NEC 747.60
    gastrointestinal 747.61
    lower limb 747.64
    renal 747.62
    specified NEC 747.69
    spinal 747.82
    upper limb 747.63
  artery (congenital) (peripheral) NEC (see also Deformity, vascular) 747.60
    acquired 447.8
    cerebral 747.81
    coronary (congenital) 746.85
      acquired (see also Ischemia, heart) 414.9
    retinal 743.9
    umbilical 747.5
  atrial septal (congenital) (heart) 745.5
  auditory canal (congenital) (external) (see also Deformity, ear) 744.3
    acquired 380.50
  auricle
    ear (congenital) (see also Deformity, ear) 744.3
      acquired 380.32
    heart (congenital) 746.9

Deformity — continued
  back (acquired) — see Deformity, spine
  Bartholin's duct (congenital) 750.9
  bile duct (congenital) 751.60
    acquired 576.8
      with calculus, choledocholithiasis, or stones — see Choledocholithiasis
  biliary duct or passage (congenital) 751.60
    acquired 576.8
      with calculus, choledocholithiasis, or stones — see Choledocholithiasis
  bladder (neck) (sphincter) (trigone) (acquired) 596.8
    congenital 753.9
  bone (acquired) NEC 738.9
    congenital 756.9
    turbinate 738.0
  boutonniere (finger) 736.21
  brain (congenital) 742.9
    acquired 348.8
    multiple 742.4
    reduction 742.2
    vessel (congenital) 747.81
  breast (acquired) 611.8
    congenital 757.9
  bronchus (congenital) 748.3
    acquired 519.19
  bursa, congenital 756.9
  canal of Nuck 752.9
  canthus (congenital) 743.9
    acquired 374.89
  capillary (acquired) 448.9
    congenital NEC (see also Deformity, vascular) 747.60
  cardiac — see Deformity, heart
  cardiovascular system (congenital) 746.9
  caruncle, lacrimal (congenital) 743.9
    acquired 375.69
  cascade, stomach 537.6
  cecum (congenital) 751.5
    acquired 569.89
  cerebral (congenital) 742.9
    acquired 348.8
  cervix (acquired) (uterus) 622.8
    congenital 752.40
  cheek (acquired) 738.19
    congenital 744.9
  chest (wall) (acquired) 738.3
    congenital 754.89
    late effect of rickets 268.1
  chin (acquired) 738.19
    congenital 744.9
  choroid (congenital) 743.9
    acquired 363.8
    plexus (congenital) 742.9
      acquired 349.2
  cicatricial — see Cicatrix
  cilia (congenital) 743.9
    acquired 374.89
  circulatory system (congenital) 747.9
  clavicle (acquired) 738.8
    congenital 755.51
  clitoris (congenital) 752.40
    acquired 624.8
  clubfoot — see Clubfoot
  coccyx (acquired) 738.6
    congenital 756.10
  colon (congenital) 751.5
    acquired 569.89
  concha (ear) (congenital) (see also Deformity, ear) 744.3
    acquired 380.32
  congenital, organ or site not listed (see also Anomaly) 759.9
  cornea (congenital) 743.9
    acquired 371.70
  coronary artery (congenital) 746.85
    acquired (see also Ischemia, heart) 414.9
  cranium (acquired) 738.19

Deformity

Deformity — continued
  cranium — continued
    congenital (see also Deformity, skull, congenital) 756.0
  cricoid cartilage (congenital) 748.3
    acquired 478.79
  cystic duct (congenital) 751.60
    acquired 575.8
  Dandy-Walker 742.3
    with spina bifida (see also Spina bifida) 741.0 ☑
  diaphragm (congenital) 756.6
    acquired 738.8
  digestive organ(s) or system (congenital) NEC 751.9
    specified type NEC 751.8
  ductus arteriosus 747.0
  duodenal bulb 537.89
  duodenum (congenital) 751.5
    acquired 537.89
  dura (congenital) 742.9
    brain 742.4
      acquired 349.2
    spinal 742.59
      acquired 349.2
  ear (congenital) 744.3
    acquired 380.32
    auricle 744.3
      causing impairment of hearing 744.02
    causing impairment of hearing 744.00
    external 744.3
      causing impairment of hearing 744.02
    internal 744.05
    lobule 744.3
    middle 744.03
      ossicles 744.04
    ossicles 744.04
  ectodermal (congenital) NEC 757.9
    specified type NEC 757.8
  ejaculatory duct (congenital) 752.9
    acquired 608.89
  elbow (joint) (acquired) 736.00
    congenital 755.50
    contraction 718.42
  endocrine gland NEC 759.2
  epididymis (congenital) 752.9
    acquired 608.89
    torsion 608.24
  epiglottis (congenital) 748.3
    acquired 478.79
  esophagus (congenital) 750.9
    acquired 530.89
  Eustachian tube (congenital) NEC 744.3
    specified type NEC 744.24
  extremity (acquired) 736.9
    congenital, except reduction deformity 755.9
      lower 755.60
      upper 755.50
    reduction — see Deformity, reduction
  eye (congenital) 743.9
    acquired 379.8
    muscle 743.9
  eyebrow (congenital) 744.89
  eyelid (congenital) 743.9
    acquired 374.89
    specified type NEC 743.62
  face (acquired) 738.19
    congenital (any part) 744.9
      due to intrauterine malposition and pressure 754.0
  fallopian tube (congenital) 752.10
    acquired 620.8
  femur (acquired) 736.89
    congenital 755.60
  fetal
    with fetopelvic disproportion 653.7 ☑
      affecting fetus or newborn 763.1
    causing obstructed labor 660.1 ☑
      affecting fetus or newborn 763.1

Deformity — continued
  fetal — continued
    known or suspected, affecting management of pregnancy 655.9 ☑
  finger (acquired) 736.20
    boutonniere type 736.21
    congenital 755.50
    flexion contracture 718.44
    swan neck 736.22
  flexion (joint) (acquired) 736.9
    congenital NEC 755.9
    hip or thigh (acquired) 736.39
      congenital (see also Subluxation, congenital, hip) 754.32
  foot (acquired) 736.70
    cavovarus 736.75
      congenital 754.59
    congenital NEC 754.70
      specified type NEC 754.79
    valgus (acquired) 736.79
      congenital 754.60
        specified type NEC 754.69
    varus (acquired) 736.79
      congenital 754.50
        specified type NEC 754.59
  forearm (acquired) 736.00
    congenital 755.50
  forehead (acquired) 738.19
    congenital (see also Deformity, skull, congenital) 756.0
  frontal bone (acquired) 738.19
    congenital (see also Deformity, skull, congenital) 756.0
  gallbladder (congenital) 751.60
    acquired 575.8
  gastrointestinal tract (congenital) NEC 751.9
    acquired 569.89
    specified type NEC 751.8
  genitalia, genital organ(s) or system NEC
    congenital 752.9
    female (congenital) 752.9
      acquired 629.89 ▲
      external 752.40
      internal 752.9
    male (congenital) 752.9
      acquired 608.89
  globe (eye) (congenital) 743.9
    acquired 360.89
  gum (congenital) 750.9
    acquired 523.9
  gunstock 736.02
  hand (acquired) 736.00
    claw 736.06
    congenital 755.50
    minus (and plus) (intrinsic) 736.09
    pill roller (intrinsic) 736.09
    plus (and minus) (intrinsic) 736.09
    swan neck (intrinsic) 736.09
  head (acquired) 738.10
    congenital (see also Deformity, skull congenital) 756.0
    specified NEC 738.19
  heart (congenital) 746.9
    auricle (congenital) 746.9
    septum 745.9
      auricular 745.5
      specified type NEC 745.8
      ventricular 745.4
    valve (congenital) NEC 746.9
      acquired — see Endocarditis
      pulmonary (congenital) 746.00
      specified type NEC 746.89
    ventricle (congenital) 746.9
  heel (acquired) 736.76
    congenital 755.67
  hepatic duct (congenital) 751.60
    acquired 576.8
      with calculus, choledocholithiasis, or stones — see Choledocholithiasis
  hip (joint) (acquired) 736.30
    congenital NEC 755.63

Deformity — continued
  hip — continued
    flexion 718.45
    congenital (see also Subluxation, congenital, hip) 754.32
  hourglass — see Contraction, hourglass
  humerus (acquired) 736.89
    congenital 755.50
  hymen (congenital) 752.40
  hypophyseal (congenital) 759.2
  ileocecal (coil) (valve) (congenital) 751.5
    acquired 569.89
  ileum (intestine) (congenital) 751.5
    acquired 569.89
  ilium (acquired) 738.6
    congenital 755.60
  integument (congenital) 757.9
  intervertebral cartilage or disc (acquired) (see also Displacement, intervertebral disc)
    congenital 756.10
  intestine (large) (small) (congenital) 751.5
    acquired 569.89
  iris (acquired) 364.75
    congenital 743.9
    prolapse 364.8
  ischium (acquired) 738.6
    congenital 755.60
  jaw (acquired) (congenital) NEC 524.9
    due to intrauterine malposition and pressure 754.0
  joint (acquired) NEC 738.8
    congenital 755.9
    contraction (abduction) (adduction) (extension) (flexion) — see Contraction, joint
  kidney(s) (calyx) (pelvis) (congenital) 753.9
    acquired 593.89
    vessel 747.62
      acquired 459.9
  Klippel-Feil (brevicollis) 756.16
  knee (acquired) NEC 736.6
    congenital 755.64
  labium (majus) (minus) (congenital) 752.40
    acquired 624.8
  lacrimal apparatus or duct (congenital) 743.9
    acquired 375.69
  larynx (muscle) (congenital) 748.3
    acquired 478.79
    web (glottic) (subglottic) 748.2
  leg (lower) (upper) (acquired) NEC 736.89
    congenital 755.60
      reduction — see Deformity, reduction, lower limb
  lens (congenital) 743.9
    acquired 379.39
  lid (fold) (congenital) 743.9
    acquired 374.89
  ligament 728.9
    congenital 756.9
  limb (acquired) 736.9
    congenital, except reduction deformity 755.9
      lower 755.60
        reduction (see also Deformity, reduction, lower limb) 755.30
      upper 755.50
        reduction (see also Deformity, reduction, upper limb) 755.20
    specified NEC 736.89
  lip (congenital) NEC 750.9
    acquired 528.5
    specified type NEC 750.26
  liver (congenital) 751.60
    acquired 573.8
    duct (congenital) 751.60

Deformity — continued
  liver — continued
    duct — continued
      acquired 576.8
        with calculus, choledocholithiasis, or stones — see Choledocholithiasis
  lower extremity — see Deformity, leg
  lumbosacral (joint) (region) (congenital) 756.10
    acquired 738.5
  lung (congenital) 748.60
    acquired 518.89
    specified type NEC 748.69
  lymphatic system, congenital 759.9
  Madelung's (radius) 755.54
  maxilla (acquired) (congenital) 524.9
  meninges or membrane (congenital) 742.9
    brain 742.4
      acquired 349.2
    spinal (cord) 742.59
      acquired 349.2
  mesentery (congenital) 751.9
    acquired 568.89
  metacarpus (acquired) 736.00
    congenital 755.50
  metatarsus (acquired) 736.70
    congenital 754.70
  middle ear, except ossicles (congenital) 744.03
    ossicles 744.04
  mitral (leaflets) (valve) (congenital) 746.9
    acquired — see Endocarditis, mitral
    Ebstein's 746.89
    parachute 746.5
    specified type NEC 746.89
    stenosis, congenital 746.5
  mouth (acquired) 528.9
    congenital NEC 750.9
      specified type NEC 750.26
  multiple, congenital NEC 759.7
    specified type NEC 759.89
  muscle (acquired) 728.9
    congenital 756.9
      specified type NEC 756.89
      sternocleidomastoid (due to intrauterine malposition and pressure) 754.1
  musculoskeletal system, congenital NEC 756.9
    specified type NEC 756.9
  nail (acquired) 703.9
    congenital 757.9
  nasal — see Deformity, nose
  neck (acquired) NEC 738.2
    congenital (any part) 744.9
      sternocleidomastoid 754.1
  nervous system (congenital) 742.9
  nipple (congenital) 757.9
    acquired 611.8
  nose, nasal (cartilage) (acquired) 738.0
    bone (turbinate) 738.0
    congenital 748.1
      bent 754.0
      squashed 754.0
    saddle 738.0
      syphilitic 090.5
    septum 470
      congenital 748.1
    sinus (wall) (congenital) 748.1
      acquired 738.0
    syphilitic (congenital) 090.5
      late 095.8
  ocular muscle (congenital) 743.9
    acquired 378.60
  opticociliary vessels (congenital) 743.9
  orbit (congenital) (eye) 743.9
    acquired NEC 376.40
      associated with craniofacial deformities 376.44
      due to
        bone disease 376.43

Deformity — *continued*
  orbit — *continued*
    acquired — *continued*
      due to — *continued*
        surgery 376.47
        trauma 376.47
  organ of Corti (congenital) 744.05
  ovary (congenital) 752.0
    acquired 620.8
  oviduct (congenital) 752.10
    acquired 620.8
  palate (congenital) 750.9
    acquired 526.89
    cleft (congenital) (*see also* Cleft, palate) 749.00
    hard, acquired 526.89
    soft, acquired 528.9
  pancreas (congenital) 751.7
    acquired 577.8
  parachute, mitral valve 746.5
  parathyroid (gland) 759.2
  parotid (gland) (congenital) 750.9
    acquired 527.8
  patella (acquired) 736.6
    congenital 755.64
  pelvis, pelvic (acquired) (bony) 738.6
    with disproportion (fetopelvic) 653.0 ☑
      affecting fetus or newborn 763.1
      causing obstructed labor 660.1 ☑
        affecting fetus or newborn 763.1
    congenital 755.60
    rachitic (late effect) 268.1
  penis (glans) (congenital) 752.9
    acquired 607.89
  pericardium (congenital) 746.9
    acquired — *see* Pericarditis
  pharynx (congenital) 750.9
    acquired 478.29
  Pierre Robin (congenital) 756.0
  pinna (acquired) 380.32
    congenital 744.3
  pituitary (congenital) 759.2
  pleural folds (congenital) 748.8
  portal vein (congenital) 747.40
  posture — *see* Curvature, spine
  prepuce (congenital) 752.9
    acquired 607.89
  prostate (congenital) 752.9
    acquired 602.8
  pulmonary valve — *see* Endocarditis, pulmonary
  pupil (congenital) 743.9
    acquired 364.75
  pylorus (congenital) 750.9
    acquired 537.89
  rachitic (acquired), healed or old 268.1
  radius (acquired) 736.00
    congenital 755.50
    reduction — *see* Deformity, reduction, upper limb
  rectovaginal septum (congenital) 752.40
    acquired 623.8
  rectum (congenital) 751.5
    acquired 569.49
  reduction (extremity) (limb) 755.4
    brain 742.2
    lower limb 755.30
      with complete absence of distal elements 755.31
      longitudinal (complete) (partial) (with distal deficiencies, incomplete) 755.32
        with complete absence of distal elements 755.31
        combined femoral, tibial, fibular (incomplete) 755.33
        femoral 755.34
        fibular 755.37
        metatarsal(s) 755.38
        phalange(s) 755.39
          meaning all digits 755.31

Deformity — *continued*
  reduction — *continued*
    lower limb — *continued*
      longitudinal — *continued*
        tarsal(s) 755.38
        tibia 755.36
        tibiofibular 755.35
      transverse 755.31
    upper limb 755.20
      with complete absence of distal elements 755.21
      longitudinal (complete) (partial) (with distal deficiencies, incomplete) 755.22
        with complete absence of distal elements 755.21
        carpal(s) 755.28
        combined humeral, radial, ulnar (incomplete) 755.23
        humeral 755.24
        metacarpal(s) 755.28
        phalange(s) 755.29
          meaning all digits 755.21
        radial 755.26
        radioulnar 755.25
        ulnar 755.27
      transverse (complete) (partial) 755.21
    renal — *see* Deformity, kidney
  respiratory system (congenital) 748.9
    specified type NEC 748.8
  rib (acquired) 738.3
    congenital 756.3
    cervical 756.2
  rotation (joint) (acquired) 736.9
    congenital 755.9
    hip or thigh 736.39
      congenital (*see also* Subluxation, congenital, hip) 754.32
  sacroiliac joint (congenital) 755.69
    acquired 738.5
  sacrum (acquired) 738.5
    congenital 756.10
  saddle
    back 737.8
    nose 738.0
      syphilitic 090.5
  salivary gland or duct (congenital) 750.9
    acquired 527.8
  scapula (acquired) 736.89
    congenital 755.50
  scrotum (congenital) 752.9
    acquired 608.89
  sebaceous gland, acquired 706.8
  seminal tract or duct (congenital) 752.9
    acquired 608.89
  septum (nasal) (acquired) 470
    congenital 748.1
  shoulder (joint) (acquired) 736.89
    congenital 755.50
      specified type NEC 755.59
    contraction 718.41
  sigmoid (flexure) (congenital) 751.5
    acquired 569.89
  sinus of Valsalva 747.29
  skin (congenital) 757.9
    acquired NEC 709.8
  skull (acquired) 738.19
    congenital 756.0
      with
        anencephalus 740.0
        encephalocele 742.0
        hydrocephalus 742.3
          with spina bifida (*see also* Spina bifida) 741.0 ☑
        microcephalus 742.1
      due to intrauterine malposition and pressure 754.0
  soft parts, organs or tissues (of pelvis)
    in pregnancy or childbirth NEC 654.9 ☑

Deformity — *continued*
  soft parts, organs or tissues — *continued*
    in pregnancy or childbirth — *continued*
      affecting fetus or newborn 763.89
      causing obstructed labor 660.2 ☑
        affecting fetus or newborn 763.1
  spermatic cord (congenital) 752.9
    acquired 608.89
      torsion 608.22 ▲
        extravaginal 608.21 ●
        intravaginal 608.22 ●
  spinal
    column — *see* Deformity, spine
    cord (congenital) 742.9
      acquired 336.8
      vessel (congenital) 747.82
    nerve root (congenital) 742.9
      acquired 724.9
  spine (acquired) NEC 738.5
    congenital 756.10
      due to intrauterine malposition and pressure 754.2
    kyphoscoliotic (*see also* Kyphoscoliosis) 737.30
    kyphotic (*see also* Kyphosis) 737.10
    lordotic (*see also* Lordosis) 737.20
    rachitic 268.1
    scoliotic (*see also* Scoliosis) 737.30
  spleen
    acquired 289.59
    congenital 759.0
  Sprengel's (congenital) 755.52
  sternum (acquired) 738.3
    congenital 756.3
  stomach (acquired) 750.9
    acquired 537.89
  submaxillary gland (congenital) 750.9
    acquired 527.8
  swan neck (acquired)
    finger 736.22
    hand 736.09
  talipes — *see* Talipes
  teeth, tooth NEC 520.9
  testis (congenital) 752.9
    acquired 608.89
      torsion 608.20 ▲
  thigh (acquired) 736.89
    congenital 755.60
  thorax (acquired) (wall) 738.3
    congenital 754.89
    late effect of rickets 268.1
  thumb (acquired) 736.20
    congenital 755.50
  thymus (tissue) (congenital) 759.2
  thyroid (gland) (congenital) 759.2
    cartilage 748.3
      acquired 478.79
  tibia (acquired) 736.89
    congenital 755.60
    saber 090.5
  toe (acquired) 735.9
    congenital 755.66
    specified NEC 735.8
  tongue (congenital) 750.10
    acquired 529.8
  tooth, teeth NEC 520.9
  trachea (rings) (congenital) 748.3
    acquired 519.19 ▲
  transverse aortic arch (congenital) 747.21
  tricuspid (leaflets) (valve) (congenital) 746.9
    acquired — *see* Endocarditis, tricuspid
    atresia or stenosis 746.1
    specified type NEC 746.89
  trunk (acquired) 738.3
    congenital 759.9
  ulna (acquired) 736.00
    congenital 755.50

Deformity — *continued*
  upper extremity — *see* Deformity, arm
  urachus (congenital) 753.7
  ureter (opening) (congenital) 753.9
    acquired 593.89
  urethra (valve) (congenital) 753.9
    acquired 599.84
  urinary tract or system (congenital) 753.9
    urachus 753.7
  uterus (congenital) 752.3
    acquired 621.8
  uvula (congenital) 750.9
    acquired 528.9
  vagina (congenital) 752.40
    acquired 623.8
  valve, valvular (heart) (congenital) 746.9
    acquired — *see* Endocarditis
    pulmonary 746.00
    specified type NEC 746.89
  vascular (congenital) (peripheral) NEC 747.60
    acquired 459.9
    gastrointestinal 747.61
    lower limb 747.64
    renal 747.62
    specified site NEC 747.69
    spinal 747.82
    upper limb 747.63
  vas deferens (congenital) 752.9
    acquired 608.89
  vein (congenital) NEC (*see also* Deformity, vascular) 747.60
    brain 747.81
    coronary 746.9
    great 747.40
  vena cava (inferior) (superior) (congenital) 747.40
  vertebra — *see* Deformity, spine
  vesicourethral orifice (acquired) 596.8
    congenital NEC 753.9
    specified type NEC 753.8
  vessels of optic papilla (congenital) 743.9
  visual field (contraction) 368.45
  vitreous humor (congenital) 743.9
    acquired 379.29
  vulva (congenital) 752.40
    acquired 624.8
  wrist (joint) (acquired) 736.00
    congenital 755.50
    contraction 718.43
    valgus 736.03
      congenital 755.59
    varus 736.04
      congenital 755.59

Degeneration, degenerative
  adrenal (capsule) (gland) 255.8
    with hypofunction 255.4
    fatty 255.8
    hyaline 255.8
    infectional 255.8
    lardaceous 277.39 ▲
  amyloid (any site) (general) 277.39 ▲
  anterior cornua, spinal cord 336.8
  aorta, aortic 440.0
    fatty 447.8
    valve (heart) (*see also* Endocarditis, aortic) 424.1
  arteriovascular — *see* Arteriosclerosis
  artery, arterial (atheromatous) (calcareous) (*see also* Arteriosclerosis)
    amyloid 277.39 ▲
    lardaceous 277.39 ▲
    medial NEC (*see also* Arteriosclerosis, extremities) 440.20
  articular cartilage NEC (*see also* Disorder, cartilage, articular) 718.0 ☑
    elbow 718.02
    knee 717.5
    patella 717.7
    shoulder 718.01
    spine (*see also* Spondylosis) 721.90

Degeneration, degenerative

Degeneration, degenerative — *continued*
- atheromatous — *see* Arteriosclerosis
- bacony (any site) 277.39 ▲
- basal nuclei or ganglia NEC 333.0
- bone 733.90
- brachial plexus 353.0
- brain (cortical) (progressive) 331.9
  - arteriosclerotic 437.0
  - childhood 330.9
    - specified type NEC 330.8
  - congenital 742.4
  - cystic 348.0
    - congenital 742.4
  - familial NEC 331.89
  - grey matter 330.8
  - heredofamilial NEC 331.89
  - in
    - alcoholism 303.9 ☑ *[331.7]*
    - beriberi 265.0 *[331.7]*
    - cerebrovascular disease 437.9 *[331.7]*
    - congenital hydrocephalus 742.3 *[331.7]*
      - with spina bifida (*see also* Spina bifida) 741.0 ☑ *[331.7]*
    - Fabry's disease 272.7 *[330.2]*
    - Gaucher's disease 272.7 *[330.2]*
    - Hunter's disease or syndrome 277.5 *[330.3]*
    - lipidosis
      - cerebral 330.1
      - generalized 272.7 *[330.2]*
    - mucopolysaccharidosis 277.5 *[330.3]*
    - myxedema (*see also* Myxedema) 244.9 *[331.7]*
    - neoplastic disease NEC (M8000/1) 239.9 *[331.7]*
    - Niemann-Pick disease 272.7 *[330.2]*
    - sphingolipidosis 272.7 *[330.2]*
    - vitamin B₁₂ deficiency 266.2 *[331.7]*
  - motor centers 331.89
  - senile 331.2
  - specified type NEC 331.89
- breast — *see* Disease, breast
- Bruch's membrane 363.40
- bundle of His 426.50
  - left 426.3
  - right 426.4
- calcareous NEC 275.49
- capillaries 448.9
  - amyloid 277.39 ▲
  - fatty 448.9
  - lardaceous 277.39 ▲
- cardiac (brown) (calcareous) (fatty) (fibrous) (hyaline) (mural) (muscular) (pigmentary) (senile) (with arteriosclerosis) (*see also* Degeneration, myocardial) 429.1
  - valve, valvular — *see* Endocarditis
- cardiorenal (*see also* Hypertension, cardiorenal) 404.90
- cardiovascular (*see also* Disease, cardiovascular) 429.2
  - renal (*see also* Hypertension, cardiorenal) 404.90
- cartilage (joint) — *see* Derangement, joint
- cerebellar NEC 334.9
  - primary (hereditary) (sporadic) 334.2
- cerebral — *see* Degeneration, brain
- cerebromacular 330.1
- cerebrovascular 437.1
  - due to hypertension 437.2
  - late effect — *see* Late effect(s) (of) cerebrovascular disease
- cervical plexus 353.2
- cervix 622.8
  - due to radiation (intended effect) 622.8

Degeneration, degenerative — *continued*
- cervix — *continued*
  - due to radiation — *continued*
    - adverse effect or misadventure 622.8
  - changes, spine or vertebra (*see also* Spondylosis) 721.90
- chitinous 277.39 ▲
- chorioretinal 363.40
  - congenital 743.53
  - hereditary 363.50
- choroid (colloid) (drusen) 363.40
  - hereditary 363.50
  - senile 363.41
    - diffuse secondary 363.42
- cochlear 386.8
- collateral ligament (knee) (medial) 717.82
  - lateral 717.81
- combined (spinal cord) (subacute) 266.2 *[336.2]*
  - with anemia (pernicious) 281.0 *[336.2]*
    - due to dietary deficiency 281.1 *[336.2]*
  - due to vitamin B₁₂ deficiency anemia (dietary) 281.1 *[336.2]*
- conjunctiva 372.50
  - amyloid 277.39 *[372.50]* ▲
- cornea 371.40
  - calcerous 371.44
  - familial (hereditary) (*see also* Dystrophy, cornea) 371.50
    - macular 371.55
    - reticular 371.54
  - hyaline (of old scars) 371.41
  - marginal (Terrien's) 371.48
  - mosaic (shagreen) 371.41
  - nodular 371.46
  - peripheral 371.48
  - senile 371.41
- cortical (cerebellar) (parenchymatous) 334.2
  - alcoholic 303.9 ☑ *[334.4]*
  - diffuse, due to arteriopathy 437.0
- corticostriatal-spinal 334.8
- cretinoid 243
- cruciate ligament (knee) (posterior) 717.84
  - anterior 717.83
- cutis 709.3
  - amyloid 277.39 ▲
- dental pulp 522.2
- disc disease — *see* Degeneration, intervertebral disc
- dorsolateral (spinal cord) — *see* Degeneration, combined
- endocardial 424.90
- extrapyramidal NEC 333.90
- eye NEC 360.40
  - macular (*see also* Degeneration, macula) 362.50
    - congenital 362.75
    - hereditary 362.76
  - fatty (diffuse) (general) 272.8
    - liver 571.8
      - alcoholic 571.0
    - localized site — *see* Degeneration, by site, fatty
    - placenta — *see* Placenta, abnormal
  - globe (eye) NEC 360.40
    - macular — *see* Degeneration, macula
- grey matter 330.8
- heart (brown) (calcareous) (fatty) (fibrous) (hyaline) (mural) (muscular) (pigmentary) (senile) (with arteriosclerosis) (*see also* Degeneration, myocardial) 429.1
  - amyloid 277.39 *[425.7]* ▲
  - atheromatous — *see* Arteriosclerosis, coronary
  - gouty 274.82
  - hypertensive (*see also* Hypertension, heart) 402.90

Degeneration, degenerative — *continued*
- heart (*see also* Degeneration, myocardial) — *continued*
  - ischemic 414.9
  - valve, valvular — *see* Endocarditis
- hepatolenticular (Wilson's) 275.1
- hepatorenal 572.4
- heredofamilial
  - brain NEC 331.89
  - spinal cord NEC 336.8
- hyaline (diffuse) (generalized) 728.9
  - localized (*see also* Degeneration, by site)
    - cornea 371.41
    - keratitis 371.41
- hypertensive vascular — *see* Hypertension
- infrapatellar fat pad 729.31
- internal semilunar cartilage 717.3
- intervertebral disc 722.6
  - with myelopathy 722.70
  - cervical, cervicothoracic 722.4
    - with myelopathy 722.71
  - lumbar, lumbosacral 722.52
    - with myelopathy 722.73
  - thoracic, thoracolumbar 722.51
    - with myelopathy 722.72
- intestine 569.89
  - amyloid 277.39 ▲
  - lardaceous 277.39 ▲
- iris (generalized) (*see also* Atrophy, iris) 364.59
  - pigmentary 364.53
  - pupillary margin 364.54
- ischemic — *see* Ischemia
- joint disease (*see also* Osteoarthrosis) 715.9 ☑
  - multiple sites 715.09
  - spine (*see also* Spondylosis) 721.90
- kidney (*see also* Sclerosis, renal) 587
  - amyloid 277.39 *[583.81]* ▲
  - cyst, cystic (multiple) (solitary) 593.2
    - congenital (*see also* Cystic, disease, kidney) 753.10
  - fatty 593.89
  - fibrocystic (congenital) 753.19
  - lardaceous 277.39 *[583.81]* ▲
  - polycystic (congenital) 753.12
    - adult type (APKD) 753.13
    - autosomal dominant 753.13
    - autosomal recessive 753.14
    - childhood type (CPKD) 753.14
    - infantile type 753.14
  - waxy 277.39 *[583.81]* ▲
- Kuhnt-Junius (retina) 362.52
- labyrinth, osseous 386.8
- lacrimal passages, cystic 375.12
- lardaceous (any site) 277.39 ▲
- lateral column (posterior), spinal cord (*see also* Degeneration, combined) 266.2 *[336.2]*
- lattice 362.63
- lens 366.9
  - infantile, juvenile, or presenile 366.00
  - senile 366.10
- lenticular (familial) (progressive) (Wilson's) (with cirrhosis of liver) 275.1
  - striate artery 437.0
- lethal ball, prosthetic heart valve 996.02
- ligament
  - collateral (knee) (medial) 717.82
    - lateral 717.81
  - cruciate (knee) (posterior) 717.84
    - anterior 717.83
- liver (diffuse) 572.8
  - amyloid 277.39 ▲
  - congenital (cystic) 751.62
  - cystic 572.8
    - congenital 751.62
  - fatty 571.8
    - alcoholic 571.0

Degeneration, degenerative — *continued*
- liver — *continued*
  - hypertrophic 572.8
  - lardaceous 277.39 ▲
  - parenchymatous, acute or subacute (*see also* Necrosis, liver) 570
  - pigmentary 572.8
  - toxic (acute) 573.8
  - waxy 277.39 ▲
- lung 518.89
- lymph gland 289.3
  - hyaline 289.3
  - lardaceous 277.39 ▲
- macula (acquired) (senile) 362.50
  - atrophic 362.51
  - Best's 362.76
  - congenital 362.75
  - cystic 362.54
  - cystoid 362.53
  - disciform 362.52
  - dry 362.51
  - exudative 362.52
  - familial pseudoinflammatory 362.77
  - hereditary 362.76
  - hole 362.54
  - juvenile (Stargardt's) 362.75
  - nonexudative 362.51
  - pseudohole 362.54
  - wet 362.52
- medullary — *see* Degeneration, brain
- membranous labyrinth, congenital (causing impairment of hearing) 744.05
- meniscus — *see* Derangement, joint
- microcystoid 362.62
- mitral — *see* Insufficiency, mitral
- Mönckeberg's (*see also* Arteriosclerosis, extremities) 440.20
- moral 301.7
- motor centers, senile 331.2
- mural (*see also* Degeneration, myocardial) 429.1
  - heart, cardiac (*see also* Degeneration, myocardial) 429.1
  - myocardium, myocardial (*see also* Degeneration, myocardial) 429.1
- muscle 728.9
  - fatty 728.9
  - fibrous 728.9
  - heart (*see also* Degeneration, myocardial) 429.1
  - hyaline 728.9
- muscular progressive 728.2
- myelin, central nervous system NEC 341.9
- myocardium, myocardial (brown) (calcareous) (fatty) (fibrous) (hyaline) (mural) (muscular) (pigmentary) (senile) (with arteriosclerosis) 429.1
  - with rheumatic fever (conditions classifiable to 390) 398.0
    - active, acute, or subacute 391.2
      - with chorea 392.0
    - inactive or quiescent (with chorea) 398.0
  - amyloid 277.39 *[425.7]* ▲
  - congenital 746.89
  - fetus or newborn 779.89
  - gouty 274.82
  - hypertensive (*see also* Hypertension, heart) 402.90
  - ischemic 414.8
  - rheumatic (*see also* Degeneration, myocardium, with rheumatic fever) 398.0
  - syphilitic 093.82
- nasal sinus (mucosa) (*see also* Sinusitis) 473.9
  - frontal 473.1
  - maxillary 473.0
- nerve — *see* Disorder, nerve

Degeneration, degenerative

Degeneration, degenerative — *continued*
- nervous system 349.89
  - amyloid 277.39 [357.4] ▲
  - autonomic (*see also* Neuropathy, peripheral, autonomic) 337.9
    - fatty 349.89
    - peripheral autonomic NEC (*see also* Neuropathy, peripheral, autonomic) 337.9
- nipple 611.9
- nose 478.19 ▲
- oculoacousticocerebral, congenital (progressive) 743.8
- olivopontocerebellar (familial) (hereditary) 333.0
- osseous labyrinth 386.8
- ovary 620.8
  - cystic 620.2
  - microcystic 620.2
- pallidal, pigmentary (progressive) 333.0
- pancreas 577.8
  - tuberculous (*see also* Tuberculosis) 017.9
- papillary muscle 429.81
- paving stone 362.61
- penis 607.89
- peritoneum 568.89
- pigmentary (diffuse) (general)
  - localized — *see* Degeneration, by site
  - pallidal (progressive) 333.0
  - secondary 362.65
- pineal gland 259.8
- pituitary (gland) 253.8
- placenta (fatty) (fibrinoid) (fibroid) — *see* Placenta, abnormal
- popliteal fat pad 729.31
- posterolateral (spinal cord) (*see also* Degeneration, combined) 266.2 [336.2]
- pulmonary valve (heart) (*see also* Endocarditis, pulmonary) 424.3
- pulp (tooth) 522.2
- pupillary margin 364.54
- renal (*see also* Sclerosis, renal) 587
  - fibrocystic 753.19
  - polycystic 753.12
    - adult type (APKD) 753.13
    - autosomal dominant 753.13
    - autosomal recessive 753.14
    - childhood type (CPKD) 753.14
    - infantile type 753.14
- reticuloendothelial system 289.89
- retina (peripheral) 362.60
  - with retinal defect (*see also* Detachment, retina, with retinal defect) 361.00
  - cystic (senile) 362.50
  - cystoid 362.53
  - hereditary (*see also* Dystrophy, retina) 362.70
    - cerebroretinal 362.71
    - congenital 362.75
    - juvenile (Stargardt's) 362.75
    - macula 362.76
    - Kuhnt-Junius 362.52
  - lattice 362.63
  - macular (*see also* Degeneration, macula) 362.50
  - microcystoid 362.62
  - palisade 362.63
  - paving stone 362.61
  - pigmentary (primary) 362.74
    - secondary 362.65
  - posterior pole (*see also* Degeneration, macula) 362.50
  - secondary 362.66
  - senile 362.60
    - cystic 362.53
    - reticular 362.64
- saccule, congenital (causing impairment of hearing) 744.05
- sacculocochlear 386.8
- senile 797

Degeneration, degenerative — *continued*
- senile — *continued*
  - brain 331.2
  - cardiac, heart, or myocardium (*see also* Degeneration, myocardial) 429.1
  - motor centers 331.2
  - reticule 362.64
  - retina, cystic 362.50
  - vascular — *see* Arteriosclerosis
- silicone rubber poppet (prosthetic valve) 996.02
- sinus (cystic) (*see also* Sinusitis) 473.9
  - polypoid 471.1
- skin 709.3
  - amyloid 277.39 ▲
  - colloid 709.3
- spinal (cord) 336.8
  - amyloid 277.39 ▲
  - column 733.90
  - combined (subacute) (*see also* Degeneration, combined) 266.2 [336.2]
    - with anemia (pernicious) 281.0 [336.2]
  - dorsolateral (*see also* Degeneration, combined) 266.2 [336.2]
  - familial NEC 336.8
  - fatty 336.8
  - funicular (*see also* Degeneration, combined) 266.2 [336.2]
  - heredofamilial NEC 336.8
  - posterolateral (*see also* Degeneration, combined) 266.2 [336.2]
  - subacute combined — *see* Degeneration, combined
  - tuberculous (*see also* Tuberculosis) 013.8 ☑
- spine 733.90
- spleen 289.59
  - amyloid 277.39 ▲
  - lardaceous 277.39 ▲
- stomach 537.89
  - lardaceous 277.39 ▲
- strionigral 333.0
- sudoriparous (cystic) 705.89
- suprarenal (capsule) (gland) 255.8
  - with hypofunction 255.4
- sweat gland 705.89
- synovial membrane (pulpy) 727.9
- tapetoretinal 362.74
  - adult or presenile form 362.50
- testis (postinfectional) 608.89
- thymus (gland) 254.8
  - fatty 254.8
  - lardaceous 277.39 ▲
- thyroid (gland) 246.8
- tricuspid (heart) (valve) — *see* Endocarditis, tricuspid
- tuberculous NEC (*see also* Tuberculosis) 011.9 ☑
- turbinate 733.90
- uterus 621.8
  - cystic 621.8
- vascular (senile) (*see also* Arteriosclerosis)
  - hypertensive — *see* Hypertension
- vitreoretinal (primary) 362.73
  - secondary 362.66
- vitreous humor (with infiltration) 379.21
- wallerian NEC — *see* Disorder, nerve
- waxy (any site) 277.39 ▲
- Wilson's hepatolenticular 275.1

Deglutition
- paralysis 784.99
  - hysterical 300.11
- pneumonia 507.0

Degos' disease or syndrome 447.8

Degradation disorder, branched-chain amino acid 270.3

Dehiscence
- anastomosis — *see* Complications, anastomosis
- cesarean wound 674.1 ☑

Dehiscence — *continued*
- episiotomy 674.2 ☑
- operation wound 998.32
  - internal 998.31
- perineal wound (postpartum) 674.2 ☑
- postoperative 998.32
  - abdomen 998.32
    - internal 998.31
  - internal 998.31
- uterine wound 674.1 ☑

Dehydration (cachexia) 276.51
- with
  - hypernatremia 276.0
  - hyponatremia 276.1
- newborn 775.5

Deiters' nucleus syndrome 386.19
Déjérine's disease 356.0
Déjérine-Klumpke paralysis 767.6
Déjérine-Roussy syndrome 338.0 ▲
Déjérine-Sottas disease or neuropathy (hypertrophic) 356.0
Déjérine-Thomas atrophy or syndrome 333.0
de Lange's syndrome (Amsterdam dwarf, mental retardation, and brachycephaly) 759.89

Delay, delayed
- adaptation, cones or rods 368.63
- any plane in pelvis
  - affecting fetus or newborn 763.1
  - complicating delivery 660.1 ☑
- birth or delivery NEC 662.1 ☑
  - affecting fetus or newborn 763.89
  - second twin, triplet, or multiple mate 662.3 ☑
- closure (*see also* Fistula)
  - cranial suture 756.0
  - fontanel 756.0
- coagulation NEC 790.92
- conduction (cardiac) (ventricular) 426.9
- delivery NEC 662.1 ☑
  - second twin, triplet, etc. 662.3 ☑
    - affecting fetus or newborn 763.89
- development
  - in childhood 783.40
    - physiological 783.40
  - intellectual NEC 315.9
  - learning NEC 315.2
  - reading 315.00
  - sexual 259.0
  - speech 315.39
    - associated with hyperkinesis 314.1
    - spelling 315.09
- gastric emptying 536.8
- menarche 256.39
  - due to pituitary hypofunction 253.4
- menstruation (cause unknown) 626.8
- milestone in childhood 783.42
- motility — *see* Hypomotility
- passage of meconium (newborn) 777.1
- primary respiration 768.9
- puberty 259.0
- separation of umbilical cord 779.83
- sexual maturation, female 259.0

Del Castillo's syndrome (germinal aplasia) 606.0
Déleage's disease 359.89
Deletion syndrome
- 5p 758.31
- 22q11.2 758.32
- autosomal NEC 758.39
- constitutional 5q deletion 758.39 ●

Delhi (boil) (button) (sore) 085.1
Delinquency (juvenile) 312.9
- group (*see also* Disturbance, conduct) 312.2 ☑
- neurotic 312.4

Delirium, delirious 780.09
- acute (psychotic) 293.0
- alcoholic 291.0
  - acute 291.0
  - chronic 291.1

Delirium, delirious — *continued*
- alcoholicum 291.0
- chronic (*see also* Psychosis) 293.89
  - due to or associated with physical condition — *see* Psychosis, organic
- drug-induced 292.81
- due to conditions classified elsewhere 293.0
- eclamptic (*see also* Eclampsia) 780.39
- exhaustion (*see also* Reaction, stress, acute) 308.9
- hysterical 300.11
- in
  - presenile dementia 290.11
  - senile dementia 290.3
- induced by drug 292.81
- manic, maniacal (acute) (*see also* Psychosis, affective) 296.0 ☑
  - recurrent episode 296.1 ☑
  - single episode 296.0 ☑
- puerperal 293.9
- senile 290.3
- subacute (psychotic) 293.1
- thyroid (*see also* Thyrotoxicosis) 242.9 ☑
- traumatic (*see also* Injury, intracranial)
  - with
    - lesion, spinal cord — *see* Injury, spinal, by site
    - shock, spinal — *see* Injury, spinal, by site
- tremens (impending) 291.0
- uremic — *see* Uremia
- withdrawal
  - alcoholic (acute) 291.0
    - chronic 291.1
  - drug 292.0

Delivery

Note — Use the following fifth-digit subclassification with categories 640–648, 651–676:

0	unspecified as to episode of care
1	delivered, with or without mention of antepartum condition
2	delivered, with mention of postpartum complication
3	antepartum condition or complication
4	postpartum condition or complication

- breech (assisted) (buttocks) (complete) (frank) (spontaneous) 652.2 ☑
  - affecting fetus or newborn 763.0
- extraction NEC 669.6 ☑
- cesarean (for) 669.7 ☑
  - abnormal
    - cervix 654.6 ☑
    - pelvic organs or tissues 654.9 ☑
    - pelvis (bony) (major) NEC 653.0 ☑
    - presentation or position 652.9 ☑
      - in multiple gestation 652.6 ☑
    - size, fetus 653.5 ☑
    - soft parts (of pelvis) 654.9 ☑
    - uterus, congenital 654.0 ☑
    - vagina 654.7 ☑
    - vulva 654.8 ☑
  - abruptio placentae 641.2 ☑
  - acromion presentation 652.8 ☑
    - affecting fetus or newborn 763.4
  - anteversion, cervix or uterus 654.4 ☑
  - atony, uterus, ▶with hemorrhage◀ 666.1 ☑
  - bicornis or bicornuate uterus 654.0 ☑
  - breech presentation (buttocks) (complete) (frank) 652.2 ☑
  - brow presentation 652.4 ☑

Index to Diseases — Delivery

Delivery — *continued*
  cesarean — *continued*
    cephalopelvic disproportion (normally formed fetus) 653.4 ☑
    chin presentation 652.4 ☑
    cicatrix of cervix 654.6 ☑
    contracted pelvis (general) 653.1 ☑
      inlet 653.2 ☑
      outlet 653.3 ☑
    cord presentation or prolapse 663.0 ☑
    cystocele 654.4 ☑
    deformity (acquired) (congenital)
      pelvic organs or tissues NEC 654.9 ☑
      pelvis (bony) NEC 653.0 ☑
    displacement, uterus NEC 654.4 ☑
    disproportion NEC 653.9 ☑
    distress
      fetal 656.8 ☑
      maternal 669.0 ☑
    eclampsia 642.6 ☑
    face presentation 652.4 ☑
    failed
      forceps 660.7 ☑
      trial of labor NEC 660.6 ☑
      vacuum extraction 660.7 ☑
      ventouse 660.7 ☑
    fetal deformity 653.7 ☑
    fetal-maternal hemorrhage 656.0 ☑
    fetus, fetal
      distress 656.8 ☑
      prematurity 656.8 ☑
    fibroid (tumor) (uterus) 654.1 ☑
    footling 652.8 ☑
      with successful version 652.1 ☑
    hemorrhage (antepartum) (intrapartum) NEC 641.9 ☑
    hydrocephalic fetus 653.6 ☑
    incarceration of uterus 654.3 ☑
    incoordinate uterine action 661.4 ☑
    inertia, uterus 661.2 ☑
      primary 661.0 ☑
      secondary 661.1 ☑
    lateroversion, uterus or cervix 654.4 ☑
    mal lie 652.9 ☑
    malposition
      fetus 652.9 ☑
        in multiple gestation 652.6 ☑
      pelvic organs or tissues NEC 654.9 ☑
      uterus NEC or cervix 654.4 ☑
    malpresentation NEC 652.9 ☑
      in multiple gestation 652.6 ☑
    maternal
      diabetes mellitus 648.0 ☑
      heart disease NEC 648.6 ☑
    meconium in liquor 656.8 ☑
      staining only 792.3
    oblique presentation 652.3 ☑
    oversize fetus 653.5 ☑
    pelvic tumor NEC 654.9 ☑
    placental insufficiency 656.5 ☑
    placenta previa 641.0 ☑
      with hemorrhage 641.1 ☑
    poor dilation, cervix 661.0 ☑
    pre-eclampsia 642.4 ☑
      severe 642.5 ☑
    previous
      cesarean delivery, section 654.2 ☑
      surgery (to)
        cervix 654.6 ☑
        gynecological NEC 654.9 ☑
        rectum 654.8 ☑
        uterus NEC 654.9 ☑
          previous cesarean delivery, section 654.2 ☑
        vagina 654.7 ☑
    prolapse
      arm or hand 652.7 ☑

Delivery — *continued*
  cesarean — *continued*
    prolapse — *continued*
      uterus 654.4 ☑
    prolonged labor 662.1 ☑
    rectocele 654.4 ☑
    retroversion, uterus or cervix 654.3 ☑
    rigid
      cervix 654.6 ☑
      pelvic floor 654.4 ☑
      perineum 654.8 ☑
      vagina 654.7 ☑
      vulva 654.8 ☑
    sacculation, pregnant uterus 654.4 ☑
    scar(s)
      cervix 654.6 ☑
      cesarean delivery, section 654.2 ☑
      uterus NEC 654.9 ☑
        due to previous cesarean delivery, section 654.2 ☑
    Shirodkar suture in situ 654.5 ☑
    shoulder presentation 652.8 ☑
    stenosis or stricture, cervix 654.6 ☑
    transverse presentation or lie 652.3 ☑
    tumor, pelvic organs or tissues NEC 654.4 ☑
    umbilical cord presentation or prolapse 663.0 ☑
  completely normal case — *see* category 650
  complicated (by) NEC 669.9 ☑
    abdominal tumor, fetal 653.7 ☑
      causing obstructed labor 660.1 ☑
    abnormal, abnormality of
      cervix 654.6 ☑
        causing obstructed labor 660.2 ☑
      forces of labor 661.9 ☑
      formation of uterus 654.0 ☑
      pelvic organs or tissues 654.9 ☑
        causing obstructed labor 660.2 ☑
      pelvis (bony) (major) NEC 653.0 ☑
        causing obstructed labor 660.1 ☑
      presentation or position NEC 652.9 ☑
        causing obstructed labor 660.0 ☑
      size, fetus 653.5 ☑
        causing obstructed labor 660.1 ☑
      soft parts (of pelvis) 654.9 ☑
        causing obstructed labor 660.2 ☑
      uterine contractions NEC 661.9 ☑
      uterus (formation) 654.0 ☑
        causing obstructed labor 660.2 ☑
      vagina 654.7 ☑
        causing obstructed labor 660.2 ☑
    abnormally formed uterus (any type) (congenital) 654.0 ☑
      causing obstructed labor 660.2 ☑
    acromion presentation 652.8 ☑
      causing obstructed labor 660.0 ☑
    adherent placenta 667.0 ☑
      with hemorrhage 666.0 ☑
    adhesions, uterus (to abdominal wall) 654.4 ☑
    advanced maternal age NEC 659.6 ☑
      multigravida 659.6 ☑
      primigravida 659.5 ☑

Delivery — *continued*
  complicated — *continued*
    air embolism 673.0 ☑
    amnionitis 658.4 ☑
    amniotic fluid embolism 673.1 ☑
    anesthetic death 668.9 ☑
    annular detachment, cervix 665.3 ☑
    antepartum hemorrhage — *see* Delivery, complicated, hemorrhage
    anteversion, cervix or uterus 654.4 ☑
      causing obstructed labor 660.2 ☑
    apoplexy 674.0 ☑
      placenta 641.2 ☑
    arrested active phase 661.1 ☑
    asymmetrical pelvis bone 653.0 ☑
      causing obstructed labor 660.1 ☑
    atony, uterus ▶with hemorrhage◀ (hypotonic) (inertia) 666.1 ☑
      hypertonic 661.4 ☑
    Bandl's ring 661.4 ☑
    battledore placenta — *see* Placenta, abnormal
    bicornis or bicornuate uterus 654.0 ☑
      causing obstructed labor 660.2 ☑
    birth injury to mother NEC 665.9 ☑
    bleeding (*see also* Delivery, complicated, hemorrhage) 641.9 ☑
    breech presentation (assisted) (buttocks) (complete) (frank) (spontaneous) 652.2 ☑
      with successful version 652.1 ☑
    brow presentation 652.4 ☑
    cephalopelvic disproportion (normally formed fetus) 653.4 ☑
      causing obstructed labor 660.1 ☑
    cerebral hemorrhage 674.0 ☑
    cervical dystocia 661.0 ☑
    chin presentation 652.4 ☑
      causing obstructed labor 660.0 ☑
    cicatrix
      cervix 654.6 ☑
        causing obstructed labor 660.2 ☑
      vagina 654.7 ☑
        causing obstructed labor 660.2 ☑
    coagulation defect 649.3 ☑ ●
    colporrhexis 665.4 ☑
      with perineal laceration 664.0 ☑
    compound presentation 652.8 ☑
      causing obstructed labor 660.0 ☑
    compression of cord (umbilical) 663.2 ☑
      around neck 663.1 ☑
      cord prolapsed 663.0 ☑
    contraction, contracted pelvis 653.1 ☑
      causing obstructed labor 660.1 ☑
      general 653.1 ☑
        causing obstructed labor 660.1 ☑
      inlet 653.2 ☑
        causing obstructed labor 660.1 ☑
      midpelvic 653.8 ☑
        causing obstructed labor 660.1 ☑
      midplane 653.8 ☑
        causing obstructed labor 660.1 ☑
      outlet 653.3 ☑
        causing obstructed labor 660.1 ☑

Delivery — *continued*
  complicated — *continued*
    contraction ring 661.4 ☑
    cord (umbilical) 663.9 ☑
      around neck, tightly or with compression 663.1 ☑
      without compression 663.3 ☑
      bruising 663.6 ☑
      complication NEC 663.9 ☑
        specified type NEC 663.8 ☑
      compression NEC 663.2 ☑
      entanglement NEC 663.3 ☑
        with compression 663.2 ☑
      forelying 663.0 ☑
      hematoma 663.6 ☑
      marginal attachment 663.8 ☑
      presentation 663.0 ☑
      prolapse (complete) (occult) (partial) 663.0 ☑
      short 663.4 ☑
      specified complication NEC 663.8 ☑
      thrombosis (vessels) 663.6 ☑
      vascular lesion 663.6 ☑
      velamentous insertion 663.8 ☑
    Couvelaire uterus 641.2 ☑
    cretin pelvis (dwarf type) (male type) 653.1 ☑
      causing obstructed labor 660.1 ☑
    crossbirth 652.3 ☑
      with successful version 652.1 ☑
      causing obstructed labor 660.0 ☑
    cyst (Gartner's duct) 654.7 ☑
    cystocele 654.4 ☑
      causing obstructed labor 660.2 ☑
    death of fetus (near term) 656.4 ☑
      early (before 22 completed weeks gestation) 632
    deformity (acquired) (congenital)
      fetus 653.7 ☑
        causing obstructed labor 660.1 ☑
      pelvic organs or tissues NEC 654.9 ☑
        causing obstructed labor 660.2 ☑
      pelvis (bony) NEC 653.0 ☑
        causing obstructed labor 660.1 ☑
    delay, delayed
      delivery in multiple pregnancy 662.3 ☑
        due to locked mates 660.5 ☑
      following rupture of membranes (spontaneous) 658.2 ☑
        artificial 658.3 ☑
    depressed fetal heart tones 659.7 ☑
    diastasis recti 665.8 ☑
    dilatation
      bladder 654.4 ☑
        causing obstructed labor 660.2 ☑
      cervix, incomplete, poor or slow 661.0 ☑
    diseased placenta 656.7 ☑
    displacement uterus NEC 654.4 ☑
      causing obstructed labor 660.2 ☑
    disproportion NEC 653.9 ☑
      causing obstructed labor 660.1 ☑
    disruptio uteri — *see* Delivery, complicated, rupture, uterus
    distress
      fetal 656.8 ☑
      maternal 669.0 ☑
    double uterus (congenital) 654.0 ☑
      causing obstructed labor 660.2 ☑
    dropsy amnion 657.0 ☑

Delivery

Delivery — continued
  complicated — continued
    dysfunction, uterus 661.9 ☑
      hypertonic 661.4 ☑
      hypotonic 661.2 ☑
        primary 661.0 ☑
        secondary 661.1 ☑
      incoordinate 661.4 ☑
    dystocia
      cervical 661.0 ☑
      fetal — *see* Delivery, complicated, abnormal, presentation
      maternal — *see* Delivery, complicated, prolonged labor
      pelvic — *see* Delivery, complicated, contraction pelvis
      positional 652.8 ☑
      shoulder girdle 660.4 ☑
    eclampsia 642.6 ☑
    ectopic kidney 654.4 ☑
      causing obstructed labor 660.2 ☑
    edema, cervix 654.6 ☑
      causing obstructed labor 660.2 ☑
    effusion, amniotic fluid 658.1 ☑
    elderly multigravida 659.6 ☑
    elderly primigravida 659.5 ☑
    embolism (pulmonary) 673.2 ☑
      air 673.0 ☑
      amniotic fluid 673.1 ☑
      blood clot 673.2 ☑
      cerebral 674.0 ☑
      fat 673.8 ☑
      pyemic 673.3 ☑
      septic 673.3 ☑
    entanglement, umbilical cord 663.3 ☑
      with compression 663.2 ☑
      around neck (with compression) 663.1 ☑
    eversion, cervix or uterus 665.2 ☑
    excessive
      fetal growth 653.5 ☑
        causing obstructed labor 660.1 ☑
      size of fetus 653.5 ☑
        causing obstructed labor 660.1 ☑
    face presentation 652.4 ☑
      causing obstructed labor 660.0 ☑
      to pubes 660.3 ☑
    failure, fetal head to enter pelvic brim 652.5 ☑
      causing obstructed labor 660.0 ☑
    female genital mutilation 660.8 ☑
    fetal
      acid-base balance 656.8 ☑
      death (near term) NEC 656.4 ☑
        early (before 22 completed weeks gestation) 632
      deformity 653.7 ☑
        causing obstructed labor 660.1 ☑
      distress 656.8 ☑
      heart rate or rhythm 659.7 ☑
      reduction of multiple fetuses reduced to single fetus 651.7 ☑
    fetopelvic disproportion 653.4 ☑
      causing obstructed labor 660.1 ☑
    fever during labor 659.2 ☑
    fibroid (tumor) (uterus) 654.1 ☑
      causing obstructed labor 660.2 ☑
    fibromyomata 654.1 ☑
      causing obstructed labor 660.2 ☑
    forelying umbilical cord 663.0 ☑
    fracture of coccyx 665.6 ☑
    hematoma 664.5 ☑

Delivery — continued
  complicated — continued
    hematoma — continued
      broad ligament 665.7 ☑
      ischial spine 665.7 ☑
      pelvic 665.7 ☑
      perineum 664.5 ☑
      soft tissues 665.7 ☑
      subdural 674.0 ☑
      umbilical cord 663.6 ☑
      vagina 665.7 ☑
      vulva or perineum 664.5 ☑
    hemorrhage (uterine) (antepartum) (intrapartum) (pregnancy) 641.9 ☑
      accidental 641.2 ☑
      associated with
        afibrinogenemia 641.3 ☑
        coagulation defect 641.3 ☑
          hyperfibrinolysis 641.3 ☑
          hypofibrinogenemia 641.3 ☑
      cerebral 674.0 ☑
      due to
        low-lying placenta 641.1 ☑
        placenta previa 641.1 ☑
        premature separation of placenta (normally implanted) 641.2 ☑
        retained placenta 666.0 ☑
        trauma 641.8 ☑
        uterine leiomyoma 641.8 ☑
      marginal sinus rupture 641.2 ☑
      placenta NEC 641.9 ☑
      postpartum (atonic) (immediate) (within 24 hours) 666.1 ☑
        with retained or trapped placenta 666.0 ☑
        delayed 666.2 ☑
        secondary 666.2 ☑
        third stage 666.0 ☑
    hourglass contraction, uterus 661.4 ☑
    hydramnios 657.0 ☑
    hydrocephalic fetus 653.6 ☑
      causing obstructed labor 660.1 ☑
    hydrops fetalis 653.7 ☑
      causing obstructed labor 660.1 ☑
    hypertension — *see* Hypertension, complicating pregnancy
    hypertonic uterine dysfunction 661.4 ☑
    hypotonic uterine dysfunction 661.2 ☑
    impacted shoulders 660.4 ☑
    incarceration, uterus 654.3 ☑
      causing obstructed labor 660.2 ☑
    incomplete dilation (cervix) 661.0 ☑
    incoordinate uterus 661.4 ☑
    indication NEC 659.9 ☑
      specified type NEC 659.8 ☑
    inertia, uterus 661.2 ☑
      hypertonic 661.4 ☑
      hypotonic 661.2 ☑
        primary 661.0 ☑
        secondary 661.1 ☑
    infantile
      genitalia 654.4 ☑
        causing obstructed labor 660.2 ☑
      uterus (os) 654.4 ☑
        causing obstructed labor 660.2 ☑
    injury (to mother) NEC 665.9 ☑
    intrauterine fetal death (near term) NEC 656.4 ☑
      early (before 22 completed weeks gestation) 632
    inversion, uterus 665.2 ☑
    kidney, ectopic 654.4 ☑

Delivery — continued
  complicated — continued
    kidney, ectopic — continued
      causing obstructed labor 660.2 ☑
    knot (true), umbilical cord 663.2 ☑
    labor, premature (before 37 completed weeks gestation) 644.2 ☑
    laceration 664.9 ☑
      anus (sphincter) 664.2 ☑
        with mucosa 664.3 ☑
      bladder (urinary) 665.5 ☑
      bowel 665.5 ☑
      central 664.4 ☑
      cervix (uteri) 665.3 ☑
      fourchette 664.0 ☑
      hymen 664.0 ☑
      labia (majora) (minora) 664.0 ☑
      pelvic
        floor 664.1 ☑
        organ NEC 665.5 ☑
      perineum, perineal 664.4 ☑
        first degree 664.0 ☑
        second degree 664.1 ☑
        third degree 664.2 ☑
        fourth degree 664.3 ☑
        central 664.4 ☑
        extensive NEC 664.4 ☑
        muscles 664.1 ☑
        skin 664.0 ☑
        slight 664.0 ☑
      peritoneum 665.5 ☑
      periurethral tissue 665.5 ☑
      rectovaginal (septum) (without perineal laceration) 665.4 ☑
        with perineum 664.2 ☑
          with anal or rectal mucosa 664.3 ☑
      skin (perineum) 664.0 ☑
      specified site or type NEC 664.8 ☑
      sphincter ani 664.2 ☑
        with mucosa 664.3 ☑
      urethra 665.5 ☑
      uterus 665.1 ☑
        before labor 665.0 ☑
      vagina, vaginal (deep) (high) (sulcus) (wall) (without perineal laceration) 665.4 ☑
        with perineum 664.0 ☑
        muscles, with perineum 664.1 ☑
      vulva 664.0 ☑
    lateroversion, uterus or cervix 654.4 ☑
      causing obstructed labor 660.2 ☑
    locked mates 660.5 ☑
    low implantation of placenta — *see* Delivery, complicated, placenta, previa
    mal lie 652.9 ☑
    malposition
      fetus NEC 652.9 ☑
        causing obstructed labor 660.0 ☑
      pelvic organs or tissues NEC 654.9 ☑
        causing obstructed labor 660.2 ☑
      placenta 641.1 ☑
        without hemorrhage 641.0 ☑
      uterus NEC or cervix 654.4 ☑
        causing obstructed labor 660.2 ☑
    malpresentation 652.9 ☑
      causing obstructed labor 660.0 ☑
    marginal sinus (bleeding) (rupture) 641.2 ☑
    maternal hypotension syndrome 669.2 ☑

Delivery — continued
  complicated — continued
    meconium in liquor 656.8 ☑
    membranes, retained — *see* Delivery, complicated, placenta, retained
    mentum presentation 652.4 ☑
      causing obstructed labor 660.0 ☑
    metrorrhagia (myopathia) — *see* Delivery, complicated, hemorrhage
    metrorrhexis — *see* Delivery, complicated, rupture, uterus
    multiparity (grand) 659.4 ☑
    myelomeningocele, fetus 653.7 ☑
      causing obstructed labor 660.1 ☑
    Nägele's pelvis 653.0 ☑
      causing obstructed labor 660.1 ☑
    nonengagement, fetal head 652.5 ☑
      causing obstructed labor 660.0 ☑
    oblique presentation 652.3 ☑
      causing obstructed labor 660.0 ☑
    obstetric
      shock 669.1 ☑
      trauma NEC 665.9 ☑
    obstructed labor 660.9 ☑
      due to
        abnormality of pelvic organs or tissues (conditions classifiable to 654.0–654.9) 660.2 ☑
        deep transverse arrest 660.3 ☑
        impacted shoulders 660.4 ☑
        locked twins 660.5 ☑
        malposition and malpresentation of fetus (conditions classifiable to 652.0–652.9) 660.0 ☑
        persistent occipitoposterior 660.3 ☑
        shoulder dystocia 660.4 ☑
    occult prolapse of umbilical cord 663.0 ☑
    oversize fetus 653.5 ☑
      causing obstructed labor 660.1 ☑
    pathological retraction ring, uterus 661.4 ☑
    pelvic
      arrest (deep) (high) (of fetal head) (transverse) 660.3 ☑
      deformity (bone) (*see also* Deformity, pelvis, with disproportion)
      soft tissue 654.9 ☑
        causing obstructed labor 660.2 ☑
      tumor NEC 654.9 ☑
        causing obstructed labor 660.2 ☑
    penetration, pregnant uterus by instrument 665.1 ☑
    perforation — *see* Delivery, complicated, laceration
    persistent
      hymen 654.8 ☑
        causing obstructed labor 660.2 ☑
      occipitoposterior 660.3 ☑
    placenta, placental
      ablatio 641.2 ☑
      abnormality 656.7 ☑
        with hemorrhage 641.2 ☑
      abruptio 641.2 ☑
      accreta 667.0 ☑
        with hemorrhage 666.0 ☑

Index to Diseases

Delivery

Delivery — *continued*
  complicated — *continued*
    placenta, placental — *continued*
      adherent (without hemorrhage) 667.0 ☑
        with hemorrhage 666.0 ☑
      apoplexy 641.2 ☑
      battledore placenta — *see* Placenta, abnormal
      detachment (premature) 641.2 ☑
      disease 656.7 ☑
      hemorrhage NEC 641.9 ☑
      increta (without hemorrhage) 667.0 ☑
        with hemorrhage 666.0 ☑
      low (implantation) 641.1 ☑
        without hemorrhage 641.0 ☑
      malformation 656.7 ☑
        with hemorrhage 641.2 ☑
      malposition 641.1 ☑
        without hemorrhage 641.0 ☑
      marginal sinus rupture 641.2 ☑
      percreta 667.0 ☑
        with hemorrhage 666.0 ☑
      premature separation 641.2 ☑
      previa (central) (lateral) (marginal) (partial) 641.1 ☑
        without hemorrhage 641.0 ☑
      retained (with hemorrhage) 666.0 ☑
        without hemorrhage 667.0 ☑
      rupture of marginal sinus 641.2 ☑
      separation (premature) 641.2 ☑
      trapped 666.0 ☑
        without hemorrhage 667.0 ☑
      vicious insertion 641.1 ☑
    polyhydramnios 657.0 ☑
    polyp, cervix 654.6 ☑
      causing obstructed labor 660.2 ☑
    precipitate labor 661.3 ☑
    premature
      labor (before 37 completed weeks gestation) 644.2 ☑
      rupture, membranes 658.1 ☑
        delayed delivery following 658.2 ☑
    presenting umbilical cord 663.0 ☑
    previous
      cesarean delivery, section 654.2 ☑
      surgery
        cervix 654.6 ☑
          causing obstructed labor 660.2 ☑
        gynecological NEC 654.9 ☑
          causing obstructed labor 660.2 ☑
        perineum 654.8 ☑
        rectum 654.8 ☑
        uterus NEC 654.9 ☑
          due to previous cesarean delivery, section 654.2 ☑
        vagina 654.7 ☑
          causing obstructed labor 660.2 ☑
        vulva 654.8 ☑
    primary uterine inertia 661.0 ☑
    primipara, elderly or old 659.5 ☑
    prolapse
      arm or hand 652.7 ☑
        causing obstructed labor 660.0 ☑
      cord (umbilical) 663.0 ☑
      fetal extremity 652.8 ☑
      foot or leg 652.8 ☑
        causing obstructed labor 660.0 ☑
      umbilical cord (complete) (occult) (partial) 663.0 ☑
      uterus 654.4 ☑

Delivery — *continued*
  complicated — *continued*
    prolapse — *continued*
      uterus — *continued*
        causing obstructed labor 660.2 ☑
    prolonged labor 662.1 ☑
      first stage 662.0 ☑
      second stage 662.2 ☑
      active phase 661.2 ☑
      due to
        cervical dystocia 661.0 ☑
        contraction ring 661.4 ☑
        tetanic uterus 661.4 ☑
        uterine inertia 661.2 ☑
          primary 661.0 ☑
          secondary 661.1 ☑
      latent phase 661.0 ☑
    pyrexia during labor 659.2 ☑
    rachitic pelvis 653.2 ☑
      causing obstructed labor 660.1 ☑
    rectocele 654.4 ☑
      causing obstructed labor 660.2 ☑
    retained membranes or portions of placenta 666.2 ☑
      without hemorrhage 667.1 ☑
    retarded (prolonged) birth 662.1 ☑
    retention secundines (with hemorrhage) 666.2 ☑
      without hemorrhage 667.1 ☑
    retroversion, uterus or cervix 654.3 ☑
      causing obstructed labor 660.2 ☑
    rigid
      cervix 654.6 ☑
        causing obstructed labor 660.2 ☑
      pelvic floor 654.4 ☑
        causing obstructed labor 660.2 ☑
      perineum or vulva 654.8 ☑
        causing obstructed labor 660.2 ☑
      vagina 654.7 ☑
        causing obstructed labor 660.2 ☑
    Robert's pelvis 653.0 ☑
      causing obstructed labor 660.1 ☑
    rupture (*see also* Delivery, complicated, laceration)
      bladder (urinary) 665.5 ☑
      cervix 665.3 ☑
      marginal sinus 641.2 ☑
      membranes, premature 658.1 ☑
      pelvic organ NEC 665.5 ☑
      perineum (without mention of other laceration) — *see* Delivery, complicated, laceration, perineum
      peritoneum 665.5 ☑
      urethra 665.5 ☑
      uterus (during labor) 665.1 ☑
        before labor 665.0 ☑
    sacculation, pregnant uterus 654.4 ☑
    sacral teratomas, fetal 653.7 ☑
      causing obstructed labor 660.1 ☑
    scar(s)
      cervix 654.6 ☑
        causing obstructed labor 660.2 ☑
      cesarean delivery, section 654.2 ☑
        causing obstructed labor 660.2 ☑
      perineum 654.8 ☑
        causing obstructed labor 660.2 ☑
      uterus NEC 654.9 ☑

Delivery — *continued*
  complicated — *continued*
    scar(s) — *continued*
      uterus — *continued*
        causing obstructed labor 660.2 ☑
        due to previous cesarean delivery, section 654.2 ☑
      vagina 654.7 ☑
        causing obstructed labor 660.2 ☑
      vulva 654.8 ☑
        causing obstructed labor 660.2 ☑
    scoliotic pelvis 653.0 ☑
      causing obstructed labor 660.1 ☑
    secondary uterine inertia 661.1 ☑
    secundines, retained — *see* Delivery, complicated, placenta, retained
    separation
      placenta (premature) 641.2 ☑
      pubic bone 665.6 ☑
      symphysis pubis 665.6 ☑
    septate vagina 654.7 ☑
      causing obstructed labor 660.2 ☑
    shock (birth) (obstetric) (puerperal) 669.1 ☑
    short cord syndrome 663.4 ☑
    shoulder
      girdle dystocia 660.4 ☑
      presentation 652.8 ☑
        causing obstructed labor 660.0 ☑
    Siamese twins 653.7 ☑
      causing obstructed labor 660.1 ☑
    slow slope active phase 661.2 ☑
    spasm
      cervix 661.4 ☑
      uterus 661.4 ☑
    spondylolisthesis, pelvis 653.3 ☑
      causing obstructed labor 660.1 ☑
    spondylolysis (lumbosacral) 653.3 ☑
      causing obstructed labor 660.1 ☑
    spondylosis 653.0 ☑
      causing obstructed labor 660.1 ☑
    stenosis or stricture
      cervix 654.6 ☑
        causing obstructed labor 660.2 ☑
      vagina 654.7 ☑
        causing obstructed labor 660.2 ☑
    sudden death, unknown cause 669.9 ☑
    tear (pelvic organ) (*see also* Delivery, complicated, laceration) 664.9 ☑
    teratomas, sacral, fetal 653.7 ☑
      causing obstructed labor 660.1 ☑
    tetanic uterus 661.4 ☑
    tipping pelvis 653.0 ☑
      causing obstructed labor 660.1 ☑
    transverse
      arrest (deep) 660.3 ☑
      presentation or lie 652.3 ☑
        with successful version 652.1 ☑
        causing obstructed labor 660.0 ☑
    trauma (obstetrical) NEC 665.9 ☑
    tumor
      abdominal, fetal 653.7 ☑
        causing obstructed labor 660.1 ☑

Delivery — *continued*
  complicated — *continued*
    tumor — *continued*
      pelvic organs or tissues NEC 654.9 ☑
        causing obstructed labor 660.2 ☑
    umbilical cord (*see also* Delivery, complicated, cord) 663.9 ☑
      around neck tightly, or with compression 663.1 ☑
      entanglement NEC 663.3 ☑
        with compression 663.2 ☑
      prolapse (complete) (occult) (partial) 663.0 ☑
    unstable lie 652.0 ☑
      causing obstructed labor 660.0 ☑
    uterine
      inertia (*see also* Delivery, complicated, inertia, uterus) 661.2 ☑
      spasm 661.4 ☑
    vasa previa 663.5 ☑
    velamentous insertion of cord 663.8 ☑
    young maternal age 659.8 ☑
  delayed NEC 662.1 ☑
    following rupture of membranes (spontaneous) 658.2 ☑
      artificial 658.3 ☑
    second twin, triplet, etc. 662.3 ☑
  difficult NEC 669.9 ☑
    previous, affecting management of pregnancy or childbirth V23.49
    specified type NEC 669.8 ☑
  early onset (spontaneous) 644.2 ☑
  footling 652.8 ☑
    with successful version 652.1 ☑
  forceps NEC 669.5 ☑
    affecting fetus or newborn 763.2
  missed (at or near term) 656.4 ☑
  multiple gestation NEC 651.9 ☑
    with fetal loss and retention of one or more fetus(es) 651.6 ☑
    following (elective) fetal reduction 651.7 ☑
    specified type NEC 651.8 ☑
      with fetal loss and retention of one or more fetus(es) 651.6 ☑
      following (elective) fetal reduction 651.7 ☑
  nonviable infant 656.4 ☑
  normal — *see* category 650
  precipitate 661.3 ☑
    affecting fetus or newborn 763.6
  premature NEC (before 37 completed weeks gestation) 644.2 ☑
    previous, affecting management of pregnancy V23.41
  quadruplet NEC 651.2 ☑
    with fetal loss and retention of one or more fetus(es) 651.5 ☑
    following (elective) fetal reduction 651.7 ☑
  quintuplet NEC 651.8 ☑
    with fetal loss and retention of one or more fetus(es) 651.6 ☑
    following (elective) fetal reduction 651.7 ☑
  sextuplet NEC 651.8 ☑
    with fetal loss and retention of one or more fetus(es) 651.6 ☑
    following (elective) fetal reduction 651.7 ☑
  specified complication NEC 669.8 ☑
  stillbirth (near term) NEC 656.4 ☑
    early (before 22 completed weeks gestation) 632
  term pregnancy (live birth) NEC — *see* category 650
    stillbirth NEC 656.4 ☑
  threatened premature 644.2 ☑

Delivery — continued
- triplets NEC 651.1 ☑
  - with fetal loss and retention of one or more fetus(es) 651.4 ☑
  - delayed delivery (one or more mates) 662.3 ☑
  - following (elective) fetal reduction 651.7 ☑
  - locked mates 660.5 ☑
- twins NEC 651.0 ☑
  - with fetal loss and retention of one fetus 651.3 ☑
  - delayed delivery (one or more mates) 662.3 ☑
  - following (elective) fetal reduction 651.7 ☑
  - locked mates 660.5 ☑
- uncomplicated — *see* category 650
- vacuum extractor NEC 669.5 ☑
  - affecting fetus or newborn 763.3
- ventouse NEC 669.5 ☑
  - affecting fetus or newborn 763.3

Dellen, cornea 371.41

Delusions (paranoid) 297.9
- grandiose 297.1
- parasitosis 300.29
- systematized 297.1

Dementia 294.8
- alcohol-induced persisting (*see also* Psychosis, alcoholic) 291.2
- Alzheimer's — *see* Alzheimer's, dementia
- arteriosclerotic (simple type) (uncomplicated) 290.40
  - with
    - acute confusional state 290.41
    - delirium 290.41
    - delusions 290.42
    - depressed mood 290.43
    - depressed type 290.43
    - paranoid type 290.42
- Binswanger's 290.12
- catatonic (acute) (*see also* Schizophrenia) 295.2 ☑
- congenital (*see also* Retardation, mental) 319
- degenerative 290.9
  - presenile-onset — *see* Dementia, presenile
  - senile-onset — *see* Dementia, senile
- developmental (*see also* Schizophrenia) 295.9 ☑
- dialysis 294.8
  - transient 293.9
- drug-induced persisting (*see also* Psychosis, drug) 292.82
- due to or associated with condition(s) classified elsewhere
  - Alzheimer's
    - with behavioral disturbance 331.0 [294.11]
    - without behavioral disturbance 331.0 [294.10]
  - cerebral lipidoses
    - with behavioral disturbance 330.1 [294.11]
    - without behavioral disturbance 330.1 [294.10]
  - epilepsy
    - with behavioral disturbance 345.9 ☑ [294.11]
    - without behavioral disturbance 345.9 ☑ [294.10]
  - hepatolenticular degeneration
    - with behavioral disturbance 275.1 [294.11]
    - without behavioral disturbance 275.1 [294.10]
  - HIV
    - with behavioral disturbance 042 [294.11]
    - without behavioral disturbance 042 [294.10]

Dementia — continued
- due to or associated with condition(s) classified elsewhere — *continued*
  - Huntington's chorea
    - with behavioral disturbance 333.4 [294.11]
    - without behavioral disturbance 333.4 [294.10]
  - Jakob-Creutzfeldt disease (new variant)
    - with behavioral disturbance 046.1 [294.11]
    - without behavioral disturbance 046.1 [294.10]
  - Lewy bodies
    - with behavioral disturbance 331.82 [294.11]
    - without behavioral disturbance 331.82 [294.10]
  - multiple sclerosis
    - with behavioral disturbance 340 [294.11]
    - without behavioral disturbance 340 [294.10]
  - neurosyphilis
    - with behavioral disturbance 094.9 [294.11]
    - without behavioral disturbance 094.9 [294.10]
  - Parkinsonism
    - with behavioral disturbance 331.82 [294.11]
    - without behavioral disturbance 331.82 [294.10]
  - Pelizaeus-Merzbacher disease
    - with behavioral disturbance 333.0 [294.11]
    - without behavioral disturbance 333.0 [294.10]
  - Pick's disease
    - with behavioral disturbance 331.11 [294.11]
    - without behavioral disturbance 331.11 [294.10]
  - polyarteritis nodosa
    - with behavioral disturbance 446.0 [294.11]
    - without behavioral disturbance 446.0 [294.10]
  - syphilis
    - with behavioral disturbance 094.1 [294.11]
    - without behavioral disturbance 094.1 [294.10]
  - Wilson's disease
    - with behavioral disturbance 275.1 [294.11]
    - without behavioral disturbance 275.1 [294.10]
- frontal 331.19
  - with behavioral disturbance 331.19 [294.11]
  - without behavioral disturbance 331.19 [294.10]
- frontotemporal 331.19
  - with behavioral disturbance 331.19 [294.11]
  - without behavioral disturbance 331.19 [294.10]
- hebephrenic (acute) 295.1 ☑
- Heller's (infantile psychosis) (*see also* Psychosis, childhood) 299.1 ☑
- idiopathic 290.9
  - presenile-onset — *see* Dementia, presenile
  - senile-onset — *see* Dementia, senile
- in
  - arteriosclerotic brain disease 290.40
  - senility 290.0
- induced by drug 292.82
- infantile, infantilia (*see also* Psychosis, childhood) 299.0 ☑
- Lewy body 331.82

Dementia — continued
- Lewy body — *continued*
  - with behavioral disturbance 331.82 [294.11]
  - without behavioral disturbance 331.82 [294.10]
- multi-infarct (cerebrovascular) (*see also* Dementia, arteriosclerotic) 290.40
- old age 290.0
- paralytica, paralytic 094.1
  - juvenilis 090.40
  - syphilitic 094.1
    - congenital 090.40
  - tabetic form 094.1
- paranoid (*see also* Schizophrenia) 295.3 ☑
- paraphrenic (*see also* Schizophrenia) 295.3 ☑
- paretic 094.1
- praecox (*see also* Schizophrenia) 295.9 ☑
- presenile 290.10
  - with
    - acute confusional state 290.11
    - delirium 290.11
    - delusional features 290.12
    - depressive features 290.13
    - depressed type 290.13
    - paranoid type 290.12
    - simple type 290.10
    - uncomplicated 290.10
- primary (acute) (*see also* Schizophrenia) 295.0 ☑
- progressive, syphilitic 094.1
- puerperal — *see* Psychosis, puerperal
- schizophrenic (*see also* Schizophrenia) 295.9 ☑
- senile 290.0
  - with
    - acute confusional state 290.3
    - delirium 290.3
    - delusional features 290.20
    - depressive features 290.21
    - depressed type 290.21
    - exhaustion 290.0
    - paranoid type 290.20
  - simple type (acute) (*see also* Schizophrenia) 295.0 ☑
- simplex (acute) (*see also* Schizophrenia) 295.0 ☑
- syphilitic 094.1
- uremic — *see* Uremia
- vascular 290.40
  - with
    - delirium 290.41
    - delusions 290.42
    - depressed mood 290.43

Demerol dependence — *see also* Dependence 304.0 ☑

Demineralization, ankle — *see also* Osteoporosis 733.00

Demodex folliculorum (infestation) 133.8

de Morgan's spots (senile angiomas) 448.1

Demyelinating
- polyneuritis, chronic inflammatory 357.81

Demyelination, demyelinization
- central nervous system 341.9
  - specified NEC 341.8
- corpus callosum (central) 341.8
- global 340

Dengue (fever) 061
- sandfly 061
- vaccination, prophylactic (against) V05.1
- virus hemorrhagic fever 065.4

Dens
- evaginatus 520.2
- in dente 520.2
- invaginatus 520.2

Density
- increased, bone (disseminated) (generalized) (spotted) 733.99

Density — continued
- lung (nodular) 518.89

Dental — *see also* condition
- examination only V72.2

Dentia praecox 520.6

Denticles (in pulp) 522.2

Dentigerous cyst 526.0

Dentin
- irregular (in pulp) 522.3
- opalescent 520.5
- secondary (in pulp) 522.3
- sensitive 521.89 ▲

Dentinogenesis imperfecta 520.5

Dentinoma (M9271/0) 213.1
- upper jaw (bone) 213.0

Dentition 520.7
- abnormal 520.6
- anomaly 520.6
- delayed 520.6
- difficult 520.7
- disorder of 520.6
- precocious 520.6
- retarded 520.6

Denture sore (mouth) 528.9

Dependence

Note — *Use the following fifth-digit subclassification with category 304:*
- 0 unspecified
- 1 continuous
- 2 episodic
- 3 in remission

- with
  - withdrawal symptoms
    - alcohol 291.81
    - drug 292.0
- 14-hydroxy-dihydromorphinone 304.0 ☑
- absinthe 304.6 ☑
- acemorphan 304.0 ☑
- acetanilid(e) 304.6 ☑
- acetophenetidin 304.6 ☑
- acetorphine 304.0 ☑
- acetyldihydrocodeine 304.0 ☑
- acetyldihydrocodeinone 304.0 ☑
- Adalin 304.1 ☑
- Afghanistan black 304.3 ☑
- agrypnal 304.1 ☑
- alcohol, alcoholic (ethyl) (methyl) (wood) 303.9 ☑
  - maternal, with suspected fetal damage affecting management of pregnancy 655.4 ☑
- allobarbitone 304.1 ☑
- allonal 304.1 ☑
- allylisopropylacetylurea 304.1 ☑
- alphaprodine (hydrochloride) 304.0 ☑
- Alurate 304.1 ☑
- Alvodine 304.0 ☑
- amethocaine 304.6 ☑
- amidone 304.0 ☑
- amidopyrine 304.6 ☑
- aminopyrine 304.6 ☑
- amobarbital 304.1 ☑
- amphetamine(s) (type) (drugs classifiable to 969.7) 304.4 ☑
- amylene hydrate 304.6 ☑
- amylobarbitone 304.1 ☑
- amylocaine 304.6 ☑
- Amytal (sodium) 304.1 ☑
- analgesic (drug) NEC 304.6 ☑
  - synthetic with morphine-like effect 304.0 ☑
- anesthetic (agent) (drug) (gas) (general) (local) NEC 304.6 ☑
- Angel dust 304.6 ☑
- anileridine 304.0 ☑
- antipyrine 304.6 ☑
- anxiolytic 304.1 ☑
- aprobarbital 304.1 ☑
- aprobarbitone 304.1 ☑
- atropine 304.6 ☑
- Avertin (bromide) 304.6 ☑

Index to Diseases — Dependence

Dependence — *continued*
- barbenyl 304.1 ☑
- barbital(s) 304.1 ☑
- barbitone 304.1 ☑
- barbiturate(s) (compounds) (drugs classifiable to 967.0) 304.1 ☑
- barbituric acid (and compounds) 304.1 ☑
- benzedrine 304.4 ☑
- benzylmorphine 304.0 ☑
- Beta-chlor 304.1 ☑
- bhang 304.3 ☑
- blue velvet 304.0 ☑
- Brevital 304.1 ☑
- bromal (hydrate) 304.1 ☑
- bromide(s) NEC 304.1 ☑
- bromine compounds NEC 304.1 ☑
- bromisovalum 304.1 ☑
- bromoform 304.1 ☑
- Bromo-seltzer 304.1 ☑
- bromural 304.1 ☑
- butabarbital (sodium) 304.1 ☑
- butabarpal 304.1 ☑
- butallylonal 304.1 ☑
- butethal 304.1 ☑
- buthalitone (sodium) 304.1 ☑
- Butisol 304.1 ☑
- butobarbitone 304.1 ☑
- butyl chloral (hydrate) 304.1 ☑
- caffeine 304.4 ☑
- cannabis (indica) (sativa) (resin) (derivatives) (type) 304.3 ☑
- carbamazepine 304.6 ☑
- Carbrital 304.1 ☑
- carbromal 304.1 ☑
- carisoprodol 304.6 ☑
- Catha (edulis) 304.4 ☑
- chloral (betaine) (hydrate) 304.1 ☑
- chloralamide 304.1 ☑
- chloralformamide 304.1 ☑
- chloralose 304.1 ☑
- chlordiazepoxide 304.1 ☑
- Chloretone 304.1 ☑
- chlorobutanol 304.1 ☑
- chlorodyne 304.1 ☑
- chloroform 304.6 ☑
- Cliradon 304.0 ☑
- coca (leaf) and derivatives 304.2 ☑
- cocaine 304.2 ☑
  - hydrochloride 304.2 ☑
  - salt (any) 304.2 ☑
- codeine 304.0 ☑
- combination of drugs (excluding morphine or opioid type drug) NEC 304.8 ☑
  - morphine or opioid type drug with any other drug 304.7 ☑
- croton-chloral 304.1 ☑
- cyclobarbital 304.1 ☑
- cyclobarbitone 304.1 ☑
- dagga 304.3 ☑
- Delvinal 304.1 ☑
- Demerol 304.0 ☑
- desocodeine 304.0 ☑
- desomorphine 304.0 ☑
- desoxyephedrine 304.4 ☑
- DET 304.5 ☑
- dexamphetamine 304.4 ☑
- dexedrine 304.4 ☑
- dextromethorphan 304.0 ☑
- dextromoramide 304.0 ☑
- dextronorpseudoephedrine 304.4 ☑
- dextrorphan 304.0 ☑
- diacetylmorphine 304.0 ☑
- Dial 304.1 ☑
- diallylbarbituric acid 304.1 ☑
- diamorphine 304.0 ☑
- diazepam 304.1 ☑
- dibucaine 304.6 ☑
- dichloroethane 304.6 ☑
- diethyl barbituric acid 304.1 ☑
- diethylsulfone-diethylmethane 304.1 ☑
- difencloxazine 304.0 ☑

Dependence — *continued*
- dihydrocodeine 304.0 ☑
- dihydrocodeinone 304.0 ☑
- dihydrohydroxycodeinone 304.0 ☑
- dihydroisocodeine 304.0 ☑
- dihydromorphine 304.0 ☑
- dihydromorphinone 304.0 ☑
- dihydroxcodeinone 304.0 ☑
- Dilaudid 304.0 ☑
- dimenhydrinate 304.6 ☑
- dimethylmeperidine 304.0 ☑
- dimethyltriptamine 304.5 ☑
- Dionin 304.0 ☑
- diphenoxylate 304.6 ☑
- dipipanone 304.0 ☑
- d-lysergic acid diethylamide 304.5 ☑
- DMT 304.5 ☑
- Dolophine 304.0 ☑
- DOM 304.2 ☑
- Doriden 304.1 ☑
- dormiral 304.1 ☑
- Dormison 304.1 ☑
- Dromoran 304.0 ☑
- drug NEC 304.9 ☑
  - analgesic NEC 304.6 ☑
  - combination (excluding morphine or opioid type drug) NEC 304.8 ☑
    - morphine or opioid type drug with any other drug 304.7 ☑
  - complicating pregnancy, childbirth, or puerperium 648.3
    - affecting fetus or newborn 779.5
  - hallucinogenic 304.5 ☑
  - hypnotic NEC 304.1 ☑
  - narcotic NEC 304.9 ☑
  - psychostimulant NEC 304.4 ☑
  - sedative 304.1 ☑
  - soporific NEC 304.1 ☑
  - specified type NEC 304.6 ☑
  - suspected damage to fetus affecting management of pregnancy 655.5 ☑
  - synthetic, with morphine-like effect 304.0 ☑
  - tranquilizing 304.1 ☑
- duboisine 304.6 ☑
- ectylurea 304.1 ☑
- Endocaine 304.6 ☑
- Equanil 304.1 ☑
- Eskabarb 304.1 ☑
- ethchlorvynol 304.1 ☑
- ether (ethyl) (liquid) (vapor) (vinyl) 304.6 ☑
- ethidene 304.6 ☑
- ethinamate 304.1 ☑
- ethoheptazine 304.6 ☑
- ethyl
  - alcohol 303.9 ☑
  - bromide 304.6 ☑
  - carbamate 304.6 ☑
  - chloride 304.6 ☑
  - morphine 304.0 ☑
- ethylene (gas) 304.6 ☑
  - dichloride 304.6 ☑
- ethylidene chloride 304.6 ☑
- etilfen 304.1 ☑
- etorphine 304.0 ☑
- etoval 304.1 ☑
- eucodal 304.0 ☑
- euneryl 304.1 ☑
- Evipal 304.1 ☑
- Evipan 304.1 ☑
- fentanyl 304.0 ☑
- ganja 304.3 ☑
- gardenal 304.1 ☑
- gardenpanyl 304.1 ☑
- gelsemine 304.6 ☑
- Gelsemium 304.6 ☑
- Gemonil 304.1 ☑
- glucochloral 304.1 ☑
- glue (airplane) (sniffing) 304.6 ☑
- glutethimide 304.1 ☑

Dependence — *continued*
- hallucinogenics 304.5 ☑
- hashish 304.3 ☑
- headache powder NEC 304.6 ☑
- Heavenly Blue 304.5 ☑
- hedonal 304.1 ☑
- hemp 304.3 ☑
- heptabarbital 304.1 ☑
- Heptalgin 304.0 ☑
- heptobarbitone 304.1 ☑
- heroin 304.0 ☑
  - salt (any) 304.0 ☑
- hexethal (sodium) 304.1 ☑
- hexobarbital 304.1 ☑
- Hycodan 304.0 ☑
- hydrocodone 304.0 ☑
- hydromorphinol 304.0 ☑
- hydromorphinone 304.0 ☑
- hydromorphone 304.0 ☑
- hydroxycodeine 304.0 ☑
- hypnotic NEC 304.1 ☑
- Indian hemp 304.3 ☑
- inhalant 304.6 ☑
- intranarcon 304.1 ☑
- Kemithal 304.1 ☑
- ketobemidone 304.0 ☑
- khat 304.4 ☑
- kif 304.3 ☑
- Lactuca (virosa) extract 304.1 ☑
- lactucarium 304.1 ☑
- laudanum 304.0 ☑
- Lebanese red 304.3 ☑
- Leritine 304.0 ☑
- lettuce opium 304.1 ☑
- Levanil 304.1 ☑
- Levo-Dromoran 304.0 ☑
- levo-iso-methadone 304.0 ☑
- levorphanol 304.0 ☑
- Librium 304.1 ☑
- Lomotil 304.6 ☑
- Lotusate 304.1 ☑
- LSD (-25) (and derivatives) 304.5 ☑
- Luminal 304.1 ☑
- lysergic acid 304.5 ☑
  - amide 304.5 ☑
- maconha 304.3 ☑
- magic mushroom 304.5 ☑
- marihuana 304.3 ☑
- MDA (methylene dioxyamphetamine) 304.4 ☑
- Mebaral 304.1 ☑
- Medinal 304.1 ☑
- Medomin 304.1 ☑
- megahallucinogenics 304.5 ☑
- meperidine 304.0 ☑
- mephobarbital 304.1 ☑
- meprobamate 304.1 ☑
- mescaline 304.5 ☑
- methadone 304.0 ☑
- methamphetamine(s) 304.4 ☑
- methaqualone 304.1 ☑
- metharbital 304.1 ☑
- methitural 304.1 ☑
- methobarbitone 304.1 ☑
- methohexital 304.1 ☑
- methopholine 304.6 ☑
- methyl
  - alcohol 303.9 ☑
  - bromide 304.6 ☑
  - morphine 304.0 ☑
  - sulfonal 304.1 ☑
- methylaparafynol 304.1 ☑
- methylated spirit 303.9 ☑
- methylbutinol 304.6 ☑
- methyldihydromorphinone 304.0 ☑
- methylene
  - chloride 304.6 ☑
  - dichloride 304.6 ☑
  - dioxyamphetamine (MDA) 304.4 ☑
- methylphenidate 304.4 ☑
- methyprylone 304.1 ☑
- metopon 304.0 ☑
- Miltown 304.1 ☑
- morning glory seeds 304.5 ☑

Dependence — *continued*
- morphinan(s) 304.0 ☑
- morphine (sulfate) (sulfite) (type) (drugs classifiable to 965.00–965.09) 304.0 ☑
- morphine or opioid type drug (drugs classifiable to 965.00–965.09) with any other drug 304.7 ☑
- morphinol(s) 304.0 ☑
- morphinon 304.0 ☑
- morpholinylethylmorphine 304.0 ☑
- mylomide 304.1 ☑
- myristicin 304.5 ☑
- narcotic (drug) NEC 304.9 ☑
- nealbarbital 304.1 ☑
- nealbarbitone 304.1 ☑
- Nembutal 304.1 ☑
- Neonal 304.1 ☑
- Neraval 304.1 ☑
- Neravan 304.1 ☑
- neurobarb 304.1 ☑
- nicotine 305.1 ☑
- Nisentil 304.0 ☑
- nitrous oxide 304.6 ☑
- Noctec 304.1 ☑
- Noludar 304.1 ☑
- nonbarbiturate sedatives and tranquilizers with similar effect 304.1 ☑
- noptil 304.1 ☑
- normorphine 304.0 ☑
- noscapine 304.0 ☑
- Novocaine 304.6 ☑
- Numorphan 304.0 ☑
- nunol 304.1 ☑
- Nupercaine 304.6 ☑
- Oblivon 304.1 ☑
- on
  - aspirator V46.0
  - hemodialysis V45.1
  - hyperbaric chamber V46.8
  - iron lung V46.11
  - machine (enabling) V46.9
    - specified type NEC V46.8
  - peritoneal dialysis V45.1
  - Possum (Patient-Operated-Selector-Mechanism) V46.8
  - renal dialysis machine V45.1
  - respirator [ventilator] V46.11
    - encounter
      - during
        - mechanical failure V46.14
        - power failure V46.12
      - for weaning V46.13
  - supplemental oxygen V46.2
- opiate 304.0 ☑
- opioids 304.0 ☑
- opioid type drug 304.0 ☑
  - with any other drug 304.7 ☑
- opium (alkaloids) (derivatives) (tincture) 304.0 ☑
- ortal 304.1 ☑
- Oxazepam 304.1 ☑
- oxycodone 304.0 ☑
- oxymorphone 304.0 ☑
- Palfium 304.0 ☑
- Panadol 304.6 ☑
- pantopium 304.0 ☑
- pantopon 304.0 ☑
- papaverine 304.0 ☑
- paracetamol 304.6 ☑
- paracodin 304.0 ☑
- paraldehyde 304.1 ☑
- paregoric 304.0 ☑
- Parzone 304.0 ☑
- PCP (phencyclidine) 304.6 ☑
- Pearly Gates 304.5 ☑
- pentazocine 304.0 ☑
- pentobarbital 304.1 ☑
- pentobarbitone (sodium) 304.1 ☑
- Pentothal 304.1 ☑
- Percaine 304.6 ☑
- Percodan 304.0 ☑
- Perichlor 304.1 ☑
- Pernocton 304.1 ☑

Dependence

Dependence — *continued*
Pernoston 304.1
peronine 304.0
pethidine (hydrochloride) 304.0
petrichloral 304.1
peyote 304.5
Phanodron 304.1
phenacetin 304.6
phenadoxone 304.0
phenaglycodol 304.1
phenazocine 304.0
phencyclidine 304.6
phenmetrazine 304.4
phenobal 304.1
phenobarbital 304.1
phenobarbitone 304.1
phenomorphan 304.0
phenonyl 304.1
phenoperidine 304.0
pholcodine 304.0
piminodine 304.0
Pipadone 304.0
Pitkin's solution 304.6
Placidyl 304.1
polysubstance 304.8
Pontocaine 304.6
pot 304.3
potassium bromide 304.1
Preludin 304.4
Prinadol 304.0
probarbital 304.1
procaine 304.6
propanal 304.1
propoxyphene 304.6
psilocibin 304.5
psilocin 304.5
psilocybin 304.5
psilocyline 304.5
psilocyn 304.5
psychedelic agents 304.5
psychostimulant NEC 304.4
psychotomimetic agents 304.5
pyrahexyl 304.3
Pyramidon 304.6
quinalbarbitone 304.1
racemoramide 304.0
racemorphan 304.0
Rela 304.6
scopolamine 304.6
secobarbital 304.1
Seconal 304.1
sedative NEC 304.1
   nonbarbiturate with barbiturate effect 304.1
Sedormid 304.1
sernyl 304.1
sodium bromide 304.1
Soma 304.6
Somnal 304.1
Somnos 304.1
Soneryl 304.1
soporific (drug) NEC 304.1
specified drug NEC 304.6
speed 304.4
spinocaine 304.6
Stovaine 304.6
STP 304.5
stramonium 304.6
Sulfonal 304.1
sulfonethylmethane 304.1
sulfonmethane 304.1
Surital 304.1
synthetic drug with morphine-like effect 304.0
talbutal 304.1
tetracaine 304.6
tetrahydrocannabinol 304.3
tetronal 304.1
THC 304.3
thebacon 304.0
thebaine 304.0
thiamil 304.1
thiamylal 304.1
thiopental 304.1

Dependence — *continued*
tobacco 305.1
toluene, toluol 304.6
tranquilizer NEC 304.1
   nonbarbiturate with barbiturate effect 304.1
tribromacetaldehyde 304.6
tribromethanol 304.6
tribromomethane 304.6
trichloroethanol 304.6
trichloroethyl phosphate 304.1
triclofos 304.1
Trional 304.1
Tuinal 304.1
Turkish Green 304.3
urethan(e) 304.6
Valium 304.1
Valmid 304.1
veganin 304.0
veramon 304.1
Veronal 304.1
versidyne 304.6
vinbarbital 304.1
vinbarbitone 304.1
vinyl bitone 304.1
vitamin B₆ 266.1
wine 303.9
Zactane 304.6
Dependency
passive 301.6
reactions 301.6
Depersonalization (episode, in neurotic state) (neurotic) (syndrome) 300.6
Depletion
carbohydrates 271.9
complement factor 279.8
extracellular fluid 276.52
plasma 276.52
potassium 276.8
   nephropathy 588.89
salt or sodium 276.1
   causing heat exhaustion or prostration 992.4
   nephropathy 593.9
volume 276.50
   extracellular fluid 276.52
   plasma 276.52
Deposit
argentous, cornea 371.16
bone, in Boeck's sarcoid 135
calcareous, calcium — *see* Calcification
cholesterol
   retina 362.82
   skin 709.3
   vitreous (humor) 379.22
conjunctival 372.56
cornea, corneal NEC 371.10
   argentous 371.16
   in
      cystinosis 270.0 [371.15]
      mucopolysaccharidosis 277.5 [371.15]
crystalline, vitreous (humor) 379.22
hemosiderin, in old scars of cornea 371.11
metallic, in lens 366.45
skin 709.3
teeth, tooth (betel) (black) (green) (materia alba) (orange) (soft) (tobacco) 523.6
urate, in kidney (*see also* Disease, renal) 593.9
Depraved appetite 307.52
Depression 311
acute (*see also* Psychosis, affective) 296.2
   recurrent episode 296.3
   single episode 296.2
agitated (*see also* Psychosis, affective) 296.2
   recurrent episode 296.3
   single episode 296.2
anaclitic 309.21
anxiety 300.4

Depression — *continued*
arches 734
   congenital 754.61
autogenous (*see also* Psychosis, affective) 296.2
   recurrent episode 296.3
   single episode 296.2
basal metabolic rate (BMR) 794.7
bone marrow 289.9
central nervous system 799.1
   newborn 779.2
cerebral 331.9
   newborn 779.2
cerebrovascular 437.8
   newborn 779.2
chest wall 738.3
endogenous (*see also* Psychosis, affective) 296.2
   recurrent episode 296.3
   single episode 296.2
functional activity 780.99
hysterical 300.11
involutional, climacteric, or menopausal (*see also* Psychosis, affective) 296.2
   recurrent episode 296.3
   single episode 296.2
manic (*see also* Psychosis, affective) 296.80
medullary 348.8
   newborn 779.2
mental 300.4
metatarsal heads — *see* Depression, arches
metatarsus — *see* Depression, arches
monopolar (*see also* Psychosis, affective) 296.2
   recurrent episode 296.3
   single episode 296.2
nervous 300.4
neurotic 300.4
nose 738.0
postpartum 648.4
psychogenic 300.4
   reactive 298.0
psychoneurotic 300.4
psychotic (*see also* Psychosis, affective) 296.2
   reactive 298.0
   recurrent episode 296.3
   single episode 296.2
reactive 300.4
   neurotic 300.4
   psychogenic 298.0
   psychoneurotic 300.4
   psychotic 298.0
recurrent 296.3
respiratory center 348.8
   newborn 770.89
scapula 736.89
senile 290.21
situational (acute) (brief) 309.0
   prolonged 309.1
skull 754.0
sternum 738.3
visual field 368.40
Depressive reaction — *see also* Reaction, depressive
acute (transient) 309.0
   with anxiety 309.28
prolonged 309.1
situational (acute) 309.0
   prolonged 309.1
Deprivation
cultural V62.4
emotional V62.89
   affecting
      adult 995.82
      infant or child 995.51
food 994.2
   specific substance NEC 269.8
protein (familial) (kwashiorkor) 260
sleep V69.4
social V62.4
   affecting
      adult 995.82

Deprivation — *continued*
social — *continued*
   affecting — *continued*
      infant or child 995.51
symptoms, syndrome
   alcohol 291.81
   drug 292.0
vitamins (*see also* Deficiency, vitamin) 269.2
water 994.3
de Quervain's
disease (tendon sheath) 727.04
thyroiditis (subacute granulomatous thyroiditis) 245.1
Derangement
ankle (internal) 718.97
   current injury (*see also* Dislocation, ankle) 837.0
   recurrent 718.37
cartilage (articular) NEC (*see also* Disorder, cartilage, articular) 718.0
   knee 717.9
      recurrent 718.36
      recurrent 718.3
collateral ligament (knee) (medial) (tibial) 717.82
   current injury 844.1
      lateral (fibular) 844.0
      lateral (fibular) 717.81
      current injury 844.0
cruciate ligament (knee) (posterior) 717.84
   anterior 717.83
      current injury 844.2
   current injury 844.2
elbow (internal) 718.92
   current injury (*see also* Dislocation, elbow) 832.00
   recurrent 718.32
gastrointestinal 536.9
heart — *see* Disease, heart
hip (joint) (internal) (old) 718.95
   current injury (*see also* Dislocation, hip) 835.00
   recurrent 718.35
intervertebral disc — *see* Displacement, intervertebral disc
joint (internal) 718.90
   ankle 718.97
   current injury (*see also* Dislocation, by site)
      knee, meniscus or cartilage (*see also* Tear, meniscus) 836.2
   elbow 718.92
   foot 718.97
   hand 718.94
   hip 718.95
   knee 717.9
   multiple sites 718.99
   pelvic region 718.95
   recurrent 718.30
      ankle 718.37
      elbow 718.32
      foot 718.37
      hand 718.34
      hip 718.35
      knee 718.36
      multiple sites 718.39
      pelvic region 718.35
      shoulder (region) 718.31
      specified site NEC 718.38
      temporomandibular (old) 524.69
      wrist 718.33
   shoulder (region) 718.91
   specified site NEC 718.98
   spine NEC 724.9
   temporomandibular 524.69
   wrist 718.93
knee (cartilage) (internal) 717.9
   current injury (*see also* Tear, meniscus) 836.2
      ligament 717.89
         capsular 717.85

Dermatitis

Derangement — *continued*
  knee — *continued*
    ligament — *continued*
      collateral — *see* Derangement, collateral ligament
      cruciate — *see* Derangement, cruciate ligament
      specified NEC 717.85
    recurrent 718.36
  low back NEC 724.9
  meniscus NEC (knee) 717.5
    current injury (*see also* Tear, meniscus) 836.2
    lateral 717.40
      anterior horn 717.42
      posterior horn 717.43
      specified NEC 717.49
    medial 717.3
      anterior horn 717.1
      posterior horn 717.2
    recurrent 718.3 ☑
    site other than knee — *see* Disorder, cartilage, articular
  mental (*see also* Psychosis) 298.9
  rotator cuff (recurrent) (tear) 726.10
    current 840.4
  sacroiliac (old) 724.6
    current — *see* Dislocation, sacroiliac
  semilunar cartilage (knee) 717.5
    current injury 836.2
      lateral 836.1
      medial 836.0
    recurrent 718.3 ☑
  shoulder (internal) 718.91
    current injury (*see also* Dislocation, shoulder) 831.00
    recurrent 718.31
  spine (recurrent) NEC 724.9
    current — *see* Dislocation, spine
  temporomandibular (internal) (joint) (old) 524.69
    current — *see* Dislocation, jaw

Dercum's disease or syndrome (adiposis dolorosa) 272.8

Derealization (neurotic) 300.6

Dermal — *see* condition

Dermaphytid — *see* Dermatophytosis

Dermatergosis — *see* Dermatitis

Dermatitis (allergic) (contact) (occupational) (venenata) 692.9
  ab igne 692.82
  acneiform 692.9
  actinic (due to sun) 692.70
    acute 692.72
    chronic NEC 692.74
    other than from sun NEC 692.82
  ambustionis
    due to
      burn or scald — *see* Burn, by site
      sunburn (*see also* Sunburn) 692.71
  amebic 006.6
  ammonia 691.0
  anaphylactoid NEC 692.9
  arsenical 692.4
  artefacta 698.4
    psychogenic 316 *[698.4]*
  asthmatic 691.8
  atopic (allergic) (intrinsic) 691.8
    psychogenic 316 *[691.8]*
  atrophicans 701.8
    diffusa 701.8
    maculosa 701.3
  berlock, berloque 692.72
  blastomycetic 116.0
  blister beetle 692.89
  Brucella NEC 023.9
  bullosa 694.9
    striata pratensis 692.6
  bullous 694.9
    mucosynechial, atrophic 694.60
      with ocular involvement 694.61
    seasonal 694.8

Dermatitis — *continued*
  calorica
    due to
      burn or scald — *see* Burn, by site
      cold 692.89
      sunburn (*see also* Sunburn) 692.71
  caterpillar 692.89
  cercarial 120.3
  combustionis
    due to
      burn or scald — *see* Burn, by site
      sunburn (*see also* Sunburn) 692.71
  congelationis 991.5
  contusiformis 695.2
  diabetic 250.8 ☑
  diaper 691.0
  diphtheritica 032.85
  due to
    acetone 692.2
    acids 692.4
    adhesive plaster 692.4
    alcohol (skin contact) (substances classifiable to 980.0–980.9) 692.4
      taken internally 693.8
    alkalis 692.4
    allergy NEC 692.9
    ammonia (household) (liquid) 692.4
    animal
      dander (cat) (dog) 692.84
      hair (cat) (dog) 692.84
    arnica 692.3
    arsenic 692.4
      taken internally 693.8
    blister beetle 692.89
    cantharides 692.3
    carbon disulphide 692.2
    caterpillar 692.89
    caustics 692.4
    cereal (ingested) 693.1
      contact with skin 692.5
    chemical(s) NEC 692.4
      internal 693.8
      irritant NEC 692.4
      taken internally 693.8
    chlorocompounds 692.2
    coffee (ingested) 693.1
      contact with skin 692.5
    cold weather 692.89
    cosmetics 692.81
    cyclohexanes 692.2
    dander, animal (cat) (dog) 692.84
    deodorant 692.81
    detergents 692.0
    dichromate 692.4
    drugs and medicinals (correct substance properly administered) (internal use) 693.0
      external (in contact with skin) 692.3
      wrong substance given or taken 976.9
        specified substance — *see* Table of Drugs and Chemicals
      wrong substance given or taken 977.9
        specified substance — *see* Table of Drugs and Chemicals
    dyes 692.89
      hair 692.89
    epidermophytosis — *see* Dermatophytosis
    esters 692.2
    external irritant NEC 692.9
      specified agent NEC 692.89
    eye shadow 692.81
    fish (ingested) 693.1
      contact with skin 692.5
    flour (ingested) 693.1
      contact with skin 692.5

Dermatitis — *continued*
  due to — *continued*
    food (ingested) 693.1
      in contact with skin 692.5
    fruit (ingested) 693.1
      contact with skin 692.5
    fungicides 692.3
    furs 692.84
    glycols 692.2
    greases NEC 692.1
    hair, animal (cat) (dog) 692.84
    hair dyes 692.89
    hot
      objects and materials — *see* Burn, by site
      weather or places 692.89
    hydrocarbons 692.2
    infrared rays, except from sun 692.82
      solar NEC (*see also* Dermatitis, due to, sun) 692.70
    ingested substance 693.9
      drugs and medicinals (*see also* Dermatitis, due to, drugs and medicinals) 693.0
      food 693.1
      specified substance NEC 693.8
    ingestion or injection of chemical 693.8
      drug (correct substance properly administered) 693.0
      wrong substance given or taken 977.9
        specified substance — *see* Table of Drugs and Chemicals
    insecticides 692.4
    internal agent 693.9
      drugs and medicinals (*see also* Dermatitis, due to, drugs and medicinals) 693.0
      food (ingested) 693.1
        in contact with skin 692.5
      specified agent NEC 693.8
    iodine 692.3
    iodoform 692.3
    irradiation 692.82
    jewelry 692.83
    keratolytics 692.3
    ketones 692.2
    lacquer tree (Rhus verniciflua) 692.6
    light (sun) NEC (*see also* Dermatitis, due to, sun) 692.70
      other 692.82
    low temperature 692.89
    mascara 692.81
    meat (ingested) 693.1
      contact with skin 692.5
    mercury, mercurials 692.3
    metals 692.83
    milk (ingested) 693.1
      contact with skin 692.5
    Neomycin 692.3
    nylon 692.4
    oils NEC 692.1
    paint solvent 692.2
    pediculocides 692.3
    petroleum products (substances classifiable to 981) 692.4
    phenol 692.3
    photosensitiveness, photosensitivity (sun) 692.72
      other light 692.82
    plants NEC 692.6
    plasters, medicated (any) 692.3
    plastic 692.4
    poison
      ivy (Rhus toxicodendron) 692.6
      oak (Rhus diversiloba) 692.6
      plant or vine 692.6
      sumac (Rhus venenata) 692.6
      vine (Rhus radicans) 692.6
    preservatives 692.89
    primrose (primula) 692.6
    primula 692.6

Dermatitis — *continued*
  due to — *continued*
    radiation 692.82
      sun NEC (*see also* Dermatitis, due to, sun) 692.70
      tanning bed 692.82
    radioactive substance 692.82
    radium 692.82
    ragweed (Senecio jacobae) 692.6
    Rhus (diversiloba) (radicans) (toxicodendron) (venenata) (verniciflua) 692.6
    rubber 692.4
    scabicides 692.3
    Senecio jacobae 692.6
    solar radiation — *see* Dermatitis, due to, sun
    solvents (any) (substances classifiable to 982.0–982.8) 692.2
      chlorocompound group 692.2
      cyclohexane group 692.2
      ester group 692.2
      glycol group 692.2
      hydrocarbon group 692.2
      ketone group 692.2
      paint 692.2
    specified agent NEC 692.89
    sun 692.70
      acute 692.72
      chronic NEC 692.74
      specified NEC 692.79
    sunburn (*see also* Sunburn) 692.71
    sunshine NEC (*see also* Dermatitis, due to, sun) 692.70
    tanning bed 692.82
    tetrachlorethylene 692.2
    toluene 692.2
    topical medications 692.3
    turpentine 692.2
    ultraviolet rays, except from sun 692.82
      sun NEC (*see also* Dermatitis, due to, sun) 692.70
    vaccine or vaccination (correct substance properly administered) 693.0
      wrong substance given or taken
        bacterial vaccine 978.8
          specified — *see* Table of Drugs and Chemicals
        other vaccines NEC 979.9
          specified — *see* Table of Drugs and Chemicals
    varicose veins (*see also* Varicose, vein, inflamed or infected) 454.1
    x-rays 692.82
  dyshydrotic 705.81
  dysmenorrheica 625.8
  eczematoid NEC 692.9
    infectious 690.8
  eczematous NEC 692.9
  epidemica 695.89
  erysipelatosa 695.81
  escharotica — *see* Burn, by site
  exfoliativa, exfoliative 695.89
    generalized 695.89
    infantum 695.81
    neonatorum 695.81
  eyelid 373.31
    allergic 373.32
    contact 373.32
    eczematous 373.31
    herpes (zoster) 053.20
      simplex 054.41
    infective 373.5
      due to
        actinomycosis 039.3 *[373.5]*
        herpes
          simplex 054.41
          zoster 053.20
        impetigo 684 *[373.5]*

Dermatitis

Dermatitis — *continued*
  eyelid — *continued*
    infective — *continued*
      due to — *continued*
        leprosy (*see also* Leprosy) 030.0 *[373.4]*
        lupus vulgaris (tuberculous) (*see also* Tuberculosis) 017.0 ☑ *[373.4]*
        mycotic dermatitis (*see also* Dermatomycosis) 111.9 *[373.5]*
        vaccinia 051.0 *[373.5]*
          postvaccination 999.0 *[373.5]*
        yaws (*see also* Yaws) 102.9 *[373.4]*
  facta, factitia 698.4
    psychogenic 316 *[698.4]*
  ficta 698.4
    psychogenic 316 *[698.4]*
  flexural 691.8
  follicularis 704.8
  friction 709.8
  fungus 111.9
    specified type NEC 111.8
  gangrenosa, gangrenous (infantum) (*see also* Gangrene) 785.4
  gestationis 646.8 ☑
  gonococcal 098.89
  gouty 274.89
  harvest mite 133.8
  heat 692.89
  herpetiformis (bullous) (erythematous) (pustular) (vesicular) 694.0
    juvenile 694.2
    senile 694.5
  hiemalis 692.89
  hypostatic, hypostatica 454.1
    with ulcer 454.2
  impetiginosa 684
  infantile (acute) (chronic) (intertriginous) (intrinsic) (seborrheic) 690.12
  infectiosa eczematoides 690.8
  infectious (staphylococcal) (streptococcal) 686.9
    eczematoid 690.8
  infective eczematoid 690.8
  Jacquet's (diaper dermatitis) 691.0
  leptus 133.8
  lichenified NEC 692.9
  lichenoid, chronic 701.0
  lichenoides purpurica pigmentosa 709.1
  meadow 692.6
  medicamentosa (correct substance properly administered) (internal use) (*see also* Dermatitis, due to, drugs or medicinals) 693.0
    due to contact with skin 692.3
  mite 133.8
  multiformis 694.0
    juvenile 694.2
    senile 694.5
  napkin 691.0
  neuro 698.3
  neurotica 694.0
  nummular NEC 692.9
  osteatosis, osteatotic 706.8
  papillaris capillitii 706.1
  pellagrous 265.2
  perioral 695.3
  perstans 696.1
  photosensitivity (sun) 692.72
    other light 692.82
  pigmented purpuric lichenoid 709.1
  polymorpha dolorosa 694.0
  primary irritant 692.9
  pruriginosa 694.0
  pruritic NEC 692.9
  psoriasiform nodularis 696.2
  psychogenic 316
  purulent 686.00
  pustular contagious 051.2
  pyococcal 686.00

Dermatitis — *continued*
  pyocyaneus 686.09
  pyogenica 686.00
  radiation 692.82
  repens 696.1
  Ritter's (exfoliativa) 695.81
  Schamberg's (progressive pigmentary dermatosis) 709.09
  schistosome 120.3
  seasonal bullous 694.8
  seborrheic 690.10
    infantile 690.12
  sensitization NEC 692.9
  septic (*see also* Septicemia) 686.00
    gonococcal 098.89
  solar, solare NEC (*see also* Dermatitis, due to, sun) 692.70
  stasis 459.81
    due to
      postphlebitic syndrome 459.12
        with ulcer 459.13
      varicose veins — *see* Varicose
    ulcerated or with ulcer (varicose) 454.2
  sunburn (*see also* Sunburn) 692.71
  suppurative 686.00
  traumatic NEC 709.8
  trophoneurotica 694.0
  ultraviolet, except from sun 692.82
    due to sun NEC (*see also* Dermatitis, due to, sun) 692.82
  varicose 454.1
    with ulcer 454.2
  vegetans 686.8
  verrucosa 117.2
  xerotic 706.8
Dermatoarthritis, lipoid 272.8 *[713.0]*
Dermatochalasia, dermatochalasis 374.87
Dermatofibroma (lenticulare) (M8832/0) — *see also* Neoplasm, skin, benign
  protuberans (M8832/1) — *see* Neoplasm, skin, uncertain behavior
Dermatofibrosarcoma (protuberans) (M8832/3) — *see* Neoplasm, skin, malignant
Dermatographia 708.3
Dermatolysis (congenital) (exfoliativa) 757.39
  acquired 701.8
  eyelids 374.34
  palpebrarum 374.34
  senile 701.8
Dermatomegaly NEC 701.8
Dermatomucomyositis 710.3
Dermatomycosis 111.9
  furfuracea 111.0
  specified type NEC 111.8
Dermatomyositis (acute) (chronic) 710.3
Dermatoneuritis of children 985.0
Dermatophiliasis 134.1
Dermatophytide — *see* Dermatophytosis
Dermatophytosis (Epidermophyton) (infection) (microsporum) (tinea) (Trichophyton) 110.9
  beard 110.0
  body 110.5
  deep seated 110.6
  fingernails 110.1
  foot 110.4
  groin 110.3
  hand 110.2
  nail 110.1
  perianal (area) 110.3
  scalp 110.0
  scrotal 110.8
  specified site NEC 110.8
  toenails 110.1
  vulva 110.8
Dermatopolyneuritis 985.0
Dermatorrhexis 756.83
  acquired 701.8
Dermatosclerosis — *see also* Scleroderma 710.1
  localized 701.0
Dermatosis 709.9

Dermatosis — *continued*
  Andrews' 686.8
  atopic 691.8
  Bowen's (M8081/2) — *see* Neoplasm, skin, in situ
  bullous 694.9
    specified type NEC 694.8
  erythematosquamous 690.8
  exfoliativa 695.89
  factitial 698.4
  gonococcal 098.89
  herpetiformis 694.0
    juvenile 694.2
    senile 694.5
  hysterical 300.11
  linear IgA 694.8
  menstrual NEC 709.8
  neutrophilic, acute febrile 695.89
  occupational (*see also* Dermatitis) 692.9
  papulosa nigra 709.8
  pigmentary NEC 709.00
    progressive 709.09
    Schamberg's 709.09
    Siemens-Bloch 757.33
  progressive pigmentary 709.09
  psychogenic 316
  pustular subcorneal 694.1
  Schamberg's (progressive pigmentary) 709.09
  senile NEC 709.3
  specified NEC 702.8
  Unna's (seborrheic dermatitis) 690.10
Dermographia 708.3
Dermographism 708.3
Dermoid (cyst) (M9084/0) — *see also* Neoplasm, by site, benign
  with malignant transformation (M9084/3) 183.0
Dermopathy
  infiltrative, with thyrotoxicosis 242.0 ☑
  senile NEC 709.3
Dermophytosis — *see* Dermatophytosis
Descemet's membrane — *see* condition
Descemetocele 371.72
Descending — *see* condition
Descensus uteri (complete) (incomplete) (partial) (without vaginal wall prolapse) 618.1
  with mention of vaginal wall prolapse — *see* Prolapse, uterovaginal
Desensitization to allergens V07.1
Desert
  rheumatism 114.0
  sore (*see also* Ulcer, skin) 707.9
Desertion (child) (newborn) 995.52
  adult 995.84
Desmoid (extra-abdominal) (tumor) (M8821/1) — *see also* Neoplasm, connective tissue, uncertain behavior
  abdominal (M8822/1) — *see* Neoplasm, connective tissue, uncertain behavior
Despondency 300.4
Desquamative dermatitis NEC 695.89
Destruction
  articular facet (*see also* Derangement, joint) 718.9 ☑
    vertebra 724.9
  bone 733.90
    syphilitic 095.5
  joint (*see also* Derangement, joint) 718.9 ☑
    sacroiliac 724.6
  kidney 593.89
  live fetus to facilitate birth NEC 763.89
  ossicles (ear) 385.24
  rectal sphincter 569.49
  septum (nasal) 478.19 ▲
  tuberculous NEC (*see also* Tuberculosis) 011.9 ☑
  tympanic membrane 384.82
  tympanum 385.89

Destruction — *continued*
  vertebral disc — *see* Degeneration, intervertebral disc
Destructiveness — *see also* Disturbance, conduct 312.9
  adjustment reaction 309.3
Detachment
  cartilage (*see also* Sprain, by site)
    knee — *see* Tear, meniscus
  cervix, annular 622.8
    complicating delivery 665.3 ☑
  choroid (old) (postinfectional) (simple) (spontaneous) 363.70
    hemorrhagic 363.72
    serous 363.71
  knee, medial meniscus (old) 717.3
    current injury 836.0
  ligament — *see* Sprain, by site
  placenta (premature) — *see* Placenta, separation
  retina (recent) 361.9
    with retinal defect (rhegmatogenous) 361.00
      giant tear 361.03
      multiple 361.02
      partial
        with
          giant tear 361.03
          multiple defects 361.02
          retinal dialysis (juvenile) 361.04
          single defect 361.01
    retinal dialysis (juvenile) 361.04
    single 361.01
    subtotal 361.05
    total 361.05
  delimited (old) (partial) 361.06
  old
    delimited 361.06
    partial 361.06
    total or subtotal 361.07
  pigment epithelium (RPE) (serous) 362.42
    exudative 362.42
    hemorrhagic 362.43
  rhegmatogenous (*see also* Detachment, retina, with retinal defect) 361.00
  serous (without retinal defect) 361.2
  specified type NEC 361.89
  traction (with vitreoretinal organization) 361.81
  vitreous humor 379.21
Detergent asthma 507.8
Deterioration
  epileptic
    with behavioral disturbance 345.9 ☑ *[294.11]*
    without behavioral disturbance 345.9 ☑ *[294.10]*
  heart, cardiac (*see also* Degeneration, myocardial) 429.1
  mental (*see also* Psychosis) 298.9
  myocardium, myocardial (*see also* Degeneration, myocardial) 429.1
  senile (simple) 797
  transplanted organ — *see* Complications, transplant, organ, by site
de Toni-Fanconi syndrome (cystinosis) 270.0
Deuteranomaly 368.52
Deuteranopia (anomalous trichromat) (complete) (incomplete) 368.52
Deutschländer's disease — *see* Fracture, foot
Development
  abnormal, bone 756.9
  arrested 783.40
    bone 733.91
    child 783.40
    due to malnutrition (protein-calorie) 263.2
    fetus or newborn 764.9 ☑
    tracheal rings (congenital) 748.3

Index to Diseases

Development — continued
  defective, congenital (see also Anomaly)
    cauda equina 742.59
    left ventricle 746.9
      with atresia or hypoplasia of aortic orifice or valve with hypoplasia of ascending aorta 746.7
      in hypoplastic left heart syndrome 746.7
  delayed (see also Delay, development) 783.40
    arithmetical skills 315.1
    language (skills) 315.31
      expressive 315.31
      mixed receptive-expressive 315.32
    learning skill, specified NEC 315.2
    mixed skills 315.5
    motor coordination 315.4
    reading 315.00
    specified
      learning skill NEC 315.2
      type NEC, except learning 315.8
    speech 315.39
      associated with hyperkinesia 314.1
      phonological 315.39
    spelling 315.09
    written expression 315.2
  imperfect, congenital (see also Anomaly)
    heart 746.9
    lungs 748.60
  improper (fetus or newborn) 764.9 ☑
  incomplete (fetus or newborn) 764.9 ☑
    affecting management of pregnancy 656.5 ☑
    bronchial tree 748.3
    organ or site not listed — see Hypoplasia
    respiratory system 748.9
  sexual, precocious NEC 259.1
  tardy, mental (see also Retardation, mental) 319
Developmental — see condition
Devergie's disease (pityriasis rubra pilaris) 696.4
Deviation
  conjugate (eye) 378.87
    palsy 378.81
    spasm, spastic 378.82
  esophagus 530.89
  eye, skew 378.87
  mandible, opening and closing 524.53
  midline (jaw) (teeth) 524.29
    specified site NEC — see Malposition
  occlusal plane 524.76
  organ or site, congenital NEC — see Malposition, congenital
  septum (acquired) (nasal) 470
    congenital 754.0
  sexual 302.9
    bestiality 302.1
    coprophilia 302.89
    ego-dystonic
      homosexuality 302.0
      lesbianism 302.0
    erotomania 302.89
      Clérambault's 297.8
    exhibitionism (sexual) 302.4
    fetishism 302.81
      transvestic 302.3
    frotteurism 302.89
    homosexuality, ego-dystonic 302.0
      pedophilic 302.2
    lesbianism, ego-dystonic 302.0
    masochism 302.83
    narcissism 302.89
    necrophilia 302.89
    nymphomania 302.89
    pederosis 302.2
    pedophilia 302.2
    sadism 302.84

Deviation — continued
  sexual — continued
    sadomasochism 302.84
    satyriasis 302.89
    specified type NEC 302.89
    transvestic fetishism 302.3
    transvestism 302.3
    voyeurism 302.82
    zoophilia (erotica) 302.1
  teeth, midline 524.29
  trachea 519.19 ▲
  ureter (congenital) 753.4
Devic's disease 341.0
Device
  cerebral ventricle (communicating) in situ V45.2
  contraceptive — see Contraceptive, device
  drainage, cerebrospinal fluid V45.2
Devil's
  grip 074.1
  pinches (purpura simplex) 287.2
Devitalized tooth 522.9
Devonshire colic 984.9
  specified type of lead — see Table of Drugs and Chemicals
Dextraposition, aorta 747.21
  with ventricular septal defect, pulmonary stenosis or atresia, and hypertrophy of right ventricle 745.2
  in tetralogy of Fallot 745.2
Dextratransposition, aorta 745.11
Dextrinosis, limit (debrancher enzyme deficiency) 271.0
Dextrocardia (corrected) (false) (isolated) (secondary) (true) 746.87
  with
    complete transposition of viscera 759.3
    situs inversus 759.3
Dextroversion, kidney (left) 753.3
Dhobie itch 110.3
Diabetes, diabetic (brittle) (congenital) (familial) (mellitus) (poorly controlled) (severe) (slight) (without complication) 250.0 ☑

Note — Use the following fifth-digit subclassification with category 250:

0 type II or unspecified type, not stated as uncontrolled

Fifth-digit 0 is for use for type II patients, even if the patient requires insulin

1 type I [juvenile type], not stated as uncontrolled

2 type II or unspecified type, uncontrolled

Fifth-digit 2 is for use for type II patients, even if the patient requires insulin

3 type I [juvenile type], uncontrolled

  with
    coma (with ketoacidosis) 250.3 ☑
      hyperosmolar (nonketotic) 250.2 ☑
    complication NEC 250.9 ☑
      specified NEC 250.8 ☑
    gangrene 250.7 ☑ [785.4]
    hyperosmolarity 250.2 ☑
    ketosis, ketoacidosis 250.1 ☑
    osteomyelitis 250.8 ☑ [731.8]
    specified manisfestations NEC 250.8 ☑
  acetonemia 250.1 ☑
  acidosis 250.1 ☑
  amyotrophy 250.6 ☑ [358.1]
  angiopathy, peripheral 250.7 ☑ [443.81]
  asymptomatic 790.29
  autonomic neuropathy (peripheral) 250.6 ☑ [337.1]

Diabetes, diabetic — continued
  bone change 250.8 ☑ [731.8]
  bronze, bronzed 275.0
  cataract 250.5 ☑ [366.41]
  chemical 790.29
    complicating pregnancy, childbirth, or puerperium 648.8 ☑
  coma (with ketoacidosis) 250.3 ☑
    hyperglycemic 250.3 ☑
    hyperosmolar (nonketotic) 250.2 ☑
    hypoglycemic 250.3 ☑
    insulin 250.3 ☑
  complicating pregnancy, childbirth, or puerperium (maternal) 648.0 ☑
    affecting fetus or newborn 775.0
  complication NEC 250.9 ☑
    specified NEC 250.8 ☑
  dorsal sclerosis 250.6 ☑ [340]
  dwarfism-obesity syndrome 258.1
  gangrene 250.7 ☑ [785.4]
  gastroparesis 250.6 ☑ [536.3]
  gestational 648.8 ☑
    complicating pregnancy, childbirth, or puerperium 648.8 ☑
  glaucoma 250.5 ☑ [365.44]
  glomerulosclerosis (intercapillary) 250.4 ☑ [581.81]
  glycogenosis, secondary 250.8 ☑ [259.8]
  hemochromatosis 275.0
  hyperosmolar coma 250.2 ☑
  hyperosmolarity 250.2 ☑
  hypertension-nephrosis syndrome 250.4 ☑ [581.81]
  hypoglycemia 250.8 ☑
  hypoglycemic shock 250.8 ☑
  insipidus 253.5
    nephrogenic 588.1
    pituitary 253.5
    vasopressin-resistant 588.1
  intercapillary glomerulosclerosis 250.4 ☑ [581.81]
  iritis 250.5 ☑ [364.42]
  ketosis, ketoacidosis 250.1 ☑
  Kimmelstiel (-Wilson) disease or syndrome (intercapillary glomerulosclerosis) 250.4 ☑ [581.81]
  Lancereaux's (diabetes mellitus with marked emaciation) 250.8 ☑ [261]
  latent (chemical) 790.29
    complicating pregnancy, childbirth, or puerperium 648.8 ☑
  lipoidosis 250.8 ☑ [272.7]
  macular edema 250.5 ☑ [362.07]
  maternal
    with manifest disease in the infant 775.1
    affecting fetus or newborn 775.0
  microaneurysms, retinal 250.5 ☑ [362.01]
  mononeuropathy 250.6 ☑ [355.9]
  neonatal, transient 775.1
  nephropathy 250.4 ☑ [583.81]
  nephrosis (syndrome) 250.4 ☑ [581.81]
  neuralgia 250.6 ☑ [357.2]
  neuritis 250.6 ☑ [357.2]
  neurogenic arthropathy 250.6 ☑ [713.5]
  neuropathy 250.6 ☑ [357.2]
  nonclinical 790.29
  osteomyelitis 250.8 ☑ [731.8]
  peripheral autonomic neuropathy 250.6 ☑ [337.1]
  phosphate 275.3
  polyneuropathy 250.6 ☑ [357.2]
  renal (true) 271.4
  retinal
    edema 250.5 ☑ [362.07]
    hemorrhage 250.5 ☑ [362.01]
    microaneurysms 250.5 ☑ [362.01]
  retinitis 250.5 ☑ [362.01]
  retinopathy 250.5 ☑ [362.01]

Diabetes, diabetic — continued
  retinopathy — continued
    background 250.5 ☑ [362.01]
    nonproliferative 250.5 ☑ [362.03]
    mild 250.5 ☑ [362.04]
    moderate 250.5 ☑ [362.05]
    severe 250.5 ☑ [362.06]
    proliferative 250.5 ☑ [362.02]
  steroid induced
    correct substance properly administered 251.8
    overdose or wrong substance given or taken 962.0
  stress 790.29
  subclinical 790.29
  subliminal 790.29
  sugar 250.0 ☑
  ulcer (skin) 250.8 ☑ [707.9]
    lower extremity 250.8 ☑ [707.10]
      ankle 250.8 ☑ [707.13]
      calf 250.8 ☑ [707.12]
      foot 250.8 ☑ [707.15]
      heel 250.8 ☑ [707.14]
      knee 250.8 ☑ [707.19]
      specified site NEC 250.8 ☑ [707.19]
      thigh 250.8 ☑ [707.11]
      toes 250.8 ☑ [707.15]
    specified site NEC 250.8 ☑ [707.8]
  xanthoma 250.8 ☑ [272.2]
Diacyclothrombopathia 287.1
Diagnosis deferred 799.9
Dialysis (intermittent) (treatment)
  anterior retinal (juvenile) (with detachment) 361.04
  extracorporeal V56.0
  hemodialysis V56.0
    status only V45.1
  peritoneal V56.8
    status only V45.1
  renal V56.0
    status only V45.1
  specified type NEC V56.8
Diamond-Blackfan anemia or syndrome (congenital hypoplastic anemia) 284.01 ▲
Diamond-Gardener syndrome (autoerythrocyte sensitization) 287.2
Diaper rash 691.0
Diaphoresis (excessive) NEC — see also Hyperhidrosis 780.8
Diaphragm — see condition
Diaphragmalgia 786.52
Diaphragmitis 519.4
Diaphyseal aclasis 756.4
Diaphysitis 733.99
Diarrhea, diarrheal (acute) (autumn) (bilious) (bloody) (catarrhal) (choleraic) (chronic) (gravis) (green) (infantile) (lienteric) (noninfectious) (presumed noninfectious) (putrefactive) (secondary) (sporadic) (summer) (symptomatic) (thermic) 787.91
  achlorhydric 536.0
  allergic 558.3
  amebic (see also Amebiasis) 006.9
    with abscess — see Abscess, amebic
    acute 006.0
    chronic 006.1
    nondysenteric 006.2
  bacillary — see Dysentery, bacillary
  bacterial NEC 008.5
  balantidial 007.0
  bile salt-induced 579.8
  cachectic NEC 787.91
  chilomastix 007.8
  choleriformis 001.1
  coccidial 007.2
  Cochin-China 579.1
    anguilluliasis 127.2
    psilosis 579.1
  Dientamoeba 007.8
  dietetic 787.91

Diarrhea, diarrheal

Diarrhea, diarrheal — continued
due to
achylia gastrica 536.8
Aerobacter aerogenes 008.2
Bacillus coli — see Enteritis, E. coli
bacteria NEC 008.5
bile salts 579.8
Capillaria
hepatica 128.8
philippinensis 127.5
Clostridium perfringens (C) (F) 008.46
Enterobacter aerogenes 008.2
enterococci 008.49
Escherichia coli — see Enteritis, E. coli
Giardia lamblia 007.1
Heterophyes heterophyes 121.6
irritating foods 787.91
Metagonimus yokogawai 121.5
Necator americanus 126.1
Paracolobactrum arizonae 008.1
Paracolon bacillus NEC 008.47
Arizona 008.1
Proteus (bacillus) (mirabilis) (Morganii) 008.3
Pseudomonas aeruginosa 008.42
S. japonicum 120.2
specified organism NEC 008.8
bacterial 008.49
viral NEC 008.69
Staphylococcus 008.41
Streptococcus 008.49
anaerobic 008.46
Strongyloides stercoralis 127.2
Trichuris trichiuria 127.3
virus NEC (see also Enteritis, viral) 008.69
dysenteric 009.2
due to specified organism NEC 008.8
dyspeptic 787.91
endemic 009.3
due to specified organism NEC 008.8
epidemic 009.2
due to specified organism NEC 008.8
fermentative 787.91
flagellate 007.9
Flexner's (ulcerative) 004.1
functional 564.5
following gastrointestinal surgery 564.4
psychogenic 306.4
giardial 007.1
Giardia lamblia 007.1
hill 579.1
hyperperistalsis (nervous) 306.4
infectious 009.2
due to specified organism NEC 008.8
presumed 009.3
inflammatory 787.91
due to specified organism NEC 008.8
malarial (see also Malaria) 084.6
mite 133.8
mycotic 117.9
nervous 306.4
neurogenic 564.5
parenteral NEC 009.2
postgastrectomy 564.4
postvagotomy 564.4
prostaglandin induced 579.8
protozoal NEC 007.9
psychogenic 306.4
septic 009.2
due to specified organism NEC 008.8
specified organism NEC 008.8
bacterial 008.49
viral NEC 008.69
Staphylococcus 008.41
Streptococcus 008.49
anaerobic 008.46

Diarrhea, diarrheal — continued
toxic 558.2
travelers' 009.2
due to specified organism NEC 008.8
trichomonal 007.3
tropical 579.1
tuberculous 014.8 ☑
ulcerative (chronic) (see also Colitis, ulcerative) 556.9
viral (see also Enteritis, viral) 008.8
zymotic NEC 009.2
Diastasis
cranial bones 733.99
congenital 756.0
joint (traumatic) — see Dislocation, by site
muscle 728.84
congenital 756.89
recti (abdomen) 728.84
complicating delivery 665.8 ☑
congenital 756.79
Diastema, teeth, tooth 524.30
Diastematomyelia 742.51
Diataxia, cerebral, infantile 343.0
Diathesis
allergic V15.09
bleeding (familial) 287.9
cystine (familial) 270.0
gouty 274.9
hemorrhagic (familial) 287.9
newborn NEC 776.0
oxalic 271.8
scrofulous (see also Tuberculosis) 017.2 ☑
spasmophilic (see also Tetany) 781.7
ulcer 536.9
uric acid 274.9
Diaz's disease or osteochondrosis 732.5
Dibothriocephaliasis 123.4
larval 123.5
Dibothriocephalus (infection) (infestation) (latus) 123.4
larval 123.5
Dicephalus 759.4
Dichotomy, teeth 520.2
Dichromat, dichromata (congenital) 368.59
Dichromatopsia (congenital) 368.59
Dichuchwa 104.0
Dicroceliasis 121.8
Didelphys, didelphic — see also Double uterus 752.2
Didymitis — see also Epididymitis 604.90
Died — see also Death
without
medical attention (cause unknown) 798.9
sign of disease 798.2
Dientamoeba diarrhea 007.8
Dietary
inadequacy or deficiency 269.9
surveillance and counseling V65.3
Dietl's crisis 593.4
Dieulafoy lesion (hemorrhagic)
of
duodenum 537.84
esophagus 530.82 ●
intestine 569.86
stomach 537.84
Difficult
birth, affecting fetus or newborn 763.9
delivery NEC 669.9 ☑
Difficulty
feeding 783.3
adult 783.3
breast 676.8 ☑
child 783.3
elderly 783.3
infant 783.3
newborn 779.3
nonorganic (infant) NEC 307.59
mechanical, gastroduodenal stoma 537.89

Difficulty — continued
reading 315.00
specific, spelling 315.09
swallowing (see also Dysphagia) 787.2
walking 719.7
Diffuse — see condition
Diffused ganglion 727.42
Di George's syndrome (thymic hypoplasia) 279.11
Digestive — see condition
Di Guglielmo's disease or syndrome (M9841/3) 207.0 ☑
Diktyoma (M9051/3) — see Neoplasm, by site, malignant
Dilaceration, tooth 520.4
Dilatation
anus 564.89
venue — see Hemorrhoids
aorta (focal) (general) (see also Aneurysm, aorta) 441.9
congenital 747.29
infectional 093.0
ruptured 441.5
syphilitic 093.0
appendix (cystic) 543.9
artery 447.8
bile duct (common) (cystic) (congenital) 751.69
acquired 576.8
bladder (sphincter) 596.8
congenital 753.8
in pregnancy or childbirth 654.4 ☑
causing obstructed labor 660.2 ☑
affecting fetus or newborn 763.1
blood vessel 459.89
bronchus, bronchi 494.0
with acute exacerbation 494.1
calyx (due to obstruction) 593.89
capillaries 448.9
cardiac (acute) (chronic) (see also Hypertrophy, cardiac) 429.3
congenital 746.89
valve NEC 746.89
pulmonary 746.09
hypertensive (see also Hypertension, heart) 402.90
cavum septi pellucidi 742.4
cecum 564.89
psychogenic 306.4
cervix (uteri) (see also Incompetency, cervix)
incomplete, poor, slow
affecting fetus or newborn 763.7
complicating delivery 661.0 ☑
affecting fetus or newborn 763.7
colon 564.7
congenital 751.3
due to mechanical obstruction 560.89
psychogenic 306.4
common bile duct (congenital) 751.69
acquired 576.8
with calculus, choledocholithiasis, or stones — see Choledocholithiasis
cystic duct 751.69
acquired (any bile duct) 575.8
duct, mammary 610.4
duodenum 564.89
esophagus 530.89
congenital 750.4
due to
achalasia 530.0
cardiospasm 530.0
Eustachian tube, congenital 744.24
fontanel 756.0
gallbladder 575.8
congenital 751.69
gastric 536.8
acute 536.1
psychogenic 306.4
heart (acute) (chronic) (see also Hypertrophy, cardiac) 429.3

Index to Diseases

Dilatation — continued
heart (see also Hypertrophy, cardiac) — continued
congenital 746.89
hypertensive (see also Hypertension, heart) 402.90
valve (see also Endocarditis)
congenital 746.89
ileum 564.89
psychogenic 306.4
inguinal rings — see Hernia, inguinal
jejunum 564.89
psychogenic 306.4
kidney (calyx) (collecting structures) (cystic) (parenchyma) (pelvis) 593.89
lacrimal passages 375.69
lymphatic vessel 457.1
mammary duct 610.4
Meckel's diverticulum (congenital) 751.0
meningeal vessels, congenital 742.8
myocardium (acute) (chronic) (see also Hypertrophy, cardiac) 429.3
organ or site, congenital NEC — see Distortion
pancreatic duct 577.8
pelvis, kidney 593.89
pericardium — see Pericarditis
pharynx 478.29
prostate 602.8
pulmonary
artery (idiopathic) 417.8
congenital 747.3
valve, congenital 746.09
pupil 379.43
rectum 564.89
renal 593.89
saccule vestibularis, congenital 744.05
salivary gland (duct) 527.8
sphincter ani 564.89
stomach 536.8
acute 536.1
psychogenic 306.4
submaxillary duct 527.8
trachea, congenital 748.3
ureter (idiopathic) 593.89
congenital 753.20
due to obstruction 593.5
urethra (acquired) 599.84
vasomotor 443.9
vein 459.89
ventricular, ventricle (acute) (chronic) (see also Hypertrophy, cardiac) 429.3
cerebral, congenital 742.4
hypertensive (see also Hypertension, heart) 402.90
venule 459.89
anus — see Hemorrhoids
vesical orifice 596.8
Dilated, dilation — see Dilatation
Diminished
hearing (acuity) (see also Deafness) 389.9
pulse pressure 785.9
vision NEC 369.9
vital capacity 794.2
Diminuta taenia 123.6
Diminution, sense or sensation (cold) (heat) (tactile) (vibratory) — see also Disturbance, sensation 782.0
Dimitri-Sturge-Weber disease (encephalocutaneous angiomatosis) 759.6
Dimple
parasacral 685.1
with abscess 685.0
pilonidal 685.1
with abscess 685.0
postanal 685.1
with abscess 685.0
Dioctophyma renale (infection) (infestation) 128.8
Dipetalonemiasis 125.4

Index to Diseases

Diphallus 752.69
Diphtheria, diphtheritic (gangrenous) (hemorrhagic) 032.9
  carrier (suspected) of V02.4
  cutaneous 032.85
  cystitis 032.84
  faucial 032.0
  infection of wound 032.85
  inoculation (anti) (not sick) V03.5
  laryngeal 032.3
  myocarditis 032.82
  nasal anterior 032.2
  nasopharyngeal 032.1
  neurological complication 032.89
  peritonitis 032.83
  specified site NEC 032.89
Diphyllobothriasis (intestine) 123.4
  larval 123.5
Diplacusis 388.41
Diplegia (upper limbs) 344.2
  brain or cerebral 437.8
  congenital 343.0
  facial 351.0
    congenital 352.6
  infantile or congenital (cerebral) (spastic) (spinal) 343.0
  lower limbs 344.1
  syphilitic, congenital 090.49
Diplococcus, diplococcal — see condition
Diplomyelia 742.59
Diplopia 368.2
  refractive 368.15
Dipsomania — see also Alcoholism 303.9 ☑
  with psychosis (see also Psychosis, alcoholic) 291.9
Dipylidiasis 123.8
  intestine 123.8
Direction, teeth, abnormal 524.30
Dirt-eating child 307.52
Disability
  heart — see Disease, heart
  learning NEC 315.2
  special spelling 315.09
Disarticulation — see also Derangement, joint 718.9 ☑
  meaning
    amputation
      status — see Absence, by site
      traumatic — see Amputation, traumatic
    dislocation, traumatic or congenital — see Dislocation
Disaster, cerebrovascular — see also Disease, cerebrovascular, acute 436
Discharge
  anal NEC 787.99
  breast (female) (male) 611.79
  conjunctiva 372.89
  continued locomotor idiopathic (see also Epilepsy) 345.5 ☑
  diencephalic autonomic idiopathic (see also Epilepsy) 345.5 ☑
  ear 388.60
    blood 388.69
    cerebrospinal fluid 388.61
  excessive urine 788.42
  eye 379.93
  nasal 478.19 ▲
  nipple 611.79
  patterned motor idiopathic (see also Epilepsy) 345.5 ☑
  penile 788.7
  postnasal — see Sinusitis
  sinus, from mediastinum 510.0
  umbilicus 789.9
  urethral 788.7
    bloody 599.84
  vaginal 623.5
Discitis 722.90
  cervical, cervicothoracic 722.91
  lumbar, lumbosacral 722.93
  thoracic, thoracolumbar 722.92

Discogenic syndrome — see Displacement, intervertebral disc
Discoid
  kidney 753.3
  meniscus, congenital 717.5
  semilunar cartilage 717.5
Discoloration
  mouth 528.9
  nails 703.8
  teeth 521.7
    due to
      drugs 521.7
      metals (copper) (silver) 521.7
      pulpal bleeding 521.7
    during formation 520.8
    extrinsic 523.6
    intrinsic posteruptive 521.7
Discomfort
  chest 786.59
  visual 368.13
Discomycosis — see Actinomycosis
Discontinuity, ossicles, ossicular chain 385.23
Discrepancy
  centric occlusion
    maximum intercuspation 524.55 ●
    of teeth 524.55
  leg length (acquired) 736.81
    congenital 755.30
  uterine size-date 649.6 ☑ ▲
Discrimination
  political V62.4
  racial V62.4
  religious V62.4
  sex V62.4
Disease, diseased — see also Syndrome
  Abrami's (acquired hemolytic jaundice) 283.9
  absorbent system 459.89
  accumulation — see Thesaurismosis
  acid-peptic 536.8
  Acosta's 993.2
  Adams-Stokes (-Morgagni) (syncope with heart block) 426.9
  Addison's (bronze) (primary adrenal insufficiency) 255.4
    anemia (pernicious) 281.0
    tuberculous (see also Tuberculosis) 017.6 ☑
  Addison-Gull — see Xanthoma
  adenoids (and tonsils) (chronic) 474.9
  adrenal (gland) (capsule) (cortex) 255.9
    hyperfunction 255.3
    hypofunction 255.4
    specified type NEC 255.8
  ainhum (dactylolysis spontanea) 136.0
  akamushi (scrub typhus) 081.2
  Akureyri (epidemic neuromyasthenia) 049.8
  Albarrán's (colibacilluria) 791.9
  Albers-Schönberg's (marble bones) 756.52
  Albert's 726.71
  Albright (-Martin) (-Bantam) 275.49
  Alibert's (mycosis fungoides) (M9700/3) 202.1 ☑
  Alibert-Bazin (M9700/3) 202.1 ☑
  alimentary canal 569.9
  alligator skin (ichthyosis congenita) 757.1
    acquired 701.1
  Almeida's (Brazilian blastomycosis) 116.1
  Alpers' 330.8
  alpine 993.2
  altitude 993.2
  alveoli, teeth 525.9
  Alzheimer's — see Alzheimer's
  amyloid (any site) 277.30 ▲
  anarthritic rheumatoid 446.5
  Anders' (adiposis tuberosa simplex) 272.8
  Andersen's (glycogenosis IV) 271.0
  Anderson's (angiokeratoma corporis diffusum) 272.7
  Andes 993.2

Disease, diseased

Disease, diseased — see also Syndrome — continued
  Andrews' (bacterid) 686.8
  angiospastic, angiospasmodic 443.9
    cerebral 435.9
      with transient neurologic deficit 435.9
    vein 459.89
  anterior
    chamber 364.9
    horn cell 335.9
      specified type NEC 335.8
  antral (chronic) 473.0
    acute 461.0
  anus NEC 569.49
  aorta (nonsyphilitic) 447.9
    syphilitic NEC 093.89
  aortic (heart) (valve) (see also Endocarditis, aortic) 424.1
  apollo 077.4
  aponeurosis 726.90
  appendix 543.9
  aqueous (chamber) 364.9
  arc-welders' lung 503
  Armenian 277.31 ▲
  Arnold-Chiari (see also Spina bifida) 741.0 ☑
  arterial 447.9
    occlusive (see also Occlusion, by site) 444.22
      with embolus or thrombus — see Occlusion, by site
      due to stricture or stenosis 447.1
    specified type NEC 447.8
  arteriocardiorenal (see also Hypertension, cardiorenal) 404.90
  arteriolar (generalized) (obliterative) 447.9
    specified type NEC 447.8
  arteriorenal — see Hypertension, kidney
  arteriosclerotic (see also Arteriosclerosis)
    cardiovascular 429.2
    coronary — see Arteriosclerosis, coronary
    heart — see Arteriosclerosis, coronary
    vascular — see Arteriosclerosis
  artery 447.9
    cerebral 437.9
    coronary — see Arteriosclerosis, coronary
    specified type NEC 447.8
  arthropod-borne NEC 088.9
    specified type NEC 088.89
  Asboe-Hansen's (incontinentia pigmenti) 757.33
  atticoantral, chronic (with posterior or superior marginal perforation of ear drum) 382.2
  auditory canal, ear 380.9
  Aujeszky's 078.89
  auricle, ear NEC 380.30
  Australian X 062.4
  autoimmune NEC 279.4
    hemolytic (cold type) (warm type) 283.0
    parathyroid 252.1
    thyroid 245.2
  aviators' (see also Effect, adverse, high altitude) 993.2
  ax(e)-grinders' 502
  Ayala's 756.89
  Ayerza's (pulmonary artery sclerosis with pulmonary hypertension) 416.0
  Azorean (of the nervous system) 334.8
  Babington's (familial hemorrhagic telangiectasia) 448.0
  back bone 733.90
  bacterial NEC 040.89
    zoonotic NEC 027.9
      specified type NEC 027.8

Disease, diseased — see also Syndrome — continued
  Baehr-Schiffrin (thrombotic thrombocytopenic purpura) 446.6
  Baelz's (cheilitis glandularis apostematosa) 528.5
  Baerensprung's (eczema marginatum) 110.3
  Balfour's (chloroma) 205.3 ☑
  balloon (see also Effect, adverse, high altitude) 993.2
  Baló's 341.1
  Bamberger (-Marie) (hypertrophic pulmonary osteoarthropathy) 731.2
  Bang's (Brucella abortus) 023.1
  Bannister's 995.1
  Banti's (with cirrhosis) (with portal hypertension) — see Cirrhosis, liver
  Barcoo (see also Ulcer, skin) 707.9
  barium lung 503
  Barlow (-Möller) (infantile scurvy) 267
  barometer makers' 985.0
  Barraquer (-Simons) (progressive lipodystrophy) 272.6
  basal ganglia 333.90
    degenerative NEC 333.0
    specified NEC 333.89
  Basedow's (exophthalmic goiter) 242.0 ☑
  basement membrane NEC 583.89
    with
      pulmonary hemorrhage (Goodpasture's syndrome) 446.21 [583.81]
  Bateman's 078.0
    purpura (senile) 287.2
  Batten's 330.1 [362.71]
  Batten-Mayou (retina) 330.1 [362.71]
  Batten-Steinert 359.2
  Battey 031.0
  Baumgarten-Cruveilhier (cirrhosis of liver) 571.5
  bauxite-workers' 503
  Bayle's (dementia paralytica) 094.1
  Bazin's (primary) (see also Tuberculosis) 017.1 ☑
  Beard's (neurasthenia) 300.5
  Beau's (see also Degeneration, myocardial) 429.1
  Bechterew's (ankylosing spondylitis) 720.0
  Becker's (idiopathic mural endomyocardial disease) 425.2
  Begbie's (exophthalmic goiter) 242.0 ☑
  Behr's 362.50
  Beigel's (white piedra) 111.2
  Bekhterev's (ankylosing spondylitis) 720.0
  Bell's (see also Psychosis, affective) 296.0 ☑
  Bennett's (leukemia) 208.9 ☑
  Benson's 379.22
  Bergeron's (hysteroepilepsy) 300.11
  Berlin's 921.3
  Bernard-Soulier (thrombopathy) 287.1
  Bernhardt (-Roth) 355.1
  beryllium 503
  Besnier-Boeck (-Schaumann) (sarcoidosis) 135
  Best's 362.76
  Beurmann's (sporotrichosis) 117.1
  Bielschowsky (-Jansky) 330.1
  Biermer's (pernicious anemia) 281.0
  Biett's (discoid lupus erythematosus) 695.4
  bile duct (see also Disease, biliary) 576.9
  biliary (duct) (tract) 576.9
    with calculus, choledocholithiasis, or stones — see Choledocholithiasis
  Billroth's (meningocele) (see also Spina bifida) 741.9 ☑
  Binswanger's 290.12

Disease, diseased — see also Syndrome — continued
- Bird's (oxaluria) 271.8
- bird fanciers' 495.2
- black lung 500
- bladder 596.9
  - specified NEC 596.8
- bleeder's 286.0
- Bloch-Sulzberger (incontinentia pigmenti) 757.33
- Blocq's (astasia-abasia) 307.9
- blood (-forming organs) 289.9
  - specified NEC 289.89
  - vessel 459.9
- Bloodgood's 610.1
- Blount's (tibia vara) 732.4
- blue 746.9
- Bodechtel-Guttmann (subacute sclerosing panencephalitis) 046.2
- Boeck's (sarcoidosis) 135
- bone 733.90
  - fibrocystic NEC 733.29
    - jaw 526.2
  - marrow 289.9
  - Paget's (osteitis deformans) 731.0
  - specified type NEC 733.99
  - von Recklinghausen's (osteitis fibrosa cystica) 252.01
- Bonfils' — see Disease, Hodgkin's
- Borna 062.9
- Bornholm (epidemic pleurodynia) 074.1
- Bostock's (see also Fever, hay) 477.9
- Bouchard's (myopathic dilatation of the stomach) 536.1
- Bouillaud's (rheumatic heart disease) 391.9
- Bourneville (-Brissaud) (tuberous sclerosis) 759.5
- Bouveret (-Hoffmann) (paroxysmal tachycardia) 427.2
- bowel 569.9
  - functional 564.9
  - psychogenic 306.4
- Bowen's (M8081/2) — see Neoplasm, skin, in situ
- Bozzolo's (multiple myeloma) (M9730/3) 203.0 ☑
- Bradley's (epidemic vomiting) 078.82
- Brailsford's 732.3
  - radius, head 732.3
  - tarsal, scaphoid 732.5
- Brailsford-Morquio (mucopolysaccharidosis IV) 277.5
- brain 348.9
  - Alzheimer's 331.0
    - with dementia — see Alzheimer's, dementia
  - arterial, artery 437.9
  - arteriosclerotic 437.0
  - congenital 742.9
  - degenerative — see Degeneration, brain
  - inflammatory (see also Encephalitis)
    - late effect — see category 326
  - organic 348.9
    - arteriosclerotic 437.0
  - parasitic NEC 123.9
  - Pick's 331.11
    - with dementia
      - with behavioral disturbance 331.11 [294.11]
      - without behavioral disturbance 331.11 [294.10]
  - senile 331.2
- braziers' 985.8
- breast 611.9
  - cystic (chronic) 610.1
  - fibrocystic 610.1
  - inflammatory 611.0
  - Paget's (M8540/3) 174.0
  - puerperal, postpartum NEC 676.3 ☑
  - specified NEC 611.8
- Breda's (see also Yaws) 102.9

Disease, diseased — see also Syndrome — continued
- Breisky's (kraurosis vulvae) 624.0
- Bretonneau's (diphtheritic malignant angina) 032.0
- Bright's (see also Nephritis) 583.9
  - arteriosclerotic (see also Hypertension, kidney) 403.90
- Brill's (recrudescent typhus) 081.1
  - flea-borne 081.0
  - louse-borne 081.1
- Brill-Symmers (follicular lymphoma) (M9690/3) 202.0 ☑
- Brill-Zinsser (recrudescent typhus) 081.1
- Brinton's (leather bottle stomach) (M8142/3) 151.9
- Brion-Kayser (see also Fever, paratyphoid) 002.9
- broad
  - beta 272.2
  - ligament, noninflammatory 620.9
    - specified NEC 620.8
- Brocq's 691.8
  - meaning
    - atopic (diffuse) neurodermatitis 691.8
    - dermatitis herpetiformis 694.0
    - lichen simplex chronicus 698.3
    - parapsoriasis 696.2
    - prurigo 698.2
- Brocq-Duhring (dermatitis herpetiformis) 694.0
- Brodie's (joint) (see also Osteomyelitis) 730.1 ☑
- bronchi 519.19 ▲
- bronchopulmonary 519.19 ▲
- bronze (Addison's) 255.4
  - tuberculous (see also Tuberculosis) 017.6 ☑
- Brown-Séquard 344.89
- Bruck's 733.99
- Bruck-de Lange (Amsterdam dwarf, mental retardation and brachycephaly) 759.89
- Bruhl's (splenic anemia with fever) 285.8
- Bruton's (X-linked agammaglobulinemia) 279.04
- buccal cavity 528.9
- Buchanan's (juvenile osteochondrosis, iliac crest) 732.1
- Buchman's (osteochondrosis juvenile) 732.1
- Budgerigar-Fanciers' 495.2
- Büdinger-Ludloff-Läwen 717.89
- Buerger's (thromboangiitis obliterans) 443.1
- Bürger-Grütz (essential familial hyperlipemia) 272.3
- Burns' (lower ulna) 732.3
- bursa 727.9
- Bury's (erythema elevatum diutinum) 695.89
- Buschke's 710.1
- Busquet's (see also Osteomyelitis) 730.1 ☑
- Busse-Buschke (cryptococcosis) 117.5
- C$_2$ (see also Alcoholism) 303.9 ☑
- Caffey's (infantile cortical hyperostosis) 756.59
- caisson 993.3
- calculous 592.9
- California 114.0
- Calvé (-Perthes) (osteochondrosis, femoral capital) 732.1
- Camurati-Engelmann (diaphyseal sclerosis) 756.59
- Canavan's 330.0
- capillaries 448.9
- Carapata 087.1
- cardiac — see Disease, heart
- cardiopulmonary, chronic 416.9

Disease, diseased — see also Syndrome — continued
- cardiorenal (arteriosclerotic) (hepatic) (hypertensive) (vascular) (see also Hypertension, cardiorenal) 404.90
- cardiovascular (arteriosclerotic) 429.2
  - congenital 746.9
  - hypertensive (see also Hypertension, heart) 402.90
    - benign 402.10
    - malignant 402.00
  - renal (see also Hypertension, cardiorenal) 404.90
  - syphilitic (asymptomatic) 093.9
- carotid gland 259.8
- Carrión's (Bartonellosis) 088.0
- cartilage NEC 733.90
  - specified NEC 733.99
- Castellani's 104.8
- cat-scratch 078.3
- Cavare's (familial periodic paralysis) 359.3
- Cazenave's (pemphigus) 694.4
- cecum 569.9
- celiac (adult) 579.0
  - infantile 579.0
- cellular tissue NEC 709.9
- central core 359.0
- cerebellar, cerebellum — see Disease, brain
- cerebral (see also Disease, brain) 348.9
  - arterial, artery 437.9
  - degenerative — see Degeneration, brain
- cerebrospinal 349.9
- cerebrovascular NEC 437.9
  - acute 436
    - embolic — see Embolism, brain
    - late effect — see Late effect(s) (of) cerebrovascular disease
    - puerperal, postpartum, childbirth 674.0 ☑
    - thrombotic — see Thrombosis, brain
  - arteriosclerotic 437.0
  - embolic — see Embolism, brain
  - ischemic, generalized NEC 437.1
  - late effect — see Late effect(s) (of) cerebrovascular disease
  - occlusive 437.1
  - puerperal, postpartum, childbirth 674.0 ☑
  - specified type NEC 437.8
  - thrombotic — see Thrombosis, brain
- ceroid storage 272.7
- cervix (uteri)
  - inflammatory 616.9
    - specified NEC 616.89 ▲
  - noninflammatory 622.9
    - specified NEC 622.8
- Chabert's 022.9
- Chagas' (see also Trypanosomiasis, American) 086.2
- Chandler's (osteochondritis dissecans, hip) 732.7
- Charcôt-Marie-Tooth 356.1
- Charcôt's (joint) 094.0 [713.5]
  - spinal cord 094.0
- Charlouis' (see also Yaws) 102.9
- Cheadle (-Möller) (-Barlow) (infantile scurvy) 267
- Chédiak-Steinbrinck (-Higashi) (congenital gigantism of peroxidase granules) 288.2
- cheek, inner 528.9
- chest 519.9
- Chiari's (hepatic vein thrombosis) 453.0
- Chicago (North American blastomycosis) 116.0
- chignon (white piedra) 111.2
- chigoe, chigo (jigger) 134.1

Disease, diseased — see also Syndrome — continued
- childhood granulomatous 288.1
- Chinese liver fluke 121.1
- chlamydial NEC 078.88
- cholecystic (see also Disease, gallbladder) 575.9
- choroid 363.9
  - degenerative (see also Degeneration, choroid) 363.40
  - hereditary (see also Dystrophy, choroid) 363.50
  - specified type NEC 363.8
- Christian's (chronic histiocytosis X) 277.89
- Christian-Weber (nodular nonsuppurative panniculitis) 729.30
- Christmas 286.1
- ciliary body 364.9
- circulatory (system) NEC 459.9
  - chronic, maternal, affecting fetus or newborn 760.3
  - specified NEC 459.89
  - syphilitic 093.9
    - congenital 090.5
- Civatte's (poikiloderma) 709.09
- climacteric 627.2
  - male 608.89
- coagulation factor deficiency (congenital) (see also Defect, coagulation) 286.9
- Coats' 362.12
- coccidioidal pulmonary 114.5
  - acute 114.0
  - chronic 114.4
  - primary 114.0
  - residual 114.4
- Cockayne's (microcephaly and dwarfism) 759.89
- Cogan's 370.52
- cold
  - agglutinin 283.0
    - or hemoglobinuria 283.0
    - paroxysmal (cold) (nocturnal) 283.2
  - hemagglutinin (chronic) 283.0
- collagen NEC 710.9
  - nonvascular 710.9
  - specified NEC 710.8
  - vascular (allergic) (see also Angiitis, hypersensitivity) 446.20
- colon 569.9
  - functional 564.9
    - congenital 751.3
  - ischemic 557.0
- combined system (of spinal cord) 266.2 [336.2]
  - with anemia (pernicious) 281.0 [336.2]
- compressed air 993.3
- Concato's (pericardial polyserositis) 423.2
  - peritoneal 568.82
  - pleural — see Pleurisy
- congenital NEC 799.89
- conjunctiva 372.9
  - chlamydial 077.98
    - specified NEC 077.8
  - specified type NEC 372.89
  - viral 077.99
    - specified NEC 077.8
- connective tissue, diffuse (see also Disease, collagen) 710.9
- Conor and Bruch's (boutonneuse fever) 082.1
- Conradi (-Hünermann) 756.59
- Cooley's (erythroblastic anemia) 282.49
- Cooper's 610.1
- Corbus' 607.1
- cork-handlers' 495.3
- cornea (see also Keratopathy) 371.9
- coronary (see also Ischemia, heart) 414.9
  - congenital 746.85
  - ostial, syphilitic 093.20

Index to Diseases — Disease, diseased

Disease, diseased — *see also* Syndrome
— *continued*
- coronary (*see also* Ischemia, heart) — *continued*
  - ostial, syphilitic — *continued*
    - aortic 093.22
    - mitral 093.21
    - pulmonary 093.24
    - tricuspid 093.23
- Corrigan's — *see* Insufficiency, aortic
- Cotugno's 724.3
- Coxsackie (virus) NEC 074.8
- cranial nerve NEC 352.9
- Creutzfeldt-Jakob (new variant) 046.1
  - with dementia
    - with behavioral disturbance 046.1 [294.11]
    - without behavioral disturbance 046.1 [294.10]
- Crigler-Najjar (congenital hyperbilirubinemia) 277.4
- Crocq's (acrocyanosis) 443.89
- Crohn's (intestine) (*see also* Enteritis, regional) 555.9
- Crouzon's (craniofacial dysostosis) 756.0
- Cruchet's (encephalitis lethargica) 049.8
- Cruveilhier's 335.21
- Cruz-Chagas (*see also* Trypanosomiasis, American) 086.2
- crystal deposition (*see also* Arthritis, due to, crystals) 712.9 ☑
- Csillag's (lichen sclerosus et atrophicus) 701.0
- Curschmann's 359.2
- Cushing's (pituitary basophilism) 255.0
- cystic
  - breast (chronic) 610.1
  - kidney, congenital (*see also* Cystic, disease, kidney) 753.10
  - liver, congenital 751.62
  - lung 518.89
    - congenital 748.4
  - pancreas 577.2
    - congenital 751.7
  - renal, congenital (*see also* Cystic, disease, kidney) 753.10
  - semilunar cartilage 717.5
- cysticercus 123.1
- cystine storage (with renal sclerosis) 270.0
- cytomegalic inclusion (generalized) 078.5
  - with
    - pneumonia 078.5 [484.1]
  - congenital 771.1
- Daae (-Finsen) (epidemic pleurodynia) 074.1
- dancing 297.8
- Danielssen's (anesthetic leprosy) 030.1
- Darier's (congenital) (keratosis follicularis) 757.39
  - erythema annulare centrifugum 695.0
  - vitamin A deficiency 264.8
- Darling's (histoplasmosis) (*see also* Histoplasmosis, American) 115.00
- Davies' 425.0
- de Beurmann-Gougerot (sporotrichosis) 117.1
- Débove's (splenomegaly) 789.2
- deer fly (*see also* Tularemia) 021.9
- deficiency 269.9
- degenerative (*see also* Degeneration)
  - disc — *see* Degeneration, intervertebral disc
- Degos' 447.8
- Déjérine (-Sottas) 356.0
- Déléage's 359.89
- demyelinating, demyelinizating (brain stem) (central nervous system) 341.9

Disease, diseased — *see also* Syndrome
— *continued*
- demyelinating, demyelinizating — *continued*
  - multiple sclerosis 340
  - specified NEC 341.8
- de Quervain's (tendon sheath) 727.04
  - thyroid (subacute granulomatous thyroiditis) 245.1
- Dercum's (adiposis dolorosa) 272.8
- Deutschländer's — *see* Fracture, foot
- Devergie's (pityriasis rubra pilaris) 696.4
- Devic's 341.0
- diaphorase deficiency 289.7
- diaphragm 519.4
- diarrheal, infectious 009.2
- diatomaceous earth 502
- Diaz's (osteochondrosis astragalus) 732.5
- digestive system 569.9
- Di Guglielmo's (erythemic myelosis) (M9841/3) 207.0 ☑
- Dimitri-Sturge-Weber (encephalocutaneous angiomatosis) 759.6
- disc, degenerative — *see* Degeneration, intervertebral disc
- discogenic (*see also* Disease, intervertebral disc) 722.90
- diverticular — *see* Diverticula
- Down's (mongolism) 758.0
- Dubini's (electric chorea) 049.8
- Dubois' (thymus gland) 090.5
- Duchenne's 094.0
  - locomotor ataxia 094.0
  - muscular dystrophy 359.1
  - paralysis 335.22
  - pseudohypertrophy, muscles 359.1
- Duchenne-Griesinger 359.1
- ductless glands 259.9
- Duhring's (dermatitis herpetiformis) 694.0
- Dukes (-Filatov) 057.8
- duodenum NEC 537.9
  - specified NEC 537.89
- Duplay's 726.2
- Dupré's (meningism) 781.6
- Dupuytren's (muscle contracture) 728.6
- Durand-Nicolas-Favre (climatic bubo) 099.1
- Duroziez's (congenital mitral stenosis) 746.5
- Dutton's (trypanosomiasis) 086.9
- Eales' 362.18
- ear (chronic) (inner) NEC 388.9
  - middle 385.9
    - adhesive (*see also* Adhesions, middle ear) 385.10
    - specified NEC 385.89
- Eberth's (typhoid fever) 002.0
- Ebstein's
  - heart 746.2
  - meaning diabetes 250.4 ☑ [581.81]
- Echinococcus (*see also* Echinococcus) 122.9
- ECHO virus NEC 078.89
- Economo's (encephalitis lethargica) 049.8
- Eddowes' (brittle bones and blue sclera) 756.51
- Edsall's 992.2
- Eichstedt's (pityriasis versicolor) 111.0
- Ellis-van Creveld (chondroectodermal dysplasia) 756.55
- endocardium — *see* Endocarditis
- endocrine glands or system NEC 259.9
  - specified NEC 259.8
- endomyocardial, idiopathic mural 425.2
- Engelmann's (diaphyseal sclerosis) 756.59
- Engel-von Recklinghausen (osteitis fibrosa cystica) 252.01
- English (rickets) 268.0

Disease, diseased — *see also* Syndrome
— *continued*
- Engman's (infectious eczematoid dermatitis) 690.8
- enteroviral, enterovirus NEC 078.89
  - central nervous system NEC 048
- epidemic NEC 136.9
- epididymis 608.9
- epigastric, functional 536.9
  - psychogenic 306.4
- Erb (-Landouzy) 359.1
- Erb-Goldflam 358.00
- Erichsen's (railway spine) 300.16
- esophagus 530.9
  - functional 530.5
  - psychogenic 306.4
- Eulenburg's (congenital paramyotonia) 359.2
- Eustachian tube 381.9
- Evans' (thrombocytopenic purpura) 287.32
- external auditory canal 380.9
- extrapyramidal NEC 333.90
- eye 379.90
  - anterior chamber 364.9
  - inflammatory NEC 364.3
  - muscle 378.9
- eyeball 360.9
- eyelid 374.9
- eyeworm of Africa 125.2
- Fabry's (angiokeratoma corporis diffusum) 272.7
- facial nerve (seventh) 351.9
  - newborn 767.5
- Fahr-Volhard (malignant nephrosclerosis) 403.00
- fallopian tube, noninflammatory 620.9
  - specified NEC 620.8
- familial periodic 277.31 ▲
  - paralysis 359.3
- Fanconi's (congenital pancytopenia) 284.09 ▲
- Farber's (disseminated lipogranulomatosis) 272.8
- fascia 728.9
  - inflammatory 728.9
- Fauchard's (periodontitis) 523.40 ▲
- Favre-Durand-Nicolas (climatic bubo) 099.1
- Favre-Racouchot (elastoidosis cutanea nodularis) 701.8
- Fede's 529.0
- Feer's 985.0
- Felix's (juvenile osteochondrosis, hip) 732.1
- Fenwick's (gastric atrophy) 537.89
- Fernels' (aortic aneurysm) 441.9
- fibrocaseous, of lung (*see also* Tuberculosis, pulmonary) 011.9 ☑
- fibrocystic (*see also* Fibrocystic, disease)
  - newborn 277.01
- Fiedler's (leptospiral jaundice) 100.0
- fifth 057.0
- Filatoff's (infectious mononucleosis) 075
- Filatov's (infectious mononucleosis) 075
- file-cutters' 984.9
  - specified type of lead — *see* Table of Drugs and Chemicals
- filterable virus NEC 078.89
- fish skin 757.1
  - acquired 701.1
- Flajani (-Basedow) (exophthalmic goiter) 242.0 ☑
- Flatau-Schilder 341.1
- flax-dressers' 504
- Fleischner's 732.3
- flint 502
- fluke — *see* Infestation, fluke
- Følling's (phenylketonuria) 270.1
- foot and mouth 078.4
- foot process 581.3
- Forbes' (glycogenosis III) 271.0

Disease, diseased — *see also* Syndrome
— *continued*
- Fordyce's (ectopic sebaceous glands) (mouth) 750.26
- Fordyce-Fox (apocrine miliaria) 705.82
- Fothergill's
  - meaning scarlatina anginosa 034.1
  - neuralgia (*see also* Neuralgia, trigeminal) 350.1
- Fournier's 608.83
- fourth 057.8
- Fox (-Fordyce) (apocrine miliaria) 705.82
- Francis' (*see also* Tularemia) 021.9
- Franklin's (heavy chain) 273.2
- Frei's (climatic bubo) 099.1
- Freiberg's (flattening metatarsal) 732.5
- Friedländer's (endarteritis obliterans) — *see* Arteriosclerosis
- Friedreich's
  - combined systemic or ataxia 334.0
  - facial hemihypertrophy 756.0
  - myoclonia 333.2
- Fröhlich's (adiposogenital dystrophy) 253.8
- Frommel's 676.6 ☑
- frontal sinus (chronic) 473.1
  - acute 461.1
- Fuller's earth 502
- fungus, fungous NEC 117.9
- Gaisböck's (polycythemia hypertonica) 289.0
- gallbladder 575.9
  - congenital 751.60
- Gamna's (siderotic splenomegaly) 289.51
- Gamstorp's (adynamia episodica hereditaria) 359.3
- Gandy-Nanta (siderotic splenomegaly) 289.51
- Gannister (occupational) 502
- Garré's (*see also* Osteomyelitis) 730.1 ☑
- gastric (*see also* Disease, stomach) 537.9
- gastrointestinal (tract) 569.9
  - amyloid 277.39 ▲
  - functional 536.9
    - psychogenic 306.4
- Gaucher's (adult) (cerebroside lipidosis) (infantile) 272.7
- Gayet's (superior hemorrhagic polioencephalitis) 265.1
- Gee (-Herter) (-Heubner) (-Thaysen) (nontropical sprue) 579.0
- generalized neoplastic (M8000/6) 199.0
- genital organs NEC
  - female 629.9
    - specified NEC 629.89 ▲
  - male 608.9
- Gerhardt's (erythromelalgia) 443.82
- Gerlier's (epidemic vertigo) 078.81
- Gibert's (pityriasis rosea) 696.3
- Gibney's (perispondylitis) 720.9
- Gierke's (glycogenosis I) 271.0
- Gilbert's (familial nonhemolytic jaundice) 277.4
- Gilchrist's (North American blastomycosis) 116.0
- Gilford (-Hutchinson) (progeria) 259.8
- Gilles de la Tourette's (motor-verbal tic) 307.23
- Giovannini's 117.9
- gland (lymph) 289.9
- Glanzmann's (hereditary hemorrhagic thrombasthenia) 287.1
- glassblowers' 527.1
- Glénard's (enteroptosis) 569.89
- Glisson's (*see also* Rickets) 268.0
- glomerular
  - membranous, idiopathic 581.1
  - minimal change 581.3

Disease, diseased — see also Syndrome — continued
- glycogen storage (Andersen's) (Cori types 1-7) (Forbes') (McArdle-Schmid-Pearson) (Pompe's) (types I-VII) 271.0
  - cardiac 271.0 [425.7]
  - generalized 271.0
  - glucose-6-phosphatase deficiency 271.0
  - heart 271.0 [425.7]
  - hepatorenal 271.0
  - liver and kidneys 271.0
  - myocardium 271.0 [425.7]
  - von Gierke's (glycogenosis I) 271.0
- Goldflam-Erb 358.00
- Goldscheider's (epidermolysis bullosa) 757.39
- Goldstein's (familial hemorrhagic telangiectasia) 448.0
- gonococcal NEC 098.0
- Goodall's (epidemic vomiting) 078.82
- Gordon's (exudative enteropathy) 579.8
- Gougerot's (trisymptomatic) 709.1
- Gougerot-Carteaud (confluent reticulate papillomatosis) 701.8
- Gougerot-Hailey-Hailey (benign familial chronic pemphigus) 757.39
- graft-versus-host (bone marrow) 996.85
  - due to organ transplant NEC — see Complications, transplant, organ
- grain-handlers' 495.8
- Grancher's (splenopneumonia) — see Pneumonia
- granulomatous (childhood) (chronic) 288.1
- graphite lung 503
- Graves' (exophthalmic goiter) 242.0 ☑
- Greenfield's 330.0
- green monkey 078.89
- Griesinger's (see also Ancylostomiasis) 126.9
- grinders' 502
- Grisel's 723.5
- Gruby's (tinea tonsurans) 110.0
- Guertin's (electric chorea) 049.8
- Guillain-Barré 357.0
- Guinon's (motor-verbal tic) 307.23
- Gull's (thyroid atrophy with myxedema) 244.8
- Gull and Sutton's — see Hypertension, kidney
- gum NEC 523.9
- Günther's (congenital erythropoietic porphyria) 277.1
- gynecological 629.9
  - specified NEC 629.89 ▲
- H 270.0
- Haas' 732.3
- Habermann's (acute parapsoriasis varioliformis) 696.2
- Haff 985.1
- Hageman (congenital factor XII deficiency) (see also Defect, congenital) 286.3
- Haglund's (osteochondrosis os tibiale externum) 732.5
- Hagner's (hypertrophic pulmonary osteoarthropathy) 731.2
- Hailey-Hailey (benign familial chronic pemphigus) 757.39
- hair (follicles) NEC 704.9
  - specified type NEC 704.8
- Hallervorden-Spatz 333.0
- Hallopeau's (lichen sclerosus et atrophicus) 701.0
- Hamman's (spontaneous mediastinal emphysema) 518.1
- hand, foot, and mouth 074.3
- Hand-Schüller-Christian (chronic histiocytosis X) 277.89
- Hanot's — see Cirrhosis, biliary
- Hansen's (leprosy) 030.9

Disease, diseased — see also Syndrome — continued
- Hansen's — continued
  - benign form 030.1
  - malignant form 030.0
- Harada's 363.22
- Harley's (intermittent hemoglobinuria) 283.2
- Hartnup (pellagra-cerebellar ataxia-renal aminoaciduria) 270.0
- Hart's (pellagra-cerebellar ataxia-renal aminoaciduria) 270.0
- Hashimoto's (struma lymphomatosa) 245.2
- Hb — see Disease, hemoglobin
- heart (organic) 429.9
  - with
    - acute pulmonary edema (see also Failure, ventricular, left) 428.1
      - hypertensive 402.91
        - with renal failure 404.93
          - benign 402.11
            - with renal failure 404.13
          - malignant 402.01
            - with renal failure 404.03
    - kidney disease — see Hypertension, cardiorenal
    - rheumatic fever (conditions classifiable to 390)
      - active 391.9
        - with chorea 392.0
      - inactive or quiescent (with chorea) 398.90
  - amyloid 277.39 [425.7] ▲
  - aortic (valve) (see also Endocarditis, aortic) 424.1
  - arteriosclerotic or sclerotic (minimal) (senile) — see Arteriosclerosis, coronary
  - artery, arterial — see Arteriosclerosis, coronary
  - atherosclerotic — see Arteriosclerosis, coronary
  - beer drinkers' 425.5
  - beriberi 265.0 [425.7]
  - black 416.0
  - congenital NEC 746.9
    - cyanotic 746.9
    - maternal, affecting fetus or newborn 760.3
    - specified type NEC 746.89
  - congestive (see also Failure, heart) 428.0
  - coronary 414.9
  - cryptogenic 429.9
  - due to
    - amyloidosis 277.39 [425.7] ▲
    - beriberi 265.0 [425.7]
    - cardiac glycogenosis 271.0 [425.7]
    - Friedreich's ataxia 334.0 [425.8]
    - gout 274.82
    - mucopolysaccharidosis 277.5 [425.7]
    - myotonia atrophica 359.2 [425.8]
    - progressive muscular dystrophy 359.1 [425.8]
    - sarcoidosis 135 [425.8]
  - fetal 746.9
    - inflammatory 746.89
  - fibroid (see also Myocarditis) 429.0
  - functional 427.9
    - postoperative 997.1
    - psychogenic 306.2
  - glycogen storage 271.0 [425.7]
  - gonococcal NEC 098.85
  - gouty 274.82
  - hypertensive (see also Hypertension, heart) 402.90
    - benign 402.10
    - malignant 402.00

Disease, diseased — see also Syndrome — continued
- heart — continued
  - hyperthyroid (see also Hyperthyroidism) 242.9 ☑ [425.7]
  - incompletely diagnosed — see Disease, heart
  - ischemic (chronic) (see also Ischemia, heart) 414.9
    - acute (see also Infarct, myocardium) 410.9 ☑
      - without myocardial infarction 411.89
        - with coronary (artery) occlusion 411.81
    - asymptomatic 412
    - diagnosed on ECG or other special investigation but currently presenting no symptoms 412
  - kyphoscoliotic 416.1
  - mitral (see also Endocarditis, mitral) 394.9
  - muscular (see also Degeneration, myocardial) 429.1
  - postpartum 674.8 ☑
  - psychogenic (functional) 306.2
  - pulmonary (chronic) 416.9
    - acute 415.0
    - specified NEC 416.8
  - rheumatic (chronic) (inactive) (old) (quiescent) (with chorea) 398.90
    - active or acute 391.9
      - with chorea (active) (rheumatic) (Sydenham's) 392.0
    - specified type NEC 391.8
  - maternal, affecting fetus or newborn 760.3
  - rheumatoid — see Arthritis, rheumatoid
  - sclerotic — see Arteriosclerosis, coronary
  - senile (see also Myocarditis) 429.0
  - specified type NEC 429.89
  - syphilitic 093.89
    - aortic 093.1
      - aneurysm 093.0
      - asymptomatic 093.89
    - congenital 090.5
  - thyroid (gland) (see also Hyperthyroidism) 242.9 ☑ [425.7]
  - thyrotoxic (see also Thyrotoxicosis) 242.9 ☑ [425.7]
  - tuberculous (see also Tuberculosis) 017.9 ☑ [425.8]
  - valve, valvular (obstructive) (regurgitant) (see also Endocarditis)
    - congenital NEC (see also Anomaly, heart, valve) 746.9
      - pulmonary 746.00
      - specified type NEC 746.89
  - vascular — see Disease, cardiovascular
- heavy-chain (gamma G) 273.2
- Heberden's 715.04
- Hebra's
  - dermatitis exfoliativa 695.89
  - erythema multiforme exudativum 695.1
  - pityriasis
    - maculata et circinata 696.3
    - rubra 695.89
      - pilaris 696.4
  - prurigo 698.2
- Heerfordt's (uveoparotitis) 135
- Heidenhain's 290.10
  - with dementia 290.10
- Heilmeyer-Schöner (M9842/3) 207.1 ☑
- Heine-Medin (see also Poliomyelitis) 045.9 ☑
- Heller's (see also Psychosis, childhood) 299.1 ☑

Disease, diseased — see also Syndrome — continued
- Heller-Döhle (syphilitic aortitis) 093.1
- hematopoietic organs 289.9
- hemoglobin (Hb) 282.7
  - with thalassemia 282.49
  - abnormal (mixed) NEC 282.7
    - with thalassemia 282.49
  - AS genotype 282.5
  - Bart's 282.49
  - C (Hb-C) 282.7
    - with other abnormal hemoglobin NEC 282.7
    - elliptocytosis 282.7
    - Hb-S (without crisis) 282.63
      - with
        - crisis 282.64
          - vaso-occlusive pain 282.64
    - sickle-cell (without crisis) 282.63
      - with
        - crisis 282.64
          - vaso-occlusive pain 282.64
    - thalassemia 282.49
  - constant spring 282.7
  - D (Hb-D) 282.7
    - with other abnormal hemoglobin NEC 282.7
    - Hb-S (without crisis) 282.68
      - with crisis 282.69
    - sickle-cell (without crisis) 282.68
      - with crisis 282.69
    - thalassemia 282.49
  - E (Hb-E) 282.7
    - with other abnormal hemoglobin NEC 282.7
    - Hb-S (without crisis) 282.68
      - with crisis 282.69
    - sickle-cell (without crisis) 282.68
      - with crisis 282.69
    - thalassemia 282.49
  - elliptocytosis 282.7
  - F (Hb-F) 282.7
  - G (Hb-G) 282.7
  - H (Hb-H) 282.49
  - hereditary persistence, fetal (HPFH) ("Swiss variety") 282.7
  - high fetal gene 282.7
  - I thalassemia 282.49
  - M 289.7
  - S (see also Disease, sickle-cell, Hb-S)
    - thalassemia (without crisis) 282.41
      - with
        - crisis 282.42
          - vaso-occlusive pain 282.42
  - spherocytosis 282.7
  - unstable, hemolytic 282.7
  - Zurich (Hb-Zurich) 282.7
- hemolytic (fetus) (newborn) 773.2
  - autoimmune (cold type) (warm type) 283.0
  - due to or with
    - incompatibility
      - ABO (blood group) 773.1
      - blood (group) (Duffy) (Kell) (Kidd) (Lewis) (M) (S) NEC 773.2
      - Rh (blood group) (factor) 773.0
    - Rh negative mother 773.0
  - unstable hemoglobin 282.7
- hemorrhagic 287.9
  - newborn 776.0
- Henoch (-Schönlein) (purpura nervosa) 287.0
- hepatic — see Disease, liver
- hepatolenticular 275.1
- heredodegenerative NEC
  - brain 331.89

Disease, diseased — see also Syndrome — continued
  heredodegenerative — continued
    spinal cord 336.8
  Hers' (glycogenosis VI) 271.0
  Herter (-Gee) (-Heubner) (nontropical sprue) 579.0
  Herxheimer's (diffuse idiopathic cutaneous atrophy) 701.8
  Heubner's 094.89
  Heubner-Herter (nontropical sprue) 579.0
  high fetal gene or hemoglobin thalassemia 282.49
  Hildenbrand's (typhus) 081.9
  hip (joint) NEC 719.95
    congenital 755.63
    suppurative 711.05
    tuberculous (see also Tuberculosis) 015.1 ☑ [730.85]
  Hippel's (retinocerebral angiomatosis) 759.6
  Hirschfeld's (acute diabetes mellitus) (see also Diabetes) 250.0 ☑
  Hirschsprung's (congenital megacolon) 751.3
  His (-Werner) (trench fever) 083.1
  HIV 042
  Hodgkin's (M9650/3) 201.9 ☑

  Note — *Use the following fifth-digit subclassification with category 201:*
  0   *unspecified site*
  1   *lymph nodes of head, face, and neck*
  2   *intrathoracic lymph nodes*
  3   *intra-abdominal lymph nodes*
  4   *lymph nodes of axilla and upper limb*
  5   *lymph nodes of inguinal region and lower limb*
  6   *intrapelvic lymph nodes*
  7   *spleen*
  8   *lymph nodes of multiple sites*

    lymphocytic
      depletion (M9653/3) 201.7 ☑
        diffuse fibrosis (M9654/3) 201.7 ☑
        reticular type (M9655/3) 201.7 ☑
      predominance (M9651/3) 201.4 ☑
    lymphocytic-histiocytic predominance (M9651/3) 201.4 ☑
    mixed cellularity (M9652/3) 201.6 ☑
    nodular sclerosis (M9656/3) 201.5 ☑
      cellular phase (M9657/3) 201.5 ☑
  Hodgson's 441.9
    ruptured 441.5
  Hoffa (-Kastert) (liposynovitis prepatellaris) 272.8
  Holla (see also Spherocytosis) 282.0
  homozygous-Hb-S 282.61
  hoof and mouth 078.4
  hookworm (see also Ancylostomiasis) 126.9
  Horton's (temporal arteritis) 446.5
  host-versus-graft (immune or nonimmune cause) 996.80
    bone marrow 996.85
    heart 996.83
    intestines 996.87
    kidney 996.81
    liver 996.82
    lung 996.84
    pancreas 996.86
    specified NEC 996.89

Disease, diseased — see also Syndrome — continued
  HPFH (hereditary persistence of fetal hemoglobin) ("Swiss variety") 282.7
  Huchard's disease (continued arterial hypertension) 401.9
  Huguier's (uterine fibroma) 218.9
  human immunodeficiency (virus) 042
  hunger 251.1
  Hunt's
    dyssynergia cerebellaris myoclonica 334.2
    herpetic geniculate ganglionitis 053.11
  Huntington's 333.4
  Huppert's (multiple myeloma) (M9730/3) 203.0 ☑
  Hurler's (mucopolysaccharidosis I) 277.5
  Hutchinson-Boeck (sarcoidosis) 135
  Hutchinson-Gilford (progeria) 259.8
  Hutchinson's, meaning
    angioma serpiginosum 709.1
    cheiropompholyx 705.81
    prurigo estivalis 692.72
  hyaline (diffuse) (generalized) 728.9
    membrane (lung) (newborn) 769
  hydatid (see also Echinococcus) 122.9
  Hyde's (prurigo nodularis) 698.3
  hyperkinetic (see also Hyperkinesia) 314.9
    heart 429.82
  hypertensive (see also Hypertension) 401.9
  hypophysis 253.9
    hyperfunction 253.1
    hypofunction 253.2
  Iceland (epidemic neuromyasthenia) 049.8
  I cell 272.7
  ill-defined 799.89
  immunologic NEC 279.9
  immunoproliferative 203.8 ☑
  inclusion 078.5
    salivary gland 078.5
  infancy, early NEC 779.9
  infective NEC 136.9
  inguinal gland 289.9
  internal semilunar cartilage, cystic 717.5
  intervertebral disc 722.90
    with myelopathy 722.70
    cervical, cervicothoracic 722.91
      with myelopathy 722.71
    lumbar, lumbosacral 722.93
      with myelopathy 722.73
    thoracic, thoracolumbar 722.92
      with myelopathy 722.72
  intestine 569.9
    functional 564.9
      congenital 751.3
      psychogenic 306.4
    lardaceous 277.39 ▲
    organic 569.9
    protozoal NEC 007.9
  iris 364.9
  iron
    metabolism 275.0
    storage 275.0
  Isambert's (see also Tuberculosis, larynx) 012.3 ☑
  Iselin's (osteochondrosis, fifth metatarsal) 732.5
  island (scrub typhus) 081.2
  itai-itai 985.5
  Jadassohn's (maculopapular erythroderma) 696.2
  Jadassohn-Pellizari's (anetoderma) 701.3
  Jakob-Creutzfeldt (new variant) 046.1
    with dementia
      with behavioral disturbance 046.1 [294.11]
      without behavioral disturbance 046.1 [294.10]

Disease, diseased — see also Syndrome — continued
  Jaksch (-Luzet) (pseudoleukemia infantum) 285.8
  Janet's 300.89
  Jansky-Bielschowsky 330.1
  jaw NEC 526.9
    fibrocystic 526.2
  Jensen's 363.05
  Jeune's (asphyxiating thoracic dystrophy) 756.4
  jigger 134.1
  Johnson-Stevens (erythema multiforme exudativum) 695.1
  joint NEC 719.9 ☑
    ankle 719.97
    Charcôt 094.0 [713.5]
    degenerative (see also Osteoarthrosis) 715.9 ☑
      multiple 715.09
      spine (see also Spondylosis) 721.90
    elbow 719.92
    foot 719.97
    hand 719.94
    hip 719.95
    hypertrophic (chronic) (degenerative) (see also Osteoarthrosis) 715.9 ☑
      spine (see also Spondylosis) 721.90
    knee 719.96
    Luschka 721.90
    multiple sites 719.99
    pelvic region 719.95
    sacroiliac 724.6
    shoulder (region) 719.91
    specified site NEC 719.98
    spine NEC 724.9
      pseudarthrosis following fusion 733.82
      sacroiliac 724.6
    wrist 719.93
  Jourdain's (acute gingivitis) 523.00 ▲
  Jüngling's (sarcoidosis) 135
  Kahler (-Bozzolo) (multiple myeloma) (M9730/3) 203.0 ☑
  Kalischer's 759.6
  Kaposi's 757.33
    lichen ruber 697.8
      acuminatus 696.4
      moniliformis 697.8
    xeroderma pigmentosum 757.33
  Kaschin-Beck (endemic polyarthritis) 716.00
    ankle 716.07
    arm 716.02
      lower (and wrist) 716.03
      upper (and elbow) 716.02
    foot (and ankle) 716.07
    forearm (and wrist) 716.03
    hand 716.04
    leg 716.06
      lower 716.06
      upper 716.05
    multiple sites 716.09
    pelvic region (hip) (thigh) 716.05
    shoulder region 716.01
    specified site NEC 716.08
  Katayama 120.2
  Kawasaki 446.1
  Kedani (scrub typhus) 081.2
  kidney (functional) (pelvis) (see also Disease, renal) 593.9
    chronic
      requiring chronic dialysis 585.6 ●
      stage
        I 585.1
        II (mild) 585.2
        III (moderate) 585.3
        IV (severe) 585.4
        V 585.5
    cystic (congenital) 753.10
      multiple 753.19

Disease, diseased — see also Syndrome — continued
  kidney (see also Disease, renal) — continued
    cystic — continued
      single 753.11
      specified NEC 753.19
    fibrocystic (congenital) 753.19
    in gout 274.10
    polycystic (congenital) 753.12
      adult type (APKD) 753.13
      autosomal dominant 753.13
      autosomal recessive 753.14
      childhood type (CPKD) 753.14
      infantile type 753.14
  Kienböck's (carpal lunate) (wrist) 732.3
  Kimmelstiel (-Wilson) (intercapillary glomerulosclerosis) 250.4 ☑ [581.81]
  Kinnier Wilson's (hepatolenticular degeneration) 275.1
  kissing 075
  Kleb's (see also Nephritis) 583.9
  Klinger's 446.4
  Klippel's 723.8
  Klippel-Feil (brevicollis) 756.16
  knight's 911.1
  Köbner's (epidermolysis bullosa) 757.39
  Koenig-Wichmann (pemphigus) 694.4
  Köhler's
    first (osteoarthrosis juvenilis) 732.5
    second (Freiberg's infraction, metatarsal head) 732.5
    patellar 732.4
    tarsal navicular (bone) (osteoarthrosis juvenilis) 732.5
  Köhler-Freiberg (infraction, metatarsal head) 732.5
  Köhler-Mouchet (osteoarthrosis juvenilis) 732.5
  Köhler-Pellegrini-Stieda (calcification, knee joint) 726.62
  Kok 759.89
  König's (osteochondritis dissecans) 732.7
  Korsakoff's (nonalcoholic) 294.0
    alcoholic 291.1
  Kostmann's (infantile genetic agranulocytosis) 288.01 ▲
  Krabbe's 330.0
  Kraepelin-Morel (see also Schizophrenia) 295.9
  Kraft-Weber-Dimitri 759.6
  Kufs' 330.1
  Kugelberg-Welander 335.11
  Kuhnt-Junius 362.52
  Kümmell's (-Verneuil) (spondylitis) 721.7
  Kundrat's (lymphosarcoma) 200.1 ☑
  kuru 046.0
  Kussmaul (-Meier) (polyarteritis nodosa) 446.0
  Kyasanur Forest 065.2
  Kyrle's (hyperkeratosis follicularis in cutem penetrans) 701.1
  labia
    inflammatory 616.9
      specified NEC 616.89 ▲
    noninflammatory 624.9
      specified NEC 624.8
  labyrinth, ear 386.8
  lacrimal system (apparatus) (passages) 375.9
    gland 375.00
    specified NEC 375.89
  Lafora's 333.2
  Lagleyze-von Hippel (retinocerebral angiomatosis) 759.6
  Lancereaux-Mathieu (leptospiral jaundice) 100.0
  Landry's 357.0
  Lane's 569.89
  lardaceous (any site) 277.39 ▲

Disease, diseased

Disease, diseased — see also Syndrome — continued
- Larrey-Weil (leptospiral jaundice) 100.0
- Larsen (-Johansson) (juvenile osteopathia patellae) 732.4
- larynx 478.70
- Lasègue's (persecution mania) 297.9
- Leber's 377.16
- Lederer's (acquired infectious hemolytic anemia) 283.19
- Legg's (capital femoral osteochondrosis) 732.1
- Legg-Calvé-Perthes (capital femoral osteochondrosis) 732.1
- Legg-Calvé-Waldenström (femoral capital osteochondrosis) 732.1
- Legg-Perthes (femoral capital osteochrondosis) 732.1
- Legionnaires' 482.84
- Leigh's 330.8
- Leiner's (exfoliative dermatitis) 695.89
- Leloir's (lupus erythematosus) 695.4
- Lenegre's 426.0
- lens (eye) 379.39
- Leriche's (osteoporosis, posttraumatic) 733.7
- Letterer-Siwe (acute histiocytosis X) (M9722/3) 202.5 ☑
- Lev's (acquired complete heart block) 426.0
- Lewandowski's (see also Tuberculosis) 017.0 ☑
- Lewandowski-Lutz (epidermodysplasia verruciformis) 078.19
- Lewy body 331.82
  - with dementia
    - with behavioral disturbance 331.82 [294.11]
    - without behavioral disturbance 331.82 [294.10]
- Leyden's (periodic vomiting) 536.2
- Libman-Sacks (verrucous endocarditis) 710.0 [424.91]
- Lichtheim's (subacute combined sclerosis with pernicious anemia) 281.0 [336.2]
- ligament 728.9
- light chain 203.0 ☑
- Lightwood's (renal tubular acidosis) 588.89
- Lignac's (cystinosis) 270.0
- Lindau's (retinocerebral angiomatosis) 759.6
- Lindau-von Hippel (angiomatosis retinocerebellosa) 759.6
- lip NEC 528.5
- lipidosis 272.7
- lipoid storage NEC 272.7
- Lipschütz's 616.50
- Little's — see Palsy, cerebral
- liver 573.9
  - alcoholic 571.3
    - acute 571.1
    - chronic 571.3
  - chronic 571.9
    - alcoholic 571.3
  - cystic, congenital 751.62
  - drug-induced 573.3
  - due to
    - chemicals 573.3
      - fluorinated agents 573.3
    - hypersensitivity drugs 573.3
    - isoniazids 573.3
  - fibrocystic (congenital) 751.62
  - glycogen storage 271.0
  - organic 573.9
  - polycystic (congenital) 751.62
- Lobo's (keloid blastomycosis) 116.2
- Lobstein's (brittle bones and blue sclera) 756.51
- locomotor system 334.9
- Lorain's (pituitary dwarfism) 253.3
- Lou Gehrig's 335.20
- Lucas-Championnière (fibrinous bronchitis) 466.0

Disease, diseased — see also Syndrome — continued
- Ludwig's (submaxillary cellulitis) 528.3
- luetic — see Syphilis
- lumbosacral region 724.6
- lung NEC 518.89
  - black 500
  - congenital 748.60
  - cystic 518.89
    - congenital 748.4
  - fibroid (chronic) (see also Fibrosis, lung) 515
  - fluke 121.2
    - oriental 121.2
  - in
    - amyloidosis 277.39 [517.8] ▲
    - polymyositis 710.4 [517.8]
    - sarcoidosis 135 [517.8]
    - Sjögren's syndrome 710.2 [517.8]
    - syphilis 095.1
    - systemic lupus erythematosus 710.0 [517.8]
    - systemic sclerosis 710.1 [517.2]
  - interstitial (chronic) 515
    - acute 136.3
  - nonspecific, chronic 496
  - obstructive (chronic) (COPD) 496
    - with
      - acute
        - bronchitis 491.22
        - exacerbation NEC 491.21
      - alveolitis, allergic (see also Alveolitis, allergic) 495.9
      - asthma (chronic) (obstructive) 493.2 ☑
      - bronchiectasis 494.0
        - with acute exacerbation 494.1
      - bronchitis (chronic) 491.20
        - with
          - acute bronchitis 491.22
          - exacerbation (acute) 491.21
      - decompensated 491.21 ●
        - with exacerbation 491.21 ●
      - emphysema NEC 492.8
    - diffuse (with fibrosis) 496
  - polycystic 518.89
    - asthma (chronic) (obstructive) 493.2 ☑
    - congenital 748.4
  - purulent (cavitary) 513.0
  - restrictive 518.89
  - rheumatoid 714.81
    - diffuse interstitial 714.81
  - specified NEC 518.89
- Lutembacher's (atrial septal defect with mitral stenosis) 745.5
- Lutz-Miescher (elastosis perforans serpiginosa) 701.1
- Lutz-Splendore-de Almeida (Brazilian blastomycosis) 116.1
- Lyell's (toxic epidermal necrolysis) 695.1
  - due to drug
    - correct substance properly administered 695.1
    - overdose or wrong substance given or taken 977.9
    - specific drug — see Table of Drugs and Chemicals
- Lyme 088.81
- lymphatic (gland) (system) 289.9
  - channel (noninfective) 457.9
  - vessel (noninfective) 457.9
  - specified NEC 457.8
- lymphoproliferative (chronic) (M9970/1) 238.79 ▲
- Machado-Joseph 334.8
- Madelung's (lipomatosis) 272.8
- Madura (actinomycotic) 039.9

Disease, diseased — see also Syndrome — continued
- Madura — continued
  - mycotic 117.4
- Magitot's 526.4
- Majocchi's (purpura annularis telangiectodes) 709.1
- malarial (see also Malaria) 084.6
- Malassez's (cystic) 608.89
- Malibu 919.8
  - infected 919.9
- malignant (M8000/3) (see also Neoplasm, by site, malignant)
  - previous, affecting management of pregnancy V23.89
- Manson's 120.1
- maple bark 495.6
- maple syrup (urine) 270.3
- Marburg (virus) 078.89
- Marchiafava (-Bignami) 341.8
- Marfan's 090.49
  - congenital syphilis 090.49
  - meaning Marfan's syndrome 759.82
- Marie-Bamberger (hypertrophic pulmonary osteoarthropathy) (secondary) 731.2
  - primary or idiopathic (acropachyderma) 757.39
  - pulmonary (hypertrophic osteoarthropathy) 731.2
- Marie-Strümpell (ankylosing spondylitis) 720.0
- Marion's (bladder neck obstruction) 596.0
- Marsh's (exophthalmic goiter) 242.0 ☑
- Martin's 715.27
- mast cell 757.33
  - systemic (M9741/3) 202.6 ☑
- mastoid (see also Mastoiditis) 383.9
  - process 385.9
- maternal, unrelated to pregnancy NEC, affecting fetus or newborn 760.9
- Mathieu's (leptospiral jaundice) 100.0
- Mauclaire's 732.3
- Mauriac's (erythema nodosum syphiliticum) 091.3
- Maxcy's 081.0
- McArdle (-Schmid-Pearson) (glycogenosis V) 271.0
- mediastinum NEC 519.3
- Medin's (see also Poliomyelitis) 045.9 ☑
- Mediterranean (with hemoglobinopathy) 282.49
- medullary center (idiopathic) (respiratory) 348.8
- Meige's (chronic hereditary edema) 757.0
- Meleda 757.39
- Ménétrier's (hypertrophic gastritis) 535.2 ☑
- Ménière's (active) 386.00
  - cochlear 386.02
  - cochleovestibular 386.01
  - inactive 386.04
  - in remission 386.04
  - vestibular 386.03
- meningeal — see Meningitis
- mental (see also Psychosis) 298.9
- Merzbacher-Pelizaeus 330.0
- mesenchymal 710.9
- mesenteric embolic 557.0
- metabolic NEC 277.9
- metastatic — see Metastasis
- Mibelli's 757.39
- microdrepanocytic 282.49
- microvascular — code to condition
- Miescher's 709.3
- Mikulicz's (dryness of mouth, absent or decreased lacrimation) 527.1
- Milkman (-Looser) (osteomalacia with pseudofractures) 268.2
- Miller's (osteomalacia) 268.2

Disease, diseased — see also Syndrome — continued
- Mills' 335.29
- Milroy's (chronic hereditary edema) 757.0
- Minamata 985.0
- Minor's 336.1
- Minot's (hemorrhagic disease, newborn) 776.0
- Minot-von Willebrand-Jürgens (angiohemophilia) 286.4
- Mitchell's (erythromelalgia) 443.82
- mitral — see Endocarditis, mitral
- Mljet (mal de Meleda) 757.39
- Möbius', Moebius' 346.8 ☑
- Moeller's 267
- Möller (-Barlow) (infantile scurvy) 267
- Mönckeberg's (see also Arteriosclerosis, extremities) 440.20
- Mondor's (thrombophlebitis of breast) 451.89
- Monge's 993.2
- Morel-Kraepelin (see also Schizophrenia) 295.9 ☑
- Morgagni's (syndrome) (hyperostosis frontalis interna) 733.3
- Morgagni-Adams-Stokes (syncope with heart block) 426.9
- Morquio (-Brailsford) (-Ullrich) (mucopolysaccharidosis IV) 277.5
- Morton's (with metatarsalgia) 355.6
- Morvan's 336.0
- motor neuron (bulbar) (mixed type) 335.20
- Mouchet's (juvenile osteochondrosis, foot) 732.5
- mouth 528.9
- Moyamoya 437.5
- Mucha's (acute parapsoriasis varioliformis) 696.2
- mu-chain 273.2
- mucolipidosis (I) (II) (III) 272.7
- Münchmeyer's (exostosis luxurians) 728.11
- Murri's (intermittent hemoglobinuria) 283.2
- muscle 359.9
  - inflammatory 728.9
  - ocular 378.9
- musculoskeletal system 729.9
- mushroom workers' 495.5
- Myà's (congenital dilation, colon) 751.3
- mycotic 117.9
- myeloproliferative (chronic) (M9960/1) 238.79 ▲
- myocardium, myocardial (see also Degeneration, myocardial) 429.1
  - hypertensive (see also Hypertension, heart 402.90
  - primary (idiopathic) 425.4
- myoneural 358.9
- Naegeli's 287.1
- nail 703.9
  - specified type NEC 703.8
- Nairobi sheep 066.1
- nasal 478.19 ▲
  - cavity NEC 478.19 ▲
  - sinus (chronic) — see Sinusitis
- navel (newborn) NEC 779.89
  - delayed separation of umbilical cord 779.83
- nemaline body 359.0
- neoplastic, generalized (M8000/6) 199.0
- nerve — see Disorder, nerve
- nervous system (central) 349.9
  - autonomic, peripheral (see also Neuropathy, peripheral, autonomic) 337.9
  - congenital 742.9
  - inflammatory — see Encephalitis
  - parasympathetic (see also Neuropathy, peripheral, autonomic) 337.9
- peripheral NEC 355.9

Index to Diseases

Disease, diseased — see also Syndrome — continued
- nervous system — continued
  - specified NEC 349.89
  - sympathetic (see also Neuropathy, peripheral, autonomic) 337.9
  - vegetative (see also Neuropathy, peripheral, autonomic) 337.9
- Nettleship's (urticaria pigmentosa) 757.33
- Neumann's (pemphigus vegetans) 694.4
- neurologic (central) NEC (see also Disease, nervous system) 349.9
  - peripheral NEC 355.9
- neuromuscular system NEC 358.9
- Newcastle 077.8
- Nicolas (-Durand) — Favre (climatic bubo) 099.1
- Niemann-Pick (lipid histiocytosis) 272.7
- nipple 611.9
  - Paget's (M8540/3) 174.0
- Nishimoto (-Takeuchi) 437.5
- nonarthropod-borne NEC 078.89
  - central nervous system NEC 049.9
  - enterovirus NEC 078.89
- nonautoimmune hemolytic NEC 283.10
- Nonne-Milroy-Meige (chronic hereditary edema) 757.0
- Norrie's (congenital progressive oculoacousticocerebral degeneration) 743.8
- nose 478.19 ▲
- nucleus pulposus — see Disease, intervertebral disc
- nutritional 269.9
  - maternal, affecting fetus or newborn 760.4
- oasthouse, urine 270.2
- obliterative vascular 447.1
- Odelberg's (juvenile osteochondrosis) 732.1
- Oguchi's (retina) 368.61
- Ohara's (see also Tularemia) 021.9
- Ollier's (chondrodysplasia) 756.4
- Opitz's (congestive splenomegaly) 289.51
- Oppenheim's 358.8
- Oppenheim-Urbach (necrobiosis lipoidica diabeticorum) 250.8 ☑ [709.3]
- optic nerve NEC 377.49
- orbit 376.9
  - specified NEC 376.89
- Oriental liver fluke 121.1
- Oriental lung fluke 121.2
- Ormond's 593.4
- Osgood-Schlatter 732.4
- Osgood's tibia (tubercle) 732.4
- Osler (-Vaquez) (polycythemia vera) (M9950/1) 238.4
- Osler-Rendu (familial hemorrhagic telangiectasia) 448.0
- osteofibrocystic 252.01
- Otto's 715.35
- outer ear 380.9
- ovary (noninflammatory) NEC 620.9
  - cystic 620.2
  - polycystic 256.4
  - specified NEC 620.8
- Owren's (congenital) (see also Defect, coagulation) 286.3
- Paas' 756.59
- Paget's (osteitis deformans) 731.0
  - with infiltrating duct carcinoma of the breast (M8541/3) — see Neoplasm, breast, malignant
  - bone 731.0
    - osteosarcoma in (M9184/3) — see Neoplasm, bone, malignant
  - breast (M8540/3) 174.0
  - extramammary (M8542/3) (see also Neoplasm, skin, malignant)

Disease, diseased — see also Syndrome — continued
- Paget's — continued
  - extramammary (see also Neoplasm, skin, malignant) — continued
    - anus 154.3
    - skin 173.5
  - malignant (M8540/3)
    - breast 174.0
    - specified site NEC (M8542/3) — see Neoplasm, skin, malignant
    - unspecified site 174.0
  - mammary (M8540/3) 174.0
  - nipple (M8540/3) 174.0
  - palate (soft) 528.9
- Paltauf-Sternberg 201.9 ☑
- pancreas 577.9
  - cystic 577.2
  - congenital 751.7
  - fibrocystic 277.00
- Panner's 732.3
  - capitellum humeri 732.3
  - head of humerus 732.3
  - tarsal navicular (bone) (osteochondrosis) 732.5
- panvalvular — see Endocarditis, mitral
- parametrium 629.9
- parasitic NEC 136.9
  - cerebral NEC 123.9
  - intestinal NEC 129
  - mouth 112.0
  - skin NEC 134.9
  - specified type — see Infestation
  - tongue 112.0
- parathyroid (gland) 252.9
  - specified NEC 252.8
- Parkinson's 332.0
- parodontal 523.9
- Parrot's (syphilitic osteochondritis) 090.0
- Parry's (exophthalmic goiter) 242.0 ☑
- Parson's (exophthalmic goiter) 242.0 ☑
- Pavy's 593.6
- Paxton's (white piedra) 111.2
- Payr's (splenic flexure syndrome) 569.89
- pearl-workers' (chronic osteomyelitis) (see also Osteomyelitis) 730.1 ☑
- Pel-Ebstein — see Disease, Hodgkin's
- Pelizaeus-Merzbacher 330.0
- Pellegrini-Stieda (calcification, knee joint) 726.62
- pelvis, pelvic
  - female NEC 629.9
    - specified NEC 629.89 ▲
  - gonococcal (acute) 098.19
    - chronic or duration of 2 months or over 098.39
  - infection (see also Disease, pelvis, inflammatory) 614.9
  - inflammatory (female) (PID) 614.9
    - with
      - abortion — see Abortion, by type, with sepsis
      - ectopic pregnancy (see also categories 633.0–633.9) 639.0
      - molar pregnancy (see also categories 630–632) 639.0
    - acute 614.3
    - chronic 614.4
    - complicating pregnancy 646.6 ☑
    - affecting fetus or newborn 760.8

Disease, diseased — see also Syndrome — continued
- pelvis, pelvic — continued
  - inflammatory — continued
    - following
      - abortion 639.0
      - ectopic or molar pregnancy 639.0
    - peritonitis (acute) 614.5
      - chronic NEC 614.7
    - puerperal, postpartum, childbirth 670.0 ☑
    - specified NEC 614.8
    - organ, female NEC 629.9
      - specified NEC 629.89 ▲
    - peritoneum, female NEC 629.9
      - specified NEC 629.89 ▲
- penis 607.9
  - inflammatory 607.2
- peptic NEC 536.9
  - acid 536.8
- periapical tissues NEC 522.9
- pericardium 423.9
  - specified type NEC 423.8
- perineum
  - female
    - inflammatory 616.9
      - specified NEC 616.89 ▲
    - noninflammatory 624.9
      - specified NEC 624.8
  - male (inflammatory) 682.2
- periodic (familial) (Reimann's) NEC 277.31
  - paralysis 359.3
- periodontal NEC 523.9
  - specified NEC 523.8
- periosteum 733.90
- peripheral
  - arterial 443.9
  - autonomic nervous system (see also Neuropathy, autonomic) 337.9
  - nerve NEC (see also Neuropathy) 356.9
  - multiple — see Polyneuropathy
  - vascular 443.9
    - specified type NEC 443.89
- peritoneum 568.9
  - pelvic, female 629.9
    - specified NEC 629.89 ▲
- Perrin-Ferraton (snapping hip) 719.65
- persistent mucosal (middle ear) (with posterior or superior marginal perforation of ear drum) 382.2
- Perthes' (capital femoral osteochondrosis) 732.1
- Petit's (see also Hernia, lumbar) 553.8
- Peutz-Jeghers 759.6
- Peyronie's 607.85
- Pfeiffer's (infectious mononucleosis) 075
- pharynx 478.20
- Phocas' 610.1
- photochromogenic (acid-fast bacilli) (pulmonary) 031.0
  - nonpulmonary 031.9
- Pick's
  - brain 331.11
    - with dementia
      - with behavioral disturbance 331.11 [294.11]
      - without behavioral disturbance 331.11 [294.10]
  - cerebral atrophy 331.11
    - with dementia
      - with behavioral disturbance 331.11 [294.11]
      - without behavioral disturbance 331.11 [294.10]
  - lipid histiocytosis 272.7
  - liver (pericardial pseudocirrhosis of liver) 423.2
  - pericardium (pericardial pseudocirrhosis of liver) 423.2
  - polyserositis (pericardial pseudocirrhosis of liver) 423.2

Disease, diseased — see also Syndrome — continued
- Pierson's (osteochondrosis) 732.1
- pigeon fanciers' or breeders' 495.2
- pineal gland 259.8
- pink 985.0
- Pinkus' (lichen nitidus) 697.1
- pinworm 127.4
- pituitary (gland) 253.9
  - hyperfunction 253.1
  - hypofunction 253.2
- pituitary snuff-takers' 495.8
- placenta
  - affecting fetus or newborn 762.2
  - complicating pregnancy or childbirth 656.7 ☑
- pleura (cavity) (see also Pleurisy) 511.0
- Plummer's (toxic nodular goiter) 242.3 ☑
- pneumatic
  - drill 994.9
  - hammer 994.9
- policeman's 729.2
- Pollitzer's (hidradenitis suppurativa) 705.83
- polycystic (congenital) 759.89
  - congenital 748.4
  - kidney or renal 753.12
    - adult type (APKD) 753.13
    - autosomal dominant 753.13
    - autosomal recessive 753.14
    - childhood type (CPKD) 753.14
    - infantile type 753.14
  - liver or hepatic 751.62
  - lung or pulmonary 518.89
  - ovary, ovaries 256.4
  - spleen 759.0
- Pompe's (glycogenosis II) 271.0
- Poncet's (tuberculous rheumatism) (see also Tuberculosis) 015.9 ☑
- Posada-Wernicke 114.9
- Potain's (pulmonary edema) 514
- Pott's (see also Tuberculosis) 015.0 [730.88]
  - osteomyelitis 015.0 ☑ [730.88]
  - paraplegia 015.0 ☑ [730.88]
  - spinal curvature 015.0 ☑ [737.43]
  - spondylitis 015.0 ☑ [720.81]
- Potter's 753.0
- Poulet's 714.2
- pregnancy NEC (see also Pregnancy) 646.9 ☑
- Preiser's (osteoporosis) 733.09
- Pringle's (tuberous sclerosis) 759.5
- Profichet's 729.9
- prostate 602.9
  - specified type NEC 602.8
- protozoal NEC 136.8
  - intestine, intestinal NEC 007.9
- pseudo-Hurler's (mucolipidosis III) 272.7
- psychiatric (see also Psychosis) 298.9
- psychotic (see also Psychosis) 298.9
- Puente's (simple glandular cheilitis) 528.5
- puerperal NEC (see also Puerperal) 674.9 ☑
- pulmonary (see also Disease, lung)
  - amyloid 277.39 [517.8] ▲
  - artery 417.9
  - circulation, circulatory 417.9
    - specified NEC 417.8
  - diffuse obstructive (chronic) 496
    - with
      - acute bronchitis 491.22
      - asthma (chronic) (obstructive) 493.2 ☑
      - exacerbation NEC (acute) 491.21
  - heart (chronic) 416.9
    - specified NEC 416.8
  - hypertensive (vascular) 416.0
    - cardiovascular 416.0
  - obstructive diffuse (chronic) 496

Disease, diseased

Disease, diseased — *see also* Syndrome — *continued*
  pulmonary (*see also* Disease, lung) — *continued*
    obstructive diffuse — *continued*
      with
        acute bronchitis 491.22
        asthma (chronic) (obstructive) 493.2 ✓
        bronchitis (chronic) 491.20
          with
            exacerbation (acute) 491.21
          acute 491.22
            exacerbation NEC (acute) 491.21
        decompensated 491.21 ●
          with exacerbation 491.21 ●
      valve (*see also* Endocarditis, pulmonary) 424.3
  pulp (dental) NEC 522.9
  pulseless 446.7
  Putnam's (subacute combined sclerosis with pernicious anemia) 281.0 [336.2]
  Pyle (-Cohn) (craniometaphyseal dysplasia) 756.89
  pyramidal tract 333.90
  Quervain's
    tendon sheath 727.04
    thyroid (subacute granulomatous thyroiditis) 245.1
  Quincke's — *see* Edema, angioneurotic
  Quinquaud (acne decalvans) 704.09
  rag sorters' 022.1
  Raynaud's (paroxysmal digital cyanosis) 443.0
  reactive airway — *see* Asthma
  Recklinghausen's (M9540/1) 237.71
    bone (osteitis fibrosa cystica) 252.01
  Recklinghausen-Applebaum (hemochromatosis) 275.0
  Reclus' (cystic) 610.1
  rectum NEC 569.49
  Refsum's (heredopathia atactica polyneuritiformis) 356.3
  Reichmann's (gastrosuccorrhea) 536.8
  Reimann's (periodic) 277.31 ▲
  Reiter's 099.3
  renal (functional) (pelvis) (*see also* Disease, kidney) 593.9
    with
      edema (*see also* Nephrosis) 581.9
      exudative nephritis 583.89
      lesion of interstitial nephritis 583.89
      stated generalized cause — *see* Nephritis
    acute 593.9
    basement membrane NEC 583.89
      with
        pulmonary hemorrhage (Goodpasture's syndrome) 446.21 [583.81]
    chronic (*see also* Disease, kidney, chronic) 593.9
    complicating pregnancy or puerperium NEC 646.2 ✓
      with hypertension — *see* Toxemia, of pregnancy
      affecting fetus or newborn 760.1
    cystic, congenital (*see also* Cystic, disease, kidney) 753.10
    diabetic 250.4 ✓ [583.81]
      due to
        amyloidosis 277.39 [583.81] ▲
        diabetes mellitus 250.4 ✓ [583.81]
        systemic lupus erythematosis 710.0 [583.81]
    end-stage 585.6
    exudative 583.89

Disease, diseased — *see also* Syndrome — *continued*
  renal (*see also* Disease, kidney) — *continued*
    fibrocystic (congenital) 753.19
    gonococcal 098.19 [583.81]
    gouty 274.10
    hypertensive (*see also* Hypertension, kidney) 403.90
    immune complex NEC 583.89
    interstitial (diffuse) (focal) 583.89
    lupus 710.0 [583.81]
    maternal, affecting fetus or newborn 760.1
      hypertensive 760.0
    phosphate-losing (tubular) 588.0
    polycystic (congenital) 753.12
      adult type (APKD) 753.13
      autosomal dominant 753.13
      autosomal recessive 753.14
      childhood type (CPKD) 753.14
      infantile type 753.14
    specified lesion or cause NEC (*see also* Glomerulonephritis) 583.89
    subacute 581.9
    syphilitic 095.4
    tuberculous (*see also* Tuberculosis) 016.0 ✓ [583.81]
    tubular (*see also* Nephrosis, tubular) 584.5
  Rendu-Osler-Weber (familial hemorrhagic telangiectasia) 448.0
  renovascular (arteriosclerotic) (*see also* Hypertension, kidney) 403.90
  respiratory (tract) 519.9
    acute or subacute (upper) NEC 465.9
      due to fumes or vapors 506.3
      multiple sites NEC 465.8
      noninfectious 478.9
      streptococcal 034.0
    chronic 519.9
      arising in the perinatal period 770.7
      due to fumes or vapors 506.4
      due to
        aspiration of liquids or solids 508.9
        external agents NEC 508.9
          specified NEC 508.8
        fumes or vapors 506.9
          acute or subacute NEC 506.3
          chronic 506.4
    fetus or newborn NEC 770.9
    obstructive 496
    specified type NEC 519.8
    upper (acute) (infectious) NEC 465.9
      multiple sites NEC 465.8
      noninfectious NEC 478.9
      streptococcal 034.0
  retina, retinal NEC 362.9
    Batten's or Batten-Mayou 330.1 [362.71]
    degeneration 362.89
    vascular lesion 362.17
  rheumatic (*see also* Arthritis) 716.8 ✓
    heart — *see* Disease, heart, rheumatic
    rheumatoid (heart) — *see* Arthritis, rheumatoid
  rickettsial NEC 083.9
    specified type NEC 083.8
  Riedel's (ligneous thyroiditis) 245.3
  Riga (-Fede) (cachectic aphthae) 529.0
  Riggs' (compound periodontitis) 523.40 ▲
  Ritter's 695.81
  Rivalta's (cervicofacial actinomycosis) 039.3
  Robles' (onchocerciasis) 125.3 [360.13]
  Roger's (congenital interventricular septal defect) 745.4
  Rokitansky's (*see also* Necrosis, liver) 570

Disease, diseased — *see also* Syndrome — *continued*
  Romberg's 349.89
  Rosenthal's (factor XI deficiency) 286.2
  Rossbach's (hyperchlorhydria) 536.8
    psychogenic 306.4
  Roth (-Bernhardt) 355.1
  Runeberg's (progressive pernicious anemia) 281.0
  Rust's (tuberculous spondylitis) (*see also* Tuberculosis) 015.0 ✓ [720.81]
  Rustitskii's (multiple myeloma) (M9730/3) 203.0 ✓
  Ruysch's (Hirschsprung's disease) 751.3
  Sachs (-Tay) 330.1
  sacroiliac NEC 724.6
  salivary gland or duct NEC 527.9
    inclusion 078.5
      streptococcal 034.0
    virus 078.5
  Sander's (paranoia) 297.1
  Sandhoff's 330.1
  sandworm 126.9
  Savill's (epidemic exfoliative dermatitis) 695.89
  Schamberg's (progressive pigmentary dermatosis) 709.09
  Schaumann's (sarcoidosis) 135
  Schenck's (sporotrichosis) 117.1
  Scheuermann's (osteochondrosis) 732.0
  Schilder (-Flatau) 341.1
  Schimmelbusch's 610.1
  Schlatter-Osgood 732.4
  Schlatter's tibia (tubercle) 732.4
  Schmorl's 722.30
    cervical 722.39
    lumbar, lumbosacral 722.32
    specified region NEC 722.39
    thoracic, thoracolumbar 722.31
  Scholz's 330.0
  Schönlein (-Henoch) (purpura rheumatica) 287.0
  Schottmüller's (*see also* Fever, paratyphoid) 002.9
  Schüller-Christian (chronic histiocytosis X) 277.89
  Schultz's (agranulocytosis) 288.09 ▲
  Schwalbe-Ziehen-Oppenheimer 333.6
  Schweninger-Buzzi (macular atrophy) 701.3
  sclera 379.19
  scrofulous (*see also* Tuberculosis) 017.2 ✓
  scrotum 608.9
  sebaceous glands NEC 706.9
  Secretan's (posttraumatic edema) 782.3
  semilunar cartilage, cystic 717.5
  seminal vesicle 608.9
  Senear-Usher (pemphigus erythematosus) 694.4
  serum NEC 999.5
  Sever's (osteochondrosis calcaneum) 732.5
  Sézary's (reticulosis) (M9701/3) 202.2 ✓
  Shaver's (bauxite pneumoconiosis) 503
  Sheehan's (postpartum pituitary necrosis) 253.2
  shimamushi (scrub typhus) 081.2
  shipyard 077.1
  sickle cell 282.60
    with
      crisis 282.62
      Hb-S disease 282.61
      other abnormal hemoglobin (Hb-D) (Hb-E) (Hb-G) (Hb-J) (Hb-K) (Hb-O) (Hb-P) (high fetal gene) (without crisis) 282.68
        with crisis 282.69

Disease, diseased — *see also* Syndrome — *continued*
  sickle cell — *continued*
    elliptocytosis 282.60
    Hb-C (without crisis) 282.63
      with
        crisis 282.64
        vaso-occlusive pain 282.64
    Hb-S 282.61
      with
        crisis 282.62
        Hb-C (without crisis) 282.63
          with
            crisis 282.64
            vaso-occlusive pain 282.64
        other abnormal hemoglobin (Hb-D) (Hb-E) (Hb-G) (Hb-J) (Hb-K) (Hb-O) (Hb-P) (high fetal gene) (without crisis) 282.68
          with crisis 282.69
    spherocytosis 282.60
    thalassemia (without crisis) 282.41
      with
        crisis 282.42
        vaso-occlusive pain 282.42
  Siegal-Cattan-Mamou (periodic) 277.31 ▲
  silo fillers' 506.9
  Simian B 054.3
  Simmonds' (pituitary cachexia) 253.2
  Simons' (progressive lipodystrophy) 272.6
  Sinding-Larsen (juvenile osteopathia patellae) 732.4
  sinus (*see also* Sinusitis)
    brain 437.9
    specified NEC 478.19 ▲
  Sirkari's 085.0
  sixth 057.8
  Sjögren (-Gougerot) 710.2
    with lung involvement 710.2 [517.8]
  Skevas-Zerfus 989.5
  skin NEC 709.9
    due to metabolic disorder 277.9
    specified type NEC 709.8
  sleeping (*see also* Narcolepsy) 347.00
    meaning sleeping sickness (*see also* Trypanosomiasis) 086.5
  small vessel 443.9
  Smith-Strang (oasthouse urine) 270.2
  Sneddon-Wilkinson (subcorneal pustular dermatosis) 694.1
  South African creeping 133.8
  Spencer's (epidemic vomiting) 078.82
  Spielmeyer-Stock 330.1
  Spielmeyer-Vogt 330.1
  spine, spinal 733.90
    combined system (*see also* Degeneration, combined) 266.2 [336.2]
      with pernicious anemia 281.0 [336.2]
    cord NEC 336.9
    congenital 742.9
    demyelinating NEC 341.8
    joint (*see also* Disease, joint, spine) 724.9
    tuberculous 015.0 ✓ [730.8] ✓
  spinocerebellar 334.9
    specified NEC 334.8
  spleen (organic) (postinfectional) 289.50
    amyloid 277.39 ▲
    lardaceous 277.39 ▲
    polycystic 759.0
    specified NEC 289.59
  sponge divers' 989.5
  Stanton's (melioidosis) 025
  Stargardt's 362.75
  Startle 759.89
  Steinert's 359.2
  Sternberg's — *see* Disease, Hodgkin's

Index to Diseases

Disease, diseased

Disease, diseased — see also Syndrome — continued
- Stevens-Johnson (erythema multiforme exudativum) 695.1
- Sticker's (erythema infectiosum) 057.0
- Stieda's (calcification, knee joint) 726.62
- Still's (juvenile rheumatoid arthritis) 714.30
- Stiller's (asthenia) 780.79
- Stokes' (exophthalmic goiter) 242.0 ☑
- Stokes-Adams (syncope with heart block) 426.9
- Stokvis (-Talma) (enterogenous cyanosis) 289.7
- stomach NEC (organic) 537.9
  - functional 536.9
    - psychogenic 306.4
  - lardaceous 277.39 ▲
- stonemasons' 502
- storage
  - glycogen (see also Disease, glycogen storage) 271.0
  - lipid 272.7
  - mucopolysaccharide 277.5
- striatopallidal system 333.90
  - specified NEC 333.89
- Strümpell-Marie (ankylosing spondylitis) 720.0
- Stuart's (congenital factor X deficiency) (see also Defect, coagulation) 286.3
- Stuart-Prower (congenital factor X deficiency) (see also Defect, coagulation) 286.3
- Sturge (-Weber) (-Dimitri) (encephalocutaneous angiomatosis) 759.6
- Stuttgart 100.89
- Sudeck's 733.7
- supporting structures of teeth NEC 525.9
- suprarenal (gland) (capsule) 255.9
  - hyperfunction 255.3
  - hypofunction 255.4
- Sutton's 709.09
- Sutton and Gull's — see Hypertension, kidney
- sweat glands NEC 705.9
  - specified type NEC 705.89
- sweating 078.2
- Sweeley-Klionsky 272.4
- Swift (-Feer) 985.0
- swimming pool (bacillus) 031.1
- swineherd's 100.89
- Sylvest's (epidemic pleurodynia) 074.1
- Symmers (follicular lymphoma) (M9690/3) 202.0 ☑
- sympathetic nervous system (see also Neuropathy, peripheral, autonomic) 337.9
- synovium 727.9
- syphilitic — see Syphilis
- systemic tissue mast cell (M9741/3) 202.6 ☑
- Taenzer's 757.4
- Takayasu's (pulseless) 446.7
- Talma's 728.85
- Tangier (familial high-density lipoprotein deficiency) 272.5
- Tarral-Besnier (pityriasis rubra pilaris) 696.4
- Taylor's 701.8
- Tay-Sachs 330.1
- tear duct 375.69
- teeth, tooth 525.9
  - hard tissues 521.9
    - specified NEC 521.89 ●
  - pulp NEC 522.9
- tendon 727.9
  - inflammatory NEC 727.9
- terminal vessel 443.9
- testis 608.9
- Thaysen-Gee (nontropical sprue) 579.0
- Thomsen's 359.2

Disease, diseased — see also Syndrome — continued
- Thomson's (congenital poikiloderma) 757.33
- Thornwaldt's, Tornwaldt's (pharyngeal bursitis) 478.29
- throat 478.20
  - septic 034.0
- thromboembolic (see also Embolism) 444.9
- thymus (gland) 254.9
  - specified NEC 254.8
- thyroid (gland) NEC 246.9
  - heart (see also Hyperthyroidism) 242.9 ☑ [425.7]
  - lardaceous 277.39 ▲
  - specified NEC 246.8
- Tietze's 733.6
- Tommaselli's
  - correct substance properly administered 599.7
  - overdose or wrong substance given or taken 961.4
- tongue 529.9
- tonsils, tonsillar (and adenoids) (chronic) 474.9
  - specified NEC 474.8
- tooth, teeth 525.9
  - hard tissues 521.9
    - specified NEC 521.89 ●
  - pulp NEC 522.9
- Tornwaldt's (pharyngeal bursitis) 478.29
- Tourette's 307.23
- trachea 519.19 ▲
- tricuspid — see Endocarditis, tricuspid
- triglyceride-storage, type I, II, III 272.7
- triple vessel (coronary arteries) — see Arteriosclerosis, coronary
- trisymptomatic, Gourgerot's 709.1
- trophoblastic (see also Hydatidiform mole) 630
  - previous, affecting management of pregnancy V23.1
- tsutsugamushi (scrub typhus) 081.2
- tube (fallopian), noninflammatory 620.9
  - specified NEC 620.8
- tuberculous NEC (see also Tuberculosis) 011.9 ☑
- tubo-ovarian
  - inflammatory (see also Salpingo-oophoritis) 614.2
  - noninflammatory 620.9
    - specified NEC 620.8
- tubotympanic, chronic (with anterior perforation of ear drum) 382.1
- tympanum 385.9
- Uhl's 746.84
- umbilicus (newborn) NEC 779.89
  - delayed separation 779.83
- Underwood's (sclerema neonatorum) 778.1
- undiagnosed 799.9
- Unna's (seborrheic dermatitis) 690.18
- unstable hemoglobin hemolytic 282.7
- Unverricht (-Lundborg) 333.2
- Urbach-Oppenheim (necrobiosis lipoidica diabeticorum) 250.8 ☑ [709.3]
- Urbach-Wiethe (lipoid proteinosis) 272.8
- ureter 593.9
- urethra 599.9
  - specified type NEC 599.84
- urinary (tract) 599.9
  - bladder 596.9
    - specified NEC 596.8
  - maternal, affecting fetus or newborn 760.1
- Usher-Senear (pemphigus erythematosus) 694.4
- uterus (organic) 621.9
  - infective (see also Endometritis) 615.9

Disease, diseased — see also Syndrome — continued
- uterus — continued
  - inflammatory (see also Endometritis) 615.9
  - noninflammatory 621.9
    - specified type NEC 621.8
- uveal tract
  - anterior 364.9
  - posterior 363.9
- vagabonds' 132.1
- vagina, vaginal
  - inflammatory 616.9
    - specified NEC 616.89 ▲
  - noninflammatory 623.9
    - specified NEC 623.8
- Valsuani's (progressive pernicious anemia, puerperal) 648.2 ☑
  - complicating pregnancy or puerperium 648.2 ☑
- valve, valvular — see Endocarditis
- van Bogaert-Nijssen (-Peiffer) 330.0
- van Creveld-von Gierke (glycogenosis I) 271.0
- van den Bergh's (enterogenous cyanosis) 289.7
- van Neck's (juvenile osteochondrosis) 732.1
- Vaquez (-Osler) (polycythemia vera) (M9950/1) 238.4
- vascular 459.9
  - arteriosclerotic — see Arteriosclerosis
  - hypertensive — see Hypertension
  - obliterative 447.1
    - peripheral 443.9
  - occlusive 459.9
  - peripheral (occlusive) 443.9
    - in diabetes mellitus 250.7 ☑ [443.81]
    - specified type NEC 443.89
- vas deferens 608.9
- vasomotor 443.9
- vasospastic 443.9
- vein 459.9
- venereal 099.9
  - chlamydial NEC 099.50
    - anus 099.52
    - bladder 099.53
    - cervix 099.53
    - epididymis 099.54
    - genitourinary NEC 099.55
      - lower 099.53
      - specified NEC 099.54
    - pelvic inflammatory disease 099.54
    - perihepatic 099.56
    - peritoneum 099.56
    - pharynx 099.51
    - rectum 099.52
    - specified site NEC 099.59
    - testis 099.54
    - vagina 099.53
    - vulva 099.53
  - complicating pregnancy, childbirth, or puerperium 647.2 ☑
  - fifth 099.1
  - sixth 099.1
  - specified nature or type NEC 099.8
    - chlamydial — see Disease, venereal, chlamydial
- Verneuil's (syphilitic bursitis) 095.7
- Verse's (calcinosis intervertebralis) 275.49 [722.90]
- vertebra, vertebral NEC 733.90
  - disc — see Disease, Intervertebral disc
- vibration NEC 994.9
- Vidal's (lichen simplex chronicus) 698.3
- Vincent's (trench mouth) 101
- Virchow's 733.99
- virus (filterable) NEC 078.89
  - arbovirus NEC 066.9
  - arthropod-borne NEC 066.9
  - central nervous system NEC 049.9

Disease, diseased — see also Syndrome — continued
- virus — continued
  - central nervous system — continued
    - specified type NEC 049.8
  - complicating pregnancy, childbirth, or puerperium 647.6 ☑
  - contact (with) V01.79
    - varicella V01.71
  - exposure to V01.79
    - varicella V01.71
  - Marburg 078.89
  - maternal
    - with fetal damage affecting management of pregnancy 655.3 ☑
  - nonarthropod-borne NEC 078.89
    - central nervous system NEC 049.9
    - specified NEC 049.8
  - vaccination, prophylactic (against) V04.89
- vitreous 379.29
- vocal cords NEC 478.5
- Vogt's (Cecile) 333.71 ▲
- Vogt-Spielmeyer 330.1
- Volhard-Fahr (malignant nephrosclerosis) 403.00
- Volkmann's
  - acquired 958.6
- von Bechterew's (ankylosing spondylitis) 720.0
- von Economo's (encephalitis lethargica) 049.8
- von Eulenburg's (congenital paramyotonia) 359.2
- von Gierke's (glycogenosis I) 271.0
- von Graefe's 378.72
- von Hippel's (retinocerebral angiomatosis) 759.6
- von Hippel-Lindau (angiomatosis retinocerebellosa) 759.6
- von Jaksch's (pseudoleukemia infantum) 285.8
- von Recklinghausen's (M9540/1) 237.71
  - bone (osteitis fibrosa cystica) 252.01
- von Recklinghausen-Applebaum (hemochromatosis) 275.0
- von Willebrand (-Jürgens) (angiohemophilia) 286.4
- von Zambusch's (lichen sclerosus et atrophicus) 701.0
- Voorhoeve's (dyschondroplasia) 756.4
- Vrolik's (osteogenesis imperfecta) 756.51
- vulva
  - inflammatory 616.9 ●
    - specified NEC 616.89 ●
  - noninflammatory 624.9
    - specified NEC 624.8
- Wagner's (colloid milium) 709.3
- Waldenström's (osteochondrosis capital femoral) 732.1
- Wallgren's (obstruction of splenic vein with collateral circulation) 459.89
- Wardrop's (with lymphangitis) 681.9
  - finger 681.02
  - toe 681.11
- Wassilieff's (leptospiral jaundice) 100.0
- wasting NEC 799.4
  - due to malnutrition 261
  - paralysis 335.21
- Waterhouse-Friderichsen 036.3
- waxy (any site) 277.39 ▲
- Weber-Christian (nodular nonsuppurative panniculitis) 729.30
- Wegner's (syphilitic osteochondritis) 090.0
- Weil's (leptospiral jaundice) 100.0
  - of lung 100.0

Disease, diseased — see also Syndrome — continued
- Weir Mitchell's (erythromelalgia) 443.82
- Werdnig-Hoffmann 335.0
- Werlhof's (see also Purpura, thrombocytopenic) 287.39
- Wermer's 258.0
- Werner's (progeria adultorum) 259.8
- Werner-His (trench fever) 083.1
- Werner-Schultz (agranulocytosis) 288.09 ▲
- Wernicke's (superior hemorrhagic polioencephalitis) 265.1
- Wernicke-Posadas 114.9
- Whipple's (intestinal lipodystrophy) 040.2
- whipworm 127.3
- White's (congenital) (keratosis follicularis) 757.39
- white
  - blood cell 288.9
    - specified NEC 288.8
  - spot 701.0
- Whitmore's (melioidosis) 025
- Widal-Abrami (acquired hemolytic jaundice) 283.9
- Wilkie's 557.1
- Wilkinson-Sneddon (subcorneal pustular dermatosis) 694.1
- Willis' (diabetes mellitus) (see also Diabetes) 250.0 ☑
- Wilson's (hepatolenticular degeneration) 275.1
- Wilson-Brocq (dermatitis exfoliativa) 695.89
- winter vomiting 078.82
- Wise's 696.2
- Wohlfart-Kugelberg-Welander 335.11
- Woillez's (acute idiopathic pulmonary congestion) 518.5
- Wolman's (primary familial xanthomatosis) 272.7
- wool-sorters' 022.1
- Zagari's (xerostomia) 527.7
- Zahorsky's (exanthem subitum) 057.8
- Ziehen-Oppenheim 333.6
- zoonotic, bacterial NEC 027.9
  - specified type NEC 027.8

Disfigurement (due to scar) 709.2
- head V48.6
- limb V49.4
- neck V48.7
- trunk V48.7

Disgerminoma — see Dysgerminoma
Disinsertion, retina 361.04
Disintegration, complete, of the body 799.89
- traumatic 869.1

Disk kidney 753.3
Dislocatable hip, congenital — see also Dislocation, hip, congenital 754.30
Dislocation (articulation) (closed) (displacement) (simple) (subluxation) 839.8

> Note — "Closed" includes simple, complete, partial, uncomplicated, and unspecified dislocation.
>
> "Open" includes dislocation specified as infected or compound and dislocation with foreign body.
>
> "Chronic," "habitual," "old," or "recurrent" dislocations should be coded as indicated under the entry "Dislocation, recurrent," and "pathological" as indicated under the entry "Dislocation, pathological."
>
> For late effect of dislocation see Late, effect, dislocation.

- with fracture — see Fracture, by site
- acromioclavicular (joint) (closed) 831.04
  - open 831.14

Dislocation — continued
- anatomical site (closed)
  - specified NEC 839.69
    - open 839.79
  - unspecified or ill-defined 839.8
    - open 839.9
- ankle (scaphoid bone) (closed) 837.0
  - open 837.1
- arm (closed) 839.8
  - open 839.9
- astragalus (closed) 837.0
  - open 837.1
- atlanto-axial (closed) 839.01
  - open 839.11
- atlas (closed) 839.01
  - open 839.11
- axis (closed) 839.02
  - open 839.12
- back (closed) 839.8
  - open 839.9
- Bell-Daly 723.8
- breast bone (closed) 839.61
  - open 839.71
- capsule, joint — see Dislocation, by site
- carpal (bone) — see Dislocation, wrist
- carpometacarpal (joint) (closed) 833.04
  - open 833.14
- cartilage (joint) (see also Dislocation, by site)
  - knee — see Tear, meniscus
- cervical, cervicodorsal, or cervicothoracic (spine) (vertebra) — see Dislocation, vertebra, cervical
- chiropractic (see also Lesion, nonallopathic) 739.9
- chondrocostal — see Dislocation, costochondral
- chronic — see Dislocation, recurrent
- clavicle (closed) 831.04
  - open 831.14
- coccyx (closed) 839.41
  - open 839.51
- collar bone (closed) 831.04
  - open 831.14
- compound (open) NEC 839.9
- congenital NEC 755.8
  - hip (see also Dislocation, hip, congenital) 754.30
  - lens 743.37
  - rib 756.3
  - sacroiliac 755.69
  - spine NEC 756.19
  - vertebra 756.19
- coracoid (closed) 831.09
  - open 831.19
- costal cartilage (closed) 839.69
  - open 839.79
- costochondral (closed) 839.69
  - open 839.79
- cricoarytenoid articulation (closed) 839.69
  - open 839.79
- cricothyroid (cartilage) articulation (closed) 839.69
  - open 839.79
- dorsal vertebrae (closed) 839.21
  - open 839.31
- ear ossicle 385.23
- elbow (closed) 832.00
  - anterior (closed) 832.01
    - open 832.11
  - congenital 754.89
  - divergent (closed) 832.09
    - open 832.19
  - lateral (closed) 832.04
    - open 832.14
  - medial (closed) 832.03
    - open 832.13
    - open 832.10
  - posterior (closed) 832.02
    - open 832.12
  - recurrent 718.32
  - specified type NEC 832.09
    - open 832.19
- eye 360.81

Dislocation — continued
- eye — continued
  - lateral 376.36
- eyeball 360.81
  - lateral 376.36
- femur
  - distal end (closed) 836.50
    - anterior 836.52
      - open 836.62
    - lateral 836.53
      - open 836.63
    - medial 836.54
      - open 836.64
    - open 836.60
    - posterior 836.51
      - open 836.61
  - proximal end (closed) 835.00
    - anterior (pubic) 835.03
      - open 835.13
    - obturator 835.02
      - open 835.12
    - open 835.10
    - posterior 835.01
      - open 835.11
- fibula
  - distal end (closed) 837.0
    - open 837.1
  - proximal end (closed) 836.59
    - open 836.69
- finger(s) (phalanx) (thumb) (closed) 834.00
  - interphalangeal (joint) 834.02
    - open 834.12
  - metacarpal (bone), distal end 834.01
    - open 834.11
  - metacarpophalangeal (joint) 834.01
    - open 834.11
  - open 834.10
  - recurrent 718.34
- foot (closed) 838.00
  - open 838.10
  - recurrent 718.37
- forearm (closed) 839.8
  - open 839.9
- fracture — see Fracture, by site
- glenoid (closed) 831.09
  - open 831.19
- habitual — see Dislocation, recurrent
- hand (closed) 839.8
  - open 839.9
- hip (closed) 835.00
  - anterior 835.03
    - obturator 835.02
      - open 835.12
    - open 835.13
  - congenital (unilateral) 754.30
    - with subluxation of other hip 754.35
    - bilateral 754.31
  - developmental 718.75
  - open 835.10
  - posterior 835.01
    - open 835.11
  - recurrent 718.35
- humerus (closed) 831.00
  - distal end (see also Dislocation, elbow) 832.00
  - open 831.10
  - proximal end (closed) 831.00
    - anterior (subclavicular) (subcoracoid) (subglenoid) (closed) 831.01
      - open 831.11
    - inferior (closed) 831.03
      - open 831.13
      - open 831.10
    - posterior (closed) 831.02
      - open 831.12
- implant — see Complications, mechanical
- incus 385.23
- infracoracoid (closed) 831.01
  - open 831.11
- innominate (pubic junction) (sacral junction) (closed) 839.69

Dislocation — continued
- innominate — continued
  - acetabulum (see also Dislocation, hip) 835.00
    - open 839.79
- interphalangeal (joint)
  - finger or hand (closed) 834.02
    - open 834.12
  - foot or toe (closed) 838.06
    - open 838.16
- jaw (cartilage) (meniscus) (closed) 830.0
  - open 830.1
  - recurrent 524.69
- joint NEC (closed) 839.8
  - developmental 718.7 ☑
  - open 839.9
  - pathological — see Dislocation, pathological
  - recurrent — see Dislocation, recurrent
- knee (closed) 836.50
  - anterior 836.51
    - open 836.61
  - congenital (with genu recurvatum) 754.41
  - habitual 718.36
  - lateral 836.54
    - open 836.64
  - medial 836.53
    - open 836.63
  - old 718.36
    - open 836.60
  - posterior 836.52
    - open 836.62
  - recurrent 718.36
  - rotatory 836.59
    - open 836.69
- lacrimal gland 375.16
- leg (closed) 839.8
  - open 839.9
- lens (crystalline) (complete) (partial) 379.32
  - anterior 379.33
  - congenital 743.37
  - ocular implant 996.53
  - posterior 379.34
  - traumatic 921.3
- ligament — see Dislocation, by site
- lumbar (vertebrae) (closed) 839.20
  - open 839.30
- lumbosacral (vertebrae) (closed) 839.20
  - congenital 756.19
  - open 839.30
- mandible (closed) 830.0
  - open 830.1
- maxilla (inferior) (closed) 830.0
  - open 830.1
- meniscus (knee) (see also Tear, meniscus)
  - other sites — see Dislocation, by site
- metacarpal (bone)
  - distal end (closed) 834.01
    - open 834.11
  - proximal end (closed) 833.05
    - open 833.15
- metacarpophalangeal (joint) (closed) 834.01
  - open 834.11
- metatarsal (bone) (closed) 838.04
  - open 838.14
- metatarsophalangeal (joint) (closed) 838.05
  - open 838.15
- midcarpal (joint) (closed) 833.03
  - open 833.13
- midtarsal (joint) (closed) 838.02
  - open 838.12
- Monteggia's — see Dislocation, hip
- multiple locations (except fingers only or toes only) (closed) 839.8
  - open 839.9
- navicular (bone) foot (closed) 837.0
  - open 837.1

Dislocation — continued
  neck (see also Dislocation, vertebra, cervical) 839.00
  Nélaton's — see Dislocation, ankle
  nontraumatic (joint) — see Dislocation, pathological
  nose (closed) 839.69
    open 839.79
  not recurrent, not current injury — see Dislocation, pathological
  occiput from atlas (closed) 839.01
    open 839.11
  old — see Dislocation, recurrent
  open (compound) NEC 839.9
  ossicle, ear 385.23
  paralytic (flaccid) (spastic) — see Dislocation, pathological
  patella (closed) 836.3
    congenital 755.64
    open 836.4
  pathological NEC 718.20
    ankle 718.27
    elbow 718.22
    foot 718.27
    hand 718.24
    hip 718.25
    knee 718.26
    lumbosacral joint 724.6
    multiple sites 718.29
    pelvic region 718.25
    sacroiliac 724.6
    shoulder (region) 718.21
    specified site NEC 718.28
    spine 724.8
      sacroiliac 724.6
    wrist 718.23
  pelvis (closed) 839.69
    acetabulum (see also Dislocation, hip) 835.00
    open 839.79
  phalanx
    foot or toe (closed) 838.09
      open 838.19
    hand or finger (see also Dislocation, finger) 834.00
  postpoliomyelitic — see Dislocation, pathological
  prosthesis, internal — see Complications, mechanical
  radiocarpal (joint) (closed) 833.02
    open 833.12
  radioulnar (joint)
    distal end (closed) 833.01
      open 833.11
    proximal end (see also Dislocation, elbow) 832.00
  radius
    distal end (closed) 833.00
      open 833.10
    proximal end (closed) 832.01
      open 832.11
  recurrent (see also Derangement, joint, recurrent) 718.3 ☑
    elbow 718.32
    hip 718.35
    joint NEC 718.38
    knee 718.36
    lumbosacral (joint) 724.6
    patella 718.36
    sacroiliac 724.6
    shoulder 718.31
    temporomandibular 524.69
  rib (cartilage) (closed) 839.69
    congenital 756.3
    open 839.79
  sacrococcygeal (closed) 839.42
    open 839.52
  sacroiliac (joint) (ligament) (closed) 839.42
    congenital 755.69
    open 839.52
    recurrent 724.6
  sacrum (closed) 839.42
    open 839.52
  scaphoid (bone)
    ankle or foot (closed) 837.0

Dislocation — continued
  scaphoid — continued
    ankle or foot — continued
      open 837.1
    wrist (closed) (see also Dislocation, wrist) 833.00
      open 833.10
  scapula (closed) 831.09
    open 831.19
  semilunar cartilage, knee — see Tear, meniscus
  septal cartilage (nose) (closed) 839.69
    open 839.79
  septum (nasal) (old) 470
  sesamoid bone — see Dislocation, by site
  shoulder (blade) (ligament) (closed) 831.00
    anterior (subclavicular) (subcoracoid) (subglenoid) (closed) 831.01
      open 831.11
    chronic 718.31
    inferior 831.03
      open 831.13
    open 831.10
    posterior (closed) 831.02
      open 831.12
    recurrent 718.31
  skull — see Injury, intracranial
  Smith's — see Dislocation, foot
  spine (articular process) (see also Dislocation, vertebra) (closed) 839.40
    atlanto-axial (closed) 839.01
      open 839.11
      recurrent 723.8
    cervical, cervicodorsal, cervicothoracic (closed) (see also Dislocation, vertebrae, cervical) 839.00
      open 839.10
      recurrent 723.8
    coccyx 839.41
      open 839.51
    congenital 756.19
    due to birth trauma 767.4
    open 839.50
    recurrent 724.9
    sacroiliac 839.42
      recurrent 724.6
    sacrum (sacrococcygeal) (sacroiliac) 839.42
      open 839.52
  spontaneous — see Dislocation, pathological
  sternoclavicular (joint) (closed) 839.61
    open 839.71
  sternum (closed) 839.61
    open 839.71
  subastragalar — see Dislocation, foot
  subglenoid (closed) 831.01
    open 831.11
  symphysis
    jaw (closed) 830.0
      open 830.1
    mandibular (closed) 830.0
      open 830.1
    pubis (closed) 839.69
      open 839.79
  tarsal (bone) (joint) 838.01
    open 838.11
  tarsometatarsal (joint) 838.03
    open 838.13
  temporomandibular (joint) (closed) 830.0
    open 830.1
    recurrent 524.69
  thigh
    distal end (see also Dislocation, femur, distal end) 836.50
    proximal end (see also Dislocation, hip) 835.00
  thoracic (vertebrae) (closed) 839.21
    open 839.31

Dislocation — continued
  thumb(s) (see also Dislocation, finger) 834.00
  thyroid cartilage (closed) 839.69
    open 839.79
  tibia
    distal end (closed) 837.0
      open 837.1
    proximal end (closed) 836.50
      anterior 836.51
        open 836.61
      lateral 836.54
        open 836.64
      medial 836.53
        open 836.63
      open 836.60
      posterior 836.52
        open 836.62
      rotatory 836.59
        open 836.69
  tibiofibular
    distal (closed) 837.0
      open 837.1
    superior (closed) 836.59
      open 836.69
  toe(s) (closed) 838.09
    open 838.19
  trachea (closed) 839.69
    open 839.79
  ulna
    distal end (closed) 833.09
      open 833.19
    proximal end — see Dislocation, elbow
  vertebra (articular process) (body) (closed) ▶(traumatic)◀ 839.40
    cervical, cervicodorsal or cervicothoracic (closed) 839.00
      first (atlas) 839.01
        open 839.11
      second (axis) 839.02
        open 839.12
      third 839.03
        open 839.13
      fourth 839.04
        open 839.14
      fifth 839.05
        open 839.15
      sixth 839.06
        open 839.16
      seventh 839.07
        open 839.17
    congenital 756.19
    multiple sites 839.08
      open 839.18
      open 839.10
    congenital 756.19
    dorsal 839.21
      open 839.31
      recurrent 724.9
    lumbar, lumbosacral 839.20
      open 839.30
    non-traumatic — see Displacement, intervertebral disc ●
    open NEC 839.50
    recurrent 724.9
    specified region NEC 839.49
      open 839.59
    thoracic 839.21
      open 839.31
  wrist (carpal bone) (scaphoid) (semilunar) (closed) 833.00
    carpometacarpal (joint) 833.04
      open 833.14
    metacarpal bone, proximal end 833.05
      open 833.15
    midcarpal (joint) 833.03
      open 833.13
    open 833.10
    radiocarpal (joint) 833.02
      open 833.12
    radioulnar (joint) 833.01
      open 833.11
    recurrent 718.33
    specified site NEC 833.09

Dislocation — continued
  wrist — continued
    specified site — continued
      open 833.19
    xiphoid cartilage (closed) 839.61
      open 839.71
Dislodgement
  artificial skin graft 996.55
  decellularized allodermis graft 996.55
Disobedience, hostile (covert) (overt) — see also Disturbance, conduct 312.0 ☑
Disorder — see also Disease
  academic underachievement, childhood and adolescence 313.83
  accommodation 367.51
    drug-induced 367.89
    toxic 367.89
  adjustment (see also Reaction, adjustment) 309.9
    with
      anxiety 309.24
      anxiety and depressed mood 309.28
      depressed mood 309.0
      disturbance of conduct 309.3
      disturbance of emotions and conduct 309.4
  adrenal (capsule) (cortex) (gland) 255.9
    specified type NEC 255.8
  adrenogenital 255.2
  affective (see also Psychosis, affective) 296.90
    atypical 296.81
  aggressive, unsocialized (see also Disturbance, conduct) 312.0 ☑
  alcohol, alcoholic (see also Alcohol) 291.9
  allergic — see Allergy
  amino acid (metabolic) (see also Disturbance, metabolism, amino acid) 270.9
    albinism 270.2
    alkaptonuria 270.2
    argininosuccinicaciduria 270.6
    beta-amino-isobutyricaciduria 277.2
    cystathioninuria 270.4
    cystinosis 270.0
    cystinuria 270.0
    glycinuria 270.0
    homocystinuria 270.4
    imidazole 270.5
    maple syrup (urine) disease 270.3
    neonatal, transitory 775.89 ▲
    oasthouse urine disease 270.2
    ochronosis 270.2
    phenylketonuria 270.1
    phenylpyruvic oligophrenia 270.1
    purine NEC 277.2
    pyrimidine NEC 277.2
    renal transport NEC 270.0
    specified type NEC 270.8
    transport NEC 270.0
      renal 270.0
    xanthinuria 277.2
  amnestic (see also Amnestic syndrome) 294.8
    alcohol-induced persisting 291.1
    drug-induced persisting 292.83
    in conditions classified elsewhere 294.0
  anaerobic glycolysis with anemia 282.3
  anxiety (see also Anxiety) 300.00
    due to or associated with physical condition 293.84
  arteriole 447.9
    specified type NEC 447.8
  artery 447.9
    specified type NEC 447.8
  articulation — see Disorder, joint
  Asperger's 299.8 ☑
  attachment of infancy or early childhood 313.89
  attention deficit 314.00

Disorder — see also Disease — continued
  attention deficit — continued
    with hyperactivity 314.01
    predominantly
      combined hyperactive/inattentive 314.01
      hyperactive/impulsive 314.01
      inattentive 314.00
    residual type 314.8
  autistic 299.0 ☑
  autoimmune NEC 279.4
    hemolytic (cold type) (warm type) 283.0
    parathyroid 252.1
    thyroid 245.2
  avoidant, childhood or adolescence 313.21
  balance
    acid-base 276.9
      mixed (with hypercapnia) 276.4
    electrolyte 276.9
    fluid 276.9
  behavior NEC (see also Disturbance, conduct) 312.9
    disruptive 312.9
  bilirubin excretion 277.4
  bipolar (affective) (alternating) 296.80

Note — Use the following fifth-digit subclassification with categories 296.0–296.6:

0	unspecified
1	mild
2	moderate
3	severe, without mention of psychotic behavior
4	severe, specified as with psychotic behavior
5	in partial or unspecified remission
6	in full remission

    atypical 296.7
    currently
      depressed 296.5 ☑
      hypomanic 296.4 ☑
      manic 296.4 ☑
      mixed 296.6 ☑
    specified type NEC 296.89
    type I 296.7
      most recent episode (or current)
        depressed 296.5 ☑
        hypomanic 296.4 ☑
        manic 296.4 ☑
        mixed 296.6 ☑
        unspecified 296.7
      single manic episode 296.0 ☑
    type II (recurrent major depressive episodes with hypomania) 296.89
  bladder 596.9
    functional NEC 596.59
    specified NEC 596.8
  bone NEC 733.90
    specified NEC 733.99
  brachial plexus 353.0
  branched-chain amino-acid degradation 270.3
  breast 611.9
    puerperal, postpartum 676.3 ☑
    specified NEC 611.8
  Briquet's 300.81
  bursa 727.9
    shoulder region 726.10
  carbohydrate metabolism, congenital 271.9
  cardiac, functional 427.9
    postoperative 997.1
    psychogenic 306.2
  cardiovascular, psychogenic 306.2
  cartilage NEC 733.90
    articular 718.00
      ankle 718.07
      elbow 718.02

Disorder — see also Disease — continued
  cartilage — continued
    articular — continued
      foot 718.07
      hand 718.04
      hip 718.05
      knee 717.9
      multiple sites 718.09
      pelvic region 718.05
      shoulder region 718.01
      specified
        site NEC 718.08
        type NEC 733.99
      wrist 718.03
  catatonic — see Catatonia
  central auditory processing 315.32
  cervical region NEC 723.9
  cervical root (nerve) NEC 353.2
  character NEC (see also Disorder, personality) 301.9
  coagulation (factor) (see also Defect, coagulation) 286.9
    factor VIII (congenital) (functional) 286.0
    factor IX (congenital) (functional) 286.1
    neonatal, transitory 776.3
  coccyx 724.70
    specified NEC 724.79
  cognitive 294.9
  colon 569.9
    functional 564.9
      congenital 751.3
  communication 307.9
  conduct (see also Disturbance, conduct) 312.9
    adjustment reaction 309.3
    adolescent onset type 312.82
    childhood onset type 312.81
    compulsive 312.30
      specified type NEC 312.39
    hyperkinetic 314.2
    onset unspecified 312.89
    socialized (type) 312.20
      aggressive 312.23
      unaggressive 312.21
    specified NEC 312.89
  conduction, heart 426.9
    specified NEC 426.89
  conflict
    sexual orientation 302.0
  congenital
    glycosylation (CDG) 271.8
  convulsive (secondary) (see also Convulsions) 780.39
    due to injury at birth 767.0
    idiopathic 780.39
  coordination 781.3
  cornea NEC 371.89
    due to contact lens 371.82
  corticosteroid metabolism NEC 255.2
  cranial nerve — see Disorder, nerve, cranial
  cyclothymic 301.13
  degradation, branched-chain amino acid 270.3
  delusional 297.1
  dentition 520.6
  depersonalization 300.6
  depressive NEC 311
    atypical 296.82
    major (see also Psychosis, affective) 296.2
      recurrent episode 296.3 ☑
      single episode 296.2 ☑
  development, specific 315.9
    associated with hyperkinesia 314.1
    coordination 315.4
    language 315.31
    learning 315.2
      arithmetical 315.1
      reading 315.00
    mixed 315.5
    motor coordination 315.4
    specified type NEC 315.8

Disorder — see also Disease — continued
  development, specific — continued
    speech 315.39
  diaphragm 519.4
  digestive 536.9
    fetus or newborn 777.9
      specified NEC 777.8
    psychogenic 306.4
  disintegrative, childhood 299.1 ☑
  dissociative 300.15
    identity 300.14
    nocturnal 307.47
  drug-related 292.9
  dysmorphic body 300.7
  dysthymic 300.4
  ear 388.9
    degenerative NEC 388.00
    external 380.9
      specified 380.89
    pinna 380.30
    specified type NEC 388.8
    vascular NEC 388.00
  eating NEC 307.50
  electrolyte NEC 276.9
    with
      abortion — see Abortion, by type, with metabolic disorder
      ectopic pregnancy (see also categories 633.0–633.9) 639.4
      molar pregnancy (see also categories 630–632) 639.4
    acidosis 276.2
      metabolic 276.2
      respiratory 276.2
    alkalosis 276.3
      metabolic 276.3
      respiratory 276.3
    following
      abortion 639.4
      ectopic or molar pregnancy 639.4
    neonatal, transitory NEC 775.5
  emancipation as adjustment reaction 309.22
  emotional (see also Disorder, mental, nonpsychotic) V40.9
  endocrine 259.9
    specified type NEC 259.8
  esophagus 530.9
    functional 530.5
    psychogenic 306.4
  explosive
    intermittent 312.34
    isolated 312.35
  expressive language 315.31
  eye 379.90
    globe — see Disorder, globe
    ill-defined NEC 379.99
    limited duction NEC 378.63
    specified NEC 379.8
  eyelid 374.9
    degenerative 374.50
    sensory 374.44
    specified type NEC 374.89
    vascular 374.85
  factitious (with combined psychological and physical signs and symptoms) (with predominantly physical signs and symptoms) 300.19
    with predominantly psychological signs and symptoms 300.16
  factor, coagulation (see also Defect, coagulation) 286.9
    IX (congenital) (funcitonal) 286.1
    VIII (congenital) (functional) 286.0
  fascia 728.9
  fatty acid oxidation 277.85
  feeding — see Feeding
  female sexual arousal 302.72
  fluid NEC 276.9
  gastric (functional) 536.9
    motility 536.8

Disorder — see also Disease — continued
  gastric — continued
    psychogenic 306.4
    secretion 536.8
  gastrointestinal (functional) NEC 536.9
    newborn (neonatal) 777.9
      specified NEC 777.8
    psychogenic 306.4
  gender (child) 302.6
    adult 302.85
  gender identity (childhood) 302.6
    adolescents 302.85
    adults (-life) 302.85
  genitourinary system, psychogenic 306.50
  globe 360.9
    degenerative 360.20
      specified NEC 360.29
    specified type NEC 360.89
  hearing (see also Deafness)
    conductive type (air) (see also Deafness, conductive) 389.00
    mixed conductive and sensorineural 389.2
    nerve, ▶bilateral◀ 389.12
    perceptive (see also Deafness, perceptive) 389.10
    sensorineural type NEC (see also Deafness, ▶sensorineural◀) 389.10
  heart action 427.9
    postoperative 997.1
  hematological, transient neonatal 776.9
    specified type NEC 776.8
  hematopoietic organs 289.9
  hemorrhagic NEC 287.9
    due to intrinsic circulating anticoagulants 286.5
    specified type NEC 287.8
  hemostasis (see also Defect, coagulation) 286.9
  homosexual conflict 302.0
  hypomanic (chronic) 301.11
  identity
    childhood and adolescence 313.82
    gender 302.6
  immune mechanism (immunity) 279.9
    single complement (C1-C9) 279.8
    specified type NEC 279.8
  impulse control (see also Disturbance, conduct, compulsive) 312.30
  infant sialic acid storage 271.8
  integument, fetus or newborn 778.9
    specified type NEC 778.8
  interactional psychotic (childhood) (see also Psychosis, childhood) 299.1 ☑
  intermittent explosive 312.34
  intervertebral disc 722.90
    cervical, cervicothoracic 722.91
    lumbar, lumbosacral 722.93
    thoracic, thoracolumbar 722.92
  intestinal 569.9
    functional NEC 564.9
      congenital 751.3
      postoperative 564.4
    psychogenic 306.4
  introverted, of childhood and adolescence 313.22
  iron, metabolism 275.0
  isolated explosive 312.35
  joint NEC 719.90
    ankle 719.97
    elbow 719.92
    foot 719.97
    hand 719.94
    hip 719.95
    knee 719.96
    multiple sites 719.99
    pelvic region 719.95
    psychogenic 306.0
    shoulder (region) 719.91
    specified site NEC 719.98

Index to Diseases

Disorder — *see also* Disease — *continued*
- joint — *continued*
  - temporomandibular 524.60
    - sounds on opening or closing 524.64
  - specified NEC 524.69
  - wrist 719.93
- kidney 593.9
  - functional 588.9
  - specified NEC 588.89
- labyrinth, labyrinthine 386.9
  - specified type NEC 386.8
- lactation 676.9 ☑
- language (developmental) (expressive) 315.31
  - mixed receptive-expressive 315.32
- learning 315.9
- ligament 728.9
- ligamentous attachments, peripheral (*see also* Enthesopathy)
  - spine 720.1
- limb NEC 729.9
  - psychogenic 306.0
- lipid
  - metabolism, congenital 272.9
  - storage 272.7
- lipoprotein deficiency (familial) 272.5
- low back NEC 724.9
  - psychogenic 306.0
- lumbosacral
  - plexus 353.1
  - root (nerve) NEC 353.4
- lymphoproliferative (chronic) NEC (M9970/1) 238.79 ▲
- major depressive (*see also* Psychosis, affective) 296.2 ☑
  - recurrent episode 296.3 ☑
  - single episode 296.2 ☑
- male erectile 607.84
  - nonorganic origin 302.72
- manic (*see also* Psychosis, affective) 296.0 ☑
  - atypical 296.81
- mathematics 315.1
- meniscus NEC (*see also* Disorder, cartilage, articular) 718.0 ☑
- menopausal 627.9
  - specified NEC 627.8
- menstrual 626.9
  - psychogenic 306.52
  - specified NEC 626.8
- mental (nonpsychotic) 300.9
  - affecting management of pregnancy, childbirth, or puerperium 648.4 ☑
  - drug-induced 292.9
    - hallucinogen persisting perception 292.89
    - specified type NEC 292.89
  - due to or associated with
    - alcoholism 291.9
    - drug consumption NEC 292.9
      - specified type NEC 292.89
    - physical condition NEC 293.9
  - induced by drug 292.9
    - specified type NEC 292.89
  - neurotic (*see also* Neurosis) 300.9
  - of infancy, childhood or adolescence 313.9
  - persistent
    - other
      - due to conditions classified elsewhere 294.8
    - unspecified
      - due to conditions classified elsewhere 294.9
  - presenile 310.1
    - psychotic NEC 290.10
  - previous, affecting management of pregnancy V23.89
  - psychoneurotic (*see also* Neurosis) 300.9
  - psychotic (*see also* Psychosis) 298.9
    - brief 298.8

Disorder — *see also* Disease — *continued*
- mental — *continued*
  - psychotic (*see also* Psychosis) — *continued*
    - senile 290.20
    - specific, following organic brain damage 310.9
      - cognitive or personality change of other type 310.1
      - frontal lobe syndrome 310.0
      - postconcussional syndrome 310.2
      - specified type NEC 310.8
  - transient
    - in conditions classified elsewhere 293.9
- metabolism NEC 277.9
  - with
    - abortion — *see* Abortion, by type, with metabolic disorder
    - ectopic pregnancy (*see also* categories 633.0–633.9) 639.4
    - molar pregnancy (*see also* categories 630–632) 639.4
  - alkaptonuria 270.2
  - amino acid (*see also* Disorder, amino acid) 270.9
    - specified type NEC 270.8
  - ammonia 270.6
  - arginine 270.6
  - argininosuccinic acid 270.6
  - basal 794.7
  - bilirubin 277.4
  - calcium 275.40
  - carbohydrate 271.9
    - specified type NEC 271.8
  - cholesterol 272.9
  - citrulline 270.6
  - copper 275.1
  - corticosteroid 255.2
  - cystine storage 270.0
  - cystinuria 270.0
  - fat 272.9
  - fatty acid oxidation 277.85
  - following
    - abortion 639.4
    - ectopic or molar pregnancy 639.4
  - fructosemia 271.2
  - fructosuria 271.2
  - fucosidosis 271.8
  - galactose-1-phosphate uridyl transferase 271.1
  - glutamine 270.7
  - glycine 270.7
  - glycogen storage NEC 271.0
    - hepatorenal 271.0
  - hemochromatosis 275.0
  - in labor and delivery 669.0 ☑
  - iron 275.0
  - lactose 271.3
  - lipid 272.9
    - specified type NEC 272.8
    - storage 272.7
  - lipoprotein (*see also* Hyperlipemia deficiency (familial)) 272.5
  - lysine 270.7
  - magnesium 275.2
  - mannosidosis 271.8
  - mineral 275.9
    - specified type NEC 275.8
  - mitochondrial 277.87
  - mucopolysaccharide 277.5
  - nitrogen 270.9
  - ornithine 270.6
  - oxalosis 271.8
  - pentosuria 271.8
  - phenylketonuria 270.1
  - phosphate 275.3
  - phosphorous 275.3
  - plasma protein 273.9
    - specified type NEC 273.8
  - porphyrin 277.1

Disorder — *see also* Disease — *continued*
- metabolism — *continued*
  - purine 277.2
  - pyrimidine 277.2
  - serine 270.7
  - sodium 276.9
  - specified type NEC 277.89
  - steroid 255.2
  - threonine 270.7
  - urea cycle 270.6
  - xylose 271.8
- micturition NEC 788.69
  - psychogenic 306.53
- misery and unhappiness, of childhood and adolescence 313.1
- mitochondrial metabolism 277.87
- mitral valve 424.0
- mood (*see also* Disorder, bipolar) 296.90
  - episodic 296.90
    - specified NEC 296.99
  - in conditions classified elsewhere 293.83
- motor tic 307.20
  - chronic 307.22
  - transient (childhood) 307.21
- movement NEC 333.90
  - hysterical 300.11
  - medication-induced 333.90
  - periodic limb 327.51
  - sleep related, unspecified 780.58
    - other organic 327.59
  - specified type NEC 333.99
  - stereotypic 307.3
- mucopolysaccharide 277.5
- muscle 728.9
  - psychogenic 306.0
  - specified type NEC 728.3
- muscular attachments, peripheral (*see also* Enthesopathy)
  - spine 720.1
- musculoskeletal system NEC 729.9
  - psychogenic 306.0
- myeloproliferative (chronic) NEC (M9960/1) 238.79 ▲
- myoneural 358.9
  - due to lead 358.2
  - specified type NEC 358.8
  - toxic 358.2
- myotonic 359.2
- neck region NEC 723.9
- nerve 349.9
  - abducens NEC 378.54
  - accessory 352.4
  - acoustic 388.5
  - auditory 388.5
  - auriculotemporal 350.8
  - axillary 353.0
  - cerebral — *see* Disorder, nerve, cranial
  - cranial 352.9
    - first 352.0
    - second 377.49
    - third
      - partial 378.51
      - total 378.52
    - fourth 378.53
    - fifth 350.9
    - sixth 378.54
    - seventh NEC 351.9
    - eighth 388.5
    - ninth 352.2
    - tenth 352.3
    - eleventh 352.4
    - twelfth 352.5
    - multiple 352.6
  - entrapment — *see* Neuropathy, entrapment
  - facial 351.9
    - specified NEC 351.8
  - femoral 355.2
  - glossopharyngeal NEC 352.2
  - hypoglossal 352.5
  - iliohypogastric 355.79
  - ilioinguinal 355.79

Disorder — *see also* Disease — *continued*
- nerve — *continued*
  - intercostal 353.8
  - lateral
    - cutaneous of thigh 355.1
    - popliteal 355.3
  - lower limb NEC 355.8
  - medial, popliteal 355.4
  - median NEC 354.1
  - obturator 355.79
  - oculomotor
    - partial 378.51
    - total 378.52
  - olfactory 352.0
  - optic 377.49
    - hypoplasia 377.43 ●
    - ischemic 377.41
    - nutritional 377.33
    - toxic 377.34
  - peroneal 355.3
  - phrenic 354.8
  - plantar 355.6
  - pneumogastric 352.3
  - posterior tibial 355.5
  - radial 354.3
  - recurrent laryngeal 352.3
  - root 353.9
    - specified NEC 353.8
  - saphenous 355.79
  - sciatic NEC 355.0
  - specified NEC 355.9
    - lower limb 355.79
    - upper limb 354.8
  - spinal 355.9
  - sympathetic NEC 337.9
  - trigeminal 350.9
    - specified NEC 350.8
  - trochlear 378.53
  - ulnar 354.2
  - upper limb NEC 354.9
  - vagus 352.3
- nervous system NEC 349.9
  - autonomic (peripheral) (*see also* Neuropathy, peripheral, autonomic) 337.9
  - cranial 352.9
  - parasympathetic (*see also* Neuropathy, peripheral, autonomic) 337.9
  - specified type NEC 349.89
  - sympathetic (*see also* Neuropathy, peripheral, autonomic) 337.9
  - vegetative (*see also* Neuropathy, peripheral, autonomic) 337.9
- neurohypophysis 253.6
- neurological NEC 781.99
  - peripheral NEC 355.9
- neuromuscular NEC 358.9
  - hereditary 359.1
  - specified NEC 358.8
  - toxic 358.2
- neurotic 300.9
  - specified type NEC 300.89
- neutrophil, polymorphonuclear (functional) 288.1
- nightmare 307.47
- night terror 307.46
- obsessive-compulsive 300.3
- oppositional defiant, childhood and adolescence 313.81
- optic
  - chiasm 377.54
    - associated with
      - inflammatory disorders 377.54
      - neoplasm NEC 377.52
        - pituitary 377.51
      - pituitary disorders 377.51
      - vascular disorders 377.53
  - nerve 377.49
  - radiations 377.63
  - tracts 377.63
- orbit 376.9
  - specified NEC 376.89

Disorder — see also Disease — continued
- orgasmic
  - female 302.73
  - male 302.74
- overanxious, of childhood and adolescence 313.0
- oxidation, fatty acid 277.85
- pancreas, internal secretion (other than diabetes mellitus) 251.9
  - specified type NEC 251.8
- panic 300.01
  - with agoraphobia 300.21
- papillary muscle NEC 429.81
- paranoid 297.9
  - induced 297.3
  - shared 297.3
- parathyroid 252.9
  - specified type NEC 252.8
- paroxysmal, mixed 780.39
- pentose phosphate pathway with anemia 282.2
- periodic limb movement 327.51
- peroxisomal 277.86
- personality 301.9
  - affective 301.10
  - aggressive 301.3
  - amoral 301.7
  - anancastic, anankastic 301.4
  - antisocial 301.7
  - asocial 301.7
  - asthenic 301.6
  - avoidant 301.82
  - borderline 301.83
  - compulsive 301.4
  - cyclothymic 301.13
  - dependent-passive 301.6
  - dyssocial 301.7
  - emotional instability 301.59
  - epileptoid 301.3
  - explosive 301.3
  - following organic brain damage 310.1
  - histrionic 301.50
  - hyperthymic 301.11
  - hypomanic (chronic) 301.11
  - hypothymic 301.12
  - hysterical 301.50
  - immature 301.89
  - inadequate 301.6
  - introverted 301.21
  - labile 301.59
  - moral deficiency 301.7
  - narcissistic 301.81
  - obsessional 301.4
  - obsessive-compulsive 301.4
  - overconscientious 301.4
  - paranoid 301.0
  - passive (-dependent) 301.6
  - passive-aggressive 301.84
  - pathological NEC 301.9
  - pseudosocial 301.7
  - psychopathic 301.9
  - schizoid 301.20
    - introverted 301.21
    - schizotypal 301.22
  - schizotypal 301.22
  - seductive 301.59
  - type A 301.4
  - unstable 301.59
- pervasive developmental 299.9 ✓
  - childhood-onset 299.8 ✓
  - specified NEC 299.8 ✓
- phonological 315.39
- pigmentation, choroid (congenital) 743.53
- pinna 380.30
  - specified type NEC 380.39
- pituitary, thalamic 253.9
  - anterior NEC 253.4
  - iatrogenic 253.7
  - postablative 253.7
  - specified NEC 253.8
- pityriasis-like NEC 696.8
- platelets (blood) 287.1

Disorder — see also Disease — continued
- polymorphonuclear neutrophils (functional) 288.1
- porphyrin metabolism 277.1
- postmenopausal 627.9
  - specified type NEC 627.8
- posttraumatic stress 309.81
- post-traumatic stress (PTSD) 309.81 ●
  - acute 309.81
  - brief 309.81
  - chronic 309.81
- premenstrual dysphoric (PMDD) 625.4
- psoriatic-like NEC 696.8
- psychic, with diseases classified elsewhere 316
- psychogenic NEC (see also condition) 300.9
  - allergic NEC
    - respiratory 306.1
  - anxiety 300.00
    - atypical 300.00
    - generalized 300.02
  - appetite 307.59
  - articulation, joint 306.0
  - asthenic 300.5
  - blood 306.8
  - cardiovascular (system) 306.2
  - compulsive 300.3
  - cutaneous 306.3
  - depressive 300.4
  - digestive (system) 306.4
  - dysmenorrheic 306.52
  - dyspneic 306.1
  - eczematous 306.3
  - endocrine (system) 306.6
  - eye 306.7
  - feeding 307.59
  - functional NEC 306.9
  - gastric 306.4
  - gastrointestinal (system) 306.4
  - genitourinary (system) 306.50
  - heart (function) (rhythm) 306.2
  - hemic 306.8
  - hyperventilatory 306.1
  - hypochondriacal 300.7
  - hysterical 300.10
  - intestinal 306.4
  - joint 306.0
  - learning 315.2
  - limb 306.0
  - lymphatic (system) 306.8
  - menstrual 306.52
  - micturition 306.53
  - monoplegic NEC 306.0
  - motor 307.9
  - muscle 306.0
  - musculoskeletal 306.0
  - neurocirculatory 306.2
  - obsessive 300.3
  - occupational 300.89
  - organ or part of body NEC 306.9
  - organs of special sense 306.7
  - paralytic NEC 306.0
  - phobic 300.20
  - physical NEC 306.9
  - pruritic 306.3
  - rectal 306.4
  - respiratory (system) 306.1
  - rheumatic 306.0
  - sexual (function) 302.70
    - specified type NEC 302.79
  - sexual orientation conflict 302.0
  - skin (allergic) (eczematous) (pruritic) 306.3
  - sleep 307.40
    - initiation or maintenance 307.41
    - persistent 307.42
    - transient 307.41
    - movement 780.58
    - sleep terror 307.46
    - specified type NEC 307.49
  - specified part of body NEC 306.8
  - stomach 306.4
- psychomotor NEC 307.9

Disorder — see also Disease — continued
- psychomotor — continued
  - hysterical 300.11
- psychoneurotic (see also Neurosis) 300.9
  - mixed NEC 300.89
- psychophysiologic (see also Disorder, psychosomatic) 306.9
- psychosexual identity (childhood) 302.6
  - adult-life 302.85
- psychosomatic NEC 306.9
  - allergic NEC
    - respiratory 306.1
  - articulation, joint 306.0
  - cardiovascular (system) 306.2
  - cutaneous 306.3
  - digestive (system) 306.4
  - dysmenorrheic 306.52
  - dyspneic 306.1
  - endocrine (system) 306.6
  - eye 306.7
  - gastric 306.4
  - gastrointestinal (system) 306.4
  - genitourinary (system) 306.50
  - heart (functional) (rhythm) 306.2
  - hyperventilatory 306.1
  - intestinal 306.4
  - joint 306.0
  - limb 306.0
  - lymphatic (system) 306.8
  - menstrual 306.52
  - micturition 306.53
  - monoplegic NEC 306.0
  - muscle 306.0
  - musculoskeletal 306.0
  - neurocirculatory 306.2
  - organs of special sense 306.7
  - paralytic NEC 306.0
  - pruritic 306.3
  - rectal 306.4
  - respiratory (system) 306.1
  - rheumatic 306.0
  - sexual (function) 302.70
  - skin 306.3
  - specified part of body NEC 306.8
  - specified type NEC 302.79
  - stomach 306.4
- psychotic (see also Psychosis) 298.9
  - brief 298.8
- purine metabolism NEC 277.2
- pyrimidine metabolism NEC 277.2
- reactive attachment of infancy or early childhood 313.89
- reading, developmental 315.00
- reflex 796.1
- REM sleep behavior 327.42
- renal function, impaired 588.9
  - specified type NEC 588.89
- renal transport NEC 588.89
- respiration, respiratory NEC 519.9
  - due to
    - aspiration of liquids or solids 508.9
    - inhalation of fumes or vapors 506.9
  - psychogenic 306.1
- retina 362.9
  - specified type NEC 362.89
- rumination 307.53
- sacroiliac joint NEC 724.6
- sacrum 724.6
- schizo-affective (see also Schizophrenia) 295.7 ✓
- schizoid, childhood or adolescence 313.22
- schizophreniform 295.4 ✓
- schizotypal personality 301.22
- secretion, thyrocalcitonin 246.0
- seizure 345.9 ✓ ▲
  - recurrent 345.9 ✓ ▲
  - epileptic — see Epilepsy
- sense of smell 781.1
  - psychogenic 306.7
- separation anxiety 309.21

Disorder — see also Disease — continued
- sexual (see also Deviation, sexual) 302.9
  - aversion 302.79
  - desire, hypoactive 302.71
  - function, psychogenic 302.70
- shyness, of childhood and adolescence 313.21
- single complement (C1-C9) 279.8
- skin NEC 709.9
  - fetus or newborn 778.9
    - specified type 778.8
  - psychogenic (allergic) (eczematous) (pruritic) 306.3
  - specified type NEC 709.8
  - vascular 709.1
- sleep 780.50
  - with apnea — see Apnea, sleep
  - alcohol induced 291.82
  - arousal 307.46
    - confusional 327.41
  - circadian rhythm 327.30
    - advanced sleep phase type 327.32
    - alcohol induced 291.82
    - delayed sleep phase type 327.31
    - drug induced 292.85
    - free running type 327.34
    - in conditions classified elsewhere 327.37
    - irregular sleep-wake type 327.33
    - jet lag type 327.35
    - other 327.39
    - shift work type 327.36
  - drug induced 292.85
  - initiation or maintenance (see also Insomnia) 780.52
    - nonorganic origin (transient) 307.41
    - persistent 307.42
  - nonorganic origin 307.40
    - specified type NEC 307.49
  - organic specified type NEC 327.8
  - periodic limb movement 327.51
  - specified NEC 780.59
  - wake
    - cycle — see Disorder, sleep, circadian rhythm
    - schedule — see Disorer, sleep, circadian rhythm
- social, of childhood and adolescence 313.22
- soft tissue 729.9
- somatization 300.81
- somatoform (atypical) (undifferentiated) 300.82
  - severe 300.81
  - specified type NEC 300.89
- speech NEC 784.5
  - nonorganic origin 307.9
- spine NEC 724.9
  - ligamentous or muscular attachments, peripheral 720.1
- steroid metabolism NEC 255.2
- stomach (functional) (see also Disorder, gastric) 536.9
  - psychogenic 306.4
- storage, iron 275.0
- stress (see also Reaction, stress, acute) 308.3
  - posttraumatic
    - acute 309.81
    - brief 309.81
    - chronic 309.81
- substitution 300.11
- suspected — see Observation
- synovium 727.9
- temperature regulation, fetus or newborn 778.4
- temporomandibular joint NEC 524.60
  - sounds on opening or closing 524.64
  - specified NEC 524.69
- tendon 727.9

Index to Diseases

Disorder — see also Disease — continued
- tendon — continued
  - shoulder region 726.10
- thoracic root (nerve) NEC 353.3
- thyrocalcitonin secretion 246.0
- thyroid (gland) NEC 246.9
  - specified type NEC 246.8
- tic 307.20
  - chronic (motor or vocal) 307.22
  - motor-verbal 307.23
  - organic origin 333.1
  - transient (of childhood) 307.21
- tooth NEC 525.9
  - development NEC 520.9
    - specified type NEC 520.8
  - eruption 520.6
  - specified type NEC 525.8
- Tourette's 307.23
- transport, carbohydrate 271.9
  - specified type NEC 271.8
- tubular, phosphate-losing 588.0
- tympanic membrane 384.9
- unaggressive, unsocialized (see also Disturbance, conduct) 312.1 ☑
- undersocialized, unsocialized (see also Disturbance, conduct)
  - aggressive (type) 312.0 ☑
  - unaggressive (type) 312.1 ☑
- vision, visual NEC 368.9
  - binocular NEC 368.30
  - cortex 377.73
    - associated with
      - inflammatory disorders 377.73
      - neoplasms 377.71
      - vascular disorders 377.72
  - pathway NEC 377.63
    - associated with
      - inflammatory disorders 377.63
      - neoplasms 377.61
      - vascular disorders 377.62
- vocal tic
  - chronic 307.22
- wakefulness (see also Hypersomnia) 780.54
  - nonorganic origin (transient) 307.43
    - persistent 307.44
- written expression 315.2

Disorganized globe 360.29

Displacement, displaced

Note — For acquired displacement of bones, cartilage, joints, tendons, due to injury, see also Dislocation.

Displacements at ages under one year should be considered congenital, provided there is no indication the condition was acquired after birth.

- acquired traumatic of bone, cartilage, joint, tendon NEC (without fracture) (see also Dislocation) 839.8
  - with fracture — see Fracture, by site
- adrenal gland (congenital) 759.1
- alveolus and teeth, vertical 524.75
- appendix, retrocecal (congenital) 751.5
- auricle (congenital) 744.29
- bladder (acquired) 596.8
  - congenital 753.8
- brachial plexus (congenital) 742.8
- brain stem, caudal 742.4
- canaliculus lacrimalis 743.65
- cardia, through esophageal hiatus 750.6
- cerebellum, caudal 742.4
- cervix ▶— see Displacement, uterus◀
- colon (congenital) 751.4
- device, implant, or graft — see Complications, mechanical
- epithelium
  - columnar of cervix 622.10

Displacement, displaced — continued
- epithelium — continued
  - cuboidal, beyond limits of external os (uterus) 752.49
  - esophageal mucosa into cardia of stomach, congenital 750.4
- esophagus (acquired) 530.89
  - congenital 750.4
- eyeball (acquired) (old) 376.36
  - congenital 743.8
  - current injury 871.3
  - lateral 376.36
- fallopian tube (acquired) 620.4
  - congenital 752.19
  - opening (congenital) 752.19
- gallbladder (congenital) 751.69
- gastric mucosa 750.7
  - into
    - duodenum 750.7
    - esophagus 750.7
    - Meckel's diverticulum, congenital 750.7
- globe (acquired) (lateral) (old) 376.36
  - current injury 871.3
- graft
  - artificial skin graft 996.55
  - decellularized allodermis graft 996.55
- heart (congenital) 746.87
  - acquired 429.89
- hymen (congenital) (upward) 752.49
- internal prosthesis NEC — see Complications, mechanical
- intervertebral disc (with neuritis, radiculitis, sciatica, or other pain) 722.2
  - with myelopathy 722.70
  - cervical, cervicodorsal, cervicothoracic 722.0
    - with myelopathy 722.71
    - due to major trauma — see Dislocation, vertebra, cervical
  - due to trauma — see Dislocation, vertebra
  - lumbar, lumbosacral 722.10
    - with myelopathy 722.73
    - due to major trauma — see Dislocation, vertebra, lumbar
  - thoracic, thoracolumbar 722.11
    - with myelopathy 722.72
    - due to major trauma — see Dislocation, vertebra, thoracic
- intrauterine device 996.32
- kidney (acquired) 593.0
  - congenital 753.3
- lacrimal apparatus or duct (congenital) 743.65
- macula (congenital) 743.55
- Meckel's diverticulum (congenital) 751.0
- nail (congenital) 757.5
  - acquired 703.8
- opening of Wharton's duct in mouth 750.26
- organ or site, congenital NEC — see Malposition, congenital
- ovary (acquired) 620.4
  - congenital 752.0
  - free in peritoneal cavity (congenital) 752.0
  - into hernial sac 620.4
- oviduct (acquired) 620.4
  - congenital 752.19
- parathyroid (gland) 252.8
- parotid gland (congenital) 750.26
- punctum lacrimale (congenital) 743.65
- sacroiliac (congenital) (joint) 755.69
  - current injury — see Dislocation, sacroiliac
  - old 724.6
- spine (congenital) 756.19
- spleen, congenital 759.0

Displacement, displaced — continued
- stomach (congenital) 750.7
  - acquired 537.89
- subglenoid (closed) 831.01
- sublingual duct (congenital) 750.26
- teeth, tooth 524.30
  - horizontal 524.33
  - vertical 524.34
- tongue (congenital) (downward) 750.19
- trachea (congenital) 748.3
- ureter or ureteric opening or orifice (congenital) 753.4
- uterine opening of oviducts or fallopian tubes 752.19
- uterus, uterine (see also Malposition, uterus) 621.6
  - congenital 752.3
- ventricular septum 746.89
  - with rudimentary ventricle 746.89
- xyphoid bone (process) 738.3

Disproportion 653.9 ☑
- affecting fetus or newborn 763.1
- caused by
  - conjoined twins 653.7 ☑
  - contraction, pelvis (general) 653.1 ☑
    - inlet 653.2 ☑
    - midpelvic 653.8 ☑
    - midplane 653.8 ☑
    - outlet 653.3 ☑
  - fetal
    - ascites 653.7 ☑
    - hydrocephalus 653.6 ☑
    - hydrops 653.7 ☑
    - meningomyelocele 653.7 ☑
    - sacral teratoma 653.7 ☑
    - tumor 653.7 ☑
  - hydrocephalic fetus 653.6 ☑
  - pelvis, pelvic, abnormality (bony) NEC 653.0 ☑
  - unusually large fetus 653.5 ☑
- causing obstructed labor 660.1 ☑
- cephalopelvic, normally formed fetus 653.4 ☑
  - causing obstructed labor 660.1 ☑
- fetal NEC 653.5 ☑
  - causing obstructed labor 660.1 ☑
- fetopelvic, normally formed fetus 653.4 ☑
  - causing obstructed labor 660.1 ☑
- mixed maternal and fetal origin, normally formed fetus 653.4 ☑
- pelvis, pelvic (bony) NEC 653.1 ☑
  - causing obstructed labor 660.1 ☑
- specified type NEC 653.8 ☑

Disruption
- cesarean wound 674.1 ☑
- family V61.0
- gastrointestinal anastomosis 997.4
- ligament(s) (see also Sprain)
  - knee
    - current injury — see Dislocation, knee
    - old 717.89
      - capsular 717.85
      - collateral (medial) 717.82
        - lateral 717.81
      - cruciate (posterior) 717.84
        - anterior 717.83
      - specified site NEC 717.85
- marital V61.10
  - involving divorce or estrangement V61.10
- operation wound (external) 998.32
  - internal 998.31
- organ transplant, anastomosis site — see Complications, transplant, organ, by site
- ossicles, ossicular chain 385.23
  - traumatic — see Fracture, skull, base
- parenchyma
  - liver (hepatic) — see Laceration, liver, major

Disruption — continued
- parenchyma — continued
  - spleen — see Laceration, spleen, parenchyma, massive
- phase-shift, of 24-hour sleep-wake cycle, unspecified 780.55
  - nonorganic origin 307.45
- sleep-wake cycle (24-hour), unspecified 780.55
  - circadian rhythm 327.33
  - nonorganic origin 307.45
- suture line (external) 998.32
  - internal 998.31
- wound
  - cesarean operation 674.1 ☑
  - episiotomy 674.2 ☑
  - operation 998.32
    - cesarean 674.1 ☑
    - internal 998.31
  - perineal (obstetric) 674.2 ☑
  - uterine 674.1 ☑

Disruptio uteri — see also Rupture, uterus
- complicating delivery — see Delivery, complicated, rupture, uterus

Dissatisfaction with
- employment V62.2
- school environment V62.3

Dissecting — see condition

Dissection
- aorta 441.00
  - abdominal 441.02
  - thoracic 441.01
  - thoracoabdominal 441.03
- artery, arterial
  - carotid 443.21
  - coronary 414.12
  - iliac 443.22
  - renal 443.23
  - specified NEC 443.29
  - vertebral 443.24
- vascular 459.9
- wound — see Wound, open, by site

Disseminated — see condition

Dissociated personality NEC 300.15

Dissociation
- auriculoventricular or atrioventricular (any degree) (AV) 426.89
  - with heart block 426.0
  - interference 426.89
  - isorhythmic 426.89
- rhythm
  - atrioventricular (AV) 426.89
  - interference 426.89

Dissociative
- identity disorder 300.14
- reaction NEC 300.15

Dissolution, vertebra — see also Osteoporosis 733.00

Distention
- abdomen (gaseous) 787.3
- bladder 596.8
- cecum 569.89
- colon 569.89
- gallbladder 575.8
- gaseous (abdomen) 787.3
- intestine 569.89
- kidney 593.89
- liver 573.9
- seminal vesicle 608.89
- stomach 536.8
  - acute 536.1
  - psychogenic 306.4
- ureter 593.5
- uterus 621.8

Distichia, distichiasis (eyelid) 743.63

Distoma hepaticum infestation 121.3

Distomiasis 121.9
- bile passages 121.3
- due to Clonorchis sinensis 121.1
- hemic 120.9
- hepatic (liver) 121.3
  - due to Clonorchis sinensis (clonorchiasis) 121.1
- intestinal 121.4
- liver 121.3

Index to Diseases

Distomiasis — continued
- liver — continued
  - due to Clonorchis sinensis 121.1
  - lung 121.2
  - pulmonary 121.2
- **Distomolar** (fourth molar) 520.1
  - causing crowding 524.31
- **Disto-occlusion** (division I) (division II) 524.22
- **Distortion** (congenital)
  - adrenal (gland) 759.1
  - ankle (joint) 755.69
  - anus 751.5
  - aorta 747.29
  - appendix 751.5
  - arm 755.59
  - artery (peripheral) NEC (see also Distortion, peripheral vascular system) 747.60
    - cerebral 747.81
    - coronary 746.85
    - pulmonary 747.3
    - retinal 743.58
    - umbilical 747.5
  - auditory canal 744.29
    - causing impairment of hearing 744.02
  - bile duct or passage 751.69
  - bladder 753.8
  - brain 742.4
  - bronchus 748.3
  - cecum 751.5
  - cervix (uteri) 752.49
  - chest (wall) 756.3
  - clavicle 755.51
  - clitoris 752.49
  - coccyx 756.19
  - colon 751.5
  - common duct 751.69
  - cornea 743.41
  - cricoid cartilage 748.3
  - cystic duct 751.69
  - duodenum 751.5
  - ear 744.29
    - auricle 744.29
      - causing impairment of hearing 744.02
    - causing impairment of hearing 744.09
    - external 744.29
      - causing impairment of hearing 744.02
    - inner 744.05
    - middle, except ossicles 744.03
      - ossicles 744.04
    - ossicles 744.04
  - endocrine (gland) NEC 759.2
  - epiglottis 748.3
  - Eustachian tube 744.24
  - eye 743.8
    - adnexa 743.69
  - face bone(s) 756.0
  - fallopian tube 752.19
  - femur 755.69
  - fibula 755.69
  - finger(s) 755.59
  - foot 755.67
  - gallbladder 751.69
  - genitalia, genital organ(s)
    - female 752.89
      - external 752.49
      - internal NEC 752.89
    - male 752.89
      - penis 752.69
  - glottis 748.3
  - gyri 742.4
  - hand bone(s) 755.59
  - heart (auricle) (ventricle) 746.89
    - valve (cusp) 746.89
  - hepatic duct 751.69
  - humerus 755.59
  - hymen 752.49
  - ileum 751.5
  - intestine (large) (small) 751.5
    - with anomalous adhesions, fixation or malrotation 751.4

Distortion — continued
- jaw NEC 524.89
- jejunum 751.5
- kidney 753.3
- knee (joint) 755.64
- labium (majus) (minus) 752.49
- larynx 748.3
- leg 755.69
- lens 743.36
- liver 751.69
- lumbar spine 756.19
  - with disproportion (fetopelvic) 653.0 ☑
    - affecting fetus or newborn 763.1
    - causing obstructed labor 660.1 ☑
- lumbosacral (joint) (region) 756.19
- lung (fissures) (lobe) 748.69
- nerve 742.8
- nose 748.1
- organ
  - of Corti 744.05
  - of site not listed — see Anomaly, specified type NEC
- ossicles, ear 744.04
- ovary 752.0
- oviduct 752.19
- pancreas 751.7
- parathyroid (gland) 759.2
- patella 755.64
- peripheral vascular system NEC 747.60
  - gastrointestinal 747.61
  - lower limb 747.64
  - renal 747.62
  - spinal 747.82
  - upper limb 747.63
- pituitary (gland) 759.2
- radius 755.59
- rectum 751.5
- rib 756.3
- sacroiliac joint 755.69
- sacrum 756.19
- scapula 755.59
- shoulder girdle 755.59
- site not listed — see Anomaly, specified type NEC
- skull bone(s) 756.0
  - with
    - anencephalus 740.0
    - encephalocele 742.0
    - hydrocephalus 742.3
      - with spina bifida (see also Spina bifida) 741.0 ☑
    - microcephalus 742.1
- spinal cord 742.59
- spine 756.19
- spleen 759.0
- sternum 756.3
- thorax (wall) 756.3
- thymus (gland) 759.2
- thyroid (gland) 759.2
  - cartilage 748.3
- tibia 755.69
- toe(s) 755.66
- tongue 750.19
- trachea (cartilage) 748.3
- ulna 755.59
- ureter 753.4
  - causing obstruction 753.20
- urethra 753.8
  - causing obstruction 753.6
- uterus 752.3
- vagina 752.49
- vein (peripheral) NEC (see also Distortion, peripheral vascular system) 747.60
  - great 747.49
  - portal 747.49
  - pulmonary 747.49
- vena cava (inferior) (superior) 747.49
- vertebra 756.19
- visual NEC 368.15
  - shape or size 368.14
- vulva 752.49
- wrist (bones) (joint) 755.59

Distress
- abdomen 789.0 ☑
- colon 564.9
- emotional V40.9
- epigastric 789.0 ☑
- fetal (syndrome) 768.4
  - affecting management of pregnancy or childbirth 656.8 ☑
  - liveborn infant 768.4
    - first noted
      - before onset of labor 768.2
      - during labor ►and◄ delivery 768.3
  - stillborn infant (death before onset of labor) 768.0
    - death during labor 768.1
- gastrointestinal (functional) 536.9
  - psychogenic 306.4
- intestinal (functional) NEC 564.9
  - psychogenic 306.4
- intrauterine — see Distress, fetal
- leg 729.5
- maternal 669.0 ☑
- mental V40.9
- respiratory 786.09
  - acute (adult) 518.82
  - adult syndrome (following shock, surgery, or trauma) 518.5
    - specified NEC 518.82
  - fetus or newborn 770.89
  - syndrome (idiopathic) (newborn) 769
- stomach 536.9
  - psychogenic 306.4

Distribution vessel, atypical NEC 747.60
- coronary artery 746.85
- spinal 747.82

Districhiasis 704.2

Disturbance — see also Disease
- absorption NEC 579.9
  - calcium 269.3
  - carbohydrate 579.8
  - fat 579.8
  - protein 579.8
  - specified type NEC 579.8
  - vitamin (see also Deficiency, vitamin) 269.2
- acid-base equilibrium 276.9
- activity and attention, simple, with hyperkinesis 314.01
- amino acid (metabolic) (see also Disorder, amino acid) 270.9
  - imidazole 270.5
  - maple syrup (urine) disease 270.3
  - transport 270.0
- assimilation, food 579.9
- attention, simple 314.00
  - with hyperactivity 314.01
- auditory, nerve, except deafness 388.5
- behavior (see also Disturbance, conduct) 312.9
- blood clotting (hypoproteinemia) (mechanism) (see also Defect, coagulation) 286.9
- central nervous system NEC 349.9
- cerebral nerve NEC 352.9
- circulatory 459.9
- conduct 312.9

Note — *Use the following fifth-digit subclassification with categories 312.0–312.2:*

0	unspecified
1	mild
2	moderate
3	severe

  - adjustment reaction 309.3
  - adolescent onset type 312.82
  - childhood onset type 312.81
  - compulsive 312.30
    - intermittent explosive disorder 312.34
    - isolated explosive disorder 312.35

Disturbance — see also Disease — continued
- conduct — continued
  - compulsive — continued
    - kleptomania 312.32
    - pathological gambling 312.31
    - pyromania 312.33
  - hyperkinetic 314.2
  - intermittent explosive 312.34
  - isolated explosive 312.35
  - mixed with emotions 312.4
  - socialized (type) 312.20
    - aggressive 312.23
    - unaggressive 312.21
  - specified type NEC 312.89
  - undersocialized, unsocialized
    - aggressive (type) 312.0 ☑
    - unaggressive (type) 312.1 ☑
- coordination 781.3
- cranial nerve NEC 352.9
- deep sensibility — see Disturbance, sensation
- digestive 536.9
  - psychogenic 306.4
- electrolyte — see Imbalance, electrolyte
- emotions specific to childhood or adolescence 313.9
  - with
    - academic underachievement 313.83
    - anxiety and fearfulness 313.0
    - elective mutism 313.23
    - identity disorder 313.82
    - jealousy 313.3
    - misery and unhappiness 313.1
    - oppositional defiant disorder 313.81
    - overanxiousness 313.0
    - sensitivity 313.21
    - shyness 313.21
    - social withdrawal 313.22
    - withdrawal reaction 313.22
  - involving relationship problems 313.3
  - mixed 313.89
  - specified type NEC 313.89
- endocrine (gland) 259.9
  - neonatal, transitory 775.9
    - specified NEC 775.89 ▲
- equilibrium 780.4
- feeding (elderly) (infant) 783.3
  - newborn 779.3
  - nonorganic origin NEC 307.59
  - psychogenic NEC 307.59
- fructose metabolism 271.2
- gait 781.2
  - hysterical 300.11
- gastric (functional) 536.9
  - motility 536.8
  - psychogenic 306.4
  - secretion 536.8
- gastrointestinal (functional) 536.9
  - psychogenic 306.4
- habit, child 307.9
- hearing, except deafness 388.40
- heart, functional (conditions classifiable to 426, 427, 428)
  - due to presence of (cardiac) prosthesis 429.4
  - postoperative (immediate) 997.1
    - long-term effect of cardiac surgery 429.4
  - psychogenic 306.2
- hormone 259.9
- innervation uterus, sympathetic, parasympathetic 621.8
- keratinization NEC
  - gingiva 523.10 ▲
  - lip 528.5
  - oral (mucosa) (soft tissue) 528.79
    - residual ridge mucosa
      - excessive 528.72
      - minimal 528.71
    - tongue 528.79

Index to Diseases

Disturbance — see also Disease — continued
  labyrinth, labyrinthine (vestibule) 386.9
  learning, specific NEC 315.2
  memory (see also Amnesia) 780.93
    mild, following organic brain damage 310.8
  mental (see also Disorder, mental) 300.9
    associated with diseases classified elsewhere 316
  metabolism (acquired) (congenital) (see also Disorder, metabolism) 277.9
    with
      abortion — see Abortion, by type, with metabolic disorder
      ectopic pregnancy (see also categories 633.0–633.9) 639.4
      molar pregnancy (see also categories 630–632) 639.4
    amino acid (see also Disorder, amino acid) 270.9
      aromatic NEC 270.2
      branched-chain 270.3
      specified type NEC 270.8
      straight-chain NEC 270.7
      sulfur-bearing 270.4
      transport 270.0
    ammonia 270.6
    arginine 270.6
    argininosuccinic acid 270.6
    carbohydrate NEC 271.9
    cholesterol 272.9
    citrulline 270.6
    cystathionine 270.4
    fat 272.9
    following
      abortion 639.4
      ectopic or molar pregnancy 639.4
    general 277.9
      carbohydrate 271.9
      iron 275.0
      phosphate 275.3
      sodium 276.9
    glutamine 270.7
    glycine 270.7
    histidine 270.5
    homocystine 270.4
    in labor or delivery 669.0 ☑
    iron 275.0
    isoleucine 270.3
    leucine 270.3
    lipoid 272.9
      specified type NEC 272.8
    lysine 270.7
    methionine 270.4
    neonatal, transitory 775.9
      specified type NEC 775.89 ▲
    nitrogen 788.9
    ornithine 270.6
    phosphate 275.3
    phosphatides 272.7
    serine 270.7
    sodium NEC 276.9
    threonine 270.7
    tryptophan 270.2
    tyrosine 270.2
    urea cycle 270.6
    valine 270.3
  motor 796.1
  nervous functional 799.2
  neuromuscular mechanism (eye) due to syphilis 094.84
  nutritional 269.9
    nail 703.8
  ocular motion 378.87
    psychogenic 306.7
  oculogyric 378.87
    psychogenic 306.7
  oculomotor NEC 378.87
    psychogenic 306.7

Disturbance — see also Disease — continued
  olfactory nerve 781.1
  optic nerve NEC 377.49
  oral epithelium, including tongue 528.79
    residual ridge mucosa
      excessive 528.72
      minimal 528.71
  personality (pattern) (trait) (see also Disorder, personality) 301.9
    following organic brain damage 310.1
  polyglandular 258.9
  psychomotor 307.9
  pupillary 379.49
  reflex 796.1
  rhythm, heart 427.9
    postoperative (immediate) 997.1
      long-term effect of cardiac surgery 429.4
    psychogenic 306.2
  salivary secretion 527.7
  sensation (cold) (heat) (localization) (tactile discrimination localization) (texture) (vibratory) NEC 782.0
    hysterical 300.11
    skin 782.0
    smell 781.1
    taste 781.1
  sensory (see also Disturbance, sensation) 782.0
    innervation 782.0
  situational (transient) (see also Reaction, adjustment) 309.9
    acute 308.3
  sleep 780.50
    with apnea — see Apnea, sleep
    initiation or maintenance (see also Insomnia) 780.52
      nonorganic origin 307.41
    nonorganic origin 307.40
      specified type NEC 307.49
    specified NEC 780.59
      nonorganic origin 307.49
    wakefulness (see also Hypersomnia) 780.54
      nonorganic origin 307.43
  sociopathic 301.7
  speech NEC 784.5
    developmental 315.39
      associated with hyperkinesis 314.1
    secondary to organic lesion 784.5
  stomach (functional) (see also Disturbance, gastric) 536.9
  sympathetic (nerve) (see also Neuropathy, peripheral, autonomic) 337.9
  temperature sense 782.0
    hysterical 300.11
  tooth
    eruption 520.6
    formation 520.4
    structure, hereditary NEC 520.5
  touch (see also Disturbance, sensation) 782.0
  vascular 459.9
    arteriosclerotic — see Arteriosclerosis
  vasomotor 443.9
  vasospastic 443.9
  vestibular labyrinth 386.9
  vision, visual NEC 368.9
    psychophysical 368.16
    specified NEC 368.8
    subjective 368.10
  voice 784.40
  wakefulness (initiation or maintenance) (see also Hypersomnia) 780.54
    nonorganic origin 307.43
Disulfiduria, beta-mercaptolactate-cysteine 270.0
Disuse atrophy, bone 733.7

Ditthomska syndrome 307.81
Diuresis 788.42
Divers'
  palsy or paralysis 993.3
  squeeze 993.3
Diverticula, diverticulosis, diverticulum (acute) (multiple) (perforated) (ruptured) 562.10
  with diverticulitis 562.11
  aorta (Kommerell's) 747.21
  appendix (noninflammatory) 543.9
  bladder (acquired) (sphincter) 596.3
    congenital 753.8
  broad ligament 620.8
  bronchus (congenital) 748.3
    acquired 494.0
      with acute exacerbation 494.1
  calyx, calyceal (kidney) 593.89
  cardia (stomach) 537.1
  cecum 562.10
    with
      diverticulitis 562.11
        with hemorrhage 562.13
      hemorrhage 562.12
    congenital 751.5
  colon (acquired) 562.10
    with
      diverticulitis 562.11
        with hemorrhage 562.13
      hemorrhage 562.12
    congenital 751.5
  duodenum 562.00
    with
      diverticulitis 562.01
        with hemorrhage 562.03
      hemorrhage 562.02
    congenital 751.5
  epiphrenic (esophagus) 530.6
  esophagus (congenital) 750.4
    acquired 530.6
    epiphrenic 530.6
    pulsion 530.6
    traction 530.6
    Zenker's 530.6
  Eustachian tube 381.89
  fallopian tube 620.8
  gallbladder (congenital) 751.69
  gastric 537.1
  heart (congenital) 746.89
  ileum 562.00
    with
      diverticulitis 562.01
        with hemorrhage 562.03
      hemorrhage 562.02
  intestine (large) 562.10
    with
      diverticulitis 562.11
        with hemorrhage 562.13
      hemorrhage 562.12
    congenital 751.5
    small 562.00
      with
        diverticulitis 562.01
          with hemorrhage 562.03
        hemorrhage 562.02
      congenital 751.5
  jejunum 562.00
    with
      diverticulitis 562.01
        with hemorrhage 562.03
      hemorrhage 562.02
  kidney (calyx) (pelvis) 593.89
    with calculus 592.0
  Kommerell's 747.21
  laryngeal ventricle (congenital) 748.3
  Meckel's (displaced) (hypertrophic) 751.0
  midthoracic 530.6
  organ or site, congenital NEC — see Distortion
  pericardium (congenital) (cyst) 746.89
    acquired (true) 423.8
  pharyngoesophageal (pulsion) 530.6
  pharynx (congenital) 750.27
  pulsion (esophagus) 530.6
  rectosigmoid 562.10

Diverticula, diverticulosis, diverticulum — continued
  rectosigmoid — continued
    with
      diverticulitis 562.11
        with hemorrhage 562.13
      hemorrhage 562.12
    congenital 751.5
  rectum 562.10
    with
      diverticulitis 562.11
        with hemorrhage 562.13
      hemorrhage 562.12
  renal (calyces) (pelvis) 593.89
    with calculus 592.0
  Rokitansky's 530.6
  seminal vesicle 608.0
  sigmoid 562.10
    with
      diverticulitis 562.11
        with hemorrhage 562.13
      hemorrhage 562.12
    congenital 751.5
  small intestine 562.00
    with
      diverticulitis 562.01
        with hemorrhage 562.03
      hemorrhage 562.02
  stomach (cardia) (juxtacardia) (juxtapyloric) (acquired) 537.1
    congenital 750.7
  subdiaphragmatic 530.6
  trachea (congenital) 748.3
    acquired 519.19 ▲
  traction (esophagus) 530.6
  ureter (acquired) 593.89
    congenital 753.4
  ureterovesical orifice 593.89
  urethra (acquired) 599.2
    congenital 753.8
  ventricle, left (congenital) 746.89
  vesical (urinary) 596.3
    congenital 753.8
  Zenker's (esophagus) 530.6
Diverticulitis (acute) — see also Diverticula 562.11
  with hemorrhage 562.13
  bladder (urinary) 596.3
  cecum (perforated) 562.11
    with hemorrhage 562.13
  colon (perforated) 562.11
    with hemorrhage 562.13
  duodenum 562.01
    with hemorrhage 562.03
  esophagus 530.6
  ileum (perforated) 562.01
    with hemorrhage 562.03
  intestine (large) (perforated) 562.11
    with hemorrhage 562.13
    small 562.01
      with hemorrhage 562.03
  jejunum (perforated) 562.01
    with hemorrhage 562.03
  Meckel's (perforated) 751.0
  pharyngoesophageal 530.6
  rectosigmoid (perforated) 562.11
    with hemorrhage 562.13
  rectum 562.11
    with hemorrhage 562.13
  sigmoid (old) (perforated) 562.11
    with hemorrhage 562.13
  small intestine (perforated) 562.01
    with hemorrhage 562.03
  vesical (urinary) 596.3
Diverticulosis — see Diverticula
Division
  cervix uteri 622.8
    external os into two openings by frenum 752.49
  external (cervical) into two openings by frenum 752.49
  glans penis 752.69
  hymen 752.49
  labia minora (congenital) 752.49
  ligament (partial or complete) (current) (see also Sprain, by site)

Division — continued

ligament (see also Sprain, by site) — continued
  with open wound — see Wound, open, by site
muscle (partial or complete) (current) (see also Sprain, by site)
  with open wound — see Wound, open, by site
nerve — see Injury, nerve, by site
penis glans 752.69
spinal cord — see Injury, spinal, by site
vein 459.9
  traumatic — see Injury, vascular, by site
Divorce V61.0
Dix-Hallpike neurolabyrinthitis 386.12
Dizziness 780.4
  hysterical 300.11
  psychogenic 306.9
Doan-Wiseman syndrome (primary splenic neutropenia) 289.53 ▲
Dog bite — see Wound, open, by site
Döhle body-panmyelopathic syndrome 288.2
Döhle-Heller aortitis 093.1
Dolichocephaly, dolichocephalus 754.0
Dolichocolon 751.5
Dolichostenomelia 759.82
Donohue's syndrome (leprechaunism) 259.8
Donor
  blood V59.01
    other blood components V59.09
    stem cells V59.02
    whole blood V59.01
  bone V59.2
    marrow V59.3
  cornea V59.5
  egg (oocyte) (ovum) V59.70
    over age 35 V59.73
      anonymous recipient V59.73
      designated recipient V59.74
    under age 35 V59.71
      anonymous recipient V59.71
      designated recipient V59.72
  heart V59.8
  kidney V59.4
  liver V59.6
  lung V59.8
  lymphocyte V59.8
  organ V59.9
    specified NEC V59.8
  potential, examination of V70.8
  skin V59.1
  specified organ or tissue NEC V59.8
  sperm V59.8
  stem cells V59.02
  tissue V59.9
    specified type NEC V59.8
Donovanosis (granuloma venereum) 099.2
DOPS (diffuse obstructive pulmonary syndrome) 496
Double
  albumin 273.8
  aortic arch 747.21
  auditory canal 744.29
  auricle (heart) 746.82
  bladder 753.8
  external (cervical) os 752.49
  kidney with double pelvis (renal) 753.3
  larynx 748.3
  meatus urinarius 753.8
  organ or site NEC — see Accessory
  orifice
    heart valve NEC 746.89
      pulmonary 746.09
  outlet, right ventricle 745.11
  pelvis (renal) with double ureter 753.4
  penis 752.69
  tongue 750.13
  ureter (one or both sides) 753.4
    with double pelvis (renal) 753.4
  urethra 753.8

Double — continued

urinary meatus 753.8
uterus (any degree) 752.2
  with doubling of cervix and vagina 752.2
  in pregnancy or childbirth 654.0 ☑
    affecting fetus or newborn 763.89
vagina 752.49
  with doubling of cervix and uterus 752.2
vision 368.2
vocal cords 748.3
vulva 752.49
whammy (syndrome) 360.81
Douglas' pouch, cul-de-sac — see condition
Down's disease or syndrome (mongolism) 758.0
Down-growth, epithelial (anterior chamber) 364.61
Dracontiasis 125.7
Dracunculiasis 125.7
Dracunculosis 125.7
Drainage
  abscess (spontaneous) — see Abscess
  anomalous pulmonary veins to hepatic veins or right atrium 747.41
  stump (amputation) (surgical) 997.62
  suprapubic, bladder 596.8
Dream state, hysterical 300.13
Drepanocytic anemia — see also Disease, sickle cell 282.60
Dresbach's syndrome (elliptocytosis) 282.1
Dreschlera (infection) 118
  hawaiiensis 117.8
Dressler's syndrome (postmyocardial infarction) 411.0
Dribbling (post-void) 788.35
Drift, ulnar 736.09
Drinking (alcohol) — see also Alcoholism
  excessive, to excess NEC (see also Abuse, drugs, nondependent) 305.0 ☑
    bouts, periodic 305.0 ☑
    continual 303.9 ☑
    episodic 305.0 ☑
    habitual 303.9 ☑
    periodic 305.0 ☑
Drip, postnasal (chronic) 784.91 ▲
  due to ●
    allergic rhinitis — see Rhinitis, allergic ●
    common cold 460 ●
    gastroesophageal reflux — see Reflux, gastroesophageal ●
    nasopharyngitis — see Nasopharyngitis ●
    other known condition — code to condition ●
    sinusitis — see Sinusitis ●
Drivers' license examination V70.3
Droop
  Cooper's 611.8
  facial 781.94
Drop
  finger 736.29
  foot 736.79
  hematocrit (precipitous) 790.01
  toe 735.8
  wrist 736.05
Dropped
  dead 798.1
  heart beats 426.6
Dropsy, dropsical — see also Edema 782.3
  abdomen 789.5
  amnion (see also Hydramnios) 657.0 ☑
  brain — see Hydrocephalus
  cardiac (see also Failure, heart) 428.0
  cardiorenal (see also Hypertension, cardiorenal) 404.90
  chest 511.9

Dropsy, dropsical — see also Edema — continued

fetus or newborn 778.0
  due to isoimmunization 773.3
gangrenous (see also Gangrene) 785.4
heart (see also Failure, heart) 428.0
hepatic — see Cirrhosis, liver
infantile — see Hydrops, fetalis
kidney (see also Nephrosis) 581.9
liver — see Cirrhosis, liver
lung 514
malarial (see also Malaria) 084.9
neonatorum — see Hydrops, fetalis
nephritic 581.9
newborn — see Hydrops, fetalis
nutritional 269.9
ovary 620.8
pericardium (see also Pericarditis) 423.9
renal (see also Nephrosis) 581.9
uremic — see Uremia
Drowned, drowning 994.1
  lung 518.5
Drowsiness 780.09
Drug — see also condition
  addiction (see also listing under Dependence) 304.9 ☑
  adverse effect NEC, correct substance properly administered 995.20 ▲
  allergy 995.27
  dependence (see also listing under Dependence) 304.9 ☑
  habit (see also listing under Dependence) 304.9 ☑
  hypersensitivity 995.27 ●
  induced
    circadian rhythm sleep disorder 292.85
    hypersomnia 292.85
    insomnia 292.85
    mental disorder 292.9
      anxiety 292.89
      mood 292.84
      sexual 292.89
      sleep 292.85
      specified type 292.89
    parasomnia 292.85
    persisting
      amnestic disorder 292.83
      dementia 292.82
    psychotic disorder
      with
        delusions 292.11
        hallucinations 292.12
    sleep disorder 292.85
  intoxication 292.89
  overdose — see Table of Drugs and Chemicals
  poisoning — see Table of Drugs and Chemicals
  therapy (maintenance) status NEC
    chemotherapy, antineoplastic V58.11
    immunotherapy, antineoplastic V58.12
    long-term (current) use V58.69
      antibiotics V58.62
      anticoagulants V58.61
      anti-inflammatories, non-steroidal (NSAID) V58.64
      antiplatelets V58.63
      antithrombotics V58.63
      aspirin V58.66
      insulin V58.67
      steroids V58.65
  wrong substance given or taken in error — see Table of Drugs and Chemicals
Drunkenness — see also Abuse, drugs, nondependent 305.0 ☑
  acute in alcoholism (see also Alcoholism) 303.0 ☑
  chronic (see also Alcoholism) 303.9 ☑
  pathologic 291.4
  simple (acute) 305.0 ☑

Drunkenness — see also Abuse, drugs, nondependent — continued

simple — continued
  in alcoholism 303.0 ☑
  sleep 307.47
Drusen
  optic disc or papilla 377.21
  retina (colloid) (hyaloid degeneration) 362.57
  hereditary 362.77
Drusenfieber 075
Dry, dryness — see also condition
  eye 375.15
    syndrome 375.15
  larynx 478.79
  mouth 527.7
  nose 478.19
  skin syndrome 701.1
  socket (teeth) 526.5
  throat 478.29
DSAP (disseminated superficial actinic porokeratosis) 692.75
Duane's retraction syndrome 378.71
Duane-Stilling-Türk syndrome (ocular retraction syndrome) 378.71
Dubini's disease (electric chorea) 049.8
Dubin-Johnson disease or syndrome 277.4
Dubois' abscess or disease 090.5
Duchenne's
  disease 094.0
    locomotor ataxia 094.0
    muscular dystrophy 359.1
    pseudohypertrophy, muscles 359.1
  paralysis 335.22
  syndrome 335.22
Duchenne-Aran myelopathic, muscular atrophy (nonprogressive) (progressive) 335.21
Duchenne-Griesinger disease 359.1
Ducrey's
  bacillus 099.0
  chancre 099.0
  disease (chancroid) 099.0
Duct, ductus — see condition
Duengero 061
Duhring's disease (dermatitis herpetiformis) 694.0
Dukes (-Filatov) disease 057.8
Dullness
  cardiac (decreased) (increased) 785.3
Dumb ague — see also Malaria 084.6
Dumbness — see also Aphasia 784.3
Dumdum fever 085.0
Dumping syndrome (postgastrectomy) 564.2
  nonsurgical 536.8
Duodenitis (nonspecific) (peptic) 535.60
  with hemorrhage 535.61
  due to
    Strongyloides stercoralis 127.2
Duodenocholangitis 575.8
Duodenum, duodenal — see condition
Duplay's disease, periarthritis, or syndrome 726.2
Duplex — see also Accessory
  kidney 753.3
  placenta — see Placenta, abnormal
  uterus 752.2
Duplication — see also Accessory
  anus 751.5
  aortic arch 747.21
  appendix 751.5
  biliary duct (any) 751.69
  bladder 753.8
  cecum 751.5
    and appendix 751.5
  clitoris 752.49
  cystic duct 751.69
  digestive organs 751.8
  duodenum 751.5
  esophagus 750.4
  fallopian tube 752.19
  frontonasal process 756.0
  gallbladder 751.69
  ileum 751.5

Index to Diseases

Duplication — see also Accessory — continued
- intestine (large) (small) 751.5
- jejunum 751.5
- kidney 753.3
- liver 751.69
- nose 748.1
- pancreas 751.7
- penis 752.69
- respiratory organs NEC 748.9
- salivary duct 750.22
- spinal cord (incomplete) 742.51
- stomach 750.7
- ureter 753.4
- vagina 752.49
- vas deferens 752.89
- vocal cords 748.3

Dupré's disease or syndrome (meningism) 781.6

Dupuytren's
- contraction 728.6
- disease (muscle contracture) 728.6
- fracture (closed) 824.4
  - ankle (closed) 824.4
    - open 824.5
  - fibula (closed) 824.4
    - open 824.5
  - radius (closed) 813.42
    - open 813.52
- muscle contracture 728.6

Durand-Nicolas-Favre disease (climatic bubo) 099.1

Duroziez's disease (congenital mitral stenosis) 746.5

Dust
- conjunctivitis 372.05
- reticulation (occupational) 504

Dutton's
- disease (trypanosomiasis) 086.9
- relapsing fever (West African) 087.1

Dwarf, dwarfism 259.4
- with infantilism (hypophyseal) 253.3
- achondroplastic 756.4
- Amsterdam 759.89
- bird-headed 759.89
- congenital 259.4
- constitutional 259.4
- hypophyseal 253.3
- infantile 259.4
- Levi type 253.3
- Lorain-Levi (pituitary) 253.3
- Lorain type (pituitary) 253.3
- metatropic 756.4
- nephrotic-glycosuric, with hypophosphatemic rickets 270.0
- nutritional 263.2
- ovarian 758.6
- pancreatic 577.8
- pituitary 253.3
- polydystrophic 277.5
- primordial 253.3
- psychosocial 259.4
- renal 588.0
  - with hypertension — see Hypertension, kidney
- Russell's (uterine dwarfism and craniofacial dysostosis) 759.89

Dyke-Young anemia or syndrome (acquired macrocytic hemolytic anemia) (secondary) (symptomatic) 283.9

Dynia abnormality — see also Defect, coagulation 286.9

Dysacousis 388.40

Dysadrenocortism 255.9
- hyperfunction 255.3
- hypofunction 255.4

Dysarthria 784.5

Dysautonomia — see also Neuropathy, peripheral, autonomic 337.9
- familial 742.8

Dysbarism 993.3

Dysbasia 719.7
- angiosclerotica intermittens 443.9
- due to atherosclerosis 440.21

Dysbasia — continued
- hysterical 300.11
- lordotica (progressiva) 333.6
- nonorganic origin 307.9
- psychogenic 307.9

Dysbetalipoproteinemia (familial) 272.2

Dyscalculia 315.1

Dyschezia — see also Constipation 564.00

Dyschondroplasia (with hemangiomata) 756.4
- Voorhoeve's 756.4

Dyschondrosteosis 756.59

Dyschromia 709.00

Dyscollagenosis 710.9

Dyscoria 743.41

Dyscraniopyophalangy 759.89

Dyscrasia
- blood 289.9
  - with antepartum hemorrhage 641.3 ☑
  - fetus or newborn NEC 776.9
  - hemorrhage, subungual 287.8
  - puerperal, postpartum 666.3 ☑
- ovary 256.8
- plasma cell 273.9
- pluriglandular 258.9
- polyglandular 258.9

Dysdiadochokinesia 781.3

Dysectasia, vesical neck 596.8

Dysendocrinism 259.9

Dysentery, dysenteric (bilious) (catarrhal) (diarrhea) (epidemic) (gangrenous) (hemorrhagic) (infectious) (sporadic) (tropical) (ulcerative) 009.0
- abscess, liver (see also Abscess, amebic) 006.3
- amebic (see also Amebiasis) 006.9
  - with abscess — see Abscess, amebic
  - acute 006.0
  - carrier (suspected) of V02.2
  - chronic 006.1
- arthritis (see also Arthritis, due to, dysentery) 009.0 [711.3] ☑
- bacillary 004.9 [711.3] ☑
- asylum 004.9
- bacillary 004.9
  - arthritis 004.9 [711.3] ☑
  - Boyd 004.2
  - Flexner 004.1
  - Schmitz (-Stutzer) 004.0
  - Shiga 004.0
  - Shigella 004.9
    - group A 004.0
    - group B 004.1
    - group C 004.2
    - group D 004.3
    - specified type NEC 004.8
  - Sonne 004.3
  - specified type NEC 004.8
- bacterium 004.9
- balantidial 007.0
- Balantidium coli 007.0
- Boyd's 004.2
- Chilomastix 007.8
- Chinese 004.9
- choleriform 001.1
- coccidial 007.2
- Dientamoeba fragilis 007.8
- due to specified organism NEC — see Enteritis, due to, by organism
- Embadomonas 007.8
- Endolimax nana — see Dysentery, amebic
- Entamoba, entamebic — see Dysentery, amebic
- Flexner's 004.1
- Flexner-Boyd 004.2
- giardial 007.1
- Giardia lamblia 007.1
- Hiss-Russell 004.1
- lamblia 007.1
- leishmanial 085.0
- malarial (see also Malaria) 084.6

Dysentery, dysenteric — continued
- metazoal 127.9
- Monilia 112.89
- protozoal NEC 007.9
- Russell's 004.8
- salmonella 003.0
- schistosomal 120.1
- Schmitz (-Stutzer) 004.0
- Shiga 004.0
- Shigella NEC (see also Dysentery, bacillary) 004.9
  - boydii 004.2
  - dysenteriae 004.0
    - Schmitz 004.0
    - Shiga 004.0
  - flexneri 004.1
  - group A 004.0
  - group B 004.1
  - group C 004.2
  - group D 004.3
    - Schmitz 004.0
    - Shiga 004.0
  - Sonnei 004.3
- Sonne 004.3
- strongyloidiasis 127.2
- trichomonal 007.3
- tuberculous (see also Tuberculosis) 014.8 ☑
- viral (see also Enteritis, viral) 008.8

Dysequilibrium 780.4

Dysesthesia 782.0
- hysterical 300.11

Dysfibrinogenemia (congenital) — see also Defect, coagulation 286.3

Dysfunction
- adrenal (cortical) 255.9
  - hyperfunction 255.3
  - hypofunction 255.4
- associated with sleep stages or arousal from sleep 780.56
  - nonorganic origin 307.47
- bladder NEC 596.59
- bleeding, uterus 626.8
- brain, minimal (see also Hyperkinesia) 314.9
- cerebral 348.30
- colon 564.9
  - psychogenic 306.4
- colostomy or enterostomy 569.62
- cystic duct 575.8
- diastolic 429.9
  - with heart failure — see Failure, heart
  - due to
    - cardiomyopathy — see Cardiomyopathy
    - hypertension — see Hypertension, heart
- endocrine NEC 259.9
- endometrium 621.8
- enteric stoma 569.62
- enterostomy 569.62
- erectile 607.84
  - nonorganic origin 302.72
- esophagostomy 530.87
- Eustachian tube 381.81
- gallbladder 575.8
- gastrointestinal 536.9
- gland, glandular NEC 259.9
- heart 427.9
  - postoperative (immediate) 997.1
  - long-term effect of cardiac surgery 429.4
- hemoglobin 289.89 ▲
- hepatic 573.9
- hepatocellular NEC 573.9
- hypophysis 253.9
  - hyperfunction 253.1
  - hypofunction 253.2
  - posterior lobe 253.6
    - hypofunction 253.5
- kidney (see also Disease, renal) 593.9
- labyrinthine 386.50
  - specified NEC 386.58
- liver 573.9
  - constitutional 277.4

Dysfunction — continued
- minimal brain (child) (see also Hyperkinesia) 314.9
- ovary, ovarian 256.9
  - hyperfunction 256.1
    - estrogen 256.0
  - hypofunction 256.39
    - postablative 256.2
  - postablative 256.2
  - specified NEC 256.8
- papillary muscle 429.81
  - with myocardial infarction 410.8 ☑
- parathyroid 252.8
  - hyperfunction 252.00
  - hypofunction 252.1
- pineal gland 259.8
- pituitary (gland) 253.9
  - hyperfunction 253.1
  - hypofunction 253.2
  - posterior 253.6
    - hypofunction 253.5
- placental — see Placenta, insufficiency
- platelets (blood) 287.1
- polyglandular 258.9
  - specified NEC 258.8
- psychosexual 302.70
  - with
    - dyspareunia (functional) (psychogenic) 302.76
    - frigidity 302.72
    - impotence 302.72
    - inhibition
      - orgasm
        - female 302.73
        - male 302.74
      - sexual
        - desire 302.71
        - excitement 302.72
    - premature ejaculation 302.75
    - sexual aversion 302.79
    - specified disorder NEC 302.79
    - vaginismus 306.51
- pylorus 537.9
- rectum 564.9
  - psychogenic 306.4
- segmental (see also Dysfunction, somatic) 739.9
- senile 797
- sexual 302.70
- sinoatrial node 427.81
- somatic 739.9
  - abdomen 739.9
  - acromioclavicular 739.7
  - cervical 739.1
  - cervicothoracic 739.1
  - costochondral 739.8
  - costovertebral 739.8
  - extremities
    - lower 739.6
    - upper 739.7
  - head 739.0
  - hip 739.5
  - lumbar, lumbosacral 739.3
  - occipitocervical 739.0
  - pelvic 739.5
  - pubic 739.5
  - rib cage 739.8
  - sacral 739.4
  - sacrococcygeal 739.4
  - sacroiliac 739.4
  - specified site NEC 739.9
  - sternochondral 739.8
  - sternoclavicular 739.7
  - temporomandibular 739.0
  - thoracic, thoracolumbar 739.2
- stomach 536.9
  - psychogenic 306.4
- suprarenal 255.9
  - hyperfunction 255.3
  - hypofunction 255.4
- symbolic NEC 784.60
  - specified type NEC 784.69
- systolic 429.9
  - with heart failure — see Failure, heart

Dysfunction

Dysfunction — *continued*
 temporomandibular (joint) (joint-pain-syndrome) NEC 524.60
  sounds on opening or closing 524.64
  specified NEC 524.69
 testicular 257.9
  hyperfunction 257.0
  hypofunction 257.2
  specified type NEC 257.8
 thymus 254.9
 thyroid 246.9
  complicating pregnancy, childbirth, or puerperium 648.1 ☑
  hyperfunction — *see* Hyperthyroidism
  hypofunction — *see* Hypothyroidism
 uterus, complicating delivery 661.9 ☑
  affecting fetus or newborn 763.7
  hypertonic 661.4 ☑
  hypotonic 661.2 ☑
   primary 661.0 ☑
   secondary 661.1 ☑
 velopharyngeal (acquired) 528.9
  congenital 750.29
 ventricular 429.9
  with congestive heart failure (*see also* Failure, heart) 428.0
  due to
   cardiomyopathy — *see* Cardiomyopathy
   hypertension — *see* Hypertension, heart
  left, reversible following sudden emotional stress 429.83 ●
 vesicourethral NEC 596.59
 vestibular 386.50
  specified type NEC 386.58
Dysgammaglobulinemia 279.06
Dysgenesis
 gonadal (due to chromosomal anomaly) 758.6
  pure 752.7
 kidney(s) 753.0
 ovarian 758.6
 renal 753.0
 reticular 279.2
 seminiferous tubules 758.6
 tidal platelet 287.31
Dysgerminoma (M9060/3)
 specified site — *see* Neoplasm, by site, malignant
 unspecified site
  female 183.0
  male 186.9
Dysgeusia 781.1
Dysgraphia 781.3
Dyshidrosis 705.81
Dysidrosis 705.81
Dysinsulinism 251.8
Dyskaryotic cervical smear 795.09
Dyskeratosis — *see also* Keratosis 701.1
 bullosa hereditaria 757.39
 cervix 622.10
 congenital 757.39
 follicularis 757.39
  vitamin A deficiency 264.8
 gingiva 523.8
 oral soft tissue NEC 528.79
 tongue 528.79
 uterus NEC 621.8
Dyskinesia 781.3
 biliary 575.8
 esophagus 530.5
 hysterical 300.11
 intestinal 564.89
 neuroleptic-induced tardive 333.85 ▲
 nonorganic origin 307.9
 orofacial 333.82
  due to drugs 333.85 ●
 psychogenic 307.9
 subacute, due to drugs 333.85 ●
 tardive (oral) 333.85 ▲
Dyslalia 784.5

Dyslalia — *continued*
 developmental 315.39
Dyslexia 784.61
 developmental 315.02
 secondary to organic lesion 784.61
Dyslipidemia 272.4
Dysmaturity — *see also* Immaturity 765.1 ☑
 lung 770.4
 pulmonary 770.4
Dysmenorrhea (essential) (exfoliative) (functional) (intrinsic) (membranous) (primary) (secondary) 625.3
 psychogenic 306.52
Dysmetabolic syndrome X 277.7
Dysmetria 781.3
Dysmorodystrophia mesodermalis congenita 759.82
Dysnomia 784.3
Dysorexia 783.0
 hysterical 300.11
Dysostosis
 cleidocranial, cleidocranialis 755.59
 craniofacial 756.0
 Fairbank's (idiopathic familial generalized osteophytosis) 756.50
 mandibularis 756.0
 mandibulofacial, incomplete 756.0
 multiplex 277.5
 orodigitofacial 759.89
Dyspareunia (female) 625.0
 male 608.89
 psychogenic 302.76
Dyspepsia (allergic) (congenital) (fermentative) (flatulent) (functional) (gastric) (gastrointestinal) (neurogenic) (occupational) (reflex) 536.8
 acid 536.8
 atonic 536.3
  psychogenic 306.4
 diarrhea 787.91
  psychogenic 306.4
 intestinal 564.89
  psychogenic 306.4
 nervous 306.4
 neurotic 306.4
 psychogenic 306.4
Dysphagia 787.2
 functional 300.11
 hysterical 300.11
 nervous 300.11
 psychogenic 306.4
 sideropenic 280.8
 spastica 530.5
Dysphagocytosis, congenital 288.1
Dysphasia 784.5
Dysphonia 784.49
 clericorum 784.49
 functional 300.11
 hysterical 300.11
 psychogenic 306.1
 spastica 478.79
Dyspigmentation — *see also* Pigmentation
 eyelid (acquired) 374.52
Dyspituitarism 253.9
 hyperfunction 253.1
 hypofunction 253.2
 posterior lobe 253.6
Dysplasia — *see also* Anomaly
 artery
  fibromuscular NEC 447.8
   carotid 447.8
   renal 447.3
 bladder 596.8
 bone (fibrous) NEC 733.29
  diaphyseal, progressive 756.59
  jaw 526.89
  monostotic 733.29
  polyostotic 756.54
  solitary 733.29
 brain 742.9
 bronchopulmonary, fetus or newborn 770.7
 cervix (uteri) 622.10

Dysplasia — *see also* Anomaly — *continued*
 cervix — *continued*
  cervical intraepithelial neoplasia I [CIN I] 622.11
  cervical intraepithelial neoplasia II [CIN II] 622.12
  cervical intraepithelial neoplasia III [CIN III] 233.1
  CIN I 622.11
  CIN II 622.12
  CIN III 233.1
  mild 622.11
  moderate 622.12
  severe 233.1
 chondroectodermal 756.55
 chondromatose 756.4
 colon 211.3
 craniocarpotarsal 759.89
 craniometaphyseal 756.89
 dentinal 520.5
 diaphyseal, progressive 756.59
 ectodermal (anhidrotic) (Bason) (Clouston's) (congenital) (Feinmesser) (hereditary) (hidrotic) (Marshall) (Robinson's) 757.31
 epiphysealis 756.9
  multiplex 756.56
  punctata 756.59
 epiphysis 756.9
  multiple 756.56
 epithelial
  epiglottis 478.79
  uterine cervix 622.10
 erythroid NEC 289.89
 eye (*see also* Microphthalmos) 743.10
 familial metaphyseal 756.89
 fibromuscular, artery NEC 447.8
  carotid 447.8
  renal 447.3
 fibrous
  bone NEC 733.29
  diaphyseal, progressive 756.59
  jaw 526.89
  monostotic 733.29
  polyostotic 756.54
  solitary 733.29
 high-grade, focal — *see* Neoplasm, by site, benign
 hip (congenital) 755.63
  with dislocation (*see also* Dislocation, hip, congenital) 754.30
 hypohidrotic ectodermal 757.31
 joint 755.8
 kidney 753.15
 leg 755.69
 linguofacialis 759.89
 lung 748.5
 macular 743.55
 mammary (benign) (gland) 610.9
  cystic 610.1
  specified type NEC 610.8
 metaphyseal 756.9
  familial 756.89
 monostotic fibrous 733.29
 muscle 756.89
 myeloid NEC 289.89
 nervous system (general) 742.9
 neuroectodermal 759.6
 oculoauriculovertebral 756.0
 oculodentodigital 759.89
 olfactogenital 253.4
 osteo-onycho-arthro (hereditary) 756.89
 periosteum 733.99
 polyostotic fibrous 756.54
 progressive diaphyseal 756.59
 prostate 602.3
  intraepithelial neoplasia I [PIN I] 602.3
  intraepithelial neoplasia II [PIN II] 602.3
  intraepithelial neoplasia III [PIN III] 233.4
 renal 753.15
 renofacialis 753.0

Dysplasia — *see also* Anomaly — *continued*
 retinal NEC 743.56
 retrolental 362.21
 spinal cord 742.9
 thymic, with immunodeficiency 279.2
 vagina 623.0
 vocal cord 478.5
 vulva 624.8
  intraepithelial neoplasia I [VIN I] 624.0 ▲
  intraepithelial neoplasia II [VIN II] 624.0 ▲
  intraepithelial neoplasia III [VIN III] 233.3
  VIN I 624.0 ▲
  VIN II 624.0 ▲
  VIN III 233.3
Dyspnea (nocturnal) (paroxysmal) 786.09
 asthmatic (bronchial) (*see also* Asthma) 493.9 ☑
  with bronchitis (*see also* Asthma) 493.9 ☑
  chronic 493.2 ☑
 cardiac (*see also* Failure, ventricular, left) 428.1
 cardiac (*see also* Failure, ventricular, left) 428.1
 functional 300.11
 hyperventilation 786.01
 hysterical 300.11
 Monday morning 504
 newborn 770.89
 psychogenic 306.1
 uremic — *see* Uremia
Dyspraxia 781.3
 syndrome 315.4
Dysproteinemia 273.8
 transient with copper deficiency 281.4
Dysprothrombinemia (constitutional) — *see also* Defect, coagulation 286.3
Dysreflexia, autonomic 337.3
Dysrhythmia
 cardiac 427.9
  postoperative (immediate) 997.1
   long-term effect of cardiac surgery 429.4
  specified type NEC 427.89
 cerebral or cortical 348.30
Dyssecretosis, mucoserous 710.2
Dyssocial reaction, without manifest psychiatric disorder
 adolescent V71.02
 adult V71.01
 child V71.02
Dyssomnia NEC 780.56
 nonorganic origin 307.47
Dyssplenism 289.4
Dyssynergia
 biliary (*see also* Disease, biliary) 576.8
 cerebellaris myoclonica 334.2
 detrusor sphincter (bladder) 596.55
 ventricular 429.89
Dystasia, hereditary areflexic 334.3
Dysthymia 300.4
Dysthymic disorder 300.4
Dysthyroidism 246.9
Dystocia 660.9 ☑
 affecting fetus or newborn 763.1
 cervical 661.0 ☑
  affecting fetus or newborn 763.7
 contraction ring 661.4 ☑
  affecting fetus or newborn 763.7
 fetal 660.9 ☑
  abnormal size 653.5 ☑
   affecting fetus or newborn 763.1
  deformity 653.7 ☑
 maternal 660.9 ☑
  affecting fetus or newborn 763.1
 positional 660.0 ☑
  affecting fetus or newborn 763.1
 shoulder (girdle) 660.4 ☑
  affecting fetus or newborn 763.1
 uterine NEC 661.4 ☑
  affecting fetus or newborn 763.7

Index to Diseases

Dystonia
  acute
    due to drugs 333.72
    neuroleptic-induced acute 333.72
  deformans progressiva 333.6
  lenticularis 333.6
  musculorum deformans 333.6
  torsion (idiopathic) 333.6
    acquired 333.79
    fragments (of) 333.89
    genetic 333.6
    symptomatic 333.79
Dystonic
  movements 781.0
Dystopia kidney 753.3
Dystrophia myotonica 359.2
Dystrophy, dystrophia 783.9
  adiposogenital 253.8
  asphyxiating thoracic 756.4
  Becker's type 359.1
  brevicollis 756.16
  Bruch's membrane 362.77
  cervical (sympathetic) NEC 337.0
  chondro-osseus with punctate epiphyseal dysplasia 756.59
  choroid (hereditary) 363.50
    central (areolar) (partial) 363.53
      total (gyrate) 363.54
    circinate 363.53
    circumpapillary (partial) 363.51
      total 363.52
    diffuse
      partial 363.56
      total 363.57
    generalized
      partial 363.56
      total 363.57
    gyrate
      central 363.54
      generalized 363.57
    helicoid 363.52
    peripapillary — see Dystrophy, choroid, circumpapillary
    serpiginous 363.54
  cornea (hereditary) 371.50
    anterior NEC 371.52
    Cogan's 371.52
    combined 371.57
    crystalline 371.56
    endothelial (Fuchs') 371.57
    epithelial 371.50
      juvenile 371.51
      microscopic cystic 371.52
    granular 371.53
    lattice 371.54
    macular 371.55
    marginal (Terrien's) 371.48
    Meesman's 371.51
    microscopic cystic (epithelial) 371.52
    nodular, Salzmann's 371.46
    polymorphous 371.58
    posterior NEC 371.58
    ring-like 371.52
    Salzmann's nodular 371.46
    stromal NEC 371.56
  dermatochondrocorneal 371.50
  Duchenne's 359.1
  due to malnutrition 263.9
  Erb's 359.1
  familial
    hyperplastic periosteal 756.59
    osseous 277.5
  foveal 362.77
  Fuchs', cornea 371.57
  Gowers' muscular 359.1
  hair 704.2
  hereditary, progressive muscular 359.1
  hypogenital, with diabetic tendency 759.81
  Landouzy-Déjérine 359.1
  Leyden-Möbius 359.1
  mesodermalis congenita 759.82
  muscular 359.1
    congenital (hereditary) 359.0

Dystrophy, dystrophia — continued
  muscular — continued
    congenital — continued
      myotonic 359.2
    distal 359.1
    Duchenne's 359.1
    Erb's 359.1
    fascioscapulohumeral 359.1
    Gowers' 359.1
    hereditary (progressive) 359.1
    Landouzy-Déjérine 359.1
    limb-girdle 359.1
    myotonic 359.2
    progressive (hereditary) 359.1
      Charcôt-Marie-Tooth 356.1
    pseudohypertrophic (infantile) 359.1
  myocardium, myocardial (see also Degeneration, myocardial) 429.1
  myotonic 359.2
  myotonica 359.2
  nail 703.8
    congenital 757.5
  neurovascular (traumatic) (see also Neuropathy, peripheral, autonomic) 337.9
  nutritional 263.9
  ocular 359.1
  oculocerebrorenal 270.8
  oculopharyngeal 359.1
  ovarian 620.8
  papillary (and pigmentary) 701.1
  pelvicrural atrophic 359.1
  pigmentary (see also Acanthosis) 701.2
  pituitary (gland) 253.8
  polyglandular 258.8
  posttraumatic sympathetic — see Dystrophy, sympathetic
  progressive ophthalmoplegic 359.1
  retina, retinal (hereditary) 362.70
    albipunctate 362.74
    Bruch's membrane 362.77
    cone, progressive 362.75
    hyaline 362.77
    in
      Bassen-Kornzweig syndrome 272.5 [362.72]
      cerebroretinal lipidosis 330.1 [362.71]
        Refsum's disease 356.3 [362.72]
        systemic lipidosis 272.7 [362.71]
    juvenile (Stargardt's) 362.75
    pigmentary 362.74
    pigment epithelium 362.76
    progressive cone (-rod) 362.75
    pseudoinflammatory foveal 362.77
    rod, progressive 362.75
    sensory 362.75
    vitelliform 362.76
  Salzmann's nodular 371.46
  scapuloperoneal 359.1
  skin NEC 709.9
  sympathetic (posttraumatic) (reflex) 337.20
    lower limb 337.22
    specified site NEC 337.29
    upper limb 337.21
  tapetoretinal NEC 362.74
  thoracic asphyxiating 756.4
  unguium 703.8
    congenital 757.5
  vitreoretinal (primary) 362.73
    secondary 362.66
  vulva 624.0
Dysuria 788.1
  psychogenic 306.53

E

Eagle-Barrett syndrome 756.71
Eales' disease (syndrome) 362.18
Ear — see also condition
  ache 388.70
    otogenic 388.71
    referred 388.72
  lop 744.29

Ear — see also condition — continued
  piercing V50.3
  swimmers' acute 380.12
  tank 380.12
  tropical 111.8 [380.15]
  wax 380.4
Earache 388.70
  otogenic 388.71
  referred 388.72
Early satiety 780.94
Eaton-Lambert syndrome — see also Neoplasm, by site, malignant 199.1 [358.1]
Eberth's disease (typhoid fever) 002.0
Ebstein's
  anomaly or syndrome (downward displacement, tricuspid valve into right ventricle) 746.2
  disease (diabetes) 250.4 [581.81]
Eccentro-osteochondrodysplasia 277.5
Ecchondroma (M9210/0) — see Neoplasm, bone, benign
Ecchondrosis (M9210/1) 238.0
Ecchordosis physaliphora 756.0
Ecchymosis (multiple) 459.89
  conjunctiva 372.72
  eye (traumatic) 921.0
  eyelids (traumatic) 921.1
  newborn 772.6
  spontaneous 782.7
  traumatic — see Contusion
Echinococciasis — see Echinococcus
Echinococcosis — see Echinococcus
Echinococcus (infection) 122.9
  granulosus 122.4
    liver 122.0
    lung 122.1
    orbit 122.3 [376.13]
    specified site NEC 122.3
    thyroid 122.2
  liver NEC 122.8
    granulosus 122.0
    multilocularis 122.5
  lung NEC 122.9
    granulosus 122.1
    multilocularis 122.6
  multilocularis 122.7
    liver 122.5
    specified site NEC 122.6
  orbit 122.9 [376.13]
    granulosus 122.3 [376.13]
    multilocularis 122.6 [376.13]
  specified site NEC 122.9
    granulosus 122.3
    multilocularis 122.6 [376.13]
  thyroid NEC 122.9
    granulosus 122.2
    multilocularis 122.6
Echinorhynchiasis 127.7
Echinostomiasis 121.8
Echolalia 784.69
ECHO virus infection NEC 079.1
Eclampsia, eclamptic (coma) (convulsions) (delirium) 780.39
  female, child-bearing age NEC — see Eclampsia, pregnancy
  gravidarum — see Eclampsia, pregnancy
  male 780.39
  not associated with pregnancy or childbirth 780.39
  pregnancy, childbirth, or puerperium 642.6
    with pre-existing hypertension 642.7
  affecting fetus or newborn 760.0
  uremic 586
Eclipse blindness (total) 363.31
Economic circumstance affecting care V60.9
  specified type NEC V60.8
Economo's disease (encephalitis lethargica) 049.8
Ectasia, ectasis
  aorta (see also Aneurysm, aorta) 441.9
    ruptured 441.5

Ectasia, ectasis — continued
  breast 610.4
  capillary 448.9
  cornea (marginal) (postinfectional) 371.71
  duct (mammary) 610.4
  kidney 593.89
  mammary duct (gland) 610.4
  papillary 448.9
  renal 593.89
  salivary gland (duct) 527.8
  scar, cornea 371.71
  sclera 379.11
Ecthyma 686.8
  contagiosum 051.2
  gangrenosum 686.09
  infectiosum 051.2
Ectocardia 746.87
Ectodermal dysplasia, congenital 757.31
Ectodermosis erosiva pluriorificialis 695.1
Ectopic, ectopia (congenital) 759.89
  abdominal viscera 751.8
    due to defect in anterior abdominal wall 756.79
  ACTH syndrome 255.0
  adrenal gland 759.1
  anus 751.5
  auricular beats 427.61
  beats 427.60
  bladder 753.5
  bone and cartilage in lung 748.69
  brain 742.4
  breast tissue 757.6
  cardiac 746.87
  cerebral 742.4
  cordis 746.87
  endometrium 617.9
  gallbladder 751.69
  gastric mucosa 750.7
  gestation — see Pregnancy, ectopic
  heart 746.87
  hormone secretion NEC 259.3
  hyperparathyroidism 259.3
  kidney (crossed) (intrathoracic) (pelvis) 753.3
    in pregnancy or childbirth 654.4
      causing obstructed labor 660.2
  lens 743.37
  lentis 743.37
  mole — see Pregnancy, ectopic
  organ or site NEC — see Malposition, congenital
  ovary 752.0
  pancreas, pancreatic tissue 751.7
  pregnancy — see Pregnancy, ectopic
  pupil 364.75
  renal 753.3
  sebaceous glands of mouth 750.26
  secretion
    ACTH 255.0
    adrenal hormone 259.3
    adrenalin 259.3
    adrenocorticotropin 255.0
    antidiuretic hormone (ADH) 259.3
    epinephrine 259.3
    hormone NEC 259.3
    norepinephrine 259.3
    pituitary (posterior) 259.3
  spleen 759.0
  testis 752.51
  thyroid 759.2
  ureter 753.4
  ventricular beats 427.69
  vesicae 753.5
Ectrodactyly 755.4
  finger (see also Absence, finger, congenital) 755.29
  toe (see also Absence, toe, congenital) 755.39
Ectromelia 755.4
  lower limb 755.30
  upper limb 755.20
Ectropion 374.10

Ectropion

Ectropion — *continued*
- anus 569.49
- cervix 622.0
  - with mention of cervicitis 616.0
- cicatricial 374.14
- congenital 743.62
- eyelid 374.10
  - cicatricial 374.14
  - congenital 743.62
  - mechanical 374.12
  - paralytic 374.12
  - senile 374.11
  - spastic 374.13
- iris (pigment epithelium) 364.54
- lip (congenital) 750.26
  - acquired 528.5
- mechanical 374.12
- paralytic 374.12
- rectum 569.49
- senile 374.11
- spastic 374.13
- urethra 599.84
- uvea 364.54

Eczema (acute) (allergic) (chronic) (erythematous) (fissum) (occupational) (rubrum) (squamous) 692.9
- asteatotic 706.8
- atopic 691.8
- contact NEC 692.9
- dermatitis NEC 692.9
- due to specified cause — *see* Dermatitis, due to
- dyshidrotic 705.81
- external ear 380.22
- flexural 691.8
- gouty 274.89
- herpeticum 054.0
- hypertrophicum 701.8
- hypostatic — *see* Varicose, vein
- impetiginous 684
- infantile (acute) (chronic) (due to any substance) (intertriginous) (seborrheic) 690.12
- intertriginous NEC 692.9
  - infantile 690.12
- intrinsic 691.8
- lichenified NEC 692.9
- marginatum 110.3
- nummular 692.9
- pustular 686.8
- seborrheic 690.18
  - infantile 690.12
- solare 692.72
- stasis (lower extremity) 454.1
  - ulcerated 454.2
- vaccination, vaccinatum 999.0
- varicose (lower extremity) — *see* Varicose, vein
- verrucosum callosum 698.3

Eczematoid, exudative 691.8

Eddowes' syndrome (brittle bones and blue sclera) 756.51

Edema, edematous 782.3
- with nephritis (*see also* Nephrosis) 581.9
- allergic 995.1
- angioneurotic (allergic) (any site) (with urticaria) 995.1
  - hereditary 277.6
- angiospastic 443.9
- Berlin's (traumatic) 921.3
- brain 348.5
  - due to birth injury 767.8
  - fetus or newborn 767.8
- cardiac (*see also* Failure, heart) 428.0
- cardiovascular (*see also* Failure, heart) 428.0
- cerebral — *see* Edema, brain
- cerebrospinal vessel — *see* Edema, brain
- cervix (acute) (uteri) 622.8
  - puerperal, postpartum 674.8 ☑
- chronic hereditary 757.0
- circumscribed, acute 995.1
  - hereditary 277.6

Edema, edematous — *continued*
- complicating pregnancy (gestational) 646.1 ☑
  - with hypertension — *see* Toxemia, of pregnancy
- conjunctiva 372.73
- connective tissue 782.3
- cornea 371.20
  - due to contact lenses 371.24
  - idiopathic 371.21
  - secondary 371.22
- cystoid macular 362.53
- due to
  - lymphatic obstruction — *see* Edema, lymphatic
  - salt retention 276.0
- epiglottis — *see* Edema, glottis
- essential, acute 995.1
  - hereditary 277.6
- extremities, lower — *see* Edema, legs
- eyelid NEC 374.82
- familial, hereditary (legs) 757.0
- famine 262
- fetus or newborn 778.5
- genital organs
  - female 629.89
  - male 608.86
- gestational 646.1 ☑
  - with hypertension — *see* Toxemia, of pregnancy
- glottis, glottic, glottides (obstructive) (passive) 478.6
  - allergic 995.1
  - hereditary 277.6
  - due to external agent — *see* Condition, respiratory, acute, due to specified agent
- heart (*see also* Failure, heart) 428.0
  - newborn 779.89
- heat 992.7
- hereditary (legs) 757.0
- inanition 262
- infectious 782.3
- intracranial 348.5
  - due to injury at birth 767.8
- iris 364.8
- joint (*see also* Effusion, joint) 719.0 ☑
- larynx (*see also* Edema, glottis) 478.6
- legs 782.3
  - due to venous obstruction 459.2
  - hereditary 757.0
- localized 782.3
  - due to venous obstruction 459.2
  - lower extremity 459.2
- lower extremities — *see* Edema, legs
- lung 514
  - acute 518.4
    - with heart disease or failure (*see also* Failure, ventricular, left) 428.1
    - congestive 428.0
  - chemical (due to fumes or vapors) 506.1
  - due to
    - external agent(s) NEC 508.9
      - specified NEC 508.8
    - fumes and vapors (chemical) (inhalation) 506.1
    - radiation 508.0
  - chemical (acute) 506.1
    - chronic 506.4
  - chronic 514
    - chemical (due to fumes or vapors) 506.4
    - due to
      - external agent(s) NEC 508.9
        - specified NEC 508.8
      - fumes or vapors (chemical) (inhalation) 506.4
      - radiation 508.1
  - due to
    - external agent 508.9
      - specified NEC 508.8
    - high altitude 993.2
    - near drowning 994.1
  - postoperative 518.4

Edema, edematous — *continued*
- lung — *continued*
  - terminal 514
- lymphatic 457.1
  - due to mastectomy operation 457.0
- macula 362.83
  - cystoid 362.53
  - diabetic 250.5 ☑ [362.07]
- malignant (*see also* Gangrene, gas) 040.0
- Milroy's 757.0
- nasopharynx 478.25
- neonatorum 778.5
- nutritional (newborn) 262
  - with dyspigmentation, skin and hair 260
- optic disc or nerve — *see* Papilledema
- orbit 376.33
  - circulatory 459.89
- palate (soft) (hard) 528.9
- pancreas 577.8
- penis 607.83
- periodic 995.1
  - hereditary 277.6
- pharynx 478.25
- pitting 782.3
- pulmonary — *see* Edema, lung
- Quincke's 995.1
  - hereditary 277.6
- renal (*see also* Nephrosis) 581.9
- retina (localized) (macular) (peripheral) 362.83
  - cystoid 362.53
  - diabetic 250.5 ☑ [362.07]
- salt 276.0
- scrotum 608.86
- seminal vesicle 608.86
- spermatic cord 608.86
- spinal cord 336.1
- starvation 262
- stasis (*see also* Hypertension, venous) 459.30
- subconjunctival 372.73
- subglottic (*see also* Edema, glottis) 478.6
- supraglottic (*see also* Edema, glottis) 478.6
- testis 608.86
- toxic NEC 782.3
- traumatic NEC 782.3
- tunica vaginalis 608.86
- vas deferens 608.86
- vocal cord — *see* Edema, glottis
- vulva (acute) 624.8

Edentia (complete) (partial) — *see also* Absence, tooth 520.0
- acquired (*see also* Edentulism) 525.40
- due to
  - caries 525.13
  - extraction 525.10
  - periodontal disease 525.12
  - specified NEC 525.19
  - trauma 525.11
- causing malocclusion 524.30
- congenital (deficiency of tooth buds) 520.0

Edentulism 525.40
- complete 525.40
  - class I 525.41
  - class II 525.42
  - class III 525.43
  - class IV 525.44
- partial 525.50
  - class I 525.51
  - class II 525.52
  - class III 525.53
  - class IV 525.54

Edsall's disease 992.2

Educational handicap V62.3

Edwards' syndrome 758.2

Effect, adverse NEC
- abnormal gravitational (G) forces or states 994.9
- air pressure — *see* Effect, adverse, atmospheric pressure

Effect, adverse — *continued*
- altitude (high) — *see* Effect, adverse, high altitude
- anesthetic
  - in labor and delivery NEC 668.9 ☑
  - affecting fetus or newborn 763.5
- antitoxin — *see* Complications, vaccination
- atmospheric pressure 993.9
  - due to explosion 993.4
  - high 993.3
  - low — *see* Effect, adverse, high altitude
  - specified effect NEC 993.8
- biological, correct substance properly administered (*see also* Effect, adverse, drug) 995.20 ▲
- blood (derivatives) (serum) (transfusion) — *see* Complications, transfusion
- chemical substance NEC 989.9
  - specified — *see* Table of Drugs and Chemicals
- cobalt, radioactive (*see also* Effect, adverse, radioactive substance) 990
- cold (temperature) (weather) 991.9
  - chilblains 991.5
  - frostbite — *see* Frostbite
  - specified effect NEC 991.8
- drugs and medicinals 995.20 ▲
  - correct substance properly administered 995.20 ▲
  - overdose or wrong substance given or taken 977.9
  - specified drug — *see* Table of Drugs and Chemicals
- electric current (shock) 994.8
  - burn — *see* Burn, by site
- electricity (electrocution) (shock) 994.8
  - burn — *see* Burn, by site
- exertion (excessive) 994.5
- exposure 994.9
  - exhaustion 994.4
- external cause NEC 994.9
- fallout (radioactive) NEC 990
- fluoroscopy NEC 990
- foodstuffs
  - allergic reaction (*see also* Allergy, food) 693.1
    - anaphylactic shock due to food NEC 995.60
  - noxious 988.9
    - specified type NEC (*see also* Poisoning, by name of noxious foodstuff) 988.8
- gases, fumes, or vapors — *see* Table of Drugs and Chemicals
- glue (airplane) sniffing 304.6 ☑
- heat — *see* Heat
- high altitude NEC 993.2
  - anoxia 993.2
  - on
    - ears 993.0
    - sinuses 993.1
  - polycythemia 289.0
- hot weather — *see* Heat
- hunger 994.2
- immersion, foot 991.4
- immunization — *see* Complications, vaccination
- immunological agents — *see* Complications, vaccination
- implantation (removable) of isotope or radium NEC 990
- infrared (radiation) (rays) NEC 990
  - burn — *see* Burn, by site
  - dermatitis or eczema 692.82
- infusion — *see* Complications, infusion
- ingestion or injection of isotope (therapeutic) NEC 990
- irradiation NEC (*see also* Effect, adverse, radiation) 990
- isotope (radioactive) NEC 990

Index to Diseases

Effect, adverse — *continued*
  lack of care (child) (infant) (newborn) 995.52
    adult 995.84
  lightning 994.0
    burn — *see* Burn, by site
  Lirugin — *see* Complications, vaccination
  medicinal substance, correct, properly administered (*see also* Effect, adverse, drugs) 995.20
  mesothorium NEC 990
  motion 994.6
  noise, inner ear 388.10
  other drug, medicinal and biological substance 995.29
  overheated places — *see* Heat
  polonium NEC 990
  psychosocial, of work environment V62.1
  radiation (diagnostic) (fallout) (infrared) (natural source) (therapeutic) (tracer) (ultraviolet) (x-ray) NEC 990
    with pulmonary manifestations
      acute 508.0
      chronic 508.1
    dermatitis or eczema 692.82
      due to sun NEC (*see also* Dermatitis, due to, sun) 692.70
    fibrosis of lungs 508.1
    maternal with suspected damage to fetus affecting management of pregnancy 655.6
    pneumonitis 508.0
  radioactive substance NEC 990
    dermatitis or eczema 692.82
  radioactivity NEC 990
  radiotherapy NEC 990
    dermatitis or eczema 692.82
  radium NEC 990
  reduced temperature 991.9
    frostbite — *see* Frostbite
    immersion, foot (hand) 991.4
    specified effect NEC 991.8
  roentgenography NEC 990
  roentgenoscopy NEC 990
  roentgen rays NEC 990
  serum (prophylactic) (therapeutic) NEC 999.5
  specified NEC 995.89
    external cause NEC 994.9
  strangulation 994.7
  submersion 994.1
  teletherapy NEC 990
  thirst 994.3
  transfusion — *see* Complications, transfusion
  ultraviolet (radiation) (rays) NEC 990
    burn (*see also* Burn, by site)
      from sun (*see also* Sunburn) 692.71
    dermatitis or eczema 692.82
      due to sun NEC (*see also* Dermatitis, due to, sun) 692.70
  uranium NEC 990
  vaccine (any) — *see* Complications, vaccination
  weightlessness 994.9
  whole blood (*see also* Complications, transfusion)
    overdose or wrong substance given (*see also* Table of Drugs and Chemicals) 964.7
  working environment V62.1
  x-rays NEC 990
    dermatitis or eczema 692.82
Effect, remote
  of cancer — *see* condition
Effects, late — *see* Late, effect (of)
Effluvium, telogen 704.02
Effort
  intolerance 306.2

Effort — *continued*
  syndrome (aviators) (psychogenic) 306.2
Effusion
  amniotic fluid (*see also* Rupture, membranes, premature) 658.1
  brain (serous) 348.5
  bronchial (*see also* Bronchitis) 490
  cerebral 348.5
  cerebrospinal (*see also* Meningitis) 322.9
    vessel 348.5
  chest — *see* Effusion, pleura
  intracranial 348.5
  joint 719.00
    ankle 719.07
    elbow 719.02
    foot 719.07
    hand 719.04
    hip 719.05
    knee 719.06
    multiple sites 719.09
    pelvic region 719.05
    shoulder (region) 719.01
    specified site NEC 719.08
    wrist 719.03
  meninges (*see also* Meningitis) 322.9
  pericardium, pericardial (*see also* Pericarditis) 423.9
    acute 420.90
  peritoneal (chronic) 568.82
  pleura, pleurisy, pleuritic, pleuropericardial 511.9
    bacterial, nontuberculous 511.1
    fetus or newborn 511.9
    malignant 197.2
    nontuberculous 511.9
      bacterial 511.1
      pneumococcal 511.1
      staphylococcal 511.1
      streptococcal 511.1
    traumatic 862.29
      with open wound 862.39
    tuberculous (*see also* Tuberculosis, pleura) 012.0
      primary progressive 010.1
  pulmonary — *see* Effusion, pleura
  spinal (*see also* Meningitis) 322.9
  thorax, thoracic — *see* Effusion, pleura
Egg (oocyte) (ovum)
  donor V59.70
    over age 35 V59.73
      anonymous recipient V59.73
      designated recipient V59.74
    under age 35 V59.71
      anonymous recipient V59.71
      designated recipient V59.72
Eggshell nails 703.8
  congenital 757.5
Ego-dystonic
  homosexuality 302.0
  lesbianism 302.0
  sexual orientation 302.0
Egyptian splenomegaly 120.1
Ehlers-Danlos syndrome 756.83
Ehrlichiosis 082.40
  chaffeensis 082.41
  specified type NEC 082.49
Eichstedt's disease (pityriasis versicolor) 111.0
Eisenmenger's complex or syndrome (ventricular septal defect) 745.4
Ejaculation, semen
  painful 608.89
    psychogenic 306.59
  premature 302.75
  retrograde 608.87
Ekbom syndrome (restless legs) 333.94
Ekman's syndrome (brittle bones and blue sclera) 756.51
Elastic skin 756.83
  acquired 701.8

Elastofibroma (M8820/0) — *see* Neoplasm, connective tissue, benign
Elastoidosis
  cutanea nodularis 701.8
  cutis cystica et comedonica 701.8
Elastoma 757.39
  juvenile 757.39
  Miescher's (elastosis perforans serpiginosa) 701.1
Elastomyofibrosis 425.3
Elastosis 701.8
  atrophicans 701.8
  perforans serpiginosa 701.1
  reactive perforating 701.1
  senilis 701.8
  solar (actinic) 692.74
Elbow — *see* condition
Electric
  current, electricity, effects (concussion) (fatal) (nonfatal) (shock) 994.8
    burn — *see* Burn, by site
  feet (foot) syndrome 266.2
Electrocution 994.8
Electrolyte imbalance 276.9
  with
    abortion — *see* Abortion, by type, with metabolic disorder
    ectopic pregnancy (*see also* categories 633.0–633.9) 639.4
    hyperemesis gravidarum (before 22 completed weeks gestation) 643.1
    molar pregnancy (*see also* categories 630–632) 639.4
  following
    abortion 639.4
    ectopic or molar pregnancy 639.4
Elephantiasis (nonfilarial) 457.1
  arabicum (*see also* Infestation, filarial) 125.9
  congenita hereditaria 757.0
  congenital (any site) 757.0
  due to
    Brugia (malayi) 125.1
    mastectomy operation 457.0
    Wuchereria (bancrofti) 125.0
    malayi 125.1
  eyelid 374.83
  filarial (*see also* Infestation, filarial) 125.9
  filariensis (*see also* Infestation, filarial) 125.9
  gingival 523.8
  glandular 457.1
  graecorum 030.9
  lymphangiectatic 457.1
  lymphatic vessel 457.1
    due to mastectomy operation 457.0
  neuromatosa 237.71
  postmastectomy 457.0
  scrotum 457.1
  streptococcal 457.1
  surgical 997.99
    postmastectomy 457.0
  telangiectodes 457.1
  vulva (nonfilarial) 624.8
Elephant man syndrome 237.71
Elevated — *see* Elevation
Elevation
  17-ketosteroids 791.9
  acid phosphatase 790.5
  alkaline phosphatase 790.5
  amylase 790.5
  antibody titers 795.79
  basal metabolic rate (BMR) 794.7
  blood pressure (*see also* Hypertension) 401.9
    reading (incidental) (isolated) (nonspecific), no diagnosis of hypertension 796.2
  body temperature (of unknown origin) — *see* Pyrexia) 780.6
  cancer antigen 125 [CA 125] 795.82
  carcinoembryonic antigen [CEA] 795.81

Elevation — *continued*
  conjugate, eye 378.81
  C-reactive protein (CRP) 790.95
  CRP (C-reactive protein) 790.95
  diaphragm, congenital 756.6
  glucose
    fasting 790.21
    tolerance test 790.22
  immunoglobulin level 795.79
  indolacetic acid 791.9
  lactic acid dehydrogenase (LDH) level 790.4
  leukocytes 288.60
  lipase 790.5
  lipoprotein a level 272.8
  liver function test (LFT) 790.6
    alkaline phosphatase 790.5
    aminotransferase 790.4
    bilirubin 782.4
    hepatic enzyme NEC 790.5
    lactate dehydrogenase 790.4
  lymphocytes 288.61
  prostate specific antigen (PSA) 790.93
  renin 790.99
    in hypertension (*see also* Hypertension, renovascular) 405.91
  Rh titer 999.7
  scapula, congenital 755.52
  sedimentation rate 790.1
  SGOT 790.4
  SGPT 790.4
  transaminase 790.4
  vanillylmandelic acid 791.9
  venous pressure 459.89
  VMA 791.9
  white blood cell count 288.60
    specified NEC 288.69
Elliptocytosis (congenital) (hereditary) 282.1
  Hb-C (disease) 282.7
  hemoglobin disease 282.7
  sickle-cell (disease) 282.60
  trait 282.5
Ellison-Zollinger syndrome (gastric hypersecretion with pancreatic islet cell tumor) 251.5
Ellis-van Creveld disease or syndrome (chondroectodermal dysplasia) 756.55
Elongation, elongated (congenital) — *see also* Distortion
  bone 756.9
  cervix (uteri) 752.49
    acquired 622.6
    hypertrophic 622.6
  colon 751.5
  common bile duct 751.69
  cystic duct 751.69
  frenulum, penis 752.69
  labia minora, acquired 624.8
  ligamentum patellae 756.89
  petiolus (epiglottidis) 748.3
  styloid bone (process) 733.99
  tooth, teeth 520.2
  uvula 750.26
    acquired 528.9
Elschnig bodies or pearls 366.51
El Tor cholera 001.1
Emaciation (due to malnutrition) 261
Emancipation disorder 309.22
Embadomoniasis 007.8
Embarrassment heart, cardiac — *see* Disease, heart
Embedded tooth, teeth 520.6
  root only 525.3
Embolic — *see* condition
Embolism 444.9
  with
    abortion — *see* Abortion, by type, with embolism
    ectopic pregnancy (*see also* categories 633.0–633.9) 639.6
    molar pregnancy (*see also* categories 630–632) 639.6
  air (any site) 958.0

Embolism

Embolism — *continued*
- air — *continued*
    - with
        - abortion — *see* Abortion, by type, with embolism
        - ectopic pregnancy (*see also* categories 633.0–633.9) 639.6
        - molar pregnancy (*see also* categories 630–632) 639.6
        - due to implanted device — *see* Complications, due to (presence of) any device, implant, or graft classified to 996.0–996.5 NEC
    - following
        - abortion 639.6
        - ectopic or molar pregnancy 639.6
    - infusion, perfusion, or transfusion 999.1
    - in pregnancy, childbirth, or puerperium 673.0 ☑
    - traumatic 958.0
- amniotic fluid (pulmonary) 673.1 ☑
    - with
        - abortion — *see* Abortion, by type, with embolism
        - ectopic pregnancy (*see also* categories 633.0–633.9) 639.6
        - molar pregnancy (*see also* categories 630–632) 639.6
    - following
        - abortion 639.6
        - ectopic or molar pregnancy 639.6
- aorta, aortic 444.1
    - abdominal 444.0
    - bifurcation 444.0
    - saddle 444.0
    - thoracic 444.1
- artery 444.9
    - auditory, internal 433.8 ☑
    - basilar (*see also* Occlusion, artery, basilar) 433.0 ☑
    - bladder 444.89
    - carotid (common) (internal) (*see also* Occlusion, artery, carotid) 433.1 ☑
    - cerebellar (anterior inferior) (posterior inferior) (superior) 433.8 ☑
    - cerebral (*see also* Embolism, brain) 434.1 ☑
    - choroidal (anterior) 433.8 ☑
    - communicating posterior 433.8 ☑
    - coronary (*see also* Infarct, myocardium) 410.9 ☑
        - without myocardial infarction 411.81
    - extremity 444.22
        - lower 444.22
        - upper 444.21
    - hypophyseal 433.8 ☑
    - mesenteric (with gangrene) 557.0
    - ophthalmic (*see also* Occlusion, retina) 362.30
    - peripheral 444.22
    - pontine 433.8 ☑
    - precerebral NEC — *see* Occlusion, artery, precerebral
    - pulmonary — *see* Embolism, pulmonary
    - renal 593.81
    - retinal (*see also* Occlusion, retina) 362.30
    - specified site NEC 444.89
    - vertebral (*see also* Occlusion, artery, vertebral) 433.2 ☑
- auditory, internal 433.8 ☑
- basilar (artery) (*see also* Occlusion, artery, basilar) 433.0 ☑
- birth, mother — *see* Embolism, obstetrical

Embolism — *continued*
- blood-clot
    - with
        - abortion — *see* Abortion, by type, with embolism
        - ectopic pregnancy (*see also* categories 633.0–633.9) 639.6
        - molar pregnancy (*see also* categories 630–632) 639.6
    - following
        - abortion 639.6
        - ectopic or molar pregnancy 639.6
    - in pregnancy, childbirth, or puerperium 673.2 ☑
- brain 434.1 ☑
    - with
        - abortion — *see* Abortion, by type, with embolism
        - ectopic pregnancy (*see also* categories 633.0–633.9) 639.6
        - molar pregnancy (*see also* categories 630–632) 639.6
    - following
        - abortion 639.6
        - ectopic or molar pregnancy 639.6
    - late effect — *see* Late effect(s) (of) cerebrovascular disease
    - puerperal, postpartum, childbirth 674.0 ☑
- capillary 448.9
- cardiac (*see also* Infarct, myocardium) 410.9 ☑
- carotid (artery) (common) (internal) (*see also* Occlusion, artery, carotid) 433.1 ☑
- cavernous sinus (venous) — *see* Embolism, intracranial venous sinus
- cerebral (*see also* Embolism, brain) 434.1 ☑
- cholesterol — *see* Atheroembolism
- choroidal (anterior) (artery) 433.8 ☑
- coronary (artery or vein) (systemic) (*see also* Infarct, myocardium) 410.9 ☑
    - without myocardial infarction 411.81
- due to (presence of) any device, implant, or graft classifiable to 996.0–996.5 — *see* Complications, due to (presence of) any device, implant, or graft classified to 996.0–996.5 NEC
- encephalomalacia (*see also* Embolism, brain) 434.1 ☑
- extremities 444.22
    - lower 444.22
    - upper 444.21
- eye 362.30
- fat (cerebral) (pulmonary) (systemic) 958.1
    - with
        - abortion — *see* Abortion, by type, with embolism
        - ectopic pregnancy (*see also* categories 633.0–633.9) 639.6
        - molar pregnancy (*see also* categories 630–632) 639.6
    - complicating delivery or puerperium 673.8 ☑
    - following
        - abortion 639.6
        - ectopic or molar pregnancy 639.6
    - in pregnancy, childbirth, or the puerperium 673.8 ☑
- femoral (artery) 444.22
    - vein 453.8
    - deep 453.41
- following
    - abortion 639.6

Embolism — *continued*
- following — *continued*
    - ectopic or molar pregnancy 639.6
    - infusion, perfusion, or transfusion
        - air 999.1
        - thrombus 999.2
- heart (fatty) (*see also* Infarct, myocardium) 410.9 ☑
- hepatic (vein) 453.0
- iliac (artery) 444.81
- iliofemoral 444.81
- in pregnancy, childbirth, or puerperium (pulmonary) — *see* Embolism, obstetrical
- intestine (artery) (vein) (with gangrene) 557.0
- intracranial (*see also* Embolism, brain) 434.1 ☑
    - venous sinus (any) 325
        - late effect — *see* category 326
        - nonpyogenic 437.6
            - in pregnancy or puerperium 671.5 ☑
- kidney (artery) 593.81
- lateral sinus (venous) — *see* Embolism, intracranial venous sinus
- longitudinal sinus (venous) — *see* Embolism, intracranial venous sinus
- lower extremity 444.22
- lung (massive) — *see* Embolism, pulmonary
- meninges (*see also* Embolism, brain) 434.1 ☑
- mesenteric (artery) (with gangrene) 557.0
- multiple NEC 444.9
- obstetrical (pulmonary) 673.2 ☑
    - air 673.0 ☑
    - amniotic fluid (pulmonary) 673.1 ☑
    - blood-clot 673.2 ☑
    - cardiac 674.8 ☑
    - fat 673.8 ☑
    - heart 674.8 ☑
    - pyemic 673.3 ☑
    - septic 673.3 ☑
    - specified NEC 674.8 ☑
- ophthalmic (*see also* Occlusion, retina) 362.30
- paradoxical NEC 444.9
- penis 607.82
- peripheral arteries NEC 444.22
    - lower 444.22
    - upper 444.21
- pituitary 253.8
- popliteal (artery) 444.22
- portal (vein) 452
- postoperative NEC 997.2
    - cerebral 997.02
    - mesenteric artery 997.71
    - other vessels 997.79
    - peripheral vascular 997.2
    - pulmonary 415.11
    - renal artery 997.72
- precerebral artery (*see also* Occlusion, artery, precerebral) 433.9 ☑
- puerperal — *see* Embolism, obstetrical
- pulmonary (artery) (vein) 415.19
    - with
        - abortion — *see* Abortion, by type, with embolism
        - ectopic pregnancy (*see also* categories 633.0–633.9) 639.6
        - molar pregnancy (*see also* categories 630–632) 639.6
    - following
        - abortion 639.6
        - ectopic or molar pregnancy 639.6
    - iatrogenic 415.11
    - in pregnancy, childbirth, or puerperium — *see* Embolism, obstetrical
    - postoperative 415.11

Embolism — *continued*
- pyemic (multiple) 038.9
    - with
        - abortion — *see* Abortion, by type, with embolism
        - ectopic pregnancy (*see also* categories 633.0–633.9) 639.6
        - molar pregnancy (*see also* categories 630–632) 639.6
    - Aerobacter aerogenes 038.49
    - enteric gram-negative bacilli 038.40
    - Enterobacter aerogenes 038.49
    - Escherichia coli 038.42
    - following
        - abortion 639.6
        - ectopic or molar pregnancy 639.6
    - Hemophilus influenzae 038.41
    - pneumococcal 038.2
    - Proteus vulgaris 038.49
    - Pseudomonas (aeruginosa) 038.43
    - puerperal, postpartum, childbirth (any organism) 673.3 ☑
    - Serratia 038.44
    - specified organism NEC 038.8
    - staphylococcal 038.10
        - aureus 038.11
        - specified organism NEC 038.19
    - streptococcal 038.0
- renal (artery) 593.81
    - vein 453.3
- retina, retinal (*see also* Occlusion, retina) 362.30
- saddle (aorta) 444.0
- septicemic — *see* Embolism, pyemic
- sinus — *see* Embolism, intracranial venous sinus
- soap
    - with
        - abortion — *see* Abortion, by type, with embolism
        - ectopic pregnancy (*see also* categories 633.0–633.9) 639.6
        - molar pregnancy (*see also* categories 630–632) 639.6
    - following
        - abortion 639.6
        - ectopic or molar pregnancy 639.6
- spinal cord (nonpyogenic) 336.1
    - in pregnancy or puerperium 671.5 ☑
    - pyogenic origin 324.1
        - late effect — *see* category 326
- spleen, splenic (artery) 444.89
- thrombus (thromboembolism) following infusion, perfusion, or transfusion 999.2
- upper extremity 444.21
- vein 453.9
    - with inflammation or phlebitis — *see* Thrombophlebitis
    - cerebral (*see also* Embolism, brain) 434.1 ☑
    - coronary (*see also* Infarct, myocardium) 410.9 ☑
        - without myocardial infarction 411.81
    - hepatic 453.0
    - lower extremity 453.8
        - deep 453.40
            - calf 453.42
            - distal (lower leg) 453.42
            - femoral 453.41
            - iliac 453.41
            - lower leg 453.42
            - peroneal 453.42
            - popliteal 453.41
            - proximal (upper leg) 453.41
            - thigh 453.41
            - tibial 453.42
    - mesenteric (with gangrene) 557.0
    - portal 452

Index to Diseases

Embolism — *continued*
  vein — *continued*
    pulmonary — *see* Embolism, pulmonary
    renal 453.3
    specified NEC 453.8
      with inflammation or phlebitis — *see* Thrombophlebitis
    vena cava (inferior) (superior) 453.2
  vessels of brain (*see also* Embolism, brain) 434.1 ☑
Embolization — *see* Embolism
Embolus — *see* Embolism
Embryoma (M9080/1) — *see also* Neoplasm, by site, uncertain behavior
  benign (M9080/0) — *see* Neoplasm, by site, benign
    kidney (M8960/3) 189.0
    liver (M8970/3) 155.0
  malignant (M9080/3) (*see also* Neoplasm, by site, malignant)
    kidney (M8960/3) 189.0
    liver (M8970/3) 155.0
    testis (M9070/3) 186.9
      undescended 186.0
    testis (M9070/3) 186.9
      undescended 186.0
Embryonic
  circulation 747.9
  heart 747.9
  vas deferens 752.89
Embryopathia NEC 759.9
Embryotomy, fetal 763.89
Embryotoxon 743.43
  interfering with vision 743.42
Emesis — *see also* Vomiting
  gravidarum — *see* Hyperemesis, gravidarum
Emissions, nocturnal (semen) 608.89
Emotional
  crisis — *see* Crisis, emotional
  disorder (*see also* Disorder, mental) 300.9
  instability (excessive) 301.3
  overlay — *see* Reaction, adjustment
  upset 300.9
Emotionality, pathological 301.3
Emotogenic disease — *see also* Disorder, psychogenic 306.9
Emphysema (atrophic) (centriacinar) (centrilobular) (chronic) (diffuse) (essential) (hypertrophic) (interlobular) (lung) (obstructive) (panlobular) (paracicatricial) (paracinar) (postural) (pulmonary) (senile) (subpleural) (traction) (unilateral) (unilobular) (vesicular) 492.8
  with bronchitis
    chronic 491.20
      with
        acute bronchitis 491.22
        exacerbation (acute) 491.21
  bullous (giant) 492.0
  cellular tissue 958.7
    surgical 998.81
  compensatory 518.2
  congenital 770.2
  conjunctiva 372.89
  connective tissue 958.7
    surgical 998.81
  due to fumes or vapors 506.4
  eye 376.89
  eyelid 374.85
    surgical 998.81
    traumatic 958.7
  fetus or newborn (interstitial) (mediastinal) (unilobular) 770.2
  heart 416.9
  interstitial 518.1
    congenital 770.2
    fetus or newborn 770.2
  laminated tissue 958.7
    surgical 998.81
  mediastinal 518.1
    fetus or newborn 770.2

Emphysema — *continued*
  newborn (interstitial) (mediastinal) (unilobular) 770.2
  obstructive diffuse with fibrosis 492.8
  orbit 376.89
  subcutaneous 958.7
    due to trauma 958.7
    nontraumatic 518.1
    surgical 998.81
  surgical 998.81
  thymus (gland) (congenital) 254.8
  traumatic 958.7
  tuberculous (*see also* Tuberculosis, pulmonary) 011.9 ☑
Employment examination (certification) V70.5
Empty sella (turcica) syndrome 253.8
Empyema (chest) (diaphragmatic) (double) (encapsulated) (general) (interlobar) (lung) (medial) (necessitatis) (perforating chest wall) (pleura) (pneumococcal) (residual) (sacculated) (streptococcal) (supradiaphragmatic) 510.9
  with fistula 510.0
  accessory sinus (chronic) (*see also* Sinusitis) 473.9
  acute 510.9
    with fistula 510.0
  antrum (chronic) (*see also* Sinusitis, maxillary) 473.0
  brain (any part) (*see also* Abscess, brain) 324.0
  ethmoidal (sinus) (chronic) (*see also* Sinusitis, ethmoidal) 473.2
  extradural (*see also* Abscess, extradural) 324.9
  frontal (sinus) (chronic) (*see also* Sinusitis, frontal) 473.1
  gallbladder (*see also* Cholecystitis, acute) 575.0
  mastoid (process) (acute) (*see also* Mastoiditis, acute) 383.00
  maxilla, maxillary 526.4
    sinus (chronic) (*see also* Sinusitis, maxillary) 473.0
  nasal sinus (chronic) (*see also* Sinusitis) 473.9
  sinus (accessory) (nasal) (*see also* Sinusitis) 473.9
  sphenoidal (chronic) (sinus) (*see also* Sinusitis, sphenoidal) 473.3
  subarachnoid (*see also* Abscess, extradural) 324.9
  subdural (*see also* Abscess, extradural) 324.9
  tuberculous (*see also* Tuberculosis, pleura) 012.0 ☑
  ureter (*see also* Ureteritis) 593.89
  ventricular (*see also* Abscess, brain) 324.0
Enameloma 520.2
Encephalitis (bacterial) (chronic) (hemorrhagic) (idiopathic) (nonepidemic) (spurious) (subacute) 323.9
  acute (*see also* Encephalitis, viral)
    disseminated (postinfectious) NEC 136.9 *[323.61]*
      postimmunization or postvaccination 323.51 ▲
    inclusional 049.8
    inclusion body 049.8
    necrotizing 049.8
  arboviral, arbovirus NEC 064
  arthropod-borne (*see also* Encephalitis, viral, arthropod-borne) 064
  Australian X 062.4
  Bwamba fever 066.3
  California (virus) 062.5
  Central European 063.2
  Czechoslovakian 063.2
  Dawson's (inclusion body) 046.2
  diffuse sclerosing 046.2
  due to
    actinomycosis 039.8 *[323.41]* ▲

Encephalitis — *continued*
  due to — *continued*
    cat-scratch disease 078.3 *[323.01]* ▲
    infection classified elsewhere 136.9 *[323.41]* ●
    infectious mononucleosis 075 *[323.01]* ▲
    malaria (*see also* Malaria) 084.6 *[323.2]* ▲
    Negishi virus 064
    ornithosis 073.7 *[323.01]* ▲
    prophylactic inoculation against smallpox 323.51 ▲
    rickettsiosis (*see also* Rickettsiosis) 083.9 *[323.1]*
    rubella 056.01
    toxoplasmosis (acquired) 130.0
      congenital (active) 771.2 *[323.41]* ▲
    typhus (fever) (*see also* Typhus) 081.9 *[323.1]*
    vaccination (smallpox) 323.51 ▲
  Eastern equine 062.2
  endemic 049.8
  epidemic 049.8
  equine (acute) (infectious) (viral) 062.9
    Eastern 062.2
    Venezuelan 066.2
    Western 062.1
  Far Eastern 063.0
  following vaccination or other immunization procedure 323.51 ▲
  herpes 054.3
  Ilheus (virus) 062.8
  inclusion body 046.2
  infectious (acute) (virus) NEC 049.8
  influenzal 487.8 *[323.41]* ▲
    lethargic 049.8
  Japanese (B type) 062.0
  La Crosse 062.5
  late effect — *see* Late, effect, encephalitis
  lead 984.9 *[323.71]* ▲
  lethargic (acute) (infectious) (influenzal) 049.8
  lethargica 049.8
  louping ill 063.1
  lupus 710.0 *[323.81]* ▲
  lymphatica 049.0
  Mengo 049.8
  meningococcal 036.1
  mumps 072.2
  Murray Valley 062.4
  myoclonic 049.8
  Negishi virus 064
  otitic NEC 382.4 *[323.41]* ▲
  parasitic NEC 123.9 *[323.41]* ▲
  periaxialis (concentrica) (diffusa) 341.1
  postchickenpox 052.0
  postexanthematous NEC 057.9 *[323.62]* ▲
  postimmunization 323.51 ▲
  postinfectious NEC 136.9 *[323.62]* ▲
  postmeasles 055.0
  posttraumatic 323.81
  postvaccinal (smallpox) 323.51 ▲
  postvaricella 052.0
  postviral NEC 079.99 *[323.62]* ▲
    postexanthematous 057.9 *[323.62]* ▲
    specified NEC 057.8 *[323.62]* ▲
  Powassan 063.8
  progressive subcortical (Binswanger's) 290.12
  Rasmussen 323.81 ●
  Rio Bravo 049.8
  rubella 056.01
  Russian
    autumnal 062.0
    spring-summer type (taiga) 063.0
  saturnine 984.9 *[323.71]* ▲
  Semliki Forest 062.8

Encephalitis — *continued*
  serous 048
  slow-acting virus NEC 046.8
  specified cause NEC 323.81 ▲
  St. Louis type 062.3
  subacute sclerosing 046.2
  subcorticalis chronica 290.12
  summer 062.0
  suppurative 324.0
  syphilitic 094.81
    congenital 090.41
  tick-borne 063.9
  torula, torular 117.5 *[323.41]* ▲
  toxic NEC 989.9 *[323.71]* ▲
  toxoplasmic (acquired) 130.0
    congenital (active) 771.2 *[323.41]* ▲
  trichinosis 124 *[323.41]* ▲
  Trypanosomiasis (*see also* Trypanosomiasis) 086.9 *[323.2]*
  tuberculous (*see also* Tuberculosis) 013.6 ☑
  type B (Japanese) 062.0
  type C 062.3
  van Bogaert's 046.2
  Venezuelan 066.2
  Vienna type 049.8
  viral, virus 049.9
    arthropod-borne NEC 064
      mosquito-borne 062.9
        Australian X disease 062.4
        California virus 062.5
        Eastern equine 062.2
        Ilheus virus 062.8
        Japanese (B type) 062.0
        Murray Valley 062.4
        specified type NEC 062.8
        St. Louis 062.3
        type B 062.0
        type C 062.3
        Western equine 062.1
      tick-borne 063.9
        biundulant 063.2
        Central European 063.2
        Czechoslovakian 063.2
        diphasic meningoencephalitis 063.2
        Far Eastern 063.0
        Langat 063.8
        louping ill 063.1
        Powassan 063.8
        Russian spring-summer (taiga) 063.0
        specified type NEC 063.8
      vector unknown 064
      Western equine 062.1
    slow acting NEC 046.8
    specified type NEC 049.8
    vaccination, prophylactic (against) V05.0
  von Economo's 049.8
  Western equine 062.1
  West Nile type 066.41
Encephalocele 742.0
  orbit 376.81
Encephalocystocele 742.0
Encephalomalacia (brain) (cerebellar) (cerebral) (cerebrospinal) — *see also* Softening, brain 434.9 ☑
  due to
    hemorrhage (*see also* Hemorrhage, brain) 431
    recurrent spasm of artery 435.9
  embolic (cerebral) (*see also* Embolism, brain) 434.1 ☑
  subcorticalis chronicus arteriosclerotica 290.12
  thrombotic (*see also* Thrombosis, brain) 434.0 ☑
Encephalomeningitis — *see* Meningoencephalitis
Encephalomeningocele 742.0
Encephalomeningomyelitis — *see* Meningoencephalitis
Encephalomeningopathy — *see also* Meningoencephalitis 349.9

Encephalomyelitis

Encephalomyelitis (chronic) (granulomatous) (hemorrhagic necrotizing, acute) (myalgic, benign) — *see also* Encephalitis 323.9
- abortive disseminated 049.8
- acute disseminated (ADEM) (postinfectious) 136.9 [323.61] ▲
    - infectious 136.9 [323.61] ▲
    - noninfectious 323.81 ▲
    - postimmunization 323.51 ▲
- due to
    - cat-scratch disease 078.3 [323.01] ●
    - infectious mononucleosis 075 [323.01] ●
    - ornithosis 073.7 [323.01] ●
    - vaccination (any) 323.51 ●
- equine (acute) (infectious) 062.9
    - Eastern 062.2
    - Venezuelan 066.2
    - Western 062.1
- funicularis infectiosa 049.8
- late effect — *see* Late, effect, encephalitis
- Munch-Peterson's 049.8
- postchickenpox 052.0
- postimmunization 323.51 ▲
- postmeasles 055.0
- postvaccinal (smallpox) 323.51 ▲
- rubella 056.01
- specified cause NEC 323.81 ▲
- syphilitic 094.81
- West Nile 066.41

Encephalomyelocele 742.0
Encephalomyelomeningitis — *see* Meningoencephalitis
Encephalomyeloneuropathy 349.9
Encephalomyelopathy 349.9
- subacute necrotizing (infantile) 330.8

Encephalomyeloradiculitis (acute) 357.0
Encephalomyeloradiculoneuritis (acute) 357.0
Encephalomyeloradiculopathy 349.9
Encephalomyocarditis 074.23
Encephalopathia hyperbilirubinemica, newborn 774.7
- due to isoimmunization (conditions classifiable to 773.0–773.2) 773.4

Encephalopathy (acute) 348.30
- alcoholic 291.2
- anoxic — *see* Damage, brain, anoxic
- arteriosclerotic 437.0
    - late effect — *see* Late effect(s) of cerebrovascular disease
- bilirubin, newborn 774.7
    - due to isoimmunization 773.4
- congenital 742.9
- demyelinating (callosal) 341.8
- due to
    - birth injury (intracranial) 767.8
    - dialysis 294.8
    - transient 293.9
    - hyperinsulinism — *see* Hyperinsulinism
    - influenza (virus) 487.8
    - lack of vitamin (*see also* Deficiency, vitamin) 269.2
    - nicotinic acid deficiency 291.2
    - serum (nontherapeutic) (therapeutic) 999.5
    - syphilis 094.81
    - trauma (postconcussional) 310.2
        - current (*see also* Concussion, brain) 850.9
            - with skull fracture — *see* Fracture, skull, by site, with intracranial injury
    - vaccination 323.51 ▲
- hepatic 572.2
- hyperbilirubinemic, newborn 774.7
    - due to isoimmunization (conditions classifiable to 773.0–773.2) 773.4
- hypertensive 437.2
- hypoglycemic 251.2
- hypoxic (*see* ▶*also*◀ Damage, brain, anoxic)
    - ischemic (HIE) 768.7 ●
- infantile cystic necrotizing (congenital) 341.8
- lead 984.9 [323.71] ▲
- leukopolio 330.0
- metabolic (*see also* Delirium) 348.31
    - toxic 349.82
- necrotizing
    - hemorrhagic 323.61 ●
    - subacute 330.8 ●
- other specified type NEC 348.39
- pellagrous 265.2
- portal-systemic 572.2
- postcontusional 310.2
- posttraumatic 310.2
- saturnine 984.9 [323.71] ▲
- septic 348.31
- spongioform, subacute (viral) 046.1
- subacute
    - necrotizing 330.8
    - spongioform 046.1
    - viral, spongioform 046.1
- subcortical progressive (Schilder) 341.1
    - chronic (Binswanger's) 290.12
- toxic 349.82
    - metabolic 349.82 ▲
- traumatic (postconcussional) 310.2
    - current (*see also* Concussion, brain) 850.9
        - with skull fracture — *see* Fracture, skull, by site, with intracranial injury
- vitamin B deficiency NEC 266.9
- Wernicke's (superior hemorrhagic polioencephalitis) 265.1

Encephalorrhagia — *see also* Hemorrhage, brain 432.9
- healed or old V12.59
- late effect — *see* Late effect(s) of cerebrovascular disease

Encephalosis, posttraumatic 310.2
Enchondroma (M9220/0) — *see also* Neoplasm, bone, benign
- multiple, congenital 756.4

Enchondromatosis (cartilaginous) (congenital) (multiple) 756.4
Enchondroses, multiple (cartilaginous) (congenital) 756.4
Encopresis — *see also* Incontinence, feces 787.6
- nonorganic origin 307.7

Encounter for — *see also* Admission for
- administrative purpose only V68.9
    - referral of patient without examination or treatment V68.81
    - specified purpose NEC V68.89
- chemotherapy, antineoplastic V58.11
- dialysis
    - extracorporeal (renal) V56.0
    - peritoneal V56.8
- end-of-life care V66.7
- hospice care V66.7
- immunotherapy, antineoplastic V58.12
- palliative care V66.7
- paternity testing V70.4
- radiotherapy V58.0
- respirator [ventilator] dependence
    - during
        - mechanical failure V46.14
        - power failure V46.12
    - for weaning V46.13
- screening mammogram NEC V76.12
    - for high-risk patient V76.11
- terminal care V66.7
- weaning from respirator [ventilator] V46.13

Encystment — *see* Cyst
Endamebiasis — *see* Amebiasis
Endamoeba — *see* Amebiasis

Endarteritis (bacterial, subacute) (infective) (septic) 447.6
- brain, cerebral or cerebrospinal 437.4
- late effect — *see* Late effect(s) of cerebrovascular disease
- coronary (artery) — *see* Arteriosclerosis, coronary
- deformans — *see* Arteriosclerosis
- embolic (*see also* Embolism) 444.9
- obliterans (*see also* Arteriosclerosis)
    - pulmonary 417.8
- pulmonary 417.8
- retina 362.18
- senile — *see* Arteriosclerosis
- syphilitic 093.89
    - brain or cerebral 094.89
    - congenital 090.5
    - spinal 094.89
- tuberculous (*see also* Tuberculosis) 017.9 ☑

Endemic — *see* condition

Endocarditis (chronic) (indeterminate) (interstitial) (marantis) (nonbacterial thrombotic) (residual) (sclerotic) (sclerous) (senile) (valvular) 424.90
- with
    - rheumatic fever (conditions classifiable to 390)
        - active — *see* Endocarditis, acute, rheumatic
        - inactive or quiescent (with chorea) 397.9
- acute or subacute 421.9
    - rheumatic (aortic) (mitral) (pulmonary) (tricuspid) 391.1
        - with chorea (acute) (rheumatic) (Sydenham's) 392.0
- aortic (heart) (nonrheumatic) (valve) 424.1
    - with
        - mitral (valve) disease 396.9
            - active or acute 391.1
                - with chorea (acute) (rheumatic) (Sydenham's) 392.0
        - bacterial 421.0
        - rheumatic fever (conditions classifiable to 390)
            - active — *see* Endocarditis, acute, rheumatic
            - inactive or quiescent (with chorea) 395.9
                - with mitral disease 396.9
    - acute or subacute 421.9
    - arteriosclerotic 424.1
    - congenital 746.89
    - hypertensive 424.1
    - rheumatic (chronic) (inactive) 395.9
        - with mitral (valve) disease 396.9
            - active or acute 391.1
                - with chorea (acute) (rheumatic) (Sydenham's) 392.0
        - active or acute 391.1
            - with chorea (acute) (rheumatic) (Sydenham's) 392.0
    - specified cause, except rheumatic 424.1
    - syphilitic 093.22
- arteriosclerotic or due to arteriosclerosis 424.99
- atypical verrucous (Libman-Sacks) 710.0 [424.91]
- bacterial (acute) (any valve) (chronic) (subacute) 421.0
- blastomycotic 116.0 [421.1]
- candidal 112.81
- congenital 425.3
- constrictive 421.0
- Coxsackie 074.22
- due to
    - blastomycosis 116.0 [421.1]
    - candidiasis 112.81
    - Coxsackie (virus) 074.22

Endocarditis — *continued*
- due to — *continued*
    - disseminated lupus erythematosus 710.0 [424.91]
    - histoplasmosis (*see also* Histoplasmosis) 115.94
    - hypertension (benign) 424.99
    - moniliasis 112.81
    - prosthetic cardiac valve 996.61
    - Q fever 083.0 [421.1]
    - serratia marcescens 421.0
    - typhoid (fever) 002.0 [421.1]
- fetal 425.3
- gonococcal 098.84
- hypertensive 424.99
- infectious or infective (acute) (any valve) (chronic) (subacute) 421.0
- lenta (acute) (any valve) (chronic) (subacute) 421.0
- Libman-Sacks 710.0 [424.91]
- Loeffler's (parietal fibroplastic) 421.0
- malignant (acute) (any valve) (chronic) (subacute) 421.0
- meningococcal 036.42
- mitral (chronic) (double) (fibroid) (heart) (inactive) (valve) (with chorea) 394.9
    - with
        - aortic (valve) disease 396.9
            - active or acute 391.1
                - with chorea (acute) (rheumatic) (Sydenham's) 392.0
            - rheumatic fever (conditions classifiable to 390)
                - active — *see* Endocarditis, acute, rheumatic
                - inactive or quiescent (with chorea) 394.9
        - with aortic valve disease 396.9
    - active or acute 391.1
        - with chorea (acute) (rheumatic) (Sydenham's) 392.0
    - bacterial 421.0
    - arteriosclerotic 424.0
    - congenital 746.89
    - hypertensive 424.0
    - nonrheumatic 424.0
        - acute or subacute 421.9
    - syphilitic 093.21
- monilial 112.81
- mycotic (acute) (any valve) (chronic) (subacute) 421.0
- pneumococcic (acute) (any valve) (chronic) (subacute) 421.0
- pulmonary (chronic) (heart) (valve) 424.3
    - with
        - rheumatic fever (conditions classifiable to 390)
            - active — *see* Endocarditis, acute, rheumatic
            - inactive or quiescent (with chorea) 397.1
    - acute or subacute 421.9
    - rheumatic 391.1
        - with chorea (acute) (rheumatic) (Sydenham's) 392.0
    - arteriosclerotic or due to arteriosclerosis 424.3
    - congenital 746.09
    - hypertensive or due to hypertension (benign) 424.3
    - rheumatic (chronic) (inactive) (with chorea) 397.1
        - active or acute 391.1
            - with chorea (acute) (rheumatic) (Sydenham's) 392.0
    - syphilitic 093.24
- purulent (acute) (any valve) (chronic) (subacute) 421.0
- rheumatic (chronic) (inactive) (with chorea) 397.9

Index to Diseases

Endocarditis — *continued*
  rheumatic — *continued*
    active or acute (aortic) (mitral)
      (pulmonary) (tricuspid) 391.1
      with chorea (acute) (rheumatic)
        (Sydenham's) 392.0
    septic (acute) (any valve) (chronic)
      (subacute) 421.0
    specified cause, except rheumatic
      424.99
    streptococcal (acute) (any valve)
      (chronic) (subacute) 421.0
    subacute — *see* Endocarditis, acute
    suppurative (any valve) (acute)
      (chronic) (subacute) 421.0
    syphilitic NEC 093.20
    toxic (*see also* Endocarditis, acute)
      421.9
    tricuspid (chronic) (heart) (inactive)
      (rheumatic) (valve) (with chorea)
      397.0
    with
      rheumatic fever (conditions
        classifiable to 390)
        active — *see* Endocarditis,
          acute, rheumatic
        inactive or quiescent (with
          chorea) 397.0
    active or acute 391.1
      with chorea (acute) (rheumatic)
        (Sydenham's) 392.0
    arteriosclerotic 424.2
    congenital 746.89
    hypertensive 424.2
    nonrheumatic 424.2
      acute or subacute 421.9
    specified cause, except rheumatic
      424.2
    syphilitic 093.23
    tuberculous (*see also* Tuberculosis)
      017.9 ☑ *[424.91]*
    typhoid 002.0 *[421.1]*
    ulcerative (acute) (any valve) (chronic)
      (subacute) 421.0
    vegetative (acute) (any valve) (chronic)
      (subacute) 421.0
    verrucous (acute) (any valve) (chronic)
      (subacute) NEC 710.0 *[424.91]*
      nonbacterial 710.0 *[424.91]*
      nonrheumatic 710.0 *[424.91]*
Endocardium, endocardial — *see also*
  condition
  cushion defect 745.60
    specified type NEC 745.69
Endocervicitis — *see also* Cervicitis
  616.0
  due to
    intrauterine (contraceptive) device
      996.65
  gonorrheal (acute) 098.15
    chronic or duration of 2 months or
      over 098.35
  hyperplastic 616.0
  syphilitic 095.8
  trichomonal 131.09
  tuberculous (*see also* Tuberculosis)
    016.7 ☑
Endocrine — *see* condition
Endocrinopathy, pluriglandular 258.9
Endodontitis 522.0
End-of-life care V66.7
Endomastoiditis — *see also* Mastoiditis
  383.9
Endometrioma 617.9
Endometriosis 617.9
  appendix 617.5
  bladder 617.8
  bowel 617.5
  broad ligament 617.3
  cervix 617.0
  colon 617.5
  cul-de-sac (Douglas') 617.3
  exocervix 617.0
  fallopian tube 617.2
  female genital organ NEC 617.8
  gallbladder 617.8

Endometriosis — *continued*
  in scar of skin 617.6
  internal 617.0
  intestine 617.5
  lung 617.8
  myometrium 617.0
  ovary 617.1
  parametrium 617.3
  pelvic peritoneum 617.3
  peritoneal (pelvic) 617.3
  rectovaginal septum 617.4
  rectum 617.5
  round ligament 617.3
  skin 617.6
  specified site NEC 617.8
  stromal (M8931/1) 236.0
  umbilicus 617.8
  uterus 617.0
    internal 617.0
  vagina 617.4
  vulva 617.8
Endometritis (nonspecific) (purulent)
  (septic) (suppurative) 615.9
  with
    abortion — *see* Abortion, by type,
      with sepsis
    ectopic pregnancy (*see also* cate-
      gories 633.0–633.9) 639.0
    molar pregnancy (*see also* cate-
      gories 630–632) 639.0
  acute 615.0
  blennorrhagic 098.16
    acute 098.16
    chronic or duration of 2 months or
      over 098.36
  cervix, cervical (*see also* Cervicitis)
    616.0
    hyperplastic 616.0
  chronic 615.1
  complicating pregnancy 646.6 ☑
    affecting fetus or newborn 760.8
  decidual 615.9
  following
    abortion 639.0
    ectopic or molar pregnancy 639.0
  gonorrheal (acute) 098.16
    chronic or duration of 2 months or
      over 098.36
  hyperplastic (*see also* Hyperplasia,
    endometrium) 621.30
    cervix 616.0
  polypoid — *see* Endometritis, hyper-
    plastic
  puerperal, postpartum, childbirth
    670.0 ☑
  senile (atrophic) 615.9
  subacute 615.0
  tuberculous (*see also* Tuberculosis)
    016.7 ☑
Endometrium — *see* condition
Endomyocardiopathy, South African
  425.2
Endomyocarditis — *see* Endocarditis
Endomyofibrosis 425.0
Endomyometritis — *see also* Endometritis 615.9
Endopericarditis — *see* Endocarditis
Endoperineuritis — *see* Disorder, nerve
Endophlebitis — *see also* Phlebitis 451.9
  leg 451.2
    deep (vessels) 451.19
    superficial (vessels) 451.0
  portal (vein) 572.1
  retina 362.18
  specified site NEC 451.89
  syphilitic 093.89
Endophthalmia — *see also* Endophthalmitis 360.00
  gonorrheal 098.42
Endophthalmitis (globe) (infective)
  (metastatic) (purulent) (subacute)
  360.00
  acute 360.01
  bleb associated 379.63 ●
  chronic 360.03
  parasitic 360.13

Endophthalmitis — *continued*
  phacoanaphylactic 360.19
  specified type NEC 360.19
  sympathetic 360.11
Endosalpingioma (M9111/1) 236.2
Endosteitis — *see* Osteomyelitis
Endothelioma, bone (M9260/3) — *see*
  Neoplasm, bone, malignant
Endotheliosis 287.8
  hemorrhagic infectional 287.8
Endotoxemia — code to condition ●
Endotoxic shock 785.52
Endotrachelitis — *see also* Cervicitis
  616.0
Enema rash 692.89
Engelmann's disease (diaphyseal sclerosis) 756.9
Engel-von Recklinghausen disease or
  syndrome (osteitis fibrosa cystica)
  252.01
English disease — *see also* Rickets
  268.0
Engman's disease (infectious eczematoid
  dermatitis) 690.8
Engorgement
  breast 611.79
    newborn 778.7
    puerperal, postpartum 676.2 ☑
  liver 573.9
  lung 514
  pulmonary 514
  retina, venous 362.37
  stomach 536.8
  venous, retina 362.37
Enlargement, enlarged — *see also* Hypertrophy
  abdomen 789.3 ☑
  adenoids 474.12
    and tonsils 474.10
  alveolar process or ridge 525.8
  apertures of diaphragm (congenital)
    756.6
  blind spot, visual field 368.42
  gingival 523.8
  heart, cardiac (*see also* Hypertrophy,
    cardiac) 429.3
  lacrimal gland, chronic 375.03
  liver (*see also* Hypertrophy, liver)
    789.1
  lymph gland or node 785.6
  orbit 376.46
  organ or site, congenital NEC — *see*
    Anomaly, specified type NEC
  parathyroid (gland) 252.01
  pituitary fossa 793.0
  prostate (simple) (soft) 600.00
    with
      other lower urinary tract ●
        symptoms (LUTS) ●
        600.01 ●
      urinary ●
        obstruction 600.01 ●
        retention 600.01 ●
  sella turcica 793.0
  spleen (*see also* Splenomegaly) 789.2
    congenital 759.0
  thymus (congenital) (gland) 254.0
  thyroid (gland) (*see also* Goiter) 240.9
  tongue 529.8
  tonsils 474.11
    and adenoids 474.10
  uterus 621.2
Enophthalmos 376.50
  due to
    atrophy of orbital tissue 376.51
    surgery 376.52
    trauma 376.52
Enostosis 526.89
Entamebiasis — *see* Amebiasis
Entamebic — *see* Amebiasis
Entanglement, umbilical cord(s)
  663.3 ☑
  with compression 663.2 ☑
  affecting fetus or newborn 762.5
  around neck with compression
    663.1 ☑

Entanglement, umbilical cord(s) —
  continued
  twins in monoamniotic sac 663.2 ☑
Enteralgia 789.0 ☑
Enteric — *see* condition
Enteritis (acute) (catarrhal) (choleraic)
  (chronic) (congestive) (diarrheal)
  (exudative) (follicular) (hemorrhagic) (infantile) (lienteric) (noninfectious) (perforative) (phlegmonous)
  (presumed noninfectious) (pseudomembranous) 558.9
  adaptive 564.9
  aertrycke infection 003.0
  allergic 558.3
  amebic (*see also* Amebiasis) 006.9
    with abscess — *see* Abscess, ame-
      bic
    acute 006.0
      with abscess — *see* Abscess,
        amebic
      nondysenteric 006.2
    chronic 006.1
      with abscess — *see* Abscess,
        amebic
      nondysenteric 006.2
    nondysenteric 006.2
  anaerobic (cocci) (gram-negative)
    (gram-positive) (mixed) NEC
    008.46
  bacillary NEC 004.9
  bacterial NEC 008.5
    specified NEC 008.49
  Bacteroides (fragilis) (melaninogenis-
    cus) (oralis) 008.46
  Butyrivibrio (fibriosolvens) 008.46
  Campylobacter 008.43
  Candida 112.85
  Chilomastix 007.8
  choleriformis 001.1
  chronic 558.9
    ulcerative (*see also* Colitis, ulcera-
      tive) 556.9
  cicatrizing (chronic) 555.0
  Clostridium
    botulinum 005.1
    difficile 008.45
    haemolyticum 008.46
    novyi 008.46
    perfringens (C) (F) 008.46
    specified type NEC 008.46
  coccidial 007.2
  dietetic 558.9
  due to
    achylia gastrica 536.8
    adenovirus 008.62
    Aerobacter aerogenes 008.2
    anaerobes (*see also* Enteritis,
      anaerobic) 008.46
    Arizona (bacillus) 008.1
    astrovirus 008.66
    Bacillus coli — *see* Enteritis, E. coli
    bacteria NEC 008.5
      specified NEC 008.49
    Bacteroides (*see also* Enteritis,
      Bacteroides) 008.46
    Butyrivibrio (fibriosolvens) 008.46
    Calcivirus 008.65
    Camplyobacter 008.43
    Clostridium — *see* Enteritis,
      Clostridium
    Cockle agent 008.64
    Coxsackie (virus) 008.67
    Ditchling agent 008.64
    ECHO virus 008.67
    Enterobacter aerogenes 008.2
    enterococci 008.49
    enterovirus NEC 008.67
    Escherichia coli — *see* Enteritis,
      E. coli
    Eubacterium 008.46
    Fusobacterium (nucleatum) 008.46
    gram-negative bacteria NEC 008.47
      anaerobic NEC 008.46
    Hawaii agent 008.63
    irritating foods 558.9

Enteritis — continued
  due to — continued
    Klebsiella aerogenes 008.47
    Marin County agent 008.66
    Montgomery County agent 008.63
    Norwalk-like agent 008.63
    Norwalk virus 008.63
    Otofuke agent 008.63
    Paracolobactrum arizonae 008.1
    paracolon bacillus NEC 008.47
      Arizona 008.1
    Paramatta agent 008.64
    Peptococcus 008.46
    Peptostreptococcus 008.46
    Proprionibacterium 008.46
    Proteus (bacillus) (mirabilis) (morganii) 008.3
    Pseudomonas aeruginosa 008.42
    Rotavirus 008.61
    Sapporo agent 008.63
    small round virus (SRV) NEC 008.64
      featureless NEC 008.63
      structured NEC 008.63
    Snow Mountain (SM) agent 008.63
    specified
      bacteria NEC 008.49
      organism, nonbacterial NEC 008.8
      virus NEC 008.69
    Staphylococcus 008.41
    Streptococcus 008.49
      anaerobic 008.46
    Taunton agent 008.63
    Torovirus 008.69
    Treponema 008.46
    Veillonella 008.46
    virus 008.8
      specified type NEC 008.69
    Wollan (W) agent 008.64
    Yersinia enterocolitica 008.44
  dysentery — see Dysentery
  E. coli 008.00
    enterohemorrhagic 008.04
    enteroinvasive 008.03
    enteropathogenic 008.01
    enterotoxigenic 008.02
    specified type NEC 008.09
  el tor 001.1
  embadomonial 007.8
  epidemic 009.0
  Eubacterium 008.46
  fermentative 558.9
  fulminant 557.0
  Fusobacterium (nucleatum) 008.46
  gangrenous (see also Enteritis, due to, by organism) 009.0
  giardial 007.1
  gram-negative bacteria NEC 008.47
    anaerobic NEC 008.46
  infectious NEC (see also Enteritis, due to, by organism) 009.0
    presumed 009.1
  influenzal 487.8
  ischemic 557.9
    acute 557.0
    chronic 557.1
      due to mesenteric artery insufficiency 557.1
  membranous 564.9
  mucous 564.9
  myxomembranous 564.9
  necrotic (see also Enteritis, due to, by organism) 009.0
  necroticans 005.2
  necrotizing of fetus or newborn 777.5
  neurogenic 564.9
  newborn 777.8
    necrotizing 777.5
  parasitic NEC 129
  paratyphoid (fever) (see also Fever, paratyphoid) 002.9
  Peptococcus 008.46
  Peptostreptococcus 008.46
  Proprionibacterium 008.46
  protozoal NEC 007.9

Enteritis — continued
  radiation 558.1
  regional (of) 555.9
    intestine
      large (bowel, colon, or rectum) 555.1
        with small intestine 555.2
      small (duodenum, ileum, or jejunum) 555.0
        with large intestine 555.2
  Salmonella infection 003.0
  salmonellosis 003.0
  segmental (see also Enteritis, regional) 555.9
  septic (see also Enteritis, due to, by organism) 009.0
  Shigella 004.9
  simple 558.9
  spasmodic 564.9
  spastic 564.9
  staphylococcal 008.41
    due to food 005.0
  streptococcal 008.49
    anaerobic 008.46
  toxic 558.2
  Treponema (denticola) (macrodentium) 008.46
  trichomonal 007.3
  tuberculous (see also Tuberculosis) 014.8 ☑
  typhosa 002.0
  ulcerative (chronic) (see also Colitis, ulcerative) 556.9
  Veillonella 008.46
  viral 008.8
    adenovirus 008.62
    enterovirus 008.67
    specified virus NEC 008.69
  Yersinia enterocolitica 008.44
  zymotic 009.0
Enteroarticular syndrome 099.3
Enterobiasis 127.4
Enterobius vermicularis 127.4
Enterocele — see also Hernia 553.9
  pelvis, pelvic (acquired) (congenital) 618.6
  vagina, vaginal (acquired) (congenital) 618.6
Enterocolitis — see also Enteritis
  fetus or newborn 777.8
    necrotizing 777.5
  fulminant 557.0
  granulomatous 555.2
  hemorrhagic (acute) 557.0
    chronic 557.1
  necrotizing (acute) (membranous) 557.0
  primary necrotizing 777.5
  pseudomembranous 008.45
  radiation 558.1
    newborn 777.5
  ulcerative 556.0
Enterocystoma 751.5
Enterogastritis — see Enteritis
Enterogenous cyanosis 289.7
Enterolith, enterolithiasis (impaction) 560.39
  with hernia (see also Hernia, by site, with obstruction)
    gangrenous — see Hernia, by site, with gangrene
Enteropathy 569.9
  exudative (of Gordon) 579.8
  gluten 579.0
  hemorrhagic, terminal 557.0
  protein-losing 579.8
Enteroperitonitis — see also Peritonitis 567.9
Enteroptosis 569.89
Enterorrhagia 578.9
Enterospasm 564.9
  psychogenic 306.4
Enterostenosis — see also Obstruction, intestine 560.9
Enterostomy status V44.4
  with complication 569.60

Enthesopathy 726.90
  ankle and tarsus 726.70
  elbow region 726.30
    specified NEC 726.39
  hip 726.5
  knee 726.60
  peripheral NEC 726.8
  shoulder region 726.10
    adhesive 726.0
  spinal 720.1
  wrist and carpus 726.4
Entrance, air into vein — see Embolism, air
Entrapment, nerve — see Neuropathy, entrapment
Entropion (eyelid) 374.00
  cicatricial 374.04
  congenital 743.62
  late effect of trachoma (healed) 139.1
  mechanical 374.02
  paralytic 374.02
  senile 374.01
  spastic 374.03
Enucleation of eye (current) (traumatic) 871.3
Enuresis 788.30
  habit disturbance 307.6
  nocturnal 788.36
    psychogenic 307.6
  nonorganic origin 307.6
  psychogenic 307.6
Enzymopathy 277.9
Eosinopenia 288.59 ▲
Eosinophilia 288.3
  allergic 288.3
  hereditary 288.3
  idiopathic 288.3
  infiltrative 518.3
  Loeffler's 518.3
  myalgia syndrome 710.5
  pulmonary (tropical) 518.3
  secondary 288.3
  tropical 518.3
Eosinophilic — see also condition
  fasciitis 728.89
  granuloma (bone) 277.89
  infiltration lung 518.3
Ependymitis (acute) (cerebral) (chronic) (granular) — see also Meningitis 322.9
Ependymoblastoma (M9392/3)
  specified site — see Neoplasm, by site, malignant
  unspecified site 191.9
Ependymoma (epithelial) (malignant) (M9391/3)
  anaplastic type (M9392/3)
    specified site — see Neoplasm, by site, malignant
    unspecified site 191.9
  benign (M9391/0)
    specified site — see Neoplasm, by site, benign
    unspecified site 225.0
  myxopapillary (M9394/1) 237.5
  papillary (M9393/1) 237.5
    specified site — see Neoplasm, by site, malignant
    unspecified site 191.9
Ependymopathy 349.2
  spinal cord 349.2
Ephelides, ephelis 709.09
Ephemeral fever — see also Pyrexia 780.6
Epiblepharon (congenital) 743.62
Epicanthus, epicanthic fold (congenital) (eyelid) 743.63
Epicondylitis (elbow) (lateral) 726.32
  medial 726.31
Epicystitis — see also Cystitis 595.9
Epidemic — see condition
Epidermidalization, cervix — see condition
Epidermidization, cervix — see condition
Epidermis, epidermal — see condition

Epidermization, cervix — see condition
Epidermodysplasia verruciformis 078.19
Epidermoid
  cholesteatoma — see Cholesteatoma
  inclusion (see also Cyst, skin) 706.2
Epidermolysis
  acuta (combustiformis) (toxica) 695.1
  bullosa 757.39
  necroticans combustiformis 695.1
    due to drug
      correct substance properly administered 695.1
      overdose or wrong substance given or taken 977.9
      specified drug — see Table of Drugs and Chemicals
Epidermophytid — see Dermatophytosis
Epidermophytosis (infected) — see Dermatophytosis
Epidermosis, ear (middle) — see also Cholesteatoma 385.30
Epididymis — see condition
Epididymitis (nonvenereal) 604.90
  with abscess 604.0
  acute 604.99
  blennorrhagic (acute) 098.0
    chronic or duration of 2 months or over 098.2
  caseous (see also Tuberculosis) 016.4 ☑
  chlamydial 099.54
  diphtheritic 032.89 [604.91]
  filarial 125.9 [604.91]
  gonococcal (acute) 098.0
    chronic or duration of 2 months or over 098.2
  recurrent 604.99
  residual 604.99
  syphilitic 095.8 [604.91]
  tuberculous (see also Tuberculosis) 016.4 ☑
Epididymo-orchitis — see also Epididymitis 604.90
  with abscess 604.0
  chlamydial 099.54
  gonococcal (acute) 098.13
    chronic or duration of 2 months or over 098.33
Epidural — see condition
Epigastric — see also Gastritis 535.5 ☑
Epigastrium, epigastric — see condition
Epigastrocele — see also Hernia, epigastric 553.29
Epiglottiditis (acute) 464.30
  with obstruction 464.31
  chronic 476.1
  viral 464.30
    with obstruction 464.31
Epiglottis — see condition
Epiglottitis (acute) 464.30
  with obstruction 464.31
  chronic 476.1
  viral 464.30
    with obstruction 464.31
Epignathus 759.4
Epilepsia
  partialis continua (see also Epilepsy) 345.7
  procursiva (see also Epilepsy) 345.8 ☑
Epilepsy, epileptic (idiopathic) 345.9 ☑

Note — use the following fifth-digit subclassification with categories 345.0, 345.1, 345.4–345.9:

0 *without mention of intractable epilepsy*

1 *with intractable epilepsy*

  abdominal 345.5 ☑
  absence (attack) 345.0 ☑
  akinetic 345.0 ☑
    psychomotor 345.4 ☑
  automatism 345.4 ☑
  autonomic diencephalic 345.5 ☑

Index to Diseases

Epilepsy, epileptic — continued
  brain 345.9 ☑
  Bravais-Jacksonian 345.5 ☑
  cerebral 345.9 ☑
  climacteric 345.9 ☑
  clonic 345.1 ☑
  clouded state 345.9 ☑
  coma 345.3
  communicating 345.4 ☑
  complicating pregnancy, childbirth, ● or the puerperium 649.4 ☑ ●
  congenital 345.9 ☑
  convulsions 345.9 ☑
  cortical (focal) (motor) 345.5 ☑
  cursive (running) 345.8 ☑
  cysticercosis 123.1
  deterioration
    with behavioral disturbance 345.9 ☑ [294.11]
    without behavioral disturbance 345.9 ☑ [294.10]
  due to syphilis 094.89
  equivalent 345.5 ☑
  fit 345.9 ☑
  focal (motor) 345.5 ☑
  gelastic 345.8 ☑
  generalized 345.9 ☑
    convulsive 345.1 ☑
    flexion 345.1 ☑
    nonconvulsive 345.0 ☑
  grand mal (idiopathic) 345.1 ☑
  Jacksonian (motor) (sensory) 345.5 ☑
  Kojevnikoff's, Kojevnikov's, Kojewnikoff's 345.7 ☑
  laryngeal 786.2
  limbic system 345.4 ☑
  localization related (focal) (partial) ● and epileptic syndromes
    with
      complex partial seizures 345.4 ☑ ●
      simple partial seizures 345.5 ☑ ●
  major (motor) 345.1 ☑
  minor 345.0 ☑
  mixed (type) 345.9 ☑
  motor partial 345.5 ☑
  musicogenic 345.1 ☑
  myoclonus, myoclonic 345.1 ☑
    progressive (familial) 333.2
  nonconvulsive, generalized 345.0 ☑
  parasitic NEC 123.9
  partial (focalized) 345.5 ☑
    with
      impairment of consciousness 345.4 ☑
      memory and ideational disturbances 345.4 ☑
      without impairment of conscious- ● ness 345.5 ☑ ●
    abdominal type 345.5 ☑
    motor type 345.5 ☑
    psychomotor type 345.4 ☑
    psychosensory type 345.4 ☑
    secondarily generalized 345.4 ☑
    sensory type 345.5 ☑
    somatomotor type 345.5 ☑
    somatosensory type 345.5 ☑
    temporal lobe type 345.4 ☑
    visceral type 345.5 ☑
    visual type 345.5 ☑
  peripheral 345.9 ☑
  petit mal 345.0 ☑
  photokinetic 345.8 ☑
  progressive myoclonic (familial) 333.2
  psychic equivalent 345.5 ☑
  psychomotor 345.4 ☑
  psychosensory 345.4 ☑
  reflex 345.1 ☑
  seizure 345.9 ☑
  senile 345.9 ☑
  sensory-induced 345.5 ☑
  sleep (see also Narcolepsy) 347.00
  somatomotor type 345.5 ☑

Epilepsy, epileptic — continued
  somatosensory 345.5 ☑
  specified type NEC 345.8 ☑
  status (grand mal) 345.3
    focal motor 345.7 ☑
    petit mal 345.2
    psychomotor 345.7 ☑
    temporal lobe 345.7 ☑
  symptomatic 345.9 ☑
  temporal lobe 345.4 ☑
  tonic (-clonic) 345.1 ☑
  traumatic (injury unspecified) 907.0
    injury specified — see Late, effect (of) specified injury
  twilight 293.0
  uncinate (gyrus) 345.4 ☑
  Unverricht (-Lundborg) (familial myoclonic) 333.2
  visceral 345.5 ☑
  visual 345.5 ☑
Epileptiform
  convulsions 780.39
  seizure 780.39
Epiloia 759.5
Epimenorrhea 626.2
Epipharyngitis — see also Nasopharyngitis 460
Epiphora 375.20
  due to
    excess lacrimation 375.21
    insufficient drainage 375.22
Epiphyseal arrest 733.91
  femoral head 732.2
Epiphyseolysis, epiphysiolysis — see also Osteochondrosis 732.9
Epiphysitis — see also Osteochondrosis 732.9
  juvenile 732.6
  marginal (Scheuermann's) 732.0
  os calcis 732.5
  syphilitic (congenital) 090.0
  vertebral (Scheuermann's) 732.0
Epiplocele — see also Hernia 553.9
Epiploitis — see also Peritonitis 567.9
Epiplosarcomphalocele — see also Hernia, umbilicus 553.1
Episcleritis 379.00
  gouty 274.89 [379.09]
  nodular 379.02
  periodica fugax 379.01
    angioneurotic — see Edema, angioneurotic
  specified NEC 379.09
  staphylococcal 379.00
  suppurative 379.00
  syphilitic 095.0
  tuberculous (see also Tuberculosis) 017.3 ☑ [379.09]
Episode
  brain (see also Disease, cerebrovascular, acute) 436
  cerebral (see also Disease, cerebrovascular, acute) 436
  depersonalization (in neurotic state) 300.6
  hyporesponsive 780.09
  psychotic (see also Psychosis) 298.9
    organic, transient 293.9
  schizophrenic (acute) NEC (see also Schizophrenia) 295.4 ☑
Epispadias
  female 753.8
  male 752.62
Episplenitis 289.59
Epistaxis (multiple) 784.7
  hereditary 448.0
  vicarious menstruation 625.8
Epithelioma (malignant) (M8011/3) — see also Neoplasm, by site, malignant
  adenoides cysticum (M8100/0) — see Neoplasm, skin, benign
  basal cell (M8090/3) — see Neoplasm, skin, malignant
  benign (M8011/0) — see Neoplasm, by site, benign

Epithelioma — see also Neoplasm, by site, malignant — continued
  Bowen's (M8081/2) — see Neoplasm, skin, in situ
  calcifying (benign) (Malherbe's) (M8110/0) — see Neoplasm, skin, benign
  external site — see Neoplasm, skin, malignant
  intraepidermal, Jadassohn (M8096/0) — see Neoplasm, skin, benign
  squamous cell (M8070/3) — see Neoplasm, by site, malignant
Epitheliopathy
  pigment, retina 363.15
  posterior multifocal placoid (acute) 363.15
Epithelium, epithelial — see condition
Epituberculosis (allergic) (with atelectasis) — see also Tuberculosis 010.8 ☑
Eponychia 757.5
Epstein's
  nephrosis or syndrome (see also Nephrosis) 581.9
  pearl (mouth) 528.4
Epstein-Barr infection (viral) 075
  chronic 780.79 [139.8]
Epulis (giant cell) (gingiva) 523.8
Equinia 024
Equinovarus (congenital) 754.51
  acquired 736.71
Equivalent
  convulsive (abdominal) (see also Epilepsy) 345.5 ☑
  epileptic (psychic) (see also Epilepsy) 345.5 ☑
Erb's
  disease 359.1
  palsy, paralysis (birth) (brachial) (newborn) 767.6
  spinal (spastic) syphilitic 094.89
  pseudohypertrophic muscular dystrophy 359.1
Erb-Goldflam disease or syndrome 358.00
Erb (-Duchenne) paralysis (birth injury) (newborn) 767.6
Erdheim's syndrome (acromegalic macrospondylitis) 253.0
Erection, painful (persistent) 607.3
Ergosterol deficiency (vitamin D) 268.9
  with
    osteomalacia 268.2
    rickets (see also Rickets) 268.0
Ergotism (ergotized grain) 988.2
  from ergot used as drug (migraine therapy)
    correct substance properly administered 349.82
    overdose or wrong substance given or taken 975.0
Erichsen's disease (railway spine) 300.16
Erlacher-Blount syndrome (tibia vara) 732.4
Erosio interdigitalis blastomycetica 112.3
Erosion
  arteriosclerotic plaque — see Arteriosclerosis, by site
  artery NEC 447.2
    without rupture 447.8
  bone 733.99
  bronchus 519.19
  cartilage (joint) 733.99
  cervix (uteri) (acquired) (chronic) (congenital) 622.0
    with mention of cervicitis 616.0
  cornea (recurrent) (see also Keratitis) 371.42
    traumatic 918.1
  dental (idiopathic) (occupational) 521.30
    extending into
      dentine 521.32

Eruption

Erosion — continued
  dental — continued
    extending into — continued
      pulp 521.33
    generalized 521.35
    limited to enamel 521.31
    localized 521.34
  duodenum, postpyloric — see Ulcer, duodenum
  esophagus 530.89
  gastric 535.4 ☑
  intestine 569.89
  lymphatic vessel 457.8
  pylorus, pyloric (ulcer) 535.4 ☑
  sclera 379.16
  spine, aneurysmal 094.89
  spleen 289.59
  stomach 535.4 ☑
  teeth (idiopathic) (occupational) (see also Erosion, dental) 521.30
    due to
      medicine 521.30
      persistent vomiting 521.30
  urethra 599.84
  uterus 621.8
  vertebra 733.99
Erotomania 302.89
  Clérambault's 297.8
Error
  in diet 269.9
  refractive 367.9
    astigmatism (see also Astigmatism) 367.20
    drug-induced 367.89
    hypermetropia 367.0
    hyperopia 367.0
    myopia 367.1
    presbyopia 367.4
    toxic 367.89
Eructation 787.3
  nervous 306.4
  psychogenic 306.4
Eruption
  creeping 126.9
  drug — see Dermatitis, due to, drug
  Hutchinson, summer 692.72
  Kaposi's varicelliform 054.0
  napkin (psoriasiform) 691.0
  polymorphous
    light (sun) 692.72
    other source 692.82
  psoriasiform, napkin 691.0
  recalcitrant pustular 694.8
  ringed 695.89
  skin (see also Dermatitis) 782.1
    creeping (meaning hookworm) 126.9
    due to
      chemical(s) NEC 692.4
        internal use 693.8
      drug — see Dermatitis, due to, drug
      prophylactic inoculation or vaccination against disease — see Dermatitis, due to, vaccine
      smallpox vaccination NEC — see Dermatitis, due to, vaccine
    erysipeloid 027.1
    feigned 698.4
    Hutchinson, summer 692.72
    Kaposi's, varicelliform 054.0
      vaccinia 999.0
    lichenoid, axilla 698.3
    polymorphous, due to light 692.72
    toxic NEC 695.0
    vesicular 709.8
  teeth, tooth
    accelerated 520.6
    delayed 520.6
    difficult 520.6
    disturbance of 520.6
    in abnormal sequence 520.6
    incomplete 520.6
    late 520.6

Eruption

Eruption — *continued*
  teeth, tooth — *continued*
    natal 520.6
    neonatal 520.6
    obstructed 520.6
    partial 520.6
    persistent primary 520.6
    premature 520.6
    prenatal 520.6
  vesicular 709.8
Erysipelas (gangrenous) (infantile) (newborn) (phlegmonous) (suppurative) 035
  external ear 035 [380.13]
  puerperal, postpartum, childbirth 670.0
Erysipelatoid (Rosenbach's) 027.1
Erysipeloid (Rosenbach's) 027.1
Erythema, erythematous (generalized) 695.9
  ab igne — *see* Burn, by site, first degree
  annulare (centrifugum) (rheumaticum) 695.0
  arthriticum epidemicum 026.1
  brucellum (*see also* Brucellosis) 023.9
  bullosum 695.1
  caloricum — *see* Burn, by site, first degree
  chronicum migrans 088.81
  circinatum 695.1
  diaper 691.0
  due to
    chemical (contact) NEC 692.4
      internal 693.8
    drug (internal use) 693.0
      contact 692.3
  elevatum diutinum 695.89
  endemic 265.2
  epidemic, arthritic 026.1
  figuratum perstans 695.0
  gluteal 691.0
  gyratum (perstans) (repens) 695.1
  heat — *see* Burn, by site, first degree
  ichthyosiforme congenitum 757.1
  induratum (primary) (scrofulosorum) (*see also* Tuberculosis) 017.1
    nontuberculous 695.2
  infantum febrile 057.8
  infectional NEC 695.9
  infectiosum 057.0
  inflammation NEC 695.9
  intertrigo 695.89
  iris 695.1
  lupus (discoid) (localized) (*see also* Lupus, erythematosus) 695.4
  marginatum 695.0
    rheumaticum — *see* Fever, rheumatic
  medicamentosum — *see* Dermatitis, due to, drug
  migrans 529.1
    chronicum 088.81
  multiforme 695.1
    bullosum 695.1
    conjunctiva 695.1
    exudativum (Hebra) 695.1
    pemphigoides 694.5
  napkin 691.0
  neonatorum 778.8
  nodosum 695.2
    tuberculous (*see also* Tuberculosis) 017.1
  nummular, nummulare 695.1
  palmar 695.0
  palmaris hereditarium 695.0
  pernio 991.5
  perstans solare 692.72
  rash, newborn 778.8
  scarlatiniform (exfoliative) (recurrent) 695.0
  simplex marginatum 057.8
  solare (*see also* Sunburn) 692.71
  streptogenes 696.5
  toxic, toxicum NEC 695.0
    newborn 778.8

Erythema, erythematous — *continued*
  tuberculous (primary) (*see also* Tuberculosis) 017.0
  venenatum 695.0
Erythematosus — *see* condition
Erythematous — *see* condition
Erythermalgia (primary) 443.82
Erythralgia 443.82
Erythrasma 039.0
Erythredema 985.0
  polyneuritica 985.0
  polyneuropathy 985.0
Erythremia (acute) (M9841/3) 207.0
  chronic (M9842/3) 207.1
  secondary 289.0
Erythroblastopenia (acquired) 284.8
  congenital 284.01
Erythroblastophthisis 284.01
Erythroblastosis (fetalis) (newborn) 773.2
  due to
    ABO
      antibodies 773.1
      incompatibility, maternal/fetal 773.1
      isoimmunization 773.1
    Rh
      antibodies 773.0
      incompatibility, maternal/fetal 773.0
      isoimmunization 773.0
Erythrocyanosis (crurum) 443.89
Erythrocythemia — *see* Erythremia
Erythrocytopenia 285.9
Erythrocytosis (megalosplenic)
  familial 289.6
  oval, hereditary (*see also* Elliptocytosis) 282.1
  secondary 289.0
  stress 289.0
Erythroderma — *see also* Erythema 695.9
  desquamativa (in infants) 695.89
  exfoliative 695.89
  ichthyosiform, congenital 757.1
  infantum 695.89
  maculopapular 696.2
  neonatorum 778.8
  psoriaticum 696.1
  secondary 695.9
Erythrogenesis imperfecta 284.09
Erythroleukemia (M9840/3) 207.0
Erythromelalgia 443.82
Erythromelia 701.8
Erythropenia 285.9
Erythrophagocytosis 289.9
Erythrophobia 300.23
Erythroplakia
  oral mucosa 528.79
  tongue 528.79
Erythroplasia (Queyrat) (M8080/2)
  specified site — *see* Neoplasm, skin, in situ
  unspecified site 233.5
Erythropoiesis, idiopathic ineffective 285.0
Escaped beats, heart 427.60
  postoperative 997.1
Esoenteritis — *see* Enteritis
Esophagalgia 530.89
Esophagectasis 530.89
  due to cardiospasm 530.0
Esophagismus 530.5
Esophagitis (alkaline) (chemical) (chronic) (infectional) (necrotic) (peptic) (postoperative) (regurgitant) 530.10
  acute 530.12
  candidal 112.84
  reflux 530.11
  specified NEC 530.19
  tuberculous (*see also* Tuberculosis) 017.8
  ulcerative 530.19
Esophagocele 530.6
Esophagodynia 530.89

Esophagomalacia 530.89
Esophagoptosis 530.89
Esophagospasm 530.5
Esophagostenosis 530.3
Esophagostomiasis 127.7
Esophagostomy
  complication 530.87
    infection 530.86
    malfunctioning 530.87
    mechanical 530.87
Esophagotracheal — *see* condition
Esophagus — *see* condition
Esophoria 378.41
  convergence, excess 378.84
  divergence, insufficiency 378.85
Esotropia (nonaccommodative) 378.00
  accommodative 378.35
  alternating 378.05
    with
      A pattern 378.06
      specified noncomitancy NEC 378.08
      V pattern 378.07
      X pattern 378.08
      Y pattern 378.08
    intermittent 378.22
  intermittent 378.20
    alternating 378.22
    monocular 378.21
  monocular 378.01
    with
      A pattern 378.02
      specified noncomitancy NEC 378.04
      V pattern 378.03
      X pattern 378.04
      Y pattern 378.04
    intermittent 378.21
Espundia 085.5
Essential — *see* condition
Esterapenia 289.89
Esthesioneuroblastoma (M9522/3) 160.0
Esthesioneurocytoma (M9521/3) 160.0
Esthesioneuroepithelioma (M9523/3) 160.0
Esthiomene 099.1
Estivo-autumnal
  fever 084.0
  malaria 084.0
Estrangement V61.0
Estriasis 134.0
Ethanolaminuria 270.8
Ethanolism — *see also* Alcoholism 303.9
Ether dependence, dependency — *see also* Dependence 304.6
Etherism — *see also* Dependence 304.6
Ethmoid, ethmoidal — *see* condition
Ethmoiditis (chronic) (nonpurulent) (purulent) — *see also* Sinusitis, ethmoidal 473.2
  influenzal 487.1
  Woakes' 471.1
Ethylism — *see also* Alcoholism 303.9
Eulenburg's disease (congenital paramyotonia) 359.2
Eunuchism 257.2
Eunuchoidism 257.2
  hypogonadotropic 257.2
European blastomycosis 117.5
Eustachian — *see* condition
Euthyroidism 244.9
Euthyroid sick syndrome 790.94
Evaluation
  fetal lung maturity 659.8
  for suspected condition (*see also* Observation) V71.9
    abuse V71.81
    exposure
      anthrax V71.82
      biologic agent NEC V71.83
      SARS V71.83
    neglect V71.81

Evaluation — *continued*
  for suspected condition (*see also* Observation) — *continued*
    newborn — *see* Observation, suspected, condition, newborn
    specified condition NEC V71.89
  mental health V70.2
    requested by authority V70.1
  nursing care V63.8
  social service V63.8
Evans' syndrome (thrombocytopenic purpura) 287.32
Eventration
  colon into chest — *see* Hernia, diaphragm
  diaphragm (congenital) 756.6
Eversion
  bladder 596.8
  cervix (uteri) 622.0
    with mention of cervicitis 616.0
  foot NEC 736.79
    congenital 755.67
  lacrimal punctum 375.51
  punctum lacrimale (postinfectional) (senile) 375.51
  ureter (meatus) 593.89
  urethra (meatus) 599.84
  uterus 618.1
    complicating delivery 665.2
      affecting fetus or newborn 763.89
    puerperal, postpartum 674.8
Evidence
  of malignancy
    cytologic
      without histologic confirmation 795.06
Evisceration
  birth injury 767.8
  bowel (congenital) — *see* Hernia, ventral
  congenital (*see also* Hernia, ventral) 553.29
  operative wound 998.32
  traumatic NEC 869.1
    eye 871.3
Evulsion — *see* Avulsion
Ewing's
  angioendothelioma (M9260/3) — *see* Neoplasm, bone, malignant
  sarcoma (M9260/3) — *see* Neoplasm, bone, malignant
  tumor (M9260/3) — *see* Neoplasm, bone, malignant
Exaggerated lumbosacral angle (with impinging spine) 756.12
Examination (general) (routine) (of) (for) V70.9
  allergy V72.7
  annual V70.0
  cardiovascular preoperative V72.81
  cervical Papanicolaou smear V76.2
    as a part of routine gynecological examination V72.31
    to confirm findings of recent normal smear following initial abnormal smear V72.32
  child care (routine) V20.2
  clinical research investigation (normal control patient) (participant) V70.7
  dental V72.2
  developmental testing (child) (infant) V20.2
  donor (potential) V70.8
  ear V72.19
  eye V72.0
  following
    accident (motor vehicle) V71.4
    alleged rape or seduction (victim or culprit) V71.5
    inflicted injury (victim or culprit) NEC V71.6
    rape or seduction, alleged (victim or culprit) V71.5
    treatment (for) V67.9

Examination — *continued*
  following — *continued*
   treatment — *continued*
    combined V67.6
    fracture V67.4
    involving high-risk medication NEC V67.51
    mental disorder V67.3
    specified condition NEC V67.59
  follow-up (routine) (following) V67.9
   cancer chemotherapy V67.2
   chemotherapy V67.2
   disease NEC V67.59
   high-risk medication NEC V67.51
   injury NEC V67.59
   population survey V70.6
   postpartum V24.2
   psychiatric V67.3
   psychotherapy V67.3
   radiotherapy V67.1
   specified surgery NEC V67.09
   surgery V67.00
    vaginal pap smear V67.01
  gynecological V72.31
   for contraceptive maintenance V25.40
    intrauterine device V25.42
    pill V25.41
    specified method NEC V25.49
  health (of)
   armed forces personnel V70.5
   checkup V70.0
   child, routine V20.2
   defined subpopulation NEC V70.5
   inhabitants of institutions V70.5
   occupational V70.5
   pre-employment screening V70.5
   preschool children V70.5
    for admission to school V70.3
   prisoners V70.5
    for entrance into prison V70.3
   prostitutes V70.5
   refugees V70.5
   school children V70.5
   students V70.5
  hearing V72.19 ▲
   following failed hearing screening ● V72.11 ●
  infant V20.2
  laboratory V72.6
  lactating mother V24.1
  medical (for) (of) V70.9
   administrative purpose NEC V70.3
   admission to
    old age home V70.3
    prison V70.3
    school V70.3
   adoption V70.3
   armed forces personnel V70.5
   at health care facility V70.0
   camp V70.3
   child, routine V20.2
   clinical research (control) (normal comparison) (participant) V70.7
   defined subpopulation NEC V70.5
   donor (potential) V70.8
   driving license V70.3
   general V70.9
    routine V70.0
    specified reason NEC V70.8
   immigration V70.3
   inhabitants of institutions V70.5
   insurance certification V70.3
   marriage V70.3
   medicolegal reasons V70.4
   naturalization V70.3
   occupational V70.5
   population survey V70.6
   pre-employment V70.5
   preschool children V70.5
    for admission to school V70.3
   prison V70.3
   prisoners V70.5
    for entrance into prison V70.3
   prostitutes V70.5

Examination — *continued*
  medical — *continued*
   refugees V70.5
   school children V70.5
   specified reason NEC V70.8
   sport competition V70.3
   students V70.5
  medicolegal reason V70.4
  pelvic (annual) (periodic) V72.31
  periodic (annual) (routine) V70.0
  postpartum
   immediately after delivery V24.0
   routine follow-up V24.2
  pregnancy (unconfirmed) (possible) V72.40
   negative result V72.41
   positive result V72.42
  prenatal V22.1
   first pregnancy V22.0
   high-risk pregnancy V23.9
    specified problem NEC V23.89
  preoperative V72.84
   cardiovascular V72.81
   respiratory V72.82
   specified NEC V72.83
  preprocedural V72.84
   cardiovascular V72.81
   general physical V72.83
   respiratory V72.82
   specified NEC V72.83
  psychiatric V70.2
   follow-up not needing further care V67.3
   requested by authority V70.1
  radiological NEC V72.5
  respiratory preoperative V72.82
  screening — *see* Screening
  sensitization V72.7
  skin V72.7
   hypersensitivity V72.7
  special V72.9
  specified type or reason NEC V72.85
   preoperative V72.83
   specified NEC V72.83
  teeth V72.2
  vaginal Papanicolaou smear V76.47
   following hysterectomy for malignant condition V67.01
  victim or culprit following
   alleged rape or seduction V71.5
   inflicted injury NEC V71.6
  vision V72.0
  well baby V20.2
Exanthem, exanthema — *see also* Rash 782.1
  Boston 048
  epidemic, with meningitis 048
  lichenoid psoriasiform 696.2
  subitum 057.8
  viral, virus NEC 057.9
   specified type NEC 057.8
Excess, excessive, excessively
  alcohol level in blood 790.3
  carbohydrate tissue, localized 278.1
  carotene (dietary) 278.3
  cold 991.9
   specified effect NEC 991.8
  convergence 378.84
  crying 780.95
   of
    adolescent 780.95 ●
    adult 780.95 ●
    baby 780.92 ●
    child 780.95 ●
    infant (baby) 780.92 ●
    newborn 780.92 ●
  development, breast 611.1
  diaphoresis (*see also* Hyperhidrosis) 780.8
  distance, interarch 524.28
  divergence 378.85
  drinking (alcohol) NEC (*see also* Abuse, drugs, nondependent) 305.0 ☑
   continual (*see also* Alcoholism) 303.9 ☑

Excess, excessive, excessively — *continued*
  drinking (*see also* Abuse, drugs, nondependent) — *continued*
   habitual (*see also* Alcoholism) 303.9 ☑
  eating 783.6
  eyelid fold (congenital) 743.62
  fat 278.02
   in heart (*see also* Degeneration, myocardial) 429.1
   tissue, localized 278.1
  foreskin 605
  gas 787.3
  gastrin 251.5
  glucagon 251.4
  heat (*see also* Heat) 992.9
  horizontal
   overjet 524.26 ●
   overlap 524.26 ●
  interarch distance 524.28
  intermaxillary vertical dimension 524.37 ●
  interocclusal distance of teeth 524.37
  large
   colon 564.7
    congenital 751.3
   fetus or infant 766.0
    with obstructed labor 660.1 ☑
     affecting management of pregnancy 656.6 ☑
    causing disproportion 653.5 ☑
    newborn (weight of 4500 grams or more) 766.0
   organ or site, congenital NEC — *see* Anomaly, specified type NEC
  lid fold (congenital) 743.62
  long
   colon 751.5
   organ or site, congenital NEC — *see* Anomaly, specified type NEC
   umbilical cord (entangled)
    affecting fetus or newborn 762.5
    in pregnancy or childbirth 663.3 ☑
     with compression 663.2 ☑
  menstruation 626.2
  number of teeth 520.1
   causing crowding 524.31
  nutrients (dietary) NEC 783.6
  potassium (K) 276.7
  salivation (*see also* Ptyalism) 527.7
  secretion (*see also* Hypersecretion)
   milk 676.6 ☑
   sputum 786.4
   sweat (*see also* Hyperhidrosis) 780.8
  short
   organ or site, congenital NEC — *see* Anomaly, specified type NEC
   umbilical cord
    affecting fetus or newborn 762.6
    in pregnancy or childbirth 663.4 ☑
  skin NEC 701.9
   eyelid 743.62
    acquired 374.30
  sodium (Na) 276.0
  spacing of teeth 524.32
  sputum 786.4
  sweating (*see also* Hyperhidrosis) 780.8
  tearing (ducts) (eye) (*see also* Epiphora) 375.20
  thirst 783.5
   due to deprivation of water 994.3
  tuberosity 524.07
  vitamin
   A (dietary) 278.2
    administered as drug (chronic) (prolonged excessive intake) 278.2

Excess, excessive, excessively — *continued*
  vitamin — *continued*
   A — *continued*
    administered as drug — *continued*
     reaction to sudden overdose 963.5
   D (dietary) 278.4
    administered as drug (chronic) (prolonged excessive intake) 278.4
    reaction to sudden overdose 963.5
  weight 278.02
   gain 783.1
    of pregnancy 646.1 ☑
   loss 783.21
Excitability, abnormal, under minor stress 309.29
Excitation
  catatonic (*see also* Schizophrenia) 295.2 ☑
  psychogenic 298.1
  reactive (from emotional stress, psychological trauma) 298.1
Excitement
  manic (*see also* Psychosis, affective) 296.0 ☑
   recurrent episode 296.1 ☑
   single episode 296.0 ☑
  mental, reactive (from emotional stress, psychological trauma) 298.1
  state, reactive (from emotional stress, psychological trauma) 298.1
Excluded pupils 364.76
Excoriation (traumatic) — *see also* Injury, superficial, by site 919.8
  neurotic 698.4
Excyclophoria 378.44
Excyclotropia 378.33
Exencephalus, exencephaly 742.0
Exercise
  breathing V57.0
  remedial NEC V57.1
  therapeutic NEC V57.1
Exfoliation, teeth due to systemic causes 525.0
Exfoliative — *see also* condition
  dermatitis 695.89
Exhaustion, exhaustive (physical NEC) 780.79
  battle (*see also* Reaction, stress, acute) 308.9
  cardiac (*see also* Failure, heart) 428.9
  delirium (*see also* Reaction, stress, acute) 308.9
  due to
   cold 991.8
   excessive exertion 994.5
   exposure 994.4
  fetus or newborn 779.89
  heart (*see also* Failure, heart) 428.9
  heat 992.5
   due to
    salt depletion 992.4
    water depletion 992.3
  manic (*see also* Psychosis, affective) 296.0 ☑
   recurrent episode 296.1 ☑
   single episode 296.0 ☑
  maternal, complicating delivery 669.8 ☑
   affecting fetus or newborn 763.89
  mental 300.5
  myocardium, myocardial (*see also* Failure, heart) 428.9
  nervous 300.5
  old age 797
  postinfectional NEC 780.79
  psychogenic 300.5
  psychosis (*see also* Reaction, stress, acute) 308.9
  senile 797
   dementia 290.0

Index to Diseases

Exhibitionism

Exhibitionism (sexual) 302.4
Exomphalos 756.79
Exophoria 378.42
  convergence, insufficiency 378.83
  divergence, excess 378.85
Exophthalmic
  cachexia 242.0 ☑
  goiter 242.0 ☑
  ophthalmoplegia 242.0 ☑ [376.22]
Exophthalmos 376.30
  congenital 743.66
  constant 376.31
  endocrine NEC 259.9 [376.22]
  hyperthyroidism 242.0 ☑ [376.21]
  intermittent NEC 376.34
  malignant 242.0 ☑ [376.21]
  pulsating 376.35
    endocrine NEC 259.9 [376.22]
  thyrotoxic 242.0 ☑ [376.21]
Exostosis 726.91
  cartilaginous (M9210/0) — see Neoplasm, bone, benign
  congenital 756.4
  ear canal, external 380.81
  gonococcal 098.89
  hip 726.5
  intracranial 733.3
  jaw (bone) 526.81
  luxurians 728.11
  multiple (cancellous) (congenital) (hereditary) 756.4
  nasal bones 726.91
  orbit, orbital 376.42
  osteocartilaginous (M9210/0) — see Neoplasm, bone, benign
  spine 721.8
    with spondylosis — see Spondylosis
  syphilitic 095.5
  wrist 726.4
Exotropia 378.10
  alternating 378.15
    with
      A pattern 378.16
      specified noncomitancy NEC 378.18
      V pattern 378.17
      X pattern 378.18
      Y pattern 378.18
    intermittent 378.24
  intermittent 378.20
    alternating 378.24
    monocular 378.23
  monocular 378.11
    with
      A pattern 378.12
      specified noncomitancy NEC 378.14
      V pattern 378.13
      X pattern 378.14
      Y pattern 378.14
    intermittent 378.23
Explanation of
  investigation finding V65.4 ☑
  medication V65.4 ☑
Exposure 994.9
  cold 991.9
    specified effect NEC 991.8
  effects of 994.9
  exhaustion due to 994.4
  to
    AIDS virus V01.79
    anthrax V01.81
    asbestos V15.84
    body fluids (hazardous) V15.85
    cholera V01.0
    communicable disease V01.9
      specified type NEC V01.89
    Escherichia coli (E. coli) V01.83
    German measles V01.4
    gonorrhea V01.6
    hazardous body fluids V15.85
    HIV V01.79
    human immunodeficiency virus V01.79
    lead V15.86

Exposure — continued
  to — continued
    meningococcus V01.84
    parasitic disease V01.89
    poliomyelitis V01.2
    potentially hazardous body fluids V15.85
    rabies V01.5
    rubella V01.4
    SARS-associated coronavirus V01.82
    smallpox V01.3
    syphilis V01.6
    tuberculosis V01.1
    varicella V01.71
    venereal disease V01.6
    viral disease NEC V01.79
      varicella V01.71
Exsanguination, fetal 772.0
Exstrophy
  abdominal content 751.8
  bladder (urinary) 753.5
Extensive — see condition
Extra — see also Accessory
  rib 756.3
    cervical 756.2
Extraction
  with hook 763.89
  breech NEC 669.6 ☑
    affecting fetus or newborn 763.0
  cataract postsurgical V45.61
  manual NEC 669.8 ☑
    affecting fetus or newborn 763.89
Extrasystole 427.60
  atrial 427.61
  postoperative 997.1
  ventricular 427.69
Extrauterine gestation or pregnancy — see Pregnancy, ectopic
Extravasation
  blood 459.0
    lower extremity 459.0
  chyle into mesentery 457.8
  pelvicalyceal 593.4
  pyelosinus 593.4
  urine 788.8
    from ureter 788.8
Extremity — see condition
Extrophy — see Exstrophy
Extroversion
  bladder 753.5
  uterus 618.1
    complicating delivery 665.2 ☑
      affecting fetus or newborn 763.89
    postpartal (old) 618.1
Extruded tooth 524.34 •
Extrusion
  alveolus and teeth 524.75
  breast implant (prosthetic) 996.54
  device, implant, or graft — see Complications, mechanical
  eye implant (ball) (globe) 996.59
  intervertebral disc — see Displacement, intervertebral disc
  lacrimal gland 375.43
  mesh (reinforcing) 996.59
  ocular lens implant 996.53
  prosthetic device NEC — see Complications, mechanical
  vitreous 379.26
Exudate, pleura — see Effusion, pleura
Exudates, retina 362.82
Exudative — see condition
Eye, eyeball, eyelid — see condition
Eyestrain 368.13
Eyeworm disease of Africa 125.2

F

Faber's anemia or syndrome (achlorhydric anemia) 280.9
Fabry's disease (angiokeratoma corporis diffusum) 272.7
Face, facial — see condition
Facet of cornea 371.44

Faciocephalalgia, autonomic — see also Neuropathy, peripheral, autonomic 337.9
Facioscapulohumeral myopathy 359.1
Factitious disorder, illness — see Illness, factitious
Factor
  deficiency — see Deficiency, factor
  psychic, associated with diseases classified elsewhere 316
  risk — see Problem
Fahr-Volhard disease (malignant nephrosclerosis) 403.00
Failure, failed
  adenohypophyseal 253.2
  attempted abortion (legal) (see also Abortion, failed) 638.9
  bone marrow (anemia) 284.9
    acquired (secondary) 284.8
    congenital 284.09 ▲
    idiopathic 284.9
  cardiac (see also Failure, heart) 428.9
    newborn 779.89
  cardiorenal (chronic) 428.9
    hypertensive (see also Hypertension, cardiorenal) 404.93
  cardiorespiratory 799.1
    specified during or due to a procedure 997.1
    long-term effect of cardiac surgery 429.4
  cardiovascular (chronic) 428.9
  cerebrovascular 437.8
  cervical dilatation in labor 661.0 ☑
    affecting fetus or newborn 763.7
  circulation, circulatory 799.89
    fetus or newborn 779.89
    peripheral 785.50
  compensation — see Disease, heart
  congestive (see also Failure, heart) 428.0
  coronary (see also Insufficiency, coronary) 411.89
  dental restoration •
    marginal integrity 525.61 •
    periodontal anatomical integrity • 525.65
  descent of head (at term) 652.5 ☑
    affecting fetus or newborn 763.1
    in labor 660.0 ☑
  device, implant, or graft — see Complications, mechanical
  engagement of head NEC 652.5 ☑
    in labor 660.0 ☑
  extrarenal 788.9
  fetal head to enter pelvic brim 652.5 ☑
    affecting fetus or newborn 763.1
    in labor 660.0 ☑
      affecting fetus or newborn 763.1
  forceps NEC 660.7 ☑
    affecting fetus or newborn 763.1
  fusion (joint) (spinal) 996.49
  growth in childhood 783.43
  heart (acute) (sudden) 428.9
    with
      abortion — see Abortion, by type, with specified complication NEC
      acute pulmonary edema (see also Failure, ventricular, left) 428.1
        with congestion (see also Failure, heart) 428.0
      decompensation (see also Failure, heart) 428.0
      dilation — see Disease, heart
      ectopic pregnancy (see also categories 633.0–633.9) 639.8
      molar pregnancy (see also categories 630–632) 639.8
    arteriosclerotic 440.9
    combined left-right sided 428.0

Failure, failed — continued
  heart — continued
    combined systolic and diastolic 428.40
      acute 428.41
      acute on chronic 428.43
      chronic 428.42
    compensated (see also Failure, heart) 428.0
    complicating
      abortion — see Abortion, by type, with specified complication NEC
      delivery (cesarean) (instrumental) 669.4 ☑
      ectopic pregnancy (see also categories 633.0–633.9) 639.8
      molar pregnancy (see also categories 630–632) 639.8
      obstetric anesthesia or sedation 668.1 ☑
      surgery 997.1
    congestive (compensated) (decompensated) (see also Failure, heart) 428.0
      with rheumatic fever (conditions classifiable to 390)
        active 391.8
        inactive or quiescent (with chorea) 398.91
      fetus or newborn 779.89
      hypertensive (see also Hypertension, heart) 402.91
        with renal disease (see also Hypertension, cardiorenal) 404.91
        with renal failure 404.93
        benign 402.11
        malignant 402.01
      rheumatic (chronic) (inactive) (with chorea) 398.91
        active or acute 391.8
          with chorea (Sydenham's) 392.0
    decompensated (see also Failure, heart) 428.0
    degenerative (see also Degeneration, myocardial) 429.1
    diastolic 428.30
      acute 428.31
      acute on chronic 428.33
      chronic 428.32
    due to presence of (cardiac) prosthesis 429.4
    fetus or newborn 779.89
    following
      abortion 639.8
      cardiac surgery 429.4
      ectopic or molar pregnancy 639.8
    high output NEC 428.9
    hypertensive (see also Hypertension, heart) 402.91
      with renal disease (see also Hypertension, cardiorenal) 404.91
      with renal failure 404.93
      benign 402.11
      malignant 402.01
    left (ventricular) (see also Failure, ventricular, left) 428.1
      with right-sided failure (see also Failure, heart) 428.0
    low output (syndrome) NEC 428.9
    organic — see Disease, heart
    postoperative (immediate) 997.1
      long term effect of cardiac surgery 429.4
    rheumatic (chronic) (congestive) (inactive) 398.91
    right (secondary to left heart failure, conditions classifiable to 428.1) (ventricular) (see also Failure, heart) 428.0
  senile 797

Index to Diseases

Failure, failed — *continued*
  heart — *continued*
    specified during or due to a procedure 997.1
      long-term effect of cardiac surgery 429.4
    systolic 428.20
      acute 428.21
      acute on chronic 428.23
      chronic 428.22
    thyrotoxic (*see also* Thyrotoxicosis) 242.9 ☑ [425.7]
    valvular — *see* Endocarditis
  hepatic 572.8
    acute 570
    due to a procedure 997.4
  hepatorenal 572.4
  hypertensive heart (*see also* Hypertension, heart) 402.91
    benign 402.11
    malignant 402.01
  induction (of labor) 659.1 ☑
    abortion (legal) (*see also* Abortion, failed) 638.9
    affecting fetus or newborn 763.89
    by oxytocic drugs 659.1 ☑
    instrumental 659.0 ☑
    mechanical 659.0 ☑
    medical 659.1 ☑
    surgical 659.0 ☑
  initial alveolar expansion, newborn 770.4
  involution, thymus (gland) 254.8
  kidney — *see* Failure, renal
  lactation 676.4 ☑
  Leydig's cell, adult 257.2
  liver 572.8
    acute 570
  medullary 799.89
  mitral — *see* Endocarditis, mitral
  myocardium, myocardial (*see also* Failure, heart) 428.9
    chronic (*see also* Failure, heart) 428.0
    congestive (*see also* Failure, heart) 428.0
  ovarian (primary) 256.39
    iatrogenic 256.2
    postablative 256.2
    postirradiation 256.2
    postsurgical 256.2
  ovulation 628.0
  prerenal 788.9
  renal 586
    with
      abortion — *see* Abortion, by type, with renal failure
      ectopic pregnancy (*see also* categories 633.0–633.9) 639.3
      edema (*see also* Nephrosis) 581.9
      hypertension (*see also* Hypertension, kidney) 403.91
      hypertensive heart disease (conditions classifiable to 402) 404.92
        with heart failure 404.93
        benign 404.12
          with heart failure 404.13
        malignant 404.02
          with heart failure 404.03
      molar pregnancy (*see also* categories 630–632) 639.3
      tubular necrosis (acute) 584.5
    acute 584.9
      with lesion of
        necrosis
          cortical (renal) 584.6
          medullary (renal) (papillary) 584.7
          tubular 584.5
      specified pathology NEC 584.8
    chronic 585.9

Failure, failed — *continued*
  renal — *continued*
    chronic — *continued*
      hypertensive or with hypertension (*see also* Hypertension, kidney) 403.91
    due to a procedure 997.5
    following
      abortion 639.3
      crushing 958.5
      ectopic or molar pregnancy 639.3
      labor and delivery (acute) 669.3 ☑
    hypertensive (*see also* Hypertension, kidney) 403.91
    puerperal, postpartum 669.3 ☑
  respiration, respiratory 518.81
    acute 518.81
    acute and chronic 518.84
    center 348.8
      newborn 770.84
    chronic 518.83
    due to trauma, surgery or shock 518.5
    newborn 770.84
  rotation
    cecum 751.4
    colon 751.4
    intestine 751.4
    kidney 753.3
  segmentation (*see also* Fusion)
    fingers (*see also* Syndactylism, fingers) 755.11
    toes (*see also* Syndactylism, toes) 755.13
  seminiferous tubule, adult 257.2
  senile (general) 797
    with psychosis 290.20
  testis, primary (seminal) 257.2
  to progress 661.2 ☑
  to thrive
    adult 783.7
    child 783.41
  transplant 996.80
    bone marrow 996.85
    organ (immune or nonimmune cause) 996.80
      bone marrow 996.85
      heart 996.83
      intestines 996.87
      kidney 996.81
      liver 996.82
      lung 996.84
      pancreas 996.86
      specified NEC 996.89
    skin 996.52
      artificial 996.55
      decellularized allodermis 996.55
      temporary allograft or pigskin graft — omit code
  trial of labor NEC 660.6 ☑
    affecting fetus or newborn 763.1
  tubal ligation 998.89
  urinary 586
  vacuum extraction
    abortion — *see* Abortion, failed
    delivery NEC 660.7 ☑
      affecting fetus or newborn 763.1
  vasectomy 998.89
  ventouse NEC 660.7 ☑
    affecting fetus or newborn 763.1
  ventricular (*see also* Failure, heart) 428.9
    left 428.1
      with rheumatic fever (conditions classifiable to 390)
        active 391.8
          with chorea 392.0
        inactive or quiescent (with chorea) 398.91
      hypertensive (*see also* Hypertension, heart) 402.91
        benign 402.11
        malignant 402.01

Failure, failed — *continued*
  ventricular (*see also* Failure, heart) — *continued*
    left — *continued*
      rheumatic (chronic) (inactive) (with chorea) 398.91
        active or acute 391.8
          with chorea 392.0
    right (*see also* Failure, heart) 428.0
  vital centers, fetus or newborn 779.89
  weight gain in childhood 783.41
Fainting (fit) (spell) 780.2
Falciform hymen 752.49
Fallen arches 734
Falling, any organ or part — *see* Prolapse
Fall, maternal, affecting fetus or newborn 760.5
Fallopian
  insufflation
    fertility testing V26.21
    following sterilization reversal V26.22
  tube — *see* condition
Fallot's
  pentalogy 745.2
  tetrad or tetralogy 745.2
  triad or trilogy 746.09
Fallout, radioactive (adverse effect) NEC 990
False — *see also* condition
  bundle branch block 426.50
  bursa 727.89
  croup 478.75
  joint 733.82
  labor (pains) 644.1 ☑
  opening, urinary, male 752.69
  passage, urethra (prostatic) 599.4
  positive
    serological test for syphilis 795.6
    Wassermann reaction 795.6
  pregnancy 300.11
Family, familial — *see also* condition
  disruption V61.0
  hemophagocytic
    lymphohistiocytosis 288.4 ●
    reticulosis 288.4 ●
  Li-Fraumeni (syndrome) V84.01
  planning advice V25.09
  problem V61.9
    specified circumstance NEC V61.8
  retinoblastoma (syndrome) 190.5
Famine 994.2
  edema 262
Fanconi's anemia (congenital pancytopenia) 284.09 ▲
Fanconi (-de Toni) (-Debré) syndrome (cystinosis) 270.0
Farber (-Uzman) syndrome or disease (disseminated lipogranulomatosis) 272.8
Farcin 024
Farcy 024
Farmers'
  lung 495.0
  skin 692.74
Farsightedness 367.0
Fascia — *see* condition
Fasciculation 781.0
Fasciculitis optica 377.32
Fasciitis 729.4
  eosinophilic 728.89
  necrotizing 728.86
  nodular 728.79
  perirenal 593.4
  plantar 728.71
  pseudosarcomatous 728.79
  traumatic (old) NEC 728.79
    current — *see* Sprain, by site
Fasciola hepatica infestation 121.3
Fascioliasis 121.3
Fasciolopsiasis (small intestine) 121.4
Fasciolopsis (small intestine) 121.4
Fast pulse 785.0

Fat
  embolism (cerebral) (pulmonary) (systemic) 958.1
    with
      abortion — *see* Abortion, by type, with embolism
      ectopic pregnancy (*see also* categories 633.0–633.9) 639.6
      molar pregnancy (*see also* categories 630–632) 639.6
      complicating delivery or puerperium 673.8 ☑
    following
      abortion 639.6
      ectopic or molar pregnancy 639.6
    in pregnancy, childbirth, or the puerperium 673.8 ☑
  excessive 278.02
    in heart (*see also* Degeneration, myocardial) 429.1
  general 278.02
  hernia, herniation 729.30
    eyelid 374.34
    knee 729.31
    orbit 374.34
    retro-orbital 374.34
    retropatellar 729.31
    specified site NEC 729.39
  indigestion 579.8
  in stool 792.1
  localized (pad) 278.1
    heart (*see also* Degeneration, myocardial) 429.1
    knee 729.31
    retropatellar 729.31
  necrosis (*see also* Fatty, degeneration)
    breast (aseptic) (segmental) 611.3
    mesentery 567.82
    omentum 567.82
    peritoneum 567.82
  pad 278.1
Fatal syncope 798.1
Fatigue 780.79
  auditory deafness (*see also* Deafness) 389.9
  chronic, syndrome 780.71
  combat (*see also* Reaction, stress, acute) 308.9
  during pregnancy 646.8 ☑
  general 780.79
    psychogenic 300.5
  heat (transient) 992.6
  muscle 729.89
  myocardium (*see also* Failure, heart) 428.9
  nervous 300.5
  neurosis 300.5
  operational 300.89
  postural 729.89
  posture 729.89
  psychogenic (general) 300.5
  senile 797
  syndrome NEC 300.5
    chronic 780.71
  undue 780.79
  voice 784.49
Fatness 278.02
Fatty — *see also* condition
  apron 278.1
  degeneration (diffuse) (general) NEC 272.8
    localized — *see* Degeneration, by site, fatty
    placenta — *see* Placenta, abnormal
  heart (enlarged) (*see also* Degeneration, myocardial) 429.1
  infiltration (diffuse) (general) (*see also* Degeneration, by site, fatty) 272.8
    heart (enlarged) (*see also* Degeneration, myocardial) 429.1
  liver 571.8
    alcoholic 571.0
  necrosis — *see* Degeneration, fatty

Fatty — see also condition — continued
  phanerosis 272.8
Fauces — see condition
Fauchard's disease (periodontitis) 523.40
Faucitis 478.29
Faulty — see also condition
  position of teeth 524.30
Favism (anemia) 282.2
Favre-Racouchot disease (elastoidosis cutanea nodularis) 701.8
Favus 110.9
  beard 110.0
  capitis 110.0
  corporis 110.5
  eyelid 110.8
  foot 110.4
  hand 110.2
  scalp 110.0
  specified site NEC 110.8
Feared complaint unfounded V65.5
Fear, fearfulness (complex) (reaction) 300.20
  child 313.0
  of
    animals 300.29
    closed spaces 300.29
    crowds 300.29
    eating in public 300.23
    heights 300.29
    open spaces 300.22
      with panic attacks 300.21
    public speaking 300.23
    streets 300.22
      with panic attacks 300.21
    travel 300.22
      with panic attacks 300.21
    washing in public 300.23
  transient 308.0
Febricula (continued) (simple) — see also Pyrexia 780.6
Febrile — see also Pyrexia 780.6
  convulsion ▶(simple)◀ 780.31
    complex 780.32 •
  seizure ▶(simple)◀ 780.31
    atypical 780.32 •
    complex 780.32 •
    complicated 780.32 •
Febris — see also Fever 780.6
  aestiva (see also Fever, hay) 477.9
  flava (see also Fever, yellow) 060.9
  melitensis 023.0
  pestis (see also Plague) 020.9
  puerperalis 672.0 ☑
  recurrens (see also Fever, relapsing) 087.9
  pediculo vestimenti 087.0
  rubra 034.1
  typhoidea 002.0
  typhosa 002.0
Fecal — see condition
Fecalith (impaction) 560.39
  with hernia (see also Hernia, by site, with obstruction)
    gangrenous — see Hernia, by site, with gangrene
  appendix 543.9
  congenital 777.1
Fede's disease 529.0
Feeble-minded 317
Feeble rapid pulse due to shock following injury 958.4
Feeding
  faulty (elderly) (infant) 783.3
    newborn 779.3
  formula check V20.2
  improper (elderly) (infant) 783.3
    newborn 779.3
  problem (elderly) (infant) 783.3
    newborn 779.3
    nonorganic origin 307.59
Feer's disease 985.0
Feet — see condition
Feigned illness V65.2

Feil-Klippel syndrome (brevicollis) 756.16
Feinmesser's (hidrotic) **ectodermal dysplasia** 757.31
Felix's disease (juvenile osteochondrosis, hip) 732.1
Felon (any digit) (with lymphangitis) 681.01
  herpetic 054.6
Felty's syndrome (rheumatoid arthritis with splenomegaly and leukopenia) 714.1
Feminism in boys 302.6
Feminization, testicular 259.5
  with pseudohermaphroditism, male 259.5
Femoral hernia — see Hernia, femoral
Femora vara 736.32
Femur, femoral — see condition
Fenestrata placenta — see Placenta, abnormal
Fenestration, fenestrated — see also Imperfect, closure
  aorta-pulmonary 745.0
  aorticopulmonary 745.0
  aortopulmonary 745.0
  cusps, heart valve NEC 746.89
    pulmonary 746.09
  hymen 752.49
  pulmonic cusps 746.09
Fenwick's disease 537.89
Fermentation (gastric) (gastrointestinal) (stomach) 536.8
  intestine 564.89
  psychogenic 306.4
  psychogenic 306.4
Fernell's disease (aortic aneurysm) 441.9
Fertile eunuch syndrome 257.2
Fertility, meaning multiparity — see Multiparity
Fetal alcohol syndrome 760.71
Fetalis uterus 752.3
Fetid
  breath 784.99 ▲
  sweat 705.89
Fetishism 302.81
  transvestic 302.3
Fetomaternal hemorrhage
  affecting management of pregnancy 656.0 ☑
  fetus or newborn 772.0
Fetus, fetal — see also condition
  papyraceous 779.89
  type lung tissue 770.4
Fever 780.6
  with chills 780.6
    in malarial regions (see also Malaria) 084.6
  abortus NEC 023.9
  aden 061
  African tick-borne 087.1
  American
    mountain tick 066.1
    spotted 082.0
  and ague (see also Malaria) 084.6
  aphthous 078.4
  arbovirus hemorrhagic 065.9
  Assam 085.0
  Australian A or Q 083.0
  Bangkok hemorrhagic 065.4
  biliary, Charcôt's intermittent — see Choledocholithiasis
  bilious, hemoglobinuric 084.8
  blackwater 084.8
  blister 054.9
  Bonvale Dam 780.79
  boutonneuse 082.1
  brain 323.9
    late effect — see category 326
  breakbone 061
  Bullis 082.8
  Bunyamwera 066.3
  Burdwan 085.0
  Bwamba (encephalitis) 066.3
  Cameroon (see also Malaria) 084.6

Fever — continued
  Canton 081.9
  catarrhal (acute) 460
    chronic 472.0
  cat-scratch 078.3
  cerebral 323.9
    late effect — see category 326
  cerebrospinal (meningococcal) (see also Meningitis, cerebrospinal) 036.0
  Chagres 084.0
  Chandipura 066.8
  changuinola 066.0
  Charcôt's (biliary) (hepatic) (intermittent) — see Choledocholithiasis
  Chikungunya (viral) 066.3
    hemorrhagic 065.4
  childbed 670.0 ☑
  Chitral 066.0
  Colombo (see also Fever, paratyphoid) 002.9
  Colorado tick (virus) 066.1
  congestive
    malarial (see also Malaria) 084.6
    remittent (see also Malaria) 084.6
  Congo virus 065.0
  continued 780.6
    malarial 084.0
  Corsican (see also Malaria) 084.6
  Crimean hemorrhagic 065.0
  Cyprus (see also Brucellosis) 023.9
  dandy 061
  deer fly (see also Tularemia) 021.9
  dehydration, newborn 778.4
  dengue (virus) 061
    hemorrhagic 065.4
  desert 114.0
  due to heat 992.0
  Dumdum 085.0
  enteric 002.0
  ephemeral (of unknown origin) (see also Pyrexia) 780.6
  epidemic, hemorrhagic of the Far East 065.0
  erysipelatous (see also Erysipelas) 035
  estivo-autumnal (malarial) 084.0
  etiocholanolone 277.31 ▲
  famine (see also Fever, relapsing)
    meaning typhus — see Typhus
  Far Eastern hemorrhagic 065.0
  five day 083.1
  Fort Bragg 100.89
  gastroenteric 002.0
  gastromalarial (see also Malaria) 084.6
  Gibraltar (see also Brucellosis) 023.9
  glandular 075
  Guama (viral) 066.3
  Haverhill 026.1
  hay (allergic) (with rhinitis) 477.9
    with
      asthma (bronchial) (see also Asthma) 493.0 ☑
      due to
        dander, animal (cat) (dog) 477.2
        dust 477.8
        fowl 477.8
        hair, animal (cat) (dog) 477.2
        pollen, any plant or tree 477.0
        specified allergen other than pollen 477.8
  heat (effects) 992.0
  hematuric, bilious 084.8
  hemoglobinuric (malarial) 084.8
    bilious 084.8
  hemorrhagic (arthropod-borne) NEC 065.9
    with renal syndrome 078.6
    arenaviral 078.7
    Argentine 078.7
    Bangkok 065.4
    Bolivian 078.7
    Central Asian 065.0
    chikungunya 065.4
    Crimean 065.0
    dengue (virus) 065.4
    Ebola 065.8

Fever — continued
  hemorrhagic — continued
    epidemic 078.6
    of Far East 065.0
    Far Eastern 065.0
    Junin virus 078.7
    Korean 078.6
    Kyasanur forest 065.2
    Machupo virus 078.7
    mite-borne NEC 065.8
    mosquito-borne 065.4
    Omsk 065.1
    Philippine 065.4
    Russian (Yaroslav) 078.6
    Singapore 065.4
    Southeast Asia 065.4
    Thailand 065.4
    tick-borne NEC 065.3
  hepatic (see also Cholecystitis) 575.8
    intermittent (Charcôt's) — see Choledocholithiasis
  herpetic (see also Herpes) 054.9
  Hyalomma tick 065.0
  icterohemorrhagic 100.0
  inanition 780.6
    newborn 778.4
  infective NEC 136.9
  intermittent (bilious) (see also Malaria) 084.6
    hepatic (Charcôt) — see Choledocholithiasis
    of unknown origin (see also Pyrexia) 780.6
    pernicious 084.0
  iodide
    correct substance properly administered 780.6
    overdose or wrong substance given or taken 975.5
  Japanese river 081.2
  jungle yellow 060.0
  Junin virus, hemorrhagic 078.7
  Katayama 120.2
  Kedani 081.2
  Kenya 082.1
  Korean hemorrhagic 078.6
  Lassa 078.89
  Lone Star 082.8
  lung — see Pneumonia
  Machupo virus, hemorrhagic 078.7
  malaria, malarial (see also Malaria) 084.6
  Malta (see also Brucellosis) 023.9
  Marseilles 082.1
  marsh (see also Malaria) 084.6
  Mayaro (viral) 066.3
  Mediterranean (see also Brucellosis) 023.9
    familial 277.31 ▲
    tick 082.1
  meningeal — see Meningitis
  metal fumes NEC 985.8
  Meuse 083.1
  Mexican — see Typhus, Mexican
  Mianeh 087.1
  miasmatic (see also Malaria) 084.6
  miliary 078.2
  milk, female 672.0 ☑
  mill 504
  mite-borne hemorrhagic 065.8
  Monday 504
  mosquito-borne NEC 066.3
    hemorrhagic NEC 065.4
  mountain 066.1
    meaning
      Rocky Mountain spotted 082.0
      undulant fever (see also Brucellosis) 023.9
    tick (American) 066.1
  Mucambo (viral) 066.3
  mud 100.89
  Neapolitan (see also Brucellosis) 023.9
  neutropenic 288.00 ▲
  nine-mile 083.0
  nonexanthematous tick 066.1
  North Asian tick-borne typhus 082.2

Fever — *continued*
 Omsk hemorrhagic 065.1
 O'nyong-nyong (viral) 066.3
 Oropouche (viral) 066.3
 Oroya 088.0
 paludal (*see also* Malaria) 084.6
 Panama 084.0
 pappataci 066.0
 paratyphoid 002.9
  A 002.1
  B (Schottmüller's) 002.2
  C (Hirschfeld) 002.3
 parrot 073.9
 periodic 277.31 ▲
 pernicious, acute 084.0
 persistent (of unknown origin) (*see also* Pyrexia) 780.6
 petechial 036.0
 pharyngoconjunctival 077.2
  adenoviral type 3 077.2
 Philippine hemorrhagic 065.4
 phlebotomus 066.0
 Piry 066.8
 Pixuna (viral) 066.3
 Plasmodium ovale 084.3
 pleural (*see also* Pleurisy) 511.0
 pneumonic — *see* Pneumonia
 polymer fume 987.8
 postoperative 998.89
  due to infection 998.59
 pretibial 100.89
 puerperal, postpartum 672.0 ☑
 putrid — *see* Septicemia
 pyemic — *see* Septicemia
 Q 083.0
  with pneumonia 083.0 [484.8]
 quadrilateral 083.0
 quartan (malaria) 084.2
 Queensland (coastal) 083.0
  seven-day 100.89
 Quintan (A) 083.1
 quotidian 084.0
 rabbit (*see also* Tularemia) 021.9
 rat-bite 026.9
  due to
   Spirillum minor or minus 026.0
   Spirochaeta morsus muris 026.0
   Streptobacillus moniliformis 026.1
 recurrent — *see* Fever, relapsing
 relapsing 087.9
  Carter's (Asiatic) 087.0
  Dutton's (West African) 087.1
  Koch's 087.9
  louse-borne (epidemic) 087.0
  Novy's (American) 087.1
  Obermeyer's (European) 087.0
  spirillum NEC 087.9
  tick-borne (endemic) 087.1
 remittent (bilious) (congestive) (gastric) (*see also* Malaria) 084.6
 rheumatic (active) (acute) (chronic) (subacute) 390
  with heart involvement 391.9
   carditis 391.9
   endocarditis (aortic) (mitral) (pulmonary) (tricuspid) 391.1
   multiple sites 391.8
   myocarditis 391.2
   pancarditis, acute 391.8
   pericarditis 391.0
   specified type NEC 391.8
   valvulitis 391.1
  cardiac hypertrophy 398.99
  inactive or quiescent
   with cardiac hypertrophy 398.99
   carditis 398.90
   endocarditis 397.9
    aortic (valve) 395.9
     with mitral (valve) disease 396.9
    mitral (valve) 394.9

Fever — *continued*
 rheumatic — *continued*
  inactive or quiescent — *continued*
   endocarditis — *continued*
    mitral — *continued*
     with aortic (valve) disease 396.9
     pulmonary (valve) 397.1
     tricuspid (valve) 397.0
    heart conditions (classifiable to 429.3, 429.6, 429.9) 398.99
     failure (congestive) (conditions classifiable to 428.0, 428.9) 398.91
     left ventricular failure (conditions classifiable to 428.1) 398.91
     myocardial degeneration (conditions classifiable to 429.1) 398.0
     myocarditis (conditions classifiable to 429.0) 398.0
    pancarditis 398.99
    pericarditis 393
 Rift Valley (viral) 066.3
 Rocky Mountain spotted 082.0
 rose 477.0
 Ross river (viral) 066.3
 Russian hemorrhagic 078.6
 sandfly 066.0
 San Joaquin (valley) 114.0
 São Paulo 082.0
 scarlet 034.1
 septic — *see* Septicemia
 seven-day 061
  Japan 100.89
  Queensland 100.89
 shin bone 083.1
 Singapore hemorrhagic 065.4
 solar 061
 sore 054.9
 South African tick-bite 087.1
 Southeast Asia hemorrhagic 065.4
 spinal — *see* Meningitis
 spirillary 026.0
 splenic (*see also* Anthrax) 022.9
 spotted (Rocky Mountain) 082.0
  American 082.0
  Brazilian 082.0
  Colombian 082.0
  meaning
   cerebrospinal meningitis 036.0
   typhus 082.9
 spring 309.23
 steroid
  correct substance properly administered 780.2
  overdose or wrong substance given or taken 962.0
 streptobacillary 026.1
 subtertian 084.0
 Sumatran mite 081.2
 sun 061
 swamp 100.89
 sweating 078.2
 swine 003.8
 sylvatic yellow 060.0
 Tahyna 062.5
 tertian — *see* Malaria, tertian
 Thailand hemorrhagic 065.4
 thermic 992.0
 three day 066.0
  with Coxsackie exanthem 074.8
 tick
  American mountain 066.1
  Colorado 066.1
  Kemerovo 066.1
  Mediterranean 082.1
  mountain 066.1
  nonxanthematous 066.1
  Quaranfil 066.1
 tick-bite NEC 066.1
 tick-borne NEC 066.1
  hemorrhagic NEC 065.3

Fever — *continued*
 transitory of newborn 778.4
 trench 083.1
 tsutsugamushi 081.2
 typhogastric 002.0
 typhoid (abortive) (ambulant) (any site) (hemorrhagic) (infection) (intermittent) (malignant) (rheumatic) 002.0
 typhomalarial (*see also* Malaria) 084.6
 typhus — *see* Typhus
 undulant (*see also* Brucellosis) 023.9
 unknown origin (*see also* Pyrexia) 780.6
 uremic — *see* Uremia
 uveoparotid 135
 valley (Coccidioidomycosis) 114.0
 Venezuelan equine 066.2
 Volhynian 083.1
 Wesselsbron (viral) 066.3
 West
  African 084.8
  Nile (viral) 066.40
   with
    cranial nerve disorders 066.42
    encephalitis 066.41
    optic neuritis 066.42
    other complications 066.49
    other neurologic manifestations 066.42
    polyradiculitis 066.42
 Whitmore's 025
 Wolhynian 083.1
 worm 128.9
 Yaroslav hemorrhagic 078.6
 yellow 060.9
  jungle 060.0
  sylvatic 060.0
  urban 060.1
  vaccination, prophylactic (against) V04.4
 Zika (viral) 066.3
Fibrillation
 atrial (established) (paroxysmal) 427.31
 auricular (atrial) (established) 427.31
 cardiac (ventricular) 427.41
 coronary (*see also* Infarct, myocardium) 410.9 ☑
 heart (ventricular) 427.41
 muscular 728.9
 postoperative 997.1
 ventricular 427.41
Fibrin
 ball or bodies, pleural (sac) 511.0
 chamber, anterior (eye) (gelatinous exudate) 364.04
Fibrinogenolysis (hemorrhagic) — *see* Fibrinolysis
Fibrinogenopenia (congenital) (hereditary) — *see also* Defect, coagulation 286.3
 acquired 286.6
Fibrinolysis (acquired) (hemorrhagic) (pathologic) 286.6
 with
  abortion — *see* Abortion, by type, with hemorrhage, delayed or excessive
  ectopic pregnancy (*see also* categories 633.0–633.9) 639.1
  molar pregnancy (*see also* categories 630–632) 639.1
 antepartum or intrapartum 641.3 ☑
  affecting fetus or newborn 762.1
 following
  abortion 639.1
  ectopic or molar pregnancy 639.1
 newborn, transient 776.2
 postpartum 666.3 ☑
Fibrinopenia (hereditary) — *see also* Defect, coagulation 286.3
 acquired 286.6
Fibrinopurulent — *see* condition
Fibrinous — *see* condition

Fibroadenoma (M9010/0)
 cellular intracanalicular (M9020/0) 217
 giant (intracanalicular) (M9020/0) 217
 intracanalicular (M9011/0)
  cellular (M9020/0) 217
  giant (M9020/0) 217
  specified site — *see* Neoplasm, by site, benign
  unspecified site 217
 juvenile (M9030/0) 217
 pericanicular (M9012/0)
  specified site — *see* Neoplasm, by site, benign
  unspecified site 217
 phyllodes (M9020/0) 217
 prostate 600.20
  with
   other lower urinary tract symptoms (LUTS) 600.21 ●
   urinary
    obstruction 600.21 ●
    retention 600.21 ●
 specified site — *see* Neoplasm, by site, benign
 unspecified site 217
Fibroadenosis, breast (chronic) (cystic) (diffuse) (periodic) (segmental) 610.2
Fibroangioma (M9160/0) — *see also* Neoplasm, by site, benign
 juvenile (M9160/0)
  specified site — *see* Neoplasm, by site, benign
  unspecified site 210.7
Fibrocellulitis progressiva ossificans 728.11
Fibrochondrosarcoma (M9220/3) — *see* Neoplasm, cartilage, malignant
Fibrocystic
 disease 277.00
  bone NEC 733.29
  breast 610.1
  jaw 526.2
  kidney (congenital) 753.19
  liver 751.62
  lung 518.89
   congenital 748.4
  pancreas 277.00
  kidney (congenital) 753.19
Fibrodysplasia ossificans multiplex (progressiva) 728.11
Fibroelastosis (cordis) (endocardial) (endomyocardial) 425.3
Fibroid (tumor) (M8890/0) — *see also* Neoplasm, connective tissue, benign
 disease, lung (chronic) (*see also* Fibrosis, lung) 515
 heart (disease) (*see also* Myocarditis) 429.0
 induration, lung (chronic) (*see also* Fibrosis, lung) 515
 in pregnancy or childbirth 654.1 ☑
  affecting fetus or newborn 763.89 ☑
  causing obstructed labor 660.2 ☑
   affecting fetus or newborn 763.1
 liver — *see* Cirrhosis, liver
 lung (*see also* Fibrosis, lung) 515
 pneumonia (chronic) (*see also* Fibrosis, lung) 515
 uterus (M8890/0) (*see also* Leiomyoma, uterus) 218.9
Fibrolipoma (M8851/0) — *see also* Lipoma, by site 214.9
Fibroliposarcoma (M8850/3) — *see* Neoplasm, connective tissue, malignant
Fibroma (M8810/0) — *see also* Neoplasm, connective tissue, benign
 ameloblastic (M9330/0) 213.1
  upper jaw (bone) 213.0
 bone (nonossifying) 733.99
  ossifying (M9262/0) — *see* Neoplasm, bone, benign

Fibroma

Fibroma — see also Neoplasm, connective tissue, benign — continued
- cementifying (M9274/0) — see Neoplasm, bone, benign
- chondromyxoid (M9241/0) — see Neoplasm, bone, benign
- desmoplastic (M8823/1) — see Neoplasm, connective tissue, uncertain behavior
- facial (M8813/0) — see Neoplasm, connective tissue, benign
- invasive (M8821/1) — see Neoplasm, connective tissue, uncertain behavior
- molle (M8851/0) (see also Lipoma, by site) 214.9
- myxoid (M8811/0) — see Neoplasm, connective tissue, benign
- nasopharynx, nasopharyngeal (juvenile) (M9160/0) 210.7
- nonosteogenic (nonossifying) — see Dysplasia, fibrous
- odontogenic (M9321/0) 213.1
  - upper jaw (bone) 213.0
- ossifying (M9262/0) — see Neoplasm, bone, benign
- periosteal (M8812/0) — see Neoplasm, bone, benign
- prostate 600.20
  - with
    - other lower urinary tract symptoms (LUTS) 600.21
    - urinary
      - obstruction 600.21
      - retention 600.21
- soft (M8851/0) (see also Lipoma, by site) 214.9

Fibromatosis 728.79
- abdominal (M8822/1) — see Neoplasm, connective tissue, uncertain behavior
- aggressive (M8821/1) — see Neoplasm, connective tissue, uncertain behavior
- congenital generalized (CGF) 759.89
- Dupuytren's 728.6
- gingival 523.8
- plantar fascia 728.71
- proliferative 728.79
- pseudosarcomatous (proliferative) (subcutaneous) 728.79
- subcutaneous pseudosarcomatous (proliferative) 728.79

Fibromyalgia 729.1

Fibromyoma (M8890/0) — see also Neoplasm, connective tissue, benign
- uterus (corpus) (see also Leiomyoma, uterus) 218.9
  - in pregnancy or childbirth 654.1
    - affecting fetus or newborn 763.89
    - causing obstructed labor 660.2
      - affecting fetus or newborn 763.1

Fibromyositis — see also Myositis 729.1
- scapulohumeral 726.2

Fibromyxolipoma (M8852/0) — see also Lipoma, by site 214.9

Fibromyxoma (M8811/0) — see Neoplasm, connective tissue, benign

Fibromyxosarcoma (M8811/3) — see Neoplasm, connective tissue, malignant

Fibro-odontoma, ameloblastic (M9290/0) 213.1
- upper jaw (bone) 213.0

Fibro-osteoma (M9262/0) — see Neoplasm, bone, benign

Fibroplasia, retrolental 362.21

Fibropurulent — see condition

Fibrosarcoma (M8810/3) — see also Neoplasm, connective tissue, malignant
- ameloblastic (M9330/3) 170.1
  - upper jaw (bone) 170.0
- congenital (M8814/3) — see Neoplasm, connective tissue, malignant
- fascial (M8813/3) — see Neoplasm, connective tissue, malignant
- infantile (M8814/3) — see Neoplasm, connective tissue, malignant
- odontogenic (M9330/3) 170.1
  - upper jaw (bone) 170.0
- periosteal (M8812/3) — see Neoplasm, bone, malignant

Fibrosclerosis
- breast 610.3
- corpora cavernosa (penis) 607.89
- familial multifocal NEC 710.8
- multifocal (idiopathic) NEC 710.8
- penis (corpora cavernosa) 607.89

Fibrosis, fibrotic
- adrenal (gland) 255.8
- alveolar (diffuse) 516.3
- amnion 658.8
- anal papillae 569.49
- anus 569.49
- appendix, appendiceal, noninflammatory 543.9
- arteriocapillary — see Arteriosclerosis
- bauxite (of lung) 503
- biliary 576.8
  - due to Clonorchis sinensis 121.1
- bladder 596.8
  - interstitial 595.1
  - localized submucosal 595.1
  - panmural 595.1
- bone, diffuse 756.59
- breast 610.3
- capillary (see also Arteriosclerosis)
  - lung (chronic) (see also Fibrosis, lung) 515
- cardiac (see also Myocarditis) 429.0
- cervix 622.8
- chorion 658.8
- corpus cavernosum 607.89
- cystic (of pancreas) 277.00
  - with
    - manifestations
      - gastrointestinal 277.03
      - pulmonary 277.02
      - specified NEC 277.09
      - meconium ileus 277.01
      - pulmonary exacerbation 277.02
- due to (presence of) any device, implant, or graft — see Complications, due to (presence of) any device, implant, or graft classified to 996.0–996.5 NEC
- ejaculatory duct 608.89
- endocardium (see also Endocarditis) 424.90
- endomyocardial (African) 425.0
- epididymis 608.89
- eye muscle 378.62
- graphite (of lung) 503
- heart (see also Myocarditis) 429.0
- hepatic (see also Cirrhosis, liver)
  - due to Clonorchis sinensis 121.1
- hepatolienal — see Cirrhosis, liver
- hepatosplenic — see Cirrhosis, liver
- infrapatellar fat pad 729.31
- interstitial pulmonary, newborn 770.7
- intrascrotal 608.89
- kidney (see also Sclerosis, renal) 587
- liver — see Cirrhosis, liver
- lung (atrophic) (capillary) (chronic) (confluent) (massive) (perialveolar) (peribronchial) 515
  - with
    - anthracosilicosis (occupational) 500
    - anthracosis (occupational) 500
    - asbestosis (occupational) 501
    - bagassosis (occupational) 495.1

Fibrosis, fibrotic — continued
- lung — continued
  - with — continued
    - bauxite 503
    - berylliosis (occupational) 503
    - byssinosis (occupational) 504
    - calcicosis (occupational) 502
    - chalicosis (occupational) 502
    - dust reticulation (occupational) 504
    - farmers' lung 495.0
    - gannister disease (occupational) 502
    - graphite 503
    - pneumoconiosis (occupational) 505
    - pneumosiderosis (occupational) 503
    - siderosis (occupational) 503
    - silicosis (occupational) 502
    - tuberculosis (see also Tuberculosis) 011.4
  - diffuse (idiopathic) (interstitial) 516.3
  - due to
    - bauxite 503
    - fumes or vapors (chemical) (inhalation) 506.4
    - graphite 503
  - following radiation 508.1
  - postinflammatory 515
  - silicotic (massive) (occupational) 502
  - tuberculous (see also Tuberculosis) 011.4
- lymphatic gland 289.3
- median bar 600.90
  - with
    - other lower urinary tract symptoms (LUTS) 600.91
    - urinary
      - obstruction 600.91
      - retention 600.91
- mediastinum (idiopathic) 519.3
- meninges 349.2
- muscle NEC 728.2
  - iatrogenic (from injection) 999.9
- myocardium, myocardial (see also Myocarditis) 429.0
- oral submucous 528.8
- ovary 620.8
- oviduct 620.8
- pancreas 577.8
  - cystic 277.00
    - with
      - manifestations
        - gastrointestinal 277.03
        - pulmonary 277.02
        - specified NEC 277.09
        - meconium ileus 277.01
        - pulmonary exacerbation 277.02
- penis 607.89
- periappendiceal 543.9
- periarticular (see also Ankylosis) 718.5
- pericardium 423.1
- perineum, in pregnancy or childbirth 654.8
  - affecting fetus or newborn 763.89
  - causing obstructed labor 660.2
    - affecting fetus or newborn 763.1
- perineural NEC 355.9
  - foot 355.6
- periureteral 593.89
- placenta — see Placenta, abnormal
- pleura 511.0
- popliteal fat pad 729.31
- preretinal 362.56
- prostate (chronic) 600.90
  - with
    - other lower urinary tract symptoms (LUTS) 600.91

Fibrosis, fibrotic — continued
- prostate — continued
  - with — continued
    - urinary
      - obstruction 600.91
      - retention 600.91
- pulmonary (chronic) (see also Fibrosis, lung) 515
  - alveolar capillary block 516.3
  - interstitial
    - diffuse (idiopathic) 516.3
    - newborn 770.7
  - radiation — see Effect, adverse, radiation
- rectal sphincter 569.49
- retroperitoneal, idiopathic 593.4
- sclerosing mesenteric (idiopathic) 567.82
- scrotum 608.89
- seminal vesicle 608.89
- senile 797
- skin NEC 709.2
- spermatic cord 608.89
- spleen 289.59
  - bilharzial (see also Schistosomiasis) 120.9
- subepidermal nodular (M8832/0) — see Neoplasm, skin, benign
- submucous NEC 709.2
  - oral 528.8
  - tongue 528.8
- syncytium — see Placenta, abnormal
- testis 608.89
  - chronic, due to syphilis 095.8
- thymus (gland) 254.8
- tunica vaginalis 608.89
- ureter 593.89
- urethra 599.84
- uterus (nonneoplastic) 621.8
  - bilharzial (see also Schistosomiasis) 120.9
  - neoplastic (see also Leiomyoma, uterus) 218.9
- vagina 623.8
- valve, heart (see also Endocarditis) 424.90
- vas deferens 608.89
- vein 459.89
  - lower extremities 459.89
- vesical 595.1

Fibrositis (periarticular) (rheumatoid) 729.6
- humeroscapular region 726.2
- nodular, chronic
  - Jaccoud's 714.4
  - rheumatoid 714.4
- ossificans 728.11
- scapulohumeral 726.2

Fibrothorax 511.0

Fibrotic — see Fibrosis

Fibrous — see condition

Fibroxanthoma (M8831/0) — see also Neoplasm, connective tissue, benign
- atypical (M8831/1) — see Neoplasm, connective tissue, uncertain behavior
- malignant (M8831/3) — see Neoplasm, connective tissue, malignant

Fibroxanthosarcoma (M8831/3) — see Neoplasm, connective tissue, malignant

Fiedler's
- disease (leptospiral jaundice) 100.0
- myocarditis or syndrome (acute isolated myocarditis) 422.91

Fiessinger-Leroy (-Reiter) syndrome 099.3

Fiessinger-Rendu syndrome (erythema multiforme exudativum) 695.1

Fifth disease (eruptive) 057.0
- venereal 099.1

Filaria, filarial — see Infestation, filarial

Filariasis — see also Infestation, filarial 125.9

Index to Diseases

Filariasis — see also Infestation, filarial — continued
- bancroftian 125.0
- Brug's 125.1
- due to
  - bancrofti 125.0
  - Brugia (Wuchereria) (malayi) 125.1
  - Loa loa 125.2
  - malayi 125.1
  - organism NEC 125.6
  - Wuchereria (bancrofti) 125.0
    - malayi 125.1
- Malayan 125.1
- ozzardi 125.5
- specified type NEC 125.6

Filatoff's, Filatov's, Filatow's disease (infectious mononucleosis) 075

File-cutters' disease 984.9
- specified type of lead — see Table of Drugs and Chemicals

Filling defect
- biliary tract 793.3
- bladder 793.5
- duodenum 793.4
- gallbladder 793.3
- gastrointestinal tract 793.4
- intestine 793.4
- kidney 793.5
- stomach 793.4
- ureter 793.5

Filtering bleb, eye (postglaucoma) (status) V45.69
- with complication or rupture 997.99
- postcataract extraction (complication) 997.99

Fimbrial cyst (congenital) 752.11
Fimbriated hymen 752.49
Financial problem affecting care V60.2

Findings, abnormal, without diagnosis (examination) (laboratory test) 796.4
- 17-ketosteroids, elevated 791.9
- acetonuria 791.6
- acid phosphatase 790.5
- albumin-globulin ratio 790.99
- albuminuria 791.0
- alcohol in blood 790.3
- alkaline phosphatase 790.5
- amniotic fluid 792.3
- amylase 790.5
- anisocytosis 790.09
- antenatal screening 796.5
- anthrax, positive 795.31
- antibody titers, elevated 795.79
- anticardiolipin antibody 795.79
- antigen-antibody reaction 795.79
- antiphospholipid antibody 795.79
- bacteriuria 791.9
- ballistocardiogram 794.39
- bicarbonate 276.9
- bile in urine 791.4
- bilirubin 277.4
- bleeding time (prolonged) 790.92
- blood culture, positive 790.7
- blood gas level (arterial) 790.91
- blood sugar level 790.29
  - high 790.29
    - fasting glucose 790.21
    - glucose tolerance test 790.22
  - low 251.2
- calcium 275.40
- cancer antigen 125 [CA 125] 795.82 ●
- carbonate 276.9
- carcinoembryonic antigen [CEA] ●
  - 795.81 ●
- casts, urine 791.7
- catecholamines 791.9
- cells, urine 791.7
- cerebrospinal fluid (color) (content) (pressure) 792.0
- cervical
  - high risk human papillomavirus (HPV) DNA test positive 795.05

Findings, abnormal, without diagnosis — continued
- cervical — continued
  - low risk human papillomavirus (HPV) DNA test positive 795.09
- chloride 276.9
- cholesterol 272.9
- chromosome analysis 795.2
- chyluria 791.1
- circulation time 794.39
- cloudy dialysis effluent 792.5
- cloudy urine 791.9
- coagulation study 790.92
- cobalt, blood 790.6
- color of urine (unusual) NEC 791.9
- copper, blood 790.6
- C-reactive protein (CRP) 790.95
- crystals, urine 791.9
- culture, positive NEC 795.39
  - blood 790.7
  - HIV V08
  - human immunodeficiency virus V08
  - nose 795.39
  - skin lesion NEC 795.39
  - spinal fluid 792.0
  - sputum 795.39
  - stool 792.1
  - throat 795.39
  - urine 791.9
  - viral
    - human immunodeficiency V08
  - wound 795.39
- echocardiogram 793.2
- echoencephalogram 794.01
- echogram NEC — see Findings, abnormal, structure
- electrocardiogram (ECG) (EKG) 794.31
- electroencephalogram (EEG) 794.02
- electrolyte level, urinary 791.9
- electromyogram (EMG) 794.17
  - ocular 794.14
- electro-oculogram (EOG) 794.12
- electroretinogram (ERG) 794.11
- enzymes, serum NEC 790.5
- fibrinogen titer coagulation study 790.92
- filling defect — see Filling defect
- function study NEC 794.9
  - auditory 794.15
  - bladder 794.9
  - brain 794.00
  - cardiac 794.30
  - endocrine NEC 794.6
    - thyroid 794.5
  - kidney 794.4
  - liver 794.8
  - nervous system
    - central 794.00
    - peripheral 794.19
    - oculomotor 794.14
  - pancreas 794.9
  - placenta 794.9
  - pulmonary 794.2
  - retina 794.11
  - special senses 794.19
  - spleen 794.9
  - vestibular 794.16
- gallbladder, nonvisualization 793.3
- glucose 790.29
  - elevated
    - fasting 790.21
    - tolerance test 790.22
- glycosuria 791.5
- heart
  - shadow 793.2
  - sounds 785.3
- hematinuria 791.2
- hematocrit
  - drop (precipitous) 790.01
  - elevated 282.7
  - low 285.9
- hematologic NEC 790.99
- hematuria 599.7

Findings, abnormal, without diagnosis — continued
- hemoglobin
  - elevated 282.7
  - low 285.9
- hemoglobinuria 791.2
- histological NEC 795.4
- hormones 259.9
- immunoglobulins, elevated 795.79
- indolacetic acid, elevated 791.9
- iron 790.6
- karyotype 795.2
- ketonuria 791.6
- lactic acid dehydrogenase (LDH) 790.4
- lead 790.6 ●
- lipase 790.5
- lipids NEC 272.9
- lithium, blood 790.6
- liver function test 790.6
- lung field (coin lesion) (shadow) 793.1
- magnesium, blood 790.6
- mammogram 793.80
  - calcification 793.89 ●
  - calculus 793.89 ●
  - microcalcification 793.81
- mediastinal shift 793.2
- melanin, urine 791.9
- microbiologic NEC 795.39
- mineral, blood NEC 790.6
- myoglobinuria 791.3
- nasal swab, anthrax 795.31
- neonatal screening 796.6
- nitrogen derivatives, blood 790.6
- nonvisualization of gallbladder 793.3
- nose culture, positive 795.39
- odor of urine (unusual) NEC 791.9
- oxygen saturation 790.91
- Papanicolaou (smear) 795.1
  - cervix 795.00
    - with
      - atypical squamous cells
        - cannot exclude high grade squamous intraepithelial lesion (ASC-H) 795.02
        - of undetermined significance (ASC-US) 795.01
      - cytologic evidence of malignancy 795.06 ●
      - high grade squamous intraepithelial lesion (HGSIL) 795.04
      - low grade squamous intraepithelial lesion (LGSIL) 795.03
    - dyskaryotic 795.09
    - nonspecific finding NEC 795.09
  - other site 795.1
- peritoneal fluid 792.9
- phonocardiogram 794.39
- phosphorus 275.3
- pleural fluid 792.9
- pneumoencephalogram 793.0
- PO$_2$-oxygen ratio 790.91
- poikilocytosis 790.09
- potassium
  - deficiency 276.8
  - excess 276.7
- PPD 795.5
- prostate specific antigen (PSA) 790.93
- protein, serum NEC 790.99
- proteinuria 791.0
- prothrombin time (partial) (prolonged) (PT) (PTT) 790.92
- pyuria 791.9
- radiologic (x-ray) 793.99 ▲
  - abdomen 793.6
  - biliary tract 793.3
  - breast 793.89
    - abnormal mammogram NOS 793.80
    - mammographic
      - calcification 793.89 ●
      - calculus 793.89 ●
      - microcalcification 793.81 ●

Findings, abnormal, without diagnosis — continued
- radiologic — continued
  - gastrointestinal tract 793.4
  - genitourinary organs 793.5
  - head 793.0
  - image test inconclusive due to ●
    - excess body fat 793.91 ●
  - intrathoracic organs NEC 793.2
  - lung 793.1
  - musculoskeletal 793.7
  - placenta 793.99 ▲
  - retroperitoneum 793.6
  - skin 793.99 ▲
  - skull 793.0
  - subcutaneous tissue 793.99 ▲
- red blood cell 790.09
  - count 790.09
  - morphology 790.09
  - sickling 790.09
  - volume 790.09
- saliva 792.4
- scan NEC 794.9
  - bladder 794.9
  - bone 794.9
  - brain 794.09
  - kidney 794.4
  - liver 794.8
  - lung 794.2
  - pancreas 794.9
  - placental 794.9
  - spleen 794.9
  - thyroid 794.5
- sedimentation rate, elevated 790.1
- semen 792.2
- serological (for)
  - human immunodeficiency virus (HIV)
    - inconclusive 795.71
    - positive V08
  - syphilis — see Findings, serology for syphilis
- serology for syphilis
  - false positive 795.6
  - positive 097.1
    - false 795.6
    - follow-up of latent syphilis — see Syphilis, latent
    - only finding — see Syphilis, latent
- serum 790.99
  - blood NEC 790.99
  - enzymes NEC 790.5
  - proteins 790.99
- SGOT 790.4
- SGPT 790.4
- sickling of red blood cells 790.09
- skin test, positive 795.79
  - tuberculin (without active tuberculosis) 795.5
- sodium 790.6
  - deficiency 276.1
  - excess 276.0
- spermatozoa 792.2
- spinal fluid 792.0
  - culture, positive 792.0
- sputum culture, positive 795.39
  - for acid-fast bacilli 795.39
- stool NEC 792.1
  - bloody 578.1
  - occult 792.1
  - color 792.1
  - culture, positive 792.1
  - occult blood 792.1
- stress test 794.39
- structure, body (echogram) (thermogram) (ultrasound) (x-ray) NEC 793.99 ▲
  - abdomen 793.6
  - breast 793.89
    - abnormal mammogram 793.80
    - mammographic
      - calcification 793.89 ●
      - calculus 793.89 ●
      - microcalcification 793.81 ●
  - gastrointestinal tract 793.4

Findings, abnormal, without diagnosis

Findings, abnormal, without diagnosis — *continued*
  structure, body — *continued*
    genitourinary organs 793.5
    head 793.0
      echogram (ultrasound) 794.01
    intrathoracic organs NEC 793.2
    lung 793.1
    musculoskeletal 793.7
    placenta 793.99 ▲
    retroperitoneum 793.6
    skin 793.99 ▲
    subcutaneous tissue NEC 793.99 ▲
  synovial fluid 792.9
  thermogram — *see* Findings, abnormal, structure
  throat culture, positive 795.39
  thyroid (function) 794.5
    metabolism (rate) 794.5
    scan 794.5
    uptake 794.5
  total proteins 790.99
  toxicology (drugs) (heavy metals) 796.0
  transaminase (level) 790.4
  triglycerides 272.9
  tuberculin skin test (without active tuberculosis) 795.5
  tumor markers NEC 795.89 ●
  ultrasound (*see also* Findings, abnormal, structure)
    cardiogram 793.2
  uric acid, blood 790.6
  urine, urinary constituents 791.9
    acetone 791.6
    albumin 791.0
    bacteria 791.9
    bile 791.4
    blood 599.7
    casts or cells 791.7
    chyle 791.1
    culture, positive 791.9
    glucose 791.5
    hemoglobin 791.2
    ketone 791.6
    protein 791.0
    pus 791.9
    sugar 791.5
  vaginal fluid 792.9
  vanillylmandelic acid, elevated 791.9
  vectorcardiogram (VCG) 794.39
  ventriculogram (cerebral) 793.0
  VMA, elevated 791.9
  Wassermann reaction
    false positive 795.6
    positive 097.1
      follow-up of latent syphilis — *see* Syphilis, latent
      only finding — *see* Syphilis, latent
  white blood cell 288.9
    count 288.9
      elevated 288.60 ▲
      low 288.50 ▲
    differential 288.9
    morphology 288.9
  wound culture 795.39
  xerography 793.89
  zinc, blood 790.6
Finger — *see* condition
Fire, St. Anthony's — *see also* Erysipelas 035
Fish
  hook stomach 537.89
  meal workers' lung 495.8
Fisher's syndrome 357.0
Fissure, fissured
  abdominal wall (congenital) 756.79
  anus, anal 565.0
    congenital 751.5
  buccal cavity 528.9
  clitoris (congenital) 752.49
  ear, lobule (congenital) 744.29
  epiglottis (congenital) 748.3
  larynx 478.79
    congenital 748.3

Fissure, fissured — *continued*
  lip 528.5
    congenital (*see also* Cleft, lip) 749.10
  nipple 611.2
    puerperal, postpartum 676.1 ☑
  palate (congenital) (*see also* Cleft, palate) 749.00
  postanal 565.0
  rectum 565.0
  skin 709.8
    streptococcal 686.9
  spine (congenital) (*see also* Spina bifida) 741.9 ☑
  sternum (congenital) 756.3
  tongue (acquired) 529.5
  tuberculous 750.13
Fistula (sinus) 686.9
  abdomen (wall) 569.81
    bladder 596.2
    intestine 569.81
    ureter 593.82
    uterus 619.2
  abdominorectal 569.81
  abdominosigmoidal 569.81
  abdominothoracic 510.0
  abdominouterine 619.2
    congenital 752.3
  abdominovesical 596.2
  accessory sinuses (*see also* Sinusitis) 473.9
  actinomycotic — *see* Actinomycosis
  alveolar
    antrum (*see also* Sinusitis, maxillary) 473.0
    process 522.7
  anorectal 565.1
  antrobuccal (*see also* Sinusitis, maxillary) 473.0
  antrum (*see also* Sinusitis, maxillary) 473.0
  anus, anal (infectional) (recurrent) 565.1
    congenital 751.5
    tuberculous (*see also* Tuberculosis) 014.8 ☑
  aortic sinus 747.29
  aortoduodenal 447.2
  appendix, appendicular 543.9
  arteriovenous (acquired) 447.0
    brain 437.3
      congenital 747.81
        ruptured (*see also* Hemorrhage, subarachnoid) 430
      ruptured (*see also* Hemorrhage, subarachnoid) 430
    cerebral 437.3
      congenital 747.81
    congenital (peripheral) 747.60
      brain — *see* Fistula, arteriovenous, brain, congenital
      coronary 746.85
      gastrointestinal 747.61
      lower limb 747.64
      pulmonary 747.3
      renal 747.62
      specified site NEC 747.69
      upper limb 747.63
    coronary 414.19
      congenital 746.85
    heart 414.19
    pulmonary (vessels) 417.0
      congenital 747.3
    surgically created (for dialysis) V45.1
      complication NEC 996.73
        atherosclerosis — *see* Arteriosclerosis, extremities
        embolism 996.74
        infection or inflammation 996.62
        mechanical 996.1
        occlusion NEC 996.74
        thrombus 996.74

Fistula — *continued*
  arteriovenous — *continued*
    traumatic — *see* Injury, blood vessel, by site
  artery 447.2
  aural 383.81
    congenital 744.49
  auricle 383.81
    congenital 744.49
  Bartholin's gland 619.8
  bile duct (*see also* Fistula, biliary) 576.4
  biliary (duct) (tract) 576.4
    congenital 751.69
  bladder (neck) (sphincter) 596.2
    into seminal vesicle 596.2
  bone 733.99
  brain 348.8
    arteriovenous — *see* Fistula, arteriovenous, brain
  branchial (cleft) 744.41
  branchiogenous 744.41
  breast 611.0
    puerperal, postpartum 675.1 ☑
  bronchial 510.0
  bronchocutaneous, bronchomediastinal, bronchopleural, bronchopleuromediastinal (infective) 510.0
    tuberculous (*see also* Tuberculosis) 011.3 ☑
  bronchoesophageal 530.89
    congenital 750.3
  buccal cavity (infective) 528.3
  canal, ear 380.89
  carotid-cavernous
    congenital 747.81
      with hemorrhage 430
    traumatic 900.82
      with hemorrhage (*see also* Hemorrhage, brain, traumatic) 853.0 ☑
      late effect 908.3
  cecosigmoidal 569.81
  cecum 569.81
  cerebrospinal (fluid) 349.81
  cervical, lateral (congenital) 744.41
  cervicoaural (congenital) 744.49
  cervicosigmoidal 619.1
  cervicovesical 619.0
  cervix 619.8
  chest (wall) 510.0
  cholecystocolic (*see also* Fistula, gallbladder) 575.5
  cholecystocolonic (*see also* Fistula, gallbladder) 575.5
  cholecystoduodenal (*see also* Fistula, gallbladder) 575.5
  cholecystoenteric (*see also* Fistula, gallbladder) 575.5
  cholecystogastric (*see also* Fistula, gallbladder) 575.5
  cholecystointestinal (*see also* Fistula, gallbladder) 575.5
  choledochoduodenal 576.4
  cholocolic (*see also* Fistula, gallbladder) 575.5
  coccyx 685.1
    with abscess 685.0
  colon 569.81
  colostomy 569.69
  colovaginal (acquired) 619.1
  common duct (bile duct) 576.4
  congenital, NEC — *see* Anomaly, specified type NEC
  cornea, causing hypotony 360.32
  coronary, arteriovenous 414.19
    congenital 746.85
  costal region 510.0
  cul-de-sac, Douglas' 619.8
  cutaneous 686.9
  cystic duct (*see also* Fistula, gallbladder) 575.5
    congenital 751.69
  dental 522.7
  diaphragm 510.0

Fistula — *continued*
  diaphragm — *continued*
    bronchovisceral 510.0
    pleuroperitoneal 510.0
    pulmonoperitoneal 510.0
  duodenum 537.4
  ear (canal) (external) 380.89
  enterocolic 569.81
  enterocutaneous 569.81
  enteroenteric 569.81
  entero-uterine 619.1
    congenital 752.3
  enterovaginal 619.1
    congenital 752.49
  enterovesical 596.1
  epididymis 608.89
    tuberculous (*see also* Tuberculosis) 016.4 ☑
  esophagobronchial 530.89
    congenital 750.3
  esophagocutaneous 530.89
  esophagopleurocutaneous 530.89
  esophagotracheal 530.84
    congenital 750.3
  esophagus 530.89
    congenital 750.4
  ethmoid (*see also* Sinusitis, ethmoidal) 473.2
  eyeball (cornea) (sclera) 360.32
  eyelid 373.11
  fallopian tube (external) 619.2
  fecal 569.81
    congenital 751.5
    from periapical lesion 522.7
  frontal sinus (*see also* Sinusitis, frontal) 473.1
  gallbladder 575.5
    with calculus, cholelithiasis, stones (*see also* Cholelithiasis) 574.2 ☑
    congenital 751.69
  gastric 537.4
  gastrocolic 537.4
    congenital 750.7
    tuberculous (*see also* Tuberculosis) 014.8 ☑
  gastroenterocolic 537.4
  gastroesophageal 537.4
  gastrojejunal 537.4
  gastrojejunocolic 537.4
  genital
    organs
      female 619.9
        specified site NEC 619.8
      male 608.89
    tract-skin (female) 619.2
  hepatopleural 510.0
  hepatopulmonary 510.0
  horseshoe 565.1
  ileorectal 569.81
  ileosigmoidal 569.81
  ileostomy 569.69
  ileovesical 596.1
  ileum 569.81
  in ano 565.1
    tuberculous (*see also* Tuberculosis) 014.8 ☑
  inner ear (*see also* Fistula, labyrinth) 386.40
  intestine 569.81
  intestinocolonic (abdominal) 569.81
  intestinoureteral 593.82
  intestinouterine 619.1
  intestinovaginal 619.1
    congenital 752.49
  intestinovesical 596.1
  involving female genital tract 619.9
    digestive-genital 619.1
    genital tract-skin 619.2
    specified site NEC 619.8
    urinary-genital 619.0
  ischiorectal (fossa) 566
  jejunostomy 569.69
  jejunum 569.81
  joint 719.80
    ankle 719.87

Index to Diseases

Fistula — *continued*
  joint — *continued*
    elbow 719.82
    foot 719.87
    hand 719.84
    hip 719.85
    knee 719.86
    multiple sites 719.89
    pelvic region 719.85
    shoulder (region) 719.81
    specified site NEC 719.88
    tuberculous — *see* Tuberculosis, joint
    wrist 719.83
  kidney 593.89
  labium (majus) (minus) 619.8
  labyrinth, labyrinthine NEC 386.40
    combined sites 386.48
    multiple sites 386.48
    oval window 386.42
    round window 386.41
    semicircular canal 386.43
  lacrimal, lachrymal (duct) (gland) (sac) 375.61
  lacrimonasal duct 375.61
  laryngotracheal 748.3
  larynx 478.79
  lip 528.5
    congenital 750.25
  lumbar, tuberculous (*see also* Tuberculosis) 015.0 ☑ *[730.8]* ☑
  lung 510.0
  lymphatic (node) (vessel) 457.8
  mamillary 611.0
  mammary (gland) 611.0
    puerperal, postpartum 675.1 ☑
  mastoid (process) (region) 383.1
  maxillary (*see also* Sinusitis, maxillary) 473.0
  mediastinal 510.0
  mediastinobronchial 510.0
  mediastinocutaneous 510.0
  middle ear 385.89
  mouth 528.3
  nasal 478.19 ▲
    sinus (*see also* Sinusitis) 473.9
  nasopharynx 478.29
  nipple — *see* Fistula, breast
  nose 478.19 ▲
  oral (cutaneous) 528.3
    maxillary (*see also* Sinusitis, maxillary) 473.0
    nasal (with cleft palate) (*see also* Cleft, palate) 749.00
  orbit, orbital 376.10
  oro-antral (*see also* Sinusitis, maxillary) 473.0
  oval window (internal ear) 386.42
  oviduct (external) 619.2
  palate (hard) 526.89
    soft 528.9
  pancreatic 577.8
  pancreaticoduodenal 577.8
  parotid (gland) 527.4
    region 528.3
  pelvoabdominointestinal 569.81
  penis 607.89
  perianal 565.1
  pericardium (pleura) (sac) (*see also* Pericarditis) 423.8
  pericecal 569.81
  perineal — *see* Fistula, perineum
  perineorectal 569.81
  perineosigmoidal 569.81
  perineo-urethroscrotal 608.89
  perineum, perineal (with urethral involvement) NEC 599.1
    tuberculous (*see also* Tuberculosis) 017.9 ☑
    ureter 593.82
  perirectal 565.1
    tuberculous (*see also* Tuberculosis) 014.8 ☑
  peritoneum (*see also* Peritonitis) 567.22
  periurethral 599.1

Fistula — *continued*
  pharyngo-esophageal 478.29
  pharynx 478.29
    branchial cleft (congenital) 744.41
  pilonidal (infected) (rectum) 685.1
    with abscess 685.0
  pleura, pleural, pleurocutaneous, pleuroperitoneal 510.0
    stomach 510.0
    tuberculous (*see also* Tuberculosis) 012.0 ☑
  pleuropericardial 423.8
  postauricular 383.81
  postoperative, persistent 998.6
  preauricular (congenital) 744.46
  prostate 602.8
  pulmonary 510.0
    arteriovenous 417.0
      congenital 747.3
    tuberculous (*see also* Tuberculosis, pulmonary) 011.9 ☑
  pulmonoperitoneal 510.0
  rectolabial 619.1
  rectosigmoid (intercommunicating) 569.81
  rectoureteral 593.82
  rectourethral 599.1
    congenital 753.8
  rectouterine 619.1
    congenital 752.3
  rectovaginal 619.1
    congenital 752.49
    old, postpartal 619.1
    tuberculous (*see also* Tuberculosis) 014.8 ☑
  rectovesical 596.1
    congenital 753.8
  rectovesicovaginal 619.1
  rectovulvar 619.1
    congenital 752.49
  rectum (to skin) 565.1
    tuberculous (*see also* Tuberculosis) 014.8 ☑
  renal 593.89
  retroauricular 383.81
  round window (internal ear) 386.41
  salivary duct or gland 527.4
    congenital 750.24
  sclera 360.32
  scrotum (urinary) 608.89
    tuberculous (*see also* Tuberculosis) 016.5 ☑
  semicircular canals (internal ear) 386.43
  sigmoid 569.81
    vesicoabdominal 596.1
  sigmoidovaginal 619.1
    congenital 752.49
  skin 686.9
    ureter 593.82
    vagina 619.2
  sphenoidal sinus (*see also* Sinusitis, sphenoidal) 473.3
  splenocolic 289.59
  stercoral 569.81
  stomach 537.4
  sublingual gland 527.4
    congenital 750.24
  submaxillary
    gland 527.4
      congenital 750.24
    region 528.3
  thoracic 510.0
    duct 457.8
  thoracoabdominal 510.0
  thoracogastric 510.0
  thoracointestinal 510.0
  thoracoabdominal 510.0
  thoracogastric 510.0
  thorax 510.0
  thyroglossal duct 759.2
  thyroid 246.8
  trachea (congenital) (external) (internal) 748.3
  tracheoesophageal 530.84
    congenital 750.3

Fistula — *continued*
  tracheoesophageal — *continued*
    following tracheostomy 519.09
  traumatic
    arteriovenous (*see also* Injury, blood vessel, by site) 904.9
    brain — *see* Injury, intracranial
  tuberculous — *see* Tuberculosis, by site
  typhoid 002.0
  umbilical 759.89
  umbilico-urinary 753.8
  urachal, urachus 753.7
  ureter (persistent) 593.82
  ureteroabdominal 593.82
  ureterocervical 593.82
  ureterorectal 593.82
  ureterosigmoido-abdominal 593.82
  ureterovaginal 619.0
  ureterovesical 596.2
  urethra 599.1
    congenital 753.8
    tuberculous (*see also* Tuberculosis) 016.3 ☑
  urethroperineal 599.1
  urethroperineovesical 596.2
  urethrorectal 599.1
    congenital 753.8
  urethroscrotal 608.89
  urethrovaginal 619.0
  urethrovesical 596.2
  urethrovesicovaginal 619.0
  urinary (persistent) (recurrent) 599.1
  uteroabdominal (anterior wall) 619.2
    congenital 752.3
  uteroenteric 619.1
  uterofecal 619.1
  uterointestinal 619.1
    congenital 752.3
  uterorectal 619.1
    congenital 752.3
  uteroureteric 619.0
  uterovaginal 619.8
  uterovesical 619.0
    congenital 752.3
  uterus 619.8
  vagina (wall) 619.8
    postpartal, old 619.8
  vaginocutaneous (postpartal) 619.2
  vaginoileal (acquired) 619.1
  vaginoperineal 619.2
  vesical NEC 596.2
  vesicoabdominal 596.2
  vesicocervicovaginal 619.0
  vesicocolic 596.1
  vesicocutaneous 596.2
  vesicoenteric 596.1
  vesicointestinal 596.1
  vesicometrorectal 619.1
  vesicoperineal 596.2
  vesicorectal 596.1
    congenital 753.8
  vesicosigmoidal 596.1
  vesicosigmoidovaginal 619.1
  vesicoureteral 596.2
  vesicoureterovaginal 619.0
  vesicourethral 596.2
  vesicourethrorectal 596.1
  vesicouterine 619.0
    congenital 752.3
  vesicovaginal 619.0
  vulvorectal 619.1
    congenital 752.49
Fit 780.39
  apoplectic (*see also* Disease, cerebrovascular, acute) 436
    late effect — *see* Late effect(s) (of) cerebrovascular disease
  epileptic (*see also* Epilepsy) 345.9 ☑
  fainting 780.2
  hysterical 300.11
  newborn 779.0
Fitting (of)
  artificial
    arm (complete) (partial) V52.0
    breast V52.4

Fitting — *continued*
  artificial — *continued*
    eye(s) V52.2
    leg(s) (complete) (partial) V52.1
  brain neuropacemaker V53.02
  cardiac pacemaker V53.31
  carotid sinus pacemaker V53.39
  cerebral ventricle (communicating) shunt V53.01
  colostomy belt V53.5
  contact lenses V53.1
  cystostomy device V53.6
  defibrillator, automatic implantable cardiac V53.32
  dentures V52.3
  device, unspecified type V53.90
    abdominal V53.5
    cardiac
      defibrillator, automatic implantable V53.32
      pacemaker V53.31
      specified NEC V53.39
    cerebral ventricle (communicating) shunt V53.01
    insulin pump V53.91
    intrauterine contraceptive V25.1
    nervous system V53.09
    orthodontic V53.4
    orthoptic V53.1
    other device V53.99
    prosthetic V52.9
      breast V52.4
      dental V52.3
      eye V52.2
      specified type NEC V52.8
    special senses V53.09
    substitution
      auditory V53.09
      nervous system V53.09
      visual V53.09
    urinary V53.6
  diaphragm (contraceptive) V25.02
  glasses (reading) V53.1
  growth rod V54.02
  hearing aid V53.2
  ileostomy device V53.5
  intestinal appliance or device NEC V53.5
  intrauterine contraceptive device V25.1
  neuropacemaker (brain) (peripheral nerve) (spinal cord) V53.02
  orthodontic device V53.4
  orthopedic (device) V53.7
    brace V53.7
    cast V53.7
    corset V53.7
    shoes V53.7
  pacemaker (cardiac) V53.31
    brain V53.02
    carotid sinus V53.39
    peripheral nerve V53.02
    spinal cord V53.02
  prosthesis V52.9
    arm (complete) (partial) V52.0
    breast V52.4
    dental V52.3
    eye V52.2
    leg (complete) (partial) V52.1
    specified type NEC V52.8
  spectacles V53.1
  wheelchair V53.8
Fitz-Hugh and Curtis syndrome 098.86
  due to
    Chlamydia trachomatis 099.56
    Neisseria gonorrhoeae (gonococcal peritonitis) 098.86
Fitz's syndrome (acute hemorrhagic pancreatitis) 577.0
Fixation
  joint — *see* Ankylosis
  larynx 478.79
  pupil 364.76
  stapes 385.22
    deafness (*see also* Deafness, conductive) 389.04

Fixation

Fixation — continued
  uterus (acquired) — see Malposition, uterus
  vocal cord 478.5
Flaccid — see also condition
  foot 736.79
  forearm 736.09
  palate, congenital 750.26
Flail
  chest 807.4
    newborn 767.3
  joint (paralytic) 718.80
    ankle 718.87
    elbow 718.82
    foot 718.87
    hand 718.84
    hip 718.85
    knee 718.86
    multiple sites 718.89
    pelvic region 718.85
    shoulder (region) 718.81
    specified site NEC 718.88
    wrist 718.83
Flajani (-Basedow) syndrome or disease (exophthalmic goiter) 242.0 ☑
Flap, liver 572.8
Flare, anterior chamber (aqueous) (eye) 364.04
Flashback phenomena (drug) (hallucinogenic) 292.89
Flat
  chamber (anterior) (eye) 360.34
  chest, congenital 754.89
  electroencephalogram (EEG) 348.8
  foot (acquired) (fixed type) (painful) (postural) (spastic) 734
    congenital 754.61
      rocker bottom 754.61
      vertical talus 754.61
    rachitic 268.1
    rocker bottom (congenital) 754.61
    vertical talus, congenital 754.61
  organ or site, congenital NEC — see Anomaly, specified type NEC
  pelvis 738.6
    with disproportion (fetopelvic) 653.2 ☑
      affecting fetus or newborn 763.1
      causing obstructed labor 660.1 ☑
        affecting fetus or newborn 763.1
    congenital 755.69
Flatau-Schilder disease 341.1
Flattening
  head, femur 736.39
  hip 736.39
  lip (congenital) 744.89
  nose (congenital) 754.0
    acquired 738.0
Flatulence 787.3
Flatus 787.3
  vaginalis 629.89
Flax dressers' disease 504
Flea bite — see Injury, superficial, by site
Fleischer (-Kayser) ring (corneal pigmentation) 275.1 [371.14]
Fleischner's disease 732.3
Fleshy mole 631
Flexibilitas cerea — see also Catalepsy 300.11
Flexion
  cervix ▶— see Flexion, uterus◀
  contracture, joint (see also Contraction, joint) 718.4 ☑
  deformity, joint (see also Contraction, joint) 736.9 ▲
    hip, congenital (see also Subluxation, congenital, hip) 754.32
  uterus (see also Malposition, uterus) 621.6
Flexner's
  bacillus 004.1
  diarrhea (ulcerative) 004.1
  dysentery 004.1

Flexner-Boyd dysentery 004.2
Flexure — see condition
Floater, vitreous 379.24
Floating
  cartilage (joint) (see also Disorder, cartilage, articular) 718.0 ☑
    knee 717.6
  gallbladder (congenital) 751.69
  kidney 593.0
    congenital 753.3
  liver (congenital) 751.69
  rib 756.3
  spleen 289.59
Flooding 626.2
Floor — see condition
Floppy
  infant NEC 781.99
  valve syndrome (mitral) 424.0
Flu — see also Influenza
  gastric NEC 008.8
Fluctuating blood pressure 796.4
Fluid
  abdomen 789.5
  chest (see also Pleurisy, with effusion) 511.9
  heart (see also Failure, heart) 428.0
  joint (see also Effusion, joint) 719.0 ☑
  loss (acute) 276.50
    with
      hypernatremia 276.0
      hyponatremia 276.1
  lung (see also Edema, lung) encysted 511.8
  peritoneal cavity 789.5
  pleural cavity (see also Pleurisy, with effusion) 511.9
  retention 276.6
Flukes NEC — see also Infestation, fluke 121.9
  blood NEC (see also Infestation, Schistosoma) 120.9
  liver 121.3
Fluor (albus) (vaginalis) 623.5
  trichomonal (Trichomonas vaginalis) 131.00
Fluorosis (dental) (chronic) 520.3
Flushing 782.62
  menopausal 627.2
Flush syndrome 259.2
Flutter
  atrial or auricular 427.32
  heart (ventricular) 427.42
    atrial 427.32
  impure 427.32
  postoperative 997.1
  ventricular 427.42
Flux (bloody) (serosanguineous) 009.0
Focal — see condition
Fochier's abscess — see Abscess, by site
Focus, Assmann's — see also Tuberculosis 011.0 ☑
Fogo selvagem 694.4
Foix-Alajouanine syndrome 336.1
Folds, anomalous — see also Anomaly, specified type NEC
  Bowman's membrane 371.31
  Descemet's membrane 371.32
  epicanthic 743.63
  heart 746.89
  posterior segment of eye, congenital 743.54
Folie à deux 297.3
Follicle
  cervix (nabothian) (ruptured) 616.0
  graafian, ruptured, with hemorrhage 620.
  nabothian 616.0
Folliclis (primary) — see also Tuberculosis 017.0 ☑
Follicular — see also condition
  cyst (atretic) 620.0
Folliculitis 704.8
  abscedens et suffodiens 704.8
  decalvans 704.09
  gonorrheal (acute) 098.0

Folliculitis — continued
  gonorrheal — continued
    chronic or duration of 2 months or more 098.2
  keloid, keloidalis 706.1
  pustular 704.8
  ulerythematosa reticulata 701.8
Folliculosis, conjunctival 372.02
Følling's disease (phenylketonuria) 270.1
Follow-up (examination) (routine) (following) V67.9
  cancer chemotherapy V67.2
  chemotherapy V67.2
  fracture V67.4
  high-risk medication V67.51
  injury NEC V67.59
  postpartum
    immediately after delivery V24.0
    routine V24.2
  psychiatric V67.3
  psychotherapy V67.3
  radiotherapy V67.1
  specified condition NEC V67.59
  specified surgery NEC V67.09
  surgery V67.00
    vaginal pap smear V67.01
  treatment V67.9
    combined NEC V67.6
    fracture V67.4
    involving high-risk medication NEC V67.51
    mental disorder V67.3
    specified NEC V67.59
Fong's syndrome (hereditary osteoonychodysplasia) 756.89
Food
  allergy 693.1
  anaphylactic shock — see Anaphylactic shock, due to, food
  asphyxia (from aspiration or inhalation) (see also Asphyxia, food) 933.1
  choked on (see also Asphyxia, food) 933.1
  deprivation 994.2
    specified kind of food NEC 269.8
  intoxication (see also Poisoning, food) 005.9
  lack of 994.2
  poisoning (see also Poisoning, food) 005.9
  refusal or rejection NEC 307.59
  strangulation or suffocation (see also Asphyxia, food) 933.1
  toxemia (see also Poisoning, food) 005.9
Foot — see also condition
  and mouth disease 078.4
  process disease 581.3
Foramen ovale (nonclosure) (patent) (persistent) 745.5
Forbes-Albright syndrome (nonpuerperal amenorrhea and lactation associated with pituitary tumor) 253.1
Forbes' (glycogen storage) disease 271.0
Forced birth or delivery NEC 669.8 ☑
  affecting fetus or newborn NEC 763.89
Forceps
  delivery NEC 669.5 ☑
    affecting fetus or newborn 763.2
Fordyce's disease (ectopic sebaceous glands) (mouth) 750.26
Fordyce-Fox disease (apocrine miliaria) 705.82
Forearm — see condition
Foreign body

Note — For foreign body with open wound, or other injury, see Wound, open, or the type of injury specified.

  accidentally left during a procedure 998.4
  anterior chamber (eye) 871.6
    magnetic 871.5

Foreign body — continued
  anterior chamber — continued
    magnetic — continued
      retained or old 360.51
    retained or old 360.61
  ciliary body (eye) 871.6
    magnetic 871.5
      retained or old 360.52
    retained or old 360.62
  entering through orifice (current) (old)
    accessory sinus 932
    air passage (upper) 933.0
      lower 934.8
    alimentary canal 938
    alveolar process 935.0
    antrum (Highmore) 932
    anus 937
    appendix 936
    asphyxia due to (see also Asphyxia, food) 933.1
    auditory canal 931
    auricle 931
    bladder 939.0
    bronchioles 934.8
    bronchus (main) 934.1
    buccal cavity 935.0
    canthus (inner) 930.1
    cecum 936
    cervix (canal) uterine 939.1
    coil, ileocecal 936
    colon 936
    conjunctiva 930.1
    conjunctival sac 930.1
    cornea 930.0
    digestive organ or tract NEC 938
    duodenum 936
    ear (external) 931
    esophagus 935.1
    eye (external) 930.9
      combined sites 930.8
      intraocular — see Foreign body, by site
      specified site NEC 930.8
    eyeball 930.8
      intraocular — see Foreign body, intraocular
    eyelid 930.1
      retained or old 374.86
    frontal sinus 932
    gastrointestinal tract 938
    genitourinary tract 939.9
    globe 930.8
      penetrating 871.6
        magnetic 871.5
          retained or old 360.50
        retained or old 360.60
    gum 935.0
    Highmore's antrum 932
    hypopharynx 933.0
    ileocecal coil 936
    ileum 936
    inspiration (of) 933.1
    intestine (large) (small) 936
    lacrimal apparatus, duct, gland, or sac 930.2
    larynx 933.1
    lung 934.8
    maxillary sinus 932
    mouth 935.0
    nasal sinus 932
    nasopharynx 933.0
    nose (passage) 932
    nostril 932
    oral cavity 935.0
    palate 935.0
    penis 939.3
    pharynx 933.0
    pyriform sinus 933.0
    rectosigmoid 937
      junction 937
    rectum 937
    respiratory tract 934.9
      specified part NEC 934.8
    sclera 930.1
    sinus 932
      accessory 932

Index to Diseases

Foreign body — *continued*
 entering through orifice — *continued*
  sinus — *continued*
   frontal 932
   maxillary 932
   nasal 932
   pyriform 933.0
  small intestine 936
  stomach (hairball) 935.2
  suffocation by (*see also* Asphyxia, food) 933.1
  swallowed 938
   tongue 933.0
  tear ducts or glands 930.2
  throat 933.0
  tongue 935.0
   swallowed 933.0
  tonsil, tonsillar 933.0
   fossa 933.0
  trachea 934.0
  ureter 939.0
  urethra 939.0
  uterus (any part) 939.1
  vagina 939.2
  vulva 939.2
  wind pipe 934.0
 granuloma (old) 728.82
  bone 733.99
  in operative wound (inadvertently left) 998.4
  due to surgical material intentionally left — *see* Complications, due to (presence of) any device, implant, or graft classified to 996.0–996.5 NEC
  muscle 728.82
  skin 709.4
  soft tissue 709.4
  subcutaneous tissue 709.4
 in
  bone (residual) 733.99
  open wound — *see* Wound, open, by site complicated
  soft tissue (residual) 729.6
 inadvertently left in operation wound (causing adhesions, obstruction, or perforation) 998.4
 ingestion, ingested NEC 938
 inhalation or inspiration (*see also* Asphyxia, food) 933.1
 internal organ, not entering through an orifice — *see* Injury, internal, by site, with open wound
 intraocular (nonmagnetic) 871.6
  combined sites 871.6
   magnetic 871.5
    retained or old 360.59
    retained or old 360.69
  magnetic 871.5
   retained or old 360.50
   retained or old 360.60
  specified site NEC 871.6
   magnetic 871.5
    retained or old 360.59
    retained or old 360.69
 iris (nonmagnetic) 871.6
  magnetic 871.5
   retained or old 360.52
   retained or old 360.62
 lens (nonmagnetic) 871.6
  magnetic 871.5
   retained or old 360.53
   retained or old 360.63
 lid, eye 930.1
 ocular muscle 870.4
  retained or old 376.6
 old or residual
  bone 733.99
  eyelid 374.86
  middle ear 385.83
  muscle 729.6
   ocular 376.6
  retrobulbar 376.6
  skin 729.6

Foreign body — *continued*
 old or residual — *continued*
  skin — *continued*
   with granuloma 709.4
  soft tissue 729.6
   with granuloma 709.4
  subcutaneous tissue 729.6
   with granuloma 709.4
 operation wound, left accidentally 998.4
 orbit 870.4
  retained or old 376.6
 posterior wall, eye 871.6
  magnetic 871.5
   retained or old 360.55
   retained or old 360.65
 respiratory tree 934.9
  specified site NEC 934.8
 retained (old) (nonmagnetic) (in)
  anterior chamber (eye) 360.61
   magnetic 360.51
  ciliary body 360.62
   magnetic 360.52
  eyelid 374.86
  globe 360.60
   magnetic 360.50
  intraocular 360.60
   magnetic 360.50
   specified site NEC 360.69
    magnetic 360.59
  iris 360.62
   magnetic 360.52
  lens 360.63
   magnetic 360.53
  muscle 729.6
  orbit 376.6
  posterior wall of globe 360.65
   magnetic 360.55
  retina 360.65
   magnetic 360.55
  retrobulbar 376.6
  skin 729.6
   with granuloma 709.4
  soft tissue 729.6
   with granuloma 709.4
  subcutaneous tissue 729.6
   with granuloma 709.4
  vitreous 360.64
   magnetic 360.54
 retina 871.6
  magnetic 871.5
   retained or old 360.55
   retained or old 360.65
 superficial, without major open wound (*see also* Injury, superficial, by site) 919.6
 swallowed NEC 938
 vitreous (humor) 871.6
  magnetic 871.5
   retained or old 360.54
   retained or old 360.64
Forking, aqueduct of Sylvius 742.3
 with spina bifida (*see also* Spina bifida) 741.0 ☑
Formation
 bone in scar tissue (skin) 709.3
 connective tissue in vitreous 379.25
 Elschnig pearls (postcataract extraction) 366.51
 hyaline in cornea 371.49
 sequestrum in bone (due to infection) (*see also* Osteomyelitis) 730.1 ☑
 valve
  colon, congenital 751.5
  ureter (congenital) 753.29
Formication 782.0
Fort Bragg fever 100.89
Fossa — *see also* condition
 pyriform — *see* condition
Foster-Kennedy syndrome 377.04
Fothergill's
 disease, meaning scarlatina anginosa 034.1
 neuralgia (*see also* Neuralgia, trigeminal) 350.1
Foul breath 784.99

Found dead (cause unknown) 798.9
Foundling V20.0
Fournier's disease (idiopathic gangrene) 608.83
Fourth
 cranial nerve — *see* condition
 disease 057.8
 molar 520.1
Foville's syndrome 344.89
Fox's
 disease (apocrine miliaria) 705.82
 impetigo (contagiosa) 684
Fox-Fordyce disease (apocrine miliaria) 705.82
Fracture (abduction) (adduction) (avulsion) (compression) (crush) (dislocation) (oblique) (separation) (closed) 829.0

> *Note* — For fracture of any of the following sites with fracture of other bones — *see* Fracture, multiple.
>
> "Closed" includes the following descriptions of fractures, with or without delayed healing, unless they are specified as open or compound:
>
> | | |
> |---|---|
> | comminuted | linear |
> | depressed | simple |
> | elevated | slipped epiphysis |
> | fissured | spiral |
> | greenstick | unspecified |
> | impacted | |
>
> "Open" includes the following descriptions of fractures, with or without delayed healing:
>
> | | |
> |---|---|
> | compound | puncture |
> | infected | with foreign body |
> | missile | |
>
> For late effect of fracture, see Late, effect, fracture, by site.

 with
  internal injuries in same region (conditions classifiable to 860–869) (*see also* Injury, internal, by site)
   pelvic region — *see* Fracture, pelvis
 acetabulum (with visceral injury) (closed) 808.0
  open 808.1
 acromion (process) (closed) 811.01
  open 811.11
 alveolus (closed) 802.8
  open 802.9
 ankle (malleolus) (closed) 824.8
  bimalleolar (Dupuytren's) (Pott's) 824.4
   open 824.5
  bone 825.21
   open 825.31
  lateral malleolus only (fibular) 824.2
   open 824.3
  medial malleolus only (tibial) 824.0
   open 824.1
   open 824.9
  pathologic 733.16
  talus 825.21
   open 825.31
  trimalleolar 824.6
   open 824.7
 antrum — *see* Fracture, skull, base
 arm (closed) 818.0
  and leg(s) (any bones) 828.0
   open 828.1
  both (any bones) (with rib(s)) (with sternum) 819.0
   open 819.1
  lower 813.80
   open 813.90

Fracture — *continued*
 arm — *continued*
  open 818.1
  upper — *see* Fracture, humerus
 astragalus (closed) 825.21
  open 825.31
 atlas — *see* Fracture, vertebra, cervical, first
 axis — *see* Fracture, vertebra, cervical, second
 back — *see* Fracture, vertebra, by site
 Barton's — *see* Fracture, radius, lower end
 basal (skull) — *see* Fracture, skull, base
 Bennett's (closed) 815.01
  open 815.11
 bimalleolar (closed) 824.4
  open 824.5
 bone (closed) NEC 829.0
  birth injury NEC 767.3
  open 829.1
  pathologic NEC (*see also* Fracture, pathologic) 733.10
  stress NEC (*see also* Fracture, stress) 733.95
 boot top — *see* Fracture, fibula
 boxers' — *see* Fracture, metacarpal bone(s)
 breast bone — *see* Fracture, sternum
 bucket handle (semilunar cartilage) — *see* Tear, meniscus
 bursting — *see* Fracture, phalanx, hand, distal
 calcaneus (closed) 825.0
  open 825.1
 capitate (bone) (closed) 814.07
  open 814.17
 capitellum (humerus) (closed) 812.49
  open 812.59
 carpal bone(s) (wrist NEC) (closed) 814.00
  open 814.10
  specified site NEC 814.09
   open 814.19
 cartilage, knee (semilunar) — *see* Tear, meniscus
 cervical — *see* Fracture, vertebra, cervical
 chauffeur's — *see* Fracture, ulna, lower end
 chisel — *see* Fracture, radius, upper end
 clavicle (interligamentous part) (closed) 810.00
  acromial end 810.03
   open 810.13
  due to birth trauma 767.2
   open 810.10
  shaft (middle third) 810.02
   open 810.12
  sternal end 810.01
   open 810.11
 clayshovelers' — *see* Fracture, vertebra, cervical
 coccyx (*see also* Fracture, vertebra, coccyx)
  complicating delivery 665.6 ☑
 collar bone — *see* Fracture, clavicle
 Colles' (reversed) (closed) 813.41
  open 813.51
 comminuted — *see* Fracture, by site
 compression (*see also* Fracture, by site)
  nontraumatic — *see* Fracture, pathologic
 congenital 756.9
 coracoid process (closed) 811.02
  open 811.12
 coronoid process (ulna) (closed) 813.02
  mandible (closed) 802.23
   open 802.33
   open 813.12
 corpus cavernosum penis 959.13

Fracture

Fracture — *continued*
  costochondral junction — *see* Fracture, rib
  costosternal junction — *see* Fracture, rib
  cranium — *see* Fracture, skull, by site
  cricoid cartilage (closed) 807.5
    open 807.6
  cuboid (ankle) (closed) 825.23
    open 825.33
  cuneiform
    foot (closed) 825.24
      open 825.34
    wrist (closed) 814.03
      open 814.13
  dental restorative material
    with loss of material 525.64
    without loss of material 525.63
  due to
    birth injury — *see* Birth injury, fracture
    gunshot — *see* Fracture, by site, open
    neoplasm — *see* Fracture, pathologic
    osteoporosis — *see* Fracture, pathologic
  Dupuytren's (ankle) (fibula) (closed) 824.4
    open 824.5
    radius 813.42
      open 813.52
  Duverney's — *see* Fracture, ilium
  elbow (*see also* Fracture, humerus, lower end)
    olecranon (process) (closed) 813.01
      open 813.11
    supracondylar (closed) 812.41
      open 812.51
  ethmoid (bone) (sinus) — *see* Fracture, skull, base
  face bone(s) (closed) NEC 802.8
    with
      other bone(s) — *see* Fracture, multiple, skull
      skull (*see also* Fracture, skull) involving other bones — *see* Fracture, multiple, skull
    open 802.9
  fatigue — *see* Fracture, march
  femur, femoral (closed) 821.00
    cervicotrochanteric 820.03
      open 820.13
    condyles, epicondyles 821.21
      open 821.31
    distal end — *see* Fracture, femur, lower end
    epiphysis (separation)
      capital 820.01
        open 820.11
      head 820.01
        open 820.11
      lower 821.22
        open 821.32
      trochanteric 820.01
        open 820.11
      upper 820.01
        open 820.11
    head 820.09
      open 820.19
    lower end or extremity (distal end) (closed) 821.20
      condyles, epicondyles 821.21
        open 821.31
      epiphysis (separation) 821.22
        open 821.32
      multiple sites 821.29
        open 821.39
      open 821.30
      specified site NEC 821.29
        open 821.39
      supracondylar 821.23
        open 821.33
      T-shaped 821.21
        open 821.31

Fracture — *continued*
  femur, femoral — *continued*
    neck (closed) 820.8
      base (cervicotrochanteric) 820.03
        open 820.13
      extracapsular 820.20
        open 820.30
      intertrochanteric (section) 820.21
        open 820.31
      intracapsular 820.00
        open 820.10
      intratrochanteric 820.21
        open 820.31
      midcervical 820.02
        open 820.12
      open 820.9
      pathologic 733.14
        specified part NEC 733.15
      specified site NEC 820.09
        open 820.19
      transcervical 820.02
        open 820.12
      transtrochanteric 820.20
        open 820.30
    open 821.10
    pathologic 733.14
      specified part NEC 733.15
    peritrochanteric (section) 820.20
      open 820.30
    shaft (lower third) (middle third) (upper third) 821.01
      open 821.11
    subcapital 820.09
      open 820.19
    subtrochanteric (region) (section) 820.22
      open 820.32
    supracondylar 821.23
      open 821.33
    transepiphyseal 820.01
      open 820.11
    trochanter (greater) (lesser) (*see also* Fracture, femur, neck, by site) 820.20
      open 820.30
    T-shaped, into knee joint 821.21
      open 821.31
    upper end 820.8
      open 820.9
  fibula (closed) 823.81
    with tibia 823.82
      open 823.92
    distal end 824.8
      open 824.9
    epiphysis
      lower 824.8
        open 824.9
      upper — *see* Fracture, fibula, upper end
    head — *see* Fracture, fibula, upper end
    involving ankle 824.2
      open 824.3
    lower end or extremity 824.8
      open 824.9
    malleolus (external) (lateral) 824.2
      open 824.3
    open NEC 823.91
    pathologic 733.16
    proximal end — *see* Fracture, fibula, upper end
    shaft 823.21
      with tibia 823.22
        open 823.32
      open 823.31
    stress 733.93
    torus 823.41
      with tibia 823.42
    upper end or extremity (epiphysis) (head) (proximal end) (styloid) 823.01
      with tibia 823.02
        open 823.12
      open 823.11

Fracture — *continued*
  finger(s), of one hand (closed) (*see also* Fracture, phalanx, hand) 816.00
    with
      metacarpal bone(s), of same hand 817.0
        open 817.1
      thumb of same hand 816.03
        open 816.13
    open 816.10
  foot, except toe(s) alone (closed) 825.20
    open 825.30
  forearm (closed) NEC 813.80
    lower end (distal end) (lower epiphysis) 813.40
      open 813.50
    open 813.90
    shaft 813.20
      open 813.30
    upper end (proximal end) (upper epiphysis) 813.00
      open 813.10
  fossa, anterior, middle, or posterior — *see* Fracture, skull, base
  Fracture (abduction) (adduction) (avulsion) (compression) (crush) (dislocation) (oblique) (separation) (closed) 829.0
  frontal (bone) (*see also* Fracture, skull, vault)
    sinus — *see* Fracture, skull, base
  Galeazzi's — *see* Fracture, radius, lower end
  glenoid (cavity) (fossa) (scapula) (closed) 811.03
    open 811.13
  Gosselin's — *see* Fracture, ankle
  greenstick — *see* Fracture, by site
  grenade-throwers' — *see* Fracture, humerus, shaft
  gutter — *see* Fracture, skull, vault
  hamate (closed) 814.08
    open 814.18
  hand, one (closed) 815.00
    carpals 814.00
      open 814.10
      specified site NEC 814.09
        open 814.19
    metacarpals 815.00
      open 815.10
    multiple, bones of one hand 817.0
      open 817.1
    open 815.10
    phalanges (*see also* Fracture, phalanx, hand) 816.00
      open 816.10
  healing
    aftercare (*see also* Aftercare, fracture) V54.89
    change of cast V54.89
    complications — *see* condition
    convalescence V66.4
    removal of
      cast V54.89
      fixation device
        external V54.89
        internal V54.01
  heel bone (closed) 825.0
    open 825.1
  hip (closed) (*see also* Fracture, femur, neck) 820.8
    open 820.9
    pathologic 733.14
  humerus (closed) 812.20
    anatomical neck 812.02
      open 812.12
    articular process (*see also* Fracture humerus, condyle(s)) 812.44
      open 812.54
    capitellum 812.49
      open 812.59
    condyle(s) 812.44
      lateral (external) 812.42
        open 812.52

Fracture — *continued*
  humerus — *continued*
    condyle(s) — *continued*
      medial (internal epicondyle) 812.43
        open 812.53
        open 812.54
    distal end — *see* Fracture, humerus, lower end
    epiphysis
      lower (*see also* Fracture, humerus, condyle(s)) 812.44
        open 812.54
      upper 812.09
        open 812.19
    external condyle 812.42
      open 812.52
    great tuberosity 812.03
      open 812.13
    head 812.09
      open 812.19
    internal epicondyle 812.43
      open 812.53
    lesser tuberosity 812.09
      open 812.19
    lower end or extremity (distal end) (*see also* Fracture, humerus, by site) 812.40
      multiple sites NEC 812.49
        open 812.59
      open 812.50
      specified site NEC 812.49
        open 812.59
    neck 812.01
      open 812.11
    open 812.30
    pathologic 733.11
    proximal end — *see* Fracture, humerus, upper end
    shaft 812.21
      open 812.31
    supracondylar 812.41
      open 812.51
    surgical neck 812.01
      open 812.11
    trochlea 812.49
      open 812.59
    T-shaped 812.44
      open 812.54
    tuberosity — *see* Fracture, humerus, upper end
    upper end or extremity (proximal end) (*see also* Fracture, humerus, by site) 812.00
      open 812.10
      specified site NEC 812.09
        open 812.19
  hyoid bone (closed) 807.5
    open 807.6
  hyperextension — *see* Fracture, radius, lower end
  ilium (with visceral injury) (closed) 808.41
    open 808.51
  impaction, impacted — *see* Fracture, by site
  incus — *see* Fracture, skull, base
  innominate bone (with visceral injury) (closed) 808.49
    open 808.59
  instep, of one foot (closed) 825.20
    with toe(s) of same foot 827.0
      open 827.1
    open 825.30
  internal
    ear — *see* Fracture, skull, base
    semilunar cartilage, knee — *see* Tear, meniscus, medial
  intertrochanteric — *see* Fracture, femur, neck, intertrochanteric
  ischium (with visceral injury) (closed) 808.42
    open 808.52
  jaw (bone) (lower) (closed) (*see also* Fracture, mandible) 802.20

Index to Diseases

Fracture

Fracture — *continued*
- jaw (see also Fracture, mandible) — *continued*
  - angle 802.25
    - open 802.35
  - open 802.30
  - upper — *see* Fracture, maxilla
- knee
  - cap (closed) 822.0
    - open 822.1
  - cartilage (semilunar) — *see* Tear, meniscus
- labyrinth (osseous) — *see* Fracture, skull, base
- larynx (closed) 807.5
  - open 807.6
- late effect — *see* Late, effects (of), fracture
- Le Fort's — *see* Fracture, maxilla
- leg (closed) 827.0
  - with rib(s) or sternum 828.0
    - open 828.1
  - both (any bones) 828.0
    - open 828.1
  - lower — *see* Fracture, tibia
    - open 827.1
  - upper — *see* Fracture, femur
- limb
  - lower (multiple) (closed) NEC 827.0
    - open 827.1
  - upper (multiple) (closed) NEC 818.0
    - open 818.1
- long bones, due to birth trauma — *see* Birth injury, fracture
- lower end or extremity (anterior lip) (posterior) 824.8
  - open 824.9
- lumbar — *see* Fracture, vertebra, lumbar
- lunate bone (closed) 814.02
  - open 814.12
- malar bone (closed) 802.4
  - open 802.5
- Malgaigne's (closed) 808.43
  - open 808.53
- malleolus (closed) 824.8
  - bimalleolar 824.4
    - open 824.5
  - lateral 824.2
    - and medial (*see also* Fracture, malleolus, bimalleolar)
      - with lip of tibia — *see* Fracture, malleolus, trimalleolar
    - open 824.3
  - medial (closed) 824.0
    - and lateral (*see also* Fracture, malleolus, bimalleolar)
      - with lip of tibia — *see* Fracture, malleolus, trimalleolar
    - open 824.1
  - open 824.9
  - trimalleolar (closed) 824.6
    - open 824.7
- malleus — *see* Fracture, skull, base
- malunion 733.81
- mandible (closed) 802.20
  - angle 802.25
    - open 802.35
  - body 802.28
    - alveolar border 802.27
      - open 802.37
    - open 802.38
    - symphysis 802.26
      - open 802.36
  - condylar process 802.21
    - open 802.31
  - coronoid process 802.23
    - open 802.33
  - multiple sites 802.29
    - open 802.39
  - open 802.30
  - ramus NEC 802.24
    - open 802.34
  - subcondylar 802.22

Fracture — *continued*
- mandible — *continued*
  - subcondylar — *continued*
    - open 802.32
  - manubrium — *see* Fracture, sternum
- march 733.95
  - fibula 733.93
  - metatarsals 733.94
  - tibia 733.93
- maxilla, maxillary (superior) (upper jaw) (closed) 802.4
  - inferior — *see* Fracture, mandible
  - open 802.5
- meniscus, knee — *see* Tear, meniscus
- metacarpus, metacarpal (bone(s)), of one hand (closed) 815.00
  - with phalanx, phalanges, hand (finger(s)) (thumb) of same hand 817.0
    - open 817.1
  - base 815.02
    - first metacarpal 815.01
      - open 815.11
    - open 815.12
    - thumb 815.01
      - open 815.11
  - multiple sites 815.09
    - open 815.19
  - neck 815.04
    - open 815.14
  - open 815.10
  - shaft 815.03
    - open 815.13
- metatarsus, metatarsal (bone(s)), of one foot (closed) 825.25
  - with tarsal bone(s) 825.29
    - open 825.39
  - open 825.35
- Monteggia's (closed) 813.03
  - open 813.13
- Moore's — *see* Fracture, radius, lower end
- multangular bone (closed)
  - larger 814.05
    - open 814.15
  - smaller 814.06
    - open 814.16
- multiple (closed) 829.0

Note — Multiple fractures of sites classifiable to the same three- or four-digit category are coded to that category, except for sites classifiable to 810–818 or 820–827 in different limbs.

Multiple fractures of sites classifiable to different fourth-digit subdivisions within the same three-digit category should be dealt with according to coding rules.

Multiple fractures of sites classifiable to different three-digit categories (identifiable from the listing under "Fracture"), and of sites classifiable to 810–818 or 820–827 in different limbs should be coded according to the following list, which should be referred to in the following priority order: skull or face bones, pelvis or vertebral column, legs, arms.

- arm (multiple bones in same arm except in hand alone) (sites classifiable to 810–817 with sites classifiable to a different three-digit category in 810–817 in same arm) (closed) 818.0
  - open 818.1
- arms, both or arm(s) with rib(s) or sternum (sites classifiable to 810–818 with sites classifiable to same range of categories in other limb or to 807) (closed) 819.0
  - open 819.1
- bones of trunk NEC (closed) 809.0
  - open 809.1

Fracture — *continued*
- multiple — *continued*
  - hand, metacarpal bone(s) with phalanx or phalanges of same hand (sites classifiable to 815 with sites classifiable to 816 in same hand) (closed) 817.0
    - open 817.1
  - leg (multiple bones in same leg) (sites classifiable to 820–826 with sites classifiable to a different three-digit category in that range in same leg) (closed) 827.0
    - open 827.1
  - legs, both or leg(s) with arm(s), rib(s), or sternum (sites classifiable to 820–827 with sites classifiable to same range of categories in other leg or to 807 or 810–819) (closed) 828.0
    - open 828.1
  - pelvis with other bones except skull or face bones (sites classifiable to 808 with sites classifiable to 805–807 or 810–829) (closed) 809.0
    - open 809.1
  - skull, specified or unspecified bones, or face bone(s) with any other bone(s) (sites classifiable to 800–803 with sites classifiable to 805–829) (closed) 804.0 ☑

Note — Use the following fifth-digit subclassification with categories 800, 801, 803, and 804:

0 *unspecified state of consciousness*

1 *with no loss of consciousness*

2 *with brief [less than one hour] loss of consciousness*

3 *with moderate [1–24 hours] loss of consciousness*

4 *with prolonged [more than 24 hours] loss of consciousness and return to pre-existing conscious level*

5 *with prolonged [more than 24 hours] loss of consciousness, without return to pre-existing conscious level*

Use fifth-digit 5 to designate when a patient is unconscious and dies before regaining consciousness, regardless of the duration of the loss of consciousness

6 *with loss of consciousness of unspecified duration*

9 *with concussion, unspecified*

- with
  - contusion, cerebral 804.1 ☑
  - epidural hemorrhage 804.2 ☑
  - extradural hemorrhage 804.2 ☑
  - hemorrhage (intracranial) NEC 804.3 ☑
  - intracranial injury NEC 804.4 ☑
  - laceration, cerebral 804.1 ☑
  - subarachnoid hemorrhage 804.2 ☑
  - subdural hemorrhage 804.2 ☑
- open 804.5 ☑
  - with
    - contusion, cerebral 804.6 ☑

Fracture — *continued*
- multiple — *continued*
  - skull, specified or unspecified bones, or face bone(s) with any other bone(s) — *continued*
    - open — *continued*
      - with — *continued*
        - epidural hemorrhage 804.7 ☑
        - extradural hemorrhage 804.7 ☑
        - hemorrhage (intracranial) NEC 804.8 ☑
        - intracranial injury NEC 804.9 ☑
        - laceration, cerebral 804.6 ☑
        - subarachnoid hemorrhage 804.7 ☑
        - subdural hemorrhage 804.7 ☑
    - vertebral column with other bones, except skull or face bones (sites classifiable to 805 or 806 with sites classifiable to 807–808 or 810–829) (closed) 809.0
      - open 809.1
- nasal (bone(s)) (closed) 802.0
  - open 802.1
  - sinus — *see* Fracture, skull, base
- navicular
  - carpal (wrist) (closed) 814.01
    - open 814.11
  - tarsal (ankle) (closed) 825.22
    - open 825.32
- neck — *see* Fracture, vertebra, cervical
- neural arch — *see* Fracture, vertebra, by site
- nonunion 733.82
- nose, nasal, (bone) (septum) (closed) 802.0
  - open 802.1
- occiput — *see* Fracture, skull, base
- odontoid process — *see* Fracture, vertebra, cervical
- olecranon (process) (ulna) (closed) 813.01
  - open 813.11
- open 829.1
- orbit, orbital (bone) (region) (closed) 802.8
  - floor (blow-out) 802.6
    - open 802.7
  - open 802.9
  - roof — *see* Fracture, skull, base
  - specified part NEC 802.8
    - open 802.9
- os
  - calcis (closed) 825.0
    - open 825.1
  - magnum (closed) 814.07
    - open 814.17
  - pubis (with visceral injury) (closed) 808.2
    - open 808.3
  - triquetrum (closed) 814.03
    - open 814.13
- osseous
  - auditory meatus — *see* Fracture, skull, base
  - labyrinth — *see* Fracture, skull, base
- ossicles, auditory (incus) (malleus) (stapes) — *see* Fracture, skull, base
- osteoporotic — *see* Fracture, pathologic
- palate (closed) 802.8
  - open 802.9
- paratrooper — *see* Fracture, tibia, lower end
- parietal bone — *see* Fracture, skull, vault

Fracture

Fracture — *continued*
  parry — *see* Fracture, Monteggia's
  patella (closed) 822.0
    open 822.1
  pathologic (cause unknown) 733.10
    ankle 733.16
    femur (neck) 733.14
      specified NEC 733.15
    fibula 733.16
    hip 733.14
    humerus 733.11
    radius (distal) 733.12
    specified site NEC 733.19
    tibia 733.16
    ulna 733.12
    vertebrae (collapse) 733.13
    wrist 733.12
  pedicle (of vertebral arch) — *see*
    Fracture, vertebra, by site
  pelvis, pelvic (bone(s)) (with visceral
      injury) (closed) 808.8
    multiple (with disruption of pelvic
        circle) 808.43
      open 808.53
    open 808.9
    rim (closed) 808.49
      open 808.59
  peritrochanteric (closed) 820.20
    open 820.30
  phalanx, phalanges, of one
      foot (closed) 826.0
    with bone(s) of same lower limb
        827.0
      open 827.1
    open 826.1
  hand (closed) 816.00
    with metacarpal bone(s) of same
        hand 817.0
      open 817.1
    distal 816.02
      open 816.12
    middle 816.01
      open 816.11
    multiple sites NEC 816.03
      open 816.13
    open 816.10
    proximal 816.01
      open 816.11
  pisiform (closed) 814.04
    open 814.14
  pond — *see* Fracture, skull, vault
  Pott's (closed) 824.4
    open 824.5
  prosthetic device, internal — *see*
    Complications, mechanical
  pubis (with visceral injury) (closed)
      808.2
    open 808.3
  Quervain's (closed) 814.01
    open 814.11
  radius (alone) (closed) 813.81
    with ulna NEC 813.83
      open 813.93
    distal end — *see* Fracture, radius,
        lower end
    epiphysis
      lower — *see* Fracture, radius,
          lower end
      upper — *see* Fracture, radius,
          upper end
    head — *see* Fracture, radius, upper
        end
    lower end or extremity (distal end)
        (lower epiphysis) 813.42
      with ulna (lower end) 813.44
        open 813.54
      open 813.52
      torus 813.45
    neck — *see* Fracture, radius, upper
        end
    open NEC 813.91
    pathologic 733.12
    proximal end — *see* Fracture, radius, upper end
    shaft (closed) 813.21
      with ulna (shaft) 813.23

Fracture — *continued*
  radius — *continued*
    shaft — *continued*
      with ulna — *continued*
        open 813.33
      open 813.31
    upper end 813.07
      with ulna (upper end) 813.08
        open 813.18
      epiphysis 813.05
        open 813.15
      head 813.05
        open 813.15
      multiple sites 813.07
        open 813.17
      neck 813.06
        open 813.16
      specified site NEC 813.07
        open 813.17
  ramus
    inferior or superior (with visceral
        injury) (closed) 808.2
      open 808.3
    ischium — *see* Fracture, ischium
    mandible 802.24
      open 802.34
  rib(s) (closed) 807.0 ☑

  *Note — Use the following fifth-digit
  subclassification with categories
  807.0–807.1:*
  0   rib(s), unspecified
  1   one rib
  2   two ribs
  3   three ribs
  4   four ribs
  5   five ribs
  6   six ribs
  7   seven ribs
  8   eight or more ribs
  9   multiple ribs, unspecified

    with flail chest (open) 807.4
      open 807.1 ☑
  root, tooth 873.63
    complicated 873.73
  sacrum — *see* Fracture, vertebra,
      sacrum
  scaphoid
    ankle (closed) 825.22
      open 825.32
    wrist (closed) 814.01
      open 814.11
  scapula (closed) 811.00
    acromial, acromion (process)
        811.01
      open 811.11
    body 811.09
      open 811.19
    coracoid process 811.02
      open 811.12
    glenoid (cavity) (fossa) 811.03
      open 811.13
    neck 811.03
      open 811.13
    open 811.10
  semilunar
    bone, wrist (closed) 814.02
      open 814.12
    cartilage (interior) (knee) — *see*
        Tear, meniscus
  sesamoid bone — *see* Fracture, by site
  Shepherd's (closed) 825.21
    open 825.31
  shoulder (*see also* Fracture, humerus,
      upper end)
    blade — *see* Fracture, scapula
    silverfork — *see* Fracture, radius,
        lower end
  sinus (ethmoid) (frontal) (maxillary)
      (nasal) (sphenoidal) — *see*
      Fracture, skull, base

Fracture — *continued*
  Skillern's — *see* Fracture, radius,
      shaft
  skull (multiple NEC) (with face bones)
      (closed) 803.0 ☑

  *Note — Use the following fifth-digit
  subclassification with categories 800,
  801, 803, and 804:*
  0   unspecified state of consciousness
  1   with no loss of consciousness
  2   with brief [less than one hour]
      loss of consciousness
  3   with moderate [1-24 hours] loss
      of consciousness
  4   with prolonged [more than 24
      hours] loss of consciousness and
      return to pre-existing conscious
      level
  5   with prolonged [more than 24
      hours] loss of consciousness,
      without return to pre-existing
      conscious level

  *Use fifth-digit 5 to designate when a
  patient is unconscious and dies before
  regaining consciousness, regardless of
  the duration of the loss of consciousness*

  6   with loss of consciousness of unspecified duration
  9   with concussion, unspecified

    with
      contusion, cerebral 803.1 ☑
      epidural hemorrhage
          803.2 ☑
      extradural hemorrhage
          803.2 ☑
      hemorrhage (intracranial)
          NEC 803.3 ☑
      intracranial injury NEC
          803.4 ☑
      laceration, cerebral 803.1 ☑
      other bones — *see* Fracture,
          multiple, skull
      subarachnoid hemorrhage
          803.2 ☑
      subdural hemorrhage
          803.2 ☑
    base (antrum) (ethmoid bone) (fossa) (internal ear) (nasal sinus) (occiput) (sphenoid)
        (temporal bone) (closed)
        801.0 ☑
      with
        contusion, cerebral
            801.1 ☑
        epidural hemorrhage
            801.2 ☑
        extradural hemorrhage
            801.2 ☑
        hemorrhage (intracranial)
            NEC 801.3 ☑
        intracranial injury NEC
            801.4 ☑
        laceration, cerebral
            801.1 ☑
        subarachnoid hemorrhage
            801.2 ☑
        subdural hemorrhage
            801.2 ☑
      open 801.5 ☑
        with
          contusion, cerebral
              801.6 ☑
          epidural hemorrhage
              801.7 ☑
          extradural hemorrhage
              801.7 ☑
          hemorrhage (intracranial) NEC
              801.8 ☑

Fracture — *continued*
  skull — *continued*
    base — *continued*
      open — *continued*
        with — *continued*
          intracranial injury NEC
              801.9 ☑
          laceration, cerebral
              801.6 ☑
          subarachnoid hemorrhage 801.7 ☑
          subdural hemorrhage
              801.7 ☑
    birth injury 767.3
    face bones — *see* Fracture, face
        bones
    open 803.5 ☑
      with
        contusion, cerebral
            803.6 ☑
        epidural hemorrhage
            803.7 ☑
        extradural hemorrhage
            803.7 ☑
        hemorrhage (intracranial)
            NEC 803.8 ☑
        intracranial injury NEC
            803.9 ☑
        laceration, cerebral
            803.6 ☑
        subarachnoid hemorrhage
            803.7 ☑
        subdural hemorrhage
            803.7 ☑
    vault (frontal bone) (parietal bone)
        (vertex) (closed) 800.0 ☑
      with
        contusion, cerebral
            800.1 ☑
        epidural hemorrhage
            800.2 ☑
        extradural hemorrhage
            800.2 ☑
        hemorrhage (intracranial)
            NEC 800.3 ☑
        intracranial injury NEC
            800.4 ☑
        laceration, cerebral
            800.1 ☑
        subarachnoid hemorrhage
            800.2 ☑
        subdural hemorrhage
            800.2 ☑
      open 800.5 ☑
        with
          contusion, cerebral
              800.6 ☑
          epidural hemorrhage
              800.7 ☑
          extradural hemorrhage
              800.7 ☑
          hemorrhage (intracranial) NEC
              800.8 ☑
          intracranial injury NEC
              800.9 ☑
          laceration, cerebral
              800.6 ☑
          subarachnoid hemorrhage 800.7 ☑
          subdural hemorrhage
              800.7 ☑
  Smith's 813.41
    open 813.51
  sphenoid (bone) (sinus) — *see* Fracture, skull, base
  spine (*see also* Fracture, vertebra, by
      site due to birth trauma) 767.4
  spinous process — *see* Fracture, vertebra, by site
  spontaneous — *see* Fracture, pathologic
  sprinters' — *see* Fracture, ilium
  stapes — *see* Fracture, skull, base

Index to Diseases

Fracture — *continued*
  stave (*see also* Fracture, metacarpus, metacarpal bone(s))
    spine — *see* Fracture, tibia, upper end
  sternum (closed) 807.2
    with flail chest (open) 807.4
    open 807.3
  Stieda's — *see* Fracture, femur, lower end
  stress 733.95
    fibula 733.93
    metatarsals 733.94
    specified site NEC 733.95
    tibia 733.93
  styloid process
    metacarpal (closed) 815.02
      open 815.12
    radius — *see* Fracture, radius, lower end
    temporal bone — *see* Fracture, skull, base
    ulna — *see* Fracture, ulna, lower end
  supracondylar, elbow 812.41
    open 812.51
  symphysis pubis (with visceral injury) (closed) 808.2
    open 808.3
  talus (ankle bone) (closed) 825.21
    open 825.31
  tarsus, tarsal bone(s) (with metatarsus) of one foot (closed) NEC 825.29
    open 825.39
  temporal bone (styloid) — *see* Fracture, skull, base
  tendon — *see* Sprain, by site
  thigh — *see* Fracture, femur, shaft
  thumb (and finger(s)) of one hand (closed) (*see also* Fracture, phalanx, hand) 816.00
    with metacarpal bone(s) of same hand 817.0
      open 817.1
    metacarpal(s) — *see* Fracture, metacarpus
    open 816.10
  thyroid cartilage (closed) 807.5
    open 807.6
  tibia (closed) 823.80
    with fibula 823.82
      open 823.92
    condyles — *see* Fracture, tibia, upper end
    distal end 824.8
      open 824.9
    epiphysis
      lower 824.8
        open 824.9
      upper — *see* Fracture, tibia, upper end
    head (involving knee joint) — *see* Fracture, tibia, upper end
    intercondyloid eminence — *see* Fracture, tibia, upper end
    involving ankle 824.0
      open 824.9
    lower end or extremity (anterior lip) (posterior lip) 824.8
      open 824.9
    malleolus (internal) (medial) 824.0
      open 824.1
    open NEC 823.90
    pathologic 733.16
    proximal end — *see* Fracture, tibia, upper end
    shaft 823.20
      with fibula 823.22
        open 823.32
      open 823.30
    spine — *see* Fracture, tibia, upper end
    stress 733.93
    torus 823.40
      with fibula 823.42

Fracture — *continued*
  tibia — *continued*
    tuberosity — *see* Fracture, tibia, upper end
    upper end or extremity (condyle) (epiphysis) (head) (spine) (proximal end) (tuberosity) 823.00
      with fibula 823.02
        open 823.12
      open 823.10
  toe(s), of one foot (closed) 826.0
    with bone(s) of same lower limb 827.0
      open 827.1
    open 826.1
  tooth (root) 873.63
    complicated 873.73
  torus
    fibula 823.41
      with tibia 823.42
    radius 813.45
    tibia 823.40
      with fibula 823.42
  trachea (closed) 807.5
    open 807.6
  transverse process — *see* Fracture, vertebra, by site
  trapezium (closed) 814.05
    open 814.15
  trapezoid bone (closed) 814.06
    open 814.16
  trimalleolar (closed) 824.6
    open 824.7
  triquetral (bone) (closed) 814.03
    open 814.13
  trochanter (greater) (lesser) (closed) (*see also* Fracture, femur, neck, by site) 820.20
    open 820.30
  trunk (bones) (closed) 809.0
    open 809.1
  tuberosity (external) — *see* Fracture, by site
  ulna (alone) (closed) 813.82
    with radius NEC 813.83
      open 813.93
    coronoid process (closed) 813.02
      open 813.12
    distal end — *see* Fracture, ulna, lower end
    epiphysis
      lower — *see* Fracture, ulna, lower end
      upper — *see* Fracture, ulna, upper end
    head — *see* Fracture, ulna, lower end
    lower end (distal end) (head) (lower epiphysis) (styloid process) 813.43
      with radius (lower end) 813.44
        open 813.54
      open 813.53
    olecranon process (closed) 813.01
      open 813.11
    open NEC 813.92
    pathologic 733.12
    proximal end — *see* Fracture, ulna, upper end
    shaft 813.22
      with radius (shaft) 813.23
        open 813.33
      open 813.32
    styloid process — *see* Fracture, ulna, lower end
    transverse — *see* Fracture, ulna, by site
    upper end (epiphysis) 813.04
      with radius (upper end) 813.08
        open 813.18
      multiple sites 813.04
        open 813.14
      specified site NEC 813.04
        open 813.14

Fracture — *continued*
  unciform (closed) 814.08
    open 814.18
  vertebra, vertebral (back) (body) (column) (neural arch) (pedicle) (spine) (spinous process) (transverse process) (closed) 805.8
    with
      hematomyelia — *see* Fracture, vertebra, by site, with spinal cord injury
      injury to
        cauda equina — *see* Fracture, vertebra, sacrum, with spinal cord injury
        nerve — *see* Fracture, vertebra, by site, with spinal cord injury
      paralysis — *see* Fracture, vertebra, by site, with spinal cord injury
      paraplegia — *see* Fracture, vertebra, by site, with spinal cord injury
      quadriplegia — *see* Fracture, vertebra, by site, with spinal cord injury
      spinal concussion — *see* Fracture, vertebra, by site, with spinal cord injury
      spinal cord injury (closed) NEC 806.8

> *Note — Use the following fifth-digit subclassification with categories 806.0–806.3:*
>
> C_1–C_4 or unspecified level and D_1–D_6 (T_1–T_6) or unspecified level with
>
> 0   unspecified spinal cord injury
> 1   complete lesion of cord
> 2   anterior cord syndrome
> 3   central cord syndrome
> 4   specified injury NEC
>
> C_5–C_7 level and D_7–D_{12} level with:
>
> 5   unspecified spinal cord injury
> 6   complete lesion of cord
> 7   anterior cord syndrome
> 8   central cord syndrome
> 9   specified injury NEC

        cervical 806.0 ☑
          open 806.1 ☑
        dorsal, dorsolumbar 806.2 ☑
          open 806.9
        thoracic, thoracolumbar 806.2 ☑
          open 806.3 ☑
    atlanto-axial — *see* Fracture, vertebra, cervical
    cervical (hangman) (teardrop) (closed) 805.00
      with spinal cord injury — *see* Fracture, vertebra, with spinal cord injury, cervical
      first (atlas) 805.01
        open 805.11
      second (axis) 805.02
        open 805.12
      third 805.03
        open 805.13
      fourth 805.04
        open 805.14
      fifth 805.05
        open 805.15
      sixth 805.06
        open 805.16
      seventh 805.07
        open 805.17
      multiple sites 805.08

Fracture — *continued*
  vertebra, vertebral — *continued*
    cervical — *continued*
      multiple sites — *continued*
        open 805.18
      open 805.10
    coccyx (closed) 805.6
      with spinal cord injury (closed) 806.60
        cauda equina injury 806.62
        complete lesion 806.61
          open 806.71
        open 806.72
        open 806.70
        specified type NEC 806.69
          open 806.79
      open 805.7
    collapsed 733.13
    compression, not due to trauma 733.13
    dorsal (closed) 805.2
      with spinal cord injury — *see* Fracture, vertebra, with spinal cord injury, dorsal
      open 805.3
    dorsolumbar (closed) 805.2
      with spinal cord injury — *see* Fracture, vertebra, with spinal cord injury, dorsal
      open 805.3
    due to osteoporosis 733.13
    fetus or newborn 767.4
    lumbar (closed) 805.4
      with spinal cord injury (closed) 806.4
        open 806.5
      open 805.5
    nontraumatic 733.13
    open NEC 805.9
    pathologic (any site) 733.13
    sacrum (closed) 805.6
      with spinal cord injury 806.60
        cauda equina injury 806.62
        complete lesion 806.61
          open 806.71
        open 806.72
        open 806.70
        specified type NEC 806.69
          open 806.79
      open 805.7
    site unspecified (closed) 805.8
      with spinal cord injury (closed) 806.8
        open 806.9
      open 805.9
    stress (any site) 733.95
    thoracic (closed) 805.2
      with spinal cord injury — *see* Fracture, vertebra, with spinal cord injury, thoracic
      open 805.3
    vertex — *see* Fracture, skull, vault
  vomer (bone) 802.0
    open 802.1
  Wagstaffe's — *see* Fracture, ankle
  wrist (closed) 814.00
    open 814.10
    pathologic 733.12
  xiphoid (process) — *see* Fracture, sternum
  zygoma (zygomatic arch) (closed) 802.4
    open 802.5

Fragile X syndrome 759.83
Fragilitas
  crinium 704.2
  hair 704.2
  ossium 756.51
    with blue sclera 756.51
  unguium 703.8
    congenital 757.5
Fragility
  bone 756.51
    with deafness and blue sclera 756.51
  capillary (hereditary) 287.8

Fragility

Fragility — continued
 hair 704.2
 nails 703.8
Fragmentation — see Fracture, by site
Frambesia, frambesial (tropica) — see also Yaws 102.9
 initial lesion or ulcer 102.0
 primary 102.0
Frambeside
 gummatous 102.4
 of early yaws 102.2
Frambesioma 102.1
Franceschetti's syndrome (mandibulofacial dysostosis) 756.0
Francis' disease — see also Tularemia 021.9
Franklin's disease (heavy chain) 273.2
Frank's essential thrombocytopenia — see also Purpura, thrombocytopenic 287.39
Fraser's syndrome 759.89
Freckle 709.09
 malignant melanoma in (M8742/3) — see Melanoma
 melanotic (of Hutchinson) (M8742/2) — see Neoplasm, skin, in situ
Freeman-Sheldon syndrome 759.89
Freezing 991.9
 specified effect NEC 991.8
Freiberg's
 disease (osteochondrosis, second metatarsal) 732.5
 infraction of metatarsal head 732.5
 osteochondrosis 732.5
Frei's disease (climatic bubo) 099.1
Fremitus, friction, cardiac 785.3
Frenulum linguae 750.0
Frenum
 external os 752.49
 tongue 750.0
Frequency (urinary) NEC 788.41
 micturition 788.41
 nocturnal 788.43
 polyuria 788.42
 psychogenic 306.53
Frey's syndrome (auriculotemporal syndrome) 705.22
Friction
 burn (see also Injury, superficial, by site) 919.0
 fremitus, cardiac 785.3
 precordial 785.3
 sounds, chest 786.7
Friderichsen-Waterhouse syndrome or disease 036.3
Friedländer's
 B (bacillus) NEC (see also condition) 041.3
 sepsis or septicemia 038.49
 disease (endarteritis obliterans) — see Arteriosclerosis
Friedreich's
 ataxia 334.0
 combined systemic disease 334.0
 disease 333.2
 combined systemic 334.0
 myoclonia 333.2
 sclerosis (spinal cord) 334.0
Friedrich-Erb-Arnold syndrome (acropachyderma) 757.39
Frigidity 302.72
 psychic or psychogenic 302.72
Fröhlich's disease or syndrome (adiposogenital dystrophy) 253.8
Froin's syndrome 336.8

Frommel-Chiari syndrome 676.6 ✓
Frommel's disease 676.6 ✓
Frontal — see also condition
 lobe syndrome 310.0
Frostbite 991.3
 face 991.0
 foot 991.2
 hand 991.1
 specified site NEC 991.3
Frotteurism 302.89
Frozen 991.9
 pelvis 620.8
 shoulder 726.0
Fructosemia 271.2
Fructosuria (benign) (essential) 271.2
Fuchs'
 black spot (myopic) 360.21
 corneal dystrophy (endothelial) 371.57
 heterochromic cyclitis 364.21
Fucosidosis 271.8
Fugue 780.99
 dissociative 300.13
 hysterical (dissociative) 300.13
 reaction to exceptional stress (transient) 308.1
Fukuhara syndrome 277.87
Fuller Albright's syndrome (osteitis fibrosa disseminata) 756.59
Fuller's earth disease 502
Fulminant, fulminating — see condition
Functional — see condition
Functioning
 borderline intellectual V62.89
Fundus — see also condition
 flavimaculatus 362.76
Fungemia 117.9
Fungus, fungous
 cerebral 348.8
 disease NEC 117.9
 infection — see Infection, fungus
 testis (see also Tuberculosis) 016.5 ✓ [608.81]
Funiculitis (acute) 608.4
 chronic 608.4
 endemic 608.4
 gonococcal (acute) 098.14
 chronic or duration of 2 months or over 098.34
 tuberculous (see also Tuberculosis) 016.5 ✓
Funnel
 breast (acquired) 738.3
 congenital 754.81
 late effect of rickets 268.1
 chest (acquired) 738.3
 congenital 754.81
 late effect of rickets 268.1
 pelvis (acquired) 738.6
 with disproportion (fetopelvic) 653.3 ✓
 affecting fetus or newborn 763.1
 causing obstructed labor 660.1 ✓
 affecting fetus or newborn 763.1
 congenital 755.69
 tuberculous (see also Tuberculosis) 016.9 ✓
FUO — see also Pyrexia 780.6
Furfur 690.18
 microsporon 111.0
Furor, paroxysmal (idiopathic) — see also Epilepsy 345.8 ✓
Furriers' lung 495.8

Furrowed tongue 529.5
 congenital 750.13
Furrowing nail(s) (transverse) 703.8
 congenital 757.5
Furuncle 680.9
 abdominal wall 680.2
 ankle 680.6
 anus 680.5
 arm (any part, above wrist) 680.3
 auditory canal, external 680.0
 axilla 680.3
 back (any part) 680.2
 breast 680.2
 buttock 680.5
 chest wall 680.2
 corpus cavernosum 607.2
 ear (any part) 680.0
 eyelid 373.13
 face (any part, except eye) 680.0
 finger (any) 680.4
 flank 680.2
 foot (any part) 680.7
 forearm 680.3
 gluteal (region) 680.5
 groin 680.2
 hand (any part) 680.4
 head (any part, except face) 680.8
 heel 680.7
 hip 680.6
 kidney (see also Abscess, kidney) 590.2
 knee 680.6
 labium (majus) (minus) 616.4
 lacrimal
 gland (see also Dacryoadenitis) 375.00
 passages (duct) (sac) (see also Dacryocystitis) 375.30
 leg, any part except foot 680.6
 malignant 022.0
 multiple sites 680.9
 neck 680.1
 nose (external) (septum) 680.0
 orbit 376.01
 partes posteriores 680.5
 pectoral region 680.2
 penis 607.2
 perineum 680.2
 pinna 680.0
 scalp (any part) 680.8
 scrotum 608.4
 seminal vesicle 608.0
 shoulder 680.3
 skin NEC 680.9
 specified site NEC 680.8
 spermatic cord 608.4
 temple (region) 680.0
 testis 604.90
 thigh 680.6
 thumb 680.4
 toe (any) 680.7
 trunk 680.2
 tunica vaginalis 608.4
 umbilicus 680.2
 upper arm 680.3
 vas deferens 608.4
 vulva 616.4
 wrist 680.4
Furunculosis — see also Furuncle 680.9
 external auditory meatus 680.0 [380.13]
Fusarium (infection) 118
Fusion, fused (congenital)
 anal (with urogenital canal) 751.5
 aorta and pulmonary artery 745.0

Fusion, fused — continued
 astragaloscaphoid 755.67
 atria 745.5
 atrium and ventricle 745.69
 auditory canal 744.02
 auricles, heart 745.5
 binocular, with defective stereopsis 368.33
 bone 756.9
 cervical spine — see Fusion, spine
 choanal 748.0
 commissure, mitral valve 746.5
 cranial sutures, premature 756.0
 cusps, heart valve NEC 746.89
 mitral 746.5
 tricuspid 746.89
 ear ossicles 744.04
 fingers (see also Syndactylism, fingers) 755.11
 hymen 752.42
 hymeno-urethral 599.89
 causing obstructed labor 660.1 ✓
 affecting fetus or newborn 763.1
 joint (acquired) (see also Ankylosis)
 congenital 755.8
 kidneys (incomplete) 753.3
 labium (majus) (minus) 752.49
 larynx and trachea 748.3
 limb 755.8
 lower 755.69
 upper 755.59
 lobe, lung 748.5
 lumbosacral (acquired) 724.6
 congenital 756.15
 surgical V45.4
 nares (anterior) (posterior) 748.0
 nose, nasal 748.0
 nostril(s) 748.0
 organ or site NEC — see Anomaly, specified type NEC
 ossicles 756.9
 auditory 744.04
 pulmonary valve segment 746.02
 pulmonic cusps 746.02
 ribs 756.3
 sacroiliac (acquired) (joint) 724.6
 congenital 755.69
 surgical V45.4
 skull, imperfect 756.0
 spine (acquired) 724.9
 arthrodesis status V45.4
 congenital (vertebra) 756.15
 postoperative status V45.4
 sublingual duct with submaxillary duct at opening in mouth 750.26
 talonavicular (bar) 755.67
 teeth, tooth 520.2
 testes 752.89
 toes (see also Syndactylism, toes) 755.13
 trachea and esophagus 750.3
 twins 759.4
 urethral-hymenal 599.89
 vagina 752.49
 valve cusps — see Fusion, cusps, heart valve
 ventricles, heart 745.4
 vertebra (arch) — see Fusion, spine
 vulva 752.49
Fusospirillosis (mouth) (tongue) (tonsil) 101
Fussy infant (baby) 780.91

Index to Diseases

G

Gafsa boil 085.1
Gain, weight (abnormal) (excessive) — *see also* Weight, gain 783.1
Gaisböck's disease or syndrome (polycythemia hypertonica) 289.0
Gait
  abnormality 781.2
    hysterical 300.11
  ataxic 781.2
    hysterical 300.11
  disturbance 781.2
    hysterical 300.11
  paralytic 781.2
  scissor 781.2
  spastic 781.2
  staggering 781.2
    hysterical 300.11
Galactocele (breast) (infected) 611.5
  puerperal, postpartum 676.8 ☑
Galactophoritis 611.0
  puerperal, postpartum 675.2 ☑
Galactorrhea 676.6 ☑
  not associated with childbirth 611.6
Galactosemia (classic) (congenital) 271.1
Galactosuria 271.1
Galacturia 791.1
  bilharziasis 120.0
Galen's vein — *see* condition
Gallbladder — *see also* condition
  acute (*see also* Disease, gallbladder) 575.0
Gall duct — *see* condition
Gallop rhythm 427.89
Gallstone (cholemic) (colic) (impacted) — *see also* Cholelithiasis
  causing intestinal obstruction 560.31
Gambling, pathological 312.31
Gammaloidosis 277.39 ▲
Gammopathy 273.9
  macroglobulinemia 273.3
  monoclonal (benign) (essential) (idiopathic) (with lymphoplasmacytic dyscrasia) 273.1
Gamna's disease (siderotic splenomegaly) 289.51
Gampsodactylia (congenital) 754.71
Gamstorp's disease (adynamia episodica hereditaria) 359.3
Gandy-Nanta disease (siderotic splenomegaly) 289.51
Gang activity, without manifest psychiatric disorder V71.09
  adolescent V71.02
  adult V71.01
  child V71.02
Gangliocytoma (M9490/0) — *see* Neoplasm, connective tissue, benign
Ganglioglioma (M9505/1) — *see* Neoplasm, by site, uncertain behavior
Ganglion 727.43
  joint 727.41
  of yaws (early) (late) 102.6
  periosteal (*see also* Periostitis) 730.3 ☑
  tendon sheath (compound) (diffuse) 727.42
  tuberculous (*see also* Tuberculosis) 015.9 ☑
Ganglioneuroblastoma (M9490/3) — *see* Neoplasm, connective tissue, malignant
Ganglioneuroma (M9490/0) — *see also* Neoplasm, connective tissue, benign
  malignant (M9490/3) — *see* Neoplasm, connective tissue, malignant
Ganglioneuromatosis (M9491/0) — *see* Neoplasm, connective tissue, benign
Ganglionitis
  fifth nerve (*see also* Neuralgia, trigeminal) 350.1
  gasserian 350.1

Ganglionitis — *continued*
  geniculate 351.1
    herpetic 053.11
    newborn 767.5
  herpes zoster 053.11
  herpetic geniculate (Hunt's syndrome) 053.11
Gangliosidosis 330.1
Gangosa 102.5
Gangrene, gangrenous (anemia) (artery) (cellulitis) (dermatitis) (dry) (infective) (moist) (pemphigus) (septic) (skin) (stasis) (ulcer) 785.4
  with
    arteriosclerosis (native artery) 440.24
      bypass graft 440.30
        autologous vein 440.31
        nonautologous biological 440.32
    diabetes (mellitus) 250.7 ☑ [785.4]
  abdomen (wall) 785.4
  adenitis 683
  alveolar 526.5
  angina 462
    diphtheritic 032.0
  anus 569.49
  appendices epiploicae — *see* Gangrene, mesentery
  appendix — *see* Appendicitis, acute
  arteriosclerotic — *see* Arteriosclerosis, with, gangrene
  auricle 785.4
  Bacillus welchii (*see also* Gangrene, gas) 040.0
  bile duct (*see also* Cholangitis) 576.8
  bladder 595.89
  bowel — *see* Gangrene, intestine
  cecum — *see* Gangrene, intestine
  Clostridium perfringens or welchii (*see also* Gangrene, gas) 040.0
  colon — *see* Gangrene, intestine
  connective tissue 785.4
  cornea 371.40
  corpora cavernosa (infective) 607.2
    noninfective 607.89
  cutaneous, spreading 785.4
  decubital (*see also* Decubitus) 707.00 [785.4]
  diabetic (any site) 250.7 ☑ [785.4]
  dropsical 785.4
  emphysematous (*see also* Gangrene, gas) 040.0
  epidemic (ergotized grain) 988.2
  epididymis (infectional) (*see also* Epididymitis) 604.99
  erysipelas (*see also* Erysipelas) 035
  extremity (lower) (upper) 785.4
  gallbladder or duct (*see also* Cholecystitis, acute) 575.0
  gas (bacillus) 040.0
    with
      abortion — *see* Abortion, by type, with sepsis
      ectopic pregnancy (*see also* categories 633.0–633.9) 639.0
      molar pregnancy (*see also* categories 630–632) 639.0
    following
      abortion 639.0
      ectopic or molar pregnancy 639.0
    puerperal, postpartum, childbirth 670.0 ☑
  glossitis 529.0
  gum 523.8
  hernia — *see* Hernia, by site, with gangrene
  hospital noma 528.1
  intestine, intestinal (acute) (hemorrhagic) (massive) 557.0
    with
      hernia — *see* Hernia, by site, with gangrene

Gangrene, gangrenous — *continued*
  intestine, intestinal — *continued*
    with — *continued*
      mesenteric embolism or infarction 557.0
      obstruction (*see also* Obstruction, intestine) 560.9
  laryngitis 464.00
    with obstruction 464.01
  liver 573.8
  lung 513.0
    spirochetal 104.8
  lymphangitis 457.2
  Meleney's (cutaneous) 686.09
  mesentery 557.0
    with
      embolism or infarction 557.0
      intestinal obstruction (*see also* Obstruction, intestine) 560.9
  mouth 528.1
  noma 528.1
  orchitis 604.90
  ovary (*see also* Salpingo-oophoritis) 614.2
  pancreas 577.0
  penis (infectional) 607.2
    noninfective 607.89
  perineum 785.4
  pharynx 462
  pneumonia 513.0
  Pott's 440.24
  presenile 443.1
  pulmonary 513.0
  pulp, tooth 522.1
  quinsy 475
  Raynaud's (symmetric gangrene) 443.0 [785.4]
  rectum 569.49
  retropharyngeal 478.24
  rupture — *see* Hernia, by site, with gangrene
  scrotum 608.4
    noninfective 608.83
  senile 440.24
  septic 034.0
  septic 034.0
  sore throat 462
  spermatic cord 608.4
    noninfective 608.89
  spine 785.4
  spirochetal NEC 104.8
  spreading cutaneous 785.4
  stomach 537.89
  stomatitis 528.1
  symmetrical 443.0 [785.4]
  testis (infectional) (*see also* Orchitis) 604.99
    noninfective 608.89
  throat 462
    diphtheritic 032.0
  thyroid (gland) 246.8
  tonsillitis (acute) 463
  tooth (pulp) 522.1
  tuberculous NEC (*see also* Tuberculosis) 011.9 ☑
  tunica vaginalis 608.4
    noninfective 608.89
  umbilicus 785.4
  uterus (*see also* Endometritis) 615.9
  uvulitis 528.3
  vas deferens 608.4
    noninfective 608.89
  vulva (*see also* Vulvitis) 616.10
Gannister disease (occupational) 502
  with tuberculosis — *see* Tuberculosis, pulmonary
Ganser's syndrome, hysterical 300.16
Gardner-Diamond syndrome (autoerythrocyte sensitization) 287.2
Gargoylism 277.5
Garré's
  disease (*see also* Osteomyelitis) 730.1 ☑
  osteitis (sclerosing) (*see also* Osteomyelitis) 730.1 ☑

Garré's — *continued*
  osteomyelitis (*see also* Osteomyelitis) 730.1 ☑
Garrod's pads, knuckle 728.79
Gartner's duct
  cyst 752.41
  persistent 752.41
Gas
  asphyxia, asphyxiation, inhalation, poisoning, suffocation NEC 987.9
    specified gas — *see* Table of Drugs and Chemicals
  bacillus gangrene or infection — *see* Gas, gangrene
  cyst, mesentery 568.89
  excessive 787.3
  gangrene 040.0
    with
      abortion — *see* Abortion, by type, with sepsis
      ectopic pregnancy (*see also* categories 633.0–633.9) 639.0
      molar pregnancy (*see also* categories 630–632) 639.0
    following
      abortion 639.0
      ectopic or molar pregnancy 639.0
    puerperal, postpartum, childbirth 670.0 ☑
  on stomach 787.3
  pains 787.3
Gastradenitis 535.0 ☑
Gastralgia 536.8
  psychogenic 307.89
Gastrectasis, gastrectasia 536.1
  psychogenic 306.4
Gastric — *see* condition
Gastrinoma (M8153/1)
  malignant (M8153/3)
    pancreas 157.4
    specified site NEC — *see* Neoplasm, by site, malignant
    unspecified site 157.4
  specified site — *see* Neoplasm, by site, uncertain behavior
  unspecified site 235.5
Gastritis 535.5 ☑

Note — Use the following fifth-digit subclassification for category 535:
0 without mention of hemorrhage
1 with hemorrhage

  acute 535.0 ☑
  alcoholic 535.3 ☑
  allergic 535.4 ☑
  antral 535.4 ☑
  atrophic 535.1 ☑
  atrophic-hyperplastic 535.1 ☑
  bile-induced 535.4 ☑
  catarrhal 535.0 ☑
  chronic (atrophic) 535.1 ☑
  cirrhotic 535.4 ☑
  corrosive (acute) 535.4 ☑
  dietetic 535.4 ☑
  due to diet deficiency 269.9 [535.4] ☑
  eosinophilic 535.4 ☑
  erosive 535.4 ☑
  follicular 535.4 ☑
    chronic 535.1 ☑
  giant hypertrophic 535.2 ☑
  glandular 535.4 ☑
    chronic 535.1 ☑
  hypertrophic (mucosa) 535.2 ☑
    chronic giant 211.1
  irritant 535.4 ☑
  nervous 306.4
  phlegmonous 535.0 ☑
  psychogenic 306.4
  sclerotic 535.4 ☑
  spastic 536.8
  subacute 535.0 ☑
  superficial 535.4 ☑

Gastritis

Gastritis — *continued*
  suppurative 535.0
  toxic 535.4
  tuberculous (*see also* Tuberculosis) 017.9
Gastrocarcinoma (M8010/3) 151.9
Gastrocolic — *see* condition
Gastrocolitis — *see* Enteritis
Gastrodisciasis 121.8
Gastroduodenitis — *see also* Gastritis 535.5
  catarrhal 535.0
  infectional 535.0
  virus, viral 008.8
    specified type NEC 008.69
Gastrodynia 536.8
Gastroenteritis (acute) (catarrhal) (congestive) (hemorrhagic) (noninfectious) — *see also* Enteritis 558.9
  aertrycke infection 003.0
  allergic 558.3
  chronic 558.9
    ulcerative (*see also* Colitis, ulcerative) 556.9
  dietetic 558.9
  due to
    food poisoning (*see also* Poisoning, food) 005.9
    radiation 558.1
  epidemic 009.0
  functional 558.9
  infectious (*see also* Enteritis, due to, by organism) 009.0
    presumed 009.1
  salmonella 003.0
  septic (*see also* Enteritis, due to, by organism) 009.0
  toxic 558.2
  tuberculous (*see also* Tuberculosis) 014.8
  ulcerative (*see also* Colitis, ulcerative) 556.9
  viral NEC 008.8
    specified type NEC 008.69
  zymotic 009.0
Gastroenterocolitis — *see* Enteritis
Gastroenteropathy, protein-losing 579.8
Gastroenteroptosis 569.89
Gastroesophageal laceration-hemorrhage syndrome 530.7
Gastroesophagitis 530.19
Gastrohepatitis — *see also* Gastritis 535.5
Gastrointestinal — *see* condition
Gastrojejunal — *see* condition
Gastrojejunitis — *see also* Gastritis 535.5
Gastrojejunocolic — *see* condition
Gastroliths 537.89
Gastromalacia 537.89
Gastroparalysis 536.3
  diabetic 250.6 [536.3]
Gastroparesis 536.3
  diabetic 250.6 [536.3]
Gastropathy 537.9
  erythematous 535.5
  exudative 579.8
Gastroptosis 537.5
Gastrorrhagia 578.0
Gastrorrhea 536.8
  psychogenic 306.4
Gastroschisis (congenital) 756.79
  acquired 569.89
Gastrospasm (neurogenic) (reflex) 536.8
  neurotic 306.4
  psychogenic 306.4
Gastrostaxis 578.0
Gastrostenosis 537.89
Gastrostomy
  attention to V55.1
  complication 536.40
    specified type 536.49
  infection 536.41
  malfunctioning 536.42
  status V44.1

Gastrosuccorrhea (continuous) (intermittent) 536.8
  neurotic 306.4
  psychogenic 306.4
Gaucher's
  disease (adult) (cerebroside lipidosis) (infantile) 272.7
  hepatomegaly 272.7
  splenomegaly (cerebroside lipidosis) 272.7
Gayet's disease (superior hemorrhagic polioencephalitis) 265.1
Gayet-Wernicke's syndrome (superior hemorrhagic polioencephalitis) 265.1
Gee (-Herter) (-Heubner) (-Thaysen) disease or syndrome (nontropical sprue) 579.0
Gélineau's syndrome — *see also* Narcolepsy 347.00
Gemination, teeth 520.2
Gemistocytoma (M9411/3)
  specified site — *see* Neoplasm, by site, malignant
  unspecified site 191.9
General, generalized — *see* condtion
Genetic
  susceptibility to
    neoplasm
      malignant, of
        breast V84.01
        endometrium V84.04
        other V84.09
        ovary V84.02
        prostate V84.03
      other disease V84.8
Genital — *see* condition
  warts 078.19
Genito-anorectal syndrome 099.1
Genitourinary system — *see* condition
Genu
  congenital 755.64
  extrorsum (acquired) 736.42
    congenital 755.64
    late effects of rickets 268.1
  introrsum (acquired) 736.41
    congenital 755.64
    late effects of rickets 268.1
  rachitic (old) 268.1
  recurvatum (acquired) 736.5
    congenital 754.40
      with dislocation of knee 754.41
    late effects of rickets 268.1
  valgum (acquired) (knock-knee) 736.41
    congenital 755.64
    late effects of rickets 268.1
  varum (acquired) (bowleg) 736.42
    congenital 755.64
    late effect of rickets 268.1
Geographic tongue 529.1
Geophagia 307.52
Geotrichosis 117.9
  intestine 117.9
  lung 117.9
  mouth 117.9
Gephyrophobia 300.29
Gerbode defect 745.4
Gerhardt's
  disease (erythromelalgia) 443.82
  syndrome (vocal cord paralysis) 478.30
Gerlier's disease (epidemic vertigo) 078.81
German measles 056.9
  exposure to V01.4
Germinoblastoma (diffuse) (M9614/3) 202.8
  follicular (M9692/3) 202.0
Germinoma (M9064/3) — *see* Neoplasm, by site, malignant
Gerontoxon 371.41
Gerstmann's syndrome (finger agnosia) 784.69
Gestation (period) — *see also* Pregnancy

Gestation — *see also* Pregnancy — *continued*
  ectopic NEC (*see also* Pregnancy, ectopic) 633.90
    with intrauterine pregnancy 633.91
Gestational proteinuria 646.2
  with hypertension — *see* Toxemia, of pregnancy
Ghon tubercle primary infection — *see also* Tuberculosis 010.0
Ghost
  teeth 520.4
  vessels, cornea 370.64
Ghoul hand 102.3
Gianotti Crosti syndrome 057.8
  due to known virus — *see* Infection, virus
  due to unknown virus 057.8
Giant
  cell
    epulis 523.8
    peripheral (gingiva) 523.8
    tumor, tendon sheath 727.02
  colon (congenital) 751.3
  esophagus (congenital) 750.4
  kidney 753.3
  urticaria 995.1
    hereditary 277.6
Giardia lamblia infestation 007.1
Giardiasis 007.1
Gibert's disease (pityriasis rosea) 696.3
Gibraltar fever — *see* Brucellosis
Giddiness 780.4
  hysterical 300.11
  psychogenic 306.9
Gierke's disease (glycogenosis I) 271.0
Gigantism (cerebral) (hypophyseal) (pituitary) 253.0
Gilbert's disease or cholemia (familial nonhemolytic jaundice) 277.4
Gilchrist's disease (North American blastomycosis) 116.0
Gilford (-Hutchinson) disease or syndrome (progeria) 259.8
Gilles de la Tourette's disease (motor-verbal tic) 307.23
Gillespie's syndrome (dysplasia oculo-dentodigitalis) 759.89
Gingivitis 523.10
  acute 523.00
    necrotizing 101
    non-plaque induced 523.01
    plaque induced 523.00
  catarrhal 523.00
  chronic 523.10
    non-plaque induced 523.11
  desquamative 523.10
  expulsiva 523.40
  hyperplastic 523.10
  marginal, simple 523.10
  necrotizing, acute 101
  non-plaque induced 523.11
  pellagrous 265.2
  plaque induced 523.10
  ulcerative 523.10
    acute necrotizing 101
  Vincent's 101
Gingivoglossitis 529.0
Gingivopericementitis 523.40
Gingivosis 523.10
Gingivostomatitis 523.10
  herpetic 054.2
Giovannini's disease 117.9
GISA (glycopeptide intermediate staphylococcus aureus) V09.8
Glanders 024
Gland, glandular — *see* condition
Glanzmann (-Naegeli) disease or thrombasthenia 287.1
Glassblowers' disease 527.1
Glaucoma (capsular) (inflammatory) (noninflammatory) (primary) 365.9
  with increased episcleral venous pressure 365.82
  absolute 360.42
  acute 365.22

Glaucoma — *continued*
  acute — *continued*
    narrow angle 365.22
    secondary 365.60
  angle closure 365.20
    acute 365.22
    chronic 365.23
    intermittent 365.21
    interval 365.21
    residual stage 365.24
    subacute 365.21
  borderline 365.00
  chronic 365.11
    noncongestive 365.11
    open angle 365.11
    simple 365.11
  closed angle — *see* Glaucoma, angle closure
  congenital 743.20
    associated with other eye anomalies 743.22
    simple 743.21
  congestive — *see* Glaucoma, narrow angle
  corticosteroid-induced (glaucomatous stage) 365.31
    residual stage 365.32
  hemorrhagic 365.60
  hypersecretion 365.81
  infantile 365.14
    congenital 743.20
      associated with other eye anomalies 743.22
      simple 743.21
  in or with
    aniridia 743.45 [365.42]
    Axenfeld's anomaly 743.44 [365.41]
    concussion of globe 921.3 [365.65]
    congenital syndromes NEC 759.89 [365.44]
    dislocation of lens
      anterior 379.33 [365.59]
      posterior 379.34 [365.59]
    disorder of lens NEC 365.59
    epithelial down-growth 364.61 [365.64]
    glaucomatocyclitic crisis 364.22 [365.62]
    hypermature cataract 366.18 [365.51]
    hyphema 364.41 [365.63]
    inflammation, ocular 365.62
    iridocyclitis 364.3 [365.62]
    iris
      anomalies NEC 743.46 [365.42]
      atrophy, essential 364.51 [365.42]
      bombé 364.74 [365.61]
      rubeosis 364.42 [365.63]
    microcornea 743.41 [365.43]
    neurofibromatosis 237.71 [365.44]
    ocular
      cysts NEC 365.64
      disorders NEC 365.60
      trauma 365.65
      tumors NEC 365.64
    postdislocation of lens
      anterior 379.33 [365.59]
      posterior 379.34 [365.59]
    pseudoexfoliation of capsule 366.11 [365.52]
    pupillary block or seclusion 364.74 [365.61]
    recession of chamber angle 364.77 [365.65]
    retinal vein occlusion 362.35 [365.63]
    Rieger's anomaly or syndrome 743.44 [365.44]
    rubeosis of iris 364.42 [365.63]
    seclusion of pupil 364.74 [365.61]
    spherophakia 743.36 [365.59]
    Sturge-Weber (-Dimitri) syndrome 759.6 [365.44]
    systemic syndrome NEC 365.44
    tumor of globe 365.64

Glaucoma — continued
  in or with — continued
    vascular disorders NEC 365.63
  juvenile 365.14
  low tension 365.12
  malignant 365.83
  narrow angle (primary) 365.20
    acute 365.22
    chronic 365.23
    intermittent 365.21
    interval 365.21
    residual stage 365.24
    subacute 365.21
  newborn 743.20
    associated with other eye anomalies 743.22
    simple 743.21
  noncongestive (chronic) 365.11
  nonobstructive (chronic) 365.11
  obstructive 365.60
    due to lens changes 365.59
  open angle 365.10
    with
      borderline intraocular pressure 365.01
        cupping of optic discs 365.01
    primary 365.11
    residual stage 365.15
  phacolytic 365.51
    with hypermature cataract 366.18 [365.51]
  pigmentary 365.13
  postinfectious 365.60
  pseudoexfoliation 365.52
    with pseudoexfoliation of capsule 366.11 [365.52]
  secondary NEC 365.60
  simple (chronic) 365.11
  simplex 365.11
  steroid responders 365.03
  suspect 365.00
  syphilitic 095.8
  traumatic NEC 365.65
    newborn 767.8
  tuberculous (see also Tuberculosis) 017.3 ☑ [365.62]
  wide angle (see also Glaucoma, open angle) 365.10
Glaucomatous flecks (subcapsular) 366.31
Glazed tongue 529.4
Gleet 098.2
Glénard's disease or syndrome (enteroptosis) 569.89
Glinski-Simmonds syndrome (pituitary cachexia) 253.2
Glioblastoma (multiforme) (M9440/3)
  with sarcomatous component (M9442/3)
    specified site — see Neoplasm, by site, malignant
    unspecified site 191.9
  giant cell (M9441/3)
    specified site — see Neoplasm, by site, malignant
    unspecified site 191.9
  specified site — see Neoplasm, by site, malignant
  unspecified site 191.9
Glioma (malignant) (M9380/3)
  astrocytic (M9400/3)
    specified site — see Neoplasm, by site, malignant
    unspecified site 191.9
  mixed (M9382/3)
    specified site — see Neoplasm, by site, malignant
    unspecified site 191.9
  nose 748.1
  specified site NEC — see Neoplasm, by site, malignant
  subependymal (M9383/1) 237.5
  unspecified site 191.9
Gliomatosis cerebri (M9381/3) 191.0
Glioneuroma (M9505/1) — see Neoplasm, by site, uncertain behavior

Gliosarcoma (M9380/3)
  specified site — see Neoplasm, by site, malignant
  unspecified site 191.9
Gliosis (cerebral) 349.89
  spinal 336.0
Glisson's
  cirrhosis — see Cirrhosis, portal
  disease (see also Rickets) 268.0
Glissonitis 573.3
Globinuria 791.2
Globus 306.4
  hystericus 300.11
Glomangioma (M8712/0) — see also Hemangioma 228.00
Glomangiosarcoma (M8710/3) — see Neoplasm, connective tissue, malignant
Glomerular nephritis — see also Nephritis 583.9
Glomerulitis — see also Nephritis 583.9
Glomerulonephritis — see also Nephritis 583.9
  with
    edema (see also Nephrosis) 581.9
    lesion of
      exudative nephritis 583.89
      interstitial nephritis (diffuse) (focal) 583.89
      necrotizing glomerulitis 583.4
        acute 580.4
        chronic 582.4
      renal necrosis 583.9
        cortical 583.6
        medullary 583.7
      specified pathology NEC 583.89
        acute 580.89
        chronic 582.89
    necrosis, renal 583.9
      cortical 583.6
      medullary (papillary) 583.7
    specified pathology or lesion NEC 583.89
  acute 580.9
    with
      exudative nephritis 580.89
      interstitial nephritis (diffuse) (focal) 580.89
      necrotizing glomerulitis 580.4
      extracapillary with epithelial crescents 580.4
      poststreptococcal 580.0
      proliferative (diffuse) 580.0
      rapidly progressive 580.4
      specified pathology NEC 580.89
    arteriolar (see also Hypertension, kidney) 403.90
    arteriosclerotic (see also Hypertension, kidney) 403.90
    ascending (see also Pyelitis) 590.80
    basement membrane NEC 583.89
      with
        pulmonary hemorrhage (Goodpasture's syndrome) 446.21 [583.81]
  chronic 582.9
    with
      exudative nephritis 582.89
      interstitial nephritis (diffuse) (focal) 582.89
      necrotizing glomerulitis 582.4
      specified pathology or lesion NEC 582.89
    endothelial 582.2
    extracapillary with epithelial crescents 582.4
    hypocomplementemic persistent 582.2
    lobular 582.2
    membranoproliferative 582.2
    membranous 582.1
      and proliferative (mixed) 582.2
      sclerosing 582.1
    mesangiocapillary 582.2
    mixed membranous and proliferative 582.2

Glomerulonephritis — see also Nephritis — continued
  chronic — continued
    proliferative (diffuse) 582.0
    rapidly progressive 582.4
    sclerosing 582.1
  cirrhotic — see Sclerosis, renal
  desquamative — see Nephrosis
  due to or associated with
    amyloidosis 277.39 [583.81] ▲
      with nephrotic syndrome 277.39 [581.81] ▲
      chronic 277.39 [582.81] ▲
    diabetes mellitus 250.4 ☑ [583.81]
      with nephrotic syndrome 250.4 ☑ [581.81]
    diphtheria 032.89 [580.81]
    gonococcal infection (acute) 098.19 [583.81]
      chronic or duration of 2 months or over 098.39 [583.81]
    infectious hepatitis 070.9 [580.81]
    malaria (with nephrotic syndrome) 084.9 [581.81]
    mumps 072.79 [580.81]
    polyarteritis (nodosa) (with nephrotic syndrome) 446.0 [581.81]
    specified pathology NEC 583.89
      acute 580.89
      chronic 582.89
    streptotrichosis 039.8 [583.81]
    subacute bacterial endocarditis 421.0 [583.81]
    syphilis (late) 095.4
      congenital 090.5 [583.81]
      early 091.69 [583.81]
    systemic lupus erythematosus 710.0 [583.81]
      with nephrotic syndrome 710.0 [581.81]
      chronic 710.0 [582.81]
    tuberculosis (see also Tuberculosis) 016.0 ☑ [583.81]
    typhoid fever 002.0 [580.81]
  extracapillary with epithelial crescents 583.4
    acute 580.4
    chronic 582.4
  exudative 583.89
    acute 580.89
    chronic 582.89
  focal (see also Nephritis) 583.9
    embolic 580.4
  granular 582.89
  granulomatous 582.89
  hydremic (see also Nephrosis) 581.9
  hypocomplementemic persistent 583.2
    with nephrotic syndrome 581.2
    chronic 582.2
  immune complex NEC 583.89
  infective (see also Pyelitis) 590.80
  interstitial (diffuse) (focal) 583.89
    with nephrotic syndrome 581.89
    acute 580.89
    chronic 582.89
  latent or quiescent 582.9
  lobular 583.2
    with nephrotic syndrome 581.2
    chronic 582.2
  membranoproliferative 583.2
    with nephrotic syndrome 581.2
    chronic 582.2
  membranous 583.1
    with nephrotic syndrome 581.1
    and proliferative (mixed) 583.2
      with nephrotic syndrome 581.2
      chronic 582.2
    chronic 582.1
    sclerosing 582.1
      with nephrotic syndrome 581.1
  mesangiocapillary 583.2
    with nephrotic syndrome 581.2
    chronic 582.2
  minimal change 581.3

Glomerulonephritis — see also Nephritis — continued
  mixed membranous and proliferative 583.2
    with nephrotic syndrome 581.2
    chronic 582.2
  necrotizing 583.4
    acute 580.4
    chronic 582.4
  nephrotic (see also Nephrosis) 581.9
  old — see Glomerulonephritis, chronic
  parenchymatous 581.89
  poststreptococcal 580.0
  proliferative (diffuse) 583.0
    with nephrotic syndrome 581.0
    acute 580.0
    chronic 582.0
  purulent (see also Pyelitis) 590.80
  quiescent — see Nephritis, chronic
  rapidly progressive 583.4
    acute 580.4
    chronic 582.4
  sclerosing membranous (chronic) 582.1
    with nephrotic syndrome 581.1
  septic (see also Pyelitis) 590.80
  specified pathology or lesion NEC 583.89
    with nephrotic syndrome 581.89
    acute 580.89
    chronic 582.89
  suppurative (acute) (disseminated) (see also Pyelitis) 590.80
  toxic — see Nephritis, acute
  tubal, tubular — see Nephrosis, tubular
  type II (Ellis) — see Nephrosis
  vascular — see Hypertension, kidney
Glomerulosclerosis — see also Sclerosis, renal 587
  focal 582.1
    with nephrotic syndrome 581.1
  intercapillary (nodular) (with diabetes) 250.4 ☑ [581.81]
Glossagra 529.6
Glossalgia 529.6
Glossitis 529.0
  areata exfoliativa 529.1
  atrophic 529.4
  benign migratory 529.1
  gangrenous 529.0
  Hunter's 529.4
  median rhomboid 529.2
  Moeller's 529.4
  pellagrous 265.2
Glossocele 529.8
Glossodynia 529.6
  exfoliativa 529.4
Glossoncus 529.8
Glossophytia 529.3
Glossoplegia 529.8
Glossoptosis 529.8
Glossopyrosis 529.6
Glossotrichia 529.3
Glossy skin 701.9
Glottis — see condition
Glottitis — see Glossitis
Glucagonoma (M8152/0)
  malignant (M8152/3)
    pancreas 157.4
    specified site NEC — see Neoplasm, by site, malignant
    unspecified site 157.4
  pancreas 211.7
  specified site NEC — see Neoplasm, by site, benign
  unspecified site 211.7
Glucoglycinuria 270.7
Glue ear syndrome 381.20
Glue sniffing (airplane glue) — see also Dependence 304.6 ☑
Glycinemia (with methylmalonic acidemia) 270.7
Glycinuria (renal) (with ketosis) 270.0

Glycogen

Glycogen
  infiltration (see also Disease, glycogen storage) 271.0
  storage disease (see also Disease, glycogen storage) 271.0
Glycogenosis — see also Disease, glycogen storage 271.0
  cardiac 271.0 [425.7]
  Cori, types I-VII 271.0
  diabetic, secondary 250.8 ☑ [259.8]
  diffuse (with hepatic cirrhosis) 271.0
  generalized 271.0
  glucose-6-phosphatase deficiency 271.0
  hepatophosphorylase deficiency 271.0
  hepatorenal 271.0
  myophosphorylase deficiency 271.0
Glycopenia 251.2
Glycopeptide
  intermediate staphylococcus aureus (GISA) V09.8 ☑
  resistant
    enterococcus V09.8 ☑
    staphylococcus aureus (GRSA) V09.8 ☑
Glycoprolinuria 270.8
Glycosuria 791.5
  renal 271.4
Gnathostoma (spinigerum) (infection) (infestation) 128.1
  wandering swellings from 128.1
Gnathostomiasis 128.1
Goiter (adolescent) (colloid) (diffuse) (dipping) (due to iodine deficiency) (endemic) (euthyroid) (heart) (hyperplastic) (internal) (intrathoracic) (juvenile) (mixed type) (nonendemic) (parenchymatous) (plunging) (sporadic) (subclavicular) (substernal) 240.9
  with
    hyperthyroidism (recurrent) (see also Goiter, toxic) 242.0 ☑
    thyrotoxicosis (see also Goiter, toxic) 242.0 ☑
  adenomatous (see also Goiter, nodular) 241.9
  cancerous (M8000/3) 193
  complicating pregnancy, childbirth, or puerperium 648.1 ☑
  congenital 246.1
  cystic (see also Goiter, nodular) 241.9
  due to enzyme defect in synthesis of thyroid hormone (butane-insoluble iodine) (coupling) (deiodinase) (iodide trapping or organification) (iodotyrosine dehalogenase) (peroxidase) 246.1
  dyshormonogenic 246.1
  exophthalmic (see also Goiter, toxic) 242.0 ☑
  familial (with deaf-mutism) 243
  fibrous 245.3
  lingual 759.2
  lymphadenoid 245.2
  malignant (M8000/3) 193
  multinodular (nontoxic) 241.1
    toxic or with hyperthyroidism (see also Goiter, toxic) 242.2 ☑
  nodular (nontoxic) 241.9
    with
      hyperthyroidism (see also Goiter, toxic) 242.3 ☑
      thyrotoxicosis (see also Goiter, toxic) 242.3 ☑
    endemic 241.9
    exophthalmic (diffuse) (see also Goiter, toxic) 242.0 ☑
    multinodular (nontoxic) 241.1
    sporadic 241.9
    toxic (see also Goiter, toxic) 242.3 ☑
    uninodular (nontoxic) 241.0
  nontoxic (nodular) 241.9
    multinodular 241.1
    uninodular 241.0

Goiter — continued
  pulsating (see also Goiter, toxic) 242.0 ☑
  simple 240.0
  toxic 242.0 ☑

Note — Use the following fifth-digit subclassification with category 242:
0 without mention of thyrotoxic crisis or storm
1 with mention of thyrotoxic crisis or storm

    adenomatous 242.3 ☑
      multinodular 242.2 ☑
      uninodular 242.1 ☑
    multinodular 242.2 ☑
    nodular 242.3 ☑
      multinodular 242.2 ☑
      uninodular 242.1 ☑
    uninodular 242.1 ☑
  uninodular (nontoxic) 241.0
  toxic or with hyperthyroidism (see also Goiter, toxic) 242.1 ☑
Goldberg (-Maxwell) (-Morris) syndrome (testicular feminization) 259.5
Goldblatt's
  hypertension 440.1
  kidney 440.1
Goldenhar's syndrome (oculoauriculovertebral dysplasia) 756.0
Goldflam-Erb disease or syndrome 358.00
Goldscheider's disease (epidermolysis bullosa) 757.39
Goldstein's disease (familial hemorrhagic telangiectasia) 448.0
Golfer's elbow 726.32
Goltz-Gorlin syndrome (dermal hypoplasia) 757.39
Gonadoblastoma (M9073/1)
  specified site — see Neoplasm, by site uncertain behavior
  unspecified site
    female 236.2
    male 236.4
Gonecystitis — see also Vesiculitis 608.0
Gongylonemiasis 125.6
  mouth 125.6
Goniosynechiae 364.73
Gonococcemia 098.89
Gonococcus, gonococcal (disease) (infection) — see also condition 098.0
  anus 098.7
  bursa 098.52
  chronic NEC 098.2
  complicating pregnancy, childbirth, or puerperium 647.1 ☑
    affecting fetus or newborn 760.2
  conjunctiva, conjunctivitis (neonatorum) 098.40
  dermatosis 098.89
  endocardium 098.84
  epididymo-orchitis 098.13
    chronic or duration of 2 months or over 098.33
  eye (newborn) 098.40
  fallopian tube (chronic) 098.37
    acute 098.17
  genitourinary (acute) (organ) (system) (tract) (see also Gonorrhea) 098.0
    lower 098.0
      chronic 098.2
    upper 098.10
      chronic 098.30
  heart NEC 098.85
  joint 098.50
  keratoderma 098.81
  keratosis (blennorrhagica) 098.81
  lymphatic (gland) (node) 098.89
  meninges 098.82
  orchitis (acute) 098.13
    chronic or duration of 2 months or over 098.33

Gonococcus, gonococcal — see also condition — continued
  pelvis (acute) 098.19
    chronic or duration of 2 months or over 098.39
  pericarditis 098.83
  peritonitis 098.86
  pharyngitis 098.6
  pharynx 098.6
  proctitis 098.7
  pyosalpinx (chronic) 098.37
    acute 098.17
  rectum 098.7
  septicemia 098.89
  skin 098.89
  specified site NEC 098.89
  synovitis 098.51
  tendon sheath 098.51
  throat 098.6
  urethra (acute) 098.0
    chronic or duration of 2 months or over 098.2
  vulva (acute) 098.0
    chronic or duration of 2 months or over 098.2
Gonocytoma (M9073/1)
  specified site — see Neoplasm, by site, uncertain behavior
  unspecified site
    female 236.2
    male 236.4
Gonorrhea 098.0
  acute 098.0
  Bartholin's gland (acute) 098.0
    chronic or duration of 2 months or over 098.2
  bladder (acute) 098.11
    chronic or duration of 2 months or over 098.31
  carrier (suspected of) V02.7
  cervix (acute) 098.15
    chronic or duration of 2 months or over 098.35
  chronic 098.2
  complicating pregnancy, childbirth, or puerperium 647.1 ☑
    affecting fetus or newborn 760.2
  conjunctiva, conjunctivitis (neonatorum) 098.40
  contact V01.6
  Cowper's gland (acute) 098.0
    chronic or duration of 2 months or over 098.2
  duration of two months or over 098.2
  exposure to V01.6
  fallopian tube (chronic) 098.37
    acute 098.17
  genitourinary (acute) (organ) (system) (tract) 098.0
    chronic 098.2
    duration of two months or over 098.2
  kidney (acute) 098.19
    chronic or duration of 2 months or over 098.39
  ovary (acute) 098.19
    chronic or duration of 2 months or over 098.39
  pelvis (acute) 098.19
    chronic or duration of 2 months or over 098.39
  penis (acute) 098.0
    chronic or duration of 2 months or over 098.2
  prostate (acute) 098.12
    chronic or duration of 2 months or over 098.32
  seminal vesicle (acute) 098.14
    chronic or duration of 2 months or over 098.34
  specified site NEC — see Gonococcus
  spermatic cord (acute) 098.14
    chronic or duration of 2 months or over 098.34
  urethra (acute) 098.0

Gonorrhea — continued
  urethra — continued
    chronic or duration of 2 months or over 098.2
  vagina (acute) 098.0
    chronic or duration of 2 months or over 098.2
  vas deferens (acute) 098.14
    chronic or duration of 2 months or over 098.34
  vulva (acute) 098.0
    chronic or duration of 2 months or over 098.2
Goodpasture's syndrome (pneumorenal) 446.21
Good's syndrome 279.06
Gopalan's syndrome (burning feet) 266.2
Gordon's disease (exudative enteropathy) 579.8
Gorlin-Chaudhry-Moss syndrome 759.89
Gougerot-Blum syndrome (pigmented purpuric lichenoid dermatitis) 709.1
Gougerot-Carteaud disease or syndrome (confluent reticulate papillomatosis) 701.8
Gougerot-Hailey-Hailey disease (benign familial chronic pemphigus) 757.39
Gougerot (-Houwer) -Sjögren syndrome (keratoconjunctivitis sicca) 710.2
Gougerot's syndrome (trisymptomatic) 709.1
Gouley's syndrome (constrictive pericarditis) 423.2
Goundou 102.6
Gout, gouty 274.9
  with specified manifestations NEC 274.89
  arthritis (acute) 274.0
  arthropathy 274.0
  degeneration, heart 274.82
  diathesis 274.9
  eczema 274.89
  episcleritis 274.89 [379.09]
  external ear (tophus) 274.81
  glomerulonephritis 274.10
  iritis 274.89 [364.11]
  joint 274.0
  kidney 274.10
  lead 984.9
    specified type of lead — see Table of Drugs and Chemicals
  nephritis 274.10
  neuritis 274.89 [357.4]
  phlebitis 274.89 [451.9]
  rheumatic 714.0
  saturnine 984.9
    specified type of lead — see Table of Drugs and Chemicals
  spondylitis 274.0
  synovitis 274.0
  syphilitic 095.8
  tophi 274.0
    ear 274.81
    heart 274.82
    specified site NEC 274.82
Gowers'
  muscular dystrophy 359.1
  syndrome (vasovagal attack) 780.2
Gowers-Paton-Kennedy syndrome 377.04
Gradenigo's syndrome 383.02
Graft-versus-host disease (bone marrow) 996.85
  due to organ transplant NEC — see Complications, transplant, organ
Graham Steell's murmur (pulmonic regurgitation) — see also Endocarditis, pulmonary 424.3
Grain-handlers' disease or lung 495.8
Grain mite (itch) 133.8
Grand
  mal (idiopathic) (see also Epilepsy) 345.1 ☑

Index to Diseases

Grand — *continued*
- mal (*see also* Epilepsy) — *continued*
  - hysteria of Charcôt 300.11
  - nonrecurrent or isolated 780.39
  - multipara
    - affecting management of labor and delivery 659.4 ☑
  - status only (not pregnant) V61.5

Granite workers' lung 502

Granular — *see also* condition
- inflammation, pharynx 472.1
- kidney (contracting) (*see also* Sclerosis, renal) 587
- liver — *see* Cirrhosis, liver
- nephritis — *see* Nephritis

Granulation tissue, abnormal — *see also* Granuloma
- abnormal or excessive 701.5
- postmastoidectomy cavity 383.33
- postoperative 701.5
- skin 701.5

Granulocytopenia, granulocytopenic (primary) 288.00 ▲
- malignant 288.09 ▲

Granuloma NEC 686.1
- abdomen (wall) 568.89
  - skin (pyogenicum) 686.1
    - from residual foreign body 709.4
- annulare 695.89
- anus 569.49
- apical 522.6
- appendix 543.9
- aural 380.23
- beryllium (skin) 709.4
  - lung 503
- bone (*see also* Osteomyelitis) 730.1 ☑
  - eosinophilic 277.89
  - from residual foreign body 733.99
- canaliculus lacrimalis 375.81
- cerebral 348.8
- cholesterin, middle ear 385.82
- coccidioidal (progressive) 114.3
  - lung 114.4
  - meninges 114.2
  - primary (lung) 114.0
- colon 569.89
- conjunctiva 372.61
- dental 522.6
- ear, middle (cholesterin) 385.82
  - with otitis media — *see* Otitis media
- eosinophilic 277.89
  - bone 277.89
  - lung 277.89
  - oral mucosa 528.9
- exuberant 701.5
- eyelid 374.89
- facial
  - lethal midline 446.3
  - malignant 446.3
- faciale 701.8
- fissuratum (gum) 523.8
- foot NEC 686.1
- foreign body (in soft tissue) NEC 728.82
  - bone 733.99
  - in operative wound 998.4
  - muscle 728.82
  - skin 709.4
  - subcutaneous tissue 709.4
- fungoides 202.1 ☑
- gangraenescens 446.3
- giant cell (central) (jaw) (reparative) 526.3
  - gingiva 523.8
  - peripheral (gingiva) 523.8
- gland (lymph) 289.3
- Hodgkin's (M9661/3) 201.1 ☑
- ileum 569.89
- infectious NEC 136.9
- inguinale (Donovan) 099.2
  - venereal 099.2
- intestine 569.89
- iridocyclitis 364.10
- jaw (bone) 526.3

Granuloma — *continued*
- jaw — *continued*
  - reparative giant cell 526.3
- kidney (*see also* Infection, kidney) 590.9
- lacrimal sac 375.81
- larynx 478.79
- lethal midline 446.3
- lipid 277.89
- lipoid 277.89
- liver 572.8
- lung (infectious) (*see also* Fibrosis, lung) 515
  - coccidioidal 114.4
  - eosinophilic 277.89
- lymph gland 289.3
- Majocchi's 110.6
- malignant, face 446.3
- mandible 526.3
- mediastinum 519.3
- midline 446.3
- monilial 112.3
- muscle 728.82
  - from residual foreign body 728.82
- nasal sinus (*see also* Sinusitis) 473.9
- operation wound 998.59
  - foreign body 998.4
  - stitch (external) 998.89
    - internal wound 998.89
  - talc 998.7
- oral mucosa, eosinophilic or pyogenic 528.9
- orbit, orbital 376.11
- paracoccidioidal 116.1
- penis, venereal 099.2
- periapical 522.6
- peritoneum 568.89
  - due to ova of helminths NEC (*see also* Helminthiasis) 128.9
- postmastoidectomy cavity 383.33
- postoperative — *see* Granuloma, operation wound
- prostate 601.8
- pudendi (ulcerating) 099.2
- pudendorum (ulcerative) 099.2
- pulp, internal (tooth) 521.49
- pyogenic, pyogenicum (skin) 686.1
  - maxillary alveolar ridge 522.6
  - oral mucosa 528.9
- rectum 569.49
- reticulohistiocytic 277.89
- rubrum nasi 705.89
- sarcoid 135
- Schistosoma 120.9
- septic (skin) 686.1
- silica (skin) 709.4
- sinus (accessory) (infectional) (nasal) (*see also* Sinusitis) 473.9
- skin (pyogenicum) 686.1
  - from foreign body or material 709.4
- sperm 608.89
- spine
  - syphilitic (epidural) 094.89
  - tuberculous (*see also* Tuberculosis) 015.0 ☑ [730.88]
- stitch (postoperative) 998.89
  - internal wound 998.89
- suppurative (skin) 686.1
- suture (postoperative) 998.89
  - internal wound 998.89
- swimming pool 031.1
- talc 728.82
  - in operation wound 998.7
- telangiectaticum (skin) 686.1
- tracheostomy 519.09
- trichophyticum 110.6
- tropicum 102.4
- umbilicus 686.1
  - newborn 771.4
- urethra 599.84
- uveitis 364.10
- vagina 099.2
- venereum 099.2
- vocal cords 478.5
- Wegener's (necrotizing respiratory) granulomatosis 446.4

Granulomatosis NEC 686.1
- disciformis chronica et progressiva 709.3
- infantiseptica 771.2
- lipoid 277.89
- lipophagic, intestinal 040.2
- miliary 027.0
- necrotizing, respiratory 446.4
- progressive, septic 288.1
- Wegener's (necrotizing respiratory) 446.4

Granulomatous tissue — *see* Granuloma
Granulosis rubra nasi 705.89
Graphite fibrosis (of lung) 503
Graphospasm 300.89
- organic 333.84

Grating scapula 733.99
Gravel (urinary) — *see also* Calculus 592.9
Graves' disease (exophthalmic goiter) — *see also* Goiter, toxic 242.0 ☑
Gravis — *see* condition
Grawitz's tumor (hypernephroma) (M8312/3) 189.0
Grayness, hair (premature) 704.3
- congenital 757.4

Gray or grey syndrome (chloramphenicol) (newborn) 779.4
Greenfield's disease 330.0
Green sickness 280.9
Greenstick fracture — *see* Fracture, by site
Greig's syndrome (hypertelorism) 756.0
Griesinger's disease — *see also* Ancylostomiasis 126.9
Grinders'
- asthma 502
- lung 502
- phthisis (*see also* Tuberculosis) 011.4 ☑

Grinding, teeth 306.8
Grip
- Dabney's 074.1
- devil's 074.1

Grippe, grippal — *see also* Influenza
- Balkan 083.0
- intestinal 487.8
- summer 074.8

Grippy cold 487.1
Grisel's disease 723.5
Groin — *see* condition
Grooved
- nails (transverse) 703.8
- tongue 529.5
  - congenital 750.13

Ground itch 126.9
Growing pains, children 781.99
Growth (fungoid) (neoplastic) (new) (M8000/1) — *see also* Neoplasm, by site, unspecified nature
- adenoid (vegetative) 474.12
- benign (M8000/0) — *see* Neoplasm, by site, benign
- fetal, poor 764.9 ☑
  - affecting management of pregnancy 656.5 ☑
- malignant (M8000/3) — *see* Neoplasm, by site, malignant
- rapid, childhood V21.0
- secondary (M8000/6) — *see* Neoplasm, by site, malignant, secondary

GRSA (glycopeptide resistant staphylococcus aureus) V09.8 ☑
Gruber's hernia — *see* Hernia, Gruber's
Gruby's disease (tinea tonsurans) 110.0
G-trisomy 758.0
Guama fever 066.3
Gubler (-Millard) paralysis or syndrome 344.89
Guérin-Stern syndrome (arthrogryposis multiplex congenita) 754.89
Guertin's disease (electric chorea) 049.8
Guillain-Barré disease or syndrome 357.0

Guinea worms (infection) (infestation) 125.7
Guinon's disease (motor-verbal tic) 307.23
Gull and Sutton's disease — *see* Hypertension, kidney
Gull's disease (thyroid atrophy with myxedema) 244.8
Gum — *see* condition
Gumboil 522.7
Gumma (syphilitic) 095.9
- artery 093.89
  - cerebral or spinal 094.89
- bone 095.5
  - of yaws (late) 102.6
- brain 094.89
- cauda equina 094.89
- central nervous system NEC 094.9
- ciliary body 095.8 [364.11]
- congenital 090.5
  - testis 090.5
- eyelid 095.8 [373.5]
- heart 093.89
- intracranial 094.89
- iris 095.8 [364.11]
- kidney 095.4
- larynx 095.8
- leptomeninges 094.2
- liver 095.3
- meninges 094.2
- myocardium 093.82
- nasopharynx 095.8
- neurosyphilitic 094.9
- nose 095.8
- orbit 095.8
- palate (soft) 095.8
- penis 095.8
- pericardium 093.81
- pharynx 095.8
- pituitary 095.8
- scrofulous (*see also* Tuberculosis) 017.0 ☑
- skin 095.8
- specified site NEC 095.8
- spinal cord 094.89
- tongue 095.8
- tonsil 095.8
- trachea 095.8
- tuberculous (*see also* Tuberculosis) 017.0 ☑
- ulcerative due to yaws 102.4
- ureter 095.8
- yaws 102.4
  - bone 102.6

Gunn's syndrome (jaw-winking syndrome) 742.8
Gunshot wound — *see also* Wound, open, by site
- fracture — *see* Fracture, by site, open
- internal organs (abdomen, chest, or pelvis) — *see* Injury, internal, by site, with open wound
- intracranial — *see* Laceration, brain, with open intracranial wound

Günther's disease or syndrome (congenital erythropoietic porphyria) 277.1
Gustatory hallucination 780.1
Gynandrism 752.7
Gynandroblastoma (M8632/1)
- specified site — *see* Neoplasm, by site, uncertain behavior
- unspecified site
  - female 236.2
  - male 236.4

Gynandromorphism 752.7
Gynatresia (congenital) 752.49
Gynecoid pelvis, male 738.6
Gynecological examination V72.31
- for contraceptive maintenance V25.40

Gynecomastia 611.1
Gynephobia 300.29
Gyrate scalp 757.39

H

Haas' disease (osteochondrosis head of humerus) 732.3

Habermann's disease

Habermann's disease (acute parapsoriasis varioliformis) 696.2
Habit, habituation
  chorea 307.22
  disturbance, child 307.9
  drug (see also Dependence) 304.9 ☑
  laxative (see also Abuse, drugs, nondependent) 305.9 ☑
  spasm 307.20
    chronic 307.22
    transient (of childhood) 307.21
  tic 307.20
    chronic 307.22
    transient (of childhood) 307.21
  use of
    nonprescribed drugs (see also Abuse, drugs, nondependent) 305.9 ☑
    patent medicines (see also Abuse, drugs, nondependent) 305.9 ☑
  vomiting 536.2
Hadfield-Clarke syndrome (pancreatic infantilism) 577.8
Haff disease 985.1
Hageman factor defect, deficiency, or disease — see also Defect, coagulation 286.3
Haglund's disease (osteochondrosis os tibiale externum) 732.5
Haglund-Läwen-Fründ syndrome 717.89
Hagner's disease (hypertrophic pulmonary osteoarthropathy) 731.2
Hag teeth, tooth 524.39
Hailey-Hailey disease (benign familial chronic pemphigus) 757.39
Hair — see also condition
  plucking 307.9
Hairball in stomach 935.2
Hairy black tongue 529.3
Half vertebra 756.14
Halitosis 784.99 ▲
Hallermann-Streiff syndrome 756.0
Hallervorden-Spatz disease or syndrome 333.0
Hallopeau's
  acrodermatitis (continua) 696.1
  disease (lichen sclerosis et atrophicus) 701.0
Hallucination (auditory) (gustatory) (olfactory) (tactile) 780.1
  alcohol-induced 291.3
  drug-induced 292.12
  visual 368.16
Hallucinosis 298.9
  alcohol-induced (acute) 291.3
  drug-induced 292.12
Hallus — see Hallux
Hallux 735.9
  malleus (acquired) 735.3
  rigidus (acquired) 735.2
    congenital 755.66
    late effects of rickets 268.1
  valgus (acquired) 735.0
    congenital 755.66
  varus (acquired) 735.1
    congenital 755.66
Halo, visual 368.15
Hamartoblastoma 759.6
Hamartoma 759.6
  epithelial (gingival), odontogenic, central, or peripheral (M9321/0) 213.1
  upper jaw (bone) 213.0
  vascular 757.32
Hamartosis, hamartoses NEC 759.6
Hamman's disease or syndrome (spontaneous mediastinal emphysema) 518.1
Hamman-Rich syndrome (diffuse interstitial pulmonary fibrosis) 516.3
Hammer toe (acquired) 735.4
  congenital 755.66
  late effects of rickets 268.1
Hand — see condition

Hand-foot syndrome 282.61
Hand-Schüller-Christian disease or syndrome (chronic histiocytosis x) 277.89
Hanging (asphyxia) (strangulation) (suffocation) 994.7
Hangnail (finger) (with lymphangitis) 681.02
Hangover (alcohol) — see also Abuse, drugs, nondependent 305.0 ☑
Hanot-Chauffard (-Troisier) syndrome (bronze diabetes) 275.0
Hanot's cirrhosis or disease — see Cirrhosis, biliary
Hansen's disease (leprosy) 030.9
  benign form 030.1
  malignant form 030.0
Harada's disease or syndrome 363.22
Hard chancre 091.0
Hardening
  artery — see Arteriosclerosis
  brain 348.8
  liver 571.8
Hard firm prostate 600.10
  with
    urinary
      obstruction 600.11 ●
      retention 600.11 ●
Harelip — see also Cleft, lip 749.10
Hare's syndrome (M8010/3) (carcinoma, pulmonary apex) 162.3
Harkavy's syndrome 446.0
Harlequin (fetus) 757.1
  color change syndrome 779.89
Harley's disease (intermittent hemoglobinuria) 283.2
Harris'
  lines 733.91
  syndrome (organic hyperinsulinism) 251.1
Hart's disease or syndrome (pellagra-cerebellar ataxia-renal aminoaciduria) 270.0
Hartmann's pouch (abnormal sacculation of gallbladder neck) 575.8
  of intestine V44.3
  attention to V55.3
Hartnup disease (pellagra-cerebellar ataxia-renal aminoaciduria) 270.0
Harvester lung 495.0
Hashimoto's disease or struma (struma lymphomatosa) 245.2
Hassall-Henle bodies (corneal warts) 371.41
Haut mal — see also Epilepsy 345.1 ☑
Haverhill fever 026.1
Hawaiian wood rose dependence 304.5 ☑
Hawkins' keloid 701.4
Hay
  asthma (see also Asthma) 493.0 ☑
  fever (allergic) (with rhinitis) 477.9
    with asthma (bronchial) (see also Asthma) 493.0 ☑
    allergic, due to grass, pollen, ragweed, or tree 477.0
    conjunctivitis 372.05
    due to
      dander, animal (cat) (dog) 477.2
      dust 477.8
      fowl 477.8
      hair, animal (cat) (dog) 477.2
      pollen 477.0
      specified allergen other than pollen 477.8
Hayem-Faber syndrome (achlorhydric anemia) 280.9
Hayem-Widal syndrome (acquired hemolytic jaundice) 283.9
Haygarth's nodosities 715.04
Hazard-Crile tumor (M8350/3) 193
Hb (abnormal)
  disease — see Disease, hemoglobin
  trait — see Trait
H disease 270.0
Head — see also condition

Head — see also condition — continued
  banging 307.3
Headache 784.0
  allergic 346.2 ☑
  cluster 346.2 ☑
  due to
    loss, spinal fluid 349.0
      lumbar puncture 349.0
      saddle block 349.0
  emotional 307.81
  histamine 346.2 ☑
  lumbar puncture 349.0
  menopausal 627.2
  migraine 346.9 ☑
  nonorganic origin 307.81
  postspinal 349.0
  psychogenic 307.81
  psychophysiologic 307.81
  sick 346.1 ☑
  spinal 349.0
    complicating labor and delivery 668.8 ☑
    postpartum 668.8 ☑
  spinal fluid loss 349.0
  tension 307.81
  vascular 784.0
    migraine type 346.9 ☑
  vasomotor 346.9 ☑
Health
  advice V65.4 ☑
  audit V70.0
  checkup V70.0
  education V65.4 ☑
  hazard (see also History of) V15.9
    falling V15.88
    specified cause NEC V15.89
  instruction V65.4 ☑
  services provided because (of)
    boarding school residence V60.6
    holiday relief for person providing home care V60.5
    inadequate
      housing V60.1
      resources V60.2
    lack of housing V60.0
    no care available in home V60.4
    person living alone V60.3
    poverty V60.3
    residence in institution V60.6
    specified cause NEC V60.8
    vacation relief for person providing home care V60.5
Healthy
  donor (see also Donor) V59.9
  infant or child
    accompanying sick mother V65.0
    receiving care V20.1
  person
    accompanying sick relative V65.0
    admitted for sterilization V25.2
    receiving prophylactic inoculation or vaccination (see also Vaccination, prophylactic) V05.9
Hearing examination V72.19 ▲
  following failed hearing screening V72.11 ●
Heart — see condition
Heartburn 787.1
  psychogenic 306.4
Heat (effects) 992.9
  apoplexy 992.0
  burn (see also Burn, by site
    from sun (see also Sunburn) 692.71
  collapse 992.1
  cramps 992.2
  dermatitis or eczema 692.89
  edema 992.7
  erythema — see Burn, by site
  excessive 992.9
    specified effect NEC 992.8
  exhaustion 992.5
    anhydrotic 992.3
    due to
      salt (and water) depletion 992.4

Heat — continued
  exhaustion — continued
    due to — continued
      water depletion 992.3
  fatigue (transient) 992.6
  fever 992.0
  hyperpyrexia 992.0
  prickly 705.1
  prostration — see Heat, exhaustion
  pyrexia 992.0
  rash 705.1
  specified effect NEC 992.8
  stroke 992.0
  sunburn (see also Sunburn) 692.71
  syncope 992.1
Heavy-chain disease 273.2
Heavy-for-dates (fetus or infant) 766.1
  4500 grams or more 766.0
  exceptionally 766.0
Hebephrenia, hebephrenic (acute) — see also Schizophrenia 295.1 ☑
  dementia (praecox) (see also Schizophrenia) 295.1 ☑
  schizophrenia (see also Schizophrenia) 295.1 ☑
Heberden's
  disease or nodes 715.04
  syndrome (angina pectoris) 413.9
Hebra's disease
  dermatitis exfoliativa 695.89
  erythema multiforme exudativum 695.1
  pityriasis 695.89
    maculata et circinata 696.3
    rubra 695.89
      pilaris 696.4
  prurigo 698.2
Hebra, nose 040.1
Hedinger's syndrome (malignant carcinoid) 259.2
Heel — see condition
Heerfordt's disease or syndrome (uveoparotitis) 135
Hegglin's anomaly or syndrome 288.2
Heidenhain's disease 290.10
  with dementia 290.10
Heilmeyer-Schöner disease (M9842/3) 207.1 ☑
Heine-Medin disease — see also Poliomyelitis 045.9 ☑
Heinz-body anemia, congenital 282.7
Heller's disease or syndrome (infantile psychosis) — see also Psychosis, childhood 299.1 ☑
H.E.L.L.P 642.5 ☑
Helminthiasis — see also Infestation, by specific parasite 128.9
  Ancylostoma (see also Ancylostoma) 126.9
  intestinal 127.9
    mixed types (types classifiable to more than one of the categories 120.0–127.7) 127.8
    specified type 127.7
  mixed types (intestinal) (types classifiable to more than one of the categories 120.0–127.7) 127.8
  Necator americanus 126.1
  specified type NEC 128.8
  Trichinella 124
Heloma 700
Hemangioblastoma (M9161/1) — see also Neoplasm, connective tissue, uncertain behavior
  malignant (M9161/3) — see Neoplasm, connective tissue, malignant
Hemangioblastomatosis, cerebelloretinal 759.6
Hemangioendothelioma (M9130/1) — see also Neoplasm, by site, uncertain behavior
  benign (M9130/0) 228.00
  bone (diffuse) (M9130/3) — see Neoplasm, bone, malignant

Hemangioendothelioma — see also
    Neoplasm, by site, uncertain
    behavior — continued
  malignant (M9130/3) — see Neo-
    plasm, connective tissue, malig-
    nant
  nervous system (M9130/0) 228.09
Hemangioendotheliosarcoma
  (M9130/3) — see Neoplasm, connective tissue, malignant
Hemangiofibroma (M9160/0) — see
  Neoplasm, by site, benign
Hemangiolipoma (M8861/0) — see
  Lipoma
Hemangioma (M9120/0) 228.00
  arteriovenous (M9123/0) — see He-
    mangioma, by site
  brain 228.02
  capillary (M9131/0) — see Heman-
    gioma, by site
  cavernous (M9121/0) — see Heman-
    gioma, by site
  central nervous system NEC 228.09
  choroid 228.09
  heart 228.09
  infantile (M9131/0) — see Heman-
    gioma, by site
  intra-abdominal structures 228.04
  intracranial structures 228.02
  intramuscular (M9132/0) — see He-
    mangioma, by site
  iris 228.09
  juvenile (M9131/0) — see Heman-
    gioma, by site
  malignant (M9120/3) — see Neo-
    plasm, connective tissue, malig-
    nant
  meninges 228.09
    brain 228.02
    spinal cord 228.09
  peritoneum 228.04
  placenta — see Placenta, abnormal
  plexiform (M9131/0) — see Heman-
    gioma, by site
  racemose (M9123/0) — see Heman-
    gioma, by site
  retina 228.03
  retroperitoneal tissue 228.04
  sclerosing (M8832/0) — see Neo-
    plasm, skin, benign
  simplex (M9131/0) — see Heman-
    gioma, by site
  skin and subcutaneous tissue 228.01
  specified site NEC 228.09
  spinal cord 228.09
  venous (M9122/0) — see Heman-
    gioma, by site
  verrucous keratotic (M9142/0) — see
    Hemangioma, by site
Hemangiomatosis (systemic) 757.32
  involving single site — see Heman-
    gioma
Hemangiopericytoma (M9150/1) — see
  also Neoplasm, connective tissue,
  uncertain behavior
  benign (M9150/0) — see Neoplasm,
    connective tissue, benign
  malignant (M9150/3) — see Neo-
    plasm, connective tissue, malig-
    nant
Hemangiosarcoma (M9120/3) — see
  Neoplasm, connective tissue, malignant
Hemarthrosis (nontraumatic) 719.10
  ankle 719.17
  elbow 719.12
  foot 719.17
  hand 719.14
  hip 719.15
  knee 719.16
  multiple sites 719.19
  pelvic region 719.15
  shoulder (region) 719.11
  specified site NEC 719.18
  traumatic — see Sprain, by site
  wrist 719.13

Hematemesis 578.0
  with ulcer — see Ulcer, by site, with
    hemorrhage
  due to S. japonicum 120.2
  Goldstein's (familial hemorrhagic
    telangiectasia) 448.0
  newborn 772.4
    due to swallowed maternal blood
      777.3
Hematidrosis 705.89
Hematinuria — see also Hemoglobinuria
  791.2
  malarial 084.8
  paroxysmal 283.2
Hematite miners' lung 503
Hematobilia 576.8
Hematocele (congenital) (diffuse) (idiopathic) 608.83
  broad ligament 620.7
  canal of Nuck 629.0
  cord, male 608.83
  fallopian tube 620.8
  female NEC 629.0
  ischiorectal 569.89
  male NEC 608.83
  ovary 629.0
  pelvis, pelvic
    female 629.0
      with ectopic pregnancy (see also
        Pregnancy, ectopic)
        633.90
        with intrauterine pregnancy
          633.91
    male 608.83
  periuterine 629.0
  retrouterine 629.0
  scrotum 608.83
  spermatic cord (diffuse) 608.83
  testis 608.84
  traumatic — see Injury, internal,
    pelvis
  tunica vaginalis 608.83
  uterine ligament 629.0
  uterus 621.4
  vagina 623.6
  vulva 624.5
Hematocephalus 742.4
Hematochezia — see also Melena 578.1
Hematochyluria — see also Infestation,
  filarial 125.9
Hematocolpos 626.8
Hematocornea 371.12
Hematogenous — see condition
Hematoma (skin surface intact) (traumatic) — see also Contusion

  Note — Hematomas are coded according
  to origin and the nature and site of the
  hematoma or the accompanying injury.
  Hematomas of unspecified origin are
  coded as injuries of the sites involved,
  except:
  (a) hematomas of genital organs
       which are coded as diseases of
       the organ involved unless they
       complicate pregnancy or delivery
  (b) hematomas of the eye which are
       coded as diseases of the eye.

  For late effect of hematoma classifiable
  to 920–924 see Late, effect, contusion
  with
    crush injury — see Crush
    fracture — see Fracture, by site
    injury of internal organs (see also
      Injury, internal, by site)
      kidney — see Hematoma, kid-
        ney traumatic
      liver — see Hematoma, liver,
        traumatic
      spleen — see Hematoma, spleen
    nerve injury — see Injury, nerve
    open wound — see Wound, open,
      by site
    skin surface intact — see Contu-
      sion

Hematoma — see also Contusion —
  continued
  abdomen (wall) — see Contusion, ab-
    domen
  amnion 658.8 ☑
  aorta, dissecting 441.00
    abdominal 441.02
    thoracic 441.01
    thoracoabdominal 441.03
  arterial (complicating trauma) 904.9
    specified site — see Injury, blood
      vessel, by site
  auricle (ear) 380.31
  birth injury 767.8
    skull 767.19
  brain (traumatic) 853.0 ☑

  Note — Use the following fifth-digit
  subclassification with categories
  851–854:
  0   unspecified state of conscious-
      ness
  1   with no loss of consciousness
  2   with brief [less than one hour]
      loss of consciousness
  3   with moderate [1–24 hours] loss
      of consciousness
  4   with prolonged [more than 24
      hours] loss of consciousness and
      return to pre–existing conscious
      level
  5   with prolonged [more than 24
      hours] loss of consciousness,
      without return to pre–existing
      conscious level

  Use fifth-digit 5 to designate when a
  patient is unconscious and dies before
  regaining consciousness, regardless of
  the duration of the loss of consciousness
  6   with loss of consciousness of un-
      specified duration
  9   with concussion, unspecified

    with
      cerebral
        contusion — see Contusion,
          brain
        laceration — see Laceration,
          brain
      open intracranial wound
        853.1 ☑
      skull fracture — see Fracture,
        skull, by site
    extradural or epidural 852.4 ☑
      with open intracranial wound
        852.5 ☑
      fetus or newborn 767.0
      nontraumatic 432.0
    fetus or newborn NEC 767.0
    nontraumatic (see also Hemor-
      rhage, brain) 431
      epidural or extradural 432.0
      newborn NEC 772.8
    subarachnoid, arachnoid, or
      meningeal (see also Hem-
      orrhage, subarachnoid)
      430
    subdural (see also Hemorrhage,
      subdural) 432.1
    subarachnoid, arachnoid, or
      meningeal 852.0 ☑
      with open intracranial wound
        852.1 ☑
      fetus or newborn 772.2
      nontraumatic (see also Hemor-
        rhage, subarachnoid) 430
    subdural 852.2 ☑
      with open intracranial wound
        852.3 ☑
      fetus or newborn (localized)
        767.0
      nontraumatic (see also Hemor-
        rhage, subdural) 432.1

Hematoma — see also Contusion —
  continued
  breast (nontraumatic) 611.8
  broad ligament (nontraumatic) 620.7
    complicating delivery 665.7 ☑
    traumatic — see Injury, internal,
      broad ligament
  calcified NEC 959.9
  capitis 920
    due to birth injury 767.19
    newborn 767.19
  cerebral — see Hematoma, brain
  cesarean section wound 674.3 ☑
  chorion — see Placenta, abnormal
  complicating delivery (perineum) (vul-
    va) 664.5 ☑
    pelvic 665.7 ☑
    vagina 665.7 ☑
  corpus
    cavernosum (nontraumatic) 607.82
    luteum (nontraumatic) (ruptured)
      620.1
  dura (mater) — see Hematoma, brain,
    subdural
  epididymis (nontraumatic) 608.83
  epidural (traumatic) (see also
    Hematoma, brain, extradural)
    spinal — see Injury, spinal, by site
  episiotomy 674.3 ☑
  external ear 380.31
  extradural (see also Hematoma, brain,
    extradural)
    fetus or newborn 767.0
    nontraumatic 432.0
      fetus or newborn 767.0
  fallopian tube 620.8
  genital organ (nontraumatic)
    female NEC 629.89
    male NEC 608.83
    traumatic (external site) 922.4
      internal — see Injury, internal,
        genital organ
  graafian follicle (ruptured) 620.0
  internal organs (abdomen, chest, or
    pelvis) (see also Injury, internal,
    by site)
    kidney — see Hematoma, kidney,
      traumatic
    liver — see Hematoma, liver, trau-
      matic
    spleen — see Hematoma, spleen
  intracranial — see Hematoma, brain
  kidney, cystic 593.81
    traumatic 866.01
      with open wound into cavity
        866.11
  labia (nontraumatic) 624.5
  lingual (and other parts of neck, scalp,
    or face, except eye) 920
  liver (subcapsular) 573.8
    birth injury 767.8
    fetus or newborn 767.8
    traumatic NEC 864.01
      with
        laceration — see Laceration,
          liver
        open wound into cavity
          864.11
  mediastinum — see Injury, internal,
    mediastinum
  meninges, meningeal (brain) (see also
    Hematoma, brain, subarach-
    noid)
    spinal — see Injury, spinal, by site
  mesosalpinx (nontraumatic) 620.8
    traumatic — see Injury, internal,
      pelvis
  muscle (traumatic) — see Contusion,
    by site
  nasal (septum) (and other part(s) of
    neck, scalp, or face, except eye)
    920
  obstetrical surgical wound 674.3 ☑
  orbit, orbital (nontraumatic) 376.32
    traumatic 921.2

Hematoma

Hematoma — see also Contusion — continued
- ovary (corpus luteum) (nontraumatic) 620.1
  - traumatic — see Injury, internal, ovary
- pelvis (female) (nontraumatic) 629.89 ▲
  - complicating delivery 665.7 ☑
  - male 608.83
  - traumatic (see also Injury, internal, pelvis)
    - specified organ NEC (see also Injury, internal, pelvis) 867.6
- penis (nontraumatic) 607.82
- pericranial (and neck, or face any part, except eye) 920
  - due to injury at birth 767.19
- perineal wound (obstetrical) 674.3 ☑
  - complicating delivery 664.5 ☑
- perirenal, cystic 593.81
- pinna 380.31
- placenta — see Placenta, abnormal
- postoperative 998.12
- retroperitoneal (nontraumatic) 568.81
  - traumatic — see Injury, internal, retroperitoneum
- retropubic, male 568.81
- scalp (and neck, or face any part, except eye) 920
  - fetus or newborn 767.19
- scrotum (nontraumatic) 608.83
  - traumatic 922.4
- seminal vesicle (nontraumatic) 608.83
  - traumatic — see Injury, internal, seminal, vesicle
- spermatic cord (see also Injury, internal, spermatic cord)
  - nontraumatic 608.83
- spinal (cord) (meninges) (see also Injury, spinal, by site)
  - fetus or newborn 767.4
  - nontraumatic 336.1
- spleen 865.01
  - with
    - laceration — see Laceration, spleen
    - open wound into cavity 865.11
- sternocleidomastoid, birth injury 767.8
- sternomastoid, birth injury 767.8
- subarachnoid (see also Hematoma, brain, subarachnoid)
  - fetus or newborn 772.2
  - nontraumatic (see also Hemorrhage, subarachnoid) 430
  - newborn 772.2
- subdural (see also Hematoma, brain, subdural)
  - fetus or newborn (localized) 767.0
  - nontraumatic (see also Hemorrhage, subdural) 432.1
- subperiosteal (syndrome) 267
  - traumatic — see Hematoma, by site
- superficial, fetus or newborn 772.6
- syncytium — see Placenta, abnormal
- testis (nontraumatic) 608.83
  - birth injury 767.8
  - traumatic 922.4
- tunica vaginalis (nontraumatic) 608.83
- umbilical cord 663.6 ☑
  - affecting fetus or newborn 762.6
- uterine ligament (nontraumatic) 620.7
  - traumatic — see Injury, internal, pelvis
- uterus 621.4
  - traumatic — see Injury, internal, pelvis
- vagina (nontraumatic) (ruptured) 623.6
  - complicating delivery 665.7 ☑
  - traumatic 922.4
- vas deferens (nontraumatic) 608.83

Hematoma — see also Contusion — continued
- vas deferens — continued
  - traumatic — see Injury, internal, vas deferens
- vitreous 379.23
- vocal cord 920
- vulva (nontraumatic) 624.5
  - complicating delivery 664.5 ☑
  - fetus or newborn 767.8
  - traumatic 922.4

Hematometra 621.4
Hematomyelia 336.1
- with fracture of vertebra (see also Fracture, vertebra, by site, with spinal cord injury) 806.8
- fetus or newborn 767.4

Hematomyelitis 323.9
- late effect — see category 326

Hematoperitoneum — see also Hemoperitoneum 568.81

Hematopneumothorax — see also Hemothorax 511.8

Hematopoiesis, cyclic 288.02 ●

Hematoporphyria (acquired) (congenital) 277.1

Hematoporphyrinuria (acquired) (congenital) 277.1

Hematorachis, hematorrhachis 336.1
- fetus or newborn 767.4

Hematosalpinx 620.8
- with
  - ectopic pregnancy (see also categories 633.0–633.9) 639.2
  - infectional (see also Salpingo-oophoritis) 614.2
  - molar pregnancy (see also categories 630–632) 639.2

Hematospermia 608.82
Hematothorax — see also Hemothorax 511.8
Hematotympanum 381.03
Hematuria (benign) (essential) (idiopathic) 599.7
- due to S. hematobium 120.0
- endemic 120.0
- intermittent 599.7
- malarial 084.8
- paroxysmal 599.7
- sulfonamide
  - correct substance properly administered 599.7
  - overdose or wrong substance given or taken 961.0
- tropical (bilharziasis) 120.0
- tuberculous (see also Tuberculosis) 016.9 ☑

Hematuric bilious fever 084.8
Hemeralopia 368.10
Hemiabiotrophy 799.89
Hemi-akinesia 781.8
Hemianalgesia — see also Disturbance, sensation 782.0
Hemianencephaly 740.0
Hemianesthesia — see also Disturbance, sensation 782.0
Hemianopia, hemianopsia (altitudinal) (homonymous) 368.46
- binasal 368.47
- bitemporal 368.47
- heteronymous 368.47
- syphilitic 095.8

Hemiasomatognosia 307.9
Hemiathetosis 781.0
Hemiatrophy 799.89
- cerebellar 334.8
- face 349.89
  - progressive 349.89
- fascia 728.9
- leg 728.2
- tongue 529.8

Hemiballism (us) 333.5
Hemiblock (cardiac) (heart) (left) 426.2
Hemicardia 746.89
Hemicephalus, hemicephaly 740.0
Hemichorea 333.5

Hemicrania 346.9 ☑
- congenital malformation 740.0
Hemidystrophy — see Hemiatrophy
Hemiectromelia 755.4
Hemihypalgesia — see also Disturbance, sensation 782.0
Hemihypertrophy (congenital) 759.89
- cranial 756.0
Hemihypesthesia — see also Disturbance, sensation 782.0
Hemi-inattention 781.8
Hemimelia 755.4
- lower limb 755.30
  - paraxial (complete) (incomplete) (intercalary) (terminal) 755.32
    - fibula 755.37
    - tibia 755.36
  - transverse (complete) (partial) 755.31
- upper limb 755.20
  - paraxial (complete) (incomplete) (intercalary) (terminal) 755.22
    - radial 755.26
    - ulnar 755.27
  - transverse (complete) (partial) 755.21

Hemiparalysis — see also Hemiplegia 342.9 ☑
Hemiparesis — see also Hemiplegia 342.9 ☑
Hemiparesthesia — see also Disturbance, sensation 782.0
Hemiplegia 342.9 ☑
- acute (see also Disease, cerebrovascular, acute) 436
- alternans facialis 344.89
- apoplectic (see also Disease, cerebrovascular, acute) 436
  - late effect or residual
    - affecting
      - dominant side 438.21
      - nondominant side 438.22
      - unspecified side 438.20
- arteriosclerotic 437.0
  - late effect or residual
    - affecting
      - dominant side 438.21
      - nondominant side 438.22
      - unspecified side 438.20
- ascending (spinal) NEC 344.89
- attack (see also Disease, cerebrovascular, acute) 436
- brain, cerebral (current episode) 437.8
  - congenital 343.1
- cerebral — see Hemiplegia, brain
- congenital (cerebral) (spastic) (spinal) 343.1
- conversion neurosis (hysterical) 300.11
- cortical — see Hemiplegia, brain
- due to
  - arteriosclerosis 437.0
    - late effect or residual
      - affecting
        - dominant side 438.21
        - nondominant side 438.22
        - unspecified side 438.20
  - cerebrovascular lesion (see also Disease, cerebrovascular, acute) 436
    - late effect
      - affecting
        - dominant side 438.21
        - nondominant side 438.22
        - unspecified side 438.20
- embolic (current) (see also Embolism, brain) 434.1
  - late effect
    - affecting
      - dominant side 438.21
      - nondominant side 438.22
      - unspecified side 438.20
- flaccid 342.0 ☑
- hypertensive (current episode) 437.8

Hemiplegia — continued
- infantile (postnatal) 343.4
- late effect
  - birth injury, intracranial or spinal 343.4
  - cerebrovascular lesion — see Late effect(s) (of) cerebrovascular disease
  - viral encephalitis 139.0
- middle alternating NEC 344.89
- newborn NEC 767.0
- seizure (current episode) (see also Disease, cerebrovascular, acute) 436
- spastic 342.1 ☑
  - congenital or infantile 343.1
- specified NEC 342.8 ☑
- thrombotic (current) (see also Thrombosis, brain) 434.0 ☑
  - late effect — see Late effect(s) (of) cerebrovascular disease

Hemisection, spinal cord — see Fracture, vertebra, by site, with spinal cord injury

Hemispasm 781.0
- facial 781.0
Hemispatial neglect 781.8
Hemisporosis 117.9
Hemitremor 781.0
Hemivertebra 756.14
Hemobilia 576.8
Hemocholecyst 575.8
Hemochromatosis (acquired) (diabetic) (hereditary) (liver) (myocardium) (primary idiopathic) (secondary) 275.0
- with refractory anemia 238.72 ▲

Hemodialysis V56.0
Hemoglobin — see also condition
- abnormal (disease) — see Disease, hemoglobin
- AS genotype 282.5
- fetal, hereditary persistence 282.7
- high-oxygen-affinity 289.0
- low NEC 285.9
- S (Hb-S), heterozygous 282.5

Hemoglobinemia 283.2
- due to blood transfusion NEC 999.8
- bone marrow 996.85
- paroxysmal 283.2

Hemoglobinopathy (mixed) — see also Disease, hemoglobin 282.7
- with thalassemia 282.49
- sickle-cell 282.60
  - with thalassemia (without crisis) 282.41
  - with
    - crisis 282.42
    - vaso-occlusive pain 282.42

Hemoglobinuria, hemoglobinuric 791.2
- with anemia, hemolytic, acquired (chronic) NEC 283.2
- cold (agglutinin) (paroxysmal) (with Raynaud's syndrome) 283.2
- due to
  - exertion 283.2
  - hemolysis (from external causes) NEC 283.2
- exercise 283.2
- fever (malaria) 084.8
- infantile 791.2
- intermittent 283.2
- malarial 084.8
- march 283.2
- nocturnal (paroxysmal) 283.2
- paroxysmal (cold) (nocturnal) 283.2

Hemolymphangioma (M9175/0) 228.1
Hemolysis
- fetal — see Jaundice, fetus or newborn
- intravascular (disseminated) NEC 286.6
- with
  - abortion — see Abortion, by type, with hemorrhage, delayed or excessive

Index to Diseases

Hemolysis — *continued*
  intravascular — *continued*
    with — *continued*
      ectopic pregnancy (*see also* categories 633.0–633.9) 639.1
      hemorrhage of pregnancy 641.3 ☑
        affecting fetus or newborn 762.1
      molar pregnancy (*see also* categories 630–632) 639.1
    acute 283.2
    following
      abortion 639.1
      ectopic or molar pregnancy 639.1
  neonatal — *see* Jaundice, fetus or newborn
  transfusion NEC 999.8
    bone marrow 996.85
Hemolytic — *see also* condition
  anemia — *see* Anemia, hemolytic
  uremic syndrome 283.11
Hemometra 621.4
Hemopericardium (with effusion) 423.0
  newborn 772.8
  traumatic (*see also* Hemothorax, traumatic) 860.2
    with open wound into thorax 860.3
Hemoperitoneum 568.81
  infectional (*see also* Peritonitis) 567.29
  traumatic — *see* Injury, internal, peritoneum
Hemophagocytic syndrome 288.4 ●
  infection-associated 288.4 ●
Hemophilia (familial) (hereditary) 286.0
  A 286.0
    carrier (asymptomatic) V83.01
      symptomatic V83.02
  acquired 286.5
  B (Leyden) 286.1
  C 286.2
  calcipriva (*see also* Fibrinolysis) 286.7
  classical 286.0
  nonfamilial 286.7
  secondary 286.5
  vascular 286.4
Hemophilus influenzae NEC 041.5
  arachnoiditis (basic) (brain) (spinal) 320.0
    late effect — *see* category 326
  bronchopneumonia 482.2
  cerebral ventriculitis 320.0
    late effect — *see* category 326
  cerebrospinal inflammation 320.0
    late effect — *see* category 326
  infection NEC 041.5
  leptomeningitis 320.0
    late effect — *see* category 326
  meningitis (cerebral) (cerebrospinal) (spinal) 320.0
    late effect — *see* category 326
  meningomyelitis 320.0
    late effect — *see* category 326
  pachymeningitis (adhesive) (fibrous) (hemorrhagic) (hypertrophic) (spinal) 320.0
    late effect — *see* category 326
  pneumonia (broncho-) 482.2
Hemophthalmos 360.43
Hemopneumothorax — *see also* Hemothorax 511.8
  traumatic 860.4
    with open wound into thorax 860.5
Hemoptysis 786.3
  due to Paragonimus (westermani) 121.2
  newborn 770.3
  tuberculous (*see also* Tuberculosis, pulmonary) 011.9 ☑
Hemorrhage, hemorrhagic (nontraumatic) 459.0
  abdomen 459.0
  accidental (antepartum) 641.2 ☑
    affecting fetus or newborn 762.1

Hemorrhage, hemorrhagic — *continued*
  adenoid 474.8
  adrenal (capsule) (gland) (medulla) 255.4
    newborn 772.5
  after labor — *see* Hemorrhage, postpartum
  alveolar
    lung, newborn 770.3
    process 525.8
  alveolus 525.8
  amputation stump (surgical) 998.11
    secondary, delayed 997.69
  anemia (chronic) 280.0
    acute 285.1
  antepartum — *see* Hemorrhage, pregnancy
  anus (sphincter) 569.3
  apoplexy (stroke) 432.9
  arachnoid — *see* Hemorrhage, subarachnoid
  artery NEC 459.0
    brain (*see also* Hemorrhage, brain) 431
    middle meningeal — *see* Hemorrhage, subarachnoid
  basilar (ganglion) (*see also* Hemorrhage, brain) 431
  bladder 596.8
  blood dyscrasia 289.9
  bowel 578.9
    newborn 772.4
  brain (miliary) (nontraumatic) 431
    with
      birth injury 767.0
    arachnoid — *see* Hemorrhage, subarachnoid
    due to
      birth injury 767.0
      rupture of aneurysm (congenital) (*see also* Hemorrhage, subarachnoid) 430
      mycotic 431
      syphilis 094.89
    epidural or extradural — *see* Hemorrhage, extradural
    fetus or newborn (anoxic) (hypoxic) (due to birth trauma) (nontraumatic) 767.0
      intraventricular 772.10
        grade I 772.11
        grade II 772.12
        grade III 772.13
        grade IV 772.14
    iatrogenic 997.02
    postoperative 997.02
    puerperal, postpartum, childbirth 674.0 ☑
    stem 431
    subarachnoid, arachnoid, or meningeal — *see* Hemorrhage, subarachnoid
    subdural — *see* Hemorrhage, subdural

Hemorrhage, hemorrhagic — *continued*
  brain — *continued*
    traumatic NEC 853.0 ☑

> Note — Use the following fifth-digit subclassification with categories 851–854:
>
> 0   unspecified state of consciousness
>
> 1   with no loss of consciousness
>
> ②   with brief [less than one hour] loss of consciousness
>
> 3   with moderate [1–24 hours] loss of consciousness
>
> 4   with prolonged [more than 24 hours] loss of consciousness and return to pre-existing conscious level
>
> 5   with prolonged [more than 24 hours] loss of consciousness, without return to pre-existing conscious level
>
> Use fifth-digit 5 to designate when a patient is unconscious and dies before regaining consciousness, regardless of the duration of the loss of consciousness
>
> 6   with loss of consciousness of unspecified duration
>
> 9   with concussion, unspecified

      with
        cerebral
          contusion — *see* Contusion, brain
          laceration — *see* Laceration, brain
        open intracranial wound 853.1 ☑
        skull fracture — *see* Fracture, skull, by site
      extradural or epidural 852.4 ☑
        with open intracranial wound 852.5 ☑
      subarachnoid 852.0 ☑
        with open intracranial wound 852.1 ☑
      subdural 852.2 ☑
        with open intracranial wound 852.3 ☑
  breast 611.79
  bronchial tube — *see* Hemorrhage, lung
  bronchopulmonary — *see* Hemorrhage, lung
  bronchus (cause unknown) (*see also* Hemorrhage, lung) 786.3
  bulbar (*see also* Hemorrhage, brain) 431
  bursa 727.89
  capillary 448.9
    primary 287.8
  capsular — *see* Hemorrhage, brain
  cardiovascular 429.89
  cecum 578.9
  cephalic (*see also* Hemorrhage, brain) 431
  cerebellar (*see also* Hemorrhage, brain) 431
  cerebellum (*see also* Hemorrhage, brain) 431
  cerebral (*see also* Hemorrhage, brain) 431
    fetus or newborn (anoxic) (traumatic) 767.0
  cerebromeningeal (*see also* Hemorrhage, brain) 431
  cerebrospinal (*see also* Hemorrhage, brain) 431
  cerebrovascular accident — *see* Hemorrhage, brain
  cerebrum (*see also* Hemorrhage, brain) 431

Hemorrhage, hemorrhagic — *continued*
  cervix (stump) (uteri) 622.8
  cesarean section wound 674.3 ☑
  chamber, anterior (eye) 364.41
  childbirth — *see* Hemorrhage, complicating, delivery
  choroid 363.61
    expulsive 363.62
  ciliary body 364.41
  cochlea 386.8
  colon — *see* Hemorrhage, intestine
  complicating
    delivery 641.9 ☑
      affecting fetus or newborn 762.1
      associated with
        afibrinogenemia 641.3 ☑
          affecting fetus or newborn 763.89
        coagulation defect 641.3 ☑
          affecting fetus or newborn 763.89
        hyperfibrinolysis 641.3 ☑
          affecting fetus or newborn 763.89
        hypofibrinogenemia 641.3 ☑
          affecting fetus or newborn 763.89
      due to
        low-lying placenta 641.1 ☑
          affecting fetus or newborn 762.0
        placenta previa 641.1 ☑
          affecting fetus or newborn 762.0
        premature separation of placenta 641.2 ☑
          affecting fetus or newborn 762.1
        retained
          placenta 666.0 ☑
          secundines 666.2 ☑
        trauma 641.8 ☑
          affecting fetus or newborn 763.89
        uterine leiomyoma 641.8 ☑
          affecting fetus or newborn 763.89
    surgical procedure 998.11
  concealed NEC 459.0
  congenital 772.9
  conjunctiva 372.72
    newborn 772.8
  cord, newborn 772.0
    slipped ligature 772.3
    stump 772.3
  corpus luteum (ruptured) 620.1
  cortical (*see also* Hemorrhage, brain) 431
  cranial 432.9
  cutaneous 782.7
    newborn 772.6
  cystitis — *see* Cystitis
  cyst, pancreas 577.2
  delayed
    with
      abortion — *see* Abortion, by type, with hemorrhage, delayed or excessive
      ectopic pregnancy (*see also* categories 633.0–633.9) 639.1
      molar pregnancy (*see also* categories 630–632) 639.1
    following
      abortion 639.1
      ectopic or molar pregnancy 639.1
    postpartum 666.2 ☑
  diathesis (familial) 287.9
    newborn 776.0
  disease 287.9
    newborn 776.0
    specified type NEC 287.8
  disorder 287.9

Hemorrhage, hemorrhagic

Hemorrhage, hemorrhagic — *continued*
- disorder — *continued*
    - due to intrinsic circulating anticoagulants 286.5
    - specified type NEC 287.8
- due to
    - any device, implant or graft (presence of) classifiable to 996.0–996.5 — *see* Complications, due to (presence of) any device, implant, or graft classified to 996.0–996.5NEC
    - intrinsic circulating anticoagulant 286.5
- duodenum, duodenal 537.89
    - ulcer — *see* Ulcer, duodenum, with hemorrhage
- dura mater — *see* Hemorrhage, subdural
- endotracheal — *see* Hemorrhage, lung
- epicranial subaponeurotic (massive) 767.11
- epidural — *see* Hemorrhage, extradural
- episiotomy 674.3 ☑
- esophagus 530.82
    - varix (*see also* Varix, esophagus, bleeding) 456.0
- excessive
    - with
        - abortion — *see* Abortion, by type, with hemorrhage, delayed or excessive
        - ectopic pregnancy (*see also* categories 633.0–633.9) 639.1
        - molar pregnancy (*see also* categories 630–632) 639.1
    - following
        - abortion 639.1
        - ectopic or molar pregnancy 639.1
- external 459.0
- extradural (traumatic) (*see also* Hemorrhage, brain, traumatic, extradural)
    - birth injury 767.0
    - fetus or newborn (anoxic) (traumatic) 767.0
    - nontraumatic 432.0
- eye 360.43
    - chamber (anterior) (aqueous) 364.41
    - fundus 362.81
- eyelid 374.81
- fallopian tube 620.8
- fetomaternal 772.0
    - affecting management of pregnancy or puerperium 656.0 ☑
- fetus, fetal 772.0
    - from
        - cut end of co-twin's cord 772.0
        - placenta 772.0
        - ruptured cord 772.0
        - vasa previa 772.0
    - into
        - co-twin 772.0
        - mother's circulation 772.0
            - affecting management of pregnancy or puerperium 656.0 ☑
- fever (*see also* Fever, hemorrhagic) 065.9
    - with renal syndrome 078.6
    - arthropod-borne NEC 065.9
    - Bangkok 065.4
    - Crimean 065.0
    - dengue virus 065.4
    - epidemic 078.6
    - Junin virus 078.7
    - Korean 078.6
    - Machupo virus 078.7
    - mite-borne 065.8
    - mosquito-borne 065.4
    - Philippine 065.4

Hemorrhage, hemorrhagic — *continued*
- fever (*see also* Fever, hemorrhagic) — *continued*
    - Russian (Yaroslav) 078.6
    - Singapore 065.4
    - southeast Asia 065.4
    - Thailand 065.4
    - tick-borne NEC 065.3
- fibrinogenolysis (*see also* Fibrinolysis) 286.6
- fibrinolytic (acquired) (*see also* Fibrinolysis) 286.6
- fontanel 767.19
- from tracheostomy stoma 519.09
- fundus, eye 362.81
- funis
    - affecting fetus or newborn 772.0
    - complicating delivery 663.8 ☑
- gastric (*see also* Hemorrhage, stomach) 578.9
- gastroenteric 578.9
    - newborn 772.4
- gastrointestinal (tract) 578.9
    - newborn 772.4
- genitourinary (tract) NEC 599.89
- gingiva 523.8
- globe 360.43
- gravidarum — *see* Hemorrhage, pregnancy
- gum 523.8
- heart 429.89
- hypopharyngeal (throat) 784.8
- intermenstrual 626.6
    - irregular 626.6
    - regular 626.5
- internal (organs) 459.0
    - capsule (*see also* Hemorrhage, brain) 431
    - ear 386.8
    - newborn 772.8
- intestine 578.9
    - congenital 772.4
    - newborn 772.4
- into
    - bladder wall 596.7
    - bursa 727.89
    - corpus luysii (*see also* Hemorrhage, brain) 431
- intra-abdominal 459.0
    - during or following surgery 998.11
- intra-alveolar, newborn (lung) 770.3
- intracerebral (*see also* Hemorrhage, brain) 431
- intracranial NEC 432.9
    - puerperal, postpartum, childbirth 674.0 ☑
    - traumatic — *see* Hemorrhage, brain, traumatic
- intramedullary NEC 336.1
- intraocular 360.43
- intraoperative 998.11
- intrapartum — *see* Hemorrhage, complicating, delivery
- intrapelvic
    - female 629.89 ▲
    - male 459.0
- intraperitoneal 459.0
- intrapontine (*see also* Hemorrhage, brain) 431
- intrauterine 621.4
    - complicating delivery — *see* Hemorrhage, complicating, delivery
    - in pregnancy or childbirth — *see* Hemorrhage, pregnancy
    - postpartum (*see also* Hemorrhage, postpartum) 666.1 ☑
- intraventricular (*see also* Hemorrhage, brain) 431
    - fetus or newborn (anoxic) (traumatic) 772.10
        - grade I 772.11
        - grade II 772.12
        - grade III 772.13
        - grade IV 772.14
- intravesical 596.7

Hemorrhage, hemorrhagic — *continued*
- iris (postinfectional) (postinflammatory) (toxic) 364.41
- joint (nontraumatic) 719.10
    - ankle 719.17
    - elbow 719.12
    - foot 719.17
    - forearm 719.13
    - hand 719.14
    - hip 719.15
    - knee 719.16
    - lower leg 719.16
    - multiple sites 719.19
    - pelvic region 719.15
    - shoulder (region) 719.11
    - specified site NEC 719.18
    - thigh 719.15
    - upper arm 719.12
    - wrist 719.13
- kidney 593.81
- knee (joint) 719.16
- labyrinth 386.8
- leg NEC 459.0
- lenticular striate artery (*see also* Hemorrhage, brain) 431
- ligature, vessel 998.11
- liver 573.8
- lower extremity NEC 459.0
- lung 786.3
    - newborn 770.3
    - tuberculous (*see also* Tuberculosis, pulmonary) 011.9 ☑
- malaria 084.8
- marginal sinus 641.2 ☑
- massive subaponeurotic, birth injury 767.11
- maternal, affecting fetus or newborn 762.1
- mediastinum 786.3
- medulla (*see also* Hemorrhage, brain) 431
- membrane (brain) (*see also* Hemorrhage, subarachnoid) 430
    - spinal cord — *see* Hemorrhage, spinal cord
- meninges, meningeal (brain) (middle) (*see also* Hemorrhage, subarachnoid) 430
    - spinal cord — *see* Hemorrhage, spinal cord
- mesentery 568.81
- metritis 626.8
- midbrain (*see also* Hemorrhage, brain) 431
- mole 631
- mouth 528.9
- mucous membrane NEC 459.0
    - newborn 772.8
- muscle 728.89
- nail (subungual) 703.8
- nasal turbinate 784.7
    - newborn 772.8
- nasopharynx 478.29
- navel, newborn 772.3
- newborn 772.9
    - adrenal 772.5
    - alveolar (lung) 770.3
    - brain (anoxic) (hypoxic) (due to birth trauma) 767.0
    - cerebral (anoxic) (hypoxic) (due to birth trauma) 767.0
    - conjunctiva 772.8
    - cutaneous 772.6
    - diathesis 776.0
    - due to vitamin K deficiency 776.0
    - epicranial subaponeurotic (massive) 767.11
    - gastrointestinal 772.4
    - internal (organs) 772.8
    - intestines 772.4
    - intra-alveolar (lung) 770.3
    - intracranial (from any perinatal cause) 767.0
    - intraventricular (from any perinatal cause) 772.10

Hemorrhage, hemorrhagic — *continued*
- newborn — *continued*
    - intraventricular — *continued*
        - grade I 772.11
        - grade II 772.12
        - grade III 772.13
        - grade IV 772.14
    - lung 770.3
    - pulmonary (massive) 770.3
    - spinal cord, traumatic 767.4
    - stomach 772.4
    - subaponeurotic (massive) 767.11
    - subarachnoid (from any perinatal cause) 772.2
    - subconjunctival 772.8
    - subgaleal 767.11
    - umbilicus 772.0
        - slipped ligature 772.3
    - vasa previa 772.0
- nipple 611.79
- nose 784.7
    - newborn 772.8
- obstetrical surgical wound 674.3 ☑
- omentum 568.89
    - newborn 772.4
- optic nerve (sheath) 377.42
- orbit 376.32
- ovary 620.1
- oviduct 620.8
- pancreas 577.8
- parathyroid (gland) (spontaneous) 252.8
- parturition — *see* Hemorrhage, complicating, delivery
- penis 607.82
- pericardium, pericarditis 423.0
- perineal wound (obstetrical) 674.3 ☑
- peritoneum, peritoneal 459.0
- peritonsillar tissue 474.8
    - after operation on tonsils 998.11
    - due to infection 475
- petechial 782.7
- pituitary (gland) 253.8
- placenta NEC 641.9 ☑
    - affecting fetus or newborn 762.1
    - from surgical or instrumental damage 641.8 ☑
        - affecting fetus or newborn 762.1
    - previa 641.1 ☑
        - affecting fetus or newborn 762.0
- pleura — *see* Hemorrhage, lung
- polioencephalitis, superior 265.1
- polymyositis — *see* Polymyositis
- pons (*see also* Hemorrhage, brain) 431
- pontine (*see also* Hemorrhage, brain) 431
- popliteal 459.0
- postcoital 626.7
- postextraction (dental) 998.11
- postmenopausal 627.1
- postnasal 784.7
- postoperative 998.11
- postpartum (atonic) (following delivery of placenta) 666.1 ☑
    - delayed or secondary (after 24 hours) 666.2 ☑
    - retained placenta 666.0 ☑
    - third stage 666.0 ☑
- pregnancy (concealed) 641.9 ☑
    - accidental 641.2 ☑
        - affecting fetus or newborn 762.1
    - affecting fetus or newborn 762.1
    - before 22 completed weeks gestation 640.9 ☑
        - affecting fetus or newborn 762.1
    - due to
        - abruptio placenta 641.2 ☑
            - affecting fetus or newborn 762.1
        - afibrinogenemia or other coagulation defect (conditions classifiable to 286.0–286.9) 641.3 ☑
            - affecting fetus or newborn 762.1

Index to Diseases

Hemorrhage, hemorrhagic — *continued*
  pregnancy — *continued*
    due to — *continued*
      coagulation defect 641.3 ☑
        affecting fetus or newborn 762.1
      hyperfibrinolysis 641.3 ☑
        affecting fetus or newborn 762.1
      hypofibrinogenemia 641.3 ☑
        affecting fetus or newborn 762.1
      leiomyoma, uterus 641.8 ☑
        affecting fetus or newborn 762.1
      low-lying placenta 641.1 ☑
        affecting fetus or newborn 762.1
      marginal sinus (rupture) 641.2 ☑
        affecting fetus or newborn 762.1
      placenta previa 641.1 ☑
        affecting fetus or newborn 762.0
      premature separation of placenta (normally implanted) 641.2 ☑
        affecting fetus or newborn 762.1
      threatened abortion 640.0 ☑
        affecting fetus or newborn 762.1
      trauma 641.8 ☑
        affecting fetus or newborn 762.1
    early (before 22 completed weeks gestation) 640.9 ☑
      affecting fetus or newborn 762.1
    previous, affecting management of pregnancy or childbirth V23.49
    unavoidable — *see* Hemorrhage, pregnancy, due to placenta previa
  prepartum (mother) — *see* Hemorrhage, pregnancy
  preretinal, cause unspecified 362.81
  prostate 602.1
  puerperal (*see also* Hemorrhage, postpartum) 666.1 ☑
  pulmonary (*see also* Hemorrhage, lung)
    newborn (massive) 770.3
    renal syndrome 446.21
  purpura (primary) (*see also* Purpura, thrombocytopenic) 287.39
  rectum (sphincter) 569.3
  recurring, following initial hemorrhage at time of injury 958.2
  renal 593.81
    pulmonary syndrome 446.21
  respiratory tract (*see also* Hemorrhage, lung) 786.3
  retina, retinal (deep) (superficial) (vessels) 362.81
    diabetic 250.5 ☑ *[362.01]*
    due to birth injury 772.8
  retrobulbar 376.89
  retroperitoneal 459.0
  retroplacental (*see also* Placenta, separation) 641.2 ☑
  scalp 459.0
    due to injury at birth 767.19
  scrotum 608.83
  secondary (nontraumatic) 459.0
    following initial hemorrhage at time of injury 958.2
  seminal vesicle 608.83
  skin 782.7
    newborn 772.6
  spermatic cord 608.83
  spinal (cord) 336.1
    aneurysm (ruptured) 336.1
    syphilitic 094.89

Hemorrhage, hemorrhagic — *continued*
  spinal — *continued*
    due to birth injury 767.4
    fetus or newborn 767.4
  spleen 289.59
  spontaneous NEC 459.0
    petechial 782.7
  stomach 578.9
    newborn 772.4
    ulcer — *see* Ulcer, stomach, with hemorrhage
  subaponeurotic, newborn 767.11
    massive (birth injury) 767.11
  subarachnoid (nontraumatic) 430
    fetus or newborn (anoxic) (traumatic) 772.2
    puerperal, postpartum, childbirth 674.0 ☑
    traumatic — *see* Hemorrhage, brain, traumatic, subarachnoid
  subconjunctival 372.72
    due to birth injury 772.8
    newborn 772.8
  subcortical (*see also* Hemorrhage, brain) 431
  subcutaneous 782.7
  subdiaphragmatic 459.0
  subdural (nontraumatic) 432.1
    due to birth injury 767.0
    fetus or newborn (anoxic) (hypoxic) (due to birth trauma) 767.0
    puerperal, postpartum, childbirth 674.0 ☑
    spinal 336.1
    traumatic — *see* Hemorrhage, brain, traumatic, subdural
  subgaleal 767.11
  subhyaloid 362.81
  subperiosteal 733.99
  subretinal 362.81
  subtentorial (*see also* Hemorrhage, subdural) 432.1
  subungual 703.8
    due to blood dyscrasia 287.8
  suprarenal (capsule) (gland) 255.4
    fetus or newborn 772.5
  tentorium (traumatic) (*see also* Hemorrhage, brain, traumatic)
    fetus or newborn 767.0
    nontraumatic — *see* Hemorrhage, brain, subdural
  testis 608.83
  thigh 459.0
  third stage 666.0 ☑
  thorax — *see* Hemorrhage, lung
  throat 784.8
  thrombocythemia 238.71 ▲
  thymus (gland) 254.8
  thyroid (gland) 246.3
    cyst 246.3
  tongue 529.8
  tonsil 474.8
    postoperative 998.11
  tooth socket (postextraction) 998.11
  trachea — *see* Hemorrhage, lung
  traumatic (*see also* nature of injury)
    brain — *see* Hemorrhage, brain, traumatic
    recurring or secondary (following initial hemorrhage at time of injury) 958.2
  tuberculous NEC (*see also* Tuberculosis, pulmonary) 011.9 ☑
  tunica vaginalis 608.83
  ulcer — *see* Ulcer, by site, with hemorrhage
  umbilicus, umbilical cord 772.0
    after birth, newborn 772.3
    complicating delivery 663.8 ☑
      affecting fetus or newborn 772.0
    slipped ligature 772.3
    stump 772.3
    unavoidable (due to placenta previa) 641.1 ☑

Hemorrhage, hemorrhagic — *continued*
  unavoidable — *continued*
    affecting fetus or newborn 762.0
  upper extremity 459.0
  urethra (idiopathic) 599.84
  uterus, uterine (abnormal) 626.9
    climacteric 627.0
    complicating delivery — *see* Hemorrhage, complicating, delivery
    due to
      intrauterine contraceptive device 996.76
        perforating uterus 996.32
    functional or dysfunctional 626.8
    in pregnancy — *see* Hemorrhage, pregnancy
    intermenstrual 626.6
      irregular 626.6
      regular 626.5
    postmenopausal 627.1
    postpartum (*see also* Hemorrhage, postpartum) 666.1 ☑
    prepubertal 626.8
    pubertal 626.3
    puerperal (immediate) 666.1 ☑
  vagina 623.8
  vasa previa 663.5 ☑
    affecting fetus or newborn 772.0
  vas deferens 608.83
  ventricular (*see also* Hemorrhage, brain) 431
  vesical 596.8
  viscera 459.0
    newborn 772.8
  vitreous (humor) (intraocular) 379.23
  vocal cord 478.5
  vulva 624.8
Hemorrhoids (anus) (rectum) (without complication) 455.6
  bleeding, prolapsed, strangulated, or ulcerated NEC 455.8
    external 455.5
    internal 455.2
  complicated NEC 455.8
  complicating pregnancy and puerperium 671.8 ☑
  external 455.3
    with complication NEC 455.5
      bleeding, prolapsed, strangulated, or ulcerated 455.5
      thrombosed 455.4
  internal 455.0
    with complication NEC 455.2
      bleeding, prolapsed, strangulated, or ulcerated 455.2
      thrombosed 455.1
  residual skin tag 455.9
  sentinel pile 455.9
  thrombosed NEC 455.7
    external 455.4
    internal 455.1
Hemosalpinx 620.8
Hemosiderosis 275.0
  dietary 275.0
  pulmonary (idiopathic) 275.0 *[516.1]*
  transfusion NEC 999.8
    bone marrow 996.85
Hemospermia 608.82
Hemothorax 511.8
  bacterial, nontuberculous 511.1
  newborn 772.8
  nontuberculous 511.8
    bacterial 511.1
  pneumococcal 511.1
  postoperative 998.11
  staphylococcal 511.1
  streptococcal 511.1
  traumatic 860.2
    with
      open wound into thorax 860.3
      pneumothorax 860.4
        with open wound into thorax 860.5
  tuberculous (*see also* Tuberculosis, pleura) 012.0 ☑

Hemotympanum 385.89
Hench-Rosenberg syndrome (palindromic arthritis) — *see also* Rheumatism, palindromic 719.3 ☑
Henle's warts 371.41
Henoch (-Schönlein)
  disease or syndrome (allergic purpura) 287.0
  purpura (allergic) 287.0
Henpue, henpuye 102.6
Heparitinuria 277.5
Hepar lobatum 095.3
Hepatalgia 573.8
Hepatic — *see also* condition
  flexure syndrome 569.89
Hepatitis 573.3
  acute (*see also* Necrosis, liver) 570
    alcoholic 571.1
    infective 070.1
      with hepatic coma 070.0
  alcoholic 571.1
  amebic — *see* Abscess, liver, amebic
  anicteric (acute) 070.1
  antigen-associated (HAA) — *see* Hepatitis, viral, type B
  Australian antigen (positive) — *see* Hepatitis, viral, type B
  autoimmune 571.49 ●
  catarrhal (acute) 070.1
    with hepatic coma 070.0
    chronic 571.40
    newborn 070.1
      with hepatic coma 070.0
  chemical 573.3
  cholangiolitic 573.8
  cholestatic 573.8
  chronic 571.40
    active 571.49
      viral — *see* Hepatitis, viral
    aggressive 571.49
    persistent 571.41
    viral — *see* Hepatitis, viral
  cytomegalic inclusion virus 078.5 *[573.1]*
  diffuse 573.3
  "dirty needle" — *see* Hepatitis, viral
  drug-induced 573.3
  due to
    Coxsackie 074.8 *[573.1]*
    cytomegalic inclusion virus 078.5 *[573.1]*
    infectious mononucleosis 075 *[573.1]*
    malaria 084.9 *[573.2]*
    mumps 072.71
    secondary syphilis 091.62
    toxoplasmosis (acquired) 130.5
      congenital (active) 771.2
  epidemic — *see* Hepatitis, viral, type A
  fetus or newborn 774.4
  fibrous (chronic) 571.49
    acute 570
  from injection, inoculation, or transfusion (blood) (other substance) (plasma) (serum) (onset within 8 months after administration) — *see* Hepatitis, viral
  fulminant (viral) (*see also* Hepatitis, viral) 070.9
    with hepatic coma 070.6
    type A 070.1
      with hepatic coma 070.0
    type B — *see* Hepatitis, viral, type B
  giant cell (neonatal) 774.4
  hemorrhagic 573.8
  history of
    B V12.09
    C V12.09
  homologous serum — *see* Hepatitis, viral
  hypertrophic (chronic) 571.49
    acute 570
  infectious, infective (acute) (chronic) (subacute) 070.1

Hepatitis

Hepatitis — *continued*
- infectious, infective — *continued*
  - with hepatic coma 070.0
  - inoculation — *see* Hepatitis, viral
- interstitial (chronic) 571.49
  - acute 570
- lupoid 571.49
- malarial 084.9 [573.2]
- malignant (*see also* Necrosis, liver) 570
- neonatal (toxic) 774.4
- newborn 774.4
- parenchymatous (acute) (*see also* Necrosis, liver) 570
- peliosis 573.3
- persistent, chronic 571.41
- plasma cell 571.49
- postimmunization — *see* Hepatitis, viral
- postnecrotic 571.49
- posttransfusion — *see* Hepatitis, viral
- recurrent 571.49
- septic 573.3
- serum — *see* Hepatitis, viral
  - carrier (suspected of) V02.61
- subacute (*see also* Necrosis, liver) 570
- suppurative (diffuse) 572.0
- syphilitic (late) 095.3
  - congenital (early) 090.0 [573.2]
    - late 090.5 [573.2]
  - secondary 091.62
- toxic (noninfectious) 573.3
  - fetus or newborn 774.4
- tuberculous (*see also* Tuberculosis) 017.9 ☑
- viral (acute) (anicteric) (cholangiolitic) (cholestatic) (chronic) (subacute) 070.9
  - with hepatic coma 070.6
  - AU-SH type virus — *see* Hepatitis, viral, type B
  - Australian antigen — *see* Hepatitis, viral, type B
  - B-antigen — *see* Hepatitis, viral, type B
  - Coxsackie 074.8 [573.1]
  - cytomegalic inclusion 078.5 [573.1]
  - IH (virus) — *see* Hepatitis, viral, type A
  - infectious hepatitis virus — *see* Hepatitis, viral, type A
  - serum hepatitis virus — *see* Hepatitis, viral, type B
  - SH — *see* Hepatitis, viral, type B
  - specified type NEC 070.59
    - with hepatic coma 070.49
  - type A 070.1
    - with hepatic coma 070.0
  - type B (acute) 070.30
    - with
      - hepatic coma 070.20
        - with hepatitis delta 070.21
      - hepatitis delta 070.31
        - with hepatic coma 070.21
    - carrier status V02.61
    - chronic 070.32
      - with
        - hepatic coma 070.22
          - with hepatitis delta 070.23
        - hepatitis delta 070.33
          - with hepatic coma 070.23
  - type C
    - acute 070.51
      - with hepatic coma 070.41
    - carrier status V02.62
    - chronic 070.54
      - with hepatic coma 070.44
      - in remission 070.54 ●
    - unspecified 070.70
      - with hepatic coma 070.71
  - type delta (with hepatitis B carrier state) 070.52

Hepatitis — *continued*
- viral — *continued*
  - type delta — *continued*
    - with
      - active hepatitis B disease — *see* Hepatitis, viral, type B
      - hepatic coma 070.42
  - type E 070.53
    - with hepatic coma 070.43
  - vaccination and inoculation (prophylactic) V05.3
  - Waldenström's (lupoid hepatitis) 571.49

Hepatization, lung (acute) — *see also* Pneumonia, lobar
- chronic (*see also* Fibrosis, lung) 515

Hepatoblastoma (M8970/3) 155.0
Hepatocarcinoma (M8170/3) 155.0
Hepatocholangiocarcinoma (M8180/3) 155.0
Hepatocholangioma, benign (M8180/0) 211.5
Hepatocholangitis 573.8
Hepatocystitis — *see also* Cholecystitis 575.10
Hepatodystrophy 570
Hepatolenticular degeneration 275.1
Hepatolithiasis — *see* Choledocholithiasis
Hepatoma (malignant) (M8170/3) 155.0
- benign (M8170/0) 211.5
- congenital (M8970/3) 155.0
- embryonal (M8970/3) 155.0

Hepatomegalia glycogenica diffusa 271.0
Hepatomegaly — *see also* Hypertrophy, liver 789.1
- congenital 751.69
- syphilitic 090.0
- due to Clonorchis sinensis 121.1
- Gaucher's 272.7
- syphilitic (congenital) 090.0

Hepatoptosis 573.8
Hepatorrhexis 573.8
Hepatosis, toxic 573.8
Hepatosplenomegaly 571.8
- due to S. japonicum 120.2
- hyperlipemic (Bürger-Grutz type) 272.3

Herald patch 696.3
Hereditary — *see* condition
Heredodegeneration 330.9
- macular 362.70

Heredopathia atactica polyneuritiformis 356.3
Heredosyphilis — *see also* Syphilis, congenital 090.9
Hermaphroditism (true) 752.7
- with specified chromosomal anomaly — *see* Anomaly, chromosomes, sex

Hernia, hernial (acquired) (recurrent) 553.9
- with
  - gangrene (obstructed) NEC 551.9
  - obstruction NEC 552.9
    - and gangrene 551.9
- abdomen (wall) — *see* Hernia, ventral
- abdominal, specified site NEC 553.8
  - with
    - gangrene (obstructed) 551.8
    - obstruction 552.8
      - and gangrene 551.8
- appendix 553.8
  - with
    - gangrene (obstructed) 551.8
    - obstruction 552.8
      - and gangrene 551.8
- bilateral (inguinal) — *see* Hernia, inguinal
- bladder (sphincter)
  - congenital (female) (male) 756.71
  - female (*see also* Cystocele, female) 618.01
  - male 596.8

Hernia, hernial — *continued*
- brain 348.4
  - congenital 742.0
- broad ligament 553.8
- cartilage, vertebral — *see* Displacement, intervertebral disc
- cerebral 348.4
  - congenital 742.0
  - endaural 742.0
- ciliary body 364.8
  - traumatic 871.1
- colic 553.9
  - with
    - gangrene (obstructed) 551.9
    - obstruction 552.9
      - and gangrene 551.9
- colon 553.9
  - with
    - gangrene (obstructed) 551.9
    - obstruction 552.9
      - and gangrene 551.9
- colostomy (stoma) 569.69
- Cooper's (retroperitoneal) 553.8
  - with
    - gangrene (obstructed) 551.8
    - obstruction 552.8
      - and gangrene 551.8
- crural — *see* Hernia, femoral
- diaphragm, diaphragmatic 553.3
  - with
    - gangrene (obstructed) 551.3
    - obstruction 552.3
      - and gangrene 551.3
  - congenital 756.6
  - due to gross defect of diaphragm 756.6
  - traumatic 862.0
    - with open wound into cavity 862.1
- direct (inguinal) — *see* Hernia, inguinal
- disc, intervertebral — *see* Displacement, intervertebral disc
- diverticulum, intestine 553.9
  - with
    - gangrene (obstructed) 551.9
    - obstruction 552.9
      - and gangrene 551.9
- double (inguinal) — *see* Hernia, inguinal
- due to adhesion with obstruction 560.81
- duodenojejunal 553.8
  - with
    - gangrene (obstructed) 551.8
    - obstruction 552.8
      - and gangrene 551.8
- en glissade — *see* Hernia, inguinal
- enterostomy (stoma) 569.69
- epigastric 553.29
  - with
    - gangrene (obstruction) 551.29
    - obstruction 552.29
      - and gangrene 551.29
  - recurrent 553.21
    - with
      - gangrene (obstructed) 551.21
      - obstruction 552.21
        - and gangrene 551.21
- esophageal hiatus (sliding) 553.3
  - with
    - gangrene (obstructed) 551.3
    - obstruction 552.3
      - and gangrene 551.3
  - congenital 750.6
- external (inguinal) — *see* Hernia, inguinal
- fallopian tube 620.4
- fascia 728.89
- fat 729.30
  - eyelid 374.34
  - orbital 374.34
  - pad 729.30
    - eye, eyelid 374.34
    - knee 729.31
    - orbit 374.34

Hernia, hernial — *continued*
- fat — *continued*
  - pad — *continued*
    - popliteal (space) 729.31
    - specified site NEC 729.39
- femoral (unilateral) 553.00
  - with
    - gangrene (obstructed) 551.00
    - obstruction 552.00
      - with gangrene 551.00
  - bilateral 553.02
    - gangrenous (obstructed) 551.02
    - obstructed 552.02
      - with gangrene 551.02
    - recurrent 553.03
      - gangrenous (obstructed) 551.03
      - obstructed 552.03
        - with gangrene 551.03
  - recurrent (unilateral) 553.01
    - bilateral 553.03
      - gangrenous (obstructed) 551.03
      - obstructed 552.03
        - with gangrene 551.01
    - gangrenous (obstructed) 551.01
    - obstructed 552.01
      - with gangrene 551.01
- foramen
  - Bochdalek 553.3
    - with
      - gangrene (obstructed) 551.3
      - obstruction 552.3
        - and gangrene 551.3
    - congenital 756.6
  - magnum 348.4
  - Morgagni, Morgagnian 553.3
    - with
      - gangrene 551.3
      - obstruction 552.3
        - and gangrene 551.3
    - congenital 756.6
- funicular (umbilical) 553.1
  - with
    - gangrene (obstructed) 551.1
    - obstruction 552.1
      - and gangrene 551.1
  - spermatic cord — *see* Hernia, inguinal
- gangrenous — *see* Hernia, by site, with gangrene
- gastrointestinal tract 553.9
  - with
    - gangrene (obstructed) 551.9
    - obstruction 552.9
      - and gangrene 551.9
- gluteal — *see* Hernia, femoral
- Gruber's (internal mesogastric) 553.8
  - with
    - gangrene (obstructed) 551.8
    - obstruction 552.8
      - and gangrene 551.8
- Hesselbach's 553.8
  - with
    - gangrene (obstructed) 551.8
    - obstruction 552.8
      - and gangrene 551.8
- hiatal (esophageal) (sliding) 553.3
  - with
    - gangrene (obstructed) 551.3
    - obstruction 552.3
      - and gangrene 551.3
  - congenital 750.6
- incarcerated (*see also* Hernia, by site, with obstruction) 552.9
  - gangrenous (*see also* Hernia, by site, with gangrene) 551.9
- incisional 553.21
  - with
    - gangrene (obstructed) 551.21
    - obstruction 552.21
      - and gangrene 551.21
- lumbar — *see* Hernia, lumbar
- recurrent 553.21
  - with
    - gangrene (obstructed) 551.21

Hernia, hernial — *continued*
　incisional — *continued*
　　recurrent — *continued*
　　　with — *continued*
　　　　obstruction 552.21
　　　　　and gangrene 551.21
　　indirect (inguinal) — *see* Hernia, inguinal
　　infantile — *see* Hernia, inguinal
　　infrapatellar fat pad 729.31
　　inguinal (direct) (double) (encysted) (external) (funicular) (indirect) (infantile) (internal) (interstitial) (oblique) (scrotal) (sliding) 550.9 ☑

> Note — Use the following fifth-digit subclassification with category 550:
> 0　unilateral or unspecified (not specified as recurrent)
> 1　unilateral or unspecified, recurrent
> 2　bilateral (not specified as recurrent)
> 3　bilateral, recurrent

　　　with
　　　　gangrene (obstructed) 550.0 ☑
　　　　obstruction 550.1 ☑
　　　　　and gangrene 550.0 ☑
　　internal 553.8
　　　with
　　　　gangrene (obstructed) 551.8
　　　　obstruction 552.8
　　　　　and gangrene 551.8
　　　inguinal — *see* Hernia, inguinal
　　interstitial 553.9
　　　with
　　　　gangrene (obstructed) 551.9
　　　　obstruction 552.9
　　　　　and gangrene 551.9
　　　inguinal — *see* Hernia, inguinal
　　intervertebral cartilage or disc — *see* Displacement, intervertebral disc
　　intestine, intestinal 553.9
　　　with
　　　　gangrene (obstructed) 551.9
　　　　obstruction 552.9
　　　　　and gangrene 551.9
　　intra-abdominal 553.9
　　　with
　　　　gangrene (obstructed) 551.9
　　　　obstruction 552.9
　　　　　and gangrene 551.9
　　intraparietal 553.9
　　　with
　　　　gangrene (obstructed) 551.9
　　　　obstruction 552.9
　　　　　and gangrene 551.9
　　iris 364.8
　　　traumatic 871.1
　　irreducible (*see also* Hernia, by site, with obstruction) 552.9
　　　gangrenous (with obstruction) (*see also* Hernia, by site, with gangrene) 551.9
　　ischiatic 553.8
　　　with
　　　　gangrene (obstructed) 551.8
　　　　obstruction 552.8
　　　　　and gangrene 551.8
　　ischiorectal 553.8
　　　with
　　　　gangrene (obstructed) 551.8
　　　　obstruction 552.8
　　　　　and gangrene 551.8
　　lens 379.32
　　　traumatic 871.1
　　linea
　　　alba — *see* Hernia, epigastric
　　　semilunaris — *see* Hernia, spigelian
　　Littre's (diverticular) 553.9
　　　with
　　　　gangrene (obstructed) 551.9

Hernia, hernial — *continued*
　Littre's — *continued*
　　with — *continued*
　　　obstruction 552.9
　　　　and gangrene 551.9
　lumbar 553.8
　　with
　　　gangrene (obstructed) 551.8
　　　obstruction 552.8
　　　　and gangrene 551.8
　lung (subcutaneous) 518.89
　　congenital 748.69
　mediastinum 519.3
　mesenteric (internal) 553.8
　　with
　　　gangrene (obstructed) 551.8
　　　obstruction 552.8
　　　　and gangrene 551.8
　mesocolon 553.8
　　with
　　　gangrene (obstructed) 551.8
　　　obstruction 552.8
　　　　and gangrene 551.8
　muscle (sheath) 728.89
　nucleus pulposus — *see* Displacement, intervertebral disc
　oblique (inguinal) — *see* Hernia, inguinal
　obstructive (*see also* Hernia, by site, with obstruction) 552.9
　　gangrenous (with obstruction) (*see also* Hernia, by site, with gangrene) 551.9
　obturator 553.8
　　with
　　　gangrene (obstructed) 551.8
　　　obstruction 552.8
　　　　and gangrene 551.8
　omental 553.8
　　with
　　　gangrene (obstructed) 551.8
　　　obstruction 552.8
　　　　and gangrene 551.8
　orbital fat (pad) 374.34
　ovary 620.4
　oviduct 620.4
　paracolostomy (stoma) 569.69
　paraduodenal 553.8
　　with
　　　gangrene (obstructed) 551.8
　　　obstruction 552.8
　　　　and gangrene 551.8
　paraesophageal 553.3
　　with
　　　gangrene (obstructed) 551.3
　　　obstruction 552.3
　　　　and gangrene 551.3
　　congenital 750.6
　parahiatal 553.3
　　with
　　　gangrene (obstructed) 551.3
　　　obstruction 552.3
　　　　and gangrene 551.3
　paraumbilical 553.1
　　with
　　　gangrene (obstructed) 551.1
　　　obstruction 552.1
　　　　and gangrene 551.1
　parietal 553.9
　　with
　　　gangrene (obstructed) 551.9
　　　obstruction 552.9
　　　　and gangrene 551.9
　perineal 553.8
　　with
　　　gangrene (obstructed) 551.8
　　　obstruction 552.8
　　　　and gangrene 551.8
　peritoneal sac, lesser 553.8
　　with
　　　gangrene (obstructed) 551.8
　　　obstruction 552.8
　　　　and gangrene 551.8
　popliteal fat pad 729.31
　postoperative 553.21

Hernia, hernial — *continued*
　postoperative — *continued*
　　with
　　　gangrene (obstructed) 551.21
　　　obstruction 552.21
　　　　and gangrene 551.21
　pregnant uterus 654.4 ☑
　prevesical 596.8
　properitoneal 553.8
　　with
　　　gangrene (obstructed) 551.8
　　　obstruction 552.8
　　　　and gangrene 551.8
　pudendal 553.8
　　with
　　　gangrene (obstructed) 551.8
　　　obstruction 552.8
　　　　and gangrene 551.8
　rectovaginal 618.6
　retroperitoneal 553.8
　　with
　　　gangrene (obstructed) 551.8
　　　obstruction 552.8
　　　　and gangrene 551.8
　Richter's (parietal) 553.9
　　with
　　　gangrene (obstructed) 551.9
　　　obstruction 552.9
　　　　and gangrene 551.9
　Rieux's, Riex's (retrocecal) 553.8
　　with
　　　gangrene (obstructed) 551.8
　　　obstruction 552.8
　　　　and gangrene 551.8
　sciatic 553.8
　　with
　　　gangrene (obstructed) 551.8
　　　obstruction 552.8
　　　　and gangrene 551.8
　scrotum, scrotal — *see* Hernia, inguinal
　sliding (inguinal) (*see also* Hernia, inguinal)
　　hiatus — *see* Hernia, hiatal
　spigelian 553.29
　　with
　　　gangrene (obstructed) 551.29
　　　obstruction 552.29
　　　　and gangrene 551.29
　spinal (*see also* Spina bifida) 741.9 ☑
　　with hydrocephalus 741.0 ☑
　strangulated (*see also* Hernia, by site, with obstruction) 552.9
　　gangrenous (with obstruction) (*see also* Hernia, by site, with gangrene) 551.9
　supraumbilicus (linea alba) — *see* Hernia, epigastric
　tendon 727.9
　testis (nontraumatic) 550.9 ☑
　　meaning
　　　scrotal hernia 550.9 ☑
　　symptomatic late syphilis 095.8
　Treitz's (fossa) 553.8
　　with
　　　gangrene (obstructed) 551.8
　　　obstruction 552.8
　　　　and gangrene 551.8
　tunica
　　albuginea 608.89
　　vaginalis 752.89
　umbilicus, umbilical 553.1
　　with
　　　gangrene (obstructed) 551.1
　　　obstruction 552.1
　　　　and gangrene 551.1
　ureter 593.89
　　with obstruction 593.4
　uterus 621.8
　　pregnant 654.4 ☑
　vaginal (posterior) 618.6
　Velpeau's (femoral) (*see also* Hernia, femoral) 553.00
　ventral 553.20
　　with
　　　gangrene (obstructed) 551.20

Hernia, hernial — *continued*
　ventral — *continued*
　　with — *continued*
　　　obstruction 552.20
　　　　and gangrene 551.20
　　incisional 553.21
　　recurrent 553.21
　　　with
　　　　gangrene (obstructed) 551.21
　　　　obstruction 552.21
　　　　　and gangrene 551.21
　vesical
　　congenital (female) (male) 756.71
　　female (*see also* Cystocele, female) 618.01
　　male 596.8
　vitreous (into anterior chamber) 379.21
　　traumatic 871.1
Herniation — *see also* Hernia
　brain (stem) 348.4
　cerebral 348.4
　gastric mucosa (into duodenal bulb) 537.89
　mediastinum 519.3
　nucleus pulposus — *see* Displacement, intervertebral disc
Herpangina 074.0
Herpes, herpetic 054.9
　auricularis (zoster) 053.71
　　simplex 054.73
　blepharitis (zoster) 053.20
　　simplex 054.41
　circinate 110.5
　circinatus 110.5
　　bullous 694.5
　conjunctiva (simplex) 054.43
　　zoster 053.21
　cornea (simplex) 054.43
　　disciform (simplex) 054.43
　　zoster 053.21
　encephalitis 054.3
　eye (zoster) 053.29
　　simplex 054.43
　eyelid (zoster) 053.20
　　simplex 054.41
　febrilis 054.9
　fever 054.9
　geniculate ganglionitis 053.11
　genital, genitalis 054.10
　　specified site NEC 054.19
　gestationis 646.8 ☑
　gingivostomatitis 054.2
　iridocyclitis (simplex) 054.44
　　zoster 053.22
　iris (any site) 695.1
　iritis (simplex) 054.44
　keratitis (simplex) 054.43
　　dendritic 054.42
　　disciform 054.43
　　interstitial 054.43
　　zoster 053.21
　keratoconjunctivitis (simplex) 054.43
　　zoster 053.21
　labialis 054.9
　　meningococcal 036.89
　lip 054.9
　meningitis (simplex) 054.72
　　zoster 053.0
　ophthalmicus (zoster) 053.20
　　simplex 054.40
　otitis externa (zoster) 053.71
　　simplex 054.73
　penis 054.13
　perianal 054.10
　pharyngitis 054.79
　progenitalis 054.10
　scrotum 054.19
　septicemia 054.5
　simplex 054.9
　　complicated 054.8
　　ophthalmic 054.40
　　　specified NEC 054.49
　　specified NEC 054.79
　　congenital 771.2
　　external ear 054.73

Herpes, herpetic

Herpes, herpetic — *continued*
  simplex — *continued*
    keratitis 054.43
      dendritic 054.42
    meningitis 054.72
    myelitis 054.74
    neuritis 054.79
    specified complication NEC 054.79
      ophthalmic 054.49
    visceral 054.71
    stomatitis 054.2
    tonsurans 110.0
      maculosus (of Hebra) 696.3
    visceral 054.71
    vulva 054.12
    vulvovaginitis 054.11
    whitlow 054.6
  zoster 053.9
    auricularis 053.71
    complicated 053.8
      specified NEC 053.79
    conjunctiva 053.21
    cornea 053.21
    ear 053.71
    eye 053.29
    geniculate 053.11
    keratitis 053.21
      interstitial 053.21
    myelitis 053.14
    neuritis 053.10
    ophthalmicus(a) 053.20
    oticus 053.71
    otitis externa 053.71
    specified complication NEC 053.79
    specified site NEC 053.9
  zosteriform, intermediate type 053.9
Herrick's
  anemia (hemoglobin S disease) 282.61
  syndrome (hemoglobin S disease) 282.61
Hers' disease (glycogenosis VI) 271.0
Herter (-Gee) disease or syndrome (nontropical sprue) 579.0
Herter's infantilism (nontropical sprue) 579.0
Herxheimer's disease (diffuse idiopathic cutaneous atrophy) 701.8
Herxheimer's reaction 995.0
Hesitancy, urinary 788.64
Hesselbach's hernia — *see* Hernia, Hesselbach's
Heterochromia (congenital) 743.46
  acquired 364.53
  cataract 366.33
  cyclitis 364.21
  hair 704.3
  iritis 364.21
  retained metallic foreign body 360.62
    magnetic 360.52
  uveitis 364.21
Heterophoria 378.40
  alternating 378.45
  vertical 378.43
Heterophyes, small intestine 121.6
Heterophyiasis 121.6
Heteropsia 368.8
Heterotopia, heterotopic — *see also* Malposition, congenital
  cerebralis 742.4
  pancreas, pancreatic 751.7
  spinalis 742.59
Heterotropia 378.30
  intermittent 378.20
    vertical 378.31
  vertical (constant) (intermittent) 378.31
Heubner's disease 094.89
Heubner-Herter disease or syndrome (nontropical sprue) 579.0
Hexadactylism 755.0 ☑
Heyd's syndrome (hepatorenal) 572.4
HGSIL (high grade squamous intraepithelial lesion) 795.04
Hibernoma (M8880/0) — *see* Lipoma
Hiccough 786.8
  epidemic 078.89

Hiccough — *continued*
  psychogenic 306.1
Hiccup — *see also* Hiccough 786.8
Hicks (-Braxton) contractures 644.1 ☑
Hidden penis 752.65
Hidradenitis (axillaris) (suppurative) 705.83
Hidradenoma (nodular) (M8400/0) — *see also* Neoplasm, skin, benign
  clear cell (M8402/0) — *see* Neoplasm, skin, benign
  papillary (M8405/0) — *see* Neoplasm, skin, benign
Hidrocystoma (M8404/0) — *see* Neoplasm, skin, benign
HIE (hypoxic-ischemic encephalopathy) 768.7
High
  A₂ anemia 282.49
  altitude effects 993.2
    anoxia 993.2
    on
      ears 993.0
      sinuses 993.1
    polycythemia 289.0
  arch
    foot 755.67
    palate 750.26
  artery (arterial) tension (*see also* Hypertension) 401.9
    without diagnosis of hypertension 796.2
  basal metabolic rate (BMR) 794.7
  blood pressure (*see also* Hypertension) 401.9
    incidental reading (isolated) (non-specific), no diagnosis of hypertension 796.2
  compliance bladder 596.4
  diaphragm (congenital) 756.6
  frequency deafness (congenital) (regional) 389.8
  head at term 652.5 ☑
    affecting fetus or newborn 763.1
  output failure (cardiac) (*see also* Failure, heart) 428.9
  oxygen-affinity hemoglobin 289.0
  palate 750.26
  risk
    behavior — *see* Problem
    cervical, human papillomavirus (HPV) DNA test positive 795.05
    family situation V61.9
      specified circumstance NEC V61.8
    individual NEC V62.89
    infant NEC V20.1
    patient taking drugs (prescribed) V67.51
      nonprescribed (*see also* Abuse, drugs, nondependent) 305.9 ☑
    pregnancy V23.89
      inadequate prenatal care V23.7
      specified problem NEC V23.89
  temperature (of unknown origin) (*see also* Pyrexia) 780.6
  thoracic rib 756.3
Hildenbrand's disease (typhus) 081.9
Hilger's syndrome 337.0
Hill diarrhea 579.1
Hilliard's lupus — *see also* Tuberculosis 017.0 ☑
Hilum — *see* condition
Hip — *see* condition
Hippel's disease (retinocerebral angiomatosis) 759.6
Hippus 379.49
Hirschfeld's disease (acute diabetes mellitus) — *see also* Diabetes 250.0 ☑
Hirschsprung's disease or megacolon (congenital) 751.3
Hirsuties — *see also* Hypertrichosis 704.1

Hirsutism — *see also* Hypertrichosis 704.1
Hirudiniasis (external) (internal) 134.2
Hiss-Russell dysentery 004.1
Histamine cephalgia 346.2 ☑
Histidinemia 270.5
Histidinuria 270.5
Histiocytic syndromes 288.4
Histiocytoma (M8832/0) — *see also* Neoplasm, skin, benign
  fibrous (M8830/0) (*see also* Neoplasm, skin, benign)
    atypical (M8830/1) — *see* Neoplasm, connective tissue, uncertain behavior
    malignant (M8830/3) — *see* Neoplasm, connective tissue, malignant
Histiocytosis (acute) (chronic) (subacute) 277.89
  acute differentiated progressive (M9722/3) 202.5 ☑
  cholesterol 277.89
  essential 277.89
  lipid, lipoid (essential) 272.7
  lipochrome (familial) 288.1
  malignant (M9720/3) 202.3 ☑
  X (chronic) 277.89
    acute (progressive) (M9722/3) 202.5 ☑
Histoplasmosis 115.90
  with
    endocarditis 115.94
    meningitis 115.91
    pericarditis 115.93
    pneumonia 115.95
    retinitis 115.92
    specified manifestation NEC 115.99
  African (due to Histoplasma duboisii) 115.10
    with
      endocarditis 115.14
      meningitis 115.11
      pericarditis 115.13
      pneumonia 115.15
      retinitis 115.12
      specified manifestation NEC 115.19
  American (due to Histoplasma capsulatum) 115.00
    with
      endocarditis 115.04
      meningitis 115.01
      pericarditis 115.03
      pneumonia 115.05
      retinitis 115.02
      specified manifestation NEC 115.09
  Darling's — *see* Histoplasmosis, American
  large form (*see also* Histoplasmosis, African) 115.10
  lung 115.05
  small form (*see also* Histoplasmosis, American) 115.00
History (personal) of
  abuse
    emotional V15.42
    neglect V15.42
    physical V15.41
    sexual V15.41
  affective psychosis V11.1
  alcoholism V11.3
    specified as drinking problem (*see also* Abuse, drugs, nondependent) 305.0 ☑
  allergy to
    analgesic agent NEC V14.6
    anesthetic NEC V14.4
    antibiotic agent NEC V14.1
      penicillin V14.0
    anti-infective agent NEC V14.3
    diathesis V15.09
    drug V14.9
      specified type NEC V14.8

History of — *continued*
  allergy to — *continued*
    eggs V15.03
    food additives V15.05
    insect bite V15.06
    latex V15.07
    medicinal agents V14.9
      specified type NEC V14.8
    milk products V15.02
    narcotic agent NEC V14.5
    nuts V15.05
      peanuts V15.01
    penicillin V14.0
    radiographic dye V15.08
    seafood V15.04
    serum V14.7
    specified food NEC V15.05
    specified nonmedicinal agents NEC V15.09
    spider bite V15.06
    sulfa V14.2
    sulfonamides V14.2
    therapeutic agent NEC V15.09
    vaccine V14.7
  anemia V12.3
  arthritis V13.4
  benign neoplasm of brain V12.41
  blood disease V12.3
  calculi, urinary V13.01
  cardiovascular disease V12.50
    myocardial infarction 412
  child abuse V15.41
  cigarette smoking V15.82
  circulatory system disease V12.50
    myocardial infarction 412
  congenital malformation V13.69
  contraception V15.7
  diathesis, allergic V15.09
  digestive system disease V12.70
    peptic ulcer V12.71
    polyps, colonic V12.72
    specified NEC V12.79
  disease (of) V13.9
    blood V12.3
    blood-forming organs V12.3
    cardiovascular system V12.50
    circulatory system V12.50
    digestive system V12.70
      peptic ulcer V12.71
      polyps, colonic V12.72
      specified NEC V12.79
    infectious V12.00
      malaria V12.03
      poliomyelitis V12.02
      specified NEC V12.09
      tuberculosis V12.01
    parasitic V12.00
      specified NEC V12.09
    respiratory system V12.60
      pneumonia V12.61
      specified NEC V12.69
    skin V13.3
    specified site NEC V13.8
    subcutaneous tissue V13.3
    trophoblastic V13.1
      affecting management of pregnancy V23.1
  disorder (of) V13.9
    endocrine V12.2
    genital system V13.29
    hematological V12.3
    immunity V12.2
    mental V11.9
      affective type V11.1
      manic-depressive V11.1
      neurosis V11.2
      schizophrenia V11.0
      specified type NEC V11.8
    metabolic V12.2
    musculoskeletal NEC V13.5
    nervous system V12.40
      specified type NEC V12.49
    obstetric V13.29
      affecting management of current pregnancy V23.49
      pre-term labor V23.41

Index to Diseases

History

History of — *continued*
  disorder — *continued*
    obstetric — *continued*
      pre-term labor V13.21
    sense organs V12.40
      specified type NEC V12.49
    specified site NEC V13.8
    urinary system V13.00
      calculi V13.01
      infection V13.02
      nephrotic syndrome V13.03
      specified NEC V13.09
  drug use
    nonprescribed (*see also* Abuse, drugs, nondependent) 305.9 ☑
    patent (*see also* Abuse, drugs, non-dependent) 305.9 ☑
  effect NEC of external cause V15.89
  embolism (pulmonary) V12.51
  emotional abuse V15.42
  encephalitis V12.42
  endocrine disorder V12.2
  extracorporeal membrane oxygenation (ECMO) V15.87
  falling V15.88
  family
    allergy V19.6
    anemia V18.2
    arteriosclerosis V17.4
    arthritis V17.7
    asthma V17.5
    blindness V19.0
    blood disorder NEC V18.3
    cardiovascular disease V17.4
    carrier, genetic disease V18.9
    cerebrovascular disease V17.1
    chronic respiratory condition NEC V17.6
    colonic polyps V18.51 ●
    congenital anomalies V19.5
    consanguinity V19.7
    coronary artery disease V17.3
    cystic fibrosis V18.1
    deafness V19.2
    diabetes mellitus V18.0
    digestive disorders V18.59 ▲
    disease or disorder (of)
      allergic V19.6
      blood NEC V18.3
      cardiovascular NEC V17.4
      cerebrovascular V17.1
      colonic polyps V18.51 ●
      coronary artery V17.3
      digestive V18.59 ▲
      ear NEC V19.3
      endocrine V18.1
      eye NEC V19.1
      genitourinary NEC V18.7
      hypertensive V17.4
      infectious V18.8
      ischemic heart V17.3
      kidney V18.69
        polycystic V18.61
      mental V17.0
      metabolic V18.1
      musculoskeletal NEC V17.89
        osteoporosis V17.81
      neurological NEC V17.2
      parasitic V18.8
      psychiatric condition V17.0
      skin condition V19.4
    ear disorder NEC V19.3
    endocrine disease V18.1
    epilepsy V17.2
    eye disorder NEC V19.1
    genetic disease carrier V18.9
    genitourinary disease NEC V18.7
    glomerulonephritis V18.69
    gout V18.1
    hay fever V17.6
    hearing loss V19.2
    hematopoietic neoplasia V16.7
    Hodgkin's disease V16.7
    Huntington's chorea V17.2
    hydrocephalus V19.5

History of — *continued*
  family — *continued*
    hypertension V17.4
    hypospadias V13.61
    infectious disease V18.8
    ischemic heart disease V17.3
    kidney disease V18.69
      polycystic V18.61
    leukemia V16.6
    lymphatic malignant neoplasia NEC V16.7
    malignant neoplasm (of) NEC V16.9
      anorectal V16.0
      anus V16.0
      appendix V16.0
      bladder V16.59
      bone V16.8
      brain V16.8
      breast V16.3
        male V16.8
      bronchus V16.1
      cecum V16.0
      cervix V16.49
      colon V16.0
      duodenum V16.0
      esophagus V16.0
      eye V16.8
      gallbladder V16.0
      gastrointestinal tract V16.0
      genital organs V16.40
      hemopoietic NEC V16.7
      ileum V16.0
      ilium V16.8
      intestine V16.0
      intrathoracic organs NEC V16.2
      kidney V16.51
      larynx V16.2
      liver V16.0
      lung V16.1
      lymphatic NEC V16.7
      ovary V16.41
      oviduct V16.41
      pancreas V16.0
      penis V16.49
      prostate V16.42
      rectum V16.0
      respiratory organs NEC V16.2
      skin V16.8
      specified site NEC V16.8
      stomach V16.0
      testis V16.43
      trachea V16.1
      ureter V16.59
      urethra V16.59
      urinary organs V16.59
      uterus V16.49
      vagina V16.49
      vulva V16.49
    mental retardation V18.4
    metabolic disease NEC V18.1
    mongolism V19.5
    multiple myeloma V16.7
    musculoskeletal disease NEC V17.89
      osteoporosis V17.81
    nephritis V18.69
    nephrosis V18.69
    osteoporosis V17.81
    parasitic disease V18.8
    polycystic kidney disease V18.61
    psychiatric disorder V17.0
    psychosis V17.0
    retardation, mental V18.4
    retinitis pigmentosa V19.1
    schizophrenia V17.0
    skin conditions V19.4
    specified condition NEC V19.8
    stroke (cerebrovascular) V17.1
    visual loss V19.0
  genital system disorder V13.29
    pre-term labor V13.21
  health hazard V15.9
    falling V15.88
    specified cause NEC V15.89
  hepatitis
    B V12.09

History of — *continued*
  hepatitis — *continued*
    C V12.09
  Hodgkin's disease V10.72
  immunity disorder V12.2
  infection
    central nervous system
    urinary (tract)
  infectious disease V12.00
    malaria V12.03
    poliomyelitis V12.02
    specified NEC V12.09
    tuberculosis V12.01
  injury NEC V15.5
  insufficient prenatal care V23.7
  irradiation V15.3
  leukemia V10.60
    lymphoid V10.61
    monocytic V10.63
    myeloid V10.62
    specified type NEC V10.69
  little or no prenatal care V23.7
  low birth weight (*see also* Status, low birth weight) V21.30
  lymphosarcoma V10.71
  malaria V12.03
  malignant neoplasm (of) V10.9
    accessory sinus V10.22
    adrenal V10.88
    anus V10.06
    bile duct V10.09
    bladder V10.51
    bone V10.81
    brain V10.85
    breast V10.3
    bronchus V10.11
    cervix uteri V10.41
    colon V10.05
    connective tissue NEC V10.89
    corpus uteri V10.42
    digestive system V10.00
      specified part NEC V10.09
    duodenum V10.09
    endocrine gland NEC V10.88
    epididymis V10.48
    esophagus V10.03
    eye V10.84
    fallopian tube V10.44
    female genital organ V10.40
      specified site NEC V10.44
    gallbladder V10.09
    gastrointestinal tract V10.00
    gum V10.02
    hematopoietic NEC V10.79
    hypopharynx V10.02
    ileum V10.09
    intrathoracic organs NEC V10.20
    jejunum V10.09
    kidney V10.52
    large intestine V10.05
    larynx V10.21
    lip V10.02
    liver V10.07
    lung V10.11
    lymphatic NEC V10.79
    lymph glands or nodes NEC V10.79
    male genital organ V10.45
      specified site NEC V10.49
    mediastinum V10.29
    melanoma (of skin) V10.82
    middle ear V10.22
    mouth V10.02
      specified part NEC V10.02
    nasal cavities V10.22
    nasopharynx V10.02
    nervous system NEC V10.86
    nose V10.22
    oropharynx V10.02
    ovary V10.43
    pancreas V10.09
    parathyroid V10.88
    penis V10.49
    pharynx V10.02
    pineal V10.88
    pituitary V10.88
    placenta V10.44

History of — *continued*
  malignant neoplasm — *continued*
    pleura V10.29
    prostate V10.46
    rectosigmoid junction V10.06
    rectum V10.06
    renal pelvis V10.53
    respiratory organs NEC V10.20
    salivary gland V10.02
    skin V10.83
      melanoma V10.82
    small intestine NEC V10.09
    soft tissue NEC V10.89
    specified site NEC V10.89
    stomach V10.04
    testis V10.47
    thymus V10.29
    thyroid V10.87
    tongue V10.01
    trachea V10.12
    ureter V10.59
    urethra V10.59
    urinary organ V10.50
    uterine adnexa V10.44
    uterus V10.42
    vagina V10.44
    vulva V10.44
  manic-depressive psychosis V11.1
  meningitis V12.42
  mental disorder V11.9
    affective type V11.1
    manic-depressive V11.1
    neurosis V11.2
    schizophrenia V11.0
    specified type NEC V11.8
  metabolic disorder V12.2
  musculoskeletal disorder NEC V13.5
  myocardial infarction 412
  neglect (emotional) V15.42
  nephrotic syndrome V13.03
  nervous system disorder V12.40
    specified type NEC V12.49
  neurosis V11.2
  noncompliance with medical treatment V15.81
  nutritional deficiency V12.1
  obstetric disorder V13.29
    affecting management of current pregnancy V23.49
      pre-term labor V23.41
    pre-term labor V13.21
  parasitic disease V12.00
    specified NEC V12.09
  perinatal problems V13.7
    low birth weight (*see also* Status, low birth weight) V21.30
  physical abuse V15.41
  poisoning V15.6
  poliomyelitis V12.02
  polyps, colonic V12.72
  poor obstetric V13.29
    affecting management of current pregnancy V23.49
      pre-term labor V23.41
    pre-term labor V13.21
  psychiatric disorder V11.9
    affective type V11.1
    manic-depressive V11.1
    neurosis V11.2
    schizophrenia V11.0
    specified type NEC V11.8
  psychological trauma V15.49
    emotional abuse V15.42
    neglect V15.42
    physical abuse V15.41
    rape V15.41
  psychoneurosis V11.2
  radiation therapy V15.3
  rape V15.41
  respiratory system disease V12.60
    pneumonia V12.61
    specified NEC V12.69
  reticulosarcoma V10.71
  schizophrenia V11.0
  skin disease V13.3
  smoking (tobacco) V15.82

History

History of — continued
  subcutaneous tissue disease V13.3
  surgery (major) to
    great vessels V15.1
    heart V15.1
    major organs NEC V15.2
  syndrome, nephrotic V13.03
  thrombophlebitis V12.52
  thrombosis V12.51
  tobacco use V15.82
  trophoblastic disease V13.1
    affecting management of pregnancy V23.1
  tuberculosis V12.01
  ulcer, peptic V12.71
  urinary system disorder V13.00
    calculi V13.01
    infection V13.02
    nephrotic syndrome V13.03
    specified NEC V13.09
His-Werner disease (trench fever) 083.1
Hives (bold) — see also Urticaria 708.9
HIV infection (disease) (illness) — see Human immunodeficiency virus (disease) (illness) (infection)
Hoarseness 784.49
Hobnail liver — see Cirrhosis, portal
Hobo, hoboism V60.0
Hodgkin's
  disease (M9650/3) 201.9 ☑
  lymphocytic
    depletion (M9653/3) 201.7 ☑
      diffuse fibrosis (M9654/3) 201.7 ☑
      reticular type (M9655/3) 201.7 ☑
    predominance (M9651/3) 201.4 ☑
  lymphocytic-histiocytic predominance (M9651/3) 201.4 ☑
  mixed cellularity (M9652/3) 201.6 ☑
  nodular sclerosis (M9656/3) 201.5 ☑
    cellular phase (M9657/3) 201.5 ☑
  granuloma (M9661/3) 201.1 ☑
  lymphogranulomatosis (M9650/3) 201.9 ☑
  lymphoma (M9650/3) 201.9 ☑
  lymphosarcoma (M9650/3) 201.9 ☑
  paragranuloma (M9660/3) 201.0 ☑
  sarcoma (M9662/3) 201.2 ☑
Hodgson's disease (aneurysmal dilatation of aorta) 441.9
  ruptured 441.5
Hodi-potsy 111.0
Hoffa (-Kastert) disease or syndrome (liposynovitis prepatellaris) 272.8
Hoffmann-Bouveret syndrome (paroxysmal tachycardia) 427.0
Hoffman's syndrome 244.9 [359.5]
Hole
  macula 362.54
  optic disc, crater-like 377.22
  retina (macula) 362.54
    round 361.31
      with detachment 361.01
Holla disease — see also Spherocytosis 282.0
Holländer-Simons syndrome (progressive lipodystrophy) 272.6
Hollow foot (congenital) 754.71
  acquired 736.73
Holmes' syndrome (visual disorientation) 368.16
Holoprosencephaly 742.2
  due to
    trisomy 13 758.1
    trisomy 18 758.2
Holthouse's hernia — see Hernia, inguinal
Homesickness 309.89
Homocystinemia 270.4
Homocystinuria 270.4

Homologous serum jaundice (prophylactic) (therapeutic) — see Hepatitis, viral
Homosexuality — omit code
  ego-dystonic 302.0
  pedophilic 302.2
  problems with 302.0
Homozygous Hb-S disease 282.61
Honeycomb lung 518.89
  congenital 748.4
Hong Kong ear 117.3
HOOD (hereditary osteo-onychodysplasia) 756.89
Hooded
  clitoris 752.49
  penis 752.69
Hookworm (anemia) (disease) (infestation) — see Ancylostomiasis
Hoppe-Goldflam syndrome 358.00
Hordeolum (external) (eyelid) 373.11
  internal 373.12
Horn
  cutaneous 702.8
    cheek 702.8
    eyelid 702.8
    penis 702.8
    iliac 756.89
    nail 703.8
      congenital 757.5
  papillary 700
Horner's
  syndrome (see also Neuropathy, peripheral, autonomic) 337.9
    traumatic 954.0
  teeth 520.4
Horseshoe kidney (congenital) 753.3
Horton's
  disease (temporal arteritis) 446.5
  headache or neuralgia 346.2 ☑
Hospice care V66.7
Hospitalism (in children) NEC 309.83
Hourglass contraction, contracture
  bladder 596.8
  gallbladder 575.2
    congenital 751.69
  stomach 536.8
    congenital 750.7
    psychogenic 306.4
  uterus 661.4 ☑
    affecting fetus or newborn 763.7
Household circumstance affecting care V60.9
  specified type NEC V60.8
Housemaid's knee 727.2
Housing circumstance affecting care V60.9
  specified type NEC V60.8
HTLV-I infection 079.51
HTLV-II infection 079.52
HTLV-III/LAV (disease) (illness) (infection) — see Human immunodeficiency virus (disease) (illness) (infection)
HTLV-III (disease) (illness) (infection) — see Human immunodeficiency virus (disease) (illness) (infection)
Huchard's disease (continued arterial hypertension) 401.9
Hudson-Ståhli lines 371.11
Huguier's disease (uterine fibroma) 218.9
Human bite (open wound) — see also Wound, open, by site
  intact skin surface — see Contusion
Human immunodeficiency virus (disease) (illness) 042
  infection V08
    with symptoms, symptomatic 042
Human immunodeficiency virus-2 infection 079.53
Human immunovirus (disease) (illness) (infection) — see Human immunodeficiency virus (disease) (illness) (infection)
Human papillomavirus 079.4

Index to Diseases

Human papillomavirus — continued
  cervical
    high risk, DNA test positive 795.05
    low risk, DNA test positive 795.09
Human T-cell lymphotrophic virus-I infection 079.51
Human T-cell lymphotrophic virus-II infection 079.52
Human T-cell lymphotrophic virus-III (disease) (illness) (infection) — see Human immunodeficiency virus (disease) (illness) (infection)
Humpback (acquired) 737.9
  congenital 756.19
Hum, venous — omit code
Hunchback (acquired) 737.9
  congenital 756.19
Hunger 994.2
  air, psychogenic 306.1
  disease 251.1
Hunner's ulcer — see also Cystitis 595.1
Hunt's
  neuralgia 053.11
  syndrome (herpetic geniculate ganglionitis) 053.11
    dyssynergia cerebellaris myoclonica 334.2
Hunter's glossitis 529.4
Hunterian chancre 091.0
Hunter (-Hurler) syndrome (mucopolysaccharidosis II) 277.5
Huntington's
  chorea 333.4
  disease 333.4
Huppert's disease (multiple myeloma) (M9730/3) 203.0 ☑
Hurler (-Hunter) disease or syndrome (mucopolysaccharidosis II) 277.5
Hürthle cell
  adenocarcinoma (M8290/3) 193
  adenoma (M8290/0) 226
  carcinoma (M8290/3) 193
  tumor (M8290/0) 226
Hutchinson's
  disease meaning
    angioma serpiginosum 709.1
    cheiropompholyx 705.81
    prurigo estivalis 692.72
    summer eruption, or summer prurigo 692.72
  incisors 090.5
  melanotic freckle (M8742/2) (see also Neoplasm, skin, in situ)
    malignant melanoma in (M8742/3) — see Melanoma
  teeth or incisors (congenital syphilis) 090.5
Hutchinson-Boeck disease or syndrome (sarcoidosis) 135
Hutchinson-Gilford disease or syndrome (progeria) 259.8
Hyaline
  degeneration (diffuse) (generalized) 728.9
  localized — see Degeneration, by site
  membrane (disease) (lung) (newborn) 769
Hyalinosis cutis et mucosae 272.8
Hyalin plaque, sclera, senile 379.16
Hyalitis (asteroid) 379.22
  syphilitic 095.8
Hydatid
  cyst or tumor (see also Echinococcus)
    fallopian tube 752.11
  mole — see Hydatidiform mole
  Morgagni (congenital) 752.89
    fallopian tube 752.11
Hydatidiform mole (benign) (complicating pregnancy) (delivered) (undelivered) 630
  invasive (M9100/1) 236.1
  malignant (M9100/1) 236.1
  previous, affecting management of pregnancy V23.1
Hydatidosis — see Echinococcus

Hyde's disease (prurigo nodularis) 698.3
Hydradenitis 705.83
Hydradenoma (M8400/0) — see Hidradenoma
Hydralazine lupus or syndrome
  correct substance properly administered 695.4
  overdose or wrong substance given or taken 972.6
Hydramnios 657.0 ☑
  affecting fetus or newborn 761.3
Hydrancephaly 742.3
  with spina bifida (see also Spina bifida) 741.0 ☑
Hydranencephaly 742.3
  with spina bifida (see also Spina bifida) 741.0 ☑
Hydrargyrism NEC 985.0
Hydrarthrosis — see also Effusion, joint 719.0 ☑
  gonococcal 098.50
  intermittent (see also Rheumatism, palindromic) 719.3 ☑
  of yaws (early) (late) 102.6
  syphilitic 095.8
    congenital 090.5
Hydremia 285.9
Hydrencephalocele (congenital) 742.0
Hydrencephalomeningocele (congenital) 742.0
Hydroa 694.0
  aestivale 692.72
  gestationis 646.8 ☑
  herpetiformis 694.0
  pruriginosa 694.0
  vacciniforme 692.72
Hydroadenitis 705.83
Hydrocalycosis — see also Hydronephrosis 591
  congenital 753.29
Hydrocalyx — see also Hydronephrosis 591
Hydrocele (calcified) (chylous) (idiopathic) (infantile) (inguinal canal) (recurrent) (senile) (spermatic cord) (testis) (tunica vaginalis) 603.9
  canal of Nuck (female) 629.1
  male 603.9
  congenital 778.6
  encysted 603.0
    congenital 778.6
  female NEC 629.89 ▲
  infected 603.1
  round ligament 629.89 ▲
  specified type NEC 603.8
    congenital 778.6
  spinalis (see also Spina bifida) 741.9 ☑
  vulva 624.8
Hydrocephalic fetus
  affecting management or pregnancy 655.0 ☑
  causing disproportion 653.6 ☑
    with obstructed labor 660.1 ☑
    affecting fetus or newborn 763.1
Hydrocephalus (acquired) (external) (internal) (malignant) (noncommunicating) (obstructive) (recurrent) 331.4
  aqueduct of Sylvius stricture 742.3
    with spina bifida (see also Spina bifida) 741.0 ☑
  chronic 742.3
    with spina bifida (see also Spina bifida) 741.0 ☑
  communicating 331.3
  congenital (external) (internal) 742.3
    with spina bifida (see also Spina bifida) 741.0 ☑
  due to
    stricture of aqueduct of Sylvius 742.3
      with spina bifida (see also Spina bifida) 741.0 ☑
    toxoplasmosis (congenital) 771.2

Hydrocephalus — *continued*
  fetal affecting management of pregnancy 655.0
  foramen Magendie block (acquired) 331.3
    congenital 742.3
      with spina bifida (*see also* Spina bifida) 741.0
  newborn 742.3
    with spina bifida (*see also* Spina bifida) 741.0
  otitic 348.2
  syphilitic, congenital 090.49
  tuberculous (*see also* Tuberculosis) 013.8
Hydrocolpos (congenital) 623.8
Hydrocystoma (M8404/0) — *see* Neoplasm, skin, benign
Hydroencephalocele (congenital) 742.0
Hydroencephalomeningocele (congenital) 742.0
Hydrohematopneumothorax — *see also* Hemothorax 511.8
Hydromeningitis — *see* Meningitis
Hydromeningocele (spinal) — *see also* Spina bifida 741.9
  cranial 742.0
Hydrometra 621.8
Hydrometrocolpos 623.8
Hydromicrocephaly 742.1
Hydromphalus (congenital) (since birth) 757.39
Hydromyelia 742.53
Hydromyelocele — *see also* Spina bifida 741.9
Hydronephrosis 591
  atrophic 591
  congenital 753.29
  due to S. hematobium 120.0
  early 591
  functionless (infected) 591
  infected 591
  intermittent 591
  primary 591
  secondary 591
  tuberculous (*see also* Tuberculosis) 016.0
Hydropericarditis — *see also* Pericarditis 423.9
Hydropericardium — *see also* Pericarditis 423.9
Hydroperitoneum 789.5
Hydrophobia 071
Hydrophthalmos — *see also* Buphthalmia 743.20
Hydropneumohemothorax — *see also* Hemothorax 511.8
Hydropneumopericarditis — *see also* Pericarditis 423.9
Hydropneumopericardium — *see also* Pericarditis 423.9
Hydropneumothorax 511.8
  nontuberculous 511.8
    bacterial 511.1
    pneumococcal 511.1
    staphylococcal 511.1
    streptococcal 511.1
  traumatic 860.0
    with open wound into thorax 860.1
  tuberculous (*see also* Tuberculosis, pleura) 012.0
Hydrops 782.3
  abdominis 789.5
  amnii (complicating pregnancy) (*see also* Hydramnios) 657.0
  articulorum intermittens (*see also* Rheumatism, palindromic) 719.3
  cardiac (*see also* Failure, heart) 428.0
  congenital — *see* Hydrops, fetalis
  endolymphatic (*see also* Disease, Ménière's) 386.00
  fetal(is) or newborn 778.0
    due to isoimmunization 773.3
    not due to isoimmunization 778.0
  gallbladder 575.3

Hydrops — *continued*
  idiopathic (fetus or newborn) 778.0
  joint (*see also* Effusion, joint) 719.0
  labyrinth (*see also* Disease, Ménière's) 386.00
  meningeal NEC 331.4
  nutritional 262
  pericardium — *see* Pericarditis
  pleura (*see also* Hydrothorax) 511.8
  renal (*see also* Nephrosis) 581.9
  spermatic cord (*see also* Hydrocele) 603.9
Hydropyonephrosis — *see also* Pyelitis 590.80
  chronic 590.00
Hydrorachis 742.53
Hydrorrhea (nasal) 478.19
  gravidarum 658.1
  pregnancy 658.1
Hydrosadenitis 705.83
Hydrosalpinx (fallopian tube) (follicularis) 614.1
Hydrothorax (double) (pleural) 511.8
  chylous (nonfilarial) 457.8
    filaria (*see also* Infestation, filarial) 125.9
  nontuberculous 511.8
    bacterial 511.1
    pneumococcal 511.1
    staphylococcal 511.1
    streptococcal 511.1
  traumatic 862.29
    with open wound into thorax 862.39
  tuberculous (*see also* Tuberculosis, pleura) 012.0
Hydroureter 593.5
  congenital 753.22
Hydroureteronephrosis — *see* Hydronephrosis 591
Hydrourethra 599.84
Hydroxykynureninuria 270.2
Hydroxyprolinemia 270.8
Hydroxyprolinuria 270.8
Hygroma (congenital) (cystic) (M9173/0) 228.1
  prepatellar 727.3
  subdural — *see* Hematoma, subdural
Hymen — *see* condition
Hymenolepiasis (diminuta) (infection) (infestation) (nana) 123.6
Hymenolepsis (diminuta) (infection) (infestation) (nana) 123.6
Hypalgesia — *see also* Disturbance, sensation 782.0
Hyperabduction syndrome 447.8
Hyperacidity, gastric 536.8
  psychogenic 306.4
Hyperactive, hyperactivity
  basal cell, uterine cervix 622.10
  bladder 596.51
  bowel (syndrome) 564.9
    sounds 787.5
  cervix epithelial (basal) 622.10
  child 314.01
  colon 564.9
  gastrointestinal 536.8
    psychogenic 306.4
  intestine 564.9
  labyrinth (unilateral) 386.51
    with loss of labyrinthine reactivity 386.58
    bilateral 386.52
  nasal mucous membrane 478.19
  stomach 536.8
  thyroid (gland) (*see also* Thyrotoxicosis) 242.9
Hyperacusis 388.42
Hyperadrenalism (cortical) 255.3
  medullary 255.6
Hyperadrenocorticism 255.3
  congenital 255.2
  iatrogenic
    correct substance properly administered 255.3

Hyperadrenocorticism — *continued*
  iatrogenic — *continued*
    overdose or wrong substance given or taken 962.0
Hyperaffectivity 301.11
Hyperaldosteronism (atypical) (hyperplastic) (normoaldosteronal) (normotensive) (primary) 255.10
  secondary 255.14
Hyperalgesia — *see also* Disturbance, sensation 782.0
Hyperalimentation 783.6
  carotene 278.3
  specified NEC 278.8
  vitamin A 278.2
  vitamin D 278.4
Hyperaminoaciduria 270.9
  arginine 270.6
  citrulline 270.6
  cystine 270.0
  glycine 270.0
  lysine 270.7
  ornithine 270.6
  renal (types I, II, III) 270.0
Hyperammonemia (congenital) 270.6
Hyperamnesia 780.99
Hyperamylasemia 790.5
Hyperaphia 782.0
Hyperazotemia 791.9
Hyperbetalipoproteinemia (acquired) (essential) (familial) (hereditary) (primary) (secondary) 272.0
  with prebetalipoproteinemia 272.2
Hyperbilirubinemia 782.4
  congenital 277.4
  constitutional 277.4
  neonatal (transient) (*see also* Jaundice, fetus or newborn) 774.6
  of prematurity 774.2
Hyperbilirubinemica encephalopathia, newborn 774.7
  due to isoimmunization 773.4
Hypercalcemia, hypercalcemic (idiopathic) 275.42
  nephropathy 588.89
Hypercalcinuria 275.40
Hypercapnia 786.09
  with mixed acid-based disorder 276.4
  fetal, affecting newborn 770.89
Hypercarotinemia 278.3
Hypercementosis 521.5
Hyperchloremia 276.9
Hyperchlorhydria 536.8
  neurotic 306.4
  psychogenic 306.4
Hypercholesterinemia — *see* Hypercholesterolemia
Hypercholesterolemia 272.0
  with hyperglyceridemia, endogenous 272.2
  essential 272.0
  familial 272.0
  hereditary 272.0
  primary 272.0
  pure 272.0
Hypercholesterolosis 272.0
Hyperchylia gastrica 536.8
Hyperchylomicronemia (familial) (with hyperbetalipoproteinemia) 272.3
Hypercoagulation syndrome (primary) 289.81
  secondary 289.82
Hypercorticosteronism
  correct substance properly administered 255.3
  overdose or wrong substance given or taken 962.0
Hypercortisonism
  correct substance properly administered 255.3
  overdose or wrong substance given or taken 962.0
Hyperdynamic beta-adrenergic state or syndrome (circulatory) 429.82
Hyperekplexia 759.89

Hyperelectrolytemia 276.9
Hyperemesis 536.2
  arising during pregnancy — *see* Hyperemesis, gravidarum
  gravidarum (mild) (before 22 completed weeks gestation) 643.0
    with
      carbohydrate depletion 643.1
      dehydration 643.1
      electrolyte imbalance 643.1
      metabolic disturbance 643.1
    affecting fetus or newborn 761.8
    severe (with metabolic disturbance) 643.1
  psychogenic 306.4
Hyperemia (acute) 780.99
  anal mucosa 569.49
  bladder 596.7
  cerebral 437.8
  conjunctiva 372.71
  ear, internal, acute 386.30
  enteric 564.89
  eye 372.71
  eyelid (active) (passive) 374.82
  intestine 564.89
  iris 364.41
  kidney 593.81
  labyrinth 386.30
  liver (active) (passive) 573.8
  lung 514
  ovary 620.8
  passive 780.99
  pulmonary 514
  renal 593.81
  retina 362.89
  spleen 289.59
  stomach 537.89
Hyperesthesia (body surface) — *see also* Disturbance, sensation 782.0
  larynx (reflex) 478.79
    hysterical 300.11
  pharynx (reflex) 478.29
Hyperestrinism 256.0
Hyperestrogenism 256.0
Hyperestrogenosis 256.0
Hyperexplexia 759.89
Hyperextension, joint 718.80
  ankle 718.87
  elbow 718.82
  foot 718.87
  hand 718.84
  hip 718.85
  knee 718.86
  multiple sites 718.89
  pelvic region 718.85
  shoulder (region) 718.81
  specified site NEC 718.88
  wrist 718.83
Hyperfibrinolysis — *see* Fibrinolysis
Hyperfolliculinism 256.0
Hyperfructosemia 271.2
Hyperfunction
  adrenal (cortex) 255.3
    androgenic, acquired benign 255.3
    medulla 255.6
    virilism 255.2
  corticoadrenal NEC 255.3
  labyrinth — *see* Hyperactive, labyrinth
  medulloadrenal 255.6
  ovary 256.1
    estrogen 256.0
  pancreas 577.8
  parathyroid (gland) 252.00
  pituitary (anterior) (gland) (lobe) 253.1
  testicular 257.0
Hypergammaglobulinemia 289.89
  monoclonal, benign (BMH) 273.1
  polyclonal 273.0
  Waldenström's 273.0
Hyperglobulinemia 273.8
Hyperglycemia 790.29
  maternal
    affecting fetus or newborn 775.0
    manifest diabetes in infant 775.1
  postpancreatectomy (complete) (partial) 251.3

Hyperglyceridemia 272.1
- endogenous 272.1
- essential 272.1
- familial 272.1
- hereditary 272.1
- mixed 272.3
- pure 272.1

Hyperglycinemia 270.7

Hypergonadism
- ovarian 256.1
- testicular (infantile) (primary) 257.0

Hyperheparinemia — see also Circulating anticoagulants 286.5

Hyperhidrosis, hyperidrosis 705.21
- axilla 705.21
- face 705.21
- focal (localized) 705.21
  - primary 705.21
    - axilla 705.21
    - face 705.21
    - palms 705.21
    - soles 705.21
  - secondary 705.22
    - axilla 705.22
    - face 705.22
    - palms 705.22
    - soles 705.22
- generalized 780.8
- palms 705.21
- psychogenic 306.3
- secondary 780.8
- soles 705.21

Hyperhistidinemia 270.5

Hyperinsulinism (ectopic) (functional) (organic) NEC 251.1
- iatrogenic 251.0
- reactive 251.2
- spontaneous 251.2
- therapeutic misadventure (from administration of insulin) 962.3

Hyperiodemia 276.9

Hyperirritability (cerebral), in newborn 779.1

Hyperkalemia 276.7

Hyperkeratosis — see also Keratosis 701.1
- cervix 622.2
- congenital 757.39
- cornea 371.89
- due to yaws (early) (late) (palmar or plantar) 102.3
- eccentrica 757.39
- figurata centrifuga atrophica 757.39
- follicularis 757.39
  - in cutem penetrans 701.1
- limbic (cornea) 371.89
- palmoplantaris climacterica 701.1
- pinta (carate) 103.1
- senile (with pruritus) 702.0
- tongue 528.79
- universalis congenita 757.1
- vagina 623.1
- vocal cord 478.5
- vulva 624.0

Hyperkinesia, hyperkinetic (disease) (reaction) (syndrome) 314.9
- with
  - attention deficit — see Disorder, attention deficit
  - conduct disorder 314.2
  - developmental delay 314.1
  - simple disturbance of activity and attention 314.01
  - specified manifestation NEC 314.8
- heart (disease) 429.82
- of childhood or adolescence NEC 314.9

Hyperlacrimation — see also Epiphora 375.20

Hyperlipemia — see also Hyperlipidemia 272.4

Hyperlipidemia 272.4
- carbohydrate-induced 272.1
- combined 272.4
- endogenous 272.1
- exogenous 272.3

Hyperlipidemia — continued
- fat-induced 272.3
- group
  - A 272.0
  - B 272.1
  - C 272.2
  - D 272.3
- mixed 272.2
- specified type NEC 272.4

Hyperlipidosis 272.7
- hereditary 272.7

Hyperlipoproteinemia (acquired) (essential) (familial) (hereditary) (primary) (secondary) 272.4
- Fredrickson type
  - I 272.3
  - IIa 272.0
  - IIb 272.2
  - III 272.2
  - IV 272.1
  - V 272.3
- low-density-lipoid-type (LDL) 272.0
- very-low-density-lipoid-type (VLDL) 272.1

Hyperlucent lung, unilateral 492.8

Hyperluteinization 256.1

Hyperlysinemia 270.7

Hypermagnesemia 275.2
- neonatal 775.5

Hypermaturity (fetus or newborn)
- post-term infant 766.21
- prolonged gestation infant 766.22

Hypermenorrhea 626.2

Hypermetabolism 794.7

Hypermethioninemia 270.4

Hypermetropia (congenital) 367.0

Hypermobility
- cecum 564.9
- coccyx 724.71
- colon 564.9
  - psychogenic 306.4
- ileum 564.89
- joint (acquired) 718.80
  - ankle 718.87
  - elbow 718.82
  - foot 718.87
  - hand 718.84
  - hip 718.85
  - knee 718.86
  - multiple sites 718.89
  - pelvic region 718.85
  - shoulder (region) 718.81
  - specified site NEC 718.88
  - wrist 718.83
- kidney, congenital 753.3
- meniscus (knee) 717.5
- scapula 718.81
- stomach 536.8
  - psychogenic 306.4
- syndrome 728.5
- testis, congenital 752.52
- urethral 599.81

Hypermotility
- gastrointestinal 536.8
- intestine 564.9
  - psychogenic 306.4
- stomach 536.8

Hypernasality 784.49

Hypernatremia 276.0
- with water depletion 276.0

Hypernephroma (M8312/3) 189.0

Hyperopia 367.0

Hyperorexia 783.6

Hyperornithinemia 270.6

Hyperosmia — see also Disturbance, sensation 781.1

Hyperosmolality 276.0

Hyperosteogenesis 733.99

Hyperostosis 733.99
- calvarial 733.3
- cortical 733.3
  - infantile 756.59
- frontal, internal of skull 733.3
- interna frontalis 733.3
- monomelic 733.99
- skull 733.3

Hyperostosis — continued
- skull — continued
  - congenital 756.0
- vertebral 721.8
  - with spondylosis — see Spondylosis
  - ankylosing 721.6

Hyperovarianism 256.1

Hyperovarism, hyperovaria 256.1

Hyperoxaluria (primary) 271.8

Hyperoxia 987.8

Hyperparathyroidism 252.00
- ectopic 259.3
- other 252.08
- primary 252.01
- secondary (of renal origin) 588.81
  - non-renal 252.02
- tertiary 252.08

Hyperpathia — see also Disturbance, sensation 782.0
- psychogenic 307.80

Hyperperistalsis 787.4
- psychogenic 306.4

Hyperpermeability, capillary 448.9

Hyperphagia 783.6

Hyperphenylalaninemia 270.1

Hyperphoria 378.40
- alternating 378.45

Hyperphosphatemia 275.3

Hyperpiesia — see also Hypertension 401.9

Hyperpiesis — see also Hypertension 401.9

Hyperpigmentation — see Pigmentation

Hyperpinealism 259.8

Hyperpipecolatemia 270.7

Hyperpituitarism 253.1

Hyperplasia, hyperplastic
- adenoids (lymphoid tissue) 474.12
  - and tonsils 474.10
- adrenal (capsule) (cortex) (gland) 255.8
  - with
    - sexual precocity (male) 255.2
    - virilism, adrenal 255.2
    - virilization (female) 255.2
  - congenital 255.2
  - due to excess ACTH (ectopic) (pituitary) 255.0
  - medulla 255.8
- alpha cells (pancreatic)
  - with
    - gastrin excess 251.5
    - glucagon excess 251.4
- appendix (lymphoid) 543.0
- artery, fibromuscular NEC 447.8
  - carotid 447.8
  - renal 447.3
- bone 733.99
  - marrow 289.9
- breast (see also Hypertrophy, breast) 611.1
- carotid artery 447.8
- cementation, cementum (teeth) (tooth) 521.5
- cervical gland 785.6
- cervix (uteri) 622.10
  - basal cell 622.10
  - congenital 752.49
  - endometrium 622.10
  - polypoid 622.10
- chin 524.05
- clitoris, congenital 752.49
- dentin 521.5
- endocervicitis 616.0
- endometrium, endometrial (adenomatous) (atypical) (cystic) (glandular) (polypoid) (uterus) 621.30
  - with atypia 621.33
  - without atypia
    - complex 621.32
    - simple 621.31
  - cervix 622.10
- epithelial 709.8
  - focal, oral, including tongue 528.79
  - mouth (focal) 528.79
  - nipple 611.8

Hyperplasia, hyperplastic — continued
- epithelial — continued
  - skin 709.8
  - tongue (focal) 528.79
  - vaginal wall 623.0
- erythroid 289.9
- fascialis ossificans (progressiva) 728.11
- fibromuscular, artery NEC 447.8
  - carotid 447.8
  - renal 447.3
- genital
  - female 629.89
  - male 608.89
- gingiva 523.8
- glandularis
  - cystica uteri 621.30
  - endometrium (uterus) 621.30
  - interstitialis uteri 621.30
- granulocytic 288.69
- gum 523.8
- hymen, congenital 752.49
- islands of Langerhans 251.1
- islet cell (pancreatic) 251.9
  - alpha cells
    - with excess
      - gastrin 251.5
      - glucagon 251.4
  - beta cells 251.1
- juxtaglomerular (complex) (kidney) 593.89
- kidney (congenital) 753.3
- liver (congenital) 751.69
- lymph node (gland) 785.6
- lymphoid (diffuse) (nodular) 785.6
  - appendix 543.0
  - intestine 569.89
- mandibular 524.02
  - alveolar 524.72
  - unilateral condylar 526.89
- Marchand multiple nodular (liver) — see Cirrhosis, postnecrotic
- maxillary 524.01
  - alveolar 524.71
- medulla, adrenal 255.8
- myometrium, myometrial 621.2
- nose (lymphoid) (polypoid) 478.19
- oral soft tissue (inflammatory) (irritative) (mucosa) NEC 528.9
  - gingiva 523.8
  - tongue 529.8
- organ or site, congenital NEC — see Anomaly, specified type NEC
- ovary 620.8
- palate, papillary 528.9
- pancreatic islet cells 251.9
  - alpha
    - with excess
      - gastrin 251.5
      - glucagon 251.4
  - beta 251.1
- parathyroid (gland) 252.01
- persistent, vitreous (primary) 743.51
- pharynx (lymphoid) 478.29
- prostate 600.90
  - with
    - other lower urinary tract symptoms (LUTS) 600.91
    - urinary
      - obstruction 600.91
      - retention 600.91
  - adenofibromatous 600.20
    - with
      - other lower urinary tract symptoms (LUTS) 600.21
      - urinary
        - obstruction 600.21
        - retention 600.21
  - nodular 600.10
    - with
      - urinary
        - obstruction 600.11

Hyperplasia, hyperplastic — continued
 prostate — continued
  nodular — continued
   with — continued
    urinary — continued
     retention 600.11
 renal artery (fibromuscular) 447.3
 reticuloendothelial (cell) 289.9
 salivary gland (any) 527.1
 Schimmelbusch's 610.1
 suprarenal (capsule) (gland) 255.8
 thymus (gland) (persistent) 254.0
 thyroid (see also Goiter) 240.9
  primary 242.0
  secondary 242.2
 tonsil (lymphoid tissue) 474.11
  and adenoids 474.10
 urethrovaginal 599.89
 uterus, uterine (myometrium) 621.2
  endometrium (see also Hyperplasia, endometrium) 621.30
 vitreous (humor), primary persistent 743.51
 vulva 624.3
 zygoma 738.11
Hyperpnea — see also Hyperventilation 786.01
Hyperpotassemia 276.7
Hyperprebetalipoproteinemia 272.1
 with chylomicronemia 272.3
 familial 272.1
Hyperprolactinemia 253.1
Hyperprolinemia 270.8
Hyperproteinemia 273.8
Hyperprothrombinemia 289.89

Hyperpselaphesia 782.0
Hyperpyrexia 780.6
 heat (effects of) 992.0
 malarial (see also Malaria) 084.6
 malignant, due to anesthetic 995.86
 rheumatic — see Fever, rheumatic
 unknown origin (see also Pyrexia) 780.6
Hyperreactor, vascular 780.2
Hyperreflexia 796.1
 bladder, autonomic 596.54
  with cauda equina 344.61
 detrusor 344.61
Hypersalivation — see also Ptyalism 527.7
Hypersarcosinemia 270.8
Hypersecretion
 ACTH 255.3
 androgens (ovarian) 256.1
 calcitonin 246.0
 corticoadrenal 255.3
 cortisol 255.0
 estrogen 256.0
 gastric 536.8
  psychogenic 306.4
 gastrin 251.5
 glucagon 251.4
 hormone
  ACTH 255.3
  anterior pituitary 253.1
  growth NEC 253.0
  ovarian androgen 256.1
  testicular 257.0
  thyroid stimulating 242.8
 insulin — see Hyperinsulinism

Hypersecretion — continued
 lacrimal glands (see also Epiphora) 375.20
 medulloadrenal 255.6
 milk 676.6
 ovarian androgens 256.1
 pituitary (anterior) 253.1
 salivary gland (any) 527.7
 testicular hormones 257.0
 thyrocalcitonin 246.0
 upper respiratory 478.9
Hypersegmentation, hereditary 288.2
 eosinophils 288.2
 neutrophil nuclei 288.2
Hypersensitive, hypersensitiveness, hypersensitivity — see also Allergy
 angiitis 446.20
  specified NEC 446.29
 carotid sinus 337.0
 colon 564.9
  psychogenic 306.4
 DNA (deoxyribonucleic acid) NEC 287.2
 drug (see also Allergy, drug) 995.27
 esophagus 530.89
 insect bites — see Injury, superficial, by site
 labyrinth 386.58
 pain (see also Disturbance, sensation) 782.0
 pneumonitis NEC 495.9
 reaction (see also Allergy) 995.3
  upper respiratory tract NEC 478.8
 stomach (allergic) (nonallergic) 536.8

Hypersensitive, hypersensitiveness, hypersensitivity — see also Allergy — continued
 stomach — continued
  psychogenic 306.4
Hypersomatotropism (classic) 253.0
Hypersomnia, unspecified 780.54
 with sleep apnea, unspecified 780.53
 alcohol induced 291.82
 drug induced 292.85
 due to
  medical condition classified elsewhere 327.14
  mental disorder 327.15
 idiopathic
  with long sleep time 327.11
  without long sleep time 327.12
 menstrual related 327.13
 nonorganic origin 307.43
  persistent (primary) 307.44
  transient 307.43
 organic 327.10
  other 327.19
  primary 327.44
 recurrent 327.13
Hypersplenia 289.4
Hypersplenism 289.4
Hypersteatosis 706.3
Hyperstimulation, ovarian 256.1
Hypersuprarenalism 255.3
Hypersusceptibility — see Allergy
Hyper-TBG-nemia 246.8
Hypertelorism 756.0
 orbit, orbital 376.41

Index to Diseases — Hypertension, hypertensive

	Malignant	Benign	Unspecified
Hypertension, hypertensive (arterial) (arteriolar) (crisis) (degeneration) (disease) (essential) (fluctuating) (idiopathic) (intermittent) (labile) (low renin) (orthostatic) (paroxysmal) (primary) (systemic) (uncontrolled) (vascular)	401.0	401.1	401.9
with			
chronic kidney disease			
stage I through stage IV, or unspecified ●	403.00	403.10	403.90
stage V or end stage renal disese ●	403.01	403.11	403.91
heart involvement (conditions classifiable to 429.0–429.3, 429.8, 429.9 due to hypertension) (see also Hypertension, heart)	402.00	402.10	402.90
with kidney involvement — see Hypertension, cardiorenal			
renal involvement (only conditions classifiable to 585, 586, 587) (excludes conditions classifiable to 584) (see also Hypertension, kidney)	403.00	403.10	403.90
with heart involvement — see Hypertension, cardiorenal			
failure (and sclerosis) (see also Hypertension, kidney)	403.01	403.11	403.91
sclerosis without failure (see also Hypertension, kidney)	403.00	403.10	403.90
accelerated (see also Hypertension, by type, malignant)	401.0	—	—
antepartum — see Hypertension, complicating pregnancy, childbirth, or the puerperium			
cardiorenal (disease)	404.00	404.10	404.90
with			
chronic kidney disease			
stage I through stage IV, or unspecified ●	404.00	404.10	404.90
and heart failure ●	404.01	404.11	404.91
stage V or end stage renal disease ●	404.02	404.12	404.92
and heart failure ●	404.03	404.13	404.93
heart failure	404.01	404.11	404.91
and chronic kidney disease	404.02	404.12	404.92
stage I through stage IV or unspecified ●	404.02	404.12	404.92
stave V or end stage renal disease ●	404.03	404.13	404.93
cardiovascular disease (arteriosclerotic) (sclerotic)	402.00	402.10	402.90
with			
heart failure	402.01	402.11	402.91
renal involvement (conditions classifiable to 403) (see also Hypertension, cardiorenal)	404.00	404.10	404.90
cardiovascular renal (disease) (sclerosis) (see also Hypertension, cardiorenal)	404.00	404.10	404.90
cerebrovascular disease NEC	437.2	437.2	437.2
complicating pregnancy, childbirth, or the puerperium	642.2 ☑	642.0 ☑	642.9 ☑
with			
albuminuria (and edema) (mild)	—	—	642.4 ☑
severe	—	—	642.5 ☑
chronic kidney disease ●	642.2 ☑	642.2 ☑	642.2 ☑
and heart disease ●	642.2 ☑	642.2 ☑	642.2 ☑
edema (mild)	—	—	642.4 ☑
severe	—	—	642.5 ☑
heart disease	642.2 ☑	642.2 ☑	642.2 ☑
and ▶chronic kidney◀ disease	642.2 ☑	642.2 ☑	642.2 ☑
renal disease	642.2 ☑	642.2 ☑	642.2 ☑
and heart disease	642.2 ☑	642.2 ☑	642.2 ☑
chronic	642.2 ☑	642.0 ☑	642.0 ☑
with pre-eclampsia or eclampsia	642.7 ☑	642.7 ☑	642.7 ☑
fetus or newborn	760.0	760.0	760.0
essential	—	642.0 ☑	642.0 ☑
with pre-eclampsia or eclampsia	—	642.7 ☑	642.7 ☑
fetus or newborn	760.0	760.0	760.0
fetus or newborn	760.0	760.0	760.0
gestational	—	—	642.3 ☑
pre-existing	642.2 ☑	642.0 ☑	642.0 ☑
with pre-eclampsia or eclampsia	642.7 ☑	642.7 ☑	642.7 ☑
fetus or newborn	760.0	760.0	760.0
secondary to renal disease	642.1 ☑	642.1 ☑	642.1 ☑
with pre-eclampsia or eclampsia	642.7 ☑	642.7 ☑	642.7 ☑
fetus or newborn	760.0	760.0	760.0
transient	—	—	642.3 ☑
due to			
aldosteronism, primary	405.09	405.19	405.99
brain tumor	405.09	405.19	405.99
bulbar poliomyelitis	405.09	405.19	405.99
calculus			
kidney	405.09	405.19	405.99
ureter	405.09	405.19	405.99
coarctation, aorta	405.09	405.19	405.99
Cushing's disease	405.09	405.19	405.99
glomerulosclerosis (see also Hypertension, kidney)	403.00	403.10	403.90
periarteritis nodosa	405.09	405.19	405.99
pheochromocytoma	405.09	405.19	405.99
polycystic kidney(s)	405.09	405.19	405.99
polycythemia	405.09	405.19	405.99
porphyria	405.09	405.19	405.99
pyelonephritis	405.09	405.19	405.99
Hypertension, hypertensive — continued			
due to — continued			
renal (artery)			
aneurysm	405.01	405.11	405.91
anomaly	405.01	405.11	405.91
embolism	405.01	405.11	405.91
fibromuscular hyperplasia	405.01	405.11	405.91
occlusion	405.01	405.11	405.91
stenosis	405.01	405.11	405.91
thrombosis	405.01	405.11	405.91
encephalopathy	437.2	437.2	437.2
gestational (transient) NEC	—	—	642.3 ☑
Goldblatt's	440.1	440.1	440.1
heart (disease) (conditions classifiable to 429.0–429.3, 429.8, 429.9 due to hypertension)	402.00	402.10	402.90
with heart failure	402.01	402.11	402.91
hypertensive kidney disease (conditions classifiable to 403) (see also Hypertension, cardiorenal)	404.00	404.10	404.90
renal sclerosis (see also Hypertension, cardiorenal)	404.00	404.10	404.90
intracranial, benign	—	348.2	—
intraocular	—	—	365.04
kidney	403.00	403.10	403.90
with			
chronic kidney disease			
stage I through stage IV, or unspecified ●	403.00	403.10	403.90
stage V or end stage renal disese ●	403.01	403.11	403.91
heart involvement (conditions classifiable to 429.0–429.3, 429.8, 429.9 due to hypertension) (see also Hypertension, cardiorenal)	404.00	404.10	404.90
hypertensive heart (disease) (conditions classifiable to 402) (see also Hypertension, cardiorenal)	404.00	404.10	404.90
lesser circulation	—	—	416.0
necrotizing	401.0	—	—
ocular	—	—	365.04
portal (due to chronic liver disease)	—	—	572.3
postoperative	—	—	997.91
psychogenic	—	—	306.2
puerperal, postpartum — see Hypertension, complicating pregnancy, childbirth, or the puerperium			
pulmonary (artery)	—	—	416.8
with cor pulmonale (chronic)	—	—	416.8
acute	—	—	415.0
idiopathic	—	—	416.0
primary	—	—	416.0
of newborn	—	—	747.83
secondary	—	—	416.8
renal (disease) (see also Hypertension, kidney)	403.00	403.10	403.90
renovascular NEC	405.01	405.11	405.91
secondary NEC	405.09	405.19	405.99
due to			
aldosteronism, primary	405.09	405.19	405.99
brain tumor	405.09	405.19	405.99
bulbar poliomyelitis	405.09	405.19	405.99
calculus			
kidney	405.09	405.19	405.99
ureter	405.09	405.19	405.99
coarctation, aorta	405.09	405.19	405.99
Cushing's disease	405.09	405.19	405.99
glomerulosclerosis (see also Hypertension, kidney)	403.00	403.10	403.90
periarteritis nodosa	405.09	405.19	405.99
pheochromocytoma	405.09	405.19	405.99
polycystic kidney(s)	405.09	405.19	405.99
polycythemia	405.09	405.19	405.99
porphyria	405.09	405.19	405.99
pyelonephritis	405.09	405.19	405.99
renal (artery)			
aneurysm	405.01	405.11	405.91
anomaly	405.01	405.11	405.91
embolism	405.01	405.11	405.91
fibromuscular hyperplasia	405.01	405.11	405.91
occlusion	405.01	405.11	405.91
stenosis	405.01	405.11	405.91
thrombosis	405.01	405.11	405.91
transient	—	—	796.2
of pregnancy	—	—	642.3 ☑
vascular degeneration	401.0	401.1	401.9
venous, chronic (asymptomatic) (idiopathic)	—	—	459.30
with			
complication, NEC	—	—	459.39
inflammation	—	—	459.32
with ulcer	—	—	459.33
ulcer	—	—	459.31
with inflammation	—	—	459.33
due to			
deep vein thrombosis (see also Syndrome, postphlebetic)	—	—	459.10

Hyperthecosis, ovary

Hyperthecosis, ovary 256.8
Hyperthermia (of unknown origin) — see also Pyrexia 780.6
  malignant (due to anesthesia) 995.86
  newborn 778.4
Hyperthymergasia — see also Psychosis, affective 296.0 ☑
  reactive (from emotional stress, psychological trauma) 298.1
  recurrent episode 296.1 ☑
  single episode 296.0 ☑
Hyperthymism 254.8
Hyperthyroid (recurrent) — see Hyperthyroidism
Hyperthyroidism (latent) (preadult) (recurrent) (without goiter) 242.9 ☑

> Note — Use the following fifth-digit subclassification with category 242:
> 0   without mention of thyrotoxic crisis or storm
> 1   with mention of thyrotoxic crisis or storm

  with
    goiter (diffuse) 242.0 ☑
      adenomatous 242.3 ☑
        multinodular 242.2 ☑
        uninodular 242.1 ☑
      nodular 242.3 ☑
        multinodular 242.2 ☑
        uninodular 242.1 ☑
      thyroid nodule 242.1 ☑
  complicating pregnancy, childbirth, or puerperium 648.1 ☑
  neonatal (transient) 775.3
Hypertonia — see Hypertonicity
Hypertonicity
  bladder 596.51
  fetus or newborn 779.89
  gastrointestinal (tract) 536.8
  infancy 779.89
    due to electrolyte imbalance 779.89
  muscle 728.85
  stomach 536.8
    psychogenic 306.4
  uterus, uterine (contractions) 661.4 ☑
    affecting fetus or newborn 763.7
Hypertony — see Hypertonicity
Hypertransaminemia 790.4
Hypertrichosis 704.1
  congenital 757.4
  eyelid 374.54
  lanuginosa 757.4
    acquired 704.1
Hypertriglyceridemia, essential 272.1
Hypertrophy, hypertrophic
  adenoids (infectional) 474.12
    and tonsils (faucial) (infective) (lingual) (lymphoid) 474.10
  adrenal 255.8
  alveolar process or ridge 525.8
  anal papillae 569.49
  apocrine gland 705.82
  artery NEC 447.8
    carotid 447.8
    congenital (peripheral) NEC 747.60
      gastrointestinal 747.61
      lower limb 747.64
      renal 747.62
      specified NEC 747.69
      spinal 747.82
      upper limb 747.63
    renal 447.3
  arthritis (chronic) (see also Osteoarthrosis) 715.9 ☑
    spine (see also Spondylosis) 721.90
  arytenoid 478.79
  asymmetrical (heart) 429.9
  auricular — see Hypertrophy, cardiac
  Bartholin's gland 624.8
  bile duct 576.8
  bladder (sphincter) (trigone) 596.8
  blind spot, visual field 368.42
  bone 733.99
  brain 348.8

Hypertrophy, hypertrophic — continued
  breast 611.1
    cystic 610.1
    fetus or newborn 778.7
    fibrocystic 610.1
    massive pubertal 611.1
    puerperal, postpartum 676.3 ☑
    senile (parenchymatous) 611.1
  cardiac (chronic) (idiopathic) 429.3
    with
      rheumatic fever (conditions classifiable to 390)
        active 391.8
          with chorea 392.0
        inactive or quiescent (with chorea) 398.99
    congenital NEC 746.89
    fatty (see also Degeneration, myocardial) 429.1
    hypertensive (see also Hypertension, heart) 402.90
    rheumatic (with chorea) 398.99
      active or acute 391.8
        with chorea 392.0
    valve (see also Endocarditis) 424.90
      congenital NEC 746.89
  cartilage 733.99
  cecum 569.89
  cervix (uteri) 622.6
    congenital 752.49
    elongation 622.6
  clitoris (cirrhotic) 624.2
    congenital 752.49
  colon 569.89
    congenital 751.3
  conjunctiva, lymphoid 372.73
  cornea 371.89
  corpora cavernosa 607.89
  duodenum 537.89
  endometrium (uterus) (see also Hyperplasia, endometrium) 621.30
    cervix 622.6
  epididymis 608.89
  esophageal hiatus (congenital) 756.6
    with hernia — see Hernia, diaphragm
  eyelid 374.30
  falx, skull 733.99
  fat pad 729.30
    infrapatellar 729.31
    knee 729.31
    orbital 374.34
    popliteal 729.31
    prepatellar 729.31
    retropatellar 729.31
    specified site NEC 729.39
  foot (congenital) 755.67
  frenum, frenulum (tongue) 529.8
    linguae 529.8
    lip 528.5
  gallbladder or cystic duct 575.8
  gastric mucosa 535.2 ☑
  gingiva 523.8
  gland, glandular (general) NEC 785.6
  gum (mucous membrane) 523.8
  heart (idiopathic) (see also Hypertrophy, cardiac)
    valve (see also Endocarditis)
      congenital NEC 746.89
  hemifacial 754.0
  hepatic — see Hypertrophy, liver
  hiatus (esophageal) 756.6
  hilus gland 785.6
  hymen, congenital 752.49
  ileum 569.89
  infrapatellar fat pad 729.31
  intestine 569.89
  jejunum 569.89
  kidney (compensatory) 593.1
    congenital 753.3
  labial frenulum 528.5
  labium (majus) (minus) 624.3
  lacrimal gland, chronic 375.03
  ligament 728.9

Hypertrophy, hypertrophic — continued
  ligament — continued
    spinal 724.8
  linguae frenulum 529.8
  lingual tonsil (infectional) 474.11
  lip (frenum) 528.5
    congenital 744.81
  liver 789.1
    acute 573.8
    cirrhotic — see Cirrhosis, liver
    congenital 751.69
    fatty — see Fatty, liver
  lymph gland 785.6
    tuberculous — see Tuberculosis, lymph gland
  mammary gland — see Hypertrophy, breast
  maxillary frenulum 528.5
  Meckel's diverticulum (congenital) 751.0
  medial meniscus, acquired 717.3
  median bar 600.90
    with
      other lower urinary tract symptoms (LUTS) 600.91
      urinary
        obstruction 600.91
        retention 600.91
  mediastinum 519.3
  meibomian gland 373.2
  meniscus, knee, congenital 755.64
  metatarsal head 733.99
  metatarsus 733.99
  mouth 528.9
  mucous membrane
    alveolar process 523.8
    nose 478.19 ▲
    turbinate (nasal) 478.0
  muscle 728.9
  muscular coat, artery NEC 447.8
    carotid 447.8
    renal 447.3
  myocardium (see also Hypertrophy, cardiac) 429.3
    idiopathic 425.4
  myometrium 621.2
  nail 703.8
    congenital 757.5
  nasal 478.19 ▲
    alae 478.19 ▲
    bone 738.0
    cartilage 478.19 ▲
    mucous membrane (septum) 478.19 ▲
    sinus (see also Sinusitis) 473.9
    turbinate 478.0
  nasopharynx, lymphoid (infectional) (tissue) (wall) 478.29
  neck, uterus 622.6
  nipple 611.1
  normal aperture diaphragm (congenital) 756.6
  nose (see also Hypertrophy, nasal) 478.19 ▲
  orbit 376.46
  organ or site, congenital NEC — see Anomaly, specified type NEC
  osteoarthropathy (pulmonary) 731.2
  ovary 620.8
  palate (hard) 526.89
    soft 528.9
  pancreas (congenital) 751.7
  papillae
    anal 569.49
    tongue 529.3
  parathyroid (gland) 252.01
  parotid gland 527.1
  penis 607.89
  phallus 607.89
    female (clitoris) 624.2
  pharyngeal tonsil 474.12
  pharyngitis 472.1
  pharynx 478.29

Hypertrophy, hypertrophic — continued
  pharynx — continued
    lymphoid (infectional) (tissue) (wall) 478.29
  pituitary (fossa) (gland) 253.8
  popliteal fat pad 729.31
  preauricular (lymph) gland (Hampstead) 785.6
  prepuce (congenital) 605
    female 624.2
  prostate (asymptomatic) (early) (recurrent) 600.90
    with
      other lower urinary tract symptlms (LUTS) 600.91 ●
      urinary
        obstruction 600.91
        retention 600.91
    adenofibromatous 600.20
      with
        other lower urinary tract symptoms (LUTS) 600.21 ●
        urinary
          obstruction 600.21
          retention 600.21
    benign 600.00
      with
        other lower urinary tract symptoms (LUTS) 600.01 ●
        urinary
          obstruction 600.01
          retention 600.01
    congenital 752.89
  pseudoedematous hypodermal 757.0
  pseudomuscular 359.1
  pylorus (muscle) (sphincter) 537.0
    congenital 750.5
    infantile 750.5
  rectal sphincter 569.49
  rectum 569.49
  renal 593.1
  rhinitis (turbinate) 472.0
  salivary duct or gland 527.1
    congenital 750.26
  scaphoid (tarsal) 733.99
  scar 701.4
  scrotum 608.89
  sella turcica 253.8
  seminal vesicle 608.89
  sigmoid 569.89
  skin condition NEC 701.9
  spermatic cord 608.89
  spinal ligament 724.8
  spleen — see Splenomegaly
  spondylitis (spine) (see also Spondylosis) 721.90
  stomach 537.89
  subaortic stenosis (idiopathic) 425.1
  sublingual gland 527.1
    congenital 750.26
  submaxillary gland 527.1
  suprarenal (gland) 255.8
  tendon 727.9
  testis 608.89
    congenital 752.89
  thymic, thymus (congenital) (gland) 254.0
  thyroid (gland) (see also Goiter) 240.9
    primary 242.0 ☑
    secondary 242.2 ☑
  toe (congenital) 755.65
    acquired 735.8
  tongue 529.8
    congenital 750.15
    frenum 529.8
    papillae (foliate) 529.3
  tonsil (faucial) (infective) (lingual) (lymphoid) 474.11
    with
      adenoiditis 474.01
      tonsillitis 474.00
        and adenoiditis 474.02
    and adenoids 474.10

Index to Diseases

Hypertrophy, hypertrophic — *continued*
- tunica vaginalis 608.89
- turbinate (mucous membrane) 478.0
- ureter 593.89
- urethra 599.84
- uterus 621.2
  - puerperal, postpartum 674.8 ☑
- uvula 528.9
- vagina 623.8
- vas deferens 608.89
- vein 459.89
- ventricle, ventricular (heart) (left) (right) (*see also* Hypertrophy, cardiac)
  - congenital 746.89
  - due to hypertension (left) (right) (*see also* Hypertension, heart) 402.90
    - benign 402.10
    - malignant 402.00
  - right with ventricular septal defect, pulmonary stenosis or atresia, and dextraposition of aorta 745.2
- verumontanum 599.89
- vesical 596.8
- vocal cord 478.5
- vulva 624.3
  - stasis (nonfilarial) 624.3

Hypertropia (intermittent) (periodic) 378.31
Hypertyrosinemia 270.2
Hyperuricemia 790.6
Hypervalinemia 270.3
Hyperventilation (tetany) 786.01
- hysterical 300.11
- psychogenic 306.1
- syndrome 306.1

Hyperviscidosis 277.00
Hyperviscosity (of serum) (syndrome) NEC 273.3
- polycythemic 289.0
- sclerocythemic 282.8

Hypervitaminosis (dietary) NEC 278.8
- A (dietary) 278.2
- D (dietary) 278.4
- from excessive administration or use of vitamin preparations (chronic) 278.8
  - reaction to sudden overdose 963.5
  - vitamin A 278.2
    - reaction to sudden overdose 963.5
  - vitamin D 278.4
    - reaction to sudden overdose 963.5
  - vitamin K
    - correct substance properly administered 278.8
    - overdose or wrong substance given or taken 964.3

Hypervolemia 276.6
Hypesthesia — *see also* Disturbance, sensation 782.0
- cornea 371.81

Hyphema (anterior chamber) (ciliary body) (iris) 364.41
- traumatic 921.3

Hyphemia — *see* Hyphema
Hypoacidity, gastric 536.8
- psychogenic 306.4

Hypoactive labyrinth (function) — *see* Hypofunction, labyrinth
Hypoadrenalism 255.4
- tuberculous (*see also* Tuberculosis) 017.6 ☑

Hypoadrenocorticism 255.4
- pituitary 253.4

Hypoalbuminemia 273.8
Hypoaldosteronism 255.4 ●
Hypoalphalipoproteinemia 272.5
Hypobarism 993.2
Hypobaropathy 993.2
Hypobetalipoproteinemia (familial) 272.5

Hypocalcemia 275.41
- cow's milk 775.4
- dietary 269.3
- neonatal 775.4
- phosphate-loading 775.4

Hypocalcification, teeth 520.4
Hypochloremia 276.9
Hypochlorhydria 536.8
- neurotic 306.4
- psychogenic 306.4

Hypocholesteremia 272.5
Hypochondria (reaction) 300.7
Hypochondriac 300.7
Hypochondriasis 300.7
Hypochromasia blood cells 280.9
Hypochromic anemia 280.9
- due to blood loss (chronic) 280.0
  - acute 285.1
- microcytic 280.9

Hypocoagulability — *see also* Defect, coagulation 286.9
Hypocomplementemia 279.8
Hypocythemia (progressive) 284.9
Hypodontia — *see also* Anodontia 520.0
Hypoeosinophilia 288.59 ▲
Hypoesthesia — *see also* Disturbance, sensation 782.0
- cornea 371.81
- tactile 782.0

Hypoestrinism 256.39
Hypoestrogenism 256.39
Hypoferremia 280.9
- due to blood loss (chronic) 280.0

Hypofertility
- female 628.9
- male 606.1

Hypofibrinogenemia 286.3
- acquired 286.6
- congenital 286.3

Hypofunction
- adrenal (gland) 255.4
  - cortex 255.4
  - medulla 255.5
  - specified NEC 255.5
- cerebral 331.9
- corticoadrenal NEC 255.4
- intestinal 564.89
- labyrinth (unilateral) 386.53
  - with loss of labyrinthine reactivity 386.55
  - bilateral 386.54
    - with loss of labyrinthine reactivity 386.56
- Leydig cell 257.2
- ovary 256.39
  - postablative 256.2
- pituitary (anterior) (gland) (lobe) 253.2
  - posterior 253.5
- testicular 257.2
  - iatrogenic 257.1
  - postablative 257.1
  - postirradiation 257.1
  - postsurgical 257.1

Hypogammaglobulinemia 279.00
- acquired primary 279.06
- non-sex-linked, congenital 279.06
- sporadic 279.06
- transient of infancy 279.09

Hypogenitalism (congenital) (female) (male) 752.89
- penis 752.69

Hypoglycemia (spontaneous) 251.2
- coma 251.0
  - diabetic 250.3 ☑
- diabetic 250.8 ☑
- due to insulin 251.0
  - therapeutic misadventure 962.3
- familial (idiopathic) 251.2
- following gastrointestinal surgery 579.3
- infantile (idiopathic) 251.2
- in infant of diabetic mother 775.0
- leucine-induced 270.3
- neonatal 775.6
- reactive 251.2
- specified NEC 251.1

Hypoglycemic shock 251.0
- diabetic 250.8 ☑
- due to insulin 251.0
- functional (syndrome) 251.1

Hypogonadism
- female 256.39
- gonadotrophic (isolated) 253.4
- hypogonadotropic (isolated) (with anosmia) 253.4
- isolated 253.4
- male 257.2
  - hereditary familial (Reifenstein's syndrome) 259.5
- ovarian (primary) 256.39
- pituitary (secondary) 253.4
- testicular (primary) (secondary) 257.2

Hypohidrosis 705.0
Hypohidrotic ectodermal dysplasia 757.31
Hypoidrosis 705.0
Hypoinsulinemia, postsurgical 251.3
- postpancreatectomy (complete) (partial) 251.3

Hypokalemia 276.8
Hypokinesia 780.99
Hypoleukia splenica 289.4
Hypoleukocytosis 288.50 ▲
Hypolipidemia 272.5
Hypolipoproteinemia 272.5
Hypomagnesemia 275.2
- neonatal 775.4

Hypomania, hypomanic reaction — *see also* Psychosis, affective 296.0 ☑
- recurrent episode 296.1 ☑
- single episode 296.0 ☑

Hypomastia (congenital) 757.6
Hypomenorrhea 626.1
Hypometabolism 783.9
Hypomotility
- gastrointestinal tract 536.8
  - psychogenic 306.4
- intestine 564.89
  - psychogenic 306.4
- stomach 536.8
  - psychogenic 306.4

Hyponasality 784.49
Hyponatremia 276.1
Hypo-ovarianism 256.39
Hypo-ovarism 256.39
Hypoparathyroidism (idiopathic) (surgically induced) 252.1
- neonatal 775.4

Hypopharyngitis 462
Hypophoria 378.40
Hypophosphatasia 275.3
Hypophosphatemia (acquired) (congenital) (familial) 275.3
- renal 275.3

Hypophyseal, hypophysis — *see also* condition
- dwarfism 253.3
- gigantism 253.0
- syndrome 253.8

Hypophyseothalamic syndrome 253.8
Hypopiesis — *see* Hypotension
Hypopigmentation 709.00
- eyelid 374.53

Hypopinealism 259.8
Hypopituitarism (juvenile) (syndrome) 253.2
- due to
  - hormone therapy 253.7
  - hypophysectomy 253.7
  - radiotherapy 253.7
- postablative 253.7
- postpartum hemorrhage 253.2

Hypoplasia, hypoplasis 759.89
- adrenal (gland) 759.1
- alimentary tract 751.8
  - lower 751.2
  - upper 750.8
- anus, anal (canal) 751.2
- aorta 747.22
- aortic
  - arch (tubular) 747.10

Hypoplasia, hypoplasis — *continued*
- aortic — *continued*
  - orifice or valve with hypoplasia of ascending aorta and defective development of left ventricle (with mitral valve atresia) 746.7
- appendix 751.2
- areola 757.6
- arm (*see also* Absence, arm, congenital) 755.20
- artery (congenital) (peripheral) 747.60
  - brain 747.81
  - cerebral 747.81
  - coronary 746.85
  - gastrointestinal 747.61
  - lower limb 747.64
  - pulmonary 747.3
  - renal 747.62
  - retinal 743.58
  - specified NEC 747.69
  - spinal 747.82
  - umbilical 747.5
  - upper limb 747.63
- auditory canal 744.29
  - causing impairment of hearing 744.02
- biliary duct (common) or passage 751.61
- bladder 753.8
- bone NEC 756.9
  - face 756.0
  - malar 756.0
  - mandible 524.04
    - alveolar 524.74
  - marrow 284.9
    - acquired (secondary) 284.8
    - congenital 284.09 ▲
    - idiopathic 284.9
  - maxilla 524.03
    - alveolar 524.73
  - skull (*see also* Hypoplasia, skull) 756.0
- brain 742.1
  - gyri 742.2
  - specified part 742.2
- breast (areola) 757.6
- bronchus (tree) 748.3
- cardiac 746.89
  - valve — *see* Hypoplasia, heart, valve
  - vein 746.89
- carpus (*see also* Absence, carpal, congenital) 755.28
- cartilaginous 756.9
- cecum 751.2
- cementum 520.4
  - hereditary 520.5
- cephalic 742.1
- cerebellum 742.2
- cervix (uteri) 752.49
- chin 524.06
- clavicle 755.51
- coccyx 756.19
- colon 751.2
- corpus callosum 742.2
- cricoid cartilage 748.3
- dermal, focal (Goltz) 757.39
- digestive organ(s) or tract NEC 751.8
  - lower 751.2
  - upper 750.8
- ear 744.29
  - auricle 744.23
  - lobe 744.29
  - middle, except ossicles 744.03
    - ossicles 744.04
  - ossicles 744.04
- enamel of teeth (neonatal) (postnatal) (prenatal) 520.4
  - hereditary 520.5
- endocrine (gland) NEC 759.2
- endometrium 621.8
- epididymis 752.89
- epiglottis 748.3
- erythroid, congenital 284.01 ▲
- erythropoietic, chronic acquired 284.8

Hypoplasia, hypoplasis

Hypoplasia, hypoplasis — *continued*
  esophagus 750.3
  Eustachian tube 744.24
  eye (*see also* Microphthalmos) 743.10
    lid 743.62
  face 744.89
    bone(s) 756.0
  fallopian tube 752.19
  femur (*see also* Absence, femur, congenital) 755.34
  fibula (*see also* Absence, fibula, congenital) 755.37
  finger (*see also* Absence, finger, congenital) 755.29
  focal dermal 757.39
  foot 755.31
  gallbladder 751.69
  genitalia, genital organ(s)
    female 752.89
      external 752.49
      internal NEC 752.89
    in adiposogenital dystrophy 253.8
    male 752.89
      penis 752.69
  glottis 748.3
  hair 757.4
  hand 755.21
  heart 746.89
    left (complex) (syndrome) 746.7
    valve NEC 746.89
      pulmonary 746.01
  humerus (*see also* Absence, humerus, congenital) 755.24
  hymen 752.49
  intestine (small) 751.1
    large 751.2
  iris 743.46
  jaw 524.09
  kidney(s) 753.0
  labium (majus) (minus) 752.49
  labyrinth, membranous 744.05
  lacrimal duct (apparatus) 743.65
  larynx 748.3
  leg (*see also* Absence, limb, congenital, lower) 755.30
  limb 755.4
    lower (*see also* Absence, limb, congenital, lower) 755.30
    upper (*see also* Absence, limb, congenital, upper) 755.20
  liver 751.69
  lung (lobe) 748.5
  mammary (areolar) 757.6
  mandibular 524.04
    alveolar 524.74
    unilateral condylar 526.89
  maxillary 524.03
    alveolar 524.73
  medullary 284.9
  megakaryocytic 287.30
  metacarpus (*see also* Absence, metacarpal, congenital) 755.28
  metatarsus (*see also* Absence, metatarsal, congenital) 755.38
  muscle 756.89
    eye 743.69
  myocardium (congenital) (Uhl's anomaly) 746.84
  nail(s) 757.5
  nasolacrimal duct 743.65
  nervous system NEC 742.8
  neural 742.8
  nose, nasal 748.1
  ophthalmic (*see also* Microphthalmos) 743.10
  optic nerve 377.43
  organ
    of Corti 744.05
    or site NEC — *see* Anomaly, by site
  osseous meatus (ear) 744.03
  ovary 752.0
  oviduct 752.19
  pancreas 751.7

Hypoplasia, hypoplasis — *continued*
  parathyroid (gland) 759.2
  parotid gland 750.26
  patella 755.64
  pelvis, pelvic girdle 755.69
  penis 752.69
  peripheral vascular system (congenital) NEC 747.60
    gastrointestinal 747.61
    lower limb 747.64
    renal 747.62
    specified NEC 747.69
    spinal 747.82
    upper limb 747.63
  pituitary (gland) 759.2
  pulmonary 748.5
    arteriovenous 747.3
    artery 747.3
    valve 746.01
  punctum lacrimale 743.65
  radioulnar (*see also* Absence, radius, congenital, with ulna) 755.25
  radius (*see also* Absence, radius, congenital) 755.26
  rectum 751.2
  respiratory system NEC 748.9
  rib 756.3
  sacrum 756.19
  scapula 755.59
  shoulder girdle 755.59
  skin 757.39
  skull (bone) 756.0
    with
      anencephalus 740.0
      encephalocele 742.0
      hydrocephalus 742.3
        with spina bifida (*see also* Spina bifida) 741.0 ☑
      microcephalus 742.1
  spinal (cord) (ventral horn cell) 742.59
    vessel 747.82
  spine 756.19
  spleen 759.0
  sternum 756.3
  tarsus (*see also* Absence, tarsal, congenital) 755.38
  testis, testicle 752.89
  thymus (gland) 279.11
  thyroid (gland) 243
    cartilage 748.3
  tibiofibular (*see also* Absence, tibia, congenital, with fibula) 755.35
  toe (*see also* Absence, toe, congenital) 755.39
  tongue 750.16
  trachea (cartilage) (rings) 748.3
  Turner's (tooth) 520.4
  ulna (*see also* Absence, ulna, congenital) 755.27
  umbilical artery 747.5
  ureter 753.29
  uterus 752.3
  vagina 752.49
  vascular (peripheral) NEC (*see also* Hypoplasia, peripheral vascular system) 747.60
    brain 747.81
  vein(s) (peripheral) NEC (*see also* Hypoplasia, peripheral vascular system) 747.60
    brain 747.81
    cardiac 746.89
    great 747.49
    portal 747.49
    pulmonary 747.49
  vena cava (inferior) (superior) 747.49
  vertebra 756.19
  vulva 752.49
  zonule (ciliary) 743.39
  zygoma 738.12
Hypopotassemia 276.8
Hypoproaccelerinemia — *see also* Defect, coagulation 286.3

Hypoproconvertinemia (congenital) — *see also* Defect, coagulation 286.3
Hypoproteinemia (essential) (hypermetabolic) (idiopathic) 273.8
Hypoproteinosis 260
Hypoprothrombinemia (congenital) (hereditary) (idiopathic) — *see also* Defect, coagulation 286.3
  acquired 286.7
  newborn 776.3
Hypopselaphesia 782.0
Hypopyon (anterior chamber) (eye) 364.05
  iritis 364.05
  ulcer (cornea) 370.04
Hypopyrexia 780.99
Hyporeflex 796.1
Hyporeninemia, extreme 790.99
  in primary aldosteronism 255.10
Hyporesponsive episode 780.09
Hyposecretion
  ACTH 253.4
  ovary 256.39
    postablative 256.2
  salivary gland (any) 527.7
Hyposegmentation of neutrophils, hereditary 288.2
Hyposiderinemia 280.9
Hyposmolality 276.1
  syndrome 276.1
Hyposomatotropism 253.3
Hyposomnia, unspecified — *see also* Insomnia 780.52
  with sleep apnea, unspecified 780.51 ▲
Hypospadias (male) 752.61
  female 753.8
Hypospermatogenesis 606.1
Hyposphagma 372.72
Hyposplenism 239.59
Hypostasis, pulmonary 514
Hypostatic — *see* condition
Hyposthenuria 593.89
Hyposuprarenalism 255.4
Hypo-TBG-nemia 246.8
Hypotension (arterial) (constitutional) 458.9
  chronic 458.1
  iatrogenic 458.29
  maternal, syndrome (following labor and delivery) 669.2 ☑
  of hemodialysis 458.21
  orthostatic (chronic) 458.0
    dysautonomic-dyskinetic syndrome 333.0
  permanent idiopathic 458.1
  postoperative 458.29
  postural 458.0
  specified type NEC 458.8
  transient 796.3
Hypothermia (accidental) 991.6
  anesthetic 995.89
  newborn NEC 778.3
  not associated with low environmental temperature 780.99
Hypothymergasia — *see also* Psychosis, affective 296.2 ☑
  recurrent episode 296.3 ☑
  single episode 296.2 ☑
Hypothyroidism (acquired) 244.9
  complicating pregnancy, childbirth, or puerperium 648.1 ☑
  congenital 243
  due to
    ablation 244.1
      radioactive iodine 244.1
      surgical 244.0
    iodine (administration) (ingestion) 244.2
      radioactive 244.1
    irradiation therapy 244.1
    p-aminosalicylic acid (PAS) 244.3
    phenylbutazone 244.3

Hypothyroidism — *continued*
  due to — *continued*
    resorcinol 244.3
    specified cause NEC 244.8
    surgery 244.0
  goitrous (sporadic) 246.1
  iatrogenic NEC 244.3
  iodine 244.2
  pituitary 244.8
  postablative NEC 244.1
  postsurgical 244.0
  primary 244.9
  secondary NEC 244.8
  specified cause NEC 244.8
  sporadic goitrous 246.1
Hypotonia, hypotonicity, hypotony 781.3
  benign congenital 358.8
  bladder 596.4
  congenital 779.89
    benign 358.8
  eye 360.30
    due to
      fistula 360.32
      ocular disorder NEC 360.33
    following loss of aqueous or vitreous 360.33
    primary 360.31
  infantile muscular (benign) 359.0
  muscle 728.9
  uterus, uterine (contractions) — *see* Inertia, uterus
Hypotrichosis 704.09
  congenital 757.4
  lid (congenital) 757.4
    acquired 374.55
  postinfectional NEC 704.09
Hypotropia 378.32
Hypoventilation 786.09
  congenital central alveolar syndrome 327.25
  idiopathic sleep related nonobstructive alveolar 327.24
  sleep related, in conditions classifiable elsewhere 327.26
Hypovitaminosis — *see also* Deficiency, vitamin 269.2
Hypovolemia 276.52
  surgical shock 998.0
  traumatic (shock) 958.4
Hypoxemia — *see also* Anoxia 799.02
  sleep related, in conditions classifiable elsewhere 327.26
Hypoxia — *see also* Anoxia 799.02
  cerebral 348.1
  during or resulting from a procedure 997.01
  newborn 770.88 ▲
    mild or moderate 768.6
    severe 768.5
  fetal, affecting newborn 770.88 ▲
    intrauterine — *see* Distress, fetal
  myocardial (*see also* Insufficiency, coronary) 411.89
    arteriosclerotic — *see* Arteriosclerosis, coronary
  newborn 770.88 ▲
  sleep related 327.24
Hypoxic-ischemic encephalopathy (HIE) 768.7 ●
Hypsarrhythmia — *see also* Epilepsy 345.6 ☑
Hysteralgia, pregnant uterus 646.8 ☑
Hysteria, hysterical 300.10
  anxiety 300.20
  Charcôt's gland 300.11
  conversion (any manifestation) 300.11
  dissociative type NEC 300.15
  psychosis, acute 298.1
Hysteroepilepsy 300.11
Hysterotomy, affecting fetus or newborn 763.89

Index to Diseases

I

Iatrogenic syndrome of excess cortisol 255.0
Iceland disease (epidemic neuromyasthenia) 049.8
Ichthyosis (congenita) 757.1
    acquired 701.1
    fetalis gravior 757.1
    follicularis 757.1
    hystrix 757.39
    lamellar 757.1
    lingual 528.6
    palmaris and plantaris 757.39
    simplex 757.1
    vera 757.1
    vulgaris 757.1
Ichthyotoxism 988.0
    bacterial (see also Poisoning, food) 005.9
Icteroanemia, hemolytic (acquired) 283.9
    congenital (see also Spherocytosis) 282.0
Icterus — see also Jaundice 782.4
    catarrhal — see Icterus, infectious
    conjunctiva 782.4
        newborn 774.6
    epidemic — see Icterus, infectious
    febrilis — see Icterus, infectious
    fetus or newborn — see Jaundice, fetus or newborn
    gravis (see also Necrosis, liver) 570
        complicating pregnancy 646.7
            affecting fetus or newborn 760.8
        fetus or newborn NEC 773.0
        obstetrical 646.7
            affecting fetus or newborn 760.8
    hematogenous (acquired) 283.9
    hemolytic (acquired) 283.9
        congenital (see also Spherocytosis) 282.0
    hemorrhagic (acute) 100.0
        leptospiral 100.0
        newborn 776.0
        spirochetal 100.0
    infectious 070.1
        with hepatic coma 070.0
        leptospiral 100.0
        spirochetal 100.0
    intermittens juvenilis 277.4
    malignant (see also Necrosis, liver) 570
    neonatorum (see also Jaundice, fetus or newborn) 774.6
    pernicious (see also Necrosis, liver) 570
    spirochetal 100.0
Ictus solaris, solis 992.0
Ideation
    suicidal V62.84
Identity disorder 313.82
    dissociative 300.14
    gender role (child) 302.6
        adult 302.85
    psychosexual (child) 302.6
        adult 302.85
Idioglossia 307.9
Idiopathic — see condition
Idiosyncrasy — see also Allergy 995.3
    drug, medicinal substance, and biological — see Allergy, drug
Idiot, idiocy (congenital) 318.2
    amaurotic (Bielschowsky) (-Jansky) (family) (infantile (late)) (juvenile (late)) (Vogt-Spielmeyer) 330.1
    microcephalic 742.1
    Mongolian 758.0
    oxycephalic 756.0
Id reaction (due to bacteria) 692.89
IgE asthma 493.0
Ileitis (chronic) — see also Enteritis 558.9
    infectious 009.0
    noninfectious 558.9
    regional (ulcerative) 555.0
        with large intestine 555.2

Ileitis — see also Enteritis — continued
    segmental 555.0
        with large intestine 555.2
    terminal (ulcerative) 555.0
        with large intestine 555.2
Ileocolitis — see also Enteritis 558.9
    infectious 009.0
    regional 555.2
    ulcerative 556.1
Ileostomy status V44.2
    with complication 569.60
Ileotyphus 002.0
Ileum — see condition
Ileus (adynamic) (bowel) (colon) (inhibitory) (intestine) (neurogenic) (paralytic) 560.1
    arteriomesenteric duodenal 537.2
    due to gallstone (in intestine) 560.31
    duodenal, chronic 537.2
    following gastrointestinal surgery 997.4
    gallstone 560.31
    mechanical (see also Obstruction, intestine) 560.9
    meconium 777.1
        due to cystic fibrosis 277.01
    myxedema 564.89
    postoperative 997.4
    transitory, newborn 777.4
Iliac — see condition
Iliotibial band friction syndrome 728.89
Illegitimacy V61.6
Ill, louping 063.1
Illness — see also Disease
    factitious 300.19
        with
            combined psychological and physical signs and symptoms 300.19
            predominantly
                physical signs and symptoms 300.19
                psychological symptoms 300.16
        chronic (with physical symptoms) 301.51
    heart — see Disease, heart
    manic-depressive (see also Psychosis, affective) 296.80
    mental (see also Disorder, mental) 300.9
Imbalance 781.2
    autonomic (see also Neuropathy, peripheral, autonomic) 337.9
    electrolyte 276.9
        with
            abortion — see Abortion, by type, with metabolic disorder
            ectopic pregnancy (see also categories 633.0–633.9) 639.4
            hyperemesis gravidarum (before 22 completed weeks gestation) 643.1
            molar pregnancy (see also categories 630–632) 639.4
        following
            abortion 639.4
            ectopic or molar pregnancy 639.4
        neonatal, transitory NEC 775.5
    endocrine 259.9
    eye muscle NEC 378.9
        heterophoria — see Heterophoria
    glomerulotubular NEC 593.89
    hormone 259.9
    hysterical (see also Hysteria) 300.10
    labyrinth NEC 386.50
    posture 729.9
    sympathetic (see also Neuropathy, peripheral, autonomic) 337.9
Imbecile, imbecility 318.0
    moral 301.7

Imbecile, imbecility — continued
    old age 290.9
    senile 290.9
    specified IQ — see IQ
    unspecified IQ 318.0
Imbedding, intrauterine device 996.32
Imbibition, cholesterol (gallbladder) 575.6
Imerslund (-Gräsbeck) syndrome (anemia due to familial selective vitamin B_{12} malabsorption) 281.1
Iminoacidopathy 270.8
Iminoglycinuria, familial 270.8
Immature — see also Immaturity
    personality 301.89
Immaturity 765.1
    extreme 765.0
    fetus or infant light-for-dates — see Light-for-dates
    lung, fetus or newborn 770.4
    organ or site NEC — see Hypoplasia
    pulmonary, fetus or newborn 770.4
    reaction 301.89
    sexual (female) (male) 259.0
Immersion 994.1
    foot 991.4
    hand 991.4
Immobile, immobility
    intestine 564.89
    joint — see Ankylosis
    syndrome (paraplegic) 728.3
Immunization
    ABO
        affecting management of pregnancy 656.2
        fetus or newborn 773.1
    complication — see Complications, vaccination
    Rh factor
        affecting management of pregnancy 656.1
        fetus or newborn 773.0
        from transfusion 999.7
Immunodeficiency 279.3
    with
        adenosine-deaminase deficiency 279.2
        defect, predominant
            B-cell 279.00
            T-cell 279.10
        hyperimmunoglobulinemia 279.2
        lymphopenia, hereditary 279.2
        thrombocytopenia and eczema 279.12
        thymic
            aplasia 279.2
            dysplasia 279.2
    autosomal recessive, Swiss-type 279.2
    common variable 279.06
    severe combined (SCID) 279.2
    to Rh factor
        affecting management of pregnancy 656.1
        fetus or newborn 773.0
    X-linked, with increased IgM 279.05
Immunotherapy, prophylactic V07.2
    antineoplastic V58.12
Impaction, impacted
    bowel, colon, rectum 560.30
        with hernia (see also Hernia, by site, with obstruction)
            gangrenous — see Hernia, by site, with gangrene
        by
            calculus 560.39
            gallstone 560.31
        fecal 560.39
        specified type NEC 560.39
    calculus — see Calculus
    cerumen (ear) (external) 380.4
    cuspid 520.6
    dental 520.6
    fecal, feces 560.39
        with hernia (see also Hernia, by site, with obstruction)

Impaction, impacted — continued
    fecal, feces — continued
        with hernia (see also Hernia, by site, with obstruction) — continued
            gangrenous — see Hernia, by site, with gangrene
    fracture — see Fracture, by site
    gallbladder — see Cholelithiasis
    gallstone(s) — see Cholelithiasis
        in intestine (any part) 560.31
    intestine(s) 560.30
        with hernia (see also Hernia, by site, with obstruction)
            gangrenous — see Hernia, by site, with gangrene
        by
            calculus 560.39
            gallstone 560.31
        fecal 560.39
        specified type NEC 560.39
    intrauterine device (IUD) 996.32
    molar 520.6
    shoulder 660.4
        affecting fetus or newborn 763.1
    tooth, teeth 520.6
    turbinate 733.99
Impaired, impairment (function)
    arm V49.1
        movement, involving
            musculoskeletal system V49.1
            nervous system V49.2
    auditory discrimination 388.43
    back V48.3
    body (entire) V49.89
    cognitive, mild, so stated 331.83
    glucose
        fasting 790.21
        tolerance test (oral) 790.22
    hearing (see also Deafness) 389.9
    heart — see Disease, heart
    kidney (see also Disease, renal) 593.9
        disorder resulting from 588.9
            specified NEC 588.89
    leg V49.1
        movement, involving
            musculoskeletal system V49.1
            nervous system V49.2
    limb V49.1
        movement, involving
            musculoskeletal system V49.1
            nervous system V49.2
    liver 573.8
    mastication 524.9
    mild cognitive, so stated 331.83
    mobility
        ear ossicles NEC 385.22
        incostapedial joint 385.22
        malleus 385.21
    myocardium, myocardial (see also Insufficiency, myocardial) 428.0
    neuromusculoskeletal NEC V49.89
        back V48.3
        head V48.2
        limb V49.2
        neck V48.3
        spine V48.3
        trunk V48.3
    rectal sphincter 787.99
    renal (see also Disease, renal) 593.9
        disorder resulting from 588.9
            specified NEC 588.89
    spine V48.3
    vision NEC 369.9
        both eyes NEC 369.3
        moderate 369.74
            both eyes 369.25
                with impairment of lesser eye (specified as)
                      blind, not further specified 369.15
                      low vision, not further specified 369.23
                      near-total 369.17
                      profound 369.18
                      severe 369.24

Impaired, impairment

Impaired, impairment — *continued*
  vision — *continued*
    moderate — *continued*
      both eyes — *continued*
        with impairment of lesser eye — *continued*
          total 369.16
      one eye 369.74
        with vision of other eye (specified as)
          near-normal 369.75
          normal 369.76
    near-total 369.64
      both eyes 369.04
        with impairment of lesser eye (specified as)
          blind, not further specified 369.02
          total 369.03
      one eye 369.64
        with vision of other eye (specified as)
          near normal 369.65
          normal 369.66
    one eye 369.60
      with low vision of other eye 369.10
  profound 369.67
    both eyes 369.08
      with impairment of lesser eye (specified as)
        blind, not further specified 369.05
        near-total 369.07
        total 369.06
    one eye 369.67
      with vision of other eye (specified as)
        near-normal 369.68
        normal 369.69
  severe 369.71
    both eyes 369.22
      with impairment of lesser eye (specified as)
        blind, not further specified 369.11
        low vision, not further specified 369.21
        near-total 369.13
        profound 369.14
        total 369.12
    one eye 369.71
      with vision of other eye (specified as)
        near-normal 369.72
        normal 369.73
  total
    both eyes 369.01
    one eye 369.61
      with vision of other eye (specified as)
        near-normal 369.62
        normal 369.63

Impaludism — *see* Malaria
Impediment, speech NEC 784.5
  psychogenic 307.9
  secondary to organic lesion 784.5
Impending
  cerebrovascular accident or attack 435.9
  coronary syndrome 411.1
  delirium tremens 291.0
  myocardial infarction 411.1
Imperception, auditory (acquired) (congenital) 389.9
Imperfect
  aeration, lung (newborn) 770.5
  closure (congenital)
    alimentary tract NEC 751.8
      lower 751.5
      upper 750.8
    atrioventricular ostium 745.69
    atrium (secundum) 745.5
      primum 745.61
    branchial cleft or sinus 744.41
    choroid 743.59

Imperfect — *continued*
  closure — *continued*
    cricoid cartilage 748.3
    cusps, heart valve NEC 746.89
      pulmonary 746.09
    ductus
      arteriosus 747.0
      Botalli 747.0
    ear drum 744.29
      causing impairment of hearing 744.03
    endocardial cushion 745.60
    epiglottis 748.3
    esophagus with communication to bronchus or trachea 750.3
    Eustachian valve 746.89
    eyelid 743.62
    face, facial (*see also* Cleft, lip) 749.10
    foramen
      Botalli 745.5
      ovale 745.5
    genitalia, genital organ(s) or system
      female 752.89
        external 752.49
        internal NEC 752.89
        uterus 752.3
      male 752.89
        penis 752.69
    glottis 748.3
    heart valve (cusps) NEC 746.89
    interatrial ostium or septum 745.5
    interauricular ostium or septum 745.5
    interventricular ostium or septum 745.4
    iris 743.46
    kidney 753.3
    larynx 748.3
    lens 743.36
    lip (*see also* Cleft, lip) 749.10
    nasal septum or sinus 748.1
    nose 748.1
    omphalomesenteric duct 751.0
    optic nerve entry 743.57
    organ or site NEC — *see* Anomaly, specified type, by site
    ostium
      interatrial 745.5
      interauricular 745.5
      interventricular 745.4
    palate (*see also* Cleft, palate) 749.00
    preauricular sinus 744.46
    retina 743.56
    roof of orbit 742.0
    sclera 743.47
    septum
      aortic 745.0
      aorticopulmonary 745.0
      atrial (secundum) 745.5
        primum 745.61
      between aorta and pulmonary artery 745.0
      heart 745.9
      interatrial (secundum) 745.5
        primum 745.61
      interauricular (secundum) 745.5
        primum 745.61
      interventricular 745.4
        with pulmonary stenosis or atresia, dextraposition of aorta, and hypertrophy of right ventricle 745.2
        in tetralogy of Fallot 745.2
      nasal 748.1
      ventricular 745.4
        with pulmonary stenosis or atresia, dextraposition of aorta, and hypertrophy of right ventricle 745.2
        in tetralogy of Fallot 745.2
    skull 756.0

Imperfect — *continued*
  closure — *continued*
    skull — *continued*
      with
        anencephalus 740.0
        encephalocele 742.0
        hydrocephalus 742.3
          with spina bifida (*see also* Spina bifida) 741.0 ☑
        microcephalus 742.1
        spine (with meningocele) (*see also* Spina bifida) 741.90
    thyroid cartilage 748.3
    trachea 748.3
    tympanic membrane 744.29
      causing impairment of hearing 744.03
    uterus (with communication to bladder, intestine, or rectum) 752.3
    uvula 749.02
      with cleft lip (*see also* Cleft, palate, with cleft lip) 749.20
    vitelline duct 751.0
  development — *see* Anomaly, by site
  erection 607.84
  fusion — *see* Imperfect, closure
  inflation lung (newborn) 770.5
  intestinal canal 751.5
  poise 729.9
  rotation — *see* Malrotation
  septum, ventricular 745.4
Imperfectly descended testis 752.51
Imperforate (congenital) — *see also* Atresia
  anus 751.2
  bile duct 751.61
  cervix (uteri) 752.49
  esophagus 750.3
  hymen 752.42
  intestine (small) 751.1
    large 751.2
  jejunum 751.1
  pharynx 750.29
  rectum 751.2
  salivary duct 750.23
  urethra 753.6
  urinary meatus 753.6
  vagina 752.49
Impervious (congenital) — *see also* Atresia
  anus 751.2
  bile duct 751.61
  esophagus 750.3
  intestine (small) 751.1
    large 751.5
  rectum 751.2
  urethra 753.6
Impetiginization of other dermatoses 684
Impetigo (any organism) (any site) (bullous) (circinate) (contagiosa) (neonatorum) (simplex) 684
  Bockhart's (superficial folliculitis) 704.8
  external ear 684 [380.13]
  eyelid 684 [373.5]
  Fox's (contagiosa) 684
  furfuracea 696.5
  herpetiformis 694.3
    nonobstetrical 694.3
  staphylococcal infection 684
  ulcerative 686.8
  vulgaris 684
Impingement, soft tissue between teeth 524.89
  anterior 524.81
  posterior 524.82
Implantation
  anomalous (*see also* Anomaly, specified type, by site)
    ureter 753.4

Implantation — *continued*
  cyst
    external area or site (skin) NEC 709.8
    iris 364.61
    vagina 623.8
    vulva 624.8
  dermoid (cyst)
    external area or site (skin) NEC 709.8
    iris 364.61
    vagina 623.8
    vulva 624.8
  placenta, low or marginal — *see* Placenta previa
Implant, endometrial 617.9
Impotence (sexual) 607.84
  organic origin NEC 607.84
  psychogenic 302.72
Impoverished blood 285.9
Impression, basilar 756.0
Imprisonment V62.5
Improper
  development, infant 764.9 ☑
Improperly tied umbilical cord (causing hemorrhage) 772.3
Impulses, obsessional 300.3
Impulsive neurosis 300.3
Inaction, kidney — *see also* Disease, renal 593.9
Inactive — *see* condition
Inadequate, inadequacy
  aesthetics of dental resoration 525.67 ●
  biologic 301.6
  cardiac and renal — *see* Hypertension, cardiorenal
  constitutional 301.6
  development
    child 783.40
    fetus 764.9 ☑
      affecting management of pregnancy 656.5 ☑
    genitalia
      after puberty NEC 259.0
      congenital — *see* Hypoplasia, genitalia
    lungs 748.5
    organ or site NEC — *see* Hypoplasia, by site
  dietary 269.9
  distance, interarch 524.28
  education V62.3
  environment
    economic problem V60.2
    household condition NEC V60.1
    poverty V60.2
    unemployment V62.0
  functional 301.6
  household care, due to
    family member
      handicapped or ill V60.4
      temporarily away from home V60.4
    on vacation V60.5
    technical defects in home V60.1
    temporary absence from home of person rendering care V60.4
  housing (heating) (space) V60.1
  interarch distance 524.28
  material resources V60.2
  mental (*see also* Retardation, mental) 319
  nervous system 799.2
  personality 301.6
  prenatal care in current pregnancy V23.7
  pulmonary
    function 786.09
      newborn 770.89
    ventilation, newborn 770.89
  respiration 786.09
    newborn 770.89
  sample, Papanicolaou smear 795.08
  social 301.6
Inanition 263.9

Inanition — continued
- with edema 262
- due to
  - deprivation of food 994.2
  - malnutrition 263.9
- fever 780.6

Inappropriate secretion
- ACTH 255.0
- antidiuretic hormone (ADH) (excessive) 253.6
  - deficiency 253.5
- ectopic hormone NEC 259.3
- pituitary (posterior) 253.6

Inattention after or at birth 995.52

Inborn errors of metabolism — see Disorder, metabolism

Incarceration, incarcerated
- bubonocele (see also Hernia, inguinal, with obstruction)
  - gangrenous — see Hernia, inguinal, with gangrene
- colon (by hernia) (see also Hernia, by site with obstruction)
  - gangrenous — see Hernia, by site, with gangrene
- enterocele 552.9
  - gangrenous 551.9
- epigastrocele 552.29
  - gangrenous 551.29
- epiplocele 552.9
  - gangrenous 551.9
- exomphalos 552.1
  - gangrenous 551.1
- fallopian tube 620.8
- hernia (see also Hernia, by site, with obstruction)
  - gangrenous — see Hernia, by site, with gangrene
- iris, in wound 871.1
- lens, in wound 871.1
- merocele (see also Hernia, femoral, with obstruction) 552.00
- omentum (by hernia) (see also Hernia, by site, with obstruction)
  - gangrenous — see Hernia, by site, with gangrene
- omphalocele 756.79
- rupture (meaning hernia) (see also Hernia, by site, with obstruction) 552.9
  - gangrenous (see also Hernia, by site, with gangrene) 551.9
- sarcoepiplocele 552.9
  - gangrenous 551.9
- sarcoepiplomphalocele 552.1
  - with gangrene 551.1
- uterus 621.8
  - gravid 654.3 ☑
    - causing obstructed labor 660.2 ☑
      - affecting fetus or newborn 763.1

Incident, cerebrovascular — see also Disease, cerebrovascular, acute 436

Incineration (entire body) (from fire, conflagration, electricity, or lightning) — see Burn, multiple, specified sites

Incised wound
- external — see Wound, open, by site
- internal organs (abdomen, chest, or pelvis) — see Injury, internal, by site, with open wound

Incision, incisional
- hernia — see Hernia, incisional
- surgical, complication — see Complications, surgical procedures
- traumatic
  - external — see Wound, open, by site
  - internal organs (abdomen, chest, or pelvis) — see Injury, internal, by site, with open wound

Inclusion
- azurophilic leukocytic 288.2

Inclusion — continued
- blennorrhea (neonatal) (newborn) 771.6
- cyst — see Cyst, skin
- gallbladder in liver (congenital) 751.69

Incompatibility
- ABO
  - affecting management of pregnancy 656.2 ☑
  - fetus or newborn 773.1
  - infusion or transfusion reaction 999.6
- blood (group) (Duffy) (E) (K(ell) (Kidd) (Lewis) (M) (N) (P) (S) NEC
  - affecting management of pregnancy 656.2 ☑
  - fetus or newborn 773.2
  - infusion or transfusion reaction 999.6
- contour of existing restoration of tooth
  - with oral health 525.65
- marital V61.10
  - involving divorce or estrangement V61.0
- Rh (blood group) (factor)
  - affecting management of pregnancy 656.1 ☑
  - fetus or newborn 773.0
  - infusion or transfusion reaction 999.7
- Rhesus — see Incompatibility, Rh

Incompetency, incompetence, incompetent
- annular
  - aortic (valve) (see also Insufficiency, aortic) 424.1
  - mitral (valve) (see also Insufficiency, mitral) 424.0
  - pulmonary valve (heart) (see also Endocarditis, pulmonary) 424.3
- aortic (valve) (see also Insufficiency, aortic) 424.1
  - syphilitic 093.22
- cardiac (orifice) 530.0
  - valve — see Endocarditis
- cervix, cervical (os) 622.5
  - in pregnancy 654.5 ☑
    - affecting fetus or newborn 761.0
- esophagogastric (junction) (sphincter) 530.0
- heart valve, congenital 746.89
- mitral (valve) — see Insufficiency, mitral
- papillary muscle (heart) 429.81
- pelvic fundus
  - pubocervical tissue 618.81
  - rectovaginal tissue 618.82
- pulmonary valve (heart) (see also Endocarditis, pulmonary) 424.3
  - congenital 746.09
- tricuspid (annular) (rheumatic) (valve) (see also Endocarditis, tricuspid) 397.0
- valvular — see Endocarditis
- vein, venous (saphenous) (varicose) (see also Varicose, vein) 454.9
- velopharyngeal (closure)
  - acquired 528.9
  - congenital 750.29

Incomplete — see also condition
- bladder emptying 788.21
- expansion lungs (newborn) 770.5
- gestation (liveborn) — see Immaturity
- rotation — see Malrotation

Incontinence 788.30
- without sensory awareness 788.34
- anal sphincter 787.6
- continuous leakage 788.37
- feces 787.6
  - due to hysteria 300.11
  - nonorganic origin 307.7
- hysterical 300.11
- mixed (male) (female) (urge and stress) 788.33

Incontinence — continued
- overflow 788.38
- paradoxical 788.39
- rectal 787.6
- specified NEC 788.39
- stress (female) 625.6
  - male NEC 788.32
- urethral sphincter 599.84
- urge 788.31
  - and stress (male) (female) 788.33
- urine 788.30
  - active 788.30
  - male 788.30
    - stress 788.32
    - and urge 788.33
  - neurogenic 788.39
  - nonorganic origin 307.6
  - stress (female) 625.6
    - male NEC 788.32
  - urge 788.31
    - and stress 788.33

Incontinentia pigmenti 757.33

Incoordinate
- uterus (action) (contractions) 661.4 ☑
  - affecting fetus or newborn 763.7

Incoordination
- esophageal-pharyngeal (newborn) 787.2
- muscular 781.3
- papillary muscle 429.81

Increase, increased
- abnormal, in development 783.9
- androgens (ovarian) 256.1
- anticoagulants (antithrombin) (anti-VIIIa) (anti-IXa) (anti-Xa) (anti-XIa) 286.5
- postpartum 666.3 ☑
- cold sense (see also Disturbance, sensation) 782.0
- estrogen 256.0
- function
  - adrenal (cortex) 255.3
    - medulla 255.6
  - pituitary (anterior) (gland) (lobe) 253.1
    - posterior 253.6
- heat sense (see also Disturbance, sensation) 782.0
- intracranial pressure 781.99
  - injury at birth 767.8
- light reflex of retina 362.13
- permeability, capillary 448.9
- pressure
  - intracranial 781.99
    - injury at birth 767.8
  - intraocular 365.00
- pulsations 785.9
- pulse pressure 785.9
- sphericity, lens 743.36
- splenic activity 289.4
- venous pressure 459.89
- portal 572.3

Incrustation, cornea, lead or zinc 930.0

Incyclophoria 378.44

Incyclotropia 378.33

Indeterminate sex 752.7

India rubber skin 756.83

Indicanuria 270.2

Indigestion (bilious) (functional) 536.8
- acid 536.8
- catarrhal 536.8
- due to decomposed food NEC 005.9
- fat 579.8
- nervous 306.4
- psychogenic 306.4

Indirect — see condition

Indolent bubo NEC 099.8

Induced
- abortion — see Abortion, induced
- birth, affecting fetus or newborn 763.89
- delivery — see Delivery
- labor — see Delivery

Induration, indurated
- brain 348.8
- breast (fibrous) 611.79

Induration, indurated — continued
- breast — continued
  - puerperal, postpartum 676.3 ☑
- broad ligament 620.8
- chancre 091.0
  - anus 091.1
  - congenital 090.0
  - extragenital NEC 091.2
- corpora cavernosa (penis) (plastic) 607.89
- liver (chronic) 573.8
  - acute 573.8
- lung (black) (brown) (chronic) (fibroid) (see also Fibrosis, lung) 515
  - essential brown 275.0 [516.1]
- penile 607.89
- phlebitic — see Phlebitis
- skin 782.8
- stomach 537.89

Induratio penis plastica 607.89

Industrial — see condition

Inebriety — see also Abuse, drugs, nondependent 305.0 ☑

Inefficiency
- kidney (see also Disease, renal) 593.9
- thyroid (acquired) (gland) 244.9

Inelasticity, skin 782.8

Inequality, leg (acquired) (length) 736.81
- congenital 755.30

Inertia
- bladder 596.4
  - neurogenic 596.54
    - with cauda equina syndrome 344.61
- stomach 536.8
  - psychogenic 306.4
- uterus, uterine 661.2 ☑
  - affecting fetus or newborn 763.7
  - primary 661.0 ☑
  - secondary 661.1 ☑
- vesical 596.4
  - neurogenic 596.54
    - with cauda equina 344.61

Infant — see also condition
- excessive crying of 780.92
- fussy (baby) 780.91
- held for adoption V68.89
- newborn — see Newborn
- post-term (gestation period over 40 completed weeks to 42 completed weeks) 766.21
- prolonged gestation of (period over 42 completed weeks) 766.22
- syndrome of diabetic mother 775.0

"Infant Hercules" syndrome 255.2

Infantile — see also condition
- genitalia, genitals 259.0
  - in pregnancy or childbirth NEC 654.4 ☑
    - affecting fetus or newborn 763.89
    - causing obstructed labor 660.2 ☑
      - affecting fetus or newborn 763.1
- heart 746.9
- kidney 753.3
- lack of care 995.52
- macula degeneration 362.75
- melanodontia 521.05
- os, uterus (see also Infantile, genitalia) 259.0
- pelvis 738.6
  - with disproportion (fetopelvic) 653.1 ☑
    - affecting fetus or newborn 763.1
    - causing obstructed labor 660.1 ☑
      - affecting fetus or newborn 763.1
- penis 259.0
- testis 257.2
- uterus (see also Infantile, genitalia) 259.0
- vulva 752.49

Infantilism 259.9

Infantilism

Infantilism — *continued*
  with dwarfism (hypophyseal) 253.3
  Brissaud's (infantile myxedema) 244.9
  celiac 579.0
  Herter's (nontropical sprue) 579.0
  hypophyseal 253.3
  hypothalamic (with obesity) 253.8
  idiopathic 259.9
  intestinal 579.0
  pancreatic 577.8
  pituitary 253.3
  renal 588.0
  sexual (with obesity) 259.0
Infants, healthy liveborn — *see* Newborn
Infarct, infarction
  adrenal (capsule) (gland) 255.4
  amnion 658.8 ☑
  anterior (with contiguous portion of intraventricular septum) NEC (*see also* Infarct, myocardium) 410.1 ☑
  appendices epiploicae 557.0
  bowel 557.0
  brain (stem) 434.91
    embolic (*see also* Embolism, brain) 434.11
    healed or old without residuals V12.59
    iatrogenic 997.02
    lacunar 434.91
    late effect — *see* Late effect(s) (of) cerebrovascular disease
    postoperative 997.02
    puerperal, postpartum, childbirth 674.0 ☑
    thrombotic (*see also* Thrombosis, brain) 434.01
  breast 611.8
  Brewer's (kidney) 593.81
  cardiac (*see also* Infarct, myocardium) 410.9 ☑
  cerebellar (*see also* Infarct, brain) 434.91
    embolic (*see also* Embolism, brain) 434.11
  cerebral (*see also* Infarct, brain) 434.91
    embolic (*see also* Embolism, brain) 434.11
    thrombotic (*see also* Infarct, brain) 434.01
  chorion 658.8 ☑
  colon (acute) (agnogenic) (embolic) (hemorrhagic) (nonocclusive) (nonthrombotic) (occlusive) (segmental) (thrombotic) (with gangrene) 557.0
  coronary artery (*see also* Infarct, myocardium) 410.9 ☑
  cortical 434.91
  embolic (*see also* Embolism) 444.9
  fallopian tube 620.8
  gallbladder 575.8
  heart (*see also* Infarct, myocardium) 410.9 ☑
  hepatic 573.4
  hypophysis (anterior lobe) 253.8
  impending (myocardium) 411.1
  intestine (acute) (agnogenic) (embolic) (hemorrhagic) (nonocclusive) (nonthrombotic) (occlusive) (thrombotic) (with gangrene) 557.0
  kidney 593.81
  lacunar 434.91
  liver 573.4
  lung (embolic) (thrombotic) 415.19
    with
      abortion — *see* Abortion, by type, with, embolism
      ectopic pregnancy (*see also* categories 633.0–633.9) 639.6
      molar pregnancy (*see also* categories 630–632) 639.6

Infarct, infarction — *continued*
  lung — *continued*
    following
      abortion 639.6
      ectopic or molar pregnancy 639.6
    iatrogenic 415.11
    in pregnancy, childbirth, or puerperium — *see* Embolism, obstetrical
    postoperative 415.11
  lymph node or vessel 457.8
  medullary (brain) — *see* Infarct, brain
  meibomian gland (eyelid) 374.85
  mesentery, mesenteric (embolic) (thrombotic) (with gangrene) 557.0
  midbrain — *see* Infarct, brain
  myocardium, myocardial (acute or with a stated duration of 8 weeks or less) (with hypertension) 410.9 ☑

Note — Use the following fifth-digit subclassification with category 410:

  0 *episode unspecified*
  1 *initial episode*
  2 *subsequent episode without recurrence*

  with symptoms after 8 weeks from date of infarction 414.8
  anterior (wall) (with contiguous portion of intraventricular septum) NEC 410.1 ☑
  anteroapical (with contiguous portion of intraventricular septum) 410.1 ☑
  anterolateral (wall) 410.0 ☑
  anteroseptal (with contiguous portion of intraventricular septum) 410.1 ☑
  apical-lateral 410.5 ☑
  atrial 410.8 ☑
  basal-lateral 410.5 ☑
  chronic (with symptoms after 8 weeks from date of infarction) 414.8
  diagnosed on ECG, but presenting no symptoms 412
  diaphragmatic wall (with contiguous portion of intraventricular septum) 410.4 ☑
  healed or old, currently presenting no symptoms 412
  high lateral 410.5 ☑
  impending 411.1
  inferior (wall) (with contiguous portion of intraventricular septum) 410.4 ☑
  inferolateral (wall) 410.2 ☑
  inferoposterior wall 410.3 ☑
  lateral wall 410.5 ☑
  non-ST elevation (NSTEMI) 410.7 ☑
  nontransmural 410.7 ☑
  papillary muscle 410.8 ☑
  past (diagnosed on ECG or other special investigation, but currently presenting no symptoms) 412
    with symptoms NEC 414.8
  posterior (strictly) (true) (wall) 410.6 ☑
  posterobasal 410.6 ☑
  posteroinferior 410.3 ☑
  posterolateral 410.5 ☑
  previous, currently presenting no symptoms 412
  septal 410.8 ☑
  specified site NEC 410.8 ☑
  ST elevation (STEMI) 410.9 ☑
    anterior (wall) 410.1 ☑
    anterolateral (wall) 410.0 ☑
    inferior (wall) 410.4 ☑
    inferolateral (wall) 410.2 ☑

Infarct, infarction — *continued*
  myocardium, myocardial — *continued*
    ST elevation — *continued*
      inferoposterior wall 410.3 ☑
      lateral wall 410.5 ☑
      posterior (strictly) (true) (wall) 410.6 ☑
      specified site NEC 410.8 ☑
      subendocardial 410.7 ☑
      syphilitic 093.82
    non-ST elevation myocardial infarction (NSTEMI) 410.7 ☑
    nontransmural 410.7 ☑
  omentum 557.0
  ovary 620.8
  pancreas 577.8
  papillary muscle (*see also* Infarct, myocardium) 410.8 ☑
  parathyroid gland 252.8
  pituitary (gland) 253.8
  placenta (complicating pregnancy) 656.7 ☑
    affecting fetus or newborn 762.2
  pontine — *see* Infarct, brain
  posterior NEC (*see also* Infarct, myocardium) 410.6 ☑
  prostate 602.8
  pulmonary (artery) (hemorrhagic) (vein) 415.19
    with
      abortion — *see* Abortion, by type, with embolism
      ectopic pregnancy (*see also* categories 633.0–633.9) 639.6
      molar pregnancy (*see also* categories 630–632) 639.6
    following
      abortion 639.6
      ectopic or molar pregnancy 639.6
    iatrogenic 415.11
    in pregnancy, childbirth, or puerperium — *see* Embolism, obstetrical
    postoperative 415.11
  renal 593.81
    embolic or thrombotic 593.81
  retina, retinal 362.84
    with occlusion — *see* Occlusion, retina
  spinal (acute) (cord) (embolic) (nonembolic) 336.1
  spleen 289.59
    embolic or thrombotic 444.89
  subchorionic — *see* Infarct, placenta
  subendocardial (*see also* Infarct, myocardium) 410.7 ☑
  suprarenal (capsule) (gland) 255.4
  syncytium — *see* Infarct, placenta
  testis 608.83
  thrombotic (*see also* Thrombosis) 453.9
    artery, arterial — *see* Embolism
  thyroid (gland) 246.3
  ventricle (heart) (*see also* Infarct, myocardium) 410.9 ☑
Infecting — *see* condition
Infection, infected, infective (opportunistic) 136.9
  with lymphangitis — *see* Lymphangitis
  abortion — *see* Abortion, by type, with, sepsis
  abscess (skin) — *see* Abscess, by site
  Absidia 117.7
  Acanthocheilonema (perstans) 125.4
    streptocerca 125.6
  accessory sinus (chronic) (*see also* Sinusitis) 473.9
  Achorion — *see* Dermatophytosis
  Acremonium falciforme 117.4
  acromioclavicular (joint) 711.91
  actinobacillus
    lignieresii 027.8
    mallei 024

Infection, infected, infective — *continued*
  actinobacillus — *continued*
    muris 026.1
  actinomadura — *see* Actinomycosis
  Actinomyces (israelii) (*see also* Actinomycosis)
    muris-ratti 026.1
  Actinomycetales (actinomadura) (Actinomyces) (Nocardia) (Streptomyces) — *see* Actinomycosis
  actinomycotic NEC (*see also* Actinomycosis) 039.9
  adenoid (chronic) 474.01
    acute 463
    and tonsil (chronic) 474.02
      acute or subacute 463
  adenovirus NEC 079.0
    in diseases classified elsewhere — *see* category 079
    unspecified nature or site 079.0
  Aerobacter aerogenes NEC 041.85
    enteritis 008.2
  aerogenes capsulatus (*see also* Gangrene, gas) 040.0
  aertrycke (*see also* Infection, Salmonella) 003.9
  ajellomyces dermatitidis 116.0
  alimentary canal NEC (*see also* Enteritis, due to, by organism) 009.0
  Alleschera boydii 117.6
  Alternaria 118
  alveolus, alveolar (process) (pulpal origin) 522.4
  ameba, amebic (histolytica) (*see also* Amebiasis) 006.9
    acute 006.0
    chronic 006.1
    free-living 136.2
    hartmanni 007.8
    specified
      site NEC 006.8
      type NEC 007.8
  amniotic fluid or cavity 658.4 ☑
    affecting fetus or newborn 762.7
  anaerobes (cocci) (gram-negative) (gram-positive) (mixed) NEC 041.84
  anal canal 569.49
  Ancylostoma braziliense 126.2
  Angiostrongylus cantonensis 128.8
  anisakiasis 127.1
  Anisakis larva 127.1
  anthrax (*see also* Anthrax) 022.9
  antrum (chronic) (*see also* Sinusitis, maxillary) 473.0
  anus (papillae) (sphincter) 569.49
  arbor virus NEC 066.9
  arbovirus NEC 066.9
  argentophil-rod 027.0
  Ascaris lumbricoides 127.0
  ascomycetes 117.4
  Aspergillus (flavus) (fumigatus) (terreus) 117.3
  atypical
    acid-fast (bacilli) (*see also* Mycobacterium, atypical) 031.9
    mycobacteria (*see also* Mycobacterium, atypical) 031.9
  auditory meatus (circumscribed) (diffuse) (external) (*see also* Otitis, externa) 380.10
  auricle (ear) (*see also* Otitis, externa) 380.10
  axillary gland 683
  Babesiasis 088.82
  Babesiosis 088.82
  Bacillus NEC 041.89
    abortus 023.1
    anthracis (*see also* Anthrax) 022.9
    cereus (food poisoning) 005.89
    coli — *see* Infection, Escherichia coli
    coliform NEC 041.85
    Ducrey's (any location) 099.0
    Flexner's 004.1

Index to Diseases

Infection, infected, infective

Infection, infected, infective — *continued*
- Bacillus — *continued*
  - Friedländer's NEC 041.3
  - fusiformis 101
  - gas (gangrene) (*see also* Gangrene, gas) 040.0
  - mallei 024
  - melitensis 023.0
  - paratyphoid, paratyphosus 002.9
    - A 002.1
    - B 002.2
    - C 002.3
  - Schmorl's 040.3
  - Shiga 004.0
  - suipestifer (*see also* Infection, Salmonella) 003.9
  - swimming pool 031.1
  - typhosa 002.0
  - welchii (*see also* Gangrene, gas) 040.0
  - Whitmore's 025
- bacterial NEC 041.9
  - specified NEC 041.89
    - anaerobic NEC 041.84
    - gram-negative NEC 041.85
      - anaerobic NEC 041.84
- Bacterium
  - paratyphosum 002.9
    - A 002.1
    - B 002.2
    - C 002.3
  - typhosum 002.0
- Bacteroides (fragilis) (melaninogenicus) (oralis) NEC 041.82
- balantidium coli 007.0
- Bartholin's gland 616.89 ▲
- Basidiobolus 117.7
- Bedsonia 079.98
  - specified NEC 079.88
- bile duct 576.1
- bladder (*see also* Cystitis) 595.9
- Blastomyces, blastomycotic 116.0
  - brasiliensis 116.1
  - dermatitidis 116.0
  - European 117.5
  - loboi 116.2
  - North American 116.0
  - South American 116.1
- bleb •
  - postprocedural 379.60 •
    - stage 1 379.61 •
    - stage 2 379.62 •
    - stage 3 379.63 •
- blood stream — *see* Septicemia
- bone 730.9 ☑
  - specified — *see* Osteomyelitis
- Bordetella 033.9
  - bronchiseptica 033.8
  - parapertussis 033.1
  - pertussis 033.0
- Borrelia
  - bergdorfi 088.81
  - vincentii (mouth) (pharynx) (tonsil) 101
- brain (*see also* Encephalitis) 323.9
  - late effect — *see* category 326
  - membranes (*see also* Meningitis) 322.9
  - septic 324.0
    - late effect — *see* category 326
    - meninges (*see also* Meningitis) 320.9
- branchial cyst 744.42
- breast 611.0
  - puerperal, postpartum 675.2 ☑
    - with nipple 675.9 ☑
      - specified type NEC 675.8 ☑
    - nonpurulent 675.2 ☑
    - purulent 675.1 ☑
- bronchus (*see also* Bronchitis) 490
  - fungus NEC 117.9
- Brucella 023.9
  - abortus 023.1
  - canis 023.3
  - melitensis 023.0

Infection, infected, infective — *continued*
- Brucella — *continued*
  - mixed 023.8
  - suis 023.2
- Brugia (Wuchereria) malayi 125.1
- bursa — *see* Bursitis
- buttocks (skin) 686.9
- Candida (albicans) (tropicalis) (*see also* Candidiasis) 112.9
  - congenital 771.7
- Candiru 136.8
- Capillaria
  - hepatica 128.8
  - philippinensis 127.5
- cartilage 733.99
- cat liver fluke 121.0
- cellulitis — *see* Cellulitis, by site
- Cephalosporum falciforme 117.4
- Cercomonas hominis (intestinal) 007.3
- cerebrospinal (*see also* Meningitis) 322.9
  - late effect — *see* category 326
- cervical gland 683
- cervix (*see also* Cervicitis) 616.0
- cesarean section wound 674.3 ☑
- Chilomastix (intestinal) 007.8
- Chlamydia 079.98
  - specified NEC 079.88
- cholera (*see also* Cholera) 001.9
- chorionic plate 658.8 ☑
- Cladosporium
  - bantianum 117.8
  - carrionii 117.2
  - mansoni 111.1
  - trichoides 117.8
  - wernecki 111.1
- Clonorchis (sinensis) (liver) 121.1
- Clostridium (haemolyticum) (novyi) NEC 041.84
  - botulinum 005.1
  - histolyticum (*see also* Gangrene, gas) 040.0
  - oedematiens (*see also* Gangrene, gas) 040.0
  - perfringens 041.83
    - due to food 005.2
  - septicum (*see also* Gangrene, gas) 040.0
  - sordellii (*see also* Gangrene, gas) 040.0
  - welchii (*see also* Gangrene, gas) 040.0
    - due to food 005.2
- Coccidioides (immitis) (*see also* Coccidioidomycosis) 114.9
- coccus NEC 041.89
- colon (*see also* Enteritis, due to, by organism) 009.0
  - bacillus — *see* Infection, Escherichia coli
- colostomy or enterostomy 569.61
- common duct 576.1
- complicating pregnancy, childbirth, or puerperium NEC 647.9 ☑
  - affecting fetus or newborn 760.2
- Condiobolus 117.7
- congenital NEC 771.89
  - Candida albicans 771.7
  - chronic 771.2
  - cytomegalovirus 771.1
  - hepatitis, viral 771.2
  - herpes simplex 771.2
  - listeriosis 771.2
  - malaria 771.2
  - poliomyelitis 771.2
  - rubella 771.0
  - toxoplasmosis 771.2
  - tuberculosis 771.2
  - urinary (tract) 771.82
  - vaccinia 771.2
- coronavirus 079.89
  - SARS-associated 079.82
- corpus luteum (*see also* Salpingo-oophoritis) 614.2

Infection, infected, infective — *continued*
- Corynebacterium diphtheriae — *see* Diphtheria
- Coxsackie (*see also* Coxsackie) 079.2
  - endocardium 074.22
  - heart NEC 074.20
  - in diseases classified elsewhere — *see* category 079 ☑
  - meninges 047.0
  - myocardium 074.23
  - pericardium 074.21
  - pharynx 074.0
  - specified disease NEC 074.8
  - unspecified nature or site 079.2
- Cryptococcus neoformans 117.5
- Cryptosporidia 007.4
- Cunninghamella 117.7
- cyst — *see* Cyst
- Cysticercus cellulosae 123.1
- cytomegalovirus 078.5
  - congenital 771.1
- dental (pulpal origin) 522.4
- deuteromycetes 117.4
- Dicrocoelium dendriticum 121.8
- Dipetalonema (perstans) 125.4
  - streptocerca 125.6
- diphtherial — *see* Diphtheria
- Diphyllobothrium (adult) (latum) (pacificum) 123.4
  - larval 123.5
- Diplogonoporus (grandis) 123.8
- Dipylidium (caninum) 123.8
- Dirofilaria 125.6
- dog tapeworm 123.8
- Dracunculus medinensis 125.7
- Dreschlera 118
  - hawaiiensis 117.8
- Ducrey's bacillus (any site) 099.0
- due to or resulting from
  - device, implant, or graft (any) (presence of) — *see* Complications, infection and inflammation, due to (presence of) any device, implant, or graft classified to 996.0–996.5 NEC
  - injection, inoculation, infusion, transfusion, or vaccination (prophylactic) (therapeutic) 999.3
  - injury NEC — *see* Wound, open, by site, complicated
  - surgery 998.59
- duodenum 535.6 ☑
- ear (*see also* Otitis)
  - external (*see also* Otitis, externa) 380.10
  - inner (*see also* Labyrinthitis) 386.30
  - middle — *see* Otitis, media
- Eaton's agent NEC 041.81
- Eberthella typhosa 002.0
- Ebola 078.89
- echinococcosis 122.9
- Echinococcus (*see also* Echinococcus) 122.9
- Echinostoma 121.8
- ECHO virus 079.1
  - in diseases classified elsewhere — *see* category 079 ☑
  - unspecified nature or site 079.1
- Ehrlichiosis 082.40
  - chaffeensis 082.41
  - specified type NEC 082.49
- Endamoeba — *see* Infection, ameba
- endocardium (*see also* Endocarditis) 421.0
- endocervix (*see also* Cervicitis) 616.0
- Entamoeba — *see* Infection, ameba
- enteric (*see also* Enteritis, due to, by organism) 009.0
- Enterobacter aerogenes NEC 041.85
- Enterobacter sakazakii 041.85
- Enterobius vermicularis 127.4
- enterococcus NEC 041.04

Infection, infected, infective — *continued*
- enterovirus NEC 079.89
  - central nervous system NEC 048
  - enteritis 008.67
  - meningitis 047.9
- Entomophthora 117.7
- Epidermophyton — *see* Dermatophytosis
- epidermophytosis — *see* Dermatophytosis
- episiotomy 674.3 ☑
- Epstein-Barr virus 075
  - chronic 780.79 [139.8]
- erysipeloid 027.1
- Erysipelothrix (insidiosa) (rhusiopathiae) 027.1
- erythema infectiosum 057.0
- Escherichia coli NEC 041.4
  - enteritis — *see* Enteritis, E. coli
  - generalized 038.42
  - intestinal — *see* Enteritis, E. coli
- esophagostomy 530.86
- ethmoidal (chronic) (sinus) (*see also* Sinusitis, ethmoidal) 473.2
- Eubacterium 041.84
- Eustachian tube (ear) 381.50
  - acute 381.51
  - chronic 381.52
- exanthema subitum 057.8
- external auditory canal (meatus) (*see also* Otitis, externa) 380.10
- eye NEC 360.00
- eyelid 373.9
  - specified NEC 373.8
- fallopian tube (*see also* Salpingo-oophoritis) 614.2
- fascia 728.89
- Fasciola
  - gigantica 121.3
  - hepatica 121.3
- Fasciolopsis (buski) 121.4
- fetus (intra-amniotic) — *see* Infection, congenital
- filarial — *see* Infestation, filarial
- finger (skin) 686.9
  - abscess (with lymphangitis) 681.00
    - pulp 681.01
  - cellulitis (with lymphangitis) 681.00
  - distal closed space (with lymphangitis) 681.00
  - nail 681.02
    - fungus 110.1
- fish tapeworm 123.4
  - larval 123.5
- flagellate, intestinal 007.9
- fluke — *see* Infestation, fluke
- focal
  - teeth (pulpal origin) 522.4
  - tonsils 474.00
    - and adenoids 474.02
- Fonsecaea
  - compactum 117.2
  - pedrosoi 117.2
- food (*see also* Poisoning, food) 005.9
- foot (skin) 686.9
  - fungus 110.4
- Francisella tularensis (*see also* Tularemia) 021.9
- frontal sinus (chronic) (*see also* Sinusitis, frontal) 473.1
- fungus NEC 117.9
  - beard 110.0
  - body 110.5
  - dermatiacious NEC 117.8
  - foot 110.4
  - groin 110.3
  - hand 110.2
  - nail 110.1
  - pathogenic to compromised host only 118
  - perianal (area) 110.3
  - scalp 110.0
  - scrotum 110.8
  - skin 111.9

Infection, infected, infective

Infection, infected, infective — *continued*
- fungus — *continued*
  - skin — *continued*
    - foot 110.4
    - hand 110.2
    - toenails 110.1
    - trachea 117.9
- Fusarium 118
- Fusobacterium 041.84
- gallbladder (*see also* Cholecystitis, acute) 575.0
- Gardnerella vaginalis 041.89
- gas bacillus (*see also* Gas, gangrene) 040.0
- gastric (*see also* Gastritis) 535.5 ☑
- Gastrodiscoides hominis 121.8
- gastroenteric (*see also* Enteritis, due to, by organism) 009.0
- gastrointestinal (*see also* Enteritis, due to, by organism) 009.0
- gastrostomy 536.41
- generalized NEC (*see also* Septicemia) 038.9
- genital organ or tract NEC
  - female 614.9
    - with
      - abortion — *see* Abortion, by type, with sepsis
      - ectopic pregnancy (*see also* categories 633.0–633.9) 639.0
      - molar pregnancy (*see also* categories 630–632) 639.0
    - complicating pregnancy 646.6 ☑
      - affecting fetus or newborn 760.8
    - following
      - abortion 639.0
      - ectopic or molar pregnancy 639.0
    - puerperal, postpartum, childbirth 670.0 ☑
      - minor or localized 646.6 ☑
        - affecting fetus or newborn 760.8
  - male 608.4
- genitourinary tract NEC 599.0
- Ghon tubercle, primary (*see also* Tuberculosis) 010.0 ☑
- Giardia lamblia 007.1
- gingival (chronic) 523.10 ▲
  - acute 523.00 ▲
  - Vincent's 101
- glanders 024
- Glenosporopsis amazonica 116.2
- Gnathostoma spinigerum 128.1
- Gongylonema 125.6
- gonococcal NEC (*see also* Gonococcus) 098.0
- gram-negative bacilli NEC 041.85
  - anaerobic 041.84
- guinea worm 125.7
- gum (*see also* Infection, gingival) 523.10 ▲
- Hantavirus 079.81
- heart 429.89
- Helicobacter pylori (H. pylori) 041.86
- helminths NEC 128.9
  - intestinal 127.9
    - mixed (types classifiable to more than one category in 120.0–127.7) 127.8
    - specified type NEC 127.7
  - specified type NEC 128.8
- Hemophilus influenzae NEC 041.5
  - generalized 038.41
- herpes (simplex) (*see also* Herpes, simplex) 054.9
  - congenital 771.2
  - zoster (*see also* Herpes, zoster) 053.9
    - eye NEC 053.29
- Heterophyes heterophyes 121.6

Infection, infected, infective — *continued*
- Histoplasma (*see also* Histoplasmosis) 115.90
  - capsulatum (*see also* Histoplasmosis, American) 115.00
  - duboisii (*see also* Histoplasmosis, African) 115.10
- HIV V08
  - with symptoms, symptomatic 042
- hookworm (*see also* Ancylostomiasis) 126.9
- human immunodeficiency virus V08
  - with symptoms, symptomatic 042
- human papillomavirus 079.4
- hydrocele 603.1
- hydronephrosis 591
- Hymenolepis 123.6
- hypopharynx 478.29
- inguinal glands 683
  - due to soft chancre 099.0
- intestine, intestinal (*see also* Enteritis, due to, by organism) 009.0
- intrauterine (*see also* Endometritis) 615.9
  - complicating delivery 646.6 ☑
- isospora belli or hominis 007.2
- Japanese B encephalitis 062.0
- jaw (bone) (acute) (chronic) (lower) (subacute) (upper) 526.4
- joint — *see* Arthritis, infectious or infective
- kidney (cortex) (hematogenous) 590.9
  - with
    - abortion — *see* Abortion, by type, with urinary tract infection
    - calculus 592.0
    - ectopic pregnancy (*see also* categories 633.0–633.9) 639.8
    - molar pregnancy (*see also* categories 630–632) 639.8
  - complicating pregnancy or puerperium 646.6 ☑
    - affecting fetus or newborn 760.1
  - following
    - abortion 639.8
    - ectopic or molar pregnancy 639.8
  - pelvis and ureter 590.3
- Klebsiella pneumoniae NEC 041.3
- knee (skin) NEC 686.9
- joint — *see* Arthritis, infectious
- Koch's (*see also* Tuberculosis, pulmonary) 011.9 ☑
- labia (majora) (minora) (*see also* Vulvitis) 616.10
- lacrimal
  - gland (*see also* Dacryoadenitis) 375.00
  - passages (duct) (sac) (*see also* Dacryocystitis) 375.30
- larynx NEC 478.79
- leg (skin) NEC 686.9
- Leishmania (*see also* Leishmaniasis) 085.9
  - braziliensis 085.5
  - donovani 085.0
  - ethiopica 085.3
  - furunculosa 085.1
  - infantum 085.0
  - mexicana 085.4
  - tropica (minor) 085.1
    - major 085.2
- Leptosphaeria senegalensis 117.4
- leptospira (*see also* Leptospirosis) 100.9
  - Australis 100.89
  - Bataviae 100.89
  - pyrogenes 100.89
  - specified type NEC 100.89
- leptospirochetal NEC (*see also* Leptospirosis) 100.9
- Leptothrix — *see* Actinomycosis

Infection, infected, infective — *continued*
- Listeria monocytogenes (listeriosis) 027.0
  - congenital 771.2
- liver fluke — *see* Infestation, fluke, liver
- Loa loa 125.2
  - eyelid 125.2 [373.6]
- Loboa loboi 116.2
- local, skin (staphylococcal) (streptococcal) NEC 686.9
  - abscess — *see* Abscess, by site
  - cellulitis — *see* Cellulitis, by site
  - ulcer (*see also* Ulcer, skin) 707.9
- Loefflerella
  - mallei 024
  - whitmori 025
- lung 518.89
  - atypical Mycobacterium 031.0
  - tuberculous (*see also* Tuberculosis, pulmonary) 011.9 ☑
  - basilar 518.89
  - chronic 518.89
  - fungus NEC 117.9
  - spirochetal 104.8
  - virus — *see* Pneumonia, virus
- lymph gland (axillary) (cervical) (inguinal) 683
  - mesenteric 289.2
- lymphoid tissue, base of tongue or posterior pharynx, NEC 474.00
- madurella
  - grisea 117.4
  - mycetomii 117.4
- major
  - with
    - abortion — *see* Abortion, by type, with sepsis
    - ectopic pregnancy (*see also* categories 633.0–633.9) 639.0
    - molar pregnancy (*see also* categories 630–632) 639.0
  - following
    - abortion 639.0
    - ectopic or molar pregnancy 639.0
  - puerperal, postpartum, childbirth 670.0 ☑
- Malassezia furfur 111.0
- Malleomyces
  - mallei 024
  - pseudomallei 025
- mammary gland 611.0
  - puerperal, postpartum 675.2 ☑
- Mansonella (ozzardi) 125.5
- mastoid (suppurative) — *see* Mastoiditis
- maxilla, maxillary 526.4
  - sinus (chronic) (*see also* Sinusitis, maxillary) 473.0
- mediastinum 519.2
- medina 125.7
- meibomian
  - cyst 373.12
  - gland 373.12
- melioidosis 025
- meninges (*see also* Meningitis) 320.9
- meningococcal (*see also* condition) 036.9
  - brain 036.1
  - cerebrospinal 036.0
  - endocardium 036.42
  - generalized 036.2
  - meninges 036.0
  - meningococcemia 036.2
  - specified site NEC 036.89
- mesenteric lymph nodes or glands NEC 289.2
- Metagonimus 121.5
- metatarsophalangeal 711.97
- microorganism resistant to drugs — *see* Resistance (to), drugs by microorganisms
- Microsporidia 136.8

Infection, infected, infective — *continued*
- microsporum, microsporic — *see* Dermatophytosis
- Mima polymorpha NEC 041.85
- mixed flora NEC 041.89
- Monilia (*see also* Candidiasis) 112.9
  - neonatal 771.7
- monkeypox 057.8
- Monosporium apiospermum 117.6
- mouth (focus) NEC 528.9
  - parasitic 136.9
- Mucor 117.7
- muscle NEC 728.89
- mycelium NEC 117.9
- mycetoma
  - actinomycotic NEC (*see also* Actinomycosis) 039.9
  - mycotic NEC 117.4
- Mycobacterium, mycobacterial (*see also* Mycobacterium) 031.9
- Mycoplasma NEC 041.81
- mycotic NEC 117.9
  - pathogenic to compromised host only 118
  - skin NEC 111.9
  - systemic 117.9
- myocardium NEC 422.90
- nail (chronic) (with lymphangitis) 681.9
  - finger 681.02
    - fungus 110.1
  - ingrowing 703.0
  - toe 681.11
    - fungus 110.1
- nasal sinus (chronic) (*see also* Sinusitis) 473.9
- nasopharynx (chronic) 478.29
  - acute 460
- navel 686.9
  - newborn 771.4
- Neisserian — *see* Gonococcus
- Neotestudina rosatii 117.4
- newborn, generalized 771.89
- nipple 611.0
  - puerperal, postpartum 675.0 ☑
    - with breast 675.9 ☑
    - specified type NEC 675.8 ☑
- Nocardia — *see* Actinomycosis
- nose 478.19 ▲
- nostril 478.19 ▲
- obstetrical surgical wound 674.3 ☑
- Oesophagostomum (apiostomum) 127.7
- Oestrus ovis 134.0
- Oidium albicans (*see also* Candidiasis) 112.9
- Onchocerca (volvulus) 125.3
  - eye 125.3 [360.13]
  - eyelid 125.3 [373.6]
- operation wound 998.59
- Opisthorchis (felineus) (tenuicollis) (viverrini) 121.0
- orbit 376.00
  - chronic 376.10
- ovary (*see also* Salpingo-oophoritis) 614.2
- Oxyuris vermicularis 127.4
- pancreas 577.0
- Paracoccidioides brasiliensis 116.1
- Paragonimus (westermani) 121.2
- parainfluenza virus 079.89
- parameningococcus NEC 036.9
  - with meningitis 036.0
- parasitic NEC 136.9
- paratyphoid 002.9
  - type A 002.1
  - type B 002.2
  - type C 002.3
- paraurethral ducts 597.89
- parotid gland 527.2
- Pasteurella NEC 027.2
  - multocida (cat-bite) (dog-bite) 027.2
  - pestis (*see also* Plague) 020.9
  - pseudotuberculosis 027.2
  - septica (cat-bite) (dog-bite) 027.2

Index to Diseases

Infection, infected, infective

Infection, infected, infective — *continued*
- Pasteurella — *continued*
  - tularensis (*see also* Tularemia) 021.9
- pelvic, female (*see also* Disease, pelvis, inflammatory) 614.9
- penis (glans) (retention) NEC 607.2
  - herpetic 054.13
- Peptococcus 041.84
- Peptostreptococcus 041.84
- periapical (pulpal origin) 522.4
- peridental 523.30 ▲
- perineal wound (obstetrical) 674.3 ☑
- periodontal 523.31 ▲
- periorbital 376.00
  - chronic 376.10
- perirectal 569.49
- perirenal (*see also* Infection, kidney) 590.9
- peritoneal (*see also* Peritonitis) 567.9
- periureteral 593.89
- periurethral 597.89
- Petriellidium boydii 117.6
- pharynx 478.29
  - Coxsackie virus 074.0
  - phlegmonous 462
  - posterior, lymphoid 474.00
- Phialophora
  - gougerotii 117.8
  - jeanselmei 117.8
  - verrucosa 117.2
- Piedraia hortai 111.3
- pinna, acute 380.11
- pinta 103.9
  - intermediate 103.1
  - late 103.2
  - mixed 103.3
  - primary 103.0
- pinworm 127.4
- pityrosporum furfur 111.0
- pleuropneumonia-like organisms NEC (PPLO) 041.81
- pneumococcal NEC 041.2
  - generalized (purulent) 038.2
- Pneumococcus NEC 041.2
- postoperative wound 998.59
- posttraumatic NEC 958.3
- postvaccinal 999.3
- prepuce NEC 607.1
- Proprionibacterium 041.84
- prostate (capsule) (*see also* Prostatitis) 601.9
- Proteus (mirabilis) (morganii) (vulgaris) NEC 041.6
  - enteritis 008.3
- protozoal NEC 136.8
  - intestinal NEC 007.9
- Pseudomonas NEC 041.7
  - mallei 024
  - pneumonia 482.1
  - pseudomallei 025
- psittacosis 073.9
- puerperal, postpartum (major) 670.0 ☑
  - minor 646.6 ☑
- pulmonary — *see* Infection, lung
- purulent — *see* Abscess
- putrid, generalized — *see* Septicemia
- pyemic — *see* Septicemia
- Pyrenochaeta romeroi 117.4
- Q fever 083.0
- rabies 071
- rectum (sphincter) 569.49
- renal (*see also* Infection, kidney) 590.9
  - pelvis and ureter 590.3
- resistant to drugs — *see* Resistance (to), drugs by microorganisms
- respiratory 519.8
  - chronic 519.8
  - influenzal (acute) (upper) 487.1
  - lung 518.89
  - rhinovirus 460
  - syncytial virus 079.6
  - upper (acute) (infectious) NEC 465.9

Infection, infected, infective — *continued*
- respiratory — *continued*
  - upper — *continued*
    - with flu, grippe, or influenza 487.1
    - influenzal 487.1
    - multiple sites NEC 465.8
    - streptococcal 034.0
    - viral NEC 465.9
- respiratory syncytial virus (RSV) 079.6
- resulting from presence of shunt or other internal prosthetic device — *see* Complications, infection and inflammation, due to (presence of) any device, implant, or graft classified to 996.0–996.5 NEC
- retroperitoneal 567.39
- retrovirus 079.50
  - human immunodeficiency virus type 2 [HIV2] 079.53
  - human T-cell lymphotrophic virus type I [HTLV-I] 079.51
  - human T-cell lymphotrophic virus type II [HTLV-II] 079.52
  - specified NEC 079.59
- Rhinocladium 117.1
- Rhinosporidium — *see beri* 117.0
- rhinovirus
  - in diseases classified elsewhere — *see* category 079 ☑
  - unspecified nature or site 079.3
- Rhizopus 117.7
- rickettsial 083.9
- rickettsialpox 083.2
- rubella (*see also* Rubella) 056.9
  - congenital 771.0
- Saccharomyces (*see also* Candidiasis) 112.9
- Saksenaea 117.7
- salivary duct or gland (any) 527.2
- Salmonella (aertrycke) (callinarum) (choleraesuis) (enteritidis) (suipestifer) (typhimurium) 003.9
  - with
    - arthritis 003.23
    - gastroenteritis 003.0
    - localized infection 003.20
      - specified type NEC 003.29
    - meningitis 003.21
    - osteomyelitis 003.24
    - pneumonia 003.22
    - septicemia 003.1
    - specified manifestation NEC 003.8
  - due to food (poisoning) (any serotype) (*see also* Poisoning, food, due to, Salmonella)
  - hirschfeldii 002.3
  - localized 003.20
    - specified type NEC 003.29
  - paratyphi 002.9
    - A 002.1
    - B 002.2
    - C 002.3
  - schottmuelleri 002.2
  - specified type NEC 003.8
  - typhi 002.0
  - typhosa 002.0
- saprophytic 136.8
- Sarcocystis, lindemanni 136.5
- SARS-associated coronavirus 079.82
- scabies 133.0
- Schistosoma — *see* Infestation, Schistosoma
- Schmorl's bacillus 040.3
- scratch or other superficial injury — *see* Injury, superficial, by site
- scrotum (acute) NEC 608.4
- secondary, burn or open wound (dislocation) (fracture) 958.3
- seminal vesicle (*see also* Vesiculitis) 608.0

Infection, infected, infective — *continued*
- septic
  - generalized — *see* Septicemia
  - localized, skin (*see also* Abscess) 682.9
- septicemic — *see* Septicemia
- seroma 998.51
- Serratia (marcescens) 041.85
  - generalized 038.44
- sheep liver fluke 121.3
- Shigella 004.9
  - boydii 004.2
  - dysenteriae 004.0
  - flexneri 004.1
  - group
    - A 004.0
    - B 004.1
    - C 004.2
    - D 004.3
  - Schmitz (-Stutzer) 004.0
  - schmitzii 004.0
  - Shiga 004.0
  - sonnei 004.3
  - specified type NEC 004.8
- Sin Nombre virus 079.81
- sinus (*see also* Sinusitis) 473.9
  - pilonidal 685.1
    - with abscess 685.0
- skin NEC 686.9
- Skene's duct or gland (*see also* Urethritis) 597.89
- skin (local) (staphylococcal) (streptococcal) NEC 686.9
  - abscess — *see* Abscess, by site
  - cellulitis — *see* Cellulitis, by site
  - due to fungus 111.9
    - specified type NEC 111.8
  - mycotic 111.9
    - specified type NEC 111.8
  - ulcer (*see also* Ulcer, skin) 707.9
- slow virus 046.9
  - specified condition NEC 046.8
- Sparganum (mansoni) (proliferum) 123.5
- spermatic cord NEC 608.4
- sphenoidal (chronic) (sinus) (*see also* Sinusitis, sphenoidal) 473.9
- Spherophorus necrophorus 040.3
- spinal cord NEC (*see also* Encephalitis) 323.9
  - abscess 324.1
    - late effect — *see* category 326
  - late effect — *see* category 326
  - meninges — *see* Meningitis
  - streptococcal 320.2
- Spirillum
  - minus or minor 026.0
  - morsus muris 026.0
  - obermeieri 087.0
- spirochetal NEC 104.9
  - lung 104.8
  - specified nature or site NEC 104.8
- spleen 289.59
- Sporothrix schenckii 117.1
- Sporotrichum (schenckii) 117.1
- Sporozoa 136.8
- staphylococcal NEC 041.10
  - aureus 041.11
  - food poisoning 005.0
  - generalized (purulent) 038.10
    - aureus 038.11
    - specified organism NEC 038.19
  - pneumonia 482.40
    - aureus 482.41
    - specified type NEC 482.49
  - septicemia 038.10
    - aureus 038.11
    - specified organism NEC 038.19
  - specified NEC 041.19
- steatoma 706.2
- Stellantchasmus falcatus 121.6
- Streptobacillus moniliformis 026.1
- streptococcal NEC 041.00
  - generalized (purulent) 038.0

Infection, infected, infective — *continued*
- streptococcal — *continued*
  - Group
    - A 041.01
    - B 041.02
    - C 041.03
    - D [enterococcus] 041.04
    - G 041.05
  - pneumonia — *see* Pneumonia, streptococcal
  - septicemia 038.0
  - sore throat 034.0
  - specified NEC 041.09
- Streptomyces — *see* Actinomycosis
- streptotrichosis — *see* Actinomycosis
- Strongyloides (stercoralis) 127.2
- stump (amputation) (posttraumatic) (surgical) 997.62
  - traumatic — *see* Amputation, traumatic, by site, complicated
- subcutaneous tissue, local NEC 686.9
- submaxillary region 528.9
- suipestifer (*see also* Infection, Salmonella) 003.9
- swimming pool bacillus 031.1
- syphilitic — *see* Syphilis
  - systemic — *see* Septicemia
- Taenia — *see* Infestation, Taenia
- Taeniarhynchus saginatus 123.2
- tapeworm — *see* Infestation, tapeworm
- tendon (sheath) 727.89
- Ternidens diminutus 127.7
- testis (*see also* Orchitis) 604.90
- thigh (skin) 686.9
- threadworm 127.4
- throat 478.29
  - pneumococcal 462
  - staphylococcal 462
  - streptococcal 034.0
  - viral NEC (*see also* Pharyngitis) 462
- thumb (skin) 686.9
  - abscess (with lymphangitis) 681.00
    - pulp 681.01
  - cellulitis (with lymphangitis) 681.00
  - nail 681.02
- thyroglossal duct 529.8
- toe (skin) 686.9
  - abscess (with lymphangitis) 681.10
  - cellulitis (with lymphangitis) 681.10
  - nail 681.11
    - fungus 110.1
- tongue NEC 529.0
  - parasitic 112.0
- tonsil (faucial) (lingual) (pharyngeal) 474.00
  - acute or subacute 463
  - and adenoid 474.02
  - tag 474.00
- tooth, teeth 522.4
  - periapical (pulpal origin) 522.4
  - peridental 523.30 ▲
  - periodontal 523.31 ▲
  - pulp 522.0
  - socket 526.5
- Torula histolytica 117.5
- Toxocara (cani) (cati) (felis) 128.0
- Toxoplasma gondii (*see also* Toxoplasmosis) 130.9
- trachea, chronic 491.8
  - fungus 117.9
- traumatic NEC 958.3
- trematode NEC 121.9
- trench fever 083.1
- Treponema
  - denticola 041.84
  - macrodenticum 041.84
  - pallidum (*see also* Syphilis) 097.9
- Trichinella (spiralis) 124
- Trichomonas 131.9
  - bladder 131.09

Infection, infected, infective

Infection, infected, infective — *continued*
- Trichomonas — *continued*
  - cervix 131.09
  - hominis 007.3
  - intestine 007.3
  - prostate 131.03
  - specified site NEC 131.8
  - urethra 131.02
  - urogenitalis 131.00
  - vagina 131.01
  - vulva 131.01
- Trichophyton, trichophytid — *see* Dermatophytosis
- Trichosporon (beigelii) cutaneum 111.2
- Trichostrongylus 127.6
- Trichuris (trichiuria) 127.3
- Trombicula (irritans) 133.8
- Trypanosoma (*see also* Trypanosomiasis) 086.9
  - cruzi 086.2
- tubal (*see also* Salpingo-oophoritis) 614.2
- tuberculous NEC (*see also* Tuberculosis) 011.9 ☑
- tubo-ovarian (*see also* Salpingo-oophoritis) 614.2
- tunica vaginalis 608.4
- tympanic membrane — *see* Myringitis
- typhoid (abortive) (ambulant) (bacillus) 002.0
- typhus 081.9
  - flea-borne (endemic) 081.0
  - louse-borne (epidemic) 080
  - mite-borne 081.2
  - recrudescent 081.1
  - tick-borne 082.9
    - African 082.1
    - North Asian 082.2
- umbilicus (septic) 686.9
  - newborn NEC 771.4
- ureter 593.89
- urethra (*see also* Urethritis) 597.80
- urinary (tract) NEC 599.0
  - with
    - abortion — *see* Abortion, by type, with urinary tract infection
    - ectopic pregnancy (*see also* categories 633.0–633.9) 639.8
    - molar pregnancy (*see also* categories 630–632) 639.8
  - candidal 112.2
  - complicating pregnancy, childbirth, or puerperium 646.6 ☑
    - affecting fetus or newborn 760.1
  - asymptomatic 646.5 ☑
    - affecting fetus or newborn 760.1
  - diplococcal (acute) 098.0
    - chronic 098.2
  - due to Trichomonas (vaginalis) 131.00
  - following
    - abortion 639.8
    - ectopic or molar pregnancy 639.8
  - gonococcal (acute) 098.0
    - chronic or duration of 2 months or over 098.2
  - newborn 771.82
  - trichomonal 131.00
  - tuberculous (*see also* Tuberculosis) 016.3 ☑
  - uterus, uterine (*see also* Endometritis) 615.9
  - utriculus masculinus NEC 597.89
  - vaccination 999.3
  - vagina (granulation tissue) (wall) (*see also* Vaginitis) 616.10
  - varicella 052.9
  - varicose veins — *see* Varicose, veins
  - variola 050.9

Infection, infected, infective — *continued*
- urinary — *continued*
  - variola — *continued*
    - major 050.0
    - minor 050.1
- vas deferens NEC 608.4
- Veillonella 041.84
- verumontanum 597.89
- vesical (*see also* Cystitis) 595.9
- Vibrio
  - cholerae 001.0
    - El Tor 001.1
  - parahaemolyticus (food poisoning) 005.4
  - vulnificus 041.85
- Vincent's (gums) (mouth) (tonsil) 101
- virus, viral 079.99
  - adenovirus
    - in diseases classified elsewhere — *see* category 079 ☑
    - unspecified nature or site 079.0
  - central nervous system NEC 049.9
    - enterovirus 048
      - meningitis 047.9
      - specified type NEC 047.8
    - slow virus 046.9
    - specified condition NEC 046.8
  - chest 519.8
  - conjunctivitis 077.99
    - specified type NEC 077.8
  - coronavirus 079.89
    - SARS-associated 079.82
  - Coxsackie (*see also* Infection, Coxsackie) 079.2
  - Ebola 065.8
  - ECHO
    - in diseases classified elsewhere — *see* category 079 ☑
    - unspecified nature or site 079.1
  - encephalitis 049.9
    - arthropod-borne NEC 064
    - tick-borne 063.9
    - specified type NEC 063.8
  - enteritis NEC (*see also* Enteritis, viral) 008.8
  - exanthem NEC 057.9
  - Hantavirus 079.81
  - human papilloma 079.4
  - in diseases classified elsewhere — *see* category 079 ☑
  - intestine (*see also* Enteritis, viral) 008.8
  - lung — *see* Pneumonia, viral
  - respiratory syncytial (RSV) 079.6
  - retrovirus 079.50
  - rhinovirus
    - in diseases classified elsewhere — *see* category 079 ☑
    - unspecified nature or site 079.3
  - salivary gland disease 078.5
  - slow 046.9
    - specified condition NEC 046.8
  - specified type NEC 079.89
    - in diseases classified elsewhere — *see* category 079 ☑
  - unspecified nature or site 079.99
  - warts NEC 078.10
- vulva (*see also* Vulvitis) 616.10
- whipworm 127.3
- Whitmore's bacillus 025
- wound (local) (posttraumatic) NEC 958.3
  - with
    - dislocation — *see* Dislocation, by site, open
    - fracture — *see* Fracture, by site, open
    - open wound — *see* Wound, open, by site, complicated
  - postoperative 998.59
  - surgical 998.59
- Wuchereria 125.0
  - bancrofti 125.0
  - malayi 125.1

Infection, infected, infective — *continued*
- yaws — *see* Yaws
- yeast (*see also* Candidiasis) 112.9
- yellow fever (*see also* Fever, yellow) 060.9
- Yersinia pestis (*see also* Plague) 020.9
- Zeis' gland 373.12
- zoonotic bacterial NEC 027.9
- Zopfia senegalensis 117.4

Infective, infectious — *see* condition

Inferiority complex 301.9
- constitutional psychopathic 301.9

Infertility
- female 628.9
  - age related 628.8
  - associated with
    - adhesions, peritubal 614.6 [628.2]
    - anomaly
      - cervical mucus 628.4
      - congenital
        - cervix 628.4
        - fallopian tube 628.2
        - uterus 628.3
        - vagina 628.4
    - anovulation 628.0
    - dysmucorrhea 628.4
    - endometritis, tuberculous (*see also* Tuberculosis) 016.7 ☑ [628.3]
    - Stein-Leventhal syndrome 256.4 [628.0]
  - due to
    - adiposogenital dystrophy 253.8 [628.1]
    - anterior pituitary disorder NEC 253.4 [628.1]
      - hyperfunction 253.1 [628.1]
    - cervical anomaly 628.4
    - fallopian tube anomaly 628.2
    - ovarian failure 256.39 [628.0]
    - Stein-Leventhal syndrome 256.4 [628.0]
    - uterine anomaly 628.3
    - vaginal anomaly 628.4
  - nonimplantation 628.3
  - origin
    - cervical 628.4
    - pituitary-hypothalamus NEC 253.8 [628.1]
      - anterior pituitary NEC 253.4 [628.1]
        - hyperfunction NEC 253.1 [628.1]
      - dwarfism 253.3 [628.1]
      - panhypopituitarism 253.2 [628.1]
    - specified NEC 628.8
    - tubal (block) (occlusion) (stenosis) 628.2
      - adhesions 614.6 [628.2]
    - uterine 628.3
    - vaginal 628.4
  - previous, requiring supervision of pregnancy V23.0
- male 606.9
  - absolute 606.0
  - due to
    - azoospermia 606.0
    - drug therapy 606.8
    - extratesticular cause NEC 606.8
    - germinal cell
      - aplasia 606.0
      - desquamation 606.1
    - hypospermatogenesis 606.1
    - infection 606.8
    - obstruction, afferent ducts 606.8
    - oligospermia 606.1
    - radiation 606.8
    - spermatogenic arrest (complete) 606.0
      - incomplete 606.1
    - systemic disease 606.8

Infestation 134.9

Infestation — *continued*
- Acanthocheilonema (perstans) 125.4
  - streptocerca 125.6
- Acariasis 133.9
  - demodex folliculorum 133.8
  - Sarcoptes scabiei 133.0
  - trombiculae 133.8
- Agamofilaria streptocerca 125.6
- Ancylostoma, Ankylostoma 126.9
  - americanum 126.1
  - braziliense 126.2
  - canium 126.8
  - ceylanicum 126.3
  - duodenale 126.0
  - new world 126.1
  - old world 126.0
- Angiostrongylus cantonensis 128.8
- anisakiasis 127.1
- Anisakis larva 127.1
- arthropod NEC 134.1
- Ascaris lumbricoides 127.0
- Bacillus fusiformis 101
- Balantidium coli 007.0
- beef tapeworm 123.2
- Bothriocephalus (latus) 123.4
  - larval 123.5
- broad tapeworm 123.4
  - larval 123.5
- Brugia malayi 125.1
- Candiru 136.8
- Capillaria
  - hepatica 128.8
  - philippinensis 127.5
- cat liver fluke 121.0
- Cercomonas hominis (intestinal) 007.3
- cestodes 123.9
  - specified type NEC 123.8
- chigger 133.8
- chigoe 134.1
- Chilomastix 007.8
- Clonorchis (sinensis) (liver) 121.1
- coccidia 007.2
- complicating pregnancy, childbirth, or puerperium 647.9 ☑
  - affecting fetus or newborn 760.8
- Cysticercus cellulosae 123.1
- Demodex folliculorum 133.8
- Dermatobia (hominis) 134.0
- Dibothriocephalus (latus) 123.4
  - larval 123.5
- Dicrocoelium dendriticum 121.8
- Diphyllobothrium (adult) (intestinal) (latum) (pacificum) 123.4
  - larval 123.5
- Diplogonoporus (grandis) 123.8
- Dipylidium (caninum) 123.8
- Distoma hepaticum 121.3
- dog tapeworm 123.8
- Dracunculus medinensis 125.7
- dragon worm 125.7
- dwarf tapeworm 123.6
- Echinococcus (*see also* Echinococcus) 122.9
- Echinostoma ilocanum 121.8
- Embadomonas 007.8
- Endamoeba (histolytica) — *see* Infection, ameba
- Entamoeba (histolytica) — *see* Infection, ameba
- Enterobius vermicularis 127.4
- Epidermophyton — *see* Dermatophytosis
- eyeworm 125.2
- Fasciola
  - gigantica 121.3
  - hepatica 121.3
- Fasciolopsis (buski) (small intestine) 121.4
  - blood NEC (*see also* Schistosomiasis) 120.9
  - cat liver 121.0
  - filarial 125.9
  - due to
    - Acanthocheilonema (perstans) 125.4
    - streptocerca 125.6

Index to Diseases

Infestation — continued
Fasciolopsis — continued
  filarial — continued
    due to — continued
      Brugia (Wuchereria) malayi 125.1
      Dracunculus medinensis 125.7
      guinea worms 125.7
      Mansonella (ozzardi) 125.5
      Onchocerca volvulus 125.3
        eye 125.3 [360.13]
        eyelid 125.3 [373.6]
      Wuchereria (bancrofti) 125.0
        malayi 125.1
    specified type NEC 125.6
fish tapeworm 123.4
  larval 123.5
fluke 121.9
  intestinal (giant) 121.4
  liver (sheep) 121.3
    cat 121.0
    Chinese 121.1
    clonorchiasis 121.1
    fascioliasis 121.3
    Oriental 121.1
  lung (oriental) 121.2
  sheep liver 121.3
fly larva 134.0
Gasterophilus (intestinalis) 134.0
Gastrodiscoides hominis 121.8
Giardia lamblia 007.1
Gnathostoma (spinigerum) 128.1
Gongylonema 125.6
guinea worm 125.7
helminth NEC 128.9
  intestinal 127.9
    mixed (types classifiable to more than one category in 120.0–127.7) 127.8
    specified type NEC 127.7
  specified type NEC 128.8
Heterophyes heterophyes (small intestine) 121.6
hookworm (see also Infestation, ancylostoma) 126.9
Hymenolepis (diminuta) (nana) 123.6
intestinal NEC 129
leeches (aquatic) (land) 134.2
Leishmania — see Leishmaniasis
lice (see also Infestation, pediculus) 132.9
Linguatulidae, linguatula (pentastoma) (serrata) 134.1
Loa loa 125.2
  eyelid 125.2 [373.6]
louse (see also Infestation, pediculus) 132.9
  body 132.1
  head 132.0
  pubic 132.2
maggots 134.0
Mansonella (ozzardi) 125.5
medina 125.7
Metagonimus yokogawai (small intestine) 121.5
Microfilaria streptocerca 125.3
  eye 125.3 [360.13]
  eyelid 125.3 [373.6]
Microsporon furfur 111.0
microsporum — see Dermatophytosis
mites 133.9
  scabic 133.0
  specified type NEC 133.8
monilia (albicans) (see also Candidiasis) 112.9
  vagina 112.1
  vulva 112.1
mouth 112.0
Necator americanus 126.1
nematode (intestinal) 127.9
  Ancylostoma (see also Ancylostoma) 126.9
  Ascaris lumbricoides 127.0
  conjunctiva NEC 128.9
  Dioctophyma 128.8

Infestation — continued
nematode — continued
  Enterobius vermicularis 127.4
  Gnathostoma spinigerum 128.1
  Oesophagostomum (apiostomum) 127.7
  Physaloptera 127.4
  specified type NEC 127.7
  Strongyloides stercoralis 127.2
  Ternidens diminutus 127.7
  Trichinella spiralis 124
  Trichostrongylus 127.6
  Trichuris (trichiuria) 127.3
Oesophagostomum (apiostomum) 127.7
Oestrus ovis 134.0
Onchocerca (volvulus) 125.3
  eye 125.3 [360.13]
  eyelid 125.3 [373.6]
Opisthorchis (felineus) (tenuicollis) (viverrini) 121.0
Oxyuris vermicularis 127.4
Paragonimus (westermani) 121.2
parasite, parasitic NEC 136.9
  eyelid 134.9 [373.6]
  intestinal 129
  mouth 112.0
  orbit 376.13
  skin 134.9
  tongue 112.0
pediculus 132.9
  capitis (humanus) (any site) 132.0
  corporis (humanus) (any site) 132.1
  eyelid 132.0 [373.6]
  mixed (classifiable to more than one category in 132.0–132.2) 132.3
  pubis (any site) 132.2
phthirus (pubis) (any site) 132.2
  with any infestation classifiable to 132.0, 132.1 and 132.3
pinworm 127.4
pork tapeworm (adult) 123.0
protozoal NEC 136.8
pubic louse 132.2
rat tapeworm 123.6
red bug 133.8
roundworm (large) NEC 127.0
sand flea 134.1
saprophytic NEC 136.8
Sarcoptes scabiei 133.0
scabies 133.0
Schistosoma 120.9
  bovis 120.8
  cercariae 120.3
  hematobium 120.0
  intercalatum 120.8
  japonicum 120.2
  mansoni 120.1
  mattheii 120.8
  specified
    site — see Schistosomiasis
    type NEC 120.8
  spindale 120.8
screw worms 134.0
skin NEC 134.9
Sparganum (mansoni) (proliferum) 123.5
  larval 123.5
specified type NEC 134.8
Spirometra larvae 123.5
Sporozoa NEC 136.8
Stellantchasmus falcatus 121.6
Strongyloides 127.2
Strongylus (gibsoni) 127.7
Taenia 123.3
  diminuta 123.6
  Echinococcus (see also Echinococcus) 122.9
  mediocanellata 123.2
  nana 123.6
  saginata (mediocanellata) 123.2
  solium (intestinal form) 123.0
    larval form 123.1
Taeniarhynchus saginatus 123.2
tapeworm 123.9

Infestation — continued
tapeworm — continued
  beef 123.2
  broad 123.4
    larval 123.5
  dog 123.8
  dwarf 123.6
  fish 123.4
    larval 123.5
  pork 123.0
  rat 123.6
Ternidens diminutus 127.7
Tetranychus molestissimus 133.8
threadworm 127.4
tongue 112.0
Toxocara (cani) (cati) (felis) 128.0
trematode(s) NEC 121.9
Trichina spiralis 124
Trichinella spiralis 124
Trichocephalus 127.3
Trichomonas 131.9
  bladder 131.09
  cervix 131.09
  intestine 007.3
  prostate 131.03
  specified site NEC 131.8
  urethra (female) (male) 131.02
  urogenital 131.00
  vagina 131.01
  vulva 131.01
Trichophyton — see Dermatophytosis
Trichostrongylus instabilis 127.6
Trichuris (trichiuria) 127.3
Trombicula (irritans) 133.8
Trypanosoma — see Trypanosomiasis
Tunga penetrans 134.1
Uncinaria americana 126.1
whipworm 127.3
worms NEC 128.9
  intestinal 127.9
Wuchereria 125.0
  bancrofti 125.0
  malayi 125.1

Infiltrate, infiltration
with an iron compound 275.0
amyloid (any site) (generalized) 277.39
calcareous (muscle) NEC 275.49
  localized — see Degeneration, by site
calcium salt (muscle) 275.49
corneal (see also Edema, cornea) 371.20
  eyelid 373.9
fatty (diffuse) (generalized) 272.8
  localized — see Degeneration, by site, fatty
glycogen, glycogenic (see also Disease, glycogen storage) 271.0
heart, cardiac
  fatty (see also Degeneration, myocardial) 429.1
  glycogenic 271.0 [425.7]
inflammatory in vitreous 379.29
kidney (see also Disease, renal) 593.9
leukemic (M9800/3) — see Leukemia
liver 573.8
  fatty — see Fatty, liver
  glycogen (see also Disease, glycogen storage) 271.0
lung (see also Infiltrate, pulmonary) 518.3
  eosinophilic 518.3
  x-ray finding only 793.1
lymphatic (see also Leukemia, lymphatic) 204.9
  gland, pigmentary 289.3
muscle, fatty 728.9
myelogenous (see also Leukemia, myeloid) 205.9
myocardium, myocardial
  fatty (see also Degeneration, myocardial) 429.1
  glycogenic 271.0 [425.7]
pulmonary 518.3

Infiltrate, infiltration — continued
pulmonary — continued
  with
    eosinophilia 518.3
    pneumonia — see Pneumonia, by type
  x-ray finding only 793.1
  Ranke's primary (see also Tuberculosis) 010.0
skin, lymphocytic (benign) 709.8
thymus (gland) (fatty) 254.8
urine 788.8
vitreous humor 379.29

Infirmity 799.89
senile 797

Inflammation, inflamed, inflammatory
(with exudation)
abducens (nerve) 378.54
accessory sinus (chronic) (see also Sinusitis) 473.9
adrenal (gland) 255.8
alimentary canal — see Enteritis
alveoli (teeth) 526.5
  scorbutic 267
amnion — see Amnionitis
anal canal 569.49
antrum (chronic) (see also Sinusitis, maxillary) 473.0
anus 569.49
appendix (see also Appendicitis) 541
arachnoid — see Meningitis
areola 611.0
  puerperal, postpartum 675.0
areolar tissue NEC 686.9
artery — see Arteritis
auditory meatus (external) (see also Otitis, externa) 380.10
Bartholin's gland 616.89
bile duct or passage 576.1
bladder (see also Cystitis) 595.9
bleb
  postprocedural 379.60
    stage 1 379.61
    stage 2 379.62
    stage 3 379.63
bone — see Osteomyelitis
bowel (see also Enteritis) 558.9
brain (see also Encephalitis) 323.9
  late effect — see category 326
  membrane — see Meningitis
breast 611.0
  puerperal, postpartum 675.2
broad ligament (see also Disease, pelvis, inflammatory) 614.4
  acute 614.3
bronchus — see Bronchitis
bursa — see Bursitis
capsule
  liver 573.3
  spleen 289.59
catarrhal (see also Catarrh) 460
  vagina 616.10
cecum (see also Appendicitis) 541
cerebral (see also Encephalitis) 323.9
  late effect — see category 326
  membrane — see Meningitis
cerebrospinal (see also Meningitis) 322.9
  late effect — see category 326
  meningococcal 036.0
  tuberculous (see also Tuberculosis) 013.6
cervix (uteri) (see also Cervicitis) 616.0
chest 519.9
choroid NEC (see also Choroiditis) 363.20
cicatrix (tissue) — see Cicatrix
colon (see also Enteritis) 558.9
  granulomatous 555.1
  newborn 558.9
connective tissue (diffuse) NEC 728.9
cornea (see also Keratitis) 370.9
  with ulcer (see also Ulcer, cornea) 370.00
corpora cavernosa (penis) 607.2

Inflammation, inflamed, inflammatory

Inflammation, inflamed, inflammatory
— *continued*
- cranial nerve — *see* Disorder, nerve, cranial
- diarrhea — *see* Diarrhea
- disc (intervertebral) (space) 722.90
  - cervical, cervicothoracic 722.91
  - lumbar, lumbosacral 722.93
  - thoracic, thoracolumbar 722.92
- Douglas' cul-de-sac or pouch (chronic) (*see also* Disease, pelvis, inflammatory) 614.4
  - acute 614.3
- due to (presence of) any device, implant, or graft classifiable to 996.0–996.5 — *see* Complications, infection and inflammation, due to (presence of) any device, implant, or graft classified to 996.0–996.5 NEC
- duodenum 535.6 ☑
- dura mater — *see* Meningitis
- ear (*see also* Otitis)
  - external (*see also* Otitis, externa) 380.10
  - inner (*see also* Labyrinthitis) 386.30
  - middle — *see* Otitis media
- esophagus 530.10
- ethmoidal (chronic) (sinus) (*see also* Sinusitis, ethmoidal) 473.2
- Eustachian tube (catarrhal) 381.50
  - acute 381.51
  - chronic 381.52
- extrarectal 569.49
- eye 379.99
- eyelid 373.9
  - specified NEC 373.8
- fallopian tube (*see also* Salpingo-oophoritis) 614.2
- fascia 728.9
- fetal membranes (acute) 658.4 ☑
  - affecting fetus or newborn 762.7
- follicular, pharynx 472.1
- frontal (chronic) (sinus) (*see also* Sinusitis, frontal) 473.1
- gallbladder (*see also* Cholecystitis, acute) 575.0
- gall duct (*see also* Cholecystitis) 575.10
- gastrointestinal (*see also* Enteritis) 558.9
- genital organ (diffuse) (internal)
  - female 614.9
    - with
      - abortion — *see* Abortion, by type, with sepsis
      - ectopic pregnancy (*see also* categories 633.0–633.9) 639.0
      - molar pregnancy (*see also* categories 630–632) 639.0
    - complicating pregnancy, childbirth, or puerperium 646.6 ☑
      - affecting fetus or newborn 760.8
    - following
      - abortion 639.0
      - ectopic or molar pregnancy 639.0
  - male 608.4
- gland (lymph) (*see also* Lymphadenitis) 289.3
- glottis (*see also* Laryngitis) 464.00
  - with obstruction 464.01
- granular, pharynx 472.1
- gum 523.10 ▲
- heart (*see also* Carditis) 429.89
- hepatic duct 576.8
- hernial sac — *see* Hernia, by site
- ileum (*see also* Enteritis) 558.9
  - terminal or regional 555.0
    - with large intestine 555.2
- intervertebral disc 722.90

Inflammation, inflamed, inflammatory
— *continued*
- intervertebral disc — *continued*
  - cervical, cervicothoracic 722.91
  - lumbar, lumbosacral 722.93
  - thoracic, thoracolumbar 722.92
- intestine (*see also* Enteritis) 558.9
- jaw (acute) (bone) (chronic) (lower) (suppurative) (upper) 526.4
- jejunum — *see* Enteritis
- joint NEC (*see also* Arthritis) 716.9 ☑
  - sacroiliac 720.2
- kidney (*see also* Nephritis) 583.9
- knee (joint) 716.66
  - tuberculous (active) (*see also* Tuberculosis) 015.2 ☑
- labium (majus) (minus) (*see also* Vulvitis) 616.10
- lacrimal
  - gland (*see also* Dacryoadenitis) 375.00
  - passages (duct) (sac) (*see also* Dacryocystitis) 375.30
- larynx (*see also* Laryngitis) 464.00
  - with obstruction 464.01
  - diphtheritic 032.3
- leg NEC 686.9
- lip 528.5
- liver (capsule) (*see also* Hepatitis) 573.3
  - acute 570
  - chronic 571.40
  - suppurative 572.0
- lung (acute) (*see also* Pneumonia) 486
  - chronic (interstitial) 518.89
- lymphatic vessel (*see also* Lymphangitis) 457.2
- lymph node or gland (*see also* Lymphadenitis) 289.3
- mammary gland 611.0
  - puerperal, postpartum 675.2 ☑
- maxilla, maxillary 526.4
  - sinus (chronic) (*see also* Sinusitis, maxillary) 473.0
- membranes of brain or spinal cord — *see* Meningitis
- meninges — *see* Meningitis
- mouth 528.00 ▲
- muscle 728.9
- myocardium (*see also* Myocarditis) 429.0
- nasal sinus (chronic) (*see also* Sinusitis) 473.9
- nasopharynx — *see* Nasopharyngitis
- navel 686.9
  - newborn NEC 771.4
- nerve NEC 729.2
- nipple 611.0
  - puerperal, postpartum 675.0 ☑
- nose 478.19 ▲
  - suppurative 472.0
- oculomotor nerve 378.51
- optic nerve 377.30
- orbit (chronic) 376.10
  - acute 376.00
  - chronic 376.10
- ovary (*see also* Salpingo-oophoritis) 614.2
- oviduct (*see also* Salpingo-oophoritis) 614.2
- pancreas — *see* Pancreatitis
- parametrium (chronic) (*see also* Disease, pelvis, inflammatory) 614.4
  - acute 614.3
- parotid region 686.9
  - gland 527.2
- pelvis, female (*see also* Disease, pelvis, inflammatory) 614.9
- penis (corpora cavernosa) 607.2
- perianal 569.49
- pericardium (*see also* Pericarditis) 423.9
- perineum (female) (male) 686.9
- perirectal 569.49
- peritoneum (*see also* Peritonitis) 567.9

Inflammation, inflamed, inflammatory
— *continued*
- periuterine (*see also* Disease, pelvis, inflammatory) 614.9
- perivesical (*see also* Cystitis) 595.9
- petrous bone (*see also* Petrositis) 383.20
- pharynx (*see also* Pharyngitis) 462
  - follicular 472.1
  - granular 472.1
- pia mater — *see* Meningitis
- pleura — *see* Pleurisy
- postmastoidectomy cavity 383.30
  - chronic 383.33
- prostate (*see also* Prostatitis) 601.9
- rectosigmoid — *see* Rectosigmoiditis
- rectum (*see also* Proctitis) 569.49
- respiratory, upper (*see also* Infection, respiratory, upper) 465.9
  - chronic, due to external agent — *see* Condition, respiratory, chronic, due to, external agent
  - due to
    - fumes or vapors (chemical) (inhalation) 506.2
    - radiation 508.1
- retina (*see also* Retinitis) 363.20
- retrocecal (*see also* Appendicitis) 541
- retroperitoneal (*see also* Peritonitis) 567.9
- salivary duct or gland (any) (suppurative) 527.2
- scorbutic, alveoli, teeth 267
- scrotum 608.4
- sigmoid — *see* Enteritis
- sinus (*see also* Sinusitis) 473.9
- Skene's duct or gland (*see also* Urethritis) 597.89
- skin 686.9
- spermatic cord 608.4
- sphenoidal (sinus) (*see also* Sinusitis, sphenoidal) 473.3
- spinal
  - cord (*see also* Encephalitis) 323.9
    - late effect — *see* category 326
  - membrane — *see* Meningitis
  - nerve — *see* Disorder, nerve
- spine (*see also* Spondylitis) 720.9
- spleen (capsule) 289.59
- stomach — *see* Gastritis
- stricture, rectum 569.49
- subcutaneous tissue NEC 686.9
- suprarenal (gland) 255.8
- synovial (fringe) (membrane) — *see* Bursitis
- tendon (sheath) NEC 726.90
- testis (*see also* Orchitis) 604.90
- thigh 686.9
- throat (*see also* Sore throat) 462
- thymus (gland) 254.8
- thyroid (gland) (*see also* Thyroiditis) 245.9
- tongue 529.0
- tonsil — *see* Tonsillitis
- trachea — *see* Tracheitis
- trochlear nerve 378.53
- tubal (*see also* Salpingo-oophoritis) 614.2
- tuberculous NEC (*see also* Tuberculosis) 011.9 ☑
- tubo-ovarian (*see also* Salpingo-oophoritis) 614.2
- tunica vaginalis 608.4
- tympanic membrane — *see* Myringitis
- umbilicus, umbilical 686.9
  - newborn NEC 771.4
- uterine ligament (*see also* Disease, pelvis, inflammatory) 614.4
  - acute 614.3
- uterus (catarrhal) (*see also* Endometritis) 615.9
- uveal tract (anterior) (*see also* Iridocyclitis) 364.3
  - posterior — *see* Chorioretinitis
  - sympathetic 360.11

Inflammation, inflamed, inflammatory
— *continued*
- vagina (*see also* Vaginitis) 616.10
- vas deferens 608.4
- vein (*see also* Phlebitis) 451.9
  - thrombotic 451.9
    - cerebral (*see also* Thrombosis, brain) 434.0 ☑
    - leg 451.2
      - deep (vessels) NEC 451.19
      - superficial (vessels) 451.0
    - lower extremity 451.2
      - deep (vessels) NEC 451.19
      - superficial (vessels) 451.0
- vocal cord 478.5
- vulva (*see also* Vulvitis) 616.10

Inflation, lung imperfect (newborn) 770.5

Influenza, influenzal 487.1
- with
  - bronchitis 487.1
  - bronchopneumonia 487.0
  - cold (any type) 487.1
  - digestive manifestations 487.8
  - hemoptysis 487.1
  - involvement of
    - gastrointestinal tract 487.8
    - nervous system 487.8
  - laryngitis 487.1
  - manifestations NEC 487.8
    - respiratory 487.1
    - pneumonia 487.0
  - pharyngitis 487.1
  - pneumonia (any form classifiable to 480–483, 485–486) 487.0
  - respiratory manifestations NEC 487.1
  - sinusitis 487.1
  - sore throat 487.1
  - tonsillitis 487.1
  - tracheitis 487.1
  - upper respiratory infection (acute) 487.1
- abdominal 487.8
- Asian 487.1
- bronchial 487.1
- bronchopneumonia 487.0
- catarrhal 487.1
- epidemic 487.1
- gastric 487.8
- intestinal 487.8
- laryngitis 487.1
- maternal affecting fetus or newborn 760.2
  - manifest influenza in infant 771.2
- pharyngitis 487.1
- pneumonia (any form) 487.0
- respiratory (upper) 487.1
- stomach 487.8
- vaccination, prophylactic (against) V04.81

Influenza-like disease 487.1

Infraction, Freiberg's (metatarsal head) 732.5

Infraeruption, teeth 524.34

Infusion complication, misadventure, or reaction — *see* Complication, infusion

Ingestion
- chemical — *see* Table of Drugs and Chemicals
- drug or medicinal substance
  - overdose or wrong substance given or taken 977.9
  - specified drug — *see* Table of Drugs and Chemicals
- foreign body NEC (*see also* Foreign body) 938

Ingrowing
- hair 704.8
- nail (finger) (toe) (infected) 703.0

Inguinal — *see also* condition
- testis 752.51

Inhalation
- carbon monoxide 986

Index to Diseases

Inhalation — *continued*
flame
lung 947.1
mouth 947.0
food or foreign body (*see also* Asphyxia, food or foreign body) 933.1
gas, fumes, or vapor (noxious) 987.9
specified agent — *see* Table of Drugs and Chemicals
liquid or vomitus (*see also* Asphyxia, food or foreign body) 933.1
lower respiratory tract NEC 934.9
meconium (fetus or newborn) 770.11
with respiratory symptoms 770.12
mucus (*see also* Asphyxia, mucus) 933.1
oil (causing suffocation) (*see also* Asphyxia, food or foreign body) 933.1
pneumonia — *see* Pneumonia, aspiration
smoke 987.9
steam 987.9
stomach contents or secretions (*see also* Asphyxia, food or foreign body) 933.1
in labor and delivery 668.0 ☑

Inhibition, inhibited
academic as adjustment reaction 309.23
orgasm
female 302.73
male 302.74
sexual
desire 302.71
excitement 302.72
work as adjustment reaction 309.23

Inhibitor, systemic lupus erythematosus (presence of) 286.5

Iniencephalus, iniencephaly 740.2

Injected eye 372.74

Injury 959.9

> *Note* — For abrasion, insect bite (nonvenomous), blister, or scratch, *see* Injury, superficial.
>
> For laceration, traumatic rupture, tear, or penetrating wound of internal organs, such as heart, lung, liver, kidney, pelvic organs, whether or not accompanied by open wound in the same region, *see* Injury, internal.
>
> For nerve injury, *see* Injury, nerve.
>
> For late effect of injuries classifiable to 850–854, 860–869, 900–919, 950–959, *see* Late, effect, injury, by type.

abdomen, abdominal (viscera) (*see also* Injury, internal, abdomen)
muscle or wall 959.12
acoustic, resulting in deafness 951.5
adenoid 959.09
adrenal (gland) — *see* Injury, internal, adrenal
alveolar (process) 959.09
ankle (and foot) (and knee) (and leg, except thigh) 959.7
anterior chamber, eye 921.3
anus 959.19
aorta (thoracic) 901.0
abdominal 902.0
appendix — *see* Injury, internal, appendix
arm, upper (and shoulder) 959.2
artery (complicating trauma) (*see also* Injury, blood vessel, by site) 904.9
cerebral or meningeal (*see also* Hemorrhage, brain, traumatic, subarachnoid) 852.0 ☑
auditory canal (external) (meatus) 959.09
auricle, auris, ear 959.09
axilla 959.2
back 959.19

Injury — *continued*
bile duct — *see* Injury, internal, bile duct
birth (*see also* Birth, injury)
canal NEC, complicating delivery 665.9 ☑
bladder (sphincter) — *see* Injury, internal, bladder
blast (air) (hydraulic) (immersion) (underwater) NEC 869.0
with open wound into cavity NEC 869.1
abdomen or thorax — *see* Injury, internal, by site
brain — *see* Concussion, brain
ear (acoustic nerve trauma) 951.5
with perforation of tympanic membrane — *see* Wound, open, ear, drum
blood vessel NEC 904.9
abdomen 902.9
multiple 902.87
specified NEC 902.89
aorta (thoracic) 901.0
abdominal 902.0
arm NEC 903.9
axillary 903.00
artery 903.01
vein 903.02
azygos vein 901.89
basilic vein 903.1
brachial (artery) (vein) 903.1
bronchial 901.89
carotid artery 900.00
common 900.01
external 900.02
internal 900.03
celiac artery 902.20
specified branch NEC 902.24
cephalic vein (arm) 903.1
colica dextra 902.26
cystic
artery 902.24
vein 902.39
deep plantar 904.6
digital (artery) (vein) 903.5
due to accidental puncture or laceration during procedure 998.2
extremity
lower 904.8
multiple 904.7
specified NEC 904.7
upper 903.9
multiple 903.8
specified NEC 903.8
femoral
artery (superficial) 904.1
above profunda origin 904.0
common 904.0
vein 904.2
gastric
artery 902.21
vein 902.39
head 900.9
intracranial — *see* Injury, intracranial
multiple 900.82
specified NEC 900.89
hemiazygos vein 901.89
hepatic
artery 902.22
vein 902.11
hypogastric 902.59
artery 902.51
vein 902.52
ileocolic
artery 902.26
vein 902.31
iliac 902.50
artery 902.53
specified branch NEC 902.59
vein 902.54
innominate
artery 901.1
vein 901.3

Injury — *continued*
blood vessel — *continued*
intercostal (artery) (vein) 901.81
jugular vein (external) 900.81
internal 900.1
leg NEC 904.8
mammary (artery) (vein) 901.82
mesenteric
artery 902.20
inferior 902.27
specified branch NEC 902.29
superior (trunk) 902.25
branches, primary 902.26
vein 902.39
inferior 902.32
superior (and primary subdivisions) 902.31
neck 900.9
multiple 900.82
specified NEC 900.89
ovarian 902.89
artery 902.81
vein 902.82
palmar artery 903.4
pelvis 902.9
multiple 902.87
specified NEC 902.89
plantar (deep) (artery) (vein) 904.6
popliteal 904.40
artery 904.41
vein 904.42
portal 902.33
pulmonary 901.40
artery 901.41
vein 901.42
radial (artery) (vein) 903.2
renal 902.40
artery 902.41
specified NEC 902.49
vein 902.42
saphenous
artery 904.7
vein (greater) (lesser) 904.3
splenic
artery 902.23
vein 902.34
subclavian
artery 901.1
vein 901.3
suprarenal 902.49
thoracic 901.9
multiple 901.83
specified NEC 901.89
tibial 904.50
artery 904.50
anterior 904.51
posterior 904.53
vein 904.50
anterior 904.52
posterior 904.54
ulnar (artery) (vein) 903.3
uterine 902.59
artery 902.55
vein 902.56
vena cava
inferior 902.10
specified branches NEC 902.19
superior 901.2
brachial plexus 953.4
newborn 767.6
brain NEC (*see also* Injury, intracranial) 854.0 ☑
breast 959.19
broad ligament — *see* Injury, internal, broad ligament
bronchus, bronchi — *see* Injury, internal, bronchus
brow 959.09
buttock 959.19
canthus, eye 921.1
cathode ray 990
cauda equina 952.4
with fracture, vertebra — *see* Fracture, vertebra, sacrum

Injury — *continued*
cavernous sinus (*see also* Injury, intracranial) 854.0 ☑
cecum — *see* Injury, internal, cecum
celiac ganglion or plexus 954.1
cerebellum (*see also* Injury, intracranial) 854.0 ☑
cervix (uteri) — *see* Injury, internal, cervix
cheek 959.09
chest (*see also* Injury, internal, chest) wall 959.11
childbirth (*see also* Birth, injury) maternal NEC 665.9 ☑
chin 959.09
choroid (eye) 921.3
clitoris 959.14
coccyx 959.19
complicating delivery 665.6 ☑
colon — *see* Injury, internal, colon
common duct — *see* Injury, internal, common duct
conjunctiva 921.1
superficial 918.2
cord
spermatic — *see* Injury, internal, spermatic cord
spinal — *see* Injury, spinal, by site
cornea 921.3
abrasion 918.1
due to contact lens 371.82
penetrating — *see* Injury, eyeball, penetrating
superficial 918.1
due to contact lens 371.82
cortex (cerebral) (*see also* Injury, intracranial) 854.0 ☑
visual 950.3
costal region 959.11
costochondral 959.11
cranial
bones — *see* Fracture, skull, by site
cavity (*see also* Injury, intracranial) 854.0 ☑
nerve — *see* Injury, nerve, cranial
crushing — *see* Crush
cutaneous sensory nerve
lower limb 956.4
upper limb 955.5
delivery (*see also* Birth, injury) maternal NEC 665.9 ☑
Descemet's membrane — *see* Injury, eyeball, penetrating
diaphragm — *see* Injury, internal, diaphragm
diffuse axonal — *see* Injury, intracranial
duodenum — *see* Injury, internal, duodenum
ear (auricle) (canal) (drum) (external) 959.09
elbow (and forearm) (and wrist) 959.3
epididymis 959.14
epigastric region 959.12
epiglottis 959.09
epiphyseal, current — *see* Fracture, by site
esophagus — *see* Injury, internal, esophagus
Eustachian tube 959.09
extremity (lower) (upper) NEC 959.8
eye 921.9
penetrating eyeball — *see* Injury, eyeball, penetrating
superficial 918.9
eyeball 921.3
penetrating 871.7
with
partial loss (of intraocular tissue) 871.2
prolapse or exposure (of intraocular tissue) 871.1
without prolapse 871.0
foreign body (nonmagnetic) 871.6

Injury

Injury — continued
 eyeball — continued
  penetrating — continued
   foreign body — continued
    magnetic 871.5
   superficial 918.9
 eyebrow 959.09
 eyelid(s) 921.1
  laceration — see Laceration, eyelid
  superficial 918.0
 face (and neck) 959.09
 fallopian tube — see Injury, internal, fallopian tube
 finger(s) (nail) 959.5
 flank 959.19
 foot (and ankle) (and knee) (and leg, except thigh) 959.7
 forceps NEC 767.9
  scalp 767.19
 forearm (and elbow) (and wrist) 959.3
 forehead 959.09
 gallbladder — see Injury, internal, gallbladder
 gasserian ganglion 951.2
 gastrointestinal tract — see Injury, internal, gastrointestinal tract
 genital organ(s)
  with
   abortion — see Abortion, by type, with, damage to pelvic organs
   ectopic pregnancy (see also categories 633.0–633.9) 639.2
   molar pregnancy (see also categories 630–632) 639.2
  external 959.14
   fracture of corpus cavernosum penis 959.13
  following
   abortion 639.2
   ectopic or molar pregnancy 639.2
  internal — see Injury, internal, genital organs
  obstetrical trauma NEC 665.9 ☑
   affecting fetus or newborn 763.89
 gland
  lacrimal 921.1
   laceration 870.8
  parathyroid 959.09
  salivary 959.09
  thyroid 959.09
 globe (eye) (see also Injury, eyeball) 921.3
 grease gun — see Wound, open, by site, complicated
 groin 959.19
 gum 959.09
 hand(s) (except fingers) 959.4
 head NEC 959.01
  with
   loss of consciousness 850.5
   skull fracture — see Fracture, skull, by site
 heart — see Injury, internal, heart
 heel 959.7
 hip (and thigh) 959.6
 hymen 959.14
 hyperextension (cervical) (vertebra) 847.0
 ileum — see Injury, internal, ileum
 iliac region 959.19
 infrared rays NEC 990
 instrumental (during surgery) 998.2
  birth injury — see Birth, injury
  nonsurgical (see also Injury, by site) 959.9
  obstetrical 665.9 ☑
   affecting fetus or newborn 763.89
   bladder 665.5 ☑
   cervix 665.3 ☑
   high vaginal 665.4 ☑
   perineal NEC 664.9 ☑

Injury — continued
 instrumental — continued
  obstetrical — continued
   urethra 665.5 ☑
   uterus 665.5 ☑
  internal 869.0

> Note — For injury of internal organ(s) by foreign body entering through a natural orifice (e.g., inhaled, ingested, or swallowed) — see Foreign body, entering through orifice.
>
> For internal injury of any of the following sites with internal injury of any other of the sites — see Injury, internal, multiple.

  with
   fracture
    pelvis — see Fracture, pelvis
    specified site, except pelvis — see Injury, internal, by site
   open wound into cavity 869.1
  abdomen, abdominal (viscera) NEC 868.00
   with
    fracture, pelvis — see Fracture, pelvis
    open wound into cavity 868.10
   specified site NEC 868.09
    with open wound into cavity 868.19
  adrenal (gland) 868.01
   with open wound into cavity 868.11
  aorta (thoracic) 901.0
   abdominal 902.0
  appendix 863.85
   with open wound into cavity 863.95
  bile duct 868.02
   with open wound into cavity 868.12
  bladder (sphincter) 867.0
   with
    abortion — see Abortion, by type, with damage to pelvic organs
    ectopic pregnancy (see also categories 633.0–633.9) 639.2
    molar pregnancy (see also categories 630–632) 639.2
    open wound into cavity 867.1
   following
    abortion 639.2
    ectopic or molar pregnancy 639.2
   obstetrical trauma 665.5 ☑
    affecting fetus or newborn 763.89
  blood vessel — see Injury, blood vessel, by site
  broad ligament 867.6
   with open wound into cavity 867.7
  bronchus, bronchi 862.21
   with open wound into cavity 862.31
  cecum 863.89
   with open wound into cavity 863.99
  cervix (uteri) 867.4
   with
    abortion — see Abortion, by type, with damage to pelvic organs
    ectopic pregnancy (see also categories 633.0–633.9) 639.2
    molar pregnancy (see also categories 630–632) 639.2
    open wound into cavity 867.5

Injury — continued
 internal — continued
  cervix — continued
   following
    abortion 639.2
    ectopic or molar pregnancy 639.2
   obstetrical trauma 665.3 ☑
    affecting fetus or newborn 763.89
  chest (see also Injury, internal, intrathoracic organs) 862.8
   with open wound into cavity 862.9
  colon 863.40
   with
    open wound into cavity 863.50
   rectum 863.46
    with open wound into cavity 863.56
   ascending (right) 863.41
    with open wound into cavity 863.51
   descending (left) 863.43
    with open wound into cavity 863.53
   multiple sites 863.46
    with open wound into cavity 863.56
   sigmoid 863.44
    with open wound into cavity 863.54
   specified site NEC 863.49
    with open wound into cavity 863.59
   transverse 863.42
    with open wound into cavity 863.52
  common duct 868.02
   with open wound into cavity 868.12
  complicating delivery 665.9 ☑
   affecting fetus or newborn 763.89
  diaphragm 862.0
   with open wound into cavity 862.1
  duodenum 863.21
   with open wound into cavity 863.31
  esophagus [intrathoracic] 862.22
   with open wound into cavity 862.32
   cervical region 874.4
    complicated 874.5
  fallopian tube 867.6
   with open wound into cavity 867.7
  gallbladder 868.02
   with open wound into cavity 868.12
  gastrointestinal tract NEC 863.80
   with open wound into cavity 863.90
  genital organ NEC 867.6
   with open wound into cavity 867.7
  heart 861.00
   with open wound into thorax 861.10
  ileum 863.29
   with open wound into cavity 863.39
  intestine NEC 863.89
   with open wound into cavity 863.99
   large NEC 863.40
    with open wound into cavity 863.50
   small NEC 863.20
    with open wound into cavity 863.30
  intra-abdominal (organ) 868.00
   with open wound into cavity 868.10

Injury — continued
 internal — continued
  intra-abdominal — continued
   multiple sites 868.09
    with open wound into cavity 868.19
   specified site NEC 868.09
    with open wound into cavity 868.19
  intrathoracic organs (multiple) 862.8
   with open wound into cavity 862.9
   diaphragm (only) — see Injury, internal, diaphragm
   heart (only) — see Injury, internal, heart
   lung (only) — see Injury, internal, lung
   specified site NEC 862.29
    with open wound into cavity 862.39
  intrauterine (see also Injury, internal, uterus) 867.4
   with open wound into cavity 867.5
  jejunum 863.29
   with open wound into cavity 863.39
  kidney (subcapsular) 866.00
   with
    disruption of parenchyma (complete) 866.03
     with open wound into cavity 866.13
    hematoma (without rupture of capsule) 866.01
     with open wound into cavity 866.11
    laceration 866.02
     with open wound into cavity 866.12
    open wound into cavity 866.10
  liver 864.00
   with
    contusion 864.01
     with open wound into cavity 864.11
    hematoma 864.01
     with open wound into cavity 864.11
    laceration 864.05
     with open wound into cavity 864.15
    major (disruption of hepatic parenchyma) 864.04
     with open wound into cavity 864.14
    minor (capsule only) 864.02
     with open wound into cavity 864.12
    moderate (involving parenchyma) 864.03
     with open wound into cavity 864.13
    multiple 864.04
    stellate 864.04
     with open wound into cavity 864.14
    open wound into cavity 864.10
  lung 861.20
   with open wound into thorax 861.30
   hemopneumothorax — see Hemopneumothorax, traumatic
   hemothorax — see Hemothorax, traumatic
   pneumohemothorax — see Pneumohemothorax, traumatic

Index to Diseases

Injury

Injury — *continued*
  internal — *continued*
    lung — *continued*
      pneumothorax — *see* Pneumothorax, traumatic
      transfusion related, acute (TRALI) 518.7 ●
    mediastinum 862.29
      with open wound into cavity 862.39
    mesentery 863.89
      with open wound into cavity 863.99
    mesosalpinx 867.6
      with open wound into cavity 867.7
    multiple 869.0

> *Note* — Multiple internal injuries of sites classifiable to the same three- or four-digit category should be classified to that category.
>
> Multiple injuries classifiable to different fourth-digit subdivisions of 861 (heart and lung injuries) should be dealt with according to coding rules.

      internal
        with open wound into cavity 869.1
      intra–abdominal organ (sites classifiable to 863–868)
        with
          intrathoracic organ(s) (sites classifiable to 861–862) 869.0
            with open wound into cavity 869.1
          other intra–abdominal organ(s) (sites classifiable to 863–868, except where classifiable to the same three–digit category) 868.09
            with open wound into cavity 868.19
      intrathoracic organ (sites classifiable to 861–862)
        with
          intra–abdominal organ(s) (sites classifiable to 863–868) 869.0
            with open wound into cavity 869.1
          other intrathoracic organ(s) (sites classifiable to 861–862, except where classifiable to the same three–digit category) 862.8
            with open wound into cavity 862.9
    myocardium — *see* Injury, internal, heart
    ovary 867.6
      with open wound into cavity 867.7
    pancreas (multiple sites) 863.84
      with open wound into cavity 863.94
      body 863.82
        with open wound into cavity 863.92
      head 863.81
        with open wound into cavity 863.91
      tail 863.83
        with open wound into cavity 863.93
    pelvis, pelvic (organs) (viscera) 867.8
      with
        fracture, pelvis — *see* Fracture, pelvis
        open wound into cavity 867.9

Injury — *continued*
  internal — *continued*
    pelvis, pelvic — *continued*
      specified site NEC 867.6
        with open wound into cavity 867.7
    peritoneum 868.03
      with open wound into cavity 868.13
    pleura 862.29
      with open wound into cavity 862.39
    prostate 867.6
      with open wound into cavity 867.7
    rectum 863.45
      with
        colon 863.46
          with open wound into cavity 863.56
        open wound into cavity 863.55
    retroperitoneum 868.04
      with open wound into cavity 868.14
    round ligament 867.6
      with open wound into cavity 867.7
    seminal vesicle 867.6
      with open wound into cavity 867.7
    spermatic cord 867.6
      with open wound into cavity 867.7
      scrotal — *see* Wound, open, spermatic cord
    spleen 865.00
      with
        disruption of parenchyma (massive) 865.04
          with open wound into cavity 865.14
        hematoma (without rupture of capsule) 865.01
          with open wound into cavity 865.11
        open wound into cavity 865.10
        tear, capsular 865.02
          with open wound into cavity 865.12
          extending into parenchyma 865.03
            with open wound into cavity 865.13
    stomach 863.0
      with open wound into cavity 863.1
    suprarenal gland (multiple) 868.01
      with open wound into cavity 868.11
    thorax, thoracic (cavity) (organs) (multiple) (*see also* Injury, internal, intrathoracic organs) 862.8
      with open wound into cavity 862.9
    thymus (gland) 862.29
      with open wound into cavity 862.39
    trachea (intrathoracic) 862.29
      with open wound into cavity 862.39
      cervical region (*see also* Wound, open, trachea) 874.02
    ureter 867.2
      with open wound into cavity 867.3
    urethra (sphincter) 867.0
      with
        abortion — *see* Abortion, by type, with damage to pelvic organs
        ectopic pregnancy (*see also* categories 633.0–633.9) 639.2

Injury — *continued*
  internal — *continued*
    urethra — *continued*
      with — *continued*
        molar pregnancy (*see also* categories 630–632) 639.2
        open wound into cavity 867.1
      following
        abortion 639.2
        ectopic or molar pregnancy 639.2
      obstetrical trauma 665.5 ☑
        affecting fetus or newborn 763.89
    uterus 867.4
      with
        abortion — *see* Abortion, by type, with damage to pelvic organs
        ectopic pregnancy (*see also* categories 633.0–633.9) 639.2
        molar pregnancy (*see also* categories 630–632) 639.2
        open wound into cavity 867.5
      following
        abortion 639.2
        ectopic or molar pregnancy 639.2
      obstetrical trauma NEC 665.5 ☑
        affecting fetus or newborn 763.89
    vas deferens 867.6
      with open wound into cavity 867.7
    vesical (sphincter) 867.0
      with open wound into cavity 867.1
    viscera (abdominal) (*see also* Injury, internal, multiple) 868.00
      with
        fracture, pelvis — *see* Fracture, pelvis
        open wound into cavity 868.10
      thoracic NEC (*see also* Injury, internal, intrathoracic organs) 862.8
        with open wound into cavity 862.9
  interscapular region 959.19
  intervertebral disc 959.19
  intestine — *see* Injury, internal, intestine
  intra-abdominal (organs) NEC — *see* Injury, internal, intra-abdominal

Injury — *continued*
  intracranial 854.0 ☑

> *Note* — Use the following fifth-digit subclassification with categories 851–854:
>
> 0   unspecified state of consciousness
>
> 1   with no loss of consciousness
>
> 2   with brief [less than one hour] loss of consciousness
>
> 3   with moderate [1–24 hours] loss of consciousness
>
> 4   with prolonged [more than 24 hours] loss of consciousness and return to pre–existing conscious level
>
> 5   with prolonged [more than 24 hours] loss of consciousness, without return to pre–existing conscious level
>
> Use fifth-digit 5 to designate when a patient is unconscious and dies before regaining consciousness, regardless of the duration of the loss of consciousness
>
> 6   with loss of consciousness of unspecified duration
>
> 9   with concussion, unspecified

    with
      open intracranial wound 854.1 ☑
      skull fracture — *see* Fracture, skull, by site
    contusion 851.8 ☑
      with open intracranial wound 851.9 ☑
      brain stem 851.4 ☑
        with open intracranial wound 851.5 ☑
      cerebellum 851.4 ☑
        with open intracranial wound 851.5 ☑
      cortex (cerebral) 851.0 ☑
        with open intracranial wound 851.2 ☑
    hematoma — *see* Injury, intracranial, hemorrhage
    hemorrhage 853.0 ☑
      with
        laceration — *see* Injury, intracranial, laceration
        open intracranial wound 853.1 ☑
      extradural 852.4 ☑
        with open intracranial wound 852.5 ☑
      subarachnoid 852.0 ☑
        with open intracranial wound 852.1 ☑
      subdural 852.2 ☑
        with open intracranial wound 852.3 ☑
    laceration 851.8 ☑
      with open intracranial wound 851.9 ☑
      brain stem 851.6 ☑
        with open intracranial wound 851.7 ☑
      cerebellum 851.6 ☑
        with open intracranial wound 851.7 ☑
      cortex (cerebral) 851.2 ☑
        with open intracranial wound 851.3 ☑
  intraocular — *see* Injury, eyeball, penetrating
  intrathoracic organs (multiple) — *see* Injury, internal, intrathoracic organs
  intrauterine — *see* Injury, internal, intrauterine

Injury

Injury — continued
- iris 921.3
  - penetrating — see Injury, eyeball, penetrating
- jaw 959.09
- jejunum — see Injury, internal, jejunum
- joint NEC 959.9
  - old or residual 718.80
    - ankle 718.87
    - elbow 718.82
    - foot 718.87
    - hand 718.84
    - hip 718.85
    - knee 718.86
    - multiple sites 718.89
    - pelvic region 718.85
    - shoulder (region) 718.81
    - specified site NEC 718.88
    - wrist 718.83
- kidney — see Injury, internal, kidney
- knee (and ankle) (and foot) (and leg, except thigh) 959.7
- labium (majus) (minus) 959.14
- labyrinth, ear 959.09
- lacrimal apparatus, gland, or sac 921.1
  - laceration 870.8
- larynx 959.09
- late effect — see Late, effects (of), injury
- leg, except thigh (and ankle) (and foot) (and knee) 959.7
  - upper or thigh 959.6
- lens, eye 921.3
  - penetrating — see Injury, eyeball, penetrating
- lid, eye — see Injury, eyelid
- lip 959.09
- liver — see Injury, internal, liver
- lobe, parietal — see Injury, intracranial
- lumbar (region) 959.19
  - plexus 953.5
- lumbosacral (region) 959.19
  - plexus 953.5
- lung — see Injury, internal, lung
- malar region 959.09
- mastoid region 959.09
- maternal, during pregnancy, affecting fetus or newborn 760.5
- maxilla 959.09
- mediastinum — see Injury, internal, mediastinum
- membrane
  - brain (see also Injury, intracranial) 854.0 ☑
  - tympanic 959.09
- meningeal artery — see Hemorrhage, brain, traumatic, subarachnoid
- meninges (cerebral) — see Injury, intracranial
- mesenteric
  - artery — see Injury, blood vessel, mesenteric, artery
  - plexus, inferior 954.1
  - vein — see Injury, blood vessel, mesenteric, vein
- mesentery — see Injury, internal, mesentery
- mesosalpinx — see Injury, internal, mesosalpinx
- middle ear 959.09
- midthoracic region 959.11
- mouth 959.09
- multiple (sites not classifiable to the same four-digit category in 959.0–959.7) 959.8
  - internal 869.0
    - with open wound into cavity 869.1
  - musculocutaneous nerve 955.4
- nail
  - finger 959.5
  - toe 959.7
- nasal (septum) (sinus) 959.09

Injury — continued
- nasopharynx 959.09
- neck (and face) 959.09
- nerve 957.9
  - abducens 951.3
  - abduscent 951.3
  - accessory 951.6
  - acoustic 951.5
  - ankle and foot 956.9
  - anterior crural, femoral 956.1
  - arm (see also Injury, nerve, upper limb) 955.9
  - auditory 951.5
  - axillary 955.0
  - brachial plexus 953.4
  - cervical sympathetic 954.0
  - cranial 951.9
    - first or olfactory 951.8
    - second or optic 950.0
    - third or oculomotor 951.0
    - fourth or trochlear 951.1
    - fifth or trigeminal 951.2
    - sixth or abducens 951.3
    - seventh or facial 951.4
    - eighth, acoustic, or auditory 951.5
    - ninth or glossopharyngeal 951.8
    - tenth, pneumogastric, or vagus 951.8
    - eleventh or accessory 951.6
    - twelfth or hypoglossal 951.7
    - newborn 767.7
  - cutaneous sensory
    - lower limb 956.4
    - upper limb 955.5
  - digital (finger) 955.6
    - toe 956.5
  - facial 951.4
    - newborn 767.5
  - femoral 956.1
  - finger 955.9
  - foot and ankle 956.9
  - forearm 955.9
  - glossopharyngeal 951.8
  - hand and wrist 955.9
  - head and neck, superficial 957.0
  - hypoglossal 951.7
  - involving several parts of body 957.8
  - leg (see also Injury, nerve, lower limb) 956.9
  - lower limb 956.9
    - multiple 956.8
    - specified site NEC 956.5
  - lumbar plexus 953.5
  - lumbosacral plexus 953.5
  - median 955.1
    - forearm 955.1
    - wrist and hand 955.1
  - multiple (in several parts of body) (sites not classifiable to the same three-digit category) 957.8
  - musculocutaneous 955.4
  - musculospiral 955.3
    - upper arm 955.3
  - oculomotor 951.0
  - olfactory 951.8
  - optic 950.0
  - pelvic girdle 956.9
    - multiple sites 956.8
    - specified site NEC 956.5
  - peripheral 957.9
    - multiple (in several regions) (sites not classifiable to the same three-digit category) 957.8
    - specified site NEC 957.1
  - peroneal 956.3
    - ankle and foot 956.3
    - lower leg 956.3
  - plantar 956.5
  - plexus 957.9
    - celiac 954.1
    - mesenteric, inferior 954.1
    - spinal 953.9

Injury — continued
- nerve — continued
  - plexus — continued
    - spinal — continued
      - brachial 953.4
      - lumbosacral 953.5
      - multiple sites 953.8
      - sympathetic NEC 954.1
  - pneumogastric 951.8
  - radial 955.3
    - wrist and hand 955.3
  - sacral plexus 953.5
  - sciatic 956.0
    - thigh 956.0
  - shoulder girdle 955.9
    - multiple 955.8
    - specified site NEC 955.7
  - specified site NEC 957.1
  - spinal 953.9
    - plexus — see Injury, nerve, plexus, spinal
    - root 953.9
      - cervical 953.0
      - dorsal 953.1
      - lumbar 953.2
      - multiple sites 953.8
      - sacral 953.3
  - splanchnic 954.1
  - sympathetic NEC 954.1
    - cervical 954.0
  - thigh 956.9
  - tibial 956.5
    - ankle and foot 956.2
    - lower leg 956.5
    - posterior 956.2
  - toe 956.9
  - trigeminal 951.2
  - trochlear 951.1
  - trunk, excluding shoulder and pelvic girdles 954.9
    - specified site NEC 954.8
    - sympathetic NEC 954.1
  - ulnar 955.2
    - forearm 955.2
    - wrist (and hand) 955.2
  - upper limb 955.9
    - multiple 955.8
    - specified site NEC 955.7
  - vagus 951.8
  - wrist and hand 955.9
- nervous system, diffuse 957.8
- nose (septum) 959.09
- obstetrical NEC 665.9 ☑
  - affecting fetus or newborn 763.89
- occipital (region) (scalp) 959.09
  - lobe (see also Injury, intracranial) 854.0 ☑
- optic 950.9
  - chiasm 950.1
  - cortex 950.3
  - nerve 950.0
  - pathways 950.2
- orbit, orbital (region) 921.2
  - penetrating 870.3
    - with foreign body 870.4
- ovary — see Injury, internal, ovary
- paint-gun — see Wound, open, by site, complicated
- palate (soft) 959.09
- pancreas — see Injury, internal, pancreas
- parathyroid (gland) 959.09
- parietal (region) (scalp) 959.09
  - lobe — see Injury, intracranial
- pelvic
  - floor 959.19
    - complicating delivery 664.1 ☑
      - affecting fetus or newborn 763.89
  - joint or ligament, complicating delivery 665.6 ☑
    - affecting fetus or newborn 763.89
  - organs (see also Injury, internal, pelvis)

Injury — continued
- pelvic — continued
  - organs (see also Injury, internal, pelvis) — continued
    - with
      - abortion — see Abortion, by type, with damage to pelvic organs
      - ectopic pregnancy (see also categories 633.0–633.9) 639.2
      - molar pregnancy (see also categories 633.0–633.9) 639.2
    - following
      - abortion 639.2
      - ectopic or molar pregnancy 639.2
    - obstetrical trauma 665.5 ☑
      - affecting fetus or newborn 763.89
- pelvis 959.19
- penis 959.14
  - fracture of corpus cavernosum 959.13
- perineum 959.14
- peritoneum — see Injury, internal, peritoneum
- periurethral tissue
  - with
    - abortion — see Abortion, by type, with damage to pelvic organs
    - ectopic pregnancy (see also categories 633.0–633.9) 639.2
    - molar pregnancy (see also categories 630–632) 639.2
  - complicating delivery 665.5 ☑
    - affecting fetus or newborn 763.89
  - following
    - abortion 639.2
    - ectopic or molar pregnancy 639.2
- phalanges
  - foot 959.7
  - hand 959.5
- pharynx 959.09
- pleura — see Injury, internal, pleura
- popliteal space 959.7
- post-cardiac surgery (syndrome) 429.4 ●
- prepuce 959.14
- prostate — see Injury, internal, prostate
- pubic region 959.19
- pudenda 959.14
- radiation NEC 990
- radioactive substance or radium NEC 990
- rectovaginal septum 959.14
- rectum — see Injury, internal, rectum
- retina 921.3
  - penetrating — see Injury, eyeball, penetrating
- retroperitoneal — see Injury, internal, retroperitoneum
- roentgen rays NEC 990
- round ligament — see Injury, internal, round ligament
- sacral (region) 959.19
  - plexus 953.5
- sacroiliac ligament NEC 959.19
- sacrum 959.19
- salivary ducts or glands 959.09
- scalp 959.09
  - due to birth trauma 767.19
  - fetus or newborn 767.19
- scapular region 959.2
- sclera 921.3
  - penetrating — see Injury, eyeball, penetrating
  - superficial 918.2
- scrotum 959.14

Index to Diseases

Injury — *continued*
  seminal vesicle — *see* Injury, internal, seminal vesicle
  shoulder (and upper arm) 959.2
  sinus
    cavernous (*see also* Injury, intracranial) 854.0 ☑
    nasal 959.09
  skeleton NEC, birth injury 767.3
  skin NEC 959.9
  skull — *see* Fracture, skull, by site
  soft tissue (of external sites) (severe) — *see* Wound, open, by site
  specified site NEC 959.8
  spermatic cord — *see* Injury, internal, spermatic cord
  spinal (cord) 952.9
    with fracture, vertebra — *see* Fracture, vertebra, by site, with spinal cord injury
    cervical (C_1-C_4) 952.00
      with
        anterior cord syndrome 952.02
        central cord syndrome 952.03
        complete lesion of cord 952.01
        incomplete lesion NEC 952.04
        posterior cord syndrome 952.04
    C_5-C_7 level 952.05
      with
        anterior cord syndrome 952.07
        central cord syndrome 952.08
        complete lesion of cord 952.06
        incomplete lesion NEC 952.09
        posterior cord syndrome 952.09
      specified type NEC 952.09
    specified type NEC 952.04
    dorsal (D_1-D_6) (T_1-T_6) (thoracic) 952.10
      with
        anterior cord syndrome 952.12
        central cord syndrome 952.13
        complete lesion of cord 952.11
        incomplete lesion NEC 952.14
        posterior cord syndrome 952.14
    D_7-D_{12} level (T_7-T_{12}) 952.15
      with
        anterior cord syndrome 952.17
        central cord syndrome 952.18
        complete lesion of cord 952.16
        incomplete lesion NEC 952.19
        posterior cord syndrome 952.19
      specified type NEC 952.19
    specified type NEC 952.14
    lumbar 952.2
    multiple sites 952.8
    nerve (root) NEC — *see* Injury, nerve, spinal, root
    plexus 953.9
      brachial 953.4
      lumbosacral 953.5
      multiple sites 953.8
    sacral 952.3
    thoracic (*see also* Injury, spinal, dorsal) 952.10
  spleen — *see* Injury, internal, spleen

Injury — *continued*
  stellate ganglion 954.1
  sternal region 959.11
  stomach — *see* Injury, internal, stomach
  subconjunctival 921.1
  subcutaneous 959.9
  subdural — *see* Injury, intracranial
  submaxillary region 959.09
  submental region 959.09
  subungual
    fingers 959.5
    toes 959.7
  superficial 919 ☑

> *Note* — Use the following fourth-digit subdivisions with categories 910–919:
>
> 0   Abrasion or friction burn without mention of infection
> 1   Abrasion or friction burn, infected
> 2   Blister without mention of infection
> 3   Blister, infected
> 4   Insect bite, nonvenomous, without mention of infection
> 5   Insect bite, nonvenomous, infected
> 6   Superficial foreign body (splinter) without major open wound and without mention of infection
> 7   Superficial foreign body (splinter) without major open wound, infected
> 8   Other and unspecified superficial injury without mention of infection
> 9   Other and unspecified superficial injury, infected
>
> *For late effects of superficial injury, see category 906.2.*

    abdomen, abdominal (muscle) (wall) (and other part(s) of trunk) 911 ☑
    ankle (and hip, knee, leg, or thigh) 916 ☑
    anus (and other part(s) of trunk) 911 ☑
    arm 913 ☑
      upper (and shoulder) 912 ☑
    auditory canal (external) (meatus) (and other part(s) of face, neck, or scalp, except eye) 910 ☑
    axilla (and upper arm) 912 ☑
    back (and other part(s) of trunk) 911 ☑
    breast (and other part(s) of trunk) 911 ☑
    brow (and other part(s) of face, neck, or scalp, except eye) 910 ☑
    buttock (and other part(s) of trunk) 911 ☑
    canthus, eye 918.0
    cheek(s) (and other part(s) of face, neck, or scalp, except eye) 910 ☑
    chest wall (and other part(s) of trunk) 911 ☑
    chin (and other part(s) of face, neck, or scalp, except eye) 910 ☑
    clitoris (and other part(s) of trunk) 911 ☑
    conjunctiva 918.2
    cornea 918.1
      due to contact lens 371.82
    costal region (and other part(s) of trunk) 911 ☑

Injury — *continued*
  superficial — *continued*
    ear(s) (auricle) (canal) (drum) (external) (and other part(s) of face, neck, or scalp, except eye) 910 ☑
    elbow (and forearm) (and wrist) 913 ☑
    epididymis (and other part(s) of trunk) 911 ☑
    epigastric region (and other part(s) of trunk) 911 ☑
    epiglottis (and other part(s) of face, neck, or scalp, except eye) 910 ☑
    eye(s) (and adnexa) NEC 918.9
    eyelid(s) (and periocular area) 918.0
    face (any part(s), except eye) (and neck or scalp) 910 ☑
    finger(s) (nail) (any) 915 ☑
    flank (and other part(s) of trunk) 911 ☑
    foot (phalanges) (and toe(s)) 917 ☑
    forearm (and elbow) (and wrist) 913 ☑
    forehead (and other part(s) of face, neck, or scalp, except eye) 910 ☑
    globe (eye) 918.9
    groin (and other part(s) of trunk) 911 ☑
    gum(s) (and other part(s) of face, neck, or scalp, except eye) 910 ☑
    hand(s) (except fingers alone) 914 ☑
    head (and other part(s) of face, neck, or scalp, except eye) 910 ☑
    heel (and foot or toe) 917 ☑
    hip (and ankle, knee, leg, or thigh) 916 ☑
    iliac region (and other part(s) of trunk) 911 ☑
    interscapular region (and other part(s) of trunk) 911 ☑
    iris 918.9
    knee (and ankle, hip, leg, or thigh) 916 ☑
    labium (majus) (minus) (and other part(s) of trunk) 911 ☑
    lacrimal (apparatus) (gland) (sac) 918.0
    leg (lower) (upper) (and ankle, hip, knee, or thigh) 916 ☑
    lip(s) (and other part(s) of face, neck, or scalp, except eye) 910 ☑
    lower extremity (except foot) 916 ☑
    lumbar region (and other part(s) of trunk) 911 ☑
    malar region (and other part(s) of face, neck, or scalp, except eye) 910 ☑
    mastoid region (and other part(s) of face, neck, or scalp, except eye) 910 ☑
    midthoracic region (and other part(s) of trunk) 911 ☑
    mouth (and other part(s) of face, neck, or scalp, except eye) 910 ☑
    multiple sites (not classifiable to the same three-digit category) 919 ☑
    nasal (septum) (and other part(s) of face, neck, or scalp, except eye) 910 ☑
    neck (and face or scalp, any part(s), except eye) 910 ☑
    nose (septum) (and other part(s) of face, neck, or scalp, except eye) 910 ☑

Injury — *continued*
  superficial — *continued*
    occipital region (and other part(s) of face, neck, or scalp, except eye) 910 ☑
    orbital region 918.0
    palate (soft) (and other part(s) of face, neck, or scalp, except eye) 910 ☑
    parietal region (and other part(s) of face, neck, or scalp, except eye) 910 ☑
    penis (and other part(s) of trunk) 911 ☑
    perineum (and other part(s) of trunk) 911 ☑
    periocular area 918.0
    pharynx (and other part(s) of face, neck, or scalp, except eye) 910 ☑
    popliteal space (and ankle, hip, leg, or thigh) 916 ☑
    prepuce (and other part(s) of trunk) 911 ☑
    pubic region (and other part(s) of trunk) 911 ☑
    pudenda (and other part(s) of trunk) 911 ☑
    sacral region (and other part(s) of trunk) 911 ☑
    salivary (ducts) (glands) (and other part(s) of face, neck, or scalp, except eye) 910 ☑
    scalp (and other part(s) of face or neck, except eye) 910 ☑
    scapular region (and upper arm) 912 ☑
    sclera 918.2
    scrotum (and other part(s) of trunk) 911 ☑
    shoulder (and upper arm) 912 ☑
    skin NEC 919 ☑
    specified site(s) NEC 919 ☑
    sternal region (and other part(s) of trunk) 911 ☑
    subconjunctival 918.2
    subcutaneous NEC 919 ☑
    submaxillary region (and other part(s) of face, neck, or scalp, except eye) 910 ☑
    submental region (and other part(s) of face, neck, or scalp, except eye) 910 ☑
    supraclavicular fossa (and other part(s) of face, neck, or scalp, except eye) 910 ☑
    supraorbital 918.0
    temple (and other part(s) of face, neck, or scalp, except eye) 910 ☑
    temporal region (and other part(s) of face, neck, or scalp, except eye) 910 ☑
    testis (and other part(s) of trunk) 911 ☑
    thigh (and ankle, hip, knee, or leg) 916 ☑
    thorax, thoracic (external) (and other part(s) of trunk) 911 ☑
    throat (and other part(s) of face, neck, or scalp, except eye) 910 ☑
    thumb(s) (nail) 915 ☑
    toe(s) (nail) (subungual) (and foot) 917 ☑
    tongue (and other part(s) of face, neck, or scalp, except eye) 910 ☑
    tooth, teeth (*see also* Abrasion, dental) 521.20
    trunk (any part(s)) 911 ☑
    tunica vaginalis 959.14

Injury

Injury — *continued*
- superficial — *continued*
  - tympanum, tympanic membrane (and other part(s) of face, neck, or scalp, except eye) 910 ☑
  - upper extremity NEC 913 ☑
  - uvula (and other part(s) of face, neck, or scalp, except eye) 910 ☑
  - vagina (and other part(s) of trunk) 911 ☑
  - vulva (and other part(s) of trunk) 911 ☑
  - wrist (and elbow) (and forearm) 913 ☑
- supraclavicular fossa 959.19
- supraorbital 959.09
- surgical complication (external or internal site) 998.2
- symphysis pubis 959.19
  - complicating delivery 665.6 ☑
    - affecting fetus or newborn 763.89
- temple 959.09
- temporal region 959.09
- testis 959.14
- thigh (and hip) 959.6
- thorax, thoracic (external) 959.11
  - cavity — *see* Injury, internal, thorax
  - internal — *see* Injury, internal, intrathoracic organs
- throat 959.09
- thumb(s) (nail) 959.5
- thymus — *see* Injury, internal, thymus
- thyroid (gland) 959.09
- toe (nail) (any) 959.7
- tongue 959.09
- tonsil 959.09
- tooth NEC 873.63
  - complicated 873.73
- trachea — *see* Injury, internal, trachea
- trunk 959.19
- tunica vaginalis 959.14
- tympanum, tympanic membrane 959.09
- ultraviolet rays NEC 990
- ureter — *see* Injury, internal, ureter
- urethra (sphincter) — *see* Injury, internal, urethra
- uterus — *see* Injury, internal, uterus
- uvula 959.09
- vagina 959.14
- vascular — *see* Injury, blood vessel
- vas deferens — *see* Injury, internal, vas deferens
- vein (*see also* Injury, blood vessel, by site) 904.9
- vena cava
  - inferior 902.10
  - superior 901.2
- vesical (sphincter) — *see* Injury, internal, vesical
- viscera (abdominal) — *see* Injury, internal, viscera
  - with fracture, pelvis — *see* Fracture, pelvis
- visual 950.9
  - cortex 950.3
- vitreous (humor) 871.2
- vulva 959.14
- whiplash (cervical spine) 847.0
- wringer — *see* Crush, by site
- wrist (and elbow) (and forearm) 959.3
- x-ray NEC 990

Inoculation — *see also* Vaccination
- complication or reaction — *see* Complication, vaccination

Insanity, insane — *see also* Psychosis 298.9
- adolescent (*see also* Schizophrenia) 295.9 ☑

Insanity, insane — *see also* Psychosis — *continued*
- alternating (*see also* Psychosis, affective, circular) 296.7
- confusional 298.9
  - acute 293.0
  - subacute 293.1
- delusional 298.9
- paralysis, general 094.1
  - progressive 094.1
- paresis, general 094.1
- senile 290.20

Insect
- bite — *see* Injury, superficial, by site
- venomous, poisoning by 989.5

Insemination, artificial V26.1

Insensitivity
- androgen 259.5
- partial 259.5

Insertion
- cord (umbilical) lateral or velamentous 663.8 ☑
  - affecting fetus or newborn 762.6
- intrauterine contraceptive device V25.1
- placenta, vicious — *see* Placenta, previa
- subdermal implantable contraceptive V25.5
- velamentous, umbilical cord 663.8 ☑
  - affecting fetus or newborn 762.6

Insolation 992.0
- meaning sunstroke 992.0

Insomnia, unspecified 780.52
- with sleep apnea, unspecified 780.51
- adjustment 307.41
- alcohol induced 291.82
- behavioral, of childhood V69.5
- drug induced 292.85
- due to
  - medical condition classified elsewhere 327.01
  - mental disorder 327.02
- idiopathic 307.42
- nonorganic origin 307.41
  - persistent (primary) 307.42
  - transient 307.41
- organic 327.00
  - other 327.09
- paradoxical 307.42
- primary 307.42
- psychophysiological 307.42
- subjective complaint 307.49

Inspiration
- food or foreign body (*see also* Asphyxia, food or foreign body) 933.1
- mucus (*see also* Asphyxia, mucus) 933.1

Inspissated bile syndrome, newborn 774.4

Instability
- detrusor 596.59
- emotional (excessive) 301.3
- joint (posttraumatic) 718.80
  - ankle 718.87
  - elbow 718.82
  - foot 718.87
  - hand 718.84
  - hip 718.85
  - knee 718.86
  - lumbosacral 724.6
  - multiple sites 718.89
  - pelvic region 718.85
  - sacroiliac 724.6
  - shoulder (region) 718.81
  - specified site NEC 718.88
  - wrist 718.83
- lumbosacral 724.6
- nervous 301.89
- personality (emotional) 301.59
- thyroid, paroxysmal 242.9 ☑
- urethral 599.83
- vasomotor 780.2

Insufficiency, insufficient
- accommodation 367.4
- adrenal (gland) (acute) (chronic) 255.4

Insufficiency, insufficient — *continued*
- adrenal — *continued*
  - medulla 255.5
  - primary 255.4
  - specified site NEC 255.5
- adrenocortical 255.4
- anterior ▶(occlusal)◀ guidance 524.54
- anus 569.49
- aortic (valve) 424.1
  - with
    - mitral (valve) disease 396.1
      - insufficiency, incompetence, or regurgitation 396.1
      - stenosis or obstruction 396.1
    - stenosis or obstruction 424.1
      - with mitral (valve) disease 396.8
  - congenital 746.4
  - rheumatic 395.1
    - with
      - mitral (valve) disease 396.1
        - insufficiency, incompetence, or regurgitation 396.3
        - stenosis or obstruction 396.1
      - stenosis or obstruction 395.2
        - with mitral (valve) disease 396.8
  - specified cause NEC 424.1
  - syphilitic 093.22
- arterial 447.1
  - basilar artery 435.0
  - carotid artery 435.8
  - cerebral 437.1
  - coronary (acute or subacute) 411.89
  - mesenteric 557.1
  - peripheral 443.9
  - precerebral 435.9
  - vertebral artery 435.1
  - vertebrobasilar 435.3
- arteriovenous 459.9
- basilar artery 435.0
- biliary 575.8
- cardiac (*see also* Insufficiency, myocardial) 428.0
  - complicating surgery 997.1
  - due to presence of (cardiac) prosthesis 429.4
  - postoperative 997.1
    - long-term effect of cardiac surgery 429.4
  - specified during or due to a procedure 997.1
    - long-term effect of cardiac surgery 429.4
- cardiorenal (*see also* Hypertension, cardiorenal) 404.90
- cardiovascular (*see also* Disease, cardiovascular) 429.2
  - renal (*see also* Hypertension, cardiorenal) 404.90
- carotid artery 435.8
- cerebral (vascular) 437.9
- cerebrovascular 437.9
  - with transient focal neurological signs and symptoms 435.9
  - acute 437.1
    - with transient focal neurological signs and symptoms 435.9
- circulatory NEC 459.9
  - fetus or newborn 779.89
- convergence 378.83
- coronary (acute or subacute) 411.89
  - chronic or with a stated duration of over 8 weeks 414.8
- corticoadrenal 255.4
- dietary 269.9
- divergence 378.85
- food 994.2
- gastroesophageal 530.89
- gonadal
  - ovary 256.39

Insufficiency, insufficient — *continued*
- gonadal — *continued*
  - testis 257.2
- gonadotropic hormone secretion 253.4
- heart (*see also* Insufficiency, myocardial)
  - fetus or newborn 779.89
  - valve (*see also* Endocarditis) 424.90
  - congenital NEC 746.89
- hepatic 573.8
- idiopathic autonomic 333.0
- interocclusal distance of teeth (ridge) 524.36
- kidney
  - acute 593.9
  - chronic 585.9
- labyrinth, labyrinthine (function) 386.53
  - bilateral 386.54
  - unilateral 386.53
- lacrimal 375.15
- liver 573.8
- lung (acute) (*see also* Insufficiency, pulmonary) 518.82
  - following trauma, surgery, or shock 518.5
  - newborn 770.89
- mental (congenital) (*see also* Retardation, mental) 319
- mesenteric 557.1
- mitral (valve) 424.0
  - with
    - aortic (valve) disease 396.3
      - insufficiency, incompetence, or regurgitation 396.3
      - stenosis or obstruction 396.2
    - obstruction or stenosis 394.2
      - with aortic valve disease 396.8
  - congenital 746.6
  - rheumatic 394.1
    - with
      - aortic (valve) disease 396.3
        - insufficiency, incompetence, or regurgitation 396.3
        - stenosis or obstruction 396.2
      - obstruction or stenosis 394.2
        - with aortic valve disease 396.8
    - active or acute 391.1
      - with chorea, rheumatic (Sydenham's) 392.0
  - specified cause, except rheumatic 424.0
- muscle
  - heart — *see* Insufficiency, myocardial
  - ocular (*see also* Strabismus) 378.9
- myocardial, myocardium (with arteriosclerosis) 428.0
  - with rheumatic fever (conditions classifiable to 390)
    - active, acute, or subacute 391.2
      - with chorea 392.0
    - inactive or quiescent (with chorea) 398.0
  - congenital 746.89
  - due to presence of (cardiac) prosthesis 429.4
  - fetus or newborn 779.89
  - following cardiac surgery 429.4
  - hypertensive (*see also* Hypertension, heart) 402.91
    - benign 402.11
    - malignant 402.01
  - postoperative 997.1
    - long-term effect of cardiac surgery 429.4
  - rheumatic 398.0
    - active, acute, or subacute 391.2
      - with chorea (Sydenham's) 392.0

Index to Diseases

Insufficiency, insufficient — *continued*
- myocardial, myocardium — *continued*
  - syphilitic 093.82
- nourishment 994.2
- organic 799.89
- ovary 256.39
  - postablative 256.2
- pancreatic 577.8
- parathyroid (gland) 252.1
- peripheral vascular (arterial) 443.9
- pituitary (anterior) 253.2
  - posterior 253.5
- placental — *see* Placenta, insufficiency
- platelets 287.5
- prenatal care in current pregnancy V23.7
- progressive pluriglandular 258.9
- pseudocholinesterase 289.89
- pulmonary (acute) 518.82
  - following
    - shock 518.5
    - surgery 518.5
    - trauma 518.5
  - newborn 770.89
  - valve (*see also* Endocarditis, pulmonary) 424.3
    - congenital 746.09
- pyloric 537.0
- renal 593.9 ▲
  - acute 593.9
  - chronic 585.9
  - due to a procedure 997.5
- respiratory 786.09
  - acute 518.82
    - following shock, surgery, or trauma 518.5
  - newborn 770.89
- rotation — *see* Malrotation
- suprarenal 255.4
  - medulla 255.5
- tarso-orbital fascia, congenital 743.66
- tear film 375.15
- testis 257.2
- thyroid (gland) (acquired) (*see also* Hypothyroidism)
  - congenital 243
- tricuspid (*see also* Endocarditis, tricuspid) 397.0
  - congenital 746.89
  - syphilitic 093.23
- urethral sphincter 599.84
- valve, valvular (heart) (*see also* Endocarditis) 424.90
- vascular 459.9
  - intestine NEC 557.9
  - mesenteric 557.1
  - peripheral 443.9
  - renal (*see also* Hypertension, kidney) 403.90
- velopharyngeal
  - acquired 528.9
  - congenital 750.29
- venous (peripheral) 459.81
- ventricular — *see* Insufficiency, myocardial
- vertebral artery 435.1
- vertebrobasilar artery 435.3
- weight gain during pregnancy 646.8 ☑
- zinc 269.3

Insufflation
- fallopian
  - fertility testing V26.21
  - following sterilization reversal V26.22
- meconium 770.11
  - with respiratory symptoms 770.12

Insular — *see* condition

Insulinoma (M8151/0)
- malignant (M8151/3)
  - pancreas 157.4
  - specified site — *see* Neoplasm, by site, malignant
  - unspecified site 157.4
- pancreas 211.7

Insulinoma — *continued*
- specified site — *see* Neoplasm, by site, benign
- unspecified site 211.7

Insuloma — *see* Insulinoma

Insult
- brain 437.9
  - acute 436
- cerebral 437.9
  - acute 436
- cerebrovascular 437.9
  - acute 436
- vascular NEC 437.9

Insurance examination (certification) V70.3

Intemperance — *see also* Alcoholism 303.9 ☑

Interception of pregnancy (menstrual extraction) V25.3

Interference
- balancing side 524.56 ●
- non-working side 524.56 ●

Intermenstrual
- bleeding 626.6
  - irregular 626.6
  - regular 626.5
- hemorrhage 626.6
  - irregular 626.6
  - regular 626.5
- pain(s) 625.2

Intermittent — *see* condition
Internal — *see* condition
Interproximal wear 521.10

Interruption
- aortic arch 747.11
- bundle of His 426.50
- fallopian tube (for sterilization) V25.2
- phase-shift, sleep cycle 307.45
- repeated REM-sleep 307.48
- sleep
  - due to perceived environmental disturbances 307.48
  - phase-shift, of 24-hour sleep-wake cycle 307.45
  - repeated REM-sleep type 307.48
- vas deferens (for sterilization) V25.2

Intersexuality 752.7
Interstitial — *see* condition
Intertrigo 695.89
- labialis 528.5

Intervertebral disc — *see* condition
Intestine, intestinal — *see also* condition
- flu 487.8

Intolerance
- carbohydrate NEC 579.8
- cardiovascular exercise, with pain (at rest) (with less than ordinary activity) (with ordinary activity) V47.2
- cold 780.99
- dissachararide (hereditary) 271.3
- drug
  - correct substance properly administered 995.27 ▲
  - wrong substance given or taken in error 977.9
  - specified drug — *see* Table of Drugs and Chemicals
- effort 306.2
- fat NEC 579.8
- foods NEC 579.8
- fructose (hereditary) 271.2
- glucose (-galactose) (congenital) 271.3
- gluten 579.0
- lactose (hereditary) (infantile) 271.3
- lysine (congenital) 270.7
- milk NEC 579.8
- protein (familial) 270.7
- starch NEC 579.8
- sucrose (-isomaltose) (congenital) 271.3

Intoxicated NEC — *see also* Alcoholism 305.0 ☑

Intoxication
- acid 276.2
- acute
  - alcoholic 305.0 ☑
    - with alcoholism 303.0 ☑
    - hangover effects 305.0 ☑
  - caffeine 305.9 ☑
  - hallucinogenic (*see also* Abuse, drugs, nondependent) 305.3 ☑
- alcohol (acute) 305.0 ☑
  - with alcoholism 303.0 ☑
  - hangover effects 305.0 ☑
  - idiosyncratic 291.4
  - pathological 291.4
- alimentary canal 558.2
- ammonia (hepatic) 572.2
- caffeine 305.9 ☑
- chemical (*see also* Table of Drugs and Chemicals)
  - via placenta or breast milk 760.70
    - alcohol 760.71
    - anticonvulsants
    - antifungals
    - anti-infective agents 760.74
    - antimetabolics
    - cocaine 760.75
    - "crack" 760.75
    - hallucinogenic agents NEC 760.73
    - medicinal agents NEC 760.79
    - narcotics 760.72
    - obstetric anesthetic or analgesic drug 763.5
    - specified agent NEC 760.79
    - suspected, affecting management of pregnancy 655.5 ☑
- cocaine, through placenta or breast milk 760.75
- delirium
  - alcohol 291.0
  - drug 292.81
- drug 292.89
  - with delirium 292.81
  - correct substance properly administered (*see also* Allergy, drug) 995.27 ▲
  - newborn 779.4
  - obstetric anesthetic or sedation 668.9 ☑
  - affecting fetus or newborn 763.5
  - overdose or wrong substance given or taken — *see* Table of Drugs and Chemicals
  - pathologic 292.2
  - specific to newborn 779.4
  - via placenta or breast milk 760.70
    - alcohol 760.71
    - anticonvulsants 760.77
    - antifungals 760.74
    - anti-infective agents 760.74
    - antimetabolics 760.78
    - cocaine 760.75
    - "crack" 760.75
    - hallucinogenic agents 760.73
    - medicinal agents NEC 760.79
    - narcotics 760.72
    - obstetric anesthetic or analgesic drug 763.5
    - specified agent NEC 760.79
    - suspected, affecting management of pregnancy 655.5 ☑
- enteric — *see* Intoxication, intestinal
- fetus or newborn, via placenta or breast milk 760.70
  - alcohol 760.71
  - anticonvulsants 760.77
  - antifungals 760.74
  - anti-infective agents 760.74
  - antimetabolics 760.78
  - cocaine 760.75
  - "crack" 760.75
  - hallucinogenic agents 760.73
  - medicinal agents NEC 760.79

Inversion

Intoxication — *continued*
- fetus or newborn, via placenta or breast milk — *continued*
  - narcotics 760.72
  - obstetric anesthetic or analgesic drug 763.5
  - specified agent NEC 760.79
  - suspected, affecting management of pregnancy 655.5 ☑
- food — *see* Poisoning, food
- gastrointestinal 558.2
- hallucinogenic (acute) 305.3 ☑
- hepatocerebral 572.2
- idiosyncratic alcohol 291.4
- intestinal 569.9
  - due to putrefaction of food 005.9
- methyl alcohol (*see also* Alcoholism) 305.0 ☑
  - with alcoholism 303.0 ☑
- pathologic 291.4
  - drug 292.2
- potassium (K) 276.7
- septic
  - with
    - abortion — *see* Abortion, by type, with sepsis
    - ectopic pregnancy (*see also* categories 633.0–633.9) 639.0
    - molar pregnancy (*see also* categories 630–632) 639.0
  - during labor 659.3 ☑
  - following
    - abortion 639.0
    - ectopic or molar pregnancy 639.0
  - generalized — *see* Septicemia
  - puerperal, postpartum, childbirth 670.0 ☑
- serum (prophylactic) (therapeutic) 999.5
- uremic — *see* Uremia
- water 276.6

Intracranial — *see* condition
Intrahepatic gallbladder 751.69
Intraligamentous — *see also* condition
- pregnancy — *see* Pregnancy, cornual

Intraocular — *see also* condition
- sepsis 360.00

Intrathoracic — *see also* condition
- kidney 753.3
- stomach — *see* Hernia, diaphragm

Intrauterine contraceptive device
- checking V25.42
- insertion V25.1
- in situ V45.51
- management V25.42
- prescription V25.02
- repeat V25.42
- reinsertion V25.42
- removal V25.42

Intraventricular — *see* condition
Intrinsic deformity — *see* Deformity
Intruded tooth 524.34 ●
Intrusion, repetitive, of sleep (due to environmental disturbances) (with atypical polysomnographic features) 307.48

Intumescent, lens (eye) NEC 366.9
- senile 366.12

Intussusception (colon) (enteric) (intestine) (rectum) 560.0
- appendix 543.9
- congenital 751.5
- fallopian tube 620.8
- ileocecal 560.0
- ileocolic 560.0
- ureter (with obstruction) 593.4

Invagination
- basilar 756.0
- colon or intestine 560.0

Invalid (since birth) 799.89
Invalidism (chronic) 799.89
Inversion
- albumin-globulin (A-G) ratio 273.8
- bladder 596.8

Inversion

Inversion — *continued*
- cecum (*see also* Intussusception) 560.0
- cervix 622.8
- nipple 611.79
  - congenital 757.6
  - puerperal, postpartum 676.3 ☑
- optic papilla 743.57
- organ or site, congenital NEC — *see* Anomaly, specified type NEC
- sleep rhythm 327.39
  - nonorganic origin 307.45
- testis (congenital) 752.51
- uterus (postinfectional) (postpartal, old) 621.7
  - chronic 621.7
  - complicating delivery 665.2 ☑
    - affecting fetus or newborn 763.89
- vagina — *see* Prolapse, vagina

Investigation
- allergens V72.7
- clinical research (control) (normal comparison) (participant) V70.7

Inviability — *see* Immaturity

Involuntary movement, abnormal 781.0

Involution, involutional — *see also* condition
- breast, cystic or fibrocystic 610.1
- depression (*see also* Psychosis, affective) 296.2 ☑
  - recurrent episode 296.3 ☑
  - single episode 296.2 ☑
- melancholia (*see also* Psychosis, affective) 296.2 ☑
  - recurrent episode 296.3 ☑
  - single episode 296.2 ☑
- ovary, senile 620.3
- paranoid state (reaction) 297.2
- paraphrenia (climacteric) (menopause) 297.2
- psychosis 298.8
- thymus failure 254.8

IQ
- under 20 318.2
- 20-34 318.1
- 35-49 318.0
- 50-70 317

IRDS 769
Irideremia 743.45
Iridis rubeosis 364.42
- diabetic 250.5 ☑ *[364.42]*

Iridochoroiditis (panuveitis) 360.12
Iridocyclitis NEC 364.3
- acute 364.00
  - primary 364.01
  - recurrent 364.02
- chronic 364.10
  - in
    - lepromatous leprosy 030.0 *[364.11]*
    - sarcoidosis 135 *[364.11]*
    - tuberculosis (*see also* Tuberculosis) 017.3 ☑ *[364.11]*
- due to allergy 364.04
- endogenous 364.01
- gonococcal 098.41
- granulomatous 364.10
- herpetic (simplex) 054.44
  - zoster 053.22
- hypopyon 364.05
- lens induced 364.23
- nongranulomatous 364.00
- primary 364.01
- recurrent 364.02
- rheumatic 364.10
- secondary 364.04
  - infectious 364.03
  - noninfectious 364.04
- subacute 364.00
  - primary 364.01
  - recurrent 364.02
- sympathetic 360.11
- syphilitic (secondary) 091.52

Iridocyclitis — *continued*
- tuberculous (chronic) (*see also* Tuberculosis) 017.3 ☑ *[364.11]*

Iridocyclochoroiditis (panuveitis) 360.12
Iridodialysis 364.76
Iridodonesis 364.8
Iridoplegia (complete) (partial) (reflex) 379.49
Iridoschisis 364.52
Iris — *see* condition
Iritis 364.3
- acute 364.00
  - primary 364.01
  - recurrent 364.02
- chronic 364.10
  - in
    - sarcoidosis 135 *[364.11]*
    - tuberculosis (*see also* Tuberculosis) 017.3 ☑ *[364.11]*
- diabetic 250.5 ☑ *[364.42]*
- due to
  - allergy 364.04
  - herpes simplex 054.44
  - leprosy 030.0 *[364.11]*
- endogenous 364.01
- gonococcal 098.41
- gouty 274.89 *[364.11]*
- granulomatous 364.10
- hypopyon 364.05
- lens induced 364.23
- nongranulomatous 364.00
- papulosa 095.8 *[364.11]*
- primary 364.01
- recurrent 364.02
- rheumatic 364.10
- secondary 364.04
  - infectious 364.03
  - noninfectious 364.04
- subacute 364.00
  - primary 364.01
  - recurrent 364.02
- sympathetic 360.11
- syphilitic (secondary) 091.52
  - congenital 090.0 *[364.11]*
  - late 095.8 *[364.11]*
- tuberculous (*see also* Tuberculosis) 017.3 ☑ *[364.11]*
- uratic 274.89 *[364.11]*

Iron
- deficiency anemia 280.9
- metabolism disease 275.0
- storage disease 275.0

Iron-miners' lung 503
Irradiated enamel (tooth, teeth) 521.89 ▲

Irradiation
- burn — *see* Burn, by site
- effects, adverse 990

Irreducible, irreducibility — *see* condition

Irregular, irregularity
- action, heart 427.9
- alveolar process 525.8
- bleeding NEC 626.4
- breathing 786.09
- colon 569.89
- contour of cornea 743.41
  - acquired 371.70
- dentin in pulp 522.3
- eye movements NEC 379.59
- menstruation (cause unknown) 626.4
- periods 626.4
- prostate 602.9
- pupil 364.75
- respiratory 786.09
- septum (nasal) 470
- shape, organ or site, congenital NEC — *see* Distortion
- sleep-wake rhythm (non-24-hour) 327.39
  - nonorganic origin 307.45
- vertebra 733.99

Irritability (nervous) 799.2
- bladder 596.8
  - neurogenic 596.54

Irritability — *continued*
- bladder — *continued*
  - neurogenic — *continued*
    - with cauda equina syndrome 344.61
- bowel (syndrome) 564.1
- bronchial (*see also* Bronchitis) 490
- cerebral, newborn 779.1
- colon 564.1
  - psychogenic 306.4
- duodenum 564.89
- heart (psychogenic) 306.2
- ileum 564.89
- jejunum 564.89
- myocardium 306.2
- rectum 564.89
- stomach 536.9
  - psychogenic 306.4
- sympathetic (nervous system) (*see also* Neuropathy, peripheral, autonomic) 337.9
- urethra 599.84
- ventricular (heart) (psychogenic) 306.2

Irritable — *see* Irritability

Irritation
- anus 569.49
- axillary nerve 353.0
- bladder 596.8
- brachial plexus 353.0
- brain (traumatic) (*see also* Injury, intracranial) 854.0 ☑
  - nontraumatic — *see* Encephalitis
- bronchial (*see also* Bronchitis) 490
- cerebral (traumatic) (*see also* Injury, intracranial) 854.0 ☑
  - nontraumatic — *see* Encephalitis
- cervical plexus 353.2
- cervix (*see also* Cervicitis) 616.0
- choroid, sympathetic 360.11
- cranial nerve — *see* Disorder, nerve, cranial
- digestive tract 536.9
  - psychogenic 306.4
- gastric 536.9
  - psychogenic 306.4
- gastrointestinal (tract) 536.9
  - functional 536.9
  - psychogenic 306.4
- globe, sympathetic 360.11
- intestinal (bowel) 564.9
- labyrinth 386.50
- lumbosacral plexus 353.1
- meninges (traumatic) (*see also* Injury, intracranial) 854.0 ☑
  - nontraumatic — *see* Meningitis
- myocardium 306.2
- nerve — *see* Disorder, nerve
- nervous 799.2
- nose 478.19 ▲
- penis 607.89
- perineum 709.9
- peripheral
  - autonomic nervous system (*see also* Neuropathy, peripheral, autonomic) 337.9
  - nerve — *see* Disorder, nerve
- peritoneum (*see also* Peritonitis) 567.9
- pharynx 478.29
- plantar nerve 355.6
- spinal (cord) (traumatic) (*see also* Injury, spinal, by site)
  - nerve (*see also* Disorder, nerve)
    - root NEC 724.9
    - traumatic — *see* Injury, nerve, spinal
  - nontraumatic — *see* Myelitis
- stomach 536.9
  - psychogenic 306.4
- sympathetic nerve NEC (*see also* Neuropathy, peripheral, autonomic) 337.9
- ulnar nerve 354.2
- vagina 623.9

Isambert's disease 012.3 ☑
Ischemia, ischemic 459.9

Ischemia, ischemic — *continued*
- basilar artery (with transient neurologic deficit) 435.0
- bone NEC 733.40
- bowel (transient) 557.9
  - acute 557.0
  - chronic 557.1
  - due to mesenteric artery insufficiency 557.1
- brain (*see also* Ischemia, cerebral)
  - recurrent focal 435.9
- cardiac (*see also* Ischemia, heart) 414.9
- cardiomyopathy 414.8
- carotid artery (with transient neurologic deficit) 435.8
- cerebral (chronic) (generalized) 437.1
  - arteriosclerotic 437.0
  - intermittent (with transient neurologic deficit) 435.9
  - newborn 779.2 ●
  - puerperal, postpartum, childbirth 674.0 ☑
  - recurrent focal (with transient neurologic deficit) 435.9
  - transient (with transient neurologic deficit) 435.9
- colon 557.9
  - acute 557.0
  - chronic 557.1
  - due to mesenteric artery insufficiency 557.1
- coronary (chronic) (*see also* Ischemia, heart) 414.9
- heart (chronic or with a stated duration of over 8 weeks) 414.9
  - acute with a stated duration of 8 weeks or less (*see also* Infarct, myocardium) 410.9 ☑
  - without myocardial infarction 411.89
    - with coronary (artery) occlusion 411.81
  - subacute 411.89
- intestine (transient) 557.9
  - acute 557.0
  - chronic 557.1
  - due to mesenteric artery insufficiency 557.1
- kidney 593.81
- labyrinth 386.50
- muscles, leg 728.89
- myocardium, myocardial (chronic or with a stated duration of over 8 weeks) 414.8
  - acute (*see also* Infarct, myocardium) 410.9 ☑
  - without myocardial infarction 411.89
    - with coronary (artery) occlusion 411.81
- renal 593.81
- retina, retinal 362.84
- small bowel 557.9
  - acute 557.0
  - chronic 557.1
  - due to mesenteric artery insufficiency 557.1
- spinal cord 336.1
- subendocardial (*see also* Insufficiency, coronary) 411.89
- vertebral artery (with transient neurologic deficit) 435.1

Ischialgia — *see also* Sciatica 724.3
Ischiopagus 759.4
Ischium, ischial — *see* condition
Ischomenia 626.8
Ischuria 788.5
Iselin's disease or osteochondrosis 732.5

Islands of
- parotid tissue in
  - lymph nodes 750.26
  - neck structures 750.26
- submaxillary glands in fascia 750.26

Index to Diseases

Islands of — *continued*
  submaxillary glands in — *continued*
    lymph nodes 750.26
    neck muscles 750.26
Islet cell tumor, pancreas (M8150/0) 211.7
Isoimmunization NEC — *see also* Incompatibility 656.2 ☑
  fetus or newborn 773.2
    ABO blood groups 773.1
    Rhesus (Rh) factor 773.0
Isolation V07.0
  social V62.4
Isosporosis 007.2
Issue
  medical certificate NEC V68.0
    cause of death V68.0
    fitness V68.0

Issue — *continued*
  medical certificate — *continued*
    incapacity V68.0
  repeat prescription NEC V68.1
    appliance V68.1
    contraceptive V25.40
      device NEC V25.49
        intrauterine V25.42
        specified type NEC V25.49
      pill V25.41
    glasses V68.1
    medicinal substance V68.1
Itch — *see also* Pruritus 698.9
  bakers' 692.89
  barbers' 110.0
  bricklayers' 692.89
  cheese 133.8
  clam diggers' 120.3
  coolie 126.9

Itch — *see also* Pruritus — *continued*
  copra 133.8
  Cuban 050.1
  dew 126.9
  dhobie 110.3
  eye 379.99
  filarial (*see also* Infestation, filarial) 125.9
  grain 133.8
  grocers' 133.8
  ground 126.9
  harvest 133.8
  jock 110.3
  Malabar 110.9
    beard 110.0
    foot 110.4
    scalp 110.0
  meaning scabies 133.0
  Norwegian 133.0

Itch — *see also* Pruritus — *continued*
  perianal 698.0
  poultrymen's 133.8
  sarcoptic 133.0
  scrub 134.1
  seven year V61.10
    meaning scabies 133.0
  straw 133.8
  swimmers' 120.3
  washerwoman's 692.4
  water 120.3
  winter 698.8
Itsenko-Cushing syndrome (pituitary basophilism) 255.0
Ivemark's syndrome (asplenia with congenital heart disease) 759.0
Ivory bones 756.52
Ixodes 134.8
Ixodiasis 134.8

Index to Diseases

J

Jaccoud's nodular fibrositis, chronic (Jaccoud's syndrome) 714.4
Jackson's
 membrane 751.4
 paralysis or syndrome 344.89
 veil 751.4
Jacksonian
 epilepsy (see also Epilepsy) 345.5 ☑
 seizures (focal) (see also Epilepsy) 345.5 ☑
Jacob's ulcer (M8090/3) — see Neoplasm, skin, malignant, by site
Jacquet's dermatitis (diaper dermatitis) 691.0
Jadassohn's
 blue nevus (M8780/0) — see Neoplasm, skin, benign
 disease (maculopapular erythroderma) 696.2
 intraepidermal epithelioma (M8096/0) — see Neoplasm, skin, benign
Jadassohn-Lewandowski syndrome (pachyonychia congenita) 757.5
Jadassohn-Pellizari's disease (anetoderma) 701.3
Jadassohn-Tièche nevus (M8780/0) — see Neoplasm, skin, benign
Jaffe-Lichtenstein (-Uehlinger) syndrome 252.01
Jahnke's syndrome (encephalocutaneous angiomatosis) 759.6
Jakob-Creutzfeldt disease (syndrome) (new variant) 046.1
 with dementia
  with behavioral disturbance 046.1 [294.11]
  without behavioral disturbance 046.1 [294.10]
Jaksch (-Luzet) disease or syndrome (pseudoleukemia infantum) 285.8
Jamaican
 neuropathy 349.82
 paraplegic tropical ataxic-spastic syndrome 349.82
Janet's disease (psychasthenia) 300.89
Janiceps 759.4
Jansky-Bielschowsky amaurotic familial idiocy 330.1
Japanese
 B type encephalitis 062.0
 river fever 081.2
 seven-day fever 100.89
Jaundice (yellow) 782.4
 acholuric (familial) (splenomegalic) (see also Spherocytosis) 282.0
 acquired 283.9
 breast milk 774.39
 catarrhal (acute) 070.1
  with hepatic coma 070.0
  chronic 571.9
  epidemic — see Jaundice, epidemic
 cholestatic (benign) 782.4
 chronic idiopathic 277.4
 epidemic (catarrhal) 070.1
  with hepatic coma 070.0
   leptospiral 100.0
   spirochetal 100.0
 febrile (acute) 070.1
  with hepatic coma 070.0
   leptospiral 100.0
   spirochetal 100.0
 fetus or newborn 774.6
  due to or associated with
   ABO
    absence or deficiency of enzyme system for bilirubin conjugation (congenital) 774.39
    antibodies 773.1
    blood group incompatibility NEC 773.2
    breast milk inhibitors to conjugation 774.39
    associated with preterm delivery 774.2
    bruising 774.1

Jaundice — continued
 fetus or newborn — continued
  due to or associated with — continued
   Crigler-Najjar syndrome 277.4 [774.31]
   delayed conjugation 774.30
    associated with preterm delivery 774.2
   development 774.39
   drugs or toxins transmitted from mother 774.1
   G-6-PD deficiency 282.2 [774.0]
   galactosemia 271.1 [774.5]
   Gilbert's syndrome 277.4 [774.31]
   hepatocellular damage 774.4
   hereditary hemolytic anemia (see also Anemia, hemolytic) 282.9 [774.0]
   hypothyroidism, congenital 243 [774.31]
   incompatibility, maternal/fetal NEC 773.2
   incompatibility, maternal/fetal 773.1
   infection 774.1
   inspissated bile syndrome 774.4
   isoimmunization NEC 773.2
   isoimmunization 773.1
   mucoviscidosis 277.01 [774.5]
   obliteration of bile duct, congenital 751.61 [774.5]
   polycythemia 774.1
   preterm delivery 774.2
   red cell defect 282.9 [774.0]
   Rh
    antibodies 773.0
    incompatibility, maternal/fetal 773.0
    isoimmunization 773.0
   spherocytosis (congenital) 282.0 [774.0]
   swallowed maternal blood 774.1
  physiological NEC 774.6
  from injection, inoculation, infusion, or transfusion (blood) (plasma) (serum) (other substance) (onset within 8 months after administration) — see Hepatitis, viral
  Gilbert's (familial nonhemolytic) 277.4
  hematogenous 283.9
  hemolytic (acquired) 283.9
   congenital (see also Spherocytosis) 282.0
  hemorrhagic (acute) 100.0
   leptospiral 100.0
   newborn 776.0
   spirochetal 100.0
  hepatocellular 573.8
  homologous (serum) — see Hepatitis, viral
  idiopathic, chronic 277.4
  infectious (acute) (subacute) 070.1
   with hepatic coma 070.0
    leptospiral 100.0
    spirochetal 100.0
   leptospiral 100.0
  malignant (see also Necrosis, liver) 570
  newborn (physiological) (see also Jaundice, fetus or newborn) 774.6
  nonhemolytic, congenital familial (Gilbert's) 277.4
  nuclear, newborn (see also Kernicterus of newborn) 774.7
  obstructive NEC (see also Obstruction, biliary) 576.8
  postimmunization — see Hepatitis, viral
  posttransfusion — see Hepatitis, viral
  regurgitation (see also Obstruction, biliary) 576.8

Jaundice — continued
 serum (homologous) (prophylactic) (therapeutic) — see Hepatitis, viral
 spirochetal (hemorrhagic) 100.0
 symptomatic 782.4
  newborn 774.6
Jaw — see condition
Jaw-blinking 374.43
 congenital 742.8
Jaw-winking phenomenon or syndrome 742.8
Jealousy
 alcoholic 291.5
 childhood 313.3
 sibling 313.3
Jejunitis — see also Enteritis 558.9
Jejunostomy status V44.4
Jejunum, jejunal — see condition
Jensen's disease 363.05
Jericho boil 085.1
Jerks, myoclonic 333.2
Jervell-Lange-Nielsen syndrome 426.82
Jeune's disease or syndrome (asphyxiating thoracic dystrophy) 756.4
Jigger disease 134.1
Job's syndrome (chronic granulomatous disease) 288.1
Jod-Basedow phenomenon 242.8 ☑
Johnson-Stevens disease (erythema multiforme exudativum) 695.1
Joint — see also condition
 Charcôt's 094.0 [713.5]
 false 733.82
 flail — see Flail, joint
 mice — see Loose, body, joint, by site
 sinus to bone 730.9 ☑
 von Gies' 095.8
Jordan's anomaly or syndrome 288.2
Josephs-Diamond-Blackfan anemia (congenital hypoplastic) 284.01 ▲
Joubert syndrome 759.89
Jumpers' knee 727.2
Jungle yellow fever 060.0
Jüngling's disease (sarcoidosis) 135
Junin virus hemorrhagic fever 078.7
Juvenile — see also condition
 delinquent 312.9
  group (see also Disturbance, conduct) 312.2 ☑
 neurotic 312.4

K

Kabuki syndrome 759.89
Kahler (-Bozzolo) disease (multiple myeloma) (M9730/3) 203.0 ☑
Kakergasia 300.9
Kakke 265.0
Kala-azar (Indian) (infantile) (Mediterranean) (Sudanese) 085.0
Kalischer's syndrome (encephalocutaneous angiomatosis) 759.6
Kallmann's syndrome (hypogonadotropic hypogonadism with anosmia) 253.4
Kanner's syndrome (autism) — see also Psychosis, childhood 299.0 ☑
Kaolinosis 502
Kaposi's
 disease 757.33
  lichen ruber 696.4
   acuminatus 696.4
   moniliformis 697.8
  xeroderma pigmentosum 757.33
 sarcoma (M9140/3) 176.9
  adipose tissue 176.1
  aponeurosis 176.1
  artery 176.1
  blood vessel 176.1
  bursa 176.1
  connective tissue 176.1
  external genitalia 176.8
  fascia 176.1
  fatty tissue 176.1
  fibrous tissue 176.1

Kaposi's — continued
 sarcoma — continued
  gastrointestinal tract NEC 176.3
  ligament 176.1
  lung 176.4
  lymph
   gland(s) 176.5
   node(s) 176.5
  lymphatic(s) NEC 176.1
  muscle (skeletal) 176.1
  oral cavity NEC 176.8
  palate 176.2
  scrotum 176.8
  skin 176.0
  soft tissue 176.1
  specified site NEC 176.8
  subcutaneous tissue 176.1
  synovia 176.1
  tendon (sheath) 176.1
  vein 176.1
  vessel 176.1
  viscera NEC 176.9
  vulva 176.8
 varicelliform eruption 054.0
 vaccinia 999.0
Kartagener's syndrome or triad (sinusitis, bronchiectasis, situs inversus) 759.3
Kasabach-Merritt syndrome (capillary hemangioma associated with thrombocytopenic purpura) 287.39
Kaschin-Beck disease (endemic polyarthritis) — see Disease, Kaschin-Beck
Kast's syndrome (dyschondroplasia with hemangiomas) 756.4
Katatonia — see Catatonia
Katayama disease or fever 120.2
Kathisophobia 781.0
Kawasaki disease 446.1
Kayser-Fleischer ring (cornea) (pseudosclerosis) 275.1 [371.14]
Kaznelson's syndrome (congenital hypoplastic anemia) 284.01 ▲
Kearns-Sayre syndrome 277.87
Kedani fever 081.2
Kelis 701.4
Kelly (-Patterson) syndrome (sideropenic dysphagia) 280.8
Keloid, cheloid 701.4
 Addison's (morphea) 701.0
 cornea 371.00
 Hawkins' 701.4
 scar 701.4
Keloma 701.4
Kenya fever 082.1
Keratectasia 371.71
 congenital 743.41
Keratinization NEC
 alveolar ridge mucosa
  excessive 528.72
  minimal 528.71
Keratitis (nodular) (nonulcerative) (simple) (zonular) NEC 370.9
 with ulceration (see also Ulcer, cornea) 370.00
 actinic 370.24
 arborescens 054.42
 areolar 370.22
 bullosa 370.8
 deep — see Keratitis, interstitial
 dendritic(a) 054.42
 desiccation 370.34
 diffuse interstitial 370.52
 disciform(is) 054.43
  varicella 052.7 [370.44]
 epithelialis vernalis 372.13 [370.32]
 exposure 370.34
 filamentary 370.23
 gonococcal (congenital) (prenatal) 098.43
 herpes, herpetic (simplex) NEC 054.43
  zoster 053.21
 hypopyon 370.04
 in
  chickenpox 052.7 [370.44]

Keratitis

Keratitis — *continued*
  in — *continued*
    exanthema (*see also* Exanthem) 057.9 *[370.44]*
    paravaccinia (*see also* Paravaccinia) 051.9 *[370.44]*
    smallpox (*see also* Smallpox) 050.9 *[370.44]*
    vernal conjunctivitis 372.13 *[370.32]*
  interstitial (nonsyphilitic) 370.50
    with ulcer (*see also* Ulcer, cornea) 370.00
    diffuse 370.52
    herpes, herpetic (simplex) 054.43
      zoster 053.21
    syphilitic (congenital) (hereditary) 090.3
    tuberculous (*see also* Tuberculosis) 017.3 ☑ *[370.59]*
  lagophthalmic 370.34
  macular 370.22
  neuroparalytic 370.35
  neurotrophic 370.35
  nummular 370.22
  oyster-shuckers' 370.8
  parenchymatous — *see* Keratitis, interstitial
  petrificans 370.8
  phlyctenular 370.31
  postmeasles 055.71
  punctata, punctate 370.21
    leprosa 030.0 *[370.21]*
    profunda 090.3
    superficial (Thygeson's) 370.21
  purulent 370.8
  pustuliformis profunda 090.3
  rosacea 695.3 *[370.49]*
  sclerosing 370.54
  specified type NEC 370.8
  stellate 370.22
  striata 370.22
  superficial 370.20
    with conjunctivitis (*see also* Keratoconjunctivitis) 370.40
    punctate (Thygeson's) 370.21
  suppurative 370.8
  syphilitic (congenital) (prenatal) 090.3
  trachomatous 076.1
    late effect 139.1
  tuberculous (phlyctenular) (*see also* Tuberculosis) 017.3 ☑ *[370.31]*
  ulcerated (*see also* Ulcer, cornea) 370.00
  vesicular 370.8
  welders' 370.24
  xerotic (*see also* Keratomalacia) 371.45
    vitamin A deficiency 264.4
Keratoacanthoma 238.2
Keratocele 371.72
Keratoconjunctivitis — *see also* Keratitis 370.40
  adenovirus type 8 077.1
  epidemic 077.1
  exposure 370.34
  gonococcal 098.43
  herpetic (simplex) 054.43
    zoster 053.21
  in
    chickenpox 052.7 *[370.44]*
    exanthema (*see also* Exanthem) 057.9 *[370.44]*
    paravaccinia (*see also* Paravaccinia) 051.9 *[370.44]*
    smallpox (*see also* Smallpox) 050.9 *[370.44]*
  infectious 077.1
  neurotrophic 370.35
  phlyctenular 370.31
  postmeasles 055.71
  shipyard 077.1
  sicca (Sjögren's syndrome) 710.2
    not in Sjögren's syndrome 370.33
  specified type NEC 370.49

Keratoconjunctivitis — *see also* Keratitis — *continued*
  tuberculous (phlyctenular) (*see also* Tuberculosis) 017.3 ☑ *[370.31]*
Keratoconus 371.60
  acute hydrops 371.62
  congenital 743.41
  stable 371.61
Keratocyst (dental) 526.0
Keratoderma, keratodermia (congenital) (palmaris et plantaris) (symmetrical) 757.39
  acquired 701.1
  blennorrhagica 701.1
    gonococcal 098.81
  climacterium 701.1
  eccentrica 757.39
  gonorrheal 098.81
  punctata 701.1
  tylodes, progressive 701.1
Keratodermatocele 371.72
Keratoglobus 371.70
  congenital 743.41
    associated with buphthalmos 743.22
Keratohemia 371.12
Keratoiritis — *see also* Iridocyclitis 364.3
  syphilitic 090.3
  tuberculous (*see also* Tuberculosis) 017.3 ☑ *[364.11]*
Keratolysis exfoliativa (congenital) 757.39
  acquired 695.89
  neonatorum 757.39
Keratoma 701.1
  congenital 757.39
  malignum congenitale 757.1
  palmaris et plantaris hereditarium 757.39
  senile 702.0
Keratomalacia 371.45
  vitamin A deficiency 264.4
Keratomegaly 743.41
Keratomycosis 111.1
  nigricans (palmaris) 111.1
Keratopathy 371.40
  band (*see also* Keratitis) 371.43
  bullous (*see also* Keratitis) 371.23
  degenerative (*see also* Degeneration, cornea) 371.40
  hereditary (*see also* Dystrophy, cornea) 371.50
  discrete colliquative 371.49
Keratoscleritis, tuberculous — *see also* Tuberculosis 017.3 ☑ *[370.31]*
Keratosis 701.1
  actinic 702.0
  arsenical 692.4
  blennorrhagica 701.1
    gonococcal 098.81
  congenital (any type) 757.39
  ear (middle) (*see also* Cholesteatoma) 385.30
  female genital (external) 629.89 ▲
  follicularis 757.39
    acquired 701.1
    congenital (acneiformis) (Siemens') 757.39
    spinulosa (decalvans) 757.39
    vitamin A deficiency 264.8
  follicular, vitamin A deficiency 264.8
    gonococcal 098.81
  larynx, laryngeal 478.79
  male genital (external) 608.89
  middle ear (*see also* Cholesteatoma) 385.30
  nigricans 701.2
    congenital 757.39
  obturans 380.21
  oral epithelium
    residual ridge mucosa
      excessive 528.72
      minimal 528.71
  palmaris et plantaris (symmetrical) 757.39

Keratosis — *continued*
  penile 607.89
  pharyngeus 478.29
  pilaris 757.39
    acquired 701.1
  punctata (palmaris et plantaris) 701.1
  scrotal 608.89
  seborrheic 702.19
    inflamed 702.11
  senilis 702.0
  solar 702.0
  suprafollicularis 757.39
  tonsillaris 478.29
  vagina 623.1
  vegetans 757.39
  vitamin A deficiency 264.8
Kerato-uveitis — *see also* Iridocyclitis 364.3
Keraunoparalysis 994.0
Kerion (celsi) 110.0
Kernicterus of newborn (not due to isoimmunization) 774.7
  due to isoimmunization (conditions classifiable to 773.0–773.2) 773.4
Ketoacidosis 276.2
  diabetic 250.1 ☑
Ketonuria 791.6
  branched-chain, intermittent 270.3
Ketosis 276.2
  diabetic 250.1 ☑
Kidney — *see* condition
Kienböck's
  disease 732.3
    adult 732.8
  osteochondrosis 732.3
Kimmelstiel (-Wilson) disease or syndrome (intercapillary glomerulosclerosis) 250.4 ☑ *[581.81]*
Kink, kinking
  appendix 543.9
  artery 447.1
  cystic duct, congenital 751.61
  hair (acquired) 704.2
  ileum or intestine (*see also* Obstruction, intestine) 560.9
  Lane's (*see also* Obstruction, intestine) 560.9
  organ or site, congenital NEC — *see* Anomaly, specified type NEC, by site
  ureter (pelvic junction) 593.3
    congenital 753.20
  vein(s) 459.2
    caval 459.2
    peripheral 459.2
Kinnier Wilson's disease (hepatolenticular degeneration) 275.1
Kissing
  osteophytes 721.5
  spine 721.5
  vertebra 721.5
Klauder's syndrome (erythema multiforme, exudativum) 695.1
Klebs' disease — *see also* Nephritis 583.9
Kleine-Levin syndrome 327.13
Klein-Waardenburg syndrome (ptosisepicanthus) 270.2
Kleptomania 312.32
Klinefelter's syndrome 758.7
Klinger's disease 446.4
Klippel's disease 723.8
Klippel-Feil disease or syndrome (brevicollis) 756.16
Klippel-Trenaunay syndrome 759.89
Klumpke (-Déjérine) palsy, paralysis (birth) (newborn) 767.6
Klüver-Bucy (-Terzian) syndrome 310.0
Knee — *see* condition
Knifegrinders' rot — *see also* Tuberculosis 011.4 ☑
Knock-knee (acquired) 736.41
  congenital 755.64
Knot
  intestinal, syndrome (volvulus) 560.2

Knot — *continued*
  umbilical cord (true) 663.2 ☑
    affecting fetus or newborn 762.5
Knots, surfer 919.8
  infected 919.9
Knotting (of)
  hair 704.2
  intestine 560.2
Knuckle pads (Garrod's) 728.79
Köbner's disease (epidermolysis bullosa) 757.39
Koch's
  infection (*see also* Tuberculosis, pulmonary) 011.9 ☑
  relapsing fever 087.9
Koch-Weeks conjunctivitis 372.03
Koenig-Wichman disease (pemphigus) 694.4
Köhler's disease (osteochondrosis) 732.5
  first (osteochondrosis juvenilis) 732.5
  second (Freiburg's infarction, metatarsal head) 732.5
  patellar 732.4
  tarsal navicular (bone) (osteoarthrosis juvenilis) 732.5
Köhler-Mouchet disease (osteoarthrosis juvenilis) 732.5
Köhler-Pellegrini-Stieda disease or syndrome (calcification, knee joint) 726.62
Koilonychia 703.8
  congenital 757.5
Kojevnikov's, Kojewnikoff's epilepsy — *see also* Epilepsy 345.7 ☑
König's
  disease (osteochondritis dissecans) 732.7
  syndrome 564.89
Koniophthisis — *see also* Tuberculosis 011.4 ☑
Koplik's spots 055.9
Kopp's asthma 254.8
Korean hemorrhagic fever 078.6
Korsakoff (-Wernicke) disease, psychosis, or syndrome (nonalcoholic) 294.0
  alcoholic 291.1
Korsakov's disease — *see* Korsakoff's disease
Korsakow's disease — *see* Korsakoff's disease
Kostmann's disease or syndrome (infantile genetic agranulocytosis) 288.01 ▲
Krabbe's
  disease (leukodystrophy) 330.0
  syndrome
    congenital muscle hypoplasia 756.89
    cutaneocerebral angioma 759.6
Kraepelin-Morel disease — *see also* Schizophrenia 295.9 ☑
Kraft-Weber-Dimitri disease 759.6
Kraurosis
  ani 569.49
  penis 607.0
  vagina 623.8
  vulva 624.0
Kreotoxism 005.9
Krukenberg's
  spindle 371.13
  tumor (M8490/6) 198.6
Kufs' disease 330.1
Kugelberg-Welander disease 335.11
Kuhnt-Junius degeneration or disease 362.52
Kulchitsky's cell carcinoma (carcinoid tumor of intestine) 259.2
Kümmell's disease or spondylitis 721.7
Kundrat's disease (lymphosarcoma) 200.1 ☑
Kunekune — *see* Dermatophytosis
Kunkel syndrome (lupoid hepatitis) 571.49
Kupffer cell sarcoma (M9124/3) 155.0
Kuru 046.0

Index to Diseases

Kussmaul's
coma (diabetic) 250.3 ☑
disease (polyarteritis nodosa) 446.0
respiration (air hunger) 786.09

Kwashiorkor (marasmus type) 260
Kyasanur Forest disease 065.2
Kyphoscoliosis, kyphoscoliotic (acquired) — *see also* Scoliosis 737.30
- congenital 756.19
- due to radiation 737.33
- heart (disease) 416.1
- idiopathic 737.30
  - infantile
    - progressive 737.32
    - resolving 737.31
- late effect of rickets 268.1 [737.43]
- specified NEC 737.39
- thoracogenic 737.34
- tuberculous (*see also* Tuberculosis) 015.9 ☑ [737.43]

Kyphosis, kyphotic (acquired) (postural) 737.10
- adolescent postural 737.0
- congenital 756.19
- dorsalis juvenilis 732.0
- due to or associated with
  - Charcôt-Marie-Tooth disease 356.1 [737.41]
  - mucopolysaccharidosis 277.5 [737.41]
  - neurofibromatosis 237.71 [737.41]
  - osteitis
    - deformans 731.0 [737.41]
    - fibrosa cystica 252.01 [737.41]
  - osteoporosis (*see also* Osteoporosis) 733.0 ☑ [737.41]
  - poliomyelitis (*see also* Poliomyelitis) 138 [737.41]
  - radiation 737.11
  - tuberculosis (*see also* Tuberculosis) 015.9 ☑ [737.41]
- Kümmell's 721.7
- late effect of rickets 268.1 [737.41]
- Morquio-Brailsford type (spinal) 277.5 [737.41]
- pelvis 738.6
- postlaminectomy 737.12
- specified cause NEC 737.19
- syphilitic, congenital 090.5 [737.41]
- tuberculous (*see also* Tuberculosis) 015.9 ☑ [737.41]

Kyrle's disease (hyperkeratosis follicularis in cutem penetrans) 701.1

L

Labia, labium — *see* condition
Labiated hymen 752.49
Labile
- blood pressure 796.2
- emotions, emotionality 301.3
- vasomotor system 443.9

Labioglossal paralysis 335.22
Labium leporinum — *see also* Cleft, lip 749.10

Labor — *see also* Delivery
- with complications — *see* Delivery, complicated
- abnormal NEC 661.9 ☑
  - affecting fetus or newborn 763.7
- arrested active phase 661.1 ☑
  - affecting fetus or newborn 763.7
- desultory 661.2 ☑
  - affecting fetus or newborn 763.7
- dyscoordinate 661.4 ☑
  - affecting fetus or newborn 763.7
- early onset (22-36 weeks gestation) 644.2 ☑
- failed
  - induction 659.1 ☑
    - mechanical 659.0 ☑
    - medical 659.1 ☑
    - surgical 659.0 ☑
  - trial (vaginal delivery) 660.6 ☑
- false 644.1 ☑

Labor — *see also* Delivery — *continued*
- forced or induced, affecting fetus or newborn 763.89
- hypertonic 661.4 ☑
  - affecting fetus or newborn 763.7
- hypotonic 661.2 ☑
  - affecting fetus or newborn 763.7
  - primary 661.0 ☑
    - affecting fetus or newborn 763.7
  - secondary 661.1 ☑
    - affecting fetus or newborn 763.7
- incoordinate 661.4 ☑
  - affecting fetus or newborn 763.7
- irregular 661.2 ☑
  - affecting fetus or newborn 763.7
- long — *see* Labor, prolonged
- missed (at or near term) 656.4 ☑
- obstructed NEC 660.9 ☑
  - affecting fetus or newborn 763.1
  - due to female genital mutilation 660.8 ☑
  - specified cause NEC 660.8 ☑
    - affecting fetus or newborn 763.1
- pains, spurious 644.1 ☑
- precipitate 661.3 ☑
  - affecting fetus or newborn 763.6
- premature 644.2 ☑
  - threatened 644.0 ☑
- prolonged or protracted 662.1 ☑
  - first stage 662.0 ☑
    - affecting fetus or newborn 763.89
  - second stage 662.2 ☑
    - affecting fetus or newborn 763.89
  - affecting fetus or newborn 763.89
- threatened NEC 644.1 ☑
- undelivered 644.1 ☑

Labored breathing — *see also* Hyperventilation 786.09

Labyrinthitis (inner ear) (destructive) (latent) 386.30
- circumscribed 386.32
- diffuse 386.31
- focal 386.32
- purulent 386.33
- serous 386.31
- suppurative 386.33
- syphilitic 095.8
- toxic 386.34
- viral 386.35

Laceration — *see also* Wound, open, by site
- accidental, complicating surgery 998.2
- Achilles tendon 845.09
  - with open wound 892.2
- anus (sphincter) 879.6
  - with
    - abortion — *see* Abortion, by type, with damage to pelvic organs
    - ectopic pregnancy (*see also* categories 633.0–633.9) 639.2
    - molar pregnancy (*see also* categories 630–632) 639.2
  - complicated 879.7
  - complicating delivery 664.2 ☑
    - with laceration of anal or rectal mucosa 664.3 ☑
  - following
    - abortion 639.2
    - ectopic or molar pregnancy 639.2
  - nontraumatic, nonpuerperal 565.0
- bladder (urinary)
  - with
    - abortion — *see* Abortion, by type, with damage to pelvic organs
    - ectopic pregnancy (*see also* categories 633.0–633.9) 639.2
    - molar pregnancy (*see also* categories 630–632) 639.2

Laceration — *see also* Wound, open, by site — *continued*
- bladder — *continued*
  - following
    - abortion 639.2
    - ectopic or molar pregnancy 639.2
  - obstetrical trauma 665.5 ☑
- blood vessel — *see* Injury, blood vessel, by site
- bowel
  - with
    - abortion — *see* Abortion, by type, with damage to pelvic organs
    - ectopic pregnancy (*see also* categories 633.0–633.9) 639.2
    - molar pregnancy (*see also* categories 630–632) 639.2
  - following
    - abortion 639.2
    - ectopic or molar pregnancy 639.2
  - obstetrical trauma 665.5 ☑
- brain (cerebral) (membrane) (with hemorrhage) 851.8 ☑

Note — Use the following fifth-digit subclassification with categories 851–854:

0	unspecified state of consciousness
1	with no loss of consciousness
2	with brief [less than one hour] loss of consciousness
3	with moderate [1–24 hours] loss of consciousness
4	with prolonged [more than 24 hours] loss of consciousness and return to pre-existing conscious level
5	with prolonged [more than 24 hours] loss of consciousness, without return to pre-existing conscious level

Use fifth-digit 5 to designate when a patient is unconscious and dies before regaining consciousness, regardless of the duration of the loss of consciousness

6	with loss of consciousness of unspecified duration
9	with concussion, unspecified

- with
  - open intracranial wound 851.9 ☑
  - skull fracture — *see* Fracture, skull, by site
- cerebellum 851.6 ☑
  - with open intracranial wound 851.7 ☑
- cortex 851.2 ☑
  - with open intracranial wound 851.3 ☑
  - during birth 767.0
- stem 851.6 ☑
  - with open intracranial wound 851.7 ☑
- broad ligament
  - with
    - abortion — *see* Abortion, by type, with damage to pelvic organs
    - ectopic pregnancy (*see also* categories 633.0–633.9) 639.2
    - molar pregnancy (*see also* categories 630–632) 639.2
  - following
    - abortion 639.2
    - ectopic or molar pregnancy 639.2

Laceration — *see also* Wound, open, by site — *continued*
- broad ligament — *continued*
  - nontraumatic 620.6
  - obstetrical trauma 665.6 ☑
  - syndrome (nontraumatic) 620.6
- capsule, joint — *see* Sprain, by site
- cardiac — *see* Laceration, heart
- causing eversion of cervix uteri (old) 622.0
- central, complicating delivery 664.4 ☑
- cerebellum — *see* Laceration, brain, cerebellum
- cerebral (*see also* Laceration, brain) during birth 767.0
- cervix (uteri)
  - with
    - abortion — *see* Abortion, by type, with damage to pelvic organs
    - ectopic pregnancy (*see also* categories 633.0–633.9) 639.2
    - molar pregnancy (*see also* categories 630–632) 639.2
  - following
    - abortion 639.2
    - ectopic or molar pregnancy 639.2
  - nonpuerperal, nontraumatic 622.3
  - obstetrical trauma (current) 665.3 ☑
  - old (postpartal) 622.3
  - traumatic — *see* Injury, internal, cervix
- chordae heart 429.5
- complicated 879.9
- cornea — *see* Laceration, eyeball
  - superficial 918.1
- cortex (cerebral) — *see* Laceration, brain, cortex
- esophagus 530.89
- eye(s) — *see* Laceration, ocular
- eyeball NEC 871.4
  - with prolapse or exposure of intraocular tissue 871.1
  - penetrating — *see* Penetrating wound, eyeball
  - specified as without prolapse of intraocular tissue 871.0
- eyelid NEC 870.8
  - full thickness 870.1
    - involving lacrimal passages 870.2
  - skin (and periocular area) 870.0
    - penetrating — *see* Penetrating wound, orbit
- fourchette
  - with
    - abortion — *see* Abortion, by type, with damage to pelvic organs
    - ectopic pregnancy (*see also* categories 633.0–633.9) 639.2
    - molar pregnancy (*see also* categories 630–632) 639.2
  - complicating delivery 664.0 ☑
  - following
    - abortion 639.2
    - ectopic or molar pregnancy 639.2
- heart (without penetration of heart chambers) 861.02
  - with
    - open wound into thorax 861.12
    - penetration of heart chambers 861.03
      - with open wound into thorax 861.13
- hernial sac — *see* Hernia, by site
- internal organ (abdomen) (chest) (pelvis) NEC — *see* Injury, internal, by site
  - NEC — *see* Injury, internal, by site
- kidney (parenchyma) 866.02

Laceration — see also Wound, open, by site — continued
- kidney — continued
  - with
    - complete disruption of parenchyma (rupture) 866.03
      - with open wound into cavity 866.13
    - open wound into cavity 866.12
- labia
  - complicating delivery 664.0 ☑
- ligament (see also Sprain, by site)
  - with open wound — see Wound, open, by site
- liver 864.05
  - with open wound into cavity 864.15
  - major (disruption of hepatic parenchyma) 864.04
    - with open wound into cavity 864.14
  - minor (capsule only) 864.02
    - with open wound into cavity 864.12
  - moderate (involving parenchyma without major disruption) 864.03
    - with open wound into cavity 864.13
  - multiple 864.04
    - with open wound into cavity 864.14
  - stellate 864.04
    - with open wound into cavity 864.14
- lung 861.22
  - with open wound into thorax 861.32
- meninges — see Laceration, brain
- meniscus (knee) (see also Tear, meniscus) 836.2
  - old 717.5
  - site other than knee (see also Sprain, by site)
    - old NEC (see also Disorder, cartilage, articular) 718.0 ☑
- muscle (see also Sprain, by site)
  - with open wound — see Wound, open, by site
- myocardium — see Laceration, heart
- nerve — see Injury, nerve, by site
- ocular NEC (see also Laceration, eyeball) 871.4
  - adnexa NEC 870.8
    - penetrating 870.3
      - with foreign body 870.4
- orbit (eye) 870.8
  - penetrating 870.3
    - with foreign body 870.4
- pelvic
  - floor (muscles)
    - with
      - abortion — see Abortion, by type, with damage to pelvic organs
      - ectopic pregnancy (see also categories 633.0–633.9) 639.2
      - molar pregnancy (see also categories 630–632) 639.2
    - complicating delivery 664.1 ☑
    - following
      - abortion 639.2
      - ectopic or molar pregnancy 639.2
    - nonpuerperal 618.7
    - old (postpartal) 618.7
  - organ NEC
    - with
      - abortion — see Abortion, by type, with damage to pelvic organs

Laceration — see also Wound, open, by site — continued
- pelvic — continued
  - organ — continued
    - with — continued
      - ectopic pregnancy (see also categories 633.0–633.9) 639.2
      - molar pregnancy (see also categories 630–632) 639.2
    - complicating delivery 665.5 ☑
      - affecting fetus or newborn 763.89
    - following
      - abortion 639.2
      - ectopic or molar pregnancy 639.2
    - obstetrical trauma 665.5 ☑
- perineum, perineal (old) (postpartal) 618.7
  - with
    - abortion — see Abortion, by type, with damage to pelvic floor
    - ectopic pregnancy (see also categories 633.0–633.9) 639.2
    - molar pregnancy (see also categories 630–632) 639.2
  - complicating delivery 664.4 ☑
    - first degree 664.0 ☑
    - second degree 664.1 ☑
    - third degree 664.2 ☑
    - fourth degree 664.3 ☑
    - central 664.4 ☑
    - involving
      - anal sphincter 664.2 ☑
      - fourchette 664.0 ☑
      - hymen 664.0 ☑
      - labia 664.0 ☑
      - pelvic floor 664.1 ☑
      - perineal muscles 664.1 ☑
      - rectovaginal septum 664.2 ☑
        - with anal mucosa 664.3 ☑
      - skin 664.0 ☑
      - sphincter (anal) 664.2 ☑
        - with anal mucosa 664.3 ☑
      - vagina 664.0 ☑
      - vaginal muscles 664.1 ☑
      - vulva 664.0 ☑
    - secondary 674.2 ☑
  - following
    - abortion 639.2
    - ectopic or molar pregnancy 639.2
  - male 879.6
    - complicated 879.7
  - muscles, complicating delivery 664.1 ☑
  - nonpuerperal, current injury 879.6
    - complicated 879.7
  - secondary (postpartal) 674.2 ☑
- peritoneum
  - with
    - abortion — see Abortion, by type, with damage to pelvic organs
    - ectopic pregnancy (see also categories 633.0–633.9) 639.2
    - molar pregnancy (see also categories 630–632) 639.2
  - following
    - abortion 639.2
    - ectopic or molar pregnancy 639.2
  - obstetrical trauma 665.5 ☑
- periurethral tissue
  - with
    - abortion — see Abortion, by type, with damage to pelvic organs

Laceration — see also Wound, open, by site — continued
- periurethral tissue — continued
  - with — continued
    - ectopic pregnancy (see also categories 633.0–633.9) 639.2
    - molar pregnancy (see also categories 630–632) 639.2
  - following
    - abortion 639.2
    - ectopic or molar pregnancy 639.2
  - obstetrical trauma 665.5 ☑
- rectovaginal (septum)
  - with
    - abortion — see Abortion, by type, with damage to pelvic organs
    - ectopic pregnancy (see also categories 633.0–633.9) 639.2
    - molar pregnancy (see also categories 630–632) 639.2
  - complicating delivery 665.4 ☑
    - with perineum 664.2 ☑
      - involving anal or rectal mucosa 664.3 ☑
  - following
    - abortion 639.2
    - ectopic or molar pregnancy 639.2
  - nonpuerperal 623.4
  - old (postpartal) 623.4
- spinal cord (meninges) (see also Injury, spinal, by site)
  - due to injury at birth 767.4
  - fetus or newborn 767.4
- spleen 865.09
  - with
    - disruption of parenchyma (massive) 865.04
      - with open wound into cavity 865.14
    - open wound into cavity 865.19
  - capsule (without disruption of parenchyma) 865.02
    - with open wound into cavity 865.12
  - parenchyma 865.03
    - with open wound into cavity 865.13
  - massive disruption (rupture) 865.04
    - with open wound into cavity 865.14
- tendon 848.9
  - with open wound — see Wound, open, by site
  - Achilles 845.09
    - with open wound 892.2
  - lower limb NEC 844.9
    - with open wound NEC 894.2
  - upper limb NEC 840.9
    - with open wound NEC 884.2
- tentorium cerebelli — see Laceration, brain, cerebellum
- tongue 873.64
  - complicated 873.74
- urethra
  - with
    - abortion — see Abortion, by type, with damage to pelvic organs
    - ectopic pregnancy (see also categories 633.0–633.9) 639.2
    - molar pregnancy (see also categories 630–632) 639.2
  - following
    - abortion 639.2
    - ectopic or molar pregnancy 639.2
  - nonpuerperal, nontraumatic 599.84
  - obstetrical trauma 665.5 ☑

Laceration — see also Wound, open, by site — continued
- uterus
  - with
    - abortion — see Abortion, by type, with damage to pelvic organs
    - ectopic pregnancy (see also categories 633.0–633.9) 639.2
    - molar pregnancy (see also categories 630–632) 639.2
  - following
    - abortion 639.2
    - ectopic or molar pregnancy 639.2
  - nonpuerperal, nontraumatic 621.8
  - obstetrical trauma NEC 665.5 ☑
  - old (postpartal) 621.8
- vagina
  - with
    - abortion — see Abortion, by type, with damage to pelvic organs
    - ectopic pregnancy (see also categories 633.0–633.9) 639.2
    - molar pregnancy (see also categories 630–632) 639.2
    - perineal involvement, complicating delivery 664.0 ☑
  - complicating delivery 665.4 ☑
    - first degree 664.0 ☑
    - second degree 664.1 ☑
    - third degree 664.2 ☑
    - fourth degree 664.3 ☑
    - high 665.4 ☑
    - muscles 664.1 ☑
    - sulcus 665.4 ☑
    - wall 665.4 ☑
  - following
    - abortion 639.2
    - ectopic or molar pregnancy 639.2
  - nonpuerperal, nontraumatic 623.4
  - old (postpartal) 623.4
- valve, heart — see Endocarditis
- vulva
  - with
    - abortion — see Abortion, by type, with damage to pelvic organs
    - ectopic pregnancy (see also categories 633.0–633.9) 639.2
    - molar pregnancy (see also categories 630–632) 639.2
  - complicating delivery 664.0 ☑
  - following
    - abortion 639.2
    - ectopic or molar pregnancy 639.2
  - nonpuerperal, nontraumatic 624.4
  - old (postpartal) 624.4

Lachrymal — see condition
Lachrymonasal duct — see condition
Lack of
- adequate intermaxillary vertical dimension 524.36 ●
- appetite (see also Anorexia) 783.0
- care
  - in home V60.4
  - of adult 995.84
  - of infant (at or after birth) 995.52
- coordination 781.3
- development (see also Hypoplasia)
  - physiological in childhood 783.40
- education V62.3
- energy 780.79
- financial resources V60.2
- food 994.2
  - in environment V60.8
- growth in childhood 783.43
- heating V60.1
- housing (permanent) (temporary) V60.0

Index to Diseases

Lack of — continued
housing — *continued*
- adequate V60.1
- material resources V60.2
- medical attention 799.89
- memory (*see also* Amnesia) 780.93
  - mild, following organic brain damage 310.1
- ovulation 628.0
- person able to render necessary care V60.4
- physical exercise V69.0
- physiologic development in childhood 783.40
- posterior occlusal support 524.57
- prenatal care in current pregnancy V23.7
- shelter V60.0
- sleep V69.4
- water 994.3

Lacrimal — *see* condition

Lacrimation, abnormal — *see also* Epiphora 375.20

Lacrimonasal duct — *see* condition

Lactation, lactating (breast) (puerperal) (postpartum)
- defective 676.4
- disorder 676.9
  - specified type NEC 676.8
- excessive 676.6
- failed 676.4
- mastitis NEC 675.2
- mother (care and/or examination) V24.1
- nonpuerperal 611.6
- suppressed 676.5

Lacticemia 271.3
- excessive 276.2

Lactosuria 271.3

Lacunar skull 756.0

Laennec's cirrhosis (alcoholic) 571.2
- nonalcoholic 571.5

Lafora's disease 333.2

Lagleyze-von Hippel disease (retinocerebral angiomatosis) 759.6

Lag, lid (nervous) 374.41

Lagophthalmos (eyelid) (nervous) 374.20
- cicatricial 374.23
- keratitis (*see also* Keratitis) 370.34
- mechanical 374.22
- paralytic 374.21

La grippe — *see* Influenza

Lahore sore 085.1

Lakes, venous (cerebral) 437.8

Laki-Lorand factor deficiency — *see also* Defect, coagulation 286.3

Lalling 307.9

Lambliasis 007.1

Lame back 724.5

Lancereaux's diabetes (diabetes mellitus with marked emaciation) 250.8 *[261]*

Landouzy-Déjérine dystrophy (fascioscapulohumeral atrophy) 359.1

Landry's disease or paralysis 357.0

Landry-Guillain-Barré syndrome 357.0

Lane's
- band 751.4
- disease 569.89
- kink (*see also* Obstruction, intestine) 560.9

Langdon Down's syndrome (mongolism) 758.0

Language abolition 784.69

Lanugo (persistent) 757.4

Laparoscopic surgical procedure converted to open procedure V64.41

Lardaceous
- degeneration (any site) 277.39 ▲
- disease 277.39 ▲
- kidney 277.39 *[583.81]* ▲
- liver 277.39 ▲

Large
- baby (regardless of gestational age) 766.1

Large — continued
baby — *continued*
- exceptionally (weight of 4500 grams or more) 766.0
- of diabetic mother 775.0
- ear 744.22
- fetus (*see also* Oversize, fetus)
  - causing disproportion 653.5
    - with obstructed labor 660.1
- for dates
  - fetus or newborn (regardless of gestational age) 766.1
    - affecting management of pregnancy 656.6
    - exceptionally (weight of 4500 grams or more) 766.0
- physiological cup 743.57
- stature 783.9
- waxy liver 277.39 ▲
- white kidney — *see* Nephrosis

Larsen-Johansson disease (juvenile osteopathia patellae) 732.4

Larsen's syndrome (flattened facies and multiple congenital dislocations) 755.8

Larva migrans
- cutaneous NEC 126.9
  - ancylostoma 126.9
- of Diptera in vitreous 128.0
- visceral NEC 128.0

Laryngeal — *see also* condition 786.2
- syncope 786.2

Laryngismus (acute) (infectious) (stridulous) 478.75
- congenital 748.3
- diphtheritic 032.3

Laryngitis (acute) (edematous) (fibrinous) (gangrenous) (infective) (infiltrative) (malignant) (membranous) (phlegmonous) (pneumococcal) (pseudomembranous) (septic) (subglottic) (suppurative) (ulcerative) (viral) 464.00
- with
  - influenza, flu, or grippe 487.1
  - obstruction 464.01
  - tracheitis (*see also* Laryngotracheitis) 464.20
    - with obstruction 464.21
    - acute 464.20
      - with obstruction 464.21
    - chronic 476.1
- atrophic 476.0
- Borrelia vincentii 101
- catarrhal 476.0
- chronic 476.0
  - with tracheitis (chronic) 476.1
  - due to external agent — *see* Condition, respiratory, chronic, due to
- diphtheritic (membranous) 032.3
- due to external agent — *see* Inflammation, respiratory, upper, due to
- Hemophilus influenzae 464.00
  - with obstruction 464.01
- H. influenzae 464.00
  - with obstruction 464.01
- hypertrophic 476.0
- influenzal 487.1
- pachydermic 478.79
- sicca 476.0
- spasmodic 478.75
  - acute 464.00
    - with obstruction 464.01
- streptococcal 034.0
- stridulous 478.75
- syphilitic 095.8
  - congenital 090.5
- tuberculous (*see also* Tuberculosis, larynx) 012.3
- Vincent's 101

Laryngocele (congenital) (ventricular) 748.3

Laryngofissure 478.79
- congenital 748.3

Laryngomalacia (congenital) 748.3

Laryngopharyngitis (acute) 465.0
- chronic 478.9
- due to external agent — *see* Condition, respiratory, chronic, due to
- due to external agent — *see* Inflammation, respiratory, upper, due to
- septic 034.0

Laryngoplegia — *see also* Paralysis, vocal cord 478.30

Laryngoptosis 478.79

Laryngospasm 478.75
- due to external agent — *see* Condition, respiratory, acute, due to

Laryngostenosis 478.74
- congenital 748.3

Laryngotracheitis (acute) (infectional) (viral) — *see also* Laryngitis 464.20
- with obstruction 464.21
- atrophic 476.1
- Borrelia vincenti 101
- catarrhal 476.1
- chronic 476.1
  - due to external agent — *see* Condition, respiratory, chronic, due to
- diphtheritic (membranous) 032.3
- due to external agent — *see* Inflammation, respiratory, upper, due to
- H. influenzae 464.20
  - with obstruction 464.21
- hypertrophic 476.1
- influenzal 487.1
- pachydermic 478.75
- sicca 476.1
- spasmodic 478.75
  - acute 464.20
    - with obstruction 464.21
- streptococcal 034.0
- stridulous 478.75
- syphilitic 095.8
  - congenital 090.5
- tuberculous (*see also* Tuberculosis, larynx) 012.3
- Vincent's 101

Laryngotracheobronchitis — *see also* Bronchitis 490
- acute 466.0
- chronic 491.8
- viral 466.0

Laryngotracheobronchopneumonitis — *see* Pneumonia, broncho-

Larynx, laryngeal — *see* condition

Lasègue's disease (persecution mania) 297.9

Lassa fever 078.89

Lassitude — *see also* Weakness 780.79

Late — *see also* condition
- effect(s) (of) (*see also* condition)
  - abscess
    - intracranial or intraspinal (conditions classifiable to 324) — *see* category 326
  - adverse effect of drug, medicinal or biological substance 909.5
  - allergic reaction 909.9
  - amputation
    - postoperative (late) 997.60
    - traumatic (injury classifiable to 885–887 and 895–897) 905.9
  - burn (injury classifiable to 948–949) 906.9
    - extremities NEC (injury classifiable to 943 or 945) 906.7
    - hand or wrist (injury classifiable to 944) 906.6
    - eye (injury classifiable to 940) 906.5
    - face, head, and neck (injury classifiable to 941) 906.5
    - specified site NEC (injury classifiable to 942 and 946–947) 906.8

Late — *see also* condition — *continued*
effect(s) (*see also* condition) — *continued*
- cerebrovascular disease (conditions classifiable to 430–437) 438.9
  - with
    - alterations of sensations 438.6
    - aphasia 438.11
    - apraxia 438.81
    - ataxia 438.84
    - cognitive deficits 438.0
    - disturbances of vision 438.7
    - dysphagia 438.82
    - dysphasia 438.12
    - facial droop 438.83
    - facial weakness 438.83
    - hemiplegia/hemiparesis affecting
      - dominant side 438.21
      - nondominant side 438.22
      - unspecified side 438.20
    - monoplegia of lower limb affecting
      - dominant side 438.41
      - nondominant side 438.42
      - unspecified side 438.40
    - monoplegia of upper limb affecting
      - dominant side 438.31
      - nondominant side 438.32
      - unspecified side 438.30
    - paralytic syndrome NEC affecting
      - bilateral 438.53
      - dominant side 438.51
      - nondominant side 438.52
      - unspecified side 438.50
    - specified type NEC 438.19
    - speech and language deficit 438.10
    - vertigo 438.85
  - specified type NEC 438.89
- childbirth complication(s) 677
- complication(s) of
  - childbirth 677
  - delivery 677
  - pregnancy 677
  - puerperium 677
  - surgical and medical care (conditions classifiable to 996–999) 909.3
  - trauma (conditions classifiable to 958) 908.6
- contusion (injury classifiable to 920–924) 906.3
- crushing (injury classifiable to 925–929) 906.4
- delivery complication(s) 677
- dislocation (injury classifiable to 830–839) 905.6
- encephalitis or encephalomyelitis (conditions classifiable to 323) — *see* category 326
- in infectious diseases 139.8
  - viral (conditions classifiable to 049.8, 049.9, 062–064) 139.0
- external cause NEC (conditions classifiable to 995) 909.9
  - certain conditions classifiable to categories 991–994 909.4
- foreign body in orifice (injury classifiable to 930–939) 908.5

Late — *see also* condition — *continued*
  effect(s) (*see also* condition) — *continued*
    fracture (multiple) (injury classifiable to 828–829) 905.5
      extremity
        lower (injury classifiable to 821–827) 905.4
        neck of femur (injury classifiable to 820) 905.3
        upper (injury classifiable to 810–819) 905.2
      face and skull (injury classifiable to 800–804) 905.0
      skull and face (injury classifiable to 800–804) 905.0
      spine and trunk (injury classifiable to 805 and 807–809) 905.1
        with spinal cord lesion (injury classifiable to 806) 907.2
    infection
      pyogenic, intracranial — *see* category 326
    infectious diseases (conditions classifiable to 001–136) NEC 139.8
    injury (injury classifiable to 959) 908.9
      blood vessel 908.3
        abdomen and pelvis (injury classifiable to 902) 908.4
        extremity (injury classifiable to 903–904) 908.3
        head and neck (injury classifiable to 900) 908.3
        intracranial (injury classifiable to 850–854) 907.0
          with skull fracture 905.0
        thorax (injury classifiable to 901) 908.4
      internal organ NEC (injury classifiable to 867 and 869) 908.2
        abdomen (injury classifiable to 863–866 and 868) 908.1
        thorax (injury classifiable to 860–862) 908.0
      intracranial (injury classifiable to 850–854) 907.0
        with skull fracture (injury classifiable to 800–801 and 803–804) 905.0
      nerve NEC (injury classifiable to 957) 907.9
        cranial (injury classifiable to 950–951) 907.1
        peripheral NEC (injury classifiable to 957) 907.9
          lower limb and pelvic girdle (injury classifiable to 956) 907.5
          upper limb and shoulder girdle (injury classifiable to 955) 907.4
        roots and plexus(es), spinal (injury classifiable to 953) 907.3
        trunk (injury classifiable to 954) 907.3
      spinal
        cord (injury classifiable to 806 and 952) 907.2
        nerve root(s) and plexus(es) (injury classifiable to 953) 907.3
      superficial (injury classifiable to 910–919) 906.2

Late — *see also* condition — *continued*
  effect(s) (*see also* condition) — *continued*
    injury — *continued*
      tendon (tendon injury classifiable to 840–848, 880–884 with .2, and 890–894 with .2) 905.8
    meningitis
      bacterial (conditions classifiable to 320) — *see* category 326
      unspecified cause (conditions classifiable to 322) — *see* category 326
    myelitis (*see also* Late, effect(s) (of), encephalitis) — *see* category 326
    parasitic diseases (conditions classifiable to 001–136 NEC) 139.8
    phlebitis or thrombophlebitis of intracranial venous sinuses (conditions classifiable to 325) — *see* category 326
    poisoning due to drug, medicinal or biological substance (conditions classifiable to 960–979) 909.0
    poliomyelitis, acute (conditions classifiable to 045) 138
    pregnancy complication(s) 677
    puerperal complication(s) 677
    radiation (conditions classifiable to 990) 909.2
    rickets 268.1
    sprain and strain without mention of tendon injury (injury classifiable to 840–848, except tendon injury) 905.7
    tendon involvement 905.8
    toxic effect of
      drug, medicinal or biological substance (conditions classifiable to 960–979) 909.0
      nonmedical substance (conditions classifiable to 980–989) 909.1
    trachoma (conditions classifiable to 076) 139.1
    tuberculosis 137.0
      bones and joints (conditions classifiable to 015) 137.3
      central nervous system (conditions classifiable to 013) 137.1
      genitourinary (conditions classifiable to 016) 137.2
      pulmonary (conditions classifiable to 010–012) 137.0
      specified organs NEC (conditions classifiable to 014, 017–018) 137.4
      viral encephalitis (conditions classifiable to 049.8, 049.9, 062–064) 139.0
    wound, open
      extremity (injury classifiable to 880–884 and 890–894, except .2) 906.1
      tendon (injury classifiable to 880–884 with .2 and 890–894 with .2) 905.8
      head, neck, and trunk (injury classifiable to 870–879) 906.0
  infant
    post-term (gestation period over 40 completed weeks to 42 completed weeks) 766.21
    prolonged gestation (period over 42 completed weeks) 766.22
Latent — *see* condition
Lateral — *see* condition

Laterocession — *see* Lateroversion
Lateroflexion — *see* Lateroversion
Lateroversion
  cervix — *see* Lateroversion, uterus
  uterus, uterine (cervix) (postinfectional) (postpartal, old) 621.6
    congenital 752.3
    in pregnancy or childbirth 654.4 ☑
      affecting fetus or newborn 763.89
Lathyrism 988.2
Launois-Bensaude's lipomatosis 272.8
Launois-Cléret syndrome (adiposogenital dystrophy) 253.8
Launois' syndrome (pituitary gigantism) 253.0
Laurence-Moon-Biedl syndrome (obesity, polydactyly, and mental retardation) 759.89
LAV (disease) (illness) (infection) — *see* Human immunodeficiency virus (disease) (illness) (infection)
LAV/HTLV-III (disease) (illness) (infection) — *see* Human immunodeficiency virus (disease) (illness) (infection)
Lawford's syndrome (encephalocutaneous angiomatosis) 759.6
Laxative habit — *see also* Abuse, drugs, nondependent 305.9 ☑
Lax, laxity — *see also* Relaxation
  ligament 728.4
  skin (acquired) 701.8
    congenital 756.83
Lazy leukocyte syndrome 288.09 ▲
LCAD (long chain/very long chain acyl CoA dehydrogenase deficiency, VLCAD) 277.85
LCHAD (long chain 3-hydroxyacyl CoA dehydrogenase deficiency) 277.85
Lead — *see also* condition
  exposure to V15.86
  incrustation of cornea 371.15
  poisoning 984.9
    specified type of lead — *see* Table of Drugs and Chemicals
Lead miners' lung 503
Leakage
  amniotic fluid 658.1 ☑
    with delayed delivery 658.2 ☑
    affecting fetus or newborn 761.1
  bile from drainage tube (T tube) 997.4
  blood (microscopic), fetal, into maternal circulation 656.0 ☑
    affecting management of pregnancy or puerperium 656.0 ☑
  device, implant, or graft — *see* Complications, mechanical
  spinal fluid at lumbar puncture site 997.09
  urine, continuous 788.37
Leaky heart — *see* Endocarditis
Learning defect, specific NEC (strephosymbolia) 315.2
Leather bottle stomach (M8142/3) 151.9
Leber's
  congenital amaurosis 362.76
  optic atrophy (hereditary) 377.16
Lederer's anemia or disease (acquired infectious hemolytic anemia) 283.19
Lederer-Brill syndrome (acquired infectious hemolytic anemia) 283.19
Leeches (aquatic) (land) 134.2
Left-sided neglect 781.8
Leg — *see* condition
Legal investigation V62.5
Legg (-Calvé) -Perthes disease or syndrome (osteochondrosis, femoral capital) 732.1
Legionnaires' disease 482.84
Leigh's disease 330.8
Leiner's disease (exfoliative dermatitis) 695.89

Leiofibromyoma (M8890/0) — *see also* Leiomyoma
  uterus (cervix) (corpus) (*see also* Leiomyoma, uterus) 218.9
Leiomyoblastoma (M8891/1) — *see* Neoplasm, connective tissue, uncertain behavior
Leiomyofibroma (M8890/0) — *see also* Neoplasm, connective tissue, benign
  uterus (cervix) (corpus) (*see also* Leiomyoma, uterus) 218.9
Leiomyoma (M8890/0) — *see also* Neoplasm, connective tissue, benign
  bizarre (M8893/0) — *see* Neoplasm, connective tissue, benign
  cellular (M8892/1) — *see* Neoplasm, connective tissue, uncertain behavior
  epithelioid (M8891/1) — *see* Neoplasm, connective tissue, uncertain behavior
  prostate (polypoid) 600.20
    with
      other lower urinary tract symptoms (LUTS) 600.21 ●
      urinary
        obstruction 600.21 ●
        retention 600.21 ●
  uterus (cervix) (corpus) 218.9
    interstitial 218.1
    intramural 218.1
    submucous 218.0
    subperitoneal 218.2
    subserous 218.2
  vascular (M8894/0) — *see* Neoplasm, connective tissue, benign
Leiomyomatosis (intravascular) (M8890/1) — *see* Neoplasm, connective tissue, uncertain behavior
Leiomyosarcoma (M8890/3) — *see also* Neoplasm, connective tissue, malignant
  epithelioid (M8891/3) — *see* Neoplasm, connective tissue, malignant
Leishmaniasis 085.9
  American 085.5
    cutaneous 085.4
    mucocutaneous 085.5
  Asian desert 085.2
  Brazilian 085.5
  cutaneous 085.9
    acute necrotizing 085.2
    American 085.4
    Asian desert 085.2
    diffuse 085.3
    dry form 085.1
    Ethiopian 085.3
    eyelid 085.5 [373.6]
    late 085.1
    lepromatous 085.3
    recurrent 085.1
    rural 085.2
    ulcerating 085.1
    urban 085.1
    wet form 085.2
    zoonotic form 085.2
  dermal (*see also* Leishmaniasis, cutaneous)
    post kala-azar 085.0
  eyelid 085.5 [373.6]
  infantile 085.0
  Mediterranean 085.0
  mucocutaneous (American) 085.5
  naso-oral 085.5
  nasopharyngeal 085.5
  Old World 085.1
  tegumentaria diffusa 085.4
  vaccination, prophylactic (against) V05.2
  visceral (Indian) 085.0
Leishmanoid, dermal — *see also* Leishmaniasis, cutaneous
  post kala-azar 085.0

Index to Diseases

Leloir's disease 695.4
Lemiere syndrome 451.89
Lenegre's disease 426.0
Lengthening, leg 736.81
Lennox-Gastaut syndrome 345.0 ☑
 with tonic seizures 345.1 ☑
Lennox's syndrome — see also Epilepsy 345.0 ☑
Lens — see condition
Lenticonus (anterior) (posterior) (congenital) 743.36
Lenticular degeneration, progressive 275.1
Lentiglobus (posterior) (congenital) 743.36
Lentigo (congenital) 709.09
 juvenile 709.09
 Maligna (M8742/2) (see also Neoplasm, skin, in situ)
  melanoma (M8742/3) — see Melanoma
 senile 709.09
Leonine leprosy 030.0
Leontiasis
 ossium 733.3
 syphilitic 095.8
  congenital 090.5
Léopold-Lévi's syndrome (paroxysmal thyroid instability) 242.9 ☑
Lepore hemoglobin syndrome 282.49
Lepothrix 039.0
Lepra 030.9
 Willan's 696.1
Leprechaunism 259.8
Lepromatous leprosy 030.0
Leprosy 030.9
 anesthetic 030.1
 beriberi 030.1
 borderline (group B) (infiltrated) (neuritic) 030.3
 cornea (see also Leprosy, by type) 030.9 [371.89]
 dimorphous (group B) (infiltrated) (lepromatous) (neuritic) (tuberculoid) 030.3
 eyelid 030.0 [373.4]
 indeterminate (group I) (macular) (neuritic) (uncharacteristic) 030.2
 leonine 030.0
 lepromatous (diffuse) (infiltrated) (macular) (neuritic) (nodular) (type L) 030.0
 macular (early) (neuritic) (simple) 030.2
 maculoanesthetic 030.1
 mixed 030.1
 neuro 030.1
 nodular 030.0
 primary neuritic 030.3
 specified type or group NEC 030.8
 tubercular 030.1
 tuberculoid (macular) (maculoanesthetic) (major) (minor) (neuritic) (type T) 030.1
Leptocytosis, hereditary 282.49
Leptomeningitis (chronic) (circumscribed) (hemorrhagic) (nonsuppurative) — see also Meningitis 322.9
 aseptic 047.9
  adenovirus 049.1
  Coxsackie virus 047.0
  ECHO virus 047.1
  enterovirus 047.9
  lymphocytic choriomeningitis 049.0
 epidemic 036.0
 late effect — see category 326
 meningococcal 036.0
 pneumococcal 320.1
 syphilitic 094.2
 tuberculous (see also Tuberculosis, meninges) 013.0 ☑
Leptomeningopathy — see also Meningitis 322.9
Leptospiral — see condition
Leptospirochetal — see condition

Leptospirosis 100.9
 autumnalis 100.89
 canicula 100.89
 grippotyphosa 100.89
 hebdomidis 100.89
 icterohemorrhagica 100.0
 nanukayami 100.89
 pomona 100.89
 Weil's disease 100.0
Leptothricosis — see Actinomycosis
Leptothrix infestation — see Actinomycosis
Leptotricosis — see Actinomycosis
Leptus dermatitis 133.8
Leriche's syndrome (aortic bifurcation occlusion) 444.0
Léris pleonosteosis 756.89
Léri-Weill syndrome 756.59
Lermoyez's syndrome — see also Disease, Ménière's 386.00
Lesbianism — omit code
 ego-dystonic 302.0
 problems with 302.0
Lesch-Nyhan syndrome (hypoxanthineguanine-phosphoribosyltransferase deficiency) 277.2
Lesion▶(s)◀
 abducens nerve 378.54
 alveolar process 525.8
 anorectal 569.49
 aortic (valve) — see Endocarditis, aortic
 auditory nerve 388.5
 basal ganglion 333.90
 bile duct (see also Disease, biliary) 576.8
 bladder 596.9
 bone 733.90
 brachial plexus 353.0
 brain 348.8
  congenital 742.9
  vascular (see also Lesion, cerebrovascular) 437.9
   degenerative 437.1
   healed or old without residuals V12.59
   hypertensive 437.2
   late effect — see Late effect(s) (of) cerebrovascular disease
 buccal 528.9
 calcified — see Calcification
 canthus 373.9
 carate — see Pinta, lesions
 cardia 537.89
 cardiac — see also Disease, heart
  congenital 746.9
  valvular — see Endocarditis
 cauda equina 344.60
  with neurogenic bladder 344.61
 cecum 569.89
 cerebral — see Lesion, brain
 cerebrovascular (see also Disease, cerebrovascular NEC) 437.9
  degenerative 437.1
  healed or old without residuals V12.59
  hypertensive 437.2
  specified type NEC 437.8
 cervical root (nerve) NEC 353.2
 chiasmal 377.54
  associated with
   inflammatory disorders 377.54
   neoplasm NEC 377.52
   pituitary 377.51
   pituitary disorders 377.51
   vascular disorders 377.53
 chorda tympani 351.8
 coin, lung 793.1
 colon 569.89
 congenital — see Anomaly
 conjunctiva 372.9
 coronary artery (see also Ischemia, heart) 414.9
 cranial nerve 352.9
  first 352.0

Lesion▶(s)◀ — continued
 cranial nerve — continued
  second 377.49
  third
   partial 378.51
   total 378.52
  fourth 378.53
  fifth 350.9
  sixth 378.54
  seventh 351.9
  eighth 388.5
  ninth 352.2
  tenth 352.3
  eleventh 352.4
  twelfth 352.5
 cystic — see Cyst
 degenerative — see Degeneration
 dermal (skin) 709.9
 Dieulafoy (hemorrhagic)
  of
   duodenum 537.84
   intestine 569.86
   stomach 537.84
 duodenum 537.89
  with obstruction 537.3
 eyelid 373.9
 gasserian ganglion 350.8
 gastric 537.89
 gastroduodenal 537.89
 gastrointestinal 569.89
 glossopharyngeal nerve 352.2
 heart (organic) (see also Disease, heart)
  vascular — see Disease, cardiovascular
 helix (ear) 709.9
 high grade myelodysplastic syndrome 238.73 ●
 hyperchromic, due to pinta (carate) 103.1
 hyperkeratotic (see also Hyperkeratosis) 701.1
 hypoglossal nerve 352.5
 hypopharynx 478.29
 hypothalamic 253.9
 ileocecal coil 569.89
 ileum 569.89
 iliohypogastric nerve 355.79
 ilioinguinal nerve 355.79
 in continuity — see Injury, nerve, by site
 inflammatory — see Inflammation
 intestine 569.89
 intracerebral — see Lesion, brain
 intrachiasmal (optic) (see also Lesion, chiasmal) 377.54
 intracranial, space-occupying NEC 784.2
 joint 719.90
  ankle 719.97
  elbow 719.92
  foot 719.97
  hand 719.94
  hip 719.95
  knee 719.96
  multiple sites 719.99
  pelvic region 719.95
  sacroiliac (old) 724.6
  shoulder (region) 719.91
  specified site NEC 719.98
  wrist 719.93
 keratotic (see also Keratosis) 701.1
 kidney (see also Disease, renal) 593.9
 laryngeal nerve (recurrent) 352.3
 leonine 030.0
 lip 528.5
 liver 573.8
 low grade myelodysplastic syndrome 238.72 ●
 lumbosacral
  plexus 353.1
  root (nerve) NEC 353.4
 lung 518.89
  coin 793.1
 maxillary sinus 473.0
 mitral — see Endocarditis, mitral

Lesion▶(s)◀ — continued
 motor cortex 348.8
 nerve (see also Disorder, nerve) 355.9
 nervous system 349.9
  congenital 742.9
 nonallopathic NEC 739.9
  in region (of)
   abdomen 739.9
   acromioclavicular 739.7
   cervical, cervicothoracic 739.1
   costochondral 739.8
   costovertebral 739.8
   extremity
    lower 739.6
    upper 739.7
   head 739.0
   hip 739.5
   lower extremity 739.6
   lumbar, lumbosacral 739.3
   occipitocervical 739.0
   pelvic 739.5
   pubic 739.5
   rib cage 739.8
   sacral, sacrococcygeal, sacroiliac 739.4
   sternochondral 739.8
   sternoclavicular 739.7
   thoracic, thoracolumbar 739.2
   upper extremity 739.7
 nose (internal) 478.19 ▲
 obstructive — see Obstruction
 obturator nerve 355.79
 occlusive
  artery — see Embolism, artery
 organ or site NEC — see Disease, by site
 osteolytic 733.90
 paramacular, of retina 363.32
 peptic 537.89
 periodontal, due to traumatic occlusion 523.8
 perirectal 569.49
 peritoneum (granulomatous) 568.89
 pigmented (skin) 709.00
 pinta — see Pinta, lesions
 polypoid — see Polyp
 prechiasmal (optic) (see also Lesion, chiasmal) 377.54
 primary (see also Syphilis, primary)
  carate 103.0
  pinta 103.0
  yaws 102.0
 pulmonary 518.89
  valve (see also Endocarditis, pulmonary) 424.3
 pylorus 537.89
 radiation NEC 990
 radium NEC 990
 rectosigmoid 569.89
 retina, retinal (see also Retinopathy)
  vascular 362.17
 retroperitoneal 568.89
 romanus 720.1
 sacroiliac (joint) 724.6
 salivary gland 527.8
  benign lymphoepithelial 527.8
 saphenous nerve 355.79
 secondary — see Syphilis, secondary
 sigmoid 569.89
 sinus (accessory) (nasal) (see also Sinusitis) 473.9
 skin 709.9
  suppurative 686.00
 SLAP (superior glenoid labrum) 840.7
 space-occupying, intracranial NEC 784.2
 spinal cord 336.9
  congenital 742.9
  traumatic (complete) (incomplete) (transverse) (see also Injury, spinal, by site)
   with
    broken
     back — see Fracture, vertebra, by site, with spinal cord injury

Lesion(s) — Lichen

Lesion(s) — continued
spinal cord — continued
  traumatic (see also Injury, spinal, by site) — continued
    with — continued
      broken — continued
        neck — see Fracture, vertebra, cervical, with spinal cord injury
      fracture, vertebra — see Fracture, vertebra, by site, with spinal cord injury
spleen 289.50
stomach 537.89
superior glenoid labrum (SLAP) 840.7
syphilitic — see Syphilis
tertiary — see Syphilis, tertiary
thoracic root (nerve) 353.3
tonsillar fossa 474.9
tooth, teeth 525.8
  white spot 521.01
traumatic NEC (see also nature and site of injury) 959.9
tricuspid (valve) — see Endocarditis, tricuspid
trigeminal nerve 350.9
ulcerated or ulcerative — see Ulcer
uterus NEC 621.9
vagina 623.8
vagus nerve 352.3
valvular — see Endocarditis
vascular 459.9
  affecting central nervous system (see also Lesion, cerebrovascular) 437.9
  following trauma (see also Injury, blood vessel, by site) 904.9
  retina 362.17
  traumatic — see Injury, blood vessel, by site
umbilical cord 663.6
  affecting fetus or newborn 762.6
visual
  cortex NEC (see also Disorder, visual, cortex) 377.73
  pathway NEC (see also Disorder, visual, pathway) 377.63
warty — see Verruca
white spot, on teeth 521.01
x-ray NEC 990
Lethargic — see condition
Lethargy 780.79
Letterer-Siwe disease (acute histiocytosis X) (M9722/3) 202.5
Leucinosis 270.3
Leucocoria 360.44
Leucosarcoma (M9850/3) 207.8
Leukasmus 270.2
Leukemia, leukemic (congenital) (M9800/3) 208.9

Note — Use the following fifth-digit subclassification for categories 203–208:
0 without mention of remission
1 with remission

acute NEC (M9801/3) 208.0
aleukemic NEC (M9804/3) 208.8
granulocytic (M9864/3) 205.8
basophilic (M9870/3) 205.1
blast (cell) (M9801/3) 208.0
blastic (M9801/3) 208.0
  granulocytic (M9861/3) 205.0
chronic NEC (M9803/3) 208.1
compound (M9810/3) 207.8
eosinophilic (M9880/3) 205.1
giant cell (M9910/3) 207.2
granulocytic (M9860/3) 205.9
  acute (M9861/3) 205.0
  aleukemic (M9864/3) 205.8
  blastic (M9861/3) 205.0
  chronic (M9863/3) 205.1
  subacute (M9862/3) 205.2
  subleukemic (M9864/3) 205.8

Leukemia, leukemic — continued
hairy cell (M9940/3) 202.4
hemoblastic (M9801/3) 208.0
histiocytic (M9890/3) 206.9
lymphatic (M9820/3) 204.9
  acute (M9821/3) 204.0
  aleukemic (M9824/3) 204.8
  chronic (M9823/3) 204.1
  subacute (M9822/3) 204.2
  subleukemic (M9824/3) 204.8
lymphoblastic (M9821/3) 204.0
lymphocytic (M9820/3) 204.9
  acute (M9821/3) 204.0
  aleukemic (M9824/3) 204.8
  chronic (M9823/3) 204.1
  subacute (M9822/3) 204.2
  subleukemic (M9824/3) 204.8
lymphogenous (M9820/3) — see Leukemia, lymphoid
lymphoid (M9820/3) 204.9
  acute (M9821/3) 204.0
  aleukemic (M9824/3) 204.8
  blastic (M9821/3) 204.0
  chronic (M9823/3) 204.1
  subacute (M9822/3) 204.2
  subleukemic (M9824/3) 204.8
lymphosarcoma cell (M9850/3) 207.8
mast cell (M9900/3) 207.8
megakaryocytic (M9910/3) 207.2
megakaryocytoid (M9910/3) 207.2
mixed (cell) (M9810/3) 207.8
monoblastic (M9891/3) 206.0
monocytic (Schilling-type) (M9890/3) 206.9
  acute (M9891/3) 206.0
  aleukemic (M9894/3) 206.8
  chronic (M9893/3) 206.1
  Naegeli-type (M9863/3) 205.1
  subacute (M9892/3) 206.2
  subleukemic (M9894/3) 206.8
monocytoid (M9890/3) 206.9
  acute (M9891/3) 206.0
  aleukemic (M9894/3) 206.8
  chronic (M9893/3) 206.1
  myelogenous (M9863/3) 205.1
  subacute (M9892/3) 206.2
  subleukemic (M9894/3) 206.8
monomyelocytic (M9860/3) — see Leukemia, myelomonocytic
myeloblastic (M9861/3) 205.0
myelocytic (M9863/3) 205.1
  acute (M9861/3) 205.0
  myelogenous (M9860/3) 205.9
  acute (M9861/3) 205.0
  aleukemic (M9864/3) 205.8
  chronic (M9863/3) 205.1
  monocytoid (M9863/3) 205.1
  subacute (M9862/3) 205.2
  subleukemic (M9864) 205.8
myeloid (M9860/3) 205.9
  acute (M9861/3) 205.0
  aleukemic (M9864/3) 205.8
  chronic (M9863/3) 205.1
  subacute (M9862/3) 205.2
  subleukemic (M9864/3) 205.8
myelomonocytic (M9860/3) 205.9
  acute (M9861/3) 205.0
  chronic (M9863/3) 205.1
Naegeli-type monocytic (M9863/3) 205.1
neutrophilic (M9865/3) 205.1
plasma cell (M9830/3) 203.1
plasmacytic (M9830/3) 203.1
prolymphocytic (M9825/3) — see Leukemia, lymphoid
promyelocytic, acute (M9866/3) 205.0
Schilling-type monocytic (M9890/3) — see Leukemia, monocytic
stem cell (M9801/3) 208.0
subacute NEC (M9802/3) 208.2
subleukemic NEC (M9804/3) 208.8
thrombocytic (M9910/3) 207.2

Leukemia, leukemic — continued
undifferentiated (M9801/3) 208.0
Leukemoid reaction (basophilic) (lymphocytic) (monocytic) (myelocytic) (neutrophilic) 288.62
Leukoclastic vasculitis 446.29
Leukocoria 360.44
Leukocythemia — see Leukemia
Leukocytopenia 288.50
Leukocytosis 288.60
  basophilic 288.8
  eosinophilic 288.3
  lymphocytic 288.8
  monocytic 288.8
  neutrophilic 288.8
Leukoderma 709.09
  syphilitic 091.3
    late 095.8
Leukodermia — see also Leukoderma 709.09
Leukodystrophy (cerebral) (globoid cell) (metachromatic) (progressive) (sudanophilic) 330.0
Leukoedema, mouth or tongue 528.79
Leukoencephalitis
  acute hemorrhagic (postinfectious) NEC 136.9 [323.61]
  postimmunization or postvaccinal 323.51
  subacute sclerosing 046.2
    van Bogaert's 046.2
  van Bogaert's (sclerosing) 046.2
Leukoencephalopathy — see also Encephalitis 323.9
  acute necrotizing hemorrhagic (postinfectious) 136.9 [323.61]
  postimmunization or postvaccinal 323.51
  metachromatic 330.0
  multifocal (progressive) 046.3
  progressive multifocal 046.3
Leukoerythroblastosis 289.9
Leukoerythrosis 289.0
Leukokeratosis — see also Leukoplakia 702.8
  mouth 528.6
  nicotina palati 528.79
  tongue 528.6
Leukokoria 360.44
Leukokraurosis vulva, vulvae 624.09
Leukolymphosarcoma (M9850/3) 207.8
Leukoma (cornea) (interfering with central vision) 371.03
  adherent 371.04
Leukomalacia, periventricular 779.7
Leukomelanopathy, hereditary 288.2
Leukonychia (punctata) (striata) 703.8
  congenital 757.5
Leukopathia
  unguium 703.8
  congenital 757.5
Leukopenia 288.50
  basophilic 288.59
  cyclic 288.02
  eosinophilic 288.59
  familial 288.59
  malignant (see also Agranulocytosis) 288.09
  periodic 288.02
  transitory neonatal 776.7
Leukopenic — see condition
Leukoplakia 702.8
  anus 569.49
  bladder (postinfectional) 596.8
  buccal 528.6
  cervix (uteri) 622.2
  esophagus 530.83
  gingiva 528.6
  kidney (pelvis) 593.89
  larynx 478.79
  lip 528.6
  mouth 528.6
  oral soft tissue (including tongue) (mucosa) 528.6

Leukoplakia — continued
palate 528.6
pelvis (kidney) 593.89
penis (infectional) 607.0
rectum 569.49
syphilitic 095.8
tongue 528.6
tonsil 478.29
ureter (postinfectional) 593.89
urethra (postinfectional) 599.84
uterus 621.8
vagina 623.1
vesical 596.8
vocal cords 478.5
vulva 624.0
Leukopolioencephalopathy 330.0
Leukorrhea (vagina) 623.5
  due to trichomonas (vaginalis) 131.00
  trichomonal (Trichomonas vaginalis) 131.00
Leukosarcoma (M9850/3) 207.8
Leukosis (M9800/3) — see Leukemia
Lev's disease or syndrome (acquired complete heart block) 426.0
Levi's syndrome (pituitary dwarfism) 253.3
Levocardia (isolated) 746.87
  with situs inversus 759.3
Levulosuria 271.2
Lewandowski's disease (primary) — see also Tuberculosis 017.0
Lewandowski-Lutz disease (epidermodysplasia verruciformis) 078.19
Lewy body dementia 331.82
Lewy body disease 331.82
Leyden's disease (periodic vomiting) 536.2
Leyden-Möbius dystrophy 359.1
Leydig cell
  carcinoma (M8650/3)
    specified site — see Neoplasm, by site, malignant
    unspecified site
      female 183.0
      male 186.9
  tumor (M8650/1)
    benign (M8650/0)
      specified site — see Neoplasm, by site, benign
      unspecified site
        female 220
        male 222.0
    malignant (M8650/3)
      specified site — see Neoplasm, by site, malignant
      unspecified site
        female 183.0
        male 186.9
    specified site — see Neoplasm, by site, uncertain behavior
    unspecified site
      female 236.2
      male 236.4
Leydig-Sertoli cell tumor (M8631/0)
  specified site — see Neoplasm, by site, benign
  unspecified site
    female 220
    male 222.0
LGSIL (low grade squamous intraepithelial lesion) 795.03
Liar, pathologic 301.7
Libman-Sacks disease or syndrome 710.0 [424.91]
Lice (infestation) 132.9
  body (pediculus corporis) 132.1
  crab 132.2
  head (pediculus capitis) 132.0
  mixed (classifiable to more than one of the categories 132.0–132.2) 132.3
  pubic (pediculus pubis) 132.2
Lichen 697.9
  albus 701.0
  annularis 695.89
  atrophicus 701.0

Index to Diseases

Lichen — continued
- corneus obtusus 698.3
- myxedematous 701.8
- nitidus 697.1
- pilaris 757.39
  - acquired 701.1
- planopilaris 697.0
- planus (acute) (chronicus) (hypertrophic) (verrucous) 697.0
  - morphoeicus 701.0
  - sclerosus (et atrophicus) 701.0
- ruber 696.4
  - acuminatus 696.4
  - moniliformis 697.8
  - obtusus corneus 698.3
  - of Wilson 697.0
  - planus 697.0
- sclerosus (et atrophicus) 701.0
- scrofulosus (primary) (see also Tuberculosis) 017.0 ☑
- simplex (Vidal's) 698.3
  - chronicus 698.3
  - circumscriptus 698.3
- spinulosus 757.39
  - mycotic 117.9
- striata 697.8
- urticatus 698.2

Lichenification 698.3
- nodular 698.3

Lichenoides tuberculosis (primary) — see also Tuberculosis 017.0 ☑

Lichtheim's disease or syndrome (subacute combined sclerosis with pernicious anemia) 281.0 [336.2]

Lien migrans 289.59

Lientery — see also Diarrhea 787.91
- infectious 009.2

Life circumstance problem NEC V62.89

Li-Fraumeni cancer syndrome V84.01

Ligament — see condition

Light-for-dates (infant) 764.0 ☑
- with signs of fetal malnutrition 764.1 ☑
- affecting management of pregnancy 656.5 ☑

Light-headedness 780.4

Lightning (effects) (shock) (stroke) (struck by) 994.0
- burn — see Burn, by site
- foot 266.2

Lightwood's disease or syndrome (renal tubular acidosis) 588.89

Lignac's disease (cystinosis) 270.0

Lignac (-Fanconi) syndrome (cystinosis) 270.0

Lignac (-de Toni) (-Fanconi) (-Debré) syndrome (cystinosis) 270.0

Ligneous thyroiditis 245.3

Likoff's syndrome (angina in menopausal women) 413.9

Limb — see condition

Limitation of joint motion — see also Stiffness, joint 719.5 ☑
- sacroiliac 724.6

Limit dextrinosis 271.0

Limited
- cardiac reserve — see Disease, heart
- duction, eye NEC 378.63
- mandibular range of motion 524.52

Lindau's disease (retinocerebral angiomatosis) 759.6

Lindau (-von Hippel) disease (angiomatosis retinocerebellosa) 759.6

Linea corneae senilis 371.41

Lines
- Beau's (transverse furrows on fingernails) 703.8
- Harris' 733.91
- Hudson-Stähli 371.11
- Stähli's 371.11

Lingua
- geographical 529.1
- nigra (villosa) 529.3
- plicata 529.5
  - congenital 750.13
- tylosis 528.6

Lingual (tongue) — see also condition
- thyroid 759.2

Linitis (gastric) 535.4 ☑
- plastica (M8142/3) 151.9

Lioderma essentialis (cum melanosis et telangiectasia) 757.33

Lip — see also condition
- biting 528.9

Lipalgia 272.8

Lipedema — see Edema

Lipemia — see also Hyperlipidemia 272.4
- retina, retinalis 272.3

Lipidosis 272.7
- cephalin 272.7
- cerebral (infantile) (juvenile) (late) 330.1
- cerebroretinal 330.1 [362.71]
- cerebroside 272.7
- cerebrospinal 272.7
- chemically-induced 272.7
- cholesterol 272.7
- diabetic 250.8 ☑ [272.7]
- dystopic (hereditary) 272.7
- glycolipid 272.7
- hepatosplenomegalic 272.3
- hereditary, dystopic 272.7
- sulfatide 330.0

Lipoadenoma (M8324/0) — see Neoplasm, by site, benign

Lipoblastoma (M8881/0) — see Lipoma, by site

Lipoblastomatosis (M8881/0) — see Lipoma, by site

Lipochondrodystrophy 277.5

Lipochrome histiocytosis (familial) 288.1

Lipodystrophia progressiva 272.6

Lipodystrophy (progressive) 272.6
- insulin 272.6
- intestinal 040.2
- mesenteric 567.82

Lipofibroma (M8851/0) — see Lipoma, by site

Lipoglycoproteinosis 272.8

Lipogranuloma, sclerosing 709.8

Lipogranulomatosis (disseminated) 272.8
- kidney 272.8

Lipoid — see also condition
- histiocytosis 272.7
- essential 272.7
- nephrosis (see also Nephrosis) 581.3
- proteinosis of Urbach 272.8

Lipoidemia — see also Hyperlipidemia 272.4

Lipoidosis — see also Lipidosis 272.7

Lipoma (M8850/0) 214.9
- breast (skin) 214.1
- face 214.0
- fetal (M8881/0) — see Lipoma, by site
  - fat cell (M8880/0) — see Lipoma, by site
- infiltrating (M8856/0) — see Lipoma, by site
- intra-abdominal 214.3
- intramuscular (M8856/0) — see Lipoma, by site
- intrathoracic 214.2
- kidney 214.3
- mediastinum 214.2
- muscle 214.8
- peritoneum 214.3
- retroperitoneum 214.3
- skin 214.1
  - face 214.0
- spermatic cord 214.4
- spindle cell (M8857/0) — see Lipoma, by site
- stomach 214.3
- subcutaneous tissue 214.1
  - face 214.0
- thymus 214.2
- thyroid gland 214.2

Lipomatosis (dolorosa) 272.8
- epidural 214.8

Lipomatosis — continued
- fetal (M8881/0) — see Lipoma, by site
- Launois-Bensaude's 272.8

Lipomyohemangioma (M8860/0)
- specified site — see Neoplasm, connective tissue, benign
- unspecified site 223.0

Lipomyoma (M8860/0)
- specified site — see Neoplasm, connective tissue, benign
- unspecified site 223.0

Lipomyxoma (M8852/0) — see Lipoma, by site

Lipomyxosarcoma (M8852/3) — see Neoplasm, connective tissue, malignant

Lipophagocytosis 289.89

Lipoproteinemia (alpha) 272.4
- broad-beta 272.2
- floating-beta 272.2
- hyper-pre-beta 272.1

Lipoproteinosis (Rössle-Urbach-Wiethe) 272.8

Liposarcoma (M8850/3) — see also Neoplasm, connective tissue, malignant
- differentiated type (M8851/3) — see Neoplasm, connective tissue, malignant
- embryonal (M8852/3) — see Neoplasm, connective tissue, malignant
- mixed type (M8855/3) — see Neoplasm, connective tissue, malignant
- myxoid (M8852/3) — see Neoplasm, connective tissue, malignant
- pleomorphic (M8854/3) — see Neoplasm, connective tissue, malignant
- round cell (M8853/3) — see Neoplasm, connective tissue, malignant
- well differentiated type (M8851/3) — see Neoplasm, connective tissue, malignant

Liposynovitis prepatellaris 272.8

Lipping
- cervix 622.0
- spine (see also Spondylosis) 721.90
- vertebra (see also Spondylosis) 721.90

Lip pits (mucus), congenital 750.25

Lipschütz disease or ulcer 616.50

Lipuria 791.1
- bilharziasis 120.0

Liquefaction, vitreous humor 379.21

Lisping 307.9

Lissauer's paralysis 094.1

Lissencephalia, lissencephaly 742.2

Listerellose 027.0

Listeriose 027.0

Listeriosis 027.0
- congenital 771.2
- fetal 771.2
- suspected fetal damage affecting management of pregnancy 655.4 ☑

Listlessness 780.79

Lithemia 790.6

Lithiasis — see also Calculus
- hepatic (duct) — see Choledocholithiasis
- urinary 592.9

Lithopedion 779.9
- affecting management of pregnancy 656.8 ☑

Lithosis (occupational) 502
- with tuberculosis — see Tuberculosis, pulmonary

Lithuria 791.9

Litigation V62.5

Little
- league elbow 718.82
- stroke syndrome 435.9

Little's disease — see Palsy, cerebral

Littre's
- gland — see condition
- hernia — see Hernia, Littre's

Littritis — see also Urethritis 597.89

Livedo 782.61
- annularis 782.61
- racemose 782.61
- reticularis 782.61

Live flesh 781.0

Liver — see also condition
- donor V59.6

Livida, asphyxia
- newborn 768.6

Living
- alone V60.3
- with handicapped person V60.4

Lloyd's syndrome 258.1

Loa loa 125.2

Loasis 125.2

Lobe, lobar — see condition

Lobo's disease or blastomycosis 116.2

Lobomycosis 116.2

Lobotomy syndrome 310.0

Lobstein's disease (brittle bones and blue sclera) 756.51

Lobster-claw hand 755.58

Lobulation (congenital) — see also Anomaly, specified type NEC, by site
- kidney, fetal 753.3
- liver, abnormal 751.69
- spleen 759.0

Lobule, lobular — see condition

Local, localized — see condition

Locked bowel or intestine — see also Obstruction, intestine 560.9

Locked-in state 344.81

Locked twins 660.5 ☑
- affecting fetus or newborn 763.1

Locking
- joint (see also Derangement, joint) 718.90
- knee 717.9

Lockjaw — see also Tetanus 037

Locomotor ataxia (progressive) 094.0

Löffler's
- endocarditis 421.0
- eosinophilia or syndrome 518.3
- pneumonia 518.3
- syndrome (eosinophilic pneumonitis) 518.3

Löfgren's syndrome (sarcoidosis) 135

Loiasis 125.2
- eyelid 125.2 [373.6]

Loneliness V62.89

Lone star fever 082.8

Longitudinal stripes or grooves, nails 703.8
- congenital 757.5

Long labor 662.1 ☑
- affecting fetus or newborn 763.89
- first stage 662.0 ☑
- second stage 662.2 ☑

Long-term (current) **drug use** V58.69
- antibiotics V58.62
- anticoagulants V58.61
- anti-inflammatories, non-steroidal (NSAID) V58.64
- antiplatelets/antithrombotics V58.63
- aspirin V58.66
- insulin V58.67
- steroids V58.65

Loop
- intestine (see also Volvulus) 560.2
- intrascleral nerve 379.29
- vascular on papilla (optic) 743.57

Loose — see also condition
- body
  - in tendon sheath 727.82
  - joint 718.10
    - ankle 718.17
    - elbow 718.12
    - foot 718.17
    - hand 718.14
    - hip 718.15
    - knee 717.6

Loose

Loose — see also condition — continued
  body — continued
    joint — continued
      multiple sites 718.19
      pelvic region 718.15
      prosthetic implant — see Complications, mechanical
      shoulder (region) 718.11
      specified site NEC 718.18
      wrist 718.13
    cartilage (joint) (see also Loose, body, joint) 718.1 ☑
      knee 717.6
    facet (vertebral) 724.9
    prosthetic implant — see Complications, mechanical
    sesamoid, joint (see also Loose, body, joint) 718.1 ☑
    tooth, teeth 525.8
  Loosening epiphysis 732.9
  Looser (-Debray) -Milkman syndrome (osteomalacia with pseudofractures) 268.2
  Lop ear (deformity) 744.29
  Lorain's disease or syndrome (pituitary dwarfism) 253.3
  Lorain-Levi syndrome (pituitary dwarfism) 253.3
  Lordosis (acquired) (postural) 737.20
    congenital 754.2
    due to or associated with
      Charcôt-Marie-Tooth disease 356.1 [737.42]
      mucopolysaccharidosis 277.5 [737.42]
      neurofibromatosis 237.71 [737.42]
      osteitis
        deformans 731.0 [737.42]
        fibrosa cystica 252.01 [737.42]
      osteoporosis (see also Osteoporosis) 733.00 [737.42]
      poliomyelitis (see also Poliomyelitis) 138 [737.42]
      tuberculosis (see also Tuberculosis) 015.0 ☑ [737.42]
    late effect of rickets 268.1 [737.42]
    postlaminectomy 737.21
    postsurgical NEC 737.22
    rachitic 268.1 [737.42]
    specified NEC 737.29
    tuberculous (see also Tuberculosis) 015.0 ☑ [737.42]
  Loss
    appetite 783.0
      hysterical 300.11
      nonorganic origin 307.59
      psychogenic 307.59
    blood — see Hemorrhage
    central vision 368.41
    consciousness 780.09
      transient 780.2
    control, sphincter, rectum 787.6
      nonorganic origin 307.7
    ear ossicle, partial 385.24
    elasticity, skin 782.8
    extremity or member, traumatic, current — see Amputation, traumatic
    fluid (acute) 276.50
      with
        hypernatremia 276.0
        hyponatremia 276.1
      fetus or newborn 775.5
    hair 704.00
    hearing (see also Deafness)
      central, ▶bilateral◀ 389.14
      conductive (air) 389.00
        with sensorineural hearing loss 389.2
        combined types 389.08
        external ear 389.01
        inner ear 389.04
        middle ear 389.03
        multiple types 389.08
        tympanic membrane 389.02

Loss — continued
  hearing (see also Deafness) — continued
    mixed type 389.2
    nerve, ▶bilateral◀ 389.12
    neural, ▶bilateral◀ 389.12
    noise-induced 388.12
    perceptive NEC (see also Loss, hearing, sensorineural) 389.10
    sensorineural 389.10
      with conductive hearing loss 389.2
      asymmetrical 389.16 ●
      central, ▶bilateral◀ 389.14
      combined types, ▶bilateral◀ 389.18
      multiple types, ▶bilateral◀ 389.18
      neural, ▶bilateral◀ 389.12
      sensory, ▶bilateral◀ 389.11
      unilateral 389.15 ●
    sensory, ▶bilateral◀ 389.11
    specified type NEC 389.8
    sudden NEC 388.2
  height 781.91
  labyrinthine reactivity (unilateral) 386.55
    bilateral 386.56
  memory (see also Amnesia) 780.93
    mild, following organic brain damage 310.1
  mind (see also Psychosis) 298.9
  occlusal vertical dimension 524.37
  organ or part — see Absence, by site, acquired
  sensation 782.0
  sense of
    smell (see also Disturbance, sensation) 781.1
    taste (see also Disturbance, sensation) 781.1
    touch (see also Disturbance, sensation) 781.1
  sight (acquired) (complete) (congenital) — see Blindness
  spinal fluid
    headache 349.0
  substance of
    bone (see also Osteoporosis) 733.00
    cartilage 733.99
    ear 380.32
    vitreous (humor) 379.26
  tooth, teeth
    acquired 525.10
      due to
        caries 525.13
        extraction 525.10
        periodontal disease 525.12
      specified NEC 525.19
      trauma 525.11
  vision, visual (see also Blindness) 369.9
    both eyes (see also Blindness, both eyes) 369.3
    complete (see also Blindness, both eyes) 369.00
    one eye 369.8
    sudden 368.11
    transient 368.12
  vitreous 379.26
  voice (see also Aphonia) 784.41
  weight (cause unknown) 783.21
Lou Gehrig's disease 335.20
Louis-Bar syndrome (ataxia-telangiectasia) 334.8
Louping ill 063.1
Lousiness — see Lice
Low
  back syndrome 724.2
  basal metabolic rate (BMR) 794.7
  birthweight 765.1 ☑
    extreme (less than 1000 grams) 765.0 ☑
    for gestational age 764.0 ☑

Low — continued
  birthweight — continued
    status (see also Status, low birth weight) V21.30
  bladder compliance 596.52
  blood pressure (see also Hypotension) 458.9
    reading (incidental) (isolated) (nonspecific) 796.3
  cardiac reserve — see Disease, heart
  compliance bladder 596.52
  frequency deafness — see Disorder, hearing
  function (see also Hypofunction)
    kidney (see also Disease, renal) 593.9
    liver 573.9
  hemoglobin 285.9
  implantation, placenta — see Placenta, previa
  insertion, placenta — see Placenta, previa
  lying
    kidney 593.0
    organ or site, congenital — see Malposition, congenital
    placenta — see Placenta, previa
  output syndrome (cardiac) (see also Failure, heart) 428.9
  platelets (blood) (see also Thrombocytopenia) 287.5
  reserve, kidney (see also Disease, renal) 593.9
  risk
    cervical, human papillomavirus (HPV) DNA test positive 795.09
  salt syndrome 593.9
  tension glaucoma 365.12
  vision 369.9
    both eyes 369.20
    one eye 369.70
Lower extremity — see condition
Lowe (-Terrey-MacLachlan) syndrome (oculocerebrorenal dystrophy) 270.8
Lown (-Ganong) -Levine syndrome (short P-R interval, normal QRS complex, and paroxysmal supraventricular tachycardia) 426.81
LSD reaction — see also Abuse, drugs, nondependent 305.3 ☑
L-shaped kidney 753.3
Lucas-Championnière disease (fibrinous bronchitis) 466.0
Lucey-Driscoll syndrome (jaundice due to delayed conjugation) 774.30
Ludwig's
  angina 528.3
  disease (submaxillary cellulitis) 528.3
Lues (venerea), **luetic** — see Syphilis
Luetscher's syndrome (dehydration) 276.51
Lumbago 724.2
  due to displacement, intervertebral disc 722.10
Lumbalgia 724.2
  due to displacement, intervertebral disc 722.10
Lumbar — see condition
Lumbarization, vertebra 756.15
Lumbermen's itch 133.8
Lump — see also Mass
  abdominal 789.3 ☑
  breast 611.72
  chest 786.6
  epigastric 789.3 ☑
  head 784.2
  kidney 753.3
  liver 789.1
  lung 786.6
  mediastinal 786.6
  neck 784.2
  nose or sinus 784.2
  pelvic 789.3 ☑

Lump — see also Mass — continued
  skin 782.2
  substernal 786.6
  throat 784.2
  umbilicus 789.3 ☑
Lunacy — see also Psychosis 298.9
Lunatomalacia 732.3
Lung — see also condition
  donor V59.8
  drug addict's 417.8
  mainliners' 417.8
  vanishing 492.0
Lupoid (miliary) **of Boeck** 135
Lupus 710.0
  anticoagulant 289.81
  Cazenave's (erythematosus) 695.4
  discoid (local) 695.4
  disseminated 710.0
  erythematodes (discoid) (local) 695.4
  erythematosus (discoid) (local) 695.4
    disseminated 710.0
    eyelid 373.34
    systemic 710.0
      with
        encephalitis 710.0 [323.81] ▲
        lung involvement 710.0 [517.8]
      inhibitor (presence of) 286.5
  exedens 017.0 ☑
  eyelid (see also Tuberculosis) 017.0 ☑ [373.4]
  Hilliard's 017.0 ☑
  hydralazine
    correct substance properly administered 695.4
    overdose or wrong substance given or taken 972.6
  miliaris disseminatus faciei 017.0 ☑
  nephritis 710.0 [583.81]
    acute 710.0 [580.81]
    chronic 710.0 [582.81]
  nontuberculous, not disseminated 695.4
  pernio (Besnier) 135
  tuberculous (see also Tuberculosis) 017.0 ☑
    eyelid (see also Tuberculosis) 017.0 ☑ [373.4]
  vulgaris 017.0 ☑
Luschka's joint disease 721.90
Luteinoma (M8610/0) 220
Lutembacher's disease or syndrome (atrial septal defect with mitral stenosis) 745.5
Luteoma (M8610/0) 220
Lutz-Miescher disease (elastosis perforans serpiginosa) 701.1
Lutz-Splendore-de Almeida disease (Brazilian blastomycosis) 116.1
Luxatio
  bulbi due to birth injury 767.8
  coxae congenita (see also Dislocation, hip, congenital) 754.30
  erecta — see Dislocation, shoulder
  imperfecta — see Sprain, by site
  perinealis — see Dislocation, hip
Luxation — see also Dislocation, by site
  eyeball 360.81
    due to birth injury 767.8
    lateral 376.36
  genital organs (external) NEC — see Wound, open, genital organs
  globe (eye) 360.81
    lateral 376.36
  lacrimal gland (postinfectional) 375.16
  lens (old) (partial) 379.32
    congenital 743.37
      syphilitic 090.49 [379.32]
    Marfan's disease 090.49
    spontaneous 379.32
  penis — see Wound, open, penis
  scrotum — see Wound, open, scrotum
  testis — see Wound, open, testis
L-xyloketosuria 271.8
Lycanthropy — see also Psychosis 298.9

Index to Diseases

Lyell's disease or syndrome (toxic epidermal necrolysis) 695.1
- due to drug
  - correct substance properly administered 695.1
  - overdose or wrong substance given or taken 977.9
    - specified drug — *see* Table of Drugs and Chemicals

Lyme disease 088.81

Lymph
- gland or node — *see* condition
- scrotum (*see also* Infestation, filarial) 125.9

Lymphadenitis 289.3
- with
  - abortion — *see* Abortion, by type, with sepsis
  - ectopic pregnancy (*see also* categories 633.0–633.9) 639.0
  - molar pregnancy (*see also* categories 630–632) 639.0
- acute 683
  - mesenteric 289.2
- any site, except mesenteric 289.3
  - acute 683
  - chronic 289.1
  - mesenteric (acute) (chronic) (nonspecific) (subacute) 289.2
  - subacute 289.1
    - mesenteric 289.2
- breast, puerperal, postpartum 675.2 ☑
- chancroidal (congenital) 099.0
- chronic 289.1
  - mesenteric 289.2
- dermatopathic 695.89
- due to
  - anthracosis (occupational) 500
  - Brugia (Wuchereria) malayi 125.1
  - diphtheria (toxin) 032.89
  - lymphogranuloma venereum 099.1
  - Wuchereria bancrofti 125.0
- following
  - abortion 639.0
  - ectopic or molar pregnancy 639.0
- generalized 289.3
- gonorrheal 098.89
- granulomatous 289.1
- infectional 683
- mesenteric (acute) (chronic) (nonspecific) (subacute) 289.2
  - due to Bacillus typhi 002.0
  - tuberculous (*see also* Tuberculosis) 014.8 ☑
- mycobacterial 031.8
- purulent 683
- pyogenic 683
- regional 078.3
- septic 683
- streptococcal 683
- subacute, unspecified site 289.1
- suppurative 683
- syphilitic (early) (secondary) 091.4
  - late 095.8
- tuberculous — *see* Tuberculosis, lymph gland
- venereal 099.1

Lymphadenoid goiter 245.2

Lymphadenopathy (general) 785.6
- due to toxoplasmosis (acquired) 130.7
- congenital (active) 771.2

Lymphadenopathy-associated virus (disease) (illness) (infection) — *see* Human immunodeficiency virus (disease) (illness) (infection)

Lymphadenosis 785.6
- acute 075

Lymphangiectasis 457.1
- conjunctiva 372.89
- postinfectional 457.1
- scrotum 457.1

Lymphangiectatic elephantiasis, non-filarial 457.1

Lymphangioendothelioma (M9170/0) 228.1

Lymphangioendothelioma — *continued*
- malignant (M9170/3) — *see* Neoplasm, connective tissue, malignant

Lymphangioma (M9170/0) 228.1
- capillary (M9171/0) 228.1
- cavernous (M9172/0) 228.1
- cystic (M9173/0) 228.1
- malignant (M9170/3) — *see* Neoplasm, connective tissue, malignant

Lymphangiomyoma (M9174/0) 228.1

Lymphangiomyomatosis (M9174/1) — *see* Neoplasm, connective tissue, uncertain behavior

Lymphangiosarcoma (M9170/3) — *see* Neoplasm, connective tissue, malignant

Lymphangitis 457.2
- with
  - abortion — *see* Abortion, by type, with sepsis
  - abscess — *see* Abscess, by site
  - cellulitis — *see* Abscess, by site
  - ectopic pregnancy (*see also* categories 633.0–633.9) 639.0
  - molar pregnancy (*see also* categories 630–632) 639.0
- acute (with abscess or cellulitis) 682.9
  - specified site — *see* Abscess, by site
- breast, puerperal, postpartum 675.2 ☑
- chancroidal 099.0
- chronic (any site) 457.2
- due to
  - Brugia (Wuchereria) malayi 125.1
  - Wuchereria bancrofti 125.0
- following
  - abortion 639.0
  - ectopic or molar pregnancy 639.0
- gangrenous 457.2
- penis
  - acute 607.2
  - gonococcal (acute) 098.0
    - chronic or duration of 2 months or more 098.2
- puerperal, postpartum, childbirth 670.0 ☑
- strumous, tuberculous (*see also* Tuberculosis) 017.2 ☑
- subacute (any site) 457.2
- tuberculous — *see* Tuberculosis, lymph gland

Lymphatic (vessel) — *see* condition

Lymphatism 254.8
- scrofulous (*see also* Tuberculosis) 017.2 ☑

Lymphectasia 457.1

Lymphedema — *see also* Elephantiasis 457.1
- acquired (chronic) 457.1
- chronic hereditary 757.0
- congenital 757.0
- idiopathic hereditary 757.0
- praecox 457.1
- secondary 457.1
- surgical NEC 997.99
- postmastectomy (syndrome) 457.0

Lymph-hemangioma (M9120/0) — *see* Hemangioma, by site

Lymphoblastic — *see* condition

Lymphoblastoma (diffuse) (M9630/3) 200.1 ☑
- giant follicular (M9690/3) 202.0 ☑
- macrofollicular (M9690/3) 202.0 ☑

Lymphoblastosis, acute benign 075

Lymphocele 457.8

Lymphocythemia 288.51 ▲

Lymphocytic — *see also* condition
- chorioencephalitis (acute) (serous) 049.0
- choriomeningitis (acute) (serous) 049.0

Lymphocytoma (diffuse) (malignant) (M9620/3) 200.1 ☑

Lymphocytomatosis (M9620/3) 200.1 ☑

Lymphocytopenia 288.51 ▲

Lymphocytosis (symptomatic) 288.61 ▲
- infectious (acute) 078.89

Lymphoepithelioma (M8082/3) — *see* Neoplasm, by site, malignant

Lymphogranuloma (malignant) (M9650/3) 201.9 ☑
- inguinale 099.1
- venereal (any site) 099.1
  - with stricture of rectum 099.1
- venereum 099.1

Lymphogranulomatosis (malignant) (M9650/3) 201.9 ☑
- benign (Boeck's sarcoid) (Schaumann's) 135
- Hodgkin's (M9650/3) 201.9 ☑

Lymphohistiocytosis, familial hemophagocytic 288.4 ●

Lymphoid — *see* condition

Lympholeukoblastoma (M9850/3) 207.8 ☑

Lympholeukosarcoma (M9850/3) 207.8 ☑

Lymphoma (malignant) (M9590/3) 202.8 ☑

Note — Use the following fifth-digit subclassification with categories 200–202:

0	unspecified site, extranodal and solid organ sites
1	lymph nodes of head, face, and neck
2	intrathoracic lymph nodes
3	intra-abdominal lymph nodes
4	lymph nodes of axilla and upper limb
5	lymph nodes of inguinal region and lower limb
6	intrapelvic lymph nodes
7	spleen
8	lymph nodes of multiple sites

- benign (M9590/0) — *see* Neoplasm, by site, benign
- Burkitt's type (lymphoblastic) (undifferentiated) (M9750/3) 200.2 ☑
- Castleman's (mediastinal lymph node hyperplasia) 785.6
- centroblastic-centrocytic
  - diffuse (M9614/3) 202.8 ☑
  - follicular (M9692/3) 202.0 ☑
- centroblastic type (diffuse) (M9632/3) 202.8 ☑
  - follicular (M9697/3) 202.0 ☑
- centrocytic (M9622/3) 202.8 ☑
- compound (M9613/3) 200.8 ☑
- convoluted cell type (lymphoblastic) (M9602/3) 202.8 ☑
- diffuse NEC (M9590/3) 202.8 ☑
- follicular (giant) (M9690/3) 202.0 ☑
  - center cell (diffuse) (M9615/3) 202.8 ☑
  - cleaved (diffuse) (M9623/3) 202.8 ☑
  - follicular (M9695/3) 202.0 ☑
  - non-cleaved (diffuse) (M9633/3) 202.8 ☑
  - follicular (M9698/3) 202.0 ☑
  - centroblastic-centrocytic (M9692/3) 202.0 ☑
  - centroblastic type (M9697/3) 202.0 ☑
  - lymphocytic
    - intermediate differentiation (M9694/3) 202.0 ☑
    - poorly differentiated (M9696/3) 202.0 ☑

Lymphoma — *continued*
- follicular — *continued*
  - mixed (cell type) (lymphocytic-histiocytic) (small cell and large cell) (M9691/3) 202.0 ☑
  - germinocytic (M9622/3) 202.8 ☑
  - giant, follicular or follicle (M9690/3) 202.0 ☑
- histiocytic (diffuse) (M9640/3) 200.0 ☑
  - nodular (M9642/3) 200.0 ☑
  - pleomorphic cell type (M9641/3) 200.0 ☑
- Hodgkin's (M9650/3) (*see also* Disease, Hodgkin's) 201.9 ☑
- immunoblastic (type) (M9612/3) 200.8 ☑
- large cell (M9640/3) 200.0 ☑
  - nodular (M9642/3) 200.0 ☑
  - pleomorphic cell type (M9641/3) 200.0 ☑
- lymphoblastic (diffuse) (M9630/3) 200.1 ☑
  - Burkitt's type (M9750/3) 200.2 ☑
  - convoluted cell type (M9602/3) 202.8 ☑
- lymphocytic (cell type) (diffuse) (M9620/3) 200.1 ☑
  - with plasmacytoid differentiation, diffuse (M9611/3) 200.8 ☑
  - intermediate differentiation (diffuse) (M9621/3) 200.1 ☑
    - follicular (M9694/3) 202.0 ☑
    - nodular (M9694/3) 202.0 ☑
    - nodular (M9690/3) 202.0 ☑
  - poorly differentiated (diffuse) (M9630/3) 200.1 ☑
    - follicular (M9696/3) 202.0 ☑
    - nodular (M9696/3) 202.0 ☑
  - well differentiated (diffuse) (M9620/3) 200.1 ☑
    - follicular (M9693/3) 202.0 ☑
    - nodular (M9693/3) 202.0 ☑
  - lymphocytic-histiocytic, mixed (diffuse) (M9613/3) 200.8 ☑
    - follicular (M9691/3) 202.0 ☑
    - nodular (M9691/3) 202.0 ☑
- lymphoplasmacytoid type (M9611/3) 200.8 ☑
- lymphosarcoma type (M9610/3) 200.1 ☑
- macrofollicular (M9690/3) 202.0 ☑
- mixed cell type (diffuse) (M9613/3) 200.8 ☑
  - follicular (M9691/3) 202.0 ☑
  - nodular (M9691/3) 202.0 ☑
- nodular (M9690/3) 202.0 ☑
  - histiocytic (M9642/3) 200.0 ☑
  - lymphocytic (M9690/3) 202.0 ☑
    - intermediate differentiation (M9694/3) 202.0 ☑
    - poorly differentiated (M9696/3) 202.0 ☑
  - mixed (cell type) (lymphocytic-histiocytic) (small cell and large cell) (M9691/3) 202.0 ☑
- non-Hodgkin's type NEC (M9591/3) 202.8 ☑
- reticulum cell (type) (M9640/3) 200.0 ☑
- small cell and large cell, mixed (diffuse) (M9613/3) 200.8 ☑
  - follicular (M9691/3) 202.0 ☑
  - nodular (9691/3) 202.0 ☑
- stem cell (type) (M9601/3) 202.8 ☑
- T-cell 202.1
- undifferentiated (cell type) (non-Burkitt's) (M9600/3) 202.8 ☑
- Burkitt's type (M9750/3) 200.2 ☑

Lymphomatosis (M9590/3) — *see also* Lymphoma
- granulomatous 099.1

Lymphopathia
- venereum 099.1
- veneris 099.1

Lymphopenia

Lymphopenia 288.51 ▲
  familial 279.2
Lymphoreticulosis, benign (of inoculation) 078.3
Lymphorrhea 457.8
Lymphosarcoma (M9610/3) 200.1 ☑
  diffuse (M9610/3) 200.1 ☑
    with plasmacytoid differentiation (M9611/3) 200.8 ☑
      lymphoplasmacytic (M9611/3) 200.8 ☑
  follicular (giant) (M9690/3) 202.0 ☑
    lymphoblastic (M9696/3) 202.0 ☑
    lymphocytic, intermediate differentiation (M9694/3) 202.0 ☑
    mixed cell type (M9691/3) 202.0 ☑
  giant follicular (M9690/3) 202.0 ☑
  Hodgkin's (M9650/3) 201.9 ☑
  immunoblastic (M9612/3) 200.8 ☑
  lymphoblastic (diffuse) (M9630/3) 200.1 ☑
    follicular (M9696/3) 202.0 ☑
    nodular (M9696/3) 202.0 ☑
  lymphocytic (diffuse) (M9620/3) 200.1 ☑
    intermediate differentiation (diffuse) (M9621/3) 200.1 ☑
      follicular (M9694/3) 202.0 ☑
      nodular (M9694/3) 202.0 ☑
  mixed cell type (diffuse) (M9613/3) 200.8 ☑
    follicular (M9691/3) 202.0 ☑
    nodular (M9691/3) 202.0 ☑
  nodular (M9690/3) 202.0 ☑
    lymphoblastic (M9696/3) 202.0 ☑
    lymphocytic, intermediate differentiation (M9694/3) 202.0 ☑
    mixed cell type (M9691/3) 202.0 ☑
  prolymphocytic (M9631/3) 200.1 ☑
  reticulum cell (M9640/3) 200.0 ☑
Lymphostasis 457.8
Lypemania — see also Melancholia 296.2 ☑
Lyssa 071

M

Macacus ear 744.29
Maceration
  fetus (cause not stated) 779.9
  wet feet, tropical (syndrome) 991.4
Machado-Joseph disease 334.8
Machupo virus hemorrhagic fever 078.7
Macleod's syndrome (abnormal transradiancy, one lung) 492.8
Macrocephalia, macrocephaly 756.0
Macrocheilia (congenital) 744.81
Macrochilia (congenital) 744.81
Macrocolon (congenital) 751.3
Macrocornea 743.41
  associated with buphthalmos 743.22
Macrocytic — see condition
Macrocytosis 289.89
Macrodactylia, macrodactylism (fingers) (thumbs) 755.57
  toes 755.65
Macrodontia 520.2
Macroencephaly 742.4
Macrogenia 524.05
Macrogenitosomia (female) (male) (praecox) 255.2
Macrogingivae 523.8
Macroglobulinemia (essential) (idiopathic) (monoclonal) (primary) (syndrome) (Waldenström's) 273.3
Macroglossia (congenital) 750.15
  acquired 529.8
Macrognathia, macrognathism (congenital) 524.00
  mandibular 524.02
    alveolar 524.72
  maxillary 524.01
    alveolar 524.71
Macrogyria (congenital) 742.4

Macrohydrocephalus — see also Hydrocephalus 331.4
Macromastia — see also Hypertrophy, breast 611.1
Macrophage activation syndrome 288.4 ●
Macropsia 368.14
Macrosigmoid 564.7
  congenital 751.3
Macrospondylitis, acromegalic 253.0
Macrostomia (congenital) 744.83
Macrotia (external ear) (congenital) 744.22
Macula
  cornea, corneal
    congenital 743.43
      interfering with vision 743.42
    interfering with central vision 371.03
    not interfering with central vision 371.02
  degeneration (see also Degeneration, macula) 362.50
  hereditary (see also Dystrophy, retina) 362.70
  edema, cystoid 362.53
Maculae ceruleae 132.1
Macules and papules 709.8
Maculopathy, toxic 362.55
Madarosis 374.55
Madelung's
  deformity (radius) 755.54
  disease (lipomatosis) 272.8
  lipomatosis 272.8
Madness — see also Psychosis 298.9
  myxedema (acute) 293.0
  subacute 293.1
Madura
  disease (actinomycotic) 039.9
    mycotic 117.4
  foot (actinomycotic) 039.9
    mycotic 117.4
Maduromycosis (actinomycotic) 039.9
  mycotic 117.4
Maffucci's syndrome (dyschondroplasia with hemangiomas) 756.4
Magenblase syndrome 306.4
Main en griffe (acquired) 736.06
  congenital 755.59
Maintenance
  chemotherapy regimen or treatment V58.11
  dialysis regimen or treatment
    extracorporeal (renal) V56.0
    peritoneal V56.8
    renal V56.0
  drug therapy or regimen
    chemotherapy, antineoplastic V58.11
    immunotherapy, antineoplastic V58.12
  external fixation NEC V54.89
  radiotherapy V58.0
  traction NEC V54.89
Majocchi's
  disease (purpura annularis telangiectodes) 709.1
  granuloma 110.6
Major — see condition
Mal
  cerebral (idiopathic) (see also Epilepsy) 345.9 ☑
  comital (see also Epilepsy) 345.9 ☑
  de los pintos (see also Pinta) 103.9
  de Meleda 757.39
  de mer 994.6
  lie — see Presentation, fetal
  perforant (see also Ulcer, lower extremity) 707.15
Malabar itch 110.9
  beard 110.0
  foot 110.4
  scalp 110.0
Malabsorption 579.9
  calcium 579.8
  carbohydrate 579.8

Malabsorption — continued
  disaccharide 271.3
  drug-induced 579.8
  due to bacterial overgrowth 579.8
  fat 579.8
  folate, congenital 281.2
  galactose 271.1
  glucose-galactose (congenital) 271.3
  intestinal 579.9
  isomaltose 271.3
  lactose (hereditary) 271.3
  methionine 270.4
  monosaccharide 271.8
  postgastrectomy 579.3
  postsurgical 579.3
  protein 579.8
  sucrose (-isomaltose) (congenital) 271.3
  syndrome 579.9
    postgastrectomy 579.3
    postsurgical 579.3
Malacia, bone 268.2
  juvenile (see also Rickets) 268.0
  Kienböck's (juvenile) (lunate) (wrist) 732.3
  adult 732.8
Malacoplakia
  bladder 596.8
  colon 569.89
  pelvis (kidney) 593.89
  ureter 593.89
  urethra 599.84
Malacosteon 268.2
  juvenile (see also Rickets) 268.0
Maladaptation — see Maladjustment
Maladie de Roger 745.4
Maladjustment
  conjugal V61.10
    involving divorce or estrangement V61.0
  educational V62.3
  family V61.9
    specified circumstance NEC V61.8
  marital V61.10
    involving divorce or estrangement V61.0
  occupational V62.2
  simple, adult (see also Reaction, adjustment) 309.9
  situational acute (see also Reaction, adjustment) 309.9
  social V62.4
Malaise 780.79
Malakoplakia — see Malacoplakia
Malaria, malarial (fever) 084.6
  algid 084.9
  any type, with
    algid malaria 084.9
    blackwater fever 084.8
    fever
      blackwater 084.8
      hemoglobinuric (bilious) 084.8
    hemoglobinuria, malarial 084.8
    hepatitis 084.9 [573.2]
    nephrosis 084.9 [581.81]
    pernicious complication NEC 084.9
      cardiac 084.9
      cerebral 084.9
  cardiac 084.9
  carrier (suspected) of V02.9
  cerebral 084.9
  complicating pregnancy, childbirth, or puerperium 647.4 ☑
  congenital 771.2
  congestion, congestive 084.6
    brain 084.9
  continued 084.0
  estivo-autumnal 084.0
  falciparum (malignant tertian) 084.0
  hematinuria 084.8
  hematuria 084.8
  hemoglobinuria 084.8
  hemorrhagic 084.6
  induced (therapeutically) 084.7
    accidental — see Malaria, by type
  liver 084.9 [573.2]

Malaria, malarial — continued
  malariae (quartan) 084.2
  malignant (tertian) 084.0
  mixed infections 084.5
  monkey 084.4
  ovale 084.3
  pernicious, acute 084.0
  Plasmodium, P.
    falciparum 084.0
    malariae 084.2
    ovale 084.3
    vivax 084.1
  quartan 084.2
  quotidian 084.0
  recurrent 084.6
    induced (therapeutically) 084.7
      accidental — see Malaria, by type
  remittent 084.6
  specified types NEC 084.4
  spleen 084.6
  subtertian 084.0
  tertian (benign) 084.1
    malignant 084.0
  tropical 084.0
  typhoid 084.6
  vivax (benign tertian) 084.1
Malassez's disease (testicular cyst) 608.89
Malassimilation 579.9
Maldescent, testis 752.51
Maldevelopment — see also Anomaly, by site
  brain 742.9
  colon 751.5
  hip (joint) 755.63
    congenital dislocation (see also Dislocation, hip, congenital) 754.30
  mastoid process 756.0
  middle ear, except ossicles 744.03
    ossicles 744.04
  newborn (not malformation) 764.9 ☑
  ossicles, ear 744.04
  spine 756.10
  toe 755.66
Male type pelvis 755.69
  with disproportion (fetopelvic) 653.2 ☑
    affecting fetus or newborn 763.1
    causing obstructed labor 660.1 ☑
      affecting fetus or newborn 763.1
Malformation (congenital) — see also Anomaly
  bone 756.9
  bursa 756.9
  Chiari
    type I 348.4
    type II (see also Spina bifida) 741.0 ☑
    type III 742.0
    type IV 742.2
  circulatory system NEC 747.9
    specified type NEC 747.89
  cochlea 744.05
  digestive system NEC 751.9
    lower 751.5
    specified type NEC 751.8
    upper 750.9
  eye 743.9
  gum 750.9
  heart NEC 746.9
    specified type NEC 746.89
    valve 746.9
  internal ear 744.05
  joint NEC 755.9
    specified type NEC 755.8
  Mondini's (congenital) (malformation, cochlea) 744.05
  muscle 756.9
  nervous system (central) 742.9
  pelvic organs or tissues
    in pregnancy or childbirth 654.9 ☑
      affecting fetus or newborn 763.1
      causing obstructed labor 660.2 ☑

Malformation — see also Anomaly — continued
  pelvic organs or tissues — continued
    in pregnancy or childbirth — continued
      causing obstructed labor — continued
        affecting fetus or newborn 763.1
  placenta (see also Placenta, abnormal) 656.7 ☑
  respiratory organs 748.9
    specified type NEC 748.8
  Rieger's 743.44
  sense organs NEC 742.9
    specified type NEC 742.8
  skin 757.9
    specified type NEC 757.8
  spinal cord 742.9
  teeth, tooth NEC 520.9
  tendon 756.9
  throat 750.9
  umbilical cord (complicating delivery) 663.9 ☑
    affecting fetus or newborn 762.6
  umbilicus 759.9
  urinary system NEC 753.9
    specified type NEC 753.8
Malfunction — see also Dysfunction
  arterial graft 996.1
  cardiac pacemaker 996.01
  catheter device — see Complications, mechanical, catheter
  colostomy 569.62
    valve 569.62
  cystostomy 997.5
  device, implant, or graft NEC — see Complications, mechanical
  enteric stoma 569.62
  enterostomy 569.62
  esophagostomy 530.87
  gastroenteric 536.8
  gastrostomy 536.42
  ileostomy
    valve 569.62
  nephrostomy 997.5
  pacemaker — see Complications, mechanical, pacemaker
  prosthetic device, internal — see Complications, mechanical
  tracheostomy 519.02
  valve
    colostomy 569.62
    ileostomy 569.62
  vascular graft or shunt 996.1
Malgaigne's fracture (closed) 808.43
  open 808.53
Malherbe's
  calcifying epithelioma (M8110/0) — see Neoplasm, skin, benign
  tumor (M8110/0) — see Neoplasm, skin, benign
Malibu disease 919.8
  infected 919.9
Malignancy (M8000/3) — see Neoplasm, by site, malignant
Malignant — see condition
Malingerer, malingering V65.2
Mallet, finger (acquired) 736.1
  congenital 755.59
  late effect of rickets 268.1
Malleus 024
Mallory's bodies 034.1
Mallory-Weiss syndrome 530.7
Malnutrition (calorie) 263.9
  complicating pregnancy 648.9 ☑
  degree
    first 263.1
    second 263.0
    third 262
    mild 263.1
    moderate 263.0
    severe 261
      protein-calorie 262
  fetus 764.2 ☑

Malnutrition — continued
  fetus — continued
    "light-for-dates" 764.1 ☑
  following gastrointestinal surgery 579.3
  intrauterine or fetal 764.2 ☑
    fetus or infant "light-for-dates" 764.1 ☑
  lack of care, or neglect (child) (infant) 995.52
    adult 995.84
  malignant 260
  mild 263.1
  moderate 263.0
  protein 260
  protein-calorie 263.9
    severe 262
    specified type NEC 263.8
  severe 261
    protein-calorie NEC 262
Malocclusion (teeth) 524.4
  angle's class I 524.21
  angle's class II 524.22
  angle's class III 524.23
  due to
    abnormal swallowing 524.59
    accessory teeth (causing crowding) 524.31
    dentofacial abnormality NEC 524.89
    impacted teeth (causing crowding) 520.6
    missing teeth 524.30
    mouth breathing 524.59
    sleep postures 524.59
    supernumerary teeth (causing crowding) 524.31
    thumb sucking 524.59
    tongue, lip, or finger habits 524.59
  temporomandibular (joint) 524.69
Malposition
  cardiac apex (congenital) 746.87
  cervix — see Malposition, uterus
  congenital
    adrenal (gland) 759.1
    alimentary tract 751.8
      lower 751.5
      upper 750.8
    aorta 747.21
    appendix 751.5
    arterial trunk 747.29
    artery (peripheral) NEC (see also Malposition, congenital, peripheral vascular system) 747.60
      coronary 746.85
      pulmonary 747.3
    auditory canal 744.29
      causing impairment of hearing 744.02
    auricle (ear) 744.29
      causing impairment of hearing 744.02
      cervical 744.43
    biliary duct or passage 751.69
    bladder (mucosa) 753.8
      exteriorized or extroverted 753.5
    brachial plexus 742.8
    brain tissue 742.4
    breast 757.6
    bronchus 748.3
    cardiac apex 746.87
    cecum 751.5
    clavicle 755.51
    colon 751.5
    digestive organ or tract NEC 751.8
      lower 751.5
      upper 750.8
    ear (auricle) (external) 744.29
      ossicles 744.04
    endocrine (gland) NEC 759.2
    epiglottis 748.3
    Eustachian tube 744.24
    eye 743.8
    facial features 744.89
    fallopian tube 752.19

Malposition — continued
  congenital — continued
    finger(s) 755.59
      supernumerary 755.01
    foot 755.67
    gallbladder 751.69
    gastrointestinal tract 751.8
    genitalia, genital organ(s) or tract
      female 752.89
        external 752.49
        internal NEC 752.89
      male 752.89
        penis 752.69
        scrotal transposition 752.81
    glottis 748.3
    hand 755.59
    heart 746.87
      dextrocardia 746.87
        with complete transposition of viscera 759.3
    hepatic duct 751.69
    hip (joint) (see also Dislocation, hip, congenital) 754.30
    intestine (large) (small) 751.5
      with anomalous adhesions, fixation, or malrotation 751.4
    joint NEC 755.8
    kidney 753.3
    larynx 748.3
    limb 755.8
      lower 755.69
      upper 755.59
    liver 751.69
    lung (lobe) 748.69
    nail(s) 757.5
    nerve 742.8
    nervous system NEC 742.8
    nose, nasal (septum) 748.1
    organ or site NEC — see Anomaly, specified type NEC, by site
    ovary 752.0
    pancreas 751.7
    parathyroid (gland) 759.2
    patella 755.64
    peripheral vascular system 747.60
      gastrointestinal 747.61
      lower limb 747.64
      renal 747.62
      specified NEC 747.69
      spinal 747.82
      upper limb 747.63
    pituitary (gland) 759.2
    respiratory organ or system NEC 748.9
    rib (cage) 756.3
      supernumerary in cervical region 756.2
    scapula 755.59
    shoulder 755.59
    spinal cord 742.59
    spine 756.19
    spleen 759.0
    sternum 756.3
    stomach 750.7
    symphysis pubis 755.69
    testis (undescended) 752.51
    thymus (gland) 759.2
    thyroid (gland) (tissue) 759.2
      cartilage 748.3
    toe(s) 755.66
      supernumerary 755.02
    tongue 750.19
    trachea 748.3
    uterus 752.3
    vein(s) (peripheral) NEC (see also Malposition, congenital, peripheral vascular system) 747.60
      great 747.49
      portal 747.49
      pulmonary 747.49
      vena cava (inferior) (superior) 747.49
  device, implant, or graft — see Complications, mechanical

Malposition — continued
  fetus NEC (see also Presentation, fetal) 652.9 ☑
    with successful version 652.1 ☑
    affecting fetus or newborn 763.1
    before labor, affecting fetus or newborn 761.7
    causing obstructed labor 660.0 ☑
    in multiple gestation (one fetus or more) 652.6 ☑
      with locking 660.5 ☑
        causing obstructed labor 660.0 ☑
  gallbladder (see also Disease, gallbladder) 575.8
  gastrointestinal tract 569.89
    congenital 751.8
  heart (see also Malposition, congenital; heart) 746.87
  intestine 569.89
    congenital 751.5
  pelvic organs or tissues
    in pregnancy or childbirth 654.4 ☑
      affecting fetus or newborn 763.89
      causing obstructed labor 660.2 ☑
        affecting fetus or newborn 763.1
  placenta — see Placenta, previa
  stomach 537.89
    congenital 750.7
  tooth, teeth 524.30
    with impaction 520.6
  uterus (acquired) (acute) (adherent) (any degree) (asymptomatic) (postinfectional) (postpartal, old) 621.6
    anteflexion or anteversion (see also Anteversion, uterus) 621.6
    congenital 752.3
    flexion 621.6
      lateral (see also Lateroversion, uterus) 621.6
    in pregnancy or childbirth 654.4 ☑
      affecting fetus or newborn 763.89
      causing obstructed labor 660.2 ☑
        affecting fetus or newborn 763.1
    inversion 621.6
    lateral (flexion) (version) (see also Lateroversion, uterus) 621.6
    lateroflexion (see also Lateroversion, uterus) 621.6
    lateroversion (see also Lateroversion, uterus) 621.6
    retroflexion or retroversion (see also Retroversion, uterus) 621.6
Malposture 729.9
Malpresentation, fetus — see also Presentation, fetal 652.9 ☑
Malrotation
  cecum 751.4
  colon 751.4
  intestine 751.4
  kidney 753.3
Malta fever — see also Brucellosis 023.9
Maltosuria 271.3
Maltreatment (of)
  adult 995.80
    emotional 995.82
    multiple forms 995.85
    neglect (nutritional) 995.84
    physical 995.81
    psychological 995.82
    sexual 995.83
  child 995.50
    emotional 995.51
    multiple forms 995.59
    neglect (nutritional) 995.52
    physical 995.54
      shaken infant syndrome 995.55
    psychological 995.51

Maltreatment — continued
child — continued
  sexual 995.53
spouse (see also Maltreatment, adult) 995.80
Malt workers' lung 495.4
Malum coxae senilis 715.25
Malunion, fracture 733.81
Mammillitis — see also Mastitis 611.0
puerperal, postpartum 675.2 ☑
Mammitis — see also Mastitis 611.0
puerperal, postpartum 675.2 ☑
Mammographic
calcification 793.89 ●
calculus 793.89 ●
microcalcification 793.81 ●
Mammoplasia 611.1
Management
contraceptive V25.9
  specified type NEC V25.8
procreative V26.9
  specified type NEC V26.8
Mangled NEC — see also nature and site of injury 959.9
Mania (monopolar) — see also Psychosis, affective 296.0 ☑
alcoholic (acute) (chronic) 291.9
Bell's — see Mania, chronic
chronic 296.0 ☑
  recurrent episode 296.1 ☑
  single episode 296.0 ☑
compulsive 300.3
delirious (acute) 296.0 ☑
  recurrent episode 296.1 ☑
  single episode 296.0 ☑
epileptic (see also Epilepsy) 345.4 ☑
hysterical 300.10
inhibited 296.89
puerperal (after delivery) 296.0 ☑
  recurrent episode 296.1 ☑
  single episode 296.0 ☑
recurrent episode 296.1 ☑
senile 290.8
single episode 296.0 ☑
stupor 296.89
stuporous 296.89
unproductive 296.89
Manic-depressive insanity, psychosis, reaction, or syndrome — see also Psychosis, affective 296.80
circular (alternating) 296.7
  currently
    depressed 296.5 ☑
    episode unspecified 296.7
    hypomanic, previously depressed 296.4 ☑
    manic 296.4 ☑
    mixed 296.6 ☑
depressed (type), depressive 296.2 ☑
  atypical 296.82
  recurrent episode 296.3 ☑
  single episode 296.2 ☑
hypomanic 296.0 ☑
  recurrent episode 296.1 ☑
  single episode 296.0 ☑
manic 296.0 ☑
  atypical 296.81
  recurrent episode 296.1 ☑
  single episode 296.0 ☑
mixed NEC 296.89
perplexed 296.89
stuporous 296.89
Manifestations, rheumatoid
lungs 714.81
pannus — see Arthritis, rheumatoid
subcutaneous nodules — see Arthritis, rheumatoid
Mankowsky's syndrome (familial dysplastic osteopathy) 731.2
Mannoheptulosuria 271.8
Mannosidosis 271.8
Manson's
disease (schistosomiasis) 120.1
pyosis (pemphigus contagiosus) 684
schistosomiasis 120.1
Mansonellosis 125.5

Manual — see condition
Maple bark disease 495.6
Maple bark-strippers' lung 495.6
Maple syrup (urine) disease or syndrome 270.3
Marable's syndrome (celiac artery compression) 447.4
Marasmus 261
brain 331.9
due to malnutrition 261
intestinal 569.89
nutritional 261
senile 797
tuberculous NEC (see also Tuberculosis) 011.9 ☑
Marble
bones 756.52
skin 782.61
Marburg disease (virus) 078.89
March
foot 733.94
hemoglobinuria 283.2
Marchand multiple nodular hyperplasia (liver) 571.5
Marchesani (-Weill) syndrome (brachymorphism and ectopia lentis) 759.89
Marchiafava (-Bignami) disease or syndrome 341.8
Marchiafava-Micheli syndrome (paroxysmal nocturnal hemoglobinuria) 283.2
Marcus Gunn's syndrome (jaw-winking syndrome) 742.8
Marfan's
congenital syphilis 090.49
disease 090.49
syndrome (arachnodactyly) 759.82
  meaning congenital syphilis 090.49
  with luxation of lens 090.49 [379.32]
Marginal
implantation, placenta — see Placenta, previa
placenta — see Placenta, previa
sinus (hemorrhage) (rupture) 641.2 ☑
  affecting fetus or newborn 762.1
Marie's
cerebellar ataxia 334.2
syndrome (acromegaly) 253.0
Marie-Bamberger disease or syndrome (hypertrophic) (pulmonary) (secondary) 731.2
idiopathic (acropachyderma) 757.39
primary (acropachyderma) 757.39
Marie-Charcôt-Tooth neuropathic atrophy, muscle 356.1
Marie-Strümpell arthritis or disease (ankylosing spondylitis) 720.0
Marihuana, marijuana
abuse (see also Abuse, drugs, nondependent) 305.2 ☑
dependence (see also Dependence) 304.3 ☑
Marion's disease (bladder neck obstruction) 596.0
Marital conflict V61.10
Mark
port wine 757.32
raspberry 757.32
strawberry 757.32
stretch 701.3
tattoo 709.09
Maroteaux-Lamy syndrome (mucopolysaccharidosis VI) 277.5
Marriage license examination V70.3
Marrow (bone)
arrest 284.9
megakaryocytic 287.30
poor function 289.9
Marseilles fever 082.1
Marshall's (hidrotic) **ectodermal dysplasia** 757.31
Marsh's disease (exophthalmic goiter) 242.0 ☑
Marsh fever — see also Malaria 084.6

Martin-Albright syndrome (pseudohypoparathyroidism) 275.49
Martin's disease 715.27
Martorell-Fabre syndrome (pulseless disease) 446.7
Masculinization, female, with adrenal hyperplasia 255.2
Masculinovoblastoma (M8670/0) 220
Masochism 302.83
Masons' lung 502
Mass
abdominal 789.3 ☑
anus 787.99
bone 733.90
breast 611.72
cheek 784.2
chest 786.6
cystic — see Cyst
ear 388.8
epigastric 789.3 ☑
eye 379.92
female genital organ 625.8
gum 784.2
head 784.2
intracranial 784.2
joint 719.60
  ankle 719.67
  elbow 719.62
  foot 719.67
  hand 719.64
  hip 719.65
  knee 719.66
  multiple sites 719.69
  pelvic region 719.65
  shoulder (region) 719.61
  specified site NEC 719.68
  wrist 719.63
kidney (see also Disease, kidney) 593.9
lung 786.6
lymph node 785.6
malignant (M8000/3) — see Neoplasm, by site, malignant
mediastinal 786.6
mouth 784.2
muscle (limb) 729.89
neck 784.2
nose or sinus 784.2
palate 784.2
pelvis, pelvic 789.3 ☑
penis 607.89
perineum 625.8
rectum 787.99
scrotum 608.89
skin 782.2
specified organ NEC — see Disease of specified organ or site
splenic 789.2
substernal 786.6
  thyroid (see also Goiter) 240.9
superficial (localized) 782.2
testes 608.89
throat 784.2
tongue 784.2
umbilicus 789.3 ☑
uterus 625.8
vagina 625.8
vulva 625.8
Massive — see condition
Mastalgia 611.71
psychogenic 307.89
Mast cell
disease 757.33
  systemic (M9741/3) 202.6 ☑
leukemia (M9900/3) 207.8 ☑
sarcoma (M9742/3) 202.6 ☑
tumor (M9740/1) 238.5
  malignant (M9740/3) 202.6 ☑
Masters-Allen syndrome 620.6
Mastitis (acute) (adolescent) (diffuse) (interstitial) (lobular) (nonpuerperal) (nonsuppurative) (parenchymatous) (phlegmonous) (simple) (subacute) (suppurative) 611.0
chronic (cystic) (fibrocystic) 610.1
cystic 610.1

Mastitis — continued
cystic — continued
  Schimmelbusch's type 610.1
fibrocystic 610.1
infective 611.0
lactational 675.2 ☑
lymphangitis 611.0
neonatal (noninfective) 778.7
  infective 771.5
periductal 610.4
plasma cell 610.4
puerperalis 675.2 ☑
puerperal, postpartum, (interstitial) (nonpurulent) (parenchymatous) 675.2 ☑
  purulent 675.1 ☑
  stagnation 676.2 ☑
retromammary 611.0
  puerperal, postpartum 675.1 ☑
submammary 611.0
  puerperal, postpartum 675.1 ☑
Mastocytoma (M9740/1) 238.5
malignant (M9740/3) 202.6 ☑
Mastocytosis 757.33
malignant (M9741/3) 202.6 ☑
systemic (M9741/3) 202.6 ☑
Mastodynia 611.71
psychogenic 307.89
Mastoid — see condition
Mastoidalgia — see also Otalgia 388.70
Mastoiditis (coalescent) (hemorrhagic) (pneumococcal) (streptococcal) (suppurative) 383.9
acute or subacute 383.00
with
  Gradenigo's syndrome 383.02
  petrositis 383.02
  specified complication NEC 383.02
  subperiosteal abscess 383.01
chronic (necrotic) (recurrent) 383.1
tuberculous (see also Tuberculosis) 015.6 ☑
Mastopathy, mastopathia 611.9
chronica cystica 610.1
diffuse cystic 610.1
estrogenic 611.8
ovarian origin 611.8
Mastoplasia 611.1
Masturbation 307.9
Maternal condition, affecting fetus or newborn
acute yellow atrophy of liver 760.8
albuminuria 760.1
anesthesia or analgesia 763.5
blood loss 762.1
chorioamnionitis 762.7
circulatory disease, chronic (conditions classifiable to 390–459, 745–747) 760.3
congenital heart disease (conditions classifiable to 745–746) 760.3
cortical necrosis of kidney 760.1
death 761.6
diabetes mellitus 775.0
  manifest diabetes in the infant 775.1
disease NEC 760.9
  circulatory system, chronic (conditions classifiable to 390–459, 745–747) 760.3
  genitourinary system (conditions classifiable to 580–599) 760.1
  respiratory (conditions classifiable to 490–519, 748) 760.3
eclampsia 760.0
hemorrhage NEC 762.1
hepatitis acute, malignant, or subacute 760.8
hyperemesis (gravidarum) 761.8
hypertension (arising during pregnancy) (conditions classifiable to 642) 760.0

Maternal condition, affecting fetus or newborn — continued
infection
disease classifiable to 001–136 ☑, 760.2
genital tract NEC 760.8
urinary tract 760.1
influenza 760.2
manifest influenza in the infant 771.2
injury (conditions classifiable to 800–996) 760.5
malaria 760.2
manifest malaria in infant or fetus 771.2
malnutrition 760.4
necrosis of liver 760.8
nephritis (conditions classifiable to 580–583) 760.1
nephrosis (conditions classifiable to 581) 760.1
noxious substance transmitted via breast milk or placenta 760.70
alcohol 760.71
anticonvulsants 760.77
antifungals 760.74
anti-infective agents 760.74
antimetabolics 760.78
cocaine 760.75
"crack" 760.75
diethylstilbestrol [DES] 760.76
hallucinogenic agents 760.73
medicinal agents NEC 760.79
narcotics 760.72
obstetric anesthetic or analgesic drug 760.72
specified agent NEC 760.79
nutritional disorder (conditions classifiable to 260–269) 760.4
operation unrelated to current delivery 760.6
pre-eclampsia 760.0
pyelitis or pyelonephritis, arising during pregnancy (conditions classifiable to 590) 760.1
renal disease or failure 760.1
respiratory disease, chronic (conditions classifiable to 490–519, 748) 760.3
rheumatic heart disease (chronic) (conditions classifiable to 393–398) 760.3
rubella (conditions classifiable to 056) 760.2
manifest rubella in the infant or fetus 771.0
surgery unrelated to current delivery 760.6
to uterus or pelvic organs 763.89
syphilis (conditions classifiable to 090–097) 760.2
manifest syphilis in the infant or fetus 090.0
thrombophlebitis 760.3
toxemia (of pregnancy) 760.0
pre-eclamptic 760.0
toxoplasmosis (conditions classifiable to 130) 760.2
manifest toxoplasmosis in the infant or fetus 771.2
transmission of chemical substance through the placenta 760.70
alcohol 760.71
anticonvulsants 760.77
antifungals 760.74
anti-infective 760.74
antimetabolics 760.78
cocaine 760.75
"crack" 760.75
diethylstilbestrol [DES] 760.76
hallucinogenic agents 760.73
narcotics 760.72
specified substance NEC 760.79
uremia 760.1
urinary tract conditions (conditions classifiable to 580–599) 760.1

Maternal condition, affecting fetus or newborn — continued
vomiting (pernicious) (persistent) (vicious) 761.8
Maternity — see Delivery
Mathieu's disease (leptospiral jaundice) 100.0
Mauclaire's disease or osteochondrosis 732.3
Maxcy's disease 081.0
Maxilla, maxillary — see condition
May (-Hegglin) anomaly or syndrome 288.2
Mayaro fever 066.3
Mazoplasia 610.8
MBD (minimal brain dysfunction), child — see also Hyperkinesia 314.9
MCAD (medium chain acyl CoA dehydrogenase deficiency) 277.85
McArdle (-Schmid-Pearson) disease or syndrome (glycogenosis V) 271.0
McCune-Albright syndrome (osteitis fibrosa disseminata) 756.59
MCLS (mucocutaneous lymph node syndrome) 446.1
McQuarrie's syndrome (idiopathic familial hypoglycemia) 251.2
Measles (black) (hemorrhagic) (suppressed) 055.9
with
encephalitis 055.0
keratitis 055.71
keratoconjunctivitis 055.71
otitis media 055.2
pneumonia 055.1
complication 055.8
specified type NEC 055.79
encephalitis 055.0
French 056.9
German 056.9
keratitis 055.71
keratoconjunctivitis 055.71
liberty 056.9
otitis media 055.2
pneumonia 055.1
specified complications NEC 055.79
vaccination, prophylactic (against) V04.2
Meatitis, urethral — see also Urethritis 597.89
Meat poisoning — see Poisoning, food
Meatus, meatal — see condition
Meat-wrappers' asthma 506.9
Meckel's
diverticulitis 751.0
diverticulum (displaced) (hypertrophic) 751.0
Meconium
aspiration 770.11
with
pneumonia 770.12
pneumonitis 770.12
respiratory symptoms 770.12
below vocal cords 770.11
with respiratory symptoms 770.12
syndrome 770.12
delayed passage in newborn 777.1
ileus 777.1
due to cystic fibrosis 277.01
in liquor 792.3
noted during delivery 656.8 ☑
insufflation 770.11
with respiratory symptoms 770.12
obstruction
fetus or newborn 777.1
in mucoviscidosis 277.01
passage of 792.3
noted during delivery 763.84
peritonitis 777.6
plug syndrome (newborn) NEC 777.1
staining 779.84
Median — see also condition
arcuate ligament syndrome 447.4
bar (prostate) 600.90

Median — see also condition — continued
bar — continued
with
other lower urinary tract symptoms (LUTS) 600.91
urinary
obstruction 600.91
retention 600.91
rhomboid glossitis 529.2
vesical orifice 600.90
with
other lower urinary tract symptoms (LUTS) 600.91
urinary
obstruction 600.91
retention 600.91
Mediastinal shift 793.2
Mediastinitis (acute) (chronic) 519.2
actinomycotic 039.8
syphilitic 095.8
tuberculous (see also Tuberculosis) 012.8 ☑
Mediastinopericarditis — see also Pericarditis 423.9
acute 420.90
chronic 423.8
rheumatic 393
rheumatic, chronic 393
Mediastinum, mediastinal — see condition
Medical services provided for — see Health, services provided because (of)
Medicine poisoning (by overdose) (wrong substance given or taken in error) 977.9
specified drug or substance — see Table of Drugs and Chemicals
Medin's disease (poliomyelitis) 045.9 ☑
Mediterranean
anemia (with other hemoglobinopathy) 282.49
disease or syndrome (hemipathic) 282.49
fever (see also Brucellosis) 023.9
familial 277.31
kala-azar 085.0
leishmaniasis 085.0
tick fever 082.1
Medulla — see condition
Medullary
cystic kidney 753.16
sponge kidney 753.17
Medullated fibers
optic (nerve) 743.57
retina 362.85
Medulloblastoma (M9470/3) 191.6
desmoplastic (M9471/3) 191.6
specified site — see Neoplasm, by site, malignant
unspecified site 191.6
Medulloepithelioma (M9501/3) — see also Neoplasm, by site, malignant
teratoid (M9502/3) — see Neoplasm, by site, malignant
Medullomyoblastoma (M9472/3)
specified site — see Neoplasm, by site, malignant
unspecified site 191.6
Meekeren-Ehlers-Danlos syndrome 756.83
Megacaryocytic — see condition
Megacolon (acquired) (functional) (not Hirschsprung's disease) 564.7
aganglionic 751.3
congenital, congenitum 751.3
Hirschsprung's (disease) 751.3
psychogenic 306.4
toxic (see also Colitis, ulcerative) 556.9
Megaduodenum 537.3
Megaesophagus (functional) 530.0
congenital 750.4

Megakaryocytic — see condition
Megalencephaly 742.4
Megalerythema (epidermicum) (infectiosum) 057.0
Megalia, cutis et ossium 757.39
Megaloappendix 751.5
Megalocephalus, megalocephaly NEC 756.0
Megalocornea 743.41
associated with buphthalmos 743.22
Megalocytic anemia 281.9
Megalodactylia (fingers) (thumbs) 755.57
toes 755.65
Megaloduodenum 751.5
Megaloesophagus (functional) 530.0
congenital 750.4
Megalogastria (congenital) 750.7
Megalomania 307.9
Megalophthalmos 743.8
Megalopsia 368.14
Megalosplenia — see also Splenomegaly 789.2
Megaloureter 593.89
congenital 753.22
Megarectum 569.49
Megasigmoid 564.7
congenital 751.3
Megaureter 593.89
congenital 753.22
Megrim 346.9 ☑
Meibomian
cyst 373.2
infected 373.12
gland — see condition
infarct (eyelid) 374.85
stye 373.11
Meibomitis 373.12
Meige
-Milroy disease (chronic hereditary edema) 757.0
syndrome (blepharospasm-oromandibular dystonia) 333.82
Melalgia, nutritional 266.2
Melancholia — see also Psychosis, affective 296.90
climacteric 296.2 ☑
recurrent episode 296.3 ☑
single episode 296.2 ☑
hypochondriac 300.7
intermittent 296.2 ☑
recurrent episode 296.3 ☑
single episode 296.2 ☑
involutional 296.2 ☑
recurrent episode 296.3 ☑
single episode 296.2 ☑
menopausal 296.2 ☑
recurrent episode 296.3 ☑
single episode 296.2 ☑
puerperal 296.2 ☑
reactive (from emotional stress, psychological trauma) 298.0
recurrent 296.3 ☑
senile 290.21
stuporous 296.2 ☑
recurrent episode 296.3 ☑
single episode 296.2 ☑
Melanemia 275.0
Melanoameloblastoma (M9363/0) — see Neoplasm, bone, benign
Melanoblastoma (M8720/3) — see Melanoma
Melanoblastosis
Block-Sulzberger 757.33
cutis linearis sive systematisata 757.33
Melanocarcinoma (M8720/3) — see Melanoma
Melanocytoma, eyeball (M8726/0) 224.0
Melanoderma, melanodermia 709.09
Addison's (primary adrenal insufficiency) 255.4
Melanodontia, infantile 521.05
Melanodontoclasia 521.05
Melanoepithelioma (M8720/3) — see Melanoma

Melanoma

Melanoma (malignant) (M8720/3) 172.9

> *Note* — Except where otherwise indicated, the morphological varieties of melanoma in the list below should be coded by site as for "Melanoma (malignant)". Internal sites should be coded to malignant neoplasm of those sites.

- abdominal wall 172.5
- ala nasi 172.3
- amelanotic (M8730/3) — *see* Melanoma, by site
- ankle 172.7
- anus, anal 154.3
  - canal 154.2
- arm 172.6
- auditory canal (external) 172.2
- auricle (ear) 172.2
- auricular canal (external) 172.2
- axilla 172.5
- axillary fold 172.5
- back 172.5
- balloon cell (M8722/3) — *see* Melanoma, by site
- benign (M8720/0) — *see* Neoplasm, skin, benign
- breast (female) (male) 172.5
- brow 172.3
- buttock 172.5
- canthus (eye) 172.1
- cheek (external) 172.3
- chest wall 172.5
- chin 172.3
- choroid 190.6
- conjunctiva 190.3
- ear (external) 172.2
- epithelioid cell (M8771/3) (*see also* Melanoma, by site)
  - and spindle cell, mixed (M8775/3) — *see* Melanoma, by site
- external meatus (ear) 172.2
- eye 190.9
- eyebrow 172.3
- eyelid (lower) (upper) 172.1
- face NEC 172.3
- female genital organ (external) NEC 184.4
- finger 172.6
- flank 172.5
- foot 172.7
- forearm 172.6
- forehead 172.3
- foreskin 187.1
- gluteal region 172.5
- groin 172.5
- hand 172.6
- heel 172.7
- helix 172.2
- hip 172.7
- in
  - giant pigmented nevus (M8761/3) — *see* Melanoma, by site
  - Hutchinson's melanotic freckle (M8742/3) — *see* Melanoma, by site
  - junctional nevus (M8740/3) — *see* Melanoma, by site
  - precancerous melanosis (M8741/3) — *see* Melanoma, by site
- interscapular region 172.5
- iris 190.0
- jaw 172.3
- juvenile (M8770/0) — *see* Neoplasm, skin, benign
- knee 172.7
- labium
  - majus 184.1
  - minus 184.2
- lacrimal gland 190.2
- leg 172.7
- lip (lower) (upper) 172.0
- liver 197.7
- lower limb NEC 172.7
- male genital organ (external) NEC 187.9
- meatus, acoustic (external) 172.2
- meibomian gland 172.1

Melanoma — *continued*
- metastatic
  - of or from specified site — *see* Melanoma, by site
  - site not of skin — *see* Neoplasm, by site, malignant, secondary
  - to specified site — *see* Neoplasm, by site, malignant, secondary
  - unspecified site 172.9
- nail 172.9
  - finger 172.6
  - toe 172.7
- neck 172.4
- nodular (M8721/3) — *see* Melanoma, by site
- nose, external 172.3
- orbit 190.1
- penis 187.4
- perianal skin 172.5
- perineum 172.5
- pinna 172.2
- popliteal (fossa) (space) 172.7
- prepuce 187.1
- pubes 172.5
- pudendum 184.4
- retina 190.5
- scalp 172.4
- scrotum 187.7
- septum nasal (skin) 172.3
- shoulder 172.6
- skin NEC 172.8
- spindle cell (M8772/3) (*see also* Melanoma, by site)
  - type A (M8773/3) 190.0
  - type B (M8774/3) 190.0
- submammary fold 172.5
- superficial spreading (M8743/3) — *see* Melanoma, by site
- temple 172.3
- thigh 172.7
- toe 172.7
- trunk NEC 172.5
- umbilicus 172.5
- upper limb NEC 172.6
- vagina vault 184.0
- vulva 184.4

Melanoplakia 528.9

Melanosarcoma (M8720/3) — *see also* Melanoma
- epithelioid cell (M8771/3) — *see* Melanoma

Melanosis 709.09
- addisonian (primary adrenal insufficiency) 255.4
  - tuberculous (*see also* Tuberculosis) 017.6 ☑
- adrenal 255.4
- colon 569.89
- conjunctiva 372.55
  - congenital 743.49
- corii degenerativa 757.33
- cornea (presenile) (senile) 371.12
  - congenital 743.43
    - interfering with vision 743.42
- eye 372.55
  - congenital 743.49
- jute spinners' 709.09
- lenticularis progressiva 757.33
- liver 573.8
- precancerous (M8741/2) (*see also* Neoplasm, skin, in situ)
  - malignant melanoma in (M8741/3) — *see* Melanoma
- prenatal 743.43
  - interfering with vision 743.42
- Riehl's 709.09
- sclera 379.19
  - congenital 743.47
- suprarenal 255.4
- tar 709.09
- toxic 709.09

Melanuria 791.9

Melasma 709.09
- adrenal (gland) 255.4
- suprarenal (gland) 255.4

Index to Diseases

MELAS syndrome (mitochondrial encephalopathy, lactic acidosis and stroke-like episodes) 277.87

Melena 578.1
- due to
  - swallowed maternal blood 777.3
  - ulcer — *see* Ulcer, by site, with hemorrhage
- newborn 772.4
  - due to swallowed maternal blood 777.3

Meleney's
- gangrene (cutaneous) 686.09
- ulcer (chronic undermining) 686.09

Melioidosis 025

Melitensis, febris 023.0

Melitococcosis 023.0

Melkersson (-Rosenthal) syndrome 351.8

Mellitus, diabetes — *see* Diabetes

Melorheostosis (bone) (leri) 733.99

Meloschisis 744.83

Melotia 744.29

Membrana
- capsularis lentis posterior 743.39
- epipapillaris 743.57

Membranacea placenta — *see* Placenta, abnormal

Membranaceous uterus 621.8

Membrane, membranous — *see also* condition
- folds, congenital — *see* Web
- Jackson's 751.4
- over face (causing asphyxia), fetus or newborn 768.9
- premature rupture — *see* Rupture, membranes, premature
- pupillary 364.74
  - persistent 743.46
- retained (complicating delivery) (with hemorrhage) 666.2 ☑
  - without hemorrhage 667.1 ☑
- secondary (eye) 366.50
- unruptured (causing asphyxia) 768.9
- vitreous humor 379.25

Membranitis, fetal 658.4 ☑
- affecting fetus or newborn 762.7

Memory disturbance, loss or lack — *see also* Amnesia 780.93
- mild, following organic brain damage 310.1

Menadione (vitamin K) **deficiency** 269.0

Menarche, precocious 259.1

Mendacity, pathologic 301.7

Mendelson's syndrome (resulting from a procedure) 997.3
- obstetric 668.0 ☑

Mende's syndrome (ptosis-epicanthus) 270.2

Ménétrier's disease or syndrome (hypertrophic gastritis) 535.2 ☑

Ménière's disease, syndrome, or vertigo 386.00
- cochlear 386.02
- cochleovestibular 386.01
- inactive 386.04
- in remission 386.04
- vestibular 386.03

Meninges, meningeal — *see* condition

Meningioma (M9530/0) — *see also* Neoplasm, meninges, benign
- angioblastic (M9535/0) — *see* Neoplasm, meninges, benign
- angiomatous (M9534/0) — *see* Neoplasm, meninges, benign
- endotheliomatous (M9531/0) — *see* Neoplasm, meninges, benign
- fibroblastic (M9532/0) — *see* Neoplasm, meninges, benign
- fibrous (M9532/0) — *see* Neoplasm, meninges, benign
- hemangioblastic (M9535/0) — *see* Neoplasm, meninges, benign
- hemangiopericytic (M9536/0) — *see* Neoplasm, meninges, benign

Meningioma — *see also* Neoplasm, meninges, benign — *continued*
- malignant (M9530/3) — *see* Neoplasm, meninges, malignant
- meningothelial (M9531/0) — *see* Neoplasm, meninges, benign
- meningotheliomatous (M9531/0) — *see* Neoplasm, meninges, benign
- mixed (M9537/0) — *see* Neoplasm, meninges, benign
- multiple (M9530/1) 237.6
- papillary (M9538/1) 237.6
- psammomatous (M9533/0) — *see* Neoplasm, meninges, benign
- syncytial (M9531/0) — *see* Neoplasm, meninges, benign
- transitional (M9537/0) — *see* Neoplasm, meninges, benign

Meningiomatosis (diffuse) (M9530/1) 237.6

Meningism — *see also* Meningismus 781.6

Meningismus (infectional) (pneumococcal) 781.6
- due to serum or vaccine 997.09 [321.8]
- influenzal NEC 487.8

Meningitis (basal) (basic) (basilar) (brain) (cerebral) (cervical) (congestive) (diffuse) (hemorrhagic) (infantile) (membranous) (metastatic) (nonspecific) (pontine) (progressive) (simple) (spinal) (subacute) (sympathetica) (toxic) 322.9
- abacterial NEC (*see also* Meningitis, aseptic) 047.9
- actinomycotic 039.8 [320.7]
- adenoviral 049.1
- Aerobacter aerogenes 320.82
- anaerobes (cocci) (gram-negative) (gram-positive) (mixed) (NEC) 320.81
- arbovirus NEC 066.9 [321.2]
  - specified type NEC 066.8 [321.2]
- aseptic (acute) NEC 047.9
  - adenovirus 049.1
  - Coxsackie virus 047.0
  - due to
    - adenovirus 049.1
    - Coxsackie virus 047.0
    - ECHO virus 047.1
    - enterovirus 047.9
    - mumps 072.1
    - poliovirus (*see also* Poliomyelitis) 045.2 ☑ [321.2]
  - ECHO virus 047.1
  - herpes (simplex) virus 054.72
  - zoster 053.0
  - leptospiral 100.81
  - lymphocytic choriomeningitis 049.0
  - noninfective 322.0
- Bacillus pyocyanus 320.89
- bacterial NEC 320.9
  - anaerobic 320.81
  - gram-negative 320.82
    - anaerobic 320.81
- Bacteroides (fragilis) (oralis) (melaninogenicus) 320.81
- cancerous (M8000/6) 198.4
- candidal 112.83
- carcinomatous (M8010/6) 198.4
- caseous (*see also* Tuberculosis, meninges) 013.0 ☑
- cerebrospinal (acute) (chronic) (diplococcal) (endemic) (epidemic) (fulminant) (infectious) (malignant) (meningococcal) (sporadic) 036.0
  - carrier (suspected) of V02.59
- chronic NEC 322.2
- clear cerebrospinal fluid NEC 322.0
- Clostridium (haemolyticum) (novyi) NEC 320.81
- coccidioidomycosis 114.2
- Coxsackie virus 047.0
- cryptococcal 117.5 [321.0]

Index to Diseases

Meningitis — *continued*
  diplococcal 036.0
    gram-negative 036.0
    gram-positive 036.1
  Diplococcus pneumoniae 320.1
  due to
    actinomycosis 039.8 *[320.7]*
    adenovirus 049.1
    coccidiomycosis 114.2
    enterovirus 047.9
      specified NEC 047.8
    histoplasmosis (*see also* Histoplasmosis) 115.91
    Listerosis 027.0 *[320.7]*
    Lyme disease 088.81 *[320.7]*
    moniliasis 112.83
    mumps 072.1
    neurosyphilis 094.2
    nonbacterial organisms NEC 321.8
    oidiomycosis 112.83
    poliovirus (*see also* Poliomyelitis) 045.2 ☑ *[321.2]*
    preventive immunization, inoculation, or vaccination 997.09 *[321.8]*
    sarcoidosis 135 *[321.4]*
    sporotrichosis 117.1 *[321.1]*
    syphilis 094.2
      acute 091.81
      congenital 090.42
      secondary 091.81
    trypanosomiasis (*see also* Trypanosomiasis) 086.9 *[321.3]*
    whooping cough 033.9 *[320.7]*
  ECHO virus 047.1
  E. coli 320.82
  endothelial-leukocytic, benign, recurrent 047.9
  Enterobacter aerogenes 320.82
  enteroviral 047.9
    specified type NEC 047.8
  enterovirus 047.9
    specified NEC 047.8
  eosinophilic 322.1
  epidemic NEC 036.0
  Escherichia coli (E. coli) 320.82
  Eubacterium 320.81
  fibrinopurulent NEC 320.9
    specified type NEC 320.89
  Friedländer (bacillus) 320.82
  fungal NEC 117.9 *[321.1]*
  Fusobacterium 320.81
  gonococcal 098.82
  gram-negative bacteria NEC 320.82
    anaerobic 320.81
    cocci 036.0
      specified NEC 320.82
    gram-negative cocci NEC 036.0
      specified NEC 320.82
    gram-positive cocci NEC 320.9
  herpes (simplex) virus 054.72
    zoster 053.0
  H. influenzae 320.0
  infectious NEC 320.9
  influenzal 320.0
  Klebsiella pneumoniae 320.82
  late effect — *see* Late, effect, meningitis
  leptospiral (aseptic) 100.81
  Listerella (monocytogenes) 027.0 *[320.7]*
  Listeria monocytogenes 027.0 *[320.7]*
  lymphocytic (acute) (benign) (serous) 049.0
    choriomeningitis virus 049.0
  meningococcal (chronic) 036.0
  Mima polymorpha 320.82
  Mollaret's 047.9
  monilial 112.83
  mumps (virus) 072.1
  mycotic NEC 117.9 *[321.1]*
  Neisseria 036.0
  neurosyphilis 094.2
  nonbacterial NEC (*see also* Meningitis, aseptic) 047.9
  nonpyogenic NEC 322.0

Meningitis — *continued*
  oidiomycosis 112.83
  ossificans 349.2
  Peptococcus 320.81
  Peptostreptococcus 320.81
  pneumococcal 320.1
  poliovirus (*see also* Poliomyelitis) 045.2 ☑ *[321.2]*
  Proprionibacterium 320.81
  Proteus morganii 320.82
  Pseudomonas (aeruginosa) (pyocyaneus) 320.82
  purulent NEC 320.9
    specified organism NEC 320.89
  pyogenic NEC 320.9
    specified organism NEC 320.89
  Salmonella 003.21
  septic NEC 320.9
    specified organism NEC 320.89
  serosa circumscripta NEC 322.0
  serous NEC (*see also* Meningitis, aseptic) 047.9
    lymphocytic 049.0
    syndrome 348.2
  Serratia (marcescens) 320.82
  specified organism NEC 320.89
  sporadic cerebrospinal 036.0
  sporotrichosis 117.1 *[321.1]*
  staphylococcal 320.3
  sterile 997.09
  streptococcal (acute) 320.2
  suppurative 320.9
    specified organism NEC 320.89
  syphilitic 094.2
    acute 091.81
    congenital 090.42
    secondary 091.81
  torula 117.5 *[321.0]*
  traumatic (complication of injury) 958.8
  Treponema (denticola) (macrodenticum) 320.81
  trypanosomiasis 086.1 *[321.3]*
  tuberculous (*see also* Tuberculosis, meninges) 013.0 ☑
  typhoid 002.0 *[320.7]*
  Veillonella 320.81
  Vibrio vulnificus 320.82
  viral, virus NEC (*see also* Meningitis, aseptic) 047.9
  Wallgren's (*see also* Meningitis, aseptic) 047.9
Meningocele (congenital) (spinal) — *see also* Spina bifida 741.9 ☑
  acquired (traumatic) 349.2
  cerebral 742.0
  cranial 742.0
Meningocerebritis — *see* Meningoencephalitis
Meningococcemia (acute) (chronic) 036.2
Meningococcus, meningococcal — *see also* condition 036.9
  adrenalitis, hemorrhagic 036.3
  carditis 036.40
  carrier (suspected) of V02.59
  cerebrospinal fever 036.0
  encephalitis 036.1
  endocarditis 036.42
  exposure to V01.84
  infection NEC 036.9
  meningitis (cerebrospinal) 036.0
  myocarditis 036.43
  optic neuritis 036.81
  pericarditis 036.41
  septicemia (chronic) 036.2
Meningoencephalitis — *see also* Encephalitis 323.9
  acute NEC 048
  bacterial, purulent, pyogenic, or septic — *see* Meningitis
  chronic NEC 094.1
  diffuse NEC 094.1
  diphasic 063.2
  due to
    actinomycosis 039.8 *[320.7]*

Meningoencephalitis — *see also* Encephalitis — *continued*
  due to — *continued*
    blastomycosis NEC (*see also* Blastomycosis) 116.0 *[323.41]* ▲
    free-living amebae 136.2
    Listeria monocytogenes 027.0 *[320.7]*
    Lyme disease 088.81 *[320.7]*
    mumps 072.2
    Naegleria (amebae) (gruberi) (organisms) 136.2
    rubella 056.01
    sporotrichosis 117.1 *[321.1]*
    toxoplasmosis (acquired) 130.0
      congenital (active) 771.2 *[323.41]* ▲
    Trypanosoma 086.1 *[323.2]*
  epidemic 036.0
  herpes 054.3
  herpetic 054.3
  H. influenzae 320.0
  infectious (acute) 048
  influenzal 320.0
  late effect — *see* category 326
  Listeria monocytogenes 027.0 *[320.7]*
  lymphocytic (serous) 049.0
  mumps 072.2
  parasitic NEC 123.9 *[323.41]* ▲
  pneumococcal 320.1
  primary amebic 136.2
  rubella 056.01
  serous 048
    lymphocytic 049.0
  specific 094.2
  staphylococcal 320.3
  streptococcal 320.2
  syphilitic 094.2
  toxic NEC 989.9 *[323.71]* ▲
    due to
      carbon tetrachloride 987.8 *[323.71]* ▲
      hydroxyquinoline derivatives poisoning 961.3 *[323.71]* ▲
      lead 984.9 *[323.71]* ▲
      mercury 985.0 *[323.71]* ▲
      thallium 985.8 *[323.71]* ▲
  toxoplasmosis (acquired) 130.0
  trypanosomic 086.1 *[323.2]*
  tuberculous (*see also* Tuberculosis, meninges) 013.0 ☑
  virus NEC 048
Meningoencephalocele 742.0
  syphilitic 094.89
  congenital 090.49
Meningoencephalomyelitis — *see also* Meningoencephalitis 323.9
  acute NEC 048
    disseminated (postinfectious) 136.9 *[323.61]* ▲
      postimmunization or postvaccination 323.51 ▲
  due to
    actinomycosis 039.8 *[320.7]*
    torula 117.5 *[323.41]* ▲
    toxoplasma or toxoplasmosis (acquired) 130.0
      congenital (active) 771.2 *[323.41]* ▲
  late effect — *see* category 326
Meningoencephalomyelopathy — *see also* Meningoencephalomyelitis 349.9
Meningoencephalopathy — *see also* Meningoencephalitis 348.39
Meningoencephalopoliomyelitis — *see also* Poliomyelitis, bulbar 045.0 ☑
  late effect 138
Meningomyelitis — *see also* Meningoencephalitis 323.9
  blastomycotic NEC (*see also* Blastomycosis) 116.0 *[323.41]* ▲
  due to
    actinomycosis 039.8 *[320.7]*

Meningomyelitis — *see also* Meningoencephalitis — *continued*
  due to — *continued*
    blastomycosis (*see also* Blastomycosis) 116.0 *[323.41]* ▲
    Meningococcus 036.0
    sporotrichosis 117.1 *[323.41]* ▲
    torula 117.5 *[323.41]* ▲
  late effect — *see* category 326
  lethargic 049.8
  meningococcal 036.0
  syphilitic 094.2
  tuberculous (*see also* Tuberculosis, meninges) 013.0 ☑
Meningomyelocele — *see also* Spina bifida 741.9 ☑
  syphilitic 094.89
Meningomyeloneuritis — *see* Meningoencephalitis
Meningoradiculitis — *see* Meningitis
Meningovascular — *see* condition
Meniscocytosis 282.60
Menkes' syndrome — *see* Syndrome, Menkes'
Menolipsis 626.0
Menometrorrhagia 626.2
Menopause, menopausal (symptoms) (syndrome) 627.2
  arthritis (any site) NEC 716.3 ☑
  artificial 627.4
  bleeding 627.0
  crisis 627.2
  depression (*see also* Psychosis, affective) 296.2 ☑
    agitated 296.2 ☑
      recurrent episode 296.3 ☑
      single episode 296.2 ☑
    psychotic 296.2 ☑
      recurrent episode 296.3 ☑
      single episode 296.2 ☑
    recurrent episode 296.3 ☑
    single episode 296.2 ☑
  melancholia (*see also* Psychosis, affective) 296.2 ☑
    recurrent episode 296.3 ☑
    single episode 296.2 ☑
  paranoid state 297.2
  paraphrenia 297.2
  postsurgical 627.4
  premature 256.31
    postirradiation 256.2
    postsurgical 256.2
  psychoneurosis 627.2
  psychosis NEC 298.8
  surgical 627.4
  toxic polyarthritis NEC 716.39
Menorrhagia (primary) 626.2
  climacteric 627.0
  menopausal 627.0
  postclimacteric 627.1
  postmenopausal 627.1
  preclimacteric 627.0
  premenopausal 627.0
  puberty (menses retained) 626.3
Menorrhalgia 625.3
Menoschesis 626.8
Menostaxis 626.2
Menses, retention 626.8
Menstrual — *see also* Menstruation
  cycle, irregular 626.4
  disorders NEC 626.9
  extraction V25.3
  fluid, retained 626.8
  molimen 625.4
  period, normal V65.5
  regulation V25.3
Menstruation
  absent 626.0
  anovulatory 628.0
  delayed 626.8
  difficult 625.3
  disorder 626.9
    psychogenic 306.52
    specified NEC 626.8
  during pregnancy 640.8 ☑

Menstruation — continued
  excessive 626.2
  frequent 626.2
  infrequent 626.1
  irregular 626.4
  latent 626.8
  membranous 626.8
  painful (primary) (secondary) 625.3
    psychogenic 306.52
  passage of clots 626.2
  precocious 626.8
  protracted 626.8
  retained 626.8
  retrograde 626.8
  scanty 626.1
  suppression 626.8
  vicarious (nasal) 625.8
Mentagra — see also Sycosis 704.8
Mental — see also condition
  deficiency (see also Retardation, mental) 319
  deterioration (see also Psychosis) 298.9
  disorder (see also Disorder, mental) 300.9
  exhaustion 300.5
  insufficiency (congenital) (see also Retardation, mental) 319
  observation without need for further medical care NEC V71.09
  retardation (see also Retardation, mental) 319
  subnormality (see also Retardation, mental) 319
    mild 317
    moderate 318.0
    profound 318.2
    severe 318.1
  upset (see also Disorder, mental) 300.9
Meralgia paresthetica 355.1
Mercurial — see condition
Mercurialism NEC 985.0
Merergasia 300.9
Merkel cell tumor — see Neoplasm, by site, malignant
Merocele — see also Hernia, femoral 553.00
Meromelia 755.4
  lower limb 755.30
    intercalary 755.32
      femur 755.34
        tibiofibular (complete) (incomplete) 755.33
      fibula 755.37
      metatarsal(s) 755.38
      tarsal(s) 755.38
      tibia 755.36
      tibiofibular 755.35
    terminal (complete) (partial) (transverse) 755.31
      longitudinal 755.32
        metatarsal(s) 755.38
        phalange(s) 755.39
        tarsal(s) 755.38
      transverse 755.31
  upper limb 755.20
    intercalary 755.22
      carpal(s) 755.28
      humeral 755.24
        radioulnar (complete) (incomplete) 755.23
      metacarpal(s) 755.28
      phalange(s) 755.29
      radial 755.26
      radioulnar 755.25
      ulnar 755.27
    terminal (complete) (partial) (transverse) 755.21
      longitudinal 755.22
        carpal(s) 755.28
        metacarpal(s) 755.28
        phalange(s) 755.29
      transverse 755.21
Merosmia 781.1

MERRF syndrome (myoclonus with epilepsy and with ragged red fibers) 277.87
Merycism — see also Vomiting
  psychogenic 307.53
Merzbacher-Pelizaeus disease 330.0
Mesaortitis — see Aortitis
Mesarteritis — see Arteritis
Mesencephalitis — see also Encephalitis 323.9
  late effect — see category 326
Mesenchymoma (M8990/1) — see also Neoplasm, connective tissue, uncertain behavior
  benign (M8990/0) — see Neoplasm, connective tissue, benign
  malignant (M8990/3) — see Neoplasm, connective tissue, malignant
Mesenteritis
  retractile 567.82
  sclerosing 567.82
Mesentery, mesenteric — see condition
Mesiodens, mesiodentes 520.1
  causing crowding 524.31
Mesio-occlusion 524.23
Mesocardia (with asplenia) 746.87
Mesocolon — see condition
Mesonephroma (malignant) (M9110/3) — see also Neoplasm, by site, malignant
  benign (M9110/0) — see Neoplasm, by site, benign
Mesophlebitis — see Phlebitis
Mesostromal dysgenesis 743.51
Mesothelioma (malignant) (M9050/3) — see also Neoplasm, by site, malignant
  benign (M9050/0) — see Neoplasm, by site, benign
  biphasic type (M9053/3) (see also Neoplasm, by site, malignant)
    benign (M9053/0) — see Neoplasm, by site, benign
  epithelioid (M9052/3) (see also Neoplasm, by site, malignant)
    benign (M9052/0) — see Neoplasm, by site, benign
  fibrous (M9051/3) (see also Neoplasm, by site, malignant)
    benign (M9051/0) — see Neoplasm, by site, benign
Metabolic syndrome 277.7
Metabolism disorder 277.9
  specified type NEC 277.89
Metagonimiasis 121.5
Metagonimus infestation (small intestine) 121.5
Metal
  pigmentation (skin) 709.00
  polishers' disease 502
Metalliferous miners' lung 503
Metamorphopsia 368.14
Metaplasia
  bone, in skin 709.3
  breast 611.8
  cervix — omit code
  endometrium (squamous) 621.8
  esophagus 530.85
  intestinal, of gastric mucosa 537.89
  kidney (pelvis) (squamous) (see also Disease, renal) 593.89
  myelogenous 289.89
  myeloid 289.89
    agnogenic 238.76
    megakaryocytic 238.76
  spleen 289.59
  squamous cell
    amnion 658.8
    bladder 596.8
    cervix — see condition
    trachea 519.19
    tracheobronchial tree 519.19
  uterus 621.8
    cervix — see condition

Metastasis, metastatic
  abscess — see Abscess
  calcification 275.40
  cancer, neoplasm, or disease
    from specified site (M8000/3) — see Neoplasm, by site, malignant
    to specified site (M8000/6) — see Neoplasm, by site, secondary
  deposits (in) (M8000/6) — see Neoplasm, by site, secondary
  pneumonia 038.8 [484.8]
  spread (to) (M8000/6) — see Neoplasm, by site, secondary
Metatarsalgia 726.70
  anterior 355.6
  due to Freiberg's disease 732.5
  Morton's 355.6
Metatarsus, metatarsal — see also condition
  abductus valgus (congenital) 754.60
  adductus varus (congenital) 754.53
  primus varus 754.52
  valgus (adductus) (congenital) 754.60
  varus (abductus) (congenital) 754.53
    primus 754.52
Methemoglobinemia 289.7
  acquired (with sulfhemoglobinemia) 289.7
  congenital 289.7
  enzymatic 289.7
  Hb-M disease 289.7
  hereditary 289.7
  toxic 289.7
Methemoglobinuria — see also Hemoglobinuria 791.2
Methicillin-resistant staphylococcus aureus (MRSA) V09.0
Methioninemia 270.4
Metritis (catarrhal) (septic) (suppurative) — see also Endometritis 615.9
  blennorrhagic 098.16
    chronic or duration of 2 months or over 098.36
  cervical (see also Cervicitis) 616.0
  gonococcal 098.16
    chronic or duration of 2 months or over 098.36
  hemorrhagic 626.8
  puerperal, postpartum, childbirth 670.0
  tuberculous (see also Tuberculosis) 016.7
Metropathia hemorrhagica 626.8
Metroperitonitis — see also Peritonitis, pelvic, female 614.5
Metrorrhagia 626.6
  arising during pregnancy — see Hemorrhage, pregnancy
  postpartum NEC 666.2
    primary 626.6
    psychogenic 306.59
  puerperal 666.2
Metrorrhexis — see Rupture, uterus
Metrosalpingitis — see also Salpingo-oophoritis 614.2
Metrostaxis 626.6
Metrovaginitis — see also Endometritis 615.9
  gonococcal (acute) 098.16
    chronic or duration of 2 months or over 098.36
Mexican fever — see Typhus, Mexican
Meyenburg-Altherr-Uehlinger syndrome 733.99
Meyer-Schwickerath and Weyers syndrome (dysplasia oculodentodigitalis) 759.89
Meynert's amentia (nonalcoholic) 294.0
  alcoholic 291.1
Mibelli's disease 757.39
Mice, joint — see also Loose, body, joint 718.1
  knee 717.6
Micheli-Rietti syndrome (thalassemia minor) 282.49

Michotte's syndrome 721.5
Micrencephalon, micrencephaly 742.1
Microalbuminuria 791.0
Microaneurysm, retina 362.14
  diabetic 250.5 [362.01]
Microangiopathy 443.9
  diabetic (peripheral) 250.7 [443.81]
    retinal 250.5 [362.01]
  peripheral 443.9
    diabetic 250.7 [443.81]
  retinal 362.18
    diabetic 250.5 [362.01]
  thrombotic 446.6
    Moschcowitz's (thrombotic thrombocytopenic purpura) 446.6
Microcalcification, mammographic 793.81
Microcephalus, microcephalic, microcephaly 742.1
  due to toxoplasmosis (congenital) 771.2
Microcheilia 744.82
Microcolon (congenital) 751.5
Microcornea (congenital) 743.41
Microcytic — see condition
Microdeletions NEC 758.33
Microdontia 520.2
Microdrepanocytosis (thalassemia-Hb-S disease) 282.49
Microembolism
  atherothrombotic — see Atheroembolism
  retina 362.33
Microencephalon 742.1
Microfilaria streptocerca infestation 125.3
Microgastria (congenital) 750.7
Microgenia 524.06
Microgenitalia (congenital) 752.89
  penis 752.64
Microglioma (M9710/3)
  specified site — see Neoplasm, by site, malignant
  unspecified site 191.9
Microglossia (congenital) 750.16
Micrognathia, micrognathism (congenital) 524.00
  mandibular 524.04
    alveolar 524.74
  maxillary 524.03
    alveolar 524.73
Microgyria (congenital) 742.2
Microinfarct, heart — see also Insufficiency, coronary 411.89
Microlithiasis, alveolar, pulmonary 516.2
Micromyelia (congenital) 742.59
Micropenis 752.64
Microphakia (congenital) 743.36
Microphthalmia (congenital) — see also Microphthalmos 743.10
Microphthalmos (congenital) 743.10
  associated with eye and adnexal anomalies NEC 743.12
  due to toxoplasmosis (congenital) 771.2
  isolated 743.11
  simple 743.11
  syndrome 759.89
Micropsia 368.14
Microsporidiosis 136.8
Microsporon furfur infestation 111.0
Microsporosis — see also Dermatophytosis 110.9
  nigra 111.1
Microstomia (congenital) 744.84
Microthelia 757.6
Microthromboembolism — see Embolism
Microtia (congenital) (external ear) 744.23
Microtropia 378.34
Micturition
  disorder NEC 788.69
    psychogenic 306.53
  frequency 788.41

Index to Diseases

Micturition — continued
  frequency — continued
    psychogenic 306.53
   nocturnal 788.43
   painful 788.1
   psychogenic 306.53
Middle
  ear — see condition
  lobe (right) syndrome 518.0
Midplane — see condition
Miescher's disease 709.3
  cheilitis 351.8
  granulomatosis disciformis 709.3
Miescher-Leder syndrome or granulomatosis 709.3
Mieten's syndrome 759.89
Migraine (idiopathic) 346.9 ☑
  with aura 346.0
  abdominal (syndrome) 346.2 ☑
  allergic (histamine) 346.2 ☑
  atypical 346.1 ☑
  basilar 346.2 ☑
  classical 346.0 ☑
  common 346.1 ☑
  hemiplegic 346.8 ☑
  lower-half 346.2 ☑
  menstrual 625.4
  ophthalmic 346.8 ☑
  ophthalmoplegic 346.8 ☑
  retinal 346.2 ☑
  variant 346.2 ☑
Migrant, social V60.0
Migratory, migrating — see also condition
  person V60.0
  testis, congenital 752.52
Mikulicz's disease or syndrome (dryness of mouth, absent or decreased lacrimation) 527.1
Milian atrophia blanche 701.3
Miliaria (crystallina) (rubra) (tropicalis) 705.1
  apocrine 705.82
Miliary — see condition
Milium — see also Cyst, sebaceous 706.2
  colloid 709.3
  eyelid 374.84
Milk
  crust 690.11
  excess secretion 676.6 ☑
  fever, female 672.0 ☑
  poisoning 988.8
  retention 676.2 ☑
  sickness 988.8
  spots 423.1
Milkers' nodes 051.1
Milk-leg (deep vessels) 671.4 ☑
  complicating pregnancy 671.3 ☑
  nonpuerperal 451.19
  puerperal, postpartum, childbirth 671.4 ☑
Milkman (-Looser) disease or syndrome (osteomalacia with pseudofractures) 268.2
Milky urine — see also Chyluria 791.1
Millar's asthma (laryngismus stridulus) 478.75
Millard-Gubler-Foville paralysis 344.89
Millard-Gubler paralysis or syndrome 344.89
Miller-Dieker syndrome 758.33
Miller's disease (osteomalacia) 268.2
Miller Fisher's syndrome 357.0
Milles' syndrome (encephalocutaneous angiomatosis) 759.6
Mills' disease 335.29
Millstone makers' asthma or lung 502
Milroy's disease (chronic hereditary edema) 757.0
Miners' — see also condition
  asthma 500
  elbow 727.2
  knee 727.2
  lung 500
  nystagmus 300.89

Miners' — see also condition — continued
  phthisis (see also Tuberculosis) 011.4 ☑
  tuberculosis (see also Tuberculosis) 011.4 ☑
Minkowski-Chauffard syndrome — see also Spherocytosis 282.0
Minor — see condition
Minor's disease 336.1
Minot's disease (hemorrhagic disease, newborn) 776.0
Minot-von Willebrand (-Jürgens) disease or syndrome (angiohemophilia) 286.4
Minus (and plus) hand (intrinsic) 736.09
Miosis (persistent) (pupil) 379.42
Mirizzi's syndrome (hepatic duct stenosis) — see also Obstruction, biliary 576.2
  with calculus, cholelithiasis, or stones — see Choledocholithiasis
Mirror writing 315.09
  secondary to organic lesion 784.69
Misadventure (prophylactic) (therapeutic) — see also Complications 999.9
  administration of insulin 962.3
  infusion — see Complications, infusion
  local applications (of fomentations, plasters, etc.) 999.9
   burn or scald — see Burn, by site
  medical care (early) (late) NEC 999.9
   adverse effect of drugs or chemicals — see Table of Drugs and Chemicals
   burn or scald — see Burn, by site
  radiation NEC 990
  radiotherapy NEC 990
  surgical procedure (early) (late) — see Complications, surgical procedure
  transfusion — see Complications, transfusion
  vaccination or other immunological procedure — see Complications, vaccination
Misanthropy 301.7
Miscarriage — see Abortion, spontaneous
Mischief, malicious, child — see also Disturbance, conduct 312.0 ☑
Misdirection
  aqueous 365.83
Mismanagement, feeding 783.3
Misplaced, misplacement
  kidney (see also Disease, renal) 593.0
   congenital 753.3
  organ or site, congenital NEC — see Malposition, congenital
Missed
  abortion 632
  delivery (at or near term) 656.4 ☑
  labor (at or near term) 656.4 ☑
Missing — see also Absence
  teeth (acquired) 525.10
   congenital (see also Anodontia) 520.0
   due to
    caries 525.13
    extraction 525.10
    periodontal disease 525.12
    specified NEC 525.19
    trauma 525.11
  vertebrae (congenital) 756.13
Misuse of drugs NEC — see also Abuse, drug, nondependent 305.9 ☑
Mitchell's disease (erythromelalgia) 443.82
Mite(s)
  diarrhea 133.8
  grain (itch) 133.8
  hair follicle (itch) 133.8
  in sputum 133.8

Mitochondrial encephalopathy, lactic acidosis and stroke-like episodes (MELAS syndrome) 277.87
Mitochondrial neurogastrointestinal encephalopathy syndrome (MNGIE) 277.87
Mitral — see condition
Mittelschmerz 625.2
Mixed — see condition
Mljet disease (mal de Meleda) 757.39
Mobile, mobility
  cecum 751.4
  coccyx 733.99
  excessive — see Hypermobility
  gallbladder 751.69
  kidney 593.0
   congenital 753.3
  organ or site, congenital NEC — see Malposition, congenital
  spleen 289.59
Mobitz heart block (atrioventricular) 426.10
  type I (Wenckebach's) 426.13
  type II 426.12
Möbius'
  disease 346.8 ☑
  syndrome
   congenital oculofacial paralysis 352.6
   ophthalmoplegic migraine 346.8 ☑
Moeller (-Barlow) disease (infantile scurvy) 267
  glossitis 529.4
Mohr's syndrome (types I and II) 759.89
Mola destruens (M9100/1) 236.1
Molarization, premolars 520.2
Molar pregnancy 631
  hydatidiform (delivered) (undelivered) 630
Molding, head (during birth) — omit code
Mold(s) in vitreous 117.9
Mole (pigmented) (M8720/0) — see also Neoplasm, skin, benign
  blood 631
  Breus' 631
  cancerous (M8720/3) — see Melanoma
  carneous 631
  destructive (M9100/1) 236.1
  ectopic — see Pregnancy, ectopic
  fleshy 631
  hemorrhagic 631
  hydatid, hydatidiform (benign) (complicating pregnancy) (delivered) (undelivered) (see also Hydatidiform mole) 630
   invasive (M9100/1) 236.1
   malignant (M9100/1) 236.1
   previous, affecting management of pregnancy V23.1
  invasive (hydatidiform) (M9100/1) 236.1
  malignant
   meaning
    malignant hydatidiform mole (9100/1) 236.1
    melanoma (M8720/3) — see Melanoma
  nonpigmented (M8730/0) — see Neoplasm, skin, benign
  pregnancy NEC 631
  skin (M8720/0) — see Neoplasm, skin, benign
  tubal — see Pregnancy, tubal
  vesicular (see also Hydatidiform mole) 630
Molimen, molimina (menstrual) 625.4
Mollaret's meningitis 047.9
Mollities (cerebellar) (cerebral) 437.8
  ossium 268.2
Molluscum
  contagiosum 078.0
  epitheliale 078.0
  fibrosum (M8851/0) — see Lipoma, by site

Molluscum — continued
  pendulum (M8851/0) — see Lipoma, by site
Mönckeberg's arteriosclerosis, degeneration, disease, or sclerosis — see also Arteriosclerosis, extremities 440.20
Monday fever 504
Monday morning dyspnea or asthma 504
Mondini's malformation (cochlea) 744.05
Mondor's disease (thrombophlebitis of breast) 451.89
Mongolian, mongolianism, mongolism, mongoloid 758.0
  spot 757.33
Monilethrix (congenital) 757.4
Monilia infestation — see Candidiasis
Moniliasis — see also Candidiasis
  neonatal 771.7
  vulvovaginitis 112.1
Monkeypox 057.8
Monoarthritis 716.60
  ankle 716.67
  arm 716.62
   lower (and wrist) 716.63
   upper (and elbow) 716.62
  foot (and ankle) 716.67
  forearm (and wrist) 716.63
  hand 716.64
  leg 716.66
   lower 716.66
   upper 716.65
  pelvic region (hip) (thigh) 716.65
  shoulder (region) 716.61
  specified site NEC 716.68
Monoblastic — see condition
Monochromatism (cone) (rod) 368.54
Monocytic — see condition
Monocytopenia 288.59 ●
Monocytosis (symptomatic) 288.63 ▲
Monofixation syndrome 378.34
Monomania — see also Psychosis 298.9
Mononeuritis 355.9
  cranial nerve — see Disorder, nerve, cranial
  femoral nerve 355.2
  lateral
   cutaneous nerve of thigh 355.1
   popliteal nerve 355.3
  lower limb 355.8
   specified nerve NEC 355.79
  medial popliteal nerve 355.4
  median nerve 354.1
  multiplex 354.5
  plantar nerve 355.6
  posterior tibial nerve 355.5
  radial nerve 354.3
  sciatic nerve 355.0
  ulnar nerve 354.2
  upper limb 354.9
   specified nerve NEC 354.8
  vestibular 388.5
Mononeuropathy — see also Mononeuritis 355.9
  diabetic NEC 250.6 ☑ [355.9]
   lower limb 250.6 ☑ [355.9]
   upper limb 250.6 ☑ [354.9]
  iliohypogastric nerve 355.79
  ilioinguinal nerve 355.79
  obturator nerve 355.79
  saphenous nerve 355.79
Mononucleosis, infectious 075
  with hepatitis 075 [573.1]
Monoplegia 344.5
  brain (current episode) (see also Paralysis, brain) 437.8
  fetus or newborn 767.8
  cerebral (current episode) (see also Paralysis, brain) 437.8
  congenital or infantile (cerebral) (spastic) (spinal) 343.3
  embolic (current) (see also Embolism, brain) 434.1 ☑

Monoplegia — *continued*
  embolic (*see also* Embolism, brain) — *continued*
    late effect — *see* Late effect(s) (of) cerebrovascular disease
  infantile (cerebral) (spastic) (spinal) 343.3
  lower limb 344.30
    affecting
      dominant side 344.31
      nondominant side 344.32
    due to late effect of cerebrovascular accident — *see* Late effect(s) (of) cerebrovascular accident
  newborn 767.8
  psychogenic 306.0
    specified as conversion reaction 300.11
  thrombotic (current) (*see also* Thrombosis, brain) 434.0 ☑
    late effect — *see* Late effect(s) (of) cerebrovascular disease
  transient 781.4
  upper limb 344.40
    affecting
      dominant side 344.41
      nondominant side 344.42
    due to late effect of cerebrovascular accident — *see* Late effect(s) (of) cerebrovascular accident
Monorchism, monorchidism 752.89
Monteggia's fracture (closed) 813.03
  open 813.13
Mood swings
  brief compensatory 296.99
  rebound 296.99
Mooren's ulcer (cornea) 370.07
Moore's syndrome — *see also* Epilepsy 345.5 ☑
Mooser bodies 081.0
Mooser-Neill reaction 081.0
Moral
  deficiency 301.7
  imbecility 301.7
Morax-Axenfeld conjunctivitis 372.03
Morbilli — *see also* Measles 055.9
Morbus
  anglicus, anglorum 268.0
  Beigel 111.2
  caducus (*see also* Epilepsy) 345.9 ☑
  caeruleus 746.89
  celiacus 579.0
  comitialis (*see also* Epilepsy) 345.9 ☑
  cordis (*see also* Disease, heart)
    valvulorum — *see* Endocarditis
  coxae 719.95
    tuberculous (*see also* Tuberculosis) 015.1 ☑
  hemorrhagicus neonatorum 776.0
  maculosus neonatorum 772.6
  renum 593.9
  senilis (*see also* Osteoarthrosis) 715.9 ☑
Morel-Kraepelin disease — *see also* Schizophrenia 295.9 ☑
Morel-Moore syndrome (hyperostosis frontalis interna) 733.3
Morel-Morgagni syndrome (hyperostosis frontalis interna) 733.3
Morgagni
  cyst, organ, hydatid, or appendage 752.89
    fallopian tube 752.11
  disease or syndrome (hyperostosis frontalis interna) 733.3
Morgagni-Adams-Stokes syndrome (syncope with heart block) 426.9
Morgagni-Stewart-Morel syndrome (hyperostosis frontalis interna) 733.3
Moria — *see also* Psychosis 298.9
Morning sickness 643.0 ☑
Moron 317
Morphea (guttate) (linear) 701.0
Morphine dependence — *see also* Dependence 304.0 ☑

Morphinism — *see also* Dependence 304.0 ☑
Morphinomania — *see also* Dependence 304.0 ☑
Morphoea 701.0
Morquio (-Brailsford) (-Ullrich) disease or syndrome (mucopolysaccharidosis IV) 277.5
  kyphosis 277.5
Morris syndrome (testicular feminization) 259.5
Morsus humanus (open wound) — *see also* Wound, open, by site
  skin surface intact — *see* Contusion
Mortification (dry) (moist) — *see also* Gangrene 785.4
Morton's
  disease 355.6
  foot 355.6
  metatarsalgia (syndrome) 355.6
  neuralgia 355.6
  neuroma 355.6
  syndrome (metatarsalgia) (neuralgia) 355.6
  toe 355.6
Morvan's disease 336.0
Mosaicism, mosaic (chromosomal) 758.9
  autosomal 758.5
  sex 758.81
Moschcowitz's syndrome (thrombotic thrombocytopenic purpura) 446.6
Mother yaw 102.0
Motion sickness (from travel, any vehicle) (from roundabouts or swings) 994.6
Mottled teeth (enamel) (endemic) (nonendemic) 520.3
Mottling enamel (endemic) (nonendemic) (teeth) 520.3
Mouchet's disease 732.5
Mould(s) (in vitreous) 117.9
Moulders'
  bronchitis 502
  tuberculosis (*see also* Tuberculosis) 011.4 ☑
Mounier-Kuhn syndrome 748.3
  with
    acute exacerbation 494.1
    bronchiectasis 494.0
      with (acute) exacerbation 494.1
  acquired 519.19 ▲
    with bronchiectasis 494.0
      with (acute) exacerbation 494.1
Mountain
  fever — *see* Fever, mountain
  sickness 993.2
    with polycythemia, acquired 289.0
    acute 289.0
  tick fever 066.1
Mouse, joint — *see also* Loose, body, joint 718.1 ☑
  knee 717.6
Mouth — *see* condition
Movable
  coccyx 724.71
  kidney (*see also* Disease, renal) 593.0
    congenital 753.3
  organ or site, congenital NEC — *see* Malposition, congenital
  spleen 289.59
Movement
  abnormal (dystonic) (involuntary) 781.0
  decreased fetal 655.7 ☑
  paradoxical facial 374.43
Moya Moya disease 437.5
Mozart's ear 744.29
MRSA (methicillin-resistant staphylococcus aureus) V09.0
Mucha's disease (acute parapsoriasis varioliformis) 696.2
Mucha-Haberman syndrome (acute parapsoriasis varioliformis) 696.2
Mu-chain disease 273.2
Mucinosis (cutaneous) (papular) 701.8

Mucocele
  appendix 543.9
  buccal cavity 528.9
  gallbladder (*see also* Disease, gallbladder) 575.3
  lacrimal sac 375.43
  orbit (eye) 376.81
  salivary gland (any) 527.6
  sinus (accessory) (nasal) 478.19 ▲
  turbinate (bone) (middle) (nasal) 478.19 ▲
  uterus 621.8
Mucocutaneous lymph node syndrome (acute) (febrile) (infantile) 446.1
Mucoenteritis 564.9
Mucolipidosis I, II, III 272.7
Mucopolysaccharidosis (types 1-6) 277.5
  cardiopathy 277.5 [425.7]
Mucormycosis (lung) 117.7
Mucositis — *see also* Inflammation, by site 528.00 ▲
  cervix (ulcerative) 616.81
  due to ●
    antineoplastic therapy (ulcerative) ● 528.01
    other drugs (ulcerative) 528.02 ●
    specified NEC 528.09 ●
  gastrointestinal (ulcerative) 538 ●
  nasal (ulcerative) 478.11 ●
  necroticans agranulocytica ▶(*see also* Agranulocytosis)◀ 288.09 ▲
  ulcerative 528.00 ●
  vagina (ulcerative) 616.81
  vulva (ulcerative) 616.81 ●
Mucous — *see also* condition
  patches (syphilitic) 091.3
  congenital 090.0
Mucoviscidosis 277.00
  with meconium obstruction 277.01
Mucus
  asphyxia or suffocation (*see also* Asphyxia, mucus) 933.1
    newborn 770.18
  in stool 792.1
  plug (*see also* Asphyxia, mucus) 933.1
    aspiration, of newborn 770.17
    tracheobronchial 519.19 ▲
      newborn 770.18
Muguet 112.0
Mulberry molars 090.5
Mullerian mixed tumor (M8950/3) — *see* Neoplasm, by site, malignant
Multicystic kidney 753.19
Multilobed placenta — *see* Placenta, abnormal
Multinodular prostate 600.10
  with
    urinary
      obstruction 600.11 ●
      retention 600.11 ●
Multiparity V61.5
  affecting
    fetus or newborn 763.89
    management of
      labor and delivery 659.4 ☑
      pregnancy V23.3
  requiring contraceptive management (*see also* Contraception) V25.9
Multipartita placenta — *see* Placenta, abnormal
Multiple, multiplex — *see also* condition
  birth
    affecting fetus or newborn 761.5
    healthy liveborn — *see* Newborn, multiple
  digits (congenital) 755.00
    fingers 755.01
    toes 755.02
  organ or site NEC — *see* Accessory
  personality 300.14
  renal arteries 747.62
Mumps 072.9
  with complication 072.8
    specified type NEC 072.79
  encephalitis 072.2

Mumps — *continued*
  hepatitis 072.71
  meningitis (aseptic) 072.1
  meningoencephalitis 072.2
  oophoritis 072.79
  orchitis 072.0
  pancreatitis 072.3
  polyneuropathy 072.72
  vaccination, prophylactic (against) V04.6
Mumu — *see also* Infestation, filarial 125.9
Münchausen syndrome 301.51
Münchmeyer's disease or syndrome (exostosis luxurians) 728.11
Mural — *see* condition
Murmur (cardiac) (heart) (nonorganic) (organic) 785.2
  abdominal 787.5
  aortic (valve) (*see also* Endocarditis, aortic) 424.1
  benign — *omit code*
  cardiorespiratory 785.2
  diastolic — *see* condition
  Flint (*see also* Endocarditis, aortic) 424.1
  functional — *omit code*
  Graham Steell (pulmonic regurgitation) (*see also* Endocarditis, pulmonary) 424.3
  innocent — *omit code*
  insignificant — *omit code*
  midsystolic 785.2
  mitral (valve) — *see* Stenosis, mitral
  physiologic — *see* condition
  presystolic, mitral — *see* Insufficiency, mitral
  pulmonic (valve) (*see also* Endocarditis, pulmonary) 424.3
  Still's (vibratory) — *omit code*
  systolic (valvular) — *see* condition
  tricuspid (valve) — *see* Endocarditis, tricuspid
  undiagnosed 785.2
  valvular — *see* condition
  vibratory — *omit code*
Murri's disease (intermittent hemoglobinuria) 283.2
Muscae volitantes 379.24
Muscle, muscular — *see* condition
Musculoneuralgia 729.1
Mushrooming hip 718.95
Mushroom workers' (pickers') lung 495.5
Mutation
  factor V leiden 289.81
  prothrombin gene 289.81
Mutism — *see also* Aphasia 784.3
  akinetic 784.3
  deaf (acquired) (congenital) 389.7
  hysterical 300.11
  selective (elective) 313.23
    adjustment reaction 309.83
Myà's disease (congenital dilation, colon) 751.3
Myalgia (intercostal) 729.1
  eosinophilia syndrome 710.5
  epidemic 074.1
    cervical 078.89
  psychogenic 307.89
  traumatic NEC 959.9
Myasthenia 358.00
  cordis — *see* Failure, heart
  gravis 358.00
    with exacerbation (acute) 358.01
    in crisis 358.01
    neonatal 775.2
    pseudoparalytica 358.00
  stomach 536.8
    psychogenic 306.4
  syndrome
    in
      botulism 005.1 [358.1]
      diabetes mellitus 250.6 ☑ [358.1]

Index to Diseases

Myasthenia — *continued*
  syndrome — *continued*
    in — *continued*
      hypothyroidism (*see also* Hypothyroidism) 244.9 *[358.1]*
      malignant neoplasm NEC 199.1 *[358.1]*
      pernicious anemia 281.0 *[358.1]*
      thyrotoxicosis (*see also* Thyrotoxicosis) 242.9 ☑ *[358.1]*
Myasthenic 728.87
Mycelium infection NEC 117.9
Mycetismus 988.1
Mycetoma (actinomycotic) 039.9
  bone 039.8
    mycotic 117.4
  foot 039.4
    mycotic 117.4
  madurae 039.9
    mycotic 117.4
  maduromycotic 039.9
    mycotic 117.4
  mycotic 117.4
  nocardial 039.9
Mycobacteriosis — *see* Mycobacterium
Mycobacterium, mycobacterial (infection) 031.9
  acid-fast (bacilli) 031.9
  anonymous (*see also* Mycobacterium, atypical) 031.9
  atypical (acid-fast bacilli) 031.9
    cutaneous 031.1
    pulmonary 031.0
      tuberculous (*see also* Tuberculosis, pulmonary) 011.9 ☑
    specified site NEC 031.8
  avium 031.0
    intracellulare complex bacteremia (MAC) 031.2
  balnei 031.1
  Battey 031.0
  cutaneous 031.1
  disseminated 031.2
    avium-intracellulare complex (DMAC) 031.2
  fortuitum 031.0
  intracellulare (battey bacillus) 031.0
  kakerifu 031.8
  kansasii 031.0
  kasongo 031.8
  leprae — *see* Leprosy
  luciflavum 031.0
  marinum 031.1
  pulmonary 031.0
    tuberculous (*see also* Tuberculosis, pulmonary) 011.9 ☑
  scrofulaceum 031.1
  tuberculosis (human, bovine) (*see also* Tuberculosis)
    avian type 031.0
  ulcerans 031.1
  xenopi 031.0
Mycosis, mycotic 117.9
  cutaneous NEC 111.9
  ear 111.8 *[380.15]*
  fungoides (M9700/3) 202.1 ☑
  mouth 112.0
  pharynx 117.9
  skin NEC 111.9
  stomatitis 112.0
  systemic NEC 117.9
  tonsil 117.9
  vagina, vaginitis 112.1
Mydriasis (persistent) (pupil) 379.43
Myelatelia 742.59
Myelinoclasis, perivascular, acute (postinfectious) NEC 136.9 *[323.61]*
  postimmunization or postvaccinal 323.51
Myelinosis, central pontine 341.8

Myelitis (ascending) (cerebellar) (childhood) (chronic) (descending) (diffuse) (disseminated) (pressure) (progressive) (spinal cord) (subacute) — *see also* Encephalitis 323.9
  acute (transverse) 341.20
    idiopathic 341.22
    in conditions classified elsewhere 341.21
  due to
    infection classified elsewhere 136.9 *[323.42]*
    specified cause NEC 323.82
    vaccination (any) 323.52
    viral diseases classified elsewhere 323.02
  herpes simplex 054.74
  herpes zoster 053.14
  late effect — *see* category 326
  optic neuritis in 341.0
  postchickenpox 052.2
  postimmunization 323.52
  postinfectious 136.9 *[323.63]*
  postvaccinal 323.52
  postvaricella 052.2
  syphilitic (transverse) 094.89
  toxic 989.9 *[323.72]*
  transverse 323.82
    acute 341.20
      idiopathic 341.22
      in conditions classified elsewhere 341.21
    idiopathic 341.22
  tuberculous (*see also* Tuberculosis) 013.6 ☑
  virus 049.9
Myeloblastic — *see* condition
Myelocele — *see also* Spina bifida 741.9 ☑
  with hydrocephalus 741.0 ☑
Myelocystocele — *see also* Spina bifida 741.9 ☑
Myelocytic — *see* condition
Myelocytoma 205.1 ☑
Myelodysplasia (spinal cord) 742.59
  meaning myelodysplastic syndrome — *see* Syndrome, myelodysplastic
Myeloencephalitis — *see* Encephalitis
Myelofibrosis 289.83
  with myeloid metaplasia 238.76
  idiopathic (chronic) 238.76
  megakaryocytic 238.79
  primary 238.76
  secondary 289.83
Myelogenous — *see* condition
Myeloid — *see* condition
Myelokathexis 288.09
Myeloleukodystrophy 330.0
Myelolipoma (M8870/0) — *see* Neoplasm, by site, benign
Myeloma (multiple) (plasma cell) (plasmacytic) (M9730/3) 203.0 ☑
  monostotic (M9731/1) 238.6
  solitary (M9731/1) 238.6
Myelomalacia 336.8
Myelomata, multiple (M9730/3) 203.0 ☑
Myelomatosis (M9730/3) 203.0 ☑
Myelomeningitis — *see* Meningoencephalitis
Myelomeningocele (spinal cord) — *see also* Spina bifida 741.9 ☑
  fetal, causing fetopelvic disproportion 653.7 ☑
Myelo-osteo-musculodysplasia hereditaria 756.89
Myelopathic — *see* condition
Myelopathy (spinal cord) 336.9
  cervical 721.1
  diabetic 250.6 ☑ *[336.3]*
  drug-induced 336.8
  due to or with
    carbon tetrachloride 987.8 *[323.72]*

Myelopathy — *continued*
  due to or with — *continued*
    degeneration or displacement, intervertebral disc 722.70
      cervical, cervicothoracic 722.71
      lumbar, lumbosacral 722.73
      thoracic, thoracolumbar 722.72
    hydroxyquinoline derivatives 961.3 *[323.72]*
    infection — *see* Encephalitis
    intervertebral disc disorder 722.70
      cervical, cervicothoracic 722.71
      lumbar, lumbosacral 722.73
      thoracic, thoracolumbar 722.72
    lead 984.9 *[323.72]*
    mercury 985.0 *[323.72]*
    neoplastic disease (*see also* Neoplasm, by site) 239.9 *[336.3]*
    pernicious anemia 281.0 *[336.3]*
    spondylosis 721.91
      cervical 721.1
      lumbar, lumbosacral 721.42
      thoracic 721.41
    thallium 985.8 *[323.72]*
  lumbar, lumbosacral 721.42
  necrotic (subacute) 336.1
  radiation-induced 336.8
  spondylogenic NEC 721.91
    cervical 721.1
    lumbar, lumbosacral 721.42
    thoracic 721.41
  thoracic 721.41
  toxic NEC 989.9 *[323.72]*
  transverse (*see also* ▶Myelitis◀) 323.82
  vascular 336.1
Myelophthisis 284.2
Myeloproliferative disease (M9960/1) 238.79
Myeloradiculitis — *see also* Polyneuropathy 357.0
Myeloradiculodysplasia (spinal) 742.59
Myelosarcoma (M9930/3) 205.3 ☑
Myelosclerosis 289.89
  with myeloid metaplasia (M9961/1) 238.76
  disseminated, of nervous system 340
  megakaryocytic (M9961/1) 238.79
Myelosis (M9860/3) — *see also* Leukemia, myeloid 205.9 ☑
  acute (M9861/3) 205.0 ☑
  aleukemic (M9864/3) 205.8 ☑
  chronic (M9863/3) 205.1 ☑
  erythremic (M9840/3) 207.0 ☑
    acute (M9841/3) 207.0 ☑
  megakaryocytic (M9920/3) 207.2 ☑
  nonleukemic (chronic) 288.8
  subacute (M9862/3) 205.2 ☑
Myesthenia — *see* Myasthenia
Myiasis (cavernous) 134.0
  orbit 134.0 *[376.13]*
Myoadenoma, prostate 600.20
  with
    other lower urinary tract symptoms (LUTS) 600.21
    urinary
      obstruction 600.21
      retention 600.21
Myoblastoma
  granular cell (M9580/0) (*see also* Neoplasm, connective tissue, benign)
    malignant (M9580/3) — *see* Neoplasm, connective tissue, malignant
  tongue (M9580/0) 210.1
Myocardial — *see* condition
Myocardiopathy (congestive) (constrictive) (familial) (hypertrophic nonobstructive) (idiopathic) (infiltrative) (obstructive) (primary) (restrictive) (sporadic) 425.4
  alcoholic 425.5
  amyloid 277.39 *[425.7]*
  beriberi 265.0 *[425.7]*

Myocardiopathy — *continued*
  cobalt-beer 425.5
  due to
    amyloidosis 277.39 *[425.7]*
    beriberi 265.0 *[425.7]*
    cardiac glycogenosis 271.0 *[425.7]*
    Chagas' disease 086.0
    Friedreich's ataxia 334.0 *[425.8]*
    influenza 487.8 *[425.8]*
    mucopolysaccharidosis 277.5 *[425.7]*
    myotonia atrophica 359.2 *[425.8]*
    progressive muscular dystrophy 359.1 *[425.8]*
    sarcoidosis 135 *[425.8]*
  glycogen storage 271.0 *[425.7]*
  hypertrophic obstructive 425.1
  metabolic NEC 277.9 *[425.7]*
  nutritional 269.9 *[425.7]*
  obscure (African) 425.2
  peripartum 674.5 ☑
  postpartum 674.5 ☑
  secondary 425.9
  thyrotoxic (*see also* Thyrotoxicosis) 242.9 ☑ *[425.7]*
  toxic NEC 425.9
Myocarditis (fibroid) (interstitial) (old) (progressive) (senile) (with arteriosclerosis) 429.0
  with
    rheumatic fever (conditions classifiable to 390) 398.0
      active (*see also* Myocarditis, acute, rheumatic) 391.2
      inactive or quiescent (with chorea) 398.0
  active (nonrheumatic) 422.90
    rheumatic 391.2
      with chorea (acute) (rheumatic) (Sydenham's) 392.0
  acute or subacute (interstitial) 422.90
    due to Streptococcus (beta-hemolytic) 391.2
    idiopathic 422.91
    rheumatic 391.2
      with chorea (acute) (rheumatic) (Sydenham's) 392.0
    specified type NEC 422.99
  aseptic of newborn 074.23
  bacterial (acute) 422.92
  chagasic 086.0
  chronic (interstitial) 429.0
  congenital 746.89
  constrictive 425.4
  Coxsackie (virus) 074.23
  diphtheritic 032.82
  due to or in
    Coxsackie (virus) 074.23
    diphtheria 032.82
    epidemic louse-borne typhus 080 *[422.0]*
    influenza 487.8 *[422.0]*
    Lyme disease 088.81 *[422.0]*
    scarlet fever 034.1 *[422.0]*
    toxoplasmosis (acquired) 130.3 *[422.0]*
    tuberculosis (*see also* Tuberculosis) 017.9 ☑ *[422.0]*
    typhoid 002.0 *[422.0]*
    typhus NEC 081.9 *[422.0]*
  eosinophilic 422.91
  epidemic of newborn 074.23
  Fiedler's (acute) (isolated) (subacute) 422.91
  giant cell (acute) (subacute) 422.91
  gonococcal 098.85
  granulomatous (idiopathic) (isolated) (nonspecific) 422.91
  hypertensive (*see also* Hypertension, heart) 402.90
  idiopathic 422.91
    granulomatous 422.91
  infective 422.92
  influenzal 487.8 *[422.0]*
  isolated (diffuse) (granulomatous) 422.91
  malignant 422.99

Myocarditis — continued
- meningococcal 036.43
- nonrheumatic, active 422.90
- parenchymatous 422.90
- pneumococcal (acute) (subacute) 422.92
- rheumatic (chronic) (inactive) (with chorea) 398.0
  - active or acute 391.2
    - with chorea (acute) (rheumatic) (Sydenham's) 392.0
- septic 422.92
- specific (giant cell) (productive) 422.91
- staphylococcal (acute) (subacute) 422.92
- suppurative 422.92
- syphilitic (chronic) 093.82
- toxic 422.93
  - rheumatic (see also Myocarditis, acute rheumatic) 391.2
- tuberculous (see also Tuberculosis) 017.9 ☑ [422.0]
- typhoid 002.0 [422.0]
- valvular — see Endocarditis
- viral, except Coxsackie 422.91
  - Coxsackie 074.23
  - of newborn (Coxsackie) 074.23

Myocardium, myocardial — see condition

Myocardosis — see also Cardiomyopathy 425.4

Myoclonia (essential) 333.2
- epileptica 333.2
- Friedrich's 333.2
- massive 333.2

Myoclonic
- epilepsy, familial (progressive) 333.2
- jerks 333.2

Myoclonus (familial essential) (multifocal) (simplex) 333.2
- with epilepsy and with ragged red fibers (MERRF syndrome) 277.87
- facial 351.8
- massive (infantile) 333.2
- pharyngeal 478.29

Myodiastasis 728.84

Myoendocarditis — see also Endocarditis
- acute or subacute 421.9

Myoepithelioma (M8982/0) — see Neoplasm, by site, benign

Myofascitis (acute) 729.1
- low back 724.2

Myofibroma (M8890/0) — see also Neoplasm, connective tissue, benign
- uterus (cervix) (corpus) (see also Leiomyoma) 218.9

Myofibromatosis ●
- infantile 759.89 ●

Myofibrosis 728.2
- heart (see also Myocarditis) 429.0
- humeroscapular region 726.2
- scapulohumeral 726.2

Myofibrositis — see also Myositis 729.1
- scapulohumeral 726.2

Myogelosis (occupational) 728.89

Myoglobinuria 791.3

Myoglobulinuria, primary 791.3

Myokymia — see also Myoclonus
- facial 351.8

Myolipoma (M8860/0)
- specified site — see Neoplasm, connective tissue, benign
- unspecified site 223.0

Myoma (M8895/0) — see also Neoplasm, connective tissue, benign
- cervix (stump) (uterus) (see also Leiomyoma) 218.9
- malignant (M8895/3) — see Neoplasm, connective tissue, malignant
- prostate 600.20

Myoma — see also Neoplasm, connective tissue, benign — continued
- prostate — continued
  - with
    - other lower urinary tract symptoms (LUTS) 600.21 ●
    - urinary ●
      - obstruction 600.21 ●
      - retention 600.21 ●
- uterus (cervix) (corpus) (see also Leiomyoma) 218.9
  - in pregnancy or childbirth 654.1 ☑
    - affecting fetus or newborn 763.89
    - causing obstructed labor 660.2 ☑
      - affecting fetus or newborn 763.1

Myomalacia 728.9
- cordis, heart (see also Degeneration, myocardial) 429.1

Myometritis — see also Endometritis 615.9

Myometrium — see condition

Myonecrosis, clostridial 040.0

Myopathy 359.9
- alcoholic 359.4
- amyloid 277.39 [359.6] ▲
- benign, congenital 359.0
- central core 359.0
- centronuclear 359.0
- congenital (benign) 359.0
- critical illness 359.81
- distal 359.1
- due to drugs 359.4
- endocrine 259.9 [359.5]
  - specified type NEC 259.8 [359.5]
- extraocular muscles 376.82
- facioscapulohumeral 359.1
- in
  - Addison's disease 255.4 [359.5]
  - amyloidosis 277.39 [359.6] ▲
  - cretinism 243 [359.5]
  - Cushing's syndrome 255.0 [359.5]
  - disseminated lupus erythematosus 710.0 [359.6]
  - giant cell arteritis 446.5 [359.6]
  - hyperadrenocorticism NEC 255.3 [359.5]
  - hyperparathyroidism 252.01 [359.5]
  - hypopituitarism 253.2 [359.5]
  - hypothyroidism (see also Hypothyroidism) 244.9 [359.5]
  - malignant neoplasm NEC (M8000/3) 199.1 [359.5]
  - myxedema (see also Myxedema) 244.9 [359.5]
  - polyarteritis nodosa 446.0 [359.6]
  - rheumatoid arthritis 714.0 [359.6]
  - sarcoidosis 135 [359.6]
  - scleroderma 710.1 [359.6]
  - Sjögren's disease 710.2 [359.6]
  - thyrotoxicosis (see also Thyrotoxicosis) 242.9 ☑ [359.5]
- inflammatory 359.89
- intensive care (ICU) 359.81
- limb-girdle 359.1
- myotubular 359.0
- necrotizing, acute 359.81
- nemaline 359.0
- ocular 359.1
- oculopharyngeal 359.1
- of critical illness 359.81
- primary 359.89
- progressive NEC 359.89
- quadriplegic, acute 359.81
- rod body 359.0
- scapulohumeral 359.1
- specified type NEC 359.89
- toxic 359.4

Myopericarditis — see also Pericarditis 423.9

Myopia (axial) (congenital) (increased curvature or refraction, nucleus of lens) 367.1
- degenerative, malignant 360.21
- malignant 360.21
- progressive high (degenerative) 360.21

Myosarcoma (M8895/3) — see Neoplasm, connective tissue, malignant

Myosis (persistent) 379.42
- stromal (endolymphatic) (M8931/1) 236.0

Myositis 729.1
- clostridial 040.0
- due to posture 729.1
- epidemic 074.1
- fibrosa or fibrous (chronic) 728.2
  - Volkmann's (complicating trauma) 958.6
- infective 728.0
- interstitial 728.81
- multiple — see Polymyositis
- occupational 729.1
- orbital, chronic 376.12
- ossificans 728.12
  - circumscribed 728.12
  - progressive 728.11
  - traumatic 728.12
- progressive fibrosing 728.11
- purulent 728.0
- rheumatic 729.1
- rheumatoid 729.1
- suppurative 728.0
- syphilitic 095.6
- traumatic (old) 729.1

Myospasia impulsiva 307.23

Myotonia (acquisita) (intermittens) 728.85
- atrophica 359.2
- congenita 359.2
- dystrophica 359.2

Myotonic pupil 379.46

Myriapodiasis 134.1

Myringitis
- with otitis media — see Otitis media
- acute 384.00
  - specified type NEC 384.09
- bullosa hemorrhagica 384.01
- bullous 384.01
- chronic 384.1

Mysophobia 300.29

Mytilotoxism 988.0

Myxadenitis labialis 528.5

Myxedema (adult) (idiocy) (infantile) (juvenile) (thyroid gland) — see also Hypothyroidism 244.9
- circumscribed 242.9 ☑
- congenital 243
- cutis 701.8
- localized (pretibial) 242.9 ☑
- madness (acute) 293.0
  - subacute 293.1
- papular 701.8
- pituitary 244.8
- postpartum 674.8 ☑
- pretibial 242.9 ☑
- primary 244.9

Myxochondrosarcoma (M9220/3) — see Neoplasm, cartilage, malignant

Myxofibroma (M8811/0) — see also Neoplasm, connective tissue, benign
- odontogenic (M9320/0) 213.1
- upper jaw (bone) 213.0

Myxofibrosarcoma (M8811/3) — see Neoplasm, connective tissue, malignant

Myxolipoma (M8852/0) — see also Lipoma, by site 214.9

Myxoliposarcoma (M8852/3) — see Neoplasm, connective tissue, malignant

Myxoma (M8840/0) — see also Neoplasm, connective tissue, benign
- odontogenic (M9320/0) 213.1
- upper jaw (bone) 213.0

Myxosarcoma (M8840/3) — see Neoplasm, connective tissue, malignant

N

Naegeli's
- disease (hereditary hemorrhagic thrombasthenia) 287.1
- leukemia, monocytic (M9863/3) 205.1 ☑
- syndrome (incontinentia pigmenti) 757.33

Naffziger's syndrome 353.0

Naga sore — see also Ulcer, skin 707.9

Nägele's pelvis 738.6
- with disproportion (fetopelvic) 653.0 ☑
  - affecting fetus or newborn 763.1
  - causing obstructed labor 660.1 ☑
    - affecting fetus or newborn 763.1

Nager-de Reynier syndrome (dysostosis mandibularis) 756.0

Nail — see also condition
- biting 307.9
- patella syndrome (hereditary osteoonychodysplasia) 756.89

Nanism, nanosomia — see also Dwarfism 259.4
- hypophyseal 253.3
- pituitary 253.3
- renis, renalis 588.0

Nanukayami 100.89

Napkin rash 691.0

Narcissism 301.81

Narcolepsy 347.00
- with cataplexy 347.01
- in conditions classified elsewhere 347.10
  - with cataplexy 347.11

Narcosis
- carbon dioxide (respiratory) 786.09
- due to drug
  - correct substance properly administered 780.09
  - overdose or wrong substance given or taken 977.9
    - specified drug — see Table of Drugs and Chemicals

Narcotism (chronic) — see also Dependence 304.9 ☑
- acute
  - correct substance properly administered 349.82
  - overdose or wrong substance given or taken 967.8
    - specified drug — see Table of Drugs and Chemicals

NARP (ataxia and retinitis pigmentosa) 277.87

Narrow
- anterior chamber angle 365.02
- pelvis (inlet) (outlet) — see Contraction, pelvis

Narrowing
- artery NEC 447.1
  - auditory, internal 433.8 ☑
  - basilar 433.0 ☑
    - with other precerebral artery 433.3 ☑
    - bilateral 433.3 ☑
  - carotid 433.1 ☑
    - with other precerebral artery 433.3 ☑
    - bilateral 433.3 ☑
  - cerebellar 433.8 ☑
  - choroidal 433.8 ☑
  - communicating posterior 433.8 ☑
  - coronary (see also Arteriosclerosis, coronary)
    - congenital 746.85
    - due to syphilis 090.5
  - hypophyseal 433.8 ☑
  - pontine 433.8 ☑
  - precerebral NEC 433.9 ☑
    - multiple or bilateral 433.3 ☑
    - specified NEC 433.8 ☑

Narrowing — continued
- artery — continued
  - vertebral 433.2
    - with other precerebral artery 433.3
      - bilateral 433.3
  - auditory canal (external) (see also Stricture, ear canal, acquired) 380.50
  - cerebral arteries 437.0
  - cicatricial — see Cicatrix
  - congenital — see Anomaly, congenital
  - coronary artery — see Narrowing, artery, coronary
  - ear, middle 385.22
  - Eustachian tube (see also Obstruction, Eustachian tube) 381.60
  - eyelid 374.46
    - congenital 743.62
  - intervertebral disc or space NEC — see Degeneration, intervertebral disc
  - joint space, hip 719.85
  - larynx 478.74
  - lids 374.46
    - congenital 743.62
  - mesenteric artery (with gangrene) 557.0
  - palate 524.89
  - palpebral fissure 374.46
  - retinal artery 362.13
  - ureter 593.3
  - urethra (see also Stricture, urethra) 598.9

Narrowness, abnormal, eyelid 743.62
Nasal — see condition
Nasolacrimal — see condition
Nasopharyngeal — see also condition
- bursa 478.29
- pituitary gland 759.2
- torticollis 723.5

Nasopharyngitis (acute) (infective) (subacute) 460
- chronic 472.2
  - due to external agent — see Condition, respiratory, chronic, due to
- due to external agent — see Condition, respiratory, due to
- septic 034.0
- streptococcal 034.0
- suppurative (chronic) 472.2
- ulcerative (chronic) 472.2

Nasopharynx, nasopharyngeal — see condition
Natal tooth, teeth 520.6
Nausea — see also Vomiting 787.02
- with vomiting 787.01
- epidemic 078.82
- gravidarum — see Hyperemesis, gravidarum
- marina 994.6

Navel — see condition
Neapolitan fever — see also Brucellosis 023.9
Nearsightedness 367.1
Near-syncope 780.2
Nebécourt's syndrome 253.3
Nebula, cornea (eye) 371.01
- congenital 743.43
  - interfering with vision 743.42

Necator americanus infestation 126.1
Necatoriasis 126.1
Neck — see condition
Necrencephalus — see also Softening, brain 437.8
Necrobacillosis 040.3
Necrobiosis 799.89
- brain or cerebral (see also Softening, brain) 437.8
- lipoidica 709.3
  - diabeticorum 250.8 [709.3]

Necrodermolysis 695.1
Necrolysis, toxic epidermal 695.1

Necrolysis, toxic epidermal — continued
- due to drug
  - correct substance properly administered 695.1
  - overdose or wrong substance given or taken 977.9
  - specified drug — see Table of Drugs and Chemicals

Necrophilia 302.89
Necrosis, necrotic
- adrenal (capsule) (gland) 255.8
- antrum, nasal sinus 478.19
- aorta (hyaline) (see also Aneurysm, aorta) 441.9
  - cystic medial 441.00
    - abdominal 441.02
    - thoracic 441.01
    - thoracoabdominal 441.03
  - ruptured 441.5
- arteritis 446.0
- artery 447.5
- aseptic, bone 733.40
  - femur (head) (neck) 733.42
    - medial condyle 733.43
  - humoral head 733.41
  - medial femoral condyle 733.43
  - specific site NEC 733.49
  - talus 733.44
- avascular, bone NEC (see also Necrosis, aseptic, bone) 733.40
- bladder (aseptic) (sphincter) 596.8
- bone (see also Osteomyelitis) 730.1
  - acute 730.0
  - aseptic or avascular 733.40
    - femur (head) (neck) 733.42
      - medial condyle 733.43
    - humoral head 733.41
    - medial femoral condyle 733.43
    - specified site NEC 733.49
    - talus 733.44
  - ethmoid 478.19
  - ischemic 733.40
  - jaw 526.4
  - marrow 289.89
  - Paget's (osteitis deformans) 731.0
  - tuberculous — see Tuberculosis, bone
- brain (softening) (see also Softening, brain) 437.8
- breast (aseptic) (fat) (segmental) 611.3
- bronchus, bronchi 519.19
- central nervous system NEC (see also Softening, brain) 437.8
- cerebellar (see also Softening, brain) 437.8
- cerebral (softening) (see also Softening, brain) 437.8
- cerebrospinal (softening) (see also Softening, brain) 437.8
- cornea (see also Keratitis) 371.40
- cortical, kidney 583.6
- cystic medial (aorta) 441.00
  - abdominal 441.02
  - thoracic 441.01
  - thoracoabdominal 441.03
- dental 521.09
  - pulp 522.1
- due to swallowing corrosive substance — see Burn, by site
- ear (ossicle) 385.24
- esophagus 530.89
- ethmoid (bone) 478.19
- eyelid 374.50
- fat, fatty (generalized) (see also Degeneration, fatty) 272.8
  - abdominal wall 567.82
  - breast (aseptic) (segmental) 611.3
  - intestine 569.89
  - localized — see Degeneration, by site, fatty
  - mesentery 567.82
  - omentum 567.82
  - pancreas 577.8
  - peritoneum 567.82
  - skin (subcutaneous) 709.3

Necrosis, necrotic — continued
- fat, fatty (see also Degeneration, fatty) — continued
  - skin — continued
    - newborn 778.1
- femur (aseptic) (avascular) 733.42
  - head 733.42
  - medial condyle 733.43
  - neck 733.42
- gallbladder (see also Cholecystitis, acute) 575.0
- gangrenous 785.4
- gastric 537.89
- glottis 478.79
- heart (myocardium) — see Infarct, myocardium
- hepatic (see also Necrosis, liver) 570
- hip (aseptic) (avascular) 733.42
- intestine (acute) (hemorrhagic) (massive) 557.0
- ischemic 785.4
- jaw 526.4
- kidney (bilateral) 583.9
  - acute 584.9
  - cortical 583.6
    - acute 584.6
      - with
        - abortion — see Abortion, by type, with renal failure
        - ectopic pregnancy (see also categories 633.0–633.9) 639.3
        - molar pregnancy (see also categories 630–632) 639.3
      - complicating pregnancy 646.2
      - affecting fetus or newborn 760.1
      - following labor and delivery 669.3
  - medullary (papillary) (see also Pyelitis) 590.80
    - in
      - acute renal failure 584.7
      - nephritis, nephropathy 583.7
  - papillary (see also Pyelitis) 590.80
    - in
      - acute renal failure 584.7
      - nephritis, nephropathy 583.7
  - tubular 584.5
    - with
      - abortion — see Abortion, by type, with renal failure
      - ectopic pregnancy (see also categories 633.0–633.9) 639.3
      - molar pregnancy (see also categories 630–632) 639.3
    - complicating
      - abortion 639.3
      - ectopic or molar pregnancy 639.3
    - pregnancy 646.2
      - affecting fetus or newborn 760.1
    - following labor and delivery 669.3
    - traumatic 958.5
- larynx 478.79
- liver (acute) (congenital) (diffuse) (massive) (subacute) 570
  - with
    - abortion — see Abortion, by type, with specified complication NEC
    - ectopic pregnancy (see also categories 633.0–633.9) 639.8
    - molar pregnancy (see also categories 630–632) 639.8
  - complicating pregnancy 646.7
  - affecting fetus or newborn 760.8

Necrosis, necrotic — continued
- liver — continued
  - following
    - abortion 639.8
    - ectopic or molar pregnancy 639.8
  - obstetrical 646.7
  - postabortal 639.8
  - puerperal, postpartum 674.8
  - toxic 573.3
- lung 513.0
- lymphatic gland 683
- mammary gland 611.3
- mastoid (chronic) 383.1
- mesentery 557.0
  - fat 567.82
- mitral valve — see Insufficiency, mitral
- myocardium, myocardial — see Infarct, myocardium
- nose (septum) 478.19
- omentum 557.0
  - with mesenteric infarction 557.0
  - fat 567.82
- orbit, orbital 376.10
- ossicles, ear (aseptic) 385.24
- ovary (see also Salpingo-oophoritis) 614.2
- pancreas (aseptic) (duct) (fat) 577.8
  - acute 577.0
  - infective 577.0
- papillary, kidney (see also Pyelitis) 590.80
- perineum 624.8
- peritoneum 557.0
  - with mesenteric infarction 557.0
  - fat 567.82
- pharynx 462
  - in granulocytopenia 288.09
- phosphorus 983.9
- pituitary (gland) (postpartum) (Sheehan) 253.2
- placenta (see also Placenta, abnormal) 656.7
- pneumonia 513.0
- pulmonary 513.0
- pulp (dental) 522.1
- pylorus 537.89
- radiation — see Necrosis, by site
- radium — see Necrosis, by site
- renal — see Necrosis, kidney
- sclera 379.19
- scrotum 608.89
- skin or subcutaneous tissue 709.8
  - due to burn — see Burn, by site
  - gangrenous 785.4
- spine, spinal (column) 730.18
  - acute 730.18
  - cord 336.1
- spleen 289.59
- stomach 537.89
- stomatitis 528.1
- subcutaneous fat 709.3
  - fetus or newborn 778.1
- subendocardial — see Infarct, myocardium
- suprarenal (capsule) (gland) 255.8
- teeth, tooth 521.09
- testis 608.89
- thymus (gland) 254.8
- tonsil 474.8
- trachea 519.19
- tuberculous NEC — see Tuberculosis
- tubular (acute) (anoxic) (toxic) 584.5
  - due to a procedure 997.5
- umbilical cord, affecting fetus or newborn 762.6
- vagina 623.8
- vertebra (lumbar) 730.18
  - acute 730.18
  - tuberculous (see also Tuberculosis) 015.0 [730.8]
- vesical (aseptic) (bladder) 596.8
- vulva 624.8
- x-ray — see Necrosis, by site

Necrospermia 606.0

Necrotizing angiitis 446.0
Negativism 301.7
Neglect (child) (newborn) NEC 995.52
    adult 995.84
        after or at birth 995.52
    hemispatial 781.8
    left-sided 781.8

Neglect — *continued*
    sensory 781.8
    visuospatial 781.8
Negri bodies 071
Neill-Dingwall syndrome (microcephaly and dwarfism) 759.89

Neisserian infection NEC — *see* Gonococcus
Nematodiasis NEC — *see also* Infestation, Nematode 127.9
    ancylostoma (*see also* Ancylostomiasis) 126.9

Neoformans cryptococcus infection 117.5
Neonatal — *see also* condition
    adrenoleukodystrophy 277.86
    teeth, tooth 520.6
Neonatorum — *see* condition

Index to Diseases

Neoplasm, blood vessel

	Malignant			Benign	Uncertain Behavior	Unspecified
	Primary	Secondary	Ca in situ			
Neoplasm, neoplastic	199.1	199.1	234.9	229.9	238.9	239.9

Notes — 1. The list below gives the code numbers for neoplasms by anatomical site. For each site there are six possible code numbers according to whether the neoplasm in question is malignant, benign, in situ, of uncertain behavior, or of unspecified nature. The description of the neoplasm will often indicate which of the six columns is appropriate; e.g., malignant melanoma of skin, benign fibroadenoma of breast, carcinoma in situ of cervix uteri.

Where such descriptors are not present, the remainder of the Index should be consulted where guidance is given to the appropriate column for each morphological (histological) variety listed; e.g., Mesonephroma — see Neoplasm, malignant; Embryoma — see also Neoplasm, uncertain behavior; Disease, Bowen's — see Neoplasm, skin, in situ. However, the guidance in the Index can be overridden if one of the descriptors mentioned above is present; e.g., malignant adenoma of colon is coded to 153.9 and not to 211.3 as the adjective "malignant" overrides the Index entry "Adenoma — see also Neoplasm, benign."

2. Sites marked with the sign * (e.g., face NEC*) should be classified to malignant neoplasm of skin of these sites if the variety of neoplasm is a squamous cell carcinoma or an epidermoid carcinoma, and to benign neoplasm of skin of these sites if the variety of neoplasm is a papilloma (any type).

	Primary	Secondary	Ca in situ	Benign	Uncertain Behavior	Unspecified
abdomen, abdominal	195.2	198.89	234.8	229.8	238.8	239.8
cavity	195.2	198.89	234.8	229.8	238.8	239.8
organ	195.2	198.89	234.8	229.8	238.8	239.8
viscera	195.2	198.89	234.8	229.8	238.8	239.8
wall	173.5	198.2	232.5	216.5	238.2	239.2
connective tissue	171.5	198.89	—	215.5	238.1	239.2
abdominopelvic	195.8	198.89	234.8	229.8	238.8	239.8
accessory sinus — see Neoplasm, sinus						
acoustic nerve	192.0	198.4	—	225.1	237.9	239.7
acromion (process)	170.4	198.5	—	213.4	238.0	239.2
adenoid (pharynx) (tissue)	147.1	198.89	230.0	210.7	235.1	239.0
adipose tissue (see also Neoplasm, connective tissue)	171.9	198.89	—	215.9	238.1	239.2
adnexa (uterine)	183.9	198.82	233.3	221.8	236.3	239.5
adrenal (cortex) (gland) (medulla)	194.0	198.7	234.8	227.0	237.2	239.7
ala nasi (external)	173.3	198.2	232.3	216.3	238.2	239.2
alimentary canal or tract NEC	159.9	197.8	230.9	211.9	235.5	239.0
alveolar	143.9	198.89	230.0	210.4	235.1	239.0
mucosa	143.9	198.89	230.0	210.4	235.1	239.0
lower	143.1	198.89	230.0	210.4	235.1	239.0
upper	143.0	198.89	230.0	210.4	235.1	239.0
ridge or process	170.1	198.5	—	213.1	238.0	239.2
carcinoma	143.9	—	—	—	—	—
lower	143.1	—	—	—	—	—
upper	143.0	—	—	—	—	—
lower	170.1	198.5	—	213.1	238.0	239.2
mucosa	143.9	198.89	230.0	210.4	235.1	239.0
lower	143.1	198.89	230.0	210.4	235.1	239.0
upper	143.0	198.89	230.0	210.4	235.1	239.0
upper	170.1	198.5	—	213.0	238.0	239.2
sulcus	145.1	198.89	230.0	210.4	235.1	239.0
alveolus	143.9	198.89	230.0	210.4	235.1	239.0
lower	143.1	198.89	230.0	210.4	235.1	239.0
upper	143.0	198.89	230.0	210.4	235.1	239.0
ampulla of Vater	156.2	197.8	230.8	211.5	235.3	239.0
ankle NEC*	195.5	198.89	232.7	229.8	238.8	239.8
anorectum, anorectal (junction)	154.8	197.5	230.7	211.4	235.2	239.0
antecubital fossa or space*	195.4	198.89	232.6	229.8	238.8	239.8
antrum (Highmore) (maxillary)	160.2	197.3	231.8	212.0	235.9	239.1
pyloric	151.2	197.8	230.2	211.1	235.2	239.0
tympanicum	160.1	197.3	231.8	212.0	235.9	239.1
anus, anal	154.3	197.5	230.6	211.4	235.5	239.0
canal	154.2	197.5	230.5	211.4	235.5	239.0
contiguous sites with rectosigmoid junction or rectum	154.8	—	—	—	—	—
margin	173.5	198.2	232.5	216.5	238.2	239.2
skin	173.5	198.2	232.5	216.5	238.2	239.2
sphincter	154.2	197.5	230.5	211.4	235.5	239.0
aorta (thoracic)	171.4	198.89	—	215.4	238.1	239.2
abdominal	171.5	198.89	—	215.5	238.1	239.2
aortic body	194.6	198.89	—	227.6	237.3	239.7
aponeurosis	171.9	198.89	—	215.9	238.1	239.2
palmar	171.2	198.89	—	215.2	238.1	239.2
plantar	171.3	198.89	—	215.3	238.1	239.2
appendix	153.5	197.5	230.3	211.3	235.2	239.0
arachnoid (cerebral)	192.1	198.4	—	225.2	237.6	239.7
spinal	192.3	198.4	—	225.4	237.6	239.7
areola (female)	174.0	198.81	233.0	217	238.3	239.3
male	175.0	198.81	233.0	217	238.3	239.3
arm NEC*	195.4	198.89	232.6	229.8	238.8	239.8
artery — see Neoplasm, connective tissue						
aryepiglottic fold	148.2	198.89	230.0	210.8	235.1	239.0
hypopharyngeal aspect	148.2	198.89	230.0	210.8	235.1	239.0
laryngeal aspect	161.1	197.3	231.0	212.1	235.6	239.1
marginal zone	148.2	198.89	230.0	210.8	235.1	239.0
arytenoid (cartilage)	161.3	197.3	231.0	212.1	235.6	239.1
fold — see Neoplasm, aryepiglottic						
atlas	170.2	198.5	—	213.2	238.0	239.2
atrium, cardiac	164.1	198.89	—	212.7	238.8	239.8
auditory canal (external) (skin)	173.2	198.2	232.2	216.2	238.2	239.2
internal	160.1	197.3	231.8	212.0	235.9	239.1
nerve	192.0	198.4	—	225.1	237.9	239.7
tube	160.1	197.3	231.8	212.0	235.9	239.1
Eustachian	160.1	197.3	231.8	212.0	235.9	239.1
opening	147.2	198.89	230.0	210.7	235.1	239.0
auricle, ear	173.2	198.2	232.2	216.2	238.2	239.2
cartilage	171.0	198.89	—	215.0	238.1	239.2
auricular canal (external)	173.2	198.2	232.2	216.2	238.2	239.2
internal	160.1	197.3	231.8	212.0	235.9	239.1
autonomic nerve or nervous system NEC	171.9	198.89	—	215.9	238.1	239.2
axilla, axillary	195.1	198.89	234.8	229.8	238.8	239.8
fold	173.5	198.2	232.5	216.5	238.2	239.2
back NEC*	195.8	198.89	232.5	229.8	238.8	239.8
Bartholin's gland	184.1	198.82	233.3	221.2	236.3	239.5
basal ganglia	191.0	198.3	—	225.0	237.5	239.6
basis pedunculi	191.7	198.3	—	225.0	237.5	239.6
bile or biliary (tract)	156.9	197.8	230.8	211.5	235.3	239.0
canaliculi (biliferi) (intrahepatic)	155.1	197.8	230.8	211.5	235.3	239.0
canals, interlobular	155.1	197.8	230.8	211.5	235.3	239.0
contiguous sites	156.8	—	—	—	—	—
duct or passage (common) (cystic) (extrahepatic)	156.1	197.8	230.8	211.5	235.3	239.0
contiguous sites with gallbladder	156.8	—	—	—	—	—
interlobular	155.1	197.8	230.8	211.5	235.3	239.0
intrahepatic	155.1	197.8	230.8	211.5	235.3	239.0
and extrahepatic	156.9	197.8	230.8	211.5	235.3	239.0
bladder (urinary)	188.9	198.1	233.7	223.3	236.7	239.4
contiguous sites	188.8	—	—	—	—	—
dome	188.1	198.1	233.7	223.3	236.7	239.4
neck	188.5	198.1	233.7	223.3	236.7	239.4
orifice	188.9	198.1	233.7	223.3	236.7	239.4
ureteric	188.6	198.1	233.7	223.3	236.7	239.4
urethral	188.5	198.1	233.7	223.3	236.7	239.4
sphincter	188.8	198.1	233.7	223.3	236.7	239.4
trigone	188.0	198.1	233.7	223.3	236.7	239.4
urachus	188.7	—	233.7	223.3	236.7	239.4
wall	188.9	198.1	233.7	223.3	236.7	239.4
anterior	188.3	198.1	233.7	223.3	236.7	239.4
lateral	188.2	198.1	233.7	223.3	236.7	239.4
posterior	188.4	198.1	233.7	223.3	236.7	239.4
blood vessel — see Neoplasm, connective tissue						

Neoplasm, bone — Index to Diseases

	Malignant			Benign	Uncertain Behavior	Unspecified
	Primary	Secondary	Ca in situ			
Neoplasm, neoplastic — *continued*						
bone (periosteum)	170.9	198.5	—	213.9	238.0	239.2

Note — Carcinomas and adenocarcinomas, of any type other than intraosseous or odontogenic, of the sites listed under "Neoplasm, bone" should be considered as constituting metastatic spread from an unspecified primary site and coded to 198.5 for morbidity coding and to 199.1 for underlying cause of death coding.

	Primary	Secondary	Ca in situ	Benign	Uncertain Behavior	Unspecified
acetabulum	170.6	198.5	—	213.6	238.0	239.2
acromion (process)	170.4	198.5	—	213.4	238.0	239.2
ankle	170.8	198.5	—	213.8	238.0	239.2
arm NEC	170.4	198.5	—	213.4	238.0	239.2
astragalus	170.8	198.5	—	213.8	238.0	239.2
atlas	170.2	198.5	—	213.2	238.0	239.2
axis	170.2	198.5	—	213.2	238.0	239.2
back NEC	170.2	198.5	—	213.2	238.0	239.2
calcaneus	170.8	198.5	—	213.8	238.0	239.2
calvarium	170.0	198.5	—	213.0	238.0	239.2
carpus (any)	170.5	198.5	—	213.5	238.0	239.2
cartilage NEC	170.9	198.5	—	213.9	238.0	239.2
clavicle	170.3	198.5	—	213.3	238.0	239.2
clivus	170.0	198.5	—	213.0	238.0	239.2
coccygeal vertebra	170.6	198.5	—	213.6	238.0	239.2
coccyx	170.6	198.5	—	213.6	238.0	239.2
costal cartilage	170.3	198.5	—	213.3	238.0	239.2
costovertebral joint	170.3	198.5	—	213.3	238.0	239.2
cranial	170.0	198.5	—	213.0	238.0	239.2
cuboid	170.8	198.5	—	213.8	238.0	239.2
cuneiform	170.9	198.5	—	213.9	238.0	239.2
ankle	170.8	198.5	—	213.8	238.0	239.2
wrist	170.5	198.5	—	213.5	238.0	239.2
digital	170.9	198.5	—	213.9	238.0	239.2
finger	170.5	198.5	—	213.5	238.0	239.2
toe	170.8	198.5	—	213.8	238.0	239.2
elbow	170.4	198.5	—	213.4	238.0	239.2
ethmoid (labyrinth)	170.0	198.5	—	213.0	238.0	239.2
face	170.0	198.5	—	213.0	238.0	239.2
lower jaw	170.1	198.5	—	213.1	238.0	239.2
femur (any part)	170.7	198.5	—	213.7	238.0	239.2
fibula (any part)	170.7	198.5	—	213.7	238.0	239.2
finger (any)	170.5	198.5	—	213.5	238.0	239.2
foot	170.8	198.5	—	213.8	238.0	239.2
forearm	170.4	198.5	—	213.4	238.0	239.2
frontal	170.0	198.5	—	213.0	238.0	239.2
hand	170.5	198.5	—	213.5	238.0	239.2
heel	170.8	198.5	—	213.8	238.0	239.2
hip	170.6	198.5	—	213.6	238.0	239.2
humerus (any part)	170.4	198.5	—	213.4	238.0	239.2
hyoid	170.0	198.5	—	213.0	238.0	239.2
ilium	170.6	198.5	—	213.6	238.0	239.2
innominate	170.6	198.5	—	213.6	238.0	239.2
intervertebral cartilage or disc	170.2	198.5	—	213.2	238.0	239.2
ischium	170.6	198.5	—	213.6	238.0	239.2
jaw (lower)	170.1	198.5	—	213.1	238.0	239.2
upper	170.0	198.5	—	213.0	238.0	239.2
knee	170.7	198.5	—	213.7	238.0	239.2
leg NEC	170.7	198.5	—	213.7	238.0	239.2
limb NEC	170.9	198.5	—	213.9	238.0	239.2
lower (long bones)	170.7	198.5	—	213.7	238.0	239.2
short bones	170.8	198.5	—	213.8	238.0	239.2
upper (long bones)	170.4	198.5	—	213.4	238.0	239.2
short bones	170.5	198.5	—	213.5	238.0	239.2
long	170.9	198.5	—	213.9	238.0	239.2
lower limbs NEC	170.7	198.5	—	213.7	238.0	239.2
upper limbs NEC	170.4	198.5	—	213.4	238.0	239.2
malar	170.0	198.5	—	213.0	238.0	239.2
mandible	170.1	198.5	—	213.1	238.0	239.2
marrow NEC	202.9 ☑	198.5	—	—	—	238.79 ▲
mastoid	170.0	198.5	—	213.0	238.0	239.2
maxilla, maxillary (superior)	170.0	198.5	—	213.0	238.0	239.2
inferior	170.1	198.5	—	213.1	238.0	239.2
metacarpus (any)	170.5	198.5	—	213.5	238.0	239.2
metatarsus (any)	170.8	198.5	—	213.8	238.0	239.2
navicular (ankle)	170.8	198.5	—	213.8	238.0	239.2
hand	170.5	198.5	—	213.5	238.0	239.2
Neoplasm, neoplastic — *continued* bone — *continued*						
nose, nasal	170.0	198.5	—	213.0	238.0	239.2
occipital	170.0	198.5	—	213.0	238.0	239.2
orbit	170.0	198.5	—	213.0	238.0	239.2
parietal	170.0	198.5	—	213.0	238.0	239.2
patella	170.8	198.5	—	213.8	238.0	239.2
pelvic	170.6	198.5	—	213.6	238.0	239.2
phalanges	170.9	198.5	—	213.9	238.0	239.2
foot	170.8	198.5	—	213.8	238.0	239.2
hand	170.5	198.5	—	213.5	238.0	239.2
pubic	170.6	198.5	—	213.6	238.0	239.2
radius (any part)	170.4	198.5	—	213.4	238.0	239.2
rib	170.3	198.5	—	213.3	238.0	239.2
sacral vertebra	170.6	198.5	—	213.6	238.0	239.2
sacrum	170.6	198.5	—	213.6	238.0	239.2
scaphoid (of hand)	170.5	198.5	—	213.5	238.0	239.2
of ankle	170.8	198.5	—	213.8	238.0	239.2
scapula (any part)	170.4	198.5	—	213.4	238.0	239.2
sella turcica	170.0	198.5	—	213.0	238.0	239.2
short	170.9	198.5	—	213.9	238.0	239.2
lower limb	170.8	198.5	—	213.8	238.0	239.2
upper limb	170.5	198.5	—	213.5	238.0	239.2
shoulder	170.4	198.5	—	213.4	238.0	239.2
skeleton, skeletal NEC	170.9	198.5	—	213.9	238.0	239.2
skull	170.0	198.5	—	213.0	238.0	239.2
sphenoid	170.0	198.5	—	213.0	238.0	239.2
spine, spinal (column)	170.2	198.5	—	213.2	238.0	239.2
coccyx	170.6	198.5	—	213.6	238.0	239.2
sacrum	170.6	198.5	—	213.6	238.0	239.2
sternum	170.3	198.5	—	213.3	238.0	239.2
tarsus (any)	170.8	198.5	—	213.8	238.0	239.2
temporal	170.0	198.5	—	213.0	238.0	239.2
thumb	170.5	198.5	—	213.5	238.0	239.2
tibia (any part)	170.7	198.5	—	213.7	238.0	239.2
toe (any)	170.8	198.5	—	213.8	238.0	239.2
trapezium	170.5	198.5	—	213.5	238.0	239.2
trapezoid	170.5	198.5	—	213.5	238.0	239.2
turbinate	170.0	198.5	—	213.0	238.0	239.2
ulna (any part)	170.4	198.5	—	213.4	238.0	239.2
unciform	170.5	198.5	—	213.5	238.0	239.2
vertebra (column)	170.2	198.5	—	213.2	238.0	239.2
coccyx	170.6	198.5	—	213.6	238.0	239.2
sacrum	170.6	198.5	—	213.6	238.0	239.2
vomer	170.0	198.5	—	213.0	238.0	239.2
wrist	170.5	198.5	—	213.5	238.0	239.2
xiphoid process	170.3	198.5	—	213.3	238.0	239.2
zygomatic	170.0	198.5	—	213.0	238.0	239.2
book-leaf (mouth)	145.8	198.89	230.0	210.4	235.1	239.0
bowel — *see* Neoplasm, intestine						
brachial plexus	171.2	198.89	—	215.2	238.1	239.2
brain NEC	191.9	198.3	—	225.0	237.5	239.6
basal ganglia	191.0	198.3	—	225.0	237.5	239.6
cerebellopontine angle	191.6	198.3	—	225.0	237.5	239.6
cerebellum NOS	191.6	198.3	—	225.0	237.5	239.6
cerebrum	191.0	198.3	—	225.0	237.5	239.6
choroid plexus	191.5	198.3	—	225.0	237.5	239.6
contiguous sites	191.8	—	—	—	—	—
corpus callosum	191.8	198.3	—	225.0	237.5	239.6
corpus striatum	191.0	198.3	—	225.0	237.5	239.6
cortex (cerebral)	191.0	198.3	—	225.0	237.5	239.6
frontal lobe	191.1	198.3	—	225.0	237.5	239.6
globus pallidus	191.0	198.3	—	225.0	237.5	239.6
hippocampus	191.2	198.3	—	225.0	237.5	239.6
hypothalamus	191.0	198.3	—	225.0	237.5	239.6
internal capsule	191.0	198.3	—	225.0	237.5	239.6
medulla oblongata	191.7	198.3	—	225.0	237.5	239.6
meninges	192.1	198.4	—	225.2	237.6	239.7
midbrain	191.7	198.3	—	225.0	237.5	239.6
occipital lobe	191.4	198.3	—	225.0	237.5	239.6
parietal lobe	191.3	198.3	—	225.0	237.5	239.6
peduncle	191.7	198.3	—	225.0	237.5	239.6
pons	191.7	198.3	—	225.0	237.5	239.6
stem	191.7	198.3	—	225.0	237.5	239.6

☑ Additional Digit Required — Refer to the Tabular List for Digit Selection
▽ Subterms under main terms may continue to next column or page

Index to Diseases

Neoplasm, cervix

	Malignant			Benign	Uncertain Behavior	Unspecified
	Primary	Secondary	Ca in situ			
Neoplasm, neoplastic — *continued*						
brain — *continued*						
tapetum	191.8	198.3	—	225.0	237.5	239.6
temporal lobe	191.2	198.3	—	225.0	237.5	239.6
thalamus	191.0	198.3	—	225.0	237.5	239.6
uncus	191.2	198.3	—	225.0	237.5	239.6
ventricle (floor)	191.5	198.3	—	225.0	237.5	239.6
branchial (cleft) (vestiges)	146.8	198.89	230.0	210.6	235.1	239.0
breast (connective tissue) (female) (glandular tissue) (soft parts)	174.9	198.81	233.0	217	238.3	239.3
areola	174.0	198.81	233.0	217	238.3	239.3
male	175.0	198.81	233.0	217	238.3	239.3
axillary tail	174.6	198.81	233.0	217	238.3	239.3
central portion	174.1	198.81	233.0	217	238.3	239.3
contiguous sites	174.8	—	—	—	—	—
ectopic sites	174.8	198.81	233.0	217	238.3	239.3
inner	174.8	198.81	233.0	217	238.3	239.3
lower	174.8	198.81	233.0	217	238.3	239.3
lower-inner quadrant	174.3	198.81	233.0	217	238.3	239.3
lower-outer quadrant	174.5	198.81	233.0	217	238.3	239.3
male	175.9	198.81	233.0	217	238.3	239.3
areola	175.0	198.81	233.0	217	238.3	239.3
ectopic tissue	175.9	198.81	233.0	217	238.3	239.3
nipple	175.0	198.81	233.0	217	238.3	239.3
mastectomy site (skin)	173.5	198.2	—	—	—	—
specified as breast tissue	174.8	198.81	—	—	—	—
midline	174.8	198.81	233.0	217	238.3	239.3
nipple	174.0	198.81	233.0	217	238.3	239.3
male	175.0	198.81	233.0	217	238.3	239.3
outer	174.8	198.81	233.0	217	238.3	239.3
skin	173.5	198.2	232.5	216.5	238.2	239.2
tail (axillary)	174.6	198.81	233.0	217	238.3	239.3
upper	174.8	198.81	233.0	217	238.3	239.3
upper-inner quadrant	174.2	198.81	233.0	217	238.3	239.3
upper-outer quadrant	174.4	198.81	233.0	217	238.3	239.3
broad ligament	183.3	198.82	233.3	221.0	236.3	239.5
bronchiogenic, bronchogenic (lung)	162.9	197.0	231.2	212.3	235.7	239.1
bronchiole	162.9	197.0	231.2	212.3	235.7	239.1
bronchus	162.9	197.0	231.2	212.3	235.7	239.1
carina	162.2	197.0	231.2	212.3	235.7	239.1
contiguous sites with lung or trachea	162.8	—	—	—	—	—
lower lobe of lung	162.5	197.0	231.2	212.3	235.7	239.1
main	162.2	197.0	231.2	212.3	235.7	239.1
middle lobe of lung	162.4	197.0	231.2	212.3	235.7	239.1
upper lobe of lung	162.3	197.0	231.2	212.3	235.7	239.1
brow	173.3	198.2	232.3	216.3	238.2	239.2
buccal (cavity)	145.9	198.89	230.0	210.4	235.1	239.0
commissure	145.0	198.89	230.0	210.4	235.1	239.0
groove (lower) (upper)	145.1	198.89	230.0	210.4	235.1	239.0
mucosa	145.0	198.89	230.0	210.4	235.1	239.0
sulcus (lower) (upper)	145.1	198.89	230.0	210.4	235.1	239.0
bulbourethral gland	189.3	198.1	233.9	223.81	236.99	239.5
bursa — *see* Neoplasm, connective tissue						
buttock NEC*	195.3	198.89	232.5	229.8	238.8	239.8
calf*	195.5	198.89	232.7	229.8	238.8	239.8
calvarium	170.0	198.5	—	213.0	238.0	239.2
calyx, renal	189.1	198.0	233.9	223.1	236.91	239.5
canal						
anal	154.2	197.5	230.5	211.4	235.5	239.0
auditory (external)	173.2	198.2	232.2	216.2	238.2	239.2
auricular (external)	173.2	198.2	232.2	216.2	238.2	239.2
canaliculi, biliary (biliferi) (intrahepatic)	155.1	197.8	230.8	211.5	235.3	239.0
Neoplasm, neoplastic — *continued*						
canthus (eye) (inner) (outer)	173.1	198.2	232.1	216.1	238.2	239.2
capillary — *see* Neoplasm, connective tissue						
caput coli	153.4	197.5	230.3	211.3	235.2	239.0
cardia (gastric)	151.0	197.8	230.2	211.1	235.2	239.0
cardiac orifice (stomach)	151.0	197.8	230.2	211.1	235.2	239.0
cardio-esophageal junction	151.0	197.8	230.2	211.1	235.2	239.0
cardio-esophagus	151.0	197.8	230.2	211.1	235.2	239.0
carina (bronchus)	162.2	197.0	231.2	212.3	235.7	239.1
carotid (artery)	171.0	198.89	—	215.0	238.1	239.2
body	194.5	198.89	—	227.5	237.3	239.7
carpus (any bone)	170.5	198.5	—	213.5	238.0	239.2
cartilage (articular) (joint) NEC (*see also* Neoplasm, bone)	170.9	198.5	—	213.9	238.0	239.2
arytenoid	161.3	197.3	231.0	212.1	235.6	239.1
auricular	171.0	198.89	—	215.0	238.1	239.2
bronchi	162.2	197.3	—	212.3	235.7	239.1
connective tissue — *see* Neoplasm, connective tissue						
costal	170.3	198.5	—	213.3	238.0	239.2
cricoid	161.3	197.3	231.0	212.1	235.6	239.1
cuneiform	161.3	197.3	231.0	212.1	235.6	239.1
ear (external)	171.0	198.89	—	215.0	238.1	239.2
ensiform	170.3	198.5	—	213.3	238.0	239.2
epiglottis	161.1	197.3	231.0	212.1	235.6	239.1
anterior surface	146.4	198.89	230.0	210.6	235.1	239.0
eyelid	171.0	198.89	—	215.0	238.1	239.2
intervertebral	170.2	198.5	—	213.2	238.0	239.2
larynx, laryngeal	161.3	197.3	231.0	212.1	235.6	239.1
nose, nasal	160.0	197.3	231.8	212.0	235.9	239.1
pinna	171.0	198.89	—	215.0	238.1	239.2
rib	170.3	198.5	—	213.3	238.0	239.2
semilunar (knee)	170.7	198.5	—	213.7	238.0	239.2
thyroid	161.3	197.3	231.0	212.1	235.6	239.1
trachea	162.0	197.3	231.1	212.2	235.7	239.1
cauda equina	192.2	198.3	—	225.3	237.5	239.7
cavity						
buccal	145.9	198.89	230.0	210.4	235.1	239.0
nasal	160.0	197.3	231.8	212.0	235.9	239.1
oral	145.9	198.89	230.0	210.4	235.1	239.0
peritoneal	158.9	197.6	—	211.8	235.4	239.0
tympanic	160.1	197.3	231.8	212.0	235.9	239.1
cecum	153.4	197.5	230.3	211.3	235.2	239.0
central						
nervous system — *see* Neoplasm, nervous system						
white matter	191.0	198.3	—	225.0	237.5	239.6
cerebellopontine (angle)	191.6	198.3	—	225.0	237.5	239.6
cerebellum, cerebellar	191.6	198.3	—	225.0	237.5	239.6
cerebrum, cerebral (cortex) (hemisphere) (white matter)	191.0	198.3	—	225.0	237.5	239.6
meninges	192.1	198.4	—	225.2	237.6	239.7
peduncle	191.7	198.3	—	225.0	237.5	239.6
ventricle (any)	191.5	198.3	—	225.0	237.5	239.6
cervical region	195.0	198.89	234.8	229.8	238.8	239.8
cervix (cervical) (uteri) (uterus)	180.9	198.82	233.1	219.0	236.0	239.5
canal	180.0	198.82	233.1	219.0	236.0	239.5
contiguous sites	180.8	—	—	—	—	—
endocervix (canal) (gland)	180.0	198.82	233.1	219.0	236.0	239.5
exocervix	180.1	198.82	233.1	219.0	236.0	239.5
external os	180.1	198.82	233.1	219.0	236.0	239.5
internal os	180.0	198.82	233.1	219.0	236.0	239.5
nabothian gland	180.0	198.82	233.1	219.0	236.0	239.5
squamocolumnar junction	180.8	198.82	233.1	219.0	236.0	239.5
stump	180.8	198.82	233.1	219.0	236.0	239.5

Neoplasm, cheek

	Malignant			Benign	Uncertain Behavior	Unspecified
	Primary	Secondary	Ca in situ			
Neoplasm, neoplastic — continued						
cheek	195.0	198.89	234.8	229.8	238.8	239.8
external	173.3	198.2	232.3	216.3	238.2	239.2
inner aspect	145.0	198.89	230.0	210.4	235.1	239.0
internal	145.0	198.89	230.0	210.4	235.1	239.0
mucosa	145.0	198.89	230.0	210.4	235.1	239.0
chest (wall) NEC	195.1	198.89	234.8	229.8	238.8	239.8
chiasma opticum	192.0	198.4	—	225.1	237.9	239.7
chin	173.3	198.2	232.3	216.3	238.2	239.2
choana	147.3	198.89	230	210.7	235.1	239.0
cholangiole	155.1	197.8	230.8	211.5	235.3	239.0
choledochal duct	156.1	197.8	230.8	211.5	235.3	239.0
choroid	190.6	198.4	234.0	224.6	238.8	239.8
plexus	191.5	198.3	—	225.0	237.5	239.6
ciliary body	190.0	198.4	234.0	224.0	238.8	239.8
clavicle	170.3	198.5	—	213.3	238.0	239.2
clitoris	184.3	198.82	233.3	221.2	236.3	239.5
clivus	170.0	198.5	—	213.0	238.0	239.2
cloacogenic zone	154.8	197.5	230.7	211.4	235.5	239.0
coccygeal						
body or glomus	194.6	198.89	—	227.6	237.3	239.7
vertebra	170.6	198.5	—	213.6	238.0	239.2
coccyx	170.6	198.5	—	213.6	238.0	239.2
colon (*see also* Neoplasm, intestine, large)						
and rectum	154.0	197.5	230.4	211.4	235.2	239.0
columnella	173.3	198.2	232.3	216.3	238.2	239.2
column, spinal — *see* Neoplasm, spine						
commissure						
labial, lip	140.6	198.89	230.0	210.4	235.1	239.0
laryngeal	161.0	197.3	231.0	212.1	235.6	239.1
common (bile) duct	156.1	197.8	230.8	211.5	235.3	239.0
concha	173.2	198.2	232.2	216.2	238.2	239.2
nose	160.0	197.3	231.8	212.0	235.9	239.1
conjunctiva	190.3	198.4	234.0	224.3	238.8	239.8
connective tissue						
NEC	171.9	198.89	—	215.9	238.1	239.2

Note — For neoplasms of connective tissue (blood vessel, bursa, fascia, ligament, muscle, peripheral nerves, sympathetic and parasympathetic nerves and ganglia, synovia, tendon, etc.) or of morphological types that indicate connective tissue, code according to the list under "Neoplasm, connective tissue"; for sites that do not appear in this list, code to neoplasm of that site; e.g.,

liposarcoma, shoulder 171.2

leiomyosarcoma, stomach 151.9

neurofibroma, chest wall 215.4

Morphological types that indicate connective tissue appear in the proper place in the alphabetic index with the instruction "see Neoplasm, connective tissue…"

	Primary	Secondary	Ca in situ	Benign	Uncertain Behavior	Unspecified
abdomen	171.5	198.89	—	215.5	238.1	239.2
abdominal wall	171.5	198.89	—	215.5	238.1	239.2
ankle	171.3	198.89	—	215.3	238.1	239.2
antecubital fossa or space	171.2	198.89	—	215.2	238.1	239.2
arm	171.2	198.89	—	215.2	238.1	239.2
auricle (ear)	171.0	198.89	—	215.0	238.1	239.2
axilla	171.4	198.89	—	215.4	238.1	239.2
back	171.7	198.89	—	215.7	238.1	239.2
breast (female) (*see also* Neoplasm, breast)	174.9	198.81	233.0	217	238.3	239.3
male	175.9	198.81	233.0	217	238.3	239.3
buttock	171.6	198.89	—	215.6	238.1	239.2
calf	171.3	198.89	—	215.3	238.1	239.2
cervical region	171.0	198.89	—	215.0	238.1	239.2
cheek	171.0	198.89	—	215.0	238.1	239.2
chest (wall)	171.4	198.89	—	215.4	238.1	239.2
chin	171.0	198.89	—	215.0	238.1	239.2
contiguous sites	171.8	—	—	—	—	—
diaphragm	171.4	198.89	—	215.4	238.1	239.2
ear (external)	171.0	198.89	—	215.0	238.1	239.2
elbow	171.2	198.89	—	215.2	238.1	239.2
extrarectal	171.6	198.89	—	215.6	238.1	239.2
extremity	171.8	198.89	—	215.8	238.1	239.2
lower	171.3	198.89	—	215.3	238.1	239.2
upper	171.2	198.89	—	215.2	238.1	239.2
Neoplasm, neoplastic — continued connective tissue — *continued*						
eyelid	171.0	198.89	—	215.0	238.1	239.2
face	171.0	198.89	—	215.0	238.1	239.2
finger	171.2	198.89	—	215.2	238.1	239.2
flank	171.7	198.89	—	215.7	238.1	239.2
foot	171.3	198.89	—	215.3	238.1	239.2
forearm	171.2	198.89	—	215.2	238.1	239.2
forehead	171.0	198.89	—	215.0	238.1	239.2
gastric	171.5	198.89	—	215.5	238.1	—
gastrointestinal	171.5	198.89	—	215.5	238.1	—
gluteal region	171.6	198.89	—	215.6	238.1	239.2
great vessels NEC	171.4	198.89	—	215.4	238.1	239.2
groin	171.6	198.89	—	215.6	238.1	239.2
hand	171.2	198.89	—	215.2	238.1	239.2
head	171.0	198.89	—	215.0	238.1	239.2
heel	171.3	198.89	—	215.3	238.1	239.2
hip	171.3	198.89	—	215.3	238.1	239.2
hypochondrium	171.5	198.89	—	215.5	238.1	239.2
iliopsoas muscle	171.6	198.89	—	215.5	238.1	239.2
infraclavicular region	171.4	198.89	—	215.4	238.1	239.2
inguinal (canal) (region)	171.6	198.89	—	215.6	238.1	239.2
intestine	171.5	198.89	—	215.5	238.1	—
intrathoracic	171.4	198.89	—	215.4	238.1	239.2
ischorectal fossa	171.6	198.89	—	215.6	238.1	239.2
jaw	143.9	198.89	230.0	210.4	235.1	239.0
knee	171.3	198.89	—	215.3	238.1	239.2
leg	171.3	198.89	—	215.3	238.1	239.2
limb NEC	171.9	198.89	—	215.8	238.1	239.2
lower	171.3	198.89	—	215.3	238.1	239.2
upper	171.2	198.89	—	215.2	238.1	239.2
nates	171.6	198.89	—	215.6	238.1	239.2
neck	171.0	198.89	—	215.0	238.1	239.2
orbit	190.1	198.4	234.0	224.1	238.8	239.8
pararectal	171.6	198.89	—	215.6	238.1	239.2
para-urethral	171.6	198.89	—	215.6	238.1	239.2
paravaginal	171.6	198.89	—	215.6	238.1	239.2
pelvis (floor)	171.6	198.89	—	215.6	238.1	239.2
pelvo-abdominal	171.8	198.89	—	215.8	238.1	239.2
perineum	171.6	198.89	—	215.6	238.1	239.2
perirectal (tissue)	171.6	198.89	—	215.6	238.1	239.2
periurethral (tissue)	171.6	198.89	—	215.6	238.1	239.2
popliteal fossa or space	171.3	198.89	—	215.3	238.1	239.2
presacral	171.6	198.89	—	215.6	238.1	239.2
psoas muscle	171.5	198.89	—	215.5	238.1	239.2
pterygoid fossa	171.0	198.89	—	215.0	238.1	239.2
rectovaginal septum or wall	171.6	198.89	—	215.6	238.1	239.2
rectovesical	171.6	198.89	—	215.6	238.1	239.2
retroperitoneum	158.0	197.6	—	211.8	235.4	239.0
sacrococcygeal region	171.6	198.89	—	215.6	238.1	239.2
scalp	171.0	198.89	—	215.0	238.1	239.2
scapular region	171.4	198.89	—	215.4	238.1	239.2
shoulder	171.2	198.89	—	215.2	238.1	239.2
skin (dermis) NEC	173.9	198.2	232.9	216.9	238.2	239.2
stomach	171.5	198.89	—	215.5	238.1	—
submental	171.0	198.89	—	215.0	238.1	239.2
supraclavicular region	171.0	198.89	—	215.0	238.1	239.2
temple	171.0	198.89	—	215.0	238.1	239.2
temporal region	171.0	198.89	—	215.0	238.1	239.2
thigh	171.3	198.89	—	215.3	238.1	239.2
thoracic (duct) (wall)	171.4	198.89	—	215.4	238.1	239.2
thorax	171.4	198.89	—	215.4	238.1	239.2
thumb	171.2	198.89	—	215.2	238.1	239.2
toe	171.3	198.89	—	215.3	238.1	239.2
trunk	171.7	198.89	—	215.7	238.1	239.2
umbilicus	171.5	198.89	—	215.5	238.1	239.2
vesicorectal	171.6	198.89	—	215.6	238.1	239.2
wrist	171.2	198.89	—	215.2	238.1	239.2
conus medullaris	192.2	198.3	—	225.3	237.5	239.7
cord (true) (vocal)	161.0	197.3	231.0	212.1	235.6	239.1

Index to Diseases

Neoplasm, fetal membrane

	Malignant			Benign	Uncertain Behavior	Unspecified
	Primary	Secondary	Ca in situ			

Neoplasm, neoplastic — continued

cord — continued
	Primary	Secondary	Ca in situ	Benign	Uncertain Behavior	Unspecified
false	161.1	197.3	231.0	212.1	235.6	239.1
spermatic	187.6	198.82	233.6	222.8	236.6	239.5
spinal (cervical) (lumbar) (thoracic)	192.2	198.3	—	225.3	237.5	239.7
cornea (limbus)	190.4	198.4	234.0	224.4	238.8	239.8
corpus						
albicans	183.0	198.6	233.3	220	236.2	239.5
callosum, brain	191.8	198.3	—	225.0	237.5	239.6
cavernosum	187.3	198.82	233.5	222.1	236.6	239.5
gastric	151.4	197.8	230.2	211.1	235.2	239.0
penis	187.3	198.82	233.5	222.1	236.6	239.5
striatum, cerebrum	191.0	198.3	—	225.0	237.5	239.6
uteri	182.0	198.82	233.2	219.1	236.0	239.5
isthmus	182.1	198.82	233.2	219.1	236.0	239.5
cortex						
adrenal	194.0	198.7	234.8	227.0	237.2	239.7
cerebral	191.0	198.3	—	225.0	237.5	239.6
costal cartilage	170.3	198.5	—	213.3	238.0	239.2
costovertebral joint	170.3	198.5	—	213.3	238.0	239.2
Cowper's gland	189.3	198.1	233.9	223.81	236.99	239.5
cranial (fossa, any)	191.9	198.3	—	225.0	237.5	239.6
meninges	192.1	198.4	—	225.2	237.6	239.7
nerve (any)	192.0	198.4	—	225.1	237.9	239.7
craniobuccal pouch	194.3	198.89	234.8	227.3	237.0	239.7
craniopharyngeal (duct) (pouch)	194.3	198.89	234.8	227.3	237.0	239.7
cricoid	148.0	198.89	230.0	210.8	235.1	239.0
cartilage	161.3	197.3	231.0	212.1	235.6	239.1
cricopharynx	148.0	198.89	230.0	210.8	235.1	239.0
crypt of Morgagni	154.8	197.5	230.7	211.4	235.2	239.0
crystalline lens	190.0	198.4	234.0	224.4	238.8	239.8
cul-de-sac (Douglas')	158.8	197.6	—	211.8	235.4	239.0
cuneiform cartilage	161.3	197.3	231.0	212.1	235.6	239.1
cutaneous — see Neoplasm, skin						
cutis — see Neoplasm, skin						
cystic (bile) duct (common)	156.1	197.8	230.8	211.5	235.3	239.0
dermis — see Neoplasm, skin						
diaphragm	171.4	198.89	—	215.4	238.1	239.2
digestive organs, system, tube, or tract NEC	159.9	197.8	230.9	211.9	235.5	239.0
contiguous sites with peritoneum	159.8	—	—	—	—	—
disc, intervertebral	170.2	198.5	—	213.2	238.0	239.2
disease, generalized	199.0	199.0	234.9	229.9	238.9	199.0
disseminated	199.0	199.0	234.9	229.9	238.9	199.0
Douglas' cul-de-sac or pouch	158.8	197.6	—	211.8	235.4	239.0
duodenojejunal junction	152.8	197.4	230.7	211.2	235.2	239.0
duodenum	152.0	197.4	230.7	211.2	235.2	239.0
dura (cranial) (mater)	192.1	198.4	—	225.2	237.6	239.7
cerebral	192.1	198.4	—	225.2	237.6	239.7
spinal	192.3	198.4	—	225.4	237.6	239.7
ear (external)	173.2	198.2	232.2	216.2	238.2	239.2
auricle or auris	173.2	198.2	232.2	216.2	238.2	239.2
canal, external	173.2	198.2	232.2	216.2	238.2	239.2
cartilage	171.0	198.89	—	215.0	238.1	239.2
external meatus	173.2	198.2	232.2	216.2	238.2	239.2
inner	160.1	197.3	231.8	212.0	235.9	239.8
lobule	173.2	198.2	232.2	216.2	238.2	239.2
middle	160.1	197.3	231.8	212.0	235.9	239.8
contiguous sites with accessory sinuses or nasal cavities	160.8	—	—	—	—	—
skin	173.2	198.2	232.2	216.2	238.2	239.2
earlobe	173.2	198.2	232.2	216.2	238.2	239.2
ejaculatory duct	187.8	198.82	233.6	222.8	236.6	239.5
elbow NEC*	195.4	198.89	232.6	229.8	238.8	239.8
endocardium	164.1	198.89	—	212.7	238.8	239.8
endocervix (canal) (gland)	180.0	198.82	233.1	219.0	236.0	239.5
endocrine gland NEC	194.9	198.89	—	227.9	237.4	239.7
pluriglandular NEC	194.8	198.89	234.8	227.8	237.4	239.7
endometrium (gland) (stroma)	182.0	198.82	233.2	219.1	236.0	239.5
ensiform cartilage	170.3	198.5	—	213.3	238.0	239.2
enteric — see Neoplasm, intestine						
ependyma (brain)	191.5	198.3	—	225.0	237.5	239.6
epicardium	164.1	198.89	—	212.7	238.8	239.8
epididymis	187.5	198.82	233.6	222.3	236.6	239.5
epidural	192.9	198.4	—	225.9	237.9	239.7
epiglottis	161.1	197.3	231.0	212.1	235.6	239.1
anterior aspect or surface	146.4	198.89	230.0	210.6	235.1	239.0
cartilage	161.3	197.3	231.0	212.1	235.6	239.1
free border (margin)	146.4	198.89	230.0	210.6	235.1	239.0
junctional region	146.5	198.89	230.0	210.6	235.1	239.0
posterior (laryngeal) surface	161.1	197.3	231.0	212.1	235.6	239.1
suprahyoid portion	161.1	197.3	231.0	212.1	235.6	239.1
esophagogastric junction	151.0	197.8	230.2	211.1	235.2	239.0
esophagus	150.9	197.8	230.1	211.0	235.5	239.0
abdominal	150.2	197.8	230.1	211.0	235.5	239.0
cervical	150.0	197.8	230.1	211.0	235.5	239.0
contiguous sites	150.8	—	—	—	—	—
distal (third)	150.5	197.8	230.1	211.0	235.5	239.0
lower (third)	150.5	197.8	230.1	211.0	235.5	239.0
middle (third)	150.4	197.8	230.1	211.0	235.5	239.0
proximal (third)	150.3	197.8	230.1	211.0	235.5	239.0
specified part NEC	150.8	197.8	230.1	211.0	235.5	239.0
thoracic	150.1	197.8	230.1	211.0	235.5	239.0
upper (third)	150.3	197.8	230.1	211.0	235.5	239.0
ethmoid (sinus)	160.3	197.3	231.8	212.0	235.9	239.1
bone or labyrinth	170.0	198.5	—	213.0	238.0	239.2
Eustachian tube	160.1	197.3	231.8	212.0	235.9	239.1
exocervix	180.1	198.82	233.1	219.0	236.0	239.5
external						
meatus (ear)	173.2	198.2	232.2	216.2	238.2	239.2
os, cervix uteri	180.1	198.82	233.1	219.0	236.0	239.5
extradural	192.9	198.4	—	225.9	237.9	239.7
extrahepatic (bile) duct	156.1	197.8	230.8	211.5	235.3	239.0
contiguous sites with gallbladder	156.8	—	—	—	—	—
extraocular muscle	190.1	198.4	234.0	224.1	238.8	239.8
extrarectal	195.3	198.89	234.8	229.8	238.8	239.8
extremity*	195.8	198.89	232.8	229.8	238.8	239.8
lower*	195.5	198.89	232.7	229.8	238.8	239.8
upper*	195.4	198.89	232.6	229.8	238.8	239.8
eye NEC	190.9	198.4	234.0	224.9	238.8	239.8
contiguous sites	190.8	—	—	—	—	—
specified sites NEC	190.8	198.4	234.0	224.8	238.8	239.8
eyeball	190.0	198.4	234.0	224.0	238.8	239.8
eyebrow	173.3	198.2	232.3	216.3	238.2	239.2
eyelid (lower) (skin) (upper)	173.1	198.2	232.1	216.1	238.2	239.2
cartilage	171.0	198.89	—	215.0	238.1	239.2
face NEC*	195.0	198.89	232.3	229.8	238.8	239.8
fallopian tube (accessory)	183.2	198.82	233.3	221.0	236.3	239.5
falx (cerebelli) (cerebri)	192.1	198.4	—	225.2	237.6	239.7
fascia (see also Neoplasm, connective tissue)						
palmar	171.2	198.89	—	215.2	238.1	239.2
plantar	171.3	198.89	—	215.3	238.1	239.2
fatty tissue — see Neoplasm, connective tissue						
fauces, faucial NEC	146.9	198.89	230.0	210.6	235.1	239.0
pillars	146.2	198.89	230.0	210.6	235.1	239.0
tonsil	146.0	198.89	230.0	210.5	235.1	239.0
femur (any part)	170.7	198.5	—	213.7	238.0	239.2
fetal membrane	181	198.82	233.2	219.8	236.1	239.5

☑ Additional Digit Required — Refer to the Tabular List for Digit Selection

▶◀ Revised Text ● New Line ▲ Revised Code

Subterms under main terms may continue to next column or page

Neoplasm, fibrous tissue

Index to Diseases

	Malignant			Benign	Uncertain Behavior	Unspecified
	Primary	Secondary	Ca in situ			

Neoplasm, neoplastic — continued						
fibrous tissue — see Neoplasm, connective tissue						
fibula (any part)	170.7	198.5	—	213.7	238.0	239.2
filum terminale	192.2	198.3	—	225.3	237.5	239.7
finger NEC*	195.4	198.89	232.6	229.8	238.8	239.8
flank NEC*	195.8	198.89	232.5	229.8	238.8	239.8
follicle, nabothian	180.0	198.82	233.1	219.0	236.0	239.5
foot NEC*	195.5	198.89	232.7	229.8	238.8	239.8
forearm NEC*	195.4	198.89	232.6	229.8	238.8	239.8
forehead (skin)	173.3	198.2	232.3	216.3	238.2	239.2
foreskin	187.1	198.82	233.5	222.1	236.6	239.5
fornix						
pharyngeal	147.3	198.89	230.0	210.7	235.1	239.0
vagina	184.0	198.82	233.3	221.1	236.3	239.5
fossa (of)						
anterior (cranial)	191.9	198.3	—	225.0	237.5	239.6
cranial	191.9	198.3	—	225.0	237.5	239.6
ischiorectal	195.3	198.89	234.8	229.8	238.8	239.8
middle (cranial)	191.9	198.3	—	225.0	237.5	239.6
pituitary	194.3	198.89	234.8	227.3	237.0	239.7
posterior (cranial)	191.9	198.3	—	225.0	237.5	239.6
pterygoid	171.0	198.89	—	215.0	238.1	239.2
pyriform	148.1	198.89	230.0	210.8	235.1	239.0
Rosenmüller	147.2	198.89	230.0	210.7	235.1	239.0
tonsillar	146.1	198.89	230.0	210.6	235.1	239.0
fourchette	184.4	198.82	233.3	221.2	236.3	239.5
frenulum						
labii — see Neoplasm, lip, internal						
linguae	141.3	198.89	230.0	210.1	235.1	239.0
frontal						
bone	170.0	198.5	—	213.0	238.0	239.2
lobe, brain	191.1	198.3	—	225.0	237.5	239.6
meninges	192.1	198.4	—	225.2	237.6	239.7
pole	191.1	198.3	—	225.0	237.5	239.6
sinus	160.4	197.3	231.8	212.0	235.9	239.1
fundus						
stomach	151.3	197.8	230.2	211.1	235.2	239.0
uterus	182.0	198.82	233.2	219.1	236.0	239.5
gallbladder	156.0	197.8	230.8	211.5	235.3	239.0
contiguous sites with extrahepatic bile ducts	156.8	—	—	—	—	—
gall duct						
(extrahepatic)	156.1	197.8	230.8	211.5	235.3	239.0
intrahepatic	155.1	197.8	230.8	211.5	235.3	239.0
ganglia (see also Neoplasm, connective tissue)	171.9	198.89	—	215.9	238.1	239.2
basal	191.0	198.3	—	225.0	237.5	239.6
ganglion (see also Neoplasm, connective tissue)	171.9	198.89	—	215.9	238.1	239.2
cranial nerve	192.0	198.4	—	225.1	237.9	239.7
Gartner's duct	184.0	198.82	233.3	221.1	236.3	239.5
gastric — see Neoplasm, stomach						
gastrocolic	159.8	197.8	230.9	211.9	235.5	239.0
gastroesophageal junction	151.0	197.8	230.2	211.1	235.2	239.0
gastrointestinal (tract) NEC	159.9	197.8	230.9	211.9	235.5	239.0
generalized	199.0	199.0	234.9	229.9	238.9	199.0
genital organ or tract						
female NEC	184.9	198.82	233.3	221.9	236.3	239.5
contiguous sites	184.8	—	—	—	—	—
specified site NEC	184.8	198.82	233.3	221.8	236.3	239.5
male NEC	187.9	198.82	233.6	222.9	236.6	239.5
contiguous sites	187.8	—	—	—	—	—
specified site NEC	187.8	198.82	233.6	222.8	236.6	239.5
genitourinary tract						
female	184.9	198.82	233.3	221.9	236.3	239.5
male	187.9	198.82	233.6	222.9	236.6	239.5

Neoplasm, neoplastic — continued						
gingiva (alveolar) (marginal)	143.9	198.89	230.0	210.4	235.1	239.0
lower	143.1	198.89	230.0	210.4	235.1	239.0
mandibular	143.1	198.89	230.0	210.4	235.1	239.0
maxillary	143.0	198.89	230.0	210.4	235.1	239.0
upper	143.0	198.89	230.0	210.4	235.1	239.0
gland, glandular (lymphatic) (system) (see also Neoplasm, lymph gland)						
endocrine NEC	194.9	198.89	—	227.9	237.4	239.7
salivary — see Neoplasm, salivary, gland						
glans penis	187.2	198.82	233.5	222.1	236.6	239.5
globus pallidus	191.0	198.3	—	225.0	237.5	239.6
glomus						
coccygeal	194.6	198.89	—	227.6	237.3	239.7
jugularis	194.6	198.89	—	227.6	237.3	239.7
glosso-epiglottic fold(s)	146.4	198.89	230.0	210.6	235.1	239.0
glossopalatine fold	146.2	198.89	230.0	210.6	235.1	239.0
glossopharyngeal sulcus	146.1	198.89	230.0	210.6	235.1	239.0
glottis	161.0	197.3	231.0	212.1	235.6	239.1
gluteal region*	195.3	198.89	232.5	229.8	238.8	239.8
great vessels NEC	171.4	198.89	—	215.4	238.1	239.2
groin NEC	195.3	198.89	232.5	229.8	238.8	239.8
gum	143.9	198.89	230.0	210.4	235.1	239.0
contiguous sites	143.8	—	—	—	—	—
lower	143.1	198.89	230.0	210.4	235.1	239.0
upper	143.0	198.89	230.0	210.4	235.1	239.0
hand NEC*	195.4	198.89	232.6	229.8	238.8	239.8
head NEC*	195.0	198.89	232.4	229.8	238.8	239.8
heart	164.1	198.89	—	212.7	238.8	239.8
contiguous sites with mediastinum or thymus	164.8					
heel NEC*	195.5	198.89	232.7	229.8	238.8	239.8
helix	173.2	198.2	232.2	216.2	238.2	239.2
hematopoietic, hemopoietic tissue NEC	202.8 ☑	198.89	—	—	—	238.79 ▲
hemisphere, cerebral	191.0	198.3	—	225.0	237.5	239.6
hemorrhoidal zone	154.2	197.5	230.5	211.4	235.5	239.0
hepatic	155.2	197.7	230.8	211.5	235.3	239.0
duct (bile)	156.1	197.8	230.8	211.5	235.3	239.0
flexure (colon)	153.0	197.5	230.3	211.3	235.2	239.0
primary	155.0	—	—	—	—	—
hilus of lung	162.2	197.0	231.2	212.3	235.7	239.1
hip NEC*	195.5	198.89	232.7	229.8	238.8	239.8
hippocampus, brain	191.2	198.3	—	225.0	237.5	239.6
humerus (any part)	170.4	198.5	—	213.4	238.0	239.2
hymen	184.0	198.82	233.3	221.1	236.3	239.5
hypopharynx, hypopharyngeal NEC	148.9	198.89	230.0	210.8	235.1	239.0
contiguous sites	148.8	—	—	—	—	—
postcricoid region	148.0	198.89	230.0	210.8	235.1	239.0
posterior wall	148.3	198.89	230.0	210.8	235.1	239.0
pyriform fossa (sinus)	148.1	198.89	230.0	210.8	235.1	239.0
specified site NEC	148.8	198.89	230.0	210.8	235.1	239.0
wall	148.9	198.89	230.0	210.8	235.1	239.0
posterior	148.3	198.89	230.0	210.8	235.1	239.0
hypophysis	194.3	198.89	234.8	227.3	237.0	239.7
hypothalamus	191.0	198.3	—	225.0	237.5	239.6
ileocecum, ileocecal (coil) (junction) (valve)	153.4	197.5	230.3	211.3	235.2	239.0
ileum	152.2	197.4	230.7	211.2	235.2	239.0
ilium	170.6	198.5	—	213.6	238.0	239.2
immunoproliferative NEC	203.8 ☑					
infraclavicular (region)*	195.1	198.89	232.5	229.8	238.8	239.8
inguinal (region)*	195.3	198.89	232.5	229.8	238.8	239.8
insula	191.0	198.3	—	225.0	237.5	239.6

Index to Diseases — Neoplasm, ligament

	Malignant			Benign	Uncertain Behavior	Unspecified
	Primary	Secondary	Ca in situ			

Neoplasm, neoplastic — *continued*						
insular tissue						
(pancreas)	157.4	197.8	230.9	211.7	235.5	239.0
brain	191.0	198.3	—	225.0	237.5	239.6
interarytenoid fold	148.2	198.89	230.0	210.8	235.1	239.0
hypopharyngeal aspect	148.2	198.89	230.0	210.8	235.1	239.0
laryngeal aspect	161.1	197.3	231.0	212.1	235.6	239.1
marginal zone	148.2	198.89	230.0	210.8	235.1	239.0
interdental papillae	143.9	198.89	230.0	210.4	235.1	239.0
lower	143.1	198.89	230.0	210.4	235.1	239.0
upper	143.0	198.89	230.0	210.4	235.1	239.0
internal						
capsule	191.0	198.3	—	225.0	237.5	239.6
os (cervix)	180.0	198.82	233.1	219.0	236.0	239.5
intervertebral cartilage or disc	170.2	198.5	—	213.2	238.0	239.2
intestine, intestinal	159.0	197.8	230.7	211.9	235.2	239.0
large	153.9	197.5	230.3	211.3	235.2	239.0
appendix	153.5	197.5	230.3	211.3	235.2	239.0
caput coli	153.4	197.5	230.3	211.3	235.2	239.0
cecum	153.4	197.5	230.3	211.3	235.2	239.0
colon	153.9	197.5	230.3	211.3	235.2	239.0
and rectum	154.0	197.5	230.4	211.4	235.2	239.0
ascending	153.6	197.5	230.3	211.3	235.2	239.0
caput	153.4	197.5	230.3	211.3	235.2	239.0
contiguous sites	153.8	—	—	—	—	—
descending	153.2	197.5	230.3	211.3	235.2	239.0
distal	153.2	197.5	230.3	211.3	235.2	239.0
left	153.2	197.5	230.3	211.3	235.2	239.0
pelvic	153.3	197.5	230.3	211.3	235.2	239.0
right	153.6	197.5	230.3	211.3	235.2	239.0
sigmoid (flexure)	153.3	197.5	230.3	211.3	235.2	239.0
transverse	153.1	197.5	230.3	211.3	235.2	239.0
contiguous sites	153.8	—	—	—	—	—
hepatic flexure	153.0	197.5	230.3	211.3	235.2	239.0
ileocecum, ileocecal (coil) (valve)	153.4	197.5	230.3	211.3	235.2	239.0
sigmoid flexure (lower) (upper)	153.3	197.5	230.3	211.3	235.2	239.0
splenic flexure	153.7	197.5	230.3	211.3	235.2	239.0
small	152.9	197.4	230.7	211.2	235.2	239.0
contiguous sites	152.8	—	—	—	—	—
duodenum	152.0	197.4	230.7	211.2	235.2	239.0
ileum	152.2	197.4	230.7	211.2	235.2	239.0
jejunum	152.1	197.4	230.7	211.2	235.2	239.0
tract NEC	159.0	197.8	230.7	211.9	235.2	239.0
intra-abdominal	195.2	198.89	234.8	229.8	238.8	239.8
intracranial NEC	191.9	198.3	—	225.0	237.5	239.6
intrahepatic (bile) duct	155.1	197.8	230.8	211.5	235.3	239.0
intraocular	190.0	198.4	234.0	224.0	238.8	239.8
intraorbital	190.1	198.4	234.0	224.1	238.8	239.8
intrasellar	194.3	198.89	234.8	227.3	237.0	239.7
intrathoracic (cavity) (organs NEC)	195.1	198.89	234.8	229.8	238.8	239.8
contiguous sites with respiratory organs	165.8	—	—	—	—	—
iris	190.0	198.4	234.0	224.0	238.8	239.8
ischiorectal (fossa)	195.3	198.89	234.8	229.8	238.8	239.8
ischium	170.6	198.5	—	213.6	238.0	239.2
island of Reil	191.0	198.3	—	225.0	237.5	239.6
islands or islets of Langerhans	157.4	197.8	230.9	211.7	235.5	239.0
isthmus uteri	182.1	198.82	233.2	219.1	236.0	239.5
jaw	195.0	198.89	234.8	229.8	238.8	239.8
bone	170.1	198.5	—	213.1	238.0	239.2
carcinoma	143.9	—	—	—	—	—
lower	143.1	—	—	—	—	—
upper	143.0	—	—	—	—	—
lower	170.1	198.5	—	213.1	238.0	239.2
upper	170.0	198.5	—	213.0	238.0	239.2
carcinoma (any type) (lower)(upper)	195.0	—	—	—	—	—
skin	173.3	198.2	232.3	216.3	238.2	239.2
jaw — *continued*						
soft tissues	143.9	198.89	230.0	210.4	235.1	239.0
lower	143.1	198.89	230.0	210.4	235.1	239.0
upper	143.0	198.89	230.0	210.4	235.1	239.0
jejunum	152.1	197.4	230.7	211.2	235.2	239.0
joint NEC (*see also* Neoplasm, bone)	170.9	198.5	—	213.9	238.0	239.2
acromioclavicular	170.4	198.5	—	213.4	238.0	239.2
bursa or synovial membrane — *see* Neoplasm, connective tissue						
costovertebral	170.3	198.5	—	213.3	238.0	239.2
sternocostal	170.3	198.5	—	213.3	238.0	239.2
temporomandibular	170.1	198.5	—	213.1	238.0	239.2
junction						
anorectal	154.8	197.5	230.7	211.4	235.5	239.0
cardioesophageal	151.0	197.8	230.2	211.1	235.2	239.0
esophagogastric	151.0	197.8	230.2	211.1	235.2	239.0
gastroesophageal	151.0	197.8	230.2	211.1	235.2	239.0
hard and soft palate	145.5	198.89	230.0	210.4	235.1	239.0
ileocecal	153.4	197.5	230.3	211.3	235.2	239.0
pelvirectal	154.0	197.5	230.4	211.4	235.2	239.0
pelviureteric	189.1	198.0	233.9	223.1	236.91	239.5
rectosigmoid	154.0	197.5	230.4	211.4	235.2	239.0
squamocolumnar, of cervix	180.8	198.82	233.1	219.0	236.0	239.5
kidney (parenchyma)	189.0	198.0	233.9	223.0	236.91	239.5
calyx	189.1	198.0	233.9	223.1	236.91	239.5
hilus	189.1	198.0	233.9	223.1	236.91	239.5
pelvis	189.1	198.0	233.9	223.1	236.91	239.5
knee NEC*	195.5	198.89	232.7	229.8	238.8	239.8
labia (skin)	184.4	198.82	233.3	221.2	236.3	239.5
majora	184.1	198.82	233.3	221.2	236.3	239.5
minora	184.2	198.82	233.3	221.2	236.3	239.5
labial (*see also* Neoplasm, lip)						
sulcus (lower) (upper)	145.1	198.89	230.0	210.4	235.1	239.0
labium (skin)	184.4	198.82	233.3	221.2	236.3	239.5
majus	184.1	198.82	233.3	221.2	236.3	239.5
minus	184.2	198.82	233.3	221.2	236.3	239.5
lacrimal						
canaliculi	190.7	198.4	234.0	224.7	238.8	239.8
duct (nasal)	190.7	198.4	234.0	224.7	238.8	239.8
gland	190.2	198.4	234.0	224.2	238.8	239.8
punctum	190.7	198.4	234.0	224.7	238.8	239.8
sac	190.7	198.4	234.0	224.7	238.8	239.8
Langerhans, islands or islets	157.4	197.8	230.9	211.7	235.5	239.0
laryngopharynx	148.9	198.89	230.0	210.8	235.1	239.0
larynx, laryngeal NEC	161.9	197.3	231.0	212.1	235.6	239.1
aryepiglottic fold	161.1	197.3	231.0	212.1	235.6	239.1
cartilage (arytenoid) (cricoid) (cuneiform) (thyroid)	161.3	197.3	231.0	212.1	235.6	239.1
commissure (anterior) (posterior)	161.0	197.3	231.0	212.1	235.6	239.1
contiguous sites	161.8	—	—	—	—	—
extrinsic NEC	161.1	197.3	231.0	212.1	235.6	239.1
meaning hypopharynx	148.9	198.89	230.0	210.8	235.1	239.0
interarytenoid fold	161.1	197.3	231.0	212.1	235.6	239.1
intrinsic	161.0	197.3	231.0	212.1	235.6	239.1
ventricular band	161.1	197.3	231.0	212.1	235.6	239.1
leg NEC*	195.5	198.89	232.7	229.8	238.8	239.8
lens, crystalline	190.0	198.4	234.0	224.0	238.8	239.8
lid (lower) (upper)	173.1	198.2	232.1	216.1	238.2	239.2
ligament (*see also* Neoplasm, connective tissue)						
broad	183.3	198.82	233.3	221.0	236.3	239.5
Mackenrodt's	183.8	198.82	233.3	221.8	236.3	239.5
non-uterine — *see* Neoplasm, connective tissue						

Neoplasm, ligament

	Malignant			Benign	Uncertain Behavior	Unspecified
	Primary	Secondary	Ca in situ			
Neoplasm, neoplastic — *continued*						
ligament (*see also* Neoplasm, connective tissue) — *continued*						
round	183.5	198.82	—	221.0	236.3	239.5
sacro-uterine	183.4	198.82	—	221.0	236.3	239.5
uterine	183.4	198.82	—	221.0	236.3	239.5
utero-ovarian	183.8	198.82	233.3	221.8	236.3	239.5
uterosacral	183.4	198.82	—	221.0	236.3	239.5
limb*	195.8	198.89	232.8	229.8	238.8	239.8
lower*	195.5	198.89	232.7	229.8	238.8	239.8
upper*	195.4	198.89	232.6	229.8	238.8	239.8
limbus of cornea	190.4	198.4	234.0	224.4	238.8	239.8
lingual NEC (*see also* Neoplasm, tongue)	141.9	198.89	230.0	210.1	235.1	239.0
lingula, lung	162.3	197.0	231.2	212.3	235.7	239.1
lip (external) (lipstick area) (vermillion border)	140.9	198.89	230.0	210.0	235.1	239.0
buccal aspect — *see* Neoplasm, lip, internal						
commissure	140.6	198.89	230.0	210.4	235.1	239.0
contiguous sites	140.8	—	—	—	—	—
with oral cavity or pharynx	149.8	—	—	—	—	—
frenulum — *see* Neoplasm, lip, internal						
inner aspect — *see* Neoplasm, lip, internal						
internal (buccal) (frenulum) (mucosa) (oral)	140.5	198.89	230.0	210.0	235.1	239.0
lower	140.4	198.89	230.0	210.0	235.1	239.0
upper	140.3	198.89	230.0	210.0	235.1	239.0
lower	140.1	198.89	230.0	210.0	235.1	239.0
internal (buccal) (frenulum) (mucosa) (oral)	140.4	198.89	230.0	210.0	235.1	239.0
mucosa — *see* Neoplasm, lip, internal						
oral aspect — *see* Neoplasm, lip, internal						
skin (commissure) (lower) (upper)	173.0	198.2	232.2	216.0	238.2	239.2
upper	140.0	198.89	230.0	210.0	235.1	239.0
internal (buccal) (frenulum) (mucosa) (oral)	140.3	198.89	230.0	210.0	235.1	239.0
liver	155.2	197.7	230.8	211.5	235.3	239.0
primary	155.0	—	—	—	—	—
lobe						
azygos	162.3	197.0	231.2	212.3	235.7	239.1
frontal	191.1	198.3	—	225.0	237.5	239.6
lower	162.5	197.0	231.2	212.3	235.7	239.1
middle	162.4	197.0	231.2	212.3	235.7	239.1
occipital	191.4	198.3	—	225.0	237.5	239.6
parietal	191.3	198.3	—	225.0	237.5	239.6
temporal	191.2	198.3	—	225.0	237.5	239.6
upper	162.3	197.0	231.2	212.3	235.7	239.1
lumbosacral plexus	171.6	198.4	—	215.6	238.1	239.2
lung	162.9	197.0	231.2	212.3	235.7	239.1
azygos lobe	162.3	197.0	231.2	212.3	235.7	239.1
carina	162.2	197.0	231.2	212.3	235.7	239.1
contiguous sites with bronchus or trachea	162.8	—	—	—	—	—
hilus	162.2	197.0	231.2	212.3	235.7	239.1
lingula	162.3	197.0	231.2	212.3	235.7	239.1
lobe NEC	162.9	197.0	231.2	212.3	235.7	239.1
lower lobe	162.5	197.0	231.2	212.3	235.7	239.1

	Malignant			Benign	Uncertain Behavior	Unspecified
	Primary	Secondary	Ca in situ			
Neoplasm, neoplastic — *continued*						
lung — *continued*						
main bronchus	162.2	197.0	231.2	212.3	235.7	239.1
middle lobe	162.4	197.0	231.2	212.3	235.7	239.1
upper lobe	162.3	197.0	231.2	212.3	235.7	239.1
lymph, lymphatic channel NEC (*see also* Neoplasm, connective tissue)	171.9	198.89	—	215.9	238.1	239.2
gland (secondary)	—	196.9	—	229.0	238.8	239.8
abdominal	—	196.2	—	229.0	238.8	239.8
aortic	—	196.2	—	229.0	238.8	239.8
arm	—	196.3	—	229.0	238.8	239.8
auricular (anterior) (posterior)	—	196.0	—	229.0	238.8	239.8
axilla, axillary	—	196.3	—	229.0	238.8	239.8
brachial	—	196.3	—	229.0	238.8	239.8
bronchial	—	196.1	—	229.0	238.8	239.8
bronchopulmonary	—	196.1	—	229.0	238.8	239.8
celiac	—	196.2	—	229.0	238.8	239.8
cervical	—	196.0	—	229.0	238.8	239.8
cervicofacial	—	196.0	—	229.0	238.8	239.8
Cloquet	—	196.5	—	229.0	238.8	239.8
colic	—	196.2	—	229.0	238.8	239.8
common duct	—	196.2	—	229.0	238.8	239.8
cubital	—	196.3	—	229.0	238.8	239.8
diaphragmatic	—	196.1	—	229.0	238.8	239.8
epigastric, inferior	—	196.6	—	229.0	238.8	239.8
epitrochlear	—	196.3	—	229.0	238.8	239.8
esophageal	—	196.1	—	229.0	238.8	239.8
face	—	196.0	—	229.0	238.8	239.8
femoral	—	196.5	—	229.0	238.8	239.8
gastric	—	196.2	—	229.0	238.8	239.8
groin	—	196.5	—	229.0	238.8	239.8
head	—	196.0	—	229.0	238.8	239.8
hepatic	—	196.2	—	229.0	238.8	239.8
hilar (pulmonary)	—	196.1	—	229.0	238.8	239.8
splenic	—	196.2	—	229.0	238.8	239.8
hypogastric	—	196.6	—	229.0	238.8	239.8
ileocolic	—	196.2	—	229.0	238.8	239.8
iliac	—	196.6	—	229.0	238.8	239.8
infraclavicular	—	196.3	—	229.0	238.8	239.8
inguina, inguinal	—	196.5	—	229.0	238.8	239.8
innominate	—	196.1	—	229.0	238.8	239.8
intercostal	—	196.1	—	229.0	238.8	239.8
intestinal	—	196.2	—	229.0	238.8	239.8
intra-abdominal	—	196.2	—	229.0	238.8	239.8
intrapelvic	—	196.6	—	229.0	238.8	239.8
intrathoracic	—	196.1	—	229.0	238.8	239.9
jugular	—	196.0	—	229.0	238.8	239.8
leg	—	196.5	—	229.0	238.8	239.8
limb						
lower	—	196.5	—	229.0	238.8	239.8
upper	—	196.3	—	229.0	238.8	239.8
lower limb	—	196.5	—	229.0	238.8	238.9
lumbar	—	196.2	—	229.0	238.8	239.8
mandibular	—	196.0	—	229.0	238.8	239.8
mediastinal	—	196.1	—	229.0	238.8	239.8
mesenteric (inferior) (superior)	—	196.2	—	229.0	238.8	239.8
midcolic	—	196.2	—	229.0	238.8	239.8
multiple sites in categories 196.0–196.6	—	196.8	—	229.0	238.8	239.8
neck	—	196.0	—	229.0	238.8	239.8
obturator	—	196.6	—	229.0	238.8	239.8
occipital	—	196.0	—	229.0	238.8	239.8
pancreatic	—	196.2	—	229.0	238.8	239.8
para-aortic	—	196.2	—	229.0	238.8	239.8
paracervical	—	196.6	—	229.0	238.8	239.8
parametrial	—	196.6	—	229.0	238.8	239.8
parasternal	—	196.1	—	229.0	238.8	239.8
parotid	—	196.0	—	229.0	238.8	239.8
pectoral	—	196.3	—	229.0	238.8	239.8
pelvic	—	196.6	—	229.0	238.8	239.8
peri-aortic	—	196.2	—	229.0	238.8	239.8

Index to Diseases

Neoplasm, nail

	Malignant			Benign	Uncertain Behavior	Unspecified
	Primary	Secondary	Ca in situ			

Neoplasm, neoplastic — *continued*
  lymph, lymphatic — *continued*
    gland — *continued*

	Primary	Secondary	Ca in situ	Benign	Uncertain Behavior	Unspecified
peripancreatic	—	196.2	—	229.0	238.8	239.8
popliteal	—	196.5	—	229.0	238.8	239.8
porta hepatis	—	196.2	—	229.0	238.8	239.8
portal	—	196.2	—	229.0	238.8	239.8
preauricular	—	196.0	—	229.0	238.8	239.8
prelaryngeal	—	196.0	—	229.0	238.8	239.8
presymphysial	—	196.6	—	229.0	238.8	239.8
pretracheal	—	196.0	—	229.0	238.8	239.8
primary (any site) NEC	202.9 ☑	—	—	—	—	—
pulmonary (hiler)	—	196.1	—	229.0	238.8	239.8
pyloric	—	196.2	—	229.0	238.8	239.8
retroperitoneal	—	196.2	—	229.0	238.8	239.8
retropharyngeal	—	196.0	—	229.0	238.8	239.8
Rosenmüller's	—	196.5	—	229.0	238.8	239.8
sacral	—	196.6	—	229.0	238.8	239.8
scalene	—	196.0	—	229.0	238.8	239.8
site NEC	—	196.9	—	229.0	238.8	239.8
splenic (hilar)	—	196.2	—	229.0	238.8	239.8
subclavicular	—	196.3	—	229.0	238.8	239.8
subinguinal	—	196.5	—	229.0	238.8	239.8
sublingual	—	196.0	—	229.0	238.8	239.8
submandibular	—	196.0	—	229.0	238.8	239.8
submaxillary	—	196.0	—	229.0	238.8	239.8
submental	—	196.0	—	229.0	238.8	239.8
subscapular	—	196.3	—	229.0	238.8	239.8
supraclavicular	—	196.0	—	229.0	238.8	239.8
thoracic	—	196.1	—	229.0	238.8	239.8
tibial	—	196.5	—	229.0	238.8	239.8
tracheal	—	196.1	—	229.0	238.8	239.8
tracheobronchial	—	196.1	—	229.0	238.8	239.8
upper limb	—	196.3	—	229.0	238.8	239.8
Virchow's	—	196.0	—	229.0	238.8	239.8
node (*see also* Neoplasm, lymph gland)						
primary NEC	202.9 ☑	—	—	—	—	—
vessel (*see also* Neoplasm, connective tissue)	171.9	198.89	—	215.9	238.1	239.2
malar	170.0	198.5	—	213.0	238.0	239.2
region — *see* Neoplasm, cheek						
mammary gland — *see* Neoplasm, breast						
mandible	170.1	198.5	—	213.1	238.0	239.2
alveolar						
mucose	143.1	198.89	230.0	210.4	235.1	239.0
ridge or process	170.1	198.5	—	213.1	238.0	239.2
carcinoma	143.1	—	—	—	—	—
carcinoma	143.1	—	—	—	—	—
marrow (bone) NEC	202.9 ☑	198.5	—	—	—	238.79 ▲
mastectomy site (skin)	173.5	198.2	—	—	—	—
specified as breast tissue	174.8	198.81	—	—	—	—
mastoid (air cells) (antrum) (cavity)	160.1	197.3	231.8	212.0	235.9	239.1
bone or process	170.0	198.5	—	213.0	238.0	239.2
maxilla, maxillary (superior)	170.0	198.5	—	213.0	238.0	239.2
alveolar						
mucosa	143.0	198.89	230.0	210.4	235.1	239.0
ridge or process	170.0	198.5	—	213.0	238.0	239.2
carcinoma	143.0	—	—	—	—	—
antrum	160.2	197.3	231.8	212.0	235.9	239.1
carcinoma	143.0	—	—	—	—	—
inferior — *see* Neoplasm, mandible						
sinus	160.2	197.3	231.8	212.0	235.9	239.1
meatus						
external (ear)	173.2	198.2	232.2	216.2	238.2	239.2
Meckel's diverticulum	152.3	197.4	230.7	211.2	235.2	239.0

Neoplasm, neoplastic — *continued*
  mediastinum,

	Primary	Secondary	Ca in situ	Benign	Uncertain Behavior	Unspecified
mediastinal	164.9	197.1	—	212.5	235.8	239.8
anterior	164.2	197.1	—	212.5	235.8	239.8
contiguous sites with heart and thymus	164.8	—	—	—	—	—
posterior	164.3	197.1	—	212.5	235.8	239.8
medulla						
adrenal	194.0	198.7	234.8	227.0	237.2	239.7
oblongata	191.7	198.3	—	225.0	237.5	239.6
meibomian gland	173.1	198.2	232.1	216.1	238.2	239.2
meninges (brain) (cerebral) (cranial) (intracranial)	192.1	198.4	—	225.2	237.6	239.7
spinal (cord)	192.3	198.4	—	225.4	237.6	239.7
meniscus, knee joint (lateral) (medial)	170.7	198.5	—	213.7	238.0	239.2
mesentery, mesenteric	158.8	197.6	—	211.8	235.4	239.0
mesoappendix	158.8	197.6	—	211.8	235.4	239.0
mesocolon	158.8	197.6	—	211.8	235.4	239.0
mesopharynx — *see* Neoplasm, oropharynx						
mesosalpinx	183.3	198.82	233.3	221.0	236.3	239.5
mesovarium	183.3	198.82	233.3	221.0	236.3	239.5
metacarpus (any bone)	170.5	198.5	—	213.5	238.0	239.2
metastatic NEC (*see also* Neoplasm, by site, secondary)	—	199.1	—	—	—	—
metatarsus (any bone)	170.8	198.5	—	213.8	238.0	239.2
midbrain	191.7	198.3	—	225.0	237.5	239.6
milk duct — *see* Neoplasm, breast						
mons						
pubis	184.4	198.82	233.3	221.2	236.3	239.5
veneris	184.4	198.82	233.3	221.2	236.3	239.5
motor tract	192.9	198.4	—	225.9	237.9	239.7
brain	191.9	198.3	—	225.0	237.5	239.6
spinal	192.2	198.3	—	225.3	237.5	239.7
mouth	145.9	198.89	230.0	210.4	235.1	239.0
contiguous sites	145.8	—	—	—	—	—
floor	144.9	198.89	230.0	210.3	235.1	239.0
anterior portion	144.0	198.89	230.0	210.3	235.1	239.0
contiguous sites	144.8	—	—	—	—	—
lateral portion	144.1	198.89	230.0	210.3	235.1	239.0
roof	145.5	198.89	230.0	210.4	235.1	239.0
specified part NEC	145.8	198.89	230.0	210.4	235.1	239.0
vestibule	145.1	198.89	230.0	210.4	235.1	239.0
mucosa						
alveolar (ridge or process)	143.9	198.89	230.0	210.4	235.1	239.0
lower	143.1	198.89	230.0	210.4	235.1	239.0
upper	143.0	198.89	230.0	210.4	235.1	239.0
buccal	145.0	198.89	230.0	210.4	235.1	239.0
cheek	145.0	198.89	230.0	210.4	235.1	239.0
lip — *see* Neoplasm, lip, internal						
nasal	160.0	197.3	231.8	212.0	235.9	239.1
oral	145.0	198.89	230.0	210.4	235.1	239.0
Müllerian duct						
female	184.8	198.82	233.3	221.8	236.3	239.5
male	187.8	198.82	233.6	222.8	236.6	239.5
multiple sites NEC	199.0	199.0	234.9	229.9	238.9	199.0
muscle (*see also* Neoplasm, connective tissue)						
extraocular	190.1	198.4	234.0	224.1	238.8	239.8
myocardium	164.1	198.89	—	212.7	238.8	239.8
myometrium	182.0	198.82	233.2	219.1	236.0	239.5
myopericardium	164.1	198.89	—	212.7	238.8	239.8
nabothian gland (follicle)	180.0	198.82	233.1	219.0	236.0	239.5
Nackenrodt's ligament	183.8	198.82	233.3	221.8	236.3	239.5
nail	173.9	198.2	232.9	216.9	238.2	239.2
finger	173.6	198.2	232.6	216.6	238.2	239.2
toe	173.7	198.2	232.7	216.7	238.2	239.2

☑ Additional Digit Required — Refer to the Tabular List for Digit Selection
▶◀ Revised Text ● New Line ▲ Revised Code
▽ Subterms under main terms may continue to next column or page

Neoplasm, nares, naris

	Malignant			Benign	Uncertain Behavior	Unspecified
	Primary	Secondary	Ca in situ			
Neoplasm, neoplastic — *continued*						
nares, naris (anterior) (posterior)	160.0	197.3	231.8	212.0	235.9	239.1
nasal — *see* Neoplasm, nose						
nasolabial groove	173.3	198.2	232.3	216.3	238.2	239.2
nasolacrimal duct	190.7	198.4	234.0	224.7	238.8	239.8
nasopharynx, nasopharyngeal	147.9	198.89	230.0	210.7	235.1	239.0
contiguous sites	147.8	—	—	—	—	—
floor	147.3	198.89	230.0	210.7	235.1	239.0
roof	147.0	198.89	230.0	210.7	235.1	239.0
specified site NEC	147.8	198.89	230.0	210.7	235.1	239.0
wall	147.9	198.89	230.0	210.7	235.1	239.0
anterior	147.3	198.89	230.0	210.7	235.1	239.0
lateral	147.2	198.89	230.0	210.7	235.1	239.0
posterior	147.1	198.89	230.0	210.7	235.1	239.0
superior	147.0	198.89	230.0	210.7	235.1	239.0
nates	173.5	198.2	232.5	216.5	238.2	239.2
neck NEC*	195.0	198.89	234.8	229.8	238.8	239.8
nerve (autonomic) (ganglion) (parasympathetic) (peripheral) (sympathetic) (*see also* Neoplasm, connective tissue)						
abducens	192.0	198.4	—	225.1	237.9	239.7
accessory (spinal)	192.0	198.4	—	225.1	237.9	239.7
acoustic	192.0	198.4	—	225.1	237.9	239.7
auditory	192.0	198.4	—	225.1	237.9	239.7
brachial	171.2	198.89	—	215.2	238.1	239.2
cranial (any)	192.0	198.4	—	225.1	237.9	239.7
facial	192.0	198.4	—	225.1	237.9	239.7
femoral	171.3	198.89	—	215.3	238.1	239.2
glossopharyngeal	192.0	198.4	—	225.1	237.9	239.7
hypoglossal	192.0	198.4	—	225.1	237.9	239.7
intercostal	171.4	198.89	—	215.4	238.1	239.2
lumbar	171.7	198.89	—	215.7	238.1	239.2
median	171.2	198.89	—	215.2	238.1	239.2
obturator	171.3	198.89	—	215.3	238.1	239.2
oculomotor	192.0	198.4	—	225.1	237.9	239.7
olfactory	192.0	198.4	—	225.1	237.9	239.7
optic	192.0	198.4	—	225.1	237.9	239.7
peripheral NEC	171.9	198.89	—	215.9	238.1	239.2
radial	171.2	198.89	—	215.2	238.1	239.2
sacral	171.6	198.89	—	215.6	238.1	239.2
sciatic	171.3	198.89	—	215.3	238.1	239.2
spinal NEC	171.9	198.89	—	215.9	238.1	239.2
trigeminal	192.0	198.4	—	225.1	237.9	239.7
trochlear	192.0	198.4	—	225.1	237.9	239.7
ulnar	171.2	198.89	—	215.2	238.1	239.2
vagus	192.0	198.4	—	225.1	237.9	239.7
nervous system (central)						
NEC	192.9	198.4	—	225.9	237.9	239.7
autonomic NEC	171.9	198.89	—	215.9	238.1	239.2
brain (*see also* Neoplasm, brain)						
membrane or meninges	192.1	198.4	—	225.2	237.6	239.7
contiguous sites	192.8	—	—	—	—	—
parasympathetic NEC	171.9	198.89	—	215.9	238.1	239.2
sympathetic NEC	171.9	198.89	—	215.9	238.1	239.2
nipple (female)	174.0	198.81	233.0	217	238.3	239.3
male	175.0	198.81	233.0	217	238.3	239.3
nose, nasal	195.0	198.89	234.8	229.8	238.8	239.8
ala (external)	173.3	198.2	232.3	216.3	238.2	239.2
bone	170.0	198.5	—	213.0	238.0	239.2
cartilage	160.0	197.3	231.8	212.0	235.9	239.1
cavity	160.0	197.3	231.8	212.0	235.9	239.1
contiguous sites with accessory sinuses or middle ear	160.8	—	—	—	—	—
choana	147.3	198.89	230.0	210.7	235.1	239.0
external (skin)	173.3	198.2	232.3	216.3	238.2	239.2
fossa	160.0	197.3	231.8	212.0	235.9	239.1
internal	160.0	197.3	231.8	212.0	235.9	239.1
Neoplasm, neoplastic — *continued*						
nose, nasal — *continued*						
mucosa	160.0	197.3	231.8	212.0	235.9	239.1
septum	160.0	197.3	231.8	212.0	235.9	239.1
posterior margin	147.3	198.89	230.0	210.7	235.1	239.0
sinus — *see* Neoplasm, sinus						
skin	173.3	198.2	232.3	216.3	238.2	239.2
turbinate (mucosa)	160.0	197.3	231.8	212.0	235.9	239.1
bone	170.0	198.5	—	213.0	238.0	239.2
vestibule	160.0	197.3	231.8	212.0	235.9	239.1
nostril	160.0	197.3	231.8	212.0	235.9	239.1
nucleus pulposus	170.2	198.5	—	213.2	238.0	239.2
occipital						
bone	170.0	198.5	—	213.0	238.0	239.2
lobe or pole, brain	191.4	198.3	—	225.0	237.5	239.6
odontogenic — *see* Neoplasm, jaw bone						
oesophagus — *see* Neoplasm, esophagus						
olfactory nerve or bulb	192.0	198.4	—	225.1	237.9	239.7
olive (brain)	191.7	198.3	—	225.0	237.5	239.6
omentum	158.8	197.6	—	211.8	235.4	239.0
operculum (brain)	191.0	198.3	—	225.0	237.5	239.6
optic nerve, chiasm, or tract	192.0	198.4	—	225.1	237.9	239.7
oral (cavity)	145.9	198.89	230.0	210.4	235.1	239.0
contiguous sites with lip or pharynx	149.8	—	—	—	—	—
ill-defined	149.9	198.89	230.0	210.4	235.1	239.0
mucosa	145.9	198.89	230.0	210.4	235.1	239.0
orbit	190.1	198.4	234.0	224.1	238.8	239.8
bone	170.0	198.5	—	213.0	238.0	239.2
eye	190.1	198.4	234.0	224.1	238.8	239.8
soft parts	190.1	198.4	234.0	224.1	238.8	239.8
organ of Zuckerkandl	194.6	198.89	—	227.6	237.3	239.7
oropharynx	146.9	198.89	230.0	210.6	235.1	239.0
branchial cleft (vestige)	146.8	198.89	230.0	210.6	235.1	239.0
contiguous sites	146.8	—	—	—	—	—
junctional region	146.5	198.89	230.0	210.6	235.1	239.0
lateral wall	146.6	198.89	230.0	210.6	235.1	239.0
pillars of fauces	146.2	198.89	230.0	210.6	235.1	239.0
posterior wall	146.7	198.89	230.0	210.6	235.1	239.0
specified part NEC	146.8	198.89	230.0	210.6	235.1	239.0
vallecula	146.3	198.89	230.0	210.6	235.1	239.0
os						
external	180.1	198.82	233.1	219	236.0	239.5
internal	180.0	198.82	233.1	219	236.0	239.5
ovary	183.0	198.6	233.3	220	236.2	239.5
oviduct	183.2	198.82	233.3	221.0	236.3	239.5
palate	145.5	198.89	230.0	210.4	235.1	239.0
hard	145.2	198.89	230.0	210.4	235.1	239.0
junction of hard and soft palate	145.5	198.89	230.0	210.4	235.1	239.0
soft	145.3	198.89	230.0	210.4	235.1	239.0
nasopharyngeal surface	147.3	198.89	230.0	210.7	235.1	239.0
posterior surface	147.3	198.89	230.0	210.7	235.1	239.0
superior surface	147.3	198.89	230.0	210.7	235.1	239.0
palatoglossal arch	146.2	198.89	230.0	210.6	235.1	239.0
palatopharyngeal arch	146.2	198.89	230.0	210.6	235.1	239.0
pallium	191.0	198.3	—	225.0	237.5	239.6
palpebra	173.1	198.2	232.1	216.1	238.2	239.2
pancreas	157.9	197.8	230.9	211.6	235.5	239.0
body	157.1	197.8	230.9	211.6	235.5	239.0
contiguous sites	157.8	—	—	—	—	—
duct (of Santorini) (of Wirsung)	157.3	197.8	230.9	211.6	235.5	239.0
ectopic tissue	157.8	197.8	230.9	211.6	235.5	239.0
head	157.0	197.8	230.9	211.6	235.5	239.0
islet cells	157.4	197.8	230.9	211.7	235.5	239.0
neck	157.8	197.8	230.9	211.6	235.5	239.0
tail	157.2	197.8	230.9	211.6	235.5	239.0
para-aortic body	194.6	198.89	—	227.6	237.3	239.7
paraganglion NEC	194.6	198.89	—	227.6	237.3	239.7

Index to Diseases

Neoplasm, retro-orbital

	Malignant			Benign	Uncertain Behavior	Unspecified
	Primary	Secondary	Ca in situ			
Neoplasm, neoplastic — continued						
parametrium	183.4	198.82	—	221.0	236.3	239.5
paranephric	158.0	197.6	—	211.8	235.4	239.0
pararectal	195.3	198.89	—	229.8	238.8	239.8
parasagittal (region)	195.0	198.89	234.8	229.8	238.8	239.8
parasellar	192.9	198.4	—	225.9	237.9	239.7
parathyroid (gland)	194.1	198.89	234.8	227.1	237.4	239.7
paraurethral	195.3	198.89	—	229.8	238.8	239.8
gland	189.4	198.1	233.9	223.89	236.99	239.5
paravaginal	195.3	198.89	—	229.8	238.8	239.8
parenchyma, kidney	189.0	198.0	233.9	223.0	236.91	239.5
parietal						
bone	170.0	198.5	—	213.0	238.0	239.2
lobe, brain	191.3	198.3	—	225.0	237.5	239.6
paroophoron	183.3	198.82	233.3	221.0	236.3	239.5
parotid (duct) (gland)	142.0	198.89	230.0	210.2	235.0	239.0
parovarium	183.3	198.82	233.3	221.0	236.3	239.5
patella	170.8	198.5	—	213.8	238.0	239.2
peduncle, cerebral	191.7	198.3	—	225.0	237.5	239.6
pelvirectal junction	154.0	197.5	230.4	211.4	235.2	239.0
pelvis, pelvic	195.3	198.89	234.8	229.8	238.8	239.8
bone	170.6	198.5	—	213.6	238.0	239.2
floor	195.3	198.89	234.8	229.8	238.8	239.8
renal	189.1	198.0	233.9	223.1	236.91	239.5
viscera	195.3	198.89	234.8	229.8	238.8	239.8
wall	195.3	198.89	234.8	229.8	238.8	239.8
pelvo-abdominal	195.8	198.89	234.8	229.8	238.8	239.8
penis	187.4	198.82	233.5	222.1	236.6	239.5
body	187.3	198.82	233.5	222.1	236.6	239.5
corpus (cavernosum)	187.3	198.82	233.5	222.1	236.6	239.5
glans	187.2	198.82	233.5	222.1	236.6	239.5
skin NEC	187.4	198.82	233.5	222.1	236.6	239.5
periadrenal (tissue)	158.0	197.6	—	211.8	235.4	239.0
perianal (skin)	173.5	198.2	232.5	216.5	238.2	239.2
pericardium	164.1	198.89	—	212.7	238.8	239.8
perinephric	158.0	197.6	—	211.8	235.4	239.0
perineum	195.3	198.89	234.8	229.8	238.8	239.8
periodontal tissue NEC	143.9	198.89	230.0	210.4	235.1	239.0
periosteum — see Neoplasm, bone						
peripancreatic	158.0	197.6	—	211.8	235.4	239.0
peripheral nerve NEC	171.9	198.89	—	215.9	238.1	239.2
perirectal (tissue)	195.3	198.89	—	229.8	238.8	239.8
perirenal (tissue)	158.0	197.6	—	211.8	235.4	239.0
peritoneum, peritoneal (cavity)	158.9	197.6	—	211.8	235.4	239.0
contiguous sites with digestive organs	158.8	—	—	—	—	—
	159.8	—	—	—	—	—
parietal	158.8	197.6	—	211.8	235.4	239.0
pelvic	158.8	197.6	—	211.8	235.4	239.0
specified part NEC	158.8	197.6	—	211.8	235.4	239.0
peritonsillar (tissue)	195.0	198.89	234.8	229.8	238.8	239.8
periurethral tissue	195.3	198.89	—	229.8	238.8	239.8
phalanges	170.9	198.5	—	213.9	238.0	239.2
foot	170.8	198.5	—	213.8	238.0	239.2
hand	170.5	198.5	—	213.5	238.0	239.2
pharynx, pharyngeal	149.0	198.89	230.0	210.9	235.1	239.0
bursa	147.1	198.89	230.0	210.7	235.1	239.0
fornix	147.3	198.89	230.0	210.7	235.1	239.0
recess	147.2	198.89	230.0	210.7	235.1	239.0
region	149.0	198.89	230.0	210.9	235.1	239.0
tonsil	147.1	198.89	230.0	210.7	235.1	239.0
wall (lateral) (posterior)	149.0	198.89	230.0	210.9	235.1	239.0
pia mater (cerebral) (cranial)	192.1	198.4	—	225.2	237.6	239.7
spinal	192.3	198.4	—	225.4	237.6	239.7
pillars of fauces	146.2	198.89	230.0	210.6	235.1	239.0
pineal (body) (gland)	194.4	198.89	234.8	227.4	237.1	239.7
pinna (ear) NEC	173.2	198.2	232.2	216.2	238.2	239.2
cartilage	171.0	198.89	—	215.0	238.1	239.2
piriform fossa or sinus	148.1	198.89	230.0	210.8	235.1	239.0
pituitary (body) (fossa) (gland) (lobe)	194.3	198.89	234.8	227.3	237.0	239.7
placenta	181	198.82	233.2	219.8	236.1	239.5
pleura, pleural (cavity)	163.9	197.2	—	212.4	235.8	239.1
contiguous sites	163.8	—	—	—	—	—
parietal	163.0	197.2	—	212.4	235.8	239.1
visceral	163.1	197.2	—	212.4	235.8	239.1
plexus						
brachial	171.2	198.89	—	215.2	238.1	239.2
cervical	171.0	198.89	—	215.0	238.1	239.2
choroid	191.5	198.3	—	225.0	237.5	239.6
lumbosacral	171.6	198.89	—	215.6	238.1	239.2
sacral	171.6	198.89	—	215.6	238.1	239.2
pluri-endocrine	194.8	198.89	234.8	227.8	237.4	239.7
pole						
frontal	191.1	198.3	—	225.0	237.5	239.6
occipital	191.4	198.3	—	225.0	237.5	239.6
pons (varolii)	191.7	198.3	—	225.0	237.5	239.6
popliteal fossa or space*	195.5	198.89	234.8	229.8	238.8	239.8
postcricoid (region)	148.0	198.89	230.0	210.8	235.1	239.0
posterior fossa (cranial)	191.9	198.3	—	225.0	237.5	239.6
postnasal space	147.9	198.89	230.0	210.7	235.1	239.0
prepuce	187.1	198.82	233.5	222.1	236.6	239.5
prepylorus	151.1	197.8	230.2	211.1	235.2	239.0
presacral (region)	195.3	198.89	—	229.8	238.8	239.8
prostate (gland)	185	198.82	233.4	222.2	236.5	239.5
utricle	189.3	198.1	233.9	223.81	236.99	239.5
pterygoid fossa	171.0	198.89	—	215.0	238.1	239.2
pubic bone	170.6	198.5	—	213.6	238.0	239.2
pudenda, pudendum (female)	184.4	198.82	233.3	221.2	236.3	239.5
pulmonary	162.9	197.0	231.2	212.3	235.7	239.1
putamen	191.0	198.3	—	225.0	237.5	239.6
pyloric						
antrum	151.2	197.8	230.2	211.1	235.2	239.0
canal	151.1	197.8	230.2	211.1	235.2	239.0
pylorus	151.1	197.8	230.2	211.1	235.2	239.0
pyramid (brain)	191.7	198.3	—	225.0	237.5	239.6
pyriform fossa or sinus	148.1	198.89	230.0	210.8	235.1	239.0
radius (any part)	170.4	198.5	—	213.4	238.0	239.2
Rathke's pouch	194.3	198.89	234.8	227.3	237.0	239.7
rectosigmoid (colon) (junction)	154.0	197.5	230.4	211.4	235.2	239.0
contiguous sites with anus or rectum	154.8	—	—	—	—	—
rectouterine pouch	158.8	197.6	—	211.8	235.4	239.0
rectovaginal septum or wall	195.3	198.89	234.8	229.8	238.8	239.8
rectovesical septum	195.3	198.89	234.8	229.8	238.8	239.8
rectum (ampulla)	154.1	197.5	230.4	211.4	235.2	239.0
and colon	154.0	197.5	230.4	211.4	235.2	239.0
contiguous sites with anus or rectosigmoid junction	154.8	—	—	—	—	—
renal	189.0	198.0	233.9	223.0	236.91	239.5
calyx	189.1	198.0	233.9	223.1	236.91	239.5
hilus	189.1	198.0	233.9	223.1	236.91	239.5
parenchyma	189.0	198.0	233.9	223.0	236.91	239.5
pelvis	189.1	198.0	233.9	223.1	236.91	239.5
respiratory						
organs or system NEC	165.9	197.3	231.9	212.9	235.9	239.1
contiguous sites with intrathoracic organs	165.8	—	—	—	—	—
specified sites NEC	165.8	197.3	231.8	212.8	235.9	239.1
tract NEC	165.9	197.3	231.9	212.9	235.9	239.1
upper	165.0	197.3	231.9	212.9	235.9	239.1
retina	190.5	198.4	234.0	224.5	238.8	239.8
retrobulbar	190.1	198.4	—	224.1	238.8	239.8
retrocecal	158.0	197.6	—	211.8	235.4	239.0
retromolar (area) (triangle) (trigone)	145.6	198.89	230.0	210.4	235.1	239.0
retro-orbital	195.0	198.89	234.8	229.8	238.8	239.8

Neoplasm, retroperitoneal

Index to Diseases

	Malignant			Benign	Uncertain Behavior	Unspecified
	Primary	Secondary	Ca in situ			
Neoplasm, neoplastic — *continued*						
retroperitoneal (space)						
(tissue)	158.0	197.6	—	211.8	235.4	239.0
contiguous sites	158.8	—	—	—	—	—
retroperitoneum	158.0	197.6	—	211.8	235.4	239.0
contiguous sites	158.8	—	—	—	—	—
retropharyngeal	149.0	198.89	230.0	210.9	235.1	239.0
retrovesical (septum)	195.3	198.89	234.8	229.8	238.8	239.8
rhinencephalon	191.0	198.3	—	225.0	237.5	239.6
rib	170.3	198.5	—	213.3	238.0	239.2
Rosenmüller's fossa	147.2	198.89	230.0	210.7	235.1	239.0
round ligament	183.5	198.82	—	221.0	236.3	239.5
sacrococcyx, sacrococcygeal	170.6	198.5	—	213.6	238.0	239.2
region	195.3	198.89	234.8	229.8	238.8	239.8
sacrouterine ligament	183.4	198.82	—	221.0	236.3	239.5
sacrum, sacral (vertebra)	170.6	198.5	—	213.6	238.0	239.2
salivary gland or duct (major)	142.9	198.89	230.0	210.2	235.0	239.0
contiguous sites	142.8	—	—	—	—	—
minor NEC	145.9	198.89	230.0	210.4	235.1	239.0
parotid	142.0	198.89	230.0	210.2	235.0	239.0
pluriglandular	142.8	198.89	—	210.2	235.0	239.0
sublingual	142.2	198.89	230.0	210.2	235.0	239.0
submandibular	142.1	198.89	230.0	210.2	235.0	239.0
submaxillary	142.1	198.89	230.0	210.2	235.0	239.0
salpinx (uterine)	183.2	198.82	233.3	221.0	236.3	239.5
Santorini's duct	157.3	197.8	230.7	211.6	235.5	239.0
scalp	173.4	198.2	232.4	216.4	238.2	239.2
scapula (any part)	170.4	198.5	—	213.4	238.0	239.2
scapular region	195.1	198.89	234.8	229.8	238.8	239.8
scar NEC (*see also* Neoplasm, skin)	173.9	198.2	232.9	216.9	238.2	239.2
sciatic nerve	171.3	198.89	—	215.3	238.1	239.2
sclera	190.0	198.4	234.0	224.0	238.8	239.8
scrotum (skin)	187.7	198.82	—	222.4	236.6	239.5
sebaceous gland — *see* Neoplasm, skin						
sella turcica	194.3	198.89	234.8	227.3	237.0	239.7
bone	170.0	198.5	—	213.0	238.0	239.2
semilunar cartilage (knee)	170.7	198.5	—	213.7	238.0	239.2
seminal vesicle	187.8	198.82	233.6	222.8	236.6	239.5
septum						
nasal	160.0	197.3	231.8	212.0	235.9	239.1
posterior margin	147.3	198.89	230.0	210.7	235.1	239.0
rectovaginal	195.3	198.89	234.8	229.8	238.8	239.8
rectovesical	195.3	198.89	234.8	229.8	238.8	239.8
urethrovaginal	184.9	198.82	233.3	221.9	236.3	239.5
vesicovaginal	184.9	198.82	233.3	221.9	236.3	239.5
shoulder NEC*	195.4	198.89	232.6	229.8	238.8	239.8
sigmoid flexure (lower) (upper)	153.3	197.5	230.3	211.3	235.2	239.0
sinus (accessory)	160.9	197.3	231.8	212.0	235.9	239.1
bone (any)	170.0	198.5	—	213.0	238.0	239.2
contiguous sites with middle ear or nasal cavities	160.8	—	—	—	—	—
ethmoidal	160.3	197.3	231.8	212.0	235.9	239.1
frontal	160.4	197.3	231.8	212.0	235.9	239.1
maxillary	160.2	197.3	231.8	212.0	235.9	239.1
nasal, paranasal NEC	160.9	197.3	231.8	212.0	235.9	239.1
pyriform	148.1	198.89	230.0	210.8	235.1	239.0
sphenoidal	160.5	197.3	231.8	212.0	235.9	239.1
skeleton, skeletal NEC	170.9	198.5	—	213.9	238.0	239.2
Skene's gland	189.4	198.1	233.9	223.89	236.99	239.5
skin NEC	173.9	198.2	232.9	216.9	238.2	239.2
abdominal wall	173.5	198.2	232.5	216.5	238.2	239.2
ala nasi	173.3	198.2	232.3	216.3	238.2	239.2
ankle	173.7	198.2	232.7	216.7	238.2	239.2
antecubital space	173.6	198.2	232.6	216.6	238.2	239.2
anus	173.5	198.2	232.5	216.5	238.2	239.2
arm	173.6	198.2	232.6	216.6	238.2	239.2
auditory canal (external)	173.2	198.2	232.2	216.2	238.2	239.2
Neoplasm, neoplastic — *continued* skin — *continued*						
auricle (ear)	173.2	198.2	232.2	216.2	238.2	239.2
auricular canal (external)	173.2	198.2	232.2	216.2	238.2	239.2
axilla, axillary fold	173.5	198.2	232.5	216.5	238.2	239.2
back	173.5	198.2	232.5	216.5	238.2	239.2
breast	173.5	198.2	232.5	216.5	238.2	239.2
brow	173.3	198.2	232.3	216.3	238.2	239.2
buttock	173.5	198.2	232.5	216.5	238.2	239.2
calf	173.7	198.2	232.7	216.7	238.2	239.2
canthus (eye) (inner) (outer)	173.1	198.2	232.1	216.1	238.2	239.2
cervical region	173.4	198.2	232.4	216.4	238.2	239.2
cheek (external)	173.3	198.2	232.3	216.3	238.2	239.2
chest (wall)	173.5	198.2	232.5	216.5	238.2	239.2
chin	173.3	198.2	232.3	216.3	238.2	239.2
clavicular area	173.5	198.2	232.5	216.5	238.2	239.2
clitoris	—	198.82	233.3	221.2	236.3	239.5
columnella	173.3	198.2	232.3	216.3	238.2	239.2
concha	173.2	198.2	232.2	216.2	238.2	239.2
contiguous sites	173.8	—	—	—	—	—
ear (external)	173.2	198.2	232.2	216.2	238.2	239.2
elbow	173.6	198.2	232.6	216.6	238.2	239.2
eyebrow	173.3	198.2	232.3	216.3	238.2	239.2
eyelid	173.1	198.2	232.1	—	238.2	239.2
face NEC	173.3	198.2	232.3	216.3	238.2	239.2
female genital organs (external)	184.4	198.82	233.3	221.2	236.3	239.5
clitoris	184.3	198.82	233.3	221.2	236.3	239.5
labium NEC	184.4	198.82	233.3	221.2	236.3	239.5
majus	184.1	198.82	233.3	221.2	236.3	239.5
minus	184.2	198.82	233.3	221.2	236.3	239.5
pudendum	184.4	198.82	233.3	221.2	236.3	239.5
vulva	184.4	198.82	233.3	221.2	236.3	239.5
finger	173.6	198.2	232.6	216.6	238.2	239.2
flank	173.5	198.2	232.5	216.5	238.2	239.2
foot	173.7	198.2	232.7	216.7	238.2	239.2
forearm	173.6	198.2	232.6	216.6	238.2	239.2
forehead	173.3	198.2	232.3	216.3	238.2	239.2
glabella	173.3	198.2	232.3	216.3	238.2	239.2
gluteal region	173.5	198.2	232.5	216.5	238.2	239.2
groin	173.5	198.2	232.5	216.5	238.2	239.2
hand	173.6	198.2	232.6	216.6	238.2	239.2
head NEC	173.4	198.2	232.4	216.4	238.2	239.2
heel	173.7	198.2	232.7	216.7	238.2	239.2
helix	173.2	198.2	—	216.2	238.2	239.2
hip	173.7	198.2	232.7	216.7	238.2	239.2
infraclavicular region	173.5	198.2	232.5	216.5	238.2	239.2
inguinal region	173.5	198.2	232.5	216.5	238.2	239.2
jaw	173.3	198.2	232.3	216.3	238.2	239.2
knee	173.7	198.2	232.7	216.7	238.2	239.2
labia						
majora	184.1	198.82	233.3	221.2	236.3	239.5
minora	184.2	198.82	233.3	221.2	236.3	239.5
leg	173.7	198.2	232.7	216.7	238.2	239.2
lid (lower) (upper)	—	198.2	232.1	216.1	238.2	239.2
limb NEC	173.9	198.2	232.9	216.9	238.2	239.2
lower	173.7	198.2	232.7	216.7	238.2	239.2
upper	173.6	198.2	232.6	216.6	238.2	239.2
lip (lower) (upper)	173.0	198.2	232.0	216.0	238.2	239.2
male genital organs	187.9	198.82	233.6	222.9	236.6	239.5
penis	187.4	198.82	233.5	222.1	236.6	239.5
prepuce	187.1	198.82	233.5	222.1	236.6	239.5
scrotum	187.7	198.82	233.6	222.4	236.6	239.5
mastectomy site	173.5	198.2	—	—	—	—
specified as breast tissue	174.8	198.81	—	—	—	—
meatus, acoustic (external)	173.2	198.2	232.2	216.2	238.2	239.2
nates	173.5	198.2	232.5	216.5	238.2	239.0
neck	173.4	198.2	232.4	216.4	238.2	239.2
nose (external)	173.3	198.2	232.3	216.3	238.2	239.2
palm	173.6	198.2	232.6	216.6	238.2	239.2
palpebra	173.1	198.2	232.1	216.1	238.2	239.2
penis NEC	187.4	198.82	233.5	222.1	236.6	239.5
perianal	173.5	198.2	232.5	216.5	238.2	239.2

☑ Additional Digit Required — Refer to the Tabular List for Digit Selection

Index to Diseases

Neoplasm, tongue

	Malignant			Benign	Uncertain Behavior	Unspecified
	Primary	Secondary	Ca in situ			
Neoplasm, neoplastic — *continued*						
skin — *continued*						
perineum	173.5	198.2	232.5	216.5	238.2	239.2
pinna	173.2	198.2	232.2	216.2	238.2	239.2
plantar	173.7	198.2	232.7	216.7	238.2	239.2
popliteal fossa or space	173.7	198.2	232.7	216.7	238.2	239.2
prepuce	187.1	198.82	233.5	222.1	236.6	239.5
pubes	173.5	198.2	232.5	216.5	238.2	239.2
sacrococcygeal region	173.5	198.2	232.5	216.5	238.2	239.2
scalp	173.4	198.2	232.4	216.4	238.2	239.2
scapular region	173.5	198.2	232.5	216.5	238.2	239.2
scrotum	187.7	198.82	233.6	222.4	236.6	239.5
shoulder	173.6	198.2	232.6	216.6	238.2	239.2
sole (foot)	173.7	198.2	232.7	216.7	238.2	239.2
specified sites NEC	173.8	198.2	232.8	216.8	232.8	239.2
submammary fold	173.5	198.2	232.5	216.5	238.2	239.2
supraclavicular region	173.4	198.2	232.4	216.4	238.2	239.2
temple	173.3	198.2	232.3	216.3	238.2	239.2
thigh	173.7	198.2	232.7	216.7	238.2	239.2
thoracic wall	173.5	198.2	232.5	216.5	238.2	239.2
thumb	173.6	198.2	232.6	216.6	238.2	239.2
toe	173.7	198.2	232.7	216.7	238.2	239.2
tragus	173.2	198.2	232.2	216.2	238.2	239.2
trunk	173.5	198.2	232.5	216.5	238.2	239.2
umbilicus	173.5	198.2	232.5	216.5	238.2	239.2
vulva	184.4	198.82	233.3	221.2	236.3	239.5
wrist	173.6	198.2	232.6	216.6	238.2	239.2
skull	170.0	198.5	—	213.0	238.0	239.2
soft parts or tissues — *see* Neoplasm, connective tissue						
specified site NEC	195.8	198.89	234.8	229.8	238.8	239.8
specified site — *see* Neoplasm, skin						
spermatic cord	187.6	198.82	233.6	222.8	236.6	239.5
sphenoid	160.5	197.3	231.8	212.0	235.9	239.1
bone	170.0	198.5	—	213.0	238.0	239.2
sinus	160.5	197.3	231.8	212.0	235.9	239.1
sphincter						
anal	154.2	197.5	230.5	211.4	235.5	239.0
of Oddi	156.1	197.8	230.8	211.5	235.3	239.0
spine, spinal (column)	170.2	198.5	—	213.2	238.0	239.2
bulb	191.7	198.3	—	225.0	237.5	239.6
coccyx	170.6	198.5	—	213.6	238.0	239.2
cord (cervical) (lumbar) (sacral) (thoracic)	192.2	198.3	—	225.3	237.5	239.7
dura mater	192.3	198.4	—	225.4	237.6	239.7
lumbosacral	170.2	198.5	—	213.2	238.0	239.2
membrane	192.3	198.4	—	225.4	237.6	239.7
meninges	192.3	198.4	—	225.4	237.6	239.7
nerve (root)	171.9	198.89	—	215.9	238.1	239.2
pia mater	192.3	198.4	—	225.4	237.6	239.7
root	171.9	198.89	—	215.9	238.1	239.2
sacrum	170.6	198.5	—	213.6	238.0	239.2
spleen, splenic NEC	159.1	197.8	230.9	211.9	235.5	239.0
flexure (colon)	153.7	197.5	230.3	211.3	235.2	239.0
stem, brain	191.7	198.3	—	225.0	237.5	239.6
Stensen's duct	142.0	198.89	230.0	210.2	235.0	239.0
sternum	170.3	198.5	—	213.3	238.0	239.2
stomach	151.9	197.8	230.2	211.1	235.2	239.0
antrum (pyloric)	151.2	197.8	230.2	211.1	235.2	239.0
body	151.4	197.8	230.2	211.1	235.2	239.0
cardia	151.0	197.8	230.2	211.1	235.2	239.0
cardiac orifice	151.0	197.8	230.2	211.1	235.2	239.0
contiguous sites	151.8	—	—	—	—	—
corpus	151.4	197.8	230.2	211.1	235.2	239.0
fundus	151.3	197.8	230.2	211.1	235.2	239.0
greater curvature NEC	151.6	197.8	230.2	211.1	235.2	239.0
lesser curvature NEC	151.5	197.8	230.2	211.1	235.2	239.0
prepylorus	151.1	197.8	230.2	211.1	235.2	239.0
pylorus	151.1	197.8	230.2	211.1	235.2	239.0
wall NEC	151.9	197.8	230.2	211.1	235.2	239.0
Neoplasm, neoplastic — *continued*						
stomach — *continued*						
wall — *continued*						
anterior NEC	151.8	197.8	230.2	211.1	235.2	239.0
posterior NEC	151.8	197.8	230.2	211.1	235.2	239.0
stroma, endometrial	182.0	198.82	233.2	219.1	236.0	239.5
stump, cervical	180.8	198.82	233.1	219.0	236.0	239.5
subcutaneous (nodule) (tissue) NEC — *see* Neoplasm, connective tissue						
subdural	192.1	198.4	—	225.2	237.6	239.7
subglottis, subglottic	161.2	197.3	231.0	212.1	235.6	239.1
sublingual	144.9	198.89	230.0	210.3	235.1	239.0
gland or duct	142.2	198.89	230.0	210.2	235.0	239.0
submandibular gland	142.1	198.89	230.0	210.2	235.0	239.0
submaxillary gland or duct	142.1	198.89	230.0	210.2	235.0	239.0
submental	195.0	198.89	234.8	229.8	238.8	239.8
subpleural	162.9	197.0	—	212.3	235.7	239.1
substernal	164.2	197.1	—	212.5	235.8	239.1
sudoriferous, sudoriparous gland, site						
unspecified	173.9	198.2	232.9	216.9	238.2	239.2
specified site — *see* Neoplasm, skin						
supraclavicular region	195.0	198.89	234.8	229.8	238.8	239.8
supraglottis	161.1	197.3	231.0	212.1	235.6	239.1
suprarenal (capsule) (cortex) (gland) (medulla)	194.0	198.7	234.8	227.0	237.2	239.7
suprasellar (region)	191.9	198.3	—	225.0	237.5	239.6
sweat gland (apocrine) (eccrine), site						
unspecified	173.9	198.2	232.9	216.9	238.2	239.2
sympathetic nerve or nervous system NEC	171.9	198.89	—	215.9	238.1	239.2
symphysis pubis	170.6	198.5	—	213.6	238.0	239.2
synovial membrane — *see* Neoplasm, connective tissue						
tapetum, brain	191.8	198.3	—	225.0	237.5	239.6
tarsus (any bone)	170.8	198.5	—	213.8	238.0	239.2
temple (skin)	173.3	198.2	232.3	216.3	238.2	239.2
temporal						
bone	170.0	198.5	—	213.0	238.0	239.2
lobe or pole	191.2	198.3	—	225.0	237.5	239.6
region	195.0	198.89	234.8	229.8	238.8	239.8
skin	173.3	198.2	232.3	216.3	238.2	239.2
tendon (sheath) — *see* Neoplasm, connective tissue						
tentorium (cerebelli)	192.1	198.4	—	225.2	237.6	239.7
testis, testes (descended) (scrotal)	186.9	198.82	233.6	222.0	236.4	239.5
ectopic	186.0	198.82	233.6	222.0	236.4	239.5
retained	186.0	198.82	233.6	222.0	236.4	239.5
undescended	186.0	198.82	233.6	222.0	236.4	239.5
thalamus	191.0	198.3	—	225.0	237.5	239.6
thigh NEC*	195.5	198.89	234.8	229.8	238.8	239.8
thorax, thoracic (cavity) (organs NEC)	195.1	198.89	234.8	229.8	238.8	239.8
duct	171.4	198.89	—	215.4	238.1	239.2
wall NEC	195.1	198.89	234.8	229.8	238.8	239.8
throat	149.0	198.89	230.0	210.9	235.1	239.0
thumb NEC*	195.4	198.89	232.6	229.8	238.8	239.8
thymus (gland)	164.0	198.89	—	212.6	235.8	239.8
contiguous sites with heart and mediastinum	164.8	—	—	—	—	—
thyroglossal duct	193	198.89	234.8	226	237.4	239.7
thyroid (gland)	193	198.89	234.8	226	237.4	239.7
cartilage	161.3	197.3	231.0	212.1	235.6	239.1
tibia (any part)	170.7	198.5	—	213.7	238.0	239.2
toe NEC*	195.5	198.89	232.7	229.8	238.8	239.8
tongue	141.9	198.89	230.0	210.1	235.1	239.0
anterior (two-thirds) NEC	141.4	198.89	230.0	210.1	235.1	239.0

Neoplasm, tongue

Index to Diseases

	Malignant			Benign	Uncertain Behavior	Unspecified
	Primary	Secondary	Ca in situ			

	Malignant			Benign	Uncertain Behavior	Unspecified
	Primary	Secondary	Ca in situ			

Neoplasm, neoplastic — continued						
tongue — continued						
anterior — continued						
dorsal surface	141.1	198.89	230.0	210.1	235.1	239.0
ventral surface	141.3	198.89	230.0	210.1	235.1	239.0
base (dorsal surface)	141.0	198.89	230.0	210.1	235.1	239.0
border (lateral)	141.2	198.89	230.0	210.1	235.1	239.0
contiguous sites	141.8	—	—	—	—	—
dorsal surface NEC	141.1	198.89	230.0	210.1	235.1	239.0
fixed part NEC	141.0	198.89	230.0	210.1	235.1	239.0
foreamen cecum	141.1	198.89	230.0	210.1	235.1	239.0
frenulum linguae	141.3	198.89	230.0	210.1	235.1	239.0
junctional zone	141.5	198.89	230.0	210.1	235.1	239.0
margin (lateral)	141.2	198.89	230.0	210.1	235.1	239.0
midline NEC	141.1	198.89	230.0	210.1	235.1	239.0
mobile part NEC	141.4	198.89	230.0	210.1	235.1	239.0
posterior (third)	141.0	198.89	230.0	210.1	235.1	239.0
root	141.0	198.89	230.0	210.1	235.1	239.0
surface (dorsal)	141.1	198.89	230.0	210.1	235.1	239.0
base	141.0	198.89	230.0	210.1	235.1	239.0
ventral	141.3	198.89	230.0	210.1	235.1	239.0
tip	141.2	198.89	230.0	210.1	235.1	239.0
tonsil	141.6	198.89	230.0	210.1	235.1	239.0
tonsil	146.0	198.89	230.0	210.5	235.1	239.0
fauces, faucial	146.0	198.89	230.0	210.5	235.1	239.0
lingual	141.6	198.89	230.0	210.1	235.1	239.0
palatine	146.0	198.89	230.0	210.5	235.1	239.0
pharyngeal	147.1	198.89	230.0	210.7	235.1	239.0
pillar (anterior) (posterior)	146.2	198.89	230.0	210.6	235.1	239.0
tonsillar fossa	146.1	198.89	230.0	210.6	235.1	239.0
tooth socket NEC	143.9	198.89	230.0	210.4	235.1	239.0
trachea (cartilage) (mucosa)	162.0	197.3	231.1	212.2	235.7	239.1
contiguous sites with bronchus or lung	162.8	—	—	—	—	—
tracheobronchial	162.8	197.3	231.1	212.2	235.7	239.1
contiguous sites with lung	162.8	—	—	—	—	—
tragus	173.2	198.2	232.2	216.2	238.2	239.2
trunk NEC*	195.8	198.89	232.5	229.8	238.8	239.8
tubo-ovarian	183.8	198.82	233.3	221.8	236.3	239.5
tunica vaginalis	187.8	198.82	233.6	222.8	236.6	239.5
turbinate (bone)	170.0	198.5	—	213.0	238.0	239.2
nasal	160.0	197.3	231.8	212.0	235.9	239.1
tympanic cavity	160.1	197.3	231.8	212.0	235.9	239.1
ulna (any part)	170.4	198.5	—	213.4	238.0	239.2
umbilicus, umbilical	173.5	198.2	232.5	216.5	238.2	239.2
uncus, brain	191.2	198.3	—	225.0	237.5	239.6
unknown site or unspecified	199.1	199.1	234.9	229.9	238.9	239.9
urachus	188.7	198.1	233.7	223.3	236.7	239.4
ureter-bladder (junction)	188.6	198.1	233.7	223.3	236.7	239.4
ureter, ureteral	189.2	198.1	233.9	223.2	236.91	239.5
orifice (bladder)	188.6	198.1	233.7	223.3	236.7	239.4
urethra, urethral (gland)	189.3	198.1	233.9	223.81	236.99	239.5
orifice, internal	188.5	198.1	233.7	223.3	236.7	239.4
urethrovaginal (septum)	184.9	198.82	233.3	221.9	236.3	239.5
urinary organ or system NEC	189.9	198.1	233.9	223.9	236.99	239.5
bladder — see Neoplasm, bladder						
contiguous sites	189.8	—	—	—	—	—
specified sites NEC	189.8	198.1	233.9	223.89	236.99	239.5
utero-ovarian	183.8	198.82	233.3	221.8	236.3	239.5
ligament	183.3	198.82	—	221.0	236.3	239.5
uterosacral ligament	183.4	198.82	—	221.0	236.3	239.5
uterus, uteri, uterine	179	198.82	233.2	219.9	236.0	239.5
adnexa NEC	183.9	198.82	233.3	221.8	236.3	239.5
contiguous sites	183.8	—	—	—	—	—
body	182.0	198.82	233.2	219.1	236.0	239.5
contiguous sites	182.8	—	—	—	—	—
cervix	180.9	198.82	233.1	219.0	236.0	239.5

Neoplasm, neoplastic — continued						
uterus, uteri, uterine — continued						
cornu	182.0	198.82	233.2	219.1	236.0	239.5
corpus	182.0	198.82	233.2	219.1	236.0	239.5
endocervix (canal) (gland)	180.0	198.82	233.1	219.0	236.0	239.5
endometrium	182.0	198.82	233.2	219.1	236.0	239.5
exocervix	180.1	198.82	233.1	219.0	236.0	239.5
external os	180.1	198.82	233.1	219.0	236.0	239.5
fundus	182.0	198.82	233.2	219.1	236.0	239.5
internal os	180.0	198.82	233.1	219.0	236.0	239.5
isthmus	182.1	198.82	233.2	219.1	236.0	239.5
ligament	183.4	198.82	—	221.0	236.3	239.5
broad	183.3	198.82	233.3	221.0	236.3	239.5
round	183.5	198.82	—	221.0	236.3	239.5
lower segment	182.1	198.82	233.2	219.1	236.0	239.5
myometrium	182.0	198.82	233.2	219.1	236.0	239.5
squamocolumnar junction	180.8	198.82	233.1	219.0	236.0	239.5
tube	183.2	198.82	233.3	221.0	236.3	239.5
utricle, prostatic	189.3	198.1	233.9	223.81	236.99	239.5
uveal tract	190.0	198.4	234.0	224.0	238.8	239.8
uvula	145.4	198.89	230	210.4	235.1	239.0
vagina, vaginal (fornix) (vault) (wall)	184.0	198.82	233.3	221.1	236.3	239.5
vaginovesical	184.9	198.82	233.3	221.9	236.3	239.5
septum	194.9	198.82	233.3	221.9	236.3	239.5
vallecula (epiglottis)	146.3	198.89	230.0	210.6	235.1	239.0
vascular — see Neoplasm, connective tissue						
vas deferens	187.6	198.82	233.6	222.8	236.6	239.5
Vater's ampulla	156.2	197.8	230.8	211.5	235.3	239.0
vein, venous — see Neoplasm, connective tissue						
vena cava (abdominal) (inferior)	171.5	198.89	—	215.5	238.1	239.2
superior	171.4	198.89	—	215.4	238.1	239.2
ventricle (cerebral) (floor) (fourth) (lateral) (third)	191.5	198.3	—	225.0	237.5	239.6
cardiac (left) (right)	164.1	198.89	—	212.7	238.8	239.8
ventricular band of larynx	161.1	197.3	231.0	212.1	235.6	239.1
ventriculus — see Neoplasm, stomach						
vermillion border — see Neoplasm, lip						
vermis, cerebellum	191.6	198.3	—	225.0	237.5	239.6
vertebra (column)	170.2	198.5	—	213.2	238.0	239.2
coccyx	170.6	198.5	—	213.6	238.0	239.2
sacrum	170.6	198.5	—	213.6	238.0	239.2
vesical — see Neoplasm, bladder						
vesicle, seminal	187.8	198.82	233.6	222.8	236.6	239.5
vesicocervical tissue	184.9	198.82	233.3	221.9	236.3	239.5
vesicorectal	195.3	198.89	234.8	229.8	238.8	239.8
vesicovaginal	184.9	198.82	233.3	221.9	236.3	239.5
septum	184.9	198.82	233.3	221.9	236.3	239.5
vessel (blood) — see Neoplasm, connective tissue						
vestibular gland, greater	184.1	198.82	233.3	221.2	236.3	239.5
vestibule						
mouth	145.1	198.89	230.0	210.4	235.1	239.0
nose	160.0	197.3	231.8	212.0	235.9	239.1
Virchow's gland	—	196.0	—	229.0	238.8	239.8
viscera NEC	195.8	198.89	234.8	229.8	238.8	239.8
vocal cords (true)	161.0	197.3	231.0	212.1	235.6	239.1
false	161.1	197.3	231.0	212.1	235.6	239.1
vomer	170.0	198.5	—	213.0	238.0	239.2
vulva	184.4	198.82	233.3	221.2	236.3	239.5
vulvovaginal gland	184.4	198.82	233.3	221.2	236.3	239.5
Waldeyer's ring	149.1	198.89	230	210.9	235.1	239.0
Wharton's duct	142.1	198.89	230.0	210.2	235.0	239.0

	Malignant			Benign	Uncertain Behavior	Unspecified
	Primary	Secondary	Ca in situ			
Neoplasm, neoplastic — *continued*						
white matter (central) (cerebral)	191.0	198.3	—	225.0	237.5	239.6
windpipe	162.0	197.3	231.1	212.2	235.7	239.1
Wirsung's duct	157.3	197.8	230.9	211.6	235.5	239.0
wolffian (body) (duct)						
female	184.8	198.82	233.3	221.8	236.3	239.5
male	187.8	198.82	233.6	222.8	236.6	239.5
womb — *see* Neoplasm, uterus						
wrist NEC*	195.4	198.89	232.6	229.8	238.8	239.8
xiphoid process	170.3	198.5	—	213.3	238.0	239.2
Zuckerkandl's organ	194.6	198.89	—	227.6	237.3	239.7

Neovascularization

Neovascularization
  choroid 362.16
  ciliary body 364.42
  cornea 370.60
    deep 370.63
    localized 370.61
  iris 364.42
  retina 362.16
  subretinal 362.16
Nephralgia 788.0
Nephritis, nephritic (albuminuric) (azotemic) (congenital) (degenerative) (diffuse) (disseminated) (epithelial) (familial) (focal) (granulomatous) (hemorrhagic) (infantile) (nonsuppurative, excretory) (uremic) 583.9
  with
    edema — see Nephrosis
    lesion of
      glomerulonephritis
        hypocomplementemic persistent 583.2
          with nephrotic syndrome 581.2
          chronic 582.2
        lobular 583.2
          with nephrotic syndrome 581.2
          chronic 582.2
        membranoproliferative 583.2
          with nephrotic syndrome 581.2
          chronic 582.2
        membranous 583.1
          with nephrotic syndrome 581.1
          chronic 582.1
        mesangiocapillary 583.2
          with nephrotic syndrome 581.2
          chronic 582.2
        mixed membranous and proliferative 583.2
          with nephrotic syndrome 581.2
          chronic 582.2
        proliferative (diffuse) 583.0
          with nephrotic syndrome 581.0
          acute 580.0
          chronic 582.0
        rapidly progressive 583.4
          acute 580.4
          chronic 582.4
      interstitial nephritis (diffuse) (focal) 583.89
        with nephrotic syndrome 581.89
        acute 580.89
        chronic 582.89
      necrotizing glomerulitis 583.4
        acute 580.4
        chronic 582.4
      renal necrosis 583.9
        cortical 583.6
        medullary 583.7
      specified pathology NEC 583.89
        with nephrotic syndrome 581.89
        acute 580.89
        chronic 582.89
    necrosis, renal 583.9
      cortical 583.6
      medullary (papillary) 583.7
    nephrotic syndrome (see also Nephrosis) 581.9
    papillary necrosis 583.7
    specified pathology NEC 583.89
  acute 580.9
    extracapillary with epithelial crescents 580.4
    hypertensive (see also Hypertension, kidney) 403.90
    necrotizing 580.4
    poststreptococcal 580.0

Nephritis, nephritic — *continued*
  acute — *continued*
    proliferative (diffuse) 580.0
    rapidly progressive 580.4
    specified pathology NEC 580.89
  amyloid 277.39 [583.81] ▲
    chronic 277.39 [582.81] ▲
  arteriolar (see also Hypertension, kidney) 403.90
  arteriosclerotic (see also Hypertension, kidney) 403.90
  ascending (see also Pyelitis) 590.80
  atrophic 582.9
  basement membrane NEC 583.89
    with
      pulmonary hemorrhage (Goodpasture's syndrome) 446.21 [583.81]
  calculus, calculous 592.0
  cardiac (see also Hypertension, kidney) 403.90
  cardiovascular (see also Hypertension, kidney) 403.90
  chronic 582.9
    arteriosclerotic (see also Hypertension, kidney) 403.90
    hypertensive (see also Hypertension, kidney) 403.90
  cirrhotic (see also Sclerosis, renal) 587
  complicating pregnancy, childbirth, or puerperium 646.2 ☑
    with hypertension 642.1 ☑
      affecting fetus or newborn 760.0
    affecting fetus or newborn 760.1
  croupous 580.9
  desquamative — see Nephrosis
  due to
    amyloidosis 277.39 [583.81] ▲
      chronic 277.39 [582.81] ▲
    arteriosclerosis (see also Hypertension, kidney) 403.90
    diabetes mellitus 250.4 ☑ [583.81]
      with nephrotic syndrome 250.4 ☑ [581.81]
    diphtheria 032.89 [580.81]
    gonococcal infection (acute) 098.19 [583.81]
      chronic or duration of 2 months or over 098.39 [583.81]
    gout 274.10
    infectious hepatitis 070.9 [580.81]
    mumps 072.79 [580.81]
    specified kidney pathology NEC 583.89
      acute 580.89
      chronic 582.89
    streptotrichosis 039.8 [583.81]
    subacute bacterial endocarditis 421.0 [580.81]
    systemic lupus erythematosus 710.0 [583.81]
      chronic 710.0 [582.81]
    typhoid fever 002.0 [580.81]
  endothelial 582.2
  end stage (chronic) (terminal) NEC 585.6
  epimembranous 581.1
  exudative 583.89
    with nephrotic syndrome 581.89
    acute 580.89
    chronic 582.89
  gonococcal (acute) 098.19 [583.81]
    chronic or duration of 2 months or over 098.39 [583.81]
  gouty 274.10
  hereditary (Alport's syndrome) 759.89
  hydremic — see Nephrosis
  hypertensive (see also Hypertension, kidney) 403.90
  hypocomplementemic persistent 583.2
    with nephrotic syndrome 581.2
    chronic 582.2
  immune complex NEC 583.89
  infective (see also Pyelitis) 590.80
  interstitial (diffuse) (focal) 583.89
    with nephrotic syndrome 581.89

Nephritis, nephritic — *continued*
  interstitial — *continued*
    acute 580.89
    chronic 582.89
  latent or quiescent — see Nephritis, chronic
  lead 984.9
    specified type of lead — see Table of Drugs and Chemicals
  lobular 583.2
    with nephrotic syndrome 581.2
    chronic 582.2
  lupus 710.0 [583.81]
    acute 710.0 [580.81]
    chronic 710.0 [582.81]
  membranoproliferative 583.2
    with nephrotic syndrome 581.2
    chronic 582.2
  membranous 583.1
    with nephrotic syndrome 581.1
    chronic 582.1
  mesangiocapillary 583.2
    with nephrotic syndrome 581.2
    chronic 582.2
  minimal change 581.3
  mixed membranous and proliferative 583.2
    with nephrotic syndrome 581.2
    chronic 582.2
  necrotic, necrotizing 583.4
    acute 580.4
    chronic 582.4
  nephrotic — see Nephrosis
  old — see Nephritis, chronic
  parenchymatous 581.89
  polycystic 753.12
    adult type (APKD) 753.13
    autosomal dominant 753.13
    autosomal recessive 753.14
    childhood type (CPKD) 753.14
    infantile type 753.14
  poststreptococcal 580.0
  pregnancy — see Nephritis, complicating pregnancy
  proliferative 583.0
    with nephrotic syndrome 581.0
    acute 580.0
    chronic 582.0
  purulent (see also Pyelitis) 590.80
  rapidly progressive 583.4
    acute 580.4
    chronic 582.4
  salt-losing or salt-wasting (see also Disease, renal) 593.9
  saturnine 984.9
    specified type of lead — see Table of Drugs and Chemicals
  septic (see also Pyelitis) 590.80
  specified pathology NEC 583.89
    acute 580.89
    chronic 582.89
  staphylococcal (see also Pyelitis) 590.80
  streptotrichosis 039.8 [583.81]
  subacute (see also Nephrosis) 581.9
  suppurative (see also Pyelitis) 590.80
  syphilitic (late) 095.4
    congenital 090.5 [583.81]
    early 091.69 [583.81]
  terminal (chronic) (end-stage) NEC 585.6
  toxic — see Nephritis, acute
  tubal, tubular — see Nephrosis, tubular
  tuberculous (see also Tuberculosis) 016.0 ☑ [583.81]
  type II (Ellis) — see Nephrosis
  vascular — see Hypertension, kidney
  war 580.9
Nephroblastoma (M8960/3) 189.0
  epithelial (M8961/3) 189.0
  mesenchymal (M8962/3) 189.0
Nephrocalcinosis 275.49
Nephrocystitis, pustular — see also Pyelitis 590.80

Nephrolithiasis (congenital) (pelvis) (recurrent) 592.0
  uric acid 274.11
Nephroma (M8960/3) 189.0
  mesoblastic (M8960/1) 236.9 ☑
Nephronephritis — see also Nephrosis 581.9
Nephronopthisis 753.16
Nephropathy — see also Nephritis 583.9
  with
    exudative nephritis 583.89
    interstitial nephritis (diffuse) (focal) 583.89
    medullary necrosis 583.7
    necrosis 583.9
      cortical 583.6
      medullary or papillary 583.7
    papillary necrosis 583.7
    specified lesion or cause NEC 583.89
  analgesic 583.89
    with medullary necrosis, acute 584.7
  arteriolar (see also Hypertension, kidney) 403.90
  arteriosclerotic (see also Hypertension, kidney) 403.90
  complicating pregnancy 646.2 ☑
  diabetic 250.4 ☑ [583.81]
  gouty 274.10
    specified type NEC 274.19
  hereditary amyloid 277.31 ●
  hypercalcemic 588.89
  hypertensive (see also Hypertension, kidney) 403.90
  hypokalemic (vacuolar) 588.89
  IgA 583.9
  obstructive 593.89
    congenital 753.20
  phenacetin 584.7
  phosphate-losing 588.0
  potassium depletion 588.89
  proliferative (see also Nephritis, proliferative) 583.0
  protein-losing 588.89
  salt-losing or salt-wasting (see also Disease, renal) 593.9
  sickle-cell (see also Disease, sickle-cell) 282.60 [583.81]
  toxic 584.5
  vasomotor 584.5
  water-losing 588.89
Nephroptosis — see also Disease, renal 593.9
  congenital (displaced) 753.3
Nephropyosis — see also Abscess, kidney 590.2
Nephrorrhagia 593.81
Nephrosclerosis (arteriolar) (arteriosclerotic) (chronic) (hyaline) — see also Hypertension, kidney 403.90
  gouty 274.10
  hyperplastic (arteriolar) (see also Hypertension, kidney) 403.90
  senile (see also Sclerosis, renal) 587
Nephrosis, nephrotic (Epstein's) (syndrome) 581.9
  with
    lesion of
      focal glomerulosclerosis 581.1
      glomerulonephritis
        endothelial 581.2
        hypocomplementemic persistent 581.2
        lobular 581.2
        membranoproliferative 581.2
        membranous 581.1
        mesangiocapillary 581.2
        minimal change 581.3
        mixed membranous and proliferative 581.2
        proliferative 581.0
        segmental hyalinosis 581.1
      specified pathology NEC 581.89
  acute — see Nephrosis, tubular
  anoxic — see Nephrosis, tubular

Index to Diseases

Nephrosis, nephrotic — *continued*
- arteriosclerotic (*see also* Hypertension, kidney) 403.90
- chemical — *see* Nephrosis, tubular
- cholemic 572.4
- complicating pregnancy, childbirth, or puerperium — *see* Nephritis, complicating pregnancy
- diabetic 250.4 ☑ *[581.81]*
- hemoglobinuric — *see* Nephrosis, tubular
- in
  - amyloidosis 277.39 *[581.81]* ▲
  - diabetes mellitus 250.4 ☑ *[581.81]*
  - epidemic hemorrhagic fever 078.6
  - malaria 084.9 *[581.81]*
  - polyarteritis 446.0 *[581.81]*
  - systemic lupus erythematosus 710.0 *[581.81]*
- ischemic — *see* Nephrosis, tubular
- lipoid 581.3
- lower nephron — *see* Nephrosis, tubular
- lupoid 710.0 *[581.81]*
- lupus 710.0 *[581.81]*
- malarial 084.9 *[581.81]*
- minimal change 581.3
- necrotizing — *see* Nephrosis, tubular
- osmotic (sucrose) 588.89
- polyarteritic 446.0 *[581.81]*
- radiation 581.9
- specified lesion or cause NEC 581.89
- syphilitic 095.4
- toxic — *see* Nephrosis, tubular
- tubular (acute) 584.5
  - due to a procedure 997.5
  - radiation 581.9

Nephrosonephritis hemorrhagic (endemic) 078.6

Nephrostomy status V44.6
- with complication 997.5

Nerve — *see* condition

Nerves 799.2

Nervous — *see also* condition 799.2
- breakdown 300.9
- heart 306.2
- stomach 306.4
- tension 799.2

Nervousness 799.2

Nesidioblastoma (M8150/0)
- pancreas 211.7
- specified site NEC — *see* Neoplasm, by site, benign
- unspecified site 211.7

Netherton's syndrome (ichthyosiform erythroderma) 757.1

Nettle rash 708.8

Nettleship's disease (urticaria pigmentosa) 757.33

Neumann's disease (pemphigus vegetans) 694.4

Neuralgia, neuralgic (acute) — *see also* Neuritis 729.2
- accessory (nerve) 352.4
- acoustic (nerve) 388.5
- ankle 355.8
- anterior crural 355.8
- anus 787.99
- arm 723.4
- auditory (nerve) 388.5
- axilla 353.0
- bladder 788.1
- brachial 723.4
- brain — *see* Disorder, nerve, cranial
- broad ligament 625.9
- cerebral — *see* Disorder, nerve, cranial
- ciliary 346.2 ☑
- cranial nerve (*see also* Disorder, nerve, cranial)
  - fifth or trigeminal (*see also* Neuralgia, trigeminal) 350.1
  - ear 388.71
    - middle 352.1
  - facial 351.8
  - finger 354.9

Neuralgia, neuralgic — *see also* Neuritis — *continued*
- flank 355.8
- foot 355.8
- forearm 354.9
- Fothergill's (*see also* Neuralgia, trigeminal) 350.1
  - postherpetic 053.12
- glossopharyngeal (nerve) 352.1
- groin 355.8
- hand 354.9
- heel 355.8
- Horton's 346.2 ☑
- Hunt's 053.11
- hypoglossal (nerve) 352.5
- iliac region 355.8
- infraorbital (*see also* Neuralgia, trigeminal) 350.1
- inguinal 355.8
- intercostal (nerve) 353.8
  - postherpetic 053.19
- jaw 352.1
- kidney 788.0
- knee 355.8
- loin 355.8
- malarial (*see also* Malaria) 084.6
- mastoid 385.89
- maxilla 352.1
- median thenar 354.1
- metatarsal 355.6
- middle ear 352.1
- migrainous 346.2 ☑
- Morton's 355.6
- nerve, cranial — *see* Disorder, nerve, cranial
- nose 352.0
- occipital 723.8
- olfactory (nerve) 352.0
- ophthalmic 377.30
  - postherpetic 053.19
- optic (nerve) 377.30
- penis 607.9
- perineum 355.8
- pleura 511.0
- postherpetic NEC 053.19
  - geniculate ganglion 053.11
  - ophthalmic 053.19
  - trifacial 053.12
  - trigeminal 053.12
- pubic region 355.8
- radial (nerve) 723.4
- rectum 787.99
- sacroiliac joint 724.3
- sciatic (nerve) 724.3
- scrotum 608.9
- seminal vesicle 608.9
- shoulder 354.9
- Sluder's 337.0
- specified nerve NEC — *see* Disorder, nerve
- spermatic cord 608.9
- sphenopalatine (ganglion) 337.0
- subscapular (nerve) 723.4
- suprascapular (nerve) 723.4
- testis 608.89
- thenar (median) 354.1
- thigh 355.8
- tongue 352.5
- trifacial (nerve) (*see also* Neuralgia, trigeminal) 350.1
- trigeminal (nerve) 350.1
  - postherpetic 053.12
- tympanic plexus 388.71
- ulnar (nerve) 723.4
- vagus (nerve) 352.3
- wrist 354.9
- writers' 300.89
  - organic 333.84

Neurapraxia — *see* Injury, nerve, by site

Neurasthenia 300.5
- cardiac 306.2
- gastric 306.4
- heart 306.2
- postfebrile 780.79
- postviral 780.79

Neurilemmoma (M9560/0) — *see also* Neoplasm, connective tissue, benign
- acoustic (nerve) 225.1
- malignant (M9560/3) (*see also* Neoplasm, connective tissue, malignant)
  - acoustic (nerve) 192.0

Neurilemmosarcoma (M9560/3) — *see* Neoplasm, connective tissue, malignant

Neurilemoma — *see* Neurilemmoma

Neurinoma (M9560/0) — *see* Neurilemmoma

Neurinomatosis (M9560/1) — *see also* Neoplasm, connective tissue, uncertain behavior
- centralis 759.5

Neuritis — *see also* Neuralgia 729.2
- abducens (nerve) 378.54
- accessory (nerve) 352.4
- acoustic (nerve) 388.5
  - syphilitic 094.86
- alcoholic 357.5
  - with psychosis 291.1
- amyloid, any site 277.39 *[357.4]* ▲
- anterior crural 355.8
- arising during pregnancy 646.4 ☑
- arm 723.4
- ascending 355.2
- auditory (nerve) 388.5
- brachial (nerve) NEC 723.4
  - due to displacement, intervertebral disc 722.0
- cervical 723.4
- chest (wall) 353.8
- costal region 353.8
- cranial nerve (*see also* Disorder, nerve, cranial)
  - first or olfactory 352.0
  - second or optic 377.30
  - third or oculomotor 378.52
  - fourth or trochlear 378.53
  - fifth or trigeminal (*see also* Neuralgia, trigeminal) 350.1
  - sixth or abducens 378.54
  - seventh or facial 351.8
    - newborn 767.5
  - eighth or acoustic 388.5
  - ninth or glossopharyngeal 352.1
  - tenth or vagus 352.3
  - eleventh or accessory 352.4
  - twelfth or hypoglossal 352.5
- Déjérine-Sottas 356.0
- diabetic 250.6 ☑ *[357.2]*
- diphtheritic 032.89 *[357.4]*
- due to
  - beriberi 265.0 *[357.4]*
  - displacement, prolapse, protrusion, or rupture of intervertebral disc 722.2
    - cervical 722.0
    - lumbar, lumbosacral 722.10
    - thoracic, thoracolumbar 722.11
  - herniation, nucleus pulposus 722.2
    - cervical 722.0
    - lumbar, lumbosacral 722.10
    - thoracic, thoracolumbar 722.11
- endemic 265.0 *[357.4]*
- facial (nerve) 351.8
  - newborn 767.5
- general — *see* Polyneuropathy
- geniculate ganglion 351.1
  - due to herpes 053.11
- glossopharyngeal (nerve) 352.1
- gouty 274.89 *[357.4]*
- hypoglossal (nerve) 352.5
- ilioinguinal (nerve) 355.8
- in diseases classified elsewhere — *see* Polyneuropathy, in
- infectious (multiple) 357.0
- intercostal (nerve) 353.8
- interstitial hypertrophic progressive NEC 356.9
- leg 355.8

Neuritis — *see also* Neuralgia — *continued*
- lumbosacral NEC 724.4
- median (nerve) 354.1
  - thenar 354.1
- multiple (acute) (infective) 356.9
  - endemic 265.0 *[357.4]*
- multiplex endemica 265.0 *[357.4]*
- nerve root (*see also* Radiculitis) 729.2
- oculomotor (nerve) 378.52
- olfactory (nerve) 352.0
- optic (nerve) 377.30
  - in myelitis 341.0
  - meningococcal 036.81
- pelvic 355.8
- peripheral (nerve) (*see also* Neuropathy, peripheral)
  - complicating pregnancy or puerperium 646.4 ☑
  - specified nerve NEC — *see* Mononeuritis
- pneumogastric (nerve) 352.3
- postchickenpox 052.7
- postherpetic 053.19
- progressive hypertrophic interstitial NEC 356.9
- puerperal, postpartum 646.4 ☑
- radial (nerve) 723.4
- retrobulbar 377.32
  - syphilitic 094.85
- rheumatic (chronic) 729.2
- sacral region 355.8
- sciatic (nerve) 724.3
  - due to displacement of intervertebral disc 722.10
- serum 999.5
- specified nerve NEC — *see* Disorder, nerve
- spinal (nerve) 355.9
  - root (*see also* Radiculitis) 729.2
- subscapular (nerve) 723.4
- suprascapular (nerve) 723.4
- syphilitic 095.8
- thenar (median) 354.1
- thoracic NEC 724.4
- toxic NEC 357.7
- trochlear (nerve) 378.53
- ulnar (nerve) 723.4
- vagus (nerve) 352.3

Neuroangiomatosis, encephalofacial 759.6

Neuroastrocytoma (M9505/1) — *see* Neoplasm, by site, uncertain behavior

Neuro-avitaminosis 269.2

Neuroblastoma (M9500/3)
- olfactory (M9522/3) 160.0
- specified site — *see* Neoplasm, by site, malignant
- unspecified site 194.0

Neurochorioretinitis — *see also* Chorioretinitis 363.20

Neurocirculatory asthenia 306.2

Neurocytoma (M9506/0) — *see* Neoplasm, by site, benign

Neurodermatitis (circumscribed) (circumscripta) (local) 698.3
- atopic 691.8
- diffuse (Brocq) 691.8
- disseminated 691.8
- nodulosa 698.3

Neuroencephalomyelopathy, optic 341.0

Neuroepithelioma (M9503/3) — *see also* Neoplasm, by site, malignant
- olfactory (M9521/3) 160.0

Neurofibroma (M9540/0) — *see also* Neoplasm, connective tissue, benign
- melanotic (M9541/0) — *see* Neoplasm, connective tissue, benign
- multiple (M9540/1) 237.70
  - type 1 237.71
  - type 2 237.72
- plexiform (M9550/0) — *see* Neoplasm, connective tissue, benign

Neurofibromatosis

Neurofibromatosis (multiple) (M9540/1) 237.70
- acoustic 237.72
- malignant (M9540/3) — see Neoplasm, connective tissue, malignant
- type 1 237.71
- type 2 237.72
- von Recklinghausen's 237.71

Neurofibrosarcoma (M9540/3) — see Neoplasm, connective tissue, malignant

Neurogenic — see also condition
- bladder (atonic) (automatic) (autonomic) (flaccid) (hypertonic) (hypotonic) (inertia) (infranuclear) (irritable) (motor) (nonreflex) (nuclear) (paralysis) (reflex) (sensory) (spastic) (supranuclear) (uninhibited) 596.54
  - with cauda equina syndrome 344.61
- bowel 564.81
- heart 306.2

Neuroglioma (M9505/1) — see Neoplasm, by site, uncertain behavior

Neurolabyrinthitis (of Dix and Hallpike) 386.12

Neurolathyrism 988.2

Neuroleprosy 030.1

Neuroleptic malignant syndrome 333.92

Neurolipomatosis 272.8

Neuroma (M9570/0) — see also Neoplasm, connective tissue, benign
- acoustic (nerve) (M9560/0) 225.1
- amputation (traumatic) (see also Injury, nerve, by site)
  - surgical complication (late) 997.61
- appendix 211.3
- auditory nerve 225.1
- digital 355.6
  - toe 355.6
- interdigital (toe) 355.6
- intermetatarsal 355.6
- Morton's 355.6
- multiple 237.70
  - type 1 237.71
  - type 2 237.72
- nonneoplastic 355.9
  - arm NEC 354.9
  - leg NEC 355.8
  - lower extremity NEC 355.8
  - specified site NEC — see Mononeuritis, by site
  - upper extremity NEC 354.9
- optic (nerve) 225.1
- plantar 355.6
- plexiform (M9550/0) — see Neoplasm, connective tissue, benign
- surgical (nonneoplastic) 355.9
  - arm NEC 354.9
  - leg NEC 355.8
  - lower extremity NEC 355.8
  - upper extremity NEC 354.9
- traumatic (see also Injury, nerve, by site)
  - old — see Neuroma, nonneoplastic

Neuromyalgia 729.1

Neuromyasthenia (epidemic) 049.8

Neuromyelitis 341.8
- ascending 357.0
- optica 341.0

Neuromyopathy NEC 358.9

Neuromyositis 729.1

Neuronevus (M8725/0) — see Neoplasm, skin, benign

Neuronitis 357.0
- ascending (acute) 355.2
- vestibular 386.12

Neuroparalytic — see condition

Neuropathy, neuropathic — see also Disorder, nerve 355.9
- acute motor 357.82
- alcoholic 357.5
  - with psychosis 291.1

Neuropathy, neuropathic — see also Disorder, nerve — continued
- arm NEC 354.9
- ataxia and retinitis pigmentosa (NARP syndrome) 277.87
- autonomic (peripheral) — see Neuropathy, peripheral, autonomic
- axillary nerve 353.0
- brachial plexus 353.0
- cervical plexus 353.2
- chronic
  - progressive segmentally demyelinating 357.89
  - relapsing demyelinating 357.89
- congenital sensory 356.2
- Déjérine-Sottas 356.0
- diabetic 250.6 ☑ [357.2]
- entrapment 355.9
  - iliohypogastric nerve 355.79
  - ilioinguinal nerve 355.79
  - lateral cutaneous nerve of thigh 355.1
  - median nerve 354.0
  - obturator nerve 355.79
  - peroneal nerve 355.3
  - posterior tibial nerve 355.5
  - saphenous nerve 355.79
  - ulnar nerve 354.2
- facial nerve 351.9
- hereditary 356.9
  - peripheral 356.0
  - sensory (radicular) 356.2
- hypertrophic
  - Charcôt-Marie-Tooth 356.1
  - Déjérine-Sottas 356.0
  - interstitial 356.9
  - Refsum 356.3
- intercostal nerve 354.8
- ischemic — see Disorder, nerve
- Jamaican (ginger) 357.7
- leg NEC 355.8
- lower extremity NEC 355.8
- lumbar plexus 353.1
- median nerve 354.1
- motor
  - acute 357.82
- multiple (acute) (chronic) (see also Polyneuropathy) 356.9
- optic 377.39
  - ischemic 377.41
  - nutritional 377.33
  - toxic 377.34
- peripheral (nerve) (see also Polyneuropathy) 356.9
  - arm NEC 354.9
  - autonomic 337.9
    - amyloid 277.39 [337.1] ▲
    - idiopathic 337.0
    - in
      - amyloidosis 277.39 [337.1] ▲
      - diabetes (mellitus) 250.6 ☑ [337.1]
      - diseases classified elsewhere 337.1
      - gout 274.89 [337.1]
      - hyperthyroidism 242.9 ☑ [337.1]
    - due to
      - antitetanus serum 357.6
      - arsenic 357.7
      - drugs 357.6
      - lead 357.7
      - organophosphate compounds 357.7
      - toxic agent NEC 357.7
  - hereditary 356.0
  - idiopathic 356.9
    - progressive 356.4
    - specified type NEC 356.8
  - in diseases classified elsewhere — see Polyneuropathy, in
  - leg NEC 355.8
  - lower extremity NEC 355.8
  - upper extremity NEC 354.9
- plantar nerves 355.6

Neuropathy, neuropathic — see also Disorder, nerve — continued
- progressive hypertrophic interstitial 356.9
- radicular NEC 729.2
  - brachial 723.4
  - cervical NEC 723.4
  - hereditary sensory 356.2
  - lumbar 724.4
  - lumbosacral 724.4
  - thoracic NEC 724.4
- sacral plexus 353.1
- sciatic 355.0
- spinal nerve NEC 355.9
  - root (see also Radiculitis) 729.2
- toxic 357.7
- trigeminal sensory 350.8
- ulnar nerve 354.2
- upper extremity NEC 354.9
- uremic 585.9 [357.4]
- vitamin B$_{12}$ 266.2 [357.4]
  - with anemia (pernicious) 281.0 [357.4]
  - due to dietary deficiency 281.1 [357.4]

Neurophthisis — see also Disorder, nerve
- diabetic 250.6 ☑ [357.2]
- peripheral 356.9

Neuropraxia — see Injury, nerve

Neuroretinitis 363.05
- syphilitic 094.85

Neurosarcoma (M9540/3) — see Neoplasm, connective tissue, malignant

Neurosclerosis — see Disorder, nerve

Neurosis, neurotic 300.9
- accident 300.16
- anancastic, anankastic 300.3
- anxiety (state) 300.00
  - generalized 300.02
  - panic type 300.01
- asthenic 300.5
- bladder 306.53
- cardiac (reflex) 306.2
- cardiovascular 306.2
- climacteric, unspecified type 627.2
- colon 306.4
- compensation 300.16
- compulsive, compulsion 300.3
- conversion 300.11
- craft 300.89
- cutaneous 306.3
- depersonalization 300.6
- depressive (reaction) (type) 300.4
- endocrine 306.6
- environmental 300.89
- fatigue 300.5
- functional (see also Disorder, psychosomatic) 306.9
- gastric 306.4
- gastrointestinal 306.4
- genitourinary 306.50
- heart 306.2
- hypochondriacal 300.7
- hysterical 300.10
  - conversion type 300.11
  - dissociative type 300.15
- impulsive 300.3
- incoordination 306.0
  - larynx 306.1
  - vocal cord 306.1
- intestine 306.4
- larynx 306.1
  - hysterical 300.11
  - sensory 306.1
- menopause, unspecified type 627.2
- mixed NEC 300.89
- musculoskeletal 306.0
- obsessional 300.3
  - phobia 300.3
- obsessive-compulsive 300.3
- occupational 300.89
- ocular 306.7
- oral 307.0

Neurosis, neurotic — continued
- organ (see also Disorder, psychosomatic) 306.9
- pharynx 306.1
- phobic 300.20
- posttraumatic (acute) (situational) 309.81
  - chronic 309.81
- psychasthenic (type) 300.89
- railroad 300.16
- rectum 306.4
- respiratory 306.1
- rumination 306.4
- senile 300.89
- sexual 302.70
- situational 300.89
- specified type NEC 300.89
- state 300.9
  - with depersonalization episode 300.6
- stomach 306.4
- vasomotor 306.2
- visceral 306.4
- war 300.16

Neurospongioblastosis diffusa 759.5

Neurosyphilis (arrested) (early) (inactive) (late) (latent) (recurrent) 094.9
- with ataxia (cerebellar) (locomotor) (spastic) (spinal) 094.0
- acute meningitis 094.2
- aneurysm 094.89
- arachnoid 094.2
- arteritis (any artery) 094.89
- asymptomatic 094.3
- congenital 090.40
- dura (mater) 094.89
- general paresis 094.1
- gumma 094.9
- hemorrhagic 094.9
- juvenile (asymptomatic) (meningeal) 090.40
- leptomeninges (aseptic) 094.2
- meningeal 094.2
- meninges (adhesive) 094.2
- meningovascular (diffuse) 094.2
- optic atrophy 094.84
- parenchymatous (degenerative) 094.1
- paresis (see also Paresis, general) 094.1
- paretic (see also Paresis, general) 094.1
- relapse 094.9
- remission in (sustained) 094.9
- serological 094.3
- specified nature or site NEC 094.89
- tabes (dorsalis) 094.0
  - juvenile 090.40
- tabetic 094.0
  - juvenile 090.40
- taboparesis 094.1
  - juvenile 090.40
- thrombosis 094.89
- vascular 094.89

Neurotic — see also Neurosis 300.9
- excoriation 698.4
- psychogenic 306.3

Neurotmesis — see Injury, nerve, by site

Neurotoxemia — see Toxemia

Neuro-occlusion 524.21

Neutropenia, neutropenic (idiopathic) (pernicious) (primary) 288.00 ▲
- chronic 288.09 ▲
  - hypoplastic 288.09 ●
- congenital (nontransient) 288.01 ▲
- cyclic 288.02 ●
- drug induced 288.03 ●
- due to infection 288.04 ●
- fever 288.00 ▲
- genetic 288.01 ●
- immune 288.09 ●
- infantile 288.01 ●
- malignant 288.09 ●
- neonatal, transitory (isoimmune) (maternal transfer) 776.7
- periodic 288.02 ●
- splenic 289.53 ●

Index to Diseases

Neutropenia, neutropenic — *continued*
  splenomegaly 289.53
  toxic 288.09
Neutrophilia, hereditary giant 288.2
Nevocarcinoma (M8720/3) — *see* Melanoma
Nevus (M8720/0) — *see also* Neoplasm, skin, benign

Note — Except where otherwise indicated, varieties of nevus in the list below that are followed by a morphology code number (M----/0) should be coded by site as for "Neoplasm, skin, benign."

  acanthotic 702.8
  achromic (M8730/0)
  amelanotic (M8730/0)
  anemic, anemicus 709.09
  angiomatous (M9120/0) (*see also* Hemangioma) 228.00
  araneus 448.1
  avasculosus 709.09
  balloon cell (M8722/0)
  bathing trunk (M8761/1) 238.2
  blue (M8780/0)
    cellular (M8790/0)
    giant (M8790/0)
    Jadassohn's (M8780/0)
    malignant (M8780/3) — *see* Melanoma
  capillary (M9131/0) (*see also* Hemangioma) 228.00
  cavernous (M9121/0) (*see also* Hemangioma) 228.00
  cellular (M8780/0)
    blue (M8790/0)
  comedonicus 757.33
  compound (M8760/0)
  conjunctiva (M8720/0) 224.3
  dermal (M8750/0)
    and epidermal (M8760/0)
  epithelioid cell (and spindle cell) (M8770/0)
  flammeus 757.32
    osteohypertrophic 759.89
  hairy (M8720/0)
  halo (M8723/0)
  hemangiomatous (M9120/0) (*see also* Hemangioma) 228.00
  intradermal (M8750/0)
  intraepidermal (M8740/0)
  involuting (M8724/0)
  Jadassohn's (blue) (M8780/0)
  junction, junctional (M8740/0)
    malignant melanoma in (M8740/3) — *see* Melanoma
  juvenile (M8770/0)
  lymphatic (M9170/0) 228.1
  magnocellular (M8726/0)
    specified site — *see* Neoplasm, by site, benign
    unspecified site 224.0
  malignant (M8720/3) — *see* Melanoma
  meaning hemangioma (M9120/0) (*see also* Hemangioma) 228.00
  melanotic (pigmented) (M8720/0)
  multiplex 759.5
  nonneoplastic 448.1
  nonpigmented (M8730/0)
  nonvascular (M8720/0)
  oral mucosa, white sponge 750.26
  osteohypertrophic, flammeus 759.89
  papillaris (M8720/0)
  papillomatosus (M8720/0)
  pigmented (M8720/0)
    giant (M8761/1) (*see also* Neoplasm, skin, uncertain behavior)
    malignant melanoma in (M8761/3) — *see* Melanoma
    systematicus 757.33
  pilosus (M8720/0)
  port wine 757.32
  sanguineous 757.32

Nevus — *see also* Neoplasm, skin, benign — *continued*
  sebaceous (senile) 702.8
  senile 448.1
  spider 448.1
  spindle cell (and epithelioid cell) (M8770/0)
  stellar 448.1
  strawberry 757.32
  syringocystadenomatous papilliferous (M8406/0)
  unius lateris 757.33
  Unna's 757.32
  vascular 757.32
  verrucous 757.33
  white sponge (oral mucosa) 750.26
Newborn (infant) (liveborn)
  affected by maternal abuse of drugs (gestational) (via placenta) (via breast milk) (*see also* Noxious, substances transmitted through placenta or breast milk affecting fetus or newborn) 760.70
  apnea 770.81
    obstructive 770.82
    specified NEC 770.82
  cardiomyopathy 425.4
    congenital 425.3
  convulsion 779.0
  electrolyte imbalance NEC (transitory) 775.5
  gestation
    24 completed weeks 765.22
    25-26 completed weeks 765.23
    27-28 completed weeks 765.24
    29-30 completed weeks 765.25
    31-32 completed weeks 765.26
    33-34 completed weeks 765.27
    35-36 completed weeks 765.28
    37 or more completed weeks 765.29
    less than 24 completed weeks 765.21
    unspecified completed weeks 765.20
  infection 771.89
    candida 771.7
    mastitis 771.5
    specified NEC 771.89
    urinary tract 771.82
  mastitis 771.5
  multiple NEC
    born in hospital (without mention of cesarean delivery or section) V37.00
    with cesarean delivery or section V37.01
    born outside hospital
      hospitalized V37.1
      not hospitalized V37.2
    mates all liveborn
      born in hospital (without mention of cesarean delivery or section) V34.00
      with cesarean delivery or section V34.01
      born outside hospital
        hospitalized V34.1
        not hospitalized V34.2
    mates all stillborn
      born in hospital (without mention of cesarean delivery or section) V35.00
      with cesarean delivery or section V35.01
      born outside hospital
        hospitalized V35.1
        not hospitalized V35.2
    mates liveborn and stillborn
      born in hospital (without mention of cesarean delivery or section) V36.00
      with cesarean delivery or section V36.01
      born outside hospital
        hospitalized V36.1

Newborn — *continued*
  multiple — *continued*
    mates liveborn and stillborn — *continued*
      born outside hospital — *continued*
        not hospitalized V36.2
  omphalitis 771.4
  seizure 779.0
  sepsis 771.81
  single
    born in hospital (without mention of cesarean delivery or section) V30.00
    with cesarean delivery or section V30.01
    born outside hospital
      hospitalized V30.1
      not hospitalized V30.2
  specified condition NEC 779.89
  twin NEC
    born in hospital (without mention of cesarean delivery or section) V33.00
    with cesarean delivery or section V33.01
    born outside hospital
      hospitalized V33.1
      not hospitalized V33.2
    mate liveborn
      born in hospital V31.0 ☑
      born outside hospital
        hospitalized V31.1
        not hospitalized V31.2
    mate stillborn
      born in hospital V32.0 ☑
      born outside hospital
        hospitalized V32.1
        not hospitalized V32.2
  unspecified as to single or multiple birth
    born in hospital (without mention of cesarean delivery or section) V39.00
    with cesarean delivery or section V39.01
    born outside hospital
      hospitalized V39.1
      not hospitalized V39.2
Newcastle's conjunctivitis or disease 077.8
Nezelof's syndrome (pure alymphocytosis) 279.13
Niacin (amide) **deficiency** 265.2
Nicolas-Durand-Favre disease (climatic bubo) 099.1
Nicolas-Favre disease (climatic bubo) 099.1
Nicotinic acid (amide) **deficiency** 265.2
Niemann-Pick disease (lipid histiocytosis) (splenomegaly) 272.7
Night
  blindness (*see also* Blindness, night) 368.60
    congenital 368.61
    vitamin A deficiency 264.5
  cramps 729.82
  sweats 780.8
  terrors, child 307.46
Nightmare 307.47
  REM-sleep type 307.47
Nipple — *see* condition
Nisbet's chancre 099.0
Nishimoto (-Takeuchi) disease 437.5
Nitritoid crisis or reaction — *see* Crisis, nitritoid
Nitrogen retention, extrarenal 788.9
Nitrosohemoglobinemia 289.89
Njovera 104.0
No
  diagnosis 799.9
  disease (found) V71.9
  room at the inn V65.0
Nocardiasis — *see* Nocardiosis
Nocardiosis 039.9
  with pneumonia 039.1

Nocardiosis — *continued*
  lung 039.1
  specified type NEC 039.8
Nocturia 788.43
  psychogenic 306.53
Nocturnal — *see also* condition
  dyspnea (paroxysmal) 786.09
  emissions 608.89
  enuresis 788.36
    psychogenic 307.6
  frequency (micturition) 788.43
    psychogenic 306.53
Nodal rhythm disorder 427.89
Nodding of head 781.0
Node(s) — *see also* Nodule(s)
  Heberden's 715.04
  larynx 478.79
  lymph — *see* condition
  milkers' 051.1
  Osler's 421.0
  rheumatic 729.89
  Schmorl's 722.30
    lumbar, lumbosacral 722.32
    specified region NEC 722.39
    thoracic, thoracolumbar 722.31
  singers' 478.5
  skin NEC 782.2
  tuberculous — *see* Tuberculosis, lymph gland
  vocal cords 478.5
Nodosities, Haygarth's 715.04
Nodule(s), nodular
  actinomycotic (*see also* Actinomycosis) 039.9
  arthritic — *see* Arthritis, nodosa
  cutaneous 782.2
  Haygarth's 715.04
  inflammatory — *see* Inflammation
  juxta-articular 102.7
    syphilitic 095.7
    yaws 102.7
  larynx 478.79
  lung, solitary 518.89
    emphysematous 492.8
  milkers' 051.1
  prostate 600.10
    with
      urinary
        obstruction 600.11
        retention 600.11
  rheumatic 729.89
  rheumatoid — *see* Arthritis, rheumatoid
  scrotum (inflammatory) 608.4
  singers' 478.5
  skin NEC 782.2
  solitary, lung 518.89
    emphysematous 492.8
  subcutaneous 782.2
  thyroid (gland) (nontoxic) (uninodular) 241.0
    with
      hyperthyroidism 242.1 ☑
      thyrotoxicosis 242.1 ☑
    toxic or with hyperthyroidism 242.1 ☑
  vocal cords 478.5
Noma (gangrenous) (hospital) (infective) 528.1
  auricle (*see also* Gangrene) 785.4
  mouth 528.1
  pudendi (*see also* Vulvitis) 616.10
  vulvae (*see also* Vulvitis) 616.10
Nomadism V60.0
Non-adherence
  artificial skin graft 996.55
  decellularized allodermis graft 996.55
Non-autoimmune hemolytic anemia NEC 283.10
Nonclosure — *see also* Imperfect, closure
  ductus
    arteriosus 747.0
    Botalli 747.0
  Eustachian valve 746.89
  foramen
    Botalli 745.5

Nonclosure — see also Imperfect, closure
— continued
  foramen — continued
    ovale 745.5
Noncompliance with medical treatment V15.81
Nondescent (congenital) — see also Malposition, congenital
  cecum 751.4
  colon 751.4
  testis 752.51
Nondevelopment
  brain 742.1
    specified part 742.2
  heart 746.89
  organ or site, congenital NEC — see Hypoplasia
Nonengagement
  head NEC 652.5 ☑
    in labor 660.1 ☑
      affecting fetus or newborn 763.1
Nonexanthematous tick fever 066.1
Nonexpansion, lung (newborn) NEC 770.4
Nonfunctioning
  cystic duct (see also Disease, gallbladder) 575.8
  gallbladder (see also Disease, gallbladder) 575.8
  kidney (see also Disease, renal) 593.9
  labyrinth 386.58
Nonhealing
  stump (surgical) 997.69
  wound, surgical 998.83
Nonimplantation of ovum, causing infertility 628.3
Noninsufflation, fallopian tube 628.2
Nonne-Milroy-Meige syndrome (chronic hereditary edema) 757.0
Nonovulation 628.0
Nonpatent fallopian tube 628.2
Nonpneumatization, lung NEC 770.4
Nonreflex bladder 596.54
  with cauda equina 344.61
Nonretention of food — see Vomiting
Nonrotation — see Malrotation
Nonsecretion, urine — see also Anuria 788.5

Nonsecretion, urine — see also Anuria — continued
  newborn 753.3
Nonunion
  fracture 733.82
  organ or site, congenital NEC — see Imperfect, closure
  symphysis pubis, congenital 755.69
  top sacrum, congenital 756.19
Nonviability 765.0 ☑
Nonvisualization, gallbladder 793.3
Nonvitalized tooth 522.9
Non-working side interference 524.56
Normal
  delivery — see category 650
  menses V65.5
  state (feared complaint unfounded) V65.5
Normoblastosis 289.89
Normocytic anemia (infectional) 285.9
  due to blood loss (chronic) 280.0
  acute 285.1
Norrie's disease (congenital) (progressive oculoacousticocerebral degeneration) 743.8
North American blastomycosis 116.0
Norwegian itch 133.0
Nosebleed 784.7
Nose, nasal — see condition
Nosomania 298.9
Nosophobia 300.29
Nostalgia 309.89
Notched lip, congenital — see also Cleft, lip 749.10
Notching nose, congenital (tip) 748.1
Notch of iris 743.46
Nothnagel's
  syndrome 378.52
  vasomotor acroparesthesia 443.89
Novy's relapsing fever (American) 087.1
Noxious
  foodstuffs, poisoning by
    fish 988.0
    fungi 988.1
    mushrooms 988.1
    plants (food) 988.2
    shellfish 988.0
    specified type NEC 988.8

Noxious — continued
  foodstuffs, poisoning by — continued
    toadstool 988.1
  substances transmitted through placenta or breast milk (affecting fetus or newborn) 760.70
    acetretin 760.78
    alcohol 760.71
    aminopterin 760.78
    antiandrogens 760.79
    anticonvulsant 760.77
    antifungal 760.74
    anti-infective agents 760.74
    antimetabolic 760.78
    atorvastatin 760.78
    carbamazepine 760.77
    cocaine 760.75
    "crack" 760.75
    diethylstilbestrol (DES) 760.76
    divalproex sodium 760.77
    endocrine disrupting chemicals 760.79
    estrogens 760.79
    etretinate 760.78
    fluconazole 760.74
    fluvastatin 760.78
    hallucinogenic agents NEC 760.73
    hormones 760.79
    lithium 760.79
    lovastatin 760.78
    medicinal agents NEC 760.79
    methotrexate 760.78
    misoprostil 760.79
    narcotics 760.72
    obstetric anesthetic or analgesic 763.5
    phenobarbital 760.77
    phenytoin 760.77
    pravastatin 760.78
    progestins 760.79
    retinoic acid 760.78
    simvastatin 760.78
    solvents 760.79
    specified agent NEC 760.79
    statins 760.78
    suspected, affecting management of pregnancy 655.5 ☑

Noxious — continued
  substances transmitted through placenta or breast milk — continued
    tetracycline 760.74
    thalidomide 760.79
    trimethadione 760.77
    valproate 760.77
    valproic acid 760.77
    vitamin A 760.78
Nuchal hitch (arm) 652.8 ☑
Nucleus pulposus — see condition
Numbness 782.0
Nuns' knee 727.2
Nursemaid's
  elbow 832.0 ☑
  shoulder 831.0 ☑
Nutmeg liver 573.8
Nutrition, deficient or insufficient (particular kind of food) 269.9
  due to
    insufficient food 994.2
    lack of
      care (child) (infant) 995.52
        adult 995.84
      food 994.2
Nyctalopia — see also Blindness, night 368.60
  vitamin A deficiency 264.5
Nycturia 788.43
  psychogenic 306.53
Nymphomania 302.89
Nystagmus 379.50
  associated with vestibular system disorders 379.54
  benign paroxysmal positional 386.11
  central positional 386.2
  congenital 379.51
  deprivation 379.53
  dissociated 379.55
  latent 379.52
  miners' 300.89
  positional
    benign paroxysmal 386.11
    central 386.2
  specified NEC 379.56
  vestibular 379.54
  visual deprivation 379.53

Index to Diseases

O

Oasthouse urine disease 270.2
Obermeyer's relapsing fever (European) 087.0
Obesity (constitutional) (exogenous) (familial) (nutritional) (simple) 278.00
- adrenal 255.8
- complicating pregnancy, childbirth, ● or puerperium 649.1 ☑
- due to hyperalimentation 278.00
- endocrine NEC 259.9
- endogenous 259.9
- Fröhlich's (adiposogenital dystrophy) 253.8
- glandular NEC 259.9
- hypothyroid (see also Hypothyroidism) 244.9
- morbid 278.01
- of pregnancy 649.1 ☑ ▲
- pituitary 253.8
- severe 278.01
- thyroid (see also Hypothyroidism) 244.9

Oblique — see also condition
- lie before labor, affecting fetus or newborn 761.7

Obliquity, pelvis 738.6

Obliteration
- abdominal aorta 446.7
- appendix (lumen) 543.9
- artery 447.1
- ascending aorta 446.7
- bile ducts 576.8
  - with calculus, choledocholithiasis, or stones — see Choledocholithiasis
  - congenital 751.61
    - jaundice from 751.61 [774.5]
- common duct 576.8
  - with calculus, choledocholithiasis, or stones — see Choledocholithiasis
  - congenital 751.61
- cystic duct 575.8
  - with calculus, choledocholithiasis, or stones — see Choledocholithiasis
- disease, arteriolar 447.1
- endometrium 621.8
- eye, anterior chamber 360.34
- fallopian tube 628.2
- lymphatic vessel 457.1
  - postmastectomy 457.0
- organ or site, congenital NEC — see Atresia
- placental blood vessels — see Placenta, abnormal
- supra-aortic branches 446.7
- ureter 593.89
- urethra 599.84
- vein 459.9
- vestibule (oral) 525.8

Observation (for) V71.9
- without need for further medical care V71.9
- accident NEC V71.4
  - at work V71.3
- criminal assault V71.6
- deleterious agent ingestion V71.89
- disease V71.9
  - cardiovascular V71.7
    - heart V71.7
  - mental V71.09
- specified condition NEC V71.89
- foreign body ingestion V71.89
- growth and development variations V21.8
- injuries (accidental) V71.4
  - inflicted NEC V71.6
    - during alleged rape or seduction V71.5
- malignant neoplasm, suspected V71.1
- postpartum
  - immediately after delivery V24.0
  - routine follow-up V24.2

Observation — continued
- pregnancy
  - high-risk V23.9
    - specified problem NEC V23.89
  - normal (without complication) V22.1
    - with nonobstetric complication V22.2
  - first V22.0
- rape or seduction, alleged V71.5
  - injury during V71.5
- suicide attempt, alleged V71.89
- suspected (undiagnosed) (unproven)
  - abuse V71.81
  - cardiovascular disease V71.7
  - child or wife battering victim V71.6
  - concussion (cerebral) V71.6
  - condition NEC V71.89
    - infant — see Observation, suspected, condition, newborn
  - newborn V29.9
    - cardiovascular disease V29.8
    - congenital anomaly V29.8
    - genetic V29.3
    - infectious V29.0
    - ingestion foreign object V29.8
    - injury V29.8
    - metabolic V29.3
    - neoplasm V29.8
    - neurological V29.1
    - poison, poisoning V29.8
    - respiratory V29.2
    - specified NEC V29.8
  - exposure
    - anthrax V71.82
    - biologic agent NEC V71.83
    - SARS V71.83
  - infectious disease not requiring isolation V71.89
  - malignant neoplasm V71.1
  - mental disorder V71.09
  - neglect V71.81
  - neoplasm
    - benign V71.89
    - malignant V71.1
  - specified condition NEC V71.89
  - tuberculosis V71.2
- tuberculosis, suspected V71.2

Obsession, obsessional 300.3
- ideas and mental images 300.3
- impulses 300.3
- neurosis 300.3
- phobia 300.3
- psychasthenia 300.3
- ruminations 300.3
- state 300.3
- syndrome 300.3

Obsessive-compulsive 300.3
- neurosis 300.3
- personality 301.4
- reaction 300.3

Obstetrical trauma NEC (complicating delivery) 665.9 ☑
- with
  - abortion — see Abortion, by type, with damage to pelvic organs
  - ectopic pregnancy (see also categories 633.0-633.9) 639.2
  - molar pregnancy (see also categories 630-632) 639.2
- affecting fetus or newborn 763.89
- following
  - abortion 639.2
  - ectopic or molar pregnancy 639.2

Obstipation — see also Constipation 564.00
- psychogenic 306.4

Obstruction, obstructed, obstructive
- airway NEC 519.8
  - with
    - allergic alveolitis NEC 495.9
    - asthma NEC (see also Asthma) 493.9 ☑
    - bronchiectasis 494.0

Obstruction, obstructed, obstructive — continued
- airway — continued
  - with — continued
    - bronchiectasis — continued
      - with acute exacerbation 494.1
    - bronchitis (chronic) (see also Bronchitis, with, obstruction) 491.20
    - emphysema NEC 492.8
  - chronic 496
    - with
      - allergic alveolitis NEC 495.5
      - asthma NEC (see also Asthma) 493.2 ☑
      - bronchiectasis 494.0
        - with acute exacerbation 494.1
      - bronchitis (chronic) (see also Bronchitis, with, obstruction) 491.20
      - emphysema NEC 492.8
    - due to
      - bronchospasm 519.11 ▲
      - foreign body 934.9
      - inhalation of fumes or vapors 506.9
      - laryngospasm 478.75
- alimentary canal (see also Obstruction, intestine) 560.9
- ampulla of Vater 576.2
  - with calculus, cholelithiasis, or stones — see Choledocholithiasis
- aortic (heart) (valve) (see also Stenosis, aortic) 424.1
  - rheumatic (see also Stenosis, aortic, rheumatic) 395.0
- aortoiliac 444.0
- aqueduct of Sylvius 331.4
  - congenital 742.3
    - with spina bifida (see also Spina bifida) 741.0 ☑
- Arnold-Chiari (see also Spina bifida) 741.0 ☑
- artery (see also Embolism, artery) 444.9
  - basilar (complete) (partial) (see also Occlusion, artery, basilar) 433.0 ☑
  - carotid (complete) (partial) (see also Occlusion, artery, carotid) 433.1 ☑
  - precerebral — see Occlusion, artery, precerebral NEC
  - retinal (central) (see also Occlusion, retina) 362.30
  - vertebral (complete) (partial) (see also Occlusion, artery, vertebral) 433.2 ☑
- asthma (chronic) (with obstructive pulmonary disease) 493.2 ☑
- band (intestinal) 560.81
- bile duct or passage (see also Obstruction, biliary) 576.2
  - congenital 751.61
    - jaundice from 751.61 [774.5]
- biliary (duct) (tract) 576.2
  - with calculus 574.51
    - with cholecystitis (chronic) 574.41
      - acute 574.31
  - congenital 751.61
    - jaundice from 751.61 [774.5]
- gallbladder 575.2
  - with calculus 574.21
    - with cholecystitis (chronic) 574.11
      - acute 574.01
- bladder neck (acquired) 596.0
  - congenital 753.6
- bowel (see also Obstruction, intestine) 560.9
- bronchus 519.19 ▲

Obstruction, obstructed, obstructive — continued
- canal, ear (see also Stricture, ear canal, acquired) 380.50
- cardia 537.89
- caval veins (inferior) (superior) 459.2
- cecum (see also Obstruction, intestine) 560.9
- circulatory 459.9
- colon (see also Obstruction, intestine) 560.9
  - sympathicotonic 560.89
- common duct (see also Obstruction, biliary) 576.2
  - congenital 751.61
- coronary (artery) (heart) (see also Arteriosclerosis, coronary)
  - acute (see also Infarct, myocardium) 410.9 ☑
    - without myocardial infarction 411.81
- cystic duct (see also Obstruction, gallbladder) 575.2
  - congenital 751.61
- device, implant, or graft — see Complications, due to (presence of) any device, implant, or graft classified to 996.0–996.5 NEC
- due to foreign body accidentally left in operation wound 998.4
- duodenum 537.3
  - congenital 751.1
  - due to
    - compression NEC 537.3
    - cyst 537.3
    - intrinsic lesion or disease NEC 537.3
    - scarring 537.3
    - torsion 537.3
    - ulcer 532.91
    - volvulus 537.3
- ejaculatory duct 608.89
- endocardium 424.90
  - arteriosclerotic 424.99
  - specified cause, except rheumatic 424.99
- esophagus 530.3
- eustachian tube (complete) (partial) 381.60
  - cartilaginous
    - extrinsic 381.63
    - intrinsic 381.62
  - due to
    - cholesteatoma 381.61
    - osseous lesion NEC 381.61
    - polyp 381.61
  - osseous 381.61
- fallopian tube (bilateral) 628.2
- fecal 560.39
  - with hernia (see also Hernia, by site, with obstruction)
    - gangrenous — see Hernia, by site, with gangrene
- foramen of Monro (congenital) 742.3
  - with spina bifida (see also Spina bifida) 741.0 ☑
- foreign body — see Foreign body
- gallbladder 575.2
  - with calculus, cholelithiasis, or stones 574.21
    - with cholecystitis (chronic) 574.11
      - acute 574.01
  - congenital 751.69
    - jaundice from 751.69 [774.5]
- gastric outlet 537.0
- gastrointestinal (see also Obstruction, intestine) 560.9
- glottis 478.79
- hepatic 573.8
  - duct (see also Obstruction, biliary) 576.2
    - congenital 751.61
  - icterus (see also Obstruction, biliary) 576.8
    - congenital 751.61

Obstruction, obstructed, obstructive — *continued*
  ileocecal coil (*see also* Obstruction, intestine) 560.9
  ileum (*see also* Obstruction, intestine) 560.9
  iliofemoral (artery) 444.81
  internal anastomosis — *see* Complications, mechanical, graft
  intestine (mechanical) (neurogenic) (paroxysmal) (postinfectional) (reflex) 560.9
    with
      adhesions (intestinal) (peritoneal) 560.81
      hernia (*see also* Hernia, by site, with obstruction)
        gangrenous — *see* Hernia, by site, with gangrene
    adynamic (*see also* Ileus) 560.1
    by gallstone 560.31
    congenital or infantile (small) 751.1
      large 751.2
    due to
      Ascaris lumbricoides 127.0
      mural thickening 560.89
      procedure 997.4
        involving urinary tract 997.5
    impaction 560.39
    infantile — *see* Obstruction, intestine, congenital
    newborn
      due to
        fecaliths 777.1
        inspissated milk 777.2
        meconium (plug) 777.1
          in mucoviscidosis 277.01
        transitory 777.4
    specified cause NEC 560.89
    transitory, newborn 777.4
    volvulus 560.2
  intracardiac ball valve prosthesis 996.02
  jaundice (*see also* Obstruction, biliary) 576.8
    congenital 751.61
  jejunum (*see also* Obstruction, intestine) 560.9
  kidney 593.89
  labor 660.9
    affecting fetus or newborn 763.1
    by
      bony pelvis (conditions classifiable to 653.0–653.9) 660.1
      deep transverse arrest 660.3
      impacted shoulder 660.4
      locked twins 660.5
      malposition (fetus) (conditions classifiable to 652.0–652.9) 660.0
      head during labor 660.3
      persistent occipitoposterior position 660.3
      soft tissue, pelvic (conditions classifiable to 654.0–654.9) 660.2
  lacrimal
    canaliculi 375.53
      congenital 743.65
    punctum 375.52
    sac 375.54
  lacrimonasal duct 375.56
    congenital 743.65
    neonatal 375.55
  lacteal, with steatorrhea 579.2
  laryngitis (*see also* Laryngitis) 464.01
  larynx 478.79
    congenital 748.3
  liver 573.8
    cirrhotic (*see also* Cirrhosis, liver) 571.5
  lung 518.89
    with
      asthma — *see* Asthma
      bronchitis (chronic) 491.20

Obstruction, obstructed, obstructive — *continued*
  lung — *continued*
    with — *continued*
      emphysema NEC 492.8
      airway, chronic 496
      chronic NEC 496
        with
          asthma (chronic) (obstructive) 493.2
      disease, chronic 496
        with
          asthma (chronic) (obstructive) 493.2
      emphysematous 492.8
  lymphatic 457.1
  meconium
    fetus or newborn 777.1
      in mucoviscidosis 277.01
    newborn due to fecaliths 777.1
  mediastinum 519.3
  mitral (rheumatic) — *see* Stenosis, mitral
  nasal 478.19 ▲
    duct 375.56
      neonatal 375.55
    sinus — *see* Sinusitis
  nasolacrimal duct 375.56
    congenital 743.65
    neonatal 375.55
  nasopharynx 478.29
  nose 478.19 ▲
  organ or site, congenital NEC — *see* Atresia
  pancreatic duct 577.8
  parotid gland 527.8
  pelviureteral junction (*see also* Obstruction, ureter) 593.4
  pharynx 478.29
  portal (circulation) (vein) 452
  prostate 600.90
    with
      other lower urinary tract symptoms (LUTS) 600.91 ●
      urinary
        obstruction 600.91 ●
        retention 600.91 ●
    valve (urinary) 596.0
  pulmonary
    valve (heart) (*see also* Endocarditis, pulmonary) 424.3
    vein, isolated 747.49
  pyemic — *see* Septicemia
  pylorus (acquired) 537.0
    congenital 750.5
    infantile 750.5
  rectosigmoid (*see also* Obstruction, intestine) 560.9
  rectum 569.49
  renal 593.89
  respiratory 519.8
    chronic 496
  retinal (artery) (vein) (central) — *see* Occlusion, retina 362.30
  salivary duct (any) 527.8
    with calculus 527.5
  sigmoid (*see also* Obstruction, intestine) 560.9
  sinus (accessory) (nasal) (*see also* Sinusitis) 473.9
  Stensen's duct 527.8
  stomach 537.89
    acute 536.1
    congenital 750.7
  submaxillary gland 527.8
    with calculus 527.5
  thoracic duct 457.1
  thrombotic — *see* Thrombosis
  tooth eruption 520.6
  trachea 519.19 ▲
  tracheostomy airway 519.09
  tricuspid — *see* Endocarditis, tricuspid
  upper respiratory, congenital 748.8
  ureter (functional) 593.4

Obstruction, obstructed, obstructive — *continued*
  ureter — *continued*
    congenital 753.20
    due to calculus 592.1
  ureteropelvic junction, congenital 753.21
  ureterovesical junction, congenital 753.22
  urethra 599.60
    congenital 753.6
  urinary (moderate) 599.60
    organ or tract (lower) 599.60
      due to
        benign prostatic hypertrophy (BPH) - see category 600
      specified NEC 599.69
        due to
          benign prostatic hypertrophy (BPH) — see category 600
    prostatic valve 596.0
  uropathy 599.60
  uterus 621.8
  vagina 623.2
  valvular — *see* Endocarditis
  vascular graft or shunt 996.1
    atherosclerosis — *see* Arteriosclerosis, coronary
    embolism 996.74
    occlusion NEC 996.74
    thrombus 996.74
  vein, venous 459.2
    caval (inferior) (superior) 459.2
    thrombotic — *see* Thrombosis
  vena cava (inferior) (superior) 459.2
  ventricular shunt 996.2
  vesical 596.0
  vesicourethral orifice 596.0
  vessel NEC 459.9
Obturator — *see* condition
Occlusal
  plane deviation 524.76
  wear, teeth 521.10
Occlusion
  anus 569.49
    congenital 751.2
    infantile 751.2
  aortoiliac (chronic) 444.0
  aqueduct of Sylvius 331.4
    congenital 742.3
      with spina bifida (*see also* Spina bifida) 741.0
  arteries of extremities, lower 444.22
    without thrombus or embolus (*see also* Arteriosclerosis, extremities) 440.20
    due to stricture or stenosis 447.1
    upper 444.21
      without thrombus or embolus (*see also* Arteriosclerosis, extremities) 440.20
      due to stricture or stenosis 447.1
  artery NEC (*see also* Embolism, artery) 444.9
    auditory, internal 433.8
    basilar 433.0
      with other precerebral artery 433.3
      bilateral 433.3
    brain or cerebral (*see also* Infarct, brain) 434.9
    carotid 433.1
      with other precerebral artery 433.3
      bilateral 433.3
    cerebellar (anterior inferior) (posterior inferior) (superior) 433.8
    cerebral (*see also* Infarct, brain) 434.9
    choroidal (anterior) 433.8
    communicating posterior 433.8

Occlusion — *continued*
  artery (*see also* Embolism, artery) — *continued*
    coronary (thrombotic) (*see also* Infarct, myocardium) 410.9
      acute 410.9
        without myocardial infarction 411.81
      healed or old 412
    hypophyseal 433.8
    iliac (artery) 444.81
    mesenteric (embolic) (thrombotic) (with gangrene) 557.0
    pontine 433.8
    precerebral NEC 433.9
      late effect — *see* Late effect(s) (of) cerebrovascular disease
      multiple or bilateral 433.3
      puerperal, postpartum, childbirth 674.0
      specified NEC 433.8
    renal 593.81
    retinal — *see* Occlusion, retina, artery
    spinal 433.8
    vertebral 433.2
      with other precerebral artery 433.3
      bilateral 433.3
  basilar (artery) — *see* Occlusion, artery, basilar
  bile duct (any) (*see also* Obstruction, biliary) 576.2
  bowel (*see also* Obstruction, intestine) 560.9
  brain (artery) (vascular) (*see also* Infarct, brain) 434.9
  breast (duct) 611.8
  carotid (artery) (common) (internal) — *see* Occlusion, artery, carotid
  cerebellar (anterior inferior) (artery) (posterior inferior) (superior) 433.8
  cerebral (artery) (*see also* Infarct, brain) 434.9
  cerebrovascular (*see also* Infarct, brain) 434.9
    diffuse 437.0
  cervical canal (*see also* Stricture, cervix) 622.4
    by falciparum malaria 084.0
  cervix (uteri) (*see also* Stricture, cervix) 622.4
  choanal 748.0
  choroidal (artery) 433.8
  colon (*see also* Obstruction, intestine) 560.9
  communicating posterior artery 433.8
  coronary (artery) (thrombotic) (*see also* Infarct, myocardium) 410.9
    without myocardial infarction 411.81
    acute 410.9
      without myocardial infarction 411.81
    healed or old 412
  cystic duct (*see also* Obstruction, gallbladder) 575.2
    congenital 751.69
  disto
    division I 524.22
    division II 524.22
  embolic — *see* Embolism
  fallopian tube 628.2
    congenital 752.19
  gallbladder (*see also* Obstruction, gallbladder) 575.2
    congenital 751.69
      jaundice from 751.69 [774.5]
  gingiva, traumatic 523.8
  hymen 623.3
    congenital 752.42
  hypophyseal (artery) 433.8
  iliac artery 444.81

Occlusion — continued
intestine (see also Obstruction, intestine) 560.9
kidney 593.89
lacrimal apparatus — see Stenosis, lacrimal
lung 518.89
lymph or lymphatic channel 457.1
mammary duct 611.8
mesenteric artery (embolic) (thrombotic) (with gangrene) 557.0
nose 478.1 ☑
  congenital 748.0
organ or site, congenital NEC — see Atresia
oviduct 628.2
  congenital 752.19
periodontal, traumatic 523.8
peripheral arteries (lower extremity) 444.22
  without thrombus or embolus (see also Arteriosclerosis, extremities) 440.20
  due to stricture or stenosis 447.1
  upper extremity 444.21
    without thrombus or embolus (see also Arteriosclerosis, extremities) 440.20
    due to stricture or stenosis 447.1
pontine (artery) 433.8 ☑
posterior lingual, of mandibular teeth 524.29
precerebral artery — see Occlusion, artery, precerebral NEC
puncta lacrimalia 375.52
pupil 364.74
pylorus (see also Stricture, pylorus) 537.0
renal artery 593.81
retina, retinal (vascular) 362.30
  artery, arterial 362.30
    branch 362.32
    central (total) 362.31
    partial 362.33
    transient 362.34
    tributary 362.32
  vein 362.30
    branch 362.36
    central (total) 362.35
    incipient 362.37
    partial 362.37
    tributary 362.36
spinal artery 433.8 ☑
stent
  coronary 996.72
teeth (mandibular) (posterior lingual) 524.29
thoracic duct 457.1
tubal 628.2
ureter (complete) (partial) 593.4
  congenital 753.29
urethra (see also Stricture, urethra) 598.9
  congenital 753.6
uterus 621.8
vagina 623.2
vascular NEC 459.9
vein — see Thrombosis
vena cava (inferior) (superior) 453.2
ventricle (brain) NEC 331.4
vertebral (artery) — see Occlusion, artery, vertebral
vessel (blood) NEC 459.9
vulva 624.8

Occlusio pupillae 364.74
Occupational
problems NEC V62.2
therapy V57.21
Ochlophobia 300.29
Ochronosis (alkaptonuric) (congenital) (endogenous) 270.2
with chloasma of eyelid 270.2
Ocular muscle — see also condition
myopathy 359.1
torticollis 781.93

Oculoauriculovertebral dysplasia 756.0
Oculogyric
crisis or disturbance 378.87
  psychogenic 306.7
Oculomotor syndrome 378.81
Oddi's sphincter spasm 576.5
Odelberg's disease (juvenile osteochondrosis) 732.1
Odontalgia 525.9
Odontoameloblastoma (M9311/0) 213.1
upper jaw (bone) 213.0
Odontoclasia 521.05
Odontoclasis 873.63
complicated 873.73
Odontodysplasia, regional 520.4
Odontogenesis imperfecta 520.5
Odontoma (M9280/0) 213.1
ameloblastic (M9311/0) 213.1
  upper jaw (bone) 213.0
calcified (M9280/0) 213.1
  upper jaw (bone) 213.0
complex (M9282/0) 213.1
  upper jaw (bone) 213.0
compound (M9281/0) 213.1
  upper jaw (bone) 213.0
fibroameloblastic (M9290/0) 213.1
  upper jaw (bone) 213.0
follicular 526.0
  upper jaw (bone) 213.0
Odontomyelitis (closed) (open) 522.0
Odontonecrosis 521.09
Odontorrhagia 525.8
Odontosarcoma, ameloblastic (M9290/3) 170.1
upper jaw (bone) 170.0
Odynophagia 787.2
Oesophagostomiasis 127.7
Oesophagostomum infestation 127.7
Oestriasis 134.0
Ogilvie's syndrome (sympathicotonic colon obstruction) 560.89
Oguchi's disease (retina) 368.61
Ohara's disease — see also Tularemia 021.9
Oidiomycosis — see also Candidiasis 112.9
Oidiomycotic meningitis 112.83
Oidium albicans infection — see also Candidiasis 112.9
Old age 797
dementia (of) 290.0
Olfactory — see condition
Oligemia 285.9
Oligergasia — see also Retardation, mental 319
Oligoamnios 658.0 ☑
affecting fetus or newborn 761.2
Oligoastrocytoma, mixed (M9382/3)
specified site — see Neoplasm, by site, malignant
unspecified site 191.9
Oligocythemia 285.9
Oligodendroblastoma (M9460/3)
specified site — see Neoplasm, by site, malignant
unspecified site 191.9
Oligodendroglioma (M9450/3)
anaplastic type (M9451/3)
  specified site — see Neoplasm, by site, malignant
  unspecified site 191.9
specified site — see Neoplasm, by site, malignant
unspecified site 191.9
Oligodendroma — see Oligodendroglioma
Oligodontia — see also Anodontia 520.0
Oligoencephalon 742.1
Oligohydramnios 658.0 ☑
affecting fetus or newborn 761.2
due to premature rupture of membranes 658.1 ☑
affecting fetus or newborn 761.2
Oligohydrosis 705.0
Oligomenorrhea 626.1

Oligophrenia — see also Retardation, mental 319
phenylpyruvic 270.1
Oligospermia 606.1
Oligotrichia 704.09
congenita 757.4
Oliguria 788.5
with
  abortion — see Abortion, by type, with renal failure
  ectopic pregnancy (see also categories 633.0–633.9) 639.3
  molar pregnancy (see also categories 630–632) 639.3
complicating
  abortion 639.3
  ectopic or molar pregnancy 639.3
  pregnancy 646.2 ☑
    with hypertension — see Toxemia, of pregnancy
  due to a procedure 997.5
  following labor and delivery 669.3 ☑
  heart or cardiac — see Failure, heart
  puerperal, postpartum 669.3 ☑
  specified due to a procedure 997.5
Ollier's disease (chondrodysplasia) 756.4
Omentitis — see also Peritonitis 567.9
Omentocele — see also Hernia, omental 553.8
Omentum, omental — see condition
Omphalitis (congenital) (newborn) 771.4
not of newborn 686.9
tetanus 771.3
Omphalocele 756.79
Omphalomesenteric duct, persistent 751.0
Omphalorrhagia, newborn 772.3
Omsk hemorrhagic fever 065.1
Onanism 307.9
Onchocerciasis 125.3
eye 125.3 [360.13]
Onchocercosis 125.3
Oncocytoma (M8290/0) — see Neoplasm, by site, benign
Ondine's curse 348.8
Oneirophrenia — see also Schizophrenia 295.4
Onychauxis 703.8
congenital 757.5
Onychia (with lymphangitis) 681.9
dermatophytic 110.1
finger 681.02
toe 681.11
Onychitis (with lymphangitis) 681.9
finger 681.02
toe 681.11
Onychocryptosis 703.0
Onychodystrophy 703.8
congenital 757.5
Onychogryphosis 703.8
Onychogryposis 703.8
Onycholysis 703.8
Onychomadesis 703.8
Onychomalacia 703.8
Onychomycosis 110.1
finger 110.1
toe 110.1
Onycho-osteodysplasia 756.89
Onychophagy 307.9
Onychoptosis 703.8
Onychorrhexis 703.8
congenital 757.5
Onychoschizia 703.8
Onychotrophia — see also Atrophy, nail 703.8
O'nyong-nyong fever 066.3
Onyxis (finger) (toe) 703.0
Onyxitis (with lymphangitis) 681.9
finger 681.02
toe 681.11
Oocyte (egg) (ovum)
donor V59.70
  over age 35 V59.73
    anonymous recipient V59.73
    designated recipient V59.74
  under age 35 V59.71

Oocyte — continued
donor — continued
  under age 35 — continued
    anonymous recipient V59.71
    designated recipient V59.72
Oophoritis (cystic) (infectional) (interstitial) — see also Salpingo-oophoritis 614.2
complicating pregnancy 646.6 ☑
fetal (acute) 752.0
gonococcal (acute) 098.19
  chronic or duration of 2 months or over 098.39
tuberculous (see also Tuberculosis) 016.6 ☑
Opacity, opacities
cornea 371.00
  central 371.03
  congenital 743.43
    interfering with vision 743.42
  degenerative (see also Degeneration, cornea) 371.40
  hereditary (see also Dystrophy, cornea) 371.50
  inflammatory (see also Keratitis) 370.9
  late effect of trachoma (healed) 139.1
  minor 371.01
  peripheral 371.02
enamel (fluoride) (nonfluoride) (teeth) 520.3
lens (see also Cataract) 366.9
snowball 379.22
vitreous (humor) 379.24
  congenital 743.51
Opalescent dentin (hereditary) 520.5
Open, opening
abnormal, organ or site, congenital — see Imperfect, closure
angle with
  borderline intraocular pressure 365.01
  cupping of discs 365.01
bite (anterior) (posterior) 524.29
false — see Imperfect, closure
margin on tooth restoration 525.61 ●
restoration margins 525.61 ●
wound — see Wound, open, by site
Operation
causing mutilation of fetus 763.89
destructive, on live fetus, to facilitate birth 763.89
for delivery, fetus or newborn 763.89
maternal, unrelated to current delivery, affecting fetus or newborn 760.6
Operational fatigue 300.89
Operative — see condition
Operculitis (chronic) 523.40 ▲
acute 523.30 ▲
Operculum, retina 361.32
with detachment 361.01
Ophiasis 704.01
Ophthalmia — see also Conjunctivitis 372.30
actinic rays 370.24
allergic (acute) 372.05
  chronic 372.14
blennorrhagic (neonatorum) 098.40
catarrhal 372.03
diphtheritic 032.81
Egyptian 076.1
electric, electrica 370.24
gonococcal (neonatorum) 098.40
metastatic 360.11
migraine 346.8 ☑
neonatorum, newborn 771.6
  gonococcal 098.40
nodosa 360.14
phlyctenular 370.31
  with ulcer (see also Ulcer, cornea) 370.00
sympathetic 360.11
Ophthalmitis — see Ophthalmia
Ophthalmocele (congenital) 743.66

Ophthalmoneuromyelitis

Ophthalmoneuromyelitis 341.0
Ophthalmopathy, infiltrative with thyrotoxicosis 242.0 ☑
Ophthalmoplegia — see also Strabismus 378.9
  anterior internuclear 378.86
  ataxia-areflexia syndrome 357.0
  bilateral 378.9
  diabetic 250.5 ☑ *[378.86]*
  exophthalmic 242.0 ☑ *[376.22]*
  external 378.55
    progressive 378.72
    total 378.56
  internal (complete) (total) 367.52
  internuclear 378.86
  migraine 346.8 ☑
  painful 378.55
  Parinaud's 378.81
  progressive external 378.72
  supranuclear, progressive 333.0
  total (external) 378.56
    internal 367.52
  unilateral 378.9
Opisthognathism 524.00
Opisthorchiasis (felineus) (tenuicollis) (viverrini) 121.0
Opisthotonos, opisthotonus 781.0
Opitz's disease (congestive splenomegaly) 289.51
Opiumism — see also Dependence 304.0 ☑
Oppenheim's disease 358.8
Oppenheim-Urbach disease or syndrome (necrobiosis lipoidica diabeticorum) 250.8 ☑ *[709.3]*
Opsoclonia 379.59
Optic nerve — see condition
Orbit — see condition
Orchioblastoma (M9071/3) 186.9
Orchitis (nonspecific) (septic) 604.90
  with abscess 604.0
  blennorrhagic (acute) 098.13
    chronic or duration of 2 months or over 098.33
  diphtheritic 032.89 *[604.91]*
  filarial 125.9 *[604.91]*
  gangrenous 604.99
  gonococcal (acute) 098.13
    chronic or duration of 2 months or over 098.33
  mumps 072.0
  parotidea 072.0
  suppurative 604.99
  syphilitic 095.8 *[604.91]*
  tuberculous (see also Tuberculosis) 016.5 ☑ *[608.81]*
Orf 051.2
Organic — see also condition
  heart — see Disease, heart
  insufficiency 799.89
Oriental
  bilharziasis 120.2
  schistosomiasis 120.2
  sore 085.1
Orientation
  ego-dystonic sexual 302.0
Orifice — see condition
Origin, both great vessels from right ventricle 745.11
Ormond's disease or syndrome 593.4
Ornithosis 073.9
  with
    complication 073.8
      specified NEC 073.7
    pneumonia 073.0
    pneumonitis (lobular) 073.0
Orodigitofacial dysostosis 759.89
Oropouche fever 066.3
Orotaciduria, oroticaciduria (congenital) (hereditary) (pyrimidine deficiency) 281.4
Oroya fever 088.0
Orthodontics V58.5
  adjustment V53.4
  aftercare V58.5
  fitting V53.4

Orthopnea 786.02
Orthoptic training V57.4
Osgood-Schlatter
  disease 732.4
  osteochondrosis 732.4
Osler's
  disease (M9950/1) (polycythemia vera) 238.4
  nodes 421.0
Osler-Rendu disease (familial hemorrhagic telangiectasia) 448.0
Osler-Vaquez disease (M9950/1) (polycythemia vera) 238.4
Osler-Weber-Rendu syndrome (familial hemorrhagic telangiectasia) 448.0
Osmidrosis 705.89
Osseous — see condition
Ossification
  artery — see Arteriosclerosis
  auricle (ear) 380.39
  bronchus 519.19 ▲
  cardiac (see also Degeneration, myocardial) 429.1
  cartilage (senile) 733.99
  coronary (artery) — see Arteriosclerosis, coronary
  diaphragm 728.10
  ear 380.39
    middle (see also Otosclerosis) 387.9
  falx cerebri 349.2
  fascia 728.10
  fontanel
    defective or delayed 756.0
    premature 756.0
  heart (see also Degeneration, myocardial) 429.1
    valve — see Endocarditis
  larynx 478.79
  ligament
    posterior longitudinal 724.8
      cervical 723.7
  meninges (cerebral) 349.2
    spinal 336.8
  multiple, eccentric centers 733.99
  muscle 728.10
    heterotopic, postoperative 728.13
  myocardial, myocardium (see also Degeneration, myocardial) 429.1
  penis 607.81
  periarticular 728.89
  sclera 379.16
  tendon 727.82
  trachea 519.19 ▲
  tympanic membrane (see also Tympanosclerosis) 385.00
  vitreous (humor) 360.44
Osteitis — see also Osteomyelitis 730.2 ☑
  acute 730.0 ☑
  alveolar 526.5
  chronic 730.1 ☑
  condensans (ilii) 733.5
  deformans (Paget's) 731.0
    due to or associated with malignant neoplasm (see also Neoplasm, bone, malignant) 170.9 *[731.1]*
  due to yaws 102.6
  fibrosa NEC 733.29
    cystica (generalisata) 252.01
    disseminata 756.59
    osteoplastica 252.01
  fragilitans 756.51
  Garré's (sclerosing) 730.1 ☑
  infectious (acute) (subacute) 730.0 ☑
    chronic or old 730.1 ☑
  jaw (acute) (chronic) (lower) (neonatal) (suppurative) (upper) 526.4
  parathyroid 252.01
  petrous bone (see also Petrositis) 383.20
  pubis 733.5
  sclerotic, nonsuppurative 730.1 ☑
  syphilitic 095.5
  tuberculosa
    cystica (of Jüngling) 135

Osteitis — see also Osteomyelitis — continued
  tuberculosa — continued
    multiplex cystoides 135
Osteoarthritica spondylitis (spine) — see also Spondylosis 721.90
Osteoarthritis — see also Osteoarthrosis 715.9 ☑
  distal interphalangeal 715.9 ☑
  hyperplastic 731.2
  interspinalis (see also Spondylosis) 721.90
  spine, spinal NEC (see also Spondylosis) 721.90
Osteoarthropathy — see also Osteoarthrosis 715.9 ☑
  chronic idiopathic hypertrophic 757.39
  familial idiopathic 757.39
  hypertrophic pulmonary 731.2
    secondary 731.2
  idiopathic hypertrophic 757.39
  primary hypertrophic 731.2
  pulmonary hypertrophic 731.2
    secondary hypertrophic 731.2
Osteoarthrosis (degenerative) (hypertrophic) (rheumatoid) 715.9 ☑

Note — Use the following fifth-digit subclassification with category 715:

0	site unspecified
1	shoulder region
2	upper arm
3	forearm
4	hand
5	pelvic region and thigh
6	lower leg
7	ankle and foot
8	other specified sites except spine
9	multiple sites

  Deformans alkaptonurica 270.2
  generalized 715.09
  juvenilis (Köhler's) 732.5
  localized 715.3 ☑
    idiopathic 715.1 ☑
    primary 715.1 ☑
    secondary 715.2 ☑
  multiple sites, not specified as generalized 715.89
  polyarticular 715.09
  spine (see also Spondylosis) 721.90
  temporomandibular joint 524.69
Osteoblastoma (M9200/0) — see Neoplasm, bone, benign
Osteochondritis — see also Osteochondrosis 732.9
  dissecans 732.7
    hip 732.7
  ischiopubica 732.1
  multiple 756.59
  syphilitic (congenital) 090.0
Osteochondrodermodysplasia 756.59
Osteochondrodystrophy 277.5
  deformans 277.5
  familial 277.5
  fetalis 756.4
Osteochondrolysis 732.7
Osteochondroma (M9210/0) — see also Neoplasm, bone, benign
  multiple, congenital 756.4
Osteochondromatosis (M9210/1) 238.0
  synovial 727.82
Osteochondromyxosarcoma (M9180/3) — see Neoplasm, bone, malignant
Osteochondropathy NEC 732.9
Osteochondrosarcoma (M9180/3) — see Neoplasm, bone, malignant
Osteochondrosis 732.9
  acetabulum 732.1
  adult spine 732.8
  astragalus 732.5
  Blount's 732.4

Osteochondrosis — continued
  Buchanan's (juvenile osteochondrosis of iliac crest) 732.1
  Buchman's (juvenile osteochondrosis) 732.1
  Burns' 732.3
  calcaneus 732.5
  capitular epiphysis (femur) 732.1
  carpal
    lunate (wrist) 732.3
    scaphoid 732.3
  coxae juvenilis 732.1
  deformans juvenilis (coxae) (hip) 732.1
    Scheuermann's 732.0
    spine 732.0
    tibia 732.4
    vertebra 732.0
  Diaz's (astragalus) 732.5
  dissecans (knee) (shoulder) 732.7
  femoral capital epiphysis 732.1
  femur (head) (juvenile) 732.1
  foot (juvenile) 732.5
  Freiberg's (disease) (second metatarsal) 732.5
  Haas' 732.3
  Haglund's (os tibiale externum) 732.5
  hand (juvenile) 732.3
  head of
    femur 732.1
    humerus (juvenile) 732.3
  hip (juvenile) 732.1
  humerus (juvenile) 732.3
  iliac crest (juvenile) 732.1
  ilium (juvenile) 732.1
  ischiopubic synchondrosis 732.1
  Iselin's (osteochondrosis fifth metatarsal) 732.5
  juvenile, juvenilis 732.6
    arm 732.3
    capital femoral epiphysis 732.1
    capitellum humeri 732.3
    capitular epiphysis 732.1
    carpal scaphoid 732.3
    clavicle, sternal epiphysis 732.6
    coxae 732.1
    deformans 732.1
    foot 732.5
    hand 732.3
    hip and pelvis 732.1
    lower extremity, except foot 732.4
    lunate, wrist 732.3
    medial cuneiform bone 732.5
    metatarsal (head) 732.5
    metatarsophalangeal 732.5
    navicular, ankle 732.5
    patella 732.4
    primary patellar center (of Köhler) 732.4
    specified site NEC 732.6
    spine 732.0
    tarsal scaphoid 732.5
    tibia (epiphysis) (tuberosity) 732.4
    upper extremity 732.3
    vertebra (body) (Calvé) 732.0
      epiphyseal plates (of Scheuermann) 732.0
  Kienböck's (disease) 732.3
  Köhler's (disease) (navicular, ankle) 732.5
    patellar 732.4
    tarsal navicular 732.5
  Legg-Calvé-Perthes (disease) 732.1
  lower extremity (juvenile) 732.4
  lunate bone 732.3
  Mauclaire's 732.3
  metacarpal heads (of Mauclaire) 732.3
  metatarsal (fifth) (head) (second) 732.5
  navicular, ankle 732.5
  os calcis 732.5
  Osgood-Schlatter 732.4
  os tibiale externum 732.5
  Panner's 732.3
  patella (juvenile) 732.4
  patellar center
    primary (of Köhler) 732.4

Index to Diseases

Osteochondrosis — *continued*
  patellar center — *continued*
    secondary (of Sinding-Larsen) 732.4
  pelvis (juvenile) 732.1
  Pierson's 732.1
  radial head (juvenile) 732.3
  Scheuermann's 732.0
  Sever's (calcaneum) 732.5
  Sinding-Larsen (secondary patellar center) 732.4
  spine (juvenile) 732.0
    adult 732.8
  symphysis pubis (of Pierson) (juvenile) 732.1
  syphilitic (congenital) 090.0
  tarsal (navicular) (scaphoid) 732.5
  tibia (proximal) (tubercle) 732.4
  tuberculous — *see* Tuberculosis, bone
  ulna 732.3
  upper extremity (juvenile) 732.3
  van Neck's (juvenile osteochondrosis) 732.1
  vertebral (juvenile) 732.0
    adult 732.8
Osteoclastoma (M9250/1) 238.0
  malignant (M9250/3) — *see* Neoplasm, bone, malignant
Osteocopic pain 733.90
Osteodynia 733.90
Osteodystrophy
  azotemic 588.0
  chronica deformans hypertrophica 731.0
  congenital 756.50
    specified type NEC 756.59
  deformans 731.0
  fibrosa localisata 731.0
  parathyroid 252.01
  renal 588.0
Osteofibroma (M9262/0) — *see* Neoplasm, bone, benign
Osteofibrosarcoma (M9182/3) — *see* Neoplasm, bone, malignant
Osteogenesis imperfecta 756.51
Osteogenic — *see* condition
Osteoma (M9180/0) — *see also* Neoplasm, bone, benign
  osteoid (M9191/0) (*see also* Neoplasm, bone, benign)
    giant (M9200/0) — *see* Neoplasm, bone, benign
Osteomalacia 268.2
  chronica deformans hypertrophica 731.0
  due to vitamin D deficiency 268.2
  infantile (*see also* Rickets) 268.0
  juvenile (*see also* Rickets) 268.0
  pelvis 268.2
  vitamin D-resistant 275.3
Osteomalacic bone 268.2
Osteomalacosis 268.2
Osteomyelitis (general) (infective) (localized) (neonatal) (purulent) (pyogenic) (septic) (staphylococcal) (streptococcal) (suppurative) (with periostitis) 730.2 ☑

Note — Use the following fifth-digit subclassification with category 730:

0   site unspecified
1   shoulder region
2   upper arm
3   forearm
4   hand
5   pelvic region and thigh
6   lower leg
7   ankle and foot
8   other specified sites
9   multiple sites

---
  acute or subacute 730.0 ☑
  chronic or old 730.1 ☑

Osteomyelitis — *continued*
  due to or associated with
    diabetes mellitus 250.8 ☑ *[731.8]*
    tuberculosis (*see also* Tuberculosis, bone) 015.9 ☑ *[730.8]* ☑
    limb bones 015.5 ☑ *[730.8]* ☑
    specified bones NEC 015.7 ☑ *[730.8]* ☑
    spine 015.0 ☑ *[730.8]* ☑
    typhoid 002.0 *[730.8]* ☑
  Garré's 730.1 ☑
  jaw (acute) (chronic) (lower) (neonatal) (suppurative) (upper) 526.4
  nonsuppurating 730.1 ☑
  orbital 376.03
  petrous bone (*see also* Petrositis) 383.20
  Salmonella 003.24
  sclerosing, nonsuppurative 730.1 ☑
  sicca 730.1 ☑
  syphilitic 095.5
    congenital 090.0 *[730.8]* ☑
  tuberculous — *see* Tuberculosis, bone
  typhoid 002.0 *[730.8]* ☑
Osteomyelofibrosis 289.89
Osteomyelosclerosis 289.89
Osteonecrosis 733.40
  meaning osteomyelitis 730.1 ☑
Osteo-onycho-arthro dysplasia 756.89
Osteo-onychodysplasia, hereditary 756.89
Osteopathia
  condensans disseminata 756.53
  hyperostotica multiplex infantilis 756.59
  hypertrophica toxica 731.2
  striata 756.4
Osteopathy resulting from poliomyelitis — *see also* Poliomyelitis 045.9 ☑ *[730.7]* ☑
  familial dysplastic 731.2
Osteopecilia 756.53
Osteopenia 733.90
Osteoperiostitis — *see also* Osteomyelitis 730.2 ☑
  ossificans toxica 731.2
  toxica ossificans 731.2
Osteopetrosis (familial) 756.52
Osteophyte — *see* Exostosis
Osteophytosis — *see* Exostosis
Osteopoikilosis 756.53
Osteoporosis (generalized) 733.00
  circumscripta 731.0
  disuse 733.03
  drug-induced 733.09
  idiopathic 733.02
  postmenopausal 733.01
  posttraumatic 733.7
  screening V82.81
  senile 733.01
  specified type NEC 733.09
Osteoporosis-osteomalacia syndrome 268.2
Osteopsathyrosis 756.51
Osteoradionecrosis, jaw 526.89
Osteosarcoma (M9180/3) — *see also* Neoplasm, bone, malignant
  chondroblastic (M9181/3) — *see* Neoplasm, bone, malignant
  fibroblastic (M9182/3) — *see* Neoplasm, bone, malignant
  in Paget's disease of bone (M9184/3) — *see* Neoplasm, bone, malignant
  juxtacortical (M9190/3) — *see* Neoplasm, bone, malignant
  parosteal (M9190/3) — *see* Neoplasm, bone, malignant
  telangiectatic (M9183/3) — *see* Neoplasm, bone, malignant
Osteosclerosis 756.52
  fragilis (generalisata) 756.52
Osteosclerotic anemia 289.89
Osteosis
  acromegaloid 757.39
  cutis 709.3

Osteosis — *continued*
  parathyroid 252.01
  renal fibrocystic 588.0
Österreicher-Turner syndrome 756.89
Ostium
  atrioventriculare commune 745.69
  primum (arteriosum) (defect) (persistent) 745.61
  secundum (arteriosum) (defect) (patent) (persistent) 745.5
Ostrum-Furst syndrome 756.59
Os, uterus — *see* condition
Otalgia 388.70
  otogenic 388.71
  referred 388.72
Othematoma 380.31
Otitic hydrocephalus 348.2
Otitis 382.9
  with effusion 381.4
    purulent 382.4
    secretory 381.4
    serous 381.4
    suppurative 382.4
  acute 382.9
  adhesive (*see also* Adhesions, middle ear) 385.10
  chronic 382.9
    with effusion 381.3
      mucoid, mucous (simple) 381.20
      purulent 382.3
      secretory 381.3
      serous 381.10
      suppurative 382.3
  diffuse parasitic 136.8
  externa (acute) (diffuse) (hemorrhagica) 380.10
    actinic 380.22
    candidal 112.82
    chemical 380.22
    chronic 380.23
      mycotic — *see* Otitis, externa, mycotic
      specified type NEC 380.23
    circumscribed 380.10
    contact 380.22
    due to
      erysipelas 035 *[380.13]*
      impetigo 684 *[380.13]*
      seborrheic dermatitis 690.10 *[380.13]*
    eczematoid 380.22
    furuncular 680.0 *[380.13]*
    infective 380.10
      chronic 380.16
    malignant 380.14
    mycotic (chronic) 380.15
      due to
        aspergillosis 117.3 *[380.15]*
        moniliasis 112.82
        otomycosis 111.8 *[380.15]*
    reactive 380.22
    specified type NEC 380.22
    tropical 111.8 *[380.15]*
  insidiosa (*see also* Otosclerosis) 387.9
  interna (*see also* Labyrinthitis) 386.30
  media (hemorrhagic) (staphylococcal) (streptococcal) 382.9
    acute 382.9
      with effusion 381.00
        allergic 381.04
          mucoid 381.05
          sanguineous 381.06
          serous 381.04
      catarrhal 381.00
      exudative 381.00
      mucoid 381.02
        allergic 381.05
      necrotizing 382.00
        with spontaneous rupture of ear drum 382.01
      in
        influenza 487.8 *[382.02]*
        measles 055.2
        scarlet fever 034.1 *[382.02]*
      nonsuppurative 381.00

Otitis — *continued*
  media — *continued*
    acute — *continued*
      purulent 382.00
        with spontaneous rupture of ear drum 382.01
      sanguineous 381.03
        allergic 381.06
      secretory 381.01
      seromucinous 381.02
      serous 381.01
        allergic 381.04
      suppurative 382.00
        with spontaneous rupture of ear drum 382.01
        due to
          influenza 487.8 *[382.02]*
          scarlet fever 034.1 *[382.02]*
      transudative 381.00
    adhesive (*see also* Adhesions, middle ear) 385.10
    allergic 381.4
      acute 381.04
        mucoid 381.05
        sanguineous 381.06
        serous 381.04
      chronic 381.3
    catarrhal 381.4
      acute 381.00
      chronic (simple) 381.10
    chronic 382.9
      with effusion 381.3
      adhesive (*see also* Adhesions, middle ear) 385.10
      allergic 381.3
      atticoantral, suppurative (with posterior or superior marginal perforation of ear drum) 382.2
      benign suppurative (with anterior or posterior perforation of ear drum) 382.1
      catarrhal 381.10
      exudative 381.3
      mucinous 381.20
      mucoid, mucous (simple) 381.20
      mucosanguineous 381.29
      nonsuppurative 381.3
      purulent 382.3
      secretory 381.3
      seromucinous 381.3
      serosanguineous 381.19
      serous (simple) 381.10
      suppurative 382.3
        atticoantral (with posterior or superior marginal perforation of ear drum) 382.2
        benign (with anterior perforation of ear drum) 382.1
        tuberculous (*see also* Tuberculosis) 017.4 ☑
      tubotympanic 382.1
      transudative 381.3
    exudative 381.4
      acute 381.00
      chronic 381.3
    fibrotic (*see also* Adhesions, middle ear) 385.10
    mucoid, mucous 381.4
      acute 381.02
      chronic (simple) 381.20
    mucosanguineous, chronic 381.29
    nonsuppurative 381.4
      acute 381.00
      chronic 381.3
    postmeasles 055.2
    purulent 382.4
      acute 382.00
        with spontaneous rupture of ear drum 382.01
      chronic 382.3
    sanguineous, acute 381.03
      allergic 381.06

Otitis

Otitis — *continued*
  media — *continued*
    secretory 381.4
      acute or subacute 381.01
      chronic 381.3
    seromucinous 381.4
      acute or subacute 381.02
      chronic 381.3
    serosanguineous, chronic 381.19
    serous 381.4
      acute or subacute 381.01
      chronic (simple) 381.10
    subacute — *see* Otitis, media, acute
    suppurative 382.4
      acute 382.00
        with spontaneous rupture of ear drum 382.01
      chronic 382.3
        atticoantral 382.2
        benign 382.1
        tuberculous (*see also* Tuberculosis) 017.4 ☑
        tubotympanic 382.1
    transudative 381.4
      acute 381.00
      chronic 381.3
    tuberculous (*see also* Tuberculosis) 017.4 ☑
  postmeasles 055.2
Otoconia 386.8
Otolith syndrome 386.19
Otomycosis 111.8 *[380.15]*
  in
    aspergillosis 117.3 *[380.15]*
    moniliasis 112.82
Otopathy 388.9
Otoporosis — *see also* Otosclerosis 387.9
Otorrhagia 388.69
  traumatic — *see* nature of injury
Otorrhea 388.60
  blood 388.69
  cerebrospinal (fluid) 388.61
Otosclerosis (general) 387.9
  cochlear (endosteal) 387.2
  involving
    otic capsule 387.2
    oval window
      nonobliterative 387.0
      obliterative 387.1
    round window 387.2
  nonobliterative 387.0
  obliterative 387.1
  specified type NEC 387.8
Otospongiosis — *see also* Otosclerosis 387.9
Otto's disease or pelvis 715.35
Outburst, aggressive — *see also* Disturbance, conduct 312.0
  in children or adolescents 313.9
Outcome of delivery
  multiple birth NEC V27.9
    all liveborn V27.5
    all stillborn V27.7
    some liveborn V27.6
    unspecified V27.9
  single V27.9
    liveborn V27.0
    stillborn V27.1
  twins V27.9
    both liveborn V27.2
    both stillborn V27.4
    one liveborn, one stillborn V27.3
Outlet — *see also* condition
  syndrome (thoracic) 353.0
Outstanding ears (bilateral) 744.29
Ovalocytosis (congenital) (hereditary) — *see also* Elliptocytosis 282.1
Ovarian — *see also* condition
  pregnancy — *see* Pregnancy, ovarian
  remnant syndrome 620.8
  vein syndrome 593.4
Ovaritis (cystic) — *see also* Salpingo-oophoritis 614.2
Ovary, ovarian — *see* condition
Overactive — *see also* Hyperfunction

Overactive — *see also* Hyperfunction — *continued*
  bladder 596.51
  eye muscle (*see also* Strabismus) 378.9
  hypothalamus 253.8
  thyroid (*see also* Thyrotoxicosis) 242.9 ☑
Overactivity, child 314.01
Overbite (deep) (excessive) (horizontal) (vertical) 524.29
Overbreathing — *see also* Hyperventilation 786.01
Overconscientious personality 301.4
Overdevelopment — *see also* Hypertrophy
  breast (female) (male) 611.1
  nasal bones 738.0
  prostate, congenital 752.89
Overdistention — *see* Distention
Overdose overdosage (drug) 977.9
  specified drug or substance — *see* Table of Drugs and Chemicals
Overeating 783.6
  nonorganic origin 307.51
Overexertion (effects) (exhaustion) 994.5
Overexposure (effects) 994.9
  exhaustion 994.4
Overfeeding — *see also* Overeating 783.6
Overfill, endodontic 526.62
Overgrowth, bone NEC 733.99
Overhanging
  tooth restoration 525.62
  unrepairable, dental restorative materials 525.62
Overheated (effects) (places) — *see* Heat
Overinhibited child 313.0
Overjet 524.29
  excessive horizontal 524.26
Overlaid, overlying (suffocation) 994.7
Overlap
  excessive horizontal 524.26
Overlapping toe (acquired) 735.8
  congenital (fifth toe) 755.66
Overload
  fluid 276.6
  potassium (K) 276.7
  sodium (Na) 276.0
Overnutrition — *see also* Hyperalimentation 783.6
Overproduction — *see also* Hypersecretion
  ACTH 255.3
  cortisol 255.0
  growth hormone 253.0
  thyroid-stimulating hormone (TSH) 242.8 ☑
Overriding
  aorta 747.21
  finger (acquired) 736.29
    congenital 755.59
  toe (acquired) 735.8
    congenital 755.66
Oversize
  fetus (weight of 4500 grams or more) 766.0
    affecting management of pregnancy 656.6 ☑
    causing disproportion 653.5 ☑
      with obstructed labor 660.1 ☑
      affecting fetus or newborn 763.1
Overstimulation, ovarian 256.1
Overstrained 780.79
  heart — *see* Hypertrophy, cardiac
Overweight — *see also* Obesity 278.00
Overwork 780.79
Oviduct — *see* condition
Ovotestis 752.7
Ovulation (cycle)
  failure or lack of 628.0
  pain 625.2
Ovum
  blighted 631
  donor V59.70
    over age 35 V59.73
      anonymous recipient V59.73

Ovum — *continued*
  donor — *continued*
    over age 35 — *continued*
      designated recipient V59.74
    under age 35 V59.71
      anonymous recipient V59.71
      designated recipient V59.72
  dropsical 631
  pathologic 631
Owren's disease or syndrome (parahemophilia) — *see also* Defect, coagulation 286.3
Oxalosis 271.8
Oxaluria 271.8
Ox heart — *see* Hypertrophy, cardiac
OX syndrome 758.6
Oxycephaly, oxycephalic 756.0
  syphilitic, congenital 090.0
Oxyuriasis 127.4
Oxyuris vermicularis (infestation) 127.4
Ozena 472.0

P

Pacemaker syndrome 429.4
Pachyderma, pachydermia 701.8
  laryngis 478.5
  laryngitis 478.79
  larynx (verrucosa) 478.79
Pachydermatitis 701.8
Pachydermatocele (congenital) 757.39
  acquired 701.8
Pachydermatosis 701.8
Pachydermoperiostitis
  secondary 731.2
Pachydermoperiostosis
  primary idiopathic 757.39
  secondary 731.2
Pachymeningitis (adhesive) (basal) (brain) (cerebral) (cervical) (chronic) (circumscribed) (external) (fibrous) (hemorrhagic) (hypertrophic) (internal) (purulent) (spinal) (suppurative) — *see also* Meningitis 322.9
  gonococcal 098.82
Pachyonychia (congenital) 757.5
  acquired 703.8
Pachyperiosteodermia
  primary or idiopathic 757.39
  secondary 731.2
Pachyperiostosis
  primary or idiopathic 757.39
  secondary 731.2
Pacinian tumor (M9507/0) — *see* Neoplasm, skin, benign
Pads, knuckle or Garrod's 728.79
Paget's disease (osteitis deformans) 731.0
  with infiltrating duct carcinoma of the breast (M8541/3) — *see* Neoplasm, breast, malignant
  bone 731.0
    osteosarcoma in (M9184/3) — *see* Neoplasm, bone, malignant
  breast (M8540/3) 174.0
  extramammary (M8542/3) (*see also* Neoplasm, skin, malignant)
    anus 154.3
    skin 173.5
  malignant (M8540/3)
    breast 174.0
    specified site NEC (M8542/3) — *see* Neoplasm, skin, malignant
    unspecified site 174.0
  mammary (M8540/3) 174.0
  necrosis of bone 731.0
  nipple (M8540/3) 174.0
  osteitis deformans 731.0
Paget-Schroetter syndrome (intermittent venous claudication) 453.8
Pain(s) 780.96
  abdominal 789.0 ☑
  acute 338.19
    due to trauma 338.11
    postoperative 338.18
      post-thoracotomy 338.12

Pain(s) — *continued*
  adnexa (uteri) 625.9
  alimentary, due to vascular insufficiency 557.9
  anginoid (*see also* Pain, precordial) 786.51
  anus 569.42
  arch 729.5
  arm 729.5
  axillary 729.5
  back (postural) 724.5
    low 724.2
      psychogenic 307.89
  bile duct 576.9
  bladder 788.9
  bone 733.90
  breast 611.71
    psychogenic 307.89
  broad ligament 625.9
  cancer associated 338.3
  cartilage NEC 733.90
  cecum 789.0 ☑
  cervicobrachial 723.3
  chest (central) 786.50
    atypical 786.59
    midsternal 786.51
    musculoskeletal 786.59
    noncardiac 786.59
    substernal 786.51
    wall (anterior) 786.52
  chronic 338.29
    associated with significant psychosocial dysfunction 338.4
    due to trauma 338.21
    postoperative 338.28
      post-thoracotomy 338.22
    syndrome 338.4
  coccyx 724.79
  colon 789.0 ☑
  common duct 576.9
  coronary — *see* Angina
  costochondral 786.52
  diaphragm 786.52
  due to (presence of) any device, implant, or graft classifiable to 996.0–996.5 — *see* Complications, due to (presence of) any device, implant, or graft classified to 996.0–996.5 NEC
    malignancy (primary) (secondary) 338.3
  ear (*see also* Otalgia) 388.70
  epigastric, epigastrium 789.06
  extremity (lower) (upper) 729.5
  eye 379.91
  face, facial 784.0
    atypical 350.2
    nerve 351.8
  false (labor) 644.1 ☑
  female genital organ NEC 625.9
    psychogenic 307.89
  finger 729.5
  flank 789.0 ☑
  foot 729.5
  gallbladder 575.9
  gas (intestinal) 787.3
  gastric 536.8
  generalized 780.96
  genital organ
    female 625.9
    male 608.9
    psychogenic 307.89
  groin 789.0 ☑
  growing 781.99
  hand 729.5
  head (*see also* Headache) 784.0
  heart (*see also* Pain, precordial) 786.51
  infraorbital (*see also* Neuralgia, trigeminal) 350.1
  intermenstrual 625.2
  jaw 526.9
  joint 719.40
    ankle 719.47
    elbow 719.42

Pain(s) — continued
  joint — continued
    foot 719.47
    hand 719.44
    hip 719.45
    knee 719.46
    multiple sites 719.49
    pelvic region 719.45
    psychogenic 307.89
    shoulder (region) 719.41
    specified site NEC 719.48
    wrist 719.43
  kidney 788.0
  labor, false or spurious 644.1 ☑
  laryngeal 784.1
  leg 729.5
  limb 729.5
  low back 724.2
  lumbar region 724.2
  mastoid (see also Otalgia) 388.70
  maxilla 526.9
  metacarpophalangeal (joint) 719.44
  metatarsophalangeal (joint) 719.47
  mouth 528.9
  muscle 729.1
    intercostal 786.59
  musculoskeletal (see also Pain, by site) 729.1 ●
  nasal 478.19 ▲
  nasopharynx 478.29
  neck NEC 723.1
    psychogenic 307.89
  neoplasm related (acute) (chronic) 338.3 ●
  nerve NEC 729.2
  neuromuscular 729.1
  nose 478.19 ▲
  ocular 379.91
  ophthalmic 379.91
  orbital region 379.91
  osteocopic 733.90
  ovary 625.9
    psychogenic 307.89
  over heart (see also Pain, precordial) 786.51
  ovulation 625.2
  pelvic (female) 625.9
    male NEC 789.0 ☑
      psychogenic 307.89
    psychogenic 307.89
  penis 607.9
    psychogenic 307.89
  pericardial (see also Pain, precordial) 786.51
  perineum
    female 625.9
    male 608.9
  pharynx 478.29
  pleura, pleural, pleuritic 786.52
  postoperative 338.18
    acute 338.18
    chronic 338.28
  post-thoracotomy 338.12
    acute 338.12
    chronic 338.22
  preauricular 388.70
  precordial (region) 786.51
    psychogenic 307.89
  psychogenic 307.80
    cardiovascular system 307.89
    gastrointestinal system 307.89
    genitourinary system 307.89
    heart 307.89
    musculoskeletal system 307.89
    respiratory system 307.89
    skin 306.3
  radicular (spinal) (see also Radiculitis) 729.2
  rectum 569.42
  respiration 786.52
  retrosternal 786.51
  rheumatic NEC 729.0
    muscular 729.1
  rib 786.50
  root (spinal) (see also Radiculitis) 729.2

Pain(s) — continued
  round ligament (stretch) 625.9
  sacroiliac 724.6
  sciatic 724.3
  scrotum 608.9
    psychogenic 307.89
  seminal vesicle 608.9
  sinus 478.19 ▲
  skin 782.0
  spermatic cord 608.9
  spinal root (see also Radiculitis) 729.2
  stomach 536.8
    psychogenic 307.89
  substernal 786.51
  temporomandibular (joint) 524.62
  temporomaxillary joint 524.62
  testis 608.9
    psychogenic 307.89
  thoracic spine 724.1
    with radicular and visceral pain 724.4
  throat 784.1
  tibia 733.90
  toe 729.5
  tongue 529.6
  tooth 525.9
  trigeminal (see also Neuralgia, trigeminal) 350.1
  tumor associated 338.3 ●
  umbilicus 789.05
  ureter 788.0
  urinary (organ) (system) 788.0
  uterus 625.9
    psychogenic 307.89
  vagina 625.9
  vertebrogenic (syndrome) 724.5
  vesical 788.9
  vulva 625.9
  xiphoid 733.90
Painful — see also Pain
  arc syndrome 726.19
  coitus
    female 625.0
    male 608.89
      psychogenic 302.76
  ejaculation (semen) 608.89
    psychogenic 302.79
  erection 607.3
  feet syndrome 266.2
  menstruation 625.3
    psychogenic 306.52
  micturition 788.1
  ophthalmoplegia 378.55
  respiration 786.52
  scar NEC 709.2
  urination 788.1
  wire sutures 998.89
Painters' colic 984.9
  specified type of lead — see Table of Drugs and Chemicals
Palate — see condition
Palatoplegia 528.9 ●
Palatoschisis — see also Cleft, palate 749.00 ●
Palilalia 784.69 ●
Palindromic arthritis — see also Rheumatism, palindromic 719.3 ☑
Palliative care V66.7
Pallor 782.61
  temporal, optic disc 377.15
Palmar — see also condition
  fascia — see condition
Palpable
  cecum 569.89
  kidney 593.89
  liver 573.9
  lymph nodes 785.6
  ovary 620.8
  prostate 602.9
  spleen (see also Splenomegaly) 789.2
  uterus 625.8
Palpitation (heart) 785.1
  psychogenic 306.2
Palsy — see also Paralysis 344.9
  atrophic diffuse 335.20
  Bell's 351.0

Palsy — see also Paralysis — continued
  Bell's — continued
    newborn 767.5
  birth 767.7
  brachial plexus 353.0
    fetus or newborn 767.6
  brain (see also Palsy, cerebral)
    noncongenital or noninfantile 344.89
      late effect — see Late effect(s) (of) cerebrovascular disease
    syphilitic 094.89
      congenital 090.49
  bulbar (chronic) (progressive) 335.22
    pseudo NEC 335.23
    supranuclear NEC 344.8 ☑
  cerebral (congenital) (infantile) (spastic) 343.9
    athetoid 333.71 ▲
    diplegic 343.0
      late effect — see Late effect(s) (of) cerebrovascular disease
    hemiplegic 343.1
    monoplegic 343.3
    noncongenital or noninfantile 437.8
      late effect — see Late effect(s) (of) cerebrovascular disease
    paraplegic 343.0
    quadriplegic 343.2
    spastic, not congenital or infantile 344.89
    syphilitic 094.89
      congenital 090.49
    tetraplegic 343.2
  cranial nerve (see also Disorder, nerve, cranial)
    multiple 352.6
  creeping 335.21
  divers' 993.3
  Erb's (birth injury) 767.6
  facial 351.0
    newborn 767.5
  glossopharyngeal 352.2
  Klumpke (-Déjérine) 767.6
  lead 984.9
    specified type of lead — see Table of Drugs and Chemicals
  median nerve (tardy) 354.0
  peroneal nerve (acute) (tardy) 355.3
  progressive supranuclear 333.0
  pseudobulbar NEC 335.23
  radial nerve (acute) 354.3
  seventh nerve 351.0
    newborn 767.5
  shaking (see also Parkinsonism) 332.0
  spastic (cerebral) (spinal) 343.9
    hemiplegic 343.1
  specified nerve NEC — see Disorder, nerve
  supranuclear NEC 356.8
    progressive 333.0
  ulnar nerve (tardy) 354.2
  wasting 335.21
Paltauf-Sternberg disease 201.9 ☑
Paludism — see Malaria
Panama fever 084.0
Panaris (with lymphangitis) 681.9
  finger 681.02
  toe 681.11
Panaritium (with lymphangitis) 681.9
  finger 681.02
  toe 681.11
Panarteritis (nodosa) 446.0
  brain or cerebral 437.4
Pancake heart 793.2
  with cor pulmonale (chronic) 416.9
Pancarditis (acute) (chronic) 429.89
  with
    rheumatic
      fever (active) (acute) (chronic) (subacute) 391.8

Pancarditis — continued
  with — continued
    rheumatic — continued
      fever — continued
        inactive or quiescent 398.99
    rheumatic, acute 391.8
    chronic or inactive 398.99
Pancoast's syndrome or tumor (carcinoma, pulmonary apex) (M8010/3) 162.3
Pancoast-Tobias syndrome (M8010/3) (carcinoma, pulmonary apex) 162.3
Pancolitis 556.6
Pancreas, pancreatic — see condition
Pancreatitis 577.0
  acute (edematous) (hemorrhagic) (recurrent) 577.0
  annular 577.0
  apoplectic 577.0
  calcerceous 577.0
  chronic (infectious) 577.1
    recurrent 577.1
  cystic 577.2
  fibrous 577.8
  gangrenous 577.0
  hemorrhagic (acute) 577.0
  interstitial (chronic) 577.1
    acute 577.0
  malignant 577.0
  mumps 072.3
  painless 577.1
  recurrent 577.1
  relapsing 577.1
  subacute 577.0
  suppurative 577.0
  syphilitic 095.8
Pancreatolithiasis 577.8
Pancytolysis 289.9
Pancytopenia (acquired) 284.1 ▲
  with malformations 284.09 ▲
  congenital 284.09 ▲
Panencephalitis — see also Encephalitis
  subacute, sclerosing 046.2
Panhematopenia 284.8
  congenital 284.09 ▲
  constitutional 284.09 ▲
  splenic, primary 289.4
Panhemocytopenia 284.8
  congenital 284.09 ▲
  constitutional 284.09 ▲
Panhypogonadism 257.2
Panhypopituitarism 253.2
  prepubertal 253.3
Panic (attack) (state) 300.01
  reaction to exceptional stress (transient) 308.0
Panmyelopathy, familial constitutional 284.09 ▲
Panmyelophthisis 284.2 ▲
  acquired (secondary) 284.8
  congenital 284.2 ▲
  idiopathic 284.9
Panmyelosis (acute) (M9951/1) 238.79 ▲
Panner's disease 732.3
  capitellum humeri 732.3
  head of humerus 732.3
  tarsal navicular (bone) (osteochondrosis) 732.5
Panneuritis endemica 265.0 [357.4]
Panniculitis 729.30
  back 724.8
  knee 729.31
  mesenteric 567.82
  neck 723.6
  nodular, nonsuppurative 729.30
  sacral 724.8
  specified site NEC 729.39
Panniculus adiposus (abdominal) 278.1
Pannus ▶(corneal)◀ 370.62
  abdominal (symptomatic) 278.1 ●
  allergic eczematous 370.62
  degenerativus 370.62
  keratic 370.62
  rheumatoid — see Arthritis, rheumatoid

Pannus

Pannus — continued
  trachomatosus, trachomatous (active) 076.1 [370.62]
    late effect 139.1
Panophthalmitis 360.02
Panotitis — see Otitis media
Pansinusitis (chronic) (hyperplastic) (nonpurulent) (purulent) 473.8
  acute 461.8
  due to fungus NEC 117.9
  tuberculous (see also Tuberculosis) 012.8 ☑
Panuveitis 360.12
  sympathetic 360.11
Panvalvular disease — see Endocarditis, mitral
Papageienkrankheit 073.9
Papanicolaou smear
  cervix (screening test) V76.2
    as part of gynecological examination V72.31
    for suspected malignant neoplasm V76.2
      no disease found V71.1
    inadequate sample 795.08
    nonspecific abnormal finding 795.00
      with
        atypical squamous cells
          cannot exclude high grade squamous intraepithelial lesion (ASC-H) 795.02
          of undetermined significance (ASC-US) 795.01
        cytologic evidence of malignancy 795.06 ●
        high grade squamous intraepithelial lesion (HGSIL) 795.04
        low grade squamous intraepithelial lesion (LGSIL) 795.03
      nonspecific finding NEC 795.09
    to confirm findings of recent normal smear following initial abnormal smear V72.32
    unsatisfactory 795.08
  other specified site (see also Screening, malignant neoplasm)
    for suspected malignant neoplasm (see also Screening, malignant neoplasm)
      no disease found V71.1
    nonspecific abnormal finding 795.1
  vagina V76.47
    following hysterectomy for malignant condition V67.01
Papilledema 377.00
  associated with
    decreased ocular pressure 377.02
    increased intracranial pressure 377.01
    retinal disorder 377.03
  choked disc 377.00
  infectional 377.00
Papillitis 377.31
  anus 569.49
  chronic lingual 529.4
  necrotizing, kidney 584.7
  optic 377.31
  rectum 569.49
  renal, necrotizing 584.7
  tongue 529.0
Papilloma (M8050/0) — see also Neoplasm, by site, benign

Note — Except where otherwise indicated, the morphological varieties of papilloma in the list below should be coded by site as for "Neoplasm, benign."

  acuminatum (female) (male) 078.11
  bladder (urinary) (transitional cell) (M8120/1) 236.7
    benign (M8120/0) 223.3

Papilloma — see also Neoplasm, by site, benign — continued
  choroid plexus (M9390/0) 225.0
    anaplastic type (M9390/3) 191.5
    malignant (M9390/3) 191.5
  ductal (M8503/0)
  dyskeratotic (M8052/0)
  epidermoid (M8052/0)
  hyperkeratotic (M8052/0)
  intracystic (M8504/0)
  intraductal (M8503/0)
  inverted (M8053/0)
  keratotic (M8052/0)
  parakeratotic (M8052/0)
  pinta (primary) 103.0
  renal pelvis (transitional cell) (M8120/1) 236.99
    benign (M8120/0) 223.1
  Schneiderian (M8121/0)
    specified site — see Neoplasm, by site, benign
    unspecified site 212.0
  serous surface (M8461/0)
    borderline malignancy (M8461/1)
      specified site — see Neoplasm, by site, uncertain behavior
      unspecified site 236.2
    specified site — see Neoplasm, by site, benign
    unspecified site 220
  squamous (cell) (M8052/0)
  transitional (cell) (M8120/0)
    bladder (urinary) (M8120/1) 236.7
    inverted type (M8121/1) — see Neoplasm, by site, uncertain behavior
    renal pelvis (M8120/1) 236.91
    ureter (M8120/1) 236.91
    ureter (transitional cell) (M8120/1) 236.91
    benign (M8120/0) 223.2
  urothelial (M8120/1) — see Neoplasm, by site, uncertain behavior
  verrucous (M8051/0)
  villous (M8261/1) — see Neoplasm, by site, uncertain behavior
  yaws, plantar or palmar 102.1
Papillomata, multiple, of yaws 102.1
Papillomatosis (M8060/0) — see also Neoplasm, by site, benign
  confluent and reticulate 701.8
  cutaneous 701.8
  ductal, breast 610.1
  Gougerot-Carteaud (confluent reticulate) 701.8
  intraductal (diffuse) (M8505/0) — see Neoplasm, by site, benign
  subareolar duct (M8506/0) 217
Papillon-Léage and Psaume syndrome (orodigitofacial dysostosis) 759.89
Papule 709.8
  carate (primary) 103.0
  fibrous, of nose (M8724/0) 216.3
  pinta (primary) 103.0
Papulosis, malignant 447.8
Papyraceous fetus 779.89
  complicating pregnancy 646.0 ☑
Paracephalus 759.7
Parachute mitral valve 746.5
Paracoccidioidomycosis 116.1
  mucocutaneous-lymphangitic 116.1
  pulmonary 116.1
  visceral 116.1
Paracoccidiomycosis — see Paracoccidioidomycosis
Paracusis 388.40
Paradentosis 523.5
Paradoxical facial movements 374.43
Paraffinoma 999.9
Paraganglioma (M8680/1)
  adrenal (M8700/0) 227.0
    malignant (M8700/3) 194.0
  aortic body (M8691/1) 237.3
    malignant (M8691/3) 194.6
  carotid body (M8692/1) 237.3

Paraganglioma — continued
  carotid body — continued
    malignant (M8692/3) 194.5
  chromaffin (M8700/0) (see also Neoplasm, by site, benign)
    malignant (M8700/3) — see Neoplasm, by site, malignant
  extra-adrenal (M8693/1)
    malignant (M8693/3)
      specified site — see Neoplasm, by site, malignant
      unspecified site 194.6
    specified site — see Neoplasm, by site, uncertain behavior
    unspecified site 237.3
  glomus jugulare (M8690/1) 237.3
    malignant (M8690/3) 194.6
  jugular (M8690/1) 237.3
    malignant (M8680/3)
      specified site — see Neoplasm, by site, malignant
      unspecified site 194.6
  nonchromaffin (M8693/1)
    malignant (M8693/3)
      specified site — see Neoplasm, by site, malignant
      unspecified site 194.6
    specified site — see Neoplasm, by site, uncertain behavior
    unspecified site 237.3
  parasympathetic (M8682/1)
    specified site — see Neoplasm, by site, uncertain behavior
    unspecified site 237.3
  specified site — see Neoplasm, by site, uncertain behavior
  sympathetic (M8681/1)
    specified site — see Neoplasm, by site, uncertain behavior
    unspecified site 237.3
  unspecified site 237.3
Parageusia 781.1
  psychogenic 306.7
Paragonimiasis 121.2
Paragranuloma, Hodgkin's (M9660/3) 201.9 ☑
Parahemophilia — see also Defect, coagulation 286.3
Parakeratosis 690.8
  psoriasiformis 696.2
  variegata 696.2
Paralysis, paralytic (complete) (incomplete) 344.9
  with
    broken
      back — see Fracture, vertebra, by site, with spinal cord injury
      neck — see Fracture, vertebra, cervical, with spinal cord injury
    fracture, vertebra — see Fracture, vertebra, by site, with spinal cord injury
    syphilis 094.89
  abdomen and back muscles 355.9
  abdominal muscles 355.9
  abducens (nerve) 378.54
  abductor 355.9
    lower extremity 355.8
    upper extremity 354.9
  accessory nerve 352.4
  accommodation 367.51
    hysterical 300.11
  acoustic nerve 388.5
  agitans 332.0
    arteriosclerotic 332.0
  alternating 344.89
    oculomotor 344.89
  amyotrophic 335.20
  ankle 355.8
  anterior serratus 355.9
  anus (sphincter) 569.49
  apoplectic (current episode) (see also Disease, cerebrovascular, acute) 436

Paralysis, paralytic — continued
  apoplectic (see also Disease, cerebrovascular, acute) — continued
    late effect — see Late effect(s) (of) cerebrovascular disease
  arm 344.40
    affecting
      dominant side 344.41
      nondominant side 344.42
    both 344.2
    hysterical 300.11
    late effect — see Late effect(s) (of) cerebrovascular disease
    psychogenic 306.0
    transient 781.4
    traumatic NEC (see also Injury, nerve, upper limb) 955.9
  arteriosclerotic (current episode) 437.0
    late effect — see Late effect(s) (of) cerebrovascular disease
  ascending (spinal), acute 357.0
  associated, nuclear 344.89
  asthenic bulbar 358.00
  ataxic NEC 334.9
    general 094.1
  athetoid 333.71 ▲
  atrophic 356.9
    infantile, acute (see also Poliomyelitis, with paralysis) 045.1 ☑
    muscle NEC 355.9
    progressive 335.21
    spinal (acute) (see also Poliomyelitis, with paralysis) 045.1 ☑
  attack (see also Disease, cerebrovascular, acute) 436
  axillary 353.0
  Babinski-Nageotte's 344.89
  Bell's 351.0
    newborn 767.5
  Benedikt's 344.89
  birth (injury) 767.7
    brain 767.0
    intracranial 767.0
    spinal cord 767.4
  bladder (sphincter) 596.53
    neurogenic 596.54
      with cauda equina syndrome 344.61
    puerperal, postpartum, childbirth 665.5 ☑
    sensory 596.54
      with cauda equina 344.61
    spastic 596.54
      with cauda equina 344.61
  bowel, colon, or intestine (see also Ileus) 560.1
  brachial plexus 353.0
    due to birth injury 767.6
    newborn 767.6
  brain
    congenital — see Palsy, cerebral
    current episode 437.8
    diplegia 344.2
    hemiplegia 342.9 ☑
      late effect — see Late effect(s) (of) cerebrovascular disease
    infantile — see Palsy, cerebral
    late effect — see Late effect(s) (of) cerebrovascular disease
    monoplegia (see also Monoplegia)
      late effect — see Late effect(s) (of) cerebrovascular disease
    paraplegia 344.1
    quadriplegia — see Quadriplegia
    syphilitic, congenital 090.49
    triplegia 344.89
  bronchi 519.19 ▲
  Brown-Séquard's 344.89
  bulbar (chronic) (progressive) 335.22
    infantile (see also Poliomyelitis, bulbar) 045.0 ☑
    poliomyelitic (see also Poliomyelitis, bulbar) 045.0 ☑

Index to Diseases

Paralysis, paralytic

Paralysis, paralytic — *continued*
- bulbar — *continued*
  - pseudo 335.23
  - supranuclear 344.89
- bulbospinal 358.00
- cardiac (*see also* Failure, heart) 428.9
- cerebral
  - current episode 437.8
  - spastic, infantile — *see* Palsy, cerebral
- cerebrocerebellar 437.8
  - diplegic infantile 343.0
- cervical
  - plexus 353.2
  - sympathetic NEC 337.0
- Céstan-Chenais 344.89
- Charcôt-Marie-Tooth type 356.1
- childhood — *see* Palsy, cerebral
- Clark's 343.9
- colon (*see also* Ileus) 560.1
- compressed air 993.3
- compression
  - arm NEC 354.9
  - cerebral — *see* Paralysis, brain
  - leg NEC 355.8
  - lower extremity NEC 355.8
  - upper extremity NEC 354.9
- congenital (cerebral) (spastic) (spinal) — *see* Palsy, cerebral
- conjugate movement (of eye) 378.81
  - cortical (nuclear) (supranuclear) 378.81
- convergence 378.83
- cordis (*see also* Failure, heart) 428.9
- cortical (*see also* Paralysis, brain) 437.8
- cranial or cerebral nerve (*see also* Disorder, nerve, cranial) 352.9
- creeping 335.21
- crossed leg 344.89
- crutch 953.4
- deglutition 784.99
  - hysterical 300.11
- dementia 094.1
- descending (spinal) NEC 335.9
- diaphragm (flaccid) 519.4
  - due to accidental section of phrenic nerve during procedure 998.2
- digestive organs NEC 564.89
- diplegic — *see* Diplegia
- divergence (nuclear) 378.85
- divers' 993.3
- Duchenne's 335.22
- due to intracranial or spinal birth injury — *see* Palsy, cerebral
- embolic (current episode) (*see also* Embolism, brain) 434.1 ☑
  - late effect — *see* Late effect(s) (of) cerebrovascular disease
- enteric (*see also* Ileus) 560.1
  - with hernia — *see* Hernia, by site, with obstruction
- Erb (-Duchenne) (birth) (newborn) 767.6
- Erb's syphilitic spastic spinal 094.89
- esophagus 530.89
- essential, infancy (*see also* Poliomyelitis) 045.9 ☑
- extremity
  - lower — *see* Paralysis, leg
  - spastic (hereditary) 343.3
    - noncongenital or noninfantile 344.1
  - transient (cause unknown) 781.4
  - upper — *see* Paralysis, arm
- eye muscle (extrinsic) 378.55
  - intrinsic 367.51
- facial (nerve) 351.0
  - birth injury 767.5
  - congenital 767.5
  - following operation NEC 998.2
  - newborn 767.5
- familial 359.3
  - periodic 359.3
  - spastic 334.1

Paralysis, paralytic — *continued*
- fauces 478.29
- finger NEC 354.9
- foot NEC 355.8
- gait 781.2
- gastric nerve 352.3
- gaze 378.81
- general 094.1
  - ataxic 094.1
  - insane 094.1
  - juvenile 090.40
  - progressive 094.1
  - tabetic 094.1
- glossopharyngeal (nerve) 352.2
- glottis (*see also* Paralysis, vocal cord) 478.30
- gluteal 353.4
- Gubler (-Millard) 344.89
- hand 354.9
  - hysterical 300.11
  - psychogenic 306.0
- heart (*see also* Failure, heart) 428.9
- hemifacial, progressive 349.89
- hemiplegic — *see* Hemiplegia
- hyperkalemic periodic (familial) 359.3
- hypertensive (current episode) 437.8
- hypoglossal (nerve) 352.5
- hypokalemic periodic 359.3
- Hyrtl's sphincter (rectum) 569.49
- hysterical 300.11
- ileus (*see also* Ileus) 560.1
- infantile (*see also* Poliomyelitis) 045.9 ☑
  - atrophic acute 045.1 ☑
  - bulbar 045.0 ☑
  - cerebral — *see* Palsy, cerebral
  - paralytic 045.1 ☑
  - progressive acute 045.9 ☑
  - spastic — *see* Palsy, cerebral
  - spinal 045.9 ☑
- infective (*see also* Poliomyelitis) 045.9 ☑
- inferior nuclear 344.9
- insane, general or progressive 094.1
- internuclear 378.86
- interosseous 355.9
- intestine (*see also* Ileus) 560.1
- intracranial (current episode) (*see also* Paralysis, brain) 437.8
  - due to birth injury 767.0
- iris 379.49
  - due to diphtheria (toxin) 032.81 [379.49]
- ischemic, Volkmann's (complicating trauma) 958.6
- isolated sleep, recurrent
- Jackson's 344.89
- jake 357.7
- Jamaica ginger (jake) 357.7
- juvenile general 090.40
- Klumpke (-Déjérine) (birth) (newborn) 767.6
- labioglossal (laryngeal) (pharyngeal) 335.22
- Landry's 357.0
- laryngeal nerve (recurrent) (superior) (*see also* Paralysis, vocal cord) 478.30
- larynx (*see also* Paralysis, vocal cord) 478.30
  - due to diphtheria (toxin) 032.3
- late effect
  - due to
    - birth injury, brain or spinal (cord) — *see* Palsy, cerebral
    - edema, brain or cerebral — *see* Paralysis, brain
    - lesion
      - late effect — *see* Late effect(s) (of) cerebrovascular disease
    - spinal (cord) — *see* Paralysis, spinal
- lateral 335.24
- lead 984.9

Paralysis, paralytic — *continued*
- lead — *continued*
  - specified type of lead — *see* Table of Drugs and Chemicals
- left side — *see* Hemiplegia
- leg 344.30
  - affecting
    - dominant side 344.31
    - nondominant side 344.32
  - both (*see also* Paraplegia) 344.1
  - crossed 344.89
  - hysterical 300.11
  - psychogenic 306.0
  - transient or transitory 781.4
    - traumatic NEC (*see also* Injury, nerve, lower limb) 956.9
- levator palpebrae superioris 374.31
- limb NEC 344.5
  - all four — *see* Quadriplegia
  - quadriplegia — *see* Quadriplegia
- lip 528.5
- Lissauer's 094.1
- local 355.9
- lower limb (*see also* Paralysis, leg)
  - both (*see also* Paraplegia) 344.1
- lung 518.89
  - newborn 770.89
- median nerve 354.1
- medullary (tegmental) 344.89
- mesencephalic NEC 344.89
  - tegmental 344.89
- middle alternating 344.89
- Millard-Gubler-Foville 344.89
- monoplegic — *see* Monoplegia
- motor NEC 344.9
  - cerebral — *see* Paralysis, brain
  - spinal — *see* Paralysis, spinal
- multiple
  - cerebral — *see* Paralysis, brain
  - spinal — *see* Paralysis, spinal
- muscle (flaccid) 359.9
  - due to nerve lesion NEC 355.9
  - eye (extrinsic) 378.55
    - intrinsic 367.51
    - oblique 378.51
  - iris sphincter 364.8
  - ischemic (complicating trauma) (Volkmann's) 958.6
  - pseudohypertrophic 359.1
- muscular (atrophic) 359.9
  - progressive 335.21
- musculocutaneous nerve 354.9
- musculospiral 354.9
- nerve (*see also* Disorder, nerve)
  - third or oculomotor (partial) 378.51
    - total 378.52
  - fourth or trochlear 378.53
  - sixth or abducens 378.54
  - seventh or facial 351.0
    - birth injury 767.5
    - due to
      - injection NEC 999.9
      - operation NEC 997.09
    - newborn 767.5
  - accessory 352.4
  - auditory 388.5
  - birth injury 767.7
  - cranial or cerebral (*see also* Disorder, nerve, cranial) 352.9
  - facial 351.0
    - birth injury 767.5
    - newborn 767.5
  - laryngeal (*see also* Paralysis, vocal cord) 478.30
  - newborn 767.7
  - phrenic 354.8
    - newborn 767.7
  - radial 354.3
    - birth injury 767.6
    - newborn 767.6
  - syphilitic 094.89
  - traumatic NEC (*see also* Injury, nerve, by site) 957.9
  - trigeminal 350.9
  - ulnar 354.2
- newborn NEC 767.0

Paralysis, paralytic — *continued*
- normokalemic periodic 359.3
- obstetrical, newborn 767.7
- ocular 378.9
- oculofacial, congenital 352.6
- oculomotor (nerve) (partial) 378.51
  - alternating 344.89
  - external bilateral 378.55
  - total 378.52
- olfactory nerve 352.0
- palate 528.9
- palatopharyngolaryngeal 352.6
- paratrigeminal 350.9
- periodic (familial) (hyperkalemic) (hypokalemic) (normokalemic) (secondary) 359.3
- peripheral
  - autonomic nervous system — *see* Neuropathy, peripheral, autonomic
  - nerve NEC 355.9
- peroneal (nerve) 355.3
- pharynx 478.29
- phrenic nerve 354.8
- plantar nerves 355.6
- pneumogastric nerve 352.3
- poliomyelitis (current) (*see also* Poliomyelitis, with paralysis) 045.1 ☑
  - bulbar 045.0 ☑
- popliteal nerve 355.3
- pressure (*see also* Neuropathy, entrapment) 355.9
- progressive 335.21
  - atrophic 335.21
  - bulbar 335.22
  - general 094.1
  - hemifacial 349.89
  - infantile, acute (*see also* Poliomyelitis) 045.9 ☑
  - multiple 335.20
- pseudobulbar 335.23
- pseudohypertrophic 359.1
  - muscle 359.1
- psychogenic 306.0
- pupil, pupillary 379.49
- quadriceps 355.8
- quadriplegic (*see also* Quadriplegia) 344.0 ☑
- radial nerve 354.3
  - birth injury 767.6
- rectum (sphincter) 569.49
- rectus muscle (eye) 378.55
- recurrent
  - isolated sleep 327.43
  - laryngeal nerve (*see also* Paralysis, vocal cord) 478.30
- respiratory (muscle) (system) (tract) 786.09
  - center NEC 344.89
    - fetus or newborn 770.87
  - congenital 768.9
  - newborn 768.9
- right side — *see* Hemiplegia
- Saturday night 354.9
- saturnine 984.9
  - specified type of lead — *see* Table of Drugs and Chemicals
- sciatic nerve 355.0
- secondary — *see* Paralysis, late effect
- seizure (cerebral) (current episode) (*see also* Disease, cerebrovascular, acute) 436
  - late effect — *see* Late effect(s) (of) cerebrovascular disease
- senile NEC 344.9
- serratus magnus 355.9
- shaking (*see also* Parkinsonism) 332.0
- shock (*see also* Disease, cerebrovascular, acute) 436
  - late effect — *see* Late effect(s) (of) cerebrovascular disease
- shoulder 354.9
- soft palate 528.9
- spasmodic — *see* Paralysis, spastic
- spastic 344.9

Paralysis, paralytic — *continued*
- spastic — *continued*
  - cerebral infantile — *see* Palsy, cerebral
  - congenital (cerebral) — *see* Palsy, cerebral
  - familial 334.1
  - hereditary 334.1
  - infantile 343.9
  - noncongenital or noninfantile, cerebral 344.9
  - syphilitic 094.0
    - spinal 094.89
- sphincter, bladder (*see also* Paralysis, bladder) 596.53
- spinal (cord) NEC 344.1
  - accessory nerve 352.4
  - acute (*see also* Poliomyelitis) 045.9
  - ascending acute 357.0
  - atrophic (acute) (*see also* Poliomyelitis, with paralysis) 045.1
    - spastic, syphilitic 094.89
  - congenital NEC 343.9
  - hemiplegic — *see* Hemiplegia
  - hereditary 336.8
  - infantile — *see also* Poliomyelitis 045.9
  - late effect NEC 344.89
  - monoplegic — *see* Monoplegia
  - nerve 355.9
  - progressive 335.10
  - quadriplegic — *see* Quadriplegia
  - spastic NEC 343.9
  - traumatic — *see* Injury, spinal, by site
- sternomastoid 352.4
- stomach 536.3
  - diabetic 250.6 [536.3]
  - nerve (nondiabetic) 352.3
- stroke (current episode) — *see* Infarct, brain
  - late effect — *see* Late effect(s) (of) cerebrovascular disease
- subscapularis 354.8
- superior nuclear NEC 334.9
- supranuclear 356.8
- sympathetic
  - cervical NEC 337.0
  - nerve NEC (*see also* Neuropathy, peripheral, autonomic) 337.9
  - nervous system — *see* Neuropathy, peripheral, autonomic
  - syndrome 344.9
    - specified NEC 344.89
- syphilitic spastic spinal (Erb's) 094.89
- tabetic general 094.1
- thigh 355.8
- throat 478.29
  - diphtheritic 032.0
  - muscle 478.29
- thrombotic (current episode) (*see also* Thrombosis, brain) 434.0
  - late effect — *see* Late effect(s) (of) cerebrovascular disease
- thumb NEC 354.9
- tick (-bite) 989.5
- Todd's (postepileptic transitory paralysis) 344.89
- toe 355.6
- tongue 529.8
- transient
  - arm or leg NEC 781.4
  - traumatic NEC (*see also* Injury, nerve, by site) 957.9
- trapezius 352.4
- traumatic, transient NEC (*see also* Injury, nerve, by site) 957.9
- trembling (*see also* Parkinsonism) 332.0
- triceps brachii 354.9
- trigeminal nerve 350.9
- trochlear nerve 378.53
- ulnar nerve 354.2
- upper limb (*see also* Paralysis, arm)
  - both (*see also* Diplegia) 344.2

Paralysis, paralytic — *continued*
- uremic — *see* Uremia
- uveoparotitic 135
- uvula 528.9
  - hysterical 300.11
  - postdiphtheritic 032.0
- vagus nerve 352.3
- vasomotor NEC 337.9
- velum palati 528.9
- vesical (*see also* Paralysis, bladder) 596.53
- vestibular nerve 388.5
- visual field, psychic 368.16
- vocal cord 478.30
  - bilateral (partial) 478.33
    - complete 478.34
  - complete (bilateral) 478.34
  - unilateral (partial) 478.31
    - complete 478.32
- Volkmann's (complicating trauma) 958.6
- wasting 335.21
- Weber's 344.89
- wrist NEC 354.9

Paramedial orifice, urethrovesical 753.8
Paramenia 626.9
Parametritis (chronic) — *see also* Disease, pelvis, inflammatory 614.4
- acute 614.3
- puerperal, postpartum, childbirth 670.0

Parametrium, parametric — *see* condition
Paramnesia — *see also* Amnesia 780.93
Paramolar 520.1
- causing crowding 524.31

Paramyloidosis 277.30
Paramyoclonus multiplex 333.2
Paramyotonia 359.2
- congenita 359.2

Paraneoplastic syndrome — *see* condition
Parangi — *see also* Yaws 102.9
Paranoia 297.1
- alcoholic 291.5
- querulans 297.8
- senile 290.20

Paranoid
- dementia (*see also* Schizophrenia) 295.3
  - praecox (acute) 295.3
  - senile 290.20
- personality 301.0
- psychosis 297.9
  - alcoholic 291.5
  - climacteric 297.2
  - drug-induced 292.11
  - involutional 297.2
  - menopausal 297.2
  - protracted reactive 298.4
  - psychogenic 298.4
    - acute 298.3
  - senile 290.20
- reaction (chronic) 297.9
  - acute 298.3
- schizophrenia (acute) (*see also* Schizophrenia) 295.3
- state 297.9
  - alcohol-induced 291.5
  - climacteric 297.2
  - drug-induced 292.11
  - due to or associated with
    - arteriosclerosis (cerebrovascular) 290.42
    - presenile brain disease 290.12
    - senile brain disease 290.20
  - involutional 297.2
  - menopausal 297.2
  - senile 290.20
  - simple 297.0
  - specified type NEC 297.8
- tendencies 301.0
- traits 301.0
- trends 301.0
- type, psychopathic personality 301.0

Paraparesis — *see also* Paralysis 344.9
Paraphasia 784.3
Paraphilia — *see also* Deviation, sexual 302.9
Paraphimosis (congenital) 605
- chancroidal 099.0

Paraphrenia, paraphrenic (late) 297.2
- climacteric 297.2
- dementia (*see also* Schizophrenia) 295.3
- involutional 297.2
- menopausal 297.2
- schizophrenia (acute) (*see also* Schizophrenia) 295.3

Paraplegia 344.1
- with
  - broken back — *see* Fracture, vertebra, by site, with spinal cord injury
  - fracture, vertebra — *see* Fracture, vertebra, by site, with spinal cord injury
- ataxic — *see* Degeneration, combined, spinal cord
- brain (current episode) (*see also* Paralysis, brain) 437.8
- cerebral (current episode) (*see also* Paralysis, brain) 437.8
- congenital or infantile (cerebral) (spastic) (spinal) 343.0
- cortical — *see* Paralysis, brain
- familial spastic 334.1
- functional (hysterical) 300.11
- hysterical 300.11
- infantile 343.0
- late effect 344.1
- Pott's (*see also* Tuberculosis) 015.0 [730.88]
- psychogenic 306.0
- spastic
  - Erb's spinal 094.89
  - hereditary 334.1
  - not infantile or congenital 344.1
- spinal (cord)
  - traumatic NEC — *see* Injury, spinal, by site
- syphilitic (spastic) 094.89
- traumatic NEC — *see* Injury, spinal, by site

Paraproteinemia 273.2
- benign (familial) 273.1
- monoclonal 273.1
- secondary to malignant or inflammatory disease 273.1

Parapsoriasis 696.2
- en plaques 696.2
- guttata 696.2
- lichenoides chronica 696.2
- retiformis 696.2
- varioliformis (acuta) 696.2

Parascarlatina 057.8
Parasitic — *see also* condition
- disease NEC (*see also* Infestation, parasitic) 136.9
- contact V01.89
- exposure to V01.89
- intestinal NEC 129
- skin NEC 134.9
- stomatitis 112.0
- sycosis 110.0
  - beard 110.0
  - scalp 110.0
- twin 759.4

Parasitism NEC 136.9
- intestinal NEC 129
- skin NEC 134.9
- specified — *see* Infestation

Parasitophobia 300.29
Parasomnia 307.47
- alcohol induced 291.82
- drug induced 292.85
- nonorganic origin 307.47
- organic 327.40
  - in conditions classified elsewhere 327.44
  - other 327.49

Paraspadias 752.69
Paraspasm facialis 351.8
Parathyroid gland — *see* condition
Parathyroiditis (autoimmune) 252.1
Parathyroprival tetany 252.1
Paratrachoma 077.0
Paratyphilitis — *see also* Appendicitis 541
Paratyphoid (fever) — *see* Fever, paratyphoid
Paratyphus — *see* Fever, paratyphoid
Paraurethral duct 753.8
Para-urethritis 597.89
- gonococcal (acute) 098.0
  - chronic or duration of 2 months or over 098.2

Paravaccinia NEC 051.9
- milkers' node 051.1

Paravaginitis — *see also* Vaginitis 616.10
Parencephalitis — *see also* Encephalitis 323.9
- late effect — *see* category 326

Parergasia 298.9
Paresis — *see also* Paralysis 344.9
- accommodation 367.51
- bladder (spastic) (sphincter) (*see also* Paralysis, bladder) 596.53
  - tabetic 094.0
- bowel, colon, or intestine (*see also* Ileus) 560.1
- brain or cerebral — *see* Paralysis, brain
- extrinsic muscle, eye 378.55
- general 094.1
  - arrested 094.1
  - brain 094.1
  - cerebral 094.1
  - insane 094.1
  - juvenile 090.40
    - remission 090.49
  - progressive 094.1
  - remission (sustained) 094.1
  - tabetic 094.1
- heart (*see also* Failure, heart) 428.9
- infantile (*see also* Poliomyelitis) 045.9
- insane 094.1
- juvenile 090.40
- late effect — *see* Paralysis, late effect
- luetic (general) 094.1
- peripheral progressive 356.9
- pseudohypertrophic 359.1
- senile NEC 344.9
- stomach 536.3
  - diabetic 250.6 [536.3]
- syphilitic (general) 094.1
  - congenital 090.40
- transient, limb 781.4
- vesical (sphincter) NEC 596.53

Paresthesia — *see also* Disturbance, sensation 782.0
- Berger's (paresthesia of lower limb) 782.0
- Bernhardt 355.1
- Magnan's 782.0

Paretic — *see* condition
Parinaud's
- conjunctivitis 372.02
- oculoglandular syndrome 372.02
- ophthalmoplegia 378.81
- syndrome (paralysis of conjugate upward gaze) 378.81

Parkes Weber and Dimitri syndrome (encephalocutaneous angiomatosis) 759.6

Parkinson's disease, syndrome, or tremor — *see* Parkinsonism
Parkinsonism (arteriosclerotic) (idiopathic) (primary) 332.0
- associated with orthostatic hypotension (idiopathic) (symptomatic) 333.0
- due to drugs 332.1
- neuroleptic-induced 332.1
- secondary 332.1

Index to Diseases

Parkinsonism — *continued*
  syphilitic 094.82
Parodontitis 523.40 ▲
Parodontosis 523.5
Paronychia (with lymphangitis) 681.9
  candidal (chronic) 112.3
  chronic 681.9
    candidal 112.3
    finger 681.02
    toe 681.11
  finger 681.02
  toe 681.11
  tuberculous (primary) (*see also* Tuberculosis) 017.0 ☑
Parorexia NEC 307.52
  hysterical 300.11
Parosmia 781.1
  psychogenic 306.7
Parotid gland — *see* condition
Parotiditis — *see also* Parotitis 527.2
  epidemic 072.9
  infectious 072.9
Parotitis 527.2
  allergic 527.2
  chronic 527.2
  epidemic (*see also* Mumps) 072.9
  infectious (*see also* Mumps) 072.9
  noninfectious 527.2
  nonspecific toxic 527.2
  not mumps 527.2
  postoperative 527.2
  purulent 527.2
  septic 527.2
  suppurative (acute) 527.2
  surgical 527.2
  toxic 527.2
Paroxysmal — *see also* condition
  dyspnea (nocturnal) 786.09
Parrot's disease (syphilitic osteochondritis) 090.0
Parrot fever 073.9
Parry's disease or syndrome (exophthalmic goiter) 242.0 ☑
Parry-Romberg syndrome 349.89
Parsonage-Aldren-Turner syndrome 353.5
Parsonage-Turner syndrome 353.5
Parson's disease (exophthalmic goiter) 242.0 ☑
Pars planitis 363.21
Particolored infant 757.39
Parturition — *see* Delivery
Passage
  false, urethra 599.4
  meconium noted during delivery 763.84
  of sounds or bougies (*see also* Attention to artificial opening) V55.9
Passive — *see* condition
Pasteurella septica 027.2
Pasteurellosis — *see also* Infection, Pasteurella 027.2
PAT (paroxysmal atrial tachycardia) 427.0
Patau's syndrome (trisomy D1) 758.1
Patch
  herald 696.3
Patches
  mucous (syphilitic) 091.3
    congenital 090.0
  smokers' (mouth) 528.6
Patellar — *see* condition
Patellofemoral syndrome 719.46
Patent — *see also* Imperfect closure
  atrioventricular ostium 745.69
  canal of Nuck 752.41
  cervix 622.5
    complicating pregnancy 654.5 ☑
      affecting fetus or newborn 761.0
  ductus arteriosus or Botalli 747.0
  Eustachian
    tube 381.7
    valve 746.89
  foramen
    Botalli 745.5
    ovale 745.5

Patent — *see also* Imperfect closure — *continued*
  interauricular septum 745.5
  interventricular septum 745.4
  omphalomesenteric duct 751.0
  os (uteri) — *see* Patent, cervix
  ostium secundum 745.5
  urachus 753.7
  vitelline duct 751.0
Paternity testing V70.4
Paterson-Kelly syndrome or web (sideropenic dysphagia) 280.8
Paterson (-Brown) (-Kelly) syndrome (sideropenic dysphagia) 280.8
Paterson's syndrome (sideropenic dysphagia) 280.8
Pathologic, pathological — *see also* condition
  asphyxia 799.01
  drunkenness 291.4
  emotionality 301.3
  fracture — *see* Fracture, pathologic
  liar 301.7
  personality 301.9
  resorption, tooth 521.40
    external 521.42
    internal 521.41
    specified NEC 521.49
  sexuality (*see also* Deviation, sexual) 302.9
Pathology (of) — *see* ▶*also*◀ Disease
  periradicular, associated with previous endodontic treatment 526.69 ●
Patterned motor discharge, idiopathic — *see also* Epilepsy 345.5 ☑
Patulous — *see also* Patent
  anus 569.49
  Eustachian tube 381.7
Pause, sinoatrial 427.81
Pavor nocturnus 307.46
Pavy's disease 593.6
Paxton's disease (white piedra) 111.2
Payr's disease or syndrome (splenic flexure syndrome) 569.89
PBA (pseudobulbar affect) 310.8
Pearls
  Elschnig 366.51
  enamel 520.2
Pearl-workers' disease (chronic osteomyelitis) — *see also* Osteomyelitis 730.1 ☑
Pectenitis 569.49
Pectenosis 569.49
Pectoral — *see* condition
Pectus
  carinatum (congenital) 754.82
    acquired 738.3
    rachitic (*see also* Rickets) 268.0
  excavatum (congenital) 754.81
    acquired 738.3
    rachitic (*see also* Rickets) 268.0
  recurvatum (congenital) 754.81
    acquired 738.3
Pedatrophia 261
Pederosis 302.2
Pediculosis (infestation) 132.9
  capitis (head louse) (any site) 132.0
  corporis (body louse) (any site) 132.1
  eyelid 132.0 [373.6]
  mixed (classifiable to more than one category in 132.0–132.2) 132.3
  pubis (pubic louse) (any site) 132.2
  vestimenti 132.1
  vulvae 132.2
Pediculus (infestation) — *see* Pediculosis
Pedophilia 302.2
Peg-shaped teeth 520.2
Pelade 704.01
Pel's crisis 094.0
Pel-Ebstein disease — *see* Disease, Hodgkin's
Pelger-Huët anomaly or syndrome (hereditary hyposegmentation) 288.2
Peliosis (rheumatica) 287.0

Pelizaeus-Merzbacher
  disease 330.0
  sclerosis, diffuse cerebral 330.0
Pellagra (alcoholic or with alcoholism) 265.2
  with polyneuropathy 265.2 [357.4]
Pellagra-cerebellar-ataxia-renal aminoaciduria syndrome 270.0
Pellegrini's disease (calcification, knee joint) 726.62
Pellegrini (-Stieda) disease or syndrome (calcification, knee joint) 726.62
Pellizzi's syndrome (pineal) 259.8
Pelvic — *see also* condition
  congestion-fibrosis syndrome 625.5
  kidney 753.3
Pelvioectasis 591
Pelviolithiasis 592.0
Pelviperitonitis
  female (*see also* Peritonitis, pelvic, female) 614.5
  male (*see also* Peritonitis) 567.21
Pelvis, pelvic — *see also* condition or type
  infantile 738.6
  Nägele's 738.6
  obliquity 738.6
  Robert's 755.69
Pemphigoid 694.5
  benign, mucous membrane 694.60
    with ocular involvement 694.61
  bullous 694.5
  cicatricial 694.60
    with ocular involvement 694.61
  juvenile 694.2
Pemphigus 694.4
  benign 694.5
    chronic familial 757.39
  Brazilian 694.4
  circinatus 694.0
  congenital, traumatic 757.39
  conjunctiva 694.61
  contagiosus 684
  erythematodes 694.4
  erythematosus 694.4
  foliaceus 694.4
  frambesiodes 694.4
  gangrenous (*see also* Gangrene) 785.4
  malignant 694.4
  neonatorum, newborn 684
  ocular 694.61
  papillaris 694.4
  seborrheic 694.4
  South American 694.4
  syphilitic (congenital) 090.0
  vegetans 694.4
  vulgaris 694.4
  wildfire 694.4
Pendred's syndrome (familial goiter with deaf-mutism) 243
Pendulous
  abdomen 701.9
    in pregnancy or childbirth 654.4 ☑
      affecting fetus or newborn 763.89
  breast 611.8
Penetrating wound — *see also* Wound, open, by site
  with internal injury — *see* Injury, internal, by site, with open wound
  eyeball 871.7
    with foreign body (nonmagnetic) 871.6
    magnetic 871.5
  ocular (*see also* Penetrating wound, eyeball) 871.7
  adnexa 870.3
    with foreign body 870.4
  orbit 870.3
    with foreign body 870.4
Penetration, pregnant uterus by instrument
  with
    abortion — *see* Abortion, by type, with damage to pelvic organs

Penetration, pregnant uterus by instrument — *continued*
  with — *continued*
    ectopic pregnancy (*see also* categories 633.0–633.9) 639.2
    molar pregnancy (*see also* categories 630–632) 639.2
  complication of delivery 665.1 ☑
    affecting fetus or newborn 763.89
  following
    abortion 639.2
    ectopic or molar pregnancy 639.2
Penfield's syndrome — *see also* Epilepsy 345.5
Penicilliosis of lung 117.3
Penis — *see* condition
Penitis 607.2
Pentalogy (of Fallot) 745.2
Penta X syndrome 758.81
Pentosuria (benign) (essential) 271.8
Peptic acid disease 536.8
Peregrinating patient V65.2
Perforated — *see* Perforation
Perforation, perforative (nontraumatic)
  antrum (*see also* Sinusitis, maxillary) 473.0
  appendix 540.0
    with peritoneal abscess 540.1
  atrial septum, multiple 745.5
  attic, ear 384.22
    healed 384.81
  bile duct, except cystic (*see also* Disease, biliary) 576.3
  cystic 575.4
  bladder (urinary) 596.6
    with
      abortion — *see* Abortion, by type, with damage to pelvic organs
      ectopic pregnancy (*see also* categories 633.0–633.9) 639.2
      molar pregnancy (*see also* categories 630–632) 639.2
    following
      abortion 639.2
      ectopic or molar pregnancy 639.2
    obstetrical trauma 665.5 ☑
  bowel 569.83
    with
      abortion — *see* Abortion, by type, with damage to pelvic organs
      ectopic pregnancy (*see also* categories 633.0–633.9) 639.2
      molar pregnancy (*see also* categories 630–632) 639.2
    fetus or newborn 777.6
    following
      abortion 639.2
      ectopic or molar pregnancy 639.2
    obstetrical trauma 665.5 ☑
  broad ligament
    with
      abortion — *see* Abortion, by type, with damage to pelvic organs
      ectopic pregnancy (*see also* categories 633.0–633.9) 639.2
      molar pregnancy (*see also* categories 630–632) 639.2
    following
      abortion 639.2
      ectopic or molar pregnancy 639.2
    obstetrical trauma 665.6 ☑
  by
    device, implant, or graft — *see* Complications, mechanical
    foreign body left accidentally in operation wound 998.4

Perforation, perforative

Perforation, perforative — *continued*
 by — *continued*
  instrument (any) during a procedure, accidental 998.2
 cecum 540.0
  with peritoneal abscess 540.1
 cervix (uteri) (*see also* Injury, internal, cervix)
  with
   abortion — *see* Abortion, by type, with damage to pelvic organs
   ectopic pregnancy (*see also* categories 633.0–633.9) 639.2
   molar pregnancy (*see also* categories 630–632) 639.2
  following
   abortion 639.2
   ectopic or molar pregnancy 639.2
  obstetrical trauma 665.3 ☑
 colon 569.83
 common duct (bile) 576.3
 cornea (*see also* Ulcer, cornea) 370.00
  due to ulceration 370.06
 cystic duct 575.4
 diverticulum (*see also* Diverticula) 562.10
  small intestine 562.00
 duodenum, duodenal (ulcer) — *see* Ulcer, duodenum, with perforation
 ear drum — *see* Perforation, tympanum
 enteritis — *see* Enteritis
 esophagus 530.4
 ethmoidal sinus (*see also* Sinusitis, ethmoidal) 473.2
 foreign body (external site) (*see also* Wound, open, by site, complicated)
  internal site, by ingested object — *see* Foreign body
 frontal sinus (*see also* Sinusitis, frontal) 473.1
 gallbladder or duct (*see also* Disease, gallbladder) 575.4
 gastric (ulcer) — *see* Ulcer, stomach, with perforation
 heart valve — *see* Endocarditis
 ileum (*see also* Perforation, intestine) 569.83
 instrumental
  external — *see* Wound, open, by site
  pregnant uterus, complicating delivery 665.9 ☑
  surgical (accidental) (blood vessel) (nerve) (organ) 998.2
 intestine 569.83
  with
   abortion — *see* Abortion, by type, with damage to pelvic organs
   ectopic pregnancy (*see also* categories 633.0–633.9) 639.2
   molar pregnancy (*see also* categories 630–632) 639.2
  fetus or newborn 777.6
  obstetrical trauma 665.5 ☑
  ulcerative NEC 569.83
 jejunum, jejunal 569.83
  ulcer — *see* Ulcer, gastrojejunal, with perforation
 mastoid (antrum) (cell) 383.89
 maxillary sinus (*see also* Sinusitis, maxillary) 473.0
 membrana tympani — *see* Perforation, tympanum
 nasal
  septum 478.19 ▲
   congenital 748.1
   syphilitic 095.8
  sinus (*see also* Sinusitis) 473.9

Perforation, perforative — *continued*
 nasal — *continued*
  sinus (*see also* Sinusitis) — *continued*
   congenital 748.1
  palate (hard) 526.89
   soft 528.9
    syphilitic 095.8
    syphilitic 095.8
  palatine vault 526.89
   syphilitic 095.8
    congenital 090.5
 pelvic
  floor
   with
    abortion — *see* Abortion, by type, with damage to pelvic organs
    ectopic pregnancy (*see also* categories 633.0–633.9) 639.2
    molar pregnancy (*see also* categories 630–632) 639.2
   obstetrical trauma 664.1 ☑
  organ
   with
    abortion — *see* Abortion, by type, with damage to pelvic organs
    ectopic pregnancy (*see also* categories 633.0–633.9) 639.2
    molar pregnancy (*see also* categories 630–632) 639.2
   following
    abortion 639.2
    ectopic or molar pregnancy 639.2
   obstetrical trauma 665.5 ☑
 perineum — *see* Laceration, perineum
 periurethral tissue
  with
   abortion — *see* Abortion, by type, with damage to pelvic organs
   ectopic pregnancy (*see also* categories 630–632) 639.2
   molar pregnancy (*see also* categories 630–632) 639.2
 pharynx 478.29
 pylorus, pyloric (ulcer) — *see* Ulcer, stomach, with perforation
 rectum 569.49
 root canal space 526.61 ●
 sigmoid 569.83
 sinus (accessory) (chronic) (nasal) (*see also* Sinusitis) 473.9
 sphenoidal sinus (*see also* Sinusitis, sphenoidal) 473.3
 stomach (due to ulcer) — *see* Ulcer, stomach, with perforation
 surgical (accidental) (by instrument) (blood vessel) (nerve) (organ) 998.2
 traumatic
  external — *see* Wound, open, by site
  eye (*see also* Penetrating wound, ocular) 871.7
  internal organ — *see* Injury, internal, by site
 tympanum (membrane) (persistent posttraumatic) (postinflammatory) 384.20
  with
   otitis media — *see* Otitis media
  attic 384.22
  central 384.21
  healed 384.81
  marginal NEC 384.23
  multiple 384.24
  pars flaccida 384.22
  total 384.25

Perforation, perforative — *continued*
 tympanum — *continued*
  traumatic — *see* Wound, open, ear, drum
 typhoid, gastrointestinal 002.0
 ulcer — *see* Ulcer, by site, with perforation
 ureter 593.89
 urethra
  with
   abortion — *see* Abortion, by type, with damage to pelvic organs
   ectopic pregnancy (*see also* categories 633.0–633.9) 639.2
   molar pregnancy (*see also* categories 630–632) 639.2
  following
   abortion 639.2
   ectopic or molar pregnancy 639.2
  obstetrical trauma 665.5 ☑
 uterus (*see also* Injury, internal, uterus)
  with
   abortion — *see* Abortion, by type, with damage to pelvic organs
   ectopic pregnancy (*see also* categories 633.0–633.9) 639.2
   molar pregnancy (*see also* categories 630–632) 639.2
  by intrauterine contraceptive device 996.32
  following
   abortion 639.2
   ectopic or molar pregnancy 639.2
  obstetrical trauma — *see* Injury, internal, uterus, obstetrical trauma
 uvula 528.9
  syphilitic 095.8
 vagina — *see* Laceration, vagina
 viscus NEC 799.89
  traumatic 868.00
   with open wound into cavity 868.10
Periadenitis mucosa necrotica recurrens 528.2
Periangiitis 446.0
Periantritis 535.4 ☑
Periappendicitis (acute) — *see also* Appendicitis 541
Periarteritis (disseminated) (infectious) (necrotizing) (nodosa) 446.0
Periarthritis (joint) 726.90
 Duplay's 726.2
 gonococcal 098.50
 humeroscapularis 726.2
 scapulohumeral 726.2
 shoulder 726.2
 wrist 726.4
Periarthrosis (angioneural) — *see* Periarthritis
Peribronchitis 491.9
 tuberculous (*see also* Tuberculosis) 011.3 ☑
Pericapsulitis, adhesive (shoulder) 726.0
Pericarditis (granular) (with decompensation) (with effusion) 423.9
 with
  rheumatic fever (conditions classifiable to 390)
   active (*see also* Pericarditis, rheumatic) 391.0
   inactive or quiescent 393
 actinomycotic 039.8 *[420.0]*
 acute (nonrheumatic) 420.90
  with chorea (acute) (rheumatic) (Sydenham's) 392.0
  bacterial 420.99
  benign 420.91

Index to Diseases

Pericarditis — *continued*
 acute — *continued*
  hemorrhagic 420.90
  idiopathic 420.91
  infective 420.90
  nonspecific 420.91
  rheumatic 391.0
   with chorea (acute) (rheumatic) (Sydenham's) 392.0
  sicca 420.90
  viral 420.91
 adhesive or adherent (external) (internal) 423.1
  acute — *see* Pericarditis, acute rheumatic (external) (internal) 393
 amebic 006.8 *[420.0]*
 bacterial (acute) (subacute) (with serous or seropurulent effusion) 420.99
 calcareous 423.2
 cholesterol (chronic) 423.8
  acute 420.90
 chronic (nonrheumatic) 423.8
  rheumatic 393
 constrictive 423.2
 Coxsackie 074.21
 due to
  actinomycosis 039.8 *[420.0]*
  amebiasis 006.8 *[420.0]*
  Coxsackie (virus) 074.21
  histoplasmosis (*see also* Histoplasmosis) 115.93
  nocardiosis 039.8 *[420.0]*
  tuberculosis (*see also* Tuberculosis) 017.9 ☑ *[420.0]*
 fibrinocaseous (*see also* Tuberculosis) 017.9 ☑ *[420.0]*
 fibrinopurulent 420.99
 fibrinous — *see* Pericarditis, rheumatic
 fibropurulent 420.99
 fibrous 423.1
 gonococcal 098.83
 hemorrhagic 423.0
 idiopathic (acute) 420.91
 infective (acute) 420.90
 meningococcal 036.41
 neoplastic (chronic) 423.8
  acute 420.90
 nonspecific 420.91
 obliterans, obliterating 423.1
 plastic 423.1
 pneumococcal (acute) 420.99
 postinfarction 411.0
 purulent (acute) 420.99
 rheumatic (active) (acute) (with effusion) (with pneumonia) 391.0
  with chorea (acute) (rheumatic) (Sydenham's) 392.0
  chronic or inactive (with chorea) 393
 septic (acute) 420.99
 serofibrinous — *see* Pericarditis, rheumatic
 staphylococcal (acute) 420.99
 streptococcal (acute) 420.99
 suppurative (acute) 420.99
 syphilitic 093.81
 tuberculous (acute) (chronic) (*see also* Tuberculosis) 017.9 ☑ *[420.0]*
 uremic 585.9 *[420.0]*
 viral (acute) 420.91
Pericardium, pericardial — *see* condition
Pericellulitis — *see also* Cellulitis 682.9
Pericementitis 523.40 ▲
 acute 523.30 ▲
 chronic (suppurative) 523.40 ▲
Pericholecystitis — *see also* Cholecystitis 575.10
Perichondritis
 auricle 380.00
  acute 380.01
  chronic 380.02
 bronchus 491.9
 ear (external) 380.00

Perichondritis — continued
  ear — continued
    acute 380.01
    chronic 380.02
  larynx 478.71
    syphilitic 095.8
    typhoid 002.0 [478.71]
  nose 478.19
  pinna 380.00
    acute 380.01
    chronic 380.02
  trachea 478.9
Periclasia 523.5
Pericolitis 569.89
Pericoronitis (chronic) 523.40
  acute 523.30
Pericystitis — see also Cystitis 595.9
Pericytoma (M9150/1) — see also Neoplasm, connective tissue, uncertain behavior
  benign (M9150/0) — see Neoplasm, connective tissue, benign
  malignant (M9150/3) — see Neoplasm, connective tissue, malignant
Peridacryocystitis, acute 375.32
Peridiverticulitis — see also Diverticulitis 562.11
Periduodenitis 535.6
Periendocarditis — see also Endocarditis 424.90
  acute or subacute 421.9
Periepididymitis — see also Epididymitis 604.90
Perifolliculitis (abscedens) 704.8
  capitis, abscedens et suffodiens 704.8
  dissecting, scalp 704.8
  scalp 704.8
  superficial pustular 704.8
Perigastritis (acute) 535.0
Perigastrojejunitis (acute) 535.0
Perihepatitis (acute) 573.3
  chlamydial 099.56
  gonococcal 098.86
Peri-ileitis (subacute) 569.89
Perilabyrinthitis (acute) — see Labyrinthitis
Perimeningitis — see Meningitis
Perimetritis — see also Endometritis 615.9
Perimetrosalpingitis — see also Salpingo-oophoritis 614.2
Perineocele 618.05
Perinephric — see condition
Perinephritic — see condition
Perinephritis — see also Infection, kidney 590.9
  purulent (see also Abscess, kidney) 590.2
Perineum, perineal — see condition
Perineuritis NEC 729.2
Periodic — see also condition
  disease (familial) 277.31
  edema 995.1
    hereditary 277.6
  fever 277.31
  limb movement disorder 327.51
  paralysis (familial) 359.3
  peritonitis 277.31
  polyserositis 277.31
  somnolence (see also Narcolepsy) 347.00
Periodontal
  cyst 522.8
  pocket 523.8
Periodontitis (chronic) (complex) (compound) (simplex) 523.40
  acute 523.33
  aggressive 523.30
    generalized 523.32
    localized 523.31
  apical 522.6
    acute (pulpal origin) 522.4
  generalized 523.42
  localized 523.41
Periodontoclasia 523.5

Periodontosis 523.5
Periods — see also Menstruation
  heavy 626.2
  irregular 626.4
Perionychia (with lymphangitis) 681.9
  finger 681.02
  toe 681.11
Perioophoritis — see also Salpingo-oophoritis 614.2
Periorchitis — see also Orchitis 604.90
Periosteum, periosteal — see condition
Periostitis (circumscribed) (diffuse) (infective) 730.3

Note — Use the following fifth-digit subclassification with category 730:

0 site unspecified
1 shoulder region
2 upper arm
3 forearm
4 hand
5 pelvic region and thigh
6 lower leg
7 ankle and foot
8 other specified sites
9 multiple sites

  with osteomyelitis (see also Osteomyelitis) 730.2
    acute or subacute 730.0
    chronic or old 730.1
  albuminosa, albuminosus 730.3
  alveolar 526.5
  alveolodental 526.5
  dental 526.5
  gonorrheal 098.89
  hyperplastica, generalized 731.2
  jaw (lower) (upper) 526.4
  monomelic 733.99
  orbital 376.02
  syphilitic 095.5
    congenital 090.0 [730.8]
    secondary 091.61
  tuberculous (see also Tuberculosis, bone) 015.9 [730.8]
  yaws (early) (hypertrophic) (late) 102.6
Periostosis — see also Periostitis 730.3
  with osteomyelitis (see also Osteomyelitis) 730.2
    acute or subacute 730.0
    chronic or old 730.1
  hyperplastic 756.59
Peripartum cardiomyopathy 674.5
Periphlebitis — see also Phlebitis 451.9
  lower extremity 451.2
    deep (vessels) 451.19
    superficial (vessels) 451.0
  portal 572.1
  retina 362.18
  superficial (vessels) 451.0
  tuberculous (see also Tuberculosis) 017.9
    retina 017.3 [362.18]
Peripneumonia — see Pneumonia
Periproctitis 569.49
Periprostatitis — see also Prostatitis 601.9
Perirectal — see condition
Perirenal — see condition
Perisalpingitis — see also Salpingo-oophoritis 614.2
Perisigmoiditis 569.89
Perisplenitis (infectional) 289.59
Perispondylitis — see Spondylitis
Peristalsis reversed or visible 787.4
Peritendinitis — see also Tenosynovitis 726.90
  adhesive (shoulder) 726.0
Perithelioma (M9150/1) — see Pericytoma
Peritoneum, peritoneal — see also condition

Peritoneum, peritoneal — see also condition — continued
  equilibration test V56.32
Peritonitis (acute) (adhesive) (fibrinous) (hemorrhagic) (idiopathic) (localized) (perforative) (primary) (with adhesions) (with effusion) 567.9
  with or following
    abortion — see Abortion, by type, with sepsis
    abscess 567.21
    appendicitis 540.0
      with peritoneal abscess 540.1
    ectopic pregnancy (see also categories 633.0–633.9) 639.0
    molar pregnancy (see also categories 630–632) 639.0
  aseptic 998.7
  bacterial 567.29
    spontaneous 567.23
  bile, biliary 567.81
  chemical 998.7
  chlamydial 099.56
  chronic proliferative 567.89
  congenital NEC 777.6
  diaphragmatic 567.22
  diffuse NEC 567.29
  diphtheritic 032.83
  disseminated NEC 567.29
  due to
    bile 567.81
    foreign
      body or object accidentally left during a procedure (instrument) (sponge) (swab) 998.4
      substance accidentally left during a procedure (chemical) (powder) (talc) 998.7
    talc 998.7
    urine 567.89
  fibrinopurulent 567.29
  fibrinous 567.29
  fibrocaseous (see also Tuberculosis) 014.0
  fibropurulent 567.29
  general, generalized (acute) 567.21
  gonococcal 098.86
  in infective disease NEC 136.9 [567.0]
  meconium (newborn) 777.6
  pancreatic 577.8
  paroxysmal, benign 277.31
  pelvic
    female (acute) 614.5
      chronic NEC 614.7
        with adhesions 614.6
      puerperal, postpartum, childbirth 670.0
    male (acute) 567.21
  periodic (familial) 277.31
  phlegmonous 567.29
  pneumococcal 567.1
  postabortal 639.0
  proliferative, chronic 567.89
  puerperal, postpartum, childbirth 670.0
  purulent 567.29
  septic 567.29
  spontaneous bacterial 567.23
  staphylococcal 567.29
  streptococcal 567.29
  subdiaphragmatic 567.29
  subphrenic 567.29
  suppurative 567.29
  syphilitic 095.2
    congenital 090.0 [567.0]
  talc 998.7
  tuberculous (see also Tuberculosis) 014.0
  urine 567.89
Peritonsillar — see condition
Peritonsillitis 475
Perityphlitis — see also Appendicitis 541
Periureteritis 593.89
Periurethral — see condition

Periurethritis (gangrenous) 597.89
Periuterine — see condition
Perivaginitis — see also Vaginitis 616.10
Perivasculitis, retinal 362.18
Perivasitis (chronic) 608.4
Periventricular leukomalacia 779.7
Perivesiculitis (seminal) — see also Vesiculitis 608.0
Perlèche 686.8
  due to
    moniliasis 112.0
    riboflavin deficiency 266.0
Pernicious — see condition
Pernio, perniosis 991.5
Persecution
  delusion 297.9
  social V62.4
Perseveration (tonic) 784.69
Persistence, persistent (congenital) 759.89
  anal membrane 751.2
  arteria stapedia 744.04
  atrioventricular canal 745.69
  bloody ejaculate 792.2
  branchial cleft 744.41
  bulbus cordis in left ventricle 745.8
  canal of Cloquet 743.51
  capsule (opaque) 743.51
  cilioretinal artery or vein 743.51
  cloaca 751.5
  communication — see Fistula, congenital
  convolutions
    aortic arch 747.21
    fallopian tube 752.19
    oviduct 752.19
    uterine tube 752.19
  double aortic arch 747.21
  ductus
    arteriosus 747.0
    Botalli 747.0
  fetal
    circulation 747.83
    form of cervix (uteri) 752.49
    hemoglobin (hereditary) ("Swiss variety") 282.7
    pulmonary hypertension 747.83
  foramen
    Botalli 745.5
    ovale 745.5
  Gartner's duct 752.41
  hemoglobin, fetal (hereditary) (HPFH) 282.7
  hyaloid
    artery (generally incomplete) 743.51
    system 743.51
  hymen (tag)
    in pregnancy or childbirth 654.8
      causing obstructed labor 660.2
  lanugo 757.4
  left
    posterior cardinal vein 747.49
    root with right arch of aorta 747.21
    superior vena cava 747.49
  Meckel's diverticulum 751.0
  mesonephric duct 752.89
    fallopian tube 752.11
  mucosal disease (middle ear) (with posterior or superior marginal perforation of ear drum) 382.2
  nail(s), anomalous 757.5
  occiput, anterior or posterior 660.3
    fetus or newborn 763.1
  omphalomesenteric duct 751.0
  organ or site NEC — see Anomaly, specified type NEC
  ostium
    atrioventriculare commune 745.69
    primum 745.61
    secundum 745.5
  ovarian rests in fallopian tube 752.19
  pancreatic tissue in intestinal tract 751.5

Persistence, persistent — continued
  primary (deciduous)
    teeth 520.6
    vitreous hyperplasia 743.51
  pulmonary hypertension 747.83
  pupillary membrane 743.46
    iris 743.46
  Rhesus (Rh) titer 999.7
  right aortic arch 747.21
  sinus
    urogenitalis 752.89
    venosus with imperfect incorporation in right auricle 747.49
  thymus (gland) 254.8
    hyperplasia 254.0
  thyroglossal duct 759.2
  thyrolingual duct 759.2
  truncus arteriosus or communis 745.0
  tunica vasculosa lentis 743.39
  umbilical sinus 753.7
  urachus 753.7
  vegetative state 780.03
  vitelline duct 751.0
  wolffian duct 752.89
Person (with)
  admitted for clinical research, as participant or control subject V70.7
  awaiting admission to adequate facility elsewhere V63.2
    undergoing social agency investigation V63.8
  concern (normal) about sick person in family V61.49
  consulting on behalf of another V65.19
    pediatric pre-birth visit for expectant mother V65.11
  feared
    complaint in whom no diagnosis was made V65.5
    condition not demonstrated V65.5
  feigning illness V65.2
  healthy, accompanying sick person V65.0
  living (in)
    without
      adequate
        financial resources V60.2
        housing (heating) (space) V60.1
      housing (permanent) (temporary) V60.0
      material resources V60.2
      person able to render necessary care V60.4
      shelter V60.0
    alone V60.3
    boarding school V60.6
    residence remote from hospital or medical care facility V63.0
    residential institution V60.6
  medical services in home not available V63.1
  on waiting list V63.2
    undergoing social agency investigation V63.8
  sick or handicapped in family V61.49
  "worried well" V65.5
Personality
  affective 301.10
  aggressive 301.3
  amoral 301.7
  anancastic, anankastic 301.4
  antisocial 301.7
  asocial 301.7
  asthenic 301.6
  avoidant 301.82
  borderline 301.83
  change 310.1
  compulsive 301.4
  cycloid 301.13
  cyclothymic 301.13
  dependent 301.6
  depressive (chronic) 301.12
  disorder, disturbance NEC 301.9

Personality — continued
  disorder, disturbance — continued
    with
      antisocial disturbance 301.7
      pattern disturbance NEC 301.9
      sociopathic disturbance 301.7
      trait disturbance 301.9
    dual 300.14
    dyssocial 301.7
    eccentric 301.89
      "haltlose" type 301.89
    emotionally unstable 301.59
    epileptoid 301.3
    explosive 301.3
    fanatic 301.0
    histrionic 301.50
    hyperthymic 301.11
    hypomanic 301.11
    hypothymic 301.12
    hysterical 301.50
    immature 301.89
    inadequate 301.6
    labile 301.59
    masochistic 301.89
    morally defective 301.7
    multiple 300.14
    narcissistic 301.81
    obsessional 301.4
    obsessive-compulsive 301.4
    overconscientious 301.4
    paranoid 301.0
    passive (-dependent) 301.6
    passive-aggressive 301.84
    pathologic NEC 301.9
    pattern defect or disturbance 301.9
    pseudosocial 301.7
    psychoinfantile 301.59
    psychoneurotic NEC 301.89
    psychopathic 301.9
      with
        amoral trend 301.7
        antisocial trend 301.7
        asocial trend 301.7
        pathologic sexuality (see also Deviation, sexual) 302.9
        mixed types 301.9
    schizoid 301.20
      with sexual deviation (see also Deviation, sexual) 302.9
        antisocial 301.7
        dyssocial 301.7
        introverted 301.21
        schizotypal 301.22
    type A 301.4
    unstable (emotional) 301.59
Perthes' disease (capital femoral osteochondrosis) 732.1
Pertussis — see also Whooping cough 033.9
  vaccination, prophylactic (against) V03.6
Peruvian wart 088.0
Perversion, perverted
  appetite 307.52
    hysterical 300.11
  function
    pineal gland 259.8
    pituitary gland 253.9
      anterior lobe
        deficient 253.2
        excessive 253.1
      posterior lobe 253.6
    placenta — see Placenta, abnormal
  sense of smell or taste 781.1
  psychogenic 306.7
  sexual (see also Deviation, sexual) 302.9
Pervious, congenital — see also Imperfect, closure
  ductus arteriosus 747.0
Pes (congenital) — see also Talipes 754.70
  abductus (congenital) 754.60
    acquired 736.79
  acquired NEC 736.79
  planus 734

Pes — see also Talipes — continued
  adductus (congenital) 754.79
    acquired 736.79
  cavus 754.71
    acquired 736.73
  planovalgus (congenital) 754.69
    acquired 736.79
  planus (acquired) (any degree) 734
    congenital 754.61
    rachitic 268.1
  valgus (congenital) 754.61
    acquired 736.79
  varus (congenital) 754.50
    acquired 736.79
Pest — see also Plague 020.9
Pestis — see also Plague 020.9
  bubonica 020.0
  fulminans 020.0
  minor 020.8
  pneumonica — see Plague, pneumonic
Petechial
  fever 036.0
  typhus 081.9
Petechia, petechiae 782.7
  fetus or newborn 772.6
Petges-Cléjat or Petges-Clégat syndrome (poikilodermatomyositis) 710.3
Petit's
  disease (see also Hernia, lumbar) 553.8
Petit mal (idiopathic) — see also Epilepsy 345.0 ☑
  status 345.2
Petrellidosis 117.6
Petrositis 383.20
  acute 383.21
  chronic 383.22
Peutz-Jeghers disease or syndrome 759.6
Peyronie's disease 607.85
Pfeiffer's disease 075
Phacentocele 379.32
  traumatic 921.3
Phacoanaphylaxis 360.19
Phacocele (old) 379.32
  traumatic 921.3
Phaehyphomycosis 117.8
Phagedena (dry) (moist) — see also Gangrene 785.4
  arteriosclerotic 440.24
  geometric 686.09
  penis 607.89
  senile 440.2 ☑ [785.4]
  sloughing 785.4
  tropical (see also Ulcer, skin) 707.9
  vulva 616.50
Phagedenic — see also condition
  abscess (see also Abscess)
    chancroid 099.0
  bubo NEC 099.8
  chancre 099.0
  ulcer (tropical) (see also Ulcer, skin) 707.9
Phagomania 307.52
Phakoma 362.89
Phantom limb (syndrome) 353.6
Pharyngeal — see also condition
  arch remnant 744.41
  pouch syndrome 279.11
Pharyngitis (acute) (catarrhal) (gangrenous) (infective) (malignant) (membranous) (phlegmonous) (pneumococcal) (pseudomembranous) (simple) (staphylococcal) (subacute) (suppurative) (ulcerative) (viral) 462
  with influenza, flu, or grippe 487.1
  aphthous 074.0
  atrophic 472.1
  chlamydial 099.51
  chronic 472.1
  Coxsackie virus 074.0
  diphtheritic (membranous) 032.0
  follicular 472.1
  fusospirochetal 101

Pharyngitis — continued
  gonococcal 098.6
  granular (chronic) 472.1
  herpetic 054.79
  hypertrophic 472.1
  infectional, chronic 472.1
  influenzal 487.1
  lymphonodular, acute 074.8
  septic 034.0
  streptococcal 034.0
  tuberculous (see also Tuberculosis) 012.8 ☑
  vesicular 074.0
Pharyngoconjunctival fever 077.2
Pharyngoconjunctivitis, viral 077.2
Pharyngolaryngitis (acute) 465.0
  chronic 478.9
  septic 034.0
Pharyngoplegia 478.29
Pharyngotonsillitis 465.8
  tuberculous 012.8 ☑
Pharyngotracheitis (acute) 465.8
  chronic 478.9
Pharynx, pharyngeal — see condition
Phase of life problem NEC V62.89
Phenomenon
  Arthus' 995.21
  flashback (drug) 292.89
  jaw-winking 742.8
  Jod-Basedow 242.8 ☑
  L. E. cell 710.0
  lupus erythematosus cell 710.0
  Pelger-Huët (hereditary hyposegmentation) 288.2
  Raynaud's (paroxysmal digital cyanosis) (secondary) 443.0
  Reilly's (see also Neuropathy, peripheral, autonomic) 337.9
  vasomotor 780.2
  vasospastic 443.9
  vasovagal 780.2
  Wenckebach's, heart block (second degree) 426.13
Phenylketonuria (PKU) 270.1
Phenylpyruvicaciduria 270.1
Pheochromoblastoma (M8700/3)
  specified site — see Neoplasm, by site, malignant
  unspecified site 194.0
Pheochromocytoma (M8700/0)
  malignant (M8700/3)
    specified site — see Neoplasm, by site, malignant
    unspecified site 194.0
  specified site — see Neoplasm, by site, benign
  unspecified site 227.0
Phimosis (congenital) 605
  chancroidal 099.0
  due to infection 605
Phlebectasia — see also Varicose, vein 454.9
  congenital NEC 747.60
  esophagus (see also Varix, esophagus) 456.1
    with hemorrhage (see also Varix, esophagus, bleeding) 456.0
Phlebitis (infective) (pyemic) (septic) (suppurative) 451.9
  antecubital vein 451.82
  arm NEC 451.84
    axillary vein 451.89
    basilic vein 451.82
    deep 451.83
    superficial 451.82
  axillary vein 451.89
  basilic vein 451.82
  blue 451.9
  brachial vein 451.83
  breast, superficial 451.89
  cavernous (venous) sinus — see Phlebitis, intracranial sinus
  cephalic vein 451.82
  cerebral (venous) sinus — see Phlebitis, intracranial sinus
  chest wall, superficial 451.89

Index to Diseases

Phlebitis — *continued*
- complicating pregnancy or puerperium 671.9 ☑
  - affecting fetus or newborn 760.3
- cranial (venous) sinus — *see* Phlebitis, intracranial sinus
- deep (vessels) 451.19
  - femoral vein 451.11
  - specified vessel NEC 451.19
- due to implanted device — *see* Complications, due to (presence of) any device, implant, or graft classified to 996.0–996.5 NEC
- during or resulting from a procedure 997.2
- femoral vein (deep) (superficial) 451.11
- femoropopliteal 451.19
- following infusion, perfusion, or transfusion 999.2
- gouty 274.89 [451.9]
- hepatic veins 451.89
- iliac vein 451.81
- iliofemoral 451.11
- intracranial sinus (any) (venous) 325
  - late effect — *see* category 326
  - nonpyogenic 437.6
    - in pregnancy or puerperium 671.5 ☑
- jugular vein 451.89
- lateral (venous) sinus — *see* Phlebitis, intracranial sinus
- leg 451.2
  - deep (vessels) 451.19
    - femoral vein 451.11
    - specified vessel NEC 451.19
  - superficial (vessels) 451.0
    - femoral vein 451.11
- longitudinal sinus — *see* Phlebitis, intracranial sinus
- lower extremity 451.2
  - deep (vessels) 451.19
    - femoral vein 451.11
    - specified vessel NEC 451.19
- migrans, migrating (superficial) 453.1
- superficial (vessels) 451.0
  - femoral vein 451.11
- pelvic
  - with
    - abortion — *see* Abortion, by type, with sepsis
    - ectopic pregnancy (*see also* categories 633.0–633.9) 639.0
    - molar pregnancy (*see also* categories 630–632) 639.0
  - following
    - abortion 639.0
    - ectopic or molar pregnancy 639.0
  - puerperal, postpartum 671.4 ☑
- popliteal vein 451.19
- portal (vein) 572.1
- postoperative 997.2
- pregnancy 671.9 ☑
  - deep 671.3 ☑
  - specified type NEC 671.5 ☑
  - superficial 671.2 ☑
- puerperal, postpartum, childbirth 671.9 ☑
  - deep 671.4 ☑
  - lower extremities 671.2 ☑
  - pelvis 671.4 ☑
  - specified site NEC 671.5 ☑
  - superficial 671.2 ☑
- radial vein 451.83
- retina 362.18
- saphenous (great) (long) 451.0
  - accessory or small 451.0
- sinus (meninges) — *see* Phlebitis, intracranial sinus
- specified site NEC 451.89
- subclavian vein 451.89
- syphilitic 093.89
- tibial vein 451.19
- ulcer, ulcerative 451.9

Phlebitis — *continued*
- ulcer, ulcerative — *continued*
  - leg 451.2
    - deep (vessels) 451.19
      - femoral vein 451.11
      - specified vessel NEC 451.19
    - superficial (vessels) 451.0
      - femoral vein 451.11
    - lower extremity 451.2
      - deep (vessels) 451.19
        - femoral vein 451.11
        - specified vessel NEC 451.19
      - superficial (vessels) 451.0
  - ulnar vein 451.83
  - umbilicus 451.89
  - upper extremity (*see also* Phlebitis, arm)
    - deep (veins) 451.83
      - brachial vein 451.83
      - radial vein 451.83
      - ulnar vein 451.83
    - superficial (veins) 451.82
      - antecubital vein 451.82
      - basilica vein 451.82
      - cephalic vein 451.82
  - uterus (septic) (*see also* Endometritis) 615.9
  - varicose (leg) (lower extremity) (*see also* Varicose, vein) 454.1

Phlebofibrosis 459.89
Phleboliths 459.89
Phlebosclerosis 459.89
Phlebothrombosis — *see* Thrombosis
Phlebotomus fever 066.0
Phlegmasia
- alba dolens (deep vessels) 451.19
  - complicating pregnancy 671.3 ☑
  - nonpuerperal 451.19
  - puerperal, postpartum, childbirth 671.4 ☑
- cerulea dolens 451.19

Phlegm, choked on 933.1
Phlegmon — *see also* Abscess 682.9
- erysipelatous (*see also* Erysipelas) 035
- iliac 682.2
  - fossa 540.1
- throat 478.29

Phlegmonous — *see* condition
Phlyctenulosis (allergic) (keratoconjunctivitis) (nontuberculous) 370.31
- cornea 370.31
  - with ulcer (*see also* Ulcer, cornea) 370.00
- tuberculous (*see also* Tuberculosis) 017.3 ☑ [370.31]

Phobia, phobic (reaction) 300.20
- animal 300.29
- isolated NEC 300.29
- obsessional 300.3
- simple NEC 300.29
- social 300.23
- specified NEC 300.29
- state 300.20

Phocas' disease 610.1
Phocomelia 755.4
- lower limb 755.32
  - complete 755.33
  - distal 755.35
  - proximal 755.34
- upper limb 755.22
  - complete 755.23
  - distal 755.25
  - proximal 755.24

Phoria — *see also* Heterophoria 378.40
Phosphate-losing tubular disorder 588.0
Phosphatemia 275.3
Phosphaturia 275.3
Photoallergic response 692.72
Photocoproporphyria 277.1
Photodermatitis (sun) 692.72
- light other than sun 692.82
Photokeratitis 370.24
Photo-ophthalmia 370.24
Photophobia 368.13
Photopsia 368.15

Photoretinitis 363.31
Photoretinopathy 363.31
Photosensitiveness (sun) 692.72
- light other than sun 692.82
Photosensitization (skin) (sun) 692.72
- light other than sun 692.82
Phototoxic response 692.72
Phrenitis 323.9
Phrynoderma 264.8
Phthiriasis (pubis) (any site) 132.2
- with any infestation classifiable to 132.0, 132.1, 132.3

Phthirus infestation — *see* Phthiriasis
Phthisis — *see also* Tuberculosis 011.9 ☑
- bulbi (infectional) 360.41
- colliers' 011.4 ☑
- cornea 371.05
- eyeball (due to infection) 360.41
- millstone makers' 011.4 ☑
- miners' 011.4 ☑
- potters' 011.4 ☑
- sandblasters' 011.4 ☑
- stonemasons' 011.4 ☑

Phycomycosis 117.7
Physalopteriasis 127.7
Physical therapy NEC V57.1
- breathing exercises V57.0

Physiological cup, optic papilla
- borderline, glaucoma suspect 365.00
- enlarged 377.14
- glaucomatous 377.14

Phytobezoar 938
- intestine 936
- stomach 935.2

Pian — *see also* Yaws 102.9
Pianoma 102.1
Piarhemia, piarrhemia — *see also* Hyperlipemia 272.4
- bilharziasis 120.9

Pica 307.52
- hysterical 300.11

Pick's
- cerebral atrophy 331.11
  - with dementia
    - with behavioral disturbance 331.11 [294.11]
    - without behavioral disturbance 331.11 [294.10]
- disease
  - brain 331.11
    - dementia in
      - with behavioral disturbance 331.11 [294.11]
      - without behavioral disturbance 331.11 [294.10]
  - lipid histiocytosis 272.7
  - liver (pericardial pseudocirrhosis of liver) 423.2
  - pericardium (pericardial pseudocirrhosis of liver) 423.2
  - polyserositis (pericardial pseudocirrhosis of liver) 423.2
- syndrome
  - heart (pericardial pseudocirrhosis of liver) 423.2
  - liver (pericardial pseudocirrhosis of liver) 423.2
- tubular adenoma (M8640/0)
  - specified site — *see* Neoplasm, by site, benign
  - unspecified site
    - female 220
    - male 222.0

Pick-Herxheimer syndrome (diffuse idiopathic cutaneous atrophy) 701.8
Pick-Niemann disease (lipid histiocytosis) 272.7
Pickwickian syndrome (cardiopulmonary obesity) 278.8
Piebaldism, classic 709.09
Piedra 111.2
- beard 111.2
  - black 111.3
  - white 111.2
- black 111.3

Piedra — *continued*
- scalp 111.3
  - black 111.3
  - white 111.2
- white 111.2

Pierre Marie-Bamberger syndrome (hypertrophic pulmonary osteoarthropathy) 731.2
Pierre Marie's syndrome (pulmonary hypertrophic osteoarthropathy) 731.2
Pierre Mauriac's syndrome (diabetes-dwarfism-obesity) 258.1
Pierre Robin deformity or syndrome (congenital) 756.0
Pierson's disease or osteochondrosis 732.1
Pigeon
- breast or chest (acquired) 738.3
  - congenital 754.82
  - rachitic (*see also* Rickets) 268.0
- breeders' disease or lung 495.2
- fanciers' disease or lung 495.2
- toe 735.8

Pigmentation (abnormal) 709.00
- anomaly 709.00
  - congenital 757.33
  - specified NEC 709.09
- conjunctiva 372.55
- cornea 371.10
  - anterior 371.11
  - posterior 371.13
  - stromal 371.12
- lids (congenital) 757.33
  - acquired 374.52
- limbus corneae 371.10
- metals 709.00
- optic papilla, congenital 743.57
- retina (congenital) (grouped) (nevoid) 743.53
  - acquired 362.74
- scrotum, congenital 757.33

Piles — *see* Hemorrhoids
Pili
- annulati or torti (congenital) 757.4
- incarnati 704.8

Pill roller hand (intrinsic) 736.09
Pilomatrixoma (M8110/0) — *see* Neoplasm, skin, benign
Pilonidal — *see* condition
Pimple 709.8
PIN I (prostatic intraepithelial neoplasia I) 602.3
PIN II (prostatic intraepithelial neoplasia II) 602.3
PIN III (prostatic intraepithelial neoplasia III) 233.4
Pinched nerve — *see* Neuropathy, entrapment
Pineal body or gland — *see* condition
Pinealoblastoma (M9362/3) 194.4
Pinealoma (M9360/1) 237.1
- malignant (M9360/3) 194.4
Pineoblastoma (M9362/3) 194.4
Pineocytoma (M9361/1) 237.1
Pinguecula 372.51
Pinhole meatus — *see also* Stricture, urethra 598.9
Pink
- disease 985.0
- eye 372.03
- puffer 492.8

Pinkus' disease (lichen nitidus) 697.1
Pinpoint
- meatus (*see also* Stricture, urethra) 598.9
- os uteri (*see also* Stricture, cervix) 622.4

Pinselhaare (congenital) 757.4
Pinta 103.9
- cardiovascular lesions 103.2
- chancre (primary) 103.0
- erythematous plaques 103.1
- hyperchromic lesions 103.1
- hyperkeratosis 103.1
- lesions 103.9

Pinta — *continued*
  lesions — *continued*
    cardiovascular 103.2
    hyperchromic 103.1
    intermediate 103.1
    late 103.2
    mixed 103.3
    primary 103.0
    skin (achromic) (cicatricial) (dyschromic) 103.2
      hyperchromic 103.1
      mixed (achromic and hyperchromic) 103.3
  papule (primary) 103.0
  skin lesions (achromic) (cicatricial) (dyschromic) 103.2
    hyperchromic 103.1
    mixed (achromic and hyperchromic) 103.3
  vitiligo 103.2
Pintid 103.0
Pinworms (disease) (infection) (infestation) 127.4
Piry fever 066.8
Pistol wound — *see* Gunshot wound
Pitchers' elbow 718.82
Pithecoid pelvis 755.69
  with disproportion (fetopelvic) 653.2
    affecting fetus or newborn 763.1
    causing obstructed labor 660.1
Pithiatism 300.11
Pit, lip (mucus), **congenital** 750.25
Pitted — *see also* Pitting
  teeth 520.4
Pitting (edema) — *see also* Edema 782.3
  lip 782.3
  nail 703.8
    congenital 757.5
Pituitary gland — *see* condition
Pituitary snuff-takers' disease 495.8
Pityriasis 696.5
  alba 696.5
  capitis 690.11
  circinata (et maculata) 696.3
  Hebra's (exfoliative dermatitis) 695.89
  lichenoides et varioliformis 696.2
  maculata (et circinata) 696.3
  nigra 111.1
  pilaris 757.39
    acquired 701.1
    Hebra's 696.4
  rosea 696.3
  rotunda 696.3
  rubra (Hebra) 695.89
    pilaris 696.4
  sicca 690.18
  simplex 690.18
  specified type NEC 696.5
  streptogenes 696.5
  versicolor 111.0
    scrotal 111.0
Placenta, placental
  ablatio 641.2
    affecting fetus or newborn 762.1
  abnormal, abnormality 656.7
    with hemorrhage 641.8
      affecting fetus or newborn 762.1
    affecting fetus or newborn 762.2
  abruptio 641.2
    affecting fetus or newborn 762.1
  accessory lobe — *see* Placenta, abnormal
  accreta (without hemorrhage) 667.0
    with hemorrhage 666.0
  adherent (without hemorrhage) 667.0
    with hemorrhage 666.0
  apoplexy — *see* Placenta, separation
  battledore — *see* Placenta, abnormal
  bilobate — *see* Placenta, abnormal
  bipartita — *see* Placenta, abnormal
  carneous mole 631
  centralis — *see* Placenta, previa
  circumvallata — *see* Placenta, abnormal

Placenta, placental — *continued*
  cyst (amniotic) — *see* Placenta, abnormal
  deficiency — *see* Placenta, insufficiency
  degeneration — *see* Placenta, insufficiency
  detachment (partial) (premature) (with hemorrhage) 641.2
    affecting fetus or newborn 762.1
  dimidiata — *see* Placenta, abnormal
  disease 656.7
    affecting fetus or newborn 762.2
  duplex — *see* Placenta, abnormal
  dysfunction — *see* Placenta, insufficiency
  fenestrata — *see* Placenta, abnormal
  fibrosis — *see* Placenta, abnormal
  fleshy mole 631
  hematoma — *see* Placenta, abnormal
  hemorrhage NEC — *see* Placenta, separation
  hormone disturbance or malfunction — *see* Placenta, abnormal
  hyperplasia — *see* Placenta, abnormal
  increta (without hemorrhage) 667.0
    with hemorrhage 666.0
  infarction 656.7
    affecting fetus or newborn 762.2
  insertion, vicious — *see* Placenta, previa
  insufficiency
    affecting
      fetus or newborn 762.2
      management of pregnancy 656.5
  lateral — *see* Placenta, previa
  low implantation or insertion — *see* Placenta, previa
  low-lying — *see* Placenta, previa
  malformation — *see* Placenta, abnormal
  malposition — *see* Placenta, previa
  marginalis, marginata — *see* Placenta, previa
  marginal sinus (hemorrhage) (rupture) 641.2
    affecting fetus or newborn 762.1
  membranacea — *see* Placenta, abnormal
  multilobed — *see* Placenta, abnormal
  multipartita — *see* Placenta, abnormal
  necrosis — *see* Placenta, abnormal
  percreta (without hemorrhage) 667.0
    with hemorrhage 666.0
  polyp 674.4
  previa (central) (centralis) (complete) (lateral) (marginal) (marginalis) (partial) (partialis) (total) (with hemorrhage) 641.1
    without hemorrhage (before labor and delivery) (during pregnancy) 641.0
    affecting fetus or newborn 762.0
    noted
      before labor, without hemorrhage (with cesarean delivery) 641.0
      during pregnancy (without hemorrhage) 641.0
  retention (with hemorrhage) 666.0
    without hemorrhage 667.0
    fragments, complicating puerperium (delayed hemorrhage) 666.2
      without hemorrhage 667.1
    postpartum, puerperal 666.2
  separation (normally implanted) (partial) (premature) (with hemorrhage) 641.2
    affecting fetus or newborn 762.1
  septuplex — *see* Placenta, abnormal
  small — *see* Placenta, insufficiency
  softening (premature) — *see* Placenta, abnormal

Placenta, placental — *continued*
  spuria — *see* Placenta, abnormal
  succenturiata — *see* Placenta, abnormal
  syphilitic 095.8
  transfusion syndromes 762.3
  transmission of chemical substance — *see* Absorption, chemical, through placenta
  trapped (with hemorrhage) 666.0
    without hemorrhage 667.0
  trilobate — *see* Placenta, abnormal
  tripartita — *see* Placenta, abnormal
  triplex — *see* Placenta, abnormal
  varicose vessel — *see* Placenta, abnormal
  vicious insertion — *see* Placenta, previa
Placentitis
  affecting fetus or newborn 762.7
  complicating pregnancy 658.4
Plagiocephaly (skull) 754.0
Plague 020.9
  abortive 020.8
  ambulatory 020.8
  bubonic 020.0
  cellulocutaneous 020.1
  lymphatic gland 020.0
  pneumonic 020.5
    primary 020.3
    secondary 020.4
  pulmonary — *see* Plague, pneumonic
  pulmonic — *see* Plague, pneumonic
  septicemic 020.2
  tonsillar 020.9
    septicemic 020.2
  vaccination, prophylactic (against) V03.3
Planning, family V25.09
  contraception V25.9
  procreation V26.4
Plaque
  artery, arterial — *see* Arteriosclerosis
  calcareous — *see* Calcification
  Hollenhorst's (retinal) 362.33
  tongue 528.6
Plasma cell myeloma 203.0
Plasmacytoma, plasmocytoma (solitary) (M9731/1) 238.6
  benign (M9731/0) — *see* Neoplasm, by site, benign
  malignant (M9731/3) 203.8
Plasmacytopenia 288.59 •
Plasmacytosis 288.64 ▲
Plaster ulcer — *see also* Decubitus 707.00
Platybasia 756.0
Platyonychia (congenital) 757.5
  acquired 703.8
Platypelloid pelvis 738.6
  with disproportion (fetopelvic) 653.2
    affecting fetus or newborn 763.1
    causing obstructed labor 660.1
      affecting fetus or newborn 763.1
  congenital 755.69
Platyspondylia 756.19
Plethora 782.62
  newborn 776.4
Pleuralgia 786.52
Pleura, pleural — *see* condition
Pleurisy (acute) (adhesive) (chronic) (costal) (diaphragmatic) (double) (dry) (fetid) (fibrinous) (fibrous) (interlobar) (latent) (lung) (old) (plastic) (primary) (residual) (sicca) (sterile) (subacute) (unresolved) (with adherent pleura) 511.0
  with
    effusion (without mention of cause) 511.9
      bacterial, nontuberculous 511.1
      nontuberculous NEC 511.9
        bacterial 511.1
      pneumococcal 511.1
      specified type NEC 511.8
      staphylococcal 511.1

Pleurisy — *continued*
  with — *continued*
    effusion — *continued*
      streptococcal 511.1
      tuberculous (*see also* Tuberculosis, pleura) 012.0
        primary, progressive 010.1
    influenza, flu, or grippe 487.1
    tuberculosis — *see* Pleurisy, tuberculous
  encysted 511.8
  exudative (*see also* Pleurisy, with effusion) 511.9
    bacterial, nontuberculous 511.1
  fibrinopurulent 510.9
    with fistula 510.0
  fibropurulent 510.9
    with fistula 510.0
  hemorrhagic 511.8
  influenzal 487.1
  pneumococcal 511.0
    with effusion 511.1
  purulent 510.9
    with fistula 510.0
  septic 510.9
    with fistula 510.0
  serofibrinous (*see also* Pleurisy, with effusion) 511.9
    bacterial, nontuberculous 511.1
  seropurulent 510.9
    with fistula 510.0
  serous (*see also* Pleurisy, with effusion) 511.9
    bacterial, nontuberculous 511.1
  staphylococcal 511.0
    with effusion 511.1
  streptococcal 511.0
    with effusion 511.1
  suppurative 510.9
    with fistula 510.0
  traumatic (post) (current) 862.29
    with open wound into cavity 862.39
  tuberculous (with effusion) (*see also* Tuberculosis, pleura) 012.0
    primary, progressive 010.1
Pleuritis sicca — *see* Pleurisy
Pleurobronchopneumonia — *see also* Pneumonia, broncho- 485
Pleurodynia 786.52
  epidemic 074.1
  viral 074.1
Pleurohepatitis 573.8
Pleuropericarditis — *see also* Pericarditis 423.9
  acute 420.90
Pleuropneumonia (acute) (bilateral) (double) (septic) — *see also* Pneumonia 486
  chronic (*see also* Fibrosis, lung) 515
Pleurorrhea — *see also* Hydrothorax 511.8
Plexitis, brachial 353.0
Plica
  knee 727.83
  polonica 132.0
  syndrome 727.83
  tonsil 474.8
Plicae dysphonia ventricularis 784.49
Plicated tongue 529.5
  congenital 750.13
Plug
  bronchus NEC 519.19 ▲
  meconium (newborn) NEC 777.1
  mucus — *see* Mucus, plug
Plumbism 984.9
  specified type of lead — *see* Table of Drugs and Chemicals
Plummer's disease (toxic nodular goiter) 242.3
Plummer-Vinson syndrome (sideropenic dysphagia) 280.8
Pluricarential syndrome of infancy 260
Pluridefeciency syndrome of infancy 260

Index to Diseases

Plus (and minus) **hand** (intrinsic) 736.09
PMDD (premenstrual dysphoric disorder) 625.4
PMS 625.4
Pneumathemia — see Air, embolism, by type
Pneumatic drill or hammer disease 994.9
Pneumatocele (lung) 518.89
   intracranial 348.8
   tension 492.0
Pneumatosis
   cystoides intestinalis 569.89
   peritonei 568.89
   pulmonum 492.8
Pneumaturia 599.84
Pneumoblastoma (M8981/3) — see Neoplasm, lung, malignant
Pneumocephalus 348.8
Pneumococcemia 038.2
Pneumococcus, pneumococcal — see condition
Pneumoconiosis (due to) (inhalation of) 505
   aluminum 503
   asbestos 501
   bagasse 495.1
   bauxite 503
   beryllium 503
   carbon electrode makers' 503
   coal
      miners' (simple) 500
      workers' (simple) 500
   cotton dust 504
   diatomite fibrosis 502
   dust NEC 504
      inorganic 503
      lime 502
      marble 502
      organic NEC 504
   fumes or vapors (from silo) 506.9
   graphite 503
   hard metal 503
   mica 502
   moldy hay 495.0
   rheumatoid 714.81
   silica NEC 502
      and carbon 500
   silicate NEC 502
   talc 502
Pneumocystis carinii pneumonia 136.3
Pneumocystis jiroveci pneumonia 136.3
Pneumocystosis 136.3
   with pneumonia 136.3
Pneumoenteritis 025
Pneumohemopericardium — see also Pericarditis 423.9
Pneumohemothorax — see also Hemothorax 511.8
   traumatic 860.4
      with open wound into thorax 860.5
Pneumohydropericardium — see also Pericarditis 423.9
Pneumohydrothorax — see also Hydrothorax 511.8
Pneumomediastinum 518.1
   congenital 770.2
   fetus or newborn 770.2
Pneumomycosis 117.9
Pneumonia (acute) (Alpenstich) (benign) (bilateral) (brain) (cerebral) (circumscribed) (congestive) (creeping) (delayed resolution) (double) (epidemic) (fever) (flash) (fulminant) (fungoid) (granulomatous) (hemorrhagic) (incipient) (infantile) (infectious) (infiltration) (insular) (intermittent) (latent) (lobe) (migratory) (newborn) (organized) (overwhelming) (primary) (progressive) (pseudolobar) (purulent) (resolved) (secondary) (senile) (septic) (suppurative) (terminal) (true) (unresolved) (vesicular) 486

Pneumonia — continued
   with influenza, flu, or grippe 487.0
   adenoviral 480.0
   adynamic 514
   alba 090.0
   allergic 518.3
   alveolar — see Pneumonia, lobar
   anaerobes 482.81
   anthrax 022.1 [484.5]
   apex, apical — see Pneumonia, lobar
   ascaris 127.0 [484.8]
   aspiration 507.0
      due to
         aspiration of microorganisms
            bacterial 482.9
               specified organism NEC 483.8
               bacterial NEC 482.89
            viral 480.9
               specified type NEC 480.8
         food (regurgitated) 507.0
         gastric secretions 507.0
         milk 507.0
         oils, essences 507.1
         solids, liquids NEC 507.8
         vomitus 507.0
      fetal 770.18
         due to
            blood 770.16
            clear amniotic fluid 770.14
            meconium 770.12
            postnatal stomach contents 770.86
      newborn 770.18
         due to
            blood 770.16
            clear amniotic fluid 770.14
            meconium 770.12
            postnatal stomach contents 770.86
   asthenic 514
   atypical (disseminated) (focal) (primary) 486
      with influenza 487.0
   bacillus 482.9
      specified type NEC 482.89
   bacterial 482.9
      specified type NEC 482.89
   Bacteroides (fragilis) (oralis) (melaninogenicus) 482.81
   basal, basic, basilar — see Pneumonia, lobar
   broncho-, bronchial (confluent) (croupous) (diffuse) (disseminated) (hemorrhagic) (involving lobes) (lobar) (terminal) 485
      with influenza 487.0
      allergic 518.3
      aspiration (see also Pneumonia, aspiration) 507.0
      bacterial 482.9
         specified type NEC 482.89
      capillary 466.19
         with bronchospasm or obstruction 466.19
      chronic (see also Fibrosis, lung) 515
      congenital (infective) 770.0
      diplococcal 481
      Eaton's agent 483.0
      Escherichia coli (E. coli) 482.82
      Friedländer's bacillus 482.0
      Hemophilus influenzae 482.2
      hiberno-vernal 083.0 [484.8]
      hypostatic 514
      influenzal 487.0
      inhalation (see also Pneumonia, aspiration) 507.0
         due to fumes or vapors (chemical) 506.0
      Klebsiella 482.0
      lipid 507.1
         endogenous 516.8
      Mycoplasma (pneumoniae) 483.0
      ornithosis 073.0

Pneumonia — continued
   broncho-, bronchial — continued
      pleuropneumonia-like organisms (PPLO) 483.0
      pneumococcal 481
      Proteus 482.83
      Pseudomonas 482.1
      specified organism NEC 483.8
         bacterial NEC 482.89
      staphylococcal 482.40
         aureus 482.41
         specified type NEC 482.49
      streptococcal — see Pneumonia, streptococcal
      typhoid 002.0 [484.8]
      viral, virus (see also Pneumonia, viral) 480.9
   Butyrivibrio (fibriosolvens) 482.81
   Candida 112.4
   capillary 466.19
      with bronchospasm or obstruction 466.19
   caseous (see also Tuberculosis) 011.6
   catarrhal — see Pneumonia, bronchocentral — see Pneumonia, lobar
   Chlamydia, chlamydial 483.1
      pneumoniae 483.1
      psittaci 073.0
      specified type NEC 483.1
      trachomatis 483.1
   cholesterol 516.8
   chronic (see also Fibrosis, lung) 515
   cirrhotic (chronic) (see also Fibrosis, lung) 515
   Clostridium (haemolyticum) (novyi) NEC 482.81
   confluent — see Pneumonia, broncho-
   congenital (infective) 770.0
      aspiration 770.18
   croupous — see Pneumonia, lobar
   cytomegalic inclusion 078.5 [484.1]
   deglutition (see also Pneumonia, aspiration) 507.0
   desquamative interstitial 516.8
   diffuse — see Pneumonia, broncho-
   diplococcal, diplococcus (broncho-) (lobar) 481
   disseminated (focal) — see Pneumonia, broncho-
   due to
      adenovirus 480.0
      anaerobes 482.81
      Bacterium anitratum 482.83
      Chlamydia, chlamydial 483.1
         pneumoniae 483.1
         psittaci 073.0
         specified type NEC 483.1
         trachomatis 483.1
      coccidioidomycosis 114.0
      Diplococcus (pneumoniae) 481
      Eaton's agent 483.0
      Escherichia coli (E. coli) 482.82
      Friedländer's bacillus 482.0
      fumes or vapors (chemical) (inhalation) 506.0
      fungus NEC 117.9 [484.7]
         coccidioidomycosis 114.0
      Hemophilus influenzae (H. influenzae) 482.2
      Herellea 482.83
      influenza 487.0
      Klebsiella pneumoniae 482.0
      Mycoplasma (pneumoniae) 483.0
      parainfluenza virus 480.2
      pleuropneumonia-like organism (PPLO) 483.0
      Pneumococcus 481
      Pneumocystis carinii 136.3
      Pneumocystis jiroveci 136.3
      Proteus 482.83
      Pseudomonas 482.1
      respiratory syncytial virus 480.1
      rickettsia 083.9 [484.8]
      SARS-associated coronavirus 480.3

Pneumonia — continued
   due to — continued
      specified
         bacteria NEC 482.89
         organism NEC 483.8
         virus NEC 480.8
      Staphylococcus 482.40
         aureus 482.41
         specified type NEC 482.49
      Streptococcus (see also Pneumonia, streptococcal)
         pneumoniae 481
      virus (see also Pneumonia, viral) 480.9
      SARS-associated coronavirus 480.3
   Eaton's agent 483.0
   embolic, embolism — (see Embolism, pulmonary
   eosinophilic 518.3
   Escherichia coli (E. coli) 482.82
   Eubacterium 482.81
   fibrinous — see Pneumonia, lobar
   fibroid (chronic) (see also Fibrosis, lung) 515
   fibrous (see also Fibrosis, lung) 515
   Friedländer's bacillus 482.0
   Fusobacterium (nucleatum) 482.81
   gangrenous 513.0
   giant cell (see also Pneumonia, viral) 480.9
   gram-negative bacteria NEC 482.83
      anaerobic 482.81
   grippal 487.0
   Hemophilus influenzae (bronchial) (lobar) 482.2
   hypostatic (broncho-) (lobar) 514
   in
      actinomycosis 039.1
      anthrax 022.1 [484.5]
      aspergillosis 117.3 [484.6]
      candidiasis 112.4
      coccidioidomycosis 114.0
      cytomegalic inclusion disease 078.5 [484.1]
      histoplasmosis (see also Histoplasmosis) 115.95
      infectious disease NEC 136.9 [484.8]
      measles 055.1
      mycosis, systemic NEC 117.9 [484.7]
      nocardiasis, nocardiosis 039.1
      ornithosis 073.0
      pneumocystosis 136.3
      psittacosis 073.0
      Q fever 083.0 [484.8]
      salmonellosis 003.22
      toxoplasmosis 130.4
      tularemia 021.2
      typhoid (fever) 002.0 [484.8]
      varicella 052.1
      whooping cough (see also Whooping cough) 033.9 [484.3]
   infective, acquired prenatally 770.0
   influenzal (broncho) (lobar) (virus) 487.0
   inhalation (see also Pneumonia, aspiration) 507.0
      fumes or vapors (chemical) 506.0
   interstitial 516.8
      with influenzal 487.0
      acute 136.3
      chronic (see also Fibrosis, lung) 515
      desquamative 516.8
      hypostatic 514
      lipoid 507.1
      lymphoid 516.8
      plasma cell 136.3
      Pseudomonas 482.1
   intrauterine (infective) 770.0
      aspiration 770.18
         blood 770.16
         clear amniotic fluid 770.14
         meconium 770.12

Pneumonia

Pneumonia — *continued*
  intrauterine — *continued*
    aspiration — *continued*
      postnatal stomach contents 770.86
  Klebsiella pneumoniae 482.0
  Legionnaires' 482.84
  lipid, lipoid (exogenous) (interstitial) 507.1
    endogenous 516.8
  lobar (diplococcal) (disseminated) (double) (interstitial) (pneumococcal, any type) 481
    with influenza 487.0
    bacterial 482.9
      specified type NEC 482.89
    chronic (*see also* Fibrosis, lung) 515
    Escherichia coli (E. coli) 482.82
    Friedländer's bacillus 482.0
    Hemophilus influenzae (H. influenzae) 482.2
    hypostatic 514
    influenzal 487.0
    Klebsiella 482.0
    ornithosis 073.0
    Proteus 482.83
    Pseudomonas 482.1
    psittacosis 073.0
    specified organism NEC 483.8
      bacterial NEC 482.89
    staphylococcal 482.40
      aureus 482.41
      specified type NEC 482.49
    streptococcal — *see* Pneumonia, streptococcal
    viral, virus (*see also* Pneumonia, viral) 480.9
  lobular (confluent) — *see* Pneumonia, broncho-
  Löffler's 518.3
  massive — *see* Pneumonia, lobar
  meconium aspiration 770.12
  metastatic NEC 038.8 [484.8]
  Mycoplasma (pneumoniae) 483.0
  necrotic 513.0
  nitrogen dioxide 506.9
  orthostatic 514
  parainfluenza virus 480.2
  parenchymatous (*see also* Fibrosis, lung) 515
  passive 514
  patchy — *see* Pneumonia, broncho-
  Peptococcus 482.81
  Peptostreptococcus 482.81
  plasma cell 136.3
  pleurolobar — *see* Pneumonia, lobar
  pleuropneumonia-like organism (PPLO) 483.0
  pneumococcal (broncho) (lobar) 481
  Pneumocystis (carinii) ▶(jiroveci)◀ 136.3
  postinfectional NEC 136.9 [484.8]
  postmeasles 055.1
  postoperative 997.3
  primary atypical 486
  Proprionibacterium 482.81
  Proteus 482.83
  Pseudomonas 482.1
  psittacosis 073.0
  radiation 508.0
  respiratory syncytial virus 480.1
  resulting from a procedure 997.3
  rheumatic 390 [517.1]
  Salmonella 003.22
  SARS-associated coronavirus 480.3
  segmented, segmental — *see* Pneumonia, broncho-
  Serratia (marcescens) 482.83
  specified
    bacteria NEC 482.89
    organism NEC 483.8
    virus NEC 480.8
  spirochetal 104.8 [484.8]
  staphylococcal (broncho) (lobar) 482.40

Pneumonia — *continued*
  staphylococcal — *continued*
    aureus 482.41
    specified type NEC 482.49
  static, stasis 514
  streptococcal (broncho) (lobar) NEC 482.30
    Group
      A 482.31
      B 482.32
      specified NEC 482.39
    pneumoniae 481
    specified type NEC 482.39
  Streptococcus pneumoniae 481
  traumatic (complication) (early) (secondary) 958.8
  tuberculous (any) (*see also* Tuberculosis) 011.6 ☑
  tularemic 021.2
  TWAR agent 483.1
  varicella 052.1
  Veillonella 482.81
  viral, virus (broncho) (interstitial) (lobar) 480.9
    with influenza, flu, or grippe 487.0
    adenoviral 480.0
    parainfluenza 480.2
    respiratory syncytial 480.1
    SARS-associated coronavirus 480.3
    specified type NEC 480.8
  white (congenital) 090.0
Pneumonic — *see* condition
Pneumonitis (acute) (primary) — *see also* Pneumonia 486
  allergic 495.9
    specified type NEC 495.8
  aspiration 507.0
    due to fumes or gases 506.0
    fetal 770.18
      due to
        blood 770.16
        clear amniotic fluid 770.14
        meconium 770.12
        postnatal stomach contents 770.86
    newborn 770.18
      due to
        blood 770.16
        clear amniotic fluid 770.14
        meconium 770.12
        postnatal stomach contents 770.86
    obstetric 668.0 ☑
  chemical 506.0
    due to fumes or gases 506.0
  cholesterol 516.8
  chronic (*see also* Fibrosis, lung) 515
  congenital rubella 771.0
  crack 506.0
  due to
    crack (cocaine) 506.0
    fumes or vapors 506.0
    inhalation
      food (regurgitated), milk, vomitus 507.0
      oils, essences 507.1
      saliva 507.0
      solids, liquids NEC 507.8
    toxoplasmosis (acquired) 130.4
      congenital (active) 771.2 [484.8]
  eosinophilic 518.3
  fetal aspiration 770.18
    due to
      blood 770.16
      clear amniotic fluid 770.14
      meconium 770.12
      postnatal stomach contents 770.86
  hypersensitivity 495.9
  interstitial (chronic) (*see also* Fibrosis, lung) 515
  lymphoid 516.8
  lymphoid, interstitial 516.8
  meconium aspiration 770.12

Pneumonitis — *see also* Pneumonia — *continued*
  postanesthetic
    correct substance properly administered 507.0
    obstetric 668.0 ☑
    overdose or wrong substance given 968.4
    specified anesthetic — *see* Table of Drugs and Chemicals
  postoperative 997.3
    obstetric 668.0 ☑
  radiation 508.0
  rubella, congenital 771.0
  "ventilation" 495.7
  wood-dust 495.8
Pneumoconiosis — *see* Pneumoconiosis
Pneumoparotid 527.8
Pneumopathy NEC 518.89
  alveolar 516.9
    specified NEC 516.8
  due to dust NEC 504
  parietoalveolar 516.9
    specified condition NEC 516.8
Pneumopericarditis — *see also* Pericarditis 423.9
  acute 420.90
Pneumopericardium — *see also* Pericarditis
  congenital 770.2
  fetus or newborn 770.2
  traumatic (post) (*see also* Pneumothorax, traumatic) 860.0
    with open wound into thorax 860.1
Pneumoperitoneum 568.89
  fetus or newborn 770.2
Pneumophagia (psychogenic) 306.4
Pneumopleurisy, pneumopleuritis — *see also* Pneumonia 486
Pneumopyopericardium 420.99
Pneumopyothorax — *see also* Pyopneumothorax 510.9
  with fistula 510.0
Pneumorrhagia 786.3
  newborn 770.3
  tuberculous (*see also* Tuberculosis, pulmonary) 011.9 ☑
Pneumosiderosis (occupational) 503
Pneumothorax (acute) (chronic) 512.8
  congenital 770.2
  due to operative injury of chest wall or lung 512.1
    accidental puncture or laceration 512.1
  fetus or newborn 770.2
  iatrogenic 512.1
  postoperative 512.1
  spontaneous 512.8
    fetus or newborn 770.2
    tension 512.0
  sucking 512.8
    iatrogenic 512.1
    postoperative 512.1
  tense valvular, infectional 512.0
  tension 512.0
    iatrogenic 512.1
    postoperative 512.1
    spontaneous 512.0
  traumatic 860.0
    with
      hemothorax 860.4
        with open wound into thorax 860.5
      open wound into thorax 860.1
    tuberculous (*see also* Tuberculosis) 011.7 ☑
Pocket(s)
  endocardial (*see also* Endocarditis) 424.90
  periodontal 523.8
Podagra 274.9
Podencephalus 759.89
Poikilocytosis 790.09
Poikiloderma 709.09
  Civatte's 709.09

Poikiloderma — *continued*
  congenital 757.33
  vasculare atrophicans 696.2
Poikilodermatomyositis 710.3
Pointed ear 744.29
Poise imperfect 729.9
Poisoned — *see* Poisoning
Poisoning (acute) — *see also* Table of Drugs and Chemicals
  Bacillus, B.
    aertrycke (*see also* Infection, Salmonella) 003.9
    botulinus 005.1
    cholerae (suis) (*see also* Infection, Salmonella) 003.9
    paratyphosus (*see also* Infection, Salmonella) 003.9
    suipestifer (*see also* Infection, Salmonella) 003.9
  bacterial toxins NEC 005.9
  berries, noxious 988.2
  blood (general) — *see* Septicemia
  botulism 005.1
  bread, moldy, mouldy — *see* Poisoning, food
  damaged meat — *see* Poisoning, food
  death-cap (Amanita phalloides) (Amanita verna) 988.1
  decomposed food — *see* Poisoning, food
  diseased food — *see* Poisoning, food
  drug — *see* Table of Drugs and Chemicals
  epidemic, fish, meat, or other food — *see* Poisoning, food
  fava bean 282.2
  fish (bacterial) (*see also* Poisoning, food)
    noxious 988.0
  food (acute) (bacterial) (diseased) (infected) NEC 005.9
    due to
      bacillus
        aertrycke (*see also* Poisoning, food, due to Salmonella) 003.9
        botulinus 005.1
        cereus 005.89
        choleraesuis (*see also* Poisoning, food, due to Salmonella) 003.9
        paratyphosus (*see also* Poisoning, food, due to Salmonella) 003.9
        suipestifer (*see also* Poisoning, food, due to Salmonella) 003.9
      Clostridium 005.3
        botulinum 005.1
        perfringens 005.2
        welchii 005.2
      Salmonella (aertrycke) (callinarum) (choleraesuis) (enteritidis) (paratyphi) (suipestifer) 003.9
        with
          gastroenteritis 003.0
          localized infection(s) (*see also* Infection, Salmonella) 003.20
          septicemia 003.1
          specified manifestation NEC 003.8
      specified bacterium NEC 005.89
      Staphylococcus 005.0
      Streptococcus 005.89
      Vibrio parahaemolyticus 005.4
      Vibrio vulnificus 005.81
    noxious or naturally toxic 988.0
      berries 988.2
      fish 988.0
      mushroom 988.1
      plants NEC 988.2
  ice cream — *see* Poisoning, food
  ichthyotoxism (bacterial) 005.9
  kreotoxism, food 005.9

Index to Diseases

Poisoning — Polyp, polypus

Poisoning — see also Table of Drugs and Chemicals — *continued*
  malarial — see Malaria
  meat — see Poisoning, food
  mushroom (noxious) 988.1
  mussel (see also Poisoning, food) noxious 988.0
  noxious foodstuffs (see also Poisoning, food, noxious) 988.9
    specified type NEC 988.8
  plants, noxious 988.2
  pork (see also Poisoning, food)
    specified NEC 988.8
    Trichinosis 124
  ptomaine — see Poisoning, food
  putrefaction, food — see Poisoning, food
  radiation 508.0
  Salmonella (see also Infection, Salmonella) 003.9
  sausage (see also Poisoning, food) Trichinosis 124
  saxitoxin 988.0
  shellfish (see also Poisoning, food) noxious 988.0
  Staphylococcus, food 005.0
  toxic, from disease NEC 799.89
  truffles — see Poisoning, food
  uremic — see Uremia
  uric acid 274.9
Poison ivy, oak, sumac or other plant dermatitis 692.6
Poker spine 720.0
Policeman's disease 729.2
Polioencephalitis (acute) (bulbar) — see also Poliomyelitis, bulbar 045.0 ☑
  inferior 335.22
  influenzal 487.8
  superior hemorrhagic (acute) (Wernicke's) 265.1
  Wernicke's (superior hemorrhagic) 265.1
Polioencephalomyelitis (acute) (anterior) (bulbar) — see also Polioencephalitis 045.0 ☑
Polioencephalopathy, superior hemorrhagic 265.1
  with
    beriberi 265.0
    pellagra 265.2
Poliomeningoencephalitis — see Meningoencephalitis
Poliomyelitis (acute) (anterior) (epidemic) 045.9 ☑

Note — Use the following fifth-digit subclassification with category 045:

0   poliovirus, unspecified type
1   poliovirus, type I
2   poliovirus, type II
3   poliovirus, type III

  with
    paralysis 045.1 ☑
      bulbar 045.0 ☑
  abortive 045.2 ☑
  ascending 045.9 ☑
    progressive 045.9 ☑
  bulbar 045.0 ☑
  cerebral 045.0 ☑
  chronic 335.21
  congenital 771.2
  contact V01.2
  deformities 138
  exposure to V01.2
  late effect 138
  nonepidemic 045.9 ☑
  nonparalytic 045.2 ☑
  old with deformity 138
  posterior, acute 053.19
  residual 138
  sequelae 138
  spinal, acute 045.9 ☑
  syphilitic (chronic) 094.89

Poliomyelitis — *continued*
  vaccination, prophylactic (against) V04.0
Poliosis (eyebrow) (eyelashes) 704.3
  circumscripta (congenital) 757.4
    acquired 704.3
  congenital 757.4
Pollakiuria 788.41
  psychogenic 306.53
Pollinosis 477.0
Pollitzer's disease (hidradenitis suppurativa) 705.83
Polyadenitis — see also Adenitis 289.3
  malignant 020.0
Polyalgia 729.9
Polyangiitis (essential) 446.0
Polyarteritis (nodosa) (renal) 446.0
Polyarthralgia 719.49
  psychogenic 306.0
Polyarthritis, polyarthropathy NEC 716.59
  due to or associated with other specified conditions — see Arthritis, due to or associated with
  endemic (see also Disease, Kaschin-Beck) 716.0 ☑
  inflammatory 714.9
    specified type NEC 714.89
  juvenile (chronic) 714.30
    acute 714.31
  migratory — see Fever, rheumatic
  rheumatic 714.0
    fever (acute) — see Fever, rheumatic
Polycarential syndrome of infancy 260
Polychondritis (atrophic) (chronic) (relapsing) 733.99
Polycoria 743.46
Polycystic (congenital) (disease) 759.89
  degeneration, kidney — see Polycystic, kidney
  kidney (congenital) 753.12
    adult type (APKD) 753.13
    autosomal dominant 753.13
    autosomal recessive 753.14
    childhood type (CPKD) 753.14
    infantile type 753.14
  liver 751.62
  lung 518.89
    congenital 748.4
  ovary, ovaries 256.4
  spleen 759.0
Polycythemia (primary) (rubra) (vera) (M9950/1) 238.4
  acquired 289.0
  benign 289.0
    familial 289.6
  due to
    donor twin 776.4
    fall in plasma volume 289.0
    high altitude 289.0
    maternal-fetal transfusion 776.4
    stress 289.0
  emotional 289.0
  erythropoietin 289.0
  familial (benign) 289.6
  Gaisböck's (hypertonica) 289.0
  high altitude 289.0
  hypertonica 289.0
  hypoxemic 289.0
  neonatorum 776.4
  nephrogenous 289.0
  relative 289.0
  secondary 289.0
  spurious 289.0
  stress 289.0
Polycytosis cryptogenica 289.0
Polydactylism, polydactyly 755.00
  fingers 755.01
  toes 755.02
Polydipsia 783.5
Polydystrophic oligophrenia 277.5
Polyembryoma (M9072/3) — see Neoplasm, by site, malignant
Polygalactia 676.6 ☑

Polyglandular
  deficiency 258.9
  dyscrasia 258.9
  dysfunction 258.9
  syndrome 258.8
Polyhydramnios — see also Hydramnios 657.0 ☑
Polymastia 757.6
Polymenorrhea 626.2
Polymicrogyria 742.2
Polymyalgia 725
  arteritica 446.5
  rheumatica 725
Polymyositis (acute) (chronic) (hemorrhagic) 710.4
  with involvement of
    lung 710.4 [517.8]
    skin 710.3
  ossificans (generalisata) (progressiva) 728.19
  Wagner's (dermatomyositis) 710.3
Polyneuritis, polyneuritic — see also Polyneuropathy 356.9
  alcoholic 357.5
    with psychosis 291.1
  cranialis 352.6
  demyelinating, chronic inflammatory 357.81
  diabetic 250.6 ☑ [357.2]
  due to lack of vitamin NEC 269.2 [357.4]
  endemic 265.0 [357.4]
  erythredema 985.0
  febrile 357.0
  hereditary ataxic 356.3
  idiopathic, acute 357.0
  infective (acute) 357.0
  nutritional 269.9 [357.4]
  postinfectious 357.0
Polyneuropathy (peripheral) 356.9
  alcoholic 357.5
  amyloid 277.39 [357.4] ▲
  arsenical 357.7
  critical illness 357.82
  diabetic 250.6 ☑ [357.2]
  due to
    antitetanus serum 357.6
    arsenic 357.7
    drug or medicinal substance 357.6
      correct substance properly administered 357.6
      overdose or wrong substance given or taken 977.9
      specified drug — see Table of Drugs and Chemicals
    lack of vitamin NEC 269.2 [357.4]
    lead 357.7
    organophosphate compounds 357.7
    pellagra 265.2 [357.4]
    porphyria 277.1 [357.4]
    serum 357.6
    toxic agent NEC 357.7
  hereditary 356.0
  idiopathic 356.9
    progressive 356.4
  in
    amyloidosis 277.39 [357.4] ▲
    avitaminosis 269.2 [357.4]
      specified NEC 269.1 [357.4]
    beriberi 265.0 [357.4]
    collagen vascular disease NEC 710.9 [357.1]
    deficiency
      B-complex NEC 266.2 [357.4]
      vitamin B 266.1 [357.4]
      vitamin B6 266.9 [357.4]
    diabetes 250.6 ☑ [357.2]
    diphtheria (see also Diphtheria) 032.89 [357.4]
    disseminated lupus erythematosus 710.1 [357.1]
    herpes zoster 053.13
    hypoglycemia 251.2 [357.4]

Polyneuropathy — *continued*
  in — *continued*
    malignant neoplasm (M8000/3) NEC 199.1 [357.3]
    mumps 072.72
    pellagra 265.2 [357.4]
    polyarteritis nodosa 446.0 [357.1]
    porphyria 277.1 [357.4]
    rheumatoid arthritis 714.0 [357.1]
    sarcoidosis 135 [357.4]
    uremia 585.9 [357.4]
  lead 357.7
  nutritional 269.9 [357.4]
    specified NEC 269.8 [357.4]
  postherpetic 053.13
  progressive 356.4
  sensory (hereditary) 356.2
Polyonychia 757.5
Polyopia 368.2
  refractive 368.15
Polyorchism, polyorchidism (three testes) 752.89
Polyorrhymenitis (peritoneal) — see also Polyserositis 568.82
  pericardial 423.2
Polyostotic fibrous dysplasia 756.54
Polyotia 744.1
Polyphagia 783.6
Polypoid — see condition
Polyposis — see also Polyp
  coli (adenomatous) (M8220/0) 211.3
    adenocarcinoma in (M8220/3) 153.9
    carcinoma in (M8220/3) 153.9
  familial (M8220/0) 211.3
  intestinal (adenomatous) (M8220/0) 211.3
  multiple (M8221/0) — see Neoplasm, by site, benign
Polyp, polypus

Note — Polyps of organs or sites that do not appear in the list below should be coded to the residual category for diseases of the organ or site concerned.

  accessory sinus 471.8
  adenoid tissue 471.0
  adenomatous (M8210/0) (see also Neoplasm, by site, benign)
    adenocarcinoma in (M8210/3) — see Neoplasm, by site, malignant
    carcinoma in (M8210/3) — see Neoplasm, by site, malignant
    multiple (M8221/0) — see Neoplasm, by site, benign
  antrum 471.8
  anus, anal (canal) (nonadenomatous) 569.0
    adenomatous 211.4
  Bartholin's gland 624.6
  bladder (M8120/1) 236.7
  broad ligament 620.8
  cervix (uteri) 622.7
    adenomatous 219.0
    in pregnancy or childbirth 654.6 ☑
      affecting fetus or newborn 763.89
      causing obstructed labor 660.2 ☑
    mucous 622.7
    nonneoplastic 622.7
  choanal 471.0
  cholesterol 575.6
  clitoris 624.6
  colon (M8210/0) (see also Polyp, adenomatous) 211.3
  corpus uteri 621.0
  dental 522.0
  ear (middle) 385.30
  endometrium 621.0
  ethmoidal (sinus) 471.8
  fallopian tube 620.8
  female genital organs NEC 624.8
  frontal (sinus) 471.8
  gallbladder 575.6
  gingiva 523.8

Polyp, polypus

Polyp, polypus — *continued*
  gum 523.8
  labia 624.6
  larynx (mucous) 478.4
  malignant (M8000/3) — *see* Neoplasm, by site, malignant
  maxillary (sinus) 471.8
  middle ear 385.30
  myometrium 621.0
  nares
    anterior 471.9
    posterior 471.0
  nasal (mucous) 471.9
    cavity 471.0
    septum 471.9
  nasopharyngeal 471.0
  neoplastic (M8210/0) — *see* Neoplasm, by site, benign
  nose (mucous) 471.9
  oviduct 620.8
  paratubal 620.8
  pharynx 478.29
    congenital 750.29
  placenta, placental 674.4 ☑
  prostate 600.20
    with
      other lower urinary tract symptoms (LUTS) 600.21 ●
      urinary
        obstruction 600.21 ●
        retention 600.21 ●
  pudenda 624.6
  pulp (dental) 522.0
  rectosigmoid 211.4
  rectum (nonadenomatous) 569.0
    adenomatous 211.4
  septum (nasal) 471.9
  sinus (accessory) (ethmoidal) (frontal) (maxillary) (sphenoidal) 471.8
  sphenoidal (sinus) 471.8
  stomach (M8210/0) 211.1
  tube, fallopian 620.8
  turbinate, mucous membrane 471.8
  ureter 593.89
  urethra 599.3
  uterine
    ligament 620.8
    tube 620.8
  uterus (body) (corpus) (mucous) 621.0
    in pregnancy or childbirth 654.1 ☑
      affecting fetus or newborn 763.89
      causing obstructed labor 660.2 ☑
  vagina 623.7
  vocal cord (mucous) 478.4
  vulva 624.6
Polyradiculitis (acute) 357.0
Polyradiculoneuropathy (acute) (segmentally demyelinating) 357.0
Polysarcia 278.00
Polyserositis (peritoneal) 568.82
  due to pericarditis 423.2
  paroxysmal (familial) 277.31 ▲
  pericardial 423.2
  periodic ▶(familial)◀ 277.31 ▲
  pleural — *see* Pleurisy
  recurrent 277.31 ▲
  tuberculous (*see also* Tuberculosis, polyserositis) 018.9 ☑
Polysialia 527.7
Polysplenia syndrome 759.0
Polythelia 757.6
Polytrichia — *see also* Hypertrichosis 704.1
Polyunguia (congenital) 757.5
  acquired 703.8
Polyuria 788.42
Pompe's disease (glycogenosis II) 271.0
Pompholyx 705.81
Poncet's disease (tuberculous rheumatism) — *see also* Tuberculosis 015.9 ☑
Pond fracture — *see* Fracture, skull, vault

Ponos 085.0
Pons, pontine — *see* condition
Poor
  aesthetics of existing restoration of tooth 525.67 ●
  contractions, labor 661.2 ☑
    affecting fetus or newborn 763.7
  fetal growth NEC 764.9 ☑
    affecting management of pregnancy 656.5 ☑
  incorporation
    artificial skin graft 996.55
    decellularized allodermis graft 996.55
  obstetrical history V13.29
    affecting management of current pregnancy V23.49
      pre-term labor V23.41
    pre-term labor V13.21
  sucking reflex (newborn) 796.1
  vision NEC 369.9
Poradenitis, nostras 099.1
Porencephaly (congenital) (developmental) (true) 742.4
  acquired 348.0
  nondevelopmental 348.0
  traumatic (post) 310.2
Porocephaliasis 134.1
Porokeratosis 757.39
  disseminated superficial actinic (DSAP) 692.75
Poroma, eccrine (M8402/0) — *see* Neoplasm, skin, benign
Porphyria (acute) (congenital) (constitutional) (erythropoietic) (familial) (hepatica) (idiopathic) (idiosyncratic) (intermittent) (latent) (mixed hepatic) (photosensitive) (South African genetic) (Swedish) 277.1
  acquired 277.1
  cutaneatarda
    hereditaria 277.1
    symptomatica 277.1
  due to drugs
    correct substance properly administered 277.1
    overdose or wrong substance given or taken 977.9
    specified drug — *see* Table of Drugs and Chemicals
  secondary 277.1
  toxic NEC 277.1
  variegata 277.1
Porphyrinuria (acquired) (congenital) (secondary) 277.1
Porphyruria (acquired) (congenital) 277.1
Portal — *see* condition
Port wine nevus or mark 757.32
Posadas-Wernicke disease 114.9
Position
  fetus, abnormal (*see also* Presentation, fetal) 652.9 ☑
  teeth, faulty (*see also* Anomaly, position tooth) 524.30
Positive
  culture (nonspecific) 795.39
    AIDS virus V08
    blood 790.7
    HIV V08
    human immunodeficiency virus V08
    nose 795.39
    skin lesion NEC 795.39
    spinal fluid 792.0
    sputum 795.39
    stool 792.1
    throat 795.39
    urine 791.9
    wound 795.39
  findings, anthrax 795.31
  HIV V08
  human immunodeficiency virus (HIV) V08
  PPD 795.5
  serology
    AIDS virus V08

Positive — *continued*
  serology — *continued*
    AIDS virus — *continued*
      inconclusive 795.71
    HIV V08
      inconclusive 795.71
    human immunodeficiency virus (HIV) V08
      inconclusive 795.71
    syphilis 097.1
      with signs or symptoms — *see* Syphilis, by site and stage
      false 795.6
    skin test 795.7 ☑
      tuberculin (without active tuberculosis) 795.5
    VDRL 097.1
      with signs or symptoms — *see* Syphilis, by site and stage
      false 795.6
    Wassermann reaction 097.1
      false 795.6
Postcardiotomy syndrome 429.4
Postcaval ureter 753.4
Postcholecystectomy syndrome 576.0
Postclimacteric bleeding 627.1
Postcommissurotomy syndrome 429.4
Postconcussional syndrome 310.2
Postcontusional syndrome 310.2
Postcricoid region — *see* condition
Post-dates (pregnancy) — *see* Pregnancy
Postencephalitic — *see also* condition
  syndrome 310.8
Posterior — *see* condition
Posterolateral sclerosis (spinal cord) — *see* Degeneration, combined
Postexanthematous — *see* condition
Postfebrile — *see* condition
Postgastrectomy dumping syndrome 564.2
Posthemiplegic chorea 344.89
Posthemorrhagic anemia (chronic) 280.0
  acute 285.1
  newborn 776.5
Posthepatitis syndrome 780.79
Postherpetic neuralgia (intercostal) (syndrome) (zoster) 053.19
  geniculate ganglion 053.11
  ophthalmica 053.19
  trigeminal 053.12
Posthitis 607.1
Postimmunization complication or reaction — *see* Complications, vaccination
Postinfectious — *see* condition
Postinfluenzal syndrome 780.79
Postlaminectomy syndrome 722.80
  cervical, cervicothoracic 722.81
  kyphosis 737.12
  lumbar, lumbosacral 722.83
  thoracic, thoracolumbar 722.82
Postleukotomy syndrome 310.0
Postlobectomy syndrome 310.0
Postmastectomy lymphedema (syndrome) 457.0
Postmaturity, postmature (fetus or newborn) (gestation period over 42 completed weeks) 766.22
  affecting management of pregnancy
    post-term pregnancy 645.1 ☑
    prolonged pregnancy 645.2 ☑
  syndrome 766.22
Postmeasles — *see also* condition
  complication 055.8
  specified NEC 055.79
Postmenopausal
  endometrium (atrophic) 627.8
    suppurative (*see also* Endometritis) 615.9
  hormone replacement therapy V07.4
  status (age related) (natural) V49.81
Postnasal drip 784.91 ▲
Postnatal — *see* condition
Postoperative — *see also* condition
  confusion state 293.9

Postoperative — *see also* condition — *continued*
  psychosis 293.9
  status NEC (*see also* Status (post)) V45.89
Postpancreatectomy hyperglycemia 251.3
Postpartum — *see also* condition
  anemia 648.2 ☑
  cardiomyopathy 674.5 ☑
  observation
    immediately after delivery V24.0
    routine follow-up V24.2
Postperfusion syndrome NEC 999.8
  bone marrow 996.85
Postpoliomyelitic — *see* condition
Postsurgery status NEC — *see also* Status (post V45.89
Post-term (pregnancy) 645.1 ☑
  infant (gestation period over 40 completed weeks to 42 completed weeks) 766.21
Posttraumatic — *see* condition
Posttraumatic brain syndrome, nonpsychotic 310.2
Post-traumatic stress disorder (PTSD) ● 309.81
Post-typhoid abscess 002.0
Postures, hysterical 300.11
Postvaccinal reaction or complication — *see* Complications, vaccination
Postvagotomy syndrome 564.2
Postvalvulotomy syndrome 429.4
Postvasectomy sperm count V25.8
Potain's disease (pulmonary edema) 514
Potain's syndrome (gastrectasis with dyspepsia) 536.1
Pott's
  curvature (spinal) (*see also* Tuberculosis) 015.0 ☑ *[737.43]*
  disease or paraplegia (*see also* Tuberculosis) 015.0 ☑ *[730.88]*
  fracture (closed) 824.4
    open 824.5
  gangrene 440.24
  osteomyelitis (*see also* Tuberculosis) 015.0 ☑ *[730.88]*
  spinal curvature (*see also* Tuberculosis) 015.0 ☑ *[737.43]*
  tumor, puffy (*see also* Osteomyelitis) 730.2 ☑
Potter's
  asthma 502
  disease 753.0
  facies 754.0
  lung 502
  syndrome (with renal agenesis) 753.0
Pouch
  bronchus 748.3
  Douglas' — *see* condition
  esophagus, esophageal (congenital) 750.4
    acquired 530.6
  gastric 537.1
  Hartmann's (abnormal sacculation of gallbladder neck) 575.8
  of intestine V44.3
    attention to V55.3
  pharynx, pharyngeal (congenital) 750.27
Poulet's disease 714.2
Poultrymen's itch 133.8
Poverty V60.2
Prader-Labhart-Willi-Fanconi syndrome (hypogenital dystrophy with diabetic tendency) 759.81
Prader-Willi syndrome (hypogenital dystrophy with diabetic tendency) 759.81
Preachers' voice 784.49
Pre-AIDS — *see* Human immunodeficiency virus (disease) (illness) (infection)
Preauricular appendage 744.1
Prebetalipoproteinemia (acquired) (essential) (familial) (hereditary) (primary) (secondary) 272.1

Index to Diseases

Pregnancy

Prebetalipoproteinemia — *continued*
　with chylomicronemia 272.3
Precipitate labor 661.3 ☑
　affecting fetus or newborn 763.6
Preclimacteric bleeding 627.0
　menorrhagia 627.0
Precocious
　adrenarche 259.1
　menarche 259.1
　menstruation 626.8
　pubarche 259.1
　puberty NEC 259.1
　sexual development NEC 259.1
　thelarche 259.1
Precocity, sexual (constitutional) (cryptogenic) (female) (idiopathic) (male) NEC 259.1
　with adrenal hyperplasia 255.2
Precordial pain 786.51
　psychogenic 307.89
Predeciduous teeth 520.2
Prediabetes, prediabetic 790.29
　complicating pregnancy, childbirth, or puerperium 648.8 ☑
　fetus or newborn 775.89 ▲
Predislocation status of hip, at birth — *see also* Subluxation, congenital, hip 754.32
Preeclampsia (mild) 642.4 ☑
　with pre-existing hypertension 642.7 ☑
　affecting fetus or newborn 760.0
　severe 642.5 ☑
　superimposed on pre-existing hypertensive disease 642.7 ☑
Preeruptive color change, teeth, tooth 520.8
Preexcitation 426.7
　atrioventricular conduction 426.7
　ventricular 426.7
Preglaucoma 365.00
Pregnancy (single) (uterine) (without sickness) V22.2

> *Note — Use the following fifth-digit subclassification with categories 640–648, 651–676:*
>
> 0　*unspecified as to episode of care*
> 1　*delivered, with or without mention of antepartum condition*
> 2　*delivered, with mention of postpartum complication*
> 3　*antepartum condition or complication*
> 4　*postpartum condition or complication*

　abdominal (ectopic) 633.00
　　with intrauterine pregnancy 633.01
　　affecting fetus or newborn 761.4
　abnormal NEC 646.9 ☑
　ampullar — *see* Pregnancy, tubal
　broad ligament — *see* Pregnancy, cornual
　cervical — *see* Pregnancy, cornual
　combined (extrauterine and intrauterine) — *see* Pregnancy, cornual
　complicated (by)
　　abnormal, abnormality NEC 646.9 ☑
　　　cervix 654.6 ☑
　　　cord (umbilical) 663.9 ☑
　　　glucose tolerance (conditions classifiable to 790.21–790.29) 648.8 ☑
　　　pelvic organs or tissues NEC 654.9 ☑
　　　pelvis (bony) 653.0 ☑
　　　perineum or vulva 654.8 ☑
　　　placenta, placental (vessel) 656.7 ☑
　　　position
　　　　cervix 654.4 ☑
　　　　placenta 641.1 ☑

Pregnancy — *continued*
　complicated — *continued*
　　abnormal, abnormality — *continued*
　　　position — *continued*
　　　　placenta — *continued*
　　　　　without hemorrhage 641.0 ☑
　　　　uterus 654.4 ☑
　　　size, fetus 653.5 ☑
　　　uterus (congenital) 654.0 ☑
　　abscess or cellulitis
　　　bladder 646.6 ☑
　　　genitourinary tract (conditions classifiable to 590, 595, 597, 599.0, 614.0–614.5, 614.7–614.9, 615) 646.6 ☑
　　　kidney 646.6 ☑
　　　urinary tract NEC 646.6 ☑
　　adhesion, pelvic peritoneal 648.9 ☑
　　air embolism 673.0 ☑
　　albuminuria 646.2 ☑
　　　with hypertension — *see* Toxemia, of pregnancy
　　amnionitis 658.4 ☑
　　amniotic fluid embolism 673.1 ☑
　　anemia (conditions classifiable to 280–285) 648.2 ☑
　　appendicitis 648.9 ☑ ●
　　atrophy, yellow (acute) (liver) (subacute) 646.7 ☑
　　bacilluria, asymptomatic 646.5 ☑
　　bacteriuria, asymptomatic 646.5 ☑
　　bariatric surgery status 649.2 ☑ ●
　　bicornis or bicornuate uterus 654.0 ☑
　　biliary problems 646.8 ☑
　　bone and joint disorders (conditions classifiable to 720–724 or conditions affecting lower limbs classifiable to 711–719, 725–738) 648.7 ☑
　　breech presentation (buttocks) (complete) (frank) 652.2 ☑
　　　with successful version 652.1 ☑
　　cardiovascular disease (conditions classifiable to 390–398, 410–429) 648.6 ☑
　　　congenital (conditions classifiable to 745–747) 648.5 ☑
　　cerebrovascular disorders (conditions classifiable to 430–434, 436–437) 674.0 ☑
　　cervicitis (conditions classifiable to 616.0) 646.6 ☑
　　chloasma (gravidarum) 646.8 ☑
　　cholelithiasis 646.8 ☑
　　chorea (gravidarum) — *see* Eclampsia, pregnancy
　　coagulation defect 649.3 ☑ ●
　　contraction, pelvis (general) 653.1 ☑
　　　inlet 653.2 ☑
　　　outlet 653.3 ☑
　　convulsions (eclamptic) (uremic) 642.6 ☑
　　　with pre-existing hypertension 642.7 ☑
　　current disease or condition (nonobstetric)
　　　abnormal glucose tolerance 648.8 ☑
　　　anemia 648.2 ☑
　　　bone and joint (lower limb) 648.7 ☑
　　　cardiovascular 648.6 ☑
　　　　congenital 648.5 ☑
　　　cerebrovascular 674.0 ☑
　　　diabetic 648.0 ☑
　　　drug dependence 648.3 ☑
　　　female genital mutilation 648.9 ☑
　　　genital organ or tract 646.6 ☑
　　　gonorrheal 647.1 ☑

Pregnancy — *continued*
　complicated — *continued*
　　current disease or condition — *continued*
　　　hypertensive 642.2 ☑
　　　　chronic kidney 642.2 ☑ ●
　　　　renal 642.1 ☑
　　　infectious 647.9 ☑
　　　　specified type NEC 647.8 ☑
　　　liver 646.7 ☑
　　　malarial 647.4 ☑
　　　nutritional deficiency 648.9 ☑
　　　parasitic NEC 647.8 ☑
　　　periodontal disease 648.9 ☑
　　　renal 646.2 ☑
　　　　hypertensive 642.1 ☑
　　　rubella 647.5 ☑
　　　specified condition NEC 648.9 ☑
　　　syphilitic 647.0 ☑
　　　thyroid 648.1 ☑
　　　tuberculous 647.3 ☑
　　　urinary 646.6 ☑
　　　venereal 647.2 ☑
　　　viral NEC 647.6 ☑
　　cystitis 646.6 ☑
　　cystocele 654.4 ☑
　　death of fetus (near term) 656.4 ☑
　　　early pregnancy (before 22 completed weeks gestation) 632
　　deciduitis 646.6 ☑
　　decreased fetal movements 655.7 ☑
　　diabetes (mellitus) (conditions classifiable to 250) 648.0 ☑
　　disorders of liver 646.7 ☑
　　displacement, uterus NEC 654.4 ☑
　　disproportion — *see* Disproportion
　　double uterus 654.0 ☑
　　drug dependence (conditions classifiable to 304) 648.3 ☑
　　dysplasia, cervix 654.6 ☑
　　early onset of delivery (spontaneous) 644.2 ☑
　　eclampsia, eclamptic (coma) (convulsions) (delirium) (nephritis) (uremia) 642.6 ☑
　　　with pre-existing hypertension 642.7 ☑
　　edema 646.1 ☑
　　　with hypertension — *see* Toxemia, of pregnancy
　　effusion, amniotic fluid 658.1 ☑
　　　delayed delivery following 658.2 ☑
　　embolism
　　　air 673.0 ☑
　　　amniotic fluid 673.1 ☑
　　　blood-clot 673.2 ☑
　　　cerebral 674.0 ☑
　　　pulmonary NEC 673.2 ☑
　　　pyemic 673.3 ☑
　　　septic 673.3 ☑
　　emesis (gravidarum) — *see* Pregnancy, complicated, vomiting
　　endometritis (conditions classifiable to 615.0–615.9) 646.6 ☑
　　　decidual 646.6 ☑
　　epilepsy 649.4 ☑ ●
　　excessive weight gain NEC 646.1 ☑
　　face presentation 652.4 ☑
　　failure, fetal head to enter pelvic brim 652.5 ☑
　　false labor (pains) 644.1 ☑
　　fatigue 646.8 ☑
　　fatty metamorphosis of liver 646.7 ☑
　　female genital mutilation 648.9 ☑
　　fetal
　　　death (near term) 656.4 ☑
　　　　early (before 22 completed weeks gestation) 632
　　　deformity 653.7 ☑
　　　distress 656.8 ☑

Pregnancy — *continued*
　complicated — *continued*
　　fetal — *continued*
　　　reduction of multiple fetuses reduced to single fetus 651.7 ☑
　　fibroid (tumor) (uterus) 654.1 ☑
　　footling presentation 652.8 ☑
　　　with successful version 652.1 ☑
　　gallbladder disease 646.8 ☑
　　gastric banding status 649.2 ☑ ●
　　gastric bypass status for obesity ●
　　goiter 648.1 ☑
　　gonococcal infection (conditions classifiable to 098) 647.1 ☑
　　gonorrhea (conditions classifiable to 098) 647.1 ☑
　　hemorrhage 641.9 ☑
　　　accidental 641.2 ☑
　　　before 22 completed weeks gestation NEC 640.9 ☑
　　　cerebrovascular 674.0 ☑
　　　due to
　　　　afibrinogenemia or other coagulation defect (conditions classifiable to 286.0–286.9) 641.3 ☑
　　　　leiomyoma, uterine 641.8 ☑
　　　　marginal sinus (rupture) 641.2 ☑
　　　　premature separation, placenta 641.2 ☑
　　　　trauma 641.8 ☑
　　　early (before 22 completed weeks gestation) 640.9 ☑
　　　threatened abortion 640.0 ☑
　　　unavoidable 641.1 ☑
　　hepatitis (acute) (malignant) (subacute) 646.7 ☑
　　　viral 647.6 ☑
　　herniation of uterus 654.4 ☑
　　high head at term 652.5 ☑
　　hydatidiform mole (delivered) (undelivered) 630
　　hydramnios 657.0 ☑
　　hydrocephalic fetus 653.6 ☑
　　hydrops amnii 657.0 ☑
　　hydrorrhea 658.1 ☑
　　hyperemesis (gravidarum) — *see* Hyperemesis, gravidarum
　　hypertension — *see* Hypertension, complicating pregnancy
　　hypertensive
　　　chronic kidney disease 642.2 ☑ ●
　　　heart and chronic kidney disease 642.2 ☑ ●
　　　heart and renal disease 642.2 ☑
　　　heart disease 642.2 ☑
　　　renal disease 642.2 ☑
　　hypertensive heart and chronic kidney disease 642.2 ☑ ●
　　hyperthyroidism 648.1 ☑
　　hypothyroidism 648.1 ☑
　　hysteralgia 646.8 ☑
　　icterus gravis 646.7 ☑
　　incarceration, uterus 654.3 ☑
　　incompetent cervix (os) 654.5 ☑
　　infection 647.9 ☑
　　　amniotic fluid 658.4 ☑
　　　bladder 646.6 ☑
　　　genital organ (conditions classifiable to 614.0–614.5, 614.7–614.9, 615) 646.6 ☑
　　　kidney (conditions classifiable to 590.0–590.9) 646.6 ☑
　　　urinary (tract) 646.6 ☑
　　　　asymptomatic 646.5 ☑
　　infective and parasitic diseases NEC 647.8 ☑
　　inflammation
　　　bladder 646.6 ☑

Pregnancy

Index to Diseases

Pregnancy — *continued*
  complicated — *continued*
    inflammation — *continued*
      genital organ (conditions classifiable to 614.0–614.5, 614.7–614.9, 615) 646.6 ☑
      urinary tract NEC 646.6 ☑
    insufficient weight gain 646.8 ☑
    intrauterine fetal death (near term) NEC 656.4 ☑
      early (before 22 completed weeks' gestation) 632
    malaria (conditions classifiable to 084) 647.4 ☑
    malformation, uterus (congenital) 654.0 ☑
    malnutrition (conditions classifiable to 260–269) 648.9 ☑
    malposition
      fetus — *see* Pregnancy, complicated, malpresentation
      uterus or cervix 654.4 ☑
    malpresentation 652.9 ☑
      with successful version 652.1 ☑
      in multiple gestation 652.6 ☑
      specified type NEC 652.8 ☑
    marginal sinus hemorrhage or rupture 641.2 ☑
    maternal obesity syndrome 646.1 ☑
    menstruation 640.8 ☑
    mental disorders (conditions classifiable to 290–303, ▶305.0, 305.2-305.9, 306–316,◀ 317–319) 648.4 ☑
    mentum presentation 652.4 ☑
    missed
      abortion 632
      delivery (at or near term) 656.4 ☑
      labor (at or near term) 656.4 ☑
    necrosis
      genital organ or tract (conditions classifiable to 614.0–614.5, 614.7–614.9, 615) 646.6 ☑
      liver (conditions classifiable to 570) 646.7 ☑
      renal, cortical 646.2 ☑
    nephritis or nephrosis (conditions classifiable to 580–589) 646.2 ☑
      with hypertension 642.1 ☑
    nephropathy NEC 646.2 ☑
    neuritis (peripheral) 646.4 ☑
    nutritional deficiency (conditions classifiable to 260–269) 648.9 ☑
    obesity 649.1 ☑ ●
      surgery status 649.2 ☑ ●
    oblique lie or presentation 652.3 ☑
      with successful version 652.1 ☑
    obstetrical trauma NEC 665.9 ☑
    oligohydramnios NEC 658.0 ☑
    onset of contractions before 37 weeks 644.0 ☑
    oversize fetus 653.5 ☑
    papyraceous fetus 646.0 ☑
    patent cervix 654.5 ☑
    pelvic inflammatory disease (conditions classifiable to 614.0–614.5, 614.7–614.9, 615) 646.6 ☑
    pelvic peritoneal adhesion 648.9 ☑
    placenta, placental
      abnormality 656.7 ☑
      abruptio or ablatio 641.2 ☑
      detachment 641.2 ☑
      disease 656.7 ☑
      infarct 656.7 ☑
      low implantation 641.1 ☑
        without hemorrhage 641.0 ☑
      malformation 656.7 ☑

Pregnancy — *continued*
  complicated — *continued*
    placenta, placental — *continued*
      malposition 641.1 ☑
        without hemorrhage 641.0 ☑
      marginal sinus hemorrhage 641.2 ☑
      previa 641.1 ☑
        without hemorrhage 641.0 ☑
      separation (premature) (undelivered) 641.2 ☑
    placentitis 658.4 ☑
    polyhydramnios 657.0 ☑
    postmaturity
      post-term 645.1 ☑
      prolonged 645.2 ☑
    prediabetes 648.8 ☑
    pre-eclampsia (mild) 642.4 ☑
      severe 642.5 ☑
      superimposed on pre-existing hypertensive disease 642.7 ☑
    premature rupture of membranes 658.1 ☑
      with delayed delivery 658.2 ☑
    previous
      infertility V23.0
      nonobstetric condition V23.89
      poor obstetrical history V23.49
      premature delivery V23.41
      trophoblastic disease (conditions classifiable to 630) V23.1
    prolapse, uterus 654.4 ☑
    proteinuria (gestational) 646.2 ☑
      with hypertension — *see* Toxemia, of pregnancy
    pruritus (neurogenic) 646.8 ☑
    psychosis or psychoneurosis 648.4 ☑
    ptyalism 646.8 ☑
    pyelitis (conditions classifiable to 590.0–590.9) 646.6 ☑
    renal disease or failure NEC 646.2 ☑
      with secondary hypertension 642.1 ☑
      hypertensive 642.2 ☑
    retention, retained dead ovum 631
    retroversion, uterus 654.3 ☑
    Rh immunization, incompatibility, or sensitization 656.1 ☑
    rubella (conditions classifiable to 056) 647.5 ☑
    rupture
      amnion (premature) 658.1 ☑
        with delayed delivery 658.2 ☑
      marginal sinus (hemorrhage) 641.2 ☑
      membranes (premature) 658.1 ☑
        with delayed delivery 658.2 ☑
      uterus (before onset of labor) 665.0 ☑
    salivation (excessive) 646.8 ☑
    salpingo–oophoritis (conditions classifiable to 614.0–614.2) 646.6 ☑
    septicemia (conditions classifiable to 038.0–038.9) 647.8 ☑
      postpartum 670.0 ☑
      puerperal 670.0 ☑
    smoking 649.0 ☑ ●
    spasms, uterus (abnormal) 646.8 ☑
    specified condition NEC 646.8 ☑
    spotting 649.5 ☑ ●
    spurious labor pains 644.1 ☑
    status post ●
      bariatric surgery 649.2 ☑ ●
      gastric banding 649.2 ☑ ●
      gastric bypass for obesity 649.2 ☑ ●

Pregnancy — *continued*
  complicated — *continued*
    status post — *continued*
      obesity surgery 649.2 ☑ ●
    superfecundation 651.9 ☑
    superfetation 651.9 ☑
    syphilis (conditions classifiable to 090–097) 647.0 ☑
    threatened
      abortion 640.0 ☑
      premature delivery 644.2 ☑
      premature labor 644.0 ☑
    thrombophlebitis (superficial) 671.2 ☑
      deep 671.3 ☑
    thrombosis 671.9 ☑
      venous (superficial) 671.2 ☑
      deep 671.3 ☑
    thyroid dysfunction (conditions classifiable to 240–246) 648.1 ☑
    thyroiditis 648.1 ☑
    thyrotoxicosis 648.1 ☑
    tobacco use disorder 649.0 ☑ ●
    torsion of uterus 654.4 ☑
    toxemia — *see* Toxemia, of pregnancy
    transverse lie or presentation 652.3 ☑
      with successful version 652.1 ☑
    trauma 648.9 ☑
      obstetrical 665.9 ☑
    tuberculosis (conditions classifiable to 010–018) 647.3 ☑
    tumor
      cervix 654.6 ☑
      ovary 654.4 ☑
      pelvic organs or tissue NEC 654.4 ☑
      uterus (body) 654.1 ☑
        cervix 654.6 ☑
      vagina 654.7 ☑
      vulva 654.8 ☑
    unstable lie 652.0 ☑
    uremia — *see* Pregnancy, complicated, renal disease
    urethritis 646.6 ☑
    vaginitis or vulvitis (conditions classifiable to 616.1) 646.6 ☑
    varicose
      placental vessels 656.7 ☑
      veins (legs) 671.0 ☑
        perineum 671.1 ☑
        vulva 671.1 ☑
    varicosity, labia or vulva 671.1 ☑
    venereal disease NEC (conditions classifiable to 099) 647.2 ☑
    viral disease NEC (conditions classifiable to 042, 050–055, 057–079) 647.6 ☑
    vomiting (incoercible) (pernicious) (persistent) (uncontrollable) (vicious) 643.9 ☑
      due to organic disease or other cause 643.8 ☑
      early — *see* Hyperemesis, gravidarum
      late (after 22 completed weeks gestation) 643.2 ☑
    young maternal age 659.8 ☑
  complications NEC 646.9 ☑
  cornual 633.80
    with intrauterine pregnancy 633.81
    affecting fetus or newborn 761.4
  death, maternal NEC 646.9 ☑
  delivered — *see* Delivery
  ectopic (ruptured) NEC 633.90
    with intrauterine pregnancy 633.91
    abdominal — *see* Pregnancy, abdominal
    affecting fetus or newborn 761.4
    combined (extrauterine and intrauterine) — *see* Pregnancy, cornual
    ovarian — *see* Pregnancy, ovarian

Pregnancy — *continued*
  ectopic — *continued*
    specified type NEC 633.80
      with intrauterine pregnancy 633.81
      affecting fetus or newborn 761.4
    tubal — *see* Pregnancy, tubal
  examination, pregnancy
    negative result V72.41
    not confirmed V72.40
    positive result V72.42
  extrauterine — *see* Pregnancy, ectopic
  fallopian — *see* Pregnancy, tubal
  false 300.11
    labor (pains) 644.1 ☑
  fatigue 646.8 ☑
  illegitimate V61.6
  incidental finding V22.2
  in double uterus 654.0 ☑
  interstitial — *see* Pregnancy, cornual
  intraligamentous — *see* Pregnancy, cornual
  intramural — *see* Pregnancy, cornual
  intraperitoneal — *see* Pregnancy, abdominal
  isthmian — *see* Pregnancy, tubal
  management affected by
    abnormal, abnormality
      fetus (suspected) 655.9 ☑
        specified NEC 655.8 ☑
      placenta 656.7 ☑
    advanced maternal age NEC 659.6 ☑
      multigravida 659.6 ☑
      primigravida 659.5 ☑
    antibodies (maternal)
      anti-c 656.1 ☑
      anti-d 656.1 ☑
      anti-e 656.1 ☑
      blood group (ABO) 656.2 ☑
        Rh(esus) 656.1 ☑
    appendicitis 648.9 ☑ ●
    bariatric surgery status 649.2 ☑●
    coagulation defect 649.3 ☑ ●
    elderly multigravida 659.6 ☑
    elderly primigravida 659.5 ☑
    epilepsy 649.4 ☑ ●
    fetal (suspected)
      abnormality 655.9 ☑
        acid-base balance 656.8 ☑
        heart rate or rhythm 659.7 ☑
        specified NEC 655.8 ☑
      acidemia 656.3 ☑
      anencephaly 655.0 ☑
      bradycardia 659.7 ☑
      central nervous system malformation 655.0 ☑
      chromosomal abnormalities (conditions classifiable to 758.0–758.9) 655.1 ☑
      damage from
        drugs 655.5 ☑
          obstetric, anesthetic, or sedative 655.5 ☑
        environmental toxins 655.8 ☑
        intrauterine contraceptive device 655.8 ☑
        maternal
          alcohol addiction 655.4 ☑
          disease NEC 655.4 ☑
          drug use 655.5 ☑
          listeriosis 655.4 ☑
          rubella 655.3 ☑
          toxoplasmosis 655.4 ☑
          viral infection 655.3 ☑
        radiation 655.6 ☑
      death (near term) 656.4 ☑
        early (before 22 completed weeks' gestation) 632
      distress 656.8 ☑
      excessive growth 656.6 ☑
      fetal-maternal hemorrhage 656.0 ☑
      growth retardation 656.5 ☑

Index to Diseases

Pregnancy — continued
- management affected by — continued
  - fetal — continued
    - hereditary disease 655.2 ☑
    - hereditary disease in family (possibly) affecting fetus 655.2 ☑
    - hydrocephalus 655.0 ☑
    - incompatibility, blood groups (ABO) 656.2 ☑
    - intrauterine death 656.4 ☑
    - poor growth 656.5 ☑
    - Rh(esus) 656.1 ☑
    - spina bifida (with myelomeningocele) 655.0 ☑
  - gastric banding status 649.2 ☑ ●
  - gastric bypass status for obesity 649.2 ☑ ●
  - insufficient prenatal care V23.7
  - intrauterine death 656.4 ☑
  - isoimmunization (ABO) 656.2 ☑
    - Rh(esus) 656.1 ☑
  - large-for-dates fetus 656.6 ☑
  - light-for-dates fetus 656.5 ☑
  - meconium in liquor 656.8 ☑
  - mental disorder (conditions classifiable to 290–303, ▶305.0, 305.2–305.9, 306–316,◀ 317–319) 648.4 ☑
  - multiparity (grand) 659.4 ☑
  - obesity 649.1 ☑ ●
    - surgery status 649.2 ☑ ●
  - poor obstetric history V23.49
    - pre-term labor V23.41
  - postmaturity
    - post-term 645.1 ☑
    - prolonged 645.2 ☑
  - post-term pregnancy 645.1 ☑
  - previous
    - abortion V23.2
      - habitual 646.3 ☑
    - cesarean delivery 654.2 ☑
    - difficult delivery V23.49
    - forceps delivery V23.49
    - habitual abortions 646.3 ☑
    - hemorrhage, antepartum or postpartum V23.49
    - hydatidiform mole V23.1
    - infertility V23.0
    - malignancy NEC V23.89
    - nonobstetrical conditions V23.8
    - premature delivery V23.41
    - trophoblastic disease (conditions in 630) V23.1
    - vesicular mole V23.1
  - prolonged pregnancy 645.2 ☑
  - small-for-dates fetus 656.5 ☑
  - smoking 649.0 ☑ ●
  - spotting 649.5 ☑ ●
  - tobacco use disorder 649.0 ☑ ●
  - young maternal age 659.8 ☑
- maternal death NEC 646.9 ☑
- mesometric (mural) — see Pregnancy, cornual
- molar 631
  - hydatidiform (see also Hydatidiform mole) 630
    - previous, affecting management of pregnancy V23.1
  - previous, affecting management of pregnancy V23.49
- multiple NEC 651.9 ☑
  - with fetal loss and retention of one or more fetus(es) 651.6 ☑
  - affecting fetus or newborn 761.5
  - following (elective) fetal reduction 651.7 ☑
  - specified type NEC 651.8 ☑
    - with fetal loss and retention of one or more fetus(es) 651.6 ☑

Pregnancy — continued
- multiple — continued
  - specified type — continued
    - following (elective) fetal reduction 651.7 ☑
  - mural — see Pregnancy, cornual
  - observation NEC V22.1
    - first pregnancy V22.0
    - high-risk V23.9
      - specified problem NEC V23.89
  - ovarian 633.20
    - with intrauterine pregnancy 633.21
    - affecting fetus or newborn 761.4
  - possible, not (yet) confirmed V72.40
  - postmature
    - post-term 645.1 ☑
    - prolonged 645.2 ☑
  - post-term 645.1 ☑
  - prenatal care only V22.1
    - first pregnancy V22.0
    - high-risk V23.9
      - specified problem NEC V23.89
  - prolonged 645.2 ☑
  - quadruplet NEC 651.2 ☑
    - with fetal loss and retention of one or more fetus(es) 651.5 ☑
    - affecting fetus or newborn 761.5
    - following (elective) fetal reduction 651.7 ☑
  - quintuplet NEC 651.8 ☑
    - with fetal loss and retention of one or more fetus(es) 651.6 ☑
    - affecting fetus or newborn 761.5
    - following (elective) fetal reduction 651.7 ☑
  - sextuplet NEC 651.8 ☑
    - with fetal loss and retention of one or more fetus(es) 651.6 ☑
    - affecting fetus or newborn 761.5
    - following (elective) fetal reduction 651.7 ☑
  - spurious 300.11
  - superfecundation NEC 651.9 ☑
    - with fetal loss and retention of one or more fetus(es) 651.6 ☑
    - following (elective) fetal reduction 651.7 ☑
  - superfetation NEC 651.9 ☑
    - with fetal loss and retention of one or more fetus(es) 651.6 ☑
    - following (elective) fetal reduction 651.7 ☑
  - supervision (of) (for) (see also Pregnancy, management affected by)
    - elderly
      - multigravida V23.82
      - primigravida V23.81
    - high-risk V23.9
      - insufficient prenatal care V23.7
      - specified problem NEC V23.89
    - multiparity V23.3
    - normal NEC V22.1
      - first V22.0
    - poor
      - obstetric history V23.49
        - pre-term labor V23.41
      - reproductive history V23.5
    - previous
      - abortion V23.2
      - hydatidiform mole V23.1
      - infertility V23.0
      - neonatal death V23.5
      - stillbirth V23.5
      - trophoblastic disease V23.1
      - vesicular mole V23.1
    - specified problem NEC V23.89
    - young
      - multigravida V23.84
      - primigravida V23.83
  - triplet NEC 651.1 ☑
    - with fetal loss and retention of one or more fetus(es) 651.4 ☑
    - affecting fetus or newborn 761.5
    - following (elective) fetal reduction 651.7 ☑
  - tubal (with rupture) 633.10

Pregnancy — continued
- tubal — continued
  - with intrauterine pregnancy 633.11
  - affecting fetus or newborn 761.4
  - twin NEC 651.0 ☑
    - with fetal loss and retention of one fetus 651.3 ☑
    - affecting fetus or newborn 761.5
    - following (elective) fetal reduction 651.7 ☑
  - unconfirmed V72.40
  - undelivered (no other diagnosis) V22.2
    - with false labor 644.1 ☑
    - high-risk V23.9
      - specified problem NEC V23.89
  - unwanted NEC V61.7
Pregnant uterus — see condition
Preiser's disease (osteoporosis) 733.09
Prekwashiorkor 260
Preleukemia 238.75 ▲
Preluxation of hip, congenital — see also Subluxation, congenital, hip 754.32
Premature — see also condition
- beats (nodal) 427.60
  - atrial 427.61
  - auricular 427.61
  - postoperative 997.1
  - specified type NEC 427.69
  - supraventricular 427.61
  - ventricular 427.69
- birth NEC 765.1 ☑
- closure
  - cranial suture 756.0
  - fontanel 756.0
  - foramen ovale 745.8
- contractions 427.60
  - atrial 427.61
  - auricular 427.61
  - auriculoventricular 427.61
  - heart (extrasystole) 427.60
  - junctional 427.60
  - nodal 427.60
  - postoperative 997.1
  - ventricular 427.69
- ejaculation 302.75
- infant NEC 765.1 ☑
  - excessive 765.0 ☑
  - light-for-dates — see Light-for-dates
- labor 644.2 ☑
  - threatened 644.0 ☑
- lungs 770.4
- menopause 256.31
- puberty 259.1
- rupture of membranes or amnion 658.1 ☑
  - affecting fetus or newborn 761.1
  - delayed delivery following 658.2 ☑
- senility (syndrome) 259.8
- separation, placenta (partial) — see Placenta, separation
- ventricular systole 427.69
Prematurity NEC 765.1 ☑
- extreme 765.0 ☑
Premenstrual syndrome 625.4
Premenstrual tension 625.4
Premolarization, cuspids 520.2
Premyeloma 273.1
Prenatal
- care, normal pregnancy V22.1
  - first V22.0
- death, cause unknown — see Death, fetus
- screening — see Antenatal, screening
- teeth 520.6 ●
Prepartum — see condition
Preponderance, left or right ventricular 429.3
Prepuce — see condition
PRES (posterior reversible encephalopathy syndrome) 348.39 ●
Presbycardia 797
- hypertensive (see also Hypertension, heart) 402.90
Presbycusis 388.01

Presbyesophagus 530.89
Presbyophrenia 310.1
Presbyopia 367.4
Prescription of contraceptives NEC V25.02
- diaphragm V25.02
- oral (pill) V25.01
  - emergency V25.03
  - postcoital V25.03
  - repeat V25.41
- repeat V25.40
  - oral (pill) V25.41
Presenile — see also condition
- aging 259.8
- dementia (see also Dementia, presenile) 290.10
Presenility 259.8
Presentation, fetal
- abnormal 652.9 ☑
  - with successful version 652.1 ☑
  - before labor, affecting fetus or newborn 761.7
  - causing obstructed labor 660.0 ☑
    - affecting fetus or newborn, any, except breech 763.1
  - in multiple gestation (one or more) 652.6 ☑
  - specified NEC 652.8 ☑
- arm 652.7 ☑
  - causing obstructed labor 660.0 ☑
- breech (buttocks) (complete) (frank) 652.2 ☑
  - with successful version 652.1 ☑
  - before labor, affecting fetus or newborn 761.7
  - before labor, affecting fetus or newborn 761.7
- brow 652.4 ☑
  - causing obstructed labor 660.0 ☑
- buttocks 652.2 ☑
- chin 652.4 ☑
- complete 652.2 ☑
- compound 652.8 ☑
- cord 663.0 ☑
- extended head 652.4 ☑
- face 652.4 ☑
  - to pubes 652.8 ☑
- footling 652.8 ☑
- frank 652.2 ☑
- hand, leg, or foot NEC 652.8 ☑
- incomplete 652.8 ☑
- mentum 652.4 ☑
- multiple gestation (one fetus or more) 652.6 ☑
- oblique 652.3 ☑
  - with successful version 652.1 ☑
- shoulder 652.8 ☑
  - affecting fetus or newborn 763.1
- transverse 652.3 ☑
  - with successful version 652.1 ☑
- umbilical cord 663.0 ☑
- unstable 652.0 ☑
Prespondylolisthesis (congenital) (lumbosacral) 756.11
Pressure
- area, skin ulcer (see also Decubitus) 707.00
- atrophy, spine 733.99
- birth, fetus or newborn NEC 767.9
- brachial plexus 353.0
- brain 348.4
  - injury at birth 767.0
- cerebral — see Pressure, brain
- chest 786.59
- cone, tentorial 348.4
  - injury at birth 767.0
- funis — see Compression, umbilical cord
- hyposystolic (see also Hypotension) 458.9
- increased
  - intracranial 781.99
    - due to
      - benign intracranial hypertension 348.2

Pressure

Pressure — *continued*
  increased — *continued*
    intracranial — *continued*
      due to — *continued*
        hydrocephalus — *see* hydrocephalus
        injury at birth 767.8
    intraocular 365.00
    lumbosacral plexus 353.1
    mediastinum 519.3
    necrosis (chronic) (skin) (*see also* Decubitus) 707.00
    nerve — *see* Compression, nerve
    paralysis (*see also* Neuropathy, entrapment) 355.9
    sore (chronic) (*see also* Decubitus) 707.00
    spinal cord 336.9
    ulcer (chronic) (*see also* Decubitus) 707.00
    umbilical cord — *see* Compression, umbilical cord
    venous, increased 459.89
Pre-syncope 780.2
Preterm infant NEC 765.1 ☑
  extreme 765.0 ☑
Priapism (penis) 607.3
Prickling sensation — *see also* Disturbance, sensation 782.0
Prickly heat 705.1
Primary — *see* condition
Primigravida, elderly
  affecting
    fetus or newborn 763.89
    management of pregnancy, labor, and delivery 659.5 ☑
Primipara, old
  affecting
    fetus or newborn 763.89
    management of pregnancy, labor, and delivery 659.5 ☑
Primula dermatitis 692.6
Primus varus (bilateral) (metatarsus) 754.52
P.R.I.N.D. 436
Pringle's disease (tuberous sclerosis) 759.5
Prinzmetal's angina 413.1
Prinzmetal-Massumi syndrome (anterior chest wall) 786.52
Prizefighter ear 738.7
Problem (with) V49.9
  academic V62.3
  acculturation V62.4
  adopted child V61.29
  aged
    in-law V61.3
    parent V61.3
    person NEC V61.8
  alcoholism in family V61.41
  anger reaction (*see also* Disturbance, conduct) 312.0 ☑
  behavioral V40.9
    specified NEC V40.3
  behavior, child 312.9
  betting V69.3
  cardiorespiratory NEC V47.2
  career choice V62.2
  care of sick or handicapped person in family or household V61.49
  communication V40.1
  conscience regarding medical care V62.6
  delinquency (juvenile) 312.9
  diet, inappropriate V69.1
  digestive NEC V47.3
  ear NEC V41.3
  eating habits, inappropriate V69.1
  economic V60.2
    affecting
      care V60.9
        specified type NEC V60.8
  educational V62.3
  enuresis, child 307.6
  exercise, lack of V69.0
  eye NEC V41.1
  family V61.9

Problem — *continued*
  family — *continued*
    specified circumstance NEC V61.8
  fear reaction, child 313.0
  feeding (elderly) (infant) 783.3
    newborn 779.3
    nonorganic 307.59
  fetal, affecting management of pregnancy 656.9 ☑
    specified type NEC 656.8 ☑
  financial V60.2
  foster child V61.29
    specified NEC V41.8
  functional V41.9
    specified type NEC V41.8
  gambling V69.3
  genital NEC V47.5
  head V48.9
    deficiency V48.0
    disfigurement V48.6
    mechanical V48.2
    motor V48.2
    movement of V48.2
    sensory V48.4
    specified condition NEC V48.8
  hearing V41.2
  high-risk sexual behavior V69.2
  identity 313.82
  influencing health status NEC V49.89
  internal organ NEC V47.9
    deficiency V47.0
    mechanical or motor V47.1
  interpersonal NEC V62.81
  jealousy, child 313.3
  learning V40.0
  legal V62.5
  life circumstance NEC V62.89
  lifestyle V69.9
    specified NEC V69.8
  limb V49.9
    deficiency V49.0
    disfigurement V49.4
    mechanical V49.1
    motor V49.2
    movement, involving
      musculoskeletal system V49.1
      nervous system V49.2
    sensory V49.3
    specified condition NEC V49.5
  litigation V62.5
  living alone V60.3
  loneliness NEC V62.89
  marital V61.10
    involving
      divorce V61.0
      estrangement V61.0
      psychosexual disorder 302.9
      sexual function V41.7
    relationship V61.10
  mastication V41.6
  medical care, within family V61.49
  mental V40.9
    specified NEC V40.2
  mental hygiene, adult V40.9
  multiparity V61.5
  nail biting, child 307.9
  neck V48.9
    deficiency V48.1
    disfigurement V48.7
    mechanical V48.3
    motor V48.3
    movement V48.3
    sensory V48.5
    specified condition NEC V48.8
  neurological NEC 781.99
  none (feared complaint unfounded) V65.5
  occupational V62.2
  parent-child V61.20
    relationship V61.20
  partner V61.10
    relationship V61.10
  personal NEC V62.89
    interpersonal conflict NEC V62.81
  personality (*see also* Disorder, personality) 301.9

Problem — *continued*
  phase of life V62.89
  placenta, affecting management of pregnancy 656.9 ☑
    specified type NEC 656.8 ☑
  poverty V60.2
  presence of sick or handicapped person in family or household V61.49
  psychiatric 300.9
  psychosocial V62.9
    specified type NEC V62.89
  relational NEC V62.81
  relationship, childhood 313.3
  religious or spiritual belief
    other than medical care V62.89
    regarding medical care V62.6
  self-damaging behavior V69.8
  sexual
    behavior, high-risk V69.2
    function NEC V41.7
  sibling
    relational V61.8
    relationship V61.8
  sight V41.0
  sleep disorder, child 307.40
  sleep, lack of V69.4
  smell V41.5
  speech V40.1
  spite reaction, child (*see also* Disturbance, conduct) 312.0 ☑
  spoiled child reaction (*see also* Disturbance, conduct) 312.1 ☑
  swallowing V41.6
  tantrum, child (*see also* Disturbance, conduct) 312.1 ☑
  taste V41.5
  thumb sucking, child 307.9
  tic (child) 307.21
  trunk V48.9
    deficiency V48.1
    disfigurement V48.7
    mechanical V48.3
    motor V48.3
    movement V48.3
    sensory V48.5
    specified condition NEC V48.8
  unemployment V62.0
  urinary NEC V47.4
  voice production V41.4
Procedure (surgical) **not done** NEC V64.3
  because of
    contraindication V64.1
    patient's decision V64.2
      for reasons of conscience or religion V62.6
    specified reason NEC V64.3
Procidentia
  anus (sphincter) 569.1
  rectum (sphincter) 569.1
  stomach 537.89
  uteri 618.1
Proctalgia 569.42
  fugax 564.6
  spasmodic 564.6
    psychogenic 307.89
Proctitis 569.49
  amebic 006.8
  chlamydial 099.52
  gonococcal 098.7
  granulomatous 555.1
  idiopathic 556.2
    with ulcerative sigmoiditis 556.3
  tuberculous (*see also* Tuberculosis) 014.8 ☑
  ulcerative (chronic) (nonspecific) 556.2
    with ulcerative sigmoiditis 556.3
Proctocele
  female (without uterine prolapse) 618.04
    with uterine prolapse 618.4
      complete 618.3
      incomplete 618.2
  male 569.49
Proctocolitis, idiopathic 556.2

Proctocolitis, idiopathic — *continued*
  with ulcerative sigmoiditis 556.3
Proctoptosis 569.1
Proctosigmoiditis 569.89
  ulcerative (chronic) 556.3
Proctospasm 564.6
  psychogenic 306.4
Prodromal-AIDS — *see* Human immunodeficiency virus (disease) (illness) (infection)
Profichet's disease or syndrome 729.9
Progeria (adultorum) (syndrome) 259.8
Prognathism (mandibular) (maxillary) 524.00
Progonoma (melanotic) (M9363/0) — *see* Neoplasm, by site, benign
Progressive — *see* condition
Prolapse, prolapsed
  anus, anal (canal) (sphincter) 569.1
  arm or hand, complicating delivery 652.7 ☑
    causing obstructed labor 660.0 ☑
      affecting fetus or newborn 763.1
    fetus or newborn 763.1
  bladder (acquired) (mucosa) (sphincter)
    congenital (female) (male) 756.71
    female (*see also* Cystocele, female) 618.01
    male 596.8
  breast implant (prosthetic) 996.54
  cecostomy 569.69
  cecum 569.89
  cervix, cervical (hypertrophied) 618.1
    anterior lip, obstructing labor 660.2 ☑
      affecting fetus or newborn 763.1
    congenital 752.49
    postpartal (old) 618.1
    stump 618.84
  ciliary body 871.1
  colon (pedunculated) 569.89
  colostomy 569.69
  conjunctiva 372.73
  cord — *see* Prolapse, umbilical cord
  disc (intervertebral) — *see* Displacement, intervertebral disc
  duodenum 537.89
  eye implant (orbital) 996.59
    lens (ocular) 996.53
  fallopian tube 620.4
  fetal extremity, complicating delivery 652.8 ☑
    causing obstructed labor 660.0 ☑
    fetus or newborn 763.1
  funis — *see* Prolapse, umbilical cord
  gastric (mucosa) 537.89
  genital, female 618.9
    specified NEC 618.89
  globe 360.81
  ileostomy bud 569.69
  intervertebral disc — *see* Displacement, intervertebral disc
  intestine (small) 569.89
  iris 364.8
    traumatic 871.1
  kidney (*see also* Disease, renal) 593.0
    congenital 753.3
  laryngeal muscles or ventricle 478.79
  leg, complicating delivery 652.8 ☑
    causing obstructed labor 660.0 ☑
    fetus or newborn 763.1
  liver 573.8
  meatus urinarius 599.5
  mitral valve 424.0
  ocular lens implant 996.53
  organ or site, congenital NEC — *see* Malposition, congenital
  ovary 620.4
  pelvic (floor), female 618.89
  perineum, female 618.89
  pregnant uterus 654.4 ☑
  rectum (mucosa) (sphincter) 569.1
    due to Trichuris trichiuria 127.3
  spleen 289.59

Prolapse, prolapsed — continued
  stomach 537.89
  umbilical cord
    affecting fetus or newborn 762.4
    complicating delivery 663.0 ☑
  ureter 593.89
    with obstruction 593.4
  ureterovesical orifice 593.89
  urethra (acquired) (infected) (mucosa) 599.5
    congenital 753.8
  uterovaginal 618.4
    complete 618.3
    incomplete 618.2
    specified NEC 618.89
  uterus (first degree) (second degree) (third degree) (complete) (without vaginal wall prolapse) 618.1
    with mention of vaginal wall prolapse — see Prolapse, uterovaginal
    congenital 752.3
    in pregnancy or childbirth 654.4 ☑
      affecting fetus or newborn 763.1
      causing obstructed labor 660.2 ☑
        affecting fetus or newborn 763.1
    postpartal (old) 618.1
  uveal 871.1
  vagina (anterior) (posterior) (vault) (wall) (without uterine prolapse) 618.00
    with uterine prolapse 618.4
      complete 618.3
      incomplete 618.2
    paravaginal 618.02
    posthysterectomy 618.5
    specified NEC 618.09
  vitreous (humor) 379.26
    traumatic 871.1
  womb — see Prolapse, uterus
Prolapsus, female 618.9
Proliferative — see condition
Prolinemia 270.8
Prolinuria 270.8
Prolonged, prolongation
  bleeding time (see also Defect, coagulation) 790.92
    "idiopathic" (in von Willebrand's disease) 286.4
  coagulation time (see also Defect, coagulation) 790.92
  gestation syndrome 766.22
  labor 662.1 ☑
    affecting fetus or newborn 763.89
    first stage 662.0 ☑
    second stage 662.2 ☑
  pregnancy 645.2 ☑
  PR interval 426.11
  prothrombin time (see also Defect, coagulation) 790.92
  QT interval 794.31
    syndrome 426.82
  rupture of membranes (24 hours or more prior to onset of labor) 658.2 ☑
  uterine contractions in labor 661.4 ☑
    affecting fetus or newborn 763.7
Prominauris 744.29
Prominence
  auricle (ear) (congenital) 744.29
    acquired 380.32
  ischial spine or sacral promontory with disproportion (fetopelvic) 653.3 ☑
    affecting fetus or newborn 763.1
    causing obstructed labor 660.1 ☑
      affecting fetus or newborn 763.1
  nose (congenital) 748.1
    acquired 738.0
Pronation
  ankle 736.79
  foot 736.79

Pronation — continued
  foot — continued
    congenital 755.67
Prophylactic
  administration of
    antibiotics V07.39
    antitoxin, any V07.2
    antivenin V07.2
    chemotherapeutic agent NEC V07.39
      fluoride V07.31
    diphtheria antitoxin V07.2
    gamma globulin V07.2
    immune sera (gamma globulin) V07.2
    RhoGAM V07.2
    tetanus antitoxin V07.2
  chemotherapy NEC V07.39
    fluoride V07.31
  hormone replacement (postmenopausal) V07.4
  immunotherapy V07.2
  measure V07.9
    specified type NEC V07.8
  postmenopausal hormone replacement V07.4
  sterilization V25.2
Proptosis (ocular) — see also Exophthalmos 376.30
  thyroid 242.0 ☑
Propulsion
  eyeball 360.81
Prosecution, anxiety concerning V62.5
Prostate, prostatic — see condition
Prostatism 600.90
  with
    other lower urinary tract symptoms (LUTS) 600.91 ●
    urinary
      obstruction 600.91 ●
      retention 600.91 ●
Prostatitis (congestive) (suppurative) 601.9
  acute 601.0
  cavitary 601.8
  chlamydial 099.54
  chronic 601.1
  diverticular 601.8
  due to Trichomonas (vaginalis) 131.03
  fibrous 600.90
    with
      other lower urinary tract symptoms (LUTS) 600.91 ●
      urinary
        obstruction 600.91 ●
        retention 600.91 ●
  gonococcal (acute) 098.12
    chronic or duration of 2 months or over 098.32
  granulomatous 601.8
  hypertrophic 600.00
    with
      other lower urinary tract symptoms (LUTS) 600.01 ●
      urinary
        obstruction 600.01 ●
        retention 600.01 ●
  specified type NEC 601.8
  subacute 601.1
  trichomonal 131.03
  tuberculous (see also Tuberculosis) 016.5 ☑ [601.4]
Prostatocystitis 601.3
Prostatorrhea 602.8
Prostatoseminovesiculitis, trichomonal 131.03
Prostration 780.79
  heat 992.5
    anhydrotic 992.3
    due to
      salt (and water) depletion 992.4
      water depletion 992.3
  nervous 300.5
  newborn 779.89

Prostration — continued
  senile 797
Protanomaly 368.51
Protanopia (anomalous trichromat) (complete) (incomplete) 368.51
Protein
  deficiency 260
  malnutrition 260
  sickness (prophylactic) (therapeutic) 999.5
Proteinemia 790.99
Proteinosis
  alveolar, lung or pulmonary 516.0
  lipid 272.8
  lipoid (of Urbach) 272.8
Proteinuria — see also Albuminuria 791.0
  Bence-Jones NEC 791.0
  gestational 646.2 ☑
    with hypertension — see Toxemia, of pregnancy
  orthostatic 593.6
  postural 593.6
Proteolysis, pathologic 286.6
Protocoproporphyria 277.1
Protoporphyria (erythrohepatic) (erythropoietic) 277.1
Protrusio acetabuli 718.65
Protrusion
  acetabulum (into pelvis) 718.65
  device, implant, or graft — see Complications, mechanical
  ear, congenital 744.29
  intervertebral disc — see Displacement, intervertebral disc
  nucleus pulposus — see Displacement, intervertebral disc
Proud flesh 701.5
Prune belly (syndrome) 756.71
Prurigo (ferox) (gravis) (Hebra's) (hebrae) (mitis) (simplex) 698.2
  agria 698.3
  asthma syndrome 691.8
  Besnier's (atopic dermatitis) (infantile eczema) 691.8
  eczematodes allergicum 691.8
  estivalis (Hutchinson's) 692.72
  Hutchinson's 692.72
  nodularis 698.3
  psychogenic 306.3
Pruritus, pruritic 698.9
  ani 698.0
    psychogenic 306.3
  conditions NEC 698.9
    psychogenic 306.3
  due to Onchocerca volvulus 125.3
  ear 698.9
  essential 698.9
  genital organ(s) 698.1
    psychogenic 306.3
  gravidarum 646.8 ☑
  hiemalis 698.8
  neurogenic (any site) 306.3
  perianal 698.0
  psychogenic (any site) 306.3
  scrotum 698.1
    psychogenic 306.3
  senile, senilis 698.8
  Trichomonas 131.9
  vulva, vulvae 698.1
    psychogenic 306.3
Psammocarcinoma (M8140/3) — see Neoplasm, by site, malignant
Pseudarthrosis, pseudoarthrosis (bone) 733.82
  joint following fusion V45.4
Pseudoacanthosis
  nigricans 701.8
Pseudoaneurysm — see Aneurysm
Pseudoangina (pectoris) — see Angina
Pseudoangioma 452
Pseudo-Argyll-Robertson pupil 379.45
Pseudoarteriosus 747.89
Pseudoarthrosis — see Pseudarthrosis
Pseudoataxia 799.89
Pseudobulbar affect (PBA) 310.8

Pseudobursa 727.89
Pseudocholera 025
Pseudochromidrosis 705.89
Pseudocirrhosis, liver, pericardial 423.2
Pseudocoarctation 747.21
Pseudocowpox 051.1
Pseudocoxalgia 732.1
Pseudocroup 478.75
Pseudocyesis 300.11
Pseudocyst
  lung 518.89
  pancreas 577.2
  retina 361.19
Pseudodementia 300.16
Pseudoelephantiasis neuroarthritica 757.0
Pseudoemphysema 518.89
Pseudoencephalitis
  superior (acute) hemorrhagic 265.1
Pseudoerosion cervix, congenital 752.49
Pseudoexfoliation, lens capsule 366.11
Pseudofracture (idiopathic) (multiple) (spontaneous) (symmetrical) 268.2
Pseudoglanders 025
Pseudoglioma 360.44
Pseudogout — see Chondrocalcinosis
Pseudohallucination 780.1
Pseudohemianesthesia 782.0
Pseudohemophilia (Bernuth's) (hereditary) (typeB) 286.4
  type A 287.8
  vascular 287.8
Pseudohermaphroditism 752.7
  with chromosomal anomaly — see Anomaly, chromosomal
  adrenal 255.2
  female (without adrenocortical disorder) 752.7
    with adrenocortical disorder 255.2
    adrenal 255.2
  male (without gonadal disorder) 752.7
    with
      adrenocortical disorder 255.2
      cleft scrotum 752.7
      feminizing testis 259.5
      gonadal disorder 257.9
    adrenal 255.2
Pseudohole, macula 362.54
Pseudo-Hurler's disease (mucolipidosis III) 272.7
Pseudohydrocephalus 348.2
Pseudohypertrophic muscular dystrophy (Erb's) 359.1
Pseudohypertrophy, muscle 359.1
Pseudohypoparathyroidism 275.49
Pseudoinfluenza 487.1
Pseudoinsomnia 307.49
Pseudoleukemia 288.8
  infantile 285.8
Pseudomembranous — see condition
Pseudomeningocele (cerebral) (infective) 349.2
  postprocedural 997.01
  spinal 349.2
Pseudomenstruation 626.8
Pseudomucinous
  cyst (ovary) (M8470/0) 220
  peritoneum 568.89
Pseudomyeloma 273.1
Pseudomyxoma peritonei (M8480/6) 197.6
Pseudoneuritis optic (nerve) 377.24
  papilla 377.24
  congenital 743.57
Pseudoneuroma — see Injury, nerve, by site
Pseudo-obstruction
  intestine (chronic) (idiopathic) (intermittent secondary) (primary) 564.89
    acute 560.89
Pseudopapilledema 377.24
Pseudoparalysis
  arm or leg 781.4

Pseudoparalysis

Pseudoparalysis — *continued*
  atonic, congenital 358.8
Pseudopelade 704.09
Pseudophakia V43.1
Pseudopolycythemia 289.0
Pseudopolyposis, colon 556.4
Pseudoporencephaly 348.0
Pseudopseudohypoparathyroidism 275.49
Pseudopsychosis 300.16
Pseudopterygium 372.52
Pseudoptosis (eyelid) 374.34
Pseudorabies 078.89
Pseudoretinitis, pigmentosa 362.65
Pseudorickets 588.0
  senile (Pozzi's) 731.0
Pseudorubella 057.8
Pseudoscarlatina 057.8
Pseudosclerema 778.1
Pseudosclerosis (brain)
  Jakob's 046.1
  of Westphal (-Strümpell) (hepatolenticular degeneration) 275.1
  spastic 046.1
    with dementia
      with behavioral disturbance 046.1 [294.11]
      without behavioral disturbance 046.1 [294.10]
Pseudoseizure 780.39
  non-psychiatric 780.39
  psychiatric 300.11
Pseudotabes 799.89
  diabetic 250.6 ☑ [337.1]
Pseudotetanus — *see also* Convulsions 780.39
Pseudotetany 781.7
  hysterical 300.11
Pseudothalassemia 285.0
Pseudotrichinosis 710.3
Pseudotruncus arteriosus 747.29
Pseudotuberculosis, pasteurella (infection) 027.2
Pseudotumor
  cerebri 348.2
  orbit (inflammatory) 376.11
Pseudo-Turner's syndrome 759.89
Pseudoxanthoma elasticum 757.39
Psilosis (sprue) (tropical) 579.1
  Monilia 112.89
  nontropical 579.0
  not sprue 704.00
Psittacosis 073.9
Psoitis 728.89
Psora NEC 696.1
Psoriasis 696.1
  any type, except arthropathic 696.1
  arthritic, arthropathic 696.0
  buccal 528.6
  flexural 696.1
  follicularis 696.1
  guttate 696.1
  inverse 696.1
  mouth 528.6
  nummularis 696.1
  psychogenic 316 [696.1]
  punctata 696.1
  pustular 696.1
  rupioides 696.1
  vulgaris 696.1
Psorospermiasis 136.4
Psorospermosis 136.4
  follicularis (vegetans) 757.39
Psychalgia 307.80
Psychasthenia 300.89
  compulsive 300.3
  mixed compulsive states 300.3
  obsession 300.3
Psychiatric disorder or problem NEC 300.9
Psychogenic — *see also* condition
  factors associated with physical conditions 316
Psychoneurosis, psychoneurotic — *see also* Neurosis 300.9
  anxiety (state) 300.00

Psychoneurosis, psychoneurotic — *see also* Neurosis — *continued*
  climacteric 627.2
  compensation 300.16
  compulsion 300.3
  conversion hysteria 300.11
  depersonalization 300.6
  depressive type 300.4
  dissociative hysteria 300.15
  hypochondriacal 300.7
  hysteria 300.10
    conversion type 300.11
    dissociative type 300.15
  mixed NEC 300.89
  neurasthenic 300.5
  obsessional 300.3
  obsessive-compulsive 300.3
  occupational 300.89
  personality NEC 301.89
  phobia 300.20
  senile NEC 300.89
Psychopathic — *see also* condition
  constitution, posttraumatic 310.2
    with psychosis 293.9
  personality 301.9
    amoral trends 301.7
    antisocial trends 301.7
    asocial trends 301.7
    mixed types 301.7
  state 301.9
Psychopathy, sexual — *see also* Deviation, sexual 302.9
Psychophysiologic, psychophysiological condition — *see* Reaction, psychophysiologic
Psychose passionelle 297.8
Psychosexual identity disorder 302.6
  adult-life 302.85
  childhood 302.6
Psychosis 298.9
  acute hysterical 298.1
  affecting management of pregnancy, childbirth, or puerperium 648.4 ☑
  affective (*see also* Disorder, mood) 296.90

Note — *Use the following fifth-digit subclassification with categories 296.0–296.6:*
  0 unspecified
  1 mild
  2 moderate
  3 severe, without mention of psychotic behavior
  4 severe, specified as with psychotic behavior
  5 in partial or unspecified remission
  6 in full remission

  drug-induced 292.84
  due to or associated with physical condition 293.83
    involutional 293.83
      recurrent episode 296.3 ☑
      single episode 296.2 ☑
    manic-depressive 296.80
      circular (alternating) 296.7
        currently depressed 296.5 ☑
        currently manic 296.4 ☑
      depressed type 296.2 ☑
        atypical 296.82
        recurrent episode 296.3 ☑
        single episode 296.2 ☑
      manic 296.0 ☑
        atypical 296.81
        recurrent episode 296.1 ☑
        single episode 296.0 ☑
      mixed type NEC 296.80
      specified type NEC 296.89
    senile 290.21
    specified type NEC 296.99
  alcoholic 291.9

Psychosis — *continued*
  alcoholic — *continued*
    with
      anxiety 291.89
      delirium tremens 291.0
      delusions 291.5
      dementia 291.2
      hallucinosis 291.3
      jealousy 291.5
      mood disturbance 291.89
      paranoia 291.5
      persisting amnesia 291.1
      sexual dysfunction 291.89
      sleep disturbance 291.89
    amnestic confabulatory 291.1
    delirium tremens 291.0
    hallucinosis 291.3
    Korsakoff's, Korsakov's, Korsakow's 291.1
    paranoid type 291.5
    pathological intoxication 291.4
    polyneuritic 291.1
    specified type NEC 291.89
  alternating (*see also* Psychosis, manic-depressive, circular) 296.7
  anergastic (*see also* Psychosis, organic) 294.9
  arteriosclerotic 290.40
    with
      acute confusional state 290.41
      delirium 290.41
      delusions 290.42
      depressed mood 290.43
      depressed type 290.43
      paranoid type 290.42
      simple type 290.40
      uncomplicated 290.40
  atypical 298.9
    depressive 296.82
    manic 296.81
  borderline (schizophrenia) (*see also* Schizophrenia) 295.5 ☑
    of childhood (*see also* Psychosis, childhood) 299.8 ☑
    prepubertal 299.8 ☑
  brief reactive 298.8
  childhood, with origin specific to 299.9 ☑

Note — *Use the following fifth-digit subclassification with category 299:*
  0 current or active state
  1 residual state

    atypical 299.8 ☑
    specified type NEC 299.8 ☑
  circular (*see also* Psychosis, manic-depressive, circular) 296.7
  climacteric (*see also* Psychosis, involutional) 298.8
  confusional 298.9
    acute 293.0
    reactive 298.2
    subacute 293.1
  depressive (*see also* Psychosis, affective) 296.2 ☑
    atypical 296.82
    involutional 296.2 ☑
      with hypomania (bipolar II) 296.89
      recurrent episode 296.3 ☑
      single episode 296.2 ☑
    psychogenic 298.0
    reactive (emotional stress) (psychological trauma) 298.0
    recurrent episode 296.3 ☑
      with hypomania (bipolar II) 296.89
    single episode 296.2 ☑
  disintegrative, childhood (*see also* Psychosis, childhood) 299.1 ☑
  drug 292.9
    with
      affective syndrome 292.84
      amnestic syndrome 292.83
      anxiety 292.89

Psychosis — *continued*
  drug — *continued*
    with — *continued*
      delirium 292.81
        withdrawal 292.0
      delusions 292.11
      dementia 292.82
      depressive state 292.84
      hallucinations 292.12
      hallucinosis 292.12
      mood disorder 292.84
      mood disturbance 292.84
      organic personality syndrome NEC 292.89
      sexual dysfunction 292.89
      sleep disturbance 292.89
      withdrawal syndrome (and delirium) 292.0
    affective syndrome 292.84
    delusions 292.11
    hallucinatory state 292.12
    hallucinosis 292.12
    paranoid state 292.11
    specified type NEC 292.89
    withdrawal syndrome (and delirium) 292.0
  due to or associated with physical condition (*see also* Psychosis, organic) 293.9
  epileptic NEC 294.8
  excitation (psychogenic) (reactive) 298.1
  exhaustive (*see also* Reaction, stress, acute) 308.9
  hypomanic (*see also* Psychosis, affective) 296.0 ☑
    recurrent episode 296.1 ☑
    single episode 296.0 ☑
  hysterical 298.8
    acute 298.1
  in
    conditions classified elsewhere
      with
        delusions 293.81
        hallucinations 293.82
      pregnancy, childbirth, or puerperium 648.4 ☑
  incipient 298.8
    schizophrenic (*see also* Schizophrenia) 295.5 ☑
  induced 297.3
  infantile (*see also* Psychosis, childhood) 299.0 ☑
  infective 293.9
    acute 293.0
    subacute 293.1
  interactional (childhood) (*see also* Psychosis, childhood) 299.1 ☑
  involutional 298.8
    depressive (*see also* Psychosis, affective) 296.2 ☑
      recurrent episode 296.3 ☑
      single episode 296.2 ☑
    melancholic 296.2 ☑
      recurrent episode 296.3 ☑
      single episode 296.2 ☑
  paranoid state 297.2
  paraphrenia 297.2
  Korsakoff's, Korakov's, Korsakow's (nonalcoholic) 294.0
    alcoholic 291.1
  mania (phase) (*see also* Psychosis, affective) 296.0 ☑
    recurrent episode 296.1 ☑
    single episode 296.0 ☑
  manic (*see also* Psychosis, affective) 296.0 ☑
    atypical 296.81
    recurrent episode 296.1 ☑
    single episode 296.0 ☑
  manic-depressive 296.80
    circular 296.7
      currently
        depressed 296.5 ☑
        manic 296.4 ☑
        mixed 296.6 ☑

Index to Diseases

Psychosis — *continued*
- manic-depressive — *continued*
  - depressive 296.2 ☑
    - recurrent episode 296.3 ☑
      - with hypomania (bipolar II) 296.89
    - single episode 296.2 ☑
  - hypomanic 296.0 ☑
    - recurrent episode 296.1 ☑
    - single episode 296.0 ☑
  - manic 296.0 ☑
    - atypical 296.81
    - recurrent episode 296.1 ☑
    - single episode 296.0 ☑
  - mixed NEC 296.89
  - perplexed 296.89
  - stuporous 296.89
- menopausal (*see also* Psychosis, involutional) 298.8
- mixed schizophrenic and affective (*see also* Schizophrenia) 295.7 ☑
- multi-infarct (cerebrovascular) (*see also* Psychosis, arteriosclerotic) 290.40
- organic NEC 294.9
  - due to or associated with
    - addiction
      - alcohol (*see also* Psychosis, alcoholic) 291.9
      - drug (*see also* Psychosis, drug) 292.9
    - alcohol intoxication, acute (*see also* Psychosis, alcoholic) 291.9
    - alcoholism (*see also* Psychosis, alcoholic) 291.9
    - arteriosclerosis (cerebral) (*see also* Psychosis, arteriosclerotic) 290.40
    - cerebrovascular disease
      - acute (psychosis) 293.0
      - arteriosclerotic (*see also* Psychosis, arteriosclerotic) 290.40
    - childbirth — *see* Psychosis, puerperal
    - dependence
      - alcohol (*see also* Psychosis, alcoholic) 291.9
      - drug 292.9
    - disease
      - alcoholic liver (*see also* Psychosis, alcoholic) 291.9
      - brain
        - arteriosclerotic (*see also* Psychosis, arteriosclerotic) 290.40
        - cerebrovascular
          - acute (psychosis) 293.0
          - arteriosclerotic (*see also* Psychosis, arteriosclerotic) 290.40
      - endocrine or metabolic 293.9
        - acute (psychosis) 293.0
        - subacute (psychosis) 293.1
      - Jakob-Creutzfeldt (new variant)
        - with behavioral disturbance 046.1 [294.11]
        - without behavioral disturbance 046.1 [294.10]
      - liver, alcoholic (*see also* Psychosis, alcoholic) 291.9
    - disorder
      - cerebrovascular
        - acute (psychosis) 293.0
      - endocrine or metabolic 293.9
        - acute (psychosis) 293.0
        - subacute (psychosis) 293.1
    - epilepsy
      - with behavioral disturbance 345.9 ☑ [294.11]
      - without behavioral disturbance 345.9 ☑ [294.10]
      - transient (acute) 293.0
    - Huntington's chorea
      - with behavioral disturbance 333.4 [294.11]
      - without behavioral disturbance 333.4 [294.10]
    - infection
      - brain 293.9
        - acute (psychosis) 293.0
        - chronic 294.8
        - subacute (psychosis) 293.1
      - intracranial NEC 293.9
        - acute (psychosis) 293.0
        - chronic 294.8
        - subacute (psychosis) 293.1
    - intoxication
      - alcoholic (acute) (*see also* Psychosis, alcoholic) 291.9
        - pathological 291.4
      - drug (*see also* Psychosis, drug) 292.2
    - ischemia
      - cerebrovascular (generalized) (*see also* Psychosis, arteriosclerotic) 290.40
    - Jakob-Creutzfeldt disease (syndrome) (new variant)
      - with behavioral disturbance 046.1 [294.11]
      - without behavioral disturbance 046.1 [294.10]
    - multiple sclerosis
      - with behavioral disturbance 340 [294.11]
      - without behavioral disturbance 340 [294.10]
    - physical condition NEC 293.9
      - with
        - delusions 293.81
        - hallucinations 293.82
    - presenility 290.10
    - puerperium — *see* Psychosis, puerperal
    - sclerosis, multiple
      - with behavioral disturbance 340 [294.11]
      - without behavioral disturbance 340 [294.10]
    - senility 290.20
    - status epilepticus
      - with behavioral disturbance 345.3 [294.11]
      - without behavioral disturbance 345.3 [294.10]
    - trauma
      - brain (birth) (from electrical current) (surgical) 293.9
        - acute (psychosis) 293.0
        - chronic 294.8
        - subacute (psychosis) 293.1
        - unspecified physical condition 293.9
          - with
            - delusion 293.81
            - hallucinations 293.82
  - infective 293.9
    - acute (psychosis) 293.0
    - subacute 293.1
  - posttraumatic 293.9
    - acute 293.0
    - subacute 293.1
  - specified type NEC 294.8
  - transient 293.9
    - with
      - anxiety 293.84
      - delusions 293.81
      - depression 293.83
      - hallucinations 293.82
    - depressive type 293.83
    - hallucinatory type 293.82
    - paranoid type 293.81
    - specified type NEC 293.89
- paranoic 297.1
- paranoid (chronic) 297.9
  - alcoholic 291.5
  - chronic 297.1
  - climacteric 297.2
  - involutional 297.2
  - menopausal 297.2
  - protracted reactive 298.4
  - psychogenic 298.4
    - acute 298.3
  - schizophrenic (*see also* Schizophrenia) 295.3 ☑
  - senile 290.20
- paroxysmal 298.9
  - senile 290.20
- polyneuritic, alcoholic 291.1
- postoperative 293.9
- postpartum — *see* Psychosis, puerperal
- prepsychotic (*see also* Schizophrenia) 295.5 ☑
- presbyophrenic (type) 290.8
- presenile (*see also* Dementia, presenile) 290.10
- prison 300.16
- psychogenic 298.8
  - depressive 298.0
  - paranoid 298.4
    - acute 298.3
- puerperal
  - specified type — *see* categories 295-298 ☑
  - unspecified type 293.89
    - acute 293.0
    - chronic 293.89
    - subacute 293.1
- reactive (emotional stress) (psychological trauma) 298.8
  - brief 298.8
  - confusion 298.2
  - depressive 298.0
  - excitation 298.1
- schizo-affective (depressed) (excited) (*see also* Schizophrenia) 295.7 ☑
- schizophrenia, schizophrenic (*see also* Schizophrenia) 295.9 ☑
  - borderline type 295.5 ☑
    - of childhood (*see also* Psychosis, childhood) 299.8 ☑
  - catatonic (excited) (withdrawn) 295.2 ☑
  - childhood type (*see also* Psychosis, childhood) 299.9 ☑
  - hebephrenic 295.1 ☑
  - incipient 295.5 ☑
  - latent 295.5 ☑
  - paranoid 295.3 ☑
  - prepsychotic 295.5 ☑
  - prodromal 295.5 ☑
  - pseudoneurotic 295.5 ☑
  - pseudopsychopathic 295.5 ☑
  - schizophreniform 295.4 ☑
  - simple 295.0 ☑
  - undifferentiated type 295.9 ☑
- schizophreniform 295.4 ☑
- senile NEC 290.20
  - with
    - delusional features 290.20
    - depressive features 290.21
  - depressed type 290.21
  - paranoid type 290.20
  - simple deterioration 290.20
- senile — *continued*
  - specified type — *see* categories 295-298 ☑
- shared 297.3
- situational (reactive) 298.8
- symbiotic (childhood) (*see also* Psychosis, childhood) 299.1 ☑
- toxic (acute) 293.9

Psychotic — *see also* condition 298.9
- episode 298.9
  - due to or associated with physical conditions (*see also* Psychosis, organic) 293.9

Pterygium (eye) 372.40
- central 372.43
- colli 744.5
- double 372.44
- peripheral (stationary) 372.41
  - progressive 372.42
- recurrent 372.45

Ptilosis 374.55

Ptomaine (poisoning) — *see also* Poisoning, food 005.9

Ptosis (adiposa) 374.30
- breast 611.8
- cecum 569.89
- colon 569.89
- congenital (eyelid) 743.61
  - specified site NEC — *see* Anomaly, specified type NEC
- epicanthus syndrome 270.2
- eyelid 374.30
  - congenital 743.61
  - mechanical 374.33
  - myogenic 374.32
  - paralytic 374.31
- gastric 537.5
- intestine 569.89
- kidney (*see also* Disease, renal) 593.0
  - congenital 753.3
- liver 573.8
- renal (*see also* Disease, renal) 593.0
  - congenital 753.3
- splanchnic 569.89
- spleen 289.59
- stomach 537.5
- viscera 569.89

PTSD (Post-traumatic stress disorder) ● 309.81 ●

Ptyalism 527.7
- hysterical 300.11
- periodic 527.2
- pregnancy 646.8 ☑
- psychogenic 306.4

Ptyalolithiasis 527.5

Pubalgia 848.8

Pubarche, precocious 259.1

Pubertas praecox 259.1

Puberty V21.1
- abnormal 259.9
- bleeding 626.3
- delayed 259.0
- precocious (constitutional) (cryptogenic) (idiopathic) NEC 259.1
  - due to
    - adrenal
      - cortical hyperfunction 255.2
      - hyperplasia 255.2
    - cortical hyperfunction 255.2
    - ovarian hyperfunction 256.1
      - estrogen 256.0
    - pineal tumor 259.8
    - testicular hyperfunction 257.0
- premature 259.1
  - due to
    - adrenal cortical hyperfunction 255.2
    - pineal tumor 259.8
    - pituitary (anterior) hyperfunction 253.1

Puckering, macula 362.56

Pudenda, pudendum — *see* condition

Puente's disease (simple glandular cheilitis) 528.5

Puerperal

Puerperal
  abscess
    areola 675.1
    Bartholin's gland 646.6
    breast 675.1
    cervix (uteri) 670.0
    fallopian tube 670.0
    genital organ 670.0
    kidney 646.6
    mammary 675.1
    mesosalpinx 670.0
    nabothian 646.6
    nipple 675.0
    ovary, ovarian 670.0
    oviduct 670.0
    parametric 670.0
    para-uterine 670.0
    pelvic 670.0
    perimetric 670.0
    periuterine 670.0
    retro-uterine 670.0
    subareolar 675.1
    suprapelvic 670.0
    tubal (ruptured) 670.0
    tubo-ovarian 670.0
    urinary tract NEC 646.6
    uterine, uterus 670.0
    vagina (wall) 646.6
    vaginorectal 646.6
    vulvovaginal gland 646.6
  accident 674.9
  adnexitis 670.0
  afibrinogenemia, or other coagulation defect 666.3
  albuminuria (acute) (subacute) 646.2
    pre-eclamptic 642.4
  anemia (conditions classifiable to 280–285) 648.2
  anuria 669.3
  apoplexy 674.0
  asymptomatic bacteriuria 646.5
  atrophy, breast 676.3
  blood dyscrasia 666.3
  caked breast 676.2
  cardiomyopathy 674.5
  cellulitis — see Puerperal, abscess
  cerebrovascular disorder (conditions classifiable to 430–434, 436–437) 674.0
  cervicitis (conditions classifiable to 616.0) 646.6
  coagulopathy (any) 666.3
  complications 674.9
    specified type NEC 674.8
  convulsions (eclamptic) (uremic) 642.6
    with pre-existing hypertension 642.7
  cracked nipple 676.1
  cystitis 646.6
  cystopyelitis 646.6
  deciduitis (acute) 670.0
  delirium NEC 293.9
  diabetes (mellitus) (conditions classifiable to 250) 648.0
  disease 674.9
    breast NEC 676.3
    cerebrovascular (acute) 674.0
    nonobstetric NEC (see also Pregnancy, complicated, current disease or condition) 648.9
    pelvis inflammatory 670.0
    renal NEC 646.2
    tubo-ovarian 670.0
    Valsuani's (progressive pernicious anemia) 648.2
  disorder
    lactation 676.9
      specified type NEC 676.8
    nonobstetric NEC (see also Pregnancy, complicated, current disease or condition) 648.9

Puerperal — continued
  disruption
    cesarean wound 674.1
    episiotomy wound 674.2
    perineal laceration wound 674.2
  drug dependence (conditions classifiable to 304) 648.3
  eclampsia 642.6
    with pre-existing hypertension 642.7
  embolism (pulmonary) 673.2
    air 673.0
    amniotic fluid 673.1
    blood-clot 673.2
    brain or cerebral 674.0
    cardiac 674.8
    fat 673.8
    intracranial sinus (venous) 671.5
    pyemic 673.3
    septic 673.3
    spinal cord 671.5
  endometritis (conditions classifiable to 615.0–615.9) 670.0
  endophlebitis — see Puerperal, phlebitis
  endotrachelitis 646.6
  engorgement, breasts 676.2
  erysipelas 670.0
  failure
    lactation 676.4
    renal, acute 669.3
  fever 670.0
    meaning pyrexia (of unknown origin) 672.0
    meaning sepsis 670.0
  fissure, nipple 676.1
  fistula
    breast 675.1
    mammary gland 675.1
    nipple 675.0
  galactophoritis 675.2
  galactorrhea 676.6
  gangrene
    gas 670.0
    uterus 670.0
  gonorrhea (conditions classifiable to 098) 647.1
  hematoma, subdural 674.0
  hematosalpinx, infectional 670.0
  hemiplegia, cerebral 674.0
  hemorrhage 666.1
    brain 674.0
    bulbar 674.0
    cerebellar 674.0
    cerebral 674.0
    cortical 674.0
    delayed (after 24 hours) (uterine) 666.2
    extradural 674.0
    internal capsule 674.0
    intracranial 674.0
    intrapontine 674.0
    meningeal 674.0
    pontine 674.0
    subarachnoid 674.0
    subcortical 674.0
    subdural 674.0
    uterine, delayed 666.2
    ventricular 674.0
  hemorrhoids 671.8
  hepatorenal syndrome 674.8
  hypertrophy
    breast 676.3
    mammary gland 676.3
  induration breast (fibrous) 676.3
  infarction
    lung — see Puerperal, embolism
    pulmonary — see Puerperal, embolism
  infection
    Bartholin's gland 646.6
    breast 675.2
      with nipple 675.9

Puerperal — continued
  infection — continued
    breast — continued
      with nipple — continued
        specified type NEC 675.8
    cervix 646.6
    endocervix 646.6
    fallopian tube 670.0
    generalized 670.0
    genital tract (major) 670.0
      minor or localized 646.6
    kidney (bacillus coli) 646.6
    mammary gland 675.2
      with nipple 675.9
        specified type NEC 675.8
    nipple 675.0
      with breast 675.9
        specified type NEC 675.8
    ovary 670.0
    pelvic 670.0
    peritoneum 670.0
    renal 646.6
    tubo-ovarian 670.0
    urinary (tract) NEC 646.6
      asymptomatic 646.5
    uterus, uterine 670.0
    vagina 646.6
  inflammation (see also Puerperal, infection)
    areola 675.1
    Bartholin's gland 646.6
    breast 675.2
    broad ligament 670.0
    cervix (uteri) 646.6
    fallopian tube 670.0
    genital organs 670.0
      localized 646.6
    mammary gland 675.2
    nipple 675.0
    ovary 670.0
    oviduct 670.0
    pelvis 670.0
    periuterine 670.0
    tubal 670.0
    vagina 646.6
    vein — see Puerperal, phlebitis
  inversion, nipple 676.3
  ischemia, cerebral 674.0
  lymphangitis 670.0
    breast 675.2
  malaria (conditions classifiable to 084) 647.4
  malnutrition 648.9
  mammillitis 675.0
  mammitis 675.2
  mania 296.0
    recurrent episode 296.1
    single episode 296.0
  mastitis 675.2
    purulent 675.1
    retromammary 675.1
    submammary 675.1
  melancholia 296.2
    recurrent episode 296.3
    single episode 296.2
  mental disorder (conditions classifiable to 290–303, ▶305.0, 305.2–305.9, 306–316◀, 317–319) 648.4
  metritis (septic) (suppurative) 670.0
  metroperitonitis 670.0
  metrorrhagia 666.2
  metrosalpingitis 670.0
  metrovaginitis 670.0
  milk leg 671.4
  monoplegia, cerebral 674.0
  necrosis
    kidney, tubular 669.3
    liver (acute) (subacute) (conditions classifiable to 570) 674.8
    ovary 670.0
    renal cortex 669.3
  nephritis or nephrosis (conditions classifiable to 580–589) 646.2

Puerperal — continued
  nephritis or nephrosis — continued
    with hypertension 642.1
  nutritional deficiency (conditions classifiable to 260–269) 648.9
  occlusion, precerebral artery 674.0
  oliguria 669.3
  oophoritis 670.0
  ovaritis 670.0
  paralysis
    bladder (sphincter) 665.5
    cerebral 674.0
  paralytic stroke 674.0
  parametritis 670.0
  paravaginitis 646.6
  pelviperitonitis 670.0
  perimetritis 670.0
  perimetrosalpingitis 670.0
  perinephritis 646.6
  perioophoritis 670.0
  periphlebitis — see Puerperal, phlebitis
  perisalpingitis 670.0
  peritoneal infection 670.0
  peritonitis (pelvic) 670.0
  perivaginitis 646.6
  phlebitis 671.9
    deep 671.4
    intracranial sinus (venous) 671.5
    pelvic 671.4
    specified site NEC 671.5
    superficial 671.2
  phlegmasia alba dolens 671.4
  placental polyp 674.4
  pneumonia, embolic — see Puerperal, embolism
  prediabetes 648.8
  pre-eclampsia (mild) 642.4
    with pre-existing hypertension 642.7
    severe 642.5
  psychosis, unspecified (see also Psychosis, puerperal) 293.89
  pyelitis 646.6
  pyelocystitis 646.6
  pyelohydronephrosis 646.6
  pyelonephritis 646.6
  pyelonephrosis 646.6
  pyemia 670.0
  pyocystitis 646.6
  pyohemia 670.0
  pyometra 670.0
  pyonephritis 646.6
  pyonephrosis 646.6
  pyo-oophoritis 670.0
  pyosalpingitis 670.0
  pyosalpinx 670.0
  pyrexia (of unknown origin) 672.0
  renal
    disease NEC 646.2
    failure, acute 669.3
  retention
    decidua (fragments) (with delayed hemorrhage) 666.2
      without hemorrhage 667.1
    placenta (fragments) (with delayed hemorrhage) 666.2
      without hemorrhage 667.1
    secundines (fragments) (with delayed hemorrhage) 666.2
      without hemorrhage 667.1
  retracted nipple 676.0
  rubella (conditions classifiable to 056) 647.5
  salpingitis 670.0
  salpingo-oophoritis 670.0
  salpingo-ovaritis 670.0
  salpingoperitonitis 670.0
  sapremia 670.0
  secondary perineal tear 674.2
  sepsis (pelvic) 670.0
  septicemia 670.0
  subinvolution (uterus) 674.8

Puerperal — *continued*
  sudden death (cause unknown) 674.9
  suppuration — *see* Puerperal, abscess
  syphilis (conditions classifiable to 090–097) 647.0 ☑
  tetanus 670.0 ☑
  thelitis 675.0 ☑
  thrombocytopenia 666.3 ☑
  thrombophlebitis (superficial) 671.2 ☑
    deep 671.4 ☑
    pelvic 671.4 ☑
    specified site NEC 671.5 ☑
  thrombosis (venous) — *see* Thrombosis, puerperal
  thyroid dysfunction (conditions classifiable to 240–246) 648.1 ☑
  toxemia (*see also* Toxemia, of pregnancy) 642.4 ☑
    eclamptic 642.6 ☑
      with pre-existing hypertension 642.7 ☑
    pre-eclamptic (mild) 642.4 ☑
      with
        convulsions 642.6 ☑
        pre-existing hypertension 642.7 ☑
      severe 642.5 ☑
  tuberculosis (conditions classifiable to 010–018) 647.3 ☑
  uremia 669.3 ☑
  vaginitis (conditions classifiable to 616.1) 646.6 ☑
  varicose veins (legs) 671.0 ☑
  vulva or perineum 671.1 ☑
  vulvitis (conditions classifiable to 616.1) 646.6 ☑
  vulvovaginitis (conditions classifiable to 616.1) 646.6 ☑
  white leg 671.4 ☑
Pulled muscle — *see* Sprain, by site
Pulmolithiasis 518.89
Pulmonary — *see* condition
Pulmonitis (unknown etiology) 486
Pulpitis (acute) (anachoretic) (chronic) (hyperplastic) (putrescent) (suppurative) (ulcerative) 522.0
Pulpless tooth 522.9
Pulse
  alternating 427.89
    psychogenic 306.2
  bigeminal 427.89
  fast 785.0
  feeble, rapid, due to shock following injury 958.4
  rapid 785.0
  slow 427.89
  strong 785.9
  trigeminal 427.89
  water-hammer (*see also* Insufficiency, aortic) 424.1
  weak 785.9
Pulseless disease 446.7
Pulsus
  alternans or trigeminy 427.89
    psychogenic 306.2
Punch drunk 310.2
Puncta lacrimalia occlusion 375.52
Punctiform hymen 752.49
Puncture (traumatic) — *see also* Wound, open, by site
  accidental, complicating surgery 998.2
  bladder, nontraumatic 596.6
  by
    device, implant, or graft — *see* Complications, mechanical
    foreign body
      internal organs (*see also* Injury, internal, by site)
        by ingested object — *see* Foreign body
      left accidentally in operation wound 998.4
    instrument (any) during a procedure, accidental 998.2

Puncture — *see also* Wound, open, by site — *continued*
  internal organs, abdomen, chest, or pelvis — *see* Injury, internal, by site
  kidney, nontraumatic 593.89
Pupil — *see* condition
Pupillary membrane 364.74
  persistent 743.46
Pupillotonia 379.46
  pseudotabetic 379.46
Purpura 287.2
  abdominal 287.0
  allergic 287.0
  anaphylactoid 287.0
  annularis telangiectodes 709.1
  arthritic 287.0
  autoerythrocyte sensitization 287.2
  autoimmune 287.0
  bacterial 287.0
  Bateman's (senile) 287.2
  capillary fragility (hereditary) (idiopathic) 287.8
  cryoglobulinemic 273.2
  devil's pinches 287.2
  fibrinolytic (*see also* Fibrinolysis) 286.6
  fulminans, fulminous 286.6
  gangrenous 287.0
  hemorrhagic (*see also* Purpura, thrombocytopenic) 287.39
    nodular 272.7
    nonthrombocytopenic 287.0
    thrombocytopenic 287.39
  Henoch's (purpura nervosa) 287.0
  Henoch-Schönlein (allergic) 287.0
  hypergammaglobulinemic (benign primary) (Waldenström's) 273.0
  idiopathic 287.31
    nonthrombocytopenic 287.0
    thrombocytopenic 287.31
  immune thrombocytopenic 287.31
  infectious 287.0
  malignant 287.0
  neonatorum 772.6
  nervosa 287.0
  newborn NEC 772.6
  nonthrombocytopenic 287.2
    hemorrhagic 287.0
    idiopathic 287.0
  nonthrombopenic 287.2
  peliosis rheumatica 287.0
  pigmentaria, progressiva 709.09
  posttransfusion 287.4
  primary 287.0
  primitive 287.0
  red cell membrane sensitivity 287.2
  rheumatica 287.0
  Schönlein (-Henoch) (allergic) 287.0
  scorbutic 267
  senile 287.2
  simplex 287.2
  symptomatica 287.0
  telangiectasia annularis 709.1
  thrombocytopenic (*see also* Thrombocytopenia) 287.30
    congenital 287.33
    essential 287.30
    hereditary 287.31
    idiopathic 287.31
    immune 287.31
    neonatal, transitory (*see also* Thrombocytopenia, neonatal transitory) 776.1
    primary 287.30
    puerperal, postpartum 666.3 ☑
    thrombotic 446.6
  thrombohemolytic (*see also* Fibrinolysis) 286.6
  thrombopenic (*see also* Thrombocytopenia) 287.30
    congenital 287.33
    essential 287.30
    thrombotic 446.6
      thrombocytic 446.6
      thrombocytopenic 446.6

Purpura — *continued*
  toxic 287.0
  variolosa 050.0
  vascular 287.0
  visceral symptoms 287.0
  Werlhof's (*see also* Purpura, thrombocytopenic) 287.39
Purpuric spots 782.7
Purulent — *see* condition
Pus
  absorption, general — *see* Septicemia
  in
    stool 792.1
    urine 791.9
  tube (rupture) (*see also* Salpingo-oophoritis) 614.2
Pustular rash 782.1
Pustule 686.9
  malignant 022.0
  nonmalignant 686.9
Putnam-Dana syndrome (subacute combined sclerosis with pernicious anemia) 281.0 [336.2]
Putnam's disease (subacute combined sclerosis with pernicious anemia) 281.0 [336.2]
Putrefaction, intestinal 569.89
Putrescent pulp (dental) 522.1
Pyarthritis — *see* Pyarthrosis
Pyarthrosis — *see also* Arthritis, pyogenic 711.0 ☑
  tuberculous — *see* Tuberculosis, joint
Pycnoepilepsy, pycnolepsy (idiopathic) — *see also* Epilepsy 345.0
Pyelectasia 593.89
Pyelectasis 593.89
Pyelitis (congenital) (uremic) 590.80
  with
    abortion — *see* Abortion, by type, with specified complication NEC
    contracted kidney 590.00
    ectopic pregnancy (*see also* categories 633.0–633.9) 639.8
    molar pregnancy (*see also* categories 630–632) 639.8
  acute 590.10
    with renal medullary necrosis 590.11
  chronic 590.00
    with
      renal medullary necrosis 590.01
    complicating pregnancy, childbirth, or puerperium 646.6 ☑
      affecting fetus or newborn 760.1
  cystica 590.3
  following
    abortion 639.8
    ectopic or molar pregnancy 639.8
  gonococcal 098.19
  chronic or duration of 2 months or over 098.39
  tuberculous (*see also* Tuberculosis) 016.0 ☑ [590.81]
Pyelocaliectasis 593.89
Pyelocystitis — *see also* Pyelitis 590.80
Pyelohydronephrosis 591
Pyelonephritis — *see also* Pyelitis 590.80
  acute 590.10
    with renal medullary necrosis 590.11
  chronic 590.00
  syphilitic (late) 095.4
  tuberculous (*see also* Tuberculosis) 016.0 ☑ [590.81]
Pyelonephrosis — *see also* Pyelitis 590.80
  chronic 590.00
Pyelophlebitis 451.89
Pyelo-ureteritis cystica 590.3
Pyemia, pyemic (purulent) — *see also* Septicemia 038.9
  abscess — *see* Abscess

Pyemia, pyemic — *see also* Septicemia — *continued*
  arthritis (*see also* Arthritis, pyogenic) 711.0 ☑
  Bacillus coli 038.42
  embolism — *see* Embolism, pyemic
  fever 038.9
  infection 038.9
  joint (*see also* Arthritis, pyogenic) 711.0 ☑
  liver 572.1
  meningococcal 036.2
  newborn 771.81
  phlebitis — *see* Phlebitis
  pneumococcal 038.2
  portal 572.1
  postvaccinal 999.3
  specified organism NEC 038.8
  staphylococcal 038.10
    aureus 038.11
    specified organism NEC 038.19
  streptococcal 038.0
  tuberculous — *see* Tuberculosis, miliary
Pygopagus 759.4
Pykno-epilepsy, pyknolepsy (idiopathic) — *see also* Epilepsy 345.0
Pyle (-Cohn) disease (craniometaphyseal dysplasia) 756.89
Pylephlebitis (suppurative) 572.1
Pylethrombophlebitis 572.1
Pylethrombosis 572.1
Pyloritis — *see also* Gastritis 535.5 ☑
Pylorospasm (reflex) 537.81
  congenital or infantile 750.5
  neurotic 306.4
  newborn 750.5
  psychogenic 306.4
Pylorus, pyloric — *see* condition
Pyoarthrosis — *see* Pyarthrosis
Pyocele
  mastoid 383.00
  sinus (accessory) (nasal) (*see also* Sinusitis) 473.9
  turbinate (bone) 473.9
  urethra (*see also* Urethritis) 597.0
Pyococcal dermatitis 686.00
Pyococcide, skin 686.00
Pyocolpos — *see also* Vaginitis 616.10
Pyocyaneus dermatitis 686.09
Pyocystitis — *see also* Cystitis 595.9
Pyoderma, pyodermia 686.00
  gangrenosum 686.01
  specified type NEC 686.09
  vegetans 686.8
Pyodermatitis 686.00
  vegetans 686.8
Pyogenic — *see* condition
Pyohemia — *see* Septicemia
Pyohydronephrosis — *see also* Pyelitis 590.80
Pyometra 615.9
Pyometritis — *see also* Endometritis 615.9
Pyometrium — *see also* Endometritis 615.9
Pyomyositis 728.0
  ossificans 728.19
  tropical (bungpagga) 040.81
Pyonephritis — *see also* Pyelitis 590.80
  chronic 590.00
Pyonephrosis (congenital) — *see also* Pyelitis 590.80
  acute 590.10
Pyo-oophoritis — *see also* Salpingo-oophoritis 614.2
Pyo-ovarium — *see also* Salpingo-oophoritis 614.2
Pyopericarditis 420.99
Pyopericardium 420.99
Pyophlebitis — *see* Phlebitis
Pyopneumopericardium 420.99
Pyopneumothorax (infectional) 510.9
  with fistula 510.0
  subdiaphragmatic (*see also* Peritonitis) 567.29

Pyopneumothorax — continued
  subphrenic (see also Peritonitis) 567.29
  tuberculous (see also Tuberculosis, pleura) 012.0 ☑
Pyorrhea (alveolar) (alveolaris) 523.40
  degenerative 523.5
Pyosalpingitis — see also Salpingo-oophoritis 614.2
Pyosalpinx — see also Salpingo-oophoritis 614.2
Pyosepticemia — see Septicemia
Pyosis
  Corlett's (impetigo) 684
  Manson's (pemphigus contagiosus) 684
Pyothorax 510.9
  with fistula 510.0
  tuberculous (see also Tuberculosis, pleura) 012.0 ☑
Pyoureter 593.89
  tuberculous (see also Tuberculosis 016.2 ☑
Pyramidopallidonigral syndrome 332.0
Pyrexia (of unknown origin) (P.U.O.) 780.6
  atmospheric 992.0
  during labor 659.2 ☑
  environmentally-induced newborn 778.4
  heat 992.0
  newborn, environmentally-induced 778.4
  puerperal 672.0 ☑
Pyroglobulinemia 273.8
Pyromania 312.33
Pyrosis 787.1
Pyrroloporphyria 277.1
Pyuria (bacterial) 791.9

Q

Q fever 083.0
  with pneumonia 083.0 [484.8]
Quadricuspid aortic valve 746.89
Quadrilateral fever 083.0
Quadriparesis — see Quadriplegia
  meaning muscle weakness 728.87
Quadriplegia 344.00
  with fracture, vertebra (process) — see Fracture, vertebra, cervical, with spinal cord injury
  brain (current episode) 437.8
  C1-C4
    complete 344.01
    incomplete 344.02
  C5-C7
    complete 344.03
    incomplete 344.04
  cerebral (current episode) 437.8
  congenital or infantile (cerebral) (spastic) (spinal) 343.2
  cortical 437.8
  embolic (current episode) (see also Embolism, brain) 434.1 ☑
  infantile (cerebral) (spastic) (spinal) 343.2
  newborn NEC 767.0
  specified NEC 344.09
  thrombotic (current episode) (see also Thrombosis, brain) 434.0 ☑
  traumatic — see Injury, spinal, cervical
Quadruplet
  affected by maternal complications of pregnancy 761.5
  healthy liveborn — see Newborn, multiple
  pregnancy (complicating delivery) NEC 651.8 ☑
    with fetal loss and retention of one or more fetus(es) 651.5 ☑
    following (elective) fetal reduction 651.7 ☑
Quarrelsomeness 301.3

Quartan
  fever 084.2
  malaria (fever) 084.2
Queensland fever 083.0
  coastal 083.0
  seven-day 100.89
Quervain's disease 727.04
  thyroid (subacute granulomatous thyroiditis) 245.1
Queyrat's erythroplasia (M8080/2)
  specified site — see Neoplasm, skin, in situ
  unspecified site 233.5
Quincke's disease or edema — see Edema, angioneurotic
Quinquaud's disease (acne decalvans) 704.09
Quinsy (gangrenous) 475
Quintan fever 083.1
Quintuplet
  affected by maternal complications of pregnancy 761.5
  healthy liveborn — see Newborn, multiple
  pregnancy (complicating delivery) NEC 651.2 ☑
    with fetal loss and retention of one or more fetus(es) 651.6 ☑
    following (elective) fetal reduction 651.7 ☑
Quotidian
  fever 084.0
  malaria (fever) 084.0

R

Rabbia 071
Rabbit fever — see also Tularemia 021.9
Rabies 071
  contact V01.5
  exposure to V01.5
  inoculation V04.5
    reaction — see Complications, vaccination
  vaccination, prophylactic (against) V04.5
Rachischisis — see also Spina bifida 741.9 ☑
Rachitic — see also condition
  deformities of spine 268.1
  pelvis 268.1
    with disproportion (fetopelvic) 653.2 ☑
      affecting fetus or newborn 763.1
    causing obstructed labor 660.1 ☑
      affecting fetus or newborn 763.1
Rachitis, rachitism — see also Rickets
  acute 268.0
  fetalis 756.4
  renalis 588.0
  tarda 268.0
Racket nail 757.5
Radial nerve — see condition
Radiation effects or sickness — see also Effect, adverse, radiation
  cataract 366.46
  dermatitis 692.82
    sunburn (see also Sunburn) 692.71
Radiculitis (pressure) (vertebrogenic) 729.2
  accessory nerve 723.4
  anterior crural 724.4
  arm 723.4
  brachial 723.4
  cervical NEC 723.4
  due to displacement of intervertebral disc — see Neuritis, due to, displacement intervertebral disc
  leg 724.4
  lumbar NEC 724.4
  lumbosacral 724.4
  rheumatic 729.2
  syphilitic 094.89
  thoracic (with visceral pain) 724.4

Radiculomyelitis 357.0
  toxic, due to
    Clostridium tetani 037
    Corynebacterium diphtheriae 032.89
Radiculopathy — see also Radiculitis 729.2
Radioactive substances, adverse effect — see Effect, adverse, radioactive substance
Radiodermal burns (acute) (chronic) (occupational) — see Burn, by site
Radiodermatitis 692.82
Radionecrosis — see Effect, adverse, radiation
Radiotherapy session V58.0
Radium, adverse effect — see Effect, adverse, radioactive substance
Raeder-Harbitz syndrome (pulseless disease) 446.7
Rage — see also Disturbance, conduct 312.0 ☑
  meaning rabies 071
Rag sorters' disease 022.1
Raillietiniasis 123.8
Railroad neurosis 300.16
Railway spine 300.16
Raised — see Elevation
Raiva 071
Rake teeth, tooth 524.39
Rales 786.7
Ramifying renal pelvis 753.3
Ramsay Hunt syndrome (herpetic geniculate ganglionitis) 053.11
  meaning dyssynergia cerebellaris myoclonica 334.2
Ranke's primary infiltration — see also Tuberculosis 010.0 ☑
Ranula 527.6
  congenital 750.26
Rape
  adult 995.83
  alleged, observation or examination V71.5
  child 995.53
Rapid
  feeble pulse, due to shock, following injury 958.4
  heart (beat) 785.0
    psychogenic 306.2
  respiration 786.06
    psychogenic 306.1
  second stage (delivery) 661.3 ☑
    affecting fetus or newborn 763.6
  time-zone change syndrome 327.35
Rarefaction, bone 733.99
Rash 782.1
  canker 034.1
  diaper 691.0
  drug (internal use) 693.0
    contact 692.3
  ECHO 9 virus 078.89
  enema 692.89
  food (see also Allergy, food) 693.1
  heat 705.1
  napkin 691.0
  nettle 708.8
  pustular 782.1
  rose 782.1
    epidemic 056.9
    of infants 057.8
  scarlet 034.1
  serum (prophylactic) (therapeutic) 999.5
  toxic 782.1
  wandering tongue 529.1
Rasmussen's aneurysm — see also Tuberculosis 011.2 ☑
Rat-bite fever 026.9
  due to Streptobacillus moniliformis 026.1
  spirochetal (morsus muris) 026.0
Rathke's pouch tumor (M9350/1) 237.0
Raymond (-Céstan) syndrome 433.8 ☑

Raynaud's
  disease or syndrome (paroxysmal digital cyanosis) 443.0
  gangrene (symmetric) 443.0 [785.4]
  phenomenon (paroxysmal digital cyanosis) (secondary) 443.0
RDS 769
Reaction
  acute situational maladjustment (see also Reaction, adjustment) 309.9
  adaptation (see also Reaction, adjustment) 309.9
  adjustment 309.9
    with
      anxious mood 309.24
        with depressed mood 309.28
      conduct disturbance 309.3
        combined with disturbance of emotions 309.4
      depressed mood 309.0
        brief 309.0
        with anxious mood 309.28
        prolonged 309.1
      elective mutism 309.83
      mixed emotions and conduct 309.4
      mutism, elective 309.83
      physical symptoms 309.82
      predominant disturbance (of)
        conduct 309.3
        emotions NEC 309.29
          mixed 309.28
        mixed, emotions and conduct 309.4
      specified type NEC 309.89
      specific academic or work inhibition 309.23
      withdrawal 309.83
    depressive 309.0
      with conduct disturbance 309.4
      brief 309.0
      prolonged 309.1
    specified type NEC 309.89
  adverse food NEC 995.7
  affective (see also Psychosis, affective) 296.90
    specified type NEC 296.99
  aggressive 301.3
    unsocialized (see also Disturbance, conduct) 312.0 ☑
  allergic (see also Allergy) 995.3
    drug, medicinal substance, and biological — see Allergy, drug
    food — see Allergy, food
    serum 999.5
  anaphylactic — see Shock, anaphylactic
  anesthesia — see Anesthesia, complication
  anger 312.0 ☑
  antisocial 301.7
  antitoxin (prophylactic) (therapeutic) — see Complications, vaccination
  anxiety 300.00
  Arthus 995.21
  asthenic 300.5
  compulsive 300.3
  conversion (anesthetic) (autonomic) (hyperkinetic) (mixed paralytic) (paresthetic) 300.11
  deoxyribonuclease (DNA) (DNase) hypersensitivity NEC 287.2
  depressive 300.4
    acute 309.0
    affective (see also Psychosis, affective) 296.2 ☑
      recurrent episode 296.3 ☑
      single episode 296.2 ☑
    brief 309.0
    manic (see also Psychosis, affective) 296.80
    neurotic 300.4
    psychoneurotic 300.4

Index to Diseases

Reaction — *continued*
- depressive — *continued*
  - psychotic 298.0
  - dissociative 300.15
- drug NEC (*see also* Table of Drugs and Chemicals) 995.20 ▲
  - allergic (*see also* Allergy, drug) 995.27
  - correct substance properly administered 995.20 ▲
  - obstetric anesthetic or analgesic NEC 668.9 ☑
    - affecting fetus or newborn 763.5
    - specified drug — *see* Table of Drugs and Chemicals
  - overdose or poisoning 977.9
    - specified drug — *see* Table of Drugs and Chemicals
  - specific to newborn 779.4
  - transmitted via placenta or breast milk — *see* Absorption, drug, through placenta
  - withdrawal NEC 292.0
    - infant of dependent mother 779.5
  - wrong substance given or taken in error 977.9
    - specified drug — *see* Table of Drugs and Chemicals
- dyssocial 301.7
- dystonic, acute, due to drugs 333.72 ●
- erysipeloid 027.1
- fear 300.20
  - child 313.0
- fluid loss, cerebrospinal 349.0
- food (*see also* Allergy, food)
  - adverse NEC 995.7
  - anaphylactic shock — *see* Anaphylactic shock, due to, food
- foreign
  - body NEC 728.82
    - in operative wound (inadvertently left) 998.4
      - due to surgical material intentionally left — *see* Complications, due to (presence of) any device, implant, or graft classified to 996.0–996.5 NEC
    - substance accidentally left during a procedure (chemical) (powder) (talc) 998.7
    - body or object (instrument) (sponge) (swab) 998.4
- graft-versus-host (GVH) 996.85
- grief (acute) (brief) 309.0
  - prolonged 309.1
- gross stress (*see also* Reaction, stress, acute) 308.9
- group delinquent (*see also* Disturbance, conduct) 312.2 ☑
- Herxheimer's 995.0
- hyperkinetic (*see also* Hyperkinesia) 314.9
- hypochondriacal 300.7
- hypoglycemic, due to insulin 251.0
  - therapeutic misadventure 962.3
- hypomanic (*see also* Psychosis, affective) 296.0 ☑
  - recurrent episode 296.1 ☑
  - single episode 296.0 ☑
- hysterical 300.10
  - conversion type 300.11
  - dissociative 300.15
- id (bacterial cause) 692.89
- immaturity NEC 301.89
  - aggressive 301.3
  - emotional instability 301.59
- immunization — *see* Complications, vaccination
- incompatibility
  - blood group (ABO) (infusion) (transfusion) 999.6
  - Rh (factor) (infusion) (transfusion) 999.7

Reaction — *continued*
- inflammatory — *see* Infection
- infusion — *see* Complications, infusion
- inoculation (immune serum) — *see* Complications, vaccination
- insulin 995.23 ▲
- involutional
  - paranoid 297.2
  - psychotic (*see also* Psychosis, affective, depressive) 296.2 ☑
- leukemoid ▶(basophilic)◀ (lymphocytic) (monocytic) (myelocytic) ▶(neutrophilic)◀ 288.62 ▲
- LSD (*see also* Abuse, drugs, nondependent) 305.3 ☑
- lumbar puncture 349.0
- manic-depressive (*see also* Psychosis, affective) 296.80
  - depressed 296.2 ☑
    - recurrent episode 296.3 ☑
    - single episode 296.2 ☑
  - hypomanic 296.0 ☑
- neurasthenic 300.5
- neurogenic (*see also* Neurosis) 300.9
- neurotic NEC 300.9
- neurotic-depressive 300.4
- nitritoid — *see* Crisis, nitritoid
- obsessive compulsive 300.3
- organic 293.9
  - acute 293.0
  - subacute 293.1
- overanxious, child or adolescent 313.0
- paranoid (chronic) 297.9
  - acute 298.3
  - climacteric 297.2
  - involutional 297.2
  - menopausal 297.2
  - senile 290.20
  - simple 297.0
- passive
  - aggressive 301.84
  - dependency 301.6
- personality (*see also* Disorder, personality) 301.9
- phobic 300.20
- postradiation — *see* Effect, adverse, radiation
- psychogenic NEC 300.9
- psychoneurotic (*see also* Neurosis) 300.9
  - anxiety 300.00
  - compulsive 300.3
  - conversion 300.11
  - depersonalization 300.6
  - depressive 300.4
  - dissociative 300.15
  - hypochondriacal 300.7
  - hysterical 300.10
    - conversion type 300.11
    - dissociative type 300.15
  - neurasthenic 300.5
  - obsessive 300.3
  - obsessive-compulsive 300.3
  - phobic 300.20
  - tension state 300.9
- psychophysiologic NEC (*see also* Disorder, psychosomatic) 306.9
  - cardiovascular 306.2
  - digestive 306.4
  - endocrine 306.6
  - gastrointestinal 306.4
  - genitourinary 306.50
  - heart 306.2
  - hemic 306.8
  - intestinal (large) (small) 306.4
  - laryngeal 306.1
  - lymphatic 306.8
  - musculoskeletal 306.0
  - pharyngeal 306.1
  - respiratory 306.1
  - skin 306.3
  - special sense organs 306.7
  - psychosomatic (*see also* Disorder, psychosomatic) 306.9
  - psychotic (*see also* Psychosis) 298.9

Reaction — *continued*
- psychotic (*see also* Psychosis) — *continued*
  - depressive 298.0
  - due to or associated with physical condition (*see also* Psychosis, organic) 293.9
  - involutional (*see also* Psychosis, affective) 296.2 ☑
    - recurrent episode 296.3 ☑
    - single episode 296.2 ☑
- pupillary (myotonic) (tonic) 379.46
- radiation — *see* Effect, adverse, radiation
- runaway (*see also* Disturbance, conduct)
  - socialized 312.2 ☑
  - undersocialized, unsocialized 312.1 ☑
- scarlet fever toxin — *see* Complications, vaccination
- schizophrenic (*see also* Schizophrenia) 295.9 ☑
  - latent 295.5 ☑
- serological for syphilis — *see* Serology for syphilis
- serum (prophylactic) (therapeutic) 999.5
  - immediate 999.4
- situational (*see also* Reaction, adjustment) 309.9
  - acute, to stress 308.3
  - adjustment (*see also* Reaction, adjustment) 309.9
- somatization (*see also* Disorder, psychosomatic) 306.9
- spinal puncture 349.0
- spite, child (*see also* Disturbance, conduct) 312.0 ☑
- stress, acute 308.9
  - with predominant disturbance (of)
    - consciousness 308.1
    - emotions 308.0
    - mixed 308.4
    - psychomotor 308.2
    - specified type NEC 308.3
  - bone or cartilage — *see* Fracture, stress
- surgical procedure — *see* Complications, surgical procedure
- tetanus antitoxin — *see* Complications, vaccination
- toxin-antitoxin — *see* Complications, vaccination
- transfusion (blood) (bone marrow) (lymphocytes) (allergic) — *see* Complications, transfusion
- tuberculin skin test, nonspecific (without active tuberculosis) 795.5
  - positive (without active tuberculosis) 795.5
- ultraviolet — *see* Effect, adverse, ultraviolet
- undersocialized, unsocialized (*see also* Disturbance, conduct)
  - aggressive (type) 312.0 ☑
  - unaggressive (type) 312.1 ☑
- vaccination (any) — *see* Complications, vaccination
- white graft (skin) 996.52
- withdrawing, child or adolescent 313.22
- x-ray — *see* Effect, adverse, x-rays

Reactive depression — *see also* Reaction, depressive 300.4
- neurotic 300.4
- psychoneurotic 300.4
- psychotic 298.0

Rebound tenderness 789.6 ☑
Recalcitrant patient V15.81
Recanalization, thrombus — *see* Thrombosis
Recession, receding
- chamber angle (eye) 364.77
- chin 524.06

Recession, receding — *continued*
- gingival (postinfective) (postoperative) 523.20
  - generalized 523.25
  - localized 523.24
  - minimal 523.21
  - moderate 523.22
  - severe 523.23

Recklinghausen-Applebaum disease (hemochromatosis) 275.0
Recklinghausen's disease (M9540/1) 237.71
- bones (osteitis fibrosa cystica) 252.01
Reclus' disease (cystic) 610.1
Recrudescent typhus (fever) 081.1
Recruitment, auditory 388.44
Rectalgia 569.42
Rectitis 569.49
Rectocele
- female (without uterine prolapse) 618.04
  - with uterine prolapse 618.4
    - complete 618.3
    - incomplete 618.2
  - in pregnancy or childbirth 654.4 ☑
    - causing obstructed labor 660.2 ☑
      - affecting fetus or newborn 763.1
- male 569.49
- vagina, vaginal (outlet) 618.04

Rectosigmoiditis 569.89
- ulcerative (chronic) 556.3

Rectosigmoid junction — *see* condition
Rectourethral — *see* condition
Rectovaginal — *see* condition
Rectovesical — *see* condition
Rectum, rectal — *see* condition
Recurrent — *see* condition
Red bugs 133.8
Red cedar asthma 495.8
Redness
- conjunctiva 379.93
- eye 379.93
- nose 478.19 ▲

Reduced ventilatory or vital capacity 794.2
Reduction
- function
  - kidney (*see also* Disease, renal) 593.9
  - liver 573.8
- ventilatory capacity 794.2
- vital capacity 794.2

Redundant, redundancy
- abdomen 701.9
- anus 751.5
- cardia 537.89
- clitoris 624.2
- colon (congenital) 751.5
- foreskin (congenital) 605
- intestine 751.5
- labia 624.3
- organ or site, congenital NEC — *see* Accessory
- panniculus (abdominal) 278.1
- prepuce (congenital) 605
- pylorus 537.89
- rectum 751.5
- scrotum 608.89
- sigmoid 751.5
- skin (of face) 701.9
  - eyelids 374.30
- stomach 537.89
- uvula 528.9
- vagina 623.8

Reduplication — *see* Duplication
Referral
- adoption (agency) V68.89
- nursing care V63.8
- patient without examination or treatment V68.81
- social services V63.8

Reflex — *see also* condition
- blink, deficient 374.45
- hyperactive gag 478.29
- neurogenic bladder NEC 596.54
  - atonic 596.54

Reflex

Reflex — see also condition — continued
  neurogenic bladder — continued
    atonic — continued
      with cauda equina syndrome 344.61
    vasoconstriction 443.9
    vasovagal 780.2
Reflux
  esophageal 530.81
    with esophagitis 530.11
  esophagitis 530.11
  gastroesophageal 530.81
  mitral — see Insufficiency, mitral
  ureteral — see Reflux, vesicoureteral
  vesicoureteral 593.70
    with
      reflux nephropathy 593.73
        bilateral 593.72
        unilateral 593.71
Reformed gallbladder 576.0
Reforming, artificial openings — see also Attention to, artificial, opening V55.9
Refractive error — see also Error, refractive 367.9
Refsum's disease or syndrome (heredopathia atactica polyneuritiformis) 356.3
Refusal of
  food 307.59
    hysterical 300.11
  treatment because of, due to
    patient's decision NEC V64.2
    reason of conscience or religion V62.6
Regaud
  tumor (M8082/3) — see Neoplasm, nasopharynx, malignant
  type carcinoma (M8082/3) — see Neoplasm, nasopharynx, malignant
Regional — see condition
Regulation feeding (elderly) (infant) 783.3
  newborn 779.3
Regurgitated
  food, choked on 933.1
  stomach contents, choked on 933.1
Regurgitation
  aortic (valve) (see also Insufficiency, aortic) 424.1
    congenital 746.4
    syphilitic 093.22
  food (see also Vomiting)
    with reswallowing — see Rumination
    newborn 779.3
  gastric contents — see Vomiting
  heart — see Endocarditis
  mitral (valve) (see also Insufficiency, mitral)
    congenital 746.6
  myocardial — see Endocarditis
  pulmonary (heart) (valve) (see also Endocarditis, pulmonary) 424.3
  stomach — see Vomiting
  tricuspid — see Endocarditis, tricuspid
  valve, valvular — see Endocarditis
  vesicoureteral — see Reflux, vesicoureteral
Rehabilitation V57.9
  multiple types V57.89
  occupational V57.21
  specified type NEC V57.89
  speech V57.3
  vocational V57.22
Reichmann's disease or syndrome (gastrosuccorrhea) 536.8
Reifenstein's syndrome (hereditary familial hypogonadism, male) 259.5
Reilly's syndrome or phenomenon — see also Neuropathy, peripheral, autonomic 337.9

Reimann's periodic disease 277.31
Reinsertion, contraceptive device V25.42
Reiter's disease, syndrome, or urethritis 099.3 [711.1]
Rejection
  food, hysterical 300.11
  transplant 996.80
    bone marrow 996.85
    corneal 996.51
    organ (immune or nonimmune cause) 996.80
      bone marrow 996.85
      heart 996.83
      intestines 996.87
      kidney 996.81
      liver 996.82
      lung 996.84
      pancreas 996.86
      specified NEC 996.89
    skin 996.52
      artificial 996.55
      decellularized allodermis 996.55
Relapsing fever 087.9
  Carter's (Asiatic) 087.0
  Dutton's (West African) 087.1
  Koch's 087.9
  louse-borne (epidemic) 087.0
  Novy's (American) 087.1
  Obermeyer's (European) 087.1
  Spirillum 087.9
  tick-borne (endemic) 087.1
Relaxation
  anus (sphincter) 569.49
    due to hysteria 300.11
  arch (foot) 734
    congenital 754.61
  back ligaments 728.4
  bladder (sphincter) 596.59
  cardio-esophageal 530.89
  cervix (see also Incompetency, cervix) 622.5
  diaphragm 519.4
  inguinal rings — see Hernia, inguinal
  joint (capsule) (ligament) (paralytic) (see also Derangement, joint) 718.90
    congenital 755.8
  lumbosacral joint 724.6
  pelvic floor 618.89
  pelvis 618.89
  perineum 618.89
  posture 729.9
  rectum (sphincter) 569.49
  sacroiliac (joint) 724.6
  scrotum 608.89
  urethra (sphincter) 599.84
  uterus (outlet) 618.89
  vagina (outlet) 618.89
  vesical 596.59
Remains
  canal of Cloquet 743.51
  capsule (opaque) 743.51
Remittent fever (malarial) 084.6
Remnant
  canal of Cloquet 743.51
  capsule (opaque) 743.51
  cervix, cervical stump (acquired) (postoperative) 622.8
  cystic duct, postcholecystectomy 576.0
  fingernail 703.8
    congenital 757.5
  meniscus, knee 717.5
  thyroglossal duct 759.2
  tonsil 474.8
    infected 474.00
  urachus 753.7
Remote effect of cancer — see condition
Removal (of)
  catheter (urinary) (indwelling) V53.6
    from artificial opening — see Attention to, artificial, opening
    non-vascular V58.82

Removal — continued
  catheter — continued
    vascular V58.81
  cerebral ventricle (communicating) shunt V53.01
  device (see also Fitting (of))
    contraceptive V25.42
    fixation
      external V54.89
      internal V54.01
    traction V54.89
  drains V58.49
  dressing
    wound V58.30
      nonsurgical V58.30
      surgical V58.31
  ileostomy V55.2
  Kirschner wire V54.89
  nonvascular catheter V58.82
  pin V54.01
  plaster cast V54.89
  plate (fracture) V54.01
  rod V54.01
  screw V54.01
  splint, external V54.89
  staples V58.32
  subdermal implantable contraceptive V25.43
  ▶sutures◀ V58.32
  traction device, external V54.89
  vascular catheter V58.81
  wound packing V58.30
    nonsurgical V58.30
    surgical V58.31
Ren
  arcuatus 753.3
  mobile, mobilis (see also Disease, renal) 593.0
    congenital 753.3
  unguliformis 753.3
Renal — see also condition
  glomerulohyalinosis-diabetic syndrome 250.4 [581.81]
Rendu-Osler-Weber disease or syndrome (familial hemorrhagic telangiectasia) 448.0
Reninoma (M8361/1) 236.91
Rénon-Delille syndrome 253.8
Repair
  pelvic floor, previous, in pregnancy or childbirth 654.4
    affecting fetus or newborn 763.89
  scarred tissue V51
Replacement by artificial or mechanical device or prosthesis of — see also Fitting (of
  artificial skin V43.83
  bladder V43.5
  blood vessel V43.4
  breast V43.82
  eye globe V43.0
  heart
    with
      assist device V43.21
      fully implantable artificial heart V43.22
    valve V43.3
  intestine V43.89
  joint V43.60
    ankle V43.66
    elbow V43.62
    finger V43.69
    hip (partial) (total) V43.64
    knee V43.65
    shoulder V43.61
    specified NEC V43.69
    wrist V43.63
  kidney V43.89
  larynx V43.81
  lens V43.1
  limb(s) V43.7
  liver V43.89
  lung V43.89
  organ NEC V43.89
  pancreas V43.89
  skin (artificial) V43.83

Index to Diseases

Replacement by artificial or mechanical device or prosthesis of — see also Fitting (of — continued
  tissue NEC V43.89
Reprogramming
  cardiac pacemaker V53.31
Request for expert evidence V68.2
Reserve, decreased or low
  cardiac — see Disease, heart
  kidney (see also Disease, renal) 593.9
Residual — see also condition
  bladder 596.8
  foreign body — see Retention, foreign body
  state, schizophrenic (see also Schizophrenia) 295.6
  urine 788.69
Resistance, resistant (to)
  activated protein C 289.81

Note — use the following subclassification for categories V09.5, V09.7, V09.8, V09.9:
  0 without mention of resistance to multiple drugs
  1 with resistance to multiple drugs
     V09.5 quinolones and fluoroquinolones
     V09.7 antimycobacterial agents
     V09.8 specified drugs NEC
     V09.9 unspecified drugs

  drugs by microorganisms V09.9
    Amikacin V09.4
    aminoglycosides V09.4
    Amodiaquine V09.5
    Amoxicillin V09.0
    Ampicillin V09.0
    antimycobacterial agents V09.7
    Azithromycin V09.2
    Azlocillin V09.0
    Aztreonam V09.1
    Bacampicillin V09.0
    Bacitracin V09.8
    Benznidazole V09.8
    B-lactam antibiotics V09.1
    Capreomycin V09.7
    Carbenicillin V09.0
    Cefaclor V09.1
    Cefadroxil V09.1
    Cefamandole V09.1
    Cefatetan V09.1
    Cefazolin V09.1
    Cefixime V09.1
    Cefonicid V09.1
    Cefoperazone V09.1
    Ceforanide V09.1
    Cefotaxime V09.1
    Cefoxitin V09.1
    Ceftazidime V09.1
    Ceftizoxime V09.1
    Ceftriaxone V09.1
    Cefuroxime V09.1
    Cephalexin V09.1
    Cephaloglycin V09.1
    Cephaloridine V09.1
    Cephalosporins V09.1
    Cephalothin V09.1
    Cephapirin V09.1
    Cephradine V09.1
    Chloramphenicol V09.8
    Chloroquine V09.5
    Chlorguanide V09.8
    Chlorproguanil V09.8
    Chlortetracycline V09.3
    Cinoxacin V09.5
    Ciprofloxacin V09.5
    Clarithromycin V09.2
    Clindamycin V09.8
    Clioquinol V09.5
    Clofazimine V09.7
    Cloxacillin V09.0

Index to Diseases

Resistance, resistant — continued
drugs by microorganisms — continued
- Cyclacillin V09.0
- Cycloserine V09.7 ☑
- Dapsone [DZ] V09.7 ☑
- Demeclocycline V09.3
- Dicloxacillin V09.0
- Doxycycline V09.3
- Enoxacin V09.5 ☑
- Erythromycin V09.2
- Ethambutol [EMB] V09.7 ☑
- Ethionamide [ETA] V09.7 ☑
- fluoroquinolones V09.5 ☑
- Gentamicin V09.4
- Halofantrine V09.8 ☑
- Imipenem V09.1
- Iodoquinol V09.5 ☑
- Isoniazid [INH] V09.7 ☑
- Kanamycin V09.4
- macrolides V09.2
- Mafenide V09.6
- MDRO (multiple drug resistant organisms) NOS V09.91
- Mefloquine V09.8 ☑
- Melasoprol V09.8 ☑
- Methacycline V09.3
- Methenamine V09.8 ☑
- Methicillin V09.0
- Metronidazole V09.8 ☑
- Mezlocillin V09.0
- Minocycline V09.3
- multiple drug resistant organisms NOS V09.91
- Nafcillin V09.0
- Nalidixic acid V09.5 ☑
- Natamycin V09.2
- Neomycin V09.4
- Netilmicin V09.4
- Nimorazole V09.8 ☑
- Nitrofurantoin V09.8 ☑
- Nitrofurtimox V09.8 ☑
- Norfloxacin V09.5 ☑
- Nystatin V09.2
- Ofloxacin V09.5 ☑
- Oleandomycin V09.2
- Oxacillin V09.0
- Oxytetracycline V09.3
- Para-amino salicylic acid [PAS] V09.7
- Paromomycin V09.4
- Penicillin (G) (V) (VK) V09.0
- penicillins V09.0
- Pentamidine V09.8 ☑
- Piperacillin V09.0
- Primaquine V09.5 ☑
- Proguanil V09.8 ☑
- Pyrazinamide [PZA] V09.7 ☑
- Pyrimethamine/Sulfalene V09.8 ☑
- Pyrimethamine/Sulfodoxine V09.8 ☑
- Quinacrine V09.5 ☑
- Quinidine V09.8 ☑
- Quinine V09.8 ☑
- quinolones V09.5 ☑
- Rifabutin V09.7 ☑
- Rifampin [RIF] V09.7 ☑
- Rifamycin V09.7 ☑
- Rolitetracycline V09.3
- specified drugs NEC V09.8 ☑
- Spectinomycin V09.8 ☑
- Spiramycin V09.2
- Streptomycin [SM] V09.4
- Sulfacetamide V09.6
- Sulfacytine V09.6
- Sulfadiazine V09.6
- Sulfadoxine V09.6
- Sulfamethoxazole V09.6
- Sulfapyridine V09.6
- Sulfasalizine V09.6
- Sulfasoxazole V09.6
- sulfonamides V09.6
- Sulfoxone V09.7 ☑
- tetracycline V09.3
- tetracyclines V09.3

Resistance, resistant — continued
drugs by microorganisms — continued
- Thiamphenicol V09.8 ☑
- Ticarcillin V09.0
- Tinidazole V09.8 ☑
- Tobramycin V09.4
- Triamphenicol V09.8 ☑
- Trimethoprim V09.8 ☑
- Vancomycin V09.8 ☑
- insulin 277.7
- thyroid hormone 246.8 ●

Resorption
- biliary 576.8
  - purulent or putrid (see also Cholecystitis) 576.8
- dental (roots) 521.40
  - alveoli 525.8
  - pathological
    - external 521.42
    - internal 521.41
    - specified NEC 521.49
- septic — see Septicemia
- teeth (roots) 521.40
  - pathological
    - external 521.42
    - internal 521.41
    - specified NEC 521.49

Respiration
- asymmetrical 786.09
- bronchial 786.09
- Cheyne-Stokes (periodic respiration) 786.04
- decreased, due to shock following injury 958.4
- disorder of 786.00
  - psychogenic 306.1
  - specified NEC 786.09
- failure 518.81
  - acute 518.81
  - acute and chronic 518.84
  - chronic 518.83
  - newborn 770.84
- insufficiency 786.09
  - acute 518.82
  - newborn NEC 770.89
- Kussmaul (air hunger) 786.09
- painful 786.52
- periodic 786.09
  - high altitude 327.22
- poor 786.09
  - newborn NEC 770.89
- sighing 786.7
- wheezing 786.07

Respiratory — see also condition
- distress 786.09
  - acute 518.82
  - fetus or newborn NEC 770.89
  - syndrome (newborn) 769
    - adult (following shock, surgery, or trauma) 518.5
    - specified NEC 518.82
- failure 518.81
  - acute 518.81
  - acute and chronic 518.84
  - chronic 518.83

Respiratory syncytial virus (RSV) 079.6
- bronchiolitis 466.11
- pneumonia 480.1
- vaccination, prophylactic (against) V04.82

Response
- photoallergic 692.72
- phototoxic 692.72

Restless legs syndrome ▶(RLS)◀ 333.94 ▲

Restlessness 799.2

Restoration of organ continuity from previous sterilization (tuboplasty) (vasoplasty) V26.0

Rest, rests
- mesonephric duct 752.89
  - fallopian tube 752.11
- ovarian, in fallopian tubes 752.19
- wolffian duct 752.89

Restriction of housing space V60.1

Restzustand, schizophrenic — see also Schizophrenia 295.6 ☑

Retained — see Retention

Retardation
- development, developmental, specific (see also Disorder, development, specific) 315.9
  - learning, specific 315.2
    - arithmetical 315.1
    - language (skills) 315.31
      - expressive 315.31
      - mixed receptive-expressive 315.32
    - mathematics 315.1
    - reading 315.00
      - phonological 315.39
    - written expression 315.2
  - motor 315.4
- endochondral bone growth 733.91
- growth (physical) in childhood 783.43
  - due to malnutrition 263.2
- fetal (intrauterine) 764.9 ☑
  - affecting management of pregnancy 656.5 ☑
- intrauterine growth 764.9 ☑
  - affecting management of pregnancy 656.5 ☑
- mental 319
  - borderline V62.89
  - mild, IQ 50-70 317
  - moderate, IQ 35-49 318.0
  - profound, IQ under 20 318.2
  - severe, IQ 20-34 318.1
- motor, specific 315.4
- physical 783.43
  - child 783.43
  - due to malnutrition 263.2
- fetus (intrauterine) 764.9 ☑
  - affecting management of pregnancy 656.5 ☑
- psychomotor NEC 307.9
- reading 315.00

Retching — see Vomiting

Retention, retained
- bladder (see also Retention, urine) 788.20
  - psychogenic 306.53
- carbon dioxide 276.2
- cyst — see Cyst
- dead
  - fetus (after 22 completed weeks gestation) 656.4 ☑
  - early fetal death (before 22 completed weeks gestation) 632
  - ovum 631
- decidua (following delivery) (fragments) (with hemorrhage) 666.2 ☑
  - without hemorrhage 667.1 ☑
- deciduous tooth 520.6
- dental root 525.3
- fecal (see also Constipation) 564.00
- fluid 276.6
- foreign body (see also Foreign body, retained)
  - bone 733.99
  - current trauma — see Foreign body, by site or type
  - middle ear 385.83
  - muscle 729.6
  - soft tissue NEC 729.6
- gastric 536.8
- membranes (following delivery) (with hemorrhage) 666.2 ☑
  - with abortion — see Abortion, by type
  - without hemorrhage 667.1 ☑
- menses 626.8
- milk (puerperal) 676.2 ☑
- nitrogen, extrarenal 788.9
- placenta (total) (with hemorrhage) 666.0 ☑
  - with abortion — see Abortion, by type
  - without hemorrhage 667.0 ☑

Retention, retained — continued
- placenta — continued
  - portions or fragments 666.2 ☑
    - without hemorrhage 667.1 ☑
- products of conception
  - early pregnancy (fetal death before 22 completed weeks gestation) 632
  - following
    - abortion — see Abortion, by type
    - delivery 666.2 ☑
      - with hemorrhage 666.2 ☑
      - without hemorrhage 667.1 ☑
- secundines (following delivery) (with hemorrhage) 666.2 ☑
  - with abortion — see Abortion, by type
  - without hemorrhage 667.1 ☑
- complicating puerperium (delayed hemorrhage) 666.2 ☑
- smegma, clitoris 624.8
- urine NEC 788.20
  - bladder, incomplete emptying 788.21
  - due to
    - benign prostatic hypertrophy (BPH) — see category 600
  - due to
    - benign prostatic hypertrophy (BPH) — see category 600
  - psychogenic 306.53
  - specified NEC 788.29
- water (in tissue) (see also Edema) 782.3

Reticulation, dust (occupational) 504

Reticulocytosis NEC 790.99

Reticuloendotheliosis
- acute infantile (M9722/3) 202.5 ☑
- leukemic (M9940/3) 202.4 ☑
- malignant (M9720/3) 202.3 ☑
- nonlipid (M9722/3) 202.5 ☑

Reticulohistiocytoma (giant cell) 277.89

Reticulohistiocytosis, multicentric 272.8

Reticulolymphosarcoma (diffuse) (M9613/3) 200.8 ☑
- follicular (M9691/3) 202.0 ☑
- nodular (M9691/3) 202.0 ☑

Reticulosarcoma (M9640/3) 200.0 ☑
- nodular (M9642/3) 200.0 ☑
- pleomorphic cell type (M9641/3) 200.0 ☑

Reticulosis (skin)
- acute of infancy (M9722/3) 202.5 ☑
- familial hemophagocytic 288.4 ●
- histiocytic medullary (M9721/3) 202.3 ☑
- lipomelanotic 695.89
- malignant (M9720/3) 202.3 ☑
- Sézary's (M9701/3) 202.2 ☑

Retina, retinal — see condition

Retinitis — see also Chorioretinitis 363.20
- albuminurica 585.9 [363.10]
- arteriosclerotic 440.8 [362.13]
- central angiospastic 362.41
- Coat's 362.12
- diabetic 250.5 ☑ [362.01]
- disciformis 362.52
- disseminated 363.10
  - metastatic 363.14
  - neurosyphilitic 094.83
  - pigment epitheliopathy 363.15
- exudative 362.12
- focal 363.00
  - in histoplasmosis 115.92
    - capsulatum 115.02
    - duboisii 115.12
  - juxtapapillary 363.05
  - macular 363.06
  - paramacular 363.06
  - peripheral 363.08
  - posterior pole NEC 363.07
- gravidarum 646.8 ☑

RETINITIS

Retinitis — see also Chorioretinitis — continued
- hemorrhagica externa 362.12
- juxtapapillary (Jensen's) 363.05
- luetic — see Retinitis, syphilitic
- metastatic 363.14
- pigmentosa 362.74
- proliferans 362.29
- proliferating 362.29
- punctata albescens 362.76
- renal 585.9 [363.13]
- syphilitic (secondary) 091.51
  - congenital 090.0 [363.13]
  - early 091.51
  - late 095.8 [363.13]
- syphilitica, central, recurrent 095.8 [363.13]
- tuberculous (see also Tuberculous) 017.3 [363.13]

Retinoblastoma (M9510/3) 190.5
- differentiated type (M9511/3) 190.5
- undifferentiated type (M9512/3) 190.5

Retinochoroiditis — see also Chorioretinitis 363.20
- central angiospastic 362.41
- disseminated 363.10
  - metastatic 363.14
  - neurosyphilitic 094.83
  - pigment epitheliopathy 363.15
  - syphilitic 094.83
- due to toxoplasmosis (acquired) (focal) 130.2
- focal 363.00
  - in histoplasmosis 115.92
    - capsulatum 115.02
    - duboisii 115.12
  - juxtapapillary (Jensen's) 363.05
  - macular 363.06
  - paramacular 363.06
  - peripheral 363.08
  - posterior pole NEC 363.07
- juxtapapillaris 363.05
- syphilitic (disseminated) 094.83

Retinopathy (background) 362.10
- arteriosclerotic 440.8 [362.13]
- atherosclerotic 440.8 [362.13]
- central serous 362.41
- circinate 362.10
- Coat's 362.12
- diabetic 250.5 ☑ [362.01]
  - nonproliferative 250.5 ☑ [362.03]
    - mild 250.5 ☑ [362.04]
    - moderate 250.5 ☑ [362.05]
    - severe 250.5 ☑ [362.06]
  - proliferative 250.5 ☑ [362.02]
- exudative 362.12
- hypertensive 362.11
- nonproliferative
  - diabetic 250.5 ☑ [362.03]
    - mild 250.5 ☑ [362.04]
    - moderate 250.5 ☑ [362.05]
    - severe 250.5 ☑ [362.06]
- of prematurity 362.21
- pigmentary, congenital 362.74
- proliferative 362.29
  - diabetic 250.5 ☑ [362.02]
  - sickle-cell 282.60 [362.29]
- solar 363.31

Retinoschisis 361.10
- bullous 361.12
- congenital 743.56
- flat 361.11
- juvenile 362.73

Retractile testis 752.52

Retraction
- cervix ▶— see Retraction, uterus◀
- drum (membrane) 384.82
- eyelid 374.41
- finger 736.29
- head 781.0
- lid 374.41
- lung 518.89
- mediastinum 519.3
- nipple 611.79
  - congenital 757.6
  - puerperal, postpartum 676.0 ☑

Retraction — continued
- palmar fascia 728.6
- pleura (see also Pleurisy) 511.0
- ring, uterus (Bandl's) (pathological) 661.4 ☑
  - affecting fetus or newborn 763.7
- sternum (congenital) 756.3
  - acquired 738.3
  - during respiration 786.9
- substernal 738.3
- supraclavicular 738.8
- syndrome (Duane's) 378.71
- uterus 621.6
- valve (heart) — see Endocarditis

Retrobulbar — see condition

Retrocaval ureter 753.4

Retrocecal — see also condition
- appendix (congenital) 751.5

Retrocession — see Retroversion

Retrodisplacement — see Retroversion

Retroflection, retroflexion — see Retroversion

Retrognathia, retrognathism (mandibular) (maxillary) 524.10

Retrograde
- ejaculation 608.87
- menstruation 626.8

Retroiliac ureter 753.4

Retroperineal — see condition

Retroperitoneal — see condition

Retroperitonitis 567.39 ▲

Retropharyngeal — see condition

Retroplacental — see condition

Retroposition — see Retroversion

Retrosternal thyroid (congenital) 759.2

Retroversion, retroverted
- cervix ▶— see Retroversion, uterus◀
- female NEC (see also Retroversion, uterus) 621.6
- iris 364.70
- testis (congenital) 752.51
- uterus, uterine (acquired) (acute) (adherent) (any degree) (asymptomatic) (cervix) (postinfectional) (postpartal, old) 621.6
  - congenital 752.3
  - in pregnancy or childbirth 654.3 ☑
    - affecting fetus or newborn 763.89
    - causing obstructed labor 660.2 ☑
      - affecting fetus or newborn 763.1

Retrusion, premaxilla (developmental) 524.04

Rett's syndrome 330.8

Reverse, reversed
- peristalsis 787.4

Reye-Sheehan syndrome (postpartum pituitary necrosis) 253.2

Reye's syndrome 331.81

Rh (factor)
- hemolytic disease 773.0
- incompatibility, immunization, or sensitization
  - affecting management of pregnancy 656.1 ☑
  - fetus or newborn 773.0
  - transfusion reaction 999.7
- negative mother, affecting fetus or newborn 773.0
- titer elevated 999.7
- transfusion reaction 999.7

Rhabdomyolysis (idiopathic) 728.88

Rhabdomyoma (M8900/0) — see also Neoplasm, connective tissue, benign
- adult (M8904/0) — see Neoplasm, connective tissue, benign
- fetal (M8903/0) — see Neoplasm, connective tissue, benign
- glycogenic (M8904/0) — see Neoplasm, connective tissue, benign

Rhabdomyosarcoma (M8900/3) — see also Neoplasm, connective tissue, malignant

Rhabdomyosarcoma — see also Neoplasm, connective tissue, malignant — continued
- alveolar (M8920/3) — see Neoplasm, connective tissue, malignant
- embryonal (M8910/3) — see Neoplasm, connective tissue, malignant
- mixed type (M8902/3) — see Neoplasm, connective tissue, malignant
- pleomorphic (M8901/3) — see Neoplasm, connective tissue, malignant

Rhabdosarcoma (M8900/3) — see Rhabdomyosarcoma

Rhesus (factor) (Rh) incompatibility — see Rh, incompatibility

Rheumaticosis — see Rheumatism

Rheumatism, rheumatic (acute NEC) 729.0
- adherent pericardium 393
- arthritis
  - acute or subacute — see Fever, rheumatic
  - chronic 714.0
    - spine 720.0
- articular (chronic) NEC (see also Arthritis) 716.9 ☑
  - acute or subacute — see Fever, rheumatic
- back 724.9
- blennorrhagic 098.59
- carditis — see Disease, heart, rheumatic
- cerebral — see Fever, rheumatic
- chorea (acute) — see Chorea, rheumatic
- chronic NEC 729.0
- coronary arteritis 391.9
  - chronic 398.99
- degeneration, myocardium (see also Degeneration, myocardium, with rheumatic fever) 398.0
- desert 114.0
- febrile — see Fever, rheumatic
- fever — see Fever, rheumatic
- gonococcal 098.59
- gout 274.0
- heart
  - disease (see also Disease, heart, rheumatic) 398.90
  - failure (chronic) (congestive) (inactive) 398.91
  - hemopericardium — see Rheumatic, pericarditis
  - hydropericardium — see Rheumatic, pericarditis
- inflammatory (acute) (chronic) (subacute) — see Fever, rheumatic
- intercostal 729.0
  - meaning Tietze's disease 733.6
- joint (chronic) NEC (see also Arthritis) 716.9 ☑
  - acute — see Fever, rheumatic
- mediastinopericarditis — see Rheumatic, pericarditis
- muscular 729.0
- myocardial degeneration (see also Degeneration, myocardium, with rheumatic fever) 398.0
- myocarditis (chronic) (inactive) (with chorea) 398.0
  - active or acute 391.2
    - with chorea (acute) (rheumatic) (Sydenham's) 392.0
- myositis 729.1
- neck 724.9
- neuralgic 729.0
- neuritis (acute) (chronic) 729.2
- neuromuscular 729.0
- nodose — see Arthritis, nodosa
- nonarticular 729.0
- palindromic 719.30
  - ankle 719.37
  - elbow 719.32

Index to Diseases

Rheumatism, rheumatic — continued
- palindromic — continued
  - foot 719.37
  - hand 719.34
  - hip 719.35
  - knee 719.36
  - multiple sites 719.39
  - pelvic region 719.35
  - shoulder (region) 719.31
  - specified site NEC 719.38
  - wrist 719.33
- pancarditis, acute 391.8
  - with chorea (acute) (rheumatic) (Sydenham's) 392.0
  - chronic or inactive 398.99
- pericarditis (active) (acute) (with effusion) (with pneumonia) 391.0
  - with chorea (acute) (rheumatic) (Sydenham's) 392.0
  - chronic or inactive 393
- pericardium — see Rheumatic, pericarditis
- pleuropericarditis — see Rheumatic, pericarditis
- pneumonia 390 [517.1]
- pneumonitis 390 [517.1]
- pneumopericarditis — see Rheumatic, pericarditis
- polyarthritis
  - acute or subacute — see Fever, rheumatic
  - chronic 714.0
- polyarticular NEC (see also Arthritis) 716.9 ☑
- psychogenic 306.0
- radiculitis 729.2
- sciatic 724.3
- septic — see Fever, rheumatic
- spine 724.9
- subacute NEC 729.0
- torticollis 723.5
- tuberculous NEC (see also Tuberculosis) 015.9 ☑
- typhoid fever 002.0

Rheumatoid — see also condition
- lungs 714.81

Rhinitis (atrophic) (catarrhal) (chronic) (croupous) (fibrinous) (hyperplastic) (hypertrophic) (membranous) (purulent) (suppurative) (ulcerative) 472.0
- with
  - hay fever (see also Fever, hay) 477.9
    - with asthma (bronchial) 493.0 ☑
  - sore throat — see Nasopharyngitis
- acute 460
- allergic (nonseasonal) (seasonal) (see also Fever, hay) 477.9
  - with asthma (see also Asthma) 493.0 ☑
  - due to food 477.1
- granulomatous 472.0
- infective 460
- obstructive 472.0
- pneumococcal 460
- syphilitic 095.8
  - congenital 090.0
- tuberculous (see also Tuberculosis) 012.8 ☑
- vasomotor (see also Fever, hay) 477.9

Rhinoantritis (chronic) 473.0
- acute 461.0

Rhinodacryolith 375.57

Rhinolalia (aperta) (clausa) (open) 784.49

Rhinolith 478.19 ▲
- nasal sinus (see also Sinusitis) 473.9

Rhinomegaly 478.19

Rhinopharyngitis (acute) (subacute) — see also Nasopharyngitis 460
- chronic 472.2
- destructive ulcerating 102.5
- mutilans 102.5

Rhinophyma 695.3

Index to Diseases

Rhinorrhea 478.19
  cerebrospinal (fluid) 349.81
  paroxysmal (see also Fever, hay) 477.9
  spasmodic (see also Fever, hay) 477.9
Rhinosalpingitis 381.50
  acute 381.51
  chronic 381.52
Rhinoscleroma 040.1
Rhinosporidiosis 117.0
Rhinovirus infection 079.3
Rhizomelic chrondrodysplasia punctata 277.86
Rhizomelique, pseudopolyarthritic 446.5
Rhoads and Bomford anemia (refractory) 238.72
Rhus
  diversiloba dermatitis 692.6
  radicans dermatitis 692.6
  toxicodendron dermatitis 692.6
  venenata dermatitis 692.6
  verniciflua dermatitis 692.6
Rhythm
  atrioventricular nodal 427.89
  disorder 427.9
    coronary sinus 427.89
    ectopic 427.89
    nodal 427.89
  escape 427.89
  heart, abnormal 427.9
    fetus or newborn — see Abnormal, heart rate
  idioventricular 426.89
    accelerated 427.89
  nodal 427.89
  sleep, inversion 327.39
    nonorganic origin 307.45
Rhytidosis facialis 701.8
Rib — see also condition
  cervical 756.2
Riboflavin deficiency 266.0
Rice bodies — see also Loose, body, joint 718.1
  knee 717.6
Richter's hernia — see Hernia, Richter's
Ricinism 988.2
Rickets (active) (acute) (adolescent) (adult) (chest wall) (congenital) (current) (infantile) (intestinal) 268.0
  celiac 579.0
  fetal 756.4
  hemorrhagic 267
  hypophosphatemic with nephrotic-glycosuric dwarfism 270.0
  kidney 588.0
  late effect 268.1
  renal 588.0
  scurvy 267
  vitamin D-resistant 275.3
Rickettsial disease 083.9
  specified type NEC 083.8
Rickettsialpox 083.2
Rickettsiosis NEC 083.9
  specified type NEC 083.8
  tick-borne 082.9
    specified type NEC 082.8
  vesicular 083.2
Ricord's chancre 091.0
Riddoch's syndrome (visual disorientation) 368.16
Rider's
  bone 733.99
  chancre 091.0
Ridge, alveolus — see also condition
  edentulous
    atrophy 525.20
      mandible 525.20
        minimal 525.21
        moderate 525.22
        severe 525.23
      maxilla 525.20
        minimal 525.24
        moderate 525.25
        severe 525.26
  flabby 525.20

Ridged ear 744.29
Riedel's
  disease (ligneous thyroiditis) 245.3
  lobe, liver 751.69
  struma (ligneous thyroiditis) 245.3
  thyroiditis (ligneous) 245.3
Rieger's anomaly or syndrome (mesodermal dysgenesis, anterior ocular segment) 743.44
Riehl's melanosis 709.09
Rietti-Greppi-Micheli anemia or syndrome 282.49
Rieux's hernia — see Hernia, Rieux's
Rift Valley fever 066.3
Riga's disease (cachectic aphthae) 529.0
Riga-Fede disease (cachectic aphthae) 529.0
Riggs' disease (compound periodontitis) 523.40
Right middle lobe syndrome 518.0
Rigid, rigidity — see also condition
  abdominal 789.4
  articular, multiple congenital 754.89
  back 724.8
  cervix uteri
    in pregnancy or childbirth 654.6
      affecting fetus or newborn 763.89
      causing obstructed labor 660.2
        affecting fetus or newborn 763.1
  hymen (acquired) (congenital) 623.3
  nuchal 781.6
  pelvic floor
    in pregnancy or childbirth 654.4
      affecting fetus or newborn 763.89
      causing obstructed labor 660.2
        affecting fetus or newborn 763.1
  perineum or vulva
    in pregnancy or childbirth 654.8
      affecting fetus or newborn 763.89
      causing obstructed labor 660.2
        affecting fetus or newborn 763.1
  spine 724.8
  vagina
    in pregnancy or childbirth 654.7
      affecting fetus or newborn 763.89
      causing obstructed labor 660.2
        affecting fetus or newborn 763.1
Rigors 780.99
Riley-Day syndrome (familial dysautonomia) 742.8
Ring(s)
  aorta 747.21
  Bandl's, complicating delivery 661.4
    affecting fetus or newborn 763.7
  contraction, complicating delivery 661.4
    affecting fetus or newborn 763.7
  esophageal (congenital) 750.3
  Fleischer (-Kayser) (cornea) 275.1 [371.14]
  hymenal, tight (acquired) (congenital) 623.3
  Kayser-Fleischer (cornea) 275.1 [371.14]
  retraction, uterus, pathological 661.4
    affecting fetus or newborn 763.7
  Schatzki's (esophagus) (congenital) (lower) 750.3
    acquired 530.3
  Soemmering's 366.51
  trachea, abnormal 748.3
  vascular (congenital) 747.21
  Vossius' 921.3

Ring(s) — continued
  Vossius' — continued
    late effect 366.21
Ringed hair (congenital) 757.4
Ringing in the ear — see also Tinnitus 388.30
Ringworm 110.9
  beard 110.0
  body 110.5
  Burmese 110.9
  corporeal 110.5
  foot 110.4
  groin 110.3
  hand 110.2
  honeycomb 110.0
  nails 110.1
  perianal (area) 110.3
  scalp 110.0
  specified site NEC 110.8
  Tokelau 110.5
Rise, venous pressure 459.89
Risk
  factor — see Problem
  falling
  suicidal 300.9
Ritter's disease (dermatitis exfoliativa neonatorum) 695.81
Rivalry, sibling 313.3
Rivalta's disease (cervicofacial actinomycosis) 039.3
River blindness 125.3 [360.13]
Robert's pelvis 755.69
  with disproportion (fetopelvic) 653.0
    affecting fetus or newborn 763.1
  causing obstructed labor 660.1
    affecting fetus or newborn 763.1
Robinson's (hidrotic) **ectodermal dysplasia** 757.31
Robin's syndrome 756.0
Robles' disease (onchocerciasis) 125.3 [360.13]
Rochalimea — see Rickettsial disease
Rocky Mountain fever (spotted) 082.0
Rodent ulcer (M8090/3) — see also Neoplasm, skin, malignant
  cornea 370.07
Roentgen ray, adverse effect — see Effect, adverse, x-ray
Roetheln 056.9
Roger's disease (congenital interventricular septal defect) 745.4
Rokitansky's
  disease (see also Necrosis, liver) 570
  tumor 620.2
Rokitansky-Aschoff sinuses (mucosal outpouching of gallbladder) — see also Disease, gallbladder 575.8
Rokitansky-Kuster-Hauser syndrome (congenital absence vagina) 752.49
Rollet's chancre (syphilitic) 091.0
Rolling of head 781.0
Romano-Ward syndrome (prolonged QT interval syndrome) 426.82
Romanus lesion 720.1
Romberg's disease or syndrome 349.89
Roof, mouth — see condition
Rosacea 695.3
  acne 695.3
  keratitis 695.3 [370.49]
Rosary, rachitic 268.0
Rose
  cold 477.0
  fever 477.0
  rash 782.1
    epidemic 056.9
    of infants 057.8
Rosenbach's erysipelatoid or erysipeloid 027.1
Rosen-Castleman-Liebow syndrome (pulmonary proteinosis) 516.0
Rosenthal's disease (factor XI deficiency) 286.2
Roseola 057.8
  infantum, infantilis 057.8
Rossbach's disease (hyperchlorhydria) 536.8

Rossbach's disease — continued
  psychogenic 306.4
Rössle-Urbach-Wiethe lipoproteinosis 272.8
Ross river fever 066.3
Rostan's asthma (cardiac) — see also Failure, ventricular, left 428.1
Rot
  Barcoo (see also Ulcer, skin) 707.9
  knife-grinders' (see also Tuberculosis) 011.4
Rotation
  anomalous, incomplete or insufficient — see Malrotation
  cecum (congenital) 751.4
  colon (congenital) 751.4
  manual, affecting fetus or newborn 763.89
  spine, incomplete or insufficient 737.8
  tooth, teeth 524.35
  vertebra, incomplete or insufficient 737.8
Rot-Bernhardt disease 355.1
Röteln 056.9
Roth-Bernhardt disease or syndrome 355.1
Roth's disease or meralgia 355.1
Rothmund (-Thomson) syndrome 757.33
Rotor's disease or syndrome (idiopathic hyperbilirubinemia) 277.4
Rotundum ulcus — see Ulcer, stomach
Round
  back (with wedging of vertebrae) 737.10
    late effect of rickets 268.1
  hole, retina 361.31
    with detachment 361.01
  ulcer (stomach) — see Ulcer, stomach
  worms (infestation) (large) NEC 127.0
Roussy-Lévy syndrome 334.3
Routine postpartum follow-up V24.2
Roy (-Jutras) syndrome (acropachyderma) 757.39
Rubella (German measles) 056.9
  complicating pregnancy, childbirth, or puerperium 647.5
  complication 056.8
    neurological 056.00
      encephalomyelitis 056.01
      specified type NEC 056.09
    specified type NEC 056.79
  congenital 771.0
  contact V01.4
  exposure to V01.4
  maternal
    with suspected fetal damage affecting management of pregnancy 655.3
      affecting fetus or newborn 760.2
    manifest rubella in infant 771.0
  specified complications NEC 056.79
  vaccination, prophylactic (against) V04.3
Rubeola (measles) — see also Measles 055.9
  complicated 055.8
  meaning rubella (see also Rubella) 056.9
  scarlatinosis 057.8
Rubeosis iridis 364.42
  diabetica 250.5 [364.42]
Rubinstein-Taybi's syndrome (brachydactylia, short stature and mental retardation) 759.89
Rudimentary (congenital) — see also Agenesis
  arm 755.22
  bone 756.9
  cervix uteri 752.49
  eye (see also Microphthalmos) 743.10
  fallopian tube 752.19
  leg 755.32
  lobule of ear 744.21
  patella 755.64

Rudimentary — see also Agenesis — continued
 respiratory organs in thoracopagus 759.4
 tracheal bronchus 748.3
 uterine horn 752.3
 uterus 752.3
  in male 752.7
  solid or with cavity 752.3
 vagina 752.49
Rud's syndrome (mental deficiency, epilepsy, and infantilism) 759.89
Ruiter-Pompen (-Wyers) syndrome (angiokeratoma corporis diffusum) 272.7
Ruled out condition — see also Observation, suspected V71.9
Rumination — see also Vomiting
 disorder 307.53
 neurotic 300.3
 obsessional 300.3
 psychogenic 307.53
Runaway reaction — see also Disturbance, conduct
 socialized 312.2 ☑
 undersocialized, unsocialized 312.1 ☑
Runeberg's disease (progressive pernicious anemia) 281.0
Runge's syndrome (postmaturity) 766.22
Rupia 091.3
 congenital 090.0
 tertiary 095.9
Rupture, ruptured 553.9
 abdominal viscera NEC 799.89
  obstetrical trauma 665.5 ☑
 abscess (spontaneous) — see Abscess, by site
 amnion — see Rupture, membranes
 aneurysm — see Aneurysm
 anus (sphincter) — see Laceration, anus
 aorta, aortic 441.5
  abdominal 441.3
  arch 441.1
  ascending 441.1
  descending 441.5
   abdominal 441.3
   thoracic 441.1
  syphilitic 093.0
  thoracoabdominal 441.6
  thorax, thoracic 441.1
  transverse 441.1
  traumatic (thoracic) 901.0
   abdominal 902.0
  valve or cusp (see also Endocarditis, aortic) 424.1
 appendix (with peritonitis) 540.0
  with peritoneal abscess 540.1
  traumatic — see Injury, internal, gastrointestinal tract
 arteriovenous fistula, brain (congenital) 430
 artery 447.2
  brain (see also Hemorrhage, brain) 431
  coronary (see also Infarct, myocardium) 410.9 ☑
  heart (see also Infarct, myocardium) 410.9 ☑
  pulmonary 417.8
  traumatic (complication) (see also Injury, blood vessel, by site) 904.9
 bile duct, except cystic (see also Disease, biliary) 576.3
  cystic 575.4
  traumatic — see Injury, internal, intra-abdominal
 bladder (sphincter) 596.6
  with
   abortion — see Abortion, by type, with damage to pelvic organs

Rupture, ruptured — continued
 bladder — continued
  with — continued
   ectopic pregnancy (see also categories 633.0–633.9) 639.2
   molar pregnancy (see also categories 630–632) 639.2
  following
   abortion 639.2
   ectopic or molar pregnancy 639.2
  nontraumatic 596.6
  obstetrical trauma 665.5 ☑
  spontaneous 596.6
  traumatic — see Injury, internal, bladder
 blood vessel (see also Hemorrhage) 459.0
 brain (see also Hemorrhage, brain) 431
 heart (see also Infarct, myocardium) 410.9 ☑
 traumatic (complication) (see also Injury, blood vessel, by site) 904.9
 bone — see Fracture, by site
 bowel 569.89
  traumatic — see Injury, internal, intestine
 Bowman's membrane 371.31
 brain
  aneurysm (congenital) (see also Hemorrhage, subarachnoid) 430
  late effect — see Late effect(s) (of) cerebrovascular disease
  syphilitic 094.87
  hemorrhagic (see also Hemorrhage, brain) 431
  injury at birth 767.0
  syphilitic 094.89
 capillaries 448.9
 cardiac (see also Infarct, myocardium) 410.9 ☑
 cartilage (articular) (current) (see also Sprain, by site)
  knee — see Tear, meniscus
  semilunar — see Tear, meniscus
 cecum (with peritonitis) 540.0
  with peritoneal abscess 540.1
  traumatic 863.89
   with open wound into cavity 863.99
 cerebral aneurysm (congenital) (see also Hemorrhage, subarachnoid) 430
 late effect — see Late effect(s) (of) cerebrovascular disease
 cervix (uteri)
  with
   abortion — see Abortion, by type, with damage to pelvic organs
   ectopic pregnancy (see also categories 633.0–633.9) 639.2
   molar pregnancy (see also categories 630–632) 639.2
  following
   abortion 639.2
   ectopic or molar pregnancy 639.2
  obstetrical trauma 665.3 ☑
  traumatic — see Injury, internal, cervix
 chordae tendineae 429.5
 choroid (direct) (indirect) (traumatic) 363.63
 circle of Willis (see also Hemorrhage, subarachnoid) 430
 late effect — see Late effect(s) (of) cerebrovascular disease
 colon 569.89

Rupture, ruptured — continued
 colon — continued
  traumatic — see Injury, internal, colon
 cornea (traumatic) (see also Rupture, eye)
  due to ulcer 370.00
 coronary (artery) (thrombotic) (see also Infarct, myocardium) 410.9 ☑
 corpus luteum (infected) (ovary) 620.1
 cyst — see Cyst
 cystic duct (see also Disease, gallbladder) 575.4
 Descemet's membrane 371.33
  traumatic — see Rupture, eye
 diaphragm (see also Hernia, diaphragm)
  traumatic — see Injury, internal, diaphragm
 diverticulum
  bladder 596.3
  intestine (large) (see also Diverticula) 562.10
  small 562.00
 duodenal stump 537.89
 duodenum (ulcer) — see Ulcer, duodenum, with perforation
 ear drum (see also Perforation, tympanum) 384.20
  with otitis media — see Otitis media
  traumatic — see Wound, open, ear
 esophagus 530.4
  traumatic 862.22
   with open wound into cavity 862.32
   cervical region — see Wound, open, esophagus
 eye (without prolapse of intraocular tissue) 871.0
  with
   exposure of intraocular tissue 871.1
   partial loss of intraocular tissue 871.2
   prolapse of intraocular tissue 871.1
  due to burn 940.5
 fallopian tube 620.8
  due to pregnancy — see Pregnancy, tubal
  traumatic — see Injury, internal, fallopian tube
 fontanel 767.3
 free wall (ventricle) (see also Infarct, myocardium) 410.9 ☑
 gallbladder or duct (see also Disease, gallbladder) 575.4
  traumatic — see Injury, internal, gallbladder
 gastric (see also Rupture, stomach) 537.89
  vessel 459.0
 globe (eye) (traumatic) — see Rupture, eye
 graafian follicle (hematoma) 620.0
 heart (auricle) (ventricle) (see also Infarct, myocardium) 410.9 ☑
  infectional 422.90
  traumatic — see Rupture, myocardium, traumatic
 hymen 623.8
 internal
  organ, traumatic (see also Injury, internal, by site)
   heart — see Rupture, myocardium, traumatic
   kidney — see Rupture, kidney
   liver — see Rupture, liver
   spleen — see Rupture, spleen, traumatic
  semilunar cartilage — see Tear, meniscus
  intervertebral disc — see Displacement, intervertebral disc

Rupture, ruptured — continued
 intervertebral disc — see Displacement, intervertebral disc — continued
  traumatic (current) — see Dislocation, vertebra
 intestine 569.89
  traumatic — see Injury, internal, intestine
 intracranial, birth injury 767.0
 iris 364.76
  traumatic — see Rupture, eye
 joint capsule — see Sprain, by site
 kidney (traumatic) 866.03
  with open wound into cavity 866.13
  due to birth injury 767.8
  nontraumatic 593.89
 lacrimal apparatus (traumatic) 870.2
 lens (traumatic) 366.20
 ligament (see also Sprain, by site)
  with open wound — see Wound, open, by site
  old (see also Disorder, cartilage, articular) 718.0 ☑
 liver 864.04
  with open wound into cavity 864.14
  due to birth injury 767.8
  nontraumatic 573.8
 lymphatic (node) (vessel) 457.8
 marginal sinus (placental) (with hemorrhage) 641.2 ☑
  affecting fetus or newborn 762.1
 meaning hernia — see Hernia
 membrana tympani (see also Perforation, tympanum) 384.20
  with otitis media — see Otitis media
  traumatic — see Wound, open, ear
 membranes (spontaneous)
  artificial
   delayed delivery following 658.3 ☑
    affecting fetus or newborn 761.1
   fetus or newborn 761.1
  delayed delivery following 658.2 ☑
   affecting fetus or newborn 761.1
  premature (less than 24 hours prior to onset of labor) 658.1 ☑
   affecting fetus or newborn 761.1
  delayed delivery following 658.2 ☑
   affecting fetus or newborn 761.1
 meningeal artery (see also Hemorrhage, subarachnoid) 430
 late effect — see Late effect(s) (of) cerebrovascular disease
 meniscus (knee) (see also Tear, meniscus)
  old (see also Derangement, meniscus) 717.5
   site other than knee — see Disorder, cartilage, articular
   site other than knee — see Sprain, by site
 mesentery 568.89
  traumatic — see Injury, internal, mesentery
 mitral — see Insufficiency, mitral
 muscle (traumatic) NEC (see also Sprain, by site)
  with open wound — see Wound, open, by site
  nontraumatic 728.83
 musculotendinous cuff (nontraumatic) (shoulder) 840.4
 mycotic aneurysm, causing cerebral hemorrhage (see also Hemorrhage, subarachnoid) 430
 late effect — see Late effect(s) (of) cerebrovascular disease
 myocardium, myocardial (see also Infarct, myocardium) 410.9 ☑

Rupture, ruptured — *continued*
- myocardium, myocardial (*see also* Infarct, myocardium) — *continued*
  - traumatic 861.03
    - with open wound into thorax 861.13
  - nontraumatic (meaning hernia) (*see also* Hernia, by site) 553.9
    - obstructed (*see also* Hernia, by site, with obstruction) 552.9
      - gangrenous (*see also* Hernia, by site, with gangrene) 551.9
- operation wound 998.32
  - internal 998.31
- ovary, ovarian 620.8
  - corpus luteum 620.1
  - follicle (graafian) 620.0
- oviduct 620.8
  - due to pregnancy — *see* Pregnancy, tubal
- pancreas 577.8
  - traumatic — *see* Injury, internal, pancreas
- papillary muscle (ventricular) 429.6
- pelvic
  - floor, complicating delivery 664.1 ☑
  - organ NEC — *see* Injury, pelvic, organs
- penis (traumatic) — *see* Wound, open, penis
- perineum 624.8
  - during delivery (*see also* Laceration, perineum, complicating delivery) 664.4 ☑
- pharynx (nontraumatic) (spontaneous) 478.29
- pregnant uterus (before onset of labor) 665.0 ☑
- prostate (traumatic) — *see* Injury, internal, prostate
- pulmonary
  - artery 417.8
  - valve (heart) (*see also* Endocarditis, pulmonary) 424.3
  - vein 417.8
  - vessel 417.8
- pupil, sphincter 364.75
- pus tube (*see also* Salpingo-oophoritis) 614.2
- pyosalpinx (*see also* Salpingo-oophoritis) 614.2
- rectum 569.49
  - traumatic — *see* Injury, internal, rectum
- retina, retinal (traumatic) (without detachment) 361.30
  - with detachment (*see also* Detachment, retina, with retinal defect) 361.00
- rotator cuff (capsule) (traumatic) 840.4
  - nontraumatic, complete 727.61
- sclera 871.0
- semilunar cartilage, knee (*see also* Tear, meniscus) 836.2

Rupture, ruptured — *continued*
- semilunar cartilage, knee (*see also* Tear, meniscus) — *continued*
  - old (*see also* Derangement, meniscus) 717.5
- septum (cardiac) 410.8 ☑
- sigmoid 569.89
  - traumatic — *see* Injury, internal, colon, sigmoid
- sinus of Valsalva 747.29
- spinal cord (*see also* Injury, spinal, by site)
  - due to injury at birth 767.4
  - fetus or newborn 767.4
  - syphilitic 094.89
  - traumatic (*see also* Injury, spinal, by site)
    - with fracture — *see* Fracture, vertebra, by site, with spinal cord injury
- spleen 289.59
  - congenital 767.8
  - due to injury at birth 767.8
  - malarial 084.9
  - nontraumatic 289.59
  - spontaneous 289.59
  - traumatic 865.04
    - with open wound into cavity 865.14
- splenic vein 459.0
- stomach 537.89
  - due to injury at birth 767.8
  - traumatic — *see* Injury, internal, stomach
  - ulcer — *see* Ulcer, stomach, with perforation
- synovium 727.50
  - specified site NEC 727.59
- tendon (traumatic) (*see also* Sprain, by site)
  - with open wound — *see* Wound, open, by site
  - Achilles 845.09
    - nontraumatic 727.67
  - ankle 845.09
    - nontraumatic 727.68
  - biceps (long head) 840.8
    - nontraumatic 727.62
  - foot 845.10
    - interphalangeal (joint) 845.13
    - metatarsophalangeal (joint) 845.12
    - nontraumatic 727.68
    - specified site NEC 845.19
    - tarsometatarsal (joint) 845.11
  - hand 842.10
    - carpometacarpal (joint) 842.11
    - interphalangeal (joint) 842.13
    - metacarpophalangeal (joint) 842.12
    - nontraumatic 727.63
      - extensors 727.63
      - flexors 727.64
    - specified site NEC 842.19
  - nontraumatic 727.60
    - specified site NEC 727.69
  - patellar 844.8

Rupture, ruptured — *continued*
- tendon (*see also* Sprain, by site) — *continued*
  - patellar — *continued*
    - nontraumatic 727.66
  - quadriceps 844.8
    - nontraumatic 727.65
  - rotator cuff (capsule) 840.4
    - nontraumatic, complete 727.61
  - wrist 842.00
    - carpal (joint) 842.01
    - nontraumatic 727.63
      - extensors 727.63
      - flexors 727.64
    - radiocarpal (joint) (ligament) 842.02
    - radioulnar (joint), distal 842.09
    - specified site NEC 842.09
- testis (traumatic) 878.2
  - complicated 878.3
  - due to syphilis 095.8
- thoracic duct 457.8
- tonsil 474.8
- traumatic
  - with open wound — *see* Wound, open, by site
  - aorta — *see* Rupture, aorta, traumatic
  - ear drum — *see* Wound, open, ear, drum
  - external site — *see* Wound, open, by site
  - eye 871.2
  - globe (eye) — *see* Wound, open, eyeball
  - internal organ (abdomen, chest, or pelvis) (*see also* Injury, internal, by site)
    - heart — *see* Rupture, myocardium, traumatic
    - kidney — *see* Rupture, kidney
    - liver — *see* Rupture, liver
    - spleen — *see* Rupture, spleen, traumatic
  - ligament, muscle, or tendon (*see also* Sprain, by site)
    - with open wound — *see* Wound, open, by site
  - meaning hernia — *see* Hernia
- tricuspid (heart) (valve) — *see* Endocarditis, tricuspid
- tube, tubal 620.8
  - abscess (*see also* Salpingo-oophoritis) 614.2
  - due to pregnancy — *see* Pregnancy, tubal
- tympanum, tympanic (membrane) (*see also* Perforation, tympanum) 384.20
  - with otitis media — *see* Otitis media
  - traumatic — *see* Wound, open, ear, drum
- umbilical cord 663.8 ☑
  - fetus or newborn 772.0
- ureter (traumatic) (*see also* Injury, internal, ureter) 867.2

Rupture, ruptured — *continued*
- ureter (*see also* Injury, internal, ureter) — *continued*
  - nontraumatic 593.89
- urethra 599.84
  - with
    - abortion — *see* Abortion, by type, with damage to pelvic organs
    - ectopic pregnancy (*see also* categories 633.0–633.9) 639.2
    - molar pregnancy (*see also* categories 630–632) 639.2
  - following
    - abortion 639.2
    - ectopic or molar pregnancy 639.2
  - obstetrical trauma 665.5 ☑
  - traumatic — *see* Injury, internal, urethra
- uterosacral ligament 620.8
- uterus (traumatic) (*see also* Injury, internal, uterus)
  - affecting fetus or newborn 763.89
  - during labor 665.1 ☑
  - nonpuerperal, nontraumatic 621.8
  - nontraumatic 621.8
  - pregnant (during labor) 665.1 ☑
    - before labor 665.0 ☑
- vagina 878.6
  - complicated 878.7
  - complicating delivery — *see* Laceration, vagina, complicating delivery
- valve, valvular (heart) — *see* Endocarditis
- varicose vein — *see* Varicose, vein
- varix — *see* Varix
- vena cava 459.0
- ventricle (free wall) (left) (*see also* Infarct, myocardium) 410.9 ☑
- vesical (urinary) 596.6
  - traumatic — *see* Injury, internal, bladder
- vessel (blood) 459.0
  - pulmonary 417.8
- viscus 799.89
- vulva 878.4
  - complicated 878.5
  - complicating delivery 664.0 ☑

Russell's dwarf (uterine dwarfism and craniofacial dysostosis) 759.89

Russell's dysentery 004.8

Russell (-Silver) syndrome (congenital hemihypertrophy and short stature) 759.89

Russian spring-summer type encephalitis 063.0

Rust's disease (tuberculous spondylitis) 015.0 ☑ *[720.81]*

Rustitskii's disease (multiple myeloma) (M9730/3) 203.0 ☑

Ruysch's disease (Hirschsprung's disease) 751.3

Rytand-Lipsitch syndrome (complete atrioventricular block) 426.0

Index to Diseases

S

Saber
  shin 090.5
  tibia 090.5
Saccharomyces infection — see also
    Candidiasis 112.9
Saccharopinuria 270.7
Saccular — see condition
Sacculation
  aorta (nonsyphilitic) (see also
      Aneurysm, aorta) 441.9
    ruptured 441.5
    syphilitic 093.0
  bladder 596.3
  colon 569.89
  intralaryngeal (congenital) (ventricular) 748.3
  larynx (congenital) (ventricular) 748.3
  organ or site, congenital — see Distortion
  pregnant uterus, complicating delivery 654.4 ☑
    affecting fetus or newborn 763.1
    causing obstructed labor 660.2 ☑
      affecting fetus or newborn 763.1
  rectosigmoid 569.89
  sigmoid 569.89
  ureter 593.89
  urethra 599.2
  vesical 596.3
Sachs (-Tay) disease (amaurotic familial idiocy) 330.1
Sacks-Libman disease 710.0 [424.91]
Sac, lacrimal — see condition
Sacralgia 724.6
Sacralization
  fifth lumbar vertebra 756.15
  incomplete (vertebra) 756.15
Sacrodynia 724.6
Sacroiliac joint — see condition
Sacroiliitis NEC 720.2
Sacrum — see condition
Saddle
  back 737.8
  embolus, aorta 444.0
  nose 738.0
    congenital 754.0
    due to syphilis 090.5
Sadism (sexual) 302.84
Saemisch's ulcer 370.04
Saenger's syndrome 379.46
Sago spleen 277.39 ▲
Sailors' skin 692.74
Saint
  Anthony's fire (see also Erysipelas) 035
  Guy's dance — see Chorea
  Louis-type encephalitis 062.3
  triad (see also Hernia, diaphragm) 553.3
  Vitus' dance — see Chorea
Salicylism
  correct substance properly administered 535.4 ☑
  overdose or wrong substance given or taken 965.1
Salivary duct or gland — see also condition
  virus disease 078.5
Salivation (excessive) — see also Ptyalism 527.7
Salmonella (aertrycke) (choleraesuis) (enteritidis) (gallinarum) (suipestifer) (typhimurium) — see also Infection, Salmonella 003.9
  arthritis 003.23
  carrier (suspected) of V02.3
  meningitis 003.21
  osteomyelitis 003.24
  pneumonia 003.22
  septicemia 003.1
  typhosa 002.0
    carrier (suspected) of V02.1

Salmonellosis 003.0
  with pneumonia 003.22
Salpingitis (catarrhal) (fallopian tube) (nodular) (pseudofollicular) (purulent) (septic) — see also Salpingo-oophoritis 614.2
  ear 381.50
    acute 381.51
    chronic 381.52
  Eustachian (tube) 381.50
    acute 381.51
    chronic 381.52
  follicularis 614.1
  gonococcal (chronic) 098.37
    acute 098.17
  interstitial, chronic 614.1
  isthmica nodosa 614.1
  old — see Salpingo-oophoritis, chronic
  puerperal, postpartum, childbirth 670.0 ☑
  specific (chronic) 098.37
    acute 098.17
  tuberculous (acute) (chronic) (see also Tuberculosis) 016.6 ☑
  venereal (chronic) 098.37
    acute 098.17
Salpingocele 620.4
Salpingo-oophoritis (catarrhal) (purulent) (ruptured) (septic) (suppurative) 614.2
  acute 614.0
    with
      abortion — see Abortion, by type, with sepsis
      ectopic pregnancy (see also categories 633.0–633.9) 639.0
      molar pregnancy (see also categories 630–632) 639.0
    following
      abortion 639.0
      ectopic or molar pregnancy 639.0
    gonococcal 098.17
    puerperal, postpartum, childbirth 670.0 ☑
    tuberculous (see also Tuberculosis) 016.6 ☑
  chronic 614.1
    gonococcal 098.37
    tuberculous (see also Tuberculosis) 016.6 ☑
  complicating pregnancy 646.6 ☑
    affecting fetus or newborn 760.8
  gonococcal (chronic) 098.37
    acute 098.17
  old — see Salpingo-oophoritis, chronic
  puerperal 670.0 ☑
  specific — see Salpingo-oophoritis, gonococcal
  subacute (see also Salpingo-oophoritis, acute) 614.0
  tuberculous (acute) (chronic) (see also Tuberculosis) 016.6 ☑
  venereal — see Salpingo-oophoritis, gonococcal
Salpingo-ovaritis — see also Salpingo-oophoritis 614.2
Salpingoperitonitis — see also Salpingo-oophoritis 614.2
Salt-losing
  nephritis (see also Disease, renal) 593.9
  syndrome (see also Disease, renal) 593.9
Salt-rheum — see also Eczema 692.9
Salzmann's nodular dystrophy 371.46
Sampson's cyst or tumor 617.1
Sandblasters'
  asthma 502
  lung 502
Sander's disease (paranoia) 297.1
Sandfly fever 066.0
Sandhoff's disease 330.1
Sanfilippo's syndrome (mucopolysaccharidosis III) 277.5

Sanger-Brown's ataxia 334.2
San Joaquin Valley fever 114.0
Sao Paulo fever or typhus 082.0
Saponification, mesenteric 567.89
Sapremia — see Septicemia
Sarcocele (benign)
  syphilitic 095.8
    congenital 090.5
Sarcoepiplocele — see also Hernia 553.9
Sarcoepiplomphalocele — see also Hernia, umbilicus 553.1
Sarcoid (any site) 135
  with lung involvement 135 [517.8]
  Boeck's 135
  Darier-Roussy 135
  Spiegler-Fendt 686.8
Sarcoidosis 135
  cardiac 135 [425.8]
  lung 135 [517.8]
Sarcoma (M8800/3) — see also Neoplasm, connective tissue, malignant
  alveolar soft part (M9581/3) — see Neoplasm, connective tissue, malignant
  ameloblastic (M9330/3) 170.1
    upper jaw (bone) 170.0
  botryoid (M8910/3) — see Neoplasm, connective tissue, malignant
  botryoides (M8910/3) — see Neoplasm, connective tissue, malignant
  cerebellar (M9480/3) 191.6
    circumscribed (arachnoidal) (M9471/3) 191.6
  circumscribed (arachnoidal) cerebellar (M9471/3) 191.6
  clear cell, of tendons and aponeuroses (M9044/3) — see Neoplasm, connective tissue, malignant
  embryonal (M8991/3) — see Neoplasm, connective tissue, malignant
  endometrial (stromal) (M8930/3) 182.0
    isthmus 182.1
  endothelial (M9130/3) (see also Neoplasm, connective tissue, malignant)
    bone (M9260/3) — see Neoplasm, bone, malignant
  epithelioid cell (M8804/3) — see Neoplasm, connective tissue, malignant
  Ewing's (M9260/3) — see Neoplasm, bone, malignant
  follicular dendritic cell 202.9 ☑
  germinoblastic (diffuse) (M9632/3) 202.8 ☑
  follicular (M9697/3) 202.0 ☑
  giant cell (M8802/3) (see also Neoplasm, connective tissue, malignant)
    bone (M9250/3) — see Neoplasm, bone, malignant
  glomoid (M8710/3) — see Neoplasm, connective tissue, malignant
  granulocytic (M9930/3) 205.3 ☑
  hemangioendothelial (M9130/3) — see Neoplasm, connective tissue, malignant
  hemorrhagic, multiple (M9140/3) — see Kaposi's, sarcoma
  Hodgkin's (M9662/3) 201.2 ☑
  immunoblastic (M9612/3) 200.8 ☑
  interdigitating dendritic cell 202.9 ☑
  Kaposi's (M9140/3) — see Kaposi's, sarcoma
  Kupffer cell (M9124/3) 155.0
  Langerhans cell 202.9 ☑
  leptomeningeal (M9530/3) — see Neoplasm, meninges, malignant
  lymphangioendothelial (M9170/3) — see Neoplasm, connective tissue, malignant

Sarcoma — see also Neoplasm, connective tissue, malignant — continued
  lymphoblastic (M9630/3) 200.1 ☑
  lymphocytic (M9620/3) 200.1 ☑
  mast cell (M9740/3) 202.6 ☑
  melanotic (M8720/3) — see Melanoma
  meningeal (M9530/3) — see Neoplasm, meninges, malignant
  meningothelial (M9530/3) — see Neoplasm, meninges, malignant
  mesenchymal (M8800/3) (see also Neoplasm, connective tissue, malignant)
    mixed (M8990/3) — see Neoplasm, connective tissue, malignant
  mesothelial (M9050/3) — see Neoplasm, by site, malignant
  monstrocellular (M9481/3)
    specified site — see Neoplasm, by site, malignant
    unspecified site 191.9
  myeloid (M9930/3) 205.3 ☑
  neurogenic (M9540/3) — see Neoplasm, connective tissue, malignant
  odontogenic (M9270/3) 170.1
    upper jaw (bone) 170.0
  osteoblastic (M9180/3) — see Neoplasm, bone, malignant
  osteogenic (M9180/3) (see also Neoplasm, bone, malignant)
    juxtacortical (M9190/3) — see Neoplasm, bone, malignant
    periosteal (M9190/3) — see Neoplasm, bone, malignant
  periosteal (M8812/3) (see also Neoplasm, bone, malignant)
    osteogenic (M9190/3) — see Neoplasm, bone, malignant
  plasma cell (M9731/3) 203.8 ☑
  pleomorphic cell (M8802/3) — see Neoplasm, connective tissue, malignant
  reticuloendothelial (M9720/3) 202.3 ☑
  reticulum cell (M9640/3) 200.0 ☑
    nodular (M9642/3) 200.0 ☑
    pleomorphic cell type (M9641/3) 200.0 ☑
  round cell (M8803/3) — see Neoplasm, connective tissue, malignant
  small cell (M8803/3) — see Neoplasm, connective tissue, malignant
  spindle cell (M8801/3) — see Neoplasm, connective tissue, malignant
  stromal (endometrial) (M8930/3) 182.0
    isthmus 182.1
  synovial (M9040/3) (see also Neoplasm, connective tissue, malignant)
    biphasic type (M9043/3) — see Neoplasm, connective tissue, malignant
    epithelioid cell type (M9042/3) — see Neoplasm, connective tissue, malignant
    spindle cell type (M9041/3) — see Neoplasm, connective tissue, malignant
Sarcomatosis
  meningeal (M9539/3) — see Neoplasm, meninges, malignant
  specified site NEC (M8800/3) — see Neoplasm, connective tissue, malignant
  unspecified site (M8800/6) 171.9
Sarcosinemia 270.8
Sarcosporidiosis 136.5
Satiety, early 780.94
Saturnine — see condition
Saturnism 984.9

Saturnism

Saturnism — *continued*
  specified type of lead — *see* Table of Drugs and Chemicals
Satyriasis 302.89
Sauriasis — *see* Ichthyosis
Sauriderma 757.39
Sauriosis — *see* Ichthyosis
Savill's disease (epidemic exfoliative dermatitis) 695.89
SBE (subacute bacterial endocarditis) 421.0
Scabies (any site) 133.0
Scabs 782.8
Scaglietti-Dagnini syndrome (acromegalic macrospondylitis) 253.0
Scald, scalded — *see also* Burn, by site
  skin syndrome 695.1
Scalenus anticus (anterior) syndrome 353.0
Scales 782.8
Scalp — *see* condition
Scaphocephaly 756.0
Scaphoiditis, tarsal 732.5
Scapulalgia 733.90
Scapulohumeral myopathy 359.1
Scarabiasis 134.1
Scarlatina 034.1
  anginosa 034.1
  maligna 034.1
  myocarditis, acute 034.1 [422.0]
    old (*see also* Myocarditis) 429.0
  otitis media 034.1 [382.02]
  ulcerosa 034.1
Scarlatinella 057.8
Scarlet fever (albuminuria) (angina) (convulsions) (lesions of lid) (rash) 034.1
Scar, scarring — *see also* Cicatrix 709.2
  adherent 709.2
  atrophic 709.2
  cervix
    in pregnancy or childbirth 654.6 ☑
      affecting fetus or newborn 763.89
      causing obstructed labor 660.2 ☑
        affecting fetus or newborn 763.1
  cheloid 701.4
  chorioretinal 363.30
    disseminated 363.35
    macular 363.32
    peripheral 363.34
    posterior pole NEC 363.33
  choroid (*see also* Scar, chorioretinal) 363.30
  compression, pericardial 423.9
  congenital 757.39
  conjunctiva 372.64
  cornea 371.00
    xerophthalmic 264.6
  due to previous cesarean delivery, complicating pregnancy or childbirth 654.2 ☑
    affecting fetus or newborn 763.89
  duodenal (bulb) (cap) 537.3
  hypertrophic 701.4
  keloid 701.4
  labia 624.4
  lung (base) 518.89
  macula 363.32
    disseminated 363.35
    peripheral 363.34
  muscle 728.89
  myocardium, myocardial 412
  painful 709.2
  papillary muscle 429.81
  posterior pole NEC 363.33
    macular — *see* Scar, macula
  postnecrotic (hepatic) (liver) 571.9
  psychic V15.49
  retina (*see also* Scar, chorioretinal) 363.30
  trachea 478.9
  uterus 621.8

Scar, scarring — *see also* Cicatrix — *continued*
  uterus — *continued*
    in pregnancy or childbirth NEC 654.9 ☑
      affecting fetus or newborn 763.89
      due to previous cesarean delivery 654.2 ☑
  vulva 624.4
Schamberg's disease, dermatitis, or dermatosis (progressive pigmentary dermatosis) 709.09
Schatzki's ring (esophagus) (lower) (congenital) 750.3
  acquired 530.3
Schaufenster krankheit 413.9
Schaumann's
  benign lymphogranulomatosis 135
  disease (sarcoidosis) 135
  syndrome (sarcoidosis) 135
Scheie's syndrome (mucopolysaccharidosis IS) 277.5
Schenck's disease (sporotrichosis) 117.1
Scheuermann's disease or osteochondrosis 732.0
Scheuthauer-Marie-Sainton syndrome (cleidocranialis dysostosis) 755.59
Schilder (-Flatau) disease 341.1
Schilling-type monocytic leukemia (M9890/3) 206.9 ☑
Schimmelbusch's disease, cystic mastitis, or hyperplasia 610.1
Schirmer's syndrome (encephalocutaneous angiomatosis) 759.6
Schistocelia 756.79
Schistoglossia 750.13
Schistosoma infestation — *see* Infestation, Schistosoma
Schistosomiasis 120.9
  Asiatic 120.2
  bladder 120.0
  chestermani 120.8
  colon 120.1
  cutaneous 120.3
  due to
    S. hematobium 120.0
    S. japonicum 120.2
    S. mansoni 120.1
    S. mattheii 120.8
  eastern 120.2
  genitourinary tract 120.0
  intestinal 120.1
  lung 120.2
  Manson's (intestinal) 120.1
  Oriental 120.2
  pulmonary 120.2
  specified type NEC 120.8
  vesical 120.0
Schizencephaly 742.4
Schizo-affective psychosis — *see also* Schizophrenia 295.7 ☑
Schizodontia 520.2
Schizoid personality 301.20
  introverted 301.21
  schizotypal 301.22
Schizophrenia, schizophrenic (reaction) 295.9 ☑

Note — Use the following fifth-digit subclassification with category 295:

0   unspecified
1   subchronic
2   chronic
3   subchronic with acute exacerbation
4   chronic with acute exacerbation
5   in remission

  acute (attack) NEC 295.8 ☑
    episode 295.4 ☑
  atypical form 295.8 ☑
  borderline 295.5 ☑
  catalepsy 295.2 ☑

Schizophrenia, schizophrenic — *continued*
  catatonic (type) (acute) (excited) (withdrawn) 295.2 ☑
  childhood (type) (*see also* Psychosis, childhood) 299.9 ☑
  chronic NEC 295.6 ☑
  coenesthesiopathic 295.8 ☑
  cyclic (type) 295.7 ☑
  disorganized (type) 295.1 ☑
  flexibilitas cerea 295.2 ☑
  hebephrenic (type) (acute) 295.1 ☑
  incipient 295.5 ☑
  latent 295.5 ☑
  paranoid (type) (acute) 295.3 ☑
  paraphrenic (acute) 295.3 ☑
  prepsychotic 295.5 ☑
  primary (acute) 295.0 ☑
  prodromal 295.5 ☑
  pseudoneurotic 295.5 ☑
  pseudopsychopathic 295.5 ☑
  reaction 295.9 ☑
  residual type (state) 295.6 ☑
  restzustand 295.6 ☑
  schizo-affective (type) (depressed) (excited) 295.7 ☑
  schizophreniform type 295.4 ☑
  simple (type) (acute) 295.0 ☑
  simplex (acute) 295.0 ☑
  specified type NEC 295.8 ☑
  syndrome of childhood NEC (*see also* Psychosis, childhood) 299.9 ☑
  undifferentiated type 295.9 ☑
    acute 295.8 ☑
    chronic 295.6 ☑
Schizothymia 301.20
  introverted 301.21
  schizotypal 301.22
Schlafkrankheit 086.5
Schlatter-Osgood disease (osteochondrosis, tibial tubercle) 732.4
Schlatter's tibia (osteochondrosis) 732.4
Schloffer's tumor — *see also* Peritonitis 567.29
Schmidt's syndrome
  sphallo-pharyngo-laryngeal hemiplegia 352.6
  thyroid-adrenocortical insufficiency 258.1
  vagoaccessory 352.6
Schmincke
  carcinoma (M8082/3) — *see* Neoplasm, nasopharynx, malignant
  tumor (M8082/3) — *see* Neoplasm, nasopharynx, malignant
Schmitz (-Stutzer) dysentery 004.0
Schmorl's disease or nodes 722.30
  lumbar, lumbosacral 722.32
  specified region NEC 722.39
  thoracic, thoracolumbar 722.31
Schneiderian
  carcinoma (M8121/3)
    specified site — *see* Neoplasm, by site, malignant
    unspecified site 160.0
  papilloma (M8121/0)
    specified site — *see* Neoplasm, by site, benign
    unspecified site 212.0
Schneider's syndrome 047.9
Schnitzler syndrome 273.1
Schoffer's tumor — *see also* Peritonitis 567.29
Scholte's syndrome (malignant carcinoid) 259.2
Scholz's disease 330.0
Scholz (-Bielschowsky-Henneberg) syndrome 330.0
Schönlein (-Henoch) disease (primary) (purpura) (rheumatic) 287.0
School examination V70.3
Schottmüller's disease — *see also* Fever, paratyphoid 002.9
Schroeder's syndrome (endocrine-hypertensive) 255.3

Schüller-Christian disease or syndrome (chronic histiocytosis X) 277.89
Schultz's disease or syndrome (agranulocytosis) 288.09 ▲
Schultze's acroparesthesia, simple 443.89
Schwalbe-Ziehen-Oppenheimer disease 333.6
Schwannoma (M9560/0) — *see also* Neoplasm, connective tissue, benign
  malignant (M9560/3) — *see* Neoplasm, connective tissue, malignant
Schwartz-Bartter syndrome (inappropriate secretion of antidiuretic hormone) 253.6
Schwartz (-Jampel) syndrome 756.89
Schweninger-Buzzi disease (macular atrophy) 701.3
Sciatic — *see* condition
Sciatica (infectional) 724.3
  due to
    displacement of intervertebral disc 722.10
    herniation, nucleus pulposus 722.10
  wallet 724.3
Scimitar syndrome (anomalous venous drainage, right lung to inferior vena cava) 747.49
Sclera — *see* condition
Sclerectasia 379.11
Scleredema
  adultorum 710.1
  Buschke's 710.1
  newborn 778.1
Sclerema
  adiposum (newborn) 778.1
  adultorum 710.1
  edematosum (newborn) 778.1
  neonatorum 778.1
  newborn 778.1
Scleriasis — *see* Scleroderma
Scleritis 379.00
  with corneal involvement 379.05
  anterior (annular) (localized) 379.03
  brawny 379.06
  granulomatous 379.09
  posterior 379.07
  specified NEC 379.09
  suppurative 379.09
  syphilitic 095.0
  tuberculous (nodular) (*see also* Tuberculosis) 017.3 ☑ [379.09]
Sclerochoroiditis — *see also* Scleritis 379.00
Scleroconjunctivitis — *see also* Scleritis 379.00
Sclerocystic ovary (syndrome) 256.4
Sclerodactylia 701.0
Scleroderma, sclerodermia (acrosclerotic) (diffuse) (generalized) (progressive) (pulmonary) 710.1
  circumscribed 701.0
  linear 701.0
  localized (linear) 701.0
  newborn 778.1
Sclerokeratitis 379.05
  meaning sclerosing keratitis 370.54
  tuberculous (*see also* Tuberculosis) 017.3 ☑ [379.09]
Scleromalacia
  multiple 731.0
  perforans 379.04
Scleroma, trachea 040.1
Scleromyxedema 701.8
Scleroperikeratitis 379.05
Sclerose en plaques 340
Sclerosis, sclerotic
  adrenal (gland) 255.8
  Alzheimer's 331.0
    with dementia — *see* Alzheimer's, dementia
  amyotrophic (lateral) 335.20

Index to Diseases

Sclerosis, sclerotic — continued
annularis fibrosi
- aortic 424.1
- mitral 424.0

aorta, aortic 440.0
- valve (see also Endocarditis, aortic) 424.1

artery, arterial, arteriolar, arteriovascular — see Arteriosclerosis
ascending multiple 340
Baló's (concentric) 341.1
basilar — see Sclerosis, brain
bone (localized) NEC 733.99
brain (general) (lobular) 341.9
- Alzheimer's — see Alzheimer's, dementia
- artery, arterial 437.0
- atrophic lobar 331.0
  - with dementia
    - with behavioral disturbance 331.0 [294.11]
    - without behavioral disturbance 331.0 [294.10]
- diffuse 341.1
  - familial (chronic) (infantile) 330.0
  - infantile (chronic) (familial) 330.0
  - Pelizaeus-Merzbacher type 330.0
- disseminated 340
- hereditary 334.2
- infantile (degenerative) (diffuse) 330.0
- insular 340
- Krabbe's 330.0
- miliary 340
- multiple 340
- Pelizaeus-Merzbacher 330.0
- progressive familial 330.0
- senile 437.0
- tuberous 759.5

bulbar, progressive 340
bundle of His 426.50
- left 426.3
- right 426.4

cardiac — see Arteriosclerosis, coronary
cardiorenal (see also Hypertension, cardiorenal) 404.90
cardiovascular (see also Disease, cardiovascular) 429.2
- renal (see also Hypertension, cardiorenal) 404.90

centrolobar, familial 330.0
cerebellar — see Sclerosis, brain
cerebral — see Sclerosis, brain
cerebrospinal 340
- disseminated 340
- multiple 340

cerebrovascular 437.0
choroid 363.40
- diffuse 363.56

combined (spinal cord) (see also Degeneration, combined)
- multiple 340

concentric, Baló's 341.1
cornea 370.54
coronary (artery) — see Arteriosclerosis, coronary
corpus cavernosum
- female 624.8
- male 607.89

Dewitzky's
- aortic 424.1
- mitral 424.0

diffuse NEC 341.1
disease, heart — see Arteriosclerosis, coronary
disseminated 340
dorsal 340
dorsolateral (spinal cord) — see Degeneration, combined
endometrium 621.8
extrapyramidal 333.90
eye, nuclear (senile) 366.16

Sclerosis, sclerotic — continued
Friedreich's (spinal cord) 334.0
funicular (spermatic cord) 608.89
gastritis 535.4 ☑
general (vascular) — see Arteriosclerosis
gland (lymphatic) 457.8
hepatic 571.9
hereditary
- cerebellar 334.2
- spinal 334.0

idiopathic cortical (Garré's) (see also Osteomyelitis) 730.1 ☑
ilium, piriform 733.5
insular 340
- pancreas 251.8

Islands of Langerhans 251.8
kidney — see Sclerosis, renal
larynx 478.79
lateral 335.24
- amyotrophic 335.20
- descending 335.24
- primary 335.24
- spinal 335.24

liver 571.9
lobar, atrophic (of brain) 331.0
- with dementia
  - with behavioral disturbance 331.0 [294.11]
  - without behavioral disturbance 331.0 [294.10]

lung (see also Fibrosis, lung) 515
mastoid 383.1
mitral — see Endocarditis, mitral
Mönckeberg's (medial) (see also Arteriosclerosis, extremities) 440.20
multiple (brain stem) (cerebral) (generalized) (spinal cord) 340
myocardium, myocardial — see Arteriosclerosis, coronary
nuclear (senile), eye 366.16
ovary 620.8
pancreas 577.8
penis 607.89
peripheral arteries (see also Arteriosclerosis, extremities) 440.20
plaques 340
pluriglandular 258.8
polyglandular 258.8
posterior (spinal cord) (syphilitic) 094.0
posterolateral (spinal cord) — see Degeneration, combined
prepuce 607.89
primary lateral 335.24
progressive systemic 710.1
pulmonary (see also Fibrosis, lung) 515
- artery 416.0
- valve (heart) (see also Endocarditis, pulmonary) 424.3

renal 587
- with
  - cystine storage disease 270.0
  - hypertension (see also Hypertension, kidney) 403.90
  - hypertensive heart disease (conditions classifiable to 402) (see also Hypertension, cardiorenal) 404.90
  - arteriolar (hyaline) (see also Hypertension, kidney) 403.90
  - hyperplastic (see also Hypertension, kidney) 403.90

retina (senile) (vascular) 362.17
rheumatic
- aortic valve 395.9
- mitral valve 394.9

Schilder's 341.1
senile — see Arteriosclerosis
spinal (cord) (general) (progressive) (transverse) 336.8
- ascending 357.0
- combined (see also Degeneration, combined)
  - multiple 340

Sclerosis, sclerotic — continued
spinal — continued
- combined (see also Degeneration, combined) — continued
  - syphilitic 094.89
- disseminated 340
- dorsolateral — see Degeneration, combined
- hereditary (Friedreich's) (mixed form) 334.0
- lateral (amyotrophic) 335.24
- multiple 340
- posterior (syphilitic) 094.0

stomach 537.89
subendocardial, congenital 425.3
systemic (progressive) 710.1
- with lung involvement 710.1 [517.2]

tricuspid (heart) (valve) — see Endocarditis, tricuspid
tuberous (brain) 759.5
tympanic membrane (see also Tympanosclerosis) 385.00
valve, valvular (heart) — see Endocarditis
vascular — see Arteriosclerosis
vein 459.89

Sclerotenonitis 379.07
Sclerotitis — see also Scleritis 379.00
- syphilitic 095.0
- tuberculous (see also Tuberculosis) 017.3 ☑ [379.09]

Scoliosis (acquired) (postural) 737.30
- congenital 754.2
- due to or associated with
  - Charcôt-Marie-Tooth disease 356.1 [737.43]
  - mucopolysaccharidosis 277.5 [737.43]
  - neurofibromatosis 237.71 [737.43]
  - osteitis
    - deformans 731.0 [737.43]
    - fibrosa cystica 252.01 [737.43]
  - osteoporosis (see also Osteoporosis) 733.00 [737.43]
  - poliomyelitis 138 [737.43]
  - radiation 737.33
  - tuberculosis (see also Tuberculosis) 015.0 ☑ [737.43]
- idiopathic 737.30
- infantile
  - progressive 737.32
  - resolving 737.31
- paralytic 737.39
- rachitic 268.1
- sciatic 724.3
- specified NEC 737.39
- thoracogenic 737.34
- tuberculous (see also Tuberculosis) 015.0 ☑ [737.43]

Scoliotic pelvis 738.6
- with disproportion (fetopelvic) 653.0 ☑
  - affecting fetus or newborn 763.1
- causing obstructed labor 660.1 ☑
  - affecting fetus or newborn 763.1

Scorbutus, scorbutic 267
- anemia 281.8

Scotoma (ring) 368.44
- arcuate 368.43
- Bjerrum 368.43
- blind spot area 368.42
- central 368.41
- centrocecal 368.41
- paracecal 368.42
- paracentral 368.41
- scintillating 368.12
- Seidel 368.43

Scratch — see Injury, superficial, by site
Screening (for) V82.9
- alcoholism V79.1
- anemia, deficiency NEC V78.1
  - iron V78.0
- anomaly, congenital V82.89
- antenatal, ▶of mother◀ V28.9
  - alphafetoprotein levels, raised V28.1

Screening — continued
antenatal, ▶of mother◀ — continued
- based on amniocentesis V28.2
  - chromosomal anomalies V28.0
  - raised alphafetoprotein levels V28.1
- fetal growth retardation using ultrasonics V28.4
- ultrasonics V28.4
- isoimmunization V28.5
- malformations using ultrasonics V28.3
- raised alphafetoprotein levels V28.1
- specified condition NEC V28.8
- Streptococcus B V28.6

arterial hypertension V81.1
arthropod-borne viral disease NEC V73.5
asymptomatic bacteriuria V81.5
bacterial
- conjunctivitis V74.4
- disease V74.9
  - specified condition NEC V74.8

bacteriuria, asymptomatic V81.5
blood disorder NEC V78.9
- specified type NEC V78.8

bronchitis, chronic V81.3
brucellosis V74.8
cancer — see Screening, malignant neoplasm
cardiovascular disease NEC V81.2
cataract V80.2
Chagas' disease V75.3
chemical poisoning V82.5
cholera V74.0
cholesterol level V77.91
chromosomal
- anomalies
  - by amniocentesis, antenatal V28.0
  - maternal postnatal V82.4
- athletes V70.3

condition
- cardiovascular NEC V81.2
- eye NEC V80.2
- genitourinary NEC V81.6
- neurological V80.0
- respiratory NEC V81.4
- skin V82.0
- specified NEC V82.89

congenital
- anomaly V82.89
- eye V80.2
- dislocation of hip V82.3
- eye condition or disease V80.2

conjunctivitis, bacterial V74.4
contamination NEC (see also Poisoning) V82.5
coronary artery disease V81.0
cystic fibrosis V77.6
deficiency anemia NEC V78.1
- iron V78.0

dengue fever V73.5
depression V79.0
developmental handicap V79.9
- in early childhood V79.3
- specified type NEC V79.8

diabetes mellitus V77.1
diphtheria V74.3
disease or disorder V82.9
- bacterial V74.9
  - specified NEC V74.8
- blood V78.9
  - specified type NEC V78.8
- blood-forming organ V78.9
  - specified type NEC V78.8
- cardiovascular NEC V81.2
  - hypertensive V81.1
  - ischemic V81.0
- Chagas' V75.3
- chlamydial V73.98
  - specified NEC V73.88
- ear NEC V80.3
- endocrine NEC V77.99
- eye NEC V80.2

Screening

Screening — *continued*
  disease or disorder — *continued*
    genitourinary NEC V81.6
    heart NEC V81.2
      hypertensive V81.1
      ischemic V81.0
    immunity NEC V77.99
    infectious NEC V75.9
    lipoid NEC V77.91
    mental V79.9
      specified type NEC V79.8
    metabolic NEC V77.99
      inborn NEC V77.7
    neurological V80.0
    nutritional NEC V77.99
    rheumatic NEC V82.2
    rickettsial V75.0
    sickle-cell V78.2
      trait V78.2
    specified type NEC V82.89
    thyroid V77.0
    vascular NEC V81.2
      ischemic V81.0
    venereal V74.5
    viral V73.99
      arthropod-borne NEC V73.5
      specified type NEC V73.89
  dislocation of hip, congenital V82.3
  drugs in athletes V70.3
  emphysema (chronic) V81.3
  encephalitis, viral (mosquito or tick borne) V73.5
  endocrine disorder NEC V77.99
  eye disorder NEC V80.2
    congenital V80.2
  fever
    dengue V73.5
    hemorrhagic V73.5
    yellow V73.4
  filariasis V75.6
  galactosemia V77.4
  genetic V82.79
    disease carrier status V82.71
  genitourinary condition NEC V81.6
  glaucoma V80.1
  gonorrhea V74.5
  gout V77.5
  Hansen's disease V74.2
  heart disease NEC V81.2
    hypertensive V81.1
    ischemic V81.0
  heavy metal poisoning V82.5
  helminthiasis, intestinal V75.7
  hematopoietic malignancy V76.89
  hemoglobinopathies NEC V78.3
  hemorrhagic fever V73.5
  Hodgkin's disease V76.89
  hormones in athletes V70.3
  hypercholesterolemia V77.91
  hyperlipidemia V77.91
  hypertension V81.1
  immunity disorder NEC V77.99
  inborn errors of metabolism NEC V77.7
  infection
    bacterial V74.9
      specified type NEC V74.8
    mycotic V75.4
    parasitic NEC V75.8
  infectious disease V75.9
    specified type NEC V75.8
  ingestion of radioactive substance V82.5
  intestinal helminthiasis V75.7
  iron deficiency anemia V78.0
  ischemic heart disease V81.0
  lead poisoning V82.5
  leishmaniasis V75.2
  leprosy V74.2
  leptospirosis V74.8
  leukemia V76.89
  lipoid disorder NEC V77.91
  lymphoma V76.89
  malaria V75.1
  malignant neoplasm (of) V76.9
    bladder V76.3

Screening — *continued*
  malignant neoplasm — *continued*
    blood V76.89
    breast V76.10
      mammogram NEC V76.12
        for high-risk patient V76.11
      specified type NEC V76.19
    cervix V76.2
    colon V76.51
    colorectal V76.51
    hematopoietic system V76.89
    intestine V76.50
      colon V76.51
      small V76.52
    lung V76.0
    lymph (glands) V76.89
    nervous system V76.81
    oral cavity V76.42
    other specified neoplasm NEC V76.89
    ovary V76.46
    prostate V76.44
    rectum V76.41
    respiratory organs V76.0
    skin V76.43
    specified sites NEC V76.49
    testis V76.45
    vagina V76.47
      following hysterectomy for malignant condition V67.01
  malnutrition V77.2
  mammogram NEC V76.12
    for high-risk patient V76.11
  maternal postnatal chromosomal anomalies V82.4
  measles V73.2
  mental
    disorder V79.9
      specified type NEC V79.8
    retardation V79.2
  metabolic disorder NEC V77.99
  metabolic errors, inborn V77.7
  mucoviscidosis V77.6
  multiphasic V82.6
  mycosis V75.4
  mycotic infection V75.4
  nephropathy V81.5
  neurological condition V80.0
  nutritional disorder V77.99
  obesity V77.8
  osteoporosis V82.81
  parasitic infection NEC V75.8
  phenylketonuria V77.3
  plague V74.8
  poisoning
    chemical NEC V82.5
    contaminated water supply V82.5
    heavy metal V82.5
  poliomyelitis V73.0
  postnatal chromosomal anomalies, maternal V82.4
  prenatal — *see* Screening, antenatal
  pulmonary tuberculosis V74.1
  radiation exposure V82.5
  renal disease V81.5
  respiratory condition NEC V81.4
  rheumatic disorder NEC V82.2
  rheumatoid arthritis V82.1
  rickettsial disease V75.0
  rubella V73.3
  schistosomiasis V75.5
  senile macular lesions of eye V80.2
  sickle-cell anemia, disease, or trait V78.2
  skin condition V82.0
  sleeping sickness V75.3
  smallpox V73.1
  special V82.9
    specified condition NEC V82.89
  specified type NEC V82.89
  spirochetal disease V74.9
    specified type NEC V74.8
  stimulants in athletes V70.3
  syphilis V74.5
  tetanus V74.8
  thyroid disorder V77.0

Screening — *continued*
  trachoma V73.6
  trypanosomiasis V75.3
  tuberculosis, pulmonary V74.1
  venereal disease V74.5
  viral encephalitis
    mosquito-borne V73.5
    tick-borne V73.5
  whooping cough V74.8
  worms, intestinal V75.7
  yaws V74.6
  yellow fever V73.4
Scrofula — *see also* Tuberculosis 017.2
Scrofulide (primary) — *see also* Tuberculosis 017.0
Scrofuloderma, scrofulodermia (any site) (primary) — *see also* Tuberculosis 017.0
Scrofulosis (universal) — *see also* Tuberculosis 017.2
Scrofulosis lichen (primary) — *see also* Tuberculosis 017.0
Scrofulous — *see* condition
Scrotal tongue 529.5
  congenital 750.13
Scrotum — *see* condition
Scurvy (gum) (infantile) (rickets) (scorbutic) 267
Sea-blue histiocyte syndrome 272.7
Seabright-Bantam syndrome (pseudohypoparathyroidism) 275.49
Seasickness 994.6
Seatworm 127.4
Sebaceous
  cyst (*see also* Cyst, sebaceous) 706.2
  gland disease NEC 706.9
Sebocystomatosis 706.2
Seborrhea, seborrheic 706.3
  adiposa 706.3
  capitis 690.11
  congestiva 695.4
  corporis 706.3
  dermatitis 690.10
    infantile 690.12
  diathesis in infants 695.89
  eczema 690.18
    infantile 690.12
  keratosis 702.19
    inflamed 702.11
  nigricans 705.89
  sicca 690.18
  wart 702.19
    inflamed 702.11
Seckel's syndrome 759.89
Seclusion pupil 364.74
Seclusiveness, child 313.22
Secondary — *see also* condition
  neoplasm — *see* Neoplasm, by site, malignant, secondary
Secretan's disease or syndrome (post-traumatic edema) 782.3
Secretion
  antidiuretic hormone, inappropriate (syndrome) 253.6
  catecholamine, by pheochromocytoma 255.6
  hormone
    antidiuretic, inappropriate (syndrome) 253.6
    by
      carcinoid tumor 259.2
      pheochromocytoma 255.6
    ectopic NEC 259.3
  urinary
    excessive 788.42
    suppression 788.5
Section
  cesarean
    affecting fetus or newborn 763.4
    post mortem, affecting fetus or newborn 761.6
    previous, in pregnancy or childbirth 654.2
      affecting fetus or newborn 763.89

Index to Diseases

Section — *continued*
  nerve, traumatic — *see* Injury, nerve, by site
Seeligmann's syndrome (ichthyosis congenita) 757.1
Segmentation, incomplete (congenital) — *see also* Fusion
  bone NEC 756.9
  lumbosacral (joint) 756.15
  vertebra 756.15
    lumbosacral 756.15
Seizure 780.39
  akinetic (idiopathic) (*see also* Epilepsy) 345.0
    psychomotor 345.4
  apoplexy, apoplectic (*see also* Disease, cerebrovascular, acute) 436
  atonic (*see also* Epilepsy) 345.0
  autonomic 300.11
  brain or cerebral (*see also* Disease, cerebrovascular, acute) 436
  convulsive (*see also* Convulsions) 780.39
  cortical (focal) (motor) (*see also* Epilepsy) 345.5
  epilepsy, epileptic (cryptogenic) (*see also* Epilepsy) 345.9
  epileptiform, epileptoid 780.39
    focal (*see also* Epilepsy) 345.5
  febrile (simple) 780.31
    with status epilepticus 345.3
    atypical 780.32
    complex 780.32
    complicated 780.32
  heart — *see* Disease, heart
  hysterical 300.11
  Jacksonian (focal) (*see also* Epilepsy) 345.5
  motor type 345.5
  sensory type 345.5
  newborn 779.0
  paralysis (*see also* Disease, cerebrovascular, acute) 436
  recurrent 345.9
    epileptic — *see* Epilepsy
  repetitive 780.39
    epileptic — *see* Epilepsy
  salaam (*see also* Epilepsy) 345.6
  uncinate (*see also* Epilepsy) 345.4
Self-mutilation 300.9
Semicoma 780.09
Semiconsciousness 780.09
Seminal
  vesicle — *see* condition
  vesiculitis (*see also* Vesiculitis) 608.0
Seminoma (M9061/3)
  anaplastic type (M9062/3)
    specified site — *see* Neoplasm, by site, malignant
    unspecified site 186.9
  specified site — *see* Neoplasm, by site, malignant
  spermatocytic (M9063/3)
    specified site — *see* Neoplasm, by site, malignant
    unspecified site 186.9
  unspecified site 186.9
Semliki Forest encephalitis 062.8
Senear-Usher disease or syndrome (pemphigus erythematosus) 694.4
Senecio jacobae dermatitis 692.6
Senectus 797
Senescence 797
Senile — *see also* condition 797
  cervix (atrophic) 622.8
  degenerative atrophy, skin 701.3
  endometrium (atrophic) 621.8
  fallopian tube (atrophic) 620.3
  heart (failure) 797
  lung 492.8
  ovary (atrophic) 620.3
  syndrome 259.8
  vagina, vaginitis (atrophic) 627.3
  wart 702.0
Senility 797

Index to Diseases

Senility — continued
with
- acute confusional state 290.3
- delirium 290.3
- mental changes 290.9
- psychosis NEC (see also Psychosis, senile) 290.20
- premature (syndrome) 259.8

Sensation
- burning (see also Disturbance, sensation) 782.0
  - tongue 529.6
- choking 784.99
- loss of (see also Disturbance, sensation) 782.0
- prickling (see also Disturbance, sensation) 782.0
- tingling (see also Disturbance, sensation) 782.0

Sense loss (touch) — see also Disturbance, sensation 782.0
- smell 781.1
- taste 781.1

Sensibility disturbance NEC (cortical) (deep) (vibratory) — see also Disturbance, sensation 782.0

Sensitive dentine 521.89

Sensitiver Beziehungswahn 297.8

Sensitivity, sensitization — see also Allergy
- autoerythrocyte 287.2
- carotid sinus 337.0
- child (excessive) 313.21
- cold, autoimmune 283.0
- methemoglobin 289.7
- suxamethonium 289.89
- tuberculin, without clinical or radiological symptoms 795.5

Sensory
- extinction 781.8
- neglect 781.8

Separation
- acromioclavicular — see Dislocation, acromioclavicular
- anxiety, abnormal 309.21
- apophysis, traumatic — see Fracture, by site
- choroid 363.70
  - hemorrhagic 363.72
  - serous 363.71
- costochondral (simple) (traumatic) — see Dislocation, costochondral
- delayed
  - umbilical cord 779.83
- epiphysis, epiphyseal
  - nontraumatic 732.9
    - upper femoral 732.2
  - traumatic — see Fracture, by site
- fracture — see Fracture, by site
- infundibulum cardiac from right ventricle by a partition 746.83
- joint (current) (traumatic) — see Dislocation, by site
- placenta (normally implanted) — see Placenta, separation
- pubic bone, obstetrical trauma 665.6
- retina, retinal (see also Detachment, retina) 361.9
  - layers 362.40
    - sensory (see also Retinoschisis) 361.10
    - pigment epithelium (exudative) 362.42
      - hemorrhagic 362.43
- sternoclavicular (traumatic) — see Dislocation, sternoclavicular
- symphysis pubis, obstetrical trauma 665.6
- tracheal ring, incomplete (congenital) 748.3

Sepsis (generalized) 995.91
with
- abortion — see Abortion, by type, with sepsis
- acute organ dysfunction 995.92

Sepsis — continued
with — continued
- ectopic pregnancy (see also categories 633.0–633.9) 639.0
- molar pregnancy (see also categories 630–632) 639.0
- multiple organ dysfunction (MOD) 995.92
- buccal 528.3
- complicating labor 659.3
- dental (pulpal origin) 522.4
- female genital organ NEC 614.9
- fetus (intrauterine) 771.81
- following
  - abortion 639.0
  - ectopic or molar pregnancy 639.0
  - infusion, perfusion, or transfusion 999.3
- Friedländer's 038.49
- intraocular 360.00
- localized
  - in operation wound 998.59
  - skin (see also Abscess) 682.9
- malleus 024
- nadir 038.9
- newborn (organism unspecified) NEC 771.81
- oral 528.3
- puerperal, postpartum, childbirth (pelvic) 670.0
- resulting from infusion, injection, transfusion, or vaccination 999.3
- severe 995.92
- skin, localized (see also Abscess) 682.9
- umbilical (newborn) (organism unspecified) 771.89
  - tetanus 771.3
- urinary 599.0
  - meaning sepsis 995.91
  - meaning urinary tract infection 599.0

Septate — see also Septum

Septic — see also condition
- adenoids 474.01
  - and tonsils 474.02
- arm (with lymphangitis) 682.3
- embolus — see Embolism
- finger (with lymphangitis) 681.00
- foot (with lymphangitis) 682.7
- gallbladder (see also Cholecystitis) 575.8
- hand (with lymphangitis) 682.4
- joint (see also Arthritis, septic) 711.0
- kidney (see also Infection, kidney) 590.9
- leg (with lymphangitis) 682.6
- mouth 528.3
- nail 681.9
  - finger 681.02
  - toe 681.11
- shock (endotoxic) 785.52
- sore (see also Abscess) 682.9
  - throat 034.0
    - milk-borne 034.0
    - streptococcal 034.0
- spleen (acute) 289.59
- teeth (pulpal origin) 522.4
- throat 034.0
- thrombus — see Thrombosis
- toe (with lymphangitis) 681.10
- tonsils 474.00
  - and adenoids 474.02
- umbilical cord (newborn) (organism unspecified) 771.89
- uterus (see also Endometritis) 615.9

Septicemia, septicemic (generalized) (suppurative) 038.9
with
- abortion — see Abortion, by type, with sepsis
- ectopic pregnancy (see also categories 633.0–633.9) 639.0

Septicemia, septicemic — continued
with — continued
- molar pregnancy (see also categories 630–632) 639.0
- Aerobacter aerogenes 038.49
- anaerobic 038.3
- anthrax 022.3
- Bacillus coli 038.42
- Bacteroides 038.3
- Clostridium 038.8
- complicating labor 659.3
- cryptogenic 038.9
- enteric gram-negative bacilli 038.40
- Enterobacter aerogenes 038.49
- Erysipelothrix (insidiosa) (rhusiopathiae) 027.1
- Escherichia coli 038.42
- following
  - abortion 639.0
  - ectopic or molar pregnancy 639.0
  - infusion, injection, transfusion, or vaccination 999.3
- Friedländer's (bacillus) 038.49
- gangrenous 038.9
- gonococcal 098.89
- gram-negative (organism) 038.40
  - anaerobic 038.3
- Hemophilus influenzae 038.41
- herpes (simplex) 054.5
- herpetic 054.5
- Listeria monocytogenes 027.0
- meningeal — see Meningitis
- meningococcal (chronic) (fulminating) 036.2
- navel, newborn (organism unspecified) 771.89
- newborn (organism unspecified) 771.81
- plague 020.2
- pneumococcal 038.2
- postabortal 639.0
- postoperative 998.59
- Proteus vulgaris 038.49
- Pseudomonas (aeruginosa) 038.43
- puerperal, postpartum 670.0
- Salmonella (aertrycke) (callinarum) (choleraesuis) (enteritidis) (suipestifer) 003.1
- Serratia 038.44
- Shigella (see also Dysentery, bacillary) 004.9
- specified organism NEC 038.8
- staphylococcal 038.10
  - aureus 038.11
  - specified organism NEC 038.19
- streptococcal (anaerobic) 038.0
- Streptococcus pneumoniae 038.2
- suipestifer 003.1
- umbilicus, newborn (organism unspecified) 771.89
- viral 079.99
- Yersinia enterocolitica 038.49

Septum, septate (congenital) — see also Anomaly, specified type NEC
- anal 751.2
- aqueduct of Sylvius 742.3
  - with spina bifida (see also Spina bifida) 741.0
- hymen 752.49
- uterus (see also Double, uterus) 752.2
- vagina 752.49
  - in pregnancy or childbirth 654.7
    - affecting fetus or newborn 763.89
  - causing obstructed labor 660.2
    - affecting fetus or newborn 763.1

Sequestration
- lung (congenital) (extralobar) (intralobar) 748.5
- orbit 376.10
- pulmonary artery (congenital) 747.3
- splenic 289.52

Sequestrum
- bone (see also Osteomyelitis) 730.1

Sequestrum — continued
- bone (see also Osteomyelitis) — continued
  - jaw 526.4
- dental 525.8
- jaw bone 526.4
- sinus (accessory) (nasal) (see also Sinusitis) 473.9
  - maxillary 473.0

Sequoiosis asthma 495.8

Serology for syphilis
- doubtful
  - with signs or symptoms — see Syphilis, by site and stage
  - follow-up of latent syphilis — see Syphilis, latent
- false positive 795.6
- negative, with signs or symptoms — see Syphilis, by site and stage
- positive 097.1
  - with signs or symptoms — see Syphilis, by site and stage
  - false 795.6
  - follow-up of latent syphilis — see Syphilis, latent
  - only finding — see Syphilis, latent
- reactivated 097.1

Seroma (postoperative) (non-infected) 998.13
- infected 998.51

Seropurulent — see condition

Serositis, multiple 569.89
- pericardial 423.2
- peritoneal 568.82
- pleural — see Pleurisy

Serotonin syndrome 333.99

Serous — see condition

Sertoli cell
- adenoma (M8640/0)
  - specified site — see Neoplasm, by site, benign
  - unspecified site
    - female 220
    - male 222.0
- carcinoma (M8640/3)
  - specified site — see Neoplasm, by site, malignant
  - unspecified site 186.9
- syndrome (germinal aplasia) 606.0
- tumor (M8640/0)
  - with lipid storage (M8641/0)
    - specified site — see Neoplasm, by site, benign
    - unspecified site
      - female 220
      - male 222.0
  - specified site — see Neoplasm, by site, benign
  - unspecified site
    - female 220
    - male 222.0

Sertoli-Leydig cell tumor (M8631/0)
- specified site — see Neoplasm, by site, benign
- unspecified site
  - female 220
  - male 222.0

Serum
- allergy, allergic reaction 999.5
  - shock 999.4
- arthritis 999.5 [713.6]
- complication or reaction NEC 999.5
- disease NEC 999.5
- hepatitis 070.3
- intoxication 999.5
- jaundice (homologous) — see Hepatitis, viral, type B
- neuritis 999.5
- poisoning NEC 999.5
- rash NEC 999.5
- reaction NEC 999.5
- sickness NEC 999.5

Sesamoiditis 733.99

Seven-day fever 061
of
- Japan 100.89

Seven-day fever — continued
of — *continued*
Queensland 100.89
Sever's disease or osteochondrosis (calcaneum) 732.5
Sex chromosome mosaics 758.81
Sextuplet
affected by maternal complications of pregnancy 761.5
healthy liveborn — *see* Newborn, multiple
pregnancy (complicating delivery) NEC 651.8 ☑
with fetal loss and retention of one or more fetus(es) 651.6 ☑
following (elective) fetal reduction 651.7 ☑
Sexual
anesthesia 302.72
deviation (*see also* Deviation, sexual) 302.9
disorder (*see also* Deviation, sexual) 302.9
frigidity (female) 302.72
function, disorder of (psychogenic) 302.70
specified type NEC 302.79
immaturity (female) (male) 259.0
impotence 607.84
organic origin NEC 607.84
psychogenic 302.72
precocity (constitutional) (cryptogenic) (female) (idiopathic) (male) NEC 259.1
with adrenal hyperplasia 255.2
sadism 302.84
Sexuality, pathological — *see also* Deviation, sexual 302.9
Sézary's disease, reticulosis, or syndrome (M9701/3) 202.2 ☑
Shadow, lung 793.1
Shaken infant syndrome 995.55
Shaking
head (tremor) 781.0
palsy or paralysis (*see also* Parkinsonism) 332.0
Shallowness, acetabulum 736.39
Shaver's disease or syndrome (bauxite pneumoconiosis) 503
Shearing
artificial skin graft 996.55
decellularized allodermis graft 996.55
Sheath (tendon) — *see* condition
Shedding
nail 703.8
teeth, premature, primary (deciduous) 520.6
Sheehan's disease or syndrome (postpartum pituitary necrosis) 253.2
Shelf, rectal 569.49
Shell
shock (current) (*see also* Reaction, stress, acute) 308.9
lasting state 300.16
teeth 520.5
Shield kidney 753.3
Shifting
pacemaker 427.89
sleep-work schedule (affecting sleep) 327.36
Shift, mediastinal 793.2
Shiga's
bacillus 004.0
dysentery 004.0
Shigella (dysentery) — *see also* Dysentery, bacillary 004.9
carrier (suspected) of V02.3
Shigellosis — *see* Dysentery, bacillary 004.9
Shingles — *see also* Herpes, zoster 053.9
eye NEC 053.29
Shin splints 844.9
Shipyard eye or disease 077.1
Shirodkar suture, in pregnancy 654.5 ☑
Shock 785.50

Shock — *continued*
with
abortion — *see* Abortion, by type, with shock
ectopic pregnancy (*see also* categories 633.0–633.9) 639.5
molar pregnancy (*see also* categories 630–632) 639.5
allergic — *see* Shock, anaphylactic
anaclitic 309.21
anaphylactic 995.0
chemical — *see* Table of Drugs and Chemicals
correct medicinal substance properly administered 995.0
drug or medicinal substance
correct substance properly administered 995.0
overdose or wrong substance given or taken 977.9
specified drug — *see* Table of Drugs and Chemicals
following sting(s) 989.5
food — *see* Anaphylactic shock, due to, food
immunization 999.4
serum 999.4
anaphylactoid — *see* Shock, anaphylactic
anesthetic
correct substance properly administered 995.4
overdose or wrong substance given 968.4
specified anesthetic — *see* Table of Drugs and Chemicals
birth, fetus or newborn NEC 779.89
cardiogenic 785.51
chemical substance — *see* Table of Drugs and Chemicals
circulatory 785.59
complicating
abortion — *see* Abortion, by type, with shock
ectopic pregnancy (*see also* categories 633.0–633.9) 639.5
labor and delivery 669.1 ☑
molar pregnancy (*see also* categories 630–632) 639.5
culture 309.29
due to
drug 995.0
correct substance properly administered 995.0
overdose or wrong substance given or taken 977.9
specified drug — *see* Table of Drugs and Chemicals
food — *see* Anaphylactic shock, due to, food
during labor and delivery 669.1 ☑
electric 994.8
endotoxic 785.52
due to surgical procedure 998.0
following
abortion 639.5
ectopic or molar pregnancy 639.5
injury (immediate) (delayed) 958.4
labor and delivery 669.1 ☑
gram-negative 785.52
hematogenic 785.59
hemorrhagic
due to
disease 785.59
surgery (intraoperative) (postoperative) 998.0
trauma 958.4
hypovolemic NEC 785.59
surgical 998.0
traumatic 958.4
insulin 251.0
therapeutic misadventure 962.3
kidney 584.5

Shock — *continued*
kidney — *continued*
traumatic (following crushing) 958.5
lightning 994.0
lung 518.5
nervous (*see also* Reaction, stress, acute) 308.9
obstetric 669.1 ☑
with
abortion — *see* Abortion, by type, with shock
ectopic pregnancy (*see also* categories 633.0–633.9) 639.5
molar pregnancy (*see also* categories 630–632) 639.5
following
abortion 639.5
ectopic or molar pregnancy 639.5
paralysis, paralytic (*see also* Disease, cerebrovascular, acute) 436
late effect — *see* Late effect(s) (of) cerebrovascular disease
pleural (surgical) 998.0
due to trauma 958.4
postoperative 998.0
with
abortion — *see* Abortion, by type, with shock
ectopic pregnancy (*see also* categories 633.0–633.9) 639.5
molar pregnancy (*see also* categories 630–632) 639.5
following
abortion 639.5
ectopic or molar pregnancy 639.5
psychic (*see also* Reaction, stress, acute) 308.9
past history (of) V15.49
psychogenic (*see also* Reaction, stress, acute) 308.9
septic 785.52
with
abortion — *see* Abortion, by type, with shock
ectopic pregnancy (*see also* categories 633.0–633.9) 639.5
molar pregnancy (*see also* categories 630–632) 639.5
due to
surgical procedure 998.0
transfusion NEC 999.8
bone marrow 996.85
following
abortion 639.5
ectopic or molar pregnancy 639.5
surgical procedure 998.0
transfusion NEC 999.8
bone marrow 996.85
spinal (*see also* Injury, spinal, by site)
with spinal bone injury — *see* Fracture, vertebra, by site, with spinal cord injury
surgical 998.0
therapeutic misadventure NEC (*see also* Complications) 998.89
thyroxin 962.7
toxic 040.82
transfusion — *see* Complications, transfusion
traumatic (immediate) (delayed) 958.4
Shoemakers' chest 738.3
Short, shortening, shortness
Achilles tendon (acquired) 727.81
arm 736.89
congenital 755.20
back 737.9
bowel syndrome 579.3
breath 786.05

Short, shortening, shortness — *continued*
chain acyl CoA dehydrogenase deficiency (SCAD) 277.85
common bile duct, congenital 751.69
cord (umbilical) 663.4 ☑
affecting fetus or newborn 762.6
cystic duct, congenital 751.69
esophagus (congenital) 750.4
femur (acquired) 736.81
congenital 755.34
frenulum linguae 750.0
frenum, lingual 750.0
hamstrings 727.81
hip (acquired) 736.39
congenital 755.63
leg (acquired) 736.81
congenital 755.30
metatarsus (congenital) 754.79
acquired 736.79
organ or site, congenital NEC — *see* Distortion
palate (congenital) 750.26
P-R interval syndrome 426.81
radius (acquired) 736.09
congenital 755.26
round ligament 629.89 ▲
sleeper 307.49
stature, constitutional (hereditary) 783.43
tendon 727.81
Achilles (acquired) 727.81
congenital 754.79
congenital 756.89
thigh (acquired) 736.81
congenital 755.34
tibialis anticus 727.81
umbilical cord 663.4 ☑
affecting fetus or newborn 762.6
urethra 599.84
uvula (congenital) 750.26
vagina 623.8
Shortsightedness 367.1
Shoshin (acute fulminating beriberi) 265.0
Shoulder — *see* condition
Shovel-shaped incisors 520.2
Shower, thromboembolic — *see* Embolism
Shunt (status)
aortocoronary bypass V45.81
arterial-venous (dialysis) V45.1
arteriovenous, pulmonary (acquired) 417.0
congenital 747.3
traumatic (complication) 901.40
cerebral ventricle (communicating) in situ V45.2
coronary artery bypass V45.81
surgical, prosthetic, with complications — *see* Complications, shunt
vascular NEC V45.89
Shutdown
renal 586
with
abortion — *see* Abortion, by type, with renal failure
ectopic pregnancy (*see also* categories 633.0–633.9) 639.3
molar pregnancy (*see also* categories 630–632) 639.3
complicating
abortion 639.3
ectopic or molar pregnancy 639.3
following labor and delivery 669.3 ☑
Shwachman's syndrome 288.02 ▲
Shy-Drager syndrome (orthostatic hypotension with multisystem degeneration) 333.0
Sialadenitis (any gland) (chronic) (suppurative) 527.2
epidemic — *see* Mumps

Index to Diseases

Sialadenosis, periodic 527.2
Sialaporia 527.7
Sialectasia 527.8
Sialitis 527.2
Sialoadenitis — see also Sialadenitis 527.2
Sialoangitis 527.2
Sialodochitis (fibrinosa) 527.2
Sialodocholithiasis 527.5
Sialolithiasis 527.5
Sialorrhea — see also Ptyalism 527.7
   periodic 527.2
Sialosis 527.8
   rheumatic 710.2
Siamese twin 759.4
Sicard's syndrome 352.6
Sicca syndrome (keratoconjunctivitis) 710.2
Sick 799.9
   cilia syndrome 759.89
   or handicapped person in family V61.49
Sickle-cell
   anemia (see also Disease, sickle-cell) 282.60
   disease (see also Disease, sickle-cell) 282.60
   hemoglobin
      C disease (without crisis) 282.63
         with
            crisis 282.64
            vaso-occlusive pain 282.64
      D disease (without crisis) 282.68
         with crisis 282.69
      E disease (without crisis) 282.68
         with crisis 282.69
      thalassemia (without crisis) 282.41
         with
            crisis 282.42
            vaso-occlusive pain 282.42
   trait 282.5
Sicklemia — see also Disease, sickle-cell 282.60
   trait 282.5
Sickness
   air (travel) 994.6
   airplane 994.6
   alpine 993.2
   altitude 993.2
   Andes 993.2
   aviators' 993.2
   balloon 993.2
   car 994.6
   compressed air 993.3
   decompression 993.3
   green 280.9
   harvest 100.89
   milk 988.8
   morning 643.0
   motion 994.6
   mountain 993.2
      acute 289.0
   protein (see also Complications, vaccination) 999.5
   radiation NEC 990
   roundabout (motion) 994.6
   sea 994.6
   serum NEC 999.5
   sleeping (African) 086.5
      by Trypanosoma 086.5
         gambiense 086.3
         rhodesiense 086.4
      Gambian 086.3
      late effect 139.8
      Rhodesian 086.4
   sweating 078.2
   swing (motion) 994.6
   train (railway) (travel) 994.6
   travel (any vehicle) 994.6
Sick sinus syndrome 427.81
Sideropenia — see also Anemia, iron deficiency 280.9
Siderosis (lung) (occupational) 503
   cornea 371.15
   eye (bulbi) (vitreous) 360.23
   lens 360.23

Siegal-Cattan-Mamou disease (periodic) 277.31
Siemens' syndrome
   ectodermal dysplasia 757.31
   keratosis follicularis spinulosa (decalvans) 757.39
Sighing respiration 786.7
Sigmoid
   flexure — see condition
   kidney 753.3
Sigmoiditis — see Enteritis
Silfverskiöld's syndrome 756.50
Silicosis, silicotic (complicated) (occupational) (simple) 502
   fibrosis, lung (confluent) (massive) (occupational) 502
   non-nodular 503
   pulmonum 502
Silicotuberculosis — see also Tuberculosis 011.4
Silo fillers' disease 506.9
Silver's syndrome (congenital hemihypertrophy and short stature) 759.89
Silver wire arteries, retina 362.13
Silvestroni-Bianco syndrome (thalassemia minima) 282.49
Simian crease 757.2
Simmonds' cachexia or disease (pituitary cachexia) 253.2
Simons' disease or syndrome (progressive lipodystrophy) 272.6
Simple, simplex — see condition
Sinding-Larsen disease (juvenile osteopathia patellae) 732.4
Singapore hemorrhagic fever 065.4
Singers' node or nodule 478.5
Single
   atrium 745.69
   coronary artery 746.85
   umbilical artery 747.5
   ventricle 745.3
Singultus 786.8
   epidemicus 078.89
Sinus — see also Fistula
   abdominal 569.81
   arrest 426.6
   arrhythmia 427.89
   bradycardia 427.89
      chronic 427.81
   branchial cleft (external) (internal) 744.41
   coccygeal (infected) 685.1
      with abscess 685.0
   dental 522.7
   dermal (congenital) 685.1
      with abscess 685.0
   draining — see Fistula
   infected, skin NEC 686.9
   marginal, ruptured or bleeding 641.2
      affecting fetus or newborn 762.1
   pause 426.6
   pericranii 742.0
   pilonidal (infected) (rectum) 685.1
      with abscess 685.0
   preauricular 744.46
   rectovaginal 619.1
   sacrococcygeal (dermoid) (infected) 685.1
      with abscess 685.0
   skin
      infected NEC 686.9
      noninfected — see Ulcer, skin
   tachycardia 427.89
   tarsi syndrome 726.79
   testis 608.89
   tract (postinfectional) — see Fistula
   urachus 753.7
Sinuses, Rokitansky-Aschoff — see also Disease, gallbladder 575.8
Sinusitis (accessory) (nasal) (hyperplastic) (nonpurulent) (purulent) (chronic) 473.9
   with influenza, flu, or grippe 487.1
   acute 461.9

Sinusitis — continued
   acute — continued
      ethmoidal 461.2
      frontal 461.1
      maxillary 461.0
      specified type NEC 461.8
      sphenoidal 461.3
   allergic (see also Fever, hay) 477.9
   antrum — see Sinusitis, maxillary
   due to
      fungus, any sinus 117.9
      high altitude 993.1
   ethmoidal 473.2
      acute 461.2
   frontal 473.1
      acute 461.1
   influenzal 478.19
   maxillary 473.0
      acute 461.0
   specified site NEC 473.8
   sphenoidal 473.3
      acute 461.3
   syphilitic, any sinus 095.8
   tuberculous, any sinus (see also Tuberculosis) 012.8
Sinusitis-bronchiectasis-situs inversus (syndrome) (triad) 759.3
Sioloangitis 527.2
Sipple's syndrome (medullary thyroid carcinoma-pheochromocytoma) 193
Sirenomelia 759.89
Siriasis 992.0
Sirkari's disease 085.0
SIRS (systemic inflammatory response syndrome) 995.90
   due to
      infectious process 995.91
         with ▶acute◀ organ dysfunction 995.92
      non-infectious process 995.93
         with ▶acute◀ organ dysfunction 995.94
Siti 104.0
Sitophobia 300.29
Situational
   disturbance (transient) (see also Reaction, adjustment) 309.9
      acute 308.3
   maladjustment, acute (see also Reaction, adjustment) 309.9
   reaction (see also Reaction, adjustment) 309.9
      acute 308.3
Situation, psychiatric 300.9
Situs inversus or transversus 759.3
   abdominalis 759.3
   thoracis 759.3
Sixth disease 057.8
Sjögren-Larsson syndrome (ichthyosis congenita) 757.1
Sjögren (-Gougerot) syndrome or disease (keratoconjunctivitis sicca) 710.2
   with lung involvement 710.2 [517.8]
Skeletal — see condition
Skene's gland — see condition
Skenitis — see also Urethritis 597.89
   gonorrheal (acute) 098.0
      chronic or duration of 2 months or over 098.2
Skerljevo 104.0
Skevas-Zerfus disease 989.5
Skin — see also condition
   donor V59.1
   hidebound 710.9
SLAP lesion (superior glenoid labrum) 840.7
Slate-dressers' lung 502
Slate-miners' lung 502
Sleep
   deprivation V69.4
   disorder 780.50
      with apnea — see Apnea, sleep
      child 307.40
      movement, unspecified 780.58
      nonorganic origin 307.40

Sleep — continued
   disorder — continued
      nonorganic origin — continued
         specified type NEC 307.49
      disturbance 780.50
         with apnea — see Apnea, sleep
         nonorganic origin 307.40
            specified type NEC 307.49
      drunkenness 307.47
      movement disorder, unspecified 780.58
      paroxysmal (see also Narcolepsy) 347.00
      related movement disorder, unspecified 780.58
      rhythm inversion 327.39
         nonorganic origin 307.45
      walking 307.46
         hysterical 300.13
Sleeping sickness 086.5
   late effect 139.8
Sleeplessness — see also Insomnia 780.52
   menopausal 627.2
   nonorganic origin 307.41
Slipped, slipping
   epiphysis (postinfectional) 732.9
      traumatic (old) 732.9
         current — see Fracture, by site
      upper femoral (nontraumatic) 732.2
   intervertebral disc — see Displacement, intervertebral disc
   ligature, umbilical 772.3
   patella 717.89
   rib 733.99
   sacroiliac joint 724.6
   tendon 727.9
   ulnar nerve, nontraumatic 354.2
   vertebra NEC (see also Spondylolisthesis) 756.12
Slocumb's syndrome 255.3
Sloughing (multiple) (skin) 686.9
   abscess — see Abscess, by site
   appendix 543.9
   bladder 596.8
   fascia 728.9
   graft — see Complications, graft
   phagedena (see also Gangrene) 785.4
   reattached extremity (see also Complications, reattached extremity) 996.90
   rectum 569.49
   scrotum 608.89
   tendon 727.9
   transplanted organ (see also Rejection, transplant, organ, by site) 996.80
   ulcer (see also Ulcer, skin) 707.9
Slow
   feeding newborn 779.3
   fetal, growth NEC 764.9
      affecting management of pregnancy 656.5
Slowing
   heart 427.89
   urinary stream 788.62
Sluder's neuralgia or syndrome 337.0
Slurred, slurring, speech 784.5
Small-for-dates — see also Light-for-dates 764.0
   affecting management of pregnancy 656.5
Smallpox 050.9
   contact V01.3
   exposure to V01.3
   hemorrhagic (pustular) 050.0
   malignant 050.0
   modified 050.2
   vaccination
      complications — see Complications, vaccination
      prophylactic (against) V04.1
Small, smallness
   cardiac reserve — see Disease, heart

Small, smallness — continued
  for dates
    fetus or newborn 764.0 ☑
      with malnutrition 764.1 ☑
      affecting management of pregnancy 656.5 ☑
    infant, term 764.0 ☑
      with malnutrition 764.1 ☑
      affecting management of pregnancy 656.5 ☑
    introitus, vagina 623.3
    kidney, unknown cause 589.9
      bilateral 589.1
      unilateral 589.0
    ovary 620.8
    pelvis
      with disproportion (fetopelvic) 653.1 ☑
        affecting fetus or newborn 763.1
      causing obstructed labor 660.1 ☑
        affecting fetus or newborn 763.1
    placenta — see Placenta, insufficiency
    uterus 621.8
    white kidney 582.9
Smith's fracture (separation) (closed) 813.41
    open 813.51
Smith-Lemli Opitz syndrome (cerebrohepatorenal syndrome) 759.89
Smith-Magenis syndrome 758.33
Smith-Strang disease (oasthouse urine) 270.2
Smokers'
    bronchitis 491.0
    cough 491.0
    syndrome (see also Abuse, drugs, nondependent) 305.1
    throat 472.1
    tongue 528.6
Smoking complicating pregnancy, childbirth, or the puerperium ● 649.0 ☑ ●
Smothering spells 786.09
Snaggle teeth, tooth 524.39
Snapping
    finger 727.05
    hip 719.65
    jaw 524.69
      temporomandibular joint sounds on opening or closing 524.64
    knee 717.9
    thumb 727.05
Sneddon-Wilkinson disease or syndrome (subcorneal pustular dermatosis) 694.1
Sneezing 784.99 ▲
    intractable 478.19 ▲
Sniffing
    cocaine (see also Dependence) 304.2 ☑
    ether (see also Dependence) 304.6 ☑
    glue (airplane) (see also Dependence) 304.6 ☑
Snoring 786.09
Snow blindness 370.24
Snuffles (nonsyphilitic) 460
    syphilitic (infant) 090.0
Social migrant V60.0
Sodoku 026.0
Soemmering's ring 366.51
Soft — see also condition
    enlarged prostate 600.00
      with
        other lower urinary tract symptoms (LUTS) 600.01 ●
        urinary
          obstruction 600.01 ●
          retention 600.01 ●
    nails 703.8
Softening
    bone 268.2
    brain (necrotic) (progressive) 434.9 ▲
      arteriosclerotic 437.0
      congenital 742.4

Softening — continued
  brain — continued
    embolic (see also Embolism, brain) 434.1 ▲
    hemorrhagic (see also Hemorrhage, brain) 431
    occlusive 434.9
    thrombotic (see also Thrombosis, brain) 434.0 ▲
  cartilage 733.92
  cerebellar — see Softening, brain
  cerebral — see Softening, brain
  cerebrospinal — see Softening, brain
  myocardial, heart (see also Degeneration, myocardial) 429.1
  nails 703.8
  spinal cord 336.8
  stomach 537.89
Solar fever 061
Soldier's
  heart 306.2
  patches 423.1
Solitary
  cyst
    bone 733.21
    kidney 593.2
  kidney (congenital) 753.0
  tubercle, brain (see also Tuberculosis, brain) 013.2 ☑
  ulcer, bladder 596.8
Somatization reaction, somatic reaction — see also Disorder, psychosomatic 306.9
  disorder 300.81
Somatoform disorder 300.82
  atypical 300.82
  severe 300.81
  undifferentiated 300.82
Somnambulism 307.46
  hysterical 300.13
Somnolence 780.09
  nonorganic origin 307.43
  periodic 349.89
Sonne dysentery 004.3
Soor 112.0
Sore
  Delhi 085.1
  desert (see also Ulcer, skin) 707.9
  eye 379.99
  Lahore 085.1
  mouth 528.9
    canker 528.2
    due to dentures 528.9
  muscle 729.1
  Naga (see also Ulcer, skin) 707.9
  oriental 085.1
  pressure (see also Decubitus) 707.00
    with gangrene (see also Decubitus) 707.00 [785.4]
  skin NEC 709.9
  soft 099.0
  throat 462
    with influenza, flu, or grippe 487.1
    acute 462
    chronic 472.1
    clergyman's 784.49
    coxsackie (virus) 074.0
    diphtheritic 032.0
    epidemic 034.0
    gangrenous 462
    herpetic 054.79
    influenzal 487.1
    malignant 462
    purulent 462
    putrid 462
    septic 034.0
    streptococcal (ulcerative) 034.0
    ulcerated 462
    viral NEC 462
      Coxsackie 074.0
  tropical (see also Ulcer, skin) 707.9
  veldt (see also Ulcer, skin) 707.9
Sotos' syndrome (cerebral gigantism) 253.0
Sounds
  friction, pleural 786.7

Sounds — continued
  succussion, chest 786.7
  temporomandibular joint
    on opening or closing 524.64
South African cardiomyopathy syndrome 425.2
South American
  blastomycosis 116.1
  trypanosomiasis — see Trypanosomiasis
Southeast Asian hemorrhagic fever 065.4
Spacing, teeth, abnormal 524.30
  excessive 524.32
Spade-like hand (congenital) 754.89
Spading nail 703.8
  congenital 757.5
Spanemia 285.9
Spanish collar 605
Sparganosis 123.5
Spasmodic — see condition
Spasmophilia — see also Tetany 781.7
Spasm, spastic, spasticity — see also condition 781.0
  accommodation 367.53
  ampulla of Vater (see also Disease, gallbladder) 576.8
  anus, ani (sphincter) (reflex) 564.6
    psychogenic 306.4
  artery NEC 443.9
    basilar 435.0
    carotid 435.8
    cerebral 435.9
      specified artery NEC 435.8
    retinal (see also Occlusion, retinal, artery) 362.30
    vertebral 435.1
    vertebrobasilar 435.3
  Bell's 351.0
  bladder (sphincter, external or internal) 596.8
  bowel 564.9
    psychogenic 306.4
  bronchus, bronchiole 519.11 ▲
  cardia 530.0
  cardiac — see Angina
  carpopedal (see also Tetany) 781.7
  cecum 564.9
    psychogenic 306.4
  cerebral (arteries) (vascular) 435.9
    specified artery NEC 435.8
  cerebrovascular 435.9
  cervix, complicating delivery 661.4 ☑
    affecting fetus or newborn 763.7
  ciliary body (of accommodation) 367.53
  colon 564.1
    psychogenic 306.4
  common duct (see also Disease, biliary) 576.8
  compulsive 307.22
  conjugate 378.82
  convergence 378.84
  coronary (artery) — see Angina
  diaphragm (reflex) 786.8
    psychogenic 306.1
  duodenum, duodenal (bulb) 564.89
  esophagus (diffuse) 530.5
    psychogenic 306.4
  facial 351.8
  fallopian tube 620.8
  gait 781.2
  gastrointestinal (tract) 536.8
    psychogenic 306.4
  glottis 478.75
    hysterical 300.11
    psychogenic 306.1
      specified as conversion reaction 300.11
    reflex through recurrent laryngeal nerve 478.75
  habit 307.20
    chronic 307.22
    transient (of childhood) 307.21
  heart — see Angina

Spasm, spastic, spasticity — see also condition — continued
  hourglass — see Contraction, hourglass
  hysterical 300.11
  infantile (see also Epilepsy) 345.6 ☑
  internal oblique, eye 378.51
  intestinal 564.9
    psychogenic 306.4
  larynx, laryngeal 478.75
    hysterical 300.11
    psychogenic 306.1
      specified as conversion reaction 300.11
  levator palpebrae superioris 333.81
  lightning (see also Epilepsy) 345.6 ☑
  mobile 781.0
  muscle 728.85
    back 724.8
    psychogenic 306.0
  nerve, trigeminal 350.1
  nervous 306.0
  nodding 307.3
    infantile (see also Epilepsy) 345.6 ☑
  occupational 300.89
  oculogyric 378.87
  ophthalmic artery 362.30
  orbicularis 781.0
  perineal 625.8
  peroneo-extensor (see also Flat, foot) 734
  pharynx (reflex) 478.29
    hysterical 300.11
    psychogenic 306.1
      specified as conversion reaction 300.11
  pregnant uterus, complicating delivery 661.4 ☑
  psychogenic 306.0
  pylorus 537.81
    adult hypertrophic 537.0
    congenital or infantile 750.5
    psychogenic 306.4
  rectum (sphincter) 564.6
    psychogenic 306.4
  retinal artery NEC (see also Occlusion, retina, artery) 362.30
  sacroiliac 724.6
  salaam (infantile) (see also Epilepsy) 345.6 ☑
  saltatory 781.0
  sigmoid 564.9
    psychogenic 306.4
  sphincter of Oddi (see also Disease, gallbladder) 576.5
  stomach 536.8
    neurotic 306.4
  throat 478.29
    hysterical 300.11
    psychogenic 306.1
      specified as conversion reaction 300.11
  tic 307.20
    chronic 307.22
    transient (of childhood) 307.21
  tongue 529.8
  torsion 333.6
  trigeminal nerve 350.1
    postherpetic 053.12
  ureter 593.89
  urethra (sphincter) 599.84
  uterus 625.8
    complicating labor 661.4 ☑
      affecting fetus or newborn 763.7
  vagina 625.1
    psychogenic 306.51
  vascular NEC 443.9
  vasomotor NEC 443.9
  vein NEC 459.89
  vesical (sphincter, external or internal) 596.8
  viscera 789.0 ☑
Spasmus nutans 307.3
Spastic — see also Spasm
  child 343.9

Index to Diseases

Spasticity — see also Spasm
 cerebral, child 343.9
Speakers' throat 784.49
Specific, specified — see condition
Speech
 defect, disorder, disturbance, impediment NEC 784.5
  psychogenic 307.9
 therapy V57.3
Spells 780.39
 breath-holding 786.9
Spencer's disease (epidemic vomiting) 078.82
Spens' syndrome (syncope with heart block) 426.9
Spermatic cord — see condition
Spermatocele 608.1
 congenital 752.89
Spermatocystitis 608.4
Spermatocytoma (M9063/3)
 specified site — see Neoplasm, by site, malignant
 unspecified site 186.9
Spermatorrhea 608.89
Sperm counts
 fertility testing V26.21
 following sterilization reversal V26.22
 postvasectomy V25.8
Sphacelus — see also Gangrene 785.4
Sphenoidal — see condition
Sphenoiditis (chronic) — see also Sinusitis, sphenoidal 473.3
Sphenopalatine ganglion neuralgia 337.0
Sphericity, increased, lens 743.36
Spherocytosis (congenital) (familial) (hereditary) 282.0
 hemoglobin disease 282.7
 sickle-cell (disease) 282.60
Spherophakia 743.36
Sphincter — see condition
Sphincteritis, sphincter of Oddi — see also Cholecystitis 576.8
Sphingolipidosis 272.7
Sphingolipodystrophy 272.7
Sphingomyelinosis 272.7
Spicule tooth 520.2
Spider
 finger 755.59
 nevus 448.1
 vascular 448.1
Spiegler-Fendt sarcoid 686.8
Spielmeyer-Stock disease 330.1
Spielmeyer-Vogt disease 330.1
Spina bifida (aperta) 741.9 ☑

> Note — Use the following fifth-digit subclassification with category 741:
> 0 unspecified region
> 1 cervical region
> 2 dorsal [thoracic] region
> 3 lumbar region

 with hydrocephalus 741.0 ☑
 fetal (suspected), affecting management of pregnancy 655.0 ☑
 occulta 756.17
Spindle, Krukenberg's 371.13
Spine, spinal — see condition
Spiradenoma (eccrine) (M8403/0) — see Neoplasm, skin, benign
Spirillosis NEC — see also Fever, relapsing 087.9
Spirillum minus 026.0
Spirillum obermeieri infection 087.0
Spirochetal — see condition
Spirochetosis 104.9
 arthritic, arthritica 104.9 [711.8] ☑
 bronchopulmonary 104.8
 icterohemorrhagica 100.0
 lung 104.8
Spitting blood — see also Hemoptysis 786.3
Splanchnomegaly 569.89
Splanchnoptosis 569.89
Spleen, splenic — see also condition

Spleen, splenic — see also condition — continued
 agenesis 759.0
 flexure syndrome 569.89
 neutropenia syndrome 289.53 ▲
 sequestration syndrome 289.52
Splenectasis — see also Splenomegaly 789.2
Splenitis (interstitial) (malignant) (nonspecific) 289.59
 malarial (see also Malaria) 084.6
 tuberculous (see also Tuberculosis) 017.7 ☑
Splenocele 289.59
Splenogalia — see Splenomegaly
Splenomegalic — see condition
Splenomegaly 789.2
 Bengal 789.2
 cirrhotic 289.51
 congenital 759.0
 congestive, chronic 289.51
 cryptogenic 789.2
 Egyptian 120.1
 Gaucher's (cerebroside lipidosis) 272.7
 idiopathic 789.2
 malarial (see also Malaria) 084.6
 neutropenic 289.53 ▲
 Niemann-Pick (lipid histiocytosis) 272.7
 siderotic 289.51
 syphilitic 095.8
  congenital 090.0
 tropical (Bengal) (idiopathic) 789.2
Splenopathy 289.50
Splenopneumonia — see Pneumonia
Splenoptosis 289.59
Splinter — see Injury, superficial, by site
Split, splitting
 heart sounds 427.89
 lip, congenital (see also Cleft, lip) 749.10
 nails 703.8
 urinary stream 788.61
Spoiled child reaction — see also Disturbance, conduct 312.1 ☑
Spondylarthritis — see also Spondylosis 721.90
Spondylarthrosis — see also Spondylosis 721.90
Spondylitis 720.9
 ankylopoietica 720.0
 ankylosing (chronic) 720.0
 atrophic 720.9
  ligamentous 720.9
 chronic (traumatic) (see also Spondylosis) 721.90
 deformans (chronic) (see also Spondylosis) 721.90
 gonococcal 098.53
 gouty 274.0
 hypertrophic (see also Spondylosis) 721.90
 infectious NEC 720.9
 juvenile (adolescent) 720.0
 Kümmell's 721.7
 Marie-Strümpell (ankylosing) 720.0
 muscularis 720.9
 ossificans ligamentosa 721.6
 osteoarthritica (see also Spondylosis) 721.90
 posttraumatic 721.7
 proliferative 720.0
 rheumatoid 720.0
 rhizomelica 720.0
 sacroiliac NEC 720.2
 senescent (see also Spondylosis) 721.90
 senile (see also Spondylosis) 721.90
 static (see also Spondylosis) 721.90
 traumatic (chronic) (see also Spondylosis) 721.90
 tuberculous (see also Tuberculosis) 015.0 ☑ [720.81]
 typhosa 002.0 [720.81]
Spondyloarthrosis — see also Spondylosis 721.90

Spondylolisthesis (congenital) (lumbosacral) 756.12
 with disproportion (fetopelvic) 653.3 ☑
  affecting fetus or newborn 763.1
  causing obstructed labor 660.1 ☑
   affecting fetus or newborn 763.1
 acquired 738.4
 degenerative 738.4
 traumatic 738.4
  acute (lumbar) — see Fracture, vertebra, lumbar
  site other than lumbosacral — see Fracture, vertebra, by site
Spondylolysis (congenital) 756.11
 acquired 738.4
 cervical 756.19
 lumbosacral region 756.11
  with disproportion (fetopelvic) 653.3 ☑
   affecting fetus or newborn 763.1
   causing obstructed labor 660.1 ☑
    affecting fetus or newborn 763.1
Spondylopathy
 inflammatory 720.9
  specified type NEC 720.89
 traumatic 721.7
Spondylose rhizomelique 720.0
Spondylosis 721.90
 with
  disproportion 653.3 ☑
   affecting fetus or newborn 763.1
   causing obstructed labor 660.1 ☑
    affecting fetus or newborn 763.1
  myelopathy NEC 721.91
 cervical, cervicodorsal 721.0
  with myelopathy 721.1
 inflammatory 720.9
 lumbar, lumbosacral 721.3
  with myelopathy 721.42
 sacral 721.3
  with myelopathy 721.42
 thoracic 721.2
  with myelopathy 721.41
 traumatic 721.7
Sponge
 divers' disease 989.5
 inadvertently left in operation wound 998.4
 kidney (medullary) 753.17
Spongioblastoma (M9422/3)
 multiforme (M9440/3)
  specified site — see Neoplasm, by site, malignant
  unspecified site 191.9
 polare (M9423/3)
  specified site — see Neoplasm, by site, malignant
  unspecified site 191.9
 primitive polar (M9443/3)
  specified site — see Neoplasm, by site, malignant
  unspecified site 191.9
 specified site — see Neoplasm, by site, malignant
 unspecified site 191.9
Spongiocytoma (M9400/3)
 specified site — see Neoplasm, by site, malignant
 unspecified site 191.9
Spongioneuroblastoma (M9504/3) — see Neoplasm, by site, malignant
Spontaneous — see also condition
 fracture — see Fracture, pathologic
Spoon nail 703.8
 congenital 757.5
Sporadic — see condition
Sporotrichosis (bones) (cutaneous) (disseminated) (epidermal) (lymphatic) (lymphocutaneous) (mucous membranes) (pulmonary) (skeletal) (visceral) 117.1

Sporotrichum schenckii infection 117.1
Spots, spotting
 atrophic (skin) 701.3
 Bitôt's (in the young child) 264.1
 café au lait 709.09
 cayenne pepper 448.1
 complicating pregnancy 649.5 ☑ ●
 cotton wool (retina) 362.83
 de Morgan's (senile angiomas) 448.1
 Fúchs' black (myopic) 360.21
 intermenstrual
  irregular 626.6
  regular 626.5
 interpalpebral 372.53
 Koplik's 055.9
 liver 709.09
 Mongolian (pigmented) 757.33
 of pregnancy 641.9 ☑
 purpuric 782.7
 ruby 448.1
Spotted fever — see Fever, spotted
Sprain, strain (joint) (ligament) (muscle) (tendon) 848.9
 abdominal wall (muscle) 848.8
 Achilles tendon 845.09
 acromioclavicular 840.0
 ankle 845.00
  and foot 845.00
 anterior longitudinal, cervical 847.0
 arm 840.9
  upper 840.9
  and shoulder 840.9
 astragalus 845.00
 atlanto-axial 847.0
 atlanto-occipital 847.0
 atlas 847.0
 axis 847.0
 back (see also Sprain, spine) 847.9
 breast bone 848.40
 broad ligament — see Injury, internal, broad ligament
 calcaneofibular 845.02
 carpal 842.01
 carpometacarpal 842.11
 cartilage
  costal, without mention of injury to sternum 848.3
   involving sternum 848.42
  ear 848.8
  knee 844.9
   with current tear (see also Tear, meniscus) 836.2
  semilunar (knee) 844.8
   with current tear (see also Tear, meniscus) 836.2
  septal, nose 848.0
  thyroid region 848.2
  xiphoid 848.49
 cervical, cervicodorsal, cervicothoracic 847.0
 chondrocostal, without mention of injury to sternum 848.3
  involving sternum 848.42
 chondrosternal 848.42
 chronic (joint) — see Derangement, joint
 clavicle 840.9
 coccyx 847.4
 collar bone 840.9
 collateral, knee (medial) (tibial) 844.1
  lateral (fibular) 844.0
  recurrent or old 717.89
   lateral 717.81
   medial 717.82
 coracoacromial 840.8
 coracoclavicular 840.1
 coracohumeral 840.2
 coracoid (process) 840.9
 coronary, knee 844.8
 costal cartilage, without mention of injury to sternum 848.3
  involving sternum 848.42
 cricoarytenoid articulation 848.2
 cricothyroid articulation 848.2

Sprain, strain — *continued*
  cruciate
    knee 844.2
    old 717.89
      anterior 717.83
      posterior 717.84
  deltoid
    ankle 845.01
    shoulder 840.8
  dorsal (spine) 847.1
  ear cartilage 848.8
  elbow 841.9
    and forearm 841.9
    specified site NEC 841.8
  femur (proximal end) 843.9
    distal end 844.9
  fibula (proximal end) 844.9
    distal end 845.00
  fibulocalcaneal 845.02
  finger(s) 842.10
  foot 845.10
    and ankle 845.00
  forearm 841.9
    and elbow 841.9
    specified site NEC 841.8
  glenoid (shoulder) (*see also* SLAP lesion) 840.8
  hand 842.10
  hip 843.9
    and thigh 843.9
  humerus (proximal end) 840.9
    distal end 841.9
  iliofemoral 843.0
  infraspinatus 840.3
  innominate
    acetabulum 843.9
    pubic junction 848.5
    sacral junction 846.1
  internal
    collateral, ankle 845.01
    semilunar cartilage 844.8
      with current tear (*see also* Tear, meniscus) 836.2
      old 717.5
  interphalangeal
    finger 842.13
    toe 845.13
  ischiocapsular 843.1
  jaw (cartilage) (meniscus) 848.1
    old 524.69
  knee 844.9
    and leg 844.9
    old 717.5
      collateral
        lateral 717.81
        medial 717.82
      cruciate
        anterior 717.83
        posterior 717.84
  late effect — *see* Late, effects (of), sprain
  lateral collateral, knee 844.0
    old 717.81
  leg 844.9
    and knee 844.9
  ligamentum teres femoris 843.8
  low back 846.9
  lumbar (spine) 847.2
  lumbosacral 846.0
    chronic or old 724.6
  mandible 848.1
    old 524.69
  maxilla 848.1
  medial collateral, knee 844.1
    old 717.82
  meniscus
    jaw 848.1
      old 524.69
    knee 844.8
      with current tear (*see also* Tear, meniscus) 836.2
      old 717.5
    mandible 848.1
      old 524.69
    specified site NEC 848.8
  metacarpal 842.10

Sprain, strain — *continued*
  metacarpal — *continued*
    distal 842.12
    proximal 842.11
  metacarpophalangeal 842.12
  metatarsal 845.10
  metatarsophalangeal 845.12
  midcarpal 842.19
  midtarsal 845.19
  multiple sites, except fingers alone or toes alone 848.8
  neck 847.0
  nose (septal cartilage) 848.0
  occiput from atlas 847.0
  old — *see* Derangement, joint
  orbicular, hip 843.9
  patella(r) 844.8
    old 717.89
  pelvis 848.5
  phalanx
    finger 842.10
    toe 845.10
  radiocarpal 842.02
  radiohumeral 841.2
  radioulnar 841.9
    distal 842.09
  radius, radial (proximal end) 841.9
    and ulna 841.9
      distal 842.09
    collateral 841.0
    distal end 842.00
  recurrent — *see* Sprain, by site
  rib (cage), without mention of injury to sternum 848.3
    involving sternum 848.42
  rotator cuff (capsule) 840.4
  round ligament (*see also* Injury, internal, round ligament)
    femur 843.8
  sacral (spine) 847.3
  sacrococcygeal 847.3
  sacroiliac (region) 846.9
    chronic or old 724.6
    ligament 846.1
    specified site NEC 846.8
  sacrospinatus 846.2
  sacrospinous 846.2
  sacrotuberous 846.3
  scaphoid bone, ankle 845.00
  scapula(r) 840.9
  semilunar cartilage (knee) 844.8
    with current tear (*see also* Tear, meniscus) 836.2
    old 717.5
  septal cartilage (nose) 848.0
  shoulder 840.9
    and arm, upper 840.9
    blade 840.9
    specified site NEC 848.8
  spine 847.9
    cervical 847.0
    coccyx 847.4
    dorsal 847.1
    lumbar 847.2
    lumbosacral 846.0
      chronic or old 724.6
    sacral 847.3
    sacroiliac (*see also* Sprain, sacroiliac) 846.9
      chronic or old 724.6
    thoracic 847.1
  sternoclavicular 848.41
  sternum 848.40
  subglenoid (*see also* SLAP lesion) 840.8
  subscapularis 840.5
  supraspinatus 840.6
  symphysis
    jaw 848.1
      old 524.69
    mandibular 848.1
      old 524.69
    pubis 848.5
  talofibular 845.09
  tarsal 845.10
  tarsometatarsal 845.11

Sprain, strain — *continued*
  temporomandibular 848.1
    old 524.69
  teres
    ligamentum femoris 843.8
    major or minor 840.8
  thigh (proximal end) 843.9
    and hip 843.9
    distal end 844.9
  thoracic (spine) 847.1
  thorax 848.8
  thumb 842.10
  thyroid cartilage or region 848.2
  tibia (proximal end) 844.9
    distal end 845.00
  tibiofibular
    distal 845.03
    superior 844.3
  toe(s) 845.10
  trachea 848.8
  trapezoid 840.8
  ulna, ulnar (proximal end) 841.9
    collateral 841.1
    distal end 842.00
  ulnohumeral 841.3
  vertebrae (*see also* Sprain, spine) 847.9
    cervical, cervicodorsal, cervicothoracic 847.0
  wrist (cuneiform) (scaphoid) (semilunar) 842.00
  xiphoid cartilage 848.49
Sprengel's deformity (congenital) 755.52
Spring fever 309.23
Sprue 579.1
  celiac 579.0
  idiopathic 579.0
  meaning thrush 112.0
  nontropical 579.0
  tropical 579.1
Spur — *see also* Exostosis
  bone 726.91
    calcaneal 726.73
  calcaneal 726.73
  iliac crest 726.5
  nose (septum) 478.19 ▲
    bone 726.91
  septal 478.19 ▲
Spuria placenta — *see* Placenta, abnormal
Spurway's syndrome (brittle bones and blue sclera) 756.51
Sputum, abnormal (amount) (color) (excessive) (odor) (purulent) 786.4
  bloody 786.3
Squamous — *see also* condition
  cell metaplasia
    bladder 596.8
    cervix — *see* condition
  epithelium in
    cervical canal (congenital) 752.49
    uterine mucosa (congenital) 752.3
  metaplasia
    bladder 596.8
    cervix — *see* condition
Squashed nose 738.0
  congenital 754.0
Squeeze, divers' 993.3
Squint — *see also* Strabismus 378.9
  accommodative (*see also* Esotropia) 378.00
  concomitant (*see also* Heterotropia) 378.30
Stab — *see also* Wound, open, by site
  internal organs — *see* Injury, internal, by site, with open wound
Staggering gait 781.2
  hysterical 300.11
Staghorn calculus 592.0
Stain, staining
  meconium 779.84
  port wine 757.32
  tooth, teeth (hard tissues) 521.7
    due to
      accretions 523.6

Stain, staining — *continued*
  tooth, teeth — *continued*
    due to — *continued*
      deposits (betel) (black) (green) (materia alba) (orange) (tobacco) 523.6
      metals (copper) (silver) 521.7
      nicotine 523.6
      pulpal bleeding 521.7
      tobacco 523.6
Stälh's
  ear 744.29
  pigment line (cornea) 371.11
Stälhi's pigment lines (cornea) 371.11
Stammering 307.0
Standstill
  atrial 426.6
  auricular 426.6
  cardiac (*see also* Arrest, cardiac) 427.5
  sinoatrial 426.6
  sinus 426.6
  ventricular (*see also* Arrest, cardiac) 427.5
Stannosis 503
Stanton's disease (melioidosis) 025
Staphylitis (acute) (catarrhal) (chronic) (gangrenous) (membranous) (suppurative) (ulcerative) 528.3
Staphylococcemia 038.10
  aureus 038.11
  specified organism NEC 038.19
Staphylococcus, staphylococcal — *see* condition
Staphyloderma (skin) 686.00
Staphyloma 379.11
  anterior, localized 379.14
  ciliary 379.11
  cornea 371.73
  equatorial 379.13
  posterior 379.12
  posticum 379.12
  ring 379.15
  sclera NEC 379.11
Starch eating 307.52
Stargardt's disease 362.75
Starvation (inanition) (due to lack of food) 994.2
  edema 262
  voluntary NEC 307.1
Stasis
  bile (duct) (*see also* Disease, biliary) 576.8
  bronchus (*see also* Bronchitis) 490
  cardiac (*see also* Failure, heart) 428.0
  cecum 564.89
  colon 564.89
  dermatitis (*see also* Varix, with stasis dermatitis) 454.1
  duodenal 536.8
  eczema (*see also* Varix, with stasis dermatitis) 454.1
  edema (*see also* Hypertension, venous) 459.30
  foot 991.4
  gastric 536.3
  ileocecal coil 564.89
  ileum 564.89
  intestinal 564.89
  jejunum 564.89
  kidney 586
  liver 571.9
    cirrhotic — *see* Cirrhosis, liver
  lymphatic 457.8
  pneumonia 514
  portal 571.9
  pulmonary 514
  rectal 564.89
  renal 586
    tubular 584.5
  stomach 536.3
  ulcer
    with varicose veins 454.0
    without varicose veins 459.81
  urine NEC (*see also* Retention, urine) 788.20
  venous 459.81

Index to Diseases

State
- affective and paranoid, mixed, organic psychotic 294.8
- agitated 307.9
  - acute reaction to stress 308.2
- anxiety (neurotic) (see also Anxiety) 300.00
  - specified type NEC 300.09
- apprehension (see also Anxiety) 300.00
  - specified type NEC 300.09
- climacteric, female 627.2
  - following induced menopause 627.4
- clouded
  - epileptic (see also Epilepsy) 345.9 ☑
  - paroxysmal (idiopathic) (see also Epilepsy) 345.9 ☑
- compulsive (mixed) (with obsession) 300.3
- confusional 298.9
  - acute 293.0
    - with
      - arteriosclerotic dementia 290.41
      - presenile brain disease 290.11
      - senility 290.3
    - alcoholic 291.0
    - drug-induced 292.81
  - epileptic 293.0
  - postoperative 293.9
  - reactive (emotional stress) (psychological trauma) 298.2
  - subacute 293.1
- constitutional psychopathic 301.9
- convulsive (see also Convulsions) 780.39
- depressive NEC 311
  - induced by drug 292.84
  - neurotic 300.4
- dissociative 300.15
- hallucinatory 780.1
  - induced by drug 292.12
- hypercoagulable (primary) 289.81
  - secondary 289.82
- hyperdynamic beta-adrenergic circulatory 429.82
- locked-in 344.81
- menopausal 627.2
  - artificial 627.4
  - following induced menopause 627.4
- neurotic NEC 300.9
  - with depersonalization episode 300.6
- obsessional 300.3
- oneiroid (see also Schizophrenia) 295.4 ☑
- panic 300.01
- paranoid 297.9
  - alcohol-induced 291.5
  - arteriosclerotic 290.42
  - climacteric 297.2
  - drug-induced 292.11
  - in
    - presenile brain disease 290.12
    - senile brain disease 290.20
  - involutional 297.2
  - menopausal 297.2
  - senile 290.20
  - simple 297.0
- postleukotomy 310.0
- pregnant (see also Pregnancy) V22.2
- psychogenic, twilight 298.2
- psychotic, organic (see also Psychosis, organic) 294.9
  - mixed paranoid and affective 294.8
  - senile or presenile NEC 290.9
- transient NEC 293.9
  - with
    - anxiety 293.84
    - delusions 293.81
    - depression 293.83
    - hallucinations 293.82

State — continued
- residual schizophrenic (see also Schizophrenia) 295.6 ☑
- tension (see also Anxiety) 300.9
- transient organic psychotic 293.9
  - anxiety type 293.84
  - depressive type 293.83
  - hallucinatory type 293.83
  - paranoid type 293.81
  - specified type NEC 293.89
- twilight
  - epileptic 293.0
  - psychogenic 298.2
- vegetative (persistent) 780.03

Status (post)
- absence
  - epileptic (see also Epilepsy) 345.2
  - of organ, acquired (postsurgical) — see Absence, by site, acquired
- anastomosis of intestine (for bypass) V45.3
- anginosus 413.9
- angioplasty, percutaneous transluminal coronary V45.82
- ankle prosthesis V43.66
- aortocoronary bypass or shunt V45.81
- arthrodesis V45.4
- artificially induced condition NEC V45.87
- artificial opening (of) V44.9
  - gastrointestinal tract NEC V44.4
  - specified site NEC V44.8
  - urinary tract NEC V44.6
  - vagina V44.7
- aspirator V46.0
- asthmaticus (see also Asthma) 493.9 ☑
- awaiting organ transplant V49.83
- bariatric surgery V45.86
  - complicating pregnancy, childbirth, or the puerperium 649.2 ☑
- bed confinement V49.84
- breast implant removal V45.83
- cardiac
  - device (in situ) V45.00
    - carotid sinus V45.09
    - fitting or adjustment V53.39
    - defibrillator, automatic implantable V45.02
    - pacemaker V45.01
      - fitting or adjustment V53.31
- carotid sinus stimulator V45.09
- cataract extraction V45.61
- chemotherapy V66.2
  - current V58.69
- circumcision, female 629.20
- clitorectomy (female genital mutilation type I) 629.21
  - with excision of labia minora (female genital mutilation type II) 629.22
- colostomy V44.3
- contraceptive device V45.59
  - intrauterine V45.51
  - subdermal V45.52
- convulsivus idiopathicus (see also Epilepsy) 345.3
- coronary artery bypass or shunt V45.81
- cutting
  - female genital 629.20
    - specified NEC 629.29
    - type I 629.21
    - type II 629.22
    - type III 629.23
    - type IV 629.29
- cystostomy V44.50
  - appendico-vesicostomy V44.52
  - cutaneous-vesicostomy V44.51
  - specified type NEC V44.59
- defibrillator, automatic implantable cardiac V45.02
- dental crowns V45.84
- dental fillings V45.84

Status — continued
- dental restoration V45.84
- dental sealant V49.82
- dialysis (hemo) (peritoneal) V45.1
- donor V59.9
- drug therapy or regimen V67.59
  - high-risk medication NEC V67.51
- elbow prosthesis V43.62
- enterostomy V44.4
- epileptic, epilepticus (absence) (grand mal) (see also Epilepsy) 345.3
  - focal motor 345.7 ☑
  - partial 345.7 ☑
  - petit mal 345.2
  - psychomotor 345.7 ☑
  - temporal lobe 345.7 ☑
- estrogen receptor
  - negative [ER-] V86.1
  - positive [ER+] V86.0
- eye (adnexa) surgery V45.69
- female genital
  - cutting 629.20
    - specified NEC 629.29
    - type I 629.21
    - type II 629.22
    - type III 629.23
    - type IV 629.29
  - mutilation 629.20
    - type I 629.21
    - type II 629.22
    - type III 629.23
    - type IV 629.29
- filtering bleb (eye) (postglaucoma) V45.69
  - with rupture or complication 997.99
  - postcataract extraction (complication) 997.99
- finger joint prosthesis V43.69
- gastric
  - banding V45.86
    - complicating pregnancy, childbirth, or the puerperium 649.2 ☑
  - bypass for obesity V45.86
    - complicating pregnancy, childbirth, or the puerperium 649.2 ☑
- gastrostomy V44.1
- grand mal 345.3
- heart valve prosthesis V43.3
- hemodialysis V45.1
- hip prosthesis (joint) (partial) (total) V43.64
- ileostomy V44.2
- infibulation (female genital mutilation type III) 629.23
- insulin pump V45.85
- intestinal bypass V45.3
- intrauterine contraceptive device V45.51
- jejunostomy V44.4
- knee joint prosthesis V43.65
- lacunaris 437.8
- lacunosis 437.8
- low birth weight V21.30
  - less than 500 grams V21.31
  - 1000–1499 grams V21.33
  - 1500–1999 grams V21.34
  - 2000–2500 grams V21.35
  - 500–999 grams V21.32
- lymphaticus 254.8
- malignant neoplasm, ablated or excised — see History, malignant neoplasm
- marmoratus 333.79 ▲
- mutilation, female 629.20
  - type I 629.21
  - type II 629.22
  - type III 629.23
  - type IV 629.29
- nephrostomy V44.6
- neuropacemaker NEC V45.89
  - brain V45.89
  - carotid sinus V45.09
  - neurologic NEC V45.89

Status — continued
- obesity surgery V45.86
  - compliating pregnancy, childbirth, or the puerperium 649.2 ☑
- organ replacement
  - by artificial or mechanical device or prosthesis of
    - artery V43.4
    - artificial skin V43.83
    - bladder V43.5
    - blood vessel V43.4
    - breast V43.82
    - eye globe V43.0
    - heart
      - assist device V43.21
      - fully implantable artificial heart V43.22
      - valve V43.3
    - intestine V43.89
    - joint V43.60
      - ankle V43.66
      - elbow V43.62
      - finger V43.69
      - hip (partial) (total) V43.64
      - knee V43.65
      - shoulder V43.61
      - specified NEC V43.69
      - wrist V43.63
    - kidney V43.89
    - larynx V43.81
    - lens V43.1
    - limb(s) V43.7
    - liver V43.89
    - lung V43.89
    - organ NEC V43.89
    - pancreas V43.89
    - skin (artificial) V43.83
    - tissue NEC V43.89
    - vein V43.4
  - by organ transplant (heterologous) (homologous) — see Status, transplant
- pacemaker
  - brain V45.89
  - cardiac V45.01
  - carotid sinus V45.09
  - neurologic NEC V45.89
  - specified site NEC V45.89
- percutaneous transluminal coronary angioplasty V45.82
- peritoneal dialysis V45.1
- petit mal 345.2
- postcommotio cerebri 310.2
- postmenopausal (age related) (natural) V49.81
- postoperative NEC V45.89
- postpartum NEC V24.2
  - care immediately following delivery V24.0
  - routine follow-up V24.2
- postsurgical NEC V45.89
- renal dialysis V45.1
- respirator [ventilator] V46.11
  - encounter
    - during
      - mechanical failure V46.14
      - power failure V46.12
    - for weaning V46.13
- reversed jejunal transposition (for bypass) V45.3
- shoulder prosthesis V43.61
- shunt
  - aortocoronary bypass V45.81
  - arteriovenous (for dialysis) V45.1
  - cerebrospinal fluid V45.2
  - vascular NEC V45.89
    - aortocoronary (bypass) V45.81
  - ventricular (communicating) (for drainage) V45.2
- sterilization
  - tubal ligation V26.51
  - vasectomy V26.52
- subdermal contraceptive device V45.52
- thymicolymphaticus 254.8

Status — continued
- thymicus 254.8
- thymolymphaticus 254.8
- tooth extraction 525.10
- tracheostomy V44.0
- transplant
  - blood vessel V42.89
  - bone V42.4
    - marrow V42.81
  - cornea V42.5
  - heart V42.1
    - valve V42.2
  - intestine V42.84
  - kidney V42.0
  - liver V42.7
  - lung V42.6
  - organ V42.9
    - specified site NEC V42.89
  - pancreas V42.83
  - peripheral stem cells V42.82
  - skin V42.3
  - stem cells, peripheral V42.82
  - tissue V42.9
    - specified type NEC V42.89
  - vessel, blood V42.89
- tubal ligation V26.51
- ureterostomy V44.6
- urethrostomy V44.6
- vagina, artificial V44.7
- vascular shunt NEC V45.89
  - aortocoronary (bypass) V45.81
- vasectomy V26.52
- ventilator [respirator] V46.11
  - encounter
    - during
      - mechanical failure V46.14
      - power failure V46.12
    - for weaning V46.13
- wrist prosthesis V43.63

Stave fracture — see Fracture, metacarpus, metacarpal bone(s)

Steal
- subclavian artery 435.2
- vertebral artery 435.1

Stealing, solitary, child problem — see also Disturbance, conduct 312.1 ☑

Steam burn — see Burn, by site

Steatocystoma multiplex 706.2

Steatoma (infected) 706.2
- eyelid (cystic) 374.84
  - infected 373.13

Steatorrhea (chronic) 579.8
- with lacteal obstruction 579.2
- idiopathic 579.0
  - adult 579.0
  - infantile 579.0
- pancreatic 579.4
- primary 579.0
- secondary 579.8
- specified cause NEC 579.8
- tropical 579.1

Steatosis 272.8
- heart (see also Degeneration, myocardial) 429.1
- kidney 593.89
- liver 571.8

Steele-Richardson (-Olszewski) Syndrome 333.0

Steinbrocker's syndrome — see also Neuropathy, peripheral, autonomic 337.9

Steinert's disease 359.2

Stein-Leventhal syndrome (polycystic ovary) 256.4

Stein's syndrome (polycystic ovary) 256.4

STEMI (ST elevation myocardial infarction — see also — Infarct, myocardium, ST elevation 410.9 ● ☑

Stenocardia — see also Angina 413.9

Stenocephaly 756.0

Stenosis (cicatricial) — see also Stricture
- ampulla of Vater 576.2
  - with calculus, cholelithiasis, or stones — see Choledocholithiasis

Stenosis — see also Stricture — continued
- anus, anal (canal) (sphincter) 569.2
  - congenital 751.2
- aorta (ascending) 747.22
  - arch 747.10
  - arteriosclerotic 440.0
  - calcified 440.0
- aortic (valve) 424.1
  - with
    - mitral (valve)
      - insufficiency or incompetence 396.2
      - stenosis or obstruction 396.0
  - atypical 396.0
  - congenital 746.3
  - rheumatic 395.0
    - with
      - insufficiency, incompetency or regurgitation 395.2
        - with mitral (valve) disease 396.8
      - mitral (valve)
        - disease (stenosis) 396.0
        - insufficiency or incompetence 396.2
        - stenosis or obstruction 396.0
  - specified cause, except rheumatic 424.1
  - syphilitic 093.22
- aqueduct of Sylvius (congenital) 742.3
  - with spina bifida (see also Spina bifida) 741.0 ☑
  - acquired 331.4
- artery NEC 447.1
  - basilar — see Narrowing, artery, basilar
  - carotid (common) (internal) — see Narrowing, artery, carotid
  - celiac 447.4
  - cerebral 437.0
    - due to
      - embolism (see also Embolism, brain) 434.1 ☑
      - thrombus (see also Thrombosis, brain) 434.0 ☑
  - precerebral — see Narrowing, artery, precerebral
  - pulmonary (congenital) 747.3
    - acquired 417.8
  - renal 440.1
  - vertebral — see Narrowing, artery, vertebral
- bile duct or biliary passage (see also Obstruction, biliary) 576.2
  - congenital 751.61
- bladder neck (acquired) 596.0
  - congenital 753.6
- brain 348.8
- bronchus 519.19 ▲
  - syphilitic 095.8
- cardia (stomach) 537.89
  - congenital 750.7
- cardiovascular (see also Disease, cardiovascular) 429.2
- carotid artery — see Narrowing, artery, carotid
- cervix, cervical (canal) 622.4
  - congenital 752.49
  - in pregnancy or childbirth 654.6 ☑
    - affecting fetus or newborn 763.89
    - causing obstructed labor 660.2 ☑
      - affecting fetus or newborn 763.1
- colon (see also Obstruction, intestine) 560.9
  - congenital 751.2
- colostomy 569.62
- common bile duct (see also Obstruction, biliary) 576.2
  - congenital 751.61
- coronary (artery) — see Arteriosclerosis, coronary

Stenosis — see also Stricture — continued
- cystic duct (see also Obstruction, gallbladder) 575.2
  - congenital 751.61
- due to (presence of) any device, implant, or graft classifiable to 996.0–996.5 — see Complications, due to (presence of) any device, implant, or graft classified to 996.0–996.5 NEC
- duodenum 537.3
  - congenital 751.1
- ejaculatory duct NEC 608.89
- endocervical os — see Stenosis, cervix
- enterostomy 569.62
- esophagostomy 530.87
- esophagus 530.3
  - congenital 750.3
  - syphilitic 095.8
    - congenital 090.5
- external ear canal 380.50
  - secondary to
    - inflammation 380.53
    - surgery 380.52
    - trauma 380.51
- gallbladder (see also Obstruction, gallbladder) 575.2
- glottis 478.74
- heart valve (acquired) (see also Endocarditis)
  - congenital NEC 746.89
    - aortic 746.3
    - mitral 746.5
    - pulmonary 746.02
    - tricuspid 746.1
- hepatic duct (see also Obstruction, biliary) 576.2
- hymen 623.3
- hypertrophic subaortic (idiopathic) 425.1
- infundibulum cardiac 746.83
- intestine (see also Obstruction, intestine) 560.9
  - congenital (small) 751.1
    - large 751.2
- lacrimal
  - canaliculi 375.53
  - duct 375.56
    - congenital 743.65
  - punctum 375.52
    - congenital 743.65
  - sac 375.54
    - congenital 743.65
- lacrimonasal duct 375.56
  - congenital 743.65
  - neonatal 375.55
- larynx 478.74
  - congenital 748.3
  - syphilitic 095.8
    - congenital 090.5
- mitral (valve) (chronic) (inactive) 394.0
  - with
    - aortic (valve)
      - disease (insufficiency) 396.1
      - insufficiency or incompetence 396.1
      - stenosis or obstruction 396.0
    - incompetency, insufficiency or regurgitation 394.2
      - with aortic valve disease 396.8
    - active or acute 391.1
      - with chorea (acute) (rheumatic) (Sydenham's) 392.0
  - congenital 746.5
  - specified cause, except rheumatic 424.0
  - syphilitic 093.21
- myocardium, myocardial (see also Degeneration, myocardial) 429.1
  - hypertrophic subaortic (idiopathic) 425.1
- nares (anterior) (posterior) 478.19 ▲
  - congenital 748.0

Stenosis — see also Stricture — continued
- nasal duct 375.56
  - congenital 743.65
- nasolacrimal duct 375.56
  - congenital 743.65
  - neonatal 375.55
- organ or site, congenital NEC — see Atresia
- papilla of Vater 576.2
  - with calculus, cholelithiasis, or stones — see Choledocholithiasis
- pulmonary (artery) (congenital) 747.3
  - with ventricular septal defect, dextraposition of aorta and hypertrophy of right ventricle 745.2
  - acquired 417.8
  - infundibular 746.83
  - in tetralogy of Fallot 745.2
  - subvalvular 746.83
  - valve (see also Endocarditis, pulmonary) 424.3
    - congenital 746.02
  - vein 747.49
    - acquired 417.8
  - vessel NEC 417.8
- pulmonic (congenital) 746.02
  - infundibular 746.83
  - subvalvular 746.83
- pylorus (hypertrophic) 537.0
  - adult 537.0
  - congenital 750.5
  - infantile 750.5
- rectum (sphincter) (see also Stricture, rectum) 569.2
- renal artery 440.1
- salivary duct (any) 527.8
- sphincter of Oddi (see also Obstruction, biliary) 576.2
- spinal 724.00
  - cervical 723.0
  - lumbar, lumbosacral 724.02
  - nerve (root) NEC 724.9
  - specified region NEC 724.09
  - thoracic, thoracolumbar 724.01
- stomach, hourglass 537.6
- subaortic 746.81
  - hypertrophic (idiopathic) 425.1
- supra (valvular)-aortic 747.22
- trachea 519.19 ▲
  - congenital 748.3
  - syphilitic 095.8
  - tuberculous (see also Tuberculosis) 012.8 ☑
- tracheostomy 519.02
- tricuspid (valve) (see also Endocarditis, tricuspid) 397.0
  - congenital 746.1
  - nonrheumatic 424.2
- tubal 628.2
- ureter (see also Stricture, ureter) 593.3
  - congenital 753.29
- urethra (see also Stricture, urethra) 598.9
- vagina 623.2
  - congenital 752.49
  - in pregnancy or childbirth 654.7 ☑
    - affecting fetus or newborn 763.89
    - causing obstructed labor 660.2 ☑
      - affecting fetus or newborn 763.1
- valve (cardiac) (heart) (see also Endocarditis) 424.90
  - congenital NEC 746.89
    - aortic 746.3
    - mitral 746.5
    - pulmonary 746.02
    - tricuspid 746.1
  - urethra 753.6
- valvular (see also Endocarditis) 424.90

Index to Diseases

Stenosis — see also Stricture — continued
  valvular (see also Endocarditis) — continued
    congenital NEC 746.89
    urethra 753.6
  vascular graft or shunt 996.1
    atherosclerosis — see Arteriosclerosis, extremities
    embolism 996.74
    occlusion NEC 996.74
    thrombus 996.74
  vena cava (inferior) (superior) 459.2
    congenital 747.49
  ventricular shunt 996.2
  vulva 624.8
Stercolith — see also Fecalith 560.39
  appendix 543.9
Stercoraceous, stercoral ulcer 569.82
  anus or rectum 569.41
Stereopsis, defective
  with fusion 368.33
  without fusion 368.32
Stereotypes NEC 307.3
Sterility
  female — see Infertility, female
  male (see also Infertility, male) 606.9
Sterilization, admission for V25.2
  status
    tubal ligation V26.51
    vasectomy V26.52
Sternalgia — see also Angina 413.9
Sternopagus 759.4
Sternum bifidum 756.3
Sternutation 784.99 ▲
Steroid
  effects (adverse) (iatrogenic)
    cushingoid
      correct substance properly administered 255.0
      overdose or wrong substance given or taken 962.0
    diabetes
      correct substance properly administered 251.8
      overdose or wrong substance given or taken 962.0
      due to
        correct substance properly administered 255.8
        overdose or wrong substance given or taken 962.0
    fever
      correct substance properly administered 780.6
      overdose or wrong substance given or taken 962.0
    withdrawal
      correct substance properly administered 255.4
      overdose or wrong substance given or taken 962.0
  responder 365.03
Stevens-Johnson disease or syndrome (erythema multiforme exudativum) 695.1
Stewart-Morel syndrome (hyperostosis frontalis interna) 733.3
Sticker's disease (erythema infectiosum) 057.
Stickler syndrome 759.89
Sticky eye 372.03
Stieda's disease (calcification, knee joint) 726.62
Stiff
  back 724.8
  neck (see also Torticollis) 723.5
Stiff-baby 759.89
Stiff-man syndrome 333.91
Stiffness, joint NEC 719.50
  ankle 719.57
  back 724.8
  elbow 719.52
  finger 719.54
  hip 719.55
  knee 719.56

Stiffness, joint — continued
  multiple sites 719.59
  sacroiliac 724.6
  shoulder 719.51
  specified site NEC 719.58
  spine 724.9
  surgical fusion V45.4
  wrist 719.53
Stigmata, congenital syphilis 090.5
Stillbirth, stillborn NEC 779.9
Still's disease or syndrome 714.30
Stiller's disease (asthenia) 780.79
Still-Felty syndrome (rheumatoid arthritis with splenomegaly and leukopenia) 714.1
Stilling-Türk-Duane syndrome (ocular retraction syndrome) 378.71
Stimulation, ovary 256.1
Sting (animal) (bee) (fish) (insect) (jellyfish) (Portuguese man-o-war) (wasp) (venomous) 989.5
  anaphylactic shock or reaction 989.5
  plant 692.6
Stippled epiphyses 756.59
Stitch
  abscess 998.59
  burst (in external operation wound) 998.32
    internal 998.31
  in back 724.5
Stojano's (subcostal) **syndrome** 098.86
Stokes-Adams syndrome (syncope with heart block) 426.9
Stokes' disease (exophthalmic goiter) 242.0 ☑
Stokvis' (-Talma) disease (enterogenous cyanosis) 289.7
Stomach — see condition
Stoma malfunction
  colostomy 569.62
  cystostomy 997.5
  enterostomy 569.62
  esophagostomy 530.87
  gastrostomy 536.42
  ileostomy 569.62
  nephrostomy 997.5
  tracheostomy 519.02
  ureterostomy 997.5
Stomatitis 528.00 ▲
  angular 528.5
    due to dietary or vitamin deficiency 266.0
  aphthous 528.2
  candidal 112.0
  catarrhal 528.00 ▲
  denture 528.9
  diphtheritic (membranous) 032.0
  due to
    dietary deficiency 266.0
    thrush 112.0
    vitamin deficiency 266.0
  epidemic 078.4
  epizootic 078.4
  follicular 528.00 ▲
  gangrenous 528.1
  herpetic 054.2
  herpetiformis 528.2
  malignant 528.00 ▲
  membranous acute 528.00 ▲
  monilial 112.0
  mycotic 112.0
  necrotic 528.1
    ulcerative 101
  necrotizing ulcerative 101
  parasitic 112.0
  septic 528.00 ▲
  specified NEC 528.09 ●
  spirochetal 101
  suppurative (acute) 528.00 ▲
  ulcerative 528.00 ▲
    necrotizing 101
  ulceromembranous 101
  vesicular 528.00 ▲
    with exanthem 074.3
  Vincent's 101
Stomatocytosis 282.8

Stomatomycosis 112.0
Stomatorrhagia 528.9
Stone(s) — see also Calculus
  bladder 594.1
    diverticulum 594.0
  cystine 270.0
  heart syndrome (see also Failure, ventricular, left) 428.1
  kidney 592.0
  prostate 602.0
  pulp (dental) 522.2
  renal 592.0
  salivary duct or gland (any) 527.5
  ureter 592.1
  urethra (impacted) 594.2
  urinary (duct) (impacted) (passage) 592.9
    bladder 594.1
      diverticulum 594.0
    lower tract NEC 594.9
    specified site 594.8
  xanthine 277.2
Stonecutters' lung 502
  tuberculous (see also Tuberculosis) 011.4 ☑
Stonemasons'
  asthma, disease, or lung 502
    tuberculous (see also Tuberculosis) 011.4 ☑
  phthisis (see also Tuberculosis) 011.4 ☑
Stoppage
  bowel (see also Obstruction, intestine) 560.9
  heart (see also Arrest, cardiac) 427.5
  intestine (see also Obstruction, intestine) 560.9
  urine NEC (see also Retention, urine) 788.20
Storm, thyroid (apathetic) — see also Thyrotoxicosis 242.9 ☑
Strabismus (alternating) (congenital) (nonparalytic) 378.9
  concomitant (see also Heterotropia) 378.30
    convergent (see also Esotropia) 378.00
    divergent (see also Exotropia) 378.10
  convergent (see also Esotropia) 378.00
  divergent (see also Exotropia) 378.10
  due to adhesions, scars — see Strabismus, mechanical
  in neuromuscular disorder NEC 378.73
  intermittent 378.20
    vertical 378.31
  latent 378.40
    convergent (esophoria) 378.41
    divergent (exophoria) 378.42
    vertical 378.43
  mechanical 378.60
    due to
      Brown's tendon sheath syndrome 378.61
      specified musculofascial disorder NEC 378.62
  paralytic 378.50
    third or oculomotor nerve (partial) 378.51
      total 378.52
    fourth or trochlear nerve 378.53
    sixth or abducens nerve 378.54
  specified type NEC 378.73
  vertical (hypertropia) 378.31
Strain — see also Sprain, by site
  eye NEC 368.13
  heart — see Disease, heart
  meaning gonorrhea — see Gonorrhea
  on urination 788.65 ●
  physical NEC V62.89
  postural 729.9
  psychological NEC V62.89
Strands
  conjunctiva 372.62
  vitreous humor 379.25

Strangulation, strangulated 994.7
  appendix 543.9
  asphyxiation or suffocation by 994.7
  bladder neck 596.0
  bowel — see Strangulation, intestine
  colon — see Strangulation, intestine
  cord (umbilical) — see Compression, umbilical cord
  due to birth injury 767.8
  food or foreign body (see also Asphyxia, food) 933.1
  hemorrhoids 455.8
    external 455.5
    internal 455.2
  hernia (see also Hernia, by site, with obstruction)
    gangrenous — see Hernia, by site, with gangrene
  intestine (large) (small) 560.2
    with hernia (see also Hernia, by site, with obstruction)
      gangrenous — see Hernia, by site, with gangrene
    congenital (small) 751.1
      large 751.2
  mesentery 560.2
  mucus (see also Asphyxia, mucus) 933.1
    newborn 770.18
  omentum 560.2
  organ or site, congenital NEC — see Atresia
  ovary 620.8
    due to hernia 620.4
  penis 607.89
    foreign body 939.3
  rupture (see also Hernia, by site, with obstruction) 552.9
    gangrenous (see also Hernia, by site, with gangrene) 551.9
  stomach, due to hernia (see also Hernia, by site, with obstruction) 552.9
    with gangrene (see also Hernia, by site, with gangrene) 551.9
  umbilical cord — see Compression, umbilical cord
  vesicourethral orifice 596.0
Strangury 788.1
Strawberry
  gallbladder (see also Disease, gallbladder) 575.6
  mark 757.32
  tongue (red) (white) 529.3
Straw itch 133.8
Streak, ovarian 752.0
Strephosymbolia 315.01
  secondary to organic lesion 784.69
Streptobacillary fever 026.1
Streptobacillus moniliformis 026.1
Streptococcemia 038.0
Streptococcicosis — see Infection, streptococcal
Streptococcus, streptococcal — see condition
Streptoderma 686.00
Streptomycosis — see Actinomycosis
Streptothricosis — see Actinomycosis
Streptothrix — see Actinomycosis
Streptotrichosis — see Actinomycosis
Stress
  fracture — see Fracture, stress
  polycythemia 289.0
  reaction (gross) (see also Reaction, stress, acute) 308.9
Stretching, nerve — see Injury, nerve, by site
Striae (albicantes) (atrophicae) (cutis distensae) (distensae) 701.3
Striations of nails 703.8
Stricture — see also Stenosis 799.89
  ampulla of Vater 576.2
    with calculus, cholelithiasis, or stones — see Choledocholithiasis
  anus (sphincter) 569.2

Stricture — see also Stenosis —
continued
- anus — *continued*
  - congenital 751.2
  - infantile 751.2
- aorta (ascending) 747.22
  - arch 747.10
  - arteriosclerotic 440.0
  - calcified 440.0
- aortic (valve) (see also Stenosis, aortic) 424.1
  - congenital 746.3
- aqueduct of Sylvius (congenital) 742.3
  - with spina bifida (see also Spina bifida) 741.0 ☑
  - acquired 331.4
- artery 447.1
  - basilar — see Narrowing, artery, basilar
  - carotid (common) (internal) — see Narrowing, artery, carotid
  - celiac 447.4
  - cerebral 437.0
    - congenital 747.81
    - due to
      - embolism (see also Embolism, brain) 434.1 ☑
      - thrombus (see also Thrombosis, brain) 434.0 ☑
  - congenital (peripheral) 747.60
    - cerebral 747.81
    - coronary 746.85
    - gastrointestinal 747.61
    - lower limb 747.64
    - renal 747.62
    - retinal 743.58
    - specified NEC 747.69
    - spinal 747.82
    - umbilical 747.5
    - upper limb 747.63
  - coronary — see Arteriosclerosis, coronary
    - congenital 746.85
  - precerebral — see Narrowing, artery, precerebral NEC
  - pulmonary (congenital) 747.3
    - acquired 417.8
  - renal 440.1
  - vertebral — see Narrowing, artery, vertebral
- auditory canal (congenital) (external) 744.02
  - acquired (see also Stricture, ear canal, acquired) 380.50
- bile duct or passage (any) (postoperative) (see also Obstruction, biliary) 576.2
  - congenital 751.61
- bladder 596.8
  - congenital 753.6
  - neck 596.0
    - congenital 753.6
- bowel (see also Obstruction, intestine) 560.9
- brain 348.8
- bronchus 519.19 ▲
  - syphilitic 095.8
- cardia (stomach) 537.89
  - congenital 750.7
- cardiac (see also Disease, heart)
  - orifice (stomach) 537.89
- cardiovascular (see also Disease, cardiovascular) 429.2
- carotid artery — see Narrowing, artery, carotid
- cecum (see also Obstruction, intestine) 560.9
- cervix, cervical (canal) 622.4
  - congenital 752.49
  - in pregnancy or childbirth 654.6 ☑
    - affecting fetus or newborn 763.89
    - causing obstructed labor 660.2 ☑
      - affecting fetus or newborn 763.1

Stricture — see also Stenosis —
continued
- colon (see also Obstruction, intestine) 560.9
  - congenital 751.2
- colostomy 569.62
- common bile duct (see also Obstruction, biliary) 576.2
  - congenital 751.61
- coronary (artery) — see Arteriosclerosis, coronary
  - congenital 746.85
- cystic duct (see also Obstruction, gallbladder) 575.2
  - congenital 751.61
- cystostomy 997.5
- digestive organs NEC, congenital 751.8
- duodenum 537.3
  - congenital 751.1
- ear canal (external) (congenital) 744.24
  - acquired 380.50
    - secondary to
      - inflammation 380.53
      - surgery 380.52
      - trauma 380.51
- ejaculatory duct 608.85
- enterostomy 569.62
- esophagostomy 530.87
- esophagus (corrosive) (peptic) 530.3
  - congenital 750.3
  - syphilitic 095.8
    - congenital 090.5
- eustachian tube (see also Obstruction, Eustachian tube) 381.60
  - congenital 744.24
- fallopian tube 628.2
  - gonococcal (chronic) 098.37
    - acute 098.17
  - tuberculous (see also Tuberculosis) 016.6 ☑
- gallbladder (see also Obstruction, gallbladder) 575.2
  - congenital 751.69
- glottis 478.74
- heart (see also Disease, heart)
  - congenital NEC 746.89
  - valve (see also Endocarditis)
    - congenital NEC 746.89
      - aortic 746.3
      - mitral 746.5
      - pulmonary 746.02
      - tricuspid 746.1
- hepatic duct (see also Obstruction, biliary) 576.2
- hourglass, of stomach 537.6
- hymen 623.3
- hypopharynx 478.29
- intestine (see also Obstruction, intestine) 560.9
  - congenital (small) 751.1
    - large 751.2
  - ischemic 557.1
- lacrimal
  - canaliculi 375.53
    - congenital 743.65
  - punctum 375.52
    - congenital 743.65
  - sac 375.54
    - congenital 743.65
- lacrimonasal duct 375.56
  - congenital 743.65
  - neonatal 375.55
- larynx 478.79
  - congenital 748.3
  - syphilitic 095.8
    - congenital 090.5
- lung 518.89
- meatus
  - ear (congenital) 744.02
    - acquired (see also Stricture, ear canal, acquired) 380.50
  - osseous (congenital) (ear) 744.03
    - acquired (see also Stricture, ear canal, acquired) 380.50

Stricture — see also Stenosis —
continued
- meatus — *continued*
  - urinarius (see also Stricture, urethra) 598.9
    - congenital 753.6
- mitral (valve) (see also Stenosis, mitral) 394.0
  - congenital 746.5
  - specified cause, except rheumatic 424.0
- myocardium, myocardial (see also Degeneration, myocardial) 429.1
  - hypertrophic subaortic (idiopathic) 425.1
- nares (anterior) (posterior) 478.19 ▲
  - congenital 748.0
- nasal duct 375.56
  - congenital 743.65
  - neonatal 375.55
- nasolacrimal duct 375.56
  - congenital 743.65
  - neonatal 375.55
- nasopharynx 478.29
  - syphilitic 095.8
- nephrostomy 997.5
- nose 478.19 ▲
  - congenital 748.0
- nostril (anterior) (posterior) 478.19 ▲
  - congenital 748.0
- organ or site, congenital NEC — see Atresia
- osseous meatus (congenital) (ear) 744.03
  - acquired (see also Stricture, ear canal, acquired) 380.50
- os uteri (see also Stricture, cervix) 622.4
- oviduct — see Stricture, fallopian tube
- pelviureteric junction 593.3
- pharynx (dilation) 478.29
- prostate 602.8
- pulmonary, pulmonic
  - artery (congenital) 747.3
    - acquired 417.8
    - noncongenital 417.8
  - infundibulum (congenital) 746.83
  - valve (see also Endocarditis, pulmonary) 424.3
    - congenital 746.02
  - vein (congenital) 747.49
    - acquired 417.8
  - vessel NEC 417.8
- punctum lacrimale 375.52
  - congenital 743.65
- pylorus (hypertrophic) 537.0
  - adult 537.0
  - congenital 750.5
  - infantile 750.5
- rectosigmoid 569.89
- rectum (sphincter) 569.2
  - congenital 751.2
  - due to
    - chemical burn 947.3
    - irradiation 569.2
    - lymphogranuloma venereum 099.1
  - gonococcal 098.7
  - inflammatory 099.1
  - syphilitic 095.8
  - tuberculous (see also Tuberculosis) 014.8 ☑
- renal artery 440.1
- salivary duct or gland (any) 527.8
- sigmoid (flexure) (see also Obstruction, intestine) 560.9
- spermatic cord 608.85
- stoma (following) (of)
  - colostomy 569.62
  - cystostomy 997.5
  - enterostomy 569.62
  - esophagostomy 530.87
  - gastrostomy 536.42
  - ileostomy 569.62

Stricture — see also Stenosis —
continued
- stoma — *continued*
  - nephrostomy 997.5
  - tracheostomy 519.02
  - ureterostomy 997.5
- stomach 537.89
  - congenital 750.7
  - hourglass 537.6
- subaortic 746.81
  - hypertrophic (acquired) (idiopathic) 425.1
- subglottic 478.74
- syphilitic NEC 095.8
- tendon (sheath) 727.81
- trachea 519.19 ▲
  - congenital 748.3
  - syphilitic 095.8
  - tuberculous (see also Tuberculosis) 012.8 ☑
- tracheostomy 519.02
- tricuspid (valve) (see also Endocarditis, tricuspid) 397.0
  - congenital 746.1
  - nonrheumatic 424.2
- tunica vaginalis 608.85
- ureter (postoperative) 593.3
  - congenital 753.29
  - tuberculous (see also Tuberculosis) 016.2 ☑
- ureteropelvic junction 593.3
  - congenital 753.21
- ureterovesical orifice 593.3
  - congenital 753.22
- urethra (anterior) (meatal) (organic) (posterior) (spasmodic) 598.9
  - associated with schistosomiasis (see also Schistosomiasis) 120.9 [598.01]
  - congenital (valvular) 753.6
  - due to
    - infection 598.00
      - syphilis 095.8 [598.01]
    - trauma 598.1
  - gonococcal 098.2 [598.01]
  - gonorrheal 098.2 [598.01]
  - infective 598.00
  - late effect of injury 598.1
  - postcatheterization 598.2
  - postobstetric 598.1
  - postoperative 598.2
  - specified cause NEC 598.8
  - syphilitic 095.8 [598.01]
  - traumatic 598.1
  - valvular, congenital 753.6
- urinary meatus (see also Stricture, urethra) 598.9
  - congenital 753.6
- uterus, uterine 621.5
  - os (external) (internal) — see Stricture, cervix
- vagina (outlet) 623.2
  - congenital 752.49
- valve (cardiac) (heart) (see also Endocarditis) 424.90
  - congenital (cardiac) (heart) NEC 746.89
    - aortic 746.3
    - mitral 746.5
    - pulmonary 746.02
    - tricuspid 746.1
  - urethra 753.6
- valvular (see also Endocarditis) 424.90
- vascular graft or shunt 996.1
  - atherosclerosis — see Arteriosclerosis, extremities
  - embolism 996.74
  - occlusion NEC 996.74
  - thrombus 996.74
- vas deferens 608.85
  - congenital 752.89
- vein 459.2
- vena cava (inferior) (superior) NEC 459.2
  - congenital 747.49

Stricture — see also Stenosis — continued
  ventricular shunt 996.2
  vesicourethral orifice 596.0
    congenital 753.6
  vulva (acquired) 624.8
Stridor 786.1
  congenital (larynx) 748.3
Stridulous — see condition
Stripping of nails 703.8
Stroke 434.91
  apoplectic (see also Disease, cerebrovascular, acute) 436
  brain — see Infarct, brain
  embolic 434.11
  epileptic — see Epilepsy
  healed or old V12.59
  heart — see Disease, heart
  heat 992.0
  hemorrhagic — see Hemorrhage, brain
  iatrogenic 997.02
  in evolution 435.9
  ischemic 434.91
  late effect — see Late effect(s) (of) cerebrovascular disease
  lightning 994.0
  paralytic — see Infarct, brain
  postoperative 997.02
  progressive 435.9
  thrombotic 434.01
Stromatosis, endometrial (M8931/1) 236.0
Strong pulse 785.9
Strongyloides stercoralis infestation 127.2
Strongyloidiasis 127.2
Strongyloidosis 127.2
Strongylus (gibsoni) infestation 127.7
Strophulus (newborn) 779.89
  pruriginosus 698.2
Struck by lightning 994.0
Struma — see also Goiter 240.9
  fibrosa 245.3
  Hashimoto (struma lymphomatosa) 245.2
  lymphomatosa 245.2
  nodosa (simplex) 241.9
    endemic 241.0
    multinodular 241.1
    sporadic 241.9
    toxic or with hyperthyroidism 242.3 ☑
      multinodular 242.2 ☑
      uninodular 242.1 ☑
    toxicosa 242.3 ☑
      multinodular 242.2 ☑
      uninodular 242.1 ☑
    uninodular 241.0
  ovarii (M9090/0) 220
    and carcinoid (M9091/1) 236.2
    malignant (M9090/3) 183.0
  Riedel's (ligneous thyroiditis) 245.3
  scrofulous (see also Tuberculosis) 017.2 ☑
  tuberculous (see also Tuberculosis) 017.2 ☑
    abscess 017.2 ☑
    adenitis 017.2 ☑
    lymphangitis 017.2 ☑
    ulcer 017.2 ☑
Strumipriva cachexia — see also Hypothyroidism 244.9
Strümpell-Marie disease or spine (ankylosing spondylitis) 720.0
Strümpell-Westphal pseudosclerosis (hepatolenticular degeneration) 275.1
Stuart's disease (congenital factor X deficiency) — see also Defect, coagulation 286.3
Stuart-Prower factor deficiency (congenital factor X deficiency) — see also Defect, coagulation 286.3
Students' elbow 727.2
Stuffy nose 478.19 ▲
Stump — see also Amputation

Stump — see also Amputation — continued
  cervix, cervical (healed) 622.8
Stupor 780.09
  catatonic (see also Schizophrenia) 295.2 ☑
  circular (see also Psychosis, manic-depressive, circular) 296.7
  manic 296.89
  manic-depressive (see also Psychosis, affective) 296.89
  mental (anergic) (delusional) 298.9
  psychogenic 298.8
  reaction to exceptional stress (transient) 308.2
  traumatic NEC (see also Injury, intracranial)
    with spinal (cord)
      lesion — see Injury, spinal, by site
      shock — see Injury, spinal, by site
Sturge (-Weber) (-Dimitri) disease or syndrome (encephalocutaneous angiomatosis) 759.6
Sturge-Kalischer-Weber syndrome (encephalocutaneous angiomatosis) 759.6
Stuttering 307.0
Sty, stye 373.11
  external 373.11
  internal 373.12
  meibomian 373.12
Subacidity, gastric 536.8
  psychogenic 306.4
Subacute — see condition
Subarachnoid — see condition
Subclavian steal syndrome 435.2
Subcortical — see condition
Subcostal syndrome 098.86
  nerve compression 354.8
Subcutaneous, subcuticular — see condition
Subdelirium 293.1
Subdural — see condition
Subendocardium — see condition
Subependymoma (M9383/1) 237.5
Suberosis 495.3
Subglossitis — see Glossitis
Subhemophilia 286.0
Subinvolution (uterus) 621.1
  breast (postlactational) (postpartum) 611.8
  chronic 621.1
  puerperal, postpartum 674.8 ☑
Sublingual — see condition
Sublinguitis 527.2
Subluxation — see also Dislocation, by site
  congenital NEC (see also Malposition, congenital)
    hip (unilateral) 754.32
      with dislocation of other hip 754.35
      bilateral 754.33
    joint
      lower limb 755.69
      shoulder 755.59
      upper limb 755.59
    lower limb (joint) 755.69
    shoulder (joint) 755.59
    upper limb (joint) 755.59
  lens 379.32
    anterior 379.33
    posterior 379.34
  rotary, cervical region of spine — see Fracture, vertebra, cervical
Submaxillary — see condition
Submersion (fatal) (nonfatal) 994.1
Submissiveness (undue), in child 313.0
Submucous — see condition
Subnormal, subnormality
  accommodation (see also Disorder, accommodation) 367.9
  mental (see also Retardation, mental) 319

Subnormal, subnormality — continued
  mental (see also Retardation, mental) — continued
    mild 317
    moderate 318.0
    profound 318.2
    severe 318.1
  temperature (accidental) 991.6
    not associated with low environmental temperature 780.99
Subphrenic — see condition
Subscapular nerve — see condition
Subseptus uterus 752.3
Subsiding appendicitis 542
Substernal thyroid — see also Goiter 240.9
  congenital 759.2
Substitution disorder 300.11
Subtentorial — see condition
Subtertian
  fever 084.0
  malaria (fever) 084.0
Subthyroidism (acquired) — see also Hypothyroidism 244.9
  congenital 243
Succenturiata placenta — see Placenta, abnormal
Succussion sounds, chest 786.7
Sucking thumb, child 307.9
Sudamen 705.1
Sudamina 705.1
Sudanese kala-azar 085.0
Sudden
  death, cause unknown (less than 24 hours) 798.1
    during childbirth 669.9 ☑
    infant 798.0
    puerperal, postpartum 674.9 ☑
  hearing loss NEC 388.2
  heart failure (see also Failure, heart) 428.9
  infant death syndrome 798.0
Sudeck's atrophy, disease, or syndrome 733.7
SUDS (sudden unexplained death) 798.2
Suffocation — see also Asphyxia 799.01
  by
    bed clothes 994.7
    bunny bag 994.7
    cave-in 994.7
    constriction 994.7
    drowning 994.1
    inhalation
      food or foreign body (see also Asphyxia, food or foreign body) 933.1
      oil or gasoline (see also Asphyxia, food or foreign body) 933.1
    overlying 994.7
    plastic bag 994.7
    pressure 994.7
    strangulation 994.7
  during birth 768.1
  mechanical 994.7
Sugar
  blood
    high 790.29
    low 251.2
  in urine 791.5
Suicide, suicidal (attempted)
  by poisoning — see Table of Drugs and Chemicals
  ideation V62.84
  risk 300.9
  tendencies 300.9
  trauma NEC (see also nature and site of injury) 959.9
Suipestifer infection — see also Infection, Salmonella 003.9
Sulfatidosis 330.0
Sulfhemoglobinemia, sulphemoglobinemia (acquired) (congenital) 289.7
Sumatran mite fever 081.2
Summer — see condition

Sunburn 692.71
  first degree 692.71
  second degree 692.76
  third degree 692.77
  dermatitis 692.71
  due to
    other ultraviolet radiation 692.82
    tanning bed 692.82
Sunken
  acetabulum 718.85
  fontanels 756.0
Sunstroke 992.0
Superfecundation 651.9 ☑
  with fetal loss and retention of one or more fetus(es) 651.6 ☑
  following (elective) fetal reduction 651.7 ☑
Superfetation 651.9 ☑
  with fetal loss and retention of one or more fetus(es) 651.6 ☑
  following (elective) fetal reduction 651.7 ☑
Superinvolution uterus 621.8
Supernumerary (congenital)
  aortic cusps 746.89
  auditory ossicles 744.04
  bone 756.9
  breast 757.6
  carpal bones 755.56
  cusps, heart valve NEC 746.89
    mitral 746.5
    pulmonary 746.09
  digit(s) 755.00
    finger 755.01
    toe 755.02
  ear (lobule) 744.1
  fallopian tube 752.19
  finger 755.01
  hymen 752.49
  kidney 753.3
  lacrimal glands 743.64
  lacrimonasal duct 743.65
  lobule (ear) 744.1
  mitral cusps 746.5
  muscle 756.82
  nipples 757.6
  organ or site NEC — see Accessory
  ossicles, auditory 744.04
  ovary 752.0
  oviduct 752.19
  pulmonic cusps 746.09
  rib 756.3
    cervical or first 756.2
      syndrome 756.2
  roots (of teeth) 520.2
  spinal vertebra 756.19
  spleen 759.0
  tarsal bones 755.67
  teeth 520.1
    causing crowding 524.31
  testis 752.89
  thumb 755.01
  toe 755.02
  uterus 752.2
  vagina 752.49
  vertebra 756.19
Supervision (of)
  contraceptive method previously prescribed V25.40
    intrauterine device V25.42
    oral contraceptive (pill) V25.41
    specified type NEC V25.49
    subdermal implantable contraceptive V25.43
  dietary (for) V65.3
    allergy (food) V65.3
    colitis V65.3
    diabetes mellitus V65.3
    food allergy intolerance V65.3
    gastritis V65.3
    hypercholesterolemia V65.3
    hypoglycemia V65.3
    intolerance (food) V65.3
    obesity V65.3
    specified NEC V65.3
  lactation V24.1

Supervision — *continued*
  pregnancy — *see* Pregnancy, supervision of
Supplemental teeth 520.1
  causing crowding 524.31
Suppression
  binocular vision 368.31
  lactation 676.5 ☑
  menstruation 626.8
  ovarian secretion 256.39
  renal 586
  urinary secretion 788.5
  urine 788.5
Suppuration, suppurative — *see also* condition
  accessory sinus (chronic) (*see also* Sinusitis) 473.9
  adrenal gland 255.8
  antrum (chronic) (*see also* Sinusitis, maxillary) 473.0
  bladder (*see also* Cystitis) 595.89
  bowel 569.89
  brain 324.0
    late effect 326
  breast 611.0
    puerperal, postpartum 675.1 ☑
  dental periosteum 526.5
  diffuse (skin) 686.00
  ear (middle) (*see also* Otitis media) 382.4
    external (*see also* Otitis, externa) 380.10
    internal 386.33
  ethmoidal (sinus) (chronic) (*see also* Sinusitis, ethmoidal) 473.2
  fallopian tube (*see also* Salpingo-oophoritis) 614.2
  frontal (sinus) (chronic) (*see also* Sinusitis, frontal) 473.1
  gallbladder (*see also* Cholecystitis, acute) 575.0
  gum 523.30 ▲
  hernial sac — *see* Hernia, by site
  intestine 569.89
  joint (*see also* Arthritis, suppurative) 711.0 ☑
  labyrinthine 386.33
  lung 513.0
  mammary gland 611.0
    puerperal, postpartum 675.1 ☑
  maxilla, maxillary 526.4
    sinus (chronic) (*see also* Sinusitis, maxillary) 473.0
  muscle 728.0
  nasal sinus (chronic) (*see also* Sinusitis) 473.9
  pancreas 577.0
  parotid gland 527.2
  pelvis, pelvic
    female (*see also* Disease, pelvis, inflammatory) 614.4
      acute 614.3
    male (*see also* Peritonitis) 567.21
  pericranial (*see also* Osteomyelitis) 730.2 ☑
  salivary duct or gland (any) 527.2
  sinus (nasal) (*see also* Sinusitis) 473.9
  sphenoidal (sinus) (chronic) (*see also* Sinusitis, sphenoidal) 473.3
  thymus (gland) 254.1
  thyroid (gland) 245.0
  tonsil 474.8
  uterus (*see also* Endometritis) 615.9
  vagina 616.10
  wound (*see also* Wound, open, by site, complicated)
    dislocation — *see* Dislocation, by site, compound
    fracture — *see* Fracture, by site, open
    scratch or other superficial injury — *see* Injury, superficial, by site
Supraeruption, teeth 524.34
Supraglottitis 464.50
  with obstruction 464.51
Suprapubic drainage 596.8
Suprarenal (gland) — *see* condition
Suprascapular nerve — *see* condition
Suprasellar — *see* condition
Supraspinatus syndrome 726.10
Surfer knots 919.8
  infected 919.9
Surgery
  cosmetic NEC V50.1
    following healed injury or operation V51
    hair transplant V50.0
  elective V50.9
    breast augmentation or reduction V50.1
    circumcision, ritual or routine (in absence of medical indication) V50.2
    cosmetic NEC V50.1
    ear piercing V50.3
    face-lift V50.1
    following healed injury or operation V51
    hair transplant V50.0
  not done because of
    contraindication V64.1
    patient's decision V64.2
    specified reason NEC V64.3
  plastic
    breast augmentation or reduction V50.1
    cosmetic V50.1
    face-lift V50.1
    following healed injury or operation V51
    repair of scarred tissue (following healed injury or operation) V51
    specified type NEC V50.8
  previous, in pregnancy or childbirth
    cervix 654.6 ☑
      affecting fetus or newborn 763.89
      causing obstructed labor 660.2 ☑
        affecting fetus or newborn 763.1
    pelvic soft tissues NEC 654.9 ☑
      affecting fetus or newborn 763.89
      causing obstructed labor 660.2 ☑
        affecting fetus or newborn 763.1
    perineum or vulva 654.8 ☑
    uterus NEC 654.9 ☑
      affecting fetus or newborn 763.89
      causing obstructed labor 660.2 ☑
        affecting fetus or newborn 763.1
      due to previous cesarean delivery 654.2 ☑
    vagina 654.7 ☑
Surgical
  abortion — *see* Abortion, legal
  emphysema 998.81
  kidney (*see also* Pyelitis) 590.80
  operation NEC 799.9
  procedures, complication or misadventure — *see* Complications, surgical procedure
  shock 998.0
Susceptibility
  genetic
    to
      neoplasm
        malignant, of
          breast V84.01
          endometrium V84.04
          other V84.09
          ovary V84.02
          prostate V84.03
        other disease V84.8
Suspected condition, ruled out — *see also* Observation, suspected V71.9
  specified condition NEC V71.89
Suspended uterus, in pregnancy or childbirth 654.4 ☑
  affecting fetus or newborn 763.89
  causing obstructed labor 660.2 ☑
    affecting fetus or newborn 763.1
Sutton and Gull's disease (arteriolar nephrosclerosis) — *see also* Hypertension, kidney 403.90
Sutton's disease 709.09
Suture
  burst (in external operation wound) 998.32
    internal 998.31
  inadvertently left in operation wound 998.4
  removal V58.32 ▲
  Shirodkar, in pregnancy (with or without cervical incompetence) 654.5 ☑
Swab inadvertently left in operation wound 998.4
Swallowed, swallowing
  difficulty (*see also* Dysphagia) 787.2
  foreign body NEC (*see also* Foreign body) 938
Swamp fever 100.89
Swan neck hand (intrinsic) 736.09
Sweat(s), sweating
  disease or sickness 078.2
  excessive (*see also* Hyperhidrosis) 780.8
  fetid 705.89
  fever 078.2
  gland disease 705.9
    specified type NEC 705.89
  miliary 078.2
  night 780.8
Sweeley-Klionsky disease (angiokeratoma corporis diffusum) 272.7
Sweet's syndrome (acute febrile neutrophilic dermatosis) 695.89
Swelling
  abdominal (not referable to specific organ) 789.3 ☑
  adrenal gland, cloudy 255.8
  ankle 719.07
  anus 787.99
  arm 729.81
  breast 611.72
  Calabar 125.2
  cervical gland 785.6
  cheek 784.2
  chest 786.6
  ear 388.8
  epigastric 789.3 ☑
  extremity (lower) (upper) 729.81
  eye 379.92
  female genital organ 625.8
  finger 729.81
  foot 729.81
  glands 785.6
  gum 784.2
  hand 729.81
  head 784.2
  inflammatory — *see* Inflammation
  joint (*see also* Effusion, joint) 719.0 ☑
    tuberculous — *see* Tuberculosis, joint
  kidney, cloudy 593.89
  leg 729.81
  limb 729.81
  liver 573.8
  lung 786.6
  lymph nodes 785.6
  mediastinal 786.6
  mouth 784.2
  muscle (limb) 729.81
  neck 784.2
  nose or sinus 784.2
  palate 784.2
  pelvis 789.3 ☑
  penis 607.83
  perineum 625.8
Swelling — *continued*
  rectum 787.99
  scrotum 608.86
  skin 782.2
  splenic (*see also* Splenomegaly) 789.2
  substernal 786.6
  superficial, localized (skin) 782.2
  testicle 608.86
  throat 784.2
  toe 729.81
  tongue 784.2
  tubular (*see also* Disease, renal) 593.9
  umbilicus 789.3 ☑
  uterus 625.8
  vagina 625.8
  vulva 625.8
  wandering, due to Gnathostoma (spinigerum) 128.1
  white — *see* Tuberculosis, arthritis
Swift's disease 985.0
Swimmers'
  ear (acute) 380.12
  itch 120.3
Swimming in the head 780.4
Swollen — *see also* Swelling
  glands 785.6
Swyer-James syndrome (unilateral hyperlucent lung) 492.8
Swyer's syndrome (XY pure gonadal dysgenesis) 752.7
Sycosis 704.8
  barbae (not parasitic) 704.8
  contagiosa 110.0
  lupoid 704.8
  mycotic 110.0
  parasitic 110.0
  vulgaris 704.8
Sydenham's chorea — *see* Chorea, Sydenham's
Sylvatic yellow fever 060.0
Sylvest's disease (epidemic pleurodynia) 074.1
Symblepharon 372.63
  congenital 743.62
Symonds' syndrome 348.2
Sympathetic — *see* condition
Sympatheticotonia — *see also* Neuropathy, peripheral, autonomic 337.9
Sympathicoblastoma (M9500/3)
  specified site — *see* Neoplasm, by site, malignant
  unspecified site 194.0
Sympathicogonioma (M9500/3) — *see* Sympathicoblastoma
Sympathoblastoma (M9500/3) — *see* Sympathicoblastoma
Sympathogonioma (M9500/3) — *see* Sympathicoblastoma
Symphalangy — *see also* Syndactylism 755.10
Symptoms, specified (general) NEC 780.99
  abdomen NEC 789.9
  bone NEC 733.90
  breast NEC 611.79
  cardiac NEC 785.9
  cardiovascular NEC 785.9
  chest NEC 786.9
  development NEC 783.9
  digestive system NEC 787.99
  eye NEC 379.99
  gastrointestinal tract NEC 787.99
  genital organs NEC
    female 625.9
    male 608.9
  head and neck NEC 784.99 ▲
  heart NEC 785.9
  joint NEC 719.60
    ankle 719.67
    elbow 719.62
    foot 719.67
    hand 719.64
    hip 719.65
    knee 719.66
    multiple sites 719.69
    pelvic region 719.65

Index to Diseases

Symptoms, specified — continued
- joint — continued
  - shoulder (region) 719.61
  - specified site NEC 719.68
  - wrist 719.63
- larynx NEC 784.99 ▲
- limbs NEC 729.89
- lymphatic system NEC 785.9
- menopausal 627.2
- metabolism NEC 783.9
- mouth NEC 528.9
- muscle NEC 728.9
- musculoskeletal NEC 781.99
  - limbs NEC 729.89
- nervous system NEC 781.99
- neurotic NEC 300.9
- nutrition, metabolism, and development NEC 783.9
- pelvis NEC 789.9
  - female 625.9
- peritoneum NEC 789.9
- respiratory system NEC 786.9
- skin and integument NEC 782.9
- subcutaneous tissue NEC 782.9
- throat NEC 784.99 ▲
- tonsil NEC 784.99 ▲
- urinary system NEC 788.9
- vascular NEC 785.9

Sympus 759.89

Synarthrosis 719.80
- ankle 719.87
- elbow 719.82
- foot 719.87
- hand 719.84
- hip 719.85
- knee 719.86
- multiple sites 719.89
- pelvic region 719.85
- shoulder (region) 719.81
- specified site NEC 719.88
- wrist 719.83

Syncephalus 759.4

Synchondrosis 756.9
- abnormal (congenital) 756.9
- ischiopubic (van Neck's) 732.1

Synchysis (senile) (vitreous humor) 379.21
- scintillans 379.22

Syncope (near) (pre-) 780.2
- anginosa 413.9
- bradycardia 427.89
- cardiac 780.2
- carotid sinus 337.0
- complicating delivery 669.2 ☑
- due to lumbar puncture 349.0
- fatal 798.1
- heart 780.2
- heat 992.1
- laryngeal 786.2
- tussive 786.2
- vasoconstriction 780.2
- vasodepressor 780.2
- vasomotor 780.2
- vasovagal 780.2

Syncytial infarct — see Placenta, abnormal

Syndactylism, syndactyly (multiple sites) 755.10
- fingers (without fusion of bone) 755.11
  - with fusion of bone 755.12
- toes (without fusion of bone) 755.13
  - with fusion of bone 755.14

Syndrome — see also Disease
- with 5q deletion 238.74 ●
- 5q minus 238.74 ●
- abdominal
  - acute 789.0 ☑
  - migraine 346.2 ☑
  - muscle deficiency 756.79
- Abercrombie's (amyloid degeneration) 277.39 ▲
- abnormal innervation 374.43
- abstinence
  - alcohol 291.81
  - drug 292.0

Syndrome — see also Disease — continued
- Abt-Letterer-Siwe (acute histiocytosis X) (M9722/3) 202.5 ☑
- Achard-Thiers (adrenogenital) 255.2
- acid pulmonary aspiration 997.3
  - obstetric (Mendelson's) 668.0 ☑
- acquired immune deficiency 042
- acquired immunodeficiency 042
- acrocephalosyndactylism 755.55
- acute abdominal 789.0 ☑
- acute chest 517.3
- acute coronary 411.1
- Adair-Dighton (brittle bones and blue sclera, deafness) 756.51
- Adams-Stokes (-Morgagni) (syncope with heart block) 426.9
- addisonian 255.4
- Adie (-Holmes) (pupil) 379.46
- adiposogenital 253.8
- adrenal
  - hemorrhage 036.3
  - meningococcic 036.3
- adrenocortical 255.3
- adrenogenital (acquired) (congenital) 255.2
  - feminizing 255.2
  - iatrogenic 760.79
  - virilism (acquired) (congenital) 255.2
- affective organic NEC 293.89
  - drug-induced 292.84
- afferent loop NEC 537.89
- African macroglobulinemia 273.3
- Ahumada-Del Castillo (nonpuerperal galactorrhea and amenorrhea) 253.1
- air blast concussion — see Injury, internal, by site
- Alagille 759.89
- Albright (-Martin) (pseudohypoparathyroidism) 275.49
- Albright-McCune-Sternberg (osteitis fibrosa disseminata) 756.59
- alcohol withdrawal 291.81
- Alder's (leukocyte granulation anomaly) 288.2
- Aldrich (-Wiskott) (eczema-thrombocytopenia) 279.12
- Alibert-Bazin (mycosis fungoides) (M9700/3) 202.1 ☑
- Alice in Wonderland 293.89
- Allen-Masters 620.6
- Alligator baby (ichthyosis congenita) 757.1
- Alport's (hereditary hematuria-nephropathy-deafness) 759.89
- Alvarez (transient cerebral ischemia) 435.9
- alveolar capillary block 516.3
- Alzheimer's 331.0
  - with dementia — see Alzheimer's, dementia
- amnestic (confabulatory) 294.0
  - alcohol-induced persisting 291.1
  - drug-induced 292.83
  - posttraumatic 294.0
- amotivational 292.89
- amyostatic 275.1
- amyotrophic lateral sclerosis 335.20
- androgen insensitivity 259.5
- Angelman 759.89
- angina (see also Angina) 413.9
- ankyloglossia superior 750.0
- anterior
  - chest wall 786.52
  - compartment (tibial) 958.8
  - spinal artery 433.8 ☑
    - compression 721.1
  - tibial (compartment) 958.8
- antibody deficiency 279.00
  - agammaglobulinemic 279.00
  - congenital 279.00
  - hypogammaglobulinemic 279.00
- anticardiolipin antibody 795.79
- antimongolism 758.39

Syndrome — see also Disease — continued
- antiphospholipid antibody 795.79
- Anton (-Babinski) (hemiasomatognosia) 307.9
- anxiety (see also Anxiety) 300.00
  - organic 293.84
- aortic
  - arch 446.7
  - bifurcation (occlusion) 444.0
  - ring 747.21
- Apert's (acrocephalosyndactyly) 755.55
- Apert-Gallais (adrenogenital) 255.2
- aphasia-apraxia-alexia 784.69
- apical ballooning 429.83 ▲
- "approximate answers" 300.16
- arcuate ligament (-celiac axis) 447.4
- arcus aortae 446.7
- arc welders' 370.24
- argentaffin, argintaffinoma 259.2
- Argonz-Del Castillo (nonpuerperal galactorrhea and amenorrhea) 253.1
- Argyll Robertson's (syphilitic) 094.89
  - nonsyphilitic 379.45
- Armenian 277.31 ●
- arm-shoulder (see also Neuropathy, peripheral, autonomic) 337.9
- Arnold-Chiari (see also Spina bifida) 741.0 ☑
  - type I 348.4
  - type II 741.0 ☑
  - type III 742.0
  - type IV 742.2
- Arrillaga-Ayerza (pulmonary artery sclerosis with pulmonary hypertension) 416.0
- arteriomesenteric duodenum occlusion 537.89
- arteriovenous steal 996.73
- arteritis, young female (obliterative brachiocephalic) 446.7
- aseptic meningitis — see Meningitis, aseptic
- Asherman's 621.5
- Asperger's 299.8 ☑
- asphyctic (see also Anxiety) 300.00
- aspiration, of newborn (massive) 770.18
  - meconium 770.12
- ataxia-telangiectasia 334.8
- Audry's (acropachyderma) 757.39
- auriculotemporal 350.8
- autosomal (see also Abnormal, autosomes NEC)
  - deletion 758.39
    - 5p 758.31
    - 22q11.2 758.32
- Avellis' 344.89
- Axenfeld's 743.44
- Ayerza (-Arrillaga) (pulmonary artery sclerosis with pulmonary hypertension) 416.0
- Baader's (erythema multiforme exudativum) 695.1
- Baastrup's 721.5
- Babinski (-Vaquez) (cardiovascular syphilis) 093.89
- Babinski-Fröhlich (adiposogenital dystrophy) 253.8
- Babinski-Nageotte 344.89
- Bagratuni's (temporal arteritis) 446.5
- Bakwin-Krida (craniometaphyseal dysplasia) 756.89
- Balint's (psychic paralysis of visual disorientation) 368.16
- Ballantyne (-Runge) (postmaturity) 766.22
- ballooning posterior leaflet 424.0
- Banti's — see Cirrhosis, liver
- Bardet-Biedl (obesity, polydactyly, and mental retardation) 759.89
- Bard-Pic's (carcinoma, head of pancreas) 157.0
- Barlow's (mitral valve prolapse) 424.0

Syndrome — see also Disease — continued
- Barlow (-Möller) (infantile scurvy) 267
- Baron Munchausen's 301.51
- Barré-Guillain 357.0
- Barré-Liéou (posterior cervical sympathetic) 723.2
- Barrett's (chronic peptic ulcer of esophagus) 530.85
- Bársony-Polgár (corkscrew esophagus) 530.5
- Bársony-Teschendorf (corkscrew esophagus) 530.5
- Barth 759.89
- Bartter's (secondary hyperaldosteronism with juxtaglomerular hyperplasia) 255.13
- Basedow's (exophthalmic goiter) 242.0
- basilar artery 435.0
- basofrontal 377.04
- Bassen-Kornzweig (abetalipoproteinemia) 272.5
- Batten-Steinert 359.2
- battered
  - adult 995.81
  - baby or child 995.54
  - spouse 995.81
- Baumgarten-Cruveilhier (cirrhosis of liver) 571.5
- Beals 759.82
- Bearn-Kunkel (-Slater) (lupoid hepatitis) 571.49
- Beau's (see also Degeneration, myocardial) 429.1
- Bechterew-Strümpell-Marie (ankylosing spondylitis) 720.0
- Beck's (anterior spinal artery occlusion) 433.8 ☑
- Beckwith (-Wiedemann) 759.89
- Behçet's 136.1
- Bekhterev-Strümpell-Marie (ankylosing spondylitis) 720.0
- Benedikt's 344.89
- Béquez César (-Steinbrinck-Chédiak-Higashi) (congenital gigantism of peroxidase granules) 288.2
- Bernard-Horner (see also Neuropathy, peripheral, autonomic) 337.9
- Bernard-Sergent (acute adrenocortical insufficiency) 255.4
- Bernhardt-Roth 355.1
- Bernheim's (see also Failure, heart) 428.0
- Bertolotti's (sacralization of fifth lumbar vertebra) 756.15
- Besnier-Boeck-Schaumann (sarcoidosis) 135
- Bianchi's (aphasia-apraxia-alexia syndrome) 784.69
- Biedl-Bardet (obesity, polydactyly, and mental retardation) 759.89
- Biemond's (obesity, polydactyly, and mental retardation) 759.89
- big spleen 289.4
- bilateral polycystic ovarian 256.4
- Bing-Horton's 346.2 ☑
- Biörck (-Thorson) (malignant carcinoid) 259.2
- Blackfan-Diamond (congenital hypoplastic anemia) 284.01 ▲
- black lung 500
- black widow spider bite 989.5
- bladder neck (see also Incontinence, urine) 788.30
- blast (concussion) — see Blast, injury
- blind loop (postoperative) 579.2
- Bloch-Siemens (incontinentia pigmenti) 757.33
- Bloch-Sulzberger (incontinentia pigmenti) 757.33
- Bloom (-Machacek) (-Torre) 757.39
- Blount-Barber (tibia vara) 732.4
- blue
  - bloater 491.20

Syndrome

Syndrome — see also Disease — continued
- blue — continued
  - bloater — continued
    - with
      - acute bronchitis 491.22
      - exacerbation (acute) 491.21
    - diaper 270.0
    - drum 381.02
    - sclera 756.51
    - toe 445.02
- Boder-Sedgwick (ataxia-telangiectasia) 334.8
- Boerhaave's (spontaneous esophageal rupture) 530.4
- Bonnevie-Ullrich 758.6
- Bonnier's 386.19
- Borjeson-Forssman-Lehmann 759.89
- Bouillaud's (rheumatic heart disease) 391.9
- Bourneville (-Pringle) (tuberous sclerosis) 759.5
- Bouveret (-Hoffmann) (paroxysmal tachycardia) 427.2
- brachial plexus 353.0
- Brachman-de Lange (Amsterdam dwarf, mental retardation, and brachycephaly) 759.89
- bradycardia-tachycardia 427.81
- Brailsford-Morquio (dystrophy) (mucopolysaccharidosis IV) 277.5
- brain (acute) (chronic) (nonpsychotic) (organic) (with behavioral reaction) (with neurotic reaction) 310.9
  - with
    - presenile brain disease (see also Dementia, presenile) 290.10
    - psychosis, psychotic reaction (see also Psychosis, organic) 294.9
  - chronic alcoholic 291.2
  - congenital (see also Retardation, mental) 319
  - postcontusional 310.2
  - posttraumatic
    - nonpsychotic 310.2
    - psychotic 293.9
      - acute 293.0
      - chronic (see also Psychosis, organic) 294.8
      - subacute 293.1
  - psycho-organic (see also Syndrome, psycho-organic) 310.9
  - psychotic (see also Psychosis, organic) 294.9
  - senile (see also Dementia, senile) 290.0
- branchial arch 744.41
- Brandt's (acrodermatitis enteropathica) 686.8
- Brennemann's 289.2
- Briquet's 300.81
- Brissaud-Meige (infantile myxedema) 244.9
- broad ligament laceration 620.6
- Brock's (atelectasis due to enlarged lymph nodes) 518.0
- broken heart 429.83
- Brown-Séquard 344.89
- brown spot 756.59
- Brown's tendon sheath 378.61
- Brugada 746.89
- Brugsch's (acropachyderma) 757.39
- bubbly lung 770.7
- Buchem's (hyperostosis corticalis) 733.3
- Budd-Chiari (hepatic vein thrombosis) 453.0
- Büdinger-Ludloff-Läwen 717.89
- bulbar 335.22
  - lateral (see also Disease, cerebrovascular, acute) 436

Syndrome — see also Disease — continued
- Bullis fever 082.8
- bundle of Kent (anomalous atrioventricular excitation) 426.7
- Bürger-Grütz (essential familial hyperlipemia) 272.3
- Burke's (pancreatic insufficiency and chronic neutropenia) 577.8
- Burnett's (milk-alkali) 275.42
- Burnier's (hypophyseal dwarfism) 253.3
- burning feet 266.2
- Bywaters' 958.5
- Caffey's (infantile cortical hyperostosis) 756.59
- Calvé-Legg-Perthes (osteochondrosis, femoral capital) 732.1
- Caplan (-Colinet) syndrome 714.81
- capsular thrombosis (see also Thrombosis, brain) 434.0
- carbohydrate-deficient glycoprotein (CDGS) 271.8
- carcinogenic thrombophlebitis 453.1
- carcinoid 259.2
- cardiac asthma (see also Failure, ventricular, left) 428.1
- cardiacos negros 416.0
- cardiopulmonary obesity 278.8
- cardiorenal (see also Hypertension, cardiorenal) 404.90
- cardiorespiratory distress (idiopathic), newborn 769
- cardiovascular renal (see also Hypertension, cardiorenal) 404.90
- cardiovasorenal 272.7
- Carini's (ichthyosis congenita) 757.1
- carotid
  - artery (internal) 435.8
  - body or sinus 337.0
- carpal tunnel 354.0
- Carpenter's 759.89
- Cassidy (-Scholte) (malignant carcinoid) 259.2
- cat-cry 758.31
- cauda equina 344.60
- causalgia 355.9
  - lower limb 355.71
  - upper limb 354.4
- cavernous sinus 437.6
- celiac 579.0
  - artery compression 447.4
  - axis 447.4
- central pain 338.0
- cerebellomedullary malformation (see also Spina bifida) 741.0
- cerebral gigantism 253.0
- cerebrohepatorenal 759.89
- cervical (root) (spine) NEC 723.8
  - disc 722.71
  - posterior, sympathetic 723.2
  - rib 353.0
  - sympathetic paralysis 337.0
  - traumatic (acute) NEC 847.0
- cervicobrachial (diffuse) 723.3
- cervicocranial 723.2
- cervicodorsal outlet 353.2
- Céstan's 344.89
- Céstan (-Raymond) 433.8
- Céstan-Chenais 344.89
- chancriform 114.1
- Charcôt's (intermittent claudication) 443.9
  - angina cruris 443.9
  - due to atherosclerosis 440.21
- Charcôt-Marie-Tooth 356.1
- Charcôt-Weiss-Baker 337.0
- CHARGE association 759.89
- Cheadle (-Möller) (-Barlow) (infantile scurvy) 267
- Chédiak-Higashi (-Steinbrinck) (congenital gigantism of peroxidase granules) 288.2
- chest wall 786.52
- Chiari's (hepatic vein thrombosis) 453.0

Syndrome — see also Disease — continued
- Chiari-Frommel 676.6
- chiasmatic 368.41
- Chilaiditi's (subphrenic displacement, colon) 751.4
- chondroectodermal dysplasia 756.55
- chorea-athetosis-agitans 275.1
- Christian's (chronic histiocytosis X) 277.89
- chromosome 4 short arm deletion 758.39
- chronic pain 338.4
- Churg-Strauss 446.4
- Clarke-Hadfield (pancreatic infantilism) 577.8
- Claude's 352.6
- Claude Bernard-Horner (see also Neuropathy, peripheral, autonomic) 337.9
- Clérambault's
  - automatism 348.8
  - erotomania 297.8
- Clifford's (postmaturity) 766.22
- climacteric 627.2
- Clouston's (hidrotic ectodermal dysplasia) 757.31
- clumsiness 315.4
- Cockayne's (microencephaly and dwarfism) 759.89
- Cockayne-Weber (epidermolysis bullosa) 757.39
- Coffin-Lowry 759.89
- Cogan's (nonsyphilitic interstitial keratitis) 370.52
- cold injury (newborn) 778.2
- Collet (-Sicard) 352.6
- combined immunity deficiency 279.2
- compartment(al) (anterior) (deep) (posterior) 958.8
  - nontraumatic
    - abdomen 729.73
    - arm 729.71
    - buttock 729.72
    - fingers 729.71
    - foot 729.72
    - forearm 729.71
    - hand 729.71
    - hip 729.72
    - leg 729.72
    - lower extremity 729.72
    - shoulder 729.71
    - specified site NEC 729.79
    - thigh 729.72
    - toes 729.72
    - upper extremity 729.71
    - wrist 729.71
  - traumatic 958.90
    - adomen 958.93
    - arm 958.91
    - buttock 958.92
    - fingers 958.91
    - foot 958.92
    - forearm 958.91
    - hand 958.91
    - hip 958.92
    - leg 958.92
    - lower extremity 958.92
    - shoulder 958.91
    - specified site NEC 958.99
    - thigh 958.92
    - tibial 958.92
    - toes 958.92
    - upper extremity 958.91
    - wrist 958.91
- compression 958.5
  - cauda equina 344.60
    - with neurogenic bladder 344.61
- concussion 310.2
- congenital
  - affecting more than one system 759.7
  - specified type NEC 759.89
  - congenital central alveolar hypoventilation 327.25
  - facial diplegia 352.6

Syndrome — see also Disease — continued
- congenital — continued
  - muscular hypertrophy-cerebral 759.89
- congestion-fibrosis (pelvic) 625.5
- conjunctivourethrosynovial 099.3
- Conn (-Louis) (primary aldosteronism) 255.12
- Conradi (-Hünermann) (chondrodysplasia calcificans congenita) 756.59
- conus medullaris 336.8
- Cooke-Apert-Gallais (adrenogenital) 255.2
- Cornelia de Lange's (Amsterdam dwarf, mental retardation, and brachycephaly) 759.8
- coronary insufficiency or intermediate 411.1
- cor pulmonale 416.9
- corticosexual 255.2
- Costen's (complex) 524.60
- costochondral junction 733.6
- costoclavicular 353.0
- costovertebral 253.0
- Cotard's (paranoia) 297.1
- Cowden 759.6
- craniovertebral 723.2
- Creutzfeldt-Jakob (new variant) 046.1
  - with dementia
    - with behavioral disturbance 046.1 [294.11]
    - without behavioral disturbance 046.1 [294.10]
- crib death 798.0
- cricopharyngeal 787.2
- cri-du-chat 758.31
- Crigler-Najjar (congenital hyperbilirubinemia) 277.4
- crocodile tears 351.8
- Cronkhite-Canada 211.3
- croup 464.4
- CRST (cutaneous systemic sclerosis) 710.1
- crush 958.5
- crushed lung (see also Injury, internal, lung) 861.20
- Cruveilhier-Baumgarten (cirrhosis of liver) 571.5
- cubital tunnel 354.2
- Cuiffini-Pancoast (M8010/3) (carcinoma, pulmonary apex) 162.3
- Curschmann (-Batten) (-Steinert) 359.2
- Cushing's (iatrogenic) (idiopathic) (pituitary basophilism) (pituitary-dependent) 255.0
  - overdose or wrong substance given or taken 962.0
- Cyriax's (slipping rib) 733.99
- cystic duct stump 576.0
- Da Costa's (neurocirculatory asthenia) 306.2
- Dameshek's (erythroblastic anemia) 282.49
- Dana-Putnam (subacute combined sclerosis with pernicious anemia) 281.0 [336.2]
- Danbolt (-Closs) (acrodermatitis enteropathica) 686.8
- Dandy-Walker (atresia, foramen of Magendie) 742.3
  - with spina bifida (see also Spina bifida) 741.0
- Danlos' 756.83
- Davies-Colley (slipping rib) 733.99
- dead fetus 641.3
- defeminization 255.2
- defibrination (see also Fibrinolysis) 286.6
- Degos' 447.8
- Deiters' nucleus 386.19
- Déjérine-Roussy 338.0
- Déjérine-Thomas 333.0

Index to Diseases

Syndrome — see also Disease — continued

de Lange's (Amsterdam dwarf, mental retardation, and brachycephaly) (Cornelia) 759.89
Del Castillo's (germinal aplasia) 606.0
deletion chromosomes 758.39
delusional
 induced by drug 292.11
dementia-aphonia, of childhood (see also Psychosis, childhood) 299.1 ☑
demyelinating NEC 341.9
denial visual hallucination 307.9
depersonalization 300.6
Dercum's (adiposis dolorosa) 272.8
de Toni-Fanconi (-Debré) (cystinosis) 270.0
diabetes-dwarfism-obesity (juvenile) 258.1
diabetes mellitus-hypertension-nephrosis 250.4 ☑ [581.81]
diabetes mellitus in newborn infant 775.1
diabetes-nephrosis 250.4 ☑ [581.81]
diabetic amyotrophy 250.6 ☑ [358.1]
Diamond-Blackfan (congenital hypoplastic anemia) 284.01 ▲
Diamond-Gardener (autoerythrocyte sensitization) 287.2
DIC (diffuse or disseminated intravascular coagulopathy) (see also Fibrinolysis) 286.6
diencephalohypophyseal NEC 253.8
diffuse cervicobrachial 723.3
diffuse obstructive pulmonary 496
DiGeorge's (thymic hypoplasia) 279.11
Dighton's 756.51
Di Guglielmo's (erythremic myelosis) (M9841/3) 207.0 ☑
disequilibrium 276.9
disseminated platelet thrombosis 446.6
Ditthomska 307.81
Doan-Wiseman (primary splenic neutropenia) 288.0 ☑
Doan-Wisemann (primary splenic neutropenia) 289.53 ●
Döhle body-panmyelopathic 288.2
Donohue's (leprechaunism) 259.8
dorsolateral medullary (see also Disease, cerebrovascular, acute) 436
double athetosis 333.71 ●
double whammy 360.81
Down's (mongolism) 758.0
Dresbach's (elliptocytosis) 282.1
Dressler's (postmyocardial infarction) 411.0
 hemoglobinuria 283.2
 postcardiotomy 429.4 ●
drug withdrawal, infant, of dependent mother 779.5
dry skin 701.1
eye 375.15
DSAP (disseminated superficial actinic porokeratosis) 692.75
Duane's (retraction) 378.71
Duane-Stilling-Türk (ocular retraction syndrome) 378.71
Dubin-Johnson (constitutional hyperbilirubinemia) 277.4
Dubin-Sprinz (constitutional hyperbilirubinemia) 277.4
Duchenne's 335.22
 due to abnormality
  autosomal NEC (see also Abnormal, autosomes NEC) 758.5
  13 758.1
  18 758.2
  21 or 22 758.0
  D1 758.1
  E3 758.2
  G 758.0
 chromosomal 758.89
 sex 758.81

Syndrome — see also Disease — continued

dumping 564.2
 nonsurgical 536.8
Duplay's 726.2
Dupré's (meningism) 781.6
Dyke-Young (acquired macrocytic hemolytic anemia) 283.9
dyspraxia 315.4
dystocia, dystrophia 654.9 ☑
Eagle-Barret 756.71
Eales' 362.18
Eaton-Lambert (see also Neoplasm, by site, malignant) 199.1 [358.1]
Ebstein's (downward displacement, tricuspid valve into right ventricle) 746.2
ectopic ACTH secretion 255.0
eczema-thrombocytopenia 279.12
Eddowes' (brittle bones and blue sclera) 756.51
Edwards' 758.2
efferent loop 537.89
effort (aviators') (psychogenic) 306.2
Ehlers-Danlos 756.83
Eisenmenger's (ventricular septal defect) 745.4
Ekbom's (restless legs) 333.94 ▲
Ekman's (brittle bones and blue sclera) 756.51
electric feet 266.2
Elephant man 237.71
Ellison-Zollinger (gastric hypersecretion with pancreatic islet cell tumor) 251.5
Ellis-van Creveld (chondroectodermal dysplasia) 756.55
embryonic fixation 270.2
empty sella (turcica) 253.8
endocrine-hypertensive 255.3
Engel-von Recklinghausen (osteitis fibrosa cystica) 252.01
enteroarticular 099.3
entrapment — see Neuropathy, entrapment
eosinophilia myalgia 710.5
epidemic vomiting 078.82
Epstein's — see Nephrosis
Erb (-Oppenheim)-Goldflam 358.00
Erdheim's (acromegalic macrospondylitis) 253.0
Erlacher-Blount (tibia vara) 732.4
erythrocyte fragmentation 283.19
euthyroid sick 790.94
Evans' (thrombocytopenic purpura) 287.32
excess cortisol, iatrogenic 255.0
exhaustion 300.5
extrapyramidal 333.90
eyelid-malar-mandible 756.0
eye retraction 378.71
Faber's (achlorhydric anemia) 280.9
Fabry (-Anderson) (angiokeratoma corporis diffusum) 272.7
facet 724.8
Fallot's 745.2
falx (see also Hemorrhage, brain) 431
familial eczema-thrombocytopenia 279.12
Fanconi (-de Toni) (-Debré) (cystinosis) 270.0
Fanconi's (anemia) (congenital pancytopenia) 284.09 ▲
Farber (-Uzman) (disseminated lipogranulomatosis) 272.8
fatigue NEC 300.5
 chronic 780.71
faulty bowel habit (idiopathic megacolon) 564.7
FDH (focal dermal hypoplasia) 757.39
fecal reservoir 560.39
Feil-Klippel (brevicollis) 756.16
Felty's (rheumatoid arthritis with splenomegaly and leukopenia) 714.1
fertile eunuch 257.2

Syndrome — see also Disease — continued

fetal alcohol 760.71
 late effect 760.71
fibrillation-flutter 427.32
fibrositis (periarticular) 729.0
Fiedler's (acute isolated myocarditis) 422.91
Fiessinger-Leroy (-Reiter) 099.3
Fiessinger-Rendu (erythema multiforme exudativum) 695.1
first arch 756.0
Fisher's 357.0
fish odor 270.8 ●
Fitz's (acute hemorrhagic pancreatitis) 577.0
Fitz-Hugh and Curtis 098.86
 due to
  Chlamydia trachomatis 099.56
  Neisseria gonorrhoeae (gonococcal peritonitis) 098.86
Flajani (-Basedow) (exophthalmic goiter) 242.0 ☑
floppy
 infant 781.99
 valve (mitral) 424.0
flush 259.2
Foix-Alajouanine 336.1
Fong's (hereditary osteo-onychodysplasia) 756.89
foramen magnum 348.4
Forbes-Albright (nonpuerperal amenorrhea and lactation associated with pituitary tumor) 253.1
Foster-Kennedy 377.04
Foville's (peduncular) 344.89
fragile X 759.83
Franceschetti's (mandibulofacial dysostosis) 756.0
Fraser's 759.89
Freeman-Sheldon 759.89
Frey's (auriculotemporal) 705.22
Friderichsen-Waterhouse 036.3
Friedrich-Erb-Arnold (acropachyderma) 757.39
Fröhlich's (adiposogenital dystrophy) 253.8
Froin's 336.8
Frommel-Chiari 676.6 ☑
frontal lobe 310.0
Fukuhara 277.87
Fuller Albright's (osteitis fibrosa disseminata) 756.59
functional
 bowel 564.9
 prepubertal castrate 752.89
Gaisböck's (polycythemia hypertonica) 289.0
ganglion (basal, brain) 333.90
 geniculi 351.1
Ganser's, hysterical 300.16
Gardner-Diamond (autoerythrocyte sensitization) 287.2
gastroesophageal junction 530.0
gastroesophageal laceration-hemorrhage 530.7
gastrojejunal loop obstruction 537.89
Gayet-Wernicke's (superior hemorrhagic polioencephalitis) 265.1
Gee-Herter-Heubner (nontropical sprue) 579.0
Gélineau's (see also Narcolepsy) 347.00
genito-anorectal 099.1
Gerhardt's (vocal cord paralysis) 478.30
Gerstmann's (finger agnosia) 784.69
Gianotti Crosti 057.8
 due to known virus — see Infection, virus
 due to unknown virus 057.8
Gilbert's 277.4
Gilford (-Hutchinson) (progeria) 259.8
Gilles de la Tourette's 307.23
Gillespie's (dysplasia oculodentodigitalis) 759.89

Syndrome — see also Disease — continued

Glénard's (enteroptosis) 569.89
Glinski-Simmonds (pituitary cachexia) 253.2
glucuronyl transferase 277.4
glue ear 381.20
Goldberg (-Maxwell) (-Morris) (testicular feminization) 259.5
Goldenhar's (oculoauriculovertebral dysplasia) 756.0
Goldflam-Erb 358.00
Goltz-Gorlin (dermal hypoplasia) 757.39
Good's 279.06
Goodpasture's (pneumorenal) 446.21
Gopalan's (burning feet) 266.2
Gorlin-Chaudhry-Moss 759.89
Gougerot-Blum (pigmented purpuric lichenoid dermatitis) 709.1
Gougerot-Carteaud (confluent reticulate papillomatosis) 701.8
Gougerot (-Houwer)-Sjögren (keratoconjunctivitis sicca) 710.2
Gouley's (constrictive pericarditis) 423.2
Gowers' (vasovagal attack) 780.2
Gowers-Paton-Kennedy 377.04
Gradenigo's 383.02
gray or grey (chloramphenicol) (newborn) 779.4
Greig's (hypertelorism) 756.0
Gubler-Millard 344.89
Guérin-Stern (arthrogryposis multiplex congenita) 754.89
Guillain-Barré (-Strohl) 357.0
Gunn's (jaw-winking syndrome) 742.8
Günther's (congenital erythropoietic porphyria) 277.1
gustatory sweating 350.8
H_2O 759.81
Hadfield-Clarke (pancreatic infantilism) 577.8
Haglund-Läwen-Fründ 717.89
hairless women 257.8
hair tourniquet (see also Injury, superficial, by site)
 finger 915.8
  infected 915.9
 penis 911.8
  infected 911.9
 toe 917.8
  infected 917.9
Hallermann-Streiff 756.0
Hallervorden-Spatz 333.0
Hamman's (spontaneous mediastinal emphysema) 518.1
Hamman-Rich (diffuse interstitial pulmonary fibrosis) 516.3
hand-foot 282.61
Hand-Schüller-Christian (chronic histiocytosis X) 277.89
Hanot-Chauffard (-Troisier) (bronze diabetes) 275.0
Harada's 363.22
Hare's (M8010/3) (carcinoma, pulmonary apex) 162.3
Harkavy's 446.0
harlequin color change 779.89
Harris' (organic hyperinsulinism) 251.1
Hart's (pellagra-cerebellar ataxia-renal aminoaciduria) 270.0
Hayem-Faber (achlorhydric anemia) 280.9
Hayem-Widal (acquired hemolytic jaundice) 283.9
Heberden's (angina pectoris) 413.9
Hedinger's (malignant carcinoid) 259.2
Hegglin's 288.2
Heller's (infantile psychosis) (see also Psychosis, childhood) 299.1 ☑
H.E.L.L.P 642.5 ☑
hemolytic-uremic (adult) (child) 283.11
hemophagocytic 288.4 ●

Syndrome — *see also* Disease — *continued*
- hemophagocytic — *continued*
  - infection-associated 288.4
- Hench-Rosenberg (palindromic arthritis) (*see also* Rheumatism, palindromic) 719.3
- Henoch-Schönlein (allergic purpura) 287.0
- hepatic flexure 569.89
- hepatorenal 572.4
  - due to a procedure 997.4
  - following delivery 674.8
- hepatourologic 572.4
- Herrick's (hemoglobin S disease) 282.61
- Herter (-Gee) (nontropical sprue) 579.0
- Heubner-Herter (nontropical sprue) 579.0
- Heyd's (hepatorenal) 572.4
- HHHO 759.81
- high grade myelodysplastic 238.73
  - with 5q deletion 238.73
- Hilger's 337.0
- histocytic 288.4
- Hoffa (-Kastert) (liposynovitis prepatellaris) 272.8
- Hoffmann's 244.9 [359.5]
- Hoffmann-Bouveret (paroxysmal tachycardia) 427.2
- Hoffmann-Werdnig 335.0
- Holländer-Simons (progressive lipodystrophy) 272.6
- Holmes' (visual disorientation) 368.16
- Holmes-Adie 379.46
- Hoppe-Goldflam 358.00
- Horner's (*see also* Neuropathy, peripheral, autonomic) 337.9
  - traumatic — *see* Injury, nerve, cervical sympathetic
- hospital addiction 301.51
- Hunt's (herpetic geniculate ganglionitis) 053.11
  - dyssynergia cerebellaris myoclonica 334.2
- Hunter (-Hurler) (mucopolysaccharidosis II) 277.5
- hunterian glossitis 529.4
- Hurler (-Hunter) (mucopolysaccharidosis II) 277.5
- Hutchinson-Boeck (sarcoidosis) 135
- Hutchinson-Gilford (progeria) 259.8
- Hutchinson's incisors or teeth 090.5
- hydralazine
  - correct substance properly administered 695.4
  - overdose or wrong substance given or taken 972.6
- hydraulic concussion (abdomen) (*see also* Injury, internal, abdomen) 868.00
- hyperabduction 447.8
- hyperactive bowel 564.9
- hyperaldosteronism with hypokalemic alkalosis (Bartter's) 255.13
- hypercalcemic 275.42
- hypercoagulation NEC 289.89
- hypereosinophilic (idiopathic) 288.3
- hyperkalemic 276.7
- hyperkinetic (*see also* Hyperkinesia) heart 429.82
- hyperlipemia-hemolytic anemia-icterus 571.1
- hypermobility 728.5
- hypernatremia 276.0
- hyperosmolarity 276.0
- hypersomnia-bulimia 349.89
- hypersplenic 289.4
- hypersympathetic (*see also* Neuropathy, peripheral, autonomic) 337.9
- hypertransfusion, newborn 776.4
- hyperventilation, psychogenic 306.1
- hyperviscosity (of serum) NEC 273.3
  - polycythemic 289.0
  - sclerothymic 282.8

Syndrome — *see also* Disease — *continued*
- hypoglycemic (familial) (neonatal) 251.2
  - functional 251.1
- hypokalemic 276.8
- hypophyseal 253.8
- hypophyseothalamic 253.8
- hypopituitarism 253.2
- hypoplastic left heart 746.7
- hypopotassemia 276.8
- hyposmolality 276.1
- hypotension, maternal 669.2
- hypotonia-hypomentia-hypogonadism-obesity 759.81
- ICF (intravascular coagulation-fibrinolysis) (*see also* Fibrinolysis) 286.6
- idiopathic cardiorespiratory distress, newborn 769
- idiopathic nephrotic (infantile) 581.9
- iliotibial band 728.89
- Imerslund (-Gräsbeck) (anemia due to familial selective vitamin B$_{12}$ malabsorption) 281.1
- immobility (paraplegic) 728.3
- immunity deficiency, combined 279.2
- impending coronary 411.1
- impingement
  - shoulder 726.2
  - vertebral bodies 724.4
- inappropriate secretion of antidiuretic hormone (ADH) 253.6
- incomplete
  - mandibulofacial 756.0
- infant
  - death, sudden (SIDS) 798.0
  - Hercules 255.2
  - of diabetic mother 775.0
  - shaken 995.55
- infantilism 253.3
- inferior vena cava 459.2
- influenza-like 487.1
- inspissated bile, newborn 774.4
- insufficient sleep 307.44
- intermediate coronary (artery) 411.1
- internal carotid artery (*see also* Occlusion, artery, carotid) 433.1
- interspinous ligament 724.8
- intestinal
  - carcinoid 259.2
  - gas 787.3
  - knot 560.2
- intravascular
  - coagulation-fibrinolysis (ICF) (*see also* Fibrinolysis) 286.6
  - coagulopathy (*see also* Fibrinolysis) 286.6
- inverted Marfan's 759.89
- IRDS (idiopathic respiratory distress, newborn) 769
- irritable
  - bowel 564.1
  - heart 306.2
  - weakness 300.5
- ischemic bowel (transient) 557.9
  - chronic 557.1
  - due to mesenteric artery insufficiency 557.1
- Itsenko-Cushing (pituitary basophilism) 255.0
- IVC (intravascular coagulopathy) (*see also* Fibrinolysis) 286.6
- Ivemark's (asplenia with congenital heart disease) 759.0
- Jaccoud's 714.4
- Jackson's 344.89
- Jadassohn-Lewandowsky (pachyonchia congenita) 757.5
- Jaffe-Lichtenstein (-Uehlinger) 252.01
- Jahnke's (encephalocutaneous angiomatosis) 759.6
- Jakob-Creutzfeldt (new variant) 046.1
  - with dementia
    - with behavioral disturbance 046.1 [294.11]

Syndrome — *see also* Disease — *continued*
- Jakob-Creutzfeldt — *continued*
  - with dementia — *continued*
    - without behavioral disturbance 046.1 [294.10]
- Jaksch's (pseudoleukemia infantum) 285.8
- Jaksch-Hayem (-Luzet) (pseudoleukemia infantum) 285.8
- jaw-winking 742.8
- jejunal 564.2
- Jervell-Lange-Nielsen 426.82
- jet lag 327.35
- Jeune's (asphyxiating thoracic dystrophy of newborn) 756.4
- Job's (chronic granulomatous disease) 288.1
- Jordan's 288.2
- Joseph-Diamond-Blackfan (congenital hypoplastic anemia) 284.01
- Joubert 759.89
- jugular foramen 352.6
- Kabuki 759.89
- Kahler's (multiple myeloma) (M9730/3) 203.0
- Kalischer's (encephalocutaneous angiomatosis) 759.6
- Kallmann's (hypogonadotropic hypogonadism with anosmia) 253.4
- Kanner's (autism) (*see also* Psychosis, childhood) 299.0
- Kartagener's (sinusitis, bronchiectasis, situs inversus) 759.3
- Kasabach-Merritt (capillary hemangioma associated with thrombocytopenic purpura) 287.39
- Kast's (dyschondroplasia with hemangiomas) 756.4
- Kaznelson's (congenital hypoplastic anemia) 284.01
- Kearns-Sayre 277.87
- Kelly's (sideropenic dysphagia) 280.8
- Kimmelstiel-Wilson (intercapillary glomerulosclerosis) 250.4 [581.81]
- Klauder's (erythema multiforme exudativum) 695.1
- Kleine-Levin 327.13
- Klein-Waardenburg (ptosis-epicanthus) 270.2
- Klinefelter's 758.7
- Klippel-Feil (brevicollis) 756.16
- Klippel-Trenaunay 759.89
- Klumpke (-Déjérine) (injury to brachial plexus at birth) 767.6
- Klüver-Bucy (-Terzian) 310.0
- Köhler-Pellegrini-Stieda (calcification, knee joint) 726.62
- König's 564.89
- Korsakoff's (nonalcoholic) 294.0
- Korsakoff (-Wernicke) (nonalcoholic) 294.0
  - alcoholic 291.1
  - alcoholic 291.1
- Kostmann's (infantile genetic agranulocytosis) 288.01
- Krabbe's
  - congenital muscle hypoplasia 756.89
  - cutaneocerebral angioma 759.6
- Kunkel (lupoid hepatitis) 571.49
- labyrinthine 386.50
- laceration, broad ligament 620.6
- Langdon Down (mongolism) 758.0
- Larsen's (flattened facies and multiple congenital dislocations) 755.8
- lateral
  - cutaneous nerve of thigh 355.1
  - medullary (*see also* Disease, cerebrovascular acute) 436
- Launois' (pituitary gigantism) 253.0
- Launois-Cléret (adiposogenital dystrophy) 253.8

Syndrome — *see also* Disease — *continued*
- Laurence-Moon (-Bardet)-Biedl (obesity, polydactyly, and mental retardation) 759.89
- Lawford's (encephalocutaneous angiomatosis) 759.6
- lazy
  - leukocyte 288.09
  - posture 728.3
- Lederer-Brill (acquired infectious hemolytic anemia) 283.19
- Legg-Calvé-Perthes (osteochondrosis capital femoral) 732.1
- Lemiere 451.89
- Lennox's (*see also* Epilepsy) 345.0
- Lennox-Gastaut syndrome 345.0
  - with tonic seizures 345.1
- lenticular 275.1
- Léopold-Lévi's (paroxysmal thyroid instability) 242.9
- Lepore hemoglobin 282.49
- Leriche's (aortic bifurcation occlusion) 444.0
- Léri-Weill 756.59
- Lermoyez's (*see also* Disease, Ménière's) 386.00
- Lesch-Nyhan (hypoxanthine-guanine-phosphoribosyltransferase deficiency) 277.2
- Lev's (acquired complete heart block) 426.0
- Levi's (pituitary dwarfism) 253.3
- Lévy-Roussy 334.3
- Lichtheim's (subacute combined sclerosis with pernicious anemia) 281.0 [336.2]
- Li-Fraumeni V84.01
- Lightwood's (renal tubular acidosis) 588.89
- Lignac (-de Toni) (-Fanconi) (-Debré) (cystinosis) 270.0
- Likoff's (angina in menopausal women) 413.9
- liver-kidney 572.4
- Lloyd's 258.1
- lobotomy 310.0
- Löffler's (eosinophilic pneumonitis) 518.3
- Löfgren's (sarcoidosis) 135
- long arm 18 or 21 deletion 758.39
- Looser (-Debray)-Milkman (osteomalacia with pseudofractures) 268.2
- Lorain-Levi (pituitary dwarfism) 253.3
- Louis-Bar (ataxia-telangiectasia) 334.8
- low
  - atmospheric pressure 993.2
  - back 724.2
    - psychogenic 306.0
  - output (cardiac) (*see also* Failure, heart) 428.9
- Lowe's (oculocerebrorenal dystrophy) 270.8
- lower radicular, newborn 767.4
- Lowe-Terrey-MacLachlan (oculocerebrorenal dystrophy) 270.8
- Lown (-Ganong)-Levine (short P-R interval, normal QRS complex, and supraventricular tachycardia) 426.81
- Lucey-Driscoll (jaundice due to delayed conjugation) 774.30
- Luetscher's (dehydration) 276.51
- lumbar vertebral 724.4
- Lutembacher's (atrial septal defect with mitral stenosis) 745.5
- Lyell's (toxic epidermal necrolysis) 695.1
  - due to drug
    - correct substance properly administered 695.1
    - overdose or wrong substance given or taken 977.9
    - specified drug — *see* Table of Drugs and Chemicals

Index to Diseases — Syndrome

Syndrome — *see also* Disease — *continued*
MacLeod's 492.8
macrogenitosomia praecox 259.8
macroglobulinemia 273.3
macrophage activation 288.4
Maffucci's (dyschondroplasia with hemangiomas) 756.4
Magenblase 306.4
magnesium-deficiency 781.7
malabsorption 579.9
    postsurgical 579.3
    spinal fluid 331.3
Mal de Debarquement 780.4
malignant carcinoid 259.2
Mallory-Weiss 530.7
mandibulofacial dysostosis 756.0
manic-depressive (*see also* Psychosis, affective) 296.80
Mankowsky's (familial dysplastic osteopathy) 731.2
maple syrup (urine) 270.3
Marable's (celiac artery compression) 447.4
Marchesani (-Weill) (brachymorphism and ectopia lentis) 759.89
Marchiafava-Bignami 341.8
Marchiafava-Micheli (paroxysmal nocturnal hemoglobinuria) 283.2
Marcus Gunn's (jaw-winking syndrome) 742.8
Marfan's (arachnodactyly) 759.82
    meaning congenital syphilis 090.49
    with luxation of lens 090.49 [379.32]
Marie's (acromegaly) 253.0
    primary or idiopathic (acropachyderma) 757.39
    secondary (hypertrophic pulmonary osteoarthropathy) 731.2
Markus-Adie 379.46
Maroteaux-Lamy (mucopolysaccharidosis VI) 277.5
Martin's 715.27
Martin-Albright (pseudohypoparathyroidism) 275.49
Martorell-Fabré (pulseless disease) 446.7
massive aspiration of newborn 770.18
Masters-Allen 620.6
mastocytosis 757.33
maternal hypotension 669.2
maternal obesity 646.1
May (-Hegglin) 288.2
McArdle (-Schmid) (-Pearson) (glycogenosis V) 271.0
McCune-Albright (osteitis fibrosa disseminata) 756.59
McQuarrie's (idiopathic familial hypoglycemia) 251.2
meconium
    aspiration 770.12
    plug (newborn) NEC 777.1
median arcuate ligament 447.4
mediastinal fibrosis 519.3
Meekeren-Ehlers-Danlos 756.83
Meige (blepharospasm-oromandibular dystonia) 333.82
  -Milroy (chronic hereditary edema) 757.0
MELAS (mitochondrial encephalopathy, lactic acidosis and stroke-like episodes) 277.87
Melkersson (-Rosenthal) 351.8
Mende's (ptosis-epicanthus) 270.2
Mendelson's (resulting from a procedure) 997.3
    during labor 668.0
    obstetric 668.0
Ménétrier's (hypertrophic gastritis) 535.2
Ménière's (*see also* Disease, Ménière's) 386.00
meningo-eruptive 047.1
Menkes' 759.89

Syndrome — *see also* Disease — *continued*
Menkes' — *continued*
    glutamic acid 759.89
    maple syrup (urine) disease 270.3
menopause 627.2
    postartificial 627.4
menstruation 625.4
MERRF (myoclonus with epilepsy and with ragged red fibers) 277.87
mesenteric
    artery, superior 557.1
    vascular insufficiency (with gangrene) 557.1
metabolic 277.7
metastatic carcinoid 259.2
Meyenburg-Altherr-Uehlinger 733.99
Meyer-Schwickerath and Weyers (dysplasia oculodentodigitalis) 759.89
Micheli-Rietti (thalassemia minor) 282.49
Michotte's 721.5
micrognathia-glossoptosis 756.0
microphthalmos (congenital) 759.89
midbrain 348.8
middle
    lobe (lung) (right) 518.0
    radicular 353.0
Miescher's
    familial acanthosis nigricans 701.2
    granulomatosis disciformis 709.3
Mieten's 759.89
migraine 346.0
Mikity-Wilson (pulmonary dysmaturity) 770.7
Mikulicz's (dryness of mouth, absent or decreased lacrimation) 527.1
milk alkali (milk drinkers') 275.42
Milkman (-Looser) (osteomalacia with pseudofractures) 268.2
Millard-Gubler 344.89
Miller-Dieker 758.33
Miller Fisher's 357.0
Milles' (encephalocutaneous angiomatosis) 759.6
Minkowski-Chauffard (*see also* Spherocytosis) 282.0
Mirizzi's (hepatic duct stenosis) 576.2
    with calculus, cholelithiasis, or stones — *see* Choledocholithiasis
mitochondrial neurogastrointestinal encephalopathy (MNGIE) 277.87
mitral
    click (-murmur) 785.2
    valve prolapse 424.0
MNGIE (mitochondrial neurogastrointestinal encephalopathy) 277.87
Möbius'
    congenital oculofacial paralysis 352.6
    ophthalmoplegic migraine 346.8
Mohr's (types I and II) 759.89
monofixation 378.34
Moore's (*see also* Epilepsy) 345.5
Morel-Moore (hyperostosis frontalis interna) 733.3
Morel-Morgagni (hyperostosis frontalis interna) 733.3
Morgagni (-Stewart-Morel) (hyperostosis frontalis interna) 733.3
Morgagni-Adams-Stokes (syncope with heart block) 426.9
Morquio (-Brailsford) (-Ullrich) (mucopolysaccharidosis IV) 277.5
Morris (testicular feminization) 259.5
Morton's (foot) (metatarsalgia) (metatarsal neuralgia) (neuralgia) (neuroma) (toe) 355.6
Moschcowitz (-Singer-Symmers) (thrombotic thrombocytopenic purpura) 446.6
Mounier-Kuhn 748.3
    with
        acute exacerbation 494.1

Syndrome — *see also* Disease — *continued*
Mounier-Kuhn — *continued*
    with — *continued*
        bronchiectasis 494.0
            with (acute) exacerbation 494.1
    acquired 519.19
        with bronchiectasis 494.0
        with (acute) exacerbation 494.1
Mucha-Haberman (acute parapsoriasis varioliformis) 696.2
mucocutaneous lymph node (acute) (febrile) (infantile) (MCLS) 446.1
multiple
    deficiency 260
    operations 301.51
Munchausen's 301.51
Münchmeyer's (exostosis luxurians) 728.11
Murchison-Sanderson — *see* Disease, Hodgkin's
myasthenic — *see* Myasthenia, syndrome
myelodysplastic 238.75
    with 5q deletion 238.74
    high grade with 5q deletion 238.73
myeloproliferative (chronic) (M9960/1) 238.79
myofascial pain NEC 729.1
Naffziger's 353.0
Nager-de Reynier (dysostosis mandibularis) 756.0
nail-patella (hereditary osteo-onychodysplasia) 756.89
NARP (neuropathy, ataxia and retinitis pigmentosa) 277.87
Nebécourt's 253.3
Neill-Dingwall (microencephaly and dwarfism) 759.89
nephrotic (*see also* Nephrosis) 581.9
    diabetic 250.4 [581.81]
Netherton's (ichthyosiform erythroderma) 757.1
neurocutaneous 759.6
neuroleptic malignant 333.92
Nezelof's (pure alymphocytosis) 279.13
Niemann-Pick (lipid histiocytosis) 272.7
Nonne-Milroy-Meige (chronic hereditary edema) 757.0
nonsense 300.16
Noonan's 759.89
Nothnagel's
    ophthalmoplegia-cerebellar ataxia 378.52
    vasomotor acroparesthesia 443.89
nucleus ambiguus-hypoglossal 352.6
OAV (oculoauriculovertebral dysplasia) 756.0
obsessional 300.3
oculocutaneous 364.24
oculomotor 378.81
oculourethroarticular 099.3
Ogilvie's (sympathicotonic colon obstruction) 560.89
ophthalmoplegia-cerebellar ataxia 378.52
Oppenheim-Urbach (necrobiosis lipoidica diabeticorum) 250.8 [709.3]
oral-facial-digital 759.89
organic
    affective NEC 293.83
        drug-induced 292.84
    anxiety 293.84
    delusional 293.81
        alcohol-induced 291.5
        drug-induced 292.11
        due to or associated with arteriosclerosis 290.42
            presenile brain disease 290.12
            senility 290.20

Syndrome — *see also* Disease — *continued*
organic — *continued*
    depressive 293.83
        drug-induced 292.84
        due to or associated with arteriosclerosis 290.43
            presenile brain disease 290.13
            senile brain disease 290.21
    hallucinosis 293.82
        drug-induced 292.84
organic affective 293.83
    induced by drug 292.84
organic personality 310.1
    induced by drug 292.89
Ormond's 593.4
orodigitofacial 759.89
orthostatic hypotensive-dysautonomic dyskinetic 333.0
Osler-Weber-Rendu (familial hemorrhagic telangiectasia) 448.0
osteodermopathic hyperostosis 757.39
osteoporosis-osteomalacia 268.2
Österreicher-Turner (hereditary osteo-onychodysplasia) 756.89
Ostrum-Furst 756.59
otolith 386.19
otopalatodigital 759.89
outlet (thoracic) 353.0
ovarian remnant 620.8
ovarian vein 593.4
Owren's (*see also* Defect, coagulation) 286.3
OX 758.6
pacemaker 429.4
Paget-Schroetter (intermittent venous claudication) 453.8
pain (*see also* Pain)
    central 338.0
    chronic 338.4
    myelopathic 338.0
    thalamic (hyperesthetic) 338.0
painful
    apicocostal vertebral (M8010/3) 162.3
    arc 726.19
    bruising 287.2
    feet 266.2
Pancoast's (carcinoma, pulmonary apex) (M8010/3) 162.3
panhypopituitary (postpartum) 253.2
papillary muscle 429.81
    with myocardial infarction 410.8
Papillon-Léage and Psaume (orodigitofacial dysostosis) 759.89
parabiotic (transfusion)
    donor (twin) 772.0
    recipient (twin) 776.4
paralysis agitans 332.0
paralytic 344.9
    specified type NEC 344.89
paraneoplastic — *see* condition
Parinaud's (paralysis of conjugate upward gaze) 378.81
    oculoglandular 372.02
Parkes Weber and Dimitri (encephalocutaneous angiomatosis) 759.6
Parkinson's (*see also* Parkinsonism) 332.0
parkinsonian (*see also* Parkinsonism) 332.0
Parry's (exophthalmic goiter) 242.0
Parry-Romberg 349.89
Parsonage-Aldren-Turner 353.5
Parsonage-Turner 353.5
Patau's (trisomy D1) 758.1
patellofemoral 719.46
Paterson (-Brown) (-Kelly) (sideropenic dysphagia) 280.8
Payr's (splenic flexure syndrome) 569.89
pectoral girdle 447.8
pectoralis minor 447.8
Pelger-Huët (hereditary hyposegmentation) 288.2

Syndrome — see also Disease — continued
  pellagra-cerebellar ataxia-renal aminoaciduria 270.0
  pellagroid 265.2
  Pellegrini-Stieda 726.62
  Pellizzi's (pineal) 259.8
  pelvic congestion (-fibrosis) 625.5
  Pendred's (familial goiter with deaf-mutism) 243
  Penfield's (see also Epilepsy) 345.5 ☑
  Penta X 758.81
  peptic ulcer — see Ulcer, peptic 533.9 ☑
  perabduction 447.8
  periodic 277.31
  periurethral fibrosis 593.4
  persistent fetal circulation 747.83
  Petges-Cléjat (poikilodermatomyositis) 710.3
  Peutz-Jeghers 759.6
  Pfeiffer (acrocephalosyndactyly) 755.55
  phantom limb 353.6
  pharyngeal pouch 279.11
  Pick's (pericardial pseudocirrhosis of liver) 423.2
    heart 423.2
    liver 423.2
  Pick-Herxheimer (diffuse idiopathic cutaneous atrophy) 701.8
  Pickwickian (cardiopulmonary obesity) 278.8
  PIE (pulmonary infiltration with eosinophilia) 518.3
  Pierre Marie-Bamberger (hypertrophic pulmonary osteoarthropathy) 731.2
  Pierre Mauriac's (diabetes-dwarfism-obesity) 258.1
  Pierre Robin 756.0
  pigment dispersion, iris 364.53
  pineal 259.8
  pink puffer 492.8
  pituitary 253.0
  placental
    dysfunction 762.2
    insufficiency 762.2
    transfusion 762.3
  plantar fascia 728.71
  plica knee 727.83
  Plummer-Vinson (sideropenic dysphagia) 280.8
  pluricarential of infancy 260
  plurideficiency of infancy 260
  pluriglandular (compensatory) 258.8
  polycarential of infancy 260
  polyglandular 258.8
  polysplenia 759.0
  pontine 433.8 ☑
  popliteal
    artery entrapment 447.8
    web 756.89
  postartificial menopause 627.4
  postcardiac injury ●
    postcardiotomy 429.4 ●
    postmyocardial infarction 411.0 ●
  postcardiotomy 429.4
  postcholecystectomy 576.0
  postcommissurotomy 429.4
  postconcussional 310.2
  postcontusional 310.2
  postencephalitic 310.8
  posterior
    cervical sympathetic 723.2
    fossa compression 348.4
    inferior cerebellar artery (see also Disease, cerebrovascular, acute) 436
    reversible encephalopathy (PRES) ● 348.39
  postgastrectomy (dumping) 564.2
  post-gastric surgery 564.2
  posthepatitis 780.79
  postherpetic (neuralgia) (zoster) 053.19

Syndrome — see also Disease — continued
  postherpetic — continued
    geniculate ganglion 053.11
    ophthalmica 053.19
  postimmunization — see Complications, vaccination
  postinfarction 411.0
  postinfluenza (asthenia) 780.79
  postirradiation 990
  postlaminectomy 722.80
    cervical, cervicothoracic 722.81
    lumbar, lumbosacral 722.83
    thoracic, thoracolumbar 722.82
  postleukotomy 310.0
  postlobotomy 310.0
  postmastectomy lymphedema 457.0
  postmature (of newborn) 766.22
  postmyocardial infarction 411.0
  postoperative NEC 998.9
    blind loop 579.2
  postpartum panhypopituitary 253.2
  postperfusion NEC 999.8
    bone marrow 996.85
  postpericardiotomy 429.4
  postphlebitic (asymptomatic) 459.10
    with
      complications NEC 459.19
      inflammation 459.12
        and ulcer 459.13
      stasis dermatitis 459.12
        with ulcer 459.13
      ulcer 459.11
        with inflammation 459.13
  postpolio (myelitis) 138
  postvagotomy 564.2
  postvalvulotomy 429.4
  postviral (asthenia) NEC 780.79
  Potain's (gastrectasis with dyspepsia) 536.1
  potassium intoxication 276.7
  Potter's 753.0
  Prader (-Labhart) -Willi (-Fanconi) 759.81
  preinfarction 411.1
  preleukemic 238.75 ▲
  premature senility 259.8
  premenstrual 625.4
  premenstrual tension 625.4
  pre ulcer 536.9
  Prinzmetal-Massumi (anterior chest wall syndrome) 786.52
  Profichet's 729.9
  progeria 259.8
  progressive pallidal degeneration 333.0
  prolonged gestation 766.22
  Proteus (dermal hypoplasia) 757.39
  prune belly 756.71
  prurigo-asthma 691.8
  pseudocarpal tunnel (sublimis) 354.0
  pseudohermaphroditism-virilism-hirsutism 255.2
  pseudoparalytica 358.00
  pseudo-Turner's 759.89
  psycho-organic 293.9
    acute 293.0
    anxiety type 293.84
    depressive type 293.83
    hallucinatory type 293.82
    nonpsychotic severity 310.1
      specified focal (partial) NEC 310.8
    paranoid type 293.81
    specified type NEC 293.89
    subacute 293.1
  pterygolymphangiectasia 758.6
  ptosis-epicanthus 270.2
  pulmonary
    arteriosclerosis 416.0
    hypoperfusion (idiopathic) 769
    renal (hemorrhagic) 446.21
  pulseless 446.7
  Putnam-Dana (subacute combined sclerosis with pernicious anemia) 281.0 [336.2]

Syndrome — see also Disease — continued
  pyloroduodenal 537.89
  pyramidopallidonigral 332.0
  pyriformis 355.0
  QT interval prolongation 426.82
  radicular NEC 729.2
    lower limbs 724.4
    upper limbs 723.4
    newborn 767.4
  Raeder-Harbitz (pulseless disease) 446.7
  Ramsay Hunt's
    dyssynergia cerebellaris myoclonica 334.2
    herpetic geniculate ganglionitis 053.11
  rapid time-zone change 327.35
  Raymond (-Céstan) 433.8 ☑
  Raynaud's (paroxysmal digital cyanosis) 443.0
  RDS (respiratory distress syndrome, newborn) 769
  Refsum's (heredopathia atactica polyneuritiformis) 356.3
  Reichmann's (gastrosuccorrhea) 536.8
  Reifenstein's (hereditary familial hypogonadism, male) 259.5
  Reilly's (see also Neuropathy, peripheral, autonomic) 337.9
  Reiter's 099.3
  renal glomerulohyalinosis-diabetic 250.4 ☑ [581.81]
  Rendu-Osler-Weber (familial hemorrhagic telangiectasia) 448.0
  renofacial (congenital biliary fibrangiomatosis) 753.0
  Rénon-Delille 253.8
  respiratory distress (idiopathic) (newborn) 769
    adult (following shock, surgery, or trauma) 518.5
    specified NEC 518.82
    type II 770.6 ●
  restless legs ▶(RLS)◀ 333.94 ▲
  retinoblastoma (familial) 190.5
  retraction (Duane's) 378.71
  retroperitoneal fibrosis 593.4
  retroviral seroconversion (acute) V08 ●
  Rett's 330.8
  Reye's 331.81
  Reye-Sheehan (postpartum pituitary necrosis) 253.2
  Riddoch's (visual disorientation) 368.16
  Ridley's (see also Failure, ventricular, left) 428.1
  Rieger's (mesodermal dysgenesis, anterior ocular segment) 743.44
  Rietti-Greppi-Micheli (thalassemia minor) 282.49
  right ventricular obstruction — see Failure, heart
  Riley-Day (familial dysautonomia) 742.8
  Robin's 756.0
  Rokitansky-Kuster-Hauser (congenital absence, vagina) 752.49
  Romano-Ward (prolonged QT interval syndrome) 426.82
  Romberg's 349.89
  Rosen-Castleman-Liebow (pulmonary proteinosis) 516.0
  rotator cuff, shoulder 726.10
  Roth's 355.1
  Rothmund's (congenital poikiloderma) 757.33
  Rotor's (idiopathic hyperbilirubinemia) 277.4
  Roussy-Lévy 334.3
  Roy (-Jutras) (acropachyderma) 757.39
  rubella (congenital) 771.0
  Rubinstein-Taybi's (brachydactylia, short stature, and mental retardation) 759.89

Syndrome — see also Disease — continued
  Rud's (mental deficiency, epilepsy, and infantilism) 759.89
  Ruiter-Pompen (-Wyers) (angiokeratoma corporis diffusum) 272.7
  Runge's (postmaturity) 766.22
  Russell (-Silver) (congenital hemihypertrophy and short stature) 759.89
  Rytand-Lipsitch (complete atrioventricular block) 426.0
  sacralization-scoliosis-sciatica 756.15
  sacroiliac 724.6
  Saenger's 379.46
  salt
    depletion (see also Disease, renal) 593.9
      due to heat NEC 992.8
        causing heat exhaustion or prostration 992.4
    low (see also Disease, renal) 593.9
  salt-losing (see also Disease, renal) 593.9
  Sanfilippo's (mucopolysaccharidosis III) 277.5
  Scaglietti-Dagnini (acromegalic macrospondylitis) 253.0
  scalded skin 695.1
  scalenus anticus (anterior) 353.0
  scapulocostal 354.8
  scapuloperoneal 359.1
  scapulovertebral 723.4
  Schaumann's (sarcoidosis) 135
  Scheie's (mucopolysaccharidosis IS) 277.5
  Scheuthauer-Marie-Sainton (cleidocranialis dysostosis) 755.59
  Schirmer's (encephalocutaneous angiomatosis) 759.6
  schizophrenic, of childhood NEC (see also Psychosis, childhood) 299.9 ☑
  Schmidt's
    sphallo-pharyngo-laryngeal hemiplegia 352.6
    thyroid-adrenocortical insufficiency 258.1
    vagoaccessory 352.6
  Schneider's 047.9
  Schnitzler 273.1
  Scholte's (malignant carcinoid) 259.2
  Scholz (-Bielschowsky-Henneberg) 330.0
  Schroeder's (endocrine-hypertensive) 255.3
  Schüller-Christian (chronic histiocytosis X) 277.89
  Schultz's (agranulocytosis) 288.09 ▲
  Schwartz (-Jampel) 756.89
  Schwartz-Bartter (inappropriate secretion of antidiuretic hormone) 253.6
  Scimitar (anomalous venous drainage, right lung to inferior vena cava) 747.49
  sclerocystic ovary 256.4
  sea-blue histiocyte 272.7
  Seabright-Bantam (pseudohypoparathyroidism) 275.49
  Seckel's 759.89
  Secretan's (posttraumatic edema) 782.2
  secretoinhibitor (keratoconjunctivitis sicca) 710.2
  Seeligmann's (ichthyosis congenita) 757.1
  Senear-Usher (pemphigus erythematosus) 694.4
  senilism 259.8
  seroconversion, retroviral (acute) V08 ●
  serotonin 333.99
  serous meningitis 348.2
  Sertoli cell (germinal aplasia) 606.0

Index to Diseases

Syndrome — see also Disease — continued
- sex chromosome mosaic 758.81
- Sézary's (reticulosis) (M9701/3) 202.2 ☑
- shaken infant 995.55
- Shaver's (bauxite pneumoconiosis) 503
- Sheehan's (postpartum pituitary necrosis) 253.2
- shock (traumatic) 958.4
  - kidney 584.5
    - following crush injury 958.5
  - lung 518.5
  - neurogenic 308.9
  - psychic 308.9
- short
  - bowel 579.3
  - P-R interval 426.81
- shoulder-arm (see also Neuropathy, peripheral, autonomic) 337.9
- shoulder-girdle 723.4
- shoulder-hand (see also Neuropathy, peripheral, autonomic) 337.9
- Shwachman's 288.02 ▲
- Shy-Drager (orthostatic hypotension with multisystem degeneration) 333.0
- Sicard's 352.6
- sicca (keratoconjunctivitis) 710.2
- sick
  - cell 276.1
  - cilia 759.89
  - sinus 427.81
- sideropenic 280.8
- Siemens
  - ectodermal dysplasia 757.31
  - keratosis follicularis spinulosa (decalvans) 757.39
- Silfverskiöld's (osteochondrodystrophy, extremities) 756.50
- Silver's (congenital hemihypertrophy and short stature) 759.89
- Silvestroni-Bianco (thalassemia minima) 282.49
- Simons' (progressive lipodystrophy) 272.6
- sinusitis-bronchiectasis-situs inversus 759.3
- sinus tarsi 726.79
- Sipple's (medullary thyroid carcinoma-pheochromocytoma) 193
- Sjögren (-Gougerot) (keratoconjunctivitis sicca) 710.2
  - with lung involvement 710.2 [517.8]
- Sjögren-Larsson (ichthyosis congenita) 757.1
- Slocumb's 255.3
- Sluder's 337.0
- Smith-Lemli-Opitz (cerebrohepatorenal syndrome) 759.89
- Smith-Magenis 758.33
- smokers' 305.1
- Sneddon-Wilkinson (subcorneal pustular dermatosis) 694.1
- Sotos' (cerebral gigantism) 253.0
- South African cardiomyopathy 425.2
- spasmodic
  - upward movement, eye(s) 378.82
  - winking 307.20
- specified NEC 528.09 ●
- Spens' (syncope with heart block) 426.9
- spherophakia-brachymorphia 759.89
- spinal cord injury (see also Injury, spinal, by site)
  - with fracture, vertebra — see Fracture, vertebra, by site, with spinal cord injury
  - cervical — see Injury, spinal, cervical
  - fluid malabsorption (acquired) 331.3
- splenic
  - agenesis 759.0

Syndrome — see also Disease — continued
- splenic — continued
  - flexure 569.89
  - neutropenia 289.53 ▲
  - sequestration 289.52
- Spurway's (brittle bones and blue sclera) 756.51
- staphylococcal scalded skin 695.1
- Stein's (polycystic ovary) 256.4
- Steinbrocker's (see also Neuropathy, peripheral, autonomic) 337.9
- Stein-Leventhal (polycystic ovary) 256.4
- Stevens-Johnson (erythema multiforme exudativum) 695.1
- Stewart-Morel (hyperostosis frontalis interna) 733.3
- Stickler 759.89
- stiff-baby 759.89
- stiff-man 333.91
- Still's (juvenile rheumatoid arthritis) 714.30
- Still-Felty (rheumatoid arthritis with splenomegaly and leukopenia) 714.1
- Stilling-Türk-Duane (ocular retraction syndrome) 378.71
- Stojano's (subcostal) 098.86
- Stokes (-Adams) (syncope with heart block) 426.9
- Stokvis-Talma (enterogenous cyanosis) 289.7
- stone heart (see also Failure, ventricular, left) 428.1
- straight-back 756.19
- stroke (see also Disease, cerebrovascular, acute) 436
  - little 435.9
- Sturge-Kalischer-Weber (encephalotrigeminal angiomatosis) 759.6
- Sturge-Weber (-Dimitri) (encephalocutaneous angiomatosis) 759.6
- subclavian-carotid obstruction (chronic) 446.7
- subclavian steal 435.2
- subcoracoid-pectoralis minor 447.8
- subcostal 098.86
  - nerve compression 354.8
- subperiosteal hematoma 267
- subphrenic interposition 751.4
- sudden infant death (SIDS) 798.0
- Sudeck's 733.7
- Sudeck-Leriche 733.7
- superior
  - cerebellar artery (see also Disease, cerebrovascular, acute) 436
  - mesenteric artery 557.1
  - pulmonary sulcus (tumor) (M8010/3) 162.3
  - vena cava 459.2
- suprarenal cortical 255.3
- supraspinatus 726.10
- swallowed blood 777.3
- sweat retention 705.1
- Sweet's (acute febrile neutrophilic dermatosis) 695.89
- Swyer's (XY pure gonadal dysgenesis) 752.7
- Swyer-James (unilateral hyperlucent lung) 492.8
- Symonds' 348.2
- sympathetic
  - cervical paralysis 337.0
  - pelvic 625.5
- syndactylic oxycephaly 755.55
- syphilitic-cardiovascular 093.89
- systemic
  - fibrosclerosing 710.8
  - inflammatory response (SIRS) 995.90
    - due to
      - infectious process 995.91
        - with ▶acute◀ organ dysfunction 995.92

Syndrome — see also Disease — continued
- systemic — continued
  - inflammatory response — continued
    - due to — continued
      - non-infectious process 995.93
        - with ▶acute◀ organ dysfunction 995.94
- systolic click (-murmur) 785.2
- Tabagism 305.1
- tachycardia-bradycardia 427.81
- Takayasu (-Onishi) (pulseless disease) 446.7
- Takotsubo 429.83 ●
- Tapia's 352.6
- tarsal tunnel 355.5
- Taussig-Bing (transposition, aorta and overriding pulmonary artery) 745.11
- Taybi's (otopalatodigital) 759.89
- Taylor's 625.5
- teething 520.7
- tegmental 344.89
- telangiectasis-pigmentation-cataract 757.33
- temporal 383.02
  - lobectomy behavior 310.0
- temporomandibular joint-pain-dysfunction [TMJ] NEC 524.60
  - specified NEC 524.69
- Terry's 362.21
- testicular feminization 259.5
- testis, nonvirilizing 257.8
- tethered (spinal) cord 742.59
- thalamic 338.0 ▲
- Thibierge-Weissenbach (cutaneous systemic sclerosis) 710.1
- Thiele 724.6
- thoracic outlet (compression) 353.0
- thoracogenous rheumatic (hypertrophic pulmonary osteoarthropathy) 731.2
- Thorn's (see also Disease, renal) 593.9
- Thorson-Biörck (malignant carcinoid) 259.2
- thrombopenia-hemangioma 287.39
- thyroid-adrenocortical insufficiency 258.1
- Tietze's 733.6
- time-zone (rapid) 327.35
- Tobias' (carcinoma, pulmonary apex) (M8010/3) 162.3
- toilet seat 926.0
- Tolosa-Hunt 378.55
- Toni-Fanconi (cystinosis) 270.0
- Touraine's (hereditary osteo-onychodysplasia) 756.89
- Touraine-Solente-Golé (acropachyderma) 757.39
- toxic
  - oil 710.5
  - shock 040.82
- transfusion
  - fetal-maternal 772.0
  - twin
    - donor (infant) 772.0
    - recipient (infant) 776.4
- transient left ventricular apical ballooning 429.83 ●
- Treacher Collins' (incomplete mandibulofacial dysostosis) 756.0
- trigeminal plate 259.8
- triple X female 758.81
- trisomy NEC 758.5
  - 13 or D_1 758.1
  - 16-18 or E 758.2
  - 18 or E_3 758.2
  - 20 758.5
  - 21 or G (mongolism) 758.0
  - 22 or G (mongolism) 758.0
  - G 758.0
- Troisier-Hanot-Chauffard (bronze diabetes) 275.0

Syndrome — see also Disease — continued
- tropical wet feet 991.4
- Trousseau's (thrombophlebitis migrans visceral cancer) 453.1
- Türk's (ocular retraction syndrome) 378.71
- Turner's 758.6
- Turner-Varny 758.6
- twin-to-twin transfusion 762.3
  - recipient twin 776.4
- Uehlinger's (acropachyderma) 757.39
- Ullrich (-Bonnevie) (-Turner) 758.6
- Ullrich-Feichtiger 759.89
- underwater blast injury (abdominal) (see also Injury, internal, abdomen) 868.00
- universal joint, cervix 620.6
- Unverricht (-Lundborg) 333.2
- Unverricht-Wagner (dermatomyositis) 710.3
- upward gaze 378.81
- Urbach-Oppenheim (necrobiosis lipoidica diabeticorum) 250.8 ☑ [709.3]
- Urbach-Wiethe (lipoid proteinosis) 272.8
- uremia, chronic 585.9
- urethral 597.81
- urethro-oculoarticular 099.3
- urethro-oculosynovial 099.3
- urohepatic 572.4
- uveocutaneous 364.24
- uveomeningeal, uveomeningitis 363.22
- vagohypoglossal 352.6
- vagovagal 780.2
- van Buchem's (hyperostosis corticalis) 733.3
- van der Hoeve's (brittle bones and blue sclera, deafness) 756.51
- van der Hoeve-Halbertsma-Waardenburg (ptosis-epicanthus) 270.2
- van der Hoeve-Waardenburg-Gualdi (ptosis-epicanthus) 270.2
- vanishing twin 651.33
- van Neck-Odelberg (juvenile osteochondrosis) 732.1
- vascular splanchnic 557.0
- vasomotor 443.9
- vasovagal 780.2
- VATER 759.89
- Velo-cardio-facial 758.32
- vena cava (inferior) (superior) (obstruction) 459.2
- Verbiest's (claudicatio intermittens spinalis) 435.1
- Vernet's 352.6
- vertebral
  - artery 435.1
    - compression 721.1
  - lumbar 724.4
  - steal 435.1
- vertebrogenic (pain) 724.5
- vertiginous NEC 386.9
- video display tube 723.8
- Villaret's 352.6
- Vinson-Plummer (sideropenic dysphagia) 280.8
- virilizing adrenocortical hyperplasia, congenital 255.2
- virus, viral 079.99
- visceral larval migrans 128.0
- visual disorientation 368.16
- vitamin B_6 deficiency 266.1
- vitreous touch 997.99
- Vogt's (corpus striatum) 333.71 ▲
- Vogt-Koyanagi 364.24
- Volkmann's 958.6
- von Bechterew-Strümpell (ankylosing spondylitis) 720.0
- von Graefe's 378.72
- von Hippel-Lindau (angiomatosis retinocerebellosa) 759.6
- von Schroetter's (intermittent venous claudication) 453.8

Syndrome

Syndrome — *see also* Disease — *continued*
- von Willebrand (-Jürgens) (angiohemophilia) 286.4
- Waardenburg-Klein (ptosis epicanthus) 270.2
- Wagner (-Unverricht) (dermatomyositis) 710.3
- Waldenström's (macroglobulinemia) 273.3
- Waldenström-Kjellberg (sideropenic dysphagia) 280.8
- Wallenberg's (posterior inferior cerebellar artery) (*see also* Disease, cerebrovascular, acute) 436
- Waterhouse (-Friderichsen) 036.3
- water retention 276.6
- Weber's 344.89
- Weber-Christian (nodular nonsuppurative panniculitis) 729.30
- Weber-Cockayne (epidermolysis bullosa) 757.39
- Weber-Dimitri (encephalocutaneous angiomatosis) 759.6
- Weber-Gubler 344.89
- Weber-Leyden 344.89
- Weber-Osler (familial hemorrhagic telangiectasia) 448.0
- Wegener's (necrotizing respiratory granulomatosis) 446.4
- Weill-Marchesani (brachymorphism and ectopia lentis) 759.89
- Weingarten's (tropical eosinophilia) 518.3
- Weiss-Baker (carotid sinus syncope) 337.0
- Weissenbach-Thibierge (cutaneous systemic sclerosis) 710.1
- Werdnig-Hoffmann 335.0
- Werlhof-Wichmann (*see also* Purpura, thrombocytopenic) 287.39
- Wermer's (polyendocrine adenomatosis) 258.0
- Werner's (progeria adultorum) 259.8
- Wernicke's (nonalcoholic) (superior hemorrhagic polioencephalitis) 265.1
- Wernicke-Korsakoff (nonalcoholic) 294.0
  - alcoholic 291.1
- Westphal-Strümpell (hepatolenticular degeneration) 275.1
- wet
  - brain (alcoholic) 303.9 ☑
  - feet (maceration) (tropical) 991.4
  - lung
    - adult 518.5
    - newborn 770.6
- whiplash 847.0
- Whipple's (intestinal lipodystrophy) 040.2
- "whistling face" (craniocarpotarsal dystrophy) 759.89
- Widal (-Abrami) (acquired hemolytic jaundice) 283.9
- Wilkie's 557.1
- Wilkinson-Sneddon (subcorneal pustular dermatosis) 694.1
- Willan-Plumbe (psoriasis) 696.1
- Willebrand (-Jürgens) (angiohemophilia) 286.4
- Willi-Prader (hypogenital dystrophy with diabetic tendency) 759.81
- Wilson's (hepatolenticular degeneration) 275.1
- Wilson-Mikity 770.7
- Wiskott-Aldrich (eczema-thrombocytopenia) 279.12
- withdrawal
  - alcohol 291.81
  - drug 292.0
    - infant of dependent mother 779.5
- Woakes' (ethmoiditis) 471.1

Syndrome — *see also* Disease — *continued*
- Wolff-Parkinson-White (anomalous atrioventricular excitation) 426.7
- Wright's (hyperabduction) 447.8
- X
  - cardiac 413.9
  - dysmetabolic 277.7
- xiphoidalgia 733.99
- XO 758.6
- XXX 758.81
- XXXXY 758.81
- XXY 758.7
- yellow vernix (placental dysfunction) 762.2
- Zahorsky's 074.0
- Zellweger 277.86
- Zieve's (jaundice, hyperlipemia and hemolytic anemia) 571.1
- Zollinger-Ellison (gastric hypersecretion with pancreatic islet cell tumor) 251.5
- Zuelzer-Ogden (nutritional megaloblastic anemia) 281.2

Synechia (iris) (pupil) 364.70
- anterior 364.72
- peripheral 364.73
- intrauterine (traumatic) 621.5
- posterior 364.71
- vulvae, congenital 752.49

Synesthesia — *see also* Disturbance, sensation 782.0

Synodontia 520.2

Synophthalmus 759.89

Synorchidism 752.89

Synorchism 752.89

Synostosis (congenital) 756.59
- astragaloscaphoid 755.67
- radioulnar 755.53
- talonavicular (bar) 755.67
- tarsal 755.67

Synovial — *see* condition

Synovioma (M9040/3) — *see also* Neoplasm, connective tissue, malignant
- benign (M9040/0) — *see* Neoplasm, connective tissue, benign

Synoviosarcoma (M9040/3) — *see* Neoplasm, connective tissue, malignant

Synovitis 727.00
- chronic crepitant, wrist 727.2
- due to crystals — *see* Arthritis, due to crystals
- gonococcal 098.51
- gouty 274.0
- syphilitic 095.7
  - congenital 090.0
- traumatic, current — *see* Sprain, by site
- tuberculous — *see* Tuberculosis, synovitis
- villonodular 719.20
  - ankle 719.27
  - elbow 719.22
  - foot 719.27
  - hand 719.24
  - hip 719.25
  - knee 719.26
  - multiple sites 719.29
  - pelvic region 719.25
  - shoulder (region) 719.21
  - specified site NEC 719.28
  - wrist 719.23

Syphilide 091.3
- congenital 090.0
- newborn 090.0
- tubercular 095.8
  - congenital 090.0

Syphilis, syphilitic (acquired) 097.9
- with lung involvement 095.1
- abdomen (late) 095.2
- acoustic nerve 094.86
- adenopathy (secondary) 091.4
- adrenal (gland) 095.8

Syphilis, syphilitic — *continued*
- adrenal — *continued*
  - with cortical hypofunction 095.8
- age under 2 years NEC (*see also* Syphilis, congenital) 090.9
  - acquired 097.9
- alopecia (secondary) 091.82
- anemia 095.8
- aneurysm (artery) (ruptured) 093.89
  - aorta 093.0
  - central nervous system 094.89
  - congenital 090.5
- anus 095.8
  - primary 091.1
  - secondary 091.3
- aorta, aortic (arch) (abdominal) (insufficiency) (pulmonary) (regurgitation) (stenosis) (thoracic) 093.89
  - aneurysm 093.0
- arachnoid (adhesive) 094.2
- artery 093.89
  - cerebral 094.89
  - spinal 094.89
- arthropathy (neurogenic) (tabetic) 094.0 [713.5]
- asymptomatic — *see* Syphilis, latent
- ataxia, locomotor (progressive) 094.0
- atrophoderma maculatum 091.3
- auricular fibrillation 093.89
- Bell's palsy 094.89
- bladder 095.8
- bone 095.5
  - secondary 091.61
- brain 094.89
- breast 095.8
- bronchus 095.8
- bubo 091.0
- bulbar palsy 094.89
- bursa (late) 095.7
- cardiac decompensation 093.89
- cardiovascular (early) (late) (primary) (secondary) (tertiary) 093.9
  - specified type and site NEC 093.89
- causing death under 2 years of age (*see also* Syphilis, congenital) 090.9
- stated to be acquired NEC 097.9
- central nervous system (any site) (early) (late) (latent) (primary) (recurrent) (relapse) (secondary) (tertiary) 094.9
  - with
    - ataxia 094.0
    - paralysis, general 094.1
      - juvenile 090.40
    - paresis (general) 094.1
      - juvenile 090.40
    - tabes (dorsalis) 094.0
      - juvenile 090.40
    - taboparesis 094.1
      - juvenile 090.40
  - aneurysm (ruptured) 094.87
  - congenital 090.40
  - juvenile 090.40
  - remission in (sustained) 094.9
  - serology doubtful, negative, or positive 094.9
  - specified nature or site NEC 094.89
  - vascular 094.89
- cerebral 094.89
  - meningovascular 094.2
  - nerves 094.89
  - sclerosis 094.89
  - thrombosis 094.89
- cerebrospinal 094.89
  - tabetic 094.0
- cerebrovascular 094.89
- cervix 095.8
- chancre (multiple) 091.0
  - extragenital 091.2
  - Rollet's 091.2
- Charcôt's joint 094.0 [713.5]
- choked disc 094.89 [377.00]
- chorioretinitis 091.51
  - congenital 090.0 [363.13]
  - late 094.83

Syphilis, syphilitic — *continued*
- choroiditis 091.51
  - congenital 090.0 [363.13]
  - late 094.83
  - prenatal 090.0 [363.13]
- choroidoretinitis (secondary) 091.51
  - congenital 090.0 [363.13]
  - late 094.83
- ciliary body (secondary) 091.52
  - late 095.8 [364.11]
- colon (late) 095.8
- combined sclerosis 094.89
- complicating pregnancy, childbirth or puerperium 647.0 ☑
  - affecting fetus or newborn 760.2
- condyloma (latum) 091.3
- congenital 090.9
  - with
    - encephalitis 090.41
    - paresis (general) 090.40
    - tabes (dorsalis) 090.40
    - taboparesis 090.40
  - chorioretinitis, choroiditis 090.0 [363.13]
  - early or less than 2 years after birth NEC 090.2
    - with manifestations 090.0
    - latent (without manifestations) 090.1
      - negative spinal fluid test 090.1
      - serology, positive 090.1
    - symptomatic 090.0
  - interstitial keratitis 090.3
  - juvenile neurosyphilis 090.40
  - late or 2 years or more after birth NEC 090.7
    - chorioretinitis, choroiditis 090.5 [363.13]
    - interstitial keratitis 090.3
    - juvenile neurosyphilis NEC 090.40
    - latent (without manifestations) 090.6
      - negative spinal fluid test 090.6
      - serology, positive 090.6
    - symptomatic or with manifestations NEC 090.5
      - interstitial keratitis 090.3
- conjugal 097.9
  - tabes 094.0
- conjunctiva 095.8 [372.10]
- contact V01.6
- cord, bladder 094.0
- cornea, late 095.8 [370.59]
- coronary (artery) 093.89
  - sclerosis 093.89
- coryza 095.8
  - congenital 090.0
- cranial nerve 094.89
- cutaneous — *see* Syphilis, skin
- dacryocystitis 095.8
- degeneration, spinal cord 094.89
- d'emblée 095.8
- dementia 094.1
  - paralytica 094.1
    - juvenilis 090.40
- destruction of bone 095.5
- dilatation, aorta 093.0
- due to blood transfusion 097.9
- dura mater 094.89
- ear 095.8
  - inner 095.8
    - nerve (eighth) 094.86
    - neurorecurrence 094.86
- early NEC 091.0
  - cardiovascular 093.9
  - central nervous system 094.9
    - paresis 094.1
    - tabes 094.0
  - latent (without manifestations) (less than 2 years after infection) 092.9
    - negative spinal fluid test 092.9

Syphilis, syphilitic — *continued*
  early — *continued*
    latent — *continued*
      serological relapse following treatment 092.0
      serology positive 092.9
    paresis 094.1
    relapse (treated, untreated) 091.7
    skin 091.3
    symptomatic NEC 091.89
      extragenital chancre 091.2
      primary, except extragenital chancre 091.0
      secondary (*see also* Syphilis, secondary) 091.3
        relapse (treated, untreated) 091.7
    tabes 094.0
    ulcer 091.3
  eighth nerve 094.86
  endemic, nonvenereal 104.0
  endocarditis 093.20
    aortic 093.22
    mitral 093.21
    pulmonary 093.24
    tricuspid 093.23
  epididymis (late) 095.8
  epiglottis 095.8
  epiphysitis (congenital) 090.0
  esophagus 095.8
  Eustachian tube 095.8
  exposure to V01.6
  eye 095.8 *[363.13]*
    neuromuscular mechanism 094.85
  eyelid 095.8 *[373.5]*
    with gumma 095.8 *[373.5]*
    ptosis 094.89
  fallopian tube 095.8
  fracture 095.5
  gallbladder (late) 095.8
  gastric 095.8
    crisis 094.0
    polyposis 095.8
  general 097.9
    paralysis 094.1
      juvenile 090.40
  genital (primary) 091.0
  glaucoma 095.8
  gumma (late) NEC 095.9
    cardiovascular system 093.9
    central nervous system 094.9
    congenital 090.5
    heart or artery 093.89
  heart 093.89
    block 093.89
    decompensation 093.89
    disease 093.89
    failure 093.89
    valve (*see also* Syphilis, endocarditis) 093.20
  hemianesthesia 094.89
  hemianopsia 095.8
  hemiparesis 094.89
  hemiplegia 094.89
  hepatic artery 093.89
  hepatitis 095.3
  hepatomegaly 095.3
    congenital 090.0
  hereditaria tarda (*see also* Syphilis, congenital, late) 090.7
  hereditary (*see also* Syphilis, congenital) 090.9
    interstitial keratitis 090.3
  Hutchinson's teeth 090.5
  hyalitis 095.8
  inactive — *see* Syphilis, latent
  infantum NEC (*see also* Syphilis, congenital) 090.9
  inherited — *see* Syphilis, congenital
  internal ear 095.8
  intestine (late) 095.8
  iris, iritis (secondary) 091.52
    late 095.8 *[364.11]*
  joint (late) 095.8

Syphilis, syphilitic — *continued*
  keratitis (congenital) (early) (interstitial) (late) (parenchymatous) (punctata profunda) 090.3
  kidney 095.4
  lacrimal apparatus 095.8
  laryngeal paralysis 095.8
  larynx 095.8
  late 097.0
    cardiovascular 093.9
    central nervous system 094.9
    latent or 2 years or more after infection (without manifestations) 096
      negative spinal fluid test 096
      serology positive 096
    paresis 094.1
    specified site NEC 095.8
    symptomatic or with symptoms 095.9
    tabes 094.0
  latent 097.1
    central nervous system 094.9
    date of infection unspecified 097.1
    early or less than 2 years after infection 092.9
    late or 2 years or more after infection 096
    serology
      doubtful
        follow-up of latent syphilis 097.1
        central nervous system 094.9
        date of infection unspecified 097.1
        early or less than 2 years after infection 092.9
        late or 2 years or more after infection 096
      positive, only finding 097.1
        date of infection unspecified 097.1
        early or less than 2 years after infection 097.1
        late or 2 years or more after infection 097.1
  lens 095.8
  leukoderma 091.3
    late 095.8
  lienis 095.8
  lip 091.3
    chancre 091.2
    late 095.8
    primary 091.2
  Lissauer's paralysis 094.1
  liver 095.3
    secondary 091.62
  locomotor ataxia 094.0
  lung 095.1
  lymphadenitis (secondary) 091.4
  lymph gland (early) (secondary) 091.4
    late 095.8
  macular atrophy of skin 091.3
    striated 095.8
  maternal, affecting fetus or newborn 760.2
    manifest syphilis in newborn — *see* Syphilis, congenital
  mediastinum (late) 095.8
  meninges (adhesive) (basilar) (brain) (spinal cord) 094.2
  meningitis 094.2
    acute 091.81
    congenital 090.42
  meningoencephalitis 094.2
  meningovascular 094.2
    congenital 090.49
  mesarteritis 093.89
    brain 094.89
    spine 094.89
  middle ear 095.8
  mitral stenosis 093.21
  monoplegia 094.89
  mouth (secondary) 091.3
    late 095.8

Syphilis, syphilitic — *continued*
  mucocutaneous 091.3
    late 095.8
  mucous
    membrane 091.3
      late 095.8
    patches 091.3
      congenital 090.0
  mulberry molars 090.5
  muscle 095.6
  myocarditis 093.82
  myositis 095.6
  nasal sinus 095.8
  neonatorum NEC (*see also* Syphilis, congenital) 090.9
  nerve palsy (any cranial nerve) 094.89
  nervous system, central 094.9
  neuritis 095.8
    acoustic nerve 094.86
  neurorecidive of retina 094.83
  neuroretinitis 094.85
  newborn (*see also* Syphilis, congenital) 090.9
  nodular superficial 095.8
  nonvenereal, endemic 104.0
  nose 095.8
    saddle back deformity 090.5
    septum 095.8
      perforated 095.8
  occlusive arterial disease 093.89
  ophthalmic 095.8 *[363.13]*
  ophthalmoplegia 094.89
  optic nerve (atrophy) (neuritis) (papilla) 094.84
  orbit (late) 095.8
  orchitis 095.8
  organic 097.9
  osseous (late) 095.5
  osteochondritis (congenital) 090.0
  osteoporosis 095.5
  ovary 095.8
  oviduct 095.8
  palate 095.8
    gumma 095.8
    perforated 090.5
  pancreas (late) 095.8
  pancreatitis 095.8
  paralysis 094.89
    general 094.1
    juvenile 090.40
  paraplegia 094.89
  paresis (general) 094.1
    juvenile 090.40
  paresthesia 094.89
  Parkinson's disease or syndrome 094.82
  paroxysmal tachycardia 093.89
  pemphigus (congenital) 090.0
  penis 091.0
    chancre 091.0
    late 095.8
  pericardium 093.81
  perichondritis, larynx 095.8
  periosteum 095.5
    congenital 090.0
    early 091.61
    secondary 091.61
  peripheral nerve 095.8
  petrous bone (late) 095.5
  pharynx 095.8
    secondary 091.3
  pituitary (gland) 095.8
  placenta 095.8
  pleura (late) 095.8
  pneumonia, white 090.0
  pontine (lesion) 094.89
  portal vein 093.89
  primary NEC 091.2
    anal 091.1
    and secondary (*see also* Syphilis, secondary) 091.9
    cardiovascular 093.9
    central nervous system 094.9
    extragenital chancre NEC 091.2
    fingers 091.2
    genital 091.0

Syphilis, syphilitic — *continued*
  primary — *continued*
    lip 091.2
    specified site NEC 091.2
    tonsils 091.2
  prostate 095.8
  psychosis (intracranial gumma) 094.89
  ptosis (eyelid) 094.89
  pulmonary (late) 095.1
    artery 093.89
  pulmonum 095.1
  pyelonephritis 095.4
  recently acquired, symptomatic NEC 091.89
  rectum 095.8
  respiratory tract 095.8
  retina
    late 094.83
    neurorecidive 094.83
  retrobulbar neuritis 094.85
  salpingitis 095.8
  sclera (late) 095.0
  sclerosis
    cerebral 094.89
    coronary 093.89
    multiple 094.89
    subacute 094.89
  scotoma (central) 095.8
  scrotum 095.8
  secondary (and primary) 091.9
    adenopathy 091.4
    anus 091.3
    bone 091.61
    cardiovascular 093.9
    central nervous system 094.9
    chorioretinitis, choroiditis 091.51
    hepatitis 091.62
    liver 091.62
    lymphadenitis 091.4
    meningitis, acute 091.81
    mouth 091.3
    mucous membranes 091.3
    periosteum 091.61
    periostitis 091.61
    pharynx 091.3
    relapse (treated) (untreated) 091.7
    skin 091.3
    specified form NEC 091.89
    tonsil 091.3
    ulcer 091.3
    viscera 091.69
    vulva 091.3
  seminal vesicle (late) 095.8
  seronegative
    with signs or symptoms — *see* Syphilis, by site or stage
  seropositive
    with signs or symptoms — *see* Syphilis, by site and stage
    follow-up of latent syphilis — *see* Syphilis, latent
    only finding — *see* Syphilis, latent
  seventh nerve (paralysis) 094.89
  sinus 095.8
  sinusitis 095.8
  skeletal system 095.5
  skin (early) (secondary) (with ulceration) 091.3
    late or tertiary 095.8
  small intestine 095.8
  spastic spinal paralysis 094.0
  spermatic cord (late) 095.8
  spinal (cord) 094.89
    with
      paresis 094.1
      tabes 094.0
  spleen 095.8
  splenomegaly 095.8
  spondylitis 095.5
  staphyloma 095.8
  stigmata (congenital) 090.5
  stomach 095.8
  synovium (late) 095.7
  tabes dorsalis (early) (late) 094.0
    juvenile 090.40

Syphilis, syphilitic — Tear, torn   Index to Diseases

Syphilis, syphilitic — *continued*
- tabetic type 094.0
  - juvenile 090.40
- taboparesis 094.1
  - juvenile 090.40
- tachycardia 093.89
- tendon (late) 095.7
- tertiary 097.0
  - with symptoms 095.8
  - cardiovascular 093.9
  - central nervous system 094.9
  - multiple NEC 095.8
  - specified site NEC 095.8
- testis 095.8
- thorax 095.8
- throat 095.8
- thymus (gland) 095.8
- thyroid (late) 095.8
- tongue 095.8
- tonsil (lingual) 095.8
  - primary 091.2
  - secondary 091.3
- trachea 095.8
- tricuspid valve 093.23
- tumor, brain 094.89
- tunica vaginalis (late) 095.8
- ulcer (any site) (early) (secondary) 091.3
  - late 095.9
  - perforating 095.9
    - foot 094.0
- urethra (stricture) 095.8
- urogenital 095.8
- uterus 095.8
- uveal tract (secondary) 091.50
  - late 095.8 [363.13]
- uveitis (secondary) 091.50
  - late 095.8 [363.13]
- uvula (late) 095.8
  - perforated 095.8
- vagina 091.0
  - late 095.8
- valvulitis NEC 093.20
- vascular 093.89
  - brain or cerebral 094.89
- vein 093.89
  - cerebral 094.89
- ventriculi 095.8
- vesicae urinariae 095.8
- viscera (abdominal) 095.2
  - secondary 091.69
- vitreous (hemorrhage) (opacities) 095.8
- vulva 091.0
  - late 095.8
  - secondary 091.3

Syphiloma 095.9
- cardiovascular system 093.9
- central nervous system 094.9
- circulatory system 093.9
- congenital 090.5

Syphilophobia 300.29

Syringadenoma (M8400/0) — *see also* Neoplasm, skin, benign
- papillary (M8406/0) — *see* Neoplasm, skin, benign

Syringobulbia 336.0

Syringocarcinoma (M8400/3) — *see* Neoplasm, skin, malignant

Syringocystadenoma (M8400/0) — *see also* Neoplasm, skin, benign
- papillary (M8406/0) — *see* Neoplasm, skin, benign

Syringocystoma (M8407/0) — *see* Neoplasm, skin, benign

Syringoma (M8407/0) — *see also* Neoplasm, skin, benign
- chondroid (M8940/0) — *see* Neoplasm, by site, benign

Syringomyelia 336.0

Syringomyelitis 323.9
- late effect — *see* category 326

Syringomyelocele — *see also* Spina bifida 741.9

Syringopontia 336.0

Syringopontia — *continued*
- disease, combined — *see* Degeneration, combined
- fibrosclerosing syndrome 710.8
- inflammatory response syndrome (SIRS) 995.90
  - due to
    - infectious process 995.91
      - with organ dysfunction 995.92
    - non-infectious process 995.93
      - with organ dysfunction 995.94
- lupus erythematosus 710.0
  - inhibitor 286.5

System, systemic — *see also* condition
- disease, combined — *see* Degeneration, combined
- fibrosclerosing syndrome 710.8
- inflammatory response syndrome (SIRS) 995.90
  - due to
    - infectious process 995.91
      - with ▶acute◀ organ dysfunction 995.92
    - non-infectious process 995.93
      - with ▶acute◀ organ dysfunction 995.94
- lupus erythematosus 710.0
  - inhibitor 286.5

T

Tab — *see* Tag
Tabacism 989.84
Tabacosis 989.84
Tabardillo 080
- flea-borne 081.0
- louse-borne 080

Tabes, tabetic
- with
  - central nervous system syphilis 094.0
  - Charcôt's joint 094.0 [713.5]
  - cord bladder 094.0
  - crisis, viscera (any) 094.0
  - paralysis, general 094.1
  - paresis (general) 094.1
  - perforating ulcer 094.0
- arthropathy 094.0 [713.5]
- bladder 094.0
- bone 094.0
- cerebrospinal 094.0
- congenital 090.40
- conjugal 094.0
- dorsalis 094.0
  - neurosyphilis 094.0
- early 094.0
- juvenile 090.40
- latent 094.0
- mesenterica (*see also* Tuberculosis) 014.8
- paralysis insane, general 094.1
- peripheral (nonsyphilitic) 799.89
- spasmodic 094.0
  - not dorsal or dorsalis 343.9
- syphilis (cerebrospinal) 094.0

Taboparalysis 094.1
Taboparesis (remission) 094.1
- with
  - Charcôt's joint 094.1 [713.5]
  - cord bladder 094.1
  - perforating ulcer 094.1
- juvenile 090.40

Tache noir 923.20
Tachyalimentation 579.3
Tachyarrhythmia, tachyrhythmia — *see also* Tachycardia
- paroxysmal with sinus bradycardia 427.81

Tachycardia 785.0
- atrial 427.89
- auricular 427.89
- AV nodal re-entry (re-entrant) 427.89
- newborn 779.82
- nodal 427.89

Tachycardia — *continued*
- nodal — *continued*
  - nonparoxysmal atrioventricular 426.89
  - nonparoxysmal atrioventricular (nodal) 426.89
- paroxysmal 427.2
  - with sinus bradycardia 427.81
  - atrial (PAT) 427.0
    - psychogenic 316 [427.0]
  - atrioventricular (AV) 427.0
    - psychogenic 316 [427.0]
  - essential 427.2
  - junctional 427.0
  - nodal 427.0
  - psychogenic 316 [427.2]
    - atrial 316 [427.0]
      - supraventricular 316 [427.0]
      - ventricular 316 [427.1]
  - supraventricular 427.0
    - psychogenic 316 [427.0]
  - ventricular 427.1
    - psychogenic 316 [427.1]
- postoperative 997.1
- psychogenic 306.2
- sick sinus 427.81
- sinoauricular 427.89
- sinus 427.89
- supraventricular 427.89
- ventricular (paroxysmal) 427.1
  - psychogenic 316 [427.1]

Tachygastria 536.8
Tachypnea 786.06
- hysterical 300.11
- newborn (idiopathic) (transitory) 770.6
- psychogenic 306.1
- transitory, of newborn 770.6

Taenia (infection) (infestation) — *see also* Infestation, taenia 123.3
- diminuta 123.6
- echinococcal infestation (*see also* Echinococcus) 122.9
- nana 123.6
- saginata infestation 123.2
- solium (intestinal form) 123.0
  - larval form 123.1

Taeniasis (intestine) — *see also* Infestation, taenia 123.3
- saginata 123.2
- solium 123.0

Taenzer's disease 757.4
Tag (hypertrophied skin) (infected) 701.9
- adenoid 474.8
- anus 455.9
- endocardial (*see also* Endocarditis) 424.90
- hemorrhoidal 455.9
- hymen 623.8
- perineal 624.8
- preauricular 744.1
- rectum 455.9
- sentinel 455.9
- skin 701.9
  - accessory 757.39
  - anus 455.9
  - congenital 757.39
  - preauricular 744.1
  - rectum 455.9
- tonsil 474.8
- urethra, urethral 599.84
- vulva 624.8

Tahyna fever 062.5
Takayasu (-Onishi) disease or syndrome (pulseless) 446.7
Takotsubo syndrome 429.83
Talc granuloma 728.82
- in operation wound 998.7

Talcosis 502
Talipes (congenital) 754.70
- acquired NEC 736.79
  - planus 734
- asymmetric 754.79
  - acquired 736.79
- calcaneovalgus 754.62
  - acquired 736.76
- calcaneovarus 754.59

Talipes — *continued*
- calcaneovarus — *continued*
  - acquired 736.76
- calcaneus 754.79
  - acquired 736.76
- cavovarus 754.59
  - acquired 736.75
- cavus 754.71
  - acquired 736.73
- equinovalgus 754.69
  - acquired 736.72
- equinovarus 754.51
  - acquired 736.71
- equinus 754.79
  - acquired, NEC 736.72
- percavus 754.71
  - acquired 736.73
- planovalgus 754.69
  - acquired 736.79
- planus (acquired) (any degree) 734
  - congenital 754.61
  - due to rickets 268.1
- valgus 754.60
  - acquired 736.79
- varus 754.50
  - acquired 736.79

Talma's disease 728.85
Talon noir 924.20
- hand 923.20
- heel 924.20
- toe 924.3

Tamponade heart (Rose's) — *see also* Pericarditis 423.9
Tanapox 078.89
Tangier disease (familial high-density lipoprotein deficiency) 272.5
Tank ear 380.12
Tantrum (childhood) — *see also* Disturbance, conduct 312.1
Tapeworm (infection) (infestation) — *see also* Infestation, tapeworm 123.9
Tapia's syndrome 352.6
Tarantism 297.8
Target-oval cell anemia 282.49
Tarlov's cyst 355.9
Tarral-Besnier disease (pityriasis rubra pilaris) 696.4
Tarsalgia 729.2
Tarsal tunnel syndrome 355.5
Tarsitis (eyelid) 373.00
- syphilitic 095.8 [373.00]
- tuberculous (*see also* Tuberculosis) 017.0 [373.4]

Tartar (teeth) 523.6
Tattoo (mark) 709.09
Taurodontism 520.2
Taussig-Bing defect, heart, or syndrome (transposition, aorta and overriding pulmonary artery) 745.11
Taybi's syndrome (otopalatodigital) 759.89
Tay's choroiditis 363.41
Taylor's
- disease (diffuse idiopathic cutaneous atrophy) 701.8
- syndrome 625.5

Tay-Sachs
- amaurotic familial idiocy 330.1
- disease 330.1

Tear stone 375.57
Tear, torn (traumatic) — *see also* Wound, open, by site
- anus, anal (sphincter) 863.89
  - with open wound in cavity 863.99
  - complicating delivery 664.2
    - with mucosa 664.3
  - nontraumatic, nonpuerperal 565.0
- articular cartilage, old (*see also* Disorder, cartilage, articular) 718.0
- bladder
  - with
    - abortion — *see* Abortion, by type, with damage to pelvic organs

Tear, torn — see also Wound, open, by site — continued
  bladder — continued
    with — continued
      ectopic pregnancy (see also categories 633.0–633.9) 639.2
      molar pregnancy (see also categories 630–632) 639.2
      following
        abortion 639.2
        ectopic or molar pregnancy 639.2
      obstetrical trauma 665.5 ☑
  bowel
    with
      abortion — see Abortion, by type, with damage to pelvic organs
      ectopic pregnancy (see also categories 633.0–633.9) 639.2
      molar pregnancy (see also categories 630–632) 639.2
      following
        abortion 639.2
        ectopic or molar pregnancy 639.2
      obstetrical trauma 665.5 ☑
  broad ligament
    with
      abortion — see Abortion, by type, with damage to pelvic organs
      ectopic pregnancy (see also categories 633.0–633.9) 639.2
      molar pregnancy (see also categories 630–632) 639.2
      following
        abortion 639.2
        ectopic or molar pregnancy 639.2
      obstetrical trauma 665.6 ☑
  bucket handle (knee) (meniscus) — see Tear, meniscus
  capsule
    joint — see Sprain, by site
    spleen — see Laceration, spleen, capsule
  cartilage (see also Sprain, by site)
    articular, old (see also Disorder, cartilage, articular) 718.0 ☑
    knee — see Tear, meniscus
    semilunar (knee) (current injury) — see Tear, meniscus
  cervix
    with
      abortion — see Abortion, by type, with damage to pelvic organs
      ectopic pregnancy (see also categories 633.0–633.9) 639.2
      molar pregnancy (see also categories 630–632) 639.2
      following
        abortion 639.2
        ectopic or molar pregnancy 639.2
      obstetrical trauma (current) 665.3 ☑
      old 622.3
  internal organ (abdomen, chest, or pelvis) — see Injury, internal, by site
  ligament (see also Sprain, by site)
    with open wound — see Wound, open by site
  meniscus (knee) (current injury) 836.2
    bucket handle 836.0
      old 717.0
    lateral 836.1
      anterior horn 836.1
        old 717.42
      bucket handle 836.1

Tear, torn — see also Wound, open, by site — continued
  meniscus — continued
    lateral — continued
      bucket handle — continued
        old 717.41
      old 717.40
      posterior horn 836.1
        old 717.43
      specified site NEC 836.1
        old 717.49
    medial 836.0
      anterior horn 836.0
        old 717.1
      bucket handle 836.0
        old 717.0
      old 717.3
      posterior horn 836.0
        old 717.2
      old NEC 717.5
    site other than knee — see Sprain, by site
  muscle (see also Sprain, by site)
    with open wound — see Wound, open by site
  pelvic
    floor, complicating delivery 664.1 ☑
    organ NEC
      with
        abortion — see Abortion, by type, with damage to pelvic organs
        ectopic pregnancy (see also categories 633.0–633.9) 639.2
        molar pregnancy (see also categories 630–632) 639.2
        following
          abortion 639.2
          ectopic or molar pregnancy 639.2
        obstetrical trauma 665.5 ☑
  perineum (see also Laceration, perineum)
    obstetrical trauma 665.5 ☑
  periurethral tissue
    with
      abortion — see Abortion, by type, with damage to pelvic organs
      ectopic pregnancy (see also categories 633.0–633.9) 639.2
      molar pregnancy (see also categories 630–632) 639.2
      following
        abortion 639.2
        ectopic or molar pregnancy 639.2
      obstetrical trauma 665.5 ☑
  rectovaginal septum — see Laceration, rectovaginal septum
  retina, retinal (recent) (with detachment) 361.00
    without detachment 361.30
    dialysis (juvenile) (with detachment) 361.04
    giant (with detachment) 361.03
    horseshoe (without detachment) 361.32
    multiple (with detachment) 361.02
      without detachment 361.33
    old
      delimited (partial) 361.06
      partial 361.06
      total or subtotal 361.07
    partial (without detachment)
      giant 361.03
      multiple defects 361.02
      old (delimited) 361.06
      single defect 361.01
    round hole (without detachment) 361.31

Tear, torn — see also Wound, open, by site — continued
  retina, retinal — continued
    single defect (with detachment) 361.01
    total or subtotal (recent) 361.05
      old 361.07
  rotator cuff (traumatic) 840.4
    current injury 840.4
    degenerative 726.10
    nontraumatic 727.61
  semilunar cartilage, knee (see also Tear, meniscus) 836.2
    old 717.5
  tendon (see also Sprain, by site)
    with open wound — see Wound, open by site
  tentorial, at birth 767.0
  umbilical cord
    affecting fetus or newborn 772.0
    complicating delivery 663.8 ☑
  urethra
    with
      abortion — see Abortion, by type, with damage to pelvic organs
      ectopic pregnancy (see also categories 633.0–633.9) 639.2
      molar pregnancy (see also categories 630–632) 639.2
      following
        abortion 639.2
        ectopic or molar pregnancy 639.2
      obstetrical trauma 665.5 ☑
  uterus — see Injury, internal, uterus
  vagina — see Laceration, vagina
  vessel, from catheter 998.2
  vulva, complicating delivery 664.0 ☑
Teething 520.7
  syndrome 520.7
Teeth, tooth — see also condition
  grinding 306.8
  prenatal 520.6 ●
Tegmental syndrome 344.89
Telangiectasia, telangiectasis (verrucous) 448.9
  ataxic (cerebellar) 334.8
  familial 448.0
  hemorrhagic, hereditary (congenital) (senile) 448.0
  hereditary hemorrhagic 448.0
  retina 362.15
  spider 448.1
Telecanthus (congenital) 743.63
Telescoped bowel or intestine — see also Intussusception 560.0
Teletherapy, adverse effect NEC 990
Telogen effluvium 704.02
Temperature
  body, high (of unknown origin) (see also Pyrexia) 780.6
  cold, trauma from 991.9
    newborn 778.2
    specified effect NEC 991.8
  high
    body (of unknown origin) (see also Pyrexia) 780.6
    trauma from — see Heat
Temper tantrum (childhood) — see also Disturbance, conduct 312.1 ☑
Temple — see condition
Temporal — see also condition
  lobe syndrome 310.0
Temporomandibular joint-pain-dysfunction syndrome 524.60
Temporosphenoidal — see condition
Tendency
  bleeding (see also Defect, coagulation) 286.9
  homosexual, ego-dystonic 302.0
  paranoid 301.0
  suicide 300.9

Tenderness
  abdominal (generalized) (localized) 789.6 ☑
  rebound 789.6 ☑
  skin 782.0
Tendinitis, tendonitis — see also Tenosynovitis 726.90
  Achilles 726.71
  adhesive 726.90
    shoulder 726.0
  calcific 727.82
    shoulder 726.11
  gluteal 726.5
  patellar 726.64
  peroneal 726.79
  pes anserinus 726.61
  psoas 726.5
  tibialis (anterior) (posterior) 726.72
  trochanteric 726.5
Tendon — see condition
Tendosynovitis — see Tenosynovitis
Tendovaginitis — see Tenosynovitis
Tenesmus 787.99
  rectal 787.99
  vesical 788.9
Tenia — see Taenia
Teniasis — see Taeniasis
Tennis elbow 726.32
Tenonitis — see also Tenosynovitis
  eye (capsule) 376.04
Tenontosynovitis — see Tenosynovitis
Tenontothecitis — see Tenosynovitis
Tenophyte 727.9
Tenosynovitis 727.00
  adhesive 726.90
    shoulder 726.0
  ankle 727.06
  bicipital (calcifying) 726.12
  buttock 727.09
  due to crystals — see Arthritis, due to crystals
  elbow 727.09
  finger 727.05
  foot 727.06
  gonococcal 098.51
  hand 727.05
  hip 727.09
  knee 727.09
  radial styloid 727.04
  shoulder 726.10
    adhesive 726.0
  spine 720.1
  supraspinatus 726.10
  toe 727.06
  tuberculous — see Tuberculosis, tenosynovitis
  wrist 727.05
Tenovaginitis — see Tenosynovitis
Tension
  arterial, high (see also Hypertension) 401.9
    without diagnosis of hypertension 796.2
  headache 307.81
  intraocular (elevated) 365.00
  nervous 799.2
  ocular (elevated) 365.00
  pneumothorax 512.0
    iatrogenic 512.1
    postoperative 512.1
    spontaneous 512.0
  premenstrual 625.4
  state 300.9
Tentorium — see condition
Teratencephalus 759.89
Teratism 759.7
Teratoblastoma (malignant) (M9080/3) — see Neoplasm, by site, malignant
Teratocarcinoma (M9081/3) — see also Neoplasm, by site, malignant
  liver 155.0
Teratoma (solid) (M9080/1) — see also Neoplasm, by site, uncertain behavior
  adult (cystic) (M9080/0) — see Neoplasm, by site, benign

Teratoma

Teratoma — see also Neoplasm, by site, uncertain behavior — continued
  and embryonal carcinoma, mixed (M9081/3) — see Neoplasm, by site, malignant
  benign (M9080/0) — see Neoplasm, by site, benign
  combined with choriocarcinoma (M9101/3) — see Neoplasm, by site, malignant
  cystic (adult) (M9080/0) — see Neoplasm, by site, benign
  differentiated type (M9080/0) — see Neoplasm, by site, benign
  embryonal (M9080/3) (see also Neoplasm, by site, malignant)
    liver 155.0
  fetal
    sacral, causing fetopelvic disproportion 653.7 ☑
  immature (M9080/3) — see Neoplasm, by site, malignant
  liver (M9080/3) 155.0
    adult, benign, cystic, differentiated type or mature (M9080/0) 211.5
  malignant (M9080/3) (see also Neoplasm, by site, malignant)
    anaplastic type (M9082/3) — see Neoplasm, by site, malignant
    intermediate type (M9083/3) — see Neoplasm, by site, malignant
    liver (M9080/3) 155.0
    trophoblastic (M9102/3)
      specified site — see Neoplasm, by site, malignant
      unspecified site 186.9
    undifferentiated type (M9082/3) — see Neoplasm, by site, malignant
  mature (M9080/0) — see Neoplasm, by site, benign
  ovary (M9080/0) 220
    embryonal, immature, or malignant (M9080/3) 183.0
  suprasellar (M9080/3) — see Neoplasm, by site, malignant
  testis (M9080/3) 186.9
    adult, benign, cystic, differentiated type or mature (M9080/0) 222.0
    undescended 186.0
Terminal care V66.7
Termination
  anomalous (see also Malposition, congenital)
    portal vein 747.49
    right pulmonary vein 747.42
  pregnancy (legal) (therapeutic) — see Abortion, legal 635.9 ☑
    fetus NEC 779.6
    illegal (see also Abortion, illegal) 636.9 ☑
Ternidens diminutus infestation 127.7
Terrors, night (child) 307.46
Terry's syndrome 362.21
Tertiary — see condition
Tessellated fundus, retina (tigroid) 362.89
Test(s)
  adequacy
    hemodialysis V56.31
    peritoneal dialysis V56.32
  AIDS virus V72.6
  allergen V72.7
  bacterial disease NEC (see also Screening, by name of disease) V74.9
  basal metabolic rate V72.6
  blood-alcohol V70.4
  blood-drug V70.4
    for therapeutic drug monitoring V58.83
  blood typing V72.86
    Rh typing V72.86
  developmental, infant or child V20.2

Test(s) — continued
  Dick V74.8
  fertility V26.21
  genetic
    female V26.32
    for genetic disease carrier status
      female V26.31
      male V26.34
    male V26.39
  hearing V72.19
    following failed hearing screening V72.11
  HIV V72.6
  human immunodeficiency virus V72.6
  Kveim V82.89
  laboratory V72.6
    for medicolegal reason V70.4
  male partner of habitual aborter V26.35
  Mantoux (for tuberculosis) V74.1
  mycotic organism V75.4
  parasitic agent NEC V75.8
  paternity V70.4
  peritoneal equilibration V56.32
  pregnancy
    negative result V72.41
    positive result V72.42
      first pregnancy V72.42
    unconfirmed V72.40
  preoperative V72.84
    cardiovascular V72.81
    respiratory V72.82
    specified NEC V72.83
  procreative management NEC V26.29
    genetic disease carrier status
      female V26.31
      male V26.34
  Rh typing V72.86
  sarcoidosis V82.89
  Schick V74.3
  Schultz-Charlton V74.8
  skin, diagnostic
    allergy V72.7
    bacterial agent NEC (see also Screening, by name of disease) V74.9
    Dick V74.8
    hypersensitivity V72.7
    Kveim V82.89
    Mantoux V74.1
    mycotic organism V75.4
    parasitic agent NEC V75.8
    sarcoidosis V82.89
    Schick V74.3
    Schultz-Charlton V74.8
    tuberculin V74.1
  specified type NEC V72.85
  tuberculin V74.1
  vision V72.0
  Wassermann
    positive (see also Serology for syphilis, positive) 097.1
    false 795.6
Testicle, testicular, testis — see also condition
  feminization (syndrome) 259.5
Tetanus, tetanic (cephalic) (convulsions) 037
  with
    abortion — see Abortion, by type, with sepsis
    ectopic pregnancy (see also categories 633.0–633.9) 639.0
    molar pregnancy — see categories 630–632 639.0
  following
    abortion 639.0
    ectopic or molar pregnancy 639.0
  inoculation V03.7
    reaction (due to serum) — see Complications, vaccination
  neonatorum 771.3
  puerperal, postpartum, childbirth 670.0 ☑
Tetany, tetanic 781.7
  alkalosis 276.3

Tetany, tetanic — continued
  associated with rickets 268.0
  convulsions 781.7
    hysterical 300.11
  functional (hysterical) 300.11
  hyperkinetic 781.7
    hysterical 300.11
  hyperpnea 786.01
    hysterical 300.11
    psychogenic 306.1
  hyperventilation 786.01
    hysterical 300.11
    psychogenic 306.1
  hypocalcemic, neonatal 775.4
  hysterical 300.11
  neonatal 775.4
  parathyroid (gland) 252.1
  parathyroprival 252.1
  postoperative 252.1
  postthyroidectomy 252.1
  pseudotetany 781.7
    hysterical 300.11
  psychogenic 306.1
    specified as conversion reaction 300.11
Tetralogy of Fallot 745.2
Tetraplegia — see Quadriplegia
Thailand hemorrhagic fever 065.4
Thalassanemia 282.49
Thalassemia (alpha) (beta) (disease) (Hb-C) (Hb-D) (Hb-E) (Hb-H) (Hb-I) (high fetal gene) (high fetal hemoglobin) (intermedia) (major) (minima) (minor) (mixed) (trait) (with other hemoglobinopathy) 282.49
  Hb-S (without crisis) 282.41
  with
    crisis 282.42
    vaso-occlusive pain 282.42
  sickle-cell (without crisis) 282.41
  with
    crisis 282.42
    vaso-occlusive pain 282.42
Thalassemic variants 282.49
Thaysen-Gee disease (nontropical sprue) 579.0
Thecoma (M8600/0) 220
  malignant (M8600/3) 183.0
Thelarche, precocious 259.1
Thelitis 611.0
  puerperal, postpartum 675.0 ☑
Therapeutic — see condition
Therapy V57.9
  blood transfusion, without reported diagnosis V58.2
  breathing V57.0
  chemotherapy, antineoplastic V58.11
    fluoride V07.31
    prophylactic NEC V07.39
  dialysis (intermittent) (treatment)
    extracorporeal V56.0
    peritoneal V56.8
    renal V56.0
    specified type NEC V56.8
  exercise NEC V57.1
    breathing V57.0
  extracorporeal dialysis (renal) V56.0
  fluoride prophylaxis V07.31
  hemodialysis V56.0
  hormone replacement (postmenopausal) V07.4
  immunotherapy antineoplastic V58.12
  long term oxygen therapy V46.2
  occupational V57.21
  orthoptic V57.4
  orthotic V57.81
  peritoneal dialysis V56.8
  physical NEC V57.1
  postmenopausal hormone replacement V07.4
  radiation V58.0
  speech V57.3
  vocational V57.22
Thermalgesia 782.0
Thermalgia 782.0
Thermanalgesia 782.0

Thermanesthesia 782.0
Thermic — see condition
Thermography (abnormal) 793.99 ▲
  breast 793.89
Thermoplegia 992.0
Thesaurismosis
  amyloid 277.39
  bilirubin 277.4
  calcium 275.40
  cystine 270.0
  glycogen (see also Disease, glycogen storage) 271.0
  kerasin 272.7
  lipoid 272.7
  melanin 255.4
  phosphatide 272.7
  urate 274.9
Thiaminic deficiency 265.1
  with beriberi 265.0
Thibierge-Weissenbach syndrome (cutaneous systemic sclerosis) 710.1
Thickened endometrium 793.5
Thickening
  bone 733.99
    extremity 733.99
  breast 611.79
  hymen 623.3
  larynx 478.79
  nail 703.8
    congenital 757.5
  periosteal 733.99
  pleura (see also Pleurisy) 511.0
  skin 782.8
  subepiglottic 478.79
  tongue 529.8
  valve, heart — see Endocarditis
Thiele syndrome 724.6
Thigh — see condition
Thinning vertebra — see also Osteoporosis 733.00
Thirst, excessive 783.5
  due to deprivation of water 994.3
Thomsen's disease 359.2
Thomson's disease (congenital poikiloderma) 757.33
Thoracic — see also condition
  kidney 753.3
  outlet syndrome 353.0
  stomach — see Hernia, diaphragm
Thoracogastroschisis (congenital) 759.89
Thoracopagus 759.4
Thoracoschisis 756.3
Thoracoscopic surgical procedure converted to open procedure V64.42
Thorax — see condition
Thorn's syndrome — see also Disease, renal 593.9
Thornwaldt's, Tornwaldt's
  bursitis (pharyngeal) 478.29
  cyst 478.26
  disease (pharyngeal bursitis) 478.29
Thorson-Biörck syndrome (malignant carcinoid) 259.2
Threadworm (infection) (infestation) 127.4
Threatened
  abortion or miscarriage 640.0 ☑
    with subsequent abortion (see also Abortion, spontaneous) 634.9 ☑
    affecting fetus 762.1
  labor 644.1 ☑
    affecting fetus or newborn 761.8
    premature 644.0 ☑
  miscarriage 640.0 ☑
    affecting fetus 762.1
  premature
    delivery 644.2 ☑
      affecting fetus or newborn 761.8
    labor 644.0 ☑
      before 22 completed weeks gestation 640.0 ☑
Three-day fever 066.0
Threshers' lung 495.0

Index to Diseases — Thrombosis, thrombotic

Thrix annulata (congenital) 757.4
Throat — see condition
Thrombasthenia (Glanzmann's) (hemorrhagic) (hereditary) 287.1
Thromboangiitis 443.1
  obliterans (general) 443.1
    cerebral 437.1
    vessels
      brain 437.1
      spinal cord 437.1
Thromboarteritis — see Arteritis
Thromboasthenia (Glanzmann's) (hemorrhagic) (hereditary) 287.1
Thrombocytasthenia (Glanzmann's) 287.1
Thrombocythemia (primary) (M9962/1) 238.71 ▲
  essential 238.71 ●
  hemorrhagic 238.71
  idiopathic ▶(hemorrhagic)◀ (M9962/1) 238.71 ▲
Thrombocytopathy (dystrophic) (granulopenic) 287.1
Thrombocytopenia, thrombocytopenic 287.5
  with
    absent radii (TAR) syndrome
    giant hemangioma
  amegakaryocytic, congenital 287.33
  congenital 287.33
  cyclic 287.39
  dilutional 287.4
  due to
    drugs 287.4
    extracorporeal circulation of blood 287.4
    massive blood transfusion 287.4
    platelet alloimmunization 287.4
  essential 287.30
  hereditary 287.30
  Kasabach-Merritt 287.39
  neonatal, transitory 776.1
    due to
      exchange transfusion 776.1
      idiopathic maternal thrombocytopenia 776.1
      isoimmunization 776.1
  primary 287.30
  puerperal, postpartum 666.3 ☑
  purpura (see also Purpura, thrombocytopenic) 287.30
    thrombotic 446.6
  secondary 287.4
  sex-linked 287.39
Thrombocytosis 238.71 ▲
  essential 238.71 ●
  primary 238.71 ●
Thromboembolism — see Embolism
Thrombopathy (Bernard-Soulier) 287.1
  constitutional 286.4
  Willebrand-Jürgens (angiohemophilia) 286.4
Thrombopenia — see also Thrombocytopenia 287.5
Thrombophlebitis 451.9
  antecubital vein 451.82
  antepartum (superficial) 671.2 ☑
    affecting fetus or newborn 760.3
    deep 671.3 ☑
  arm 451.89
    deep 451.83
    superficial 451.82
  breast, superficial 451.89
  cavernous (venous) sinus — see Thrombophlebitis, intracranial venous sinus
  cephalic vein 451.82
  cerebral (sinus) (vein) 325
    late effect — see category 326
    nonpyogenic 437.6
      in pregnancy or puerperium 671.5 ☑
      late effect — see Late effect(s) (of) cerebrovascular disease

Thrombophlebitis — continued
  due to implanted device — see Complications, due to (presence of) any device, implant or graft classified to 996.0–996.5 NEC
  during or resulting from a procedure NEC 997.2
  femoral 451.11
  femoropopliteal 451.19
  following infusion, perfusion, or transfusion 999.2
  hepatic (vein) 451.89
  idiopathic, recurrent 453.1
  iliac vein 451.81
  iliofemoral 451.11
  intracranial venous sinus (any) 325
    late effect — see category 326
    nonpyogenic 437.6
      in pregnancy or puerperium 671.5 ☑
      late effect — see Late effect(s) (of) cerebrovascular disease
  jugular vein 451.89
  lateral (venous) sinus — see Thrombophlebitis, intracranial venous sinus
  leg 451.2
    deep (vessels) 451.19
      femoral vein 451.11
      specified vessel NEC 451.19
    superficial (vessels) 451.0
    femoral vein 451.11
  longitudinal (venous) sinus — see Thrombophlebitis, intracranial venous sinus
  lower extremity 451.2
    deep (vessels) 451.19
      femoral vein 451.11
      specified vessel NEC 451.19
    superficial (vessels) 451.0
  migrans, migrating 453.1
  pelvic
    with
      abortion — see Abortion, by type, with sepsis
      ectopic pregnancy (see also categories 633.0–633.9) 639.0
      molar pregnancy (see also categories 630–632) 639.0
    following
      abortion 639.0
      ectopic or molar pregnancy 639.0
    puerperal 671.4 ☑
  popliteal vein 451.19
  portal (vein) 572.1
  postoperative 997.2
  pregnancy (superficial) 671.2 ☑
    affecting fetus or newborn 760.3
    deep 671.3 ☑
  puerperal, postpartum, childbirth (extremities) (superficial) 671.2 ☑
    deep 671.4 ☑
    pelvic 671.4 ☑
    specified site NEC 671.5 ☑
  radial vein 451.83
  saphenous (greater) (lesser) 451.0
  sinus (intracranial) — see Thrombophlebitis, intracranial venous sinus
  specified site NEC 451.89
  tibial vein 451.19
Thrombosis, thrombotic (marantic) (multiple) (progressive) (septic) (vein) (vessel) 453.9
  with childbirth or during the puerperium — see Thrombosis, puerperal, postpartum
  antepartum — see Thrombosis, pregnancy
  aorta, aortic 444.1
    abdominal 444.0
    bifurcation 444.0

Thrombosis, thrombotic — continued
  aorta, aortic — continued
    saddle 444.0
    terminal 444.0
    thoracic 444.1
    valve — see Endocarditis, aortic
  apoplexy (see also Thrombosis, brain) 434.0 ☑
    late effect — see Late effect(s) (of) cerebrovascular disease
  appendix, septic — see Appendicitis, acute
  arteriolar-capillary platelet, disseminated 446.6
  artery, arteries (postinfectional) 444.9
    auditory, internal 433.8 ☑
    basilar (see also Occlusion, artery, basilar) 433.0 ☑
    carotid (common) (internal) (see also Occlusion, artery, carotid) 433.1 ☑
      with other precerebral artery 433.3 ☑
    cerebellar (anterior inferior) (posterior inferior) (superior) 433.8 ☑
    cerebral (see also Thrombosis, brain) 434.0 ☑
    choroidal (anterior) 433.8 ☑
    communicating posterior 433.8 ☑
    coronary (see also Infarct, myocardium) 410.9 ☑
      without myocardial infarction 411.81
      due to syphilis 093.89
      healed or specified as old 412
    extremities 444.22
      lower 444.22
      upper 444.21
    femoral 444.22
    hepatic 444.89
    hypophyseal 433.8 ☑
    meningeal, anterior or posterior 433.8 ☑
    mesenteric (with gangrene) 557.0
    ophthalmic (see also Occlusion, retina) 362.30
    pontine 433.8 ☑
    popliteal 444.22
    precerebral — see Occlusion, artery, precerebral NEC
    pulmonary 415.19
      iatrogenic 415.11
      postoperative 415.11
    renal 593.81
    retinal (see also Occlusion, retina) 362.30
    specified site NEC 444.89
    spinal, anterior or posterior 433.8 ☑
    traumatic (complication) (early) (see also Injury, blood vessel, by site) 904.9
    vertebral (see also Occlusion, artery, vertebral) 433.2 ☑
      with other precerebral artery 433.3 ☑
  atrial (endocardial) 424.90
    without endocarditis 429.89 ●
    due to syphilis 093.89
  auricular (see also Infarct, myocardium) 410.9 ☑
  axillary (vein) 453.8
  basilar (artery) (see also Occlusion, artery, basilar) 433.0 ☑
  bland NEC 453.9
  brain (artery) (stem) 434.0 ☑
    due to syphilis 094.89
    iatrogenic 997.02
    late effect — see Late effect(s) (of) cerebrovascular disease
    postoperative 997.02
    puerperal, postpartum, childbirth 674.0 ☑

Thrombosis, thrombotic — continued
  brain — continued
    sinus (see also Thrombosis, intracranial venous sinus) 325
  capillary 448.9
    arteriolar, generalized 446.6
  cardiac (see also Infarct, myocardium) 410.9 ☑
    due to syphilis 093.89
    healed or specified as old 412
    valve — see Endocarditis
  carotid (artery) (common) (internal) (see also Occlusion, artery, carotid) 433.1 ☑
    with other precerebral artery 433.3 ☑
  cavernous sinus (venous) — see Thrombosis, intracranial venous sinus
  cerebellar artery (anterior inferior) (posterior inferior) (superior) 433.8 ☑
    late effect — see Late effect(s) (of) cerebrovascular disease
  cerebral (arteries) (see also Thrombosis, brain) 434.0 ☑
    late effect — see Late effect(s) (of) cerebrovascular disease
  coronary (artery) (see also Infarct, myocardium) 410.9 ☑
    without myocardial infarction 411.81
    due to syphilis 093.89
    healed or specified as old 412
  corpus cavernosum 607.82
  cortical (see also Thrombosis, brain) 434.0 ☑
  due to (presence of) any device, implant, or graft classifiable to 996.0–996.5 — see Complications, due to (presence of) any device, implant, or graft classified to 996.0–996.5 NEC
  effort 453.8
  endocardial — see Infarct, myocardium
  eye (see also Occlusion, retina) 362.30
  femoral (vein) 453.8
    with inflammation or phlebitis 451.11
    artery 444.22
    deep 453.41
  genital organ, male 608.83
  heart (chamber) (see also Infarct, myocardium) 410.9 ☑
  hepatic (vein) 453.0
    artery 444.89
    infectional or septic 572.1
  iliac (vein) 453.8
    with inflammation or phlebitis 451.81
    artery (common) (external) (internal) 444.81
  inflammation, vein — see Thrombophlebitis
  internal carotid artery (see also Occlusion, artery, carotid) 433.1 ☑
    with other precerebral artery 433.3 ☑
  intestine (with gangrene) 557.0
  intracranial (see also Thrombosis, brain) 434.0 ☑
    venous sinus (any) 325
      nonpyogenic origin 437.6
        in pregnancy or puerperium 671.5 ☑
  intramural (see also Infarct, myocardium) 410.9 ☑
    without
      cardiac condition 429.89
      coronary artery disease 429.89
      myocardial infarction 429.89
    healed or specified as old 412
  jugular (bulb) 453.8
  kidney 593.81

Thrombosis, thrombotic — continued
kidney — continued
  artery 593.81
lateral sinus (venous) — see Thrombosis, intracranial venous sinus
leg 453.8
  with inflammation or phlebitis — see Thrombophlebitis
  deep (vessels) 453.40
    lower (distal) 453.42
    upper (proximal) 453.41
  superficial (vessels) 453.8
liver (venous) 453.0
  artery 444.89
  infectional or septic 572.1
  portal vein 452
longitudinal sinus (venous) — see Thrombosis, intracranial venous sinus
lower extremity 453.8
  deep vessels 453.40
    calf 453.42
    distal (lower leg) 453.42
    femoral 453.41
    iliac 453.41
    lower leg 453.42
    peroneal 453.42
    popliteal 453.41
    proximal (upper leg) 453.41
    thigh 453.41
    tibial 453.42
lung 415.19
  iatrogenic 415.11
  postoperative 415.11
marantic, dural sinus 437.6
meninges (brain) (see also Thrombosis, brain) 434.0 ☑
mesenteric (artery) (with gangrene) 557.0
  vein (inferior) (superior) 557.0
mitral — see Insufficiency, mitral
mural (heart chamber) (see also Infarct, myocardium) 410.9 ☑
  without
    cardiac condition 429.89
    coronary artery disease 429.89
    myocardial infarction 429.89
  due to syphilis 093.89
  following myocardial infarction 429.79
  healed or specified as old 412
omentum (with gangrene) 557.0
ophthalmic (artery) (see also Occlusion, retina) 362.30
pampiniform plexus (male) 608.83
  female 620.8
parietal (see also Infarct, myocardium) 410.9 ☑
penis, penile 607.82
peripheral arteries 444.22
  lower 444.22
  upper 444.21
platelet 446.6
portal 452
  due to syphilis 093.89
  infectional or septic 572.1
precerebral artery (see also Occlusion, artery, precerebral NEC)
pregnancy 671.9 ☑
  deep (vein) 671.3 ☑
  superficial (vein) 671.2 ☑
puerperal, postpartum, childbirth 671.9 ☑
  brain (artery) 674.0 ☑
    venous 671.5 ☑
  cardiac 674.8 ☑
  cerebral (artery) 674.0 ☑
    venous 671.5 ☑
  deep (vein) 671.4 ☑
  intracranial sinus (nonpyogenic) (venous) 671.5 ☑
  pelvic 671.4 ☑
  pulmonary (artery) 673.2 ☑
  specified site NEC 671.5 ☑
  superficial 671.2 ☑

Thrombosis, thrombotic — continued
pulmonary (artery) (vein) 415.19
  iatrogenic 415.11
  postoperative 415.11
renal (artery) 593.81
  vein 453.3
resulting from presence of shunt or other internal prosthetic device — see Complications, due to (presence of) any device, implant, or graft classified to 996.0–996.5 NEC
retina, retinal (artery) 362.30
  arterial branch 362.32
  central 362.31
  partial 362.33
  vein
    central 362.35
    tributary (branch) 362.36
scrotum 608.83
seminal vesicle 608.83
sigmoid (venous) sinus — see Thrombosis, intracranial venous sinus 325
silent NEC 453.9
sinus, intracranial (venous) (any) (see also Thrombosis, intracranial venous sinus) 325
softening, brain (see also Thrombosis, brain) 434.0 ☑
specified site NEC 453.8
spermatic cord 608.83
spinal cord 336.1
  due to syphilis 094.89
  in pregnancy or puerperium 671.5 ☑
  pyogenic origin 324.1
  late effect — see category 326
spleen, splenic 289.59
  artery 444.89
testis 608.83
traumatic (complication) (early) (see also Injury, blood vessel, by site) 904.9
tricuspid — see Endocarditis, tricuspid
tumor — see Neoplasm, by site
tunica vaginalis 608.83
umbilical cord (vessels) 663.6 ☑
  affecting fetus or newborn 762.6
vas deferens 608.83
vein
  deep 453.40
  lower extremity — see Thrombosis, lower extremity
vena cava (inferior) (superior) 453.2
Thrombus — see Thrombosis
Thrush 112.0
  newborn 771.7
Thumb — see also condition
  gamekeeper's 842.12
  sucking (child problem) 307.9
Thygeson's superficial punctate keratitis 370.21
Thymergasia — see also Psychosis, affective 296.80
Thymitis 254.8
Thymoma (benign) (M8580/0) 212.6
  malignant (M8580/3) 164.0
Thymus, thymic (gland) — see condition
Thyrocele — see also Goiter 240.9
Thyroglossal — see also condition
  cyst 759.2
  duct, persistent 759.2
Thyroid (body) (gland) — see also condition
  hormone resistance 246.8
  lingual 759.2
Thyroiditis 245.9
  acute (pyogenic) (suppurative) 245.0
    nonsuppurative 245.0
  autoimmune 245.2
  chronic (nonspecific) (sclerosing) 245.8
    fibrous 245.3
    lymphadenoid 245.2

Thyroiditis — continued
chronic — continued
  lymphocytic 245.2
  lymphoid 245.2
  complicating pregnancy, childbirth, or puerperium 648.1 ☑
de Quervain's (subacute granulomatous) 245.1
fibrous (chronic) 245.3
giant (cell) (follicular) 245.1
granulomatous (de Quervain's) (subacute) 245.1
Hashimoto's (struma lymphomatosa) 245.2
iatrogenic 245.4
invasive (fibrous) 245.3
ligneous 245.3
lymphocytic (chronic) 245.2
lymphoid 245.2
lymphomatous 245.2
pseudotuberculous 245.1
pyogenic 245.0
radiation 245.4
Riedel's (ligneous) 245.3
subacute 245.1
suppurative 245.0
tuberculous (see also Tuberculosis) 017.5 ☑
viral 245.1
woody 245.3
Thyrolingual duct, persistent 759.2
Thyromegaly 240.9
Thyrotoxic
  crisis or storm (see also Thyrotoxicosis) 242.9 ☑
  heart failure (see also Thyrotoxicosis) 242.9 ☑ [425.7]
Thyrotoxicosis 242.9 ☑

Note — Use the following fifth-digit subclassification with category 242:
0 without mention of thyrotoxic crisis or storm
1 with mention of thyrotoxic crisis or storm

with
  goiter (diffuse) 242.0 ☑
    adenomatous 242.3 ☑
      multinodular 242.2 ☑
      uninodular 242.1 ☑
    nodular 242.3 ☑
      multinodular 242.2 ☑
      uninodular 242.1 ☑
  infiltrative
    dermopathy 242.0 ☑
    ophthalmopathy 242.0 ☑
  thyroid acropachy 242.0 ☑
  complicating pregnancy, childbirth, or puerperium 648.1 ☑
  due to
    ectopic thyroid nodule 242.4 ☑
    ingestion of (excessive) thyroid material 242.8 ☑
    specified cause NEC 242.8 ☑
  factitia 242.8 ☑
  heart 242.9 ☑ [425.7]
  neonatal (transient) 775.3
TIA (transient ischemic attack) 435.9
  with transient neurologic deficit 435.9
  late effect — see Late effect(s) (of) cerebrovascular disease
Tibia vara 732.4
Tic 307.20
  breathing 307.20
  child problem 307.21
  compulsive 307.22
  convulsive 307.20
  degenerative (generalized) (localized) 333.3
    facial 351.8
  douloureux (see also Neuralgia, trigeminal) 350.1
    atypical 350.2
  habit 307.20
    chronic (motor or vocal) 307.22

Tic — continued
habit — continued
  transient (of childhood) 307.21
lid 307.20
  transient (of childhood) 307.21
motor-verbal 307.23
occupational 300.89
orbicularis 307.20
  transient (of childhood) 307.21
organic origin 333.3
postchoreic — see Chorea
psychogenic 307.20
  compulsive 307.22
salaam 781.0
spasm 307.20
  chronic (motor or vocal) 307.22
  transient (of childhood) 307.21
Tick-bite fever NEC 066.1
  African 087.1
  Colorado (virus) 066.1
  Rocky Mountain 082.0
Tick (-borne) **fever** NEC 066.1
  American mountain 066.1
  Colorado 066.1
  hemorrhagic NEC 065.3
    Crimean 065.0
    Kyasanur Forest 065.2
    Omsk 065.1
  mountain 066.1
  nonexanthematous 066.1
Tick paralysis 989.5
Tics and spasms, compulsive 307.22
Tietze's disease or syndrome 733.6
Tight, tightness
  anus 564.89
  chest 786.59
  fascia (lata) 728.9
  foreskin (congenital) 605
  hymen 623.3
  introitus (acquired) (congenital) 623.3
  rectal sphincter 564.89
  tendon 727.81
    Achilles (heel) 727.81
  urethral sphincter 598.9
Tilting vertebra 737.9
Timidity, child 313.21
Tinea (intersecta) (tarsi) 110.9
  amiantacea 110.0
  asbestina 110.0
  barbae 110.0
  beard 110.0
  black dot 110.0
  blanca 111.2
  capitis 110.0
  corporis 110.5
  cruris 110.3
  decalvans 704.09
  flava 111.0
  foot 110.4
  furfuracea 111.0
  imbricata (Tokelau) 110.5
  lepothrix 039.0
  manuum 110.2
  microsporic (see also Dermatophytosis) 110.9
  nigra 111.1
  nodosa 111.2
  pedis 110.4
  scalp 110.0
  specified site NEC 110.8
  sycosis 110.0
  tonsurans 110.0
  trichophytic (see also Dermatophytosis) 110.9
  unguium 110.1
  versicolor 111.0
Tingling sensation — see also Disturbance, sensation 782.0
Tin-miners' lung 503
Tinnitus (aurium) 388.30
  audible 388.32
  objective 388.32
  subjective 388.31
Tipped, teeth 524.33
Tipping
  pelvis 738.6

Index to Diseases

Tipping — *continued*
  pelvis — *continued*
    with disproportion (fetopelvic) 653.0 ☑
      affecting fetus or newborn 763.1
      causing obstructed labor 660.1 ☑
        affecting fetus or newborn 763.1
  teeth 524.33
Tiredness 780.79
Tissue — *see* condition
Tobacco
  abuse (affecting health) NEC (*see also* Abuse, drugs, nondependent) 305.1
  heart 989.84
  use disorder complicating pregnancy, childbirth, or the puerperium 649.0 ☑
Tobias' syndrome (carcinoma, pulmonary apex) (M8010/3) 162.3
Tocopherol deficiency 269.1
Todd's
  cirrhosis — *see* Cirrhosis, biliary
  paralysis (postepileptic transitory paralysis) 344.89
Toe — *see* condition
Toilet, artificial opening — *see also* Attention to, artificial, opening V55.9
Tokelau ringworm 110.5
Tollwut 071
Tolosa-Hunt syndrome 378.55
Tommaselli's disease
  correct substance properly administered 599.7
  overdose or wrong substance given or taken 961.4
Tongue — *see also* condition
  worms 134.1
Tongue tie 750.0
Tonic pupil 379.46
Toni-Fanconi syndrome (cystinosis) 270.0
Tonsil — *see* condition
Tonsillitis (acute) (catarrhal) (croupous) (follicular) (gangrenous) (infective) (lacunar) (lingual) (malignant) (membranous) (phlegmonous) (pneumococcal) (pseudomembranous) (purulent) (septic) (staphylococcal) (subacute) (suppurative) (toxic) (ulcerative) (vesicular) (viral) 463
  with influenza, flu, or grippe 487.1
  chronic 474.00
  diphtheritic (membranous) 032.0
  hypertrophic 474.00
  influenzal 487.1
  parenchymatous 475
  streptococcal 034.0
  tuberculous (*see also* Tuberculosis) 012.8 ☑
  Vincent's 101
Tonsillopharyngitis 465.8
Toothache 525.9
Tooth, teeth — *see* condition
Topagnosis 782.0
Tophi (gouty) 274.0
  ear 274.81
  heart 274.82
  specified site NEC 274.82
Torn — *see* Tear, torn
Tornwaldt's bursitis (disease) (pharyngeal bursitis) 478.29
  cyst 478.26
Torpid liver 573.9
Torsion
  accessory tube 620.5
  adnexa (female) 620.5
  aorta (congenital) 747.29
    acquired 447.1
  appendix
    epididymis 608.24 ●
    testis 608.23 ●

Torsion — *continued*
  bile duct 576.8
    with calculus, choledocholithiasis or stones — *see* Choledocholithiasis
    congenital 751.69
  bowel, colon, or intestine 560.2
  cervix ▶— *see* Malposition, uterus◀
  duodenum 537.3
  dystonia — *see* Dystonia, torsion
  epididymis 608.24 ▲
    appendix 608.24 ▲
  fallopian tube 620.5
  gallbladder (*see also* Disease, gallbladder) 575.8
    congenital 751.69
  gastric 537.89
  hydatid of Morgagni (female) 620.5
  kidney (pedicle) 593.89
  Meckel's diverticulum (congenital) 751.0
  mesentery 560.2
  omentum 560.2
  organ or site, congenital NEC — *see* Anomaly, specified type NEC
  ovary (pedicle) 620.5
    congenital 752.0
  oviduct 620.5
  penis 607.89
    congenital 752.69
  renal 593.89
  spasm — *see* Dystonia, torsion
  spermatic cord 608.22 ▲
    extravaginal 608.21 ●
    intravaginal 608.22 ●
  spleen 289.59
  testicle, testis 608.20 ▲
    appendix 608.23 ●
  tibia 736.89
  umbilical cord — *see* Compression, umbilical cord
  uterus (*see also* Malposition, uterus) 621.6
Torticollis (intermittent) (spastic) 723.5
  congenital 754.1
    sternomastoid 754.1
  due to birth injury 767.8
  hysterical 300.11
  ocular 781.93
  psychogenic 306.0
    specified as conversion reaction 300.11
  rheumatic 723.5
  rheumatoid 714.0
  spasmodic 333.83
  traumatic, current NEC 847.0
Tortuous
  artery 447.1
  fallopian tube 752.19
  organ or site, congenital NEC — *see* Distortion
  renal vessel (congenital) 747.62
  retina vessel (congenital) 743.58
    acquired 362.17
  ureter 593.4
  urethra 599.84
  vein — *see* Varicose, vein
Torula, torular (infection) 117.5
  histolytica 117.5
  lung 117.5
Torulosis 117.5
Torus
  fracture
    fibula 823.41
      with tibia 823.42
    radius 813.45
    tibia 823.40
      with fibula 823.42
  mandibularis 526.81
  palatinus 526.81
Touch, vitreous 997.99
Touraine-Solente-Golé syndrome (acropachyderma) 757.39
Touraine's syndrome (hereditary osteo-onychodysplasia) 756.89

Tourette's disease (motor-verbal tic) 307.23
Tower skull 756.0
  with exophthalmos 756.0
Toxemia 799.89
  with
    abortion — *see* Abortion, by type, with toxemia
  bacterial — *see* Septicemia
  biliary (*see also* Disease, biliary) 576.8
  burn — *see* Burn, by site
  congenital NEC 779.89
  eclamptic 642.6 ☑
    with pre-existing hypertension 642.7 ☑
  erysipelatous (*see also* Erysipelas) 035
  fatigue 799.89
  fetus or newborn NEC 779.89
  food (*see also* Poisoning, food) 005.9
  gastric 537.89
  gastrointestinal 558.2
  intestinal 558.2
  kidney (*see also* Disease, renal) 593.9
  lung 518.89
  malarial NEC (*see also* Malaria) 084.6
  maternal (of pregnancy), affecting fetus or newborn 760.0
  myocardial — *see* Myocarditis, toxic
  of pregnancy (mild) (pre-eclamptic) 642.4 ☑
    with
      convulsions 642.6 ☑
      pre-existing hypertension 642.7 ☑
    affecting fetus or newborn 760.0
    severe 642.5 ☑
  pre-eclamptic — *see* Toxemia, of pregnancy
  puerperal, postpartum — *see* Toxemia, of pregnancy
  pulmonary 518.89
  renal (*see also* Disease, renal) 593.9
  septic (*see also* Septicemia) 038.9
  small intestine 558.2
  staphylococcal 038.10
    aureus 038.11
    due to food 005.0
    specified organism NEC 038.19
  stasis 799.89
  stomach 537.89
  uremic (*see also* Uremia) 586
  urinary 586
Toxemica cerebropathia psychica (nonalcoholic) 294.0
  alcoholic 291.1
Toxic (poisoning) — *see also* condition
  from drug or poison — *see* Table of Drugs and Chemicals
  oil syndrome 710.5
  shock syndrome 040.82
  thyroid (gland) (*see also* Thyrotoxicosis) 242.9 ☑
Toxicemia — *see* Toxemia
Toxicity
  dilantin
    asymptomatic 796.0
    symptomatic — *see* Table of Drugs and Chemicals
  drug
    asymptomatic 796.0
    symptomatic — *see* Table of Drugs and Chemicals
  fava bean 282.2
  from drug or poison
    asymptomatic 796.0
    symptomatic — *see* Table of Drugs and Chemicals
Toxicosis — *see also* Toxemia 799.89
  capillary, hemorrhagic 287.0
Toxinfection 799.89
  gastrointestinal 558.2
Toxocariasis 128.0
Toxoplasma infection, generalized 130.9
Toxoplasmosis (acquired) 130.9
  with pneumonia 130.4

Toxoplasmosis — *continued*
  congenital, active 771.2
  disseminated (multisystemic) 130.8
  maternal
    with suspected damage to fetus affecting management of pregnancy 655.4 ☑
    affecting fetus or newborn 760.2
    manifest toxoplasmosis in fetus or newborn 771.2
  multiple sites 130.8
  multisystemic disseminated 130.8
  specified site NEC 130.7
Trabeculation, bladder 596.8
Trachea — *see* condition
Tracheitis (acute) (catarrhal) (infantile) (membranous) (plastic) (pneumococcal) (septic) (suppurative) (viral) 464.10
  with
    bronchitis 490
      acute or subacute 466.0
      chronic 491.8
      tuberculosis — *see* Tuberculosis, pulmonary
    laryngitis (acute) 464.20
      with obstruction 464.21
      chronic 476.1
      tuberculous (*see also* Tuberculosis, larynx) 012.3 ☑
    obstruction 464.11
  chronic 491.8
    with
      bronchitis (chronic) 491.8
      laryngitis (chronic) 476.1
      due to external agent — *see* Condition, respiratory, chronic, due to
  diphtheritic (membranous) 032.3
  due to external agent — *see* Inflammation, respiratory, upper, due to
  edematous 464.11
  influenzal 487.1
  streptococcal 034.0
  syphilitic 095.8
  tuberculous (*see also* Tuberculosis) 012.8 ☑
Trachelitis (nonvenereal) — *see also* Cervicitis 616.0
  trichomonal 131.09
Tracheobronchial — *see* condition
Tracheobronchitis — *see also* Bronchitis 490
  acute or subacute 466.0
    with bronchospasm or obstruction 466.0
  chronic 491.8
  influenzal 487.1
  senile 491.8
Tracheobronchomegaly (congenital) 748.3
  with bronchiectasis 494.0
    with (acute) exacerbation 494.1
  acquired 519.19 ▲
    with bronchiectasis 494.0
      with (acute) exacerbation 494.1
Tracheobronchopneumonitis — *see* Pneumonia, broncho
Tracheocele (external) (internal) 519.19 ▲
  congenital 748.3
Tracheomalacia 519.19 ▲
  congenital 748.3
Tracheopharyngitis (acute) 465.8
  chronic 478.9
  due to external agent — *see* Condition, respiratory, chronic, due to
  due to external agent — *see* Inflammation, respiratory, upper, due to
Tracheostenosis 519.19 ▲
  congenital 748.3
Tracheostomy
  attention to V55.0
  complication 519.00

Tracheostomy

Tracheostomy — *continued*
  granuloma 519.09
  hemorrhage 519.09
  infection 519.01
  malfunctioning 519.02
  obstruction 519.09
  sepsis 519.01
  status V44.0
  stenosis 519.02
Trachoma, trachomatous 076.9
  active (stage) 076.1
  contraction of conjunctiva 076.1
  dubium 076.0
  healed or late effect 139.1
  initial (stage) 076.0
  Türck's (chronic catarrhal laryngitis) 476.0
Trachyphonia 784.49
Training
  insulin pump V65.46
  orthoptic V57.4
  orthotic V57.81
Train sickness 994.6
Trait
  hemoglobin
    abnormal NEC 282.7
      with thalassemia 282.49
    C (*see also* Disease, hemoglobin, C) 282.7
      with elliptocytosis 282.7
    S (Hb-S) 282.5
  Lepore 282.49
    with other abnormal hemoglobin NEC 282.49
  paranoid 301.0
  sickle-cell 282.5
    with
      elliptocytosis 282.5
      spherocytosis 282.5
Traits, paranoid 301.0
Tramp V60.0
Trance 780.09
  hysterical 300.13
Transaminasemia 790.4
Transfusion, blood
  without reported diagnosis V58.2
  donor V59.01
    stem cells V59.02
  incompatible 999.6
  reaction or complication — *see* Complications, transfusion
  related acute lung injury (TRALI) 518.7 ●
  syndrome
    fetomaternal 772.0
    twin-to-twin
      blood loss (donor twin) 772.0
      recipient twin 776.4
Transient — *see also* condition
  alteration of awareness 780.02
  blindness 368.12
  deafness (ischemic) 388.02
  global amnesia 437.7
  person (homeless) NEC V60.0
Transitional, lumbosacral joint of vertebra 756.19
Translocation
  autosomes NEC 758.5
    13-15 758.1
    16-18 758.2
    21 or 22 758.0
    balanced in normal individual 758.4
    D$_1$ 758.1
    E$_3$ 758.2
    G 758.0
  balanced autosomal in normal individual 758.4
  chromosomes NEC 758.89
  Down's syndrome 758.0
Translucency, iris 364.53
Transmission of chemical substances through the placenta (affecting fetus or newborn) 760.70
  alcohol 760.71
  anticonvulsants 760.77

Transmission of chemical substances through the placenta — *continued*
  antifungals 760.74
  anti-infective agents 760.74
  antimetabolics 760.78
  cocaine 760.75
  "crack" 760.75
  diethylstilbestrol [DES] 760.76
  hallucinogenic agents 760.73
  medicinal agents NEC 760.79
  narcotics 760.72
  obstetric anesthetic or analgesic drug 763.5
  specified agent NEC 760.79
  suspected, affecting management of pregnancy 655.5 ☑
Transplant(ed)
  bone V42.4
    marrow V42.81
  complication (*see also* Complications, due to (presence of) any device, implant, or graft classified to 996.0–996.5 NEC)
    bone marrow 996.85
    corneal graft NEC 996.79
      infection or inflammation 996.69
      reaction 996.51
      rejection 996.51
    organ (failure) (immune or nonimmune cause) (infection) (rejection) 996.80
      bone marrow 996.85
      heart 996.83
      intestines 996.87
      kidney 996.81
      liver 996.82
      lung 996.84
      pancreas 996.86
      specified NEC 996.89
    skin NEC 996.79
      infection or inflammation 996.69
      rejection 996.52
        artificial 996.55
        decellularized allodermis 996.55
  cornea V42.5
  hair V50.0
  heart V42.1
    valve V42.2
  intestine V42.84
  kidney V42.0
  liver V42.7
  lung V42.6
  organ V42.9
    specified NEC V42.89
  pancreas V42.83
  peripheral stem cells V42.82
  skin V42.3
  stem cells, peripheral V42.82
  tissue V42.9
    specified NEC V42.89
Transplants, ovarian, endometrial 617.1
Transposed — *see* Transposition
Transposition (congenital) — *see also* Malposition, congenital
  abdominal viscera 759.3
  aorta (dextra) 745.11
  appendix 751.5
  arterial trunk 745.10
  colon 751.5
  great vessels (complete) 745.10
    both originating from right ventricle 745.11
    corrected 745.12
    double outlet right ventricle 745.11
    incomplete 745.11
    partial 745.11
    specified type NEC 745.19
  heart 746.87
    with complete transposition of viscera 759.3
  intestine (large) (small) 751.5

Transposition — *see also* Malposition, congenital — *continued*
  pulmonary veins 747.49
  reversed jejunal (for bypass) (status) V45.3
  scrotal 752.81
  stomach 750.7
    with general transposition of viscera 759.3
  teeth, tooth 524.30
  vessels (complete) 745.10
    partial 745.11
  viscera (abdominal) (thoracic) 759.3
Trans-sexualism 302.50
  with
    asexual history 302.51
    heterosexual history 302.53
    homosexual history 302.52
Transverse — *see also* condition
  arrest (deep), in labor 660.3 ☑
    affecting fetus or newborn 763.1
  lie 652.3 ☑
    before labor, affecting fetus or newborn 761.7
    causing obstructed labor 660.0 ☑
      affecting fetus or newborn 763.1
    during labor, affecting fetus or newborn 763.1
Transvestism, transvestitism (transvestic fetishism) 302.3
Trapped placenta (with hemorrhage) 666.0 ☑
  without hemorrhage 667.0 ☑
Traumatic — *see* condition
Trauma, traumatism — *see also* Injury, by site 959.9
  birth — *see* Birth, injury NEC
  causing hemorrhage of pregnancy or delivery 641.8 ☑
  complicating
    abortion — *see* Abortion, by type, with damage to pelvic organs
    ectopic pregnancy (*see also* categories 633.0–633.9) 639.2
    molar pregnancy (*see also* categories 630–632) 639.2
  during delivery NEC 665.9 ☑
  following
    abortion 639.2
    ectopic or molar pregnancy 639.2
  maternal, during pregnancy, affecting fetus or newborn 760.5
  neuroma — *see* Injury, nerve, by site
  previous major, affecting management of pregnancy, childbirth, or puerperium V23.89
  psychic (current) (*see also* Reaction, adjustment)
    previous (history) V15.49
  psychologic, previous (affecting health) V15.49
  transient paralysis — *see* Injury, nerve, by site
Treacher Collins' syndrome (incomplete facial dysostosis) 756.0
Treitz's hernia — *see* Hernia, Treitz's
Trematode infestation NEC 121.9
Trematodiasis NEC 121.9
Trembles 988.8
Trembling paralysis — *see also* Parkinsonism 332.0
Tremor 781.0
  essential (benign) 333.1
  familial 333.1
  flapping (liver) 572.8
  hereditary 333.1
  hysterical 300.11
  intention 333.1
  medication-induced postural 333.1
  mercurial 985.0
  muscle 728.85
  Parkinson's (*see also* Parkinsonism) 332.0
  psychogenic 306.0
    specified as conversion reaction 300.11

Tremor — *continued*
  senilis 797
  specified type NEC 333.1
Trench
  fever 083.1
  foot 991.4
  mouth 101
  nephritis — *see* Nephritis, acute
Treponema pallidum infection — *see also* Syphilis 097.9
Treponematosis 102.9
  due to
    T. pallidum — *see* Syphilis
    T. pertenue (yaws) (*see also* Yaws) 102.9
Triad
  Kartagener's 759.3
  Reiter's (complete) (incomplete) 099.3
  Saint's (*see also* Hernia, diaphragm) 553.3
Trichiasis 704.2
  cicatricial 704.2
  eyelid 374.05
    with entropion (*see also* Entropion) 374.00
Trichinella spiralis (infection) (infestation) 124
Trichinelliasis 124
Trichinellosis 124
Trichiniasis 124
Trichinosis 124
Trichobezoar 938
  intestine 936
  stomach 935.2
Trichocephaliasis 127.3
Trichocephalosis 127.3
Trichocephalus infestation 127.3
Trichoclasis 704.2
Trichoepithelioma (M8100/0) — *see also* Neoplasm, skin, benign
  breast 217
  genital organ NEC — *see* Neoplasm, by site, benign
  malignant (M8100/3) — *see* Neoplasm, skin, malignant
Trichofolliculoma (M8101/0) — *see* Neoplasm, skin, benign
Tricholemmoma (M8102/0) — *see* Neoplasm, skin, benign
Trichomatosis 704.2
Trichomoniasis 131.9
  bladder 131.09
  cervix 131.09
  intestinal 007.3
  prostate 131.03
  seminal vesicle 131.09
  specified site NEC 131.8
  urethra 131.02
  urogenitalis 131.00
  vagina 131.01
  vulva 131.01
  vulvovaginal 131.01
Trichomycosis 039.0
  axillaris 039.0
  nodosa 111.2
  nodularis 111.2
  rubra 039.0
Trichonocardiosis (axillaris) (palmellina) 039.0
Trichonodosis 704.2
Trichophytide — *see* Dermatophytosis
Trichophytid, trichophyton infection — *see also* Dermatophytosis 110.9
Trichophytobezoar 938
  intestine 936
  stomach 935.2
Trichophytosis — *see* Dermatophytosis
Trichoptilosis 704.2
Trichorrhexis (nodosa) 704.2
Trichosporosis nodosa 111.2
Trichostasis spinulosa (congenital) 757.4
Trichostrongyliasis (small intestine) 127.6
Trichostrongylosis 127.6

Index to Diseases

Trichostrongylus (instabilis) infection 127.6
Trichotillomania 312.39
Trichromat, anomalous (congenital) 368.59
Trichromatopsia, anomalous (congenital) 368.59
Trichuriasis 127.3
Trichuris trichiuria (any site) (infection) (infestation) 127.3
Tricuspid (valve) — see condition
Trifid — see also Accessory
  kidney (pelvis) 753.3
  tongue 750.13
Trigeminal neuralgia — see also Neuralgia, trigeminal 350.1
Trigeminoencephaloangiomatosis 759.6
Trigeminy 427.89
  postoperative 997.1
Trigger finger (acquired) 727.03
  congenital 756.89
Trigonitis (bladder) (chronic) (pseudomembranous) 595.3
  tuberculous (see also Tuberculosis) 016.1 ☑
Trigonocephaly 756.0
Trihexosidosis 272.7
Trilobate placenta — see Placenta, abnormal
Trilocular heart 745.8
Trimethylaminuria 270.8 ●
Tripartita placenta — see Placenta, abnormal
Triple — see also Accessory
  kidneys 753.3
  uteri 752.2
  X female 758.81
Triplegia 344.89
  congenital or infantile 343.8
Triplet
  affected by maternal complications of pregnancy 761.5
  healthy liveborn — see Newborn, multiple
  pregnancy (complicating delivery) NEC 651.1 ☑
    with fetal loss and retention of one or more fetus(es) 651.4 ☑
    following (elective) fetal reduction 651.7 ☑
Triplex placenta — see Placenta, abnormal
Triplication — see Accessory
Trismus 781.0
  neonatorum 771.3
  newborn 771.3
Trisomy (syndrome) NEC 758.5
  13 (partial) 758.1
  16-18 758.2
  18 (partial) 758.2
  21 (partial) 758.0
  22 758.0
  autosomes NEC 758.5
  D₁ 758.1
  E₃ 758.2
  G (group) 758.0
    group D₁ 758.1
    group E 758.2
    group G 758.0
Tritanomaly 368.53
Tritanopia 368.53
Troisier-Hanot-Chauffard syndrome (bronze diabetes) 275.0
Trombidiosis 133.8
Trophedema (hereditary) 757.0
  congenital 757.0
Trophoblastic disease — see also Hydatidiform mole 630
  previous, affecting management of pregnancy V23.1
Tropholymphedema 757.0
Trophoneurosis NEC 356.9
  arm NEC 354.9
  disseminated 710.1
  facial 349.89

Trophoneurosis — continued
  leg NEC 355.8
  lower extremity NEC 355.8
  upper extremity NEC 354.9
Tropical — see also condition
  maceration feet (syndrome) 991.4
  wet foot (syndrome) 991.4
Trouble — see also Disease
  bowel 569.9
  heart — see Disease, heart
  intestine 569.9
  kidney (see also Disease, renal) 593.9
  nervous 799.2
  sinus (see also Sinusitis) 473.9
Trousseau's syndrome (thrombophlebitis migrans) 453.1
Truancy, childhood — see also Disturbance, conduct
  socialized 312.2 ☑
  undersocialized, unsocialized 312.1 ☑
Truncus
  arteriosus (persistent) 745.0
  common 745.0
  communis 745.0
Trunk — see condition
Trychophytide — see Dermatophytosis
Trypanosoma infestation — see Trypanosomiasis
Trypanosomiasis 086.9
  with meningoencephalitis 086.9 [323.2]
  African 086.5
    due to Trypanosoma 086.5
      gambiense 086.3
      rhodesiense 086.4
  American 086.2
    with
      heart involvement 086.0
      other organ involvement 086.1
      without mention of organ involvement 086.2
  Brazilian — see Trypanosomiasis, American
  Chagas' — see Trypanosomiasis, American
  due to Trypanosoma
    cruzi — see Trypanosomiasis, American
    gambiense 086.3
    rhodesiense 086.4
  gambiensis, Gambian 086.3
  North American — see Trypanosomiasis, American
  rhodesiensis, Rhodesian 086.4
  South American — see Trypanosomiasis, American
T-shaped incisors 520.2
Tsutsugamushi fever 081.2
Tubercle — see also Tuberculosis
  brain, solitary 013.2 ☑
  Darwin's 744.29
  epithelioid noncaseating 135
  Ghon, primary infection 010.0 ☑
Tuberculid, tuberculide (indurating) (lichenoid) (miliary) (papulonecrotic) (primary) (skin) (subcutaneous) — see also Tuberculosis 017.0 ☑
Tuberculoma — see also Tuberculosis
  brain (any part) 013.2 ☑
  meninges (cerebral) (spinal) 013.1 ☑
  spinal cord 013.4 ☑

Tuberculosis, tubercular, tuberculous (calcification) (calcified) (caseous) (chromogenic acid-fast bacilli) (congenital) (degeneration) (disease) (fibrocaseous) (fistula) (gangrene) (interstitial) (isolated circumscribed lesions) (necrosis) (parenchymatous) (ulcerative) 011.9 ☑

> *Note* — *Use the following fifth-digit subclassification with categories 010–018:*
>
> 0 *unspecified*
>
> 1 *bacteriological or histological examination not done*
>
> 2 *bacteriological or histological examination unknown (at present)*
>
> 3 *tubercle bacilli found (in sputum) by microscopy*
>
> 4 *tubercle bacilli not found (in sputum) by microscopy, but found by bacterial culture*
>
> 5 *tubercle bacilli not found by bacteriological exam–ination, but tuberculosis confirmed histologically*
>
> 6 *tubercle bacilli not found by bacteriological or histological examination, but tuberculosis confirmed by other methods [inoculation of animals]*
>
> *For tuberculous conditions specified as late effects or sequelae, see category 137.*

  abdomen 014.8 ☑
    lymph gland 014.8 ☑
  abscess 011.9 ☑
    arm 017.9 ☑
    bone (see also Osteomyelitis, due to, tuberculosis) 015.9 ☑ [730.8]
      hip 015.1 ☑ [730.85]
      knee 015.2 ☑ [730.86]
      sacrum 015.0 ☑ [730.88]
      specified site NEC 015.7 ☑ [730.88]
      spinal 015.0 ☑ [730.88]
      vertebra 015.0 ☑ [730.88]
    brain 013.3 ☑
    breast 017.9 ☑
    Cowper's gland 016.5 ☑
    dura (mater) 013.8 ☑
      brain 013.3 ☑
      spinal cord 013.5 ☑
    epidural 013.8 ☑
      brain 013.3 ☑
      spinal cord 013.5 ☑
    frontal sinus — see Tuberculosis, sinus
    genital organs NEC 016.9 ☑
      female 016.7 ☑
      male 016.5 ☑
    genitourinary NEC 016.9 ☑
    gland (lymphatic) — see Tuberculosis, lymph gland
    hip 015.1 ☑
    iliopsoas 015.0 ☑ [730.88]
    intestine 014.8 ☑
    ischiorectal 014.8 ☑
    joint 015.9 ☑
      hip 015.1 ☑
      knee 015.2 ☑
      specified joint NEC 015.8 ☑
      vertebral 015.0 ☑ [730.88]
    kidney 016.0 ☑ [590.81]
    knee 015.2 ☑
    lumbar 015.0 ☑ [730.88]
    lung 011.2 ☑
      primary, progressive 010.8 ☑
    meninges (cerebral) (spinal) 013.0 ☑
    pelvic 016.9 ☑

Tuberculosis, tubercular, tuberculous — continued
  abscess — continued
    pelvic — continued
      female 016.7 ☑
      male 016.5 ☑
    perianal 014.8 ☑
      fistula 014.8 ☑
    perinephritic 016.0 ☑ [590.81]
    perineum 017.9 ☑
    perirectal 014.8 ☑
    psoas 015.0 ☑ [730.88]
    rectum 014.8 ☑
    retropharyngeal 012.8 ☑
    sacrum 015.0 ☑ [730.88]
    scrofulous 017.2 ☑
    scrotum 016.5 ☑
    skin 017.0 ☑
      primary 017.0 ☑
    spinal cord 013.5 ☑
    spine or vertebra (column) 015.0 ☑ [730.88]
    strumous 017.2 ☑
    subdiaphragmatic 014.8 ☑
    testis 016.5 ☑
    thigh 017.9 ☑
    urinary 016.3 ☑
      kidney 016.0 ☑ [590.81]
    uterus 016.7 ☑
  accessory sinus — see Tuberculosis, sinus
  Addison's disease 017.6 ☑
  adenitis (see also Tuberculosis, lymph gland) 017.2 ☑
  adenoids 012.8 ☑
  adenopathy (see also Tuberculosis, lymph gland) 017.2 ☑
    tracheobronchial 012.1 ☑
      primary progressive 010.8 ☑
  adherent pericardium 017.9 ☑ [420.0]
  adnexa (uteri) 016.7 ☑
  adrenal (capsule) (gland) 017.6 ☑
  air passage NEC 012.8 ☑
  alimentary canal 014.8 ☑
  anemia 017.9 ☑
  ankle (joint) 015.8 ☑
    bone 015.5 ☑ [730.87]
  anus 014.8 ☑
  apex (see also Tuberculosis, pulmonary) 011.9 ☑
  apical (see also Tuberculosis, pulmonary) 011.9 ☑
  appendicitis 014.8 ☑
  appendix 014.8 ☑
  arachnoid 013.0 ☑
  artery 017.9 ☑
  arthritis (chronic) (synovial) 015.9 ☑ [711.40]
    ankle 015.8 ☑ [730.87]
    hip 015.1 ☑ [711.45]
    knee 015.2 ☑ [711.46]
    specified site NEC 015.8 ☑ [711.48]
    spine or vertebra (column) 015.0 ☑ [720.81]
    wrist 015.8 ☑ [730.83]
  articular — see Tuberculosis, joint
  ascites 014.0 ☑
  asthma (see also Tuberculosis, pulmonary) 011.9 ☑
  axilla, axillary 017.2 ☑
    gland 017.2 ☑
  bilateral (see also Tuberculosis, pulmonary) 011.9 ☑
  bladder 016.1 ☑
  bone (see also Osteomyelitis, due to, tuberculosis) 015.9 ☑ [730.8]
    hip 015.1 ☑ [730.85]
    knee 015.2 ☑ [730.86]
    limb NEC 015.5 ☑ [730.88]
    sacrum 015.0 ☑ [730.88]
    specified site NEC 015.7 ☑ [730.88]
    spinal or vertebral column 015.0 ☑ [730.88]
  bowel 014.8 ☑

Tuberculosis, tubercular, tuberculous

Tuberculosis, tubercular, tuberculous — *continued*
- bowel — *continued*
  - miliary 018.9 ☑
- brain 013.2 ☑
- breast 017.9 ☑
- broad ligament 016.7 ☑
- bronchi, bronchial, bronchus 011.3 ☑
  - ectasia, ectasis 011.5 ☑
  - fistula 011.3 ☑
    - primary, progressive 010.8 ☑
  - gland 012.1 ☑
    - primary, progressive 010.8 ☑
  - isolated 012.2 ☑
  - lymph gland or node 012.1 ☑
    - primary, progressive 010.8 ☑
- bronchiectasis 011.5 ☑
- bronchitis 011.3 ☑
- bronchopleural 012.0 ☑
- bronchopneumonia, bronchopneumonic 011.6 ☑
- bronchorrhagia 011.3 ☑
- bronchotracheal 011.3 ☑
  - isolated 012.2 ☑
- bronchus — *see* Tuberculosis, bronchi
- bronze disease (Addison's) 017.6 ☑
- buccal cavity 017.9 ☑
- bulbourethral gland 016.5 ☑
- bursa (*see also* Tuberculosis, joint) 015.9 ☑
- cachexia NEC (*see also* Tuberculosis, pulmonary) 011.9 ☑
- cardiomyopathy 017.9 ☑ [425.8]
- caries (*see also* Tuberculosis, bone) 015.9 ☑ [730.8]
- cartilage (*see also* Tuberculosis, bone) 015.9 ☑ [730.8]
  - intervertebral 015.0 ☑ [730.88]
- catarrhal (*see also* Tuberculosis, pulmonary) 011.9 ☑
- cecum 014.8 ☑
- cellular tissue (primary) 017.0 ☑
- cellulitis (primary) 017.0 ☑
- central nervous system 013.9 ☑
  - specified site NEC 013.8 ☑
- cerebellum (current) 013.2 ☑
- cerebral (current) 013.2 ☑
  - meninges 013.0 ☑
- cerebrospinal 013.6 ☑
  - meninges 013.0 ☑
- cerebrum (current) 013.2 ☑
- cervical 017.2 ☑
  - gland 017.2 ☑
  - lymph nodes 017.2 ☑
- cervicitis (uteri) 016.7 ☑
- cervix 016.7 ☑
- chest (*see also* Tuberculosis, pulmonary) 011.9 ☑
- childhood type or first infection 010.0 ☑
- choroid 017.3 ☑ [363.13]
- choroiditis 017.3 ☑ [363.13]
- ciliary body 017.3 ☑ [364.11]
- colitis 014.8 ☑
- colliers' 011.4 ☑
- colliquativa (primary) 017.0 ☑
- colon 014.8 ☑
  - ulceration 014.8 ☑
- complex, primary 010.0 ☑
- complicating pregnancy, childbirth, or puerperium 647.3 ☑
  - affecting fetus or newborn 760.2
- congenital 771.2
- conjunctiva 017.3 ☑ [370.31]
- connective tissue 017.9 ☑
  - bone — *see* Tuberculosis, bone
- contact V01.1
- converter (tuberculin skin test) (without disease) 795.5
- cornea (ulcer) 017.3 ☑ [370.31]
- Cowper's gland 016.5 ☑
- coxae 015.1 ☑ [730.85]
- coxalgia 015.1 ☑ [730.85]
- cul-de-sac of Douglas 014.8 ☑

Tuberculosis, tubercular, tuberculous — *continued*
- curvature, spine 015.0 ☑ [737.40]
- cutis (colliquativa) (primary) 017.0 ☑
- cystitis 016.1 ☑
- cyst, ovary 016.6 ☑
- dacryocystitis 017.3 ☑ [375.32]
- dactylitis 015.5 ☑
- diarrhea 014.8 ☑
- diffuse (*see also* Tuberculosis, miliary) 018.9 ☑
  - lung — *see* Tuberculosis, pulmonary
  - meninges 013.0 ☑
- digestive tract 014.8 ☑
- disseminated (*see also* Tuberculosis, miliary) 018.9 ☑
  - meninges 013.0 ☑
- duodenum 014.8 ☑
- dura (mater) 013.9 ☑
  - abscess 013.8 ☑
    - cerebral 013.3 ☑
    - spinal 013.5 ☑
- dysentery 014.8 ☑
- ear (inner) (middle) 017.4 ☑
  - bone 015.6 ☑
  - external (primary) 017.0 ☑
  - skin (primary) 017.0 ☑
- elbow 015.8 ☑
- emphysema — *see* Tuberculosis, pulmonary
- empyema 012.0 ☑
- encephalitis 013.6 ☑
- endarteritis 017.9 ☑
- endocarditis (any valve) 017.9 ☑ [424.91]
- endocardium (any valve) 017.9 ☑ [424.91]
- endocrine glands NEC 017.9 ☑
- endometrium 016.7 ☑
- enteric, enterica 014.8 ☑
- enteritis 014.8 ☑
- enterocolitis 014.8 ☑
- epididymis 016.4 ☑
- epididymitis 016.4 ☑
- epidural abscess 013.8 ☑
  - brain 013.3 ☑
  - spinal cord 013.5 ☑
- epiglottis 012.3 ☑
- episcleritis 017.3 ☑ [379.00]
- erythema (induratum) (nodosum) (primary) 017.1 ☑
- esophagus 017.8 ☑
- Eustachian tube 017.4 ☑
- exposure to V01.1
- exudative 012.0 ☑
  - primary, progressive 010.1 ☑
- eye 017.3 ☑
  - glaucoma 017.3 ☑ [365.62]
- eyelid (primary) 017.0 ☑
  - lupus 017.0 ☑ [373.4]
- fallopian tube 016.6 ☑
- fascia 017.9 ☑
- fauces 012.8 ☑
- finger 017.9 ☑
- first infection 010.0 ☑
- fistula, perirectal 014.8 ☑
- Florida 011.6 ☑
- foot 017.9 ☑
- funnel pelvis 137.3
- gallbladder 017.9 ☑
- galloping (*see also* Tuberculosis, pulmonary) 011.9 ☑
- ganglionic 015.9 ☑
- gastritis 017.9 ☑
- gastrocolic fistula 014.8 ☑
- gastroenteritis 014.8 ☑
- gastrointestinal tract 014.8 ☑
- general, generalized 018.9 ☑
  - acute 018.0 ☑
  - chronic 018.8 ☑
- genital organs NEC 016.9 ☑
  - female 016.7 ☑
  - male 016.5 ☑

Tuberculosis, tubercular, tuberculous — *continued*
- genitourinary NEC 016.9 ☑
- genu 015.2 ☑
- glandulae suprarenalis 017.6 ☑
- glandular, general 017.2 ☑
- glottis 012.3 ☑
- grinders' 011.4 ☑
- groin 017.2 ☑
- gum 017.9 ☑
- hand 017.9 ☑
- heart 017.9 ☑ [425.8]
- hematogenous — *see* Tuberculosis, miliary
- hemoptysis (*see also* Tuberculosis, pulmonary) 011.9 ☑
- hemorrhage NEC (*see also* Tuberculosis, pulmonary) 011.9 ☑
- hemothorax 012.0 ☑
- hepatitis 017.9 ☑
- hilar lymph nodes 012.1 ☑
  - primary, progressive 010.8 ☑
- hip (disease) (joint) 015.1 ☑
  - bone 015.1 ☑ [730.85]
- hydrocephalus 013.8 ☑
- hydropneumothorax 012.0 ☑
- hydrothorax 012.0 ☑
- hypoadrenalism 017.6 ☑
- hypopharynx 012.8 ☑
- ileocecal (hyperplastic) 014.8 ☑
- ileocolitis 014.8 ☑
- ileum 014.8 ☑
- iliac spine (superior) 015.0 ☑ [730.88]
- incipient NEC (*see also* Tuberculosis, pulmonary) 011.9 ☑
- indurativa (primary) 017.1 ☑
- infantile 010.0 ☑
- infection NEC 011.9 ☑
  - without clinical manifestation 010.0 ☑
- infraclavicular gland 017.2 ☑
- inguinal gland 017.2 ☑
- inguinalis 017.2 ☑
- intestine (any part) 014.8 ☑
- iris 017.3 ☑ [364.11]
- iritis 017.3 ☑ [364.11]
- ischiorectal 014.8 ☑
- jaw 015.7 ☑ [730.88]
- jejunum 014.8 ☑
- joint 015.9 ☑
  - hip 015.1 ☑
  - knee 015.2 ☑
  - specified site NEC 015.8 ☑
  - vertebral 015.0 ☑ [730.88]
- keratitis 017.3 ☑ [370.31]
  - interstitial 017.3 ☑ [370.59]
- keratoconjunctivitis 017.3 ☑ [370.31]
- kidney 016.0 ☑
- knee (joint) 015.2 ☑
- kyphoscoliosis 015.0 ☑ [737.43]
- kyphosis 015.0 ☑ [737.41]
- lacrimal apparatus, gland 017.3 ☑
- laryngitis 012.3 ☑
- larynx 012.3 ☑
- leptomeninges, leptomeningitis (cerebral) (spinal) 013.0 ☑
- lichenoides (primary) 017.0 ☑
- linguae 017.9 ☑
- lip 017.9 ☑
- liver 017.9 ☑
- lordosis 015.0 ☑ [737.42]
- lung — *see* Tuberculosis, pulmonary
- luposa 017.0 ☑
  - eyelid 017.0 ☑ [373.4]
- lymphadenitis — *see* Tuberculosis, lymph gland
- lymphangitis — *see* Tuberculosis, lymph gland
- lymphatic (gland) (vessel) — *see* Tuberculosis, lymph gland
- lymph gland or node (peripheral) 017.2 ☑
  - abdomen 014.8 ☑
  - bronchial 012.1 ☑

Tuberculosis, tubercular, tuberculous — *continued*
- lymph gland or node — *continued*
  - bronchial — *continued*
    - primary, progressive 010.8 ☑
  - cervical 017.2 ☑
  - hilar 012.1 ☑
    - primary, progressive 010.8 ☑
  - intrathoracic 012.1 ☑
    - primary, progressive 010.8 ☑
  - mediastinal 012.1 ☑
    - primary, progressive 010.8 ☑
  - mesenteric 014.8 ☑
  - peripheral 017.2 ☑
  - retroperitoneal 014.8 ☑
  - tracheobronchial 012.1 ☑
    - primary, progressive 010.8 ☑
- malignant NEC (*see also* Tuberculosis, pulmonary) 011.9 ☑
- mammary gland 017.9 ☑
- marasmus NEC (*see also* Tuberculosis, pulmonary) 011.9 ☑
- mastoiditis 015.6 ☑
- maternal, affecting fetus or newborn 760.2
- mediastinal (lymph) gland or node 012.1 ☑
  - primary, progressive 010.8 ☑
- mediastinitis 012.8 ☑
  - primary, progressive 010.8 ☑
- mediastinopericarditis 017.9 ☑ [420.0]
- mediastinum 012.8 ☑
  - primary, progressive 010.8 ☑
- medulla 013.9 ☑
  - brain 013.2 ☑
  - spinal cord 013.4 ☑
- melanosis, Addisonian 017.6 ☑
- membrane, brain 013.0 ☑
- meninges (cerebral) (spinal) 013.0 ☑
- meningitis (basilar) (brain) (cerebral) (cerebrospinal) (spinal) 013.0 ☑
- meningoencephalitis 013.0 ☑
- mesentery, mesenteric 014.8 ☑
  - lymph gland or node 014.8 ☑
- miliary (any site) 018.9 ☑
  - acute 018.0 ☑
  - chronic 018.8 ☑
  - specified type NEC 018.8 ☑
- millstone makers' 011.4 ☑
- miners' 011.4 ☑
- moulders' 011.4 ☑
- mouth 017.9 ☑
- multiple 018.9 ☑
  - acute 018.0 ☑
  - chronic 018.8 ☑
- muscle 017.9 ☑
- myelitis 013.6 ☑
- myocarditis 017.9 ☑ [422.0]
- myocardium 017.9 ☑ [422.0]
- nasal (passage) (sinus) 012.8 ☑
- nasopharynx 012.8 ☑
- neck gland 017.2 ☑
- nephritis 016.0 ☑ [583.81]
- nerve 017.9 ☑
- nose (septum) 012.8 ☑
- ocular 017.3 ☑
- old NEC 137.0
  - without residuals V12.01
- omentum 014.8 ☑
- oophoritis (acute) (chronic) 016.6 ☑
- optic 017.3 ☑ [377.39]
  - nerve trunk 017.3 ☑ [377.39]
  - papilla, papillae 017.3 ☑ [377.39]
- orbit 017.3 ☑
- orchitis 016.5 ☑ [608.81]
- organ, specified NEC 017.9 ☑
- orificialis (primary) 017.0 ☑
- osseous (*see also* Tuberculosis, bone) 015.9 ☑ [730.8]
- osteitis (*see also* Tuberculosis, bone) 015.9 ☑ [730.8]
- osteomyelitis (*see also* Tuberculosis, bone) 015.9 ☑ [730.8]
- otitis (media) 017.4 ☑

Tuberculosis, tubercular, tuberculous — continued

ovaritis (acute) (chronic) 016.6 ☑
ovary (acute) (chronic) 016.6 ☑
oviducts (acute) (chronic) 016.6 ☑
pachymeningitis 013.0 ☑
palate (soft) 017.9 ☑
pancreas 017.9 ☑
papulonecrotic (primary) 017.0 ☑
parathyroid glands 017.9 ☑
paronychia (primary) 017.0 ☑
parotid gland or region 017.9 ☑
pelvic organ NEC 016.9 ☑
    female 016.7 ☑
    male 016.5 ☑
pelvis (bony) 015.7 ☑ [730.85]
penis 016.5 ☑
peribronchitis 011.3 ☑
pericarditis 017.9 ☑ [420.0]
pericardium 017.9 ☑ [420.0]
perichondritis, larynx 012.3 ☑
perineum 017.9 ☑
periostitis (see also Tuberculosis, bone) 015.9 ☑ [730.8]
periphlebitis 017.9 ☑
    eye vessel 017.3 ☑ [362.18]
    retina 017.3 ☑ [362.18]
perirectal fistula 014.8 ☑
peritoneal gland 014.8 ☑
peritoneum 014.0 ☑
peritonitis 014.0 ☑
pernicious NEC (see also Tuberculosis, pulmonary) 011.9 ☑
pharyngitis 012.8 ☑
pharynx 012.8 ☑
phlyctenulosis (conjunctiva) 017.3 ☑ [370.31]
phthisis NEC (see also Tuberculosis, pulmonary) 011.9 ☑
pituitary gland 017.9 ☑
placenta 016.7 ☑
pleura, pleural, pleurisy, pleuritis (fibrinous) (obliterative) (purulent) (simple plastic) (with effusion) 012.0 ☑
    primary, progressive 010.1 ☑
pneumonia, pneumonic 011.6 ☑
pneumothorax 011.7 ☑
polyserositis 018.9 ☑
    acute 018.0 ☑
    chronic 018.8 ☑
potters' 011.4 ☑
prepuce 016.5 ☑
primary 010.9 ☑
    complex 010.0 ☑
    complicated 010.8 ☑
        with pleurisy or effusion 010.1 ☑
        progressive 010.8 ☑
            with pleurisy or effusion 010.1 ☑
    skin 017.0 ☑
proctitis 014.8 ☑
prostate 016.5 ☑ [601.4]
prostatitis 016.5 ☑ [601.4]
pulmonaris (see also Tuberculosis, pulmonary) 011.9 ☑
pulmonary (artery) (incipient) (malignant) (multiple round foci) (pernicious) (reinfection stage) 011.9 ☑
    cavitated or with cavitation 011.2 ☑
        primary, progressive 010.8 ☑
    childhood type or first infection 010.0 ☑
    chromogenic acid-fast bacilli 795.39
    fibrosis or fibrotic 011.4 ☑
    infiltrative 011.0 ☑
        primary, progressive 010.9 ☑
    nodular 011.1 ☑
    specified NEC 011.8 ☑
    sputum positive only 795.39

Tuberculosis, tubercular, tuberculous — continued

pulmonary — continued
    status following surgical collapse of lung NEC 011.9 ☑
pyelitis 016.0 ☑ [590.81]
pyelonephritis 016.0 ☑ [590.81]
pyemia — see Tuberculosis, miliary
pyonephrosis 016.0 ☑
pyopneumothorax 012.0 ☑
pyothorax 012.0 ☑
rectum (with abscess) 014.8 ☑
    fistula 014.8 ☑
reinfection stage (see also Tuberculosis, pulmonary) 011.9 ☑
renal 016.0 ☑
renis 016.0 ☑
reproductive organ 016.7 ☑
respiratory NEC (see also Tuberculosis, pulmonary) 011.9 ☑
    specified site NEC 012.8 ☑
retina 017.3 ☑ [363.13]
retroperitoneal (lymph gland or node) 014.8 ☑
    gland 014.8 ☑
retropharyngeal abscess 012.8 ☑
rheumatism 015.9 ☑
rhinitis 012.8 ☑
sacroiliac (joint) 015.8 ☑
sacrum 015.0 ☑ [730.88]
salivary gland 017.9 ☑
salpingitis (acute) (chronic) 016.6 ☑
sandblasters' 011.4 ☑
sclera 017.3 ☑ [379.09]
scoliosis 015.0 ☑ [737.43]
scrofulous 017.2 ☑
scrotum 016.5 ☑
seminal tract or vesicle 016.5 ☑ [608.81]
senile NEC (see also Tuberculosis, pulmonary) 011.9 ☑
septic NEC (see also Tuberculosis, miliary) 018.9 ☑
shoulder 015.8 ☑
    blade 015.7 ☑ [730.8]
sigmoid 014.8 ☑
sinus (accessory) (nasal) 012.8 ☑
    bone 015.7 ☑ [730.88]
    epididymis 016.4 ☑
skeletal NEC (see also Osteomyelitis, due to tuberculosis) 015.9 ☑ [730.8]
skin (any site) (primary) 017.0 ☑
small intestine 014.8 ☑
soft palate 017.9 ☑
spermatic cord 016.5 ☑
spinal
    column 015.0 ☑ [730.88]
    cord 013.4 ☑
    disease 015.0 ☑ [730.88]
    medulla 013.4 ☑
    membrane 013.0 ☑
    meninges 013.0 ☑
spine 015.0 ☑ [730.88]
spleen 017.7 ☑
splenitis 017.7 ☑
spondylitis 015.0 ☑ [720.81]
spontaneous pneumothorax — see Tuberculosis, pulmonary
sternoclavicular joint 015.8 ☑
stomach 017.9 ☑
stonemasons' 011.4 ☑
struma 017.2 ☑
subcutaneous tissue (cellular) (primary) 017.0 ☑
subcutis (primary) 017.0 ☑
subdeltoid bursa 017.9 ☑
submaxillary 017.9 ☑
    region 017.9 ☑
supraclavicular gland 017.2 ☑
suprarenal (capsule) (gland) 017.6 ☑
swelling, joint (see also Tuberculosis, joint) 015.9 ☑
symphysis pubis 015.7 ☑ [730.88]

Tuberculosis, tubercular, tuberculous — continued

synovitis 015.9 ☑ [727.01]
    hip 015.1 ☑ [727.01]
    knee 015.2 ☑ [727.01]
    specified site NEC 015.8 ☑ [727.01]
    spine or vertebra 015.0 ☑ [727.01]
systemic — see Tuberculosis, miliary
tarsitis (eyelid) 017.0 ☑ [373.4]
    ankle (bone) 015.5 ☑ [730.87]
tendon (sheath) — see Tuberculosis, tenosynovitis
tenosynovitis 015.9 ☑ [727.01]
    hip 015.1 ☑ [727.01]
    knee 015.2 ☑ [727.01]
    specified site NEC 015.8 ☑ [727.01]
    spine or vertebra 015.0 ☑ [727.01]
testis 016.5 ☑ [608.81]
throat 012.8 ☑
thymus gland 017.9 ☑
thyroid gland 017.5 ☑
toe 017.9 ☑
tongue 017.9 ☑
tonsil (lingual) 012.8 ☑
tonsillitis 012.8 ☑
trachea, tracheal 012.8 ☑
    gland 012.1 ☑
        primary, progressive 010.8 ☑
    isolated 012.2 ☑
tracheobronchial 011.3 ☑
    glandular 012.1 ☑
        primary, progressive 010.8 ☑
    isolated 012.2 ☑
    lymph gland or node 012.1 ☑
        primary, progressive 010.8 ☑
tubal 016.6 ☑
tunica vaginalis 016.5 ☑
typhlitis 014.8 ☑
ulcer (primary) (skin) 017.0 ☑
    bowel or intestine 014.8 ☑
    specified site NEC — see Tuberculosis, by site
unspecified site — see Tuberculosis, pulmonary
ureter 016.2 ☑
urethra, urethral 016.3 ☑
urinary organ or tract 016.3 ☑
    kidney 016.0 ☑
uterus 016.7 ☑
uveal tract 017.3 ☑ [363.13]
uvula 017.9 ☑
vaccination, prophylactic (against) V03.2
vagina 016.7 ☑
vas deferens 016.5 ☑
vein 017.9 ☑
verruca (primary) 017.0 ☑
verrucosa (cutis) (primary) 017.0 ☑
vertebra (column) 015.0 ☑ [730.88]
vesiculitis 016.5 ☑ [608.81]
viscera NEC 014.8 ☑
vulva 016.7 ☑ [616.51]
wrist (joint) 015.8 ☑
    bone 015.5 ☑ [730.83]

Tuberculum
    auriculae 744.29
    occlusal 520.2
    paramolare 520.2

Tuberosity
    jaw, excessive 524.07 ●
    maxillary, entire 524.07 ●

Tuberous sclerosis (brain) 759.5

Tube, tubal, tubular — see also condition
    ligation, admission for V25.2

Tubo-ovarian — see condition

Tuboplasty, after previous sterilization V26.0

Tubotympanitis 381.10

Tularemia 021.9
    with
        conjunctivitis 021.3
        pneumonia 021.2
    bronchopneumonic 021.2
    conjunctivitis 021.3

Tularemia — continued

cryptogenic 021.1
disseminated 021.8
enteric 021.1
generalized 021.8
glandular 021.8
intestinal 021.1
oculoglandular 021.3
ophthalmic 021.3
pneumonia 021.2
pulmonary 021.2
specified NEC 021.8
typhoidal 021.1
ulceroglandular 021.0
vaccination, prophylactic (against) V03.4

Tularensis conjunctivitis 021.3

Tumefaction — see also Swelling
    liver (see also Hypertrophy, liver) 789.1

Tumor (M8000/1) — see also Neoplasm, by site, unspecified nature
Abrikossov's (M9580/0) (see also Neoplasm, connective tissue, benign)
    malignant (M9580/3) — see Neoplasm, connective tissue, malignant
acinar cell (M8550/1) — see Neoplasm, by site, uncertain behavior
acinic cell (M8550/1) — see Neoplasm, by site, uncertain behavior
adenomatoid (M9054/0) (see also Neoplasm, by site, benign)
    odontogenic (M9300/0) 213.1
        upper jaw (bone) 213.0
adnexal (skin) (M8390/0) — see Neoplasm, skin, benign
adrenal
    cortical (benign) (M8370/0) 227.0
        malignant (M8370/3) 194.0
    rest (M8671/0) — see Neoplasm, by site, benign
alpha cell (M8152/0)
    malignant (M8152/3)
        pancreas 157.4
        specified site NEC — see Neoplasm, by site, malignant
        unspecified site 157.4
    pancreas 211.7
    specified site NEC — see Neoplasm, by site, benign
    unspecified site 211.7
aneurysmal (see also Aneurysm) 442.9
aortic body (M8691/1) 237.3
    malignant (M8691/3) 194.6
argentaffin (M8241/1) — see Neoplasm, by site, uncertain behavior
basal cell (M8090/1) (see also Neoplasm, skin, uncertain behavior)
benign (M8000/0) — see Neoplasm, by site, benign
beta cell (M8151/0)
    malignant (M8151/3)
        pancreas 157.4
        specified site — see Neoplasm, by site, malignant
        unspecified site 157.4
    pancreas 211.7
    specified site NEC — see Neoplasm, by site, benign
    unspecified site 211.7
blood — see Hematoma
Brenner (M9000/0) 220
    borderline malignancy (M9000/1) 236.2
    malignant (M9000/3) 183.0
    proliferating (M9000/1) 236.2
Brooke's (M8100/0) — see Neoplasm, skin, benign
brown fat (M8880/0) — see Lipoma, by site
Burkitt's (M9750/3) 200.2 ☑

Tumor — see also Neoplasm, by site, unspecified nature — continued
- calcifying epithelial odontogenic (M9340/0) 213.1
  - upper jaw (bone) 213.0
- carcinoid (M8240/1) — see Carcinoid
- carotid body (M8692/1) 237.3
  - malignant (M8692/3) 194.5
- Castleman's (mediastinal lymph node hyperplasia) 785.6
- cells (M8001/1) (see also Neoplasm, by site, unspecified nature)
  - benign (M8001/0) — see Neoplasm, by site, benign
  - malignant (M8001/3) — see Neoplasm, by site, malignant
  - uncertain whether benign or malignant (M8001/1) — see Neoplasm, by site, uncertain nature
- cervix
  - in pregnancy or childbirth 654.6 ☑
    - affecting fetus or newborn 763.89
    - causing obstructed labor 660.2 ☑
      - affecting fetus or newborn 763.1
- chondromatous giant cell (M9230/0) — see Neoplasm, bone, benign
- chromaffin (M8700/0) (see also Neoplasm, by site, benign)
  - malignant (M8700/3) — see Neoplasm, by site, malignant
- Cock's peculiar 706.2
- Codman's (benign chondroblastoma) (M9230/0) — see Neoplasm, bone, benign
- dentigerous, mixed (M9282/0) 213.1
  - upper jaw (bone) 213.0
- dermoid (M9084/0) — see Neoplasm, by site, benign
  - with malignant transformation (M9084/3) 183.0
- desmoid (extra-abdominal) (M8821/1) (see also Neoplasm, connective tissue, uncertain behavior)
  - abdominal (M8822/1) — see Neoplasm, connective tissue, uncertain behavior
- embryonal (mixed) (M9080/1) (see also Neoplasm, by site, uncertain behavior)
  - liver (M9080/3) 155.0
- endodermal sinus (M9071/3)
  - specified site — see Neoplasm, by site, malignant
  - unspecified site
    - female 183.0
    - male 186.9
- epithelial
  - benign (M8010/0) — see Neoplasm, by site, benign
  - malignant (M8010/3) — see Neoplasm, by site, malignant
- Ewing's (M9260/3) — see Neoplasm, bone, malignant
- fatty — see Lipoma
- fetal, causing disproportion 653.7 ☑
  - causing obstructed labor 660.1 ☑
- fibroid (M8890/0) — see Leiomyoma
- G cell (M8153/1)
  - malignant (M8153/3)
    - pancreas 157.4
    - specified site NEC — see Neoplasm, by site, malignant
    - unspecified site 157.4
  - specified site — see Neoplasm, by site, uncertain behavior
  - unspecified site 235.5
- giant cell (type) (M8003/1) (see also Neoplasm, by site, unspecified nature)
  - bone (M9250/1) 238.0

Tumor — see also Neoplasm, by site, unspecified nature — continued
- giant cell (see also Neoplasm, by site, unspecified nature) — continued
  - bone — continued
    - malignant (M9250/3) — see Neoplasm, bone, malignant
    - chondromatous (M9230/0) — see Neoplasm, bone, benign
    - malignant (M8003/3) — see Neoplasm, by site, malignant
    - peripheral (gingiva) 523.8
  - soft parts (M9251/1) (see also Neoplasm, connective tissue, uncertain behavior)
    - malignant (M9251/3) — see Neoplasm, connective tissue, malignant
  - tendon sheath 727.02
- glomus (M8711/0) (see also Hemangioma, by site)
  - jugulare (M8690/1) 237.3
    - malignant (M8690/3) 194.6
- gonadal stromal (M8590/1) — see Neoplasm, by site, uncertain behavior
- granular cell (M9580/0) (see also Neoplasm, connective tissue, benign)
  - malignant (M9580/3) — see Neoplasm, connective tissue, malignant
- granulosa cell (M8620/1) 236.2
  - malignant (M8620/3) 183.0
- granulosa cell-theca cell (M8621/1) 236.2
  - malignant (M8621/3) 183.0
- Grawitz's (hypernephroma) (M8312/3) 189.0
- hazard-crile (M8350/3) 193
- hemorrhoidal — see Hemorrhoids
- hilar cell (M8660/0) 220
- Hürthle cell (benign) (M8290/0) 226
  - malignant (M8290/3) 193
- hydatid (see also Echinococcus) 122.9
- hypernephroid (M8311/1) (see also Neoplasm, by site, uncertain behavior)
- interstitial cell (M8650/1) (see also Neoplasm, by site, uncertain behavior)
  - benign (M8650/0) — see Neoplasm, by site, benign
  - malignant (M8650/3) — see Neoplasm, by site, malignant
- islet cell (M8150/0)
  - malignant (M8150/3)
    - pancreas 157.4
    - specified site — see Neoplasm, by site, malignant
    - unspecified site 157.4
  - pancreas 211.7
  - specified site NEC — see Neoplasm, by site, benign
  - unspecified site 211.7
- juxtaglomerular (M8361/1) 236.91
- Krukenberg's (M8490/6) 198.6
- Leydig cell (M8650/1)
  - benign (M8650/0)
    - specified site — see Neoplasm, by site, benign
    - unspecified site
      - female 220
      - male 222.0
  - malignant (M8650/3)
    - specified site — see Neoplasm, by site, malignant
    - unspecified site
      - female 183.0
      - male 186.9
  - specified site — see Neoplasm, by site, uncertain behavior
  - unspecified site
    - female 236.2

Tumor — see also Neoplasm, by site, unspecified nature — continued
- Leydig cell — continued
  - unspecified site — continued
    - male 236.4
- lipid cell, ovary (M8670/0) 220
- lipoid cell, ovary (M8670/0) 220
- lymphomatous, benign (M9590/0) (see also Neoplasm, by site, benign)
- Malherbe's (M8110/0) — see Neoplasm, skin, benign
- malignant (M8000/3) (see also Neoplasm, by site, malignant)
  - fusiform cell (type) (M8004/3) — see Neoplasm, by site, malignant
  - giant cell (type) (M8003/3) — see Neoplasm, by site, malignant
  - mixed NEC (M8940/3) — see Neoplasm, by site, malignant
  - small cell (type) (M8002/3) — see Neoplasm, by site, malignant
  - spindle cell (type) (M8004/3) — see Neoplasm, by site, malignant
- mast cell (M9740/1) 238.5
  - malignant (M9740/3) 202.6 ☑
- melanotic, neuroectodermal (M9363/0) — see Neoplasm, by site, benign
- Merkel cell — see Neoplasm, by site, malignant
- mesenchymal
  - malignant (M8800/3) — see Neoplasm, connective tissue, malignant
  - mixed (M8990/1) — see Neoplasm, connective tissue, uncertain behavior
- mesodermal, mixed (M8951/3) (see also Neoplasm, by site, malignant)
  - liver 155.0
- mesonephric (M9110/1) (see also Neoplasm, by site, uncertain behavior)
  - malignant (M9110/3) — see Neoplasm, by site, malignant
- metastatic
  - from specified site (M8000/3) — see Neoplasm, by site, malignant
  - to specified site (M8000/6) — see Neoplasm, by site, malignant, secondary
- mixed NEC (M8940/0) (see also Neoplasm, by site, benign)
  - malignant (M8940/3) — see Neoplasm, by site, malignant
- mucocarcinoid, malignant (M8243/3) — see Neoplasm, by site, malignant
- mucoepidermoid (M8430/1) — see Neoplasm, by site, uncertain behavior
- Mullerian, mixed (M8950/3) — see Neoplasm, by site, malignant
- myoepithelial (M8982/0) — see Neoplasm, by site, benign
- neurogenic olfactory (M9520/3) 160.0
- nonencapsulated sclerosing (M8350/3) 193
- odontogenic (M9270/1) 238.0
  - adenomatoid (M9300/0) 213.1
    - upper jaw (bone) 213.0
  - benign (M9270/0) 213.1
    - upper jaw (bone) 213.0
  - calcifying epithelial (M9340/0) 213.1
    - upper jaw (bone) 213.0
  - malignant (M9270/3) 170.1
    - upper jaw (bone) 170.0
  - squamous (M9312/0) 213.1
    - upper jaw (bone) 213.0
- ovarian stromal (M8590/1) 236.2
- ovary
  - in pregnancy or childbirth 654.4 ☑

Tumor — see also Neoplasm, by site, unspecified nature — continued
- ovary — continued
  - in pregnancy or childbirth — continued
    - affecting fetus or newborn 763.89
    - causing obstructed labor 660.2 ☑
      - affecting fetus or newborn 763.1
- pacinian (M9507/0) — see Neoplasm, skin, benign
- Pancoast's (M8010/3) 162.3
- papillary — see Papilloma
- pelvic, in pregnancy or childbirth 654.9 ☑
  - affecting fetus or newborn 763.89
  - causing obstructed labor 660.2 ☑
    - affecting fetus or newborn 763.1
- phantom 300.11
- plasma cell (M9731/1) 238.6
  - benign (M9731/0) — see Neoplasm, by site, benign
  - malignant (M9731/3) 203.8 ☑
- polyvesicular vitelline (M9071/3)
  - specified site — see Neoplasm, by site, malignant
  - unspecified site
    - female 183.0
    - male 186.9
- Pott's puffy (see also Osteomyelitis) 730.2
- Rathke's pouch (M9350/1) 237.0
- regaud's (M8082/3) — see Neoplasm, nasopharynx, malignant
- rete cell (M8140/0) 222.0
- retinal anlage (M9363/0) — see Neoplasm, by site, benign
- Rokitansky's 620.2
- salivary gland type, mixed (M8940/0) (see also Neoplasm, by site, benign)
  - malignant (M8940/3) — see Neoplasm, by site, malignant
- Sampson's 617.1
- Schloffer's (see also Peritonitis) 567.29
- Schmincke (M8082/3) — see Neoplasm, nasopharynx, malignant
- sebaceous (see also Cyst, sebaceous) 706.2
- secondary (M8000/6) — see Neoplasm, by site, secondary
- Sertoli cell (M8640/0)
  - with lipid storage (M8641/0)
    - specified site — see Neoplasm, by site, benign
    - unspecified site
      - female 220
      - male 222.0
  - specified site — see Neoplasm, by site, benign
  - unspecified site
    - female 220
    - male 222.0
- Sertoli-Leydig cell (M8631/0)
  - specified site — see Neoplasm, by site, benign
  - unspecified site
    - female 220
    - male 222.0
- sex cord (-stromal) (M8590/1) — see Neoplasm, by site, uncertain behavior
- skin appendage (M8390/0) — see Neoplasm, skin, benign
- soft tissue
  - benign (M8800/0) — see Neoplasm, connective tissue, benign
  - malignant (M8800/3) — see Neoplasm, connective tissue, malignant
- sternomastoid 754.1

Index to Diseases

Tumor — see also Neoplasm, by site, unspecified nature — continued
  stromal
    abdomen
      benign 215.5
      malignant 171.5
      uncertain behavior 238.1
    digestive system 238.1
      benign 215.5
      malignant 171.5
      uncertain behavior 238.1
    gastric 238.1
      benign 215.5
      malignant 171.5
      uncertain behavior 238.1
    gastrointestinal 238.1
      benign 215.5
      malignant 171.5
      uncertain behavior 238.1
    intestine ▶(small) (large)◀ 238.1
      benign 215.5
      malignant 171.5
      uncertain behavior 238.1
    stomach 238.1
      benign 215.5
      malignant 171.5
      uncertain behavior 238.1
  superior sulcus (lung) (pulmonary) (syndrome) (M8010/3) 162.3
  suprasulcus (M8010/3) 162.3
  sweat gland (M8400/1) (see also Neoplasm, skin, uncertain behavior)
    benign (M8400/0) — see Neoplasm, skin, benign
    malignant (M8400/3) — see Neoplasm, skin, malignant
  syphilitic brain 094.89
    congenital 090.49
  testicular stromal (M8590/1) 236.4
  theca cell (M8600/0) 220
  theca cell-granulosa cell (M8621/1) 236.2
  theca-lutein (M8610/0) 220
  turban (M8200/0) 216.4
  uterus
    in pregnancy or childbirth 654.1 ☑
      affecting fetus or newborn 763.89
      causing obstructed labor 660.2 ☑
        affecting fetus or newborn 763.1
  vagina
    in pregnancy or childbirth 654.7 ☑
      affecting fetus or newborn 763.89
      causing obstructed labor 660.2 ☑
        affecting fetus or newborn 763.1
  varicose (see also Varicose, vein) 454.9
  von Recklinghausen's (M9540/1) 237.71
  vulva
    in pregnancy or childbirth 654.8 ☑
      affecting fetus or newborn 763.89
      causing obstructed labor 660.2 ☑
        affecting fetus or newborn 763.1
  Warthin's (salivary gland) (M8561/0) 210.2
  white (see also Tuberculosis, arthritis)
  White-Darier 757.39
  Wilms' (nephroblastoma) (M8960/3) 189.0
  yolk sac (M9071/3)
    specified site — see Neoplasm, by site, malignant
    unspecified site
      female 183.0
      male 186.9
Tumorlet (M8040/1) — see Neoplasm, by site, uncertain behavior
Tungiasis 134.1
Tunica vasculosa lentis 743.39
Tunnel vision 368.45
Turban tumor (M8200/0) 216.4
Türck's trachoma (chronic catarrhal laryngitis) 476.0
Türk's syndrome (ocular retraction syndrome) 378.71
Turner's
  hypoplasia (tooth) 520.4
  syndrome 758.6
  tooth 520.4
Turner-Kieser syndrome (hereditary osteo-onychodysplasia) 756.89
Turner-Varny syndrome 758.6
Turricephaly 756.0
Tussis convulsiva — see also Whooping cough 033.9
Twin
  affected by maternal complications of pregnancy 761.5
  conjoined 759.4
  healthy liveborn — see Newborn, twin
  pregnancy (complicating delivery) NEC 651.0 ☑
    with fetal loss and retention of one fetus 651.3 ☑
    following (elective) fetal reduction
Twinning, teeth 520.2
Twist, twisted
  bowel, colon, or intestine 560.2
  hair (congenital) 757.4
  mesentery 560.2
  omentum 560.2
  organ or site, congenital NEC — see Anomaly, specified type NEC
  ovarian pedicle 620.5
    congenital 752.0
  umbilical cord — see Compression, umbilical cord
Twitch 781.0
Tylosis 700
  buccalis 528.6
  gingiva 523.8
  linguae 528.6
  palmaris et plantaris 757.39
Tympanism 787.3
Tympanites (abdominal) (intestine) 787.3
Tympanitis — see Myringitis
Tympanosclerosis 385.00
  involving
    combined sites NEC 385.09
      with tympanic membrane 385.03
    tympanic membrane 385.01
      with ossicles 385.02
        and middle ear 385.03
Tympanum — see condition
Tympany
  abdomen 787.3
  chest 786.7
Typhlitis — see also Appendicitis 541
Typhoenteritis 002.0
Typhogastric fever 002.0
Typhoid (abortive) (ambulant) (any site) (fever) (hemorrhagic) (infection) (intermittent) (malignant) (rheumatic) 002.0
  with pneumonia 002.0 [484.8]
  abdominal 002.0
  carrier (suspected) of V02.1
  cholecystitis (current) 002.0
  clinical (Widal and blood test negative) 002.0
  endocarditis 002.0 [421.1]
  inoculation reaction — see Complications, vaccination
  meningitis 002.0 [320.7]
  mesenteric lymph nodes 002.0
  myocarditis 002.0 [422.0]
  osteomyelitis (see also Osteomyelitis, due to, typhoid) 002.0 [730.8] ☑
  perichondritis, larynx 002.0 [478.71]
  pneumonia 002.0 [484.8]
  spine 002.0 [720.81]
  ulcer (perforating) 002.0
Typhoid — continued
  vaccination, prophylactic (against) V03.1
  Widal negative 002.0
Typhomalaria (fever) — see also Malaria 084.6
Typhomania 002.0
Typhoperitonitis 002.0
Typhus (fever) 081.9
  abdominal, abdominalis 002.0
  African tick 082.1
  amarillic (see also Fever, Yellow) 060.9
  brain 081.9
  cerebral 081.9
  classical 081.9
  endemic (flea-borne) 081.0
  epidemic (louse-borne) 080
  exanthematic NEC 080
  exanthematicus SAI 080
    brillii SAI 081.1
    Mexicanus SAI 081.0
    pediculo vestimenti causa 080
    typhus murinus 081.0
  flea-borne 081.0
  Indian tick 082.1
  Kenya tick 082.1
  louse-borne 080
  Mexican 081.0
    flea-borne 081.0
    louse-borne 080
    tabardillo 080
  mite-borne 081.2
  murine 081.0
  North Asian tick-borne 082.2
  petechial 081.9
  Queensland tick 082.3
  rat 081.0
  recrudescent 081.1
  recurrent (see also Fever, relapsing) 087.9
  São Paulo 082.0
  scrub (China) (India) (Malaya) (New Guinea) 081.2
  shop (of Malaya) 081.0
  Siberian tick 082.2
  tick-borne NEC 082.9
  tropical 081.2
  vaccination, prophylactic (against) V05.8
Tyrosinemia 270.2
  neonatal 775.89
Tyrosinosis (Medes) (Sakai) 270.2
Tyrosinuria 270.2
Tyrosyluria 270.2

U

Uehlinger's syndrome (acropachyderma) 757.39
Uhl's anomaly or disease (hypoplasia of myocardium, right ventricle) 746.84
Ulcerosa scarlatina 034.1
Ulcer, ulcerated, ulcerating, ulceration, ulcerative 707.9
  with gangrene 707.9 [785.4]
  abdomen (wall) (see also Ulcer, skin) 707.8
  ala, nose 478.19
  alveolar process 526.5
  amebic (intestine) 006.9
    skin 006.6
  anastomotic — see Ulcer, gastrojejunal
  anorectal 569.41
  antral — see Ulcer, stomach
  anus (sphincter) (solitary) 569.41
    varicose — see Varicose, ulcer, anus
  aorta — see Aneurysm
  aphthous (oral) (recurrent) 528.2
    genital organ(s)
      female 616.89
      male 608.89
    mouth 528.2
  arm (see also Ulcer, skin) 707.8
Ulcer, ulcerated, ulcerating, ulceration, ulcerative — continued
  arteriosclerotic plaque — see Arteriosclerosis, by site
  artery NEC 447.2
    without rupture 447.8
  atrophic NEC — see Ulcer, skin
  Barrett's (chronic peptic ulcer of esophagus) 530.85
  bile duct 576.8
  bladder (solitary) (sphincter) 596.8
    bilharzial (see also Schistosomiasis) 120.9 [595.4]
    submucosal (see also Cystitis) 595.1
    tuberculous (see also Tuberculosis) 016.1 ☑
  bleeding NEC — see Ulcer, peptic, with hemorrhage
  bone 730.9 ☑
  bowel (see also Ulcer, intestine) 569.82
  breast 611.0
  bronchitis 491.8
  bronchus 519.19
  buccal (cavity) (traumatic) 528.9
  burn (acute) — see Ulcer, duodenum
  Buruli 031.1
  buttock (see also Ulcer, skin) 707.8
    decubitus (see also Ulcer, decubitus) 707.0
  cancerous (M8000/3) — see Neoplasm, by site, malignant
  cardia — see Ulcer, stomach
  cardio-esophageal (peptic) 530.20
    with bleeding 530.21
  cecum (see also Ulcer, intestine) 569.82
  cervix (uteri) (trophic) 622.0
    with mention of cervicitis 616.0
  chancroidal 099.0
  chest (wall) (see also Ulcer, skin) 707.8
  Chiclero 085.4
  chin (pyogenic) (see also Ulcer, skin) 707.8
  chronic (cause unknown) (see also Ulcer, skin)
    penis 607.89
  Cochin-China 085.1
  colitis — see Colitis, ulcerative
  colon (see also Ulcer, intestine) 569.82
  conjunctiva (acute) (postinfectional) 372.00
  cornea (infectional) 370.00
    with perforation 370.06
    annular 370.02
    catarrhal 370.01
    central 370.03
    dendritic 054.42
    marginal 370.01
    mycotic 370.05
    phlyctenular, tuberculous (see also Tuberculosis) 017.3 ☑ [370.31]
    ring 370.02
    rodent 370.07
    serpent, serpiginous 370.04
    superficial marginal 370.01
    tuberculous (see also Tuberculosis) 017.3 ☑ [370.31]
  corpus cavernosum (chronic) 607.89
  crural — see Ulcer, lower extremity
  Curling's — see Ulcer, duodenum
  Cushing's — see Ulcer, peptic
  cystitis (interstitial) 595.1
  decubitus (unspecified site) 707.00
    with gangrene 707.00 [785.4]
    ankle 707.06
    back
      lower 707.03
      upper 707.02
    buttock 707.05
    elbow 707.01
    head 707.09
    heel 707.07

Ulcer, ulcerated, ulcerating

Ulcer, ulcerated, ulcerating, ulceration, ulcerative — *continued*
- decubitus — *continued*
  - hip 707.04
  - other site 707.09
  - sacrum 707.03
  - shoulder blades 707.02
- dendritic 054.42
- diabetes, diabetic (mellitus) 250.8 ☑ [707.9]
  - lower limb 250.8 ☑ [707.10]
    - ankle 250.8 ☑ [707.13]
    - calf 250.8 ☑ [707.12]
    - foot 250.8 ☑ [707.15]
    - heel 250.8 ☑ [707.14]
    - knee 250.8 ☑ [707.19]
    - specified site NEC 250.8 ☑ [707.19]
    - thigh 250.8 ☑ [707.11]
    - toes 250.8 ☑ [707.15]
  - specified site NEC 250.8 ☑ [707.8]
- Dieulafoy — *see* Lesion, Dieulafoy
- due to
  - infection NEC — *see* Ulcer, skin
  - radiation, radium — *see* Ulcer, by site
  - trophic disturbance (any region) — *see* Ulcer, skin
  - x-ray — *see* Ulcer, by site
- duodenum, duodenal (eroded) (peptic) 532.9 ☑

Note — Use the following fifth-digit subclassification with categories 531–534:
- 0   without mention of obstruction
- 1   with obstruction

  - with
    - hemorrhage (chronic) 532.4 ☑
      - and perforation 532.6 ☑
    - perforation (chronic) 532.5 ☑
      - and hemorrhage 532.6 ☑
  - acute 532.3 ☑
    - with
      - hemorrhage 532.0 ☑
        - and perforation 532.2 ☑
      - perforation 532.1 ☑
        - and hemorrhage 532.2 ☑
  - bleeding (recurrent) — *see* Ulcer, duodenum, with hemorrhage
  - chronic 532.7 ☑
    - with
      - hemorrhage 532.4 ☑
        - and perforation 532.6 ☑
      - perforation 532.5 ☑
        - and hemorrhage 532.6 ☑
  - penetrating — *see* Ulcer, duodenum, with perforation
  - perforating — *see* Ulcer, duodenum, with perforation
- dysenteric NEC 009.0
- elusive 595.1
- endocarditis (any valve) (acute) (chronic) (subacute) 421.0
- enteritis — *see* Colitis, ulcerative
- enterocolitis 556.0
- epiglottis 478.79
- esophagus (peptic) 530.20
  - with bleeding 530.21
  - due to ingestion
    - aspirin 530.20
    - chemicals 530.20
    - medicinal agents 530.20
  - fungal 530.20
  - infectional 530.20
  - varicose (*see also* Varix, esophagus) 456.1
    - bleeding (*see also* Varix, esophagus, bleeding) 456.0
- eye NEC 360.00
  - dendritic 054.42
- eyelid (region) 373.01
- face (*see also* Ulcer, skin) 707.8
- fauces 478.29

Ulcer, ulcerated, ulcerating, ulceration, ulcerative — *continued*
- Fenwick (-Hunner) (solitary) (*see also* Cystitis) 595.1
- fistulous NEC — *see* Ulcer, skin
- foot (indolent) (*see also* Ulcer, lower extremity) 707.15
  - perforating 707.15
    - leprous 030.1
    - syphilitic 094.0
  - trophic 707.15
  - varicose 454.0
    - inflamed or infected 454.2
- frambesial, initial or primary 102.0
- gallbladder or duct 575.8
- gall duct 576.8
- gangrenous (*see also* Gangrene) 785.4
- gastric — *see* Ulcer, stomach
- gastrocolic — *see* Ulcer, gastrojejunal
- gastroduodenal — *see* Ulcer, peptic
- gastroesophageal — *see* Ulcer, stomach
- gastrohepatic — *see* Ulcer, stomach
- gastrointestinal — *see* Ulcer, gastrojejunal
- gastrojejunal (eroded) (peptic) 534.9 ☑

Note — Use the following fifth-digit subclassification with categories 531–534:
- 0   without mention of obstruction
- 1   with obstruction

  - with
    - hemorrhage (chronic) 534.4 ☑
      - and perforation 534.6 ☑
    - perforation 534.5 ☑
      - and hemorrhage 534.6 ☑
  - acute 534.3 ☑
    - with
      - hemorrhage 534.0 ☑
        - and perforation 534.2 ☑
      - perforation 534.1 ☑
        - and hemorrhage 534.2 ☑
  - bleeding (recurrent) — *see* Ulcer, gastrojejunal, with hemorrhage
  - chronic 534.7 ☑
    - with
      - hemorrhage 534.4 ☑
        - and perforation 534.6 ☑
      - perforation 534.5 ☑
        - and hemorrhage 534.6 ☑
  - penetrating — *see* Ulcer, gastrojejunal, with perforation
  - perforating — *see* Ulcer, gastrojejunal, with perforation
- gastrojejunocolic — *see* Ulcer, gastrojejunal
- genital organ
  - female 629.89 ▲
  - male 608.89
- gingiva 523.8
- gingivitis 523.10 ▲
- glottis 478.79
- granuloma of pudenda 099.2
- groin (*see also* Ulcer, skin) 707.8
- gum 523.8
- gumma, due to yaws 102.4
- hand (*see also* Ulcer, skin) 707.8
- hard palate 528.9
- heel (*see also* Ulcer, lower extremity) 707.14
  - decubitus (*see also* Ulcer, decubitus) 707.07
- hemorrhoids 455.8
  - external 455.5
  - internal 455.2
- hip (*see also* Ulcer, skin) 707.8
  - decubitus (*see also* Ulcer, decubitus) 707.04
- Hunner's 595.1
- hypopharynx 478.29
- hypopyon (chronic) (subacute) 370.04
- hypostaticum — *see* Ulcer, varicose
- ileocolitis 556.1

Ulcer, ulcerated, ulcerating, ulceration, ulcerative — *continued*
- ileum (*see also* Ulcer, intestine) 569.82
  - with perforation 569.83
  - amebic 006.9
  - duodenal — *see* Ulcer, duodenum
  - granulocytopenic (with hemorrhage) 288.09 ▲
  - marginal 569.82
  - perforating 569.83
  - small, primary 569.82
  - stercoraceous 569.82
  - stercoral 569.82
  - tuberculous (*see also* Tuberculosis) 014.8 ☑
  - typhoid (fever) 002.0
  - varicose 456.8
- ischemic 707.9
  - lower extremity (*see also* Ulcer, lower extremity) 707.10
    - ankle 707.13
    - calf 707.12
    - foot 707.15
    - heel 707.14
    - knee 707.19
    - specified site NEC 707.19
    - thigh 707.11
    - toes 707.15
- jejunum, jejunal — *see* Ulcer, gastrojejunal
- keratitis (*see also* Ulcer, cornea) 370.00
- knee — *see* Ulcer, lower extremity
- labium (majus) (minus) 616.50
- laryngitis (*see also* Laryngitis) 464.00
  - with obstruction 464.01
- larynx (aphthous) (contact) 478.79
  - diphtheritic 032.3
- leg — *see* Ulcer, lower extremity
- lip 528.5
- Lipschütz's 616.50
- lower extremity (atrophic) (chronic) (neurogenic) (perforating) (pyogenic) (trophic) (tropical) 707.10
  - with gangrene (*see also* Ulcer, lower extremity) 707.10 [785.4]
    - arteriosclerotic 440.24
  - ankle 707.13
  - arteriosclerotic 440.23
    - with gangrene 440.24
  - calf 707.12
  - decubitus 707.00
    - with gangrene 707.00 [785.4]
    - ankle 707.06
    - buttock 707.05
    - heel 707.07
    - hip 707.04
  - foot 707.15
  - heel 707.14
  - knee 707.19
  - specified site NEC 707.19
  - thigh 707.11
  - toes 707.15
  - varicose 454.0
    - inflamed or infected 454.2
- luetic — *see* Ulcer, syphilitic
- lung 518.89
  - tuberculous (*see also* Tuberculosis) 011.2 ☑
- malignant (M8000/3) — *see* Neoplasm, by site, malignant
- marginal NEC — *see* Ulcer, gastrojejunal
- meatus (urinarius) 597.89
- Meckel's diverticulum 751.0
- Meleney's (chronic undermining) 686.09
- Mooren's (cornea) 370.07
- mouth (traumatic) 528.9
- mycobacterial (skin) 031.1
- nasopharynx 478.29
- navel cord (newborn) 771.4
- neck (*see also* Ulcer, skin) 707.8
- uterus 622.0

Ulcer, ulcerated, ulcerating, ulceration, ulcerative — *continued*
- neurogenic NEC — *see* Ulcer, skin
- nose, nasal (infectional) (passage) 478.19 ▲
  - septum 478.19 ▲
  - varicose 456.8
- skin — *see* Ulcer, skin
- spirochetal NEC 104.8
- oral mucosa (traumatic) 528.9
- palate (soft) 528.9
- penetrating NEC — *see* Ulcer, peptic, with perforation
- penis (chronic) 607.89
- peptic (site unspecified) 533.9 ☑

Note — Use the following fifth-digit subclassification with categories 531–534:
- 0   without mention of obstruction
- 1   with obstruction

  - with
    - hemorrhage 533.4 ☑
      - and perforation 533.6 ☑
    - perforation (chronic) 533.5 ☑
      - and hemorrhage 533.6 ☑
  - acute 533.3 ☑
    - with
      - hemorrhage 533.0 ☑
        - and perforation 533.2 ☑
      - perforation 533.1 ☑
        - and hemorrhage 533.2 ☑
  - bleeding (recurrent) — *see* Ulcer, peptic, with hemorrhage
  - chronic 533.7 ☑
    - with
      - hemorrhage 533.4 ☑
        - and perforation 533.6 ☑
      - perforation 533.5 ☑
        - and hemorrhage 533.6 ☑
  - penetrating — *see* Ulcer, peptic, with perforation
  - perforating NEC (*see also* Ulcer, peptic, with perforation) 533.5 ☑
- skin 707.9
- perineum (*see also* Ulcer, skin) 707.8
- peritonsillar 474.8
- phagedenic (tropical) NEC — *see* Ulcer, skin
- pharynx 478.29
- phlebitis — *see* Phlebitis
- plaster (*see also* Ulcer, decubitus) 707.00
- popliteal space — *see* Ulcer, lower extremity
- postpyloric — *see* Ulcer, duodenum
- prepuce 607.89
- prepyloric — *see* Ulcer, stomach
- pressure (*see also* Ulcer, decubitus) 707.00
- primary of intestine 569.82
  - with perforation 569.83
- proctitis 556.2
  - with ulcerative sigmoiditis 556.3
- prostate 601.8
- pseudopeptic — *see* Ulcer, peptic
- pyloric — *see* Ulcer, stomach
- rectosigmoid 569.82
  - with perforation 569.83
- rectum (sphincter) (solitary) 569.41
  - stercoraceous, stercoral 569.41
  - varicose — *see* Varicose, ulcer, anus
- retina (*see also* Chorioretinitis) 363.20
- rodent (M8090/3) (*see also* Neoplasm, skin, malignant)
  - cornea 370.07
- round — *see* Ulcer, stomach
- sacrum (region) (*see also* Ulcer, skin) 707.8
- Saemisch's 370.04
- scalp (*see also* Ulcer, skin) 707.8
- sclera 379.09
- scrofulous (*see also* Tuberculosis) 017.2 ☑

Index to Diseases

Ulcer, ulcerated, ulcerating, ulceration, ulcerative — continued
- scrotum 608.89
  - tuberculous (see also Tuberculosis) 016.5 ☑
  - varicose 456.4
- seminal vesicle 608.89
- sigmoid 569.82
  - with perforation 569.83
- skin (atrophic) (chronic) (neurogenic) (non-healing) (perforating) (pyogenic) (trophic) 707.9
  - with gangrene 707.9 [785.4]
  - amebic 006.6
  - decubitus (see also Ulcer, decubitus) 707.00
    - with gangrene 707.00 [785.4]
  - in granulocytopenia 288.09
  - lower extremity (see also Ulcer, lower extremity) 707.10
    - with gangrene 707.10 [785.4]
    - arteriosclerotic 440.24
    - ankle 707.13
      - arteriosclerotic 440.23
        - with gangrene 440.24
    - calf 707.12
    - foot 707.15
    - heel 707.14
    - knee 707.19
    - specified site NEC 707.19
    - thigh 707.11
    - toes 707.15
  - mycobacterial 031.1
  - syphilitic (early) (secondary) 091.3
  - tuberculous (primary) (see also Tuberculosis) 017.0 ☑
  - varicose — see Ulcer, varicose
- sloughing NEC — see Ulcer, skin
- soft palate 528.9
- solitary, anus or rectum (sphincter) 569.41
- sore throat 462
  - streptococcal 034.0
- spermatic cord 608.89
- spine (tuberculous) 015.0 ☑ [730.88]
- stasis (leg) (venous) 454.0
  - with varicose veins 454.0
  - without varicose veins 459.81
  - inflamed or infected 454.2
- stercoral, stercoraceous 569.82
  - with perforation 569.83
- anus or rectum 569.41
- stomach (eroded) (peptic) (round) 531.9 ☑

Note — Use the following fifth-digit subclassification with categories 531–534:
- 0 without mention of obstruction
- 1 with obstruction

  - with
    - hemorrhage 531.4 ☑
      - and perforation 531.6 ☑
    - perforation (chronic) 531.5 ☑
      - and hemorrhage 531.6 ☑
    - acute 531.3 ☑
      - with
        - hemorrhage 531.0 ☑
          - and perforation 531.2 ☑
        - perforation 531.1 ☑
          - and hemorrhage 531.2 ☑
    - bleeding (recurrent) — see Ulcer, stomach, with hemorrhage
    - chronic 531.7 ☑
      - with
        - hemorrhage 531.4 ☑
          - and perforation 531.6 ☑
        - perforation 531.5 ☑
          - and hemorrhage 531.6 ☑
    - penetrating — see Ulcer, stomach, with perforation
    - perforating — see Ulcer, stomach, with perforation
- stoma, stomal — see Ulcer, gastrojejunal

Ulcer, ulcerated, ulcerating, ulceration, ulcerative — continued
- stomatitis 528.00
- stress — see Ulcer, peptic
- strumous (tuberculous) (see also Tuberculosis) 017.2 ☑
- submental (see also Ulcer, skin) 707.8
- submucosal, bladder 595.1
- syphilitic (any site) (early) (secondary) 091.3
  - late 095.9
  - perforating 095.9
    - foot 094.0
- testis 608.89
- thigh — see Ulcer, lower extremity
- throat 478.29
  - diphtheritic 032.0
- toe — see Ulcer, lower extremity
- tongue (traumatic) 529.0
- tonsil 474.8
  - diphtheritic 032.0
- trachea 519.19
- trophic — see Ulcer, skin
- tropical NEC (see also Ulcer, skin) 707.9
- tuberculous — see Tuberculosis, ulcer
- tunica vaginalis 608.89
- turbinate 730.9 ☑
- typhoid (fever) 002.0
  - perforating 002.0
- umbilicus (newborn) 771.4
- unspecified site NEC — see Ulcer, skin
- urethra (meatus) (see also Urethritis) 597.89
- uterus 621.8
  - cervix 622.0
    - with mention of cervicitis 616.0
  - neck 622.0
    - with mention of cervicitis 616.0
- vagina 616.89
- valve, heart 421.0
- varicose (lower extremity, any part) 454.0
  - anus — see Varicose, ulcer, anus
  - broad ligament 456.5
  - esophagus (see also Varix, esophagus) 456.1
    - bleeding (see also Varix, esophagus, bleeding) 456.0
  - inflamed or infected 454.2
  - nasal septum 456.8
  - perineum 456.6
  - rectum — see Varicose, ulcer, anus
  - scrotum 456.4
  - specified site NEC 456.8
  - sublingual 456.3
  - vulva 456.6
- vas deferens 608.89
- vesical (see also Ulcer, bladder) 596.8
- vulva (acute) (infectional) 616.50
  - Behçet's syndrome 136.1 [616.51]
  - herpetic 054.12
  - tuberculous 016.7 ☑ [616.51]
- vulvobuccal, recurring 616.50
- x-ray — see Ulcer, by site
- yaws 102.4

Ulcus — see also Ulcer
- cutis tuberculosum (see also Tuberculosis) 017.0 ☑
- duodeni — see Ulcer, duodenum
- durum 091.0
  - extragenital 091.2
- gastrojejunale — see Ulcer, gastrojejunal
- hypostaticum — see Ulcer, varicose
- molle (cutis) (skin) 099.0
- serpens corneae (pneumococcal) 370.04
- ventriculi — see Ulcer, stomach

Ulegyria 742.4

Ulerythema
- acneiforma 701.8
- centrifugum 695.4
- ophryogenes 757.4

Ullrich-Feichtiger syndrome 759.89

Ullrich (-Bonnevie) (-Turner) syndrome 758.6

Ulnar — see condition

Ulorrhagia 523.8

Ulorrhea 523.8

Umbilicus, umbilical — see also condition
- cord necrosis, affecting fetus or newborn 762.6

Unacceptable
- existing dental restoration
  - contours 525.65
  - morphology 525.65

Unavailability of medical facilities (at) V63.9
- due to
  - investigation by social service agency V63.8
  - lack of services at home V63.1
  - remoteness from facility V63.0
  - waiting list V63.2
- home V63.1
- outpatient clinic V63.0
- specified reason NEC V63.8

Uncinaria americana infestation 126.1

Uncinariasis — see also Ancylostomiasis 126.9

Unconscious, unconsciousness 780.09

Underdevelopment — see also Undeveloped
- sexual 259.0

Underfill, endodontic 526.63

Undernourishment 269.9

Undernutrition 269.9

Under observation — see Observation

Underweight 783.22
- for gestational age — see Light-for-dates

Underwood's disease (sclerema neonatorum) 778.1

Undescended — see also Malposition, congenital
- cecum 751.4
- colon 751.4
- testis 752.51

Undetermined diagnosis or cause 799.9

Undeveloped, undevelopment — see also Hypoplasia
- brain (congenital) 742.1
- cerebral (congenital) 742.1
- fetus or newborn 764.9 ☑
- heart 746.89
- lung 748.5
- testis 257.2
- uterus 259.0

Undiagnosed (disease) 799.9

Undulant fever — see also Brucellosis 023.9

Unemployment, anxiety concerning V62.0

Unequal leg (acquired) (length) 736.81
- congenital 755.30

Unerupted teeth, tooth 520.6

Unextracted dental root 525.3

Unguis incarnatus 703.0

Unicornis uterus 752.3

Unicorporeus uterus 752.3

Uniformis uterus 752.3

Unilateral — see also condition
- development, breast 611.8
- organ or site, congenital NEC — see Agenesis
- vagina 752.49

Unilateralis uterus 752.3

Unilocular heart 745.8

Uninhibited bladder 596.54
- with cauda equina syndrome 344.61
- neurogenic — see also Neurogenic, bladder 596.54

Union, abnormal — see also Fusion
- divided tendon 727.89
- larynx and trachea 748.3

Universal
- joint, cervix 620.6
- mesentery 751.4

Unknown
- cause of death 799.9
- diagnosis 799.9

Unna's disease (seborrheic dermatitis) 690.10

Unresponsiveness, adrenocorticotropin (ACTH) 255.4

Unsatisfactory
- restoration, tooth (existing) 525.60
  - specified NEC 525.69
- smear 795.08

Unsoundness of mind — see also Psychosis 298.9

Unspecified cause of death 799.9

Unstable
- back NEC 724.9
- colon 569.89
- joint — see Instability, joint
- lie 652.0 ☑
  - affecting fetus or newborn (before labor) 761.7
  - causing obstructed labor 660.0 ☑
    - affecting fetus or newborn 763.1
- lumbosacral joint (congenital) 756.19
  - acquired 724.6
- sacroiliac 724.6
- spine NEC 724.9

Untruthfulness, child problem — see also Disturbance, conduct 312.0 ☑

Unverricht (-Lundborg) disease, syndrome, or epilepsy 333.2

Unverricht-Wagner syndrome (dermatomyositis) 710.3

Upper respiratory — see condition

Upset
- gastric 536.8
  - psychogenic 306.4
- gastrointestinal 536.8
  - psychogenic 306.4
  - virus (see also Enteritis, viral) 008.8
- intestinal (large) (small) 564.9
  - psychogenic 306.4
- menstruation 626.9
- mental 300.9
- stomach 536.8
  - psychogenic 306.4

Urachus — see also condition
- patent 753.7
- persistent 753.7

Uratic arthritis 274.0

Urbach's lipoid proteinosis 272.8

Urbach-Oppenheim disease or syndrome (necrobiosis lipoidica diabeticorum) 250.8 ☑ [709.3]

Urbach-Wiethe disease or syndrome (lipoid proteinosis) 272.8

Urban yellow fever 060.1

Urea, blood, high — see Uremia

Uremia, uremic (absorption) (amaurosis) (amblyopia) (aphasia) (apoplexy) (coma) (delirium) (dementia) (dropsy) (dyspnea) (fever) (intoxication) (mania) (paralysis) (poisoning) (toxemia) (vomiting) 586
- with
  - abortion — see Abortion, by type, with renal failure
  - ectopic pregnancy (see also categories 633.0–633.9) 639.3
  - hypertension (see also Hypertension, kidney) 403.91
  - molar pregnancy (see also categories 630–632) 639.3
- chronic 585.9
- complicating
  - abortion 639.3
  - ectopic or molar pregnancy 639.3
  - hypertension (see also Hypertension, kidney) 403.91
  - labor and delivery 669.3 ☑
- congenital 779.89
- extrarenal 788.9
- hypertensive (chronic) (see also Hypertension, kidney) 403.91

Uremia, uremic — continued
  maternal NEC, affecting fetus or newborn 760.1
  neuropathy 585.9 *[357.4]*
  pericarditis 585.9 *[420.0]*
  prerenal 788.9
  pyelitic (see also Pyelitis) 590.80
Ureteralgia 788.0
Ureterectasis 593.89
Ureteritis 593.89
  cystica 590.3
  due to calculus 592.1
  gonococcal (acute) 098.19
    chronic or duration of 2 months or over 098.39
  nonspecific 593.89
Ureterocele (acquired) 593.89
  congenital 753.23
Ureterolith 592.1
Ureterolithiasis 592.1
Ureterostomy status V44.6
  with complication 997.5
Ureter, ureteral — see condition
Urethralgia 788.9
Urethra, urethral — see condition
Urethritis (abacterial) (acute) (allergic) (anterior) (chronic) (nonvenereal) (posterior) (recurrent) (simple) (subacute) (ulcerative) (undifferentiated) 597.80
  diplococcal (acute) 098.0
    chronic or duration of 2 months or over 098.2
  due to Trichomonas (vaginalis) 131.02
  gonococcal (acute) 098.0
    chronic or duration of 2 months or over 098.2
  nongonococcal (sexually transmitted) 099.40
    Chlamydia trachomatis 099.41
    Reiter's 099.3
    specified organism NEC 099.49
  nonspecific (sexually transmitted) (see also Urethritis, nongonococcal) 099.40
  not sexually transmitted 597.80
  Reiter's 099.3
  trichomonal or due to Trichomonas (vaginalis) 131.02
  tuberculous (see also Tuberculosis) 016.3 ☑
  venereal NEC (see also Urethritis, nongonococcal) 099.40
Urethrocele
  female 618.03
    with uterine prolapse 618.4
      complete 618.3
      incomplete 618.2
  male 599.5
Urethrolithiasis 594.2

Urethro-oculoarticular syndrome 099.3
Urethro-oculosynovial syndrome 099.3
Urethrorectal — see condition
Urethrorrhagia 599.84
Urethrorrhea 788.7
Urethrostomy status V44.6
  with complication 997.5
Urethrotrigonitis 595.3
Urethrovaginal — see condition
Urhidrosis, uridrosis 705.89
Uric acid
  diathesis 274.9
  in blood 790.6
Uricacidemia 790.6
Uricemia 790.6
Uricosuria 791.9
Urination
  frequent 788.41
  painful 788.1
  urgency 788.63
Urinemia — see Uremia
Urine, urinary — see also condition
  abnormality NEC 788.69
  blood in (see also Hematuria) 599.7
  discharge, excessive 788.42
  enuresis 788.30
    nonorganic origin 307.6
  extravasation 788.8
  frequency 788.41
  hesitancy 788.64
  incontinence 788.30
    active 788.30
    female 788.30
      stress 625.6
      and urge 788.33
    male 788.30
      stress 788.32
      and urge 788.33
    mixed (stress and urge) 788.33
    neurogenic 788.39
    nonorganic origin 307.6
    overflow 788.38
    stress (female) 625.6
      male NEC 788.32
  intermittent stream 788.61
  pus in 791.9
  retention or stasis NEC 788.20
    bladder, incomplete emptying 788.21
    psychogenic 306.53
    specified NEC 788.29
  secretion
    deficient 788.5
    excessive 788.42
    frequency 788.41
  strain 788.65
  stream
    intermittent 788.61
    slowing 788.62
    splitting 788.61

Urine, urinary — see also condition — continued
  stream — continued
    weak 788.62
    urgency 788.63
Urinoma NEC 599.9
  bladder 596.8
  kidney 593.89
  renal 593.89
  ureter 593.89
  urethra 599.84
Uroarthritis, infectious 099.3
Urodialysis 788.5
Urolithiasis 592.9
Uronephrosis 593.89
Uropathy 599.9
  obstructive 599.60
Urosepsis 599.0
  meaning sepsis 995.91
  meaning urinary tract infection 599.0
Urticaria 708.9
  with angioneurotic edema 995.1
    hereditary 277.6
  allergic 708.0
  cholinergic 708.5
  chronic 708.8
  cold, familial 708.2
  dermatographic 708.3
  due to
    cold or heat 708.2
    drugs 708.0
    food 708.0
    inhalants 708.0
    plants 708.8
    serum 999.5
  factitial 708.3
  giant 995.1
    hereditary 277.6
  gigantea 995.1
    hereditary 277.6
  idiopathic 708.1
  larynx 995.1
    hereditary 277.6
  neonatorum 778.8
  nonallergic 708.1
  papulosa (Hebra) 698.2
  perstans hemorrhagica 757.39
  pigmentosa 757.33
  recurrent periodic 708.8
  serum 999.5
  solare 692.72
  specified type NEC 708.8
  thermal (cold) (heat) 708.2
  vibratory 708.4
Urticarioides acarodermatitis 133.9
Use of
  nonprescribed drugs (see also Abuse, drugs, nondependent) 305.9 ☑
  patent medicines (see also Abuse, drugs, nondependent) 305.9 ☑

Usher-Senear disease (pemphigus erythematosus) 694.4
Uta 085.5
Uterine size-date discrepancy 649.6 ☑ ▲
Uteromegaly 621.2
Uterovaginal — see condition
Uterovesical — see condition
Uterus — see condition
Utriculitis (utriculus prostaticus) 597.89
Uveal — see condition
Uveitis (anterior) — see also Iridocyclitis 364.3
  acute or subacute 364.00
    due to or associated with
      gonococcal infection 098.41
      herpes (simplex) 054.44
        zoster 053.22
    primary 364.01
    recurrent 364.02
  secondary (noninfectious) 364.04
    infectious 364.03
  allergic 360.11
  chronic 364.10
    due to or associated with
      sarcoidosis 135 *[364.11]*
      tuberculosis (see also Tuberculosis) 017.3 ☑ *[364.11]*
  due to
    operation 360.11
    toxoplasmosis (acquired) 130.2
      congenital (active) 771.2
  granulomatous 364.10
  heterochromic 364.21
  lens-induced 364.23
  nongranulomatous 364.00
  posterior 363.20
    disseminated — see Chorioretinitis, disseminated
    focal — see Chorioretinitis, focal
  recurrent 364.02
  sympathetic 360.11
  syphilitic (secondary) 091.50
    congenital 090.0 *[363.13]*
    late 095.8 *[363.13]*
  tuberculous (see also Tuberculosis) 017.3 ☑ *[364.11]*
Uveoencephalitis 363.22
Uveokeratitis — see also Iridocyclitis 364.3
Uveoparotid fever 135
Uveoparotitis 135
Uvula — see condition
Uvulitis (acute) (catarrhal) (chronic) (gangrenous) (membranous) (suppurative) (ulcerative) 528.3

Index to Diseases

V

Vaccination
complication or reaction — see Complications, vaccination
not carried out V64.00
because of
acute illness V64.01
allergy to vaccine or component V64.04
caregiver refusal V64.05
chronic illness V64.02
immune compromised state V64.03
patient had disease being vaccinated against V64.08
patient refusal V64.06
reason NEC V64.09
religious reasons V64.07
prophylactic (against) V05.9
arthropod-borne viral
disease NEC V05.1
encephalitis V05.0
chickenpox V05.4
cholera (alone) V03.0
with typhoid-paratyphoid (cholera + TAB) V06.0
common cold V04.7
diphtheria (alone) V03.5
with
poliomyelitis (DTP+ polio) V06.3
tetanus V06.5
pertussis combined (DTP) (DTaP) V06.1
typhoid-paratyphoid (DTP + TAB) V06.2
disease (single) NEC V05.9
bacterial NEC V03.9
specified type NEC V03.89
combination NEC V06.9
specified type NEC V06.8
specified type NEC V05.8
encephalitis, viral, arthropod-borne V05.0
Hemophilus influenzae, type B [Hib] V03.81
hepatitis, viral V05.3
influenza V04.81
with
Streptococcus pneumoniae [pneumococcus] V06.6
leishmaniasis V05.2
measles (alone) V04.2
with mumps-rubella (MMR) V06.4
mumps (alone) V04.6
with measles and rubella (MMR) V06.4
pertussis alone V03.6
plague V03.3
poliomyelitis V04.0
with diphtheria-tetanus-pertussis (DTP + polio) V06.3
rabies V04.5
respiratory syncytial virus (RSV) V04.82
rubella (alone) V04.3
with measles and mumps (MMR) V06.4
smallpox V04.1
Streptococcus pneumoniae [pneumococcus] V03.82
with
influenza V06.6
tetanus toxoid (alone) V03.7
with diphtheria [Td] [DT] V06.5
with
pertussis (DTP) (DTaP) V06.1
with poliomyelitis (DTP+polio) V06.3
tuberculosis (BCG) V03.2
tularemia V03.4
typhoid-paratyphoid (TAB) (alone) V03.1

Vaccination — continued
prophylactic — continued
typhoid-paratyphoid — continued
with diphtheria-tetanus-pertussis (TAB + DTP) V06.2
varicella V05.4
viral
disease NEC V04.89
encephalitis, arthropod-borne V05.0
hepatitis V05.3
yellow fever V04.4
Vaccinia (generalized) 999.0
without vaccination 051.0
congenital 771.2
conjunctiva 999.3
eyelids 999.0 *[373.5]*
localized 999.0
nose 999.3
not from vaccination 051.0
eyelid 051.0 *[373.5]*
sine vaccinatione 051.0
Vacuum
extraction of fetus or newborn 763.3
in sinus (accessory) (nasal) (see also Sinusitis) 473.9
Vagabond V60.0
Vagabondage V60.0
Vagabonds' disease 132.1
Vaginalitis (tunica) 608.4
Vagina, vaginal — see condition
Vaginismus (reflex) 625.1
functional 306.51
hysterical 300.11
psychogenic 306.51
Vaginitis (acute) (chronic) (circumscribed) (diffuse) (emphysematous) (Hemophilus vaginalis) (nonspecific) (nonvenereal) (ulcerative) 616.10
with
abortion — see Abortion, by type, with sepsis
ectopic pregnancy (see also categories 633.0–633.9) 639.0
molar pregnancy (see also categories 630–632) 639.0
adhesive, congenital 752.49
atrophic, postmenopausal 627.3
bacterial 616.10
blennorrhagic (acute) 098.0
chronic or duration of 2 months or over 098.2
candidal 112.1
chlamydial 099.53
complicating pregnancy or puerperium 646.6
affecting fetus or newborn 760.8
congenital (adhesive) 752.49
due to
C. albicans 112.1
Trichomonas (vaginalis) 131.01
following
abortion 639.0
ectopic or molar pregnancy 639.0
gonococcal (acute) 098.0
chronic or duration of 2 months or over 098.2
granuloma 099.2
Monilia 112.1
mycotic 112.1
pinworm 127.4 *[616.11]*
postirradiation 616.10
postmenopausal atrophic 627.3
senile (atrophic) 627.3
syphilitic (early) 091.0
late 095.8
trichomonal 131.01
tuberculous (see also Tuberculosis) 016.7
venereal NEC 099.8
Vaginosis — see Vaginitis
Vagotonia 352.3
Vagrancy V60.0
Vallecula — see condition
Valley fever 114.0

Valsuani's disease (progressive pernicious anemia, puerperal) 648.2
Valve, valvular (formation) — see also condition
cerebral ventricle (communicating) in situ V45.2
cervix, internal os 752.49
colon 751.5
congenital NEC — see Atresia
formation, congenital NEC — see Atresia
heart defect — see Anomaly, heart, valve
ureter 753.29
pelvic junction 753.21
vesical orifice 753.22
urethra 753.6
Valvulitis (chronic) — see also Endocarditis 424.90
rheumatic (chronic) (inactive) (with chorea) 397.9
active or acute (aortic) (mitral) (pulmonary) (tricuspid) 391.1
syphilitic NEC 093.20
aortic 093.22
mitral 093.21
pulmonary 093.24
tricuspid 093.23
Valvulopathy — see Endocarditis
van Bogaert-Nijssen (-Peiffer) disease 330.0
van Bogaert's leukoencephalitis (sclerosing) (subacute) 046.2
van Buchem's syndrome (hyperostosis corticalis) 733.3
Vancomycin (glycopeptide)
intermediate staphylococcus aureus (VISA/GISA) V09.8
resistant
enterococcus (VRE) V09.8
staphylococcus aureus (VRSA/GRSA) V09.8
van Creveld-von Gierke disease (glycogenosis I) 271.0
van den Bergh's disease (enterogenous cyanosis) 289.7
van der Hoeve-Halbertsma-Waardenburg syndrome (ptosis-epicanthus) 270.2
van der Hoeve-Waardenburg-Gualdi syndrome (ptosis epicanthus) 270.2
van der Hoeve's syndrome (brittle bones and blue sclera, deafness) 756.51
Vanillism 692.89
Vanishing lung 492.0
Vanishing twin 651.33
van Neck (-Odelberg) disease or syndrome (juvenile osteochondrosis) 732.1
Vapor asphyxia or suffocation NEC 987.9
specified agent — see Table of Drugs and Chemicals
Vaquez's disease (M9950/1) 238.4
Vaquez-Osler disease (polycythemia vera) (M9950/1) 238.4
Variance, lethal ball, prosthetic heart valve 996.02
Variants, thalassemic 282.49
Variations in hair color 704.3
Varicella 052.9
with
complication 052.8
specified NEC 052.7
pneumonia 052.1
vaccination and inoculation (prophylactic) V05.4
exposure to V01.71
vaccination and inoculation (against) (prophylactic) V05.4
Varices — see Varix
Varicocele (scrotum) (thrombosed) 456.4
ovary 456.5
perineum 456.6
spermatic cord (ulcerated) 456.4

Varicose
aneurysm (ruptured) (see also Aneurysm) 442.9
dermatitis (lower extremity) — see Varicose, vein, inflamed or infected
eczema — see Varicose, vein
phlebitis — see Varicose, vein, inflamed or infected
placental vessel — see Placenta, abnormal
tumor — see Varicose, vein
ulcer (lower extremity, any part) 454.0
anus 455.8
external 455.5
internal 455.2
esophagus (see also Varix, esophagus) 456.1
bleeding (see also Varicose, esophagus, bleeding) 456.0
inflamed or infected 454.2
nasal septum 456.8
perineum 456.6
rectum — see Varicose, ulcer, anus
scrotum 456.4
specified site NEC 456.8
vein (lower extremity) (ruptured) (see also Varix) 454.9
with
complications NEC 454.8
edema 454.8
inflammation or infection 454.1
ulcerated 454.2
pain 454.8
stasis dermatitis 454.1
with ulcer 454.2
swelling 454.8
ulcer 454.0
inflamed or infected 454.2
anus — see Hemorrhoids
broad ligament 456.5
congenital (peripheral) 747.60
gastrointestinal 747.61
lower limb 747.64
renal 747.62
specified NEC 747.69
upper limb 747.63
esophagus (ulcerated) (see also Varix, esophagus) 456.1
bleeding (see also Varix, esophagus, bleeding) 456.0
inflamed or infected 454.1
with ulcer 454.2
in pregnancy or puerperium 671.0
vulva or perineum 671.1
nasal septum (with ulcer) 456.8
pelvis 456.5
perineum 456.6
in pregnancy, childbirth, or puerperium 671.1
rectum — see Hemorrhoids
scrotum (ulcerated) 456.4
specified site NEC 456.8
sublingual 456.3
ulcerated 454.0
inflamed or infected 454.2
umbilical cord, affecting fetus or newborn 762.6
urethra 456.8
vulva 456.6
in pregnancy, childbirth, or puerperium 671.1
vessel (see also Varix)
placenta — see Placenta, abnormal
Varicosis, varicosities, varicosity — see also Varix 454.9
Variola 050.9
hemorrhagic (pustular) 050.0
major 050.0
minor 050.1
modified 050.2
Varioloid 050.2
Variolosa, purpura 050.0
Varix (lower extremity) (ruptured) 454.9

Varix

Varix — *continued*
with
complications NEC 454.8
edema 454.8
inflammation or infection 454.1
with ulcer 454.2
pain 454.8
stasis dermatitis 454.1
with ulcer 454.2
swelling 454.8
ulcer 454.0
with inflammation or infection 454.2
aneurysmal (*see also* Aneurysm) 442.9
anus — *see* Hemorrhoids
arteriovenous (congenital) (peripheral) NEC 747.60
gastrointestinal 747.61
lower limb 747.64
renal 747.62
specified NEC 747.69
spinal 747.82
upper limb 747.63
bladder 456.5
broad ligament 456.5
congenital (peripheral) 747.60
esophagus (ulcerated) 456.1
bleeding 456.0
in
cirrhosis of liver 571.5 [456.20]
portal hypertension 572.3 [456.20]
congenital 747.69
in
cirrhosis of liver 571.5 [456.21]
with bleeding 571.5 [456.20]
portal hypertension 572.3 [456.21]
with bleeding 572.3 [456.20]
gastric 456.8
inflamed or infected 454.1
ulcerated 454.2
in pregnancy or puerperium 671.0 ☑
perineum 671.1 ☑
vulva 671.1 ☑
labia (majora) 456.6
orbit 456.8
congenital 747.69
ovary 456.5
papillary 448.1
pelvis 456.5
perineum 456.6
in pregnancy or puerperium 671.1 ☑
pharynx 456.8
placenta — *see* Placenta, abnormal
prostate 456.8
rectum — *see* Hemorrhoids
renal papilla 456.8
retina 362.17
scrotum (ulcerated) 456.4
sigmoid colon 456.8
specified site NEC 456.8
spinal (cord) (vessels) 456.8
spleen, splenic (vein) (with phlebolith) 456.8
sublingual 456.3
ulcerated 454.0
inflamed or infected 454.2
umbilical cord, affecting fetus or newborn 762.6
uterine ligament 456.5
vocal cord 456.8
vulva 456.6
in pregnancy, childbirth, or puerperium 671.1 ☑
Vasa previa 663.5 ☑
affecting fetus or newborn 762.6
hemorrhage from, affecting fetus or newborn 772.0
Vascular — *see also* condition
loop on papilla (optic) 743.57

Vascular — *see also* condition — *continued*
sheathing, retina 362.13
spasm 443.9
spider 448.1
Vascularity, pulmonary, congenital 747.3
Vascularization
choroid 362.16
cornea 370.60
deep 370.63
localized 370.61
retina 362.16
subretinal 362.16
Vasculitis 447.6
allergic 287.0
cryoglobulinemic 273.2
disseminated 447.6
kidney 447.8
leukocytoclastic 446.29
nodular 695.2
retinal 362.18
rheumatic — *see* Fever, rheumatic
Vasculopathy
cardiac allograft 996.83
Vas deferens — *see* condition
Vas deferentitis 608.4
Vasectomy, admission for V25.2
Vasitis 608.4
nodosa 608.4
scrotum 608.4
spermatic cord 608.4
testis 608.4
tuberculous (*see also* Tuberculosis) 016.5 ☑
tunica vaginalis 608.4
vas deferens 608.4
Vasodilation 443.9
Vasomotor — *see* condition
Vasoplasty, after previous sterilization V26.0
Vasoplegia, splanchnic — *see also* Neuropathy, peripheral, autonomic 337.9
Vasospasm 443.9
cerebral (artery) 435.9
with transient neurologic deficit 435.9
coronary 413.1
nerve
arm NEC 354.9
autonomic 337.9
brachial plexus 353.0
cervical plexus 353.2
leg NEC 355.8
lower extremity NEC 355.8
peripheral NEC 355.9
spinal NEC 355.9
sympathetic 337.9
upper extremity NEC 354.9
peripheral NEC 443.9
retina (artery) (*see also* Occlusion, retinal, artery) 362.30
Vasospastic — *see* condition
Vasovagal attack (paroxysmal) 780.2
psychogenic 306.2
Vater's ampulla — *see* condition
VATER syndrome 759.89
Vegetation, vegetative
adenoid (nasal fossa) 474.2
consciousness (persistent) 780.03
endocarditis (acute) (any valve) (chronic) (subacute) 421.0
heart (mycotic) (valve) 421.0
state (persistent) 780.03
Veil
Jackson's 751.4
over face (causing asphyxia) 768.9
Vein, venous — *see* condition
Veldt sore — *see also* Ulcer, skin 707.9
Velo-cardio-facial syndrome 758.32
Velpeau's hernia — *see* Hernia, femoral
Venereal
balanitis NEC 099.8
bubo 099.1
disease 099.9

Venereal — *continued*
disease — *continued*
specified nature or type NEC 099.8
granuloma inguinale 099.2
lymphogranuloma (Durand-Nicolas-Favre), any site 099.1
salpingitis 098.37
urethritis (*see also* Urethritis, non-gonococcal) 099.40
vaginitis NEC 099.8
warts 078.19
Vengefulness, in child — *see also* Disturbance, conduct 312.0 ☑
Venofibrosis 459.89
Venom, venomous
bite or sting (animal or insect) 989.5
poisoning 989.5
Venous — *see* condition
Ventouse delivery NEC 669.5 ☑
affecting fetus or newborn 763.3
Ventral — *see* condition
Ventricle, ventricular — *see also* condition
escape 427.69
standstill (*see also* Arrest, cardiac) 427.5
Ventriculitis, cerebral — *see also* Meningitis 322.9
Ventriculostomy status V45.2
Verbiest's syndrome (claudicatio intermittens spinalis) 435.1
Vernet's syndrome 352.6
Verneuil's disease (syphilitic bursitis) 095.7
Verruca (filiformis) 078.10
acuminata (any site) 078.11
necrogenica (primary) (*see also* Tuberculosis) 017.0 ☑
peruana 088.0
peruviana 088.0
plana (juvenilis) 078.19
plantaris 078.19
seborrheica 702.19
inflamed 702.11
senilis 702.0
tuberculosa (primary) (*see also* Tuberculosis) 017.0 ☑
venereal 078.19
viral NEC 078.10
Verrucosities — *see also* Verruca 078.10
Verrucous endocarditis (acute) (any valve) (chronic) (subacute) 710.0 [424.91]
nonbacterial 710.0 [424.91]
Verruga
peruana 088.0
peruviana 088.0
Verse's disease (calcinosis intervertebralis) 275.49 [722.90]
Version
before labor, affecting fetus or newborn 761.7
cephalic (correcting previous malposition) 652.1 ☑
affecting fetus or newborn 763.1
cervix ▶ — *see* Version,◀ uterus
uterus (postinfectional) (postpartal, old) (*see also* Malposition, uterus) 621.6
forward — *see* Anteversion, uterus
lateral — *see* Lateroversion, uterus
Vertebra, vertebral — *see* condition
Vertigo 780.4
auditory 386.19
aural 386.19
benign paroxysmal positional 386.11
central origin 386.2
cerebral 386.2
Dix and Hallpike (epidemic) 386.12
endemic paralytic 078.81
epidemic 078.81
Dix and Hallpike 386.12
Gerlier's 078.81
Pedersen's 386.12
vestibular neuronitis 386.12
epileptic — *see* Epilepsy

Vertigo — *continued*
Gerlier's (epidemic) 078.81
hysterical 300.11
labyrinthine 386.10
laryngeal 786.2
malignant positional 386.2
Ménière's (*see also* Disease, Ménière's) 386.00
menopausal 627.2
otogenic 386.19
paralytic 078.81
paroxysmal positional, benign 386.11
Pedersen's (epidemic) 386.12
peripheral 386.10
specified type NEC 386.19
positional
benign paroxysmal 386.11
malignant 386.2
Verumontanitis (chronic) — *see also* Urethritis 597.89
Vesania — *see also* Psychosis 298.9
Vesical — *see* condition
Vesicle
cutaneous 709.8
seminal — *see* condition
skin 709.8
Vesicocolic — *see* condition
Vesicoperineal — *see* condition
Vesicorectal — *see* condition
Vesicourethrorectal — *see* condition
Vesicovaginal — *see* condition
Vesicular — *see* condition
Vesiculitis (seminal) 608.0
amebic 006.8
gonorrheal (acute) 098.14
chronic or duration of 2 months or over 098.34
trichomonal 131.09
tuberculous (*see also* Tuberculosis) 016.5 ☑ [608.81]
Vestibulitis (ear) — *see also* Labyrinthitis 386.30
nose (external) 478.19 ▲
vulvar 616.10
Vestibulopathy, acute peripheral (recurrent) 386.12
Vestige, vestigial — *see also* Persistence
branchial 744.41
structures in vitreous 743.51
Vibriosis NEC 027.9
Vidal's disease (lichen simplex chronicus) 698.3
Video display tube syndrome 723.8
Vienna-type encephalitis 049.8
Villaret's syndrome 352.6
Villous — *see* condition
VIN I (vulvar intraepithelial neoplasia I) 624.0 ▲
VIN II (vulvar intraepithelial neoplasia II) 624.0 ▲
VIN III (vulvar intraepithelial neoplasia III) 233.3
Vincent's
angina 101
bronchitis 101
disease 101
gingivitis 101
infection (any site) 101
laryngitis 101
stomatitis 101
tonsillitis 101
Vinson-Plummer syndrome (sideropenic dysphagia) 280.8
Viosterol deficiency — *see also* Deficiency, calciferol 268.9
Virchow's disease 733.99
Viremia 790.8
Virilism (adrenal) (female) NEC 255.2
with
3-beta-hydroxysteroid dehydrogenase defect 255.2
11-hydroxylase defect 255.2
21-hydroxylase defect 255.2
adrenal
hyperplasia 255.2
insufficiency (congenital) 255.2

Index to Diseases

Weak, weakness

Virilism — *continued*
 with — *continued*
  cortical hyperfunction 255.2
Virilization (female) (suprarenal) — *see also* Virilism 255.2
 isosexual 256.4
Virulent bubo 099.0
Virus, viral — *see also* condition
 infection NEC (*see also* Infection, viral) 079.99
 septicemia 079.99
VISA (vancomycin intermediate staphylococcus aureus) V09.8 ☑
Viscera, visceral — *see* condition
Visceroptosis 569.89
Visible peristalsis 787.4
Vision, visual
 binocular, suppression 368.31
 blurred, blurring 368.8
  hysterical 300.11
 defect, defective (*see also* Impaired, vision) 369.9
 disorientation (syndrome) 368.16
 disturbance NEC (*see also* Disturbance, vision) 368.9
  hysterical 300.11
 examination V72.0
 field, limitation 368.40
 fusion, with defective steropsis 368.33
 hallucinations 368.16
 halos 368.16
 loss 369.9
  both eyes (*see also* Blindness, both eyes) 369.3
  complete (*see also* Blindness, both eyes) 369.00
  one eye 369.8
  sudden 368.16
 low (both eyes) 369.20
  one eye (other eye normal) (*see also* Impaired, vision) 369.70
   blindness, other eye 369.10
 perception, simultaneous without fusion 368.32
 tunnel 368.45
Vitality, lack or want of 780.79
 newborn 779.89
Vitamin deficiency NEC — *see also* Deficiency, vitamin 269.2
Vitelline duct, persistent 751.0
Vitiligo 709.01
 due to pinta (carate) 103.2
 eyelid 374.53
 vulva 624.8
Vitium cordis — *see* Disease, heart
Vitreous — *see also* condition
 touch syndrome 997.99
VLCAD (long chain/very long chain acyl CoA dehydrogenase deficiency, LCAD) 277.85
Vocal cord — *see* condition
Vocational rehabilitation V57.22
Vogt's (Cecile) disease or syndrome 333.7 ☑
Vogt-Koyanagi syndrome 364.24
Vogt-Spielmeyer disease (amaurotic familial idiocy) 330.1
Voice
 change (*see also* Dysphonia) 784.49
 loss (*see also* Aphonia) 784.41
Volhard-Fahr disease (malignant nephrosclerosis) 403.00
Volhynian fever 083.1
Volkmann's ischemic contracture or paralysis (complicating trauma) 958.6
Voluntary starvation 307.1
Volvulus (bowel) (colon) (intestine) 560.2
 with
  hernia (*see also* Hernia, by site, with obstruction)
   gangrenous — *see* Hernia, by site, with gangrene
  perforation 560.2
 congenital 751.5
 duodenum 537.3

Volvulus — *continued*
 fallopian tube 620.5
 oviduct 620.5
 stomach (due to absence of gastrocolic ligament) 537.89
Vomiting 787.03
 with nausea 787.01
 allergic 535.4 ☑
 asphyxia 933.1
 bilious (cause unknown) 787.0 ☑
  following gastrointestinal surgery 564.3
 blood (*see also* Hematemesis) 578.0
 causing asphyxia, choking, or suffocation (*see also* Asphyxia, food) 933.1
 cyclical 536.2
  psychogenic 306.4
 epidemic 078.82
 fecal matter 569.89
 following gastrointestinal surgery 564.3
 functional 536.8
  psychogenic 306.4
 habit 536.2
  hysterical 300.11
 nervous 306.4
 neurotic 306.4
 newborn 779.3
 of or complicating pregnancy 643.9 ☑
  due to
   organic disease 643.8 ☑
   specific cause NEC 643.8 ☑
  early — *see* Hyperemesis, gravidarum
  late (after 22 completed weeks of gestation) 643.2 ☑
  pernicious or persistent 536.2
   complicating pregnancy — *see* Hyperemesis, gravidarum
   psychogenic 306.4
 physiological 787.0 ☑
 psychic 306.4
 psychogenic 307.54
 stercoral 569.89
 uncontrollable 536.2
  psychogenic 306.4
 uremic — *see* Uremia
 winter 078.82
von Bechterew (-Strumpell) disease or syndrome (ankylosing spondylitis) 720.0
von Bezold's abscess 383.01
von Economo's disease (encephalitis lethargica) 049.8
von Eulenburg's disease (congenital paramyotonia) 359.2
von Gierke's disease (glycogenosis I) 271.0
von Gies' joint 095.8
von Graefe's disease or syndrome 378.72
von Hippel (-Lindau) disease or syndrome (retinocerebral angiomatosis) 759.6
von Jaksch's anemia or disease (pseudoleukemia infantum) 285.8
von Recklinghausen-Applebaum disease (hemochromatosis) 275.0
von Recklinghausen's
 disease or syndrome (nerves) (skin) (M9540/1) 237.71
  bones (osteitis fibrosa cystica) 252.01
 tumor (M9540/1) 237.71
von Schroetter's syndrome (intermittent venous claudication) 453.8
von Willebrand (-Jürgens) (-Minot) disease or syndrome (angiohemophilia) 286.4
von Zambusch's disease (lichen sclerosus et atrophicus) 701.0
Voorhoeve's disease or dyschondroplasia 756.4
Vossius' ring 921.3
 late effect 366.21

Voyeurism 302.82
VRE (vancomycin resistant enterococcus) V09.8 ☑
Vrolik's disease (osteogenesis imperfecta) 756.51
VRSA (vancomycin resistant staphylococcus aureus) V09.8 ☑
Vulva — *see* condition
Vulvismus 625.1
Vulvitis (acute) (allergic) (aphthous) (chronic) (gangrenous) (hypertrophic) (intertriginous) 616.10
 with
  abortion — *see* Abortion, by type, with sepsis
  ectopic pregnancy (*see also* categories 633.0–633.9) 639.0
  molar pregnancy (*see also* categories 630–632) 639.0
 adhesive, congenital 752.49
 blennorrhagic (acute) 098.0
  chronic or duration of 2 months or over 098.2
 chlamydial 099.53
 complicating pregnancy or puerperium 646.6 ☑
 due to Ducrey's bacillus 099.0
 following
  abortion 639.0
  ectopic or molar pregnancy 639.0
 gonococcal (acute) 098.0
  chronic or duration of 2 months or over 098.2
 herpetic 054.11
 leukoplakic 624.0
 monilial 112.1
 puerperal, postpartum, childbirth 646.6 ☑
 syphilitic (early) 091.0
  late 095.8
 trichomonal 131.01
Vulvodynia 625.9
Vulvorectal — *see* condition
Vulvovaginitis — *see also* Vulvitis 616.10
 amebic 006.8
 chlamydial 099.53
 gonococcal (acute) 098.0
  chronic or duration of 2 months or over 098.2
 herpetic 054.11
 monilial 112.1
 trichomonal (Trichomonas vaginalis) 131.01

W

Waardenburg-Klein syndrome (ptosis-epicanthus) 270.2
Waardenburg's syndrome 756.89
 meaning ptosis-epicanthus 270.2
Wagner's disease (colloid milium) 709.3
Wagner (-Unverricht) syndrome (dermatomyositis) 710.3
Waiting list, person on V63.2
 undergoing social agency investigation V63.8
Wakefulness disorder — *see also* Hypersomnia 780.54
 nonorganic origin 307.43
Waldenström's
 disease (osteochondrosis, capital femoral) 732.1
 hepatitis (lupoid hepatitis) 571.49
 hypergammaglobulinemia 273.0
 macroglobulinemia 273.3
 purpura, hypergammaglobulinemic 273.0
 syndrome (macroglobulinemia) 273.3
Waldenström-Kjellberg syndrome (sideropenic dysphagia) 280.8
Walking
 difficulty 719.7
  psychogenic 307.9
 sleep 307.46
  hysterical 300.13
Wall, abdominal — *see* condition

Wallenberg's syndrome (posterior inferior cerebellar artery) — *see also* Disease, cerebrovascular, acute 436
Wallgren's
 disease (obstruction of splenic vein with collateral circulation) 459.89
 meningitis (*see also* Meningitis, aseptic) 047.9
Wandering
 acetabulum 736.39
 gallbladder 751.69
 kidney, congenital 753.3
 organ or site, congenital NEC — *see* Malposition, congenital
 pacemaker (atrial) (heart) 427.89
 spleen 289.59
Wardrop's disease (with lymphangitis) 681.9
 finger 681.02
 toe 681.11
War neurosis 300.16
Wart (common) (digitate) (filiform) (infectious) (viral) 078.10
 external genital organs (venereal) 078.19
 fig 078.19
 Hassall-Henle's (of cornea) 371.41
 Henle's (of cornea) 371.41
 juvenile 078.19
 moist 078.10
 Peruvian 088.0
 plantar 078.19
 prosector (*see also* Tuberculosis) 017.0 ☑
 seborrheic 702.19
  inflamed 702.11
 senile 702.0
 specified NEC 078.19
 syphilitic 091.3
 tuberculous (*see also* Tuberculosis) 017.0 ☑
 venereal (female) (male) 078.19
Warthin's tumor (salivary gland) (M8561/0) 210.2
Washerwoman's itch 692.4
Wassilieff's disease (leptospiral jaundice) 100.0
Wasting
 disease 799.4
  due to malnutrition 261
 extreme (due to malnutrition) 261
 muscular NEC 728.2
 palsy, paralysis 335.21
 pelvic muscle 618.83
Water
 clefts 366.12
 deprivation of 994.3
 in joint (*see also* Effusion, joint) 719.0 ☑
 intoxication 276.6
 itch 120.3
 lack of 994.3
 loading 276.6
 on
  brain — *see* Hydrocephalus
  chest 511.8
 poisoning 276.6
Waterbrash 787.1
Water-hammer pulse — *see also* Insufficiency, aortic 424.1
Waterhouse (-Friderichsen) disease or syndrome 036.3
Water-losing nephritis 588.89
Wax in ear 380.4
Waxy
 degeneration, any site 277.39 ▲
 disease 277.39 ▲
 kidney 277.39 [583.81] ▲
 liver (large) 277.39 ▲
 spleen 277.39 ▲
Weak, weakness (generalized) 780.79
 arches (acquired) 734
  congenital 754.61
 bladder sphincter 596.59

Weak, weakness

Weak, weakness — *continued*
  congenital 779.89
  eye muscle — *see* Strabismus
  facial 781.94
  foot (double) — *see* Weak, arches
  heart, cardiac (*see also* Failure, heart) 428.9
    congenital 746.9
  mind 317
  muscle (generalized) 728.87
  myocardium (*see also* Failure, heart) 428.9
  newborn 779.89
  pelvic fundus
    pubocervical tissue 618.81
    rectovaginal tissue 618.82
  pulse 785.9
  senile 797
  urinary stream 788.62
  valvular — *see* Endocarditis
Wear, worn, tooth, teeth (approximal) (hard tissues) (interproximal) (occlusal) — *see also* Attrition, teeth 521.10
Weather, weathered
  effects of
    cold NEC 991.9
      specified effect NEC 991.8
    hot (*see also* Heat) 992.9
  skin 692.74
Weber-Christian disease or syndrome (nodular nonsuppurative panniculitis) 729.30
Weber-Cockayne syndrome (epidermolysis bullosa) 757.39
Weber-Dimitri syndrome 759.6
Weber-Gubler syndrome 344.89
Weber-Leyden syndrome 344.89
Weber-Osler syndrome (familial hemorrhagic telangiectasia) 448.0
Weber's paralysis or syndrome 344.89
Web, webbed (congenital) — *see also* Anomaly, specified type NEC
  canthus 743.63
  digits (*see also* Syndactylism) 755.10
  duodenal 751.5
  esophagus 750.3
  fingers (*see also* Syndactylism, fingers) 755.11
  larynx (glottic) (subglottic) 748.2
  neck (pterygium colli) 744.5
  Paterson-Kelly (sideropenic dysphagia) 280.8
  popliteal syndrome 756.89
  toes (*see also* Syndactylism, toes) 755.13
Wedge-shaped or wedging vertebra — *see also* Osteoporosis 733.00
Wegener's granulomatosis or syndrome 446.4
Wegner's disease (syphilitic osteochondritis) 090.0
Weight
  gain (abnormal) (excessive) 783.1
    during pregnancy 646.1 ☑
      insufficient 646.8 ☑
    less than 1000 grams at birth 765.0 ☑
  loss (cause unknown) 783.21
Weightlessness 994.9
Weil's disease (leptospiral jaundice) 100.0
Weill-Marchesani syndrome (brachymorphism and ectopia lentis) 759.89
Weingarten's syndrome (tropical eosinophilia) 518.3
Weir Mitchell's disease (erythromelalgia) 443.82
Weiss-Baker syndrome (carotid sinus syncope) 337.0
Weissenbach-Thibierge syndrome (cutaneous systemic sclerosis) 710.1
Wen — *see also* Cyst, sebaceous 706.2
Wenckebach's phenomenon, heart block (second degree) 426.13
Werdnig-Hoffmann syndrome (muscular atrophy) 335.0

Werlhof-Wichmann syndrome — *see also* Purpura, thrombocytopenic 287.39
Werlhof's disease — *see also* Purpura, thrombocytopenic 287.39
Wermer's syndrome or disease (polyendocrine adenomatosis) 258.0
Werner's disease or syndrome (progeria adultorum) 259.8
Werner-His disease (trench fever) 083.1
Werner-Schultz disease (agranulocytosis) 288.09 ▲
Wernicke's encephalopathy, disease, or syndrome (superior hemorrhagic polioencephalitis) 265.1
Wernicke-Korsakoff syndrome or psychosis (nonalcoholic) 294.0
  alcoholic 291.1
Wernicke-Posadas disease — *see also* Coccidioidomycosis 114.9
Wesselsbron fever 066.3
West African fever 084.8
West Nile
  encephalitis 066.41
  encephalomyelitis 066.41
  fever 066.40
    with
      cranial nerve disorders 066.42
      encephalitis 066.41
      optic neuritis 066.42
      other complications 066.49
      other neurologic manifestations 066.42
      polyradiculitis 066.42
  virus 066.40
Westphal-Strümpell syndrome (hepatolenticular degeneration) 275.1
Wet
  brain (alcoholic) (*see also* Alcoholism) 303.9 ☑
  feet, tropical (syndrome) (maceration) 991.4
  lung (syndrome)
    adult 518.5
    newborn 770.6
Wharton's duct — *see* condition
Wheal 709.8
Wheezing 786.07
Whiplash injury or syndrome 847.0
Whipple's disease or syndrome (intestinal lipodystrophy) 040.2
Whipworm 127.3
"Whistling face" syndrome (craniocarpotarsal dystrophy) 759.89
White — *see also* condition
  kidney
    large — *see* Nephrosis
    small 582.9
  leg, puerperal, postpartum, childbirth 671.4 ☑
    nonpuerperal 451.19
  mouth 112.0
  patches of mouth 528.6
  sponge nevus of oral mucosa 750.26
  spot lesions, teeth 521.01
White's disease (congenital) (keratosis follicularis) 757.39
Whitehead 706.2
Whitlow (with lymphangitis) 681.01
  herpetic 054.6
Whitmore's disease or fever (melioidosis) 025
Whooping cough 033.9
  with pneumonia 033.9 [484.3]
  due to
    Bordetella
      bronchoseptica 033.8
        with pneumonia 033.8 [484.3]
      parapertussis 033.1
        with pneumonia 033.1 [484.3]
      pertussis 033.0
        with pneumonia 033.0 [484.3]

Whooping cough — *continued*
  due to — *continued*
    specified organism NEC 033.8
      with pneumonia 033.8 [484.3]
  vaccination, prophylactic (against) V03.6
Wichmann's asthma (laryngismus stridulus) 478.75
Widal (-Abrami) syndrome (acquired hemolytic jaundice) 283.9
Widening aorta — *see also* Aneurysm, aorta 441.9
  ruptured 441.5
Wilkie's disease or syndrome 557.1
Wilkinson-Sneddon disease or syndrome (subcorneal pustular dermatosis) 694.1
Willan's lepra 696.1
Willan-Plumbe syndrome (psoriasis) 696.1
Willebrand (-Jürgens) syndrome or thrombopathy (angiohemophilia) 286.4
Willi-Prader syndrome (hypogenital dystrophy with diabetic tendency) 759.81
Willis' disease (diabetes mellitus) — *see also* Diabetes 250.0 ☑
Wilms' tumor or neoplasm (nephroblastoma) (M8960/3) 189.0
Wilson's
  disease or syndrome (hepatolenticular degeneration) 275.1
  hepatolenticular degeneration 275.1
  lichen ruber 697.0
Wilson-Brocq disease (dermatitis exfoliativa) 695.89
Wilson-Mikity syndrome 770.7
Window — *see also* Imperfect, closure
  aorticopulmonary 745.0
Winged scapula 736.89
Winter — *see also* condition
  vomiting disease 078.82
Wise's disease 696.2
Wiskott-Aldrich syndrome (eczema-thrombocytopenia) 279.12
Withdrawal symptoms, syndrome
  alcohol 291.81
    delirium (acute) 291.0
      chronic 291.1
    newborn 760.71
  drug or narcotic 292.0
  newborn, infant of dependent mother 779.5
  steroid NEC
    correct substance properly administered 255.4
    overdose or wrong substance given or taken 962.0
Withdrawing reaction, child or adolescent 313.22
Witts' anemia (achlorhydric anemia) 280.9
Witzelsucht 301.9
Woakes' syndrome (ethmoiditis) 471.1
Wohlfart-Kugelberg-Welander disease 335.11
Woillez's disease (acute idiopathic pulmonary congestion) 518.5
Wolff-Parkinson-White syndrome (anomalous atrioventricular excitation) 426.7
Wolhynian fever 083.1
Wolman's disease (primary familial xanthomatosis) 272.7
Wood asthma 495.8
Woolly, wooly hair (congenital) (nevus) 757.4
Wool-sorters' disease 022.1
Word
  blindness (congenital) (developmental) 315.01
    secondary to organic lesion 784.61
  deafness (secondary to organic lesion) 784.69
  developmental 315.31

Worm(s) (colic) (fever) (infection) (infestation) — *see also* Infestation 128.9
  guinea 125.7
  in intestine NEC 127.9
Worm-eaten soles 102.3
Worn out — *see* Exhaustion 780.79
"Worried well" V65.5
Wound, open (by cutting or piercing instrument) (by firearms) (cut) (dissection) (incised) (laceration) (penetration) (perforating) (puncture) (with initial hemorrhage, not internal) 879.8

> *Note* — For fracture with open wound, see Fracture.
>
> For laceration, traumatic rupture, tear or penetrating wound of internal organs, such as heart, lung, liver, kidney, pelvic organs, etc., whether or not accompanied by open wound or fracture in the same region, see Injury, internal.
>
> For contused wound, see Contusion. For crush injury, see Crush. For abrasion, insect bite (nonvenomous), blister, or scratch, see Injury, superficial.
>
> Complicated includes wounds with:
>   delayed healing
>   delayed treatment
>   foreign body
>   primary infection
>
> For late effect of open wound, see Late, effect, wound, open, by site.

  abdomen, abdominal (external) (muscle) 879.2
    complicated 879.3
    wall (anterior) 879.2
      complicated 879.3
      lateral 879.4
        complicated 879.5
  alveolar (process) 873.62
    complicated 873.72
  ankle 891.0
    with tendon involvement 891.2
    complicated 891.1
  anterior chamber, eye (*see also* Wound, open, intraocular) 871.9
  anus 879.6
    complicated 879.7
  arm 884.0
    with tendon involvement 884.2
    complicated 884.1
    forearm 881.00
      with tendon involvement 881.20
      complicated 881.10
    multiple sites — *see* Wound, open, multiple, upper limb
    upper 880.03
      with tendon involvement 880.23
      complicated 880.13
      multiple sites (with axillary or shoulder regions) 880.09
        with tendon involvement 880.29
        complicated 880.19
  artery — *see* Injury, blood vessel, by site
  auditory
    canal (external) (meatus) 872.02
      complicated 872.12
    ossicles (incus) (malleus) (stapes) 872.62
      complicated 872.72
  auricle, ear 872.01
    complicated 872.11
  axilla 880.02
    with tendon involvement 880.22
    complicated 880.12
      with tendon involvement 880.29
    involving other sites of upper arm 880.09
    complicated 880.19
  back 876.0

Index to Diseases

Wound, open

Wound, open — continued
- back — continued
  - complicated 876.1
- bladder — see Injury, internal, bladder
- blood vessel — see Injury, blood vessel, by site
- brain — see Injury, intracranial, with open intracranial wound
- breast 879.0
  - complicated 879.1
- brow 873.42
  - complicated 873.52
- buccal mucosa 873.61
  - complicated 873.71
- buttock 877.0
  - complicated 877.1
- calf 891.0
  - with tendon involvement 891.2
  - complicated 891.1
- canaliculus lacrimalis 870.8
  - with laceration of eyelid 870.2
- canthus, eye 870.8
  - laceration — see Laceration, eyelid
- cavernous sinus — see Injury, intracranial
- cerebellum — see Injury, intracranial
- cervical esophagus 874.4
  - complicated 874.5
- cervix — see Injury, internal, cervix
- cheek(s) (external) 873.41
  - complicated 873.51
  - internal 873.61
    - complicated 873.71
- chest (wall) (external) 875.0
  - complicated 875.1
- chin 873.44
  - complicated 873.54
- choroid 363.63
- ciliary body (eye) (see also Wound, open, intraocular) 871.9
- clitoris 878.8
  - complicated 878.9
- cochlea 872.64
  - complicated 872.74
- complicated 879.9
- conjunctiva — see Wound, open, intraocular
- cornea (nonpenetrating) (see also Wound, open, intraocular) 871.9
- costal region 875.0
  - complicated 875.1
- Descemet's membrane (see also Wound, open, intraocular) 871.9
- digit(s)
  - foot 893.0
    - with tendon involvement 893.2
    - complicated 893.1
  - hand 883.0
    - with tendon involvement 883.2
    - complicated 883.1
- drumhead, ear 872.61
  - complicated 872.71
- ear 872.8
  - canal 872.02
    - complicated 872.12
  - complicated 872.9
  - drum 872.61
    - complicated 872.71
  - external 872.00
    - complicated 872.10
  - multiple sites 872.69
    - complicated 872.79
  - ossicles (incus) (malleus) (stapes) 872.62
    - complicated 872.72
  - specified part NEC 872.69
    - complicated 872.79
- elbow 881.01
  - with tendon involvement 881.21
  - complicated 881.11
- epididymis 878.2
  - complicated 878.3
- epigastric region 879.2
  - complicated 879.3
- epiglottis 874.01

Wound, open — continued
- epiglottis — continued
  - complicated 874.11
- esophagus (cervical) 874.4
  - complicated 874.5
  - thoracic — see Injury, internal, esophagus
- Eustachian tube 872.63
  - complicated 872.73
- extremity
  - lower (multiple) NEC 894.0
    - with tendon involvement 894.2
    - complicated 894.1
  - upper (multiple) NEC 884.0
    - with tendon involvement 884.2
    - complicated 884.1
- eye(s) (globe) — see Wound, open, intraocular
- eyeball NEC 871.9
  - laceration (see also Laceration, eyeball) 871.4
  - penetrating (see also Penetrating wound, eyeball) 871.7
- eyebrow 873.42
  - complicated 873.52
- eyelid NEC 870.8
  - laceration — see Laceration, eyelid
- face 873.40
  - complicated 873.50
  - multiple sites 873.49
    - complicated 873.59
  - specified part NEC 873.49
    - complicated 873.59
- fallopian tube — see Injury, internal, fallopian tube
- finger(s) (nail) (subungual) 883.0
  - with tendon involvement 883.2
  - complicated 883.1
- flank 879.4
  - complicated 879.5
- foot (any part except toe(s) alone) 892.0
  - with tendon involvement 892.2
  - complicated 892.1
- forearm 881.00
  - with tendon involvement 881.20
  - complicated 881.10
- forehead 873.42
  - complicated 873.52
- genital organs (external) NEC 878.8
  - complicated 878.9
  - internal — see Injury, internal, by site
- globe (eye) (see also Wound, open, eyeball) 871.9
- groin 879.4
  - complicated 879.5
- gum(s) 873.62
  - complicated 873.72
- hand (except finger(s) alone) 882.0
  - with tendon involvement 882.2
  - complicated 882.1
- head NEC 873.8
  - with intracranial injury — see Injury, intracranial
  - due to or associated with skull fracture — see Fracture, skull
  - complicated 873.9
  - scalp — see Wound, open, scalp
- heel 892.0
  - with tendon involvement 892.2
  - complicated 892.1
- high-velocity (grease gun) — see Wound, open, complicated, by site
- hip 890.0
  - with tendon involvement 890.2
  - complicated 890.1
- hymen 878.6
  - complicated 878.7
- hypochondrium 879.4
  - complicated 879.5
- hypogastric region 879.2
  - complicated 879.3
- iliac (region) 879.4

Wound, open — continued
- iliac — continued
  - complicated 879.5
- incidental to
  - dislocation — see Dislocation, open, by site
  - fracture — see Fracture, open, by site
  - intracranial injury — see Injury, intracranial, with open intracranial wound
  - nerve injury — see Injury, nerve, by site
- inguinal region 879.4
  - complicated 879.5
- instep 892.0
  - with tendon involvement 892.2
  - complicated 892.1
- interscapular region 876.0
  - complicated 876.1
- intracranial — see Injury, intracranial, with open intracranial wound
- intraocular 871.9
  - with
    - partial loss (of intraocular tissue) 871.2
    - prolapse or exposure (of intraocular tissue) 871.1
    - without prolapse (of intraocular tissue) 871.0
  - laceration (see also Laceration, eyeball) 871.4
  - penetrating 871.7
    - with foreign body (nonmagnetic) 871.6
    - magnetic 871.5
- iris (see also Wound, open, eyeball) 871.9
- jaw (fracture not involved) 873.44
  - with fracture — see Fracture, jaw
  - complicated 873.54
- knee 891.0
  - with tendon involvement 891.2
  - complicated 891.1
- labium (majus) (minus) 878.4
  - complicated 878.5
- lacrimal apparatus, gland, or sac 870.8
  - with laceration of eyelid 870.2
- larynx 874.01
  - with trachea 874.00
    - complicated 874.10
  - complicated 874.11
- leg (multiple) 891.0
  - with tendon involvement 891.2
  - complicated 891.1
  - lower 891.0
    - with tendon involvement 891.2
    - complicated 891.1
  - thigh 890.0
    - with tendon involvement 890.2
    - complicated 890.1
  - upper 890.0
    - with tendon involvement 890.2
    - complicated 890.1
- lens (eye) (alone) (see also Cataract, traumatic) 366.20
  - with involvement of other eye structures — see Wound, open, eyeball
- limb
  - lower (multiple) NEC 894.0
    - with tendon involvement 894.2
    - complicated 894.1
  - upper (multiple) NEC 884.0
    - with tendon involvement 884.2
    - complicated 884.1
- lip 873.43
  - complicated 873.53
- loin 876.0
  - complicated 876.1
- lumbar region 876.0
  - complicated 876.1
- malar region 873.41
  - complicated 873.51
- mastoid region 873.49

Wound, open — continued
- mastoid region — continued
  - complicated 873.59
- mediastinum — see Injury, internal, mediastinum
- midthoracic region 875.0
  - complicated 875.1
- mouth 873.60
  - complicated 873.70
  - floor 873.64
    - complicated 873.74
  - multiple sites 873.69
    - complicated 873.79
  - specified site NEC 873.69
    - complicated 873.79
- multiple, unspecified site(s) 879.8

> Note — Multiple open wounds of sites classifiable to the same four-digit category should be classified to that category unless they are in different limbs.
>
> Multiple open wounds of sites classifiable to different four-digit categories, or to different limbs, should be coded separately.

  - complicated 879.9
  - lower limb(s) (one or both) (sites classifiable to more than one three-digit category in 890 to 893) 894.0
    - with tendon involvement 894.2
    - complicated 894.1
  - upper limb(s) (one or both) (sites classifiable to more than one three-digit category in 880 to 883) 884.0
    - with tendon involvement 884.2
    - complicated 884.1
- muscle — see Sprain, by site
- nail
  - finger(s) 883.0
    - complicated 883.1
  - thumb 883.0
    - complicated 883.1
  - toe(s) 893.0
    - complicated 893.1
- nape (neck) 874.8
  - complicated 874.9
  - specified part NEC 874.8
    - complicated 874.9
- nasal (see also Wound, open, nose)
  - cavity 873.22
    - complicated 873.32
  - septum 873.21
    - complicated 873.31
  - sinuses 873.23
    - complicated 873.33
- nasopharynx 873.22
  - complicated 873.32
- neck 874.8
  - complicated 874.9
  - nape 874.8
    - complicated 874.9
  - specified part NEC 874.8
    - complicated 874.9
- nerve — see Injury, nerve, by site
- non-healing surgical 998.83
- nose 873.20
  - complicated 873.30
  - multiple sites 873.29
    - complicated 873.39
  - septum 873.21
    - complicated 873.31
  - sinuses 873.23
    - complicated 873.33
- occipital region — see Wound, open, scalp
- ocular NEC 871.9
  - adnexa 870.9
    - specified region NEC 870.8
  - laceration (see also Laceration, ocular) 871.4
  - muscle (extraocular) 870.3
    - with foreign body 870.4
    - eyelid 870.1

Wound, open

Wound, open — *continued*
- ocular — *continued*
  - muscle — *continued*
    - intraocular — *see* Wound, open, eyeball
  - penetrating (*see also* Penetrating wound, ocular) 871.7
- orbit 870.8
  - penetrating 870.3
    - with foreign body 870.4
- orbital region 870.9
- ovary — *see* Injury, internal, pelvic organs
- palate 873.65
  - complicated 873.75
- palm 882.0
  - with tendon involvement 882.2
  - complicated 882.1
- parathyroid (gland) 874.2
  - complicated 874.3
- parietal region — *see* Wound, open, scalp
- pelvic floor or region 879.6
  - complicated 879.7
- penis 878.0
  - complicated 878.1
- perineum 879.6
  - complicated 879.7
- periocular area 870.8
  - laceration of skin 870.0
- pharynx 874.4
  - complicated 874.5
- pinna 872.01
  - complicated 872.11
- popliteal space 891.0
  - with tendon involvement 891.2
  - complicated 891.1
- prepuce 878.0
  - complicated 878.1
- pubic region 879.2
  - complicated 879.3
- pudenda 878.8
  - complicated 878.9
- rectovaginal septum 878.8
  - complicated 878.9
- sacral region 877.0
  - complicated 877.1
- sacroiliac region 877.0
  - complicated 877.1
- salivary (ducts) (glands) 873.69
  - complicated 873.79
- scalp 873.0
  - complicated 873.1
- scalpel, fetus or newborn 767.8
- scapular region 880.01
  - with tendon involvement 880.21
  - complicated 880.11
  - involving other sites of upper arm 880.09
    - with tendon involvement 880.29
    - complicated 880.19
- sclera (*see also* Wound, open, intraocular) 871.9
- scrotum 878.2
  - complicated 878.3
- seminal vesicle — *see* Injury, internal, pelvic organs
- shin 891.0
  - with tendon involvement 891.2
  - complicated 891.1
- shoulder 880.00
  - with tendon involvement 880.20
  - complicated 880.10
  - involving other sites of upper arm 880.09
    - with tendon involvement 880.29
    - complicated 880.19
- skin NEC 879.8
  - complicated 879.9
- skull (*see also* Injury, intracranial, with open intracranial wound)
  - with skull fracture — *see* Fracture, skull
- spermatic cord (scrotal) 878.2
  - complicated 878.3

Wound, open — *continued*
- spermatic cord — *continued*
  - pelvic region — *see* Injury, internal, spermatic cord
- spinal cord — *see* Injury, spinal
- sternal region 875.0
  - complicated 875.1
- subconjunctival — *see* Wound, open, intraocular
- subcutaneous NEC 879.8
  - complicated 879.9
- submaxillary region 873.44
  - complicated 873.54
- submental region 873.44
  - complicated 873.54
- subungual
  - finger(s) (thumb) — *see* Wound, open, finger
  - toe(s) — *see* Wound, open, toe
- supraclavicular region 874.8
  - complicated 874.9
- supraorbital 873.42
  - complicated 873.52
- surgical, non-healing 998.83
- temple 873.49
  - complicated 873.59
- temporal region 873.49
  - complicated 873.59
- testis 878.2
  - complicated 878.3
- thigh 890.0
  - with tendon involvement 890.2
  - complicated 890.1
- thorax, thoracic (external) 875.0
  - complicated 875.1
- throat 874.8
  - complicated 874.9
- thumb (nail) (subungual) 883.0
  - with tendon involvement 883.2
  - complicated 883.1
- thyroid (gland) 874.2
  - complicated 874.3
- toe(s) (nail) (subungual) 893.0
  - with tendon involvement 893.2
  - complicated 893.1
- tongue 873.64
  - complicated 873.74
- tonsil — *see* Wound, open, neck
- trachea (cervical region) 874.02
  - with larynx 874.00
    - complicated 874.10
  - complicated 874.12
  - intrathoracic — *see* Injury, internal, trachea
- trunk (multiple) NEC 879.6
  - complicated 879.7
  - specified site NEC 879.6
    - complicated 879.7
- tunica vaginalis 878.2
  - complicated 878.3
- tympanic membrane 872.61
  - complicated 872.71
- tympanum 872.61
  - complicated 872.71
- umbilical region 879.2
  - complicated 879.3
- ureter — *see* Injury, internal, ureter
- urethra — *see* Injury, internal, urethra
- uterus — *see* Injury, internal, uterus
- uvula 873.69
  - complicated 873.79
- vagina 878.6
  - complicated 878.7
- vas deferens — *see* Injury, internal, vas deferens
- vitreous (humor) 871.2
- vulva 878.4
  - complicated 878.5
- wrist 881.02
  - with tendon involvement 881.22
  - complicated 881.12

Wright's syndrome (hyperabduction) 447.8
- pneumonia 390 [517.1]

Wringer injury — *see* Crush injury, by site
Wrinkling of skin 701.8
Wrist — *see also* condition
- drop (acquired) 736.05
Wrong drug (given in error) NEC 977.9
- specified drug or substance — *see* Table of Drugs and Chemicals
Wry neck — *see also* Torticollis
- congenital 754.1
Wuchereria infestation 125.0
- bancrofti 125.0
- Brugia malayi 125.1
- malayi 125.1
Wuchereriasis 125.0
Wuchereriosis 125.0
Wuchernde struma langhans (M8332/3) 193

X

Xanthelasma 272.2
- eyelid 272.2 [374.51]
- palpebrarum 272.2 [374.51]
Xanthelasmatosis (essential) 272.2
Xanthelasmoidea 757.33
Xanthine stones 277.2
Xanthinuria 277.2
Xanthofibroma (M8831/0) — *see* Neoplasm, connective tissue, benign
Xanthoma(s), xanthomatosis 272.2
- with
  - hyperlipoproteinemia
    - type I 272.3
    - type III 272.2
    - type IV 272.1
    - type V 272.3
- bone 272.7
- craniohypophyseal 277.89
- cutaneotendinous 272.7
- diabeticorum 250.8 ☑ [272.2]
- disseminatum 272.7
- eruptive 272.2
- eyelid 272.2 [374.51]
- familial 272.7
- hereditary 272.7
- hypercholesterinemic 272.0
- hypercholesterolemic 272.0
- hyperlipemic 272.4
- hyperlipidemic 272.4
- infantile 272.7
- joint 272.7
- juvenile 272.7
- multiple 272.7
- multiplex 272.7
- primary familial 272.7
- tendon (sheath) 272.7
- tuberosum 272.2
- tuberous 272.2
- tubo-eruptive 272.2
Xanthosis 709.09
- surgical 998.81
Xenophobia 300.29
Xeroderma (congenital) 757.39
- acquired 701.1
- eyelid 373.33
- eyelid 373.33
- pigmentosum 757.33
- vitamin A deficiency 264.8
Xerophthalmia 372.53
- vitamin A deficiency 264.7
Xerosis
- conjunctiva 372.53
  - with Bitôt's spot 372.53
    - vitamin A deficiency 264.1
  - vitamin A deficiency 264.0
- cornea 371.40
  - with corneal ulceration 370.00
    - vitamin A deficiency 264.3
  - vitamin A deficiency 264.2
- cutis 706.8
- skin 706.8
Xerostomia 527.7
Xiphodynia 733.90
Xiphoidalgia 733.90
Xiphoiditis 733.99
Xiphopagus 759.4

XO syndrome 758.6
X-ray
- effects, adverse, NEC 990
- of chest
  - for suspected tuberculosis V71.2
  - routine V72.5
XXX syndrome 758.81
XXXXY syndrome 758.81
XXY syndrome 758.7
Xyloketosuria 271.8
Xylosuria 271.8
Xylulosuria 271.8
XYY syndrome 758.81

Y

Yawning 786.09
- psychogenic 306.1
Yaws 102.9
- bone or joint lesions 102.6
- butter 102.1
- chancre 102.0
- cutaneous, less than five years after infection 102.2
- early (cutaneous) (macular) (maculopapular) (micropapular) (papular) 102.2
  - frambeside 102.2
  - skin lesions NEC 102.2
- eyelid 102.9 [373.4]
- ganglion 102.6
- gangosis, gangosa 102.5
- gumma, gummata 102.4
  - bone 102.6
- gummatous
  - frambeside 102.4
  - osteitis 102.6
  - periostitis 102.6
- hydrarthrosis 102.6
- hyperkeratosis (early) (late) (palmar) (plantar) 102.3
- initial lesions 102.0
- joint lesions 102.6
- juxta-articular nodules 102.7
- late nodular (ulcerated) 102.4
- latent (without clinical manifestations) (with positive serology) 102.8
- mother 102.0
- mucosal 102.7
- multiple papillomata 102.1
- nodular, late (ulcerated) 102.4
- osteitis 102.6
- papilloma, papillomata (palmar) (plantar) 102.1
- periostitis (hypertrophic) 102.6
- ulcers 102.4
- wet crab 102.1
Yeast infection — *see also* Candidiasis 112.9
Yellow
- atrophy (liver) 570
  - chronic 571.8
  - resulting from administration of blood, plasma, serum, or other biological substance (within 8 months of administration) — *see* Hepatitis, viral
- fever — *see* Fever, yellow
- jack (*see also* Fever, yellow) 060.9
- jaundice (*see also* Jaundice) 782.4
- vernix syndrome 762.2
Yersinia septica 027.8

Z

Zagari's disease (xerostomia) 527.7
Zahorsky's disease (exanthema subitum) 057.8
- syndrome (herpangina) 074.0
Zellweger syndrome 277.86
Zenker's diverticulum (esophagus) 530.6
Ziehen-Oppenheim disease 333.6
Zieve's syndrome (jaundice, hyperlipemia, and hemolytic anemia) 571.1
Zika fever 066.3

Index to Diseases

Zollinger-Ellison syndrome (gastric hypersecretion with pancreatic islet cell tumor) 251.5
Zona — see also Herpes, zoster 053.9
Zoophilia (erotica) 302.1
Zoophobia 300.29
Zoster (herpes) — see also Herpes, zoster 053.9
Zuelzer (-Ogden) **anemia or syndrome** (nutritional megaloblastic anemia) 281.2
Zygodactyly — see also Syndactylism 755.10
Zygomycosis 117.7
Zymotic — see condition

SECTION 2

Alphabetic Index to Poisoning and External Causes of Adverse Effects of Drugs and Other Chemical Substances

TABLE OF DRUGS AND CHEMICALS

This table contains a classification of drugs and other chemical substances to identify poisoning states and external causes of adverse effects.

Each of the listed substances in the table is assigned a code according to the poisoning classification (960-989). These codes are used when there is a statement of poisoning, overdose, wrong substance given or taken, or intoxication.

The table also contains a listing of external causes of adverse effects. An adverse effect is a pathologic manifestation due to ingestion or exposure to drugs or other chemical substances (e.g., dermatitis, hypersensitivity reaction, aspirin gastritis). The adverse effect is to be identified by the appropriate code found in Section 1, Index to Diseases and Injuries. An external cause code can then be used to identify the circumstances involved. The table headings pertaining to external causes are defined below:

Accidental poisoning (E850-E869) — accidental overdose of drug, wrong substance given or taken, drug taken inadvertently, accidents in the usage of drugs and biologicals in medical and surgical procedures, and to show external causes of poisonings classifiable to 980-989.

Therapeutic use (E930-E949) — a correct substance properly administered in therapeutic or prophylactic dosage as the external cause of adverse effects.

Suicide attempt (E950-E952) — instances in which self-inflicted injuries or poisonings are involved.

Assault (E961-E962) — injury or poisoning inflicted by another person with the intent to injure or kill.

Undetermined (E980-E982) — to be used when the intent of the poisoning or injury cannot be determined whether it was intentional or accidental.

The American Hospital Formulary Service list numbers are included in the table to help classify new drugs not identified in the table by name. The AHFS list numbers are keyed to the continually revised American Hospital Formulary Service (AHFS).* These listings are found in the table under the main term **Drug**.

Excluded from the table are radium and other radioactive substances. The classification of adverse effects and complications pertaining to these substances will be found in Section 1, Index to Diseases and Injuries, and Section 3, Index to External Causes of Injuries.

Although certain substances are indexed with one or more subentries, the majority are listed according to one use or state. It is recognized that many substances may be used in various ways, in medicine and in industry, and may cause adverse effects whatever the state of the agent (solid, liquid, or fumes arising from a liquid). In cases in which the reported data indicates a use or state not in the table, or which is clearly different from the one listed, an attempt should be made to classify the substance in the form which most nearly expresses the reported facts.

*American Hospital Formulary Service, 2 vol. (Washington, D.C.: American Society of Hospital Pharmacists, 1959-)

Table of Drugs and Chemicals

	Poisoning	Accident	Therapeutic Use	Suicide Attempt	Assault	Undetermined
1-propanol	980.3	E860.4	—	E950.9	E962.1	E980.9
2-propanol	980.2	E860.3	—	E950.9	E962.1	E980.9
2, 4-D (dichlorophenoxyacetic acid)	989.4	E863.5	—	E950.6	E962.1	E980.7
2, 4-toluene diisocyanate	983.0	E864.0	—	E950.7	E962.1	E980.6
2, 4, 5-T (trichlorophenoxyacetic acid)	989.2	E863.5	—	E950.6	E962.1	E980.7
14-hydroxydihydromorphinone	965.09	E850.2	E935.2	E950.0	E962.0	E980.0
ABOB	961.7	E857	E931.7	E950.4	E962.0	E980.4
Abrus (seed)	988.2	E865.3	—	E950.9	E962.1	E980.9
Absinthe	980.0	E860.1	—	E950.9	E962.1	E980.9
beverage	980.0	E860.0	—	E950.9	E962.1	E980.9
Acenocoumarin, acenocoumarol	964.2	E858.2	E934.2	E950.4	E962.0	E980.4
Acepromazine	969.1	E853.0	E939.1	E950.3	E962.0	E980.3
Acetal	982.8	E862.4	—	E950.9	E962.1	E980.9
Acetaldehyde (vapor)	987.8	E869.8	—	E952.8	E962.2	E982.8
liquid	989.89	E866.8	—	E950.9	E962.1	E980.9
Acetaminophen	965.4	E850.4	E935.4	E950.0	E962.0	E980.0
Acetaminosalol	965.1	E850.3	E935.3	E950.0	E962.0	E980.0
Acetanilid(e)	965.4	E850.4	E935.4	E950.0	E962.0	E980.0
Acetarsol, acetarsone	961.1	E857	E931.1	E950.4	E962.0	E980.4
Acetazolamide	974.2	E858.5	E944.2	E950.4	E962.0	E980.4
Acetic						
acid	983.1	E864.1	—	E950.7	E962.1	E980.6
with sodium acetate (ointment)	976.3	E858.7	E946.3	E950.4	E962.0	E980.4
irrigating solution	974.5	E858.5	E944.5	E950.4	E962.0	E980.4
lotion	976.2	E858.7	E946.2	E950.4	E962.0	E980.4
anhydride	983.1	E864.1	—	E950.7	E962.1	E980.6
ether (vapor)	982.8	E862.4	—	E950.9	E962.1	E980.9
Acetohexamide	962.3	E858.0	E932.3	E950.4	E962.0	E980.4
Acetomenaphthone	964.3	E858.2	E934.3	E950.4	E962.0	E980.4
Acetomorphine	965.01	E850.0	E935.0	E950.0	E962.0	E980.0
Acetone (oils) (vapor)	982.8	E862.4	—	E950.9	E962.1	E980.9
Acetophenazine (maleate)	969.1	E853.0	E939.1	E950.3	E962.0	E980.3
Acetophenetidin	965.4	E850.4	E935.4	E950.0	E962.0	E980.0
Acetophenone	982.0	E862.4	—	E950.9	E962.1	E980.9
Acetorphine	965.09	E850.2	E935.2	E950.0	E962.0	E980.0
Acetosulfone (sodium)	961.8	E857	E931.8	E950.4	E962.0	E980.4
Acetrizoate (sodium)	977.8	E858.8	E947.8	E950.4	E962.0	E980.4
Acetylcarbromal	967.3	E852.2	E937.3	E950.2	E962.0	E980.2
Acetylcholine (chloride)	971.0	E855.3	E941.0	E950.4	E962.0	E980.4
Acetylcysteine	975.5	E858.6	E945.5	E950.4	E962.0	E980.4
Acetyldigitoxin	972.1	E858.3	E942.1	E950.4	E962.0	E980.4
Acetyldihydrocodeine	965.09	E850.2	E935.2	E950.0	E962.0	E980.0
Acetyldihydrocodeinone	965.09	E850.2	E935.2	E950.0	E962.0	E980.0
Acetylene (gas) (industrial)	987.1	E868.1	—	E951.8	E962.2	E981.8
incomplete combustion of — see Carbon monoxide, fuel, utility						
tetrachloride (vapor)	982.3	E862.4	—	E950.9	E962.1	E980.9
Acetyliodosalicylic acid	965.1	E850.3	E935.3	E950.0	E962.0	E980.0
Acetylphenylhydrazine	965.8	E850.8	E935.8	E950.0	E962.0	E980.0
Acetylsalicylic acid	965.1	E850.3	E935.3	E950.0	E962.0	E980.0
Achromycin	960.4	E856	E930.4	E950.4	E962.0	E980.4
ophthalmic preparation	976.5	E858.7	E946.5	E950.4	E962.0	E980.4
topical NEC	976.0	E858.7	E946.0	E950.4	E962.0	E980.4
Acidifying agents	963.2	E858.1	E933.2	E950.4	E962.0	E980.4
Acids (corrosive) NEC	983.1	E864.1	—	E950.7	E962.1	E980.6
Aconite (wild)	988.2	E865.4	—	E950.9	E962.1	E980.9
Aconitine (liniment)	976.8	E858.7	E946.8	E950.4	E962.0	E980.4
Aconitum ferox	988.2	E865.4	—	E950.9	E962.1	E980.9
Acridine	983.0	E864.0	—	E950.7	E962.1	E980.6
vapor	987.8	E869.8	—	E952.8	E962.2	E982.8
Acriflavine	961.9	E857	E931.9	E950.4	E962.0	E980.4
Acrisorcin	976.0	E858.7	E946.0	E950.4	E962.0	E980.4
Acrolein (gas)	987.8	E869.8	—	E952.8	E962.2	E982.8
liquid	989.89	E866.8	—	E950.9	E962.1	E980.9
Actaea spicata	988.2	E865.4	—	E950.9	E962.1	E980.9
Acterol	961.5	E857	E931.5	E950.4	E962.0	E980.4
ACTH	962.4	E858.0	E932.4	E950.4	E962.0	E980.4
Acthar	962.4	E858.0	E932.4	E950.4	E962.0	E980.4
Actinomycin (C) (D)	960.7	E856	E930.7	E950.4	E962.0	E980.4
Adalin (acetyl)	967.3	E852.2	E937.3	E950.2	E962.0	E980.2
Adenosine (phosphate)	977.8	E858.8	E947.8	E950.4	E962.0	E980.4
ADH	962.5	E858.0	E932.5	E950.4	E962.0	E980.4
Adhesives	989.89	E866.6	—	E950.9	E962.1	E980.9
Adicillin	960.0	E856	E930.0	E950.4	E962.0	E980.4
Adiphenine	975.1	E855.6	E945.1	E950.4	E962.0	E980.4
Adjunct, pharmaceutical	977.4	E858.8	E947.4	E950.4	E962.0	E980.4
Adrenal (extract, cortex or medulla) (glucocorticoids) (hormones) (mineralocorticoids)	962.0	E858.0	E932.0	E950.4	E962.0	E980.4
ENT agent	976.6	E858.7	E946.6	E950.4	E962.0	E980.4
ophthalmic preparation	976.5	E858.7	E946.5	E950.4	E962.0	E980.4
topical NEC	976.0	E858.7	E946.0	E950.4	E962.0	E980.4
Adrenalin	971.2	E855.5	E941.2	E950.4	E962.0	E980.4
Adrenergic blocking agents	971.3	E855.6	E941.3	E950.4	E962.0	E980.4
Adrenergics	971.2	E855.5	E941.2	E950.4	E962.0	E980.4
Adrenochrome (derivatives)	972.8	E858.3	E942.8	E950.4	E962.0	E980.4
Adrenocorticotropic hormone	962.4	E858.0	E932.4	E950.4	E962.0	E980.4
Adrenocorticotropin	962.4	E858.0	E932.4	E950.4	E962.0	E980.4
Adriamycin	960.7	E856	E930.7	E950.4	E962.0	E980.4
Aerosol spray — see Sprays						
Aerosporin	960.8	E856	E930.8	E950.4	E962.0	E980.4
ENT agent	976.6	E858.7	E946.6	E950.4	E962.0	E980.4
ophthalmic preparation	976.5	E858.7	E946.5	E950.4	E962.0	E980.4
topical NEC	976.0	E858.7	E946.0	E950.4	E962.0	E980.4
Aethusa cynapium	988.2	E865.4	—	E950.9	E962.1	E980.9
Afghanistan black	969.6	E854.1	E939.6	E950.3	E962.0	E980.3
Aflatoxin	989.7	E865.9	—	E950.9	E962.1	E980.9
African boxwood	988.2	E865.4	—	E950.9	E962.1	E980.9
Agar (-agar)	973.3	E858.4	E943.3	E950.4	E962.0	E980.4
Agricultural agent NEC	989.89	E863.9	—	E950.6	E962.1	E980.7
Agrypnal	967.0	E851	E937.0	E950.1	E962.0	—
Air contaminant(s), source or type not specified	987.9	E869.9	—	E952.9	E962.2	E982.9
specified type — see specific substance						
Akee	988.2	E865.4	—	E950.9	E962.1	E980.9
Akrinol	976.0	E858.7	E946.0	E950.4	E962.0	E980.4
Alantolactone	961.6	E857	E931.6	E950.4	E962.0	E980.4
Albamycin	960.8	E856	E930.8	E950.4	E962.0	E980.4
Albumin (normal human serum)	964.7	E858.2	E934.7	E950.4	E962.0	E980.4
Albuterol	975.7	E858.6	E945.7	E950.4	E962.0	E980.4
Alcohol	980.9	E860.9	—	E950.9	E962.1	E980.9
absolute	980.0	E860.1	—	E950.9	E962.1	E980.9
beverage	980.0	E860.0	E947.8	E950.9	E962.1	E980.9
amyl	980.3	E860.4	—	E950.9	E962.1	E980.9
antifreeze	980.1	E860.2	—	E950.9	E962.1	E980.9
butyl	980.3	E860.4	—	E950.9	E962.1	E980.9
dehydrated	980.0	E860.1	—	E950.9	E962.1	E980.9
beverage	980.0	E860.0	E947.8	E950.9	E962.1	E980.9
denatured	980.0	E860.1	—	E950.9	E962.1	E980.9
deterrents	977.3	E858.8	E947.3	E950.4	E962.0	E980.4
diagnostic (gastric function)	977.8	E858.8	E947.8	E950.4	E962.0	E980.4
ethyl	980.0	E860.1	—	E950.9	E962.1	E980.9
beverage	980.0	E860.0	E947.8	E950.9	E962.1	E980.9
grain	980.0	E860.1	—	E950.9	E962.1	E980.9
beverage	980.0	E860.0	E947.8	E950.9	E962.1	E980.9
industrial	980.9	E860.9	—	E950.9	E962.1	E980.9
isopropyl	980.2	E860.3	—	E950.9	E962.1	E980.9
methyl	980.1	E860.2	—	E950.9	E962.1	E980.9
preparation for consumption	980.0	E860.0	E947.8	E950.9	E962.1	E980.9
propyl	980.3	E860.4	—	E950.9	E962.1	E980.9
secondary	980.2	E860.3	—	E950.9	E962.1	E980.9
radiator	980.1	E860.2	—	E950.9	E962.1	E980.9
rubbing	980.2	E860.3	—	E950.9	E962.1	E980.9
specified type NEC	980.8	E860.8	—	E950.9	E962.1	E980.9
surgical	980.9	E860.9	—	E950.9	E962.1	E980.9
vapor (from any type of alcohol)	987.8	E869.8	—	E952.8	E962.2	E982.8
wood	980.1	E860.2	—	E950.9	E962.1	E980.9
Alcuronium chloride	975.2	E858.6	E945.2	E950.4	E962.0	E980.4
Aldactone	974.4	E858.5	E944.4	E950.4	E962.0	E980.4
Aldicarb	989.3	E863.2	—	E950.6	E962.1	E980.7
Aldomet	972.6	E858.3	E942.6	E950.4	E962.0	E980.4
Aldosterone	962.0	E858.0	E932.0	E950.4	E962.0	E980.4
Aldrin (dust)	989.2	E863.0	—	E950.6	E962.1	E980.7
Algeldrate	973.0	E858.4	E943.0	E950.4	E962.0	E980.4
Alidase	963.4	E858.1	E933.4	E950.4	E962.0	E980.4
Aliphatic thiocyanates	989.0	E866.8	—	E950.9	E962.1	E980.9
Alkaline antiseptic solution (aromatic)	976.6	E858.7	E946.6	E950.4	E962.0	E980.4

Table of Drugs and Chemicals

	Poisoning	External Cause (E-Code)						Poisoning	External Cause (E-Code)				
		Accident	Therapeutic Use	Suicide Attempt	Assault	Undetermined			Accident	Therapeutic Use	Suicide Attempt	Assault	Undetermined
Alkalinizing agents							**Ammoniated mercury**	976.0	E858.7	E946.0	E950.4	E962.0	E980.4
(medicinal)	963.3	E858.1	E933.3	E950.4	E962.0	E980.4	**Ammonium**						
Alkalis, caustic	983.2	E864.2	—	E950.7	E962.1	E980.6	carbonate	983.2	E864.2	—	E950.7	E962.1	E980.6
Alkalizing agents							chloride (acidifying agent)	963.2	E858.1	E933.2	E950.4	E962.0	E980.4
(medicinal)	963.3	E858.1	E933.3	E950.4	E962.0	E980.4	expectorant	975.5	E858.6	E945.5	E950.4	E962.0	E980.4
Alka-seltzer	965.1	E850.3	E935.3	E950.0	E962.0	E980.0	compounds (household)						
Alkavervir	972.6	E858.3	E942.6	E950.4	E962.0	E980.4	NEC	983.2	E861.4	—	E950.7	E962.1	E980.6
Allegron	969.0	E854.0	E939.0	E950.3	E962.0	E980.3	fumes (any usage)	987.8	E869.8	—	E952.8	E962.2	E982.8
Alleve — Naproxen							industrial	983.2	E864.2	—	E950.7	E962.1	E980.6
Allobarbital,							ichthyosulfonate	976.4	E858.7	E946.4	E950.4	E962.0	E980.4
allobarbitone	967.0	E851	E937.0	E950.1	E962.0	E980.1	mandelate	961.9	E857	E931.9	E950.4	E962.0	E980.4
Allopurinol	974.7	E858.5	E944.7	E950.4	E962.0	E980.4	Amobarbital	967.0	E851	E937.0	E950.1	E962.0	E980.1
Allylestrenol	962.2	E858.0	E932.2	E950.4	E962.0	E980.4	Amodiaquin(e)	961.4	E857	E931.4	E950.4	E962.0	E980.4
Allylisopropylacetylurea	967.8	E852.8	E937.8	E950.2	E962.0	E980.2	Amopyroquin(e)	961.4	E857	E931.4	E950.4	E962.0	E980.4
Allylisopropylmalonylurea	967.0	E851	E937.0	E950.1	E962.0	E980.1	Amphenidone	969.5	E853.8	E939.5	E950.3	E962.0	E980.3
Allyltribromide	967.3	E852.2	E937.3	E950.2	E962.0	E980.2	Amphetamine	969.7	E854.2	E939.7	E950.3	E962.0	E980.3
Aloe, aloes, aloin	973.1	E858.4	E943.1	E950.4	E962.0	E980.4	Amphomycin	960.8	E856	E930.8	E950.4	E962.0	E980.4
Alosetron	973.8	E858.4	E943.8	E950.4	E962.0	E980.4	Amphotericin B	960.1	E856	E930.1	E950.4	E962.0	E980.4
Aloxidone	966.0	E855.0	E936.0	E950.4	E962.0	E980.4	topical	976.0	E858.7	E946.0	E950.4	E962.0	E980.4
Aloxiprin	965.1	E850.3	E935.3	E950.0	E962.0	E980.0	Ampicillin	960.0	E856	E930.0	E950.4	E962.0	E980.4
Alpha amylase	963.4	E858.1	E933.4	E950.4	E962.0	E980.4	Amprotropine	971.1	E855.4	E941.1	E950.4	E962.0	E980.4
Alphaprodine							Amygdalin	977.8	E858.8	E947.8	E950.4	E962.0	E980.4
(hydrochloride)	965.09	E850.2	E935.2	E950.0	E962.0	E980.0	**Amyl**						
Alpha tocopherol	963.5	E858.1	E933.5	E950.4	E962.0	E980.4	acetate (vapor)	982.8	E862.4	—	E950.9	E962.1	E980.9
Alseroxylon	972.6	E858.3	E942.6	E950.4	E962.0	E980.4	alcohol	980.3	E860.4	—	E950.9	E962.1	E980.9
Alum (ammonium)							nitrite (medicinal)	972.4	E858.3	E942.4	E950.4	E962.0	E980.4
(potassium)	983.2	E864.2	—	E950.7	E962.1	E980.6	**Amylase** (alpha)	963.4	E858.1	E933.4	E950.4	E962.0	E980.4
medicinal (astringent) NEC	976.2	E858.7	E946.2	E950.4	E962.0	E980.4	Amylene hydrate	980.8	E860.8	—	E950.9	E962.1	E980.9
Aluminium, aluminum (gel)							Amylobarbitone	967.0	E851	E937.0	E950.1	E962.0	E980.1
(hydroxide)	973.0	E858.4	E943.0	E950.4	E962.0	E980.4	Amylocaine	968.9	E855.2	E938.9	E950.4	E962.0	E980.4
acetate solution	976.2	E858.7	E946.2	E950.4	E962.0	E980.4	infiltration (subcutaneous)	968.5	E855.2	E938.5	E950.4	E962.0	E980.4
aspirin	965.1	E850.3	E935.3	E950.0	E962.0	E980.0	nerve block (peripheral)						
carbonate	973.0	E858.4	E943.0	E950.4	E962.0	E980.4	(plexus)	968.6	E855.2	E938.6	E950.4	E962.0	E980.4
glycinate	973.0	E858.4	E943.0	E950.4	E962.0	E980.4	spinal	968.7	E855.2	E938.7	E950.4	E962.0	E980.4
nicotinate	972.2	E858.3	E942.2	E950.4	E962.0	E980.4	topical (surface)	968.5	E855.2	E938.5	E950.4	E962.0	E980.4
ointment (surgical) (topical)	976.3	E858.7	E946.3	E950.4	E962.0	E980.4	**Amytal** (sodium)	967.0	E851	E937.0	E950.1	E962.0	E980.1
phosphate	973.0	E858.4	E943.0	E950.4	E962.0	E980.4	Analeptics	970.0	E854.3	E940.0	E950.4	E962.0	E980.4
subacetate	976.2	E858.7	E946.2	E950.4	E962.0	E980.4	Analgesics	965.9	E850.9	E935.9	E950.0	E962.0	E980.0
topical NEC	976.3	E858.7	E946.3	E950.4	E962.0	E980.4	aromatic NEC	965.4	E850.4	E935.4	E950.0	E962.0	E980.0
Alurate	967.0	E851	E937.0	E950.1	E962.0	E980.1	non-narcotic NEC	965.7	E850.7	E935.7	E950.0	E962.0	E980.0
Alverine (citrate)	975.1	E858.6	E945.1	E950.4	E962.0	E980.4	specified NEC	965.8	E850.8	E935.8	E950.0	E962.0	E980.0
Alvodine	965.09	E850.2	E935.2	E950.0	E962.0	E980.0	Anamirta cocculus	988.2	E865.3	—	E950.9	E962.1	E980.9
Amanita phalloides	988.1	E865.5	—	E950.9	E962.1	E980.9	Ancillin	960.0	E856	E930.0	E950.4	E962.0	E980.4
Amantadine (hydrochloride)	966.4	E855.0	E936.4	E950.4	E962.0	E980.4	**Androgens** (anabolic						
Ambazone	961.9	E857	E931.9	E950.4	E962.0	E980.4	congeners)	962.1	E858.0	E932.1	E950.4	E962.0	E980.4
Ambenonium	971.0	E855.3	E941.0	E950.4	E962.0	E980.4	Androstalone	962.1	E858.0	E932.1	E950.4	E962.0	E980.4
Ambutonium bromide	971.1	E855.4	E941.1	E950.4	E962.0	E980.4	Androsterone	962.1	E858.0	E932.1	E950.4	E962.0	E980.4
Ametazole	977.8	E858.8	E947.8	E950.4	E962.0	E980.4	Anemone pulsatilla	988.2	E865.4	—	E950.9	E962.1	E980.9
Amethocaine (infiltration)							**Anesthesia, anesthetic** (general)						
(topical)	968.5	E855.2	E938.5	E950.4	E962.0	E980.4	NEC	968.4	E855.1	E938.4	E950.4	E962.0	E980.4
nerve block (peripheral)							block (nerve) (plexus)	968.6	E855.2	E938.6	E950.4	E962.0	E980.4
(plexus)	968.6	E855.2	E938.6	E950.4	E962.0	E980.4	gaseous NEC	968.2	E855.1	E938.2	E950.4	E962.0	E980.4
spinal	968.7	E855.2	E938.7	E950.4	E962.0	E980.4	halogenated hydrocarbon						
Amethopterin	963.1	E858.1	E933.1	E950.4	E962.0	E980.4	derivatives NEC	968.2	E855.1	E938.2	E950.4	E962.0	E980.4
Amfepramone	977.0	E858.8	E947.0	E950.4	E962.0	E980.4	infiltration (intradermal)						
Amidon	965.02	E850.1	E935.1	E950.0	E962.0	E980.0	(subcutaneous)						
Amidopyrine	965.5	E850.5	E935.5	E950.0	E962.0	E980.0	(submucosal)	968.5	E855.2	E938.5	E950.4	E962.0	E980.4
Aminacrine	976.0	E858.7	E946.0	E950.4	E962.0	E980.4	intravenous	968.3	E855.1	E938.3	E950.4	E962.0	E980.4
Aminitrozole	961.5	E857	E931.5	E950.4	E962.0	E980.4	local NEC	968.9	E855.2	E938.9	E950.4	E962.0	E980.4
Aminoacetic acid	974.5	E858.5	E944.5	E950.4	E962.0	E980.4	nerve blocking (peripheral)						
Amino acids	974.5	E858.5	E944.5	E950.4	E962.0	E980.4	(plexus)	968.6	E855.2	E938.6	E950.4	E962.0	E980.4
Aminocaproic acid	964.4	E858.2	E934.4	E950.4	E962.0	E980.4	rectal NEC	968.3	E855.1	E938.3	E950.4	E962.0	E980.4
Aminoethylisothiourium	963.8	E858.1	E933.8	E950.4	E962.0	E980.4	spinal	968.7	E855.2	E938.7	E950.4	E962.0	E980.4
Aminoglutethimide	966.3	E855.0	E936.3	E950.4	E962.0	E980.4	surface	968.5	E855.2	E938.5	E950.4	E962.0	E980.4
Aminometradine	974.3	E858.5	E944.3	E950.4	E962.0	E980.4	topical	968.5	E855.2	E938.5	E950.4	E962.0	E980.4
Aminopentamide	971.1	E855.4	E941.1	E950.4	E962.0	E980.4	Aneurine	963.5	E858.1	E933.5	E950.4	E962.0	E980.4
Aminophenazone	965.5	E850.5	E935.5	E950.0	E962.0	E980.0	Anginine — see Glyceryl						
Aminophenol	983.0	E864.0	—	E950.7	E962.1	E980.6	trinitrate						
Aminophenylpyridone	969.5	E853.8	E939.5	E950.3	E962.0	E980.3	Angio-Conray	977.8	E858.8	E947.8	E950.4	E962.0	E980.4
Aminophyllin	975.7	E858.6	E945.7	E950.4	E962.0	E980.4	Angiotensin	971.2	E855.5	E941.2	E950.4	E962.0	E980.4
Aminopterin	963.1	E858.1	E933.1	E950.4	E962.0	E980.4	Anhydrohydroxyprogesterone	962.2	E858.0	E932.2	E950.4	E962.0	E980.4
Aminopyrine	965.5	E850.5	E935.5	E950.0	E962.0	E980.0	Anhydron	974.3	E858.5	E944.3	E950.4	E962.0	E980.4
Aminosalicylic acid	961.8	E857	E931.8	E950.4	E962.0	E980.4	Anileridine	965.09	E850.2	E935.2	E950.0	E962.0	E980.0
Amiphenazole	970.1	E854.3	E940.1	E950.4	E962.0	E980.4	Aniline (dye) (liquid)	983.0	E864.0	—	E950.7	E962.1	E980.6
Amiquinsin	972.6	E858.3	E942.6	E950.4	E962.0	E980.4	analgesic	965.4	E850.4	E935.4	E950.0	E962.0	E980.0
Amisometradine	974.3	E858.5	E944.3	E950.4	E962.0	E980.4	derivatives, therapeutic						
Amitriptyline	969.0	E854.0	E939.0	E950.3	E962.0	E980.3	NEC	965.4	E850.4	E935.4	E950.0	E962.0	E980.0
Ammonia (fumes) (gas)							vapor	987.8	E869.8	—	E952.8	E962.2	E982.8
(vapor)	987.8	E869.8	—	E952.8	E962.2	E982.8	Aniscoropine	971.1	E855.4	E941.1	E950.4	E962.0	E980.4
liquid (household) NEC	983.2	E861.4	—	E950.7	E962.1	E980.6	Anisindione	964.2	E858.2	E934.2	E950.4	E962.0	E980.4
spirit, aromatic	970.8	E854.3	E940.8	E950.4	E962.0	E980.4	**Anorexic agents**	977.0	E858.8	E947.0	E950.4	E962.0	E980.4

☑ Additional Digit Required — Refer to the Tabular List for Digit Selection

▶◀ Revised Text   ● New Line   ▲ Revised Code

Subterms under main terms may continue to next column or page

Table of Drugs and Chemicals

			External Cause (E-Code)			
	Poisoning	Accident	Therapeutic Use	Suicide Attempt	Assault	Undetermined
Ant (bite) (sting)	—	E905.5	—	E950.9	E962.1	E980.9
Antabuse	977.3	E858.8	E947.3	E950.4	E962.0	E980.4
Antacids	973.0	E858.4	E943.0	E950.4	E962.0	E980.4
Antazoline	963.0	E858.1	E933.0	E950.4	E962.0	E980.4
Anthralin	976.4	E858.7	E946.4	E950.4	E962.0	E980.4
Anthramycin	960.7	E856	E930.7	E950.4	E962.0	E980.4
Antiadrenergics	971.3	E855.6	E941.3	E950.4	E962.0	E980.4
Antiallergic agents	963.0	E858.1	E933.0	E950.4	E962.0	E980.4
Antianemic agents NEC	964.1	E858.2	E934.1	E950.4	E962.0	E980.4
Antiaris toxicaria	988.2	E865.4	—	E950.9	E962.1	E980.9
Antiarteriosclerotic agents	972.2	E858.3	E942.2	E950.4	E962.0	E980.4
Antiasthmatics	975.7	E858.6	E945.7	E950.4	E962.0	E980.4
Antibiotics	960.9	E856	E930.9	E950.4	E962.0	E980.4
antifungal	960.1	E856	E930.1	E950.4	E962.0	E980.4
antimycobacterial	960.6	E856	E930.6	E950.4	E962.0	E980.4
antineoplastic	960.7	E856	E930.7	E950.4	E962.0	E980.4
cephalosporin (group)	960.5	E856	E930.5	E950.4	E962.0	E980.4
chloramphenicol (group)	960.2	E856	E930.2	E950.4	E962.0	E980.4
macrolides	960.3	E856	E930.3	E950.4	E962.0	E980.4
specified NEC	960.8	E856	E930.8	E950.4	E962.0	E980.4
tetracycline (group)	960.4	E856	E930.4	E950.4	E962.0	E980.4
Anticancer agents NEC	963.1	E858.1	E933.1	E950.4	E962.0	E980.4
antibiotics	960.7	E856	E930.7	E950.4	E962.0	E980.4
Anticholinergics	971.1	E855.4	E941.1	E950.4	E962.0	E980.4
Anticholinesterase (organophosphorus) (reversible)	971.0	E855.3	E941.0	E950.4	E962.0	E980.4
Anticoagulants	964.2	E858.2	E934.2	E950.4	E962.0	E980.4
antagonists	964.5	E858.2	E934.5	E950.4	E962.0	E980.4
Anti-common cold agents NEC	975.6	E858.6	E945.6	E950.4	E962.0	E980.4
Anticonvulsants NEC	966.3	E855.0	E936.3	E950.4	E962.0	E980.4
Antidepressants	969.0	E854.0	E939.0	E950.3	E962.0	E980.3
Antidiabetic agents	962.3	E858.0	E932.3	E950.4	E962.0	E980.4
Antidiarrheal agents	973.5	E858.4	E943.5	E950.4	E962.0	E980.4
Antidiuretic hormone	962.5	E858.0	E932.5	E950.4	E962.0	E980.4
Antidotes NEC	977.2	E858.8	E947.2	E950.4	E962.0	E980.4
Antiemetic agents	963.0	E858.1	E933.0	E950.4	E962.0	E980.4
Antiepilepsy agent NEC	966.3	E855.0	E936.3	E950.4	E962.0	E980.4
Antifertility pills	962.2	E858.0	E932.2	E950.4	E962.0	E980.4
Antiflatulents	973.8	E858.4	E943.8	E950.4	E962.0	E980.4
Antifreeze	989.89	E866.8	—	E950.9	E962.1	E980.9
alcohol	980.1	E860.2	—	E950.9	E962.1	E980.9
ethylene glycol	982.8	E862.4	—	E950.9	E962.1	E980.9
Antifungals (nonmedicinal) (sprays)	989.4	E863.6	—	E950.6	E962.1	E980.7
medicinal NEC	961.9	E857	E931.9	E950.4	E962.0	E980.4
antibiotic	960.1	E856	E930.1	E950.4	E962.0	E980.4
topical	976.0	E858.7	E946.0	E950.4	E962.0	E980.4
Antigastric secretion agents	973.0	E858.4	E943.0	E950.4	E962.0	E980.4
Antihelmintics	961.6	E857	E931.6	E950.4	E962.0	E980.4
Antihemophilic factor (human)	964.7	E858.2	E934.7	E950.4	E962.0	E980.4
Antihistamine	963.0	E858.1	E933.0	E950.4	E962.0	E980.4
Antihypertensive agents NEC	972.6	E858.3	E942.6	E950.4	E962.0	E980.4
Anti-infectives NEC	961.9	E857	E931.9	E950.4	E962.0	E980.4
antibiotics	960.9	E856	E930.9	E950.4	E962.0	E980.4
specified NEC	960.8	E856	E930.8	E950.4	E962.0	E980.4
antihelmintic	961.6	E857	E931.6	E950.4	E962.0	E980.4
antimalarial	961.4	E857	E931.4	E950.4	E962.0	E980.4
antimycobacterial NEC	961.8	E857	E931.8	E950.4	E962.0	E980.4
antibiotics	960.6	E856	E930.6	E950.4	E962.0	E980.4
antiprotozoal NEC	961.5	E857	E931.5	E950.4	E962.0	—
blood	961.4	E857	E931.4	E950.4	E962.0	E980.4
antiviral	961.7	E857	E931.7	E950.4	E962.0	E980.4
arsenical	961.1	E857	E931.1	E950.4	E962.0	E980.4
ENT agents	976.6	E858.7	E946.6	E950.4	E962.0	E980.4
heavy metals NEC	961.2	E857	E931.2	E950.4	E962.0	E980.4
local	976.0	E858.7	E946.0	E950.4	E962.0	E980.4
ophthalmic preparation	976.5	E858.7	E946.5	E950.4	E962.0	E980.4
topical NEC	976.0	E858.7	E946.0	E950.4	E962.0	E980.4
Anti-inflammatory agents (topical)	976.0	E858.7	E946.0	E950.4	E962.0	E980.4
Antiknock (tetraethyl lead)	984.1	E862.1	—	E950.9	—	E980.9
Antilipemics	972.2	E858.3	E942.2	E950.4	E962.0	E980.4
Antimalarials	961.4	E857	E931.4	E950.4	E962.0	E980.4
Antimony (compounds) (vapor) NEC	985.4	E866.2	—	E950.9	E962.1	E980.9
Antimony (compounds) (vapor) — continued						
anti-infectives	961.2	E857	E931.2	E950.4	E962.0	E980.4
pesticides (vapor)	985.4	E863.4	—	E950.6	E962.2	E980.7
potassium tartrate	961.2	E857	E931.2	E950.4	E962.0	E980.4
tartrated	961.2	E857	E931.2	E950.4	E962.0	E980.4
Antimuscarinic agents	971.1	E855.4	E941.1	E950.4	E962.0	E980.4
Antimycobacterials NEC	961.8	E857	E931.8	E950.4	E962.0	E980.4
antibiotics	960.6	E856	E930.6	E950.4	E962.0	E980.4
Antineoplastic agents	963.1	E858.1	E933.1	E950.4	E962.0	E980.4
antibiotics	960.7	E856	E930.7	E950.4	E962.0	E980.4
Anti-Parkinsonism agents	966.4	E855.0	E936.4	E950.4	E962.0	E980.4
Antiphlogistics	965.69	E850.6	E935.6	E950.0	E962.0	E980.0
Antiprotozoals NEC	961.5	E857	E931.5	E950.4	E962.0	E980.4
blood	961.4	E857	E931.4	E950.4	E962.0	E980.4
Antipruritics (local)	976.1	E858.7	E946.1	E950.4	E962.0	E980.4
Antipsychotic agents NEC	969.3	E853.8	E939.3	E950.3	E962.0	E980.3
Antipyretics	965.9	E850.9	E935.9	E950.0	E962.0	E980.0
specified NEC	965.8	E850.8	E935.8	E950.0	E962.0	E980.0
Antipyrine	965.5	E850.5	E935.5	E950.0	E962.0	E980.0
Antirabies serum (equine)	979.9	E858.8	E949.9	E950.4	E962.0	E980.4
Antirheumatics	965.69	E850.6	E935.6	E950.0	E962.0	E980.0
Antiseborrheics	976.4	E858.7	E946.4	E950.4	E962.0	E980.4
Antiseptics (external) (medicinal)	976.0	E858.7	E946.0	E950.4	E962.0	E980.4
Antistine	963.0	E858.1	E933.0	E950.4	E962.0	E980.4
Antithyroid agents	962.8	E858.0	E932.8	E950.4	E962.0	E980.4
Antitoxin, any	979.9	E858.8	E949.9	E950.4	E962.0	E980.4
Antituberculars	961.8	E857	E931.8	E950.4	E962.0	E980.4
antibiotics	960.6	E856	E930.6	E950.4	E962.0	E980.4
Antitussives	975.4	E858.6	E945.4	E950.4	E962.0	E980.4
Antivaricose agents (sclerosing)	972.7	E858.3	E942.7	E950.4	E962.0	E980.4
Antivenin (crotaline) (spider-bite)	979.9	E858.8	E949.9	E950.4	E962.0	E980.4
Antivert	963.0	E858.1	E933.0	E950.4	E962.0	E980.4
Antivirals NEC	961.7	E857	E931.7	E950.4	E962.0	E980.4
Ant poisons — see Pesticides						
Antrol	989.4	E863.4	—	E950.6	E962.1	E980.7
fungicide	989.4	E863.6	—	E950.6	E962.1	E980.7
Apomorphine hydrochloride (emetic)	973.6	E858.4	E943.6	E950.4	E962.0	E980.4
Appetite depressants, central	977.0	E858.8	E947.0	E950.4	E962.0	E980.4
Apresoline	972.6	E858.3	E942.6	E950.4	E962.0	E980.4
Aprobarbital, aprobarbitone	967.0	E851	E937.0	E950.1	E962.0	E980.1
Apronalide	967.8	E852.8	E937.8	E950.2	E962.0	E980.2
Aqua fortis	983.1	E864.1	—	E950.7	E962.1	E980.6
Arachis oil (topical)	976.3	E858.7	E946.3	E950.4	E962.0	E980.4
cathartic	973.2	E858.4	E943.2	E950.4	E962.0	E980.4
Aralen	961.4	E857	E931.4	E950.4	E962.0	E980.4
Arginine salts	974.5	E858.5	E944.5	E950.4	E962.0	E980.4
Argyrol	976.0	E858.7	E946.0	E950.4	E962.0	E980.4
ENT agent	976.6	E858.7	E946.6	E950.4	E962.0	E980.4
ophthalmic preparation	976.5	E858.7	E946.5	E950.4	E962.0	E980.4
Aristocort	962.0	E858.0	E932.0	E950.4	E962.0	E980.4
ENT agent	976.6	E858.7	E946.6	E950.4	E962.0	E980.4
ophthalmic preparation	976.5	E858.7	E946.5	E950.4	E962.0	E980.4
topical NEC	976.0	E858.7	E946.0	E950.4	E962.0	E980.4
Aromatics, corrosive	983.0	E864.0	—	E950.7	E962.1	E980.6
disinfectants	983.0	E861.4	—	E950.7	E962.1	E980.6
Arsenate of lead (insecticide)	985.1	E863.4	—	E950.8	E962.1	E980.8
herbicide	985.1	E863.5	—	E950.8	E962.1	E980.8
Arsenic, arsenicals (compounds) (dust) (fumes) (vapor) NEC	985.1	E866.3	—	E950.8	E962.1	E980.8
anti-infectives	961.1	E857	E931.1	E950.4	E962.0	E980.4
pesticide (dust) (fumes)	985.1	E863.4	—	E950.8	E962.1	E980.8
Arsine (gas)	985.1	E866.3	—	E950.8	E962.1	E980.8
Arsphenamine (silver)	961.1	E857	E931.1	E950.4	E962.0	E980.4
Arsthinol	961.1	E857	E931.1	E950.4	E962.0	E980.4
Artane	971.1	E855.4	E941.1	E950.4	E962.0	E980.4
Arthropod (venomous) NEC	989.5	E905.5	—	E950.9	E962.1	E980.9
Asbestos	989.81	E866.8	—	E950.9	E962.1	E980.9
Ascaridole	961.6	E857	E931.6	E950.4	E962.0	E980.4
Ascorbic acid	963.5	E858.1	E933.5	E950.4	E962.0	E980.4
Asiaticoside	976.0	E858.7	E946.0	E950.4	E962.0	E980.4
Aspidium (oleoresin)	961.6	E857	E931.6	E950.4	E962.0	E980.4

Table of Drugs and Chemicals

	Poisoning	Accident	Therapeutic Use	Suicide Attempt	Assault	Undetermined
Aspirin	965.1	E850.3	E935.3	E950.0	E962.0	E980.0
Astringents (local)	976.2	E858.7	E946.2	E950.4	E962.0	E980.4
Atabrine	961.3	E857	E931.3	E950.4	E962.0	E980.4
Atactics	969.5	E853.8	E939.5	E950.3	E962.0	E980.3
Atonia drug, intestinal	973.3	E858.4	E943.3	E950.4	E962.0	E980.4
Atophan	974.7	E858.5	E944.7	E950.4	E962.0	E980.4
Atropine	971.1	E855.4	E941.1	E950.4	E962.0	E980.4
Attapulgite	973.5	E858.4	E943.5	E950.4	E962.0	E980.4
Attenuvax	979.4	E858.8	E949.4	E950.4	E962.0	E980.4
Aureomycin	960.4	E856	E930.4	E950.4	E962.0	E980.4
ophthalmic preparation	976.5	E858.7	E946.5	E950.4	E962.0	E980.4
topical NEC	976.0	E858.7	E946.0	E950.4	E962.0	E980.4
Aurothioglucose	965.69	E850.6	E935.6	E950.0	E962.0	E980.0
Aurothioglycanide	965.69	E850.6	E935.6	E950.0	E962.0	E980.0
Aurothiomalate	965.69	E850.6	E935.6	E950.0	E962.0	E980.0
Automobile fuel	981	E862.1	—	E950.9	E962.1	E980.9
Autonomic nervous system agents NEC	971.9	E855.9	E941.9	E950.4	E962.0	E980.4
Avlosulfon	961.8	E857	E931.8	E950.4	E962.0	E980.4
Avomine	967.8	E852.8	E937.8	E950.2	E962.0	E980.2
Azacyclonol	969.5	E853.8	E939.5	E950.3	E962.0	E980.3
Azapetine	971.3	E855.6	E941.3	E950.4	E962.0	E980.4
Azaribine	963.1	E858.1	E933.1	E950.4	E962.0	E980.4
Azaserine	960.7	E856	E930.7	E950.4	E962.0	E980.4
Azathioprine	963.1	E858.1	E933.1	E950.4	E962.0	E980.4
Azosulfamide	961.0	E857	E931.0	E950.4	E962.0	E980.4
Azulfidine	961.0	E857	E931.0	E950.4	E962.0	E980.4
Azuresin	977.8	E858.8	E947.8	E950.4	E962.0	E980.4
Bacimycin	976.0	E858.7	E946.0	E950.4	E962.0	E980.4
ophthalmic preparation	976.5	E858.7	E946.5	E950.4	E962.0	E980.4
Bacitracin	960.8	E856	E930.8	E950.4	E962.0	E980.4
ENT agent	976.6	E858.7	E946.6	E950.4	E962.0	E980.4
ophthalmic preparation	976.5	E858.7	E946.5	E950.4	E962.0	E980.4
topical NEC	976.0	E858.7	E946.0	E950.4	E962.0	E980.4
Baking soda	963.3	E858.1	E933.3	E950.4	E962.0	E980.4
BAL	963.8	E858.1	E933.8	E950.4	E962.0	E980.4
Bamethan (sulfate)	972.5	E858.3	E942.5	E950.4	E962.0	E980.4
Bamipine	963.0	E858.1	E933.0	E950.4	E962.0	E980.4
Baneberry	988.2	E865.4	—	E950.9	E962.1	E980.9
Banewort	988.2	E865.4	—	E950.9	E962.1	E980.9
Barbenyl	967.0	E851	E937.0	E950.1	E962.0	E980.1
Barbital, barbitone	967.0	E851	E937.0	E950.1	E962.0	E980.1
Barbiturates, barbituric acid	967.0	E851	E937.0	E950.1	E962.0	E980.1
anesthetic (intravenous)	968.3	E855.1	E938.3	E950.4	E962.0	E980.4
Barium (carbonate) (chloride) (sulfate)	985.8	E866.4	—	E950.9	E962.1	E980.9
diagnostic agent	977.8	E858.8	E947.8	E950.4	E962.0	E980.4
pesticide	985.8	E863.4	—	E950.6	E962.1	E980.7
rodenticide	985.8	E863.7	—	E950.6	E962.1	E980.7
Barrier cream	976.3	E858.7	E946.3	E950.4	E962.0	E980.4
Battery acid or fluid	983.1	E864.1	—	E950.7	E962.1	E980.6
Bay rum	980.8	E860.8	—	E950.9	E962.1	E980.9
BCG vaccine	978.0	E858.8	E948.0	E950.4	E962.0	E980.4
Bearsfoot	988.2	E865.4	—	E950.9	E962.1	E980.9
Beclamide	966.3	E855.0	E936.3	E950.4	E962.0	E980.4
Bee (sting) (venom)	989.5	E905.3	—	E950.9	E962.1	E980.9
Belladonna (alkaloids)	971.1	E855.4	E941.1	E950.4	E962.0	E980.4
Bemegride	970.0	E854.3	E940.0	E950.4	E962.0	E980.4
Benactyzine	969.8	E855.8	E939.8	E950.3	E962.0	E980.3
Benadryl	963.0	E858.1	E933.0	E950.4	E962.0	E980.4
Bendrofluazide	974.3	E858.5	E944.3	E950.4	E962.0	E980.4
Bendroflumethiazide	974.3	E858.5	E944.3	E950.4	E962.0	E980.4
Benemid	974.7	E858.5	E944.7	E950.4	E962.0	E980.4
Benethamine penicillin G	960.0	E856	E930.0	E950.4	E962.0	E980.4
Benisone	976.0	E858.7	E946.0	E950.4	E962.0	E980.4
Benoquin	976.8	E858.7	E946.8	E950.4	E962.0	E980.4
Benoxinate	968.5	E855.2	E938.5	E950.4	E962.0	E980.4
Bentonite	976.3	E858.7	E946.3	E950.4	E962.0	E980.4
Benzalkonium (chloride)	976.0	E858.7	E946.0	E950.4	E962.0	E980.4
ophthalmic preparation	976.5	E858.7	E946.5	E950.4	E962.0	E980.4
Benzamidosalicylate (calcium)	961.8	E857	E931.8	E950.4	E962.0	E980.4
Benzathine penicillin	960.0	E856	E930.0	E950.4	E962.0	E980.4
Benzcarbimine	963.1	E858.1	E933.1	E950.4	E962.0	E980.4
Benzedrex	971.2	E855.5	E941.2	E950.4	E962.0	E980.4
Benzedrine (amphetamine)	969.7	E854.2	E939.7	E950.3	E962.0	E980.3
Benzene (acetyl) (dimethyl) (methyl) (solvent) (vapor)	982.0	E862.4	—	E950.9	E962.1	E980.9
hexachloride (gamma) (insecticide) (vapor)	989.2	E863.0	—	E950.6	E962.1	E980.7
Benzethonium	976.0	E858.7	E946.0	E950.4	E962.0	E980.4
Benzhexol (chloride)	966.4	E855.0	E936.4	E950.4	E962.0	E980.4
Benzilonium	971.1	E855.4	E941.1	E950.4	E962.0	E980.4
Benzin(e) — see Ligroin						
Benziodarone	972.4	E858.3	E942.4	E950.4	E962.0	E980.4
Benzocaine	968.5	E855.2	E938.5	E950.4	E962.0	E980.4
Benzodiapin	969.4	E853.2	E939.4	E950.3	E962.0	E980.3
Benzodiazepines (tranquilizers) NEC	969.4	E853.2	E939.4	E950.3	E962.0	E980.3
Benzoic acid (with salicylic acid) (anti-infective)	976.0	E858.7	E946.0	E950.4	E962.0	E980.4
Benzoin	976.3	E858.7	E946.3	E950.4	E962.0	E980.4
Benzol (vapor)	982.0	E862.4	—	E950.9	E962.1	E980.9
Benzomorphan	965.09	E850.2	E935.2	E950.0	E962.0	E980.0
Benzonatate	975.4	E858.6	E945.4	E950.4	E962.0	E980.4
Benzothiadiazides	974.3	E858.5	E944.3	E950.4	E962.0	E980.4
Benzoylpas	961.8	E857	E931.8	E950.4	E962.0	E980.4
Benzperidol	969.5	E853.8	E939.5	E950.3	E962.0	E980.3
Benzphetamine	977.0	E858.8	E947.0	E950.4	E962.0	E980.4
Benzpyrinium	971.0	E855.3	E941.0	E950.4	E962.0	E980.4
Benzquinamide	963.0	E858.1	E933.0	E950.4	E962.0	E980.4
Benzthiazide	974.3	E858.5	E944.3	E950.4	E962.0	E980.4
Benztropine	971.1	E855.4	E941.1	E950.4	E962.0	E980.4
Benzyl						
acetate	982.8	E862.4	—	E950.9	E962.1	E980.9
benzoate (anti-infective)	976.0	E858.7	E946.0	E950.4	E962.0	E980.4
morphine	965.09	E850.2	E935.2	E950.0	E962.0	E980.0
penicillin	960.0	E856	E930.0	E950.4	E962.0	E980.4
Bephenium hydroxynapthoate	961.6	E857	E931.6	E950.4	E962.0	E980.4
Bergamot oil	989.89	E866.8	—	E950.9	E962.1	E980.9
Berries, poisonous	988.2	E865.3	—	E950.9	E962.1	E980.9
Beryllium (compounds) (fumes)	985.3	E866.4	—	E950.9	E962.1	E980.9
Beta-carotene	976.3	E858.7	E946.3	E950.4	E962.0	E980.4
Beta-Chlor	967.1	E852.0	E937.1	E950.2	E962.0	E980.2
Betamethasone	962.0	E858.0	E932.0	E950.4	E962.0	E980.4
topical	976.0	E858.7	E946.0	E950.4	E962.0	E980.4
Betazole	977.8	E858.8	E947.8	E950.4	E962.0	E980.4
Bethanechol	971.0	E855.3	E941.0	E950.4	E962.0	E980.4
Bethanidine	972.6	E858.3	E942.6	E950.4	E962.0	E980.4
Betula oil	976.3	E858.7	E946.3	E950.4	E962.0	E980.4
Bhang	969.6	E854.1	E939.6	E950.3	E962.0	E980.3
Bialamicol	961.5	E857	E931.5	E950.4	E962.0	E980.4
Bichloride of mercury — see Mercury, chloride						
Bichromates (calcium) (crystals) (potassium) (sodium)	983.9	E864.3	—	E950.7	E962.1	E980.6
fumes	987.8	E869.8	—	E952.8	E962.2	E982.8
Biguanide derivatives, oral	962.3	E858.0	E932.3	E950.4	E962.0	E980.4
Biligrafin	977.8	E858.8	E947.8	E950.4	E962.0	E980.4
Bilopaque	977.8	E858.8	E947.8	E950.4	E962.0	E980.4
Bioflavonoids	972.8	E858.3	E942.8	E950.4	E962.0	E980.4
Biological substance NEC	979.9	E858.8	E949.9	E950.4	E962.0	E980.4
Biperiden	966.4	E855.0	E936.4	E950.4	E962.0	E980.4
Bisacodyl	973.1	E858.4	E943.1	E950.4	E962.0	E980.4
Bishydroxycoumarin	964.2	E858.2	E934.2	E950.4	E962.0	E980.4
Bismarsen	961.1	E857	E931.1	E950.4	E962.0	E980.4
Bismuth (compounds) NEC	985.8	E866.4	—	E950.9	E962.1	E980.9
anti-infectives	961.2	E857	E931.2	E950.4	E962.0	E980.4
subcarbonate	973.5	E858.4	E943.5	E950.4	E962.0	E980.4
sulfarsphenamine	961.1	E857	E931.1	E950.4	E962.0	E980.4
Bithionol	961.6	E857	E931.6	E950.4	E962.0	E980.4
Bitter almond oil	989.0	E866.8	—	E950.9	E962.1	E980.9
Bittersweet	988.2	E865.4	—	E950.9	E962.1	E930.9
Black						
flag	989.4	E863.4	—	E950.6	E962.1	E980.7
henbane	988.2	E865.4	—	E950.9	E962.1	E980.9
leaf (40)	989.4	E863.4	—	E950.6	E962.1	E980.7
widow spider (bite)	989.5	E905.1	—	E950.9	E962.1	E980.9
antivenin	979.9	E858.8	E949.9	E950.4	E962.0	E980.4
Blast furnace gas (carbon monoxide from)	986	E868.8	—	E952.1	E962.2	E982.1
Bleach NEC	983.9	E864.3	—	E950.7	E962.1	E980.6
Bleaching solutions	983.9	E864.3	—	E950.7	E962.1	E980.6
Bleomycin (sulfate)	960.7	E856	E930.7	E950.4	E962.0	E980.4
Blockain	968.9	E855.2	E938.9	E950.4	E962.0	E980.4
infiltration (subcutaneous)	968.5	E855.2	E938.5	E950.4	E962.0	E980.4

Blockain — Table of Drugs and Chemicals

		External Cause (E-Code)				
	Poisoning	Accident	Therapeutic Use	Suicide Attempt	Assault	Undetermined
Blockain — continued						
nerve block (peripheral)						
(plexus)	968.6	E855.2	E938.6	E950.4	E962.0	E980.4
topical (surface)	968.5	E855.2	E938.5	E950.4	E962.0	E980.4
Blood (derivatives) (natural)						
(plasma) (whole)	964.7	E858.2	E934.7	E950.4	E962.0	E980.4
affecting agent	964.9	E858.2	E934.9	E950.4	E962.0	E980.4
specified NEC	964.8	E858.2	E934.8	E950.4	E962.0	E980.4
substitute						
(macromolecular)	964.8	E858.2	E934.8	E950.4	E962.0	E980.4
Blue velvet	965.09	E850.2	E935.2	E950.0	E962.0	E980.0
Bone meal	989.89	E866.5	—	E950.9	E962.1	E980.9
Bonine	963.0	E858.1	E933.0	E950.4	E962.0	E980.4
Boracic acid	976.0	E858.7	E946.0	E950.4	E962.0	E980.4
ENT agent	976.6	E858.7	E946.6	E950.4	E962.0	E980.4
ophthalmic preparation	976.5	E858.7	E946.5	E950.4	E962.0	E980.4
Borate (cleanser) (sodium)	989.6	E861.3	—	E950.9	E962.1	E980.9
Borax (cleanser)	989.6	E861.3	—	E950.9	E962.1	E980.9
Boric acid	976.0	E858.7	E946.0	E950.4	E962.0	E980.4
ENT agent	976.6	E858.7	E946.6	E950.4	E962.0	E980.4
ophthalmic preparation	976.5	E858.7	E946.5	E950.4	E962.0	E980.4
Boron hydride NEC	989.89	E866.8	—	E950.9	E962.1	E980.9
fumes or gas	987.8	E869.8	—	E952.8	E962.2	E982.8
Botox	975.3	E858.6	E945.3	E950.4	E962.0	E980.4
Brake fluid vapor	987.8	E869.8	—	E952.8	E962.2	E982.8
Brass (compounds) (fumes)	985.8	E866.4	—	E950.9	E962.1	E980.9
Brasso	981	E861.3	—	E950.9	E962.1	E980.9
Bretylium (tosylate)	972.6	E858.3	E942.6	E950.4	E962.0	E980.4
Brevital (sodium)	968.3	E855.1	E938.3	E950.4	E962.0	E980.4
British antilewisite	963.8	E858.1	E933.8	E950.4	E962.0	E980.4
Bromal (hydrate)	967.3	E852.2	E937.3	E950.2	E962.0	E980.2
Bromelains	963.4	E858.1	E933.4	E950.4	E962.0	E980.4
Bromides NEC	967.3	E852.2	E937.3	E950.2	E962.0	E980.2
Bromine (vapor)	987.8	E869.8	—	E952.8	E962.2	E982.8
compounds (medicinal)	967.3	E852.2	E937.3	E950.2	E962.0	E980.2
Bromisovalum	967.3	E852.2	E937.3	E950.2	E962.0	E980.2
Bromobenzyl cyanide	987.5	E869.3	—	E952.8	E962.2	E982.8
Bromodiphenhydramine	963.0	E858.1	E933.0	E950.4	E962.0	E980.4
Bromoform	967.3	E852.2	E937.3	E950.2	E962.0	E980.2
Bromophenol blue						
reagent	977.8	E858.8	E947.8	E950.4	E962.0	E980.4
Bromosalicylhydroxamic						
acid	961.8	E857	E931.8	E950.4	E962.0	E980.4
Bromo-seltzer	965.4	E850.4	E935.4	E950.0	E962.0	E980.0
Brompheniramine	963.0	E858.1	E933.0	E950.4	E962.0	E980.4
Bromural	967.3	E852.2	E937.3	E950.2	E962.0	E980.2
Brown spider (bite) (venom)	989.5	E905.1	—	E950.9	E962.1	E980.9
Brucia	988.2	E865.3	—	E950.9	E962.1	E980.9
Brucine	989.1	E863.7	—	E950.6	E962.1	E980.7
Brunswick green — see Copper						
Bruten — see Ibuprofen						
Bryonia (alba) (dioica)	988.2	E865.4	—	E950.9	E962.1	E980.9
Buclizine	969.5	E853.8	E939.5	E950.3	E962.0	E980.3
Bufferin	965.1	E850.3	E935.3	E950.0	E962.0	E980.0
Bufotenine	969.6	E854.1	E939.6	E950.3	E962.0	E980.3
Buphenine	971.2	E855.5	E941.2	E950.4	E962.0	E980.4
Bupivacaine	968.9	E855.2	E938.9	E950.4	E962.0	E980.4
infiltration (subcutaneous)	968.5	E855.2	E938.5	E950.4	E962.0	E980.4
nerve block (peripheral)						
(plexus)	968.6	E855.2	E938.6	E950.4	E962.0	E980.4
Busulfan	963.1	E858.1	E933.1	E950.4	E962.0	E980.4
Butabarbital (sodium)	967.0	E851	E937.0	E950.1	E962.0	E980.1
Butabarbitone	967.0	E851	E937.0	E950.1	E962.0	E980.1
Butabarpal	967.0	E851	E937.0	E950.1	E962.0	E980.1
Butacaine	968.5	E855.2	E938.5	E950.4	E962.0	E980.4
Butallylonal	967.0	E851	E937.0	E950.1	E962.0	E980.1
Butane (distributed in mobile						
container)	987.0	E868.0	—	E951.1	E962.2	E981.1
distributed through pipes	987.0	E867	—	E951.0	E962.2	E981.0
incomplete combustion of — see						
Carbon monoxide, butane						
Butanol	980.3	E860.4	—	E950.9	E962.1	E980.9
Butanone	982.8	E862.4	—	E950.9	E962.1	E980.9
Butaperazine	969.1	E853.0	E939.1	E950.3	E962.0	E980.3
Butazolidin	965.5	E850.5	E935.5	E950.0	E962.0	E980.0
Butethal	967.0	E851	E937.0	E950.1	E962.0	E980.1
Butethamate	971.1	E855.4	E941.1	E950.4	E962.0	E980.4
Buthalitone (sodium)	968.3	E855.1	E938.3	E950.4	E962.0	E980.4
Butisol (sodium)	967.0	E851	E937.0	E950.1	E962.0	E980.1
Butobarbital,						
butobarbitone	967.0	E851	E937.0	E950.1	E962.0	E980.1
Butriptyline	969.0	E854.0	E939.0	E950.3	E962.0	E980.3
Buttercups	988.2	E865.4	—	E950.9	E962.1	E980.9
Butter of antimony — see Antimony						
Butyl						
acetate (secondary)	982.8	E862.4	—	E950.9	E962.1	E980.9
alcohol	980.3	E860.4	—	E950.9	E962.1	E980.9
carbinol	980.8	E860.8	—	E950.9	E962.1	E980.9
carbitol	982.8	E862.4	—	E950.9	E962.1	E980.9
cellosolve	982.8	E862.4	—	E950.9	E962.1	E980.9
chloral (hydrate)	967.1	E852.0	E937.1	E950.2	E962.0	E980.2
formate	982.8	E862.4	—	E950.9	E962.1	E980.9
scopolammonium bromide	971.1	E855.4	E941.1	E950.4	E962.0	E980.4
Butyn	968.5	E855.2	E938.5	E950.4	E962.0	E980.4
Butyrophenone (-based tranquilizers)	969.2	E853.1	E939.2	E950.3	E962.0	E980.3
Cacodyl, cacodylic acid — see Arsenic						
Cactinomycin	960.7	E856	E930.7	E950.4	E962.0	E980.4
Cade oil	976.4	E858.7	E946.4	E950.4	E962.0	E980.4
Cadmium (chloride) (compounds)						
(dust) (fumes) (oxide)	985.5	E866.4	—	E950.9	E962.1	E980.9
sulfide (medicinal) NEC	976.4	E858.7	E946.4	E950.4	E962.0	E980.4
Caffeine	969.7	E854.2	E939.7	E950.3	E962.0	E980.3
Calabar bean	988.2	E865.4	—	E950.9	E962.1	E980.9
Caladium seguinium	988.2	E865.4	—	E950.9	E962.1	E980.9
Calamine (liniment) (lotion)	976.3	E858.7	E946.3	E950.4	E962.0	E980.4
Calciferol	963.5	E858.1	E933.5	E950.4	E962.0	E980.4
Calcium (salts) NEC	974.5	E858.5	E944.5	E950.4	E962.0	E980.4
acetylsalicylate	965.1	E850.3	E935.3	E950.0	E962.0	E980.0
benzamidosalicylate	961.8	E857	E931.8	E950.4	E962.0	E980.4
carbaspirin	965.1	E850.3	E935.3	E950.0	E962.0	E980.0
carbimide (citrated)	977.3	E858.8	E947.3	E950.4	E962.0	E980.4
carbonate (antacid)	973.0	E858.4	E943.0	E950.4	E962.0	E980.4
cyanide (citrated)	977.3	E858.8	E947.3	E950.4	E962.0	E980.4
dioctyl sulfosuccinate	973.2	E858.4	E943.2	E950.4	E962.0	E980.4
disodium edathamil	963.8	E858.1	E933.8	E950.4	E962.0	E980.4
disodium edetate	963.8	E858.1	E933.8	E950.4	E962.0	E980.4
EDTA	963.8	E858.1	E933.8	E950.4	E962.0	E980.4
hydrate, hydroxide	983.2	E864.2	—	E950.7	E962.1	E980.6
mandelate	961.9	E857	E931.9	E950.4	E962.0	E980.4
oxide	983.2	E864.2	—	E950.7	E962.1	E980.6
Calomel — see Mercury, chloride						
Caloric agents NEC	974.5	E858.5	E944.5	E950.4	E962.0	E980.4
Calusterone	963.1	E858.1	E933.1	E950.4	E962.0	E980.4
Camoquin	961.4	E857	E931.4	E950.4	E962.0	E980.4
Camphor (oil)	976.1	E858.7	E946.1	E950.4	E962.0	E980.4
Candeptin	976.0	E858.7	E946.0	E950.4	E962.0	E980.4
Candicidin	976.0	E858.7	E946.0	E950.4	E962.0	E980.4
Cannabinols	969.6	E854.1	E939.6	E950.3	E962.0	E980.3
Cannabis (derivatives) (indica)						
(sativa)	969.6	E854.1	E939.6	E950.3	E962.0	E980.3
Canned heat	980.1	E860.2	—	E950.9	E962.1	E980.9
Cantharides, cantharidin, cantharis	976.8	E858.7	E946.8	E950.4	E962.0	E980.4
Capillary agents	972.8	E858.3	E942.8	E950.4	E962.0	E980.4
Capreomycin	960.6	E856	E930.6	E950.4	E962.0	E980.4
Captodiame, captodiamine	969.5	E853.8	E939.5	E950.3	E962.0	E980.3
Caramiphen (hydrochloride)	971.1	E855.4	E941.1	E950.4	E962.0	E980.4
Carbachol	971.0	E855.3	E941.0	E950.4	E962.0	E980.4
Carbacrylamine resins	974.5	E858.5	E944.5	E950.4	E962.0	E980.4
Carbamate (sedative)	967.8	E852.8	E937.8	E950.2	E962.0	E980.2
herbicide	989.3	E863.5	—	E950.6	E962.1	E980.7
insecticide	989.3	E863.2	—	E950.6	E962.1	E980.7
Carbamazepine	966.3	E855.0	E936.3	E950.4	E962.0	E980.4
Carbamic esters	967.8	E852.8	E937.8	E950.2	E962.0	E980.2
Carbamide	974.4	E858.5	E944.4	E950.4	E962.0	E980.4
topical	976.8	E858.7	E946.8	E950.4	E962.0	E980.4
Carbamylcholine chloride	971.0	E855.3	E941.0	E950.4	E962.0	E980.4
Carbarsone	961.1	E857	E931.1	E950.4	E962.0	E980.4
Carbaryl	989.3	E863.2	—	E950.6	E962.1	E980.7
Carbaspirin	965.1	E850.3	E935.3	E950.0	E962.0	E980.0
Carbazochrome	972.8	E858.3	E942.8	E950.4	E962.0	E980.4
Carbenicillin	960.0	E856	E930.0	E950.4	E962.0	E980.4
Carbenoxolone	973.8	E858.4	E943.8	E950.4	E962.0	E980.4
Carbetapentane	975.4	E858.6	E945.4	E950.4	E962.0	E980.4
Carbimazole	962.8	E858.0	E932.8	E950.4	E962.0	E980.4
Carbinol	980.1	E860.2	—	E950.9	E962.1	E980.9
Carbinoxamine	963.0	E858.1	E933.0	E950.4	E962.0	E980.4
Carbitol	982.8	E862.4	—	E950.9	E962.1	E980.9

Table of Drugs and Chemicals

	Poisoning	Accident	Therapeutic Use	Suicide Attempt	Assault	Undetermined
Carbocaine	968.9	E855.2	E938.9	E950.4	E962.0	E980.4
infiltration (subcutaneous)	968.5	E855.2	E938.5	E950.4	E962.0	E980.4
nerve block (peripheral) (plexus)	968.6	E855.2	E938.6	E950.4	E962.0	E980.4
topical (surface)	968.5	E855.2	E938.5	E950.4	E962.0	E980.4
Carbol-fuchsin solution	976.0	E858.7	E946.0	E950.4	E962.0	E980.4
Carbolic acid — see also Phenol	983.0	E864.0	—	E950.7	E962.1	E980.6
Carbomycin	960.8	E856	E930.8	E950.4	E962.0	E980.4
Carbon						
bisulfide (liquid) (vapor)	982.2	E862.4	—	E950.9	E962.1	E980.9
dioxide (gas)	987.8	E869.8	—	E952.8	E962.2	E982.8
disulfide (liquid) (vapor)	982.2	E862.4	—	E950.9	E962.1	E980.9
monoxide (from incomplete combustion of) (in)						
NEC	986	E868.9	—	E952.1	E962.2	E982.1
blast furnace gas	986	E868.8	—	E952.1	E962.2	E982.1
butane (distributed in mobile container)	986	E868.0	—	E951.1	E962.2	E981.1
distributed through pipes	986	E867	—	E951.0	E962.2	E981.0
charcoal fumes	986	E868.3	—	E952.1	E962.2	E982.1
coal						
gas (piped)	986	E867	—	E951.0	E962.2	E981.0
solid (in domestic stoves, fireplaces)	986	E868.3	—	E952.1	E962.2	E982.1
coke (in domestic stoves, fireplaces)	986	E868.3	—	E952.1	E962.2	E982.1
exhaust gas (motor) not in transit	986	E868.2	—	E952.0	E962.2	E982.0
combustion engine, any not in watercraft	986	E868.2	—	E952.0	E962.2	E982.0
farm tractor, not in transit	986	E868.2	—	E952.0	E962.2	E982.0
gas engine	986	E868.2	—	E952.0	E962.2	E982.0
motor pump	986	E868.2	—	E952.0	E962.2	E982.0
motor vehicle, not in transit	986	E868.2	—	E952.0	E962.2	E982.0
fuel (in domestic use)	986	E868.3	—	E952.1	E962.2	E982.1
gas (piped)	986	E867	—	E951.0	E962.2	E981.0
in mobile container	986	E868.0	—	E951.1	E962.2	E981.1
utility	986	E868.1	—	E951.8	E962.2	E981.1
in mobile container	986	E868.0	—	E951.1	E962.2	E981.1
piped (natural)	986	E867	—	E951.0	E962.2	E981.0
illuminating gas	986	E868.1	—	E951.8	E962.2	E981.8
industrial fuels or gases, any	986	E868.8	—	E952.1	E962.2	E982.1
kerosene (in domestic stoves, fireplaces)	986	E868.3	—	E952.1	E962.2	E982.1
kiln gas or vapor	986	E868.8	—	E952.1	E962.2	E982.1
motor exhaust gas, not in transit	986	E868.2	—	E952.0	E962.2	E982.0
piped gas (manufactured) (natural)	986	E867	—	E951.0	E962.2	E981.0
producer gas	986	E868.8	—	E952.1	E962.2	E982.1
propane (distributed in mobile container)	986	E868.0	—	E951.1	E962.2	E981.1
distributed through pipes	986	E867	—	E951.0	E962.2	E981.0
specified source NEC	986	E868.8	—	E952.1	E962.2	E982.1
stove gas	986	E868.1	—	E951.8	E962.2	E981.8
piped	986	E867	—	E951.0	E962.2	E981.0
utility gas	986	E868.1	—	E951.8	E962.2	E981.8
piped	986	E867	—	E951.0	E962.2	E981.0
water gas	986	E868.1	—	E951.8	E962.2	E981.8
wood (in domestic stoves, fireplaces)	986	E868.3	—	E952.1	E962.2	E982.1
tetrachloride (vapor) NEC	987.8	E869.8	—	E952.8	E962.2	E982.8
liquid (cleansing agent) NEC	982.1	E861.3	—	E950.9	E962.1	E980.9
solvent	982.1	E862.4	—	E950.9	E962.1	E980.9
Carbonic acid (gas)	987.8	E869.8	—	E952.8	E962.2	E982.8
anhydrase inhibitors	974.2	E858.5	E944.2	E950.4	E962.0	E980.4
Carbowax	976.3	E858.7	E946.3	E950.4	E962.0	E980.4
Carbrital	967.0	E851	E937.0	E950.1	E962.0	E980.1
Carbromal (derivatives)	967.3	E852.2	E937.3	E950.2	E962.0	E980.2
Cardiac						
depressants	972.0	E858.3	E942.0	E950.4	E962.0	E980.4
rhythm regulators	972.0	E858.3	E942.0	E950.4	E962.0	E980.4
Cardiografin	977.8	E858.8	E947.8	E950.4	E962.0	E980.4
Cardio-green	977.8	E858.8	E947.8	E950.4	E962.0	E980.4
Cardiotonic glycosides	972.1	E858.3	E942.1	E950.4	E962.0	E980.4
Cardiovascular agents NEC	972.9	E858.3	E942.9	E950.4	E962.0	E980.4
Cardrase	974.2	E858.5	E944.2	E950.4	E962.0	E980.4
Carfusin	976.0	E858.7	E946.0	E950.4	E962.0	E980.4
Carisoprodol	968.0	E855.1	E938.0	E950.4	E962.0	E980.4
Carmustine	963.1	E858.1	E933.1	E950.4	E962.0	E980.4
Carotene	963.5	E858.1	E933.5	E950.4	E962.0	E980.4
Carphenazine (maleate)	969.1	E853.0	E939.1	E950.3	E962.0	E980.3
Carter's Little Pills	973.1	E858.4	E943.1	E950.4	E962.0	E980.4
Cascara (sagrada)	973.1	E858.4	E943.1	E950.4	E962.0	E980.4
Cassava	988.2	E865.4	—	E950.9	E962.1	E980.9
Castellani's paint	976.0	E858.7	E946.0	E950.4	E962.0	E980.4
Castor						
bean	988.2	E865.3	—	E950.9	E962.1	E980.9
oil	973.1	E858.4	E943.1	E950.4	E962.0	E980.4
Caterpillar (sting)	989.5	E905.5	—	E950.9	E962.1	E980.9
Catha (edulis)	970.8	E854.3	E940.8	E950.4	E962.0	E980.4
Cathartics NEC	973.3	E858.4	E943.3	E950.4	E962.0	E980.4
contact	973.1	E858.4	E943.1	E950.4	E962.0	E980.4
emollient	973.2	E858.4	E943.2	E950.4	E962.0	E980.4
intestinal irritants	973.1	E858.4	E943.1	E950.4	E962.0	E980.4
saline	973.3	E858.4	E943.3	E950.4	E962.0	E980.4
Cathomycin	960.8	E856	E930.8	E950.4	E962.0	E980.4
Caustic(s)	983.9	E864.4	—	E950.7	E962.1	E980.6
alkali	983.2	E864.2	—	E950.7	E962.1	E980.6
hydroxide	983.2	E864.2	—	E950.7	E962.1	E980.6
potash	983.2	E864.2	—	E950.7	E962.1	E980.6
soda	983.2	E864.2	—	E950.7	E962.1	E980.6
specified NEC	983.9	E864.3	—	E950.7	E962.1	E980.6
Ceepryn	976.0	E858.7	E946.0	E950.4	E962.0	E980.4
ENT agent	976.6	E858.7	E946.6	E950.4	E962.0	E980.4
lozenges	976.6	E858.7	E946.6	E950.4	E962.0	E980.4
Celestone	962.0	E858.0	E932.0	E950.4	E962.0	E980.4
topical	976.0	E858.7	E946.0	E950.4	E962.0	E980.4
Cellosolve	982.8	E862.4	—	E950.9	E962.1	E980.9
Cell stimulants and proliferants	976.8	E858.7	E946.8	E950.4	E962.0	E980.4
Cellulose derivatives,						
cathartic	973.3	E858.4	E943.3	E950.4	E962.0	E980.4
nitrates (topical)	976.3	E858.7	E946.3	E950.4	E962.0	E980.4
Centipede (bite)	989.5	E905.4	—	E950.9	E962.1	E980.9
Central nervous system						
depressants	968.4	E855.1	E938.4	E950.4	E962.0	E980.4
anesthetic (general) NEC	968.4	E855.1	E938.4	E950.4	E962.0	E980.4
gases NEC	968.2	E855.1	E938.2	E950.4	E962.0	E980.4
intravenous	968.3	E855.1	E938.3	E950.4	E962.0	E980.4
barbiturates	967.0	E851	E937.0	E950.1	E962.0	E980.1
bromides	967.3	E852.2	E937.3	E950.2	E962.0	E980.2
cannabis sativa	969.6	E854.1	E939.6	E950.3	E962.0	E980.3
chloral hydrate	967.1	E852.0	E937.1	E950.2	E962.0	E980.2
hallucinogenics	969.6	E854.1	E939.6	E950.3	E962.0	E980.3
hypnotics	967.9	E852.9	E937.9	E950.2	E962.0	E980.2
specified NEC	967.8	E852.8	E937.8	E950.2	E962.0	E980.2
muscle relaxants	968.0	E855.1	E938.0	E950.4	E962.0	E980.4
paraldehyde	967.2	E852.1	E937.2	E950.2	E962.0	E980.2
sedatives	967.9	E852.9	E937.9	E950.2	E962.0	E980.2
mixed NEC	967.6	E852.5	E937.6	E950.2	E962.0	E980.2
specified NEC	967.8	E852.8	E937.8	E950.2	E962.0	E980.2
muscle-tone depressants	—	—	—	—	—	E980.4
stimulants	970.9	E854.3	E940.9	E950.4	E962.0	E980.4
amphetamines	969.7	E854.2	E939.7	E950.3	E962.0	E980.3
analeptics	970.0	E854.3	E940.0	E950.4	E962.0	E980.4
antidepressants	969.0	E854.0	E939.0	E950.3	E962.0	E980.3
opiate antagonists	970.1	E854.3	E940.1	E950.4	E962.0	E980.4
specified NEC	970.8	E854.3	E940.8	E950.4	E962.0	E980.4
Cephalexin	960.5	E856	E930.5	E950.4	E962.0	E980.4
Cephaloglycin	960.5	E856	E930.5	E950.4	E962.0	E980.4
Cephaloridine	960.5	E856	E930.5	E950.4	E962.0	E980.4
Cephalosporins NEC	960.5	E856	E930.5	E950.4	E962.0	E980.4
N (adicillin)	960.0	E856	E930.0	E950.4	E962.0	E980.4
Cephalothin (sodium)	960.5	E856	E930.5	E950.4	E962.0	E980.4
Cerbera (odallam)	988.2	E865.4	—	E950.9	E962.1	E980.9
Cerberin	972.1	E858.3	E942.1	E950.4	E962.0	E980.4
Cerebral stimulants	970.9	E854.3	E940.9	E950.4	E962.0	E980.4
psychotherapeutic	969.7	E854.2	E939.7	E950.3	E962.0	E980.3
specified NEC	970.8	E854.3	E940.8	E950.4	E962.0	E980.4
Cetalkonium (chloride)	976.0	E858.7	E946.0	E950.4	E962.0	E980.4
Cetoxime	963.0	E858.1	E933.0	E950.4	E962.0	E980.4
Cetrimide	976.2	E858.7	E946.2	E950.4	E962.0	E980.4
Cetylpyridinium	976.0	E858.7	E946.0	E950.4	E962.0	E980.4
ENT agent	976.6	E858.7	E946.6	E950.4	E962.0	E980.4

Cetylpyridinium — Table of Drugs and Chemicals

	Poisoning	External Cause (E-Code)				
		Accident	Therapeutic Use	Suicide Attempt	Assault	Undetermined
Cetylpyridinium — continued						
lozenges	976.6	E858.7	E946.6	E950.4	E962.0	E980.4
Cevadilla — see Sabadilla						
Cevitamic acid	963.5	E858.1	E933.5	E950.4	E962.0	E980.4
Chalk, precipitated	973.0	E858.4	E943.0	E950.4	E962.0	E980.4
Charcoal						
fumes (carbon monoxide)	986	E868.3	—	E952.1	E962.2	E982.1
industrial	986	E868.8	—	E952.1	E962.2	E982.1
medicinal (activated)	973.0	E858.4	E943.0	E950.4	E962.0	E980.4
Chelating agents NEC	977.2	E858.8	E947.2	E950.4	E962.0	E980.4
Chelidonium majus	988.2	E865.4	—	E950.9	E962.1	E980.9
Chemical substance	989.9	E866.9	—	E950.9	E962.1	E980.9
specified NEC	989.89	E866.8	—	E950.9	E962.1	E980.9
Chemotherapy, antineoplastic	963.1	E858.1	E933.1	E950.4	E962.0	E980.4
Chenopodium (oil)	961.6	E857	E931.6	E950.4	E962.0	E980.4
Cherry laurel	988.2	E865.4	—	E950.9	E962.1	E980.9
Chiniofon	961.3	E857	E931.3	E950.4	E962.0	E980.4
Chlophedianol	975.4	E858.6	E945.4	E950.4	E962.0	E980.4
Chloral (betaine) (formamide) (hydrate)	967.1	E852.0	E937.1	E950.2	E962.0	E980.2
Chloralamide	967.1	E852.0	E937.1	E950.2	E962.0	E980.2
Chlorambucil	963.1	E858.1	E933.1	E950.4	E962.0	E980.4
Chloramphenicol	960.2	E856	E930.2	E950.4	E962.0	E980.4
ENT agent	976.6	E858.7	E946.6	E950.4	E962.0	E980.4
ophthalmic preparation	976.5	E858.7	E946.5	E950.4	E962.0	E980.4
topical NEC	976.0	E858.7	E946.0	E950.4	E962.0	E980.4
Chlorate(s) (potassium) (sodium) NEC	983.9	E864.3	—	E950.7	E962.1	E980.6
herbicides	989.4	E863.5	—	E950.6	E962.1	E980.7
Chlorcyclizine	963.0	E858.1	E933.0	E950.4	E962.0	E980.4
Chlordan(e) (dust)	989.2	E863.0	—	E950.6	E962.1	E980.7
Chlordantoin	976.0	E858.7	E946.0	E950.4	E962.0	E980.4
Chlordiazepoxide	969.4	E853.2	E939.4	E950.3	E962.0	E980.3
Chloresium	976.8	E858.7	E946.8	E950.4	E962.0	E980.4
Chlorethiazol	967.1	E852.0	E937.1	E950.2	E962.0	E980.2
Chlorethyl — see Ethyl, chloride						
Chloretone	967.1	E852.0	E937.1	E950.2	E962.0	E980.2
Chlorex	982.3	E862.4	—	E950.9	E962.1	E980.9
Chlorhexadol	967.1	E852.0	E937.1	E950.2	E962.0	E980.2
Chlorhexidine (hydrochloride)	976.0	E858.7	E946.0	E950.4	E962.0	E980.4
Chlorhydroxyquinolin	976.0	E858.7	E946.0	E950.4	E962.0	E980.4
Chloride of lime (bleach)	983.9	E864.3	—	E950.7	E962.1	E980.6
Chlorinated						
camphene	989.2	E863.0	—	E950.6	E962.1	E980.7
diphenyl	989.89	E866.8	—	E950.9	E962.1	E980.9
hydrocarbons NEC	989.2	E863.0	—	E950.6	E962.1	E980.7
solvent	982.3	E862.4	—	E950.9	E962.1	E980.9
lime (bleach)	983.9	E864.3	—	E950.7	E962.1	E980.6
naphthalene — see Naphthalene						
pesticides NEC	989.2	E863.0	—	E950.6	E962.1	E980.7
soda — see Sodium, hypochlorite						
Chlorine (fumes) (gas)	987.6	E869.8	—	E952.8	E962.2	E982.8
bleach	983.9	E864.3	—	E950.7	E962.1	E980.6
compounds NEC	983.9	E864.3	—	E950.7	E962.1	E980.6
disinfectant	983.9	E861.4	—	E950.7	E962.1	E980.6
releasing agents NEC	983.9	E864.3	—	E950.7	E962.1	E980.6
Chlorisondamine	972.3	E858.3	E942.3	E950.4	E962.0	E980.4
Chlormadinone	962.2	E858.0	E932.2	E950.4	E962.0	E980.4
Chlormerodrin	974.0	E858.5	E944.0	E950.4	E962.0	E980.4
Chlormethiazole	967.1	E852.0	E937.1	E950.2	E962.0	E980.2
Chlormethylenecycline	960.4	E856	E930.4	E950.4	E962.0	E980.4
Chlormezanone	969.5	E853.8	E939.5	E950.3	E962.0	E980.3
Chloroacetophenone	987.5	E869.3	—	E952.8	E962.2	E982.8
Chloroaniline	983.0	E864.0	—	E950.7	E962.1	E980.6
Chlorobenzene, chlorobenzol	982.0	E862.4	—	E950.9	E962.1	E980.9
Chlorobutanol	967.1	E852.0	E937.1	E950.2	E962.0	E980.2
Chlorodinitrobenzene	983.0	E864.0	—	E950.7	E962.1	E980.6
dust or vapor	987.8	E869.8	—	E952.8	E962.2	E982.8
Chloroethane — see Ethyl, chloride						
Chloroform (fumes) (vapor)	987.8	E869.8	—	E952.8	E962.2	E982.8
anesthetic (gas)	968.2	E855.1	E938.2	E950.4	E962.0	E980.4
liquid NEC	968.4	E855.1	E938.4	E950.4	E962.0	E980.4
solvent	982.3	E862.4	—	E950.9	E962.1	E980.9
Chloroguanide	961.4	E857	E931.4	E950.4	E962.0	E980.4
Chloromycetin	960.2	E856	E930.2	E950.4	E962.0	E980.4
Chloromycetin — continued						
ENT agent	976.6	E858.7	E946.6	E950.4	E962.0	E980.4
ophthalmic preparation	976.5	E858.7	E946.5	E950.4	E962.0	E980.4
otic solution	976.6	E858.7	E946.6	E950.4	E962.0	E980.4
topical NEC	976.0	E858.7	E946.0	E950.4	E962.0	E980.4
Chloronitrobenzene	983.0	E864.0	—	E950.7	E962.1	E980.6
dust or vapor	987.8	E869.8	—	E952.8	E962.2	E982.8
Chlorophenol	983.0	E864.0	—	E950.7	E962.1	E980.6
Chlorophenothane	989.2	E863.0	—	E950.6	E962.1	E980.7
Chlorophyll (derivatives)	976.8	E858.7	E946.8	E950.4	E962.0	E980.4
Chloropicrin (fumes)	987.8	E869.8	—	E952.8	E962.2	E982.8
fumigant	989.4	E863.8	—	E950.6	E962.1	E980.7
fungicide	989.4	E863.6	—	E950.6	E962.1	E980.7
pesticide (fumes)	989.4	E863.4	—	E950.6	E962.1	E980.7
Chloroprocaine	968.9	E855.2	E938.9	E950.4	E962.0	E980.4
infiltration (subcutaneous)	968.5	E855.2	E938.5	E950.4	E962.0	E980.4
nerve block (peripheral) (plexus)	968.6	E855.2	E938.6	E950.4	E962.0	E980.4
Chloroptic	976.5	E858.7	E946.5	E950.4	E962.0	E980.4
Chloropurine	963.1	E858.1	E933.1	E950.4	E962.0	E980.4
Chloroquine (hydrochloride) (phosphate)	961.4	E857	E931.4	E950.4	E962.0	E980.4
Chlorothen	963.0	E858.1	E933.0	E950.4	E962.0	E980.4
Chlorothiazide	974.3	E858.5	E944.3	E950.4	E962.0	E980.4
Chlorotrianisene	962.2	E858.0	E932.2	E950.4	E962.0	E980.4
Chlorovinyldichloroarsine	985.1	E866.3	—	E950.8	E962.1	E980.8
Chloroxylenol	976.0	E858.7	E946.0	E950.4	E962.0	E980.4
Chlorphenesin (carbamate)	968.0	E855.1	E938.0	E950.4	E962.0	E980.4
topical (antifungal)	976.0	E858.7	E946.0	E950.4	E962.0	E980.4
Chlorpheniramine	963.0	E858.1	E933.0	E950.4	E962.0	E980.4
Chlorphenoxamine	966.4	E855.0	E936.4	E950.4	E962.0	E980.4
Chlorphentermine	977.0	E858.8	E947.0	E950.4	E962.0	E980.4
Chlorproguanil	961.4	E857	E931.4	E950.4	E962.0	E980.4
Chlorpromazine	969.1	E853.0	E939.1	E950.3	E962.0	E980.3
Chlorpropamide	962.3	E858.0	E932.3	E950.4	E962.0	E980.4
Chlorprothixene	969.3	E853.8	E939.3	E950.3	E962.0	E980.3
Chlorquinaldol	976.0	E858.7	E946.0	E950.4	E962.0	E980.4
Chlortetracycline	960.4	E856	E930.4	E950.4	E962.0	E980.4
Chlorthalidone	974.4	E858.5	E944.4	E950.4	E962.0	E980.4
Chlortrianisene	962.2	E858.0	E932.2	E950.4	E962.0	E980.4
Chlor-Trimeton	963.0	E858.1	E933.0	E950.4	E962.0	E980.4
Chlorzoxazone	968.0	E855.1	E938.0	E950.4	E962.0	E980.4
Choke damp	987.8	E869.8	—	E952.8	E962.2	E982.8
Cholebrine	977.8	E858.8	E947.8	E950.4	E962.0	E980.4
Cholera vaccine	978.2	E858.8	E948.2	E950.4	E962.0	E980.4
Cholesterol-lowering agents	972.2	E858.3	E942.2	E950.4	E962.0	E980.4
Cholestyramine (resin)	972.2	E858.3	E942.2	E950.4	E962.0	E980.4
Cholic acid	973.4	E858.4	E943.4	E950.4	E962.0	E980.4
Choline						
dihydrogen citrate	977.1	E858.8	E947.1	E950.4	E962.0	E980.4
salicylate	965.1	E850.3	E935.3	E950.0	E962.0	E980.0
theophyllinate	974.1	E858.5	E944.1	E950.4	E962.0	E980.4
Cholinergics	971.0	E855.3	E941.0	E950.4	E962.0	E980.4
Cholografin	977.8	E858.8	E947.8	E950.4	E962.0	E980.4
Chorionic gonadotropin	962.4	E858.0	E932.4	E950.4	E962.0	E980.4
Chromates	983.9	E864.3	—	E950.7	E962.1	E980.6
dust or mist	987.8	E869.8	—	E952.8	E962.2	E982.8
lead	984.0	E866.0	—	E950.9	E962.1	E980.9
paint	984.0	E861.5	—	E950.9	E962.1	E980.9
Chromic acid	983.9	E864.3	—	E950.7	E962.1	E980.6
dust or mist	987.8	E869.8	—	E952.8	E962.2	E982.8
Chromium	985.6	E866.4	—	E950.9	E962.1	E980.9
compounds — see Chromates						
Chromonar	972.4	E858.3	E942.4	E950.4	E962.0	E980.4
Chromyl chloride	983.9	E864.3	—	E950.7	E962.1	E980.6
Chrysarobin (ointment)	976.4	E858.7	E946.4	E950.4	E962.0	E980.4
Chrysazin	973.1	E858.4	E943.1	E950.4	E962.0	E980.4
Chymar	963.4	E858.1	E933.4	E950.4	E962.0	E980.4
ophthalmic preparation	976.5	E858.7	E946.5	E950.4	E962.0	E980.4
Chymotrypsin	963.4	E858.1	E933.4	E950.4	E962.0	E980.4
ophthalmic preparation	976.5	E858.7	E946.5	E950.4	E962.0	E980.4
Cicuta maculata or virosa	988.2	E865.4	—	E950.9	E962.1	E980.9
Cigarette lighter fluid	981	E862.1	—	E950.9	E962.1	E980.9
Cinchocaine (spinal)	968.7	E855.2	E938.7	E950.4	E962.0	E980.4
topical (surface)	968.5	E855.2	E938.5	E950.4	E962.0	E980.4
Cinchona	961.4	E857	E931.4	E950.4	E962.0	E980.4
Cinchonine alkaloids	961.4	E857	E931.4	E950.4	E962.0	E980.4
Cinchophen	974.7	E858.5	E944.7	E950.4	E962.0	E980.4
Cinnarizine	963.0	E858.1	E933.0	E950.4	E962.0	E980.4
Citanest	968.9	E855.2	E938.9	E950.4	E962.0	E980.4

Table of Drugs and Chemicals

	Poisoning	External Cause (E-Code)				
		Accident	Therapeutic Use	Suicide Attempt	Assault	Undetermined
Citanest — *continued*						
infiltration (subcutaneous)	968.5	E855.2	E938.5	E950.4	E962.0	E980.4
nerve block (peripheral) (plexus)	968.6	E855.2	E938.6	E950.4	E962.0	E980.4
Citric acid	989.89	E866.8	—	E950.9	E962.1	E980.9
Citrovorum factor	964.1	E858.2	E934.1	E950.4	E962.0	E980.4
Claviceps purpurea	988.2	E865.4	—	E950.9	E962.1	E980.9
Cleaner, cleansing agent						
NEC	989.89	E861.3	—	E950.9	E962.1	E980.9
of paint or varnish	982.8	E862.9	—	E950.9	E962.1	E980.9
Clematis vitalba	988.2	E865.4	—	E950.9	E962.1	E980.9
Clemizole	963.0	E858.1	E933.0	E950.4	E962.0	E980.4
penicillin	960.0	E856	E930.0	E950.4	E962.0	E980.4
Clidinium	971.1	E855.4	E941.1	E950.4	E962.0	E980.4
Clindamycin	960.8	E856	E930.8	E950.4	E962.0	E980.4
Cliradon	965.09	E850.2	E935.2	E950.0	E962.0	E980.0
Clocortolone	962.0	E858.0	E932.0	E950.4	E962.0	E980.4
Clofedanol	975.4	E858.6	E945.4	E950.4	E962.0	E980.4
Clofibrate	972.2	E858.3	E942.2	E950.4	E962.0	E980.4
Clomethiazole	967.1	E852.0	E937.1	E950.2	E962.0	E980.2
Clomiphene	977.8	E858.8	E947.8	E950.4	E962.0	E980.4
Clonazepam	969.4	E853.2	E939.4	E950.3	E962.0	E980.3
Clonidine	972.6	E858.3	E942.6	E950.4	E962.0	E980.4
Clopamide	974.3	E858.5	E944.3	E950.4	E962.0	E980.4
Clorazepate	969.4	E853.2	E939.4	E950.3	E962.0	E980.3
Clorexolone	974.4	E858.5	E944.4	E950.4	E962.0	E980.4
Clorox (bleach)	983.9	E864.3	—	E950.7	E962.1	E980.6
Clortermine	977.0	E858.8	E947.0	E950.4	E962.0	E980.4
Clotrimazole	976.0	E858.7	E946.0	E950.4	E962.0	E980.4
Cloxacillin	960.0	E856	E930.0	E950.4	E962.0	E980.4
Coagulants NEC	964.5	E858.2	E934.5	E950.4	E962.0	E980.4
Coal (carbon monoxide from) — *see also* Carbon, monoxide, coal						
oil — *see* Kerosene						
tar NEC	983.0	E864.0	—	E950.7	E962.1	E980.6
fumes	987.8	E869.8	—	E952.8	E962.2	E982.8
medicinal (ointment)	976.4	E858.7	E946.4	E950.4	E962.0	E980.4
analgesics NEC	965.5	E850.5	E935.5	E950.0	E962.0	E980.0
naphtha (solvent)	981	E862.0	—	E950.9	E962.1	E980.9
Cobalt (fumes) (industrial)	985.8	E866.4	—	E950.9	E962.1	E980.9
Cobra (venom)	989.5	E905.0	—	E950.9	E962.1	E980.9
Coca (leaf)	970.8	E854.3	E940.8	E950.4	E962.0	E980.4
Cocaine (hydrochloride) (salt)	970.8	E854.3	E940.8	E950.4	E962.0	E980.4
topical anesthetic	968.5	E855.2	E938.5	E950.4	E962.0	E980.4
Coccidioidin	977.8	E858.8	E947.8	E950.4	E962.0	E980.4
Cocculus indicus	988.2	E865.3	—	E950.9	E962.1	E980.9
Cochineal	989.89	E866.8	—	E950.9	E962.1	E980.9
medicinal products	977.4	E858.8	E947.4	E950.4	E962.0	E980.4
Codeine	965.09	E850.2	E935.2	E950.0	E962.0	E980.0
Coffee	989.89	E866.8	—	E950.9	E962.1	E980.9
Cogentin	971.1	E855.4	E941.1	E950.4	E962.0	E980.4
Coke fumes or gas (carbon monoxide)	986	E868.3	—	E952.1	E962.2	E982.1
industrial use	986	E868.8	—	E952.1	E962.2	E982.1
Colace	973.2	E858.4	E943.2	E950.4	E962.0	E980.4
Colchicine	974.7	E858.5	E944.7	E950.4	E962.0	E980.4
Colchicum	988.2	E865.3	—	E950.9	E962.1	E980.9
Cold cream	976.3	E858.7	E946.3	E950.4	E962.0	E980.4
Colestipol	972.2	E858.3	E942.2	E950.4	E962.0	E980.4
Colistimethate	960.8	E856	E930.8	E950.4	E962.0	E980.4
Colistin	960.8	E856	E930.8	E950.4	E962.0	E980.4
Collagen	977.8	E866.8	E947.8	E950.9	E962.1	E980.9
Collagenase	976.8	E858.7	E946.8	E950.4	E962.0	E980.4
Collodion (flexible)	976.3	E858.7	E946.3	E950.4	E962.0	E980.4
Colocynth	973.1	E858.4	E943.1	E950.4	E962.0	E980.4
Coloring matter — *see* Dye(s)						
Combustion gas — *see* Carbon, monoxide						
Compazine	969.1	E853.0	E939.1	E950.3	E962.0	E980.3
Compound						
42 (warfarin)	989.4	E863.7	—	E950.6	E962.1	E980.7
269 (endrin)	989.2	E863.0	—	E950.6	E962.1	E980.7
497 (dieldrin)	989.2	E863.0	—	E950.6	E962.1	E980.7
1080 (sodium fluoroacetate)	989.4	E863.7	—	E950.6	E962.1	E980.7
3422 (parathion)	989.3	E863.1	—	E950.6	E962.1	E980.7
3911 (phorate)	989.3	E863.1	—	E950.6	E962.1	E980.7
3956 (toxaphene)	989.2	E863.0	—	E950.6	E962.1	E980.7
4049 (malathion)	989.3	E863.1	—	E950.6	E962.1	E980.7
Compound — *continued*						
4124 (dicapthon)	989.4	E863.4	—	E950.6	E962.1	E980.7
E (cortisone)	962.0	E858.0	E932.0	E950.4	E962.0	E980.4
F (hydrocortisone)	962.0	E858.0	E932.0	E950.4	E962.0	E980.4
Congo red	977.8	E858.8	E947.8	E950.4	E962.0	E980.4
Coniine, conine	965.7	E850.7	E935.7	E950.0	E962.0	E980.0
Conium (maculatum)	988.2	E865.4	—	E950.9	E962.1	E980.9
Conjugated estrogens (equine)	962.2	E858.0	E932.2	E950.4	E962.0	E980.4
Contac	975.6	E858.6	E945.6	E950.4	E962.0	E980.4
Contact lens solution	976.5	E858.7	E946.5	E950.4	E962.0	E980.4
Contraceptives (oral)	962.2	E858.0	E932.2	E950.4	E962.0	E980.4
vaginal	976.8	E858.7	E946.8	E950.4	E962.0	E980.4
Contrast media (roentgenographic)	977.8	E858.8	E947.8	E950.4	E962.0	E980.4
Convallaria majalis	988.2	E865.4	—	E950.9	E962.1	E980.9
Copper (dust) (fumes) (salts)						
NEC	985.8	E866.4	—	E950.9	E962.1	E980.9
arsenate, arsenite	985.1	E866.3	—	E950.8	E962.1	E980.8
insecticide	985.1	E863.4	—	E950.8	E962.1	E980.8
emetic	973.6	E858.4	E943.6	E950.4	E962.0	E980.4
fungicide	985.8	E863.6	—	E950.6	E962.1	E980.7
insecticide	985.8	E863.4	—	E950.6	E962.1	E980.7
oleate	976.0	E858.7	E946.0	E950.4	E962.0	E980.4
sulfate	983.9	E864.3	—	E950.7	E962.1	E980.6
cupric	973.6	E858.4	E943.6	E950.4	E962.0	E980.4
cuprous	983.9	E864.3	—	E950.7	E962.1	E980.6
fungicide	983.9	E863.6	—	E950.7	E962.1	E980.6
Copperhead snake (bite) (venom)	989.5	E905.0	—	E950.9	E962.1	E980.9
Coral (sting)	989.5	E905.6	—	E950.9	E962.1	E980.9
snake (bite) (venom)	989.5	E905.0	—	E950.9	E962.1	E980.9
Cordran	976.0	E858.7	E946.0	E950.4	E962.0	E980.4
Corn cures	976.4	E858.7	E946.4	E950.4	E962.0	E980.4
Cornhusker's lotion	976.3	E858.7	E946.3	E950.4	E962.0	E980.4
Corn starch	976.3	E858.7	E946.3	E950.4	E962.0	E980.4
Corrosive	983.9	E864.4	—	E950.7	E962.1	E980.6
acids NEC	983.1	E864.1	—	E950.7	E962.1	E980.6
aromatics	983.0	E864.0	—	E950.7	E962.1	E980.6
disinfectant	983.0	E861.4	—	E950.7	E962.1	E980.6
fumes NEC	987.9	E869.9	—	E952.9	E962.2	E982.9
specified NEC	983.9	E864.3	—	E950.7	E962.1	E980.6
sublimate — *see* Mercury, chloride						
Cortate	962.0	E858.0	E932.0	E950.4	E962.0	E980.4
Cort-Dome	962.0	E858.0	E932.0	E950.4	E962.0	E980.4
ENT agent	976.6	E858.7	E946.6	E950.4	E962.0	E980.4
ophthalmic preparation	976.5	E858.7	E946.5	E950.4	E962.0	E980.4
topical NEC	976.0	E858.7	E946.0	E950.4	E962.0	E980.4
Cortef	962.0	E858.0	E932.0	E950.4	E962.0	E980.4
ENT agent	976.6	E858.7	E946.6	E950.4	E962.0	E980.4
ophthalmic preparation	976.5	E858.7	E946.5	E950.4	E962.0	E980.4
topical NEC	976.0	E858.7	E946.0	E950.4	E962.0	E980.4
Corticosteroids (fluorinated)	962.0	E858.0	E932.0	E950.4	E962.0	E980.4
ENT agent	976.6	E858.7	E946.6	E950.4	E962.0	E980.4
ophthalmic preparation	976.5	E858.7	E946.5	E950.4	E962.0	E980.4
topical NEC	976.0	E858.7	E946.0	E950.4	E962.0	E980.4
Corticotropin	962.4	E858.0	E932.4	E950.4	E962.0	E980.4
Cortisol	962.0	E858.0	E932.0	E950.4	E962.0	E980.4
ENT agent	976.6	E858.7	E946.6	E950.4	E962.0	E980.4
ophthalmic preparation	976.5	E858.7	E946.5	E950.4	E962.0	E980.4
topical NEC	976.0	E858.7	E946.0	E950.4	E962.0	E980.4
Cortisone derivatives (acetate)	962.0	E858.0	E932.0	E950.4	E962.0	E980.4
ENT agent	976.6	E858.7	E946.6	E950.4	E962.0	E980.4
ophthalmic preparation	976.5	E858.7	E946.5	E950.4	E962.0	E980.4
topical NEC	976.0	E858.7	E946.0	E950.4	E962.0	E980.4
Cortogen	962.0	E858.0	E932.0	E950.4	E962.0	E980.4
ENT agent	976.6	E858.7	E946.6	E950.4	E962.0	E980.4
ophthalmic preparation	976.5	E858.7	E946.5	E950.4	E962.0	E980.4
Cortone	962.0	E858.0	E932.0	E950.4	E962.0	E980.4
ENT agent	976.6	E858.7	E946.6	E950.4	E962.0	E980.4
ophthalmic preparation	976.5	E858.7	E946.5	E950.4	E962.0	E980.4
Cortril	962.0	E858.0	E932.0	E950.4	E962.0	E980.4
ENT agent	976.6	E858.7	E946.6	E950.4	E962.0	E980.4
ophthalmic preparation	976.5	E858.7	E946.5	E950.4	E962.0	E980.4
topical NEC	976.0	E858.7	E946.0	E950.4	E962.0	E980.4
Cosmetics	989.89	E866.7	—	E950.9	E962.1	E980.9
Cosyntropin	977.8	E858.8	E947.8	E950.4	E962.0	E980.4
Cotarnine	964.5	E858.2	E934.5	E950.4	E962.0	E980.4

Cottonseed oil

Table of Drugs and Chemicals

	Poisoning	Accident	Therapeutic Use	Suicide Attempt	Assault	Undetermined
Cottonseed oil	976.3	E858.7	E946.3	E950.4	E962.0	E980.4
Cough mixtures						
(antitussives)	975.4	E858.6	E945.4	E950.4	E962.0	E980.4
containing opiates	965.09	E850.2	E935.2	E950.0	E962.0	E980.0
expectorants	975.5	E858.6	E945.5	E950.4	E962.0	E980.4
Coumadin	964.2	E858.2	E934.2	E950.4	E962.0	E980.4
rodenticide	989.4	E863.7	—	E950.6	E962.1	E980.7
Coumarin	964.2	E858.2	E934.2	E950.4	E962.0	E980.4
Coumetarol	964.2	E858.2	E934.2	E950.4	E962.0	E980.4
Cowbane	988.2	E865.4	—	E950.9	E962.1	E980.9
Cozyme	963.5	E858.1	E933.5	E950.4	E962.0	E980.4
Crack	970.8	E854.3	E940.8	E950.4	E962.0	E980.4
Creolin	983.0	E864.0	—	E950.7	E962.1	E980.6
disinfectant	983.0	E861.4	—	E950.7	E962.1	E980.6
Creosol (compound)	983.0	E864.0	—	E950.7	E962.1	E980.6
Creosote (beechwood) (coal tar)	983.0	E864.0	—	E950.7	E962.1	E980.6
medicinal (expectorant)	975.5	E858.6	E945.5	E950.4	E962.0	E980.4
syrup	975.5	E858.6	E945.5	E950.4	E962.0	E980.4
Cresol	983.0	E864.0	—	E950.7	E962.1	E980.6
disinfectant	983.0	E861.4	—	E950.7	E962.1	E980.6
Cresylic acid	983.0	E864.0	—	E950.7	E962.1	E980.6
Cropropamide	965.7	E850.7	E935.7	E950.0	E962.0	E980.0
with crotethamide	970.0	E854.3	E940.0	E950.4	E962.0	E980.4
Crotamiton	976.0	E858.7	E946.0	E950.4	E962.0	E980.4
Crotethamide	965.7	E850.7	E935.7	E950.0	E962.0	E980.0
with cropropamide	970.0	E854.3	E940.0	E950.4	E962.0	E980.4
Croton (oil)	973.1	E858.4	E943.1	E950.4	E962.0	E980.4
chloral	967.1	E852.0	E937.1	E950.2	E962.0	E980.2
Crude oil	981	E862.1	—	E950.9	E962.1	E980.9
Cryogenine	965.8	E850.8	E935.8	E950.0	E962.0	E980.0
Cryolite (pesticide)	989.4	E863.4	—	E950.6	E962.1	E980.7
Cryptenamine	972.6	E858.3	E942.6	E950.4	E962.0	E980.4
Crystal violet	976.0	E858.7	E946.0	E950.4	E962.0	E980.4
Cuckoopint	988.2	E865.4	—	E950.9	E962.1	E980.9
Cumetharol	964.2	E858.2	E934.2	E950.4	E962.0	E980.4
Cupric sulfate	973.6	E858.4	E943.6	E950.4	E962.0	E980.4
Cuprous sulfate	983.9	E864.3	—	E950.7	E962.1	E980.6
Curare, curarine	975.2	E858.6	E945.2	E950.4	E962.0	E980.4
Cyanic acid — see Cyanide(s)						
Cyanide(s) (compounds) (hydrogen) (potassium) (sodium) NEC	989.0	E866.8	—	E950.9	E962.1	E980.9
dust or gas (inhalation) NEC	987.7	E869.8	—	E952.8	E962.2	E982.8
fumigant	989.0	E863.8	—	E950.6	E962.1	E980.7
mercuric — see Mercury						
pesticide (dust) (fumes)	989.0	E863.4	—	E950.6	E962.1	E980.7
Cyanocobalamin	964.1	E858.2	E934.1	E950.4	E962.0	E980.4
Cyanogen (chloride) (gas) NEC	987.8	E869.8	—	E952.8	E962.2	E982.8
Cyclaine	968.5	E855.2	E938.5	E950.4	E962.0	E980.4
Cyclamen europaeum	988.2	E865.4	—	E950.9	E962.1	E980.9
Cyclandelate	972.5	E858.3	E942.5	E950.4	E962.0	E980.4
Cyclazocine	965.09	E850.2	E935.2	E950.0	E962.0	E980.0
Cyclizine	963.0	E858.1	E933.0	E950.4	E962.0	E980.4
Cyclobarbital, cyclobarbitone	967.0	E851	E937.0	E950.1	E962.0	E980.1
Cycloguanil	961.4	E857	E931.4	E950.4	E962.0	E980.4
Cyclohexane	982.0	E862.4	—	E950.9	E962.1	E980.9
Cyclohexanol	980.8	E860.8	—	E950.9	E962.1	E980.9
Cyclohexanone	982.8	E862.4	—	E950.9	E962.1	E980.9
Cyclomethycaine	968.5	E855.2	E938.5	E950.4	E962.0	E980.4
Cyclopentamine	971.2	E855.5	E941.2	E950.4	E962.0	E980.4
Cyclopenthiazide	974.3	E858.5	E944.3	E950.4	E962.0	E980.4
Cyclopentolate	971.1	E855.4	E941.1	E950.4	E962.0	E980.4
Cyclophosphamide	963.1	E858.1	E933.1	E950.4	E962.0	E980.4
Cyclopropane	968.2	E855.1	E938.2	E950.4	E962.0	E980.4
Cycloserine	960.6	E856	E930.6	E950.4	E962.0	E980.4
Cyclothiazide	974.3	E858.5	E944.3	E950.4	E962.0	E980.4
Cycrimine	966.4	E855.0	E936.4	E950.4	E962.0	E980.4
Cymarin	972.1	E858.3	E942.1	E950.4	E962.0	E980.4
Cyproheptadine	963.0	E858.1	E933.0	E950.4	E962.0	E980.4
Cyprolidol	969.0	E854.0	E939.0	E950.3	E962.0	E980.3
Cytarabine	963.1	E858.1	E933.1	E950.4	E962.0	E980.4
Cytisus						
laburnum	988.2	E865.4	—	E950.9	E962.1	E980.9
scoparius	988.2	E865.4	—	E950.9	E962.1	E980.9
Cytomel	962.7	E858.0	E932.7	E950.4	E962.0	E980.4
Cytosine (antineoplastic)	963.1	E858.1	E933.1	E950.4	E962.0	E980.4
Cytoxan	963.1	E858.1	E933.1	E950.4	E962.0	E980.4

	Poisoning	Accident	Therapeutic Use	Suicide Attempt	Assault	Undetermined
Dacarbazine	963.1	E858.1	E933.1	E950.4	E962.0	E980.4
Dactinomycin	960.7	E856	E930.7	E950.4	E962.0	E980.4
DADPS	961.8	E857	E931.8	E950.4	E962.0	E980.4
Dakin's solution (external)	976.0	E858.7	E946.0	E950.4	E962.0	E980.4
Dalmane	969.4	E853.2	E939.4	E950.3	E962.0	E980.3
DAM	977.2	E858.8	E947.2	E950.4	E962.0	E980.4
Danilone	964.2	E858.2	E934.2	E950.4	E962.0	E980.4
Danthron	973.1	E858.4	E943.1	E950.4	E962.0	E980.4
Dantrolene	975.2	E858.6	E945.2	E950.4	E962.0	E980.4
Daphne (gnidium) (mezereum)	988.2	E865.4	—	E950.9	E962.1	E980.9
berry	988.2	E865.3	—	E950.9	E962.1	E980.9
Dapsone	961.8	E857	E931.8	E950.4	E962.0	E980.4
Daraprim	961.4	E857	E931.4	E950.4	E962.0	E980.4
Darnel	988.2	E865.3	—	E950.9	E962.1	E980.9
Darvon	965.8	E850.8	E935.8	E950.0	E962.0	E980.0
Daunorubicin	960.7	E856	E930.7	E950.4	E962.0	E980.4
DBI	962.3	E858.0	E932.3	E950.4	E962.0	E980.4
D-Con (rodenticide)	989.4	E863.7	—	E950.6	E962.1	E980.7
DDS	961.8	E857	E931.8	E950.4	E962.0	E980.4
DDT	989.2	E863.0	—	E950.6	E962.1	E980.7
Deadly nightshade	988.2	E865.4	—	E950.9	E962.1	E980.9
berry	988.2	E865.3	—	E950.9	E962.1	E980.9
Deanol	969.7	E854.2	E939.7	E950.3	E962.0	E980.3
Debrisoquine	972.6	E858.3	E942.6	E950.4	E962.0	E980.4
Decaborane	989.89	E866.8	—	E950.9	E962.1	E980.9
fumes	987.8	E869.8	—	E952.8	E962.2	E982.8
Decadron	962.0	E858.0	E932.0	E950.4	E962.0	E980.4
ENT agent	976.6	E858.7	E946.6	E950.4	E962.0	E980.4
ophthalmic preparation	976.5	E858.7	E946.5	E950.4	E962.0	E980.4
topical NEC	976.0	E858.7	E946.0	E950.4	E962.0	E980.4
Decahydronaphthalene	982.0	E862.4	—	E950.9	E962.1	E980.9
Decalin	982.0	E862.4	—	E950.9	E962.1	E980.9
Decamethonium	975.2	E858.6	E945.2	E950.4	E962.0	E980.4
Decholin	973.4	E858.4	E943.4	E950.4	E962.0	E980.4
sodium (diagnostic)	977.8	E858.8	E947.8	E950.4	E962.0	E980.4
Declomycin	960.4	E856	E930.4	E950.4	E962.0	E980.4
Deferoxamine	963.8	E858.1	E933.8	E950.4	E962.0	E980.4
Dehydrocholic acid	973.4	E858.4	E943.4	E950.4	E962.0	E980.4
DeKalin	982.0	E862.4	—	E950.9	E962.1	E980.9
Delalutin	962.2	E858.0	E932.2	E950.4	E962.0	E980.4
Delphinium	988.2	E865.3	—	E950.9	E962.1	E980.9
Deltasone	962.0	E858.0	E932.0	E950.4	E962.0	E980.4
Deltra	962.0	E858.0	E932.0	E950.4	E962.0	E980.4
Delvinal	967.0	E851	E937.0	E950.1	E962.0	E980.1
Demecarium (bromide)	971.0	E855.3	E941.0	E950.4	E962.0	E980.4
Demeclocycline	960.4	E856	E930.4	E950.4	E962.0	E980.4
Demecolcine	963.1	E858.1	E933.1	E950.4	E962.0	E980.4
Demelanizing agents	976.8	E858.7	E946.8	E950.4	E962.0	E980.4
Demerol	965.09	E850.2	E935.2	E950.0	E962.0	E980.0
Demethylchlortetracycline	960.4	E856	E930.4	E950.4	E962.0	E980.4
Demethyltetracycline	960.4	E856	E930.4	E950.4	E962.0	E980.4
Demeton	989.3	E863.1	—	E950.6	E962.1	E980.7
Demulcents	976.3	E858.7	E946.3	E950.4	E962.0	E980.4
Demulen	962.2	E858.0	E932.2	E950.4	E962.0	E980.4
Denatured alcohol	980.0	E860.1	—	E950.9	E962.1	E980.9
Dendrid	976.5	E858.7	E946.5	E950.4	E962.0	E980.4
Dental agents, topical	976.7	E858.7	E946.7	E950.4	E962.0	E980.4
Deodorant spray (feminine hygiene)	976.8	E858.7	E946.8	E950.4	E962.0	E980.4
Deoxyribonuclease	963.4	E858.1	E933.4	E950.4	E962.0	E980.4
Depressants						
appetite, central	977.0	E858.8	E947.0	E950.4	E962.0	E980.4
cardiac	972.0	E858.3	E942.0	E950.4	E962.0	E980.4
central nervous system (anesthetic)	968.4	E855.1	E938.4	E950.4	E962.0	E980.4
psychotherapeutic	969.5	E853.9	E939.5	E950.3	E962.0	E980.3
Dequalinium	976.0	E858.7	E946.0	E950.4	E962.0	E980.4
Dermolate	976.2	E858.7	E946.2	E950.4	E962.0	E980.4
DES	962.2	E858.0	E932.2	E950.4	E962.0	E980.4
Desenex	976.0	E858.7	E946.0	E950.4	E962.0	E980.4
Deserpidine	972.6	E858.3	E942.6	E950.4	E962.0	E980.4
Desipramine	969.0	E854.0	E939.0	E950.3	E962.0	E980.3
Deslanoside	972.1	E858.3	E942.1	E950.4	E962.0	E980.4
Desocodeine	965.09	E850.2	E935.2	E950.0	E962.0	E980.0
Desomorphine	965.09	E850.2	E935.2	E950.0	E962.0	E980.0
Desonide	976.0	E858.7	E946.0	E950.4	E962.0	E980.4
Desoxycorticosterone derivatives	962.0	E858.0	E932.0	E950.4	E962.0	E980.4
Desoxyephedrine	969.7	E854.2	E939.7	E950.3	E962.0	E980.3
DET	969.6	E854.1	E939.6	E950.3	E962.0	E980.3

Table of Drugs and Chemicals

	Poisoning	External Cause (E-Code)				
		Accident	Therapeutic Use	Suicide Attempt	Assault	Undetermined
Detergents (ingested)						
(synthetic)	989.6	E861.0	—	E950.9	E962.1	E980.9
ENT agent	976.6	E858.7	E946.6	E950.4	E962.0	E980.4
external medication	976.2	E858.7	E946.2	E950.4	E962.0	E980.4
ophthalmic preparation	976.5	E858.7	E946.5	E950.4	E962.0	E980.4
topical NEC	976.0	E858.7	E946.0	E950.4	E962.0	E980.4
Deterrent, alcohol	977.3	E858.8	E947.3	E950.4	E962.0	E980.4
Dethyronine	962.7	E858.0	E932.7	E950.4	E962.0	E980.4
Dettol (external medication)	976.0	E858.7	E946.0	E950.4	E962.0	E980.4
Dexamethasone	962.0	E858.0	E932.0	E950.4	E962.0	E980.4
Dexamphetamine	969.7	E854.2	E939.7	E950.3	E962.0	E980.3
Dexedrine	969.7	E854.2	E939.7	E950.3	E962.0	E980.3
Dexpanthenol	963.5	E858.1	E933.5	E950.4	E962.0	E980.4
Dextran	964.8	E858.2	E934.8	E950.4	E962.0	E980.4
Dextriferron	964.0	E858.2	E934.0	E950.4	E962.0	E980.4
Dextroamphetamine	969.7	E854.2	E939.7	E950.3	E962.0	E980.3
Dextro calcium pantothenate	963.5	E858.1	E933.5	E950.4	E962.0	E980.4
Dextromethorphan	975.4	E858.6	E945.4	E950.4	E962.0	E980.4
Dextromoramide	965.09	E850.2	E935.2	E950.0	E962.0	E980.0
Dextro pantothenyl alcohol	963.5	E858.1	E933.5	E950.4	E962.0	E980.4
topical	976.8	E858.7	E946.8	E950.4	E962.0	E980.4
Dextropropoxyphene (hydrochloride)	965.8	E850.8	E935.8	E950.0	E962.0	E980.0
Dextrorphan	965.09	E850.2	E935.2	E950.0	E962.0	E980.0
Dextrose NEC	974.5	E858.5	E944.5	E950.4	E962.0	E980.4
Dextrothyroxin	962.7	E858.0	E932.7	E950.4	E962.0	E980.4
DFP	971.0	E855.3	E941.0	E950.4	E962.0	E980.4
DHE-45	972.9	E858.3	E942.9	E950.4	E962.0	E980.4
Diabinese	962.3	E858.0	E932.3	E950.4	E962.0	E980.4
Diacetyl monoxime	977.2	E858.8	E947.2	E950.4	E962.0	E980.4
Diacetylmorphine	965.01	E850.0	E935.0	E950.0	E962.0	E980.0
Diagnostic agents	977.8	E858.8	E947.8	E950.4	E962.0	E980.4
Dial (soap)	976.2	E858.7	E946.2	E950.4	E962.0	E980.4
sedative	967.0	E851	E937.0	E950.1	E962.0	E980.1
Diallylbarbituric acid	967.0	E851	E937.0	E950.1	E962.0	E980.1
Diaminodiphenylsulfone	961.8	E857	E931.8	E950.4	E962.0	E980.4
Diamorphine	965.01	E850.0	E935.0	E950.0	E962.0	E980.0
Diamox	974.2	E858.5	E944.2	E950.4	E962.0	E980.4
Diamthazole	976.0	E858.7	E946.0	E950.4	E962.0	E980.4
Diaphenylsulfone	961.8	E857	E931.8	E950.4	E962.0	E980.4
Diasone (sodium)	961.8	E857	E931.8	E950.4	E962.0	E980.4
Diazepam	969.4	E853.2	E939.4	E950.3	E962.0	E980.3
Diazinon	989.3	E863.1	—	E950.6	E962.1	E980.7
Diazomethane (gas)	987.8	E869.8	—	E952.8	E962.2	E982.8
Diazoxide	972.5	E858.3	E942.5	E950.4	E962.0	E980.4
Dibenamine	971.3	E855.6	E941.3	E950.4	E962.0	E980.4
Dibenzheptropine	963.0	E858.1	E933.0	E950.4	E962.0	E980.4
Dibenzyline	971.3	E855.6	E941.3	E950.4	E962.0	E980.4
Diborane (gas)	987.8	E869.8	—	E952.8	E962.2	E982.8
Dibromomannitol	963.1	E858.1	E933.1	E950.4	E962.0	E980.4
Dibucaine (spinal)	968.7	E855.2	E938.7	E950.4	E962.0	E980.4
topical (surface)	968.5	E855.2	E938.5	E950.4	E962.0	E980.4
Dibunate sodium	975.4	E858.6	E945.4	E950.4	E962.0	E980.4
Dibutoline	971.1	E855.4	E941.1	E950.4	E962.0	E980.4
Dicapthon	989.4	E863.4	—	E950.6	E962.1	E980.7
Dichloralphenazone	967.1	E852.0	E937.1	E950.2	E962.0	E980.2
Dichlorodifluoromethane	987.4	E869.2	—	E952.8	E962.2	E982.8
Dichloroethane	982.3	E862.4	—	E950.9	E962.1	E980.9
Dichloroethylene	982.3	E862.4	—	E950.9	E962.1	E980.9
Dichloroethyl sulfide	987.8	E869.8	—	E952.8	E962.2	E982.8
Dichlorohydrin	982.3	E862.4	—	E950.9	E962.1	E980.9
Dichloromethane (solvent) (vapor)	982.3	E862.4	—	E950.9	E962.1	E980.9
Dichlorophen(e)	961.6	E857	E931.6	E950.4	E962.0	E980.4
Dichlorphenamide	974.2	E858.5	E944.2	E950.4	E962.0	E980.4
Dichlorvos	989.3	E863.1	—	E950.6	E962.1	E980.7
Diclofenac sodium	965.69	E850.6	E935.6	E950.0	E962.0	E980.0
Dicoumarin, dicumarol	964.2	E858.2	E934.2	E950.4	E962.0	E980.4
Dicyanogen (gas)	987.8	E869.8	—	E952.8	E962.2	E982.8
Dicyclomine	971.1	E855.4	E941.1	E950.4	E962.0	E980.4
Dieldrin (vapor)	989.2	E863.0	—	E950.6	E962.1	E980.7
Dienestrol	962.2	E858.0	E932.2	E950.4	E962.0	E980.4
Dietetics	977.0	E858.8	E947.0	E950.4	E962.0	E980.4
Diethazine	966.4	E855.0	E936.4	E950.4	E962.0	E980.4
Diethyl						
barbituric acid	967.0	E851	E937.0	E950.1	E962.0	E980.1
carbamazine	961.6	E857	E931.6	E950.4	E962.0	E980.4
carbinol	980.8	E860.8	—	E950.9	E962.1	E980.9
carbonate	982.8	E862.4	—	E950.9	E962.1	E980.9

	Poisoning	External Cause (E-Code)				
		Accident	Therapeutic Use	Suicide Attempt	Assault	Undetermined
Diethyl — continued						
dioxide	982.8	E862.4	—	E950.9	E962.1	E980.9
ether (vapor) — see ther(s)						
glycol (monoacetate) (monoethyl ether)	982.8	E862.4	—	E950.9	E962.1	E980.9
propion	977.0	E858.8	E947.0	E950.4	E962.0	E980.4
stilbestrol	962.2	E858.0	E932.2	E950.4	E962.0	E980.4
Diethylene						
Diethylsulfone-diethylmethane	967.8	E852.8	E937.8	E950.2	E962.0	E980.2
Difencloxazine	965.09	E850.2	E935.2	E950.0	E962.0	E980.0
Diffusin	963.4	E858.1	E933.4	E950.4	E962.0	E980.4
Diflos	971.0	E855.3	E941.0	E950.4	E962.0	E980.4
Digestants	973.4	E858.4	E943.4	E950.4	E962.0	E980.4
Digitalin(e)	972.1	E858.3	E942.1	E950.4	E962.0	E980.4
Digitalis glycosides	972.1	E858.3	E942.1	E950.4	E962.0	E980.4
Digitoxin	972.1	E858.3	E942.1	E950.4	E962.0	E980.4
Digoxin	972.1	E858.3	E942.1	E950.4	E962.0	E980.4
Dihydrocodeine	965.09	E850.2	E935.2	E950.0	E962.0	E980.0
Dihydrocodeinone	965.09	E850.2	E935.2	E950.0	E962.0	E980.0
Dihydroergocristine	972.9	E858.3	E942.9	E950.4	E962.0	E980.4
Dihydroergotamine	972.9	E858.3	E942.9	E950.4	E962.0	E980.4
Dihydroergotoxine	972.9	E858.3	E942.9	E950.4	E962.0	E980.4
Dihydrohydroxycodeinone	965.09	E850.2	E935.2	E950.0	E962.0	E980.0
Dihydrohydroxymorphinone	965.09	E850.2	E935.2	E950.0	E962.0	E980.0
Dihydroisocodeine	965.09	E850.2	E935.2	E950.0	E962.0	E980.0
Dihydromorphine	965.09	E850.2	E935.2	E950.0	E962.0	E980.0
Dihydromorphinone	965.09	E850.2	E935.2	E950.0	E962.0	E980.0
Dihydrostreptomycin	960.6	E856	E930.6	E950.4	E962.0	E980.4
Dihydrotachysterol	962.6	E858.0	E932.6	E950.4	E962.0	E980.4
Dihydroxyanthraquinone	973.1	E858.4	E943.1	E950.4	E962.0	E980.4
Dihydroxycodeinone	965.09	E850.2	E935.2	E950.0	E962.0	E980.0
Diiodohydroxyquin	961.3	E857	E931.3	E950.4	E962.0	E980.4
topical	976.0	E858.7	E946.0	E950.4	E962.0	E980.4
Diiodohydroxyquinoline	961.3	E857	E931.3	E950.4	E962.0	E980.4
Dilantin	966.1	E855.0	E936.1	E950.4	E962.0	E980.4
Dilaudid	965.09	E850.2	E935.2	E950.0	E962.0	E980.0
Diloxanide	961.5	E857	E931.5	E950.4	E962.0	E980.4
Dimefline	970.0	E854.3	E940.0	E950.4	E962.0	E980.4
Dimenhydrinate	963.0	E858.1	E933.0	E950.4	E962.0	E980.4
Dimercaprol	963.8	E858.1	E933.8	E950.4	E962.0	E980.4
Dimercaptopropanol	963.8	E858.1	E933.8	E950.4	E962.0	E980.4
Dimetane	963.0	E858.1	E933.0	E950.4	E962.0	E980.4
Dimethicone	976.3	E858.7	E946.3	E950.4	E962.0	E980.4
Dimethindene	963.0	E858.1	E933.0	E950.4	E962.0	E980.4
Dimethisoquin	968.5	E855.2	E938.5	E950.4	E962.0	E980.4
Dimethisterone	962.2	E858.0	E932.2	E950.4	E962.0	E980.4
Dimethoxanate	975.4	E858.6	E945.4	E950.4	E962.0	E980.4
Dimethyl						
arsine, arsinic acid — see Arsenic						
carbinol	980.2	E860.3	—	E950.9	E962.1	E980.9
diguanide	962.3	E858.0	E932.3	E950.4	E962.0	E980.4
ketone	982.8	E862.4	—	E950.9	E962.1	E980.9
vapor	987.8	E869.8	—	E952.8	E962.2	E982.8
meperidine	965.09	E850.2	E935.2	E950.0	E962.0	E980.0
parathion	989.3	E863.1	—	E950.6	E962.1	E980.7
polysiloxane	973.8	E858.4	E943.8	E950.4	E962.0	E980.4
sulfate (fumes)	987.8	E869.8	—	E952.8	E962.2	E982.8
liquid	983.9	E864.3	—	E950.7	E962.1	E980.6
sulfoxide NEC	982.8	E862.4	—	E950.9	E962.1	E980.9
medicinal	976.4	E858.7	E946.4	E950.4	E962.0	E980.4
triptamine	969.6	E854.1	E939.6	E950.3	E962.0	E980.3
tubocurarine	975.2	E858.6	E945.2	E950.4	E962.0	E980.4
Dindevan	964.2	E858.2	E934.2	E950.4	E962.0	E980.4
Dinitrobenzene	983.0	E864.0	—	E950.7	E962.1	E980.6
vapor	987.8	E869.8	—	E952.8	E962.2	E982.8
Dinitro (-ortho-) cresol						
(herbicide) (spray)	989.4	E863.5	—	E950.6	E962.1	E980.7
insecticide	989.4	E863.4	—	E950.6	E962.1	E980.7
Dinitro-orthocresol						
(herbicide)	989.4	E863.5	—	E950.6	E962.1	E980.7
insecticide	989.4	E863.4	—	E950.6	E962.1	E980.7
Dinitrophenol (herbicide)						
(spray)	989.4	E863.5	—	E950.6	E962.1	E980.7
insecticide	989.4	E863.4	—	E950.6	E962.1	E980.7
Dinoprost	975.0	E858.6	E945.0	E950.4	E962.0	E980.4
Dioctyl sulfosuccinate (calcium) (sodium)	973.2	E858.4	E943.2	E950.4	E962.0	E980.4
Diodoquin	961.3	E857	E931.3	E950.4	E962.0	E980.4
Dione derivatives NEC	966.3	E855.0	E936.3	E950.4	E962.0	E980.4
Dionin	965.09	E850.2	E935.2	E950.0	E962.0	E980.0

Dioxane — Table of Drugs and Chemicals

		External Cause (E-Code)							External Cause (E-Code)			
	Poisoning	Accident	Therapeutic Use	Suicide Attempt	Assault	Undetermined		Poisoning	Accident	Therapeutic Use	Suicide Attempt	Assault	Undetermined
Dioxane	982.8	E862.4	—	E950.9	E962.1	E980.9	**Drug** — continued						
Dioxin — see Herbicide							AHFS List						
Dioxyline	972.5	E858.3	E942.5	E950.4	E962.0	E980.4	4:00 antihistamine drugs	963.0	E858.1	E933.0	E950.4	E962.0	E980.4
Dipentene	982.8	E862.4	—	E950.9	E962.1	E980.9	8:04 amebacides	961.5	E857	E931.5	E950.4	E962.0	E980.4
Diphemanil	971.1	E855.4	E941.1	E950.4	E962.0	E980.4	arsenical anti-infectives	961.1	E857	E931.1	E950.4	E962.0	E980.4
Diphenadione	964.2	E858.2	E934.2	E950.4	E962.0	E980.4	quinoline derivatives	961.3	E857	E931.3	E950.4	E962.0	E980.4
Diphenhydramine	963.0	E858.1	E933.0	E950.4	E962.0	E980.4	8:08 anthelmintics	961.6	E857	E931.6	E950.4	E962.0	E980.4
Diphenidol	963.0	E858.1	E933.0	E950.4	E962.0	E980.4	quinoline derivatives	961.3	E857	E931.3	E950.4	E962.0	E980.4
Diphenoxylate	973.5	E858.4	E943.5	E950.4	E962.0	E980.4	8:12.04 antifungal						
Diphenylchloroarsine	985.1	E866.3	—	E950.8	E962.1	E980.8	antibiotics	960.1	E856	E930.1	E950.4	E962.0	E980.4
Diphenylhydantoin							8:12.06 cephalosporins	960.5	E856	E930.5	E950.4	E962.0	E980.4
(sodium)	966.1	E855.0	E936.1	E950.4	E962.0	E980.4	8:12.08 chloramphenicol	960.2	E856	E930.2	E950.4	E962.0	E980.4
Diphenylpyraline	963.0	E858.1	E933.0	E950.4	E962.0	E980.4	8:12.12 erythromycins	960.3	E856	E930.3	E950.4	E962.0	E980.4
Diphtheria							8:12.16 penicillins	960.0	E856	E930.0	E950.4	E962.0	E980.4
antitoxin	979.9	E858.8	E949.9	E950.4	E962.0	E980.4	8:12.20 streptomycins	960.6	E856	E930.6	E950.4	E962.0	E980.4
toxoid	978.5	E858.8	E948.5	E950.4	E962.0	E980.4	8:12.24 tetracyclines	960.4	E856	E930.4	E950.4	E962.0	E980.4
with tetanus toxoid	978.9	E858.8	E948.9	E950.4	E962.0	E980.4	8:12.28 other antibiotics	960.8	E856	E930.8	E950.4	E962.0	E980.4
with pertussis component	978.6	E858.8	E948.6	E950.4	E962.0	E980.4	antimycobacterial	960.6	E856	E930.6	E950.4	E962.0	E980.4
vaccine	978.5	E858.8	E948.5	E950.4	E962.0	E980.4	macrolides	960.3	E856	E930.3	E950.4	E962.0	E980.4
Dipipanone	965.09	E850.2	E935.2	E950.0	E962.0	E980.0	8:16 antituberculars	961.8	E857	E931.8	E950.4	E962.0	E980.4
Diplovax	979.5	E858.8	E949.5	E950.4	E962.0	E980.4	antibiotics	960.6	E856	E930.6	E950.4	E962.0	E980.4
Diprophylline	975.1	E858.6	E945.1	E950.4	E962.0	E980.4	8:18 antivirals	961.7	E857	E931.7	E950.4	E962.0	E980.4
Dipyridamole	972.4	E858.3	E942.4	E950.4	E962.0	E980.4	8:20 plasmodicides (antimalarials)	961.4	E857	E931.4	E950.4	E962.0	E980.4
Dipyrone	965.5	E850.5	E935.5	E950.0	E962.0	E980.0	8:24 sulfonamides	961.0	E857	E931.0	E950.4	E962.0	E980.4
Diquat	989.4	E863.5	—	E950.6	E962.1	E980.7	8:26 sulfones	961.8	E857	E931.8	E950.4	E962.0	E980.4
Disinfectant NEC	983.9	E861.4	—	E950.7	E962.1	E980.6	8:28 treponemicides	961.2	E857	E931.2	E950.4	E962.0	E980.4
alkaline	983.2	E861.4	—	E950.7	E962.1	E980.6	8:32 trichomonacides	961.5	E857	E931.5	E950.4	E962.0	E980.4
aromatic	983.0	E861.4	—	E950.7	E962.1	E980.6	nitrofuran derivatives	961.9	E857	E931.9	E950.4	E962.0	E980.4
Disipal	966.4	E855.0	E936.4	E950.4	E962.0	E980.4	quinoline derivatives	961.3	E857	E931.3	E950.4	E962.0	E980.4
Disodium edetate	963.8	E858.1	E933.8	E950.4	E962.0	E980.4	8:36 urinary germicides	961.9	E857	E931.9	E950.4	E962.0	E980.4
Disulfamide	974.4	E858.5	E944.4	E950.4	E962.0	E980.4	quinoline derivatives	961.3	E857	E931.3	E950.4	E962.0	E980.4
Disulfanilamide	961.0	E857	E931.0	E950.4	E962.0	E980.4	8:40 other anti-infectives	961.9	E857	E931.9	E950.4	E962.0	E980.4
Disulfiram	977.3	E858.8	E947.3	E950.4	E962.0	E980.4	10:00 antineoplastic agents	963.1	E858.1	E933.1	E950.4	E962.0	E980.4
Dithiazanine	961.6	E857	E931.6	E950.4	E962.0	E980.4	antibiotics	960.7	E856	E930.7	E950.4	E962.0	E980.4
Dithioglycerol	963.8	E858.1	E933.8	E950.4	E962.0	E980.4	progestogens	962.2	E858.0	E932.2	E950.4	E962.0	E980.4
Dithranol	976.4	E858.7	E946.4	E950.4	E962.0	E980.4	12:04 parasympathomimetic (cholinergic) agents	971.0	E855.3	E941.0	E950.4	E962.0	E980.4
Diucardin	974.3	E858.5	E944.3	E950.4	E962.0	E980.4	12:08 parasympatholytic (cholinergic-blocking) agents	971.1	E855.4	E941.1	E950.4	E962.0	E980.4
Diupres	974.3	E858.5	E944.3	E950.4	E962.0	E980.4	12:12 Sympathomimetic (adrenergic) agents	971.2	E855.5	E941.2	E950.4	E962.0	E980.4
Diuretics NEC	974.4	E858.5	E944.4	E950.4	E962.0	E980.4	12:16 sympatholytic (adrenergic-blocking) agents	971.3	E855.6	E941.3	E950.4	E962.0	E980.4
carbonic acid anhydrase inhibitors	974.2	E858.5	E944.2	E950.4	E962.0	E980.4	12:20 skeletal muscle relaxants						
mercurial	974.0	E858.5	E944.0	E950.4	E962.0	E980.4	central nervous system muscle-tone depressants	968.0	E855.1	E938.0	E950.4	E962.0	E980.4
osmotic	974.4	E858.5	E944.4	E950.4	E962.0	E980.4	myoneural blocking agents	975.2	E858.6	E945.2	E950.4	E962.0	E980.4
purine derivatives	974.1	E858.5	E944.1	E950.4	E962.0	E980.4	16:00 blood derivatives	964.7	E858.2	E934.7	E950.4	E962.0	E980.4
saluretic	974.3	E858.5	E944.3	E950.4	E962.0	E980.4	20:04.04 iron preparations	964.0	E858.2	E934.0	E950.4	E962.0	E980.4
Diuril	974.3	E858.5	E944.3	E950.4	E962.0	E980.4	20:04.08 liver and stomach preparations	964.1	E858.2	E934.1	E950.4	E962.0	E980.4
Divinyl ether	968.2	E855.1	E938.2	E950.4	E962.0	E980.4	20:04 antianemia drugs	964.1	E858.2	E934.1	E950.4	E962.0	E980.4
D-lysergic acid diethylamide	969.6	E854.1	E939.6	E950.3	E962.0	E980.3	20:12.04 anticoagulants	964.2	E858.2	E934.2	E950.4	E962.0	E980.4
DMCT	960.4	E856	E930.4	E950.4	E962.0	E980.4	20:12.08 antiheparin agents	964.5	E858.2	E934.5	E950.4	E962.0	E980.4
DMSO	982.8	E862.4	—	E950.9	E962.1	E980.9	20:12.12 coagulants	964.5	E858.2	E934.5	E950.4	E962.0	E980.4
DMT	969.6	E854.1	E939.6	E950.3	E962.0	E980.3	20:12.16 hemostatics NEC	964.5	E858.2	E934.5	E950.4	E962.0	E980.4
DNOC	989.4	E863.5	—	E950.6	E962.1	E980.7	capillary active drugs	972.8	E858.3	E942.8	E950.4	E962.0	E980.4
DOCA	962.0	E858.0	E932.0	E950.4	E962.0	E980.4	24:04 cardiac drugs	972.9	E858.3	E942.9	E950.4	E962.0	E980.4
Dolophine	965.02	E850.1	E935.1	E950.0	E962.0	E980.0	cardiotonic agents	972.1	E858.3	E942.1	E950.4	E962.0	E980.4
Doloxene	965.8	E850.8	E935.8	E950.0	E962.0	E980.0	rhythm regulators	972.0	E858.3	E942.0	E950.4	E962.0	E980.4
DOM	969.6	E854.1	E939.6	E950.3	E962.0	E980.3	24:06 antilipemic agents	972.2	E858.3	E942.2	E950.4	E962.0	E980.4
Domestic gas — see Gas, utility							thyroid derivatives	962.7	E858.0	E932.7	E950.4	E962.0	E980.4
Domiphen (bromide) (lozenges)	976.6	E858.7	E946.6	E950.4	E962.0	E980.4	24:08 hypotensive agents	972.6	E858.3	E942.6	E950.4	E962.0	E980.4
Dopa (levo)	966.4	E855.0	E936.4	E950.4	E962.0	E980.4	adrenergic blocking agents	971.3	E855.6	E941.3	E950.4	E962.0	E980.4
Dopamine	971.2	E855.5	E941.2	E950.4	E962.0	E980.4	ganglion blocking agents	972.3	E858.3	E942.3	E950.4	E962.0	E980.4
Doriden	967.5	E852.4	E937.5	E950.2	E962.0	E980.2	vasodilators	972.5	E858.3	E942.5	E950.4	E962.0	E980.4
Dormiral	967.0	E851	E937.0	E950.1	E962.0	E980.1	24:12 vasodilating agents NEC	972.5	E858.3	E942.5	E950.4	E962.0	E980.4
Dormison	967.8	E852.8	E937.8	E950.2	E962.0	E980.2	coronary	972.4	E858.3	E942.4	E950.4	E962.0	E980.4
Dornase	963.4	E858.1	E933.4	E950.4	E962.0	E980.4	nicotinic acid derivatives	972.2	E858.3	E942.2	E950.4	E962.0	E980.4
Dorsacaine	968.5	E855.2	E938.5	E950.4	E962.0	E980.4	24:16 sclerosing agents	972.7	E858.3	E942.7	E950.4	E962.0	E980.4
Dothiepin hydrochloride	969.0	E854.0	E939.0	E950.3	E962.0	E980.3	28:04 general anesthetics	968.4	E855.1	E938.4	E950.4	E962.0	E980.4
Doxapram	970.0	E854.3	E940.0	E950.4	E962.0	E980.4	gaseous anesthetics	968.2	E855.1	E938.2	E950.4	E962.0	E980.4
Doxepin	969.0	E854.0	E939.0	E950.3	E962.0	E980.3	halothane	968.1	E855.1	E938.1	E950.4	E962.0	E980.4
Doxorubicin	960.7	E856	E930.7	E950.4	E962.0	E980.4							
Doxycycline	960.4	E856	E930.4	E950.4	E962.0	E980.4							
Doxylamine	963.0	E858.1	E933.0	E950.4	E962.0	E980.4							
Dramamine	963.0	E858.1	E933.0	E950.4	E962.0	E980.4							
Drano (drain cleaner)	983.2	E864.2	—	E950.7	E962.1	E980.6							
Dromoran	965.09	E850.2	E935.2	E950.0	E962.0	E980.0							
Dromostanolone	962.1	E858.0	E932.1	E950.4	E962.0	E980.4							
Droperidol	969.2	E853.1	E939.2	E950.3	E962.0	E980.3							
Drotrecogin alfa	964.2	E858.2	E934.2	E950.4	E962.0	E980.4							
Drug	977.9	E858.9	E947.9	E950.5	E962.0	E980.5							

Table of Drugs and Chemicals

Drug	External Cause (E-Code)						Drug	External Cause (E-Code)				
	Poisoning	Accident	Therapeutic Use	Suicide Attempt	Assault	Undetermined		Poisoning	Accident	Therapeutic Use	Suicide Attempt	Assault	Undetermined
Drug — *continued*							**Drug** — *continued*						
28:04 general anesthetics — *continued*							40:40 uricosuric agents	974.7	E858.5	E944.7	E950.4	E962.0	E980.4
intravenous anesthetics	968.3	E855.1	E938.3	E950.4	E962.0	E980.4	44:00 enzymes	963.4	E858.1	E933.4	E950.4	E962.0	E980.4
28:08 analgesics and							fibrinolysis-affecting agents	964.4	E858.2	E934.4	E950.4	E962.0	E980.4
antipyretics	965.9	E850.9	E935.9	E950.0	E962.0	E980.0	gastric agents	973.4	E858.4	E943.4	E950.4	E962.0	E980.4
antirheumatics	965.69	E850.6	E935.6	E950.0	E962.0	E980.0	48:00 expectorants and cough preparations						
aromatic analgesics	965.4	E850.4	E935.4	E950.0	E962.0	E980.0	antihistamine agents	963.0	E858.1	E933.0	E950.4	E962.0	E980.4
non-narcotic NEC	965.7	E850.7	E935.7	E950.0	E962.0	E980.0	antitussives	975.4	E858.6	E945.4	E950.4	E962.0	E980.4
opium alkaloids	965.00	E850.2	E935.2	E950.0	E962.0	E980.0	codeine derivatives	965.09	E850.2	E935.2	E950.0	E962.0	E980.0
heroin	965.01	E850.0	E935.0	E950.0	E962.0	E980.0	expectorants	975.5	E858.6	E945.5	E950.4	E962.0	E980.4
methadone	965.02	E850.1	E935.1	E950.0	E962.0	E980.0	narcotic agents NEC	965.09	E850.2	E935.2	E950.0	E962.0	E980.0
specified type NEC	965.09	E850.2	E935.2	E950.0	E962.0	E980.0	52:04.04 antibiotics (EENT)						
pyrazole derivatives	965.5	E850.5	E935.5	E950.0	E962.0	E980.0	ENT agent	976.6	E858.7	E946.6	E950.4	E962.0	E980.4
salicylates	965.1	E850.3	E935.3	E950.0	E962.0	E980.0	ophthalmic preparation	976.5	E858.7	E946.5	E950.4	E962.0	E980.4
specified NEC	965.8	E850.8	E935.8	E950.0	E962.0	E980.0	52:04.06 antivirals (EENT)						
28:10 narcotic antagonists	970.1	E854.3	E940.1	E950.4	E962.0	E980.4	ENT agent	976.6	E858.7	E946.6	E950.4	E962.0	E980.4
28:12 anticonvulsants	966.3	E855.0	E936.3	E950.4	E962.0	E980.4	ophthalmic preparation	976.5	E858.7	E946.5	E950.4	E962.0	E980.4
barbiturates	967.0	E851	E937.0	E950.1	E962.0	E980.1	52:04.08 sulfonamides (EENT)						
benzodiazepine-based tranquilizers	969.4	E853.2	E939.4	E950.3	E962.0	E980.3	ENT agent	976.6	E858.7	E946.6	E950.4	E962.0	E980.4
bromides	967.3	E852.2	E937.3	E950.2	E962.0	E980.2	ophthalmic preparation	976.5	E858.7	E946.5	E950.4	E962.0	E980.4
hydantoin derivatives	966.1	E855.0	E936.1	E950.4	E962.0	E980.4	52:04.12 miscellaneous anti-infectives (EENT)						
oxazolidine (derivatives)	966.0	E855.0	E936.0	E950.4	E962.0	E980.4	ENT agent	976.6	E858.7	E946.6	E950.4	E962.0	E980.4
succinimides	966.2	E855.0	E936.2	E950.4	E962.0	E980.4	ophthalmic preparation	976.5	E858.7	E946.5	E950.4	E962.0	E980.4
28:16.04 antidepressants	969.0	E854.0	E939.0	E950.3	E962.0	E980.3	52:04 anti-infectives (EENT)						
28:16.08 tranquilizers	969.5	E853.9	E939.5	E950.3	E962.0	E980.3	ENT agent	976.6	E858.7	E946.6	E950.4	E962.0	E980.4
benzodiazepine-based	969.4	E853.2	E939.4	E950.3	E962.0	E980.3	ophthalmic preparation	976.5	E858.7	E946.5	E950.4	E962.0	E980.4
butyrophenone-based	969.2	E853.1	E939.2	E950.3	E962.0	E980.3	52:08 anti-inflammatory agents (EENT)						
major NEC	969.3	E853.8	E939.3	E950.3	E962.0	E980.3	ENT agent	976.6	E858.7	E946.6	E950.4	E962.0	E980.4
phenothiazine-based	969.1	E853.0	E939.1	E950.3	E962.0	E980.3	ophthalmic preparation	976.5	E858.7	E946.5	E950.4	E962.0	E980.4
28:16.12 other psychotherapeutic agents	969.8	E855.8	E939.8	E950.3	E962.0	E980.3	52:10 carbonic anhydrase inhibitors	974.2	E858.5	E944.2	E950.4	E962.0	E980.4
28:20 respiratory and cerebral							52:12 contact lens solutions	976.5	E858.7	E946.5	E950.4	E962.0	E980.4
stimulants	970.9	E854.3	E940.9	E950.4	E962.0	E980.4	52:16 local anesthetics (EENT)	968.5	E855.2	E938.5	E950.4	E962.0	E980.4
analeptics	970.0	E854.3	E940.0	E950.4	E962.0	E980.4	52:20 miotics	971.0	E855.3	E941.0	E950.4	E962.0	E980.4
anorexigenic agents	977.0	E858.8	E947.0	E950.4	E962.0	E980.4	52:24 mydriatics						
psychostimulants	969.7	E854.2	E939.7	E950.3	E962.0	E980.3	adrenergics	971.2	E855.5	E941.2	E950.4	E962.0	E980.4
specified NEC	970.8	E854.3	E940.8	E950.4	E962.0	E980.4	anticholinergics	971.1	E855.4	E941.1	E950.4	E962.0	E980.4
28:24 sedatives and							antimuscarinics	971.1	E855.4	E941.1	E950.4	E962.0	E980.4
hypnotics	967.9	E852.9	E937.9	E950.2	E962.0	E980.2	parasympatholytics	971.1	E855.4	E941.1	E950.4	E962.0	E980.4
barbiturates	967.0	E851	E937.0	E950.1	E962.0	E980.1	spasmolytics	971.1	E855.4	E941.1	E950.4	E962.0	E980.4
benzodiazepine-based tranquilizers	969.4	E853.2	E939.4	E950.3	E962.0	E980.3	sympathomimetics	971.2	E855.5	E941.2	E950.4	E962.0	E980.4
chloral hydrate (group)	967.1	E852.0	E937.1	E950.2	E962.0	E980.2	52:28 mouth washes and gargles	976.6	E858.7	E946.6	E950.4	E962.0	E980.4
glutethamide group	967.5	E852.4	E937.5	E950.2	E962.0	E980.2	52:32 vasoconstrictors (EENT)	971.2	E855.5	E941.2	E950.4	E962.0	E980.4
intravenous anesthetics	968.3	E855.1	E938.3	E950.4	E962.0	E980.4	52:36 unclassified agents (EENT)						
methaqualone (compounds)	967.4	E852.3	E937.4	E950.2	E962.0	E980.2	ENT agent	976.6	E858.7	E946.6	E950.4	E962.0	E980.4
paraldehyde	967.2	E852.1	E937.2	E950.2	E962.0	E980.2	ophthalmic preparation	976.5	E858.7	E946.5	E950.4	E962.0	E980.4
phenothiazine-based tranquilizers	969.1	E853.0	E939.1	E950.3	E962.0	E980.3	56:04 antacids and adsorbents	973.0	E858.4	E943.0	E950.4	E962.0	E980.4
specified NEC	967.8	E852.8	E937.8	E950.2	E962.0	E980.2	56:08 antidiarrhea agents	973.5	E858.4	E943.5	E950.4	E962.0	E980.4
thiobarbiturates	968.3	E855.1	E938.3	E950.4	E962.0	E980.4	56:10 antiflatulents	973.8	E858.4	E943.8	E950.4	E962.0	E980.4
tranquilizer NEC	969.5	E853.9	E939.5	E950.3	E962.0	E980.3	56:12 cathartics NEC	973.3	E858.4	E943.3	E950.4	E962.0	E980.4
36:04 to 36:88 diagnostic agents	977.8	E858.8	E947.8	E950.4	E962.0	E980.4	emollients	973.2	E858.4	E943.2	E950.4	E962.0	E980.4
40:00 electrolyte, caloric, and water balance agents							irritants	973.1	E858.4	E943.1	E950.4	E962.0	E980.4
NEC	974.5	E858.5	E944.5	E950.4	E962.0	E980.4	56:16 digestants	973.4	E858.4	E943.4	E950.4	E962.0	E980.4
40:04 acidifying agents	963.2	E858.1	E933.2	E950.4	E962.0	E980.4	56:20 emetics and antiemetics						
40:08 alkalinizing agents	963.3	E858.1	E933.3	E950.4	E962.0	E980.4	antiemetics	963.0	E858.1	E933.0	E950.4	E962.0	E980.4
40:10 ammonia detoxicants	974.5	E858.5	E944.5	E950.4	E962.0	E980.4	emetics	973.6	E858.4	E943.6	E950.4	E962.0	E980.4
40:12 replacement solutions	974.5	E858.5	E944.5	E950.4	E962.0	E980.4	56:24 lipotropic agents	977.1	E858.8	E947.1	E950.4	E962.0	E980.4
plasma expanders	964.8	E858.2	E934.8	E950.4	E962.0	E980.4	56:40 miscellaneous G.I. drugs	973.8	E858.4	E943.8	E950.4	E962.0	E980.4
40:16 sodium-removing resins	974.5	E858.5	E944.5	E950.4	E962.0	E980.4	60:00 gold compounds	965.69	E850.6	E935.6	E950.0	E962.0	E980.0
40:18 potassium-removing resins	974.5	E858.5	E944.5	E950.4	E962.0	E980.4	64:00 heavy metal antagonists	963.8	E858.1	E933.8	E950.4	E962.0	E980.4
40:20 caloric agents	974.5	E858.5	E944.5	E950.4	E962.0	E980.4	68:04 adrenals	962.0	E858.0	E932.0	E950.4	E962.0	E980.4
40:24 salt and sugar substitutes	974.5	E858.5	E944.5	E950.4	E962.0	E980.4	68:08 androgens	962.1	E858.0	E932.1	E950.4	E962.0	E980.4
40:28 diuretics NEC	974.4	E858.5	E944.4	E950.4	E962.0	E980.4	68:12 contraceptives, oral	962.2	E858.0	E932.2	E950.4	E962.0	E980.4
carbonic acid anhydrase inhibitors	974.2	E858.5	E944.2	E950.4	E962.0	E980.4	68:16 estrogens	962.2	E858.0	E932.2	E950.4	E962.0	E980.4
mercurials	974.0	E858.5	E944.0	E950.4	E962.0	E980.4	68:18 gonadotropins	962.4	E858.0	E932.4	E950.4	E962.0	E980.4
purine derivatives	974.1	E858.5	E944.1	E950.4	E962.0	E980.4	68:20.08 insulins	962.3	E858.0	E932.3	E950.4	E962.0	E980.4
saluretics	974.3	E858.5	E944.3	E950.4	E962.0	E980.4	68:20 insulins and antidiabetic agents	962.3	E858.0	E932.3	E950.4	E962.0	E980.4
thiazides	974.3	E858.5	E944.3	E950.4	E962.0	E980.4	68:24 parathyroid	962.6	E858.0	E932.6	E950.4	E962.0	E980.4
40:36 irrigating solutions	974.5	E858.5	E944.5	E950.4	E962.0	E980.4	68:28 pituitary (posterior)	962.5	E858.0	E932.5	E950.4	E962.0	E980.4
							anterior	962.4	E858.0	E932.4	E950.4	E962.0	E980.4

Drug — Table of Drugs and Chemicals

Drug	Poisoning	Accident	Therapeutic Use	Suicide Attempt	Assault	Undetermined
Drug — continued						
68:32 progestogens	962.2	E858.0	E932.2	E950.4	E962.0	E980.4
68:34 other corpus luteum hormones NEC	962.2	E858.0	E932.2	E950.4	E962.0	E980.4
68:36 thyroid and antithyroid						
antithyroid	962.8	E858.0	E932.8	E950.4	E962.0	E980.4
thyroid (derivatives)	962.7	E858.0	E932.7	E950.4	E962.0	E980.4
72:00 local anesthetics						
NEC	968.9	E855.2	E938.9	E950.4	E962.0	E980.4
infiltration (intradermal) (subcutaneous) (submucosal)	968.5	E855.2	E938.5	E950.4	E962.0	E980.4
nerve blocking (peripheral) (plexus) (regional)	968.6	E855.2	E938.6	E950.4	E962.0	E980.4
spinal	968.7	E855.2	E938.7	E950.4	E962.0	E980.4
topical (surface)	968.5	E855.2	E938.5	E950.4	E962.0	E980.4
76:00 oxytocics	975.0	E858.6	E945.0	E950.4	E962.0	E980.4
78:00 radioactive agents	990	—	—	—	—	—
80:04 serums NEC	979.9	E858.8	E949.9	E950.4	E962.0	E980.4
immune gamma globulin (human)	964.6	E858.2	E934.6	E950.4	E962.0	E980.4
80:08 toxoids NEC	978.8	E858.8	E948.8	E950.4	E962.0	E980.4
diphtheria	978.5	E858.8	E948.5	E950.4	E962.0	E980.4
and diphtheria	978.9	E858.8	E948.9	E950.4	E962.0	E980.4
with pertussis component	978.6	E858.8	E948.6	E950.4	E962.0	E980.4
and tetanus	978.9	E858.8	E948.9	E950.4	E962.0	E980.4
with pertussis component	978.6	E858.8	E948.6	E950.4	E962.0	E980.4
tetanus	978.4	E858.8	E948.4	E950.4	E962.0	E980.4
80:12 vaccines	979.9	E858.8	E949.9	E950.4	E962.0	E980.4
bacterial NEC	978.8	E858.8	E948.8	E950.4	E962.0	E980.4
with other bacterial components	978.9	E858.8	E948.9	E950.4	E962.0	E980.4
pertussis component	978.6	E858.8	E948.6	E950.4	E962.0	E980.4
viral and rickettsial components	979.7	E858.8	E949.7	E950.4	E962.0	E980.4
rickettsial NEC	979.6	E858.8	E949.6	E950.4	E962.0	E980.4
with bacterial component	979.7	E858.8	E949.7	E950.4	E962.0	E980.4
pertussis component	978.6	E858.8	E948.6	E950.4	E962.0	E980.4
viral component	979.7	E858.8	E949.7	E950.4	E962.0	E980.4
viral NEC	979.6	E858.8	E949.6	E950.4	E962.0	E980.4
with bacterial component	979.7	E858.8	E949.7	E950.4	E962.0	E980.4
pertussis component	978.6	E858.8	E948.6	E950.4	E962.0	E980.4
rickettsial component	979.7	E858.8	E949.7	E950.4	E962.0	E980.4
84:04.04 antibiotics (skin and mucous membrane)	976.0	E858.7	E946.0	E950.4	E962.0	E980.4
84:04.08 fungicides (skin and mucous membrane)	976.0	E858.7	E946.0	E950.4	E962.0	E980.4
84:04.12 scabicides and pediculicides (skin and mucous membrane)	976.0	E858.7	E946.0	E950.4	E962.0	E980.4
84:04.16 miscellaneous local anti-infectives (skin and mucous membrane)	976.0	E858.7	E946.0	E950.4	E962.0	E980.4
84:06 anti-inflammatory agents (skin and mucous membrane)	976.0	E858.7	E946.0	E950.4	E962.0	E980.4
84:08 antipruritics and local anesthetics						
antipruritics	976.1	E858.7	E946.1	E950.4	E962.0	E980.4
local anesthetics	968.5	E855.2	E938.5	E950.4	E962.0	E980.4
84:12 astringents	976.2	E858.7	E946.2	E950.4	E962.0	E980.4
84:16 cell stimulants and proliferants	976.8	E858.7	E946.8	E950.4	E962.0	E980.4
84:20 detergents	976.2	E858.7	E946.2	E950.4	E962.0	E980.4
84:24 emollients, demulcents, and protectants	976.3	E858.7	E946.3	E950.4	E962.0	E980.4
84:28 keratolytic agents	976.4	E858.7	E946.4	E950.4	E962.0	E980.4
84:32 keratoplastic agents	976.4	E858.7	E946.4	E950.4	E962.0	E980.4
84:36 miscellaneous agents (skin and mucous membrane)	976.8	E858.7	E946.8	E950.4	E962.0	E980.4
86:00 spasmolytic agents	975.1	E858.6	E945.1	E950.4	E962.0	E980.4
antiasthmatics	975.7	E858.6	E945.7	E950.4	E962.0	E980.4
papaverine	972.5	E858.3	E942.5	E950.4	E962.0	E980.4
theophylline	974.1	E858.6	E944.1	E950.4	E962.0	E980.4
88:04 vitamin A	963.5	E858.1	E933.5	E950.4	E962.0	E980.4
88:08 vitamin B complex	963.5	E858.1	E933.5	E950.4	E962.0	E980.4
hematopoietic vitamin	964.1	E858.2	E934.1	E950.4	E962.0	E980.4
nicotinic acid derivatives	972.2	E858.3	E942.2	E950.4	E962.0	E980.4
88:12 vitamin C	963.5	E858.1	E933.5	E950.4	E962.0	E980.4
88:16 vitamin D	963.5	E858.1	E933.5	E950.4	E962.0	E980.4
88:20 vitamin E	963.5	E858.1	E933.5	E950.4	E962.0	E980.4
88:24 vitamin K activity	964.3	E858.2	E934.3	E950.4	E962.0	E980.4
88:28 multivitamin preparations	963.5	E858.1	E933.5	E950.4	E962.0	E980.4
92:00 unclassified therapeutic agents	977.8	E858.8	E947.8	E950.4	E962.0	E980.4
specified NEC	977.8	E858.8	E947.8	E950.4	E962.0	E980.4
Duboisine	971.1	E855.4	E941.1	E950.4	E962.0	E980.4
Dulcolax	973.1	E858.4	E943.1	E950.4	E962.0	E980.4
Duponol (C) (EP)	976.2	E858.7	E946.2	E950.4	E962.0	E980.4
Durabolin	962.1	E858.0	E932.1	E950.4	E962.0	E980.4
Dyclone	968.5	E855.2	E938.5	E950.4	E962.0	E980.4
Dyclonine	968.5	E855.2	E938.5	E950.4	E962.0	E980.4
Dydrogesterone	962.2	E858.0	E932.2	E950.4	E962.0	E980.4
Dyes NEC	989.89	E866.8	—	E950.9	E962.1	E980.9
diagnostic agents	977.8	E858.8	E947.8	E950.4	E962.0	E980.4
pharmaceutical NEC	977.4	E858.8	E947.4	E950.4	E962.0	E980.4
Dyfols	971.0	E855.3	E941.0	E950.4	E962.0	E980.4
Dymelor	962.3	E858.0	E932.3	E950.4	E962.0	E980.4
Dynamite	989.89	E866.8	—	E950.9	E962.1	E980.9
fumes	987.8	E869.8	—	E952.8	E962.2	E982.8
Dyphylline	975.1	E858.6	E945.1	E950.4	E962.0	E980.4
Ear preparations	976.6	E858.7	E946.6	E950.4	E962.0	E980.4
Echothiopate, ecothiopate	971.0	E855.3	E941.0	E950.4	E962.0	E980.4
Ecstasy	969.7	E854.2	E939.7	E950.3	E962.0	E980.3
Ectylurea	967.8	E852.8	E937.8	E950.2	E962.0	E980.2
Edathamil disodium	963.8	E858.1	E933.8	E950.4	E962.0	E980.4
Edecrin	974.4	E858.5	E944.4	E950.4	E962.0	E980.4
Edetate, disodium (calcium)	963.8	E858.1	E933.8	E950.4	E962.0	E980.4
Edrophonium	971.0	E855.3	E941.0	E950.4	E962.0	E980.4
Elase	976.8	E858.7	E946.8	E950.4	E962.0	E980.4
Elaterium	973.1	E858.4	E943.1	E950.4	E962.0	E980.4
Elder	988.2	E865.4	—	E950.9	E962.1	E980.9
berry (unripe)	988.2	E865.3	—	E950.9	E962.1	E980.9
Electrolytes NEC	974.5	E858.5	E944.5	E950.4	E962.0	E980.4
Electrolytic agent NEC	974.5	E858.5	E944.5	E950.4	E962.0	E980.4
Embramine	963.0	E858.1	E933.0	E950.4	E962.0	E980.4
Emetics	973.6	E858.4	E943.6	E950.4	E962.0	E980.4
Emetine (hydrochloride)	961.5	E857	E931.5	E950.4	E962.0	E980.4
Emollients	976.3	E858.7	E946.3	E950.4	E962.0	E980.4
Emylcamate	969.5	E853.8	E939.5	E950.3	E962.0	E980.3
Encyprate	969.0	E854.0	E939.0	E950.3	E962.0	E980.3
Endocaine	968.5	E855.2	E938.5	E950.4	E962.0	E980.4
Endrin	989.2	E863.0	—	E950.6	E962.1	E980.7
Enflurane	968.2	E855.1	E938.2	E950.4	E962.0	E980.4
Enovid	962.2	E858.0	E932.2	E950.4	E962.0	E980.4
ENT preparations (anti-infectives)	976.6	E858.7	E946.6	E950.4	E962.0	E980.4
Enzodase	963.4	E858.1	E933.4	E950.4	E962.0	E980.4
Enzymes NEC	963.4	E858.1	E933.4	E950.4	E962.0	E980.4
Epanutin	966.1	E855.0	E936.1	E950.4	E962.0	E980.4
Ephedra (tincture)	971.2	E855.5	E941.2	E950.4	E962.0	E980.4
Ephedrine	971.2	E855.5	E941.2	E950.4	E962.0	E980.4
Epiestriol	962.2	E858.0	E932.2	E950.4	E962.0	E980.4
Epilim — see Sodium valproate						
Epinephrine	971.2	E855.5	E941.2	E950.4	E962.0	E980.4
Epsom salt	973.3	E858.4	E943.3	E950.4	E962.0	E980.4
Equanil	969.5	E853.8	E939.5	E950.3	E962.0	E980.3
Equisetum (diuretic)	974.4	E858.5	E944.4	E950.4	E962.0	E980.4
Ergometrine	975.0	E858.6	E945.0	E950.4	E962.0	E980.4
Ergonovine	975.0	E858.6	E945.0	E950.4	E962.0	E980.4
Ergot NEC	988.2	E865.4	—	E950.9	E962.1	E980.9
medicinal (alkaloids)	975.0	E858.6	E945.0	E950.4	E962.0	E980.4
Ergotamine (tartrate) (for migraine) NEC	972.9	E858.3	E942.9	E950.4	E962.0	E980.4
Ergotrate	975.0	E858.6	E945.0	E950.4	E962.0	E980.4
Erythrityl tetranitrate	972.4	E858.3	E942.4	E950.4	E962.0	E980.4
Erythrol tetranitrate	972.4	E858.3	E942.4	E950.4	E962.0	E980.4
Erythromycin	960.3	E856	E930.3	E950.4	E962.0	E980.4
ophthalmic preparation	976.5	E858.7	E946.5	E950.4	E962.0	E980.4

Table of Drugs and Chemicals

	Poisoning	External Cause (E-Code)				
		Accident	Therapeutic Use	Suicide Attempt	Assault	Undetermined
Erythromycin — *continued*						
topical NEC	976.0	E858.7	E946.0	E950.4	E962.0	E980.4
Eserine	971.0	E855.3	E941.0	E950.4	E962.0	E980.4
Eskabarb	967.0	E851	E937.0	E950.1	E962.0	E980.1
Eskalith	969.8	E855.8	E939.8	E950.3	E962.0	E980.3
Estradiol (cypionate) (dipropionate)						
(valerate)	962.2	E858.0	E932.2	E950.4	E962.0	E980.4
Estriol	962.2	E858.0	E932.2	E950.4	E962.0	E980.4
Estrogens (with						
progestogens)	962.2	E858.0	E932.2	E950.4	E962.0	E980.4
Estrone	962.2	E858.0	E932.2	E950.4	E962.0	E980.4
Etafedrine	971.2	E855.5	E941.2	E950.4	E962.0	E980.4
Ethacrynate sodium	974.4	E858.5	E944.4	E950.4	E962.0	E980.4
Ethacrynic acid	974.4	E858.5	E944.4	E950.4	E962.0	E980.4
Ethambutol	961.8	E857	E931.8	E950.4	E962.0	E980.4
Ethamide	974.2	E858.5	E944.2	E950.4	E962.0	E980.4
Ethamivan	970.0	E854.3	E940.0	E950.4	E962.0	E980.4
Ethamsylate	964.5	E858.2	E934.5	E950.4	E962.0	E980.4
Ethanol	980.0	E860.1	—	E950.9	E962.1	E980.9
beverage	980.0	E860.0	—	E950.9	E962.1	E980.9
Ethchlorvynol	967.8	E852.8	E937.8	E950.2	E962.0	E980.2
Ethebenecid	974.7	E858.5	E944.7	E950.4	E962.0	E980.4
Ether(s) (diethyl) (ethyl)						
(vapor)	987.8	E869.8	—	E952.8	E962.2	E982.8
anesthetic	968.2	E855.1	E938.2	E950.4	E962.0	E980.4
petroleum — see Ligroin						
solvent	982.8	E862.4	—	E950.9	E962.1	E980.9
Ethidine chloride (vapor)	987.8	E869.8	—	E952.8	E962.2	E982.8
liquid (solvent)	982.3	E862.4	—	E950.9	E962.1	E980.9
Ethinamate	967.8	E852.8	E937.8	E950.2	E962.0	E980.2
Ethinylestradiol	962.2	E858.0	E932.2	E950.4	E962.0	E980.4
Ethionamide	961.8	E857	E931.8	E950.4	E962.0	E980.4
Ethisterone	962.2	E858.0	E932.2	E950.4	E962.0	E980.4
Ethobral	967.0	E851	E937.0	E950.1	E962.0	E980.1
Ethocaine (infiltration)						
(topical)	968.5	E855.2	E938.5	E950.4	E962.0	E980.4
nerve block (peripheral)						
(plexus)	968.6	E855.2	E938.6	E950.4	E962.0	E980.4
spinal	968.7	E855.2	E938.7	E950.4	E962.0	E980.4
Ethoheptazine (citrate)	965.7	E850.7	E935.7	E950	E962.0	E980.0
Ethopropazine	966.4	E855.0	E936.4	E950.4	E962.0	E980.4
Ethosuximide	966.2	E855.0	E936.2	E950.4	E962.0	E980.4
Ethotoin	966.1	E855.0	E936.1	E950.4	E962.0	E980.4
Ethoxazene	961.9	E857	E931.9	E950.4	E962.0	E980.4
Ethoxzolamide	974.2	E858.5	E944.2	E950.4	E962.0	E980.4
Ethyl						
acetate (vapor)	982.8	E862.4	—	E950.9	E962.1	E980.9
alcohol	980.0	E860.1	—	E950.9	E962.1	E980.9
beverage	980.0	E860.0	—	E950.9	E962.1	E980.9
aldehyde (vapor)	987.8	E869.8	—	E952.8	E962.2	E982.8
liquid	989.89	E866.8	—	E950.9	E962.1	E980.9
aminobenzoate	968.5	E855.2	E938.5	E950.4	E962.0	E980.4
biscoumacetate	964.2	E858.2	E934.2	E950.4	E962.0	E980.4
bromide (anesthetic)	968.2	E855.1	E938.2	E950.4	E962.0	E980.4
carbamate (antineoplastic)	963.1	E858.1	E933.1	E950.4	E962.0	E980.4
carbinol	980.3	E860.4	—	E950.9	E962.1	E980.9
chaulmoograte	961.8	E857	E931.8	E950.4	E962.0	E980.4
chloride (vapor)	987.8	E869.8	—	E952.8	E962.2	E982.8
anesthetic (local)	968.5	E855.2	E938.5	E950.4	E962.0	E980.4
inhaled	968.2	E855.1	E938.2	E950.4	E962.0	E980.4
solvent	982.3	E862.4	—	E950.9	E962.1	E980.9
estranol	962.1	E858.0	E932.1	E950.4	E962.0	E980.4
ether — see Ether(s)						
formate (solvent) NEC	982.8	E862.4	—	E950.9	E962.1	E980.9
iodoacetate	987.5	E869.3	—	E952.8	E962.2	E982.8
lactate (solvent) NEC	982.8	E862.4	—	E950.9	E962.1	E980.9
methylcarbinol	980.8	E860.8	—	E950	E962.1	E980.9
morphine	965.09	E850.2	E935.2	E950.0	E962.0	E980.0
Ethylene (gas)	987.1	E869.8	—	E952.8	E962.2	E982.8
anesthetic (general)	968.2	E855.1	E938.2	E950.4	E962.0	E980.4
chlorohydrin (vapor)	982.3	E862.4	—	E950.9	E962.1	E980.9
dichloride (vapor)	982.3	E862.4	—	E950.9	E962.1	E980.9
glycol(s) (any) (vapor)	982.8	E862.4	—	E950.9	E962.1	E980.9
Ethylidene						
chloride NEC	982.3	E862.4	—	E950.9	E962.1	E980.9
diethyl ether	982.8	E862.4	—	E950.9	E962.1	E980.9
Ethynodiol	962.2	E858.0	E932.2	E950.4	E962.0	E980.4
Etidocaine	968.9	E855.2	E938.9	E950.4	E962.0	E980.4
infiltration (subcutaneous)	968.5	E855.2	E938.5	E950.4	E962.0	E980.4
nerve (peripheral) (plexus)	968.6	E855.2	E938.6	E950.4	E962.0	E980.4
Etilfen	967.0	E851	E937.0	E950.1	E962.0	E980.1
Etomide	965.7	E850.7	E935.7	E950.0	E962.0	E980.0
Etorphine	965.09	E850.2	E935.2	E950.0	E962.0	E980.0
Etoval	967.0	E851	E937.0	E950.1	E962.0	E980.1
Etryptamine	969.0	E854.0	E939.0	E950.3	E962.0	E980.3
Eucaine	968.5	E855.2	E938.5	E950.4	E962.0	E980.4
Eucalyptus (oil) NEC	975.5	E858.6	E945.5	E950.4	E962.0	E980.4
Eucatropine	971.1	E855.4	E941.1	E950.4	E962.0	E980.4
Eucodal	965.09	E850.2	E935.2	E950.0	E962.0	E980.0
Euneryl	967.0	E851	E937.0	E950.1	E962.0	E980.1
Euphthalmine	971.1	E855.4	E941.1	E950.4	E962.0	E980.4
Eurax	976.0	E858.7	E946.0	E950.4	E962.0	E980.4
Euresol	976.4	E858.7	E946.4	E950.4	E962.0	E980.4
Euthroid	962.7	E858.0	E932.7	E950.4	E962.0	E980.4
Evans blue	977.8	E858.8	E947.8	E950.4	E962.0	E980.4
Evipal	967.0	E851	E937.0	E950.1	E962.0	E980.1
sodium	968.3	E855.1	E938.3	E950.4	E962.0	E980.4
Evipan	967.0	E851	E937.0	E950.1	E962.0	E980.1
sodium	968.3	E855.1	E938.3	E950.4	E962.0	E980.4
Exalgin	965.4	E850.4	E935.4	E950.0	E962.0	E980.0
Excipients,						
pharmaceutical	977.4	E858.8	E947.4	E950.4	E962.0	E980.4
Exhaust gas — *see* Carbon, monoxide						
Ex-Lax (phenolphthalein)	973.1	E858.4	E943.1	E950.4	E962.0	E980.4
Expectorants	975.5	E858.6	E945.5	E950.4	E962.0	E980.4
External medications (skin)						
(mucous membrane)	976.9	E858.7	E946.9	E950.4	E962.0	E980.4
dental agent	976.7	E858.7	E946.7	E950.4	E962.0	E980.4
ENT agent	976.6	E858.7	E946.6	E950.4	E962.0	E980.4
ophthalmic preparation	976.5	E858.7	E946.5	E950.4	E962.0	E980.4
specified NEC	976.8	E858.7	E946.8	E950.4	E962.0	E980.4
Eye agents (anti-infective)	976.5	E858.7	E946.5	E950.4	E962.0	E980.4
Factor IX complex (human)	964.5	E858.2	E934.5	E950.4	E962.0	E980.4
Fecal softeners	973.2	E858.4	E943.2	E950.4	E962.0	E980.4
Fenbutrazate	977.0	E858.8	E947.0	E950.4	E962.0	E980.4
Fencamfamin	970.8	E854.3	E940.8	E950.4	E962.0	E980.4
Fenfluramine	977.0	E858.8	E947.0	E950.4	E962.0	E980.4
Fenoprofen	965.61	E850.6	E935.6	E950.0	E962.0	E980.0
Fentanyl	965.09	E850.2	E935.2	E950.0	E962.0	E980.0
Fentazin	969.1	E853.0	E939.1	E950.3	E962.0	E980.3
Fenticlor, fentichlor	976.0	E858.7	E946.0	E950.4	E962.0	E980.4
Fer de lance (bite) (venom)	989.5	E905.0	—	E950.9	E962.1	E980.9
Ferric — *see* Iron						
Ferrocholinate	964.0	E858.2	E934.0	E950.4	E962.0	E980.4
Ferrous fumerate, gluconate, lactate, salt NEC, sulfate						
(medicinal)	964.0	E858.2	E934.0	E950.4	E962.0	E980.4
Ferrum — *see* Iron						
Fertilizers NEC	989.89	E866.5	—	E950.9	E962.1	E980.4
with herbicide mixture	989.4	E863.5	—	E950.6	E962.1	E980.7
Fibrinogen (human)	964.7	E858.2	E934.7	E950.4	E962.0	E980.4
Fibrinolysin	964.4	E858.2	E934.4	E950.4	E962.0	E980.4
Fibrinolysis-affecting						
agents	964.4	E858.2	E934.4	E950.4	E962.0	E980.4
Filix mas	961.6	E857	E931.6	E950.4	E962.0	E980.4
Fiorinal	965.1	E850.3	E935.3	E950.0	E962.0	E980.0
Fire damp	987.1	E869.8	—	E952.8	E962.2	E982.8
Fish, nonbacterial or						
noxious	988.0	E865.2	—	E950.9	E962.1	E980.9
shell	988.0	E865.1	—	E950.9	E962.1	E980.9
Flagyl	961.5	E857	E931.5	E950.4	E962.0	E980.4
Flavoxate	975.1	E858.6	E945.1	E950.4	E962.0	E980.4
Flaxedil	975.2	E858.6	E945.2	E950.4	E962.0	E980.4
Flaxseed (medicinal)	976.3	E858.7	E946.3	E950.4	E962.0	E980.4
Florantyrone	973.4	E858.4	E943.4	E950.4	E962.0	E980.4
Floraquin	961.3	E857	E931.3	E950.4	E962.0	E980.4
Florinef	962.0	E858.0	E932.0	E950.4	E962.0	E980.4
ENT agent	976.6	E858.7	E946.6	E950.4	E962.0	E980.4
ophthalmic preparation	976.5	E858.7	E946.5	E950.4	E962.0	E980.4
topical NEC	976.0	E858.7	E946.0	E950.4	E962.0	E980.4
Flowers of sulfur	976.4	E858.7	E946.4	E950.4	E962.0	E980.4
Floxuridine	963.1	E858.1	E933.1	E950.4	E962.0	E980.4
Flucytosine	961.9	E857	E931.9	E950.4	E962.0	E980.4
Fludrocortisone	962.0	E858.0	E932.0	E950.4	E962.0	E980.4
ENT agent	976.6	E858.7	E946.6	E950.4	E962.0	E980.4
ophthalmic preparation	976.5	E858.7	E946.5	E950.4	E962.0	E980.4
topical NEC	976.0	E858.7	E946.0	E950.4	E962.0	E980.4
Flumethasone	976.0	E858.7	E946.0	E950.4	E962.0	E980.4
Flumethiazide	974.3	E858.5	E944.3	E950.4	E962.0	E980.4
Flumidin	961.7	E857	E931.7	E950.4	E962.0	E980.4
Flunitrazepam	969.4	E853.2	E939.4	E950.3	E962.0	E980.3

Table of Drugs and Chemicals

Fluocinolone — Gas

	Poisoning	Accident	Therapeutic Use	Suicide Attempt	Assault	Undetermined
Fluocinolone	976.0	E858.7	E946.0	E950.4	E962.0	E980.4
Fluocortolone	962.0	E858.0	E932.0	E950.4	E962.0	E980.4
Fluohydrocortisone	962.0	E858.0	E932.0	E950.4	E962.0	E980.4
ENT agent	976.6	E858.7	E946.6	E950.4	E962.0	E980.4
ophthalmic preparation	976.5	E858.7	E946.5	E950.4	E962.0	E980.4
topical NEC	976.0	E858.7	E946.0	E950.4	E962.0	E980.4
Fluonid	976.0	E858.7	E946.0	E950.4	E962.0	E980.4
Fluopromazine	969.1	E853.0	E939.1	E950.3	E962.0	E980.3
Fluoracetate	989.4	E863.7	—	E950.6	E962.1	E980.7
Fluorescein (sodium)	977.8	E858.8	E947.8	E950.4	E962.0	E980.4
Fluoride(s) (pesticides) (sodium)						
NEC	989.4	E863.4	—	E950.6	E962.1	E980.7
hydrogen — see Hydrofluoric acid						
medicinal	976.7	E858.7	E946.7	E950.4	E962.0	E980.4
not pesticide NEC	983.9	E864.4	—	E950.7	E962.1	E980.6
stannous	976.7	E858.7	E946.7	E950.4	E962.0	E980.4
Fluorinated						
corticosteroids	962.0	E858.0	E932.0	E950.4	E962.0	E980.4
Fluorine (compounds) (gas)	987.8	E869.8	—	E952.8	E962.2	E982.8
salt — see Fluoride(s)						
Fluoristan	976.7	E858.7	E946.7	E950.4	E962.0	E980.4
Fluoroacetate	989.4	E863.7	—	E950.6	E962.1	E980.7
Fluorodeoxyuridine	963.1	E858.1	E933.1	E950.4	E962.0	E980.4
Fluorometholone (topical)						
NEC	976.0	E858.7	E946.0	E950.4	E962.0	E980.4
ophthalmic preparation	976.5	E858.7	E946.5	E950.4	E962.0	E980.4
Fluorouracil	963.1	E858.1	E933.1	E950.4	E962.0	E980.4
Fluothane	968.1	E855.1	E938.1	E950.4	E962.0	E980.4
Fluoxetine hydrochloride	969.0	E854.0	E939.0	E950.3	E962.0	E980.3
Fluoxymesterone	962.1	E858.0	E932.1	E950.4	E962.0	E980.4
Fluphenazine	969.1	E853.0	E939.1	E950.3	E962.0	E980.3
Fluprednisolone	962.0	E858.0	E932.0	E950.4	E962.0	E980.4
Flurandrenolide	976.0	E858.7	E946.0	E950.4	E962.0	E980.4
Flurazepam (hydrochloride)	969.4	E853.2	E939.4	E950.3	E962.0	E980.3
Flurbiprofen	965.61	E850.6	E935.6	E950.0	E962.0	E980.0
Flurobate	976.0	E858.7	E946.0	E950.4	E962.0	E980.4
Flurothyl	969.8	E855.8	E939.8	E950.3	E962.0	E980.3
Fluroxene	968.2	E855.1	E938.2	E950.4	E962.0	E980.4
Folacin	964.1	E858.2	E934.1	E950.4	E962.0	E980.4
Folic acid	964.1	E858.2	E934.1	E950.4	E962.0	E980.4
Follicle stimulating						
hormone	962.4	E858.0	E932.4	E950.4	E962.0	E980.4
Food, foodstuffs, nonbacterial						
or noxious	988.9	E865.9	—	E950.9	E962.1	E980.9
berries, seeds	988.2	E865.3	—	E950.9	E962.1	E980.9
fish	988.0	E865.2	—	E950.9	E962.1	E980.9
mushrooms	988.1	E865.5	—	E950.9	E962.1	E980.9
plants	988.2	E865.9	—	E950.9	E962.1	E980.9
specified type NEC	988.2	E865.4	—	E950.9	E962.1	E980.9
shellfish	988.0	E865.1	—	E950.9	E962.1	E980.9
specified NEC	988.8	E865.8	—	E950.9	E962.1	E980.9
Fool's parsley	988.2	E865.4	—	E950.9	E962.1	E980.9
Formaldehyde (solution)	989.89	E861.4	—	E950.9	E962.1	E980.9
fungicide	989.4	E863.6	—	E950.6	E962.1	E980.7
gas or vapor	987.8	E869.8	—	E952.8	E962.2	E982.8
Formalin	989.89	E861.4	—	E950.9	E962.1	E980.9
fungicide	989.4	E863.6	—	E950.6	E962.1	E980.7
vapor	987.8	E869.8	—	E952.8	E962.2	E982.8
Formic acid	983.1	E864.1	—	E950.7	E962.1	E980.6
automobile	981	E862.1	—	E950.9	E962.1	E980.9
exhaust gas, not in transit	986	E868.2	—	E952.0	E962.2	E982.0
vapor NEC	987.1	E869.8	—	E952.8	E962.2	E982.8
gas (domestic use) (see also Carbon, monoxide, fuel)						
utility	987.1	E868.1	—	E951.8	E962.2	E981.8
incomplete combustion of — see Carbon, monoxide, fuel, utility						
in mobile container	987.0	E868.0	—	E951.1	E962.2	E981.1
piped (natural)	987.1	E867	—	E951.0	E962.2	E981.0
industrial, incomplete combustion	986	E868.3	—	E952.1	E962.2	E982.1
vapor	987.8	E869.8	—	E952.8	E962.2	E982.8
Fowler's solution	985.1	E866.3	—	E950.8	E962.1	E980.8
Foxglove	988.2	E865.4	—	E950.9	E962.1	E980.9
Fox green	977.8	E858.8	E947.8	E950.4	E962.0	E980.4
Framycetin	960.8	E856	E930.8	E950.4	E962.0	E980.4
Frangula (extract)	973.1	E858.4	E943.1	E950.4	E962.0	E980.4
Frei antigen	977.8	E858.8	E947.8	E950.4	E962.0	E980.4
Freons	987.4	E869.2	—	E952.8	E962.2	E982.8
Fructose	974.5	E858.5	E944.5	E950.4	E962.0	E980.4
Frusemide	974.4	E858.5	E944.4	E950.4	E962.0	E980.4
FSH	962.4	E858.0	E932.4	E950.4	E962.0	E980.4
Fuel						
Fugillin	960.8	E856	E930.8	E950.4	E962.0	E980.4
Fulminate of mercury	985.0	E866.1	—	E950.9	E962.1	E980.9
Fulvicin	960.1	E856	E930.1	E950.4	E962.0	E980.4
Fumadil	960.8	E856	E930.8	E950.4	E962.0	E980.4
Fumagillin	960.8	E856	E930.8	E950.4	E962.0	E980.4
Fumes (from)	987.9	E869.9	—	E952.9	E962.2	E982.9
carbon monoxide — see Carbon, monoxide						
charcoal (domestic use)	986	E868.3	—	E952.1	E962.2	E982.1
chloroform — see Chloroform						
coke (in domestic stoves, fireplaces)	986	E868.3	—	E952.1	E962.2	E982.1
corrosive NEC	987.8	E869.8	—	E952.8	E962.2	E982.8
ether — see Ether(s)						
freons	987.4	E869.2	—	E952.8	E962.2	E982.8
hydrocarbons	987.1	E869.8	—	E952.8	E962.2	E982.8
petroleum (liquefied)	987.0	E868.0	—	E951.1	E962.2	E981.1
distributed through pipes (pure or mixed with air)	987.0	E867	—	E951.0	E962.2	E981.0
lead — see Lead						
metals — see specified metal						
nitrogen dioxide	987.2	E869.0	—	E952.8	E962.2	E982.8
pesticides — see Pesticides						
petroleum (liquefied)	987.0	E868.0	—	E951.1	E962.2	E981.1
distributed through pipes (pure or mixed with air)	987.0	E867	—	E951.0	E962.2	E981.0
polyester	987.8	E869.8	—	E952.8	E962.2	E982.8
specified, source other (see also substance specified)	987.8	E869.8	—	E952.8	E962.2	E982.8
sulfur dioxide	987.3	E869.1	—	E952.8	E962.2	E982.8
Fumigants	989.4	E863.8	—	E950.6	E962.1	E980.7
Fungicides — see also						
Antifungals	989.4	E863.6	—	E950.6	E962.1	E980.7
Fungi, noxious, used as						
food	988.1	E865.5	—	E950.9	E962.1	E980.9
Fungizone	960.1	E856	E930.1	E950.4	E962.0	E980.4
topical	976.0	E858.7	E946.0	E950.4	E962.0	E980.4
Furacin	976.0	E858.7	E946.0	E950.4	E962.0	E980.4
Furadantin	961.9	E857	E931.9	E950.4	E962.0	E980.4
Furazolidone	961.9	E857	E931.9	E950.4	E962.0	E980.4
Furnace (coal burning) (domestic),						
gas from	986	E868.3	—	E952.1	E962.2	E982.1
industrial	986	E868.8	—	E952.1	E962.2	E982.1
Furniture polish	989.89	E861.2	—	E950.9	E962.1	E980.9
Furosemide	974.4	E858.5	E944.4	E950.4	E962.0	E980.4
Furoxone	961.9	E857	E931.9	E950.4	E962.0	E980.4
Fusel oil (amyl) (butyl) (propyl)	980.3	E860.4	—	E950.9	E962.1	E980.9
Fusidic acid	960.8	E856	E930.8	E950.4	E962.0	E980.4
Gallamine	975.2	E858.6	E945.2	E950.4	E962.0	E980.4
Gallotannic acid	976.2	E858.7	E946.2	E950.4	E962.0	E980.4
Gamboge	973.1	E858.4	E943.1	E950.4	E962.0	E980.4
Gamimune	964.6	E858.2	E934.6	E950.4	E962.0	E980.4
Gamma-benzene hexachloride						
(vapor)	989.2	E863.0	—	E950.6	E962.1	E980.7
Gamma globulin	964.6	E858.2	E934.6	E950.4	E962.0	E980.4
Gamma hydroxy butyrate						
(GHB)	968.4	E855.1	E938.4	E950.4	E962.0	E980.4
Gamulin	964.6	E858.2	E934.6	E950.4	E962.0	E980.4
Ganglionic blocking						
agents	972.3	E858.3	E942.3	E950.4	E962.0	E980.4
Ganja	969.6	E854.1	E939.6	E950.3	E962.0	E980.3
Garamycin	960.8	E856	E930.8	E950.4	E962.0	E980.4
ophthalmic preparation	976.5	E858.7	E946.5	E950.4	E962.0	E980.4
topical NEC	976.0	E858.7	E946.0	E950.4	E962.0	E980.4
Gardenal	967.0	E851	E937.0	E950.1	E962.0	E980.1
Gardepanyl	967.0	E851	E937.0	E950.1	E962.0	E980.1
Gas	987.9	E869.9	—	E952.9	E962.2	E982.9
acetylene	987.1	E868.1	—	E951.8	E962.2	E981.8
incomplete combustion of — see Carbon, monoxide, fuel, utility						
air contaminants, source or type not specified	987.9	E869.9	—	E952.9	E962.2	E982.9
anesthetic (general) NEC	968.2	E855.1	E938.2	E950.4	E962.0	E980.4

Table of Drugs and Chemicals — Hashish

	Poisoning	Accident	Therapeutic Use	Suicide Attempt	Assault	Undetermined
Gas — *continued*						
blast furnace	986	E868.8	—	E952.1	E962.2	E982.1
butane — *see* Butane						
carbon monoxide — *see* Carbon, monoxide						
chlorine	987.6	E869.8	—	E952.8	E962.2	E982.8
coal — *see* Carbon, monoxide, coal						
cyanide	987.7	E869.8	—	E952.8	E962.2	E982.8
dicyanogen	987.8	E869.8	—	E952.8	E962.2	E982.8
domestic — *see* Gas, utility						
exhaust — *see* Carbon, monoxide, exhaust gas						
from wood- or coal-burning stove or fireplace	986	E868.3	—	E952.1	E962.2	E982.1
fuel (domestic use) (*see also* Carbon, monoxide, fuel)						
industrial use	986	E868.8	—	E952.1	E962.2	E982.1
utility	987.1	E868.1	—	E951.8	E962.2	E981.8
incomplete combustion of — *see* Carbon, monoxide, fuel, utility						
in mobile container	987.0	E868.0	—	E951.1	E962.2	E981.1
piped (natural)	987.1	E867	—	E951.0	E962.2	E981.0
garage	986	E868.2	—	E952.0	E962.2	E982.0
hydrocarbon NEC	987.1	E869.8	—	E952.8	E962.2	E982.8
incomplete combustion of — *see* Carbon, monoxide, fuel, utility						
liquefied (mobile container)	987.0	E868.0	—	E951.1	E962.2	E981.1
piped	987.0	E867	—	E951.0	E962.2	E981.0
hydrocyanic acid	987.7	E869.8	—	E952.8	E962.2	E982.8
illuminating — *see* Gas, utility						
incomplete combustion, any — *see* Carbon, monoxide						
kiln	986	E868.8	—	E952.1	E962.2	E982.1
lacrimogenic	987.5	E869.3	—	E952.8	E962.2	E982.8
marsh	987.1	E869.8	—	E952.8	E962.2	E982.8
motor exhaust, not in transit	986	E868.8	—	E952.1	E962.2	E982.1
mustard — *see* Mustard, gas						
natural	987.1	E867	—	E951.0	E962.2	E981.0
nerve (war)	987.9	E869.9	—	E952.9	E962.2	E982.9
oils	981	E862.1	—	E950.9	E962.1	E980.9
petroleum (liquefied) (distributed in mobile containers)	987.0	E868.0	—	E951.1	E962.2	E981.1
piped (pure or mixed with air)	987.0	E867	—	E951.1	E962.2	E981.1
piped (manufactured) (natural) NEC	987.1	E867	—	E951.0	E962.2	E981.0
producer	986	E868.8	—	E952.1	E962.2	E982.1
propane — *see* Propane						
refrigerant (freon)	987.4	E869.2	—	E952.8	E962.2	E982.8
not freon	987.9	E869.9	—	E952.9	E962.2	E982.9
sewer	987.8	E869.8	—	E952.8	E962.2	E982.8
specified source NEC (*see also* substance specified)	987.8	E869.8	—	E952.8	E962.2	E982.8
stove — *see* Gas, utility						
tear	987.5	E869.3	—	E952.8	E962.2	E982.8
utility (for cooking, heating, or lighting) (piped) NEC	987.1	E868.1	—	E951.8	E962.2	E981.8
incomplete combustion of — *see* Carbon, monoxide, fuel, utilty						
in mobile container	987.0	E868.0	—	E951.1	E962.2	E981.1
piped (natural)	987.1	E867	—	E951.0	E962.2	E981.0
water	987.1	E868.1	—	E951.8	E962.2	E981.8
incomplete combustion of — *see* Carbon, monoxide, fuel, utility						
Gaseous substance — *see* Gas						
Gasoline, gasolene	981	E862.1	—	E950.9	E962.1	E980.9
vapor	987.1	E869.8	—	E952.8	E962.2	E982.8
Gastric enzymes	973.4	E858.4	E943.4	E950.4	E962.0	E980.4
Gastrografin	977.8	E858.8	E947.8	E950.4	E962.0	E980.4
Gastrointestinal agents	973.9	E858.4	E943.9	E950.4	E962.0	E980.4
specified NEC	973.8	E858.4	E943.8	E950.4	E962.0	E980.4
Gaultheria procumbens	988.2	E865.4	—	E950.9	E962.1	E980.9
Gelatin (intravenous)	964.8	E858.2	E934.8	E950.4	E962.0	E980.4
absorbable (sponge)	964.5	E858.2	E934.5	E950.4	E962.0	E980.4
Gelfilm	976.8	E858.7	E946.8	E950.4	E962.0	E980.4
Gelfoam	964.5	E858.2	E934.5	E950.4	E962.0	E980.4
Gelsemine	970.8	E854.3	E940.8	E950.4	E962.0	E980.4
Gelsemium (sempervirens)	988.2	E865.4	—	E950.9	E962.1	E980.9
Gemonil	967.0	E851	E937.0	E950.1	E962.0	E980.1
Gentamicin	960.8	E856	E930.8	E950.4	E962.0	E980.4
ophthalmic preparation	976.5	E858.7	E946.5	E950.4	E962.0	E980.4
topical NEC	976.0	E858.7	E946.0	E950.4	E962.0	E980.4
Gentian violet	976.0	E858.7	E946.0	E950.4	E962.0	E980.4
Gexane	976.0	E858.7	E946.0	E950.4	E962.0	E980.4
Gila monster (venom)	989.5	E905.0	—	E950.9	E962.1	E980.9
Ginger, Jamaica	989.89	E866.8	—	E950.9	E962.1	E980.9
Gitalin	972.1	E858.3	E942.1	E950.4	E962.0	E980.4
Gitoxin	972.1	E858.3	E942.1	E950.4	E962.0	E980.4
Glandular extract (medicinal) NEC	977.9	E858.9	E947.9	E950.5	E962.0	E980.5
Glaucarubin	961.5	E857	E931.5	E950.4	E962.0	E980.4
Globin zinc insulin	962.3	E858.0	E932.3	E950.4	E962.0	E980.4
Glucagon	962.3	E858.0	E932.3	E950.4	E962.0	E980.4
Glucochloral	967.1	E852.0	E937.1	E950.2	E962.0	E980.2
Glucocorticoids	962.0	E858.0	E932.0	E950.4	E962.0	E980.4
Glucose	974.5	E858.5	E944.5	E950.4	E962.0	E980.4
oxidase reagent	977.8	E858.8	E947.8	E950.4	E962.0	E980.4
Glucosulfone sodium	961.8	E857	E931.8	E950.4	E962.0	E980.4
Glue(s)	989.89	E866.6	—	E950.9	E962.1	E980.9
Glutamic acid (hydrochloride)	973.4	E858.4	E943.4	E950.4	E962.0	E980.4
Glutaraldehyde	989.89	E861.4	—	E950.9	E962.1	E980.9
Glutathione	963.8	E858.1	E933.8	E950.4	E962.0	E980.4
Glutethimide (group)	967.5	E852.4	E937.5	E950.2	E962.0	E980.2
Glycerin (lotion)	976.3	E858.7	E946.3	E950.4	E962.0	E980.4
Glycerol (topical)	976.3	E858.7	E946.3	E950.4	E962.0	E980.4
Glyceryl						
guaiacolate	975.5	E858.6	E945.5	E950.4	E962.0	E980.4
triacetate (topical)	976.0	E858.7	E946.0	E950.4	E962.0	E980.4
trinitrate	972.4	E858.3	E942.4	E950.4	E962.0	E980.4
Glycine	974.5	E858.5	E944.5	E950.4	E962.0	E980.4
Glycobiarsol	961.1	E857	E931.1	E950.4	E962.0	E980.4
Glycols (ether)	982.8	E862.4	—	E950.9	E962.1	E980.9
Glycopyrrolate	971.1	E855.4	E941.1	E950.4	E962.0	E980.4
Glymidine	962.3	E858.0	E932.3	E950.4	E962.0	E980.4
Gold (compounds) (salts)	965.69	E850.6	E935.6	E950.0	E962.0	E980.0
Golden sulfide of antimony	985.4	E866.2	—	E950.9	E962.1	E980.9
Goldylocks	988.2	E865.4	—	E950.9	E962.1	E980.9
Gonadal tissue extract	962.9	E858.0	E932.9	E950.4	E962.0	E980.4
beverage	980.0	E860.0	—	E950.9	E962.1	E980.9
female	962.2	E858.0	E932.2	E950.4	E962.0	E980.4
male	962.1	E858.0	E932.1	E950.4	E962.0	E980.4
Gonadotropin	962.4	E858.0	E932.4	E950.4	E962.0	E980.4
Grain alcohol	980.0	E860.1	—	E950.9	E962.1	E980.9
Gramicidin	960.8	E856	E930.8	E950.4	E962.0	E980.4
Gratiola officinalis	988.2	E865.4	—	E950.9	E962.1	E980.9
Grease	989.89	E866.8	—	E950.9	E962.1	E980.9
Green hellebore	988.2	E865.4	—	E950.9	E962.1	E980.9
Green soap	976.2	E858.7	E946.2	E950.4	E962.0	E980.4
Grifulvin	960.1	E856	E930.1	E950.4	E962.0	E980.4
Griseofulvin	960.1	E856	E930.1	E950.4	E962.0	E980.4
Growth hormone	962.4	E858.0	E932.4	E950.4	E962.0	E980.4
Guaiacol	975.5	E858.6	E945.5	E950.4	E962.0	E980.4
Guaiac reagent	977.8	E858.8	E947.8	E950.4	E962.0	E980.4
Guaifenesin	975.5	E858.6	E945.5	E950.4	E962.0	E980.4
Guaiphenesin	975.5	E858.6	E945.5	E950.4	E962.0	E980.4
Guanatol	961.4	E857	E931.4	E950.4	E962.0	E980.4
Guanethidine	972.6	E858.3	E942.6	E950.4	E962.0	E980.4
Guano	989.89	E866.5	—	E950.9	E962.1	E980.9
Guanochlor	972.6	E858.3	E942.6	E950.4	E962.0	E980.4
Guanoctine	972.6	E858.3	E942.6	E950.4	E962.0	E980.4
Guanoxan	972.6	E858.3	E942.6	E950.4	E962.0	E980.4
Hair treatment agent NEC	976.4	E858.7	E946.4	E950.4	E962.0	E980.4
Halcinonide	976.0	E858.7	E946.0	E950.4	E962.0	E980.4
Halethazole	976.0	E858.7	E946.0	E950.4	E962.0	E980.4
Hallucinogens	969.6	E854.1	E939.6	E950.3	E962.0	E980.3
Haloperidol	969.2	E853.1	E939.2	E950.3	E962.0	E980.3
Haloprogin	976.0	E858.7	E946.0	E950.4	E962.0	E980.4
Halotex	976.0	E858.7	E946.0	E950.4	E962.0	E980.4
Halothane	968.1	E855.1	E938.1	E950.4	E962.0	E980.4
Halquinols	976.0	E858.7	E946.0	E950.4	E962.0	E980.4
Harmonyl	972.6	E858.3	E942.6	E950.4	E962.0	E980.4
Hartmann's solution	974.5	E858.5	E944.5	E950.4	E962.0	E980.4
Hashish	969.6	E854.1	E939.6	E950.3	E962.0	E980.3

Hawaiian wood rose seeds — Table of Drugs and Chemicals

Substance	Poisoning	Accident	Therapeutic Use	Suicide Attempt	Assault	Undetermined
Hawaiian wood rose seeds	969.6	E854.1	E939.6	E950.3	E962.0	E980.3
Headache cures, drugs, powders NEC	977.9	E858.9	E947.9	E950.5	E962.0	E980.9
Heavenly Blue (morning glory)	969.6	E854.1	E939.6	E950.3	E962.0	E980.3
Heavy metal antagonists	963.8	E858.1	E933.8	E950.4	E962.0	E980.4
anti-infectives	961.2	E857	E931.2	E950.4	E962.0	E980.4
Hedaquinium	976.0	E858.7	E946.0	E950.4	E962.0	E980.4
Hedge hyssop	988.2	E865.4	—	E950.9	E962.1	E980.9
Heet	976.8	E858.7	E946.8	E950.4	E962.0	E980.4
Helenin	961.6	E857	E931.6	E950.4	E962.0	E980.4
Hellebore (black) (green) (white)	988.2	E865.4	—	E950.9	E962.1	E980.9
Hemlock	988.2	E865.4	—	E950.9	E962.1	E980.9
Hemostatics	964.5	E858.2	E934.5	E950.4	E962.0	E980.4
capillary active drugs	972.8	E858.3	E942.8	E950.4	E962.0	E980.4
Henbane	988.2	E865.4	—	E950.9	E962.1	E980.9
Heparin (sodium)	964.2	E858.2	E934.2	E950.4	E962.0	E980.4
Heptabarbital, heptabarbitone	967.0	E851	E937.0	E950.1	E962.0	E980.1
Heptachlor	989.2	E863.0	—	E950.6	E962.1	E980.7
Heptalgin	965.09	E850.2	E935.2	E950.0	E962.0	E980.0
Herbicides	989.4	E863.5	—	E950.6	E962.1	E980.7
Heroin	965.01	E850.0	E935.0	E950.0	E962.0	E980.0
Herplex	976.5	E858.7	E946.5	E950.4	E962.0	E980.4
HES	964.8	E858.2	E934.8	E950.4	E962.0	E980.4
Hetastarch	964.8	E858.2	E934.8	E950.4	E962.0	E980.4
Hexachlorocyclohexane	989.2	E863.0	—	E950.6	E962.1	E980.7
Hexachlorophene	976.2	E858.7	E946.2	E950.4	E962.0	E980.4
Hexadimethrine (bromide)	964.5	E858.2	E934.5	E950.4	E962.0	E980.4
Hexafluorenium	975.2	E858.6	E945.2	E950.4	E962.0	E980.4
Hexa-germ	976.2	E858.7	E946.2	E950.4	E962.0	E980.4
Hexahydrophenol	980.8	E860.8	—	E950.9	E962.1	E980.9
Hexalin	980.8	E860.8	—	E950.9	E962.1	E980.9
Hexamethonium	972.3	E858.3	E942.3	E950.4	E962.0	E980.4
Hexamethyleneamine	961.9	E857	E931.9	E950.4	E962.0	E980.4
Hexamine	961.9	E857	E931.9	E950.4	E962.0	E980.4
Hexanone	982.8	E862.4	—	E950.9	E962.1	E980.9
Hexapropymate	967.8	E852.8	E937.8	E950.2	E962.0	E980.2
Hexestrol	962.2	E858.0	E932.2	E950.4	E962.0	E980.4
Hexethal (sodium)	967.0	E851	E937.0	E950.1	E962.0	E980.1
Hexetidine	976.0	E858.7	E946.0	E950.4	E962.0	E980.4
Hexobarbital, hexobarbitone	967.0	E851	E937.0	E950.1	E962.0	E980.1
sodium (anesthetic)	968.3	E855.1	E938.3	E950.4	E962.0	E980.4
soluble	968.3	E855.1	E938.3	E950.4	E962.0	E980.4
Hexocyclium	971.1	E855.4	E941.1	E950.4	E962.0	E980.4
Hexoestrol	962.2	E858.0	E932.2	E950.4	E962.0	E980.4
Hexone	982.8	E862.4	—	E950.9	E962.1	E980.9
Hexylcaine	968.5	E855.2	E938.5	E950.4	E962.0	E980.4
Hexylresorcinol	961.6	E857	E931.6	E950.4	E962.0	E980.4
Hinkle's pills	973.1	E858.4	E943.1	E950.4	E962.0	E980.4
Histalog	977.8	E858.8	E947.8	E950.4	E962.0	E980.4
Histamine (phosphate)	972.5	E858.3	E942.5	E950.4	E962.0	E980.4
Histoplasmin	977.8	E858.8	E947.8	E950.4	E962.0	E980.4
Holly berries	988.2	E865.3	—	E950.9	E962.1	E980.9
Homatropine	971.1	E855.4	E941.1	E950.4	E962.0	E980.4
Homo-tet	964.6	E858.2	E934.6	E950.4	E962.0	E980.4
Hormones (synthetic substitute) NEC	962.9	E858.0	E932.9	E950.4	E962.0	E980.4
adrenal cortical steroids	962.0	E858.0	E932.0	E950.4	E962.0	E980.4
antidiabetic agents	962.3	E858.0	E932.3	E950.4	E962.0	E980.4
follicle stimulating	962.4	E858.0	E932.4	E950.4	E962.0	E980.4
gonadotropic	962.4	E858.0	E932.4	E950.4	E962.0	E980.4
growth	962.4	E858.0	E932.4	E950.4	E962.0	E980.4
ovarian (substitutes)	962.2	E858.0	E932.2	E950.4	E962.0	E980.4
parathyroid (derivatives)	962.6	E858.0	E932.6	E950.4	E962.0	E980.4
pituitary (posterior)	962.5	E858.0	E932.5	E950.4	E962.0	E980.4
anterior	962.4	E858.0	E932.4	E950.4	E962.0	E980.4
thyroid (derivative)	962.7	E858.0	E932.7	E950.4	E962.0	E980.4
Hornet (sting)	989.5	E905.3	—	E950.9	E962.1	E980.9
Horticulture agent NEC	989.4	E863.9	—	E950.6	E962.1	E980.7
Hyaluronidase	963.4	E858.1	E933.4	E950.4	E962.0	E980.4
Hyazyme	963.4	E858.1	E933.4	E950.4	E962.0	E980.4
Hycodan	965.09	E850.2	E935.2	E950.0	E962.0	E980.0
Hydantoin derivatives	966.1	E855.0	E936.1	E950.4	E962.0	E980.4
Hydeltra	962.0	E858.0	E932.0	E950.4	E962.0	E980.4
Hydergine	971.3	E855.6	E941.3	E950.4	E962.0	E980.4
Hydrabamine penicillin	960.0	E856	E930.0	E950.4	E962.0	E980.4
Hydralazine, hydrallazine	972.6	E858.3	E942.6	E950.4	E962.0	E980.4
Hydrargaphen	976.0	E858.7	E946.0	E950.4	E962.0	E980.4
Hydrazine	983.9	E864.3	—	E950.7	E962.1	E980.6
Hydriodic acid	975.5	E858.6	E945.5	E950.4	E962.0	E980.4
Hydrocarbon gas	987.1	E869.8	—	E952.8	E962.2	E982.8
incomplete combustion of — see Carbon, monoxide, fuel, utility						
liquefied (mobile container)	987.0	E868.0	—	E951.1	E962.2	E981.1
piped (natural)	987.0	E867	—	E951.0	E962.2	E981.0
Hydrochloric acid (liquid)	983.1	E864.1	—	E950.7	E962.1	E980.6
medicinal	973.4	E858.4	E943.4	E950.4	E962.0	E980.4
vapor	987.8	E869.8	—	E952.8	E962.2	E982.8
Hydrochlorothiazide	974.3	E858.5	E944.3	E950.4	E962.0	E980.4
Hydrocodone	965.09	E850.2	E935.2	E950.0	E962.0	E980.0
Hydrocortisone	962.0	E858.0	E932.0	E950.4	E962.0	E980.4
ENT agent	976.6	E858.7	E946.6	E950.4	E962.0	E980.4
ophthalmic preparation	976.5	E858.7	E946.5	E950.4	E962.0	E980.4
topical NEC	976.0	E858.7	E946.0	E950.4	E962.0	E980.4
Hydrocortone	962.0	E858.0	E932.0	E950.4	E962.0	E980.4
ENT agent	976.6	E858.7	E946.6	E950.4	E962.0	E980.4
ophthalmic preparation	976.5	E858.7	E946.5	E950.4	E962.0	E980.4
topical NEC	976.0	E858.7	E946.0	E950.4	E962.0	E980.4
Hydrocyanic acid — see Cyanide(s)						
Hydroflumethiazide	974.3	E858.5	E944.3	E950.4	E962.0	E980.4
Hydrofluoric acid (liquid)	983.1	E864.1	—	E950.7	E962.1	E980.6
vapor	987.8	E869.8	—	E952.8	E962.2	E982.8
Hydrogen	987.8	E869.8	—	E952.8	E962.2	E982.8
arsenide	985.1	E866.3	—	E950.8	E962.1	E980.8
arseniureted	985.1	E866.3	—	E950.8	E962.1	E980.8
cyanide (salts)	989.0	E866.8	—	E950.9	E962.1	E980.9
gas	987.7	E869.8	—	E952.8	E962.2	E982.8
fluoride (liquid)	983.1	E864.1	—	E950.7	E962.1	E980.6
vapor	987.8	E869.8	—	E952.8	E962.2	E982.8
peroxide (solution)	976.6	E858.7	E946.6	E950.4	E962.0	E980.4
phosphureted	987.8	E869.8	—	E952.8	E962.2	E982.8
sulfide (gas)	987.8	E869.8	—	E952.8	E962.2	E982.8
arseniureted	985.1	E866.3	—	E950.8	E962.1	E980.8
sulfureted	987.8	E869.8	—	E952.8	E962.2	E982.8
Hydromorphinol	965.09	E850.2	E935.2	E950.0	E962.0	E980.0
Hydromorphinone	965.09	E850.2	E935.2	E950.0	E962.0	E980.0
Hydromorphone	965.09	E850.2	E935.2	E950.0	E962.0	E980.0
Hydromox	974.3	E858.5	E944.3	E950.4	E962.0	E980.4
Hydrophilic lotion	976.3	E858.7	E946.3	E950.4	E962.0	E980.4
Hydroquinone	983.0	E864.0	—	E950.7	E962.1	E980.6
vapor	987.8	E869.8	—	E952.8	E962.2	E982.8
Hydrosulfuric acid (gas)	987.8	E869.8	—	E952.8	E962.2	E982.8
Hydrous wool fat (lotion)	976.3	E858.7	E946.3	E950.4	E962.0	E980.4
Hydroxide, caustic	983.2	E864.2	—	E950.7	E962.1	E980.6
Hydroxocobalamin	964.1	E858.2	E934.1	E950.4	E962.0	E980.4
Hydroxyamphetamine	971.2	E855.5	E941.2	E950.4	E962.0	E980.4
Hydroxychloroquine	961.4	E857	E931.4	E950.4	E962.0	E980.4
Hydroxydihydrocodeinone	965.09	E850.2	E935.2	E950.0	E962.0	E980.0
Hydroxyethyl starch	964.8	E858.2	E934.8	E950.4	E962.0	E980.4
Hydroxyphenamate	969.5	E853.8	E939.8	E950.3	E962.0	E980.3
Hydroxyphenylbutazone	965.5	E850.5	E935.5	E950.0	E962.0	E980.0
Hydroxyprogesterone	962.2	E858.0	E932.2	E950.4	E962.0	E980.4
Hydroxyquinoline derivatives	961.3	E857	E931.3	E950.4	E962.0	E980.4
Hydroxystilbamidine	961.5	E857	E931.5	E950.4	E962.0	E980.4
Hydroxyurea	963.1	E858.1	E933.1	E950.4	E962.0	E980.4
Hydroxyzine	969.5	E853.8	E939.5	E950.3	E962.0	E980.3
Hyoscine (hydrobromide)	971.1	E855.4	E941.1	E950.4	E962.0	E980.4
Hyoscyamine	971.1	E855.4	E941.1	E950.4	E962.0	E980.4
Hyoscyamus (albus) (niger)	988.2	E865.4	—	E950.9	E962.1	E980.9
Hypaque	977.8	E858.8	E947.8	E950.4	E962.0	E980.4
Hypertussis	964.6	E858.2	E934.6	E950.4	E962.0	E980.4
Hypnotics NEC	967.9	E852.9	E937.9	E950.2	E962.0	E980.2
Hypochlorites — see Sodium, hypochlorite						
Hypotensive agents NEC	972.6	E858.3	E942.6	E950.4	E962.0	E980.4
Ibufenac	965.69	E850.6	E935.6	E950.0	E962.0	E980.0
Ibuprofen	965.61	E850.6	E935.6	E950.0	E962.0	E980.0
ICG	977.8	E858.8	E947.8	E950.4	E962.0	E980.4
Ichthammol	976.4	E858.7	E946.4	E950.4	E962.0	E980.4
Ichthyol	976.4	E858.7	E946.4	E950.4	E962.0	E980.4
Idoxuridine	976.5	E858.7	E946.5	E950.4	E962.0	E980.4
IDU	976.5	E858.7	E946.5	E950.4	E962.0	E980.4
Iletin	962.3	E858.0	E932.3	E950.4	E962.0	E980.4
Ilex	988.2	E865.4	—	E950.9	E962.1	E980.9

Table of Drugs and Chemicals

	Poisoning	Accident	Therapeutic Use	Suicide Attempt	Assault	Undetermined
Illuminating gas — see Gas, utility						
Ilopan	963.5	E858.1	E933.5	E950.4	E962.0	E980.4
Ilotycin	960.3	E856	E930.3	E950.4	E962.0	E980.4
ophthalmic preparation	976.5	E858.7	E946.5	E950.4	E962.0	E980.4
topical NEC	976.0	E858.7	E946.0	E950.4	E962.0	E980.4
Imipramine	969.0	E854.0	E939.0	E950.3	E962.0	E980.3
Immu-G	964.6	E858.2	E934.6	E950.4	E962.0	E980.4
Immuglobin	964.6	E858.2	E934.6	E950.4	E962.0	E980.4
Immune serum globulin	964.6	E858.2	E934.6	E950.4	E962.0	E980.4
Immunosuppressive agents	963.1	E858.1	E933.1	E950.4	E962.0	E980.4
Immu-tetanus	964.6	E858.2	E934.6	E950.4	E962.0	E980.4
Indandione (derivatives)	964.2	E858.2	E934.2	E950.4	E962.0	E980.4
Inderal	972.0	E858.3	E942.0	E950.4	E962.0	E980.4
Indian						
hemp	969.6	E854.1	E939.6	E950.3	E962.0	E980.3
tobacco	988.2	E865.4	—	E950.9	E962.1	E980.9
Indigo carmine	977.8	E858.8	E947.8	E950.4	E962.0	E980.4
Indocin	965.69	E850.6	E935.6	E950.0	E962.0	E980.0
Indocyanine green	977.8	E858.8	E947.8	E950.4	E962.0	E980.4
Indomethacin	965.69	E850.6	E935.6	E950.0	E962.0	E980.0
Industrial						
alcohol	980.9	E860.9	—	E950.9	E962.1	E980.9
fumes	987.8	E869.8	—	E952.8	E962.2	E982.8
solvents (fumes) (vapors)	982.8	E862.9	—	E950.9	E962.1	E980.9
Influenza vaccine	979.6	E858.8	E949.6	E950.4	E962.0	E982.8
Ingested substances NEC	989.9	E866.9	—	E950.9	E962.1	E980.9
INH (isoniazid)	961.8	E857	E931.8	E950.4	E962.0	E980.4
Inhalation, gas (noxious) — see Gas						
Ink	989.89	E866.8	—	E950.9	E962.1	E980.9
Innovar	967.6	E852.5	E937.6	E950.2	E962.0	E980.2
Inositol niacinate	972.2	E858.3	E942.2	E950.4	E962.0	E980.4
Inproquone	963.1	E858.1	E933.1	E950.4	E962.0	E980.4
Insecticides — see also Pesticides	989.4	E863.4	—	E950.6	E962.1	E980.7
chlorinated	989.2	E863.0	—	E950.6	E962.1	E980.7
mixtures	989.4	E863.3	—	E950.6	E962.1	E980.7
organochlorine (compounds)	989.2	E863.0	—	E950.6	E962.1	E980.7
organophosphorus (compounds)	989.3	E863.1	—	E950.6	E962.1	E980.7
Insect (sting), venomous	989.5	E905.5	—	E950.9	E962.1	E980.9
Insular tissue extract	962.3	E858.0	E932.3	E950.4	E962.0	E980.4
Insulin (amorphous) (globin) (isophane) (Lente) (NPH) (protamine) (Semilente) (Ultralente) (zinc)	962.3	E858.0	E932.3	E950.4	E962.0	E980.4
Intranarcon	968.3	E855.1	E938.3	E950.4	E962.0	E980.4
Inulin	977.8	E858.8	E947.8	E950.4	E962.0	E980.4
Invert sugar	974.5	E858.5	E944.5	E950.4	E962.0	E980.4
Inza — see Naproxen						
Iodide NEC — see also						
iodine	976.0	E858.7	E946.0	E950.4	E962.0	E980.4
mercury (ointment)	976.0	E858.7	E946.0	E950.4	E962.0	E980.4
methylate	976.0	E858.7	E946.0	E950.4	E962.0	E980.4
potassium (expectorant) NEC	975.5	E858.6	E945.5	E950.4	E962.0	E980.4
Iodinated glycerol	975.5	E858.6	E945.5	E950.4	E962.0	E980.4
Iodine (antiseptic, external) (tincture) NEC	976.0	E858.7	E946.0	E950.4	E962.0	E980.4
diagnostic	977.8	E858.8	E947.8	E950.4	E962.0	E980.4
for thyroid conditions (antithyroid)	962.8	E858.0	E932.8	E950.4	E962.0	E980.4
vapor	987.8	E869.8	—	E952.8	E962.2	E982.8
Iodized oil	977.8	E858.8	E947.8	E950.4	E962.0	E980.4
Iodobismitol	961.2	E857	E931.2	E950.4	E962.0	E980.4
Iodochlorhydroxyquin	961.3	E857	E931.3	E950.4	E962.0	E980.4
topical	976.0	E858.7	E946.0	E950.4	E962.0	E980.4
Iodoform	976.0	E858.7	E946.0	E950.4	E962.0	E980.4
Iodopanoic acid	977.8	E858.8	E947.8	E950.4	E962.0	E980.4
Iodophthalein	977.8	E858.8	E947.8	E950.4	E962.0	E980.4
Ion exchange resins	974.5	E858.5	E944.5	E950.4	E962.0	E980.4
Iopanoic acid	977.8	E858.8	E947.8	E950.4	E962.0	E980.4
Iophendylate	977.8	E858.8	E947.8	E950.4	E962.0	E980.4
Iothiouracil	962.8	E858.0	E932.8	E950.4	E962.0	E980.4
Ipecac	973.6	E858.4	E943.6	E950.4	E962.0	E980.4
Ipecacuanha	973.6	E858.4	E943.6	E950.4	E962.0	E980.4
Ipodate	977.8	E858.8	E947.8	E950.4	E962.0	E980.4
Ipral	967.0	E851	E937.0	E950.1	E962.0	E980.1
Ipratropium	975.1	E858.6	E945.1	E950.4	E962.0	E980.4
Iproniazid	969.0	E854.0	E939.0	E950.3	E962.0	E980.3
Iron (compounds) (medicinal) (preparations)	964.0	E858.2	E934.0	E950.4	E962.0	E980.4
dextran	964.0	E858.2	E934.0	E950.4	E962.0	E980.4
nonmedicinal (dust) (fumes) NEC	985.8	E866.4	—	E950.9	E962.1	E980.9
Irritant drug	977.9	E858.9	E947.9	E950.5	E962.0	E980.5
Ismelin	972.6	E858.3	E942.6	E950.4	E962.0	E980.4
Isoamyl nitrite	972.4	E858.3	E942.4	E950.4	E962.0	E980.4
Isobutyl acetate	982.8	E862.4	—	E950.9	E962.1	E980.9
Isocarboxazid	969.0	E854.0	E939.0	E950.3	E962.0	E980.3
Isoephedrine	971.2	E855.5	E941.2	E950.4	E962.0	E980.4
Isoetharine	971.2	E855.5	E941.2	E950.4	E962.0	E980.4
Isofluorophate	971.0	E855.3	E941.0	E950.4	E962.0	E980.4
Isoniazid (INH)	961.8	E857	E931.8	E950.4	E962.0	E980.4
Isopentaquine	961.4	E857	E931.4	E950.4	E962.0	E980.4
Isophane insulin	962.3	E858.0	E932.3	E950.4	E962.0	E980.4
Isopregnenone	962.2	E858.0	E932.2	E950.4	E962.0	E980.4
Isoprenaline	971.2	E855.5	E941.2	E950.4	E962.0	E980.4
Isopropamide	971.1	E855.4	E941.1	E950.4	E962.0	E980.4
Isopropanol	980.2	E860.3	—	E950.9	E962.1	E980.9
topical (germicide)	976.0	E858.7	E946.0	E950.4	E962.0	E980.4
Isopropyl						
acetate	982.8	E862.4	—	E950.9	E962.1	E980.9
alcohol	980.2	E860.3	—	E950.9	E962.1	E980.9
topical (germicide)	976.0	E858.7	E946.0	E950.4	E962.0	E980.4
ether	982.8	E862.4	—	E950.9	E962.1	E980.9
Isoproterenol	971.2	E855.5	E941.2	E950.4	E962.0	E980.4
Isosorbide dinitrate	972.4	E858.3	E942.4	E950.4	E962.0	E980.4
Isothipendyl	963.0	E858.1	E933.0	E950.4	E962.0	E980.4
Isoxazolyl penicillin	960.0	E856	E930.0	E950.4	E962.0	E980.4
Isoxsuprine hydrochloride	972.5	E858.3	E942.5	E950.4	E962.0	E980.4
l-thyroxine sodium	962.7	E858.0	E932.7	E950.4	E962.0	E980.4
Jaborandi (pilocarpus) (extract)	971.0	E855.3	E941.0	E950.4	E962.0	E980.4
Jalap	973.1	E858.4	E943.1	E950.4	E962.0	E980.4
Jamaica						
dogwood (bark)	965.7	E850.7	E935.7	E950.0	E962.0	E980.0
ginger	989.89	E866.8	—	E950.9	E962.1	E980.9
Jatropha	988.2	E865.4	—	E950.9	E962.1	E980.9
curcas	988.2	E865.3	—	E950.9	E962.1	E980.9
Jectofer	964.0	E858.2	E934.0	E950.4	E962.0	E980.4
Jellyfish (sting)	989.5	E905.6	—	E950.9	E962.1	E980.9
Jequirity (bean)	988.2	E865.3	—	E950.9	E962.1	E980.9
Jimson weed	988.2	E865.4	—	E950.9	E962.1	E980.9
seeds	988.2	E865.3	—	E950.9	E962.1	E980.9
Juniper tar (oil) (ointment)	976.4	E858.7	E946.4	E950.4	E962.0	E980.4
Kallikrein	972.5	E858.3	E942.5	E950.4	E962.0	E980.4
Kanamycin	960.6	E856	E930.6	E950.4	E962.0	E980.4
Kantrex	960.6	E856	E930.6	E950.4	E962.0	E980.4
Kaolin	973.5	E858.4	E943.5	E950.4	E962.0	E980.4
Karaya (gum)	973.3	E858.4	E943.3	E950.4	E962.0	E980.4
Kemithal	968.3	E855.1	E938.3	E950.4	E962.0	E980.4
Kenacort	962.0	E858.0	E932.0	E950.4	E962.0	E980.4
Keratolytics	976.4	E858.7	E946.4	E950.4	E962.0	E980.4
Keratoplastics	976.4	E858.7	E946.4	E950.4	E962.0	E980.4
Kerosene, kerosine (fuel) (solvent) NEC	981	E862.1	—	E950.9	E962.1	E980.9
insecticide	981	E863.4	—	E950.6	E962.1	E980.7
vapor	987.1	E869.8	—	E952.8	E962.2	E982.8
Ketamine	968.3	E855.1	E938.3	E950.4	E962.0	E980.4
Ketobemidone	965.09	E850.2	E935.2	E950.0	E962.0	E980.0
Ketols	982.8	E862.4	—	E950.9	E962.1	E980.9
Ketone oils	982.8	E862.4	—	E950.9	E962.1	E980.9
Ketoprofen	965.61	E850.6	E935.6	E950.0	E962.0	E980.0
Kiln gas or vapor (carbon monoxide)	986	E868.8	—	E952.1	E962.2	E982.1
Konsyl	973.3	E858.4	E943.3	E950.4	E962.0	E980.4
Kosam seed	988.2	E865.3	—	E950.9	E962.1	E980.9
Krait (venom)	989.5	E905.0	—	E950.9	E962.1	E980.9
Kwell (insecticide)	989.2	E863.0	—	E950.6	E962.1	E980.7
anti-infective (topical)	976.0	E858.7	E946.0	E950.4	E962.0	E980.4
Laburnum (flowers) (seeds)	988.2	E865.3	—	E950.9	E962.1	E980.9
leaves	988.2	E865.4	—	E950.9	E962.1	E980.9
Lacquers	989.89	E861.6	—	E950.9	E962.1	E980.9
Lacrimogenic gas	987.5	E869.3	—	E952.8	E962.2	E982.8
Lactic acid	983.1	E864.1	—	E950.7	E962.1	E980.6
Lactobacillus acidophilus	973.5	E858.4	E943.5	E950.4	E962.0	E980.4
Lactoflavin	963.5	E858.1	E933.5	E950.4	E962.0	E980.4
Lactuca (virosa) (extract)	967.8	E852.8	E937.8	E950.2	E962.0	E980.2

Lactucarium

Table of Drugs and Chemicals

		External Cause (E-Code)							External Cause (E-Code)			
	Poisoning	Accident	Therapeutic Use	Suicide Attempt	Assault	Undetermined		Poisoning	Accident	Therapeutic Use	Suicide Attempt	Assault	Undetermined
Lactucarium	967.8	E852.8	E937.8	E950.2	E962.0	E980.2	Lignocaine — continued						
Laevulose	974.5	E858.5	E944.5	E950.4	E962.0	E980.4	spinal	968.7	E855.2	E938.7	E950.4	E962.0	E980.4
Lanatoside (C)	972.1	E858.3	E942.1	E950.4	E962.0	E980.4	Ligroin(e) (solvent)	981	E862.0	—	E950.9	E962.1	E980.9
Lanolin (lotion)	976.3	E858.7	E946.3	E950.4	E962.0	E980.4	vapor	987.1	E869.8	—	E952.8	E962.2	E982.8
Largactil	969.1	E853.0	E939.1	E950.3	E962.0	E980.3	Ligustrum vulgare	988.2	E865.3	—	E950.9	E962.1	E980.9
Larkspur	988.2	E865.3	—	E950.9	E962.1	E980.9	Lily of the valley	988.2	E865.4	—	E950.9	E962.1	E980.9
Laroxyl	969.0	E854.0	E939.0	E950.3	E962.0	E980.3	Lime (chloride)	983.2	E864.2	—	E950.7	E962.1	E980.6
Lasix	974.4	E858.5	E944.4	E950.4	E962.0	E980.4	solution, sulferated	976.4	E858.7	E946.4	E950.4	E962.0	E980.4
Latex	989.82	E866.8	—	E950.9	E962.1	E980.9	Limonene	982.8	E862.4	—	E950.9	E962.1	E980.9
Lathyrus (seed)	988.2	E865.3	—	E950.9	E962.1	E980.9	Lincomycin	960.8	E856	E930.8	E950.4	E962.0	E980.4
Laudanum	965.09	E850.2	E935.2	E950.0	E962.0	E980.0	Lindane (insecticide)(vapor)	989.2	E863.0	—	E950.6	E962.1	E980.7
Laudexium	975.2	E858.6	E945.2	E950.4	E962.0	E980.4	anti-infective (topical)	976.0	E858.7	E946.0	E950.4	E962.0	E980.4
Laurel, black or cherry	988.2	E865.4	—	E950.9	E962.1	E980.9	Liniments NEC	976.9	E858.7	E946.9	E950.4	E962.0	E980.4
Laurolinium	976.0	E858.7	E946.0	E950.4	E962.0	E980.4	Linoleic acid	972.2	E858.3	E942.2	E950.4	E962.0	E980.4
Lauryl sulfoacetate	976.2	E858.7	E946.2	E950.4	E962.0	E980.4	Liothyronine	962.7	E858.0	E932.7	E950.4	E962.0	E980.4
Laxatives NEC	973.3	E858.4	E943.3	E950.4	E962.0	E980.4	Liotrix	962.7	E858.0	E932.7	E950.4	E962.0	E980.4
emollient	973.2	E858.4	E943.2	E950.4	E962.0	E980.4	Lipancreatin	973.4	E858.4	E943.4	E950.4	E962.0	E980.4
L-dopa	966.4	E855.0	E936.4	E950.4	E962.0	E980.4	Lipo-Lutin	962.2	E858.0	E932.2	E950.4	E962.0	E980.4
Lead (dust) (fumes) (vapor)							Lipotropic agents	977.1	E858.8	E947.1	E950.4	E962.0	E980.4
NEC	984.9	E866.0	—	E950.9	E962.1	E980.9	Liquefied petroleum						
acetate (dust)	984.1	E866.0	—	E950.9	E962.1	E980.9	gases	987.0	E868.0	—	E951.1	E962.2	E981.1
anti-infectives	961.2	E857	E931.2	E950.4	E962.0	E980.4	piped (pure or mixed with						
antiknock compound							air)	987.0	E867	—	E951.0	E962.2	E981.0
(tetraethyl)	984.1	E862.1	—	E950.9	E962.1	E980.9	Liquid petrolatum	973.2	E858.4	E943.2	E950.4	E962.0	E980.4
arsenate, arsenite (dust)							substance	989.9	E866.9	—	E950.9	E962.1	E980.9
(insecticide) (vapor)	985.1	E863.4	—	E950.8	E962.1	E980.8	specified NEC	989.89	E866.8	—	E950.9	E962.1	E980.9
herbicide	985.1	E863.5	—	E950.8	E962.1	E980.8	Lirugen	979.4	E858.8	E949.4	E950.4	E962.0	E980.4
carbonate	984.0	E866.0	—	E950.9	E962.1	E980.9	Lithane	969.8	E855.8	E939.8	E950.3	E962.0	E980.3
paint	984.0	E861.5	—	E950.9	E962.1	E980.9	Lithium	985.8	E866.4	—	E950.9	E962.1	E980.9
chromate	984.0	E866.0	—	E950.9	E962.1	E980.9	carbonate	969.8	E855.8	E939.8	E950.3	E962.0	E980.3
paint	984.0	E861.5	—	E950.9	E962.1	E980.9	Lithonate	969.8	E855.8	E939.8	E950.3	E962.0	E980.3
dioxide	984.0	E866.0	—	E950.9	E962.1	E980.9	Liver (extract) (injection)						
inorganic (compound)	984.0	E866.0	—	E950.9	E962.1	E980.9	(preparations)	964.1	E858.2	E934.1	E950.4	E962.0	E980.4
paint	984.0	E861.5	—	E950.9	E962.1	E980.9	Lizard (bite) (venom)	989.5	E905.0	—	E950.9	E962.1	E980.9
iodide	984.0	E866.0	—	E950.9	E962.1	E980.9	LMD	964.8	E858.2	E934.8	E950.4	E962.0	E980.4
pigment (paint)	984.0	E861.5	—	E950.9	E962.1	E980.9	Lobelia	988.2	E865.4	—	E950.9	E962.1	E980.9
monoxide (dust)	984.0	E866.0	—	E950.9	E962.1	E980.9	Lobeline	970.0	E854.3	E940.0	E950.4	E962.0	E980.4
paint	984.0	E861.5	—	E950.9	E962.1	E980.9	Locorten	976.0	E858.7	E946.0	E950.4	E962.0	E980.4
organic	984.1	E866.0	—	E950.9	E962.1	E980.9	Lolium temulentum	988.2	E865.3	—	E950.9	E962.1	E980.9
oxide	984.0	E866.0	—	E950.9	E962.1	E980.9	Lomotil	973.5	E858.4	E943.5	E950.4	E962.0	E980.4
paint	984.0	E861.5	—	E950.9	E962.1	E980.9	Lomustine	963.1	E858.1	E933.1	E950.4	E962.0	E980.4
paint	984.0	E861.5	—	E950.9	E962.1	E980.9	Lophophora williamsii	969.6	E854.1	E939.6	E950.3	E962.0	E980.3
salts	984.0	E866.0	—	E950.9	E962.1	E980.9	Lorazepam	969.4	E853.2	E939.4	E950.3	E962.0	E980.3
specified compound NEC	984.8	E866.0	—	E950.9	E962.1	E980.9	Lotions NEC	976.9	E858.7	E946.9	E950.4	E962.0	E980.4
tetra-ethyl	984.1	E862.1	—	E950.9	E962.1	E980.9	Lotronex	973.8	E858.4	E943.8	E950.4	E962.0	E980.4
Lebanese red	969.6	E854.1	E939.6	E950.3	E962.0	E980.3	Lotusate	967.0	E851	E937.0	E950.1	E962.0	E980.1
Lente Iletin (insulin)	962.3	E858.0	E932.3	E950.4	E962.0	E980.4	Lowila	976.2	E858.7	E946.2	E950.4	E962.0	E980.4
Leptazol	970.0	E854.3	E940.0	E950.4	E962.0	E980.4	Loxapine	969.3	E853.8	E939.3	E950.3	E962.0	E980.3
Leritine	965.09	E850.2	E935.2	E950.0	E962.0	E980.0	Lozenges (throat)	976.6	E858.7	E946.6	E950.4	E962.0	E980.4
Letter	962.7	E858.0	E932.7	E950.4	E962.0	E980.4	LSD (25)	969.6	E854.1	E939.6	E950.3	E962.0	E980.3
Lettuce opium	967.8	E852.8	E937.8	E950.2	E962.0	E980.2	L-Tryptophan — see amino acid						
Leucovorin (factor)	964.1	E858.2	E934.1	E950.4	E962.0	E980.4	Lubricating oil NEC	981	E862.2	—	E950.9	E962.1	E980.9
Leukeran	963.1	E858.1	E933.1	E950.4	E962.0	E980.4	Lucanthone	961.6	E857	E931.6	E950.4	E962.0	E980.4
Levalbuterol	975.7	E858.6	E945.7	E950.4	E962.0	E980.4	Luminal	967.0	E851	E937.0	E950.1	E962.0	E980.1
Levallorphan	970.1	E854.3	E940.1	E950.4	E962.0	E980.4	Lung irritant (gas) NEC	987.9	E869.9	—	E952.9	E962.2	E982.9
Levanil	967.8	E852.8	E937.8	E950.2	E962.0	E980.2	Lutocylol	962.2	E858.0	E932.2	E950.4	E962.0	E980.4
Levarterenol	971.2	E855.5	E941.2	E950.4	E962.0	E980.4	Lutromone	962.2	E858.0	E932.2	E950.4	E962.0	E980.4
Levodopa	966.4	E855.0	E936.4	E950.4	E962.0	E980.4	Lututrin	975.0	E858.6	E945.0	E950.4	E962.0	E980.4
Levo-dromoran	965.09	E850.2	E935.2	E950.0	E962.0	E980.0	Lye (concentrated)	983.2	E864.2	—	E950.7	E962.1	E980.6
Levoid	962.7	E858.0	E932.7	E950.4	E962.0	E980.4	Lygranum (skin test)	977.8	E858.8	E947.8	E950.4	E962.0	E980.4
Levo-iso-methadone	965.02	E850.1	E935.1	E950.0	E962.0	E980.0	Lymecycline	960.4	E856	E930.4	E950.4	E962.0	E980.4
Levomepromazine	967.8	E852.8	E937.8	E950.2	E962.0	E980.2	Lymphogranuloma venereum						
Levoprome	967.8	E852.8	E937.8	E950.2	E962.0	E980.2	antigen	977.8	E858.8	E947.8	E950.4	E962.0	E980.4
Levopropoxyphene	975.4	E858.6	E945.4	E950.4	E962.0	E980.4	Lynestrenol	962.2	E858.0	E932.2	E950.4	E962.0	E980.4
Levorphan, levophanol	965.09	E850.2	E935.2	E950.0	E962.0	E980.0	Lyovac Sodium Edecrin	974.4	E858.5	E944.4	E950.4	E962.0	E980.4
Levothyroxine (sodium)	962.7	E858.0	E932.7	E950.4	E962.0	E980.4	Lypressin	962.5	E858.0	E932.5	E950.4	E962.0	E980.4
Levsin	971.1	E855.4	E941.1	E950.4	E962.0	E980.4	Lysergic acid (amide)						
Levulose	974.5	E858.5	E944.5	E950.4	E962.0	E980.4	(diethylamide)	969.6	E854.1	E939.6	E950.3	E962.0	E980.3
Lewisite (gas)	985.1	E866.3	—	E950.8	E962.1	E980.8	Lysergide	969.6	E854.1	E939.6	E950.3	E962.0	E980.3
Librium	969.4	E853.2	E939.4	E950.3	E962.0	E980.3	Lysine vasopressin	962.5	E858.0	E932.5	E950.4	E962.0	E980.4
Lidex	976.0	E858.7	E946.0	E950.4	E962.0	E980.4	Lysol	983.0	E864.0	—	E950.7	E962.1	E980.6
Lidocaine (infiltration)							Lytta (vitatta)	976.8	E858.7	E946.8	E950.4	E962.0	E980.4
(topical)	968.5	E855.2	E938.5	E950.4	E962.0	E980.4	Mace	987.5	E869.3	—	E952.8	E962.2	E982.8
nerve block (peripheral)							Macrolides (antibiotics)	960.3	E856	E930.3	E950.4	E962.0	E980.4
(plexus)	968.6	E855.2	E938.6	E950.4	E962.0	E980.4	Mafenide	976.0	E858.7	E946.0	E950.4	E962.0	E980.4
spinal	968.7	E855.2	E938.7	E950.4	E962.0	E980.4	Magaldrate	973.0	E858.4	E943.0	E950.4	E962.0	E980.4
Lighter fluid	981	E862.1	—	E950.9	E962.1	E980.9	Magic mushroom	969.6	E854.1	E939.6	E950.3	E962.0	E980.3
Lignocaine (infiltration)							Magnamycin	960.8	E856	E930.8	E950.4	E962.0	E980.4
(topical)	968.5	E855.2	E938.5	E950.4	E962.0	E980.4	Magnesia magma	973.0	E858.4	E943.0	E950.4	E962.0	E980.4
nerve block (peripheral)							Magnesium (compounds)						
(plexus)	968.6	E855.2	E938.6	E950.4	E962.0	E980.4	(fumes) NEC	985.8	E866.4	—	E950.9	E962.1	E980.9

Table of Drugs and Chemicals

	Poisoning	Accident	Therapeutic Use	Suicide Attempt	Assault	Undetermined
Magnesium (compounds) (fumes) — continued						
antacid	973.0	E858.4	E943.0	E950.4	E962.0	E980.4
carbonate	973.0	E858.4	E943.0	E950.4	E962.0	E980.4
cathartic	973.3	E858.4	E943.3	E950.4	E962.0	E980.4
citrate	973.3	E858.4	E943.3	E950.4	E962.0	E980.4
hydroxide	973.0	E858.4	E943.0	E950.4	E962.0	E980.4
oxide	973.0	E858.4	E943.0	E950.4	E962.0	E980.4
sulfate (oral)	973.3	E858.4	E943.3	E950.4	E962.0	E980.4
intravenous	966.3	E855.0	E936.3	E950.4	E962.0	E980.4
trisilicate	973.0	E858.4	E943.0	E950.4	E962.0	E980.4
Malathion (insecticide)	989.3	E863.1	—	E950.6	E962.1	E980.7
Male fern (oleoresin)	961.6	E857	E931.6	E950.4	E962.0	E980.4
Mandelic acid	961.9	E857	E931.9	E950.4	E962.0	E980.4
Manganese compounds (fumes) NEC	985.2	E866.4	—	E950.9	E962.1	E980.9
Mannitol (diuretic) (medicinal) NEC	974.4	E858.5	E944.4	E950.4	E962.0	E980.4
hexanitrate	972.4	E858.3	E942.4	E950.4	E962.0	E980.4
mustard	963.1	E858.1	E933.1	E950.4	E962.0	E980.4
Mannomustine	963.1	E858.1	E933.1	E950.4	E962.0	E980.4
MAO inhibitors	969.0	E854.0	E939.0	E950.3	E962.0	E980.3
Mapharsen	961.1	E857	E931.1	E950.4	E962.0	E980.4
Marcaine	968.9	E855.2	E938.9	E950.4	E962.0	E980.4
infiltration (subcutaneous)	968.5	E855.2	E938.5	E950.4	E962.0	E980.4
nerve block (peripheral) (plexus)	968.6	E855.2	E938.6	E950.4	E962.0	E980.4
Marezine	963.0	E858.1	E933.0	E950.4	E962.0	E980.4
Marihuana, marijuana (derivatives)	969.6	E854.1	E939.6	E950.3	E962.0	E980.3
Marine animals or plants (sting)	989.5	E905.6	—	E950.9	E962.1	E980.9
Marplan	969.0	E854.0	E939.0	E950.3	E962.0	E980.3
Marsh gas	987.1	E869.8	—	E952.8	E962.2	E982.8
Marsilid	969.0	E854.0	E939.0	E950.3	E962.0	E980.3
Matulane	963.1	E858.1	E933.1	E950.4	E962.0	E980.4
Mazindol	977.0	E858.8	E947.0	E950.4	E962.0	E980.4
MDMA	969.7	E854.2	E939.7	E950.3	E962.0	E980.3
Meadow saffron	988.2	E865.3	—	E950.9	E962.1	E980.9
Measles vaccine	979.4	E858.8	E949.4	E950.4	E962.0	E980.4
Meat, noxious or nonbacterial	988.8	E865.0	—	E950.9	E962.1	E980.9
Mebanazine	969.0	E854.0	E939.0	E950.3	E962.0	E980.3
Mebaral	967.0	E851	E937.0	E950.1	E962.0	E980.1
Mebendazole	961.6	E857	E931.6	E950.4	E962.0	E980.4
Mebeverine	975.1	E858.6	E945.1	E950.4	E962.0	E980.4
Mebhydroline	963.0	E858.1	E933.0	E950.4	E962.0	E980.4
Mebrophenhydramine	963.0	E858.1	E933.0	E950.4	E962.0	E980.4
Mebutamate	969.5	E853.8	E939.5	E950.3	E962.0	E980.3
Mecamylamine (chloride)	972.3	E858.3	E942.3	E950.4	E962.0	E980.4
Mechlorethamine hydrochloride	963.1	E858.1	E933.1	E950.4	E962.0	E980.4
Meclizene (hydrochloride)	963.0	E858.1	E933.0	E950.4	E962.0	E980.4
Meclofenoxate	970.0	E854.3	E940.0	E950.4	E962.0	E980.4
Meclozine (hydrochloride)	963.0	E858.1	E933.0	E950.4	E962.0	E980.4
Medazepam	969.4	E853.2	E939.4	E950.3	E962.0	E980.3
Medicine, medicinal substance	977.9	E858.9	E947.9	E950.5	E962.0	E980.5
specified NEC	977.8	E858.8	E947.8	E950.4	E962.0	E980.4
Medinal	967.0	E851	E937.0	E950.1	E962.0	E980.1
Medomin	967.0	E851	E937.0	E950.1	E962.0	E980.1
Medroxyprogesterone	962.2	E858.0	E932.2	E950.4	E962.0	E980.4
Medrysone	976.5	E858.7	E946.5	E950.4	E962.0	E980.4
Mefenamic acid	965.7	E850.7	E935.7	E950.0	E962.0	E980.0
Megahallucinogen	969.6	E854.1	E939.6	E950.3	E962.0	E980.3
Megestrol	962.2	E858.0	E932.2	E950.4	E962.0	E980.4
Meglumine	977.8	E858.8	E947.8	E950.4	E962.0	E980.4
Meladinin	976.3	E858.7	E946.3	E950.4	E962.0	E980.4
Melanizing agents	976.3	E858.7	E946.3	E950.4	E962.0	E980.4
Melarsoprol	961.1	E857	E931.1	E950.4	E962.0	E980.4
Melia azedarach	988.2	E865.3	—	E950.9	E962.1	E980.9
Mellaril	969.1	E853.0	E939.1	E950.3	E962.0	E980.3
Meloxine	976.3	E858.7	E946.3	E950.4	E962.0	E980.4
Melphalan	963.1	E858.1	E933.1	E950.4	E962.0	E980.4
Menadiol sodium diphosphate	964.3	E858.2	E934.3	E950.4	E962.0	E980.4
Menadione (sodium bisulfite)	964.3	E858.2	E934.3	E950.4	E962.0	E980.4
Menaphthone	964.3	E858.2	E934.3	E950.4	E962.0	E980.4
Meningococcal vaccine	978.8	E858.8	E948.8	E950.4	E962.0	E980.4
Menningovax-C	978.8	E858.8	E948.8	E950.4	E962.0	E980.4
Menotropins	962.4	E858.0	E932.4	E950.4	E962.0	E980.4
Menthol NEC	976.1	E858.7	E946.1	E950.4	E962.0	E980.4
Mepacrine	961.3	E857	E931.3	E950.4	E962.0	E980.4
Meparfynol	967.8	E852.8	E937.8	E950.2	E962.0	E980.2
Mepazine	969.1	E853.0	E939.1	E950.3	E962.0	E980.3
Mepenzolate	971.1	E855.4	E941.1	E950.4	E962.0	E980.4
Meperidine	965.09	E850.2	E935.2	E950.0	E962.0	E980.0
Mephenamin(e)	966.4	E855.0	E936.4	E950.4	E962.0	E980.4
Mephenesin (carbamate)	968.0	E855.1	E938.0	E950.4	E962.0	E980.4
Mephenoxalone	969.5	E853.8	E939.5	E950.3	E962.0	E980.3
Mephentermine	971.2	E855.5	E941.2	E950.4	E962.0	E980.4
Mephenytoin	966.1	E855.0	E936.1	E950.4	E962.0	E980.4
Mephobarbital	967.0	E851	E937.0	E950.1	E962.0	E980.1
Mepiperphenidol	971.1	E855.4	E941.1	E950.4	E962.0	E980.4
Mepivacaine	968.9	E855.2	E938.9	E950.4	E962.0	E980.4
infiltration (subcutaneous)	968.5	E855.2	E938.5	E950.4	E962.0	E980.4
nerve block (peripheral) (plexus)	968.6	E855.2	E938.6	E950.4	E962.0	E980.4
topical (surface)	968.5	E855.2	E938.5	E950.4	E962.0	E980.4
Meprednisone	962.0	E858.0	E932.0	E950.4	E962.0	E980.4
Meprobam	969.5	E853.8	E939.5	E950.3	E962.0	E980.3
Meprobamate	969.5	E853.8	E939.5	E950.3	E962.0	E980.3
Mepyramine (maleate)	963.0	E858.1	E933.0	E950.4	E962.0	E980.4
Meralluride	974.0	E858.5	E944.0	E950.4	E962.0	E980.4
Merbaphen	974.0	E858.5	E944.0	E950.4	E962.0	E980.4
Merbromin	976.0	E858.7	E946.0	E950.4	E962.0	E980.4
Mercaptomerin	974.0	E858.5	E944.0	E950.4	E962.0	E980.4
Mercaptopurine	963.1	E858.1	E933.1	E950.4	E962.0	E980.4
Mercumatilin	974.0	E858.5	E944.0	E950.4	E962.0	E980.4
Mercuramide	974.0	E858.5	E944.0	E950.4	E962.0	E980.4
Mercuranin	976.0	E858.7	E946.0	E950.4	E962.0	E980.4
Mercurochrome	976.0	E858.7	E946.0	E950.4	E962.0	E980.4
Mercury, mercuric, mercurous (compounds) (cyanide) (fumes) (nonmedicinal) (vapor) NEC	985.0	E866.1	—	E950.9	E962.1	E980.9
ammoniated	976.0	E858.7	E946.0	E950.4	E962.0	E980.4
anti-infective	961.2	E857	E931.2	E950.4	E962.0	E980.4
topical	976.0	E858.7	E946.0	E950.4	E962.0	E980.4
chloride (antiseptic) NEC	976.0	E858.7	E946.0	E950.4	E962.0	E980.4
fungicide	985.0	E863.6	—	E950.6	E962.1	E980.7
diuretic compounds	974.0	E858.5	E944.0	E950.4	E962.0	E980.4
fungicide	985.0	E863.6	—	E950.6	E962.1	E980.7
organic (fungicide)	985.0	E863.6	—	E950.6	E962.1	E980.7
Merethoxylline	974.0	E858.5	E944.0	E950.4	E962.0	E980.4
Mersalyl	974.0	E858.5	E944.0	E950.4	E962.0	E980.4
Merthiolate (topical)	976.0	E858.7	E946.0	E950.4	E962.0	E980.4
ophthalmic preparation	976.5	E858.7	E946.5	E950.4	E962.0	E980.4
Meruvax	979.4	E858.8	E949.4	E950.4	E962.0	E980.4
Mescal buttons	969.6	E854.1	E939.6	E950.3	E962.0	E980.3
Mescaline (salts)	969.6	E854.1	E939.6	E950.3	E962.0	E980.3
Mesoridazine besylate	969.1	E853.0	E939.1	E950.3	E962.0	E980.3
Mestanolone	962.1	E858.0	E932.1	E950.4	E962.0	E980.4
Mestranol	962.2	E858.0	E932.2	E950.4	E962.0	E980.4
Metacresylacetate	976.0	E858.7	E946.0	E950.4	E962.0	E980.4
Metaldehyde (snail killer) NEC	989.4	E863.4	—	E950.6	E962.1	E980.7
Metals (heavy) (nonmedicinal) NEC	985.9	E866.4	—	E950.9	E962.1	E980.9
dust, fumes, or vapor NEC	985.9	E866.4	—	E950.9	E962.1	E980.9
light NEC	985.9	E866.4	—	E950.9	E962.1	E980.9
dust, fumes, or vapor NEC	985.9	E866.4	—	E950.9	E962.1	E980.9
pesticides (dust) (vapor)	985.9	E863.4	—	E950.6	E962.1	E980.7
Metamucil	973.3	E858.4	E943.3	E950.4	E962.0	E980.4
Metaphen	976.0	E858.7	E946.0	E950.4	E962.0	E980.4
Metaproterenol	975.1	E858.6	E945.1	E950.4	E962.0	E980.4
Metaraminol	972.8	E858.3	E942.8	E950.4	E962.0	E980.4
Metaxalone	968.0	E855.1	E938.0	E950.4	E962.0	E980.4
Metformin	962.3	E858.0	E932.3	E950.4	E962.0	E980.4
Methacycline	960.4	E856	E930.4	E950.4	E962.0	E980.4
Methadone	965.02	E850.1	E935.1	E950.0	E962.0	E980.0
Methallenestril	962.2	E858.0	E932.2	E950.4	E962.0	E980.4
Methamphetamine	969.7	E854.2	E939.7	E950.3	E962.0	E980.3
Methandienone	962.1	E858.0	E932.1	E950.4	E962.0	E980.4
Methandriol	962.1	E858.0	E932.1	E950.4	E962.0	E980.4
Methandrostenolone	962.1	E858.0	E932.1	E950.4	E962.0	E980.4
Methane gas	987.1	E869.8	—	E952.8	E962.2	E982.8
Methanol	980.1	E860.2	—	E950.9	E962.1	E980.9
vapor	987.8	E869.8	—	E952.8	E962.2	E982.8
Methantheline	971.1	E855.4	E941.1	E950.4	E962.0	E980.4

Methaphenilene — Mumps

Table of Drugs and Chemicals

	Poisoning	Accident	Therapeutic Use	Suicide Attempt	Assault	Undetermined
Methaphenilene	963.0	E858.1	E933.0	E950.4	E962.0	E980.4
Methapyrilene	963.0	E858.1	E933.0	E950.4	E962.0	E980.4
Methaqualone (compounds)	967.4	E852.3	E937.4	E950.2	E962.0	E980.2
Metharbital, metharbitone	967.0	E851	E937.0	E950.1	E962.0	E980.1
Methazolamide	974.2	E858.5	E944.2	E950.4	E962.0	E980.4
Methdilazine	963.0	E858.1	E933.0	E950.4	E962.0	E980.4
Methedrine	969.7	E854.2	E939.7	E950.3	E962.0	E980.3
Methenamine (mandelate)	961.9	E857	E931.9	E950.4	E962.0	E980.4
Methenolone	962.1	E858.0	E932.1	E950.4	E962.0	E980.4
Methergine	975.0	E858.6	E945.0	E950.4	E962.0	E980.4
Methiacil	962.8	E858.0	E932.8	E950.4	E962.0	E980.4
Methicillin (sodium)	960.0	E856	E930.0	E950.4	E962.0	E980.4
Methimazole	962.8	E858.0	E932.8	E950.4	E962.0	E980.4
Methionine	977.1	E858.8	E947.1	E950.4	E962.0	E980.4
Methisazone	961.7	E857	E931.7	E950.4	E962.0	E980.4
Methitural	967.0	E851	E937.0	E950.1	E962.0	E980.1
Methixene	971.1	E855.4	E941.1	E950.4	E962.0	E980.4
Methobarbital, methobarbitone	967.0	E851	E937.0	E950.1	E962.0	E980.1
Methocarbamol	968.0	E855.1	E938.0	E950.4	E962.0	E980.4
Methohexital, methohexitone (sodium)	968.3	E855.1	E938.3	E950.4	E962.0	E980.4
Methoin	966.1	E855.0	E936.1	E950.4	E962.0	E980.4
Methopholine	965.7	E850.7	E935.7	E950.0	E962.0	E980.0
Methorate	975.4	E858.6	E945.4	E950.4	E962.0	E980.4
Methoserpidine	972.6	E858.3	E942.6	E950.4	E962.0	E980.4
Methotrexate	963.1	E858.1	E933.1	E950.4	E962.0	E980.4
Methotrimeprazine	967.8	E852.8	E937.8	E950.2	E962.0	E980.2
Methoxa-Dome	976.3	E858.7	E946.3	E950.4	E962.0	E980.4
Methoxamine	971.2	E855.5	E941.2	E950.4	E962.0	E980.4
Methoxsalen	976.3	E858.7	E946.3	E950.4	E962.0	E980.4
Methoxybenzyl penicillin	960.0	E856	E930.0	E950.4	E962.0	E980.4
Methoxychlor	989.2	E863.0	—	E950.6	E962.1	E980.7
Methoxyflurane	968.2	E855.1	E938.2	E950.4	E962.0	E980.4
Methoxyphenamine	971.2	E855.5	E941.2	E950.4	E962.0	E980.4
Methoxypromazine	969.1	E853.0	E939.1	E950.3	E962.0	E980.3
Methoxypsoralen	976.3	E858.7	E946.3	E950.4	E962.0	E980.4
Methscopolamine (bromide)	971.1	E855.4	E941.1	E950.4	E962.0	E980.4
Methsuximide	966.2	E855.0	E936.2	E950.4	E962.0	E980.4
Methyclothiazide	974.3	E858.5	E944.3	E950.4	E962.0	E980.4
Methyl						
acetate	982.8	E862.4	—	E950.9	E962.1	E980.9
acetone	982.8	E862.4	—	E950.9	E962.1	E980.9
alcohol	980.1	E860.2	—	E950.9	E962.1	E980.9
amphetamine	969.7	E854.2	E939.7	E950.3	E962.0	E980.3
androstanolone	962.1	E858.0	E932.1	E950.4	E962.0	E980.4
atropine	971.1	E855.4	E941.1	E950.4	E962.0	E980.4
benzene	982.0	E862.4	—	E950.9	E962.1	E980.9
bromide (gas)	987.8	E869.8	—	E952.8	E962.2	E982.8
fumigant	987.8	E863.8	—	E950.6	E962.2	E980.7
butanol	980.8	E860.8	—	E950.9	E962.1	E980.9
carbinol	980.1	E860.2	—	E950.9	E962.1	E980.9
cellosolve	982.8	E862.4	—	E950.9	E962.1	E980.9
cellulose	973.3	E858.4	E943.3	E950.4	E962.0	E980.4
chloride (gas)	987.8	E869.8	—	E952.8	E962.2	E982.8
cyclohexane	982.8	E862.4	—	E950.9	E962.1	E980.9
cyclohexanone	982.8	E862.4	—	E950.9	E962.1	E980.9
dihydromorphinone	965.09	E850.2	E935.2	E950.0	E962.0	E980.0
ergometrine	975.0	E858.6	E945.0	E950.4	E962.0	E980.4
ergonovine	975.0	E858.6	E945.0	E950.4	E962.0	E980.4
ethyl ketone	982.8	E862.4	—	E950.9	E962.1	E980.9
hydrazine	983.9	E864.3	—	E950.7	E962.1	E980.6
isobutyl ketone	982.8	E862.4	—	E950.9	E962.1	E980.9
morphine NEC	965.09	E850.2	E935.2	E950.0	E962.0	E980.0
parafynol	967.8	E852.8	E937.8	E950.2	E962.0	E980.2
parathion	989.3	E863.1	—	E950.6	E962.1	E980.7
pentynol NEC	967.8	E852.8	E937.8	E950.2	E962.0	E980.2
peridol	969.2	E853.1	E939.2	E950.3	E962.0	E980.3
phenidate	969.7	E854.2	E939.7	E950.3	E962.0	E980.3
prednisolone	962.0	E858.0	E932.0	E950.4	E962.0	E980.4
ENT agent	976.6	E858.7	E946.6	E950.4	E962.0	E980.4
ophthalmic preparation	976.5	E858.7	E946.5	E950.4	E962.0	E980.4
topical NEC	976.0	E858.7	E946.0	E950.4	E962.0	E980.4
propylcarbinol	980.8	E860.8	—	E950.9	E962.1	E980.9
rosaniline NEC	976.0	E858.7	E946.0	E950.4	E962.0	E980.4
salicylate NEC	976.3	E858.7	E946.3	E950.4	E962.0	E980.4
sulfate (fumes)	987.8	E869.8	—	E952.8	E962.2	E982.8
liquid	983.9	E864.3	—	E950.7	E962.1	E980.6
sulfonal	967.8	E852.8	E937.8	E950.2	E962.0	E980.2
testosterone	962.1	E858.0	E932.1	E950.4	E962.0	E980.4
Methyl — continued						
thiouracil	962.8	E858.0	E932.8	E950.4	E962.0	E980.4
Methylated spirit	980.0	E860.1	—	E950.9	E962.1	E980.9
Methyldopa	972.6	E858.3	E942.6	E950.4	E962.0	E980.4
Methylene						
blue	961.9	E857	E931.9	E950.4	E962.0	E980.4
chloride or dichloride (solvent) NEC	982.3	E862.4	—	E950.9	E962.1	E980.9
Methylhexabital	967.0	E851	E937.0	E950.1	E962.0	E980.1
Methylparaben (ophthalmic)	976.5	E858.7	E946.5	E950.4	E962.0	E980.4
Methyprylon	967.5	E852.4	E937.5	E950.2	E962.0	E980.2
Methysergide	971.3	E855.6	E941.3	E950.4	E962.0	E980.4
Metoclopramide	963.0	E858.1	E933.0	E950.4	E962.0	E980.4
Metofoline	965.7	E850.7	E935.7	E950.0	E962.0	E980.0
Metopon	965.09	E850.2	E935.2	E950.0	E962.0	E980.0
Metronidazole	961.5	E857	E931.5	E950.4	E962.0	E980.4
Metycaine	968.9	E855.2	E938.9	E950.4	E962.0	E980.4
infiltration (subcutaneous)	968.5	E855.2	E938.5	E950.4	E962.0	E980.4
nerve block (peripheral) (plexus)	968.6	E855.2	E938.6	E950.4	E962.0	E980.4
topical (surface)	968.5	E855.2	E938.5	E950.4	E962.0	E980.4
Metyrapone	977.8	E858.8	E947.8	E950.4	E962.0	E980.4
Mevinphos	989.3	E863.1	—	E950.6	E962.1	E980.7
Mezereon (berries)	988.2	E865.3	—	E950.9	E962.1	E980.9
Micatin	976.0	E858.7	E946.0	E950.4	E962.0	E980.4
Miconazole	976.0	E858.7	E946.0	E950.4	E962.0	E980.4
Midol	965.1	E850.3	E935.3	E950.0	E962.0	E980.0
Mifepristone	962.9	E858.0	E932.9	E950.4	E962.0	E980.4
Milk of magnesia	973.0	E858.4	E943.0	E950.4	E962.0	E980.4
Millipede (tropical) (venomous)	989.5	E905.4	—	E950.9	E962.1	E980.9
Miltown	969.5	E853.8	E939.5	E950.3	E962.0	E980.3
Mineral						
oil (medicinal)	973.2	E858.4	E943.2	E950.4	E962.0	E980.4
nonmedicinal	981	E862.1	—	E950.9	E962.1	E980.9
topical	976.3	E858.7	E946.3	E950.4	E962.0	E980.4
salts NEC	974.6	E858.5	E944.6	E950.4	E962.0	E980.4
spirits	981	E862.0	—	E950.9	E962.1	E980.9
Minocycline	960.4	E856	E930.4	E950.4	E962.0	E980.4
Mithramycin (antineoplastic)	960.7	E856	E930.7	E950.4	E962.0	E980.4
Mitobronitol	963.1	E858.1	E933.1	E950.4	E962.0	E980.4
Mitomycin (antineoplastic)	960.7	E856	E930.7	E950.4	E962.0	E980.4
Mitotane	963.1	E858.1	E933.1	E950.4	E962.0	E980.4
Moderil	972.6	E858.3	E942.6	E950.4	E962.0	E980.4
Mogadon — see Nitrazepam						
Molindone	969.3	E853.8	E939.3	E950.3	E962.0	E980.3
Monistat	976.0	E858.7	E946.0	E950.4	E962.0	E980.4
Monkshood	988.2	E865.4	—	E950.9	E962.1	E980.9
Monoamine oxidase inhibitors	969.0	E854.0	E939.0	E950.3	E962.0	E980.3
Monochlorobenzene	982.0	E862.4	—	E950.9	E962.1	E980.9
Monosodium glutamate	989.89	E866.8	—	E950.9	E962.1	E980.9
Monoxide, carbon — see Carbon, monoxide						
Moperone	969.2	E853.1	E939.2	E950.3	E962.0	E980.3
Morning glory seeds	969.6	E854.1	E939.6	E950.3	E962.0	E980.3
Moroxydine (hydrochloride)	961.7	E857	E931.7	E950.4	E962.0	E980.4
Morphazinamide	961.8	E857	E931.8	E950.4	E962.0	E980.4
Morphinans	965.09	E850.2	E935.2	E950.0	E962.0	E980.0
Morphine NEC	965.09	E850.2	E935.2	E950.0	E962.0	E980.0
antagonists	970.1	E854.3	E940.1	E950.4	E962.0	E980.4
Morpholinylethylmorphine	965.09	E850.2	E935.2	E950.0	E962.0	E980.0
Morrhuate sodium	972.7	E858.3	E942.7	E950.4	E962.0	E980.4
Moth balls — see also Pesticides	989.4	E863.4	—	E950.6	E962.1	E980.7
naphthalene	983.0	E863.4	—	E950.7	E962.1	E980.6
Motor exhaust gas — see Carbon, monoxide, exhaust gas						
Mouth wash	976.6	E858.7	E946.6	E950.4	E962.0	E980.4
Mucolytic agent	975.5	E858.6	E945.5	E950.4	E962.0	E980.4
Mucomyst	975.5	E858.6	E945.5	E950.4	E962.0	E980.4
Mucous membrane agents (external)	976.9	E858.7	E946.9	E950.4	E962.0	E980.4
specified NEC	976.8	E858.7	E946.8	E950.4	E962.0	E980.4
Mumps						
immune globulin (human)	964.6	E858.2	E934.6	E950.4	E962.0	E980.4
skin test antigen	977.8	E858.8	E947.8	E950.4	E962.0	E980.4
vaccine	979.6	E858.8	E949.6	E950.4	E962.0	E980.4

Table of Drugs and Chemicals

Substance	Poisoning	Accident	Therapeutic Use	Suicide Attempt	Assault	Undetermined
Mumpsvax	979.6	E858.8	E949.6	E950.4	E962.0	E980.4
Muriatic acid — see Hydrochloric acid						
Muscarine	971.0	E855.3	E941.0	E950.4	E962.0	E980.4
Muscle affecting agents						
NEC	975.3	E858.6	E945.3	E950.4	E962.0	E980.4
oxytocic	975.0	E858.6	E945.0	E950.4	E962.0	E980.4
relaxants	975.3	E858.6	E945.3	E950.4	E962.0	E980.4
central nervous system	968.0	E855.1	E938.0	E950.4	E962.0	E980.4
skeletal	975.2	E858.6	E945.2	E950.4	E962.0	E980.4
smooth	975.1	E858.6	E945.1	E950.4	E962.0	E980.4
Mushrooms, noxious	988.1	E865.5	—	E950.9	E962.1	E980.9
Mussel, noxious	988.0	E865.1	—	E950.9	E962.1	E980.9
Mustard (emetic)	973.6	E858.4	E943.6	E950.4	E962.0	E980.4
gas	987.8	E869.8	—	E952.8	E962.2	E982.8
nitrogen	963.1	E858.1	E933.1	E950.4	E962.0	E980.4
Mustine	963.1	E858.1	E933.1	E950.4	E962.0	E980.4
M-vac	979.4	E858.8	E949.4	E950.4	E962.0	E980.4
Mycifradin	960.8	E856	E930.8	E950.4	E962.0	E980.4
topical	976.0	E858.7	E946.0	E950.4	E962.0	E980.4
Mycitracin	960.8	E856	E930.8	E950.4	E962.0	E980.4
ophthalmic preparation	976.5	E858.7	E946.5	E950.4	E962.0	E980.4
Mycostatin	960.1	E856	E930.1	E950.4	E962.0	E980.4
topical	976.0	E858.7	E946.0	E950.4	E962.0	E980.4
Mydriacyl	971.1	E855.4	E941.1	E950.4	E962.0	E980.4
Myelobromal	963.1	E858.1	E933.1	E950.4	E962.0	E980.4
Myleran	963.1	E858.1	E933.1	E950.4	E962.0	E980.4
Myochrysin(e)	965.69	E850.6	E935.6	E950.0	E962.0	E980.0
Myoneural blocking agents	975.2	E858.6	E945.2	E950.4	E962.0	E980.4
Myristica fragrans	988.2	E865.3	—	E950.9	E962.1	E980.9
Myristicin	988.2	E865.3	—	E950.9	E962.1	E980.9
Mysoline	966.3	E855.0	E936.3	E950.4	E962.0	E980.4
Nafcillin (sodium)	960.0	E856	E930.0	E950.4	E962.0	E980.4
Nail polish remover	982.8	E862.4	—	E950.9	E962.1	E908.9
Nalidixic acid	961.9	E857	E931.9	E950.4	E962.0	E980.4
Nalorphine	970.1	E854.3	E940.1	E950.4	E962.0	E980.4
Naloxone	970.1	E854.3	E940.1	E950.4	E962.0	E980.4
Nandrolone (decanoate) (phenproprioate)	962.1	E858.0	E932.1	E950.4	E962.0	E980.4
Naphazoline	971.2	E855.5	E941.2	E950.4	E962.0	E980.4
Naphtha (painter's)						
(petroleum)	981	E862.0	—	E950.9	E962.1	E980.9
solvent	981	E862.0	—	E950.9	E962.1	E980.9
vapor	987.1	E869.8	—	E952.8	E962.2	E982.8
Naphthalene (chlorinated)	983.0	E864.0	—	E950.7	E962.1	E980.6
insecticide or moth repellent	983.0	E863.4	—	E950.7	E962.1	E980.6
vapor	987.8	E869.8	—	E952.8	E962.2	E982.8
Naphthol	983.0	E864.0	—	E950.7	E962.1	E980.6
Naphthylamine	983.0	E864.0	—	E950.7	E962.1	E980.6
Naprosyn — see Naproxen						
Naproxen	965.61	E850.6	E935.6	E950.0	E962.0	E980.0
Narcotic (drug)	967.9	E852.9	E937.9	E950.2	E962.0	E980.2
analgesic NEC	965.8	E850.8	E935.8	E950.0	E962.0	E980.0
antagonist	970.1	E854.3	E940.1	E950.4	E962.0	E980.4
specified NEC	967.8	E852.8	E937.8	E950.2	E962.0	E980.2
Narcotine	975.4	E858.6	E945.4	E950.4	E962.0	E980.4
Nardil	969.0	E854.0	E939.0	E950.3	E962.0	E980.3
Natrium cyanide — see Cyanide(s)						
Natural						
blood (product)	964.7	E858.2	E934.7	E950.4	E962.0	E980.4
gas (piped)	987.1	E867	—	E951.0	E962.2	E981.0
incomplete combustion	986	E867	—	E951.0	E962.2	E981.0
Nealbarbital, nealbarbitone	967.0	E851	E937.0	E950.1	E962.0	E980.1
Nectadon	975.4	E858.6	E945.4	E950.4	E962.0	E980.4
Nematocyst (sting)	989.5	E905.6	—	E950.9	E962.1	E980.9
Nembutal	967.0	E851	E937.0	E950.1	E962.0	E980.1
Neoarsphenamine	961.1	E857	E931.1	E950.4	E962.0	E980.4
Neocinchophen	974.7	E858.5	E944.7	E950.4	E962.0	E980.4
Neomycin	960.8	E856	E930.8	E950.4	E962.0	E980.4
ENT agent	976.6	E858.7	E946.6	E950.4	E962.0	E980.4
ophthalmic preparation	976.5	E858.7	E946.5	E950.4	E962.0	E980.4
topical NEC	976.0	E858.7	E946.0	E950.4	E962.0	E980.4
Neonal	967.0	E851	E937.0	E950.1	E962.0	E980.1
Neoprontosil	961.0	E857	E931.0	E950.4	E962.0	E980.4
Neosalvarsan	961.1	E857	E931.1	E950.4	E962.0	E980.4
Neosilversalvarsan	961.1	E857	E931.1	E950.4	E962.0	E980.4
Neosporin	960.8	E856	E930.8	E950.4	E962.0	E980.4
Neosporin — continued						
ENT agent	976.6	E858.7	E946.6	E950.4	E962.0	E980.4
opthalmic preparation	976.5	E858.7	E946.5	E950.4	E962.0	E980.4
topical NEC	976.0	E858.7	E946.0	E950.4	E962.0	E980.4
Neostigmine	971.0	E855.3	E941.0	E950.4	E962.0	E980.4
Neraval	967.0	E851	E937.0	E950.1	E962.0	E980.1
Neravan	967.0	E851	E937.0	E950.1	E962.0	E980.1
Nerium oleander	988.2	E865.4	—	E950.9	E962.1	E980.9
Nerve gases (war)	987.9	E869.9	—	E952.9	E962.2	E982.9
Nesacaine	968.9	E855.2	E938.9	E950.4	E962.0	E980.4
infiltration (subcutaneous)	968.5	E855.2	E938.5	E950.4	E962.0	E980.4
nerve block (peripheral) (plexus)	968.6	E855.2	E938.6	E950.4	E962.0	E980.4
Neurobarb	967.0	E851	E937.0	E950.1	E962.0	E980.1
Neuroleptics NEC	969.3	E853.8	E939.3	E950.3	E962.0	E980.3
Neuroprotective agent	977.8	E858.8	E947.8	E950.4	E962.0	E980.4
Neutral spirits	980.0	E860.1	—	E950.9	E962.1	E980.9
beverage	980.0	E860.0	—	E950.9	E962.1	E980.9
Niacin, niacinamide	972.2	E858.3	E942.2	E950.4	E962.0	E980.4
Nialamide	969.0	E854.0	E939.0	E950.3	E962.0	E980.3
Nickle (carbonyl) (compounds) (fumes) (tetracarbonyl) (vapor)	985.8	E866.4	—	E950.9	E962.1	E980.9
Niclosamide	961.6	E857	E931.6	E950.4	E962.0	E980.4
Nicomorphine	965.09	E850.2	E935.2	E950.0	E962.0	E980.0
Nicotinamide	972.2	E858.3	E942.2	E950.4	E962.0	E980.4
Nicotine (insecticide) (spray) (sulfate) NEC	989.4	E863.4	—	E950.6	E962.1	E980.7
not insecticide	989.89	E866.8	—	E950.9	E962.1	E980.9
Nicotinic acid (derivatives)	972.2	E858.3	E942.2	E950.4	E962.0	E980.4
Nicotinyl alcohol	972.2	E858.3	E942.2	E950.4	E962.0	E980.4
Nicoumalone	964.2	E858.2	E934.2	E950.4	E962.0	E980.4
Nifenazone	965.5	E850.5	E935.5	E950.0	E962.0	E980.0
Nifuraldezone	961.9	E857	E931.9	E950.4	E962.0	E980.4
Nightshade (deadly)	988.2	E865.4	—	E950.9	E962.1	E980.9
Nikethamide	970.0	E854.3	E940.0	E950.4	E962.0	E980.4
Nilstat	960.1	E856	E930.1	E950.4	E962.0	E980.4
topical	976.0	E858.7	E946.0	E950.4	E962.0	E980.4
Nimodipine	977.8	E858.8	E947.8	E950.4	E962.0	E980.4
Niridazole	961.6	E857	E931.6	E950.4	E962.0	E980.4
Nisentil	965.09	E850.2	E935.2	E950.0	E962.0	E980.0
Nitrates	972.4	E858.3	E942.4	E950.4	E962.0	E980.4
Nitrazepam	969.4	E853.2	E939.4	E950.3	E962.0	E980.3
Nitric						
acid (liquid)	983.1	E864.1	—	E950.7	E962.1	E980.6
vapor	987.8	E869.8	—	E952.8	E962.2	E982.8
oxide (gas)	987.2	E869.0	—	E952.8	E962.2	E982.8
Nitrite, amyl (medicinal) (vapor)	972.4	E858.3	E942.4	E950.4	E962.0	E980.4
Nitroaniline	983.0	E864.0	—	E950.7	E962.1	E980.6
vapor	987.8	E869.8	—	E952.8	E962.2	E982.8
Nitrobenzene, nitrobenzol	983.0	E864.0	—	E950.7	E962.1	E980.6
vapor	987.8	E869.8	—	E952.8	E962.2	E982.8
Nitrocellulose	976.3	E858.7	E946.3	E950.4	E962.0	E980.4
Nitrofuran derivatives	961.9	E857	E931.9	E950.4	E962.0	E980.4
Nitrofurantoin	961.9	E857	E931.9	E950.4	E962.0	E980.4
Nitrofurazone	976.0	E858.7	E946.0	E950.4	E962.0	E980.4
Nitrogen (dioxide) (gas) (oxide)	987.2	E869.0	—	E952.8	E962.2	E982.8
mustard (antineoplastic)	963.1	E858.1	E933.1	E950.4	E962.0	E980.4
nonmedicinal	989.89	E866.8	—	E950.9	E962.1	E980.9
fumes	987.8	E869.8	—	E952.8	E962.2	E982.8
Nitroglycerin, nitroglycerol (medicinal)	972.4	E858.3	E942.4	E950.4	E962.0	E980.4
Nitrohydrochloric acid	983.1	E864.1	—	E950.7	E962.1	E980.6
Nitromersol	976.0	E858.7	E946.0	E950.4	E962.0	E980.4
Nitronaphthalene	983.0	E864.0	—	E950.7	E962.2	E980.6
Nitrophenol	983.0	E864.0	—	E950.7	E962.1	E980.6
Nitrothiazol	961.6	E857	E931.6	E950.4	E962.0	E980.4
Nitrotoluene, nitrotoluol	983.0	E864.0	—	E950.7	E962.1	E980.6
vapor	987.8	E869.8	—	E952.8	E962.2	E982.8
Nitrous	968.2	E855.1	E938.2	E950.4	E962.0	E980.4
acid (liquid)	983.1	E864.1	—	E950.7	E962.1	E980.6
fumes	987.2	E869.0	—	E952.8	E962.2	E982.8
oxide (anesthetic) NEC	968.2	E855.1	E938.2	E950.4	E962.0	E980.4
Nitrozone	976.0	E858.7	E946.0	E950.4	E962.0	E980.4
Noctec	967.1	E852.0	E937.1	E950.2	E962.0	E980.2
Noludar	967.5	E852.4	E937.5	E950.2	E962.0	E980.2
Noptil	967.0	E851	E937.0	E950.1	E962.0	E980.1
Noradrenalin	971.2	E855.5	E941.2	E950.4	E962.0	E980.4
Noramidopyrine	965.5	E850.5	E935.5	E950.0	E962.0	E980.0

Norepinephrine — Table of Drugs and Chemicals

	Poisoning	Accident	Therapeutic Use	Suicide Attempt	Assault	Undetermined
Norepinephrine	971.2	E855.5	E941.2	E950.4	E962.0	E980.4
Norethandrolone	962.1	E858.0	E932.1	E950.4	E962.0	E980.4
Norethindrone	962.2	E858.0	E932.2	E950.4	E962.0	E980.4
Norethisterone	962.2	E858.0	E932.2	E950.4	E962.0	E980.4
Norethynodrel	962.2	E858.0	E932.2	E950.4	E962.0	E980.4
Norlestrin	962.2	E858.0	E932.2	E950.4	E962.0	E980.4
Norlutin	962.2	E858.0	E932.2	E950.4	E962.0	E980.4
Normison — see Benzodiazepines						
Normorphine	965.09	E850.2	E935.2	E950.0	E962.0	E980.0
Nortriptyline	969.0	E854.0	E939.0	E950.3	E962.0	E980.3
Noscapine	975.4	E858.6	E945.4	E950.4	E962.0	E980.4
Nose preparations	976.6	E858.7	E946.6	E950.4	E962.0	E980.4
Novobiocin	960.8	E856	E930.8	E950.4	E962.0	E980.4
Novocain (infiltration)						
(topical)	968.5	E855.2	E938.5	E950.4	E962.0	E980.4
nerve block (peripheral) (plexus)	968.6	E855.2	E938.6	E950.4	E962.0	E980.4
spinal	968.7	E855.2	E938.7	E950.4	E962.0	E980.4
Noxythiolin	961.9	E857	E931.9	E950.4	E962.0	E980.4
NPH Iletin (insulin)	962.3	E858.0	E932.3	E950.4	E962.0	E980.4
Numorphan	965.09	E850.2	E935.2	E950.0	E962.0	E980.0
Nunol	967.0	E851	E937.0	E950.1	E962.0	E980.1
Nupercaine (spinal anesthetic)	968.7	E855.2	E938.7	E950.4	E962.0	E980.4
topical (surface)	968.5	E855.2	E938.5	E950.4	E962.0	E980.4
Nutmeg oil (liniment)	976.3	E858.7	E946.3	E950.4	E962.0	E980.4
Nux vomica	989.1	E863.7	—	E950.6	E962.1	E980.7
Nydrazid	961.8	E857	E931.8	E950.4	E962.0	E980.4
Nylidrin	971.2	E855.5	E941.2	E950.4	E962.0	E980.4
Nystatin	960.1	E856	E930.1	E950.4	E962.0	E980.4
topical	976	E858.7	E946.0	E950.4	E962.0	E980.4
Nytol	963.0	E858.1	E933.0	E950.4	E962.0	E980.4
Oblivion	967.8	E852.8	E937.8	E950.2	E962.0	E980.2
Octyl nitrite	972.4	E858.3	E942.4	E950.4	E962.0	E980.4
Oestradiol (cypionate) (dipropionate) (valerate)	962.2	E858.0	E932.2	E950.4	E962.0	E980.4
Oestriol	962.2	E858.0	E932.2	E950.4	E962.0	E980.4
Oestrone	962.2	E858.0	E932.2	E950.4	E962.0	E980.4
Oil (of) NEC	989.89	E866.8	—	E950.9	E962.1	E980.9
bitter almond	989.0	E866.8	—	E950.9	E962.1	E980.9
camphor	976.1	E858.7	E946.1	E950.4	E962.0	E980.4
colors	989.89	E861.6	—	E950.9	E962.1	E980.9
fumes	987.8	E869.8	—	E952.8	E962.2	E982.8
lubricating	981	E862.2	—	E950.9	E962.1	E980.9
specified source, other — see substance specified						
vitriol (liquid)	983.1	E864.1	—	E950.7	E962.1	E980.6
fumes	987.8	E869.8	—	E952.8	E962.2	E982.8
wintergreen (bitter) NEC	976.3	E858.7	E946.3	E950.4	E962.0	E980.4
Ointments NEC	976.9	E858.7	E946.9	E950.4	E962.0	E980.4
Oleander	988.2	E865.4	—	E950.9	E962.1	E980.9
Oleandomycin	960.3	E856	E930.3	E950.4	E962.0	E980.4
Oleovitamin A	963.5	E858.1	E933.5	E950.4	E962.0	E980.4
Oleum ricini	973.1	E858.4	E943.1	E950.4	E962.0	E980.4
Olive oil (medicinal) NEC	973.2	E858.4	E943.2	E950.4	E962.0	E980.4
OMPA	989.3	E863.1	—	E950.6	E962.1	E980.7
Oncovin	963.1	E858.1	E933.1	E950.4	E962.0	E980.4
Ophthaine	968.5	E855.2	E938.5	E950.4	E962.0	E980.4
Ophthetic	968.5	E855.2	E938.5	E950.4	E962.0	E980.4
Opiates, opioids, opium NEC	965.00	E850.2	E935.2	E950.0	E962.0	E980.0
antagonists	970.1	E854.3	E940.1	E950.4	E962.0	E980.4
Oracon	962.2	E858.0	E932.2	E950.4	E962.0	E980.4
Oragrafin	977.8	E858.8	E947.8	E950.4	E962.0	E980.4
Oral contraceptives	962.2	E858.0	E932.2	E950.4	E962.0	E980.4
Orciprenaline	975.1	E858.6	E945.1	E950.4	E962.0	E980.4
Organidin	975.5	E858.6	E945.5	E950.4	E962.0	E980.4
Organophosphates	989.3	E863.1	—	E950.6	E962.1	E980.7
Orimune	979.5	E858.8	E949.5	E950.4	E962.0	E980.4
Orinase	962.3	E858.0	E932.3	E950.4	E962.0	E980.4
Orphenadrine	966.4	E855.0	E936.4	E950.4	E962.0	E980.4
Ortal (sodium)	967.0	E851	E937.0	E950.1	E962.0	E980.1
Orthoboric acid	976.0	E858.7	E946.0	E950.4	E962.0	E980.4
ENT agent	976.6	E858.7	E946.6	E950.4	E962.0	E980.4
ophthalmic preparation	976.5	E858.7	E946.5	E950.4	E962.0	E980.4
Orthocaine	968.5	E855.2	E938.5	E950.4	E962.0	E980.4
Ortho-Novum	962.2	E858.0	E932.2	E950.4	E962.0	E980.4
Orthotolidine (reagent)	977.8	E858.8	E947.8	E950.4	E962.0	E980.4
Osmic acid (liquid)	983.1	E864.1	—	E950.7	E962.1	E980.6
fumes	987.8	E869.8	—	E952.8	E962.2	E982.8
Osmotic diuretics	974.4	E858.5	E944.4	E950.4	E962.0	E980.4
Ouabain	972.1	E858.3	E942.1	E950.4	E962.0	E980.4
Ovarian hormones (synthetic substitutes)	962.2	E858.0	E932.2	E950.4	E962.0	E980.4
Ovral	962.2	E858.0	E932.2	E950.4	E962.0	E980.4
Ovulation suppressants	962.2	E858.0	E932.2	E950.4	E962.0	E980.4
Ovulen	962.2	E858.0	E932.2	E950.4	E962.0	E980.4
Oxacillin (sodium)	960.0	E856	E930.0	E950.4	E962.0	E980.4
Oxalic acid	983.1	E864.1	—	E950.7	E962.1	E980.6
Oxanamide	969.5	E853.8	E939.5	E950.3	E962.0	E980.3
Oxandrolone	962.1	E858.0	E932.1	E950.4	E962.0	E980.4
Oxaprozin	965.61	E850.6	E935.6	E950.0	E962.0	E980.0
Oxazepam	969.4	E853.2	E939.4	E950.3	E962.0	E980.3
Oxazolidine derivatives	966.0	E855.0	E936.0	E950.4	E962.0	E980.4
Ox bile extract	973.4	E858.4	E943.4	E950.4	E962.0	E980.4
Oxedrine	971.2	E855.5	E941.2	E950.4	E962.0	E980.4
Oxeladin	975.4	E858.6	E945.4	E950.4	E962.0	E980.4
Oxethazaine NEC	968.5	E855.2	E938.5	E950.4	E962.0	E980.4
Oxidizing agents NEC	983.9	E864.3	—	E950.7	E962.1	E980.6
Oxolinic acid	961.3	E857	E931.3	E950.4	E962.0	E980.4
Oxophenarsine	961.1	E857	E931.1	E950.4	E962.0	E980.4
Oxsoralen	976.3	E858.7	E946.3	E950.4	E962.0	E980.4
Oxtriphylline	975.7	E858.6	E945.7	E950.4	E962.0	E980.4
Oxybuprocaine	968.5	E855.2	E938.5	E950.4	E962.0	E980.4
Oxybutynin	975.1	E858.6	E945.1	E950.4	E962.0	E980.4
Oxycodone	965.09	E850.2	E935.2	E950.0	E962.0	E980.0
Oxygen	987.8	E869.8	—	E952.8	E962.2	E982.8
Oxylone	976	E858.7	E946.0	E950.4	E962.0	E980.4
ophthalmic preparation	976.5	E858.7	E946.5	E950.4	E962.0	E980.4
Oxymesterone	962.1	E858.0	E932.1	E950.4	E962.0	E980.4
Oxymetazoline	971.2	E855.5	E941.2	E950.4	E962.0	E980.4
Oxymetholone	962.1	E858.0	E932.1	E950.4	E962.0	E980.4
Oxymorphone	965.09	E850.2	E935.2	E950.0	E962.0	E980.0
Oxypertine	969.0	E854.0	E939.0	E950.3	E962.0	E980.3
Oxyphenbutazone	965.5	E850.5	E935.5	E950.0	E962.0	E980.0
Oxyphencyclimine	971.1	E855.4	E941.1	E950.4	E962.0	E980.4
Oxyphenisatin	973.1	E858.4	E943.1	E950.4	E962.0	E980.4
Oxyphenonium	971.1	E855.4	E941.1	E950.4	E962.0	E980.4
Oxyquinoline	961.3	E857	E931.3	E950.4	E962.0	E980.4
Oxytetracycline	960.4	E856	E930.4	E950.4	E962.0	E980.4
Oxytocics	975.0	E858.6	E945.0	E950.4	E962.0	E980.4
Oxytocin	975.0	E858.6	E945.0	E950.4	E962.0	E980.4
Ozone	987.8	E869.8	—	E952.8	E962.2	E982.8
PABA	976.3	E858.7	E946.3	E950.4	E962.0	E980.4
Packed red cells	964.7	E858.2	E934.7	E950.4	E962.0	E980.4
Paint NEC	989.89	E861.6	—	E950.9	E962.1	E980.9
cleaner	982.8	E862.9	—	E950.9	E962.1	E980.9
fumes NEC	987.8	E869.8	—	E952.8	E962.1	E982.8
lead (fumes)	984.0	E861.5	—	E950.9	E962.1	E980.9
solvent NEC	982.8	E862.9	—	E950.9	E962.1	E980.9
stripper	982.8	E862.9	—	E950.9	E962.1	E980.9
Palfium	965.09	E850.2	E935.2	E950.0	E962.0	E980.0
Palivizumab	979.9	E858.8	E949.6	E950.4	E962.0	E980.4
Paludrine	961.4	E857	E931.4	E950.4	E962.0	E980.4
PAM	977.2	E855.8	E947.2	E950.4	E962.0	E980.4
Pamaquine (naphthoate)	961.4	E857	E931.4	E950.4	E962.0	E980.4
Pamprin	965.1	E850.3	E935.3	E950.0	E962.0	E980.0
Panadol	965.4	E850.4	E935.4	E950.0	E962.0	E980.0
Pancreatic dornase (mucolytic)	963.4	E858.1	E933.4	E950.4	E962.0	E980.4
Pancreatin	973.4	E858.4	E943.4	E950.4	E962.0	E980.4
Pancrelipase	973.4	E858.4	E943.4	E950.4	E962.0	E980.4
Pangamic acid	963.5	E858.1	E933.5	E950.4	E962.0	E980.4
Panthenol	963.5	E858.1	E933.5	E950.4	E962.0	E980.4
topical	976.8	E858.7	E946.8	E950.4	E962.0	E980.4
Pantopaque	977.8	E858.8	E947.8	E950.4	E962.0	E980.4
Pantopon	965.00	E850.2	E935.2	E950.0	E962.0	E980.0
Pantothenic acid	963.5	E858.1	E933.5	E950.4	E962.0	E980.4
Panwarfin	964.2	E858.2	E934.2	E950.4	E962.0	E980.4
Papain	973.4	E858.4	E943.4	E950.4	E962.0	E980.4
Papaverine	972.5	E858.3	E942.5	E950.4	E962.0	E980.4
Para-aminobenzoic acid	976.3	E858.7	E946.3	E950.4	E962.0	E980.4
Para-aminophenol derivatives	965.4	E850.4	E935.4	E950.0	E962.0	E980.0
Para-aminosalicylic acid (derivatives)	961.8	E857	E931.8	E950.4	E962.0	E980.4
Paracetaldehyde (medicinal)	967.2	E852.1	E937.2	E950.2	E962.0	E980.2
Paracetamol	965.4	E850.4	E935.4	E950.0	E962.0	E980.0
Paracodin	965.09	E850.2	E935.2	E950.0	E962.0	E980.0
Paradione	966.0	E855.0	E936.0	E950.4	E962.0	E980.4

Table of Drugs and Chemicals

	Poisoning	External Cause (E-Code)				
		Accident	Therapeutic Use	Suicide Attempt	Assault	Undetermined
Paraffin(s) (wax)	981	E862.3	—	E950.9	E962.1	E980.9
liquid (medicinal)	973.2	E858.4	E943.2	E950.4	E962.0	E980.4
nonmedicinal (oil)	981	E962.1	—	E950.9	E962.1	E980.9
Paraldehyde (medicinal)	967.2	E852.1	E937.2	E950.2	E962.0	E980.2
Paramethadione	966.0	E855.0	E936.0	E950.4	E962.0	E980.4
Paramethasone	962.0	E858.0	E932.0	E950.4	E962.0	E980.4
Paraquat	989.4	E863.5	—	E950.6	E962.1	E980.7
Parasympatholytics	971.1	E855.4	E941.1	E950.4	E962.0	E980.4
Parasympathomimetics	971.0	E855.3	E941.0	E950.4	E962.0	E980.4
Parathion	989.3	E863.1	—	E950.6	E962.1	E980.7
Parathormone	962.6	E858.0	E932.6	E950.4	E962.0	E980.4
Parathyroid (derivatives)	962.6	E858.0	E932.6	E950.4	E962.0	E980.4
Paratyphoid vaccine	978.1	E858.8	E948.1	E950.4	E962.0	E980.4
Paredrine	971.2	E855.5	E941.2	E950.4	E962.0	E980.4
Paregoric	965.00	E850.2	E935.2	E950.0	E962.0	E980.0
Pargyline	972.3	E858.3	E942.3	E950.4	E962.0	E980.4
Paris green	985.1	E866.3	—	E950.8	E962.1	E980.8
insecticide	985.1	E863.4	—	E950.8	E962.1	E980.8
Parnate	969.0	E854.0	E939.0	E950.3	E962.0	E980.3
Paromomycin	960.8	E856	E930.8	E950.4	E962.0	E980.4
Paroxypropione	963.1	E858.1	E933.1	E950.4	E962.0	E980.4
Parzone	965.09	E850.2	E935.2	E950.0	E962.0	E980.0
PAS	961.8	E857	E931.8	E950.4	E962.0	E980.4
PCBs	981	E862.3	—	E950.9	E962.1	E980.9
PCP (pentachlorophenol)	989.4	E863.6	—	E950.6	E962.1	E980.7
herbicide	989.4	E863.5	—	E950.6	E962.1	E980.7
insecticide	989.4	E863.4	—	E950.6	E962.1	E980.7
phencyclidine	968.3	E855.1	E938.3	E950.4	E962.0	E980.4
Peach kernel oil (emulsion)	973.2	E858.4	E943.2	E950.4	E962.0	E980.4
Peanut oil (emulsion) NEC	973.2	E858.4	E943.2	E950.4	E962.0	E980.4
topical	976.3	E858.7	E946.3	E950.4	E962.0	E980.4
Pearly Gates (morning glory seeds)	969.6	E854.1	E939.6	E950.3	E962.0	E980.3
Pecazine	969.1	E853.0	E939.1	E950.3	E962.0	E980.3
Pecilocin	960.1	E856	E930.1	E950.4	E962.0	E980.4
Pectin (with kaolin) NEC	973.5	E858.4	E943.5	E950.4	E962.0	E980.4
Pelletierine tannate	961.6	E857	E931.6	E950.4	E962.0	E980.4
Pemoline	969.7	E854.2	E939.7	E950.3	E962.0	E980.3
Pempidine	972.3	E858.3	E942.3	E950.4	E962.0	E980.4
Penamecillin	960.0	E856	E930.0	E950.4	E962.0	E980.4
Penethamate hydriodide	960.0	E856	E930.0	E950.4	E962.0	E980.4
Penicillamine	963.8	E858.1	E933.8	E950.4	E962.0	E980.4
Penicillin (any type)	960.0	E856	E930.0	E950.4	E962.0	E980.4
Penicillinase	963.4	E858.1	E933.4	E950.4	E962.0	E980.4
Pentachlorophenol (fungicide)	989.4	E863.6	—	E950.6	E962.1	E980.7
herbicide	989.4	E863.5	—	E950.6	E962.1	E980.7
insecticide	989.4	E863.4	—	E950.6	E962.1	E980.7
Pentaerythritol	972.4	E858.3	E942.4	E950.4	E962.0	E980.4
chloral	967.1	E852.0	E937.1	E950.2	E962.0	E980.2
tetranitrate NEC	972.4	E858.3	E942.4	E950.4	E962.0	E980.4
Pentagastrin	977.8	E858.8	E947.8	E950.4	E962.0	E980.4
Pentalin	982.3	E862.4	—	E950.9	E962.1	E980.9
Pentamethonium (bromide)	972.3	E858.3	E942.3	E950.4	E962.0	E980.4
Pentamidine	961.5	E857	E931.5	E950.4	E962.0	E980.4
Pentanol	980.8	E860.8	—	E950.9	E962.1	E980.9
Pentaquine	961.4	E857	E931.4	E950.4	E962.0	E980.4
Pentazocine	965.8	E850.8	E935.8	E950.0	E962.0	E980.0
Penthienate	971.1	E855.4	E941.1	E950.4	E962.0	E980.4
Pentobarbital, pentobarbitone (sodium)	967.0	E851	E937.0	E950.1	E962.0	E980.1
Pentolinium (tartrate)	972.3	E858.3	E942.3	E950.4	E962.0	E980.4
Pentothal	968.3	E855.1	E938.3	E950.4	E962.0	E980.4
Pentylenetetrazol	970.0	E854.3	E940.0	E950.4	E962.0	E980.4
Pentylsalicylamide	961.8	E857	E931.8	E950.4	E962.0	E980.4
Pepsin	973.4	E858.4	E943.4	E950.4	E962.0	E980.4
Peptavlon	977.8	E858.8	E947.8	E950.4	E962.0	E980.4
Percaine (spinal)	968.7	E855.2	E938.7	E950.4	E962.0	E980.4
topical (surface)	968.5	E855.2	E938.5	E950.4	E962.0	E980.4
Perchloroethylene (vapor)	982.3	E862.4	—	E950.9	E962.1	E980.9
medicinal	961.6	E857	E931.6	E950.4	E962.0	E980.4
Percodan	965.09	E850.2	E935.2	E950.0	E962.0	E980.0
Percogesic	965.09	E850.2	E935.2	E950.0	E962.0	E980.0
Percorten	962.0	E858.0	E932.0	E950.4	E962.0	E980.4
Pergonal	962.4	E858.0	E932.4	E950.4	E962.0	E980.4
Perhexiline	972.4	E858.3	E942.4	E950.4	E962.0	E980.4
Periactin	963.0	E858.1	E933.0	E950.4	E962.0	E980.4
Periclor	967.1	E852.0	E937.1	E950.2	E962.0	E980.2
Pericyazine	969.1	E853.0	E939.1	E950.3	E962.0	E980.3
Peritrate	972.4	E858.3	E942.4	E950.4	E962.0	E980.4
Permanganates NEC	983.9	E864.3	—	E950.7	E962.1	E980.6
Permanganates — continued potassium (topical)	976.0	E858.7	E946.0	E950.4	E962.0	E980.4
Pernocton	967.0	E851	E937.0	E950.1	E962.0	E980.1
Pernoston	967.0	E851	E937.0	E950.1	E962.0	E980.1
Peronin(e)	965.09	E850.2	E935.2	E950.0	E962.0	E980.0
Perphenazine	969.1	E853.0	E939.1	E950.3	E962.0	E980.3
Pertofrane	969.0	E854.0	E939.0	E950.3	E962.0	E980.3
Pertussis immune serum (human)	964.6	E858.2	E934.6	E950.4	E962.0	E980.4
vaccine (with diphtheria toxoid) (with tetanus toxoid)	978.6	E858.8	E948.6	E950.4	E962.0	E980.4
Peruvian balsam	976.8	E858.7	E946.8	E950.4	E962.0	E980.4
Pesticides (dust) (fumes) (vapor)	989.4	E863.4	—	E950.6	E962.1	E980.7
arsenic	985.1	E863.4	—	E950.8	E962.1	E980.8
chlorinated	989.2	E863.0	—	E950.6	E962.1	E980.7
cyanide	989.0	E863.4	—	E950.6	E962.1	E980.7
kerosene	981	E863.4	—	E950.6	E962.1	E980.7
mixture (of compounds)	989.4	E863.3	—	E950.6	E962.1	E980.7
naphthalene	983.0	E863.4	—	E950.7	E962.1	E980.6
organochlorine (compounds)	989.2	E863.0	—	E950.6	E962.1	E980.7
petroleum (distillate) (products) NEC	981	E863.4	—	E950.6	E962.1	E980.7
specified ingredient NEC	989.4	E863.4	—	E950.6	E962.1	E980.7
strychnine	989.1	E863.4	—	E950.6	E962.1	E980.7
thallium	985.8	E863.7	—	E950.6	E962.1	E980.7
Pethidine (hydrochloride)	965.09	E850.2	E935.2	E950.0	E962.0	E980.0
Petrichloral	967.1	E852.0	E937.1	E950.2	E962.0	E980.2
Petrol	981	E862.1	—	E950.9	E962.1	E980.9
vapor	987.1	E869.8	—	E952.8	E962.2	E982.8
Petrolatum (jelly) (ointment)	976.3	E858.7	E946.3	E950.4	E962.0	E980.4
hydrophilic	976.3	E858.7	E946.3	E950.4	E962.0	E980.4
liquid	973.2	E858.4	E943.2	E950.4	E962.0	E980.4
topical	976.3	E858.7	E946.3	E950.4	E962.0	E980.4
nonmedicinal	981	E862.1	—	E950.9	E962.1	E980.9
Petroleum (cleaners) (fuels) (products) NEC	981	E862.1	—	E950.9	E962.1	E980.9
benzin(e) — see Ligroin						
ether — see Ligroin						
jelly — see Petrolatum						
naphtha — see Ligroin						
pesticide	981	E863.4	—	E950.6	E962.1	E980.7
solids	981	E862.3	—	E950.9	E962.1	E980.9
solvents	981	E862.0	—	E950.9	E962.1	E980.9
vapor	987.1	E869.8	—	E952.8	E962.2	E982.8
Peyote	969.6	E854.1	E939.6	E950.3	E962.0	E980.3
Phanodorm, phanodorn	967.0	E851	E937.0	E950.1	E962.0	E980.1
Phanquinone, phanquone	961.5	E857	E931.5	E950.4	E962.0	E980.4
Pharmaceutical excipient or adjunct	977.4	E858.8	E947.4	E950.4	E962.0	E980.4
Phenacemide	966.3	E855.0	E936.3	E950.4	E962.0	E980.4
Phenacetin	965.4	E850.4	E935.4	E950.0	E962.0	E980.0
Phenadoxone	965.09	E850.2	E935.2	E950.0	E962.0	E980.0
Phenaglycodol	969.5	E853.8	E939.5	E950.3	E962.0	E980.3
Phenantoin	966.1	E855.0	E936.1	E950.4	E962.0	E980.4
Phenaphthazine reagent	977.8	E858.8	E947.8	E950.4	E962.0	E980.4
Phenazocine	965.09	E850.2	E935.2	E950.0	E962.0	E980.0
Phenazone	965.5	E850.5	E935.5	E950.0	E962.0	E980.0
Phenazopyridine	976.1	E858.7	E946.1	E950.4	E962.0	E980.4
Phenbenicillin	960.0	E856	E930.0	E950.4	E962.0	E980.4
Phenbutrazate	977.0	E858.8	E947.0	E950.4	E962.0	E980.4
Phencyclidine	968.3	E855.1	E938.3	E950.4	E962.0	E980.4
Phendimetrazine	977.0	E858.8	E947.0	E950.4	E962.0	E980.4
Phenelzine	969.0	E854.0	E939.0	E950.3	E962.0	E980.3
Phenergan	967.8	E852.8	E937.8	E950.2	E962.0	E980.2
Phenethicillin (potassium)	960.0	E856	E930.0	E950.4	E962.0	E980.4
Phenetsal	965.1	E850.3	E935.3	E950.0	E962.0	E980.0
Pheneturide	966.3	E855.0	E936.3	E950.4	E962.0	E980.4
Phenformin	962.3	E858.0	E932.3	E950.4	E962.0	E980.4
Phenglutarimide	971.1	E855.4	E941.1	E950.4	E962.0	E980.4
Phenicarbazide	965.8	E850.8	E935.8	E950.0	E962.0	E980.0
Phenindamine (tartrate)	963.0	E858.1	E933.0	E950.4	E962.0	E980.4
Phenindione	964.2	E858.2	E934.2	E950.4	E962.0	E980.4
Pheniprazine	969.0	E854.0	E939.0	E950.3	E962.0	E980.3
Pheniramine (maleate)	963.0	E858.1	E933.0	E950.4	E962.0	E980.4
Phenmetrazine	977.0	E858.8	E947.0	E950.4	E962.0	E980.4
Phenobal	967.0	E851	E937.0	E950.1	E962.0	E980.1
Phenobarbital	967.0	E851	E937.0	E950.1	E962.0	E980.1
Phenobarbitone	967.0	E851	E937.0	E950.1	E962.0	E980.1
Phenoctide	976.0	E858.7	E946.0	E950.4	E962.0	E980.4

Table of Drugs and Chemicals

			External Cause (E-Code)			
	Poisoning	Accident	Therapeutic Use	Suicide Attempt	Assault	Undetermined
Phenol (derivatives) NEC	983.0	E864.0	—	E950.7	E962.1	E980.6
disinfectant	983.0	E864.0	—	E950.7	E962.1	E980.6
pesticide	989.4	E863.4	—	E950.6	E962.1	E980.7
red	977.8	E858.8	E947.8	E950.4	E962.0	E980.4
Phenolphthalein	973.1	E858.4	E943.1	E950.4	E962.0	E980.4
Phenolsulfonphthalein	977.8	E858.8	E947.8	E950.4	E962.0	E980.4
Phenomorphan	965.09	E850.2	E935.2	E950.0	E962.0	E980.0
Phenonyl	967.0	E851	E937.0	E950.1	E962.0	E980.1
Phenoperidine	965.09	E850.2	E935.2	E950.0	E962.0	E980.0
Phenoquin	974.7	E858.5	E944.7	E950.4	E962.0	E980.4
Phenothiazines (tranquilizers)						
NEC	969.1	E853.0	E939.1	E950.3	E962.0	E980.3
insecticide	989.3	E863.4	—	E950.6	E962.1	E980.7
Phenoxybenzamine	971.3	E855.6	E941.3	E950.4	E962.0	E980.4
Phenoxymethyl penicillin	960.0	E856	E930.0	E950.4	E962.0	E980.4
Phenprocoumon	964.2	E858.2	E934.2	E950.4	E962.0	E980.4
Phensuximide	966.2	E855.0	E936.2	E950.4	E962.0	E980.4
Phentermine	977.0	E858.8	E947.0	E950.4	E962.0	E980.4
Phentolamine NEC	971.3	E855.6	E941.3	E950.4	E962.0	E980.4
Phenyl						
butazone	965.5	E850.5	E935.5	E950.0	E962.0	E980.0
enediamine	983.0	E864.0	—	E950.7	E962.1	E980.6
hydrazine	983.0	E864.0	—	E950.7	E962.1	E980.6
antineoplastic	963.1	E858.1	E933.1	E950.4	E962.0	E980.4
mercuric compounds — see Mercury						
salicylate	976.3	E858.7	E946.3	E950.4	E962.0	E980.4
Phenylephrin	971.2	E855.5	E941.2	E950.4	E962.0	E980.4
Phenylethylbiguanide	962.3	E858.0	E932.3	E950.4	E962.0	E980.4
Phenylpropanolamine	971.2	E855.5	E941.2	E950.4	E962.0	E980.4
Phenylsulfthion	989.3	E863.1	—	E950.6	E962.1	E980.7
Phenyramidol, phenyramidon	965.7	E850.7	E935.7	E950.0	E962.0	E980.0
Phenytoin	966.1	E855.0	E936.1	E950.4	E962.0	E980.4
pHisoHex	976.2	E858.7	E946.2	E950.4	E962.0	E980.4
Pholcodine	965.09	E850.2	E935.2	E950.0	E962.0	E980.0
Phorate	989.3	E863.1	—	E950.6	E962.1	E980.7
Phosdrin	989.3	E863.1	—	E950.6	E962.1	E980.7
Phosgene (gas)	987.8	E869.8	—	E952.8	E962.2	E982.8
Phosphate (tricresyl)	989.89	E866.8	—	E950.9	E962.1	E980.9
organic	989.3	E863.1	—	E950.6	E962.1	E980.7
solvent	982.8	E862.4	—	E950.9	E926.1	E980.9
Phosphine	987.8	E869.8	—	E952.8	E962.2	E982.8
fumigant	987.8	E863.8	—	E950.6	E962.2	E980.7
Pholpholine	971.0	E855.3	E941.0	E950.4	E962.0	E980.4
Phosphoric acid	983.1	E864.1	—	E950.7	E962.1	E980.6
Phosphorus (compounds) NEC	983.9	E864.3	—	E950.7	E962.1	E980.6
rodenticide	983.9	E863.7	—	E950.7	E962.1	E980.6
Phthalimidoglutarimide	967.8	E852.8	E937.8	E950.2	E962.0	E980.2
Phthalylsulfathiazole	961.0	E857	E931.0	E950.4	E962.0	E980.4
Phylloquinone	964.3	E858.2	E934.3	E950.4	E962.0	E980.4
Physeptone	965.02	E850.1	E935.1	E950.0	E962.0	E980.0
Physostigma venenosum	988.2	E865.4	—	E950.9	E962.1	E980.9
Physostigmine	971.0	E855.3	E941.0	E950.4	E962.0	E980.4
Phytolacca decandra	988.2	E865.4	—	E950.9	E962.1	E980.9
Phytomenadione	964.3	E858.2	E934.3	E950.4	E962.0	E980.4
Phytonadione	964.3	E858.2	E934.3	E950.4	E962.0	E980.4
Picric (acid)	983.0	E864.0	—	E950.7	E962.1	E980.6
Picrotoxin	970.0	E854.3	E940.0	E950.4	E962.0	E980.4
Pilocarpine	971.0	E855.3	E941.0	E950.4	E962.0	E980.4
Pilocarpus (jaborandi) extract	971.0	E855.3	E941.0	E950.4	E962.0	E980.4
Pimaricin	960.1	E856	E930.1	E950.4	E962.0	E980.4
Piminodine	965.09	E850.2	E935.2	E950.0	E962.0	E980.0
Pine oil, pinesol (disinfectant)	983.9	E861.4	—	E950.7	E962.1	E980.6
Pinkroot	961.6	E857	E931.6	E950.4	E962.0	E980.4
Pipadone	965.09	E850.2	E935.2	E950.0	E962.0	E980.0
Pipamazine	963.0	E858.1	E933.0	E950.4	E962.0	E980.4
Pipazethate	975.4	E858.6	E945.4	E950.4	E962.0	E980.4
Pipenzolate	971.1	E855.4	E941.1	E950.4	E962.0	E980.4
Piperacetazine	969.1	E853.0	E939.1	E950.3	E962.0	E980.3
Piperazine NEC	961.6	E857	E931.6	E950.4	E962.0	E980.4
estrone sulfate	962.2	E858.0	E932.2	E950.4	E962.0	E980.4
Piper cubeba	988.2	E865.4	—	E950.9	E962.1	E980.9
Piperidione	975.4	E858.6	E945.4	E950.4	E962.0	E980.4
Piperidolate	971.1	E855.4	E941.1	E950.4	E962.0	E980.4
Piperocaine	968.9	E855.2	E938.9	E950.4	E962.0	E980.4
infiltration (subcutaneous)	968.5	E855.2	E938.5	E950.4	E962.0	E980.4
Piperocaine — continued						
nerve block (peripheral) (plexus)	968.6	E855.2	E938.6	E950.4	E962.0	E980.4
topical (surface)	968.5	E855.2	E938.5	E950.4	E962.0	E980.4
Pipobroman	963.1	E858.1	E933.1	E950.4	E962.0	E980.4
Pipradrol	970.8	E854.3	E940.8	E950.4	E962.0	E980.4
Piscidia (bark) (erythrina)	965.7	E850.7	E935.7	E950.0	E962.0	E980.0
Pitch	983.0	E864.0	—	E950.7	E962.1	E980.6
Pitkin's solution	968.7	E855.2	E938.7	E950.4	E962.0	E980.4
Pitocin	975.0	E858.6	E945.0	E950.4	E962.0	E980.4
Pitressin (tannate)	962.5	E858.0	E932.5	E950.4	E962.0	E980.4
Pituitary extracts (posterior)	962.5	E858.0	E932.5	E950.4	E962.0	E980.4
anterior	962.4	E858.0	E932.4	E950.4	E962.0	E980.4
Pituitrin	962.5	E858.0	E932.5	E950.4	E962.0	E980.4
Placental extract	962.9	E858.0	E932.9	E950.4	E962.0	E980.4
Placidyl	967.8	E852.8	E937.8	E950.2	E962.0	E980.2
Plague vaccine	978.3	E858.8	E948.3	E950.4	E962.0	E980.4
Plant foods or fertilizers NEC	989.89	E866.5	—	E950.9	E962.1	E980.9
mixed with herbicides	989.4	E863.5	—	E950.6	E962.1	E980.7
Plants, noxious, used as food	988.2	E865.9	—	E950.9	E962.1	E980.9
berries and seeds	988.2	E865.3	—	E950.9	E962.1	E980.9
specified type NEC	988.2	E865.4	—	E950.9	E962.1	E980.9
Plasma (blood)	964.7	E858.2	E934.7	E950.4	E962.0	E980.4
expanders	964.8	E858.2	E934.8	E950.4	E962.0	E980.4
Plasmanate	964.7	E858.2	E934.7	E950.4	E962.0	E980.4
Plegicil	969.1	E853.0	E939.1	E950.3	E962.0	E980.3
Podophyllin	976.4	E858.7	E946.4	E950.4	E962.0	E980.4
Podophyllum resin	976.4	E858.7	E946.4	E950.4	E962.0	E980.4
Poison NEC	989.9	E866.9	—	E950.9	E962.1	E980.9
Poisonous berries	988.2	E865.3	—	E950.9	E962.1	E980.9
Pokeweed (any part)	988.2	E865.4	—	E950.9	E962.1	E980.9
Poldine	971.1	E855.4	E941.1	E950.4	E962.0	E980.4
Poliomyelitis vaccine	979.5	E858.8	E949.5	E950.4	E962.0	E980.4
Poliovirus vaccine	979.5	E858.8	E949.5	E950.4	E962.0	E980.4
Polish (car) (floor) (furniture) (metal) (silver)	989.89	E861.2	—	E950.9	E962.1	E980.9
abrasive	989.89	E861.3	—	E950.9	E962.1	E980.9
porcelain	989.89	E861.3	—	E950.9	E962.1	E980.9
Poloxalkol	973.2	E858.4	E943.2	E950.4	E962.0	E980.4
Polyaminostyrene resins	974.5	E858.5	E944.5	E950.4	E962.0	E980.4
Polychlorinated biphenyl — see PCBs						
Polycycline	960.4	E856	E930.4	E950.4	E962.0	E980.4
Polyester resin hardener	982.8	E862.4	—	E950.9	E962.1	E980.9
fumes	987.8	E869.8	—	E952.8	E962.2	E982.8
Polyestradiol (phosphate)	962.2	E858.0	E932.2	E950.4	E962.0	E980.4
Polyethanolamine alkyl sulfate	976.2	E858.7	E946.2	E950.4	E962.0	E980.4
Polyethylene glycol	976.3	E858.7	E946.3	E950.4	E962.0	E980.4
Polyferose	964.0	E858.2	E934.0	E950.4	E962.0	E980.4
Polymyxin B	960.8	E856	E930.8	E950.4	E962.0	E980.4
ENT agent	976.6	E858.7	E946.6	E950.4	E962.0	E980.4
ophthalmic preparation	976.5	E858.7	E946.5	E950.4	E962.0	E980.4
topical NEC	976.0	E858.7	E946.0	E950.4	E962.0	E980.4
Polynoxylin(e)	976.0	E858.7	E946.0	E950.4	E962.0	E980.4
Polyoxymethyleneurea	976.0	E858.7	E946.0	E950.4	E962.0	E980.4
Polytetrafluoroethylene (inhaled)	987.8	E869.8	—	E952.8	E962.2	E982.8
Polythiazide	974.3	E858.5	E944.3	E950.4	E962.0	E980.4
Polyvinylpyrrolidone	964.8	E858.2	E934.8	E950.4	E962.0	E980.4
Pontocaine (hydrochloride) (infiltration) (topical)	968.5	E855.2	E938.5	E950.4	E962.0	E980.4
nerve block (peripheral) (plexus)	968.6	E855.2	E938.6	E950.4	E962.0	E980.4
spinal	968.7	E855.2	E938.7	E950.4	E962.0	E980.4
Pot	969.6	E854.1	E939.6	E950.3	E962.0	E980.3
Potash (caustic)	983.2	E864.2	—	E950.7	E962.1	E980.6
Potassic saline injection (lactated)	974.5	E858.5	E944.5	E950.4	E962.0	E980.4
Potassium (salts) NEC	974.5	E858.5	E944.5	E950.4	E962.0	E980.4
aminosalicylate	961.8	E857	E931.8	E950.4	E962.0	E980.4
arsenite (solution)	985.1	E866.3	—	E950.8	E962.1	E980.8
bichromate	983.9	E864.3	—	E950.7	E962.1	E980.6
bisulfate	983.9	E864.3	—	E950.7	E962.1	E980.6
bromide (medicinal) NEC	967.3	E852.2	E937.3	E950.2	E962.0	E980.2
carbonate	983.2	E864.2	—	E950.7	E962.1	E980.6
chlorate NEC	983.9	E864.3	—	E950.7	E962.1	E980.6
cyanide — see Cyanide						

Table of Drugs and Chemicals

	Poisoning	Accident	Therapeutic Use	Suicide Attempt	Assault	Undetermined
Potassium (salts) — continued						
hydroxide	983.2	E864.2	—	E950.7	E962.1	E980.6
iodide (expectorant) NEC	975.5	E858.6	E945.5	E950.4	E962.0	E980.4
nitrate	989.89	E866.8	—	E950.9	E962.1	E980.9
oxalate	983.9	E864.3	—	E950.7	E962.1	E980.6
perchlorate NEC	977.8	E858.8	E947.8	E950.4	E962.0	E980.4
antithyroid	962.8	E858.0	E932.8	E950.4	E962.0	E980.4
permanganate	976.0	E858.7	E946.0	E950.4	E962.0	E980.4
nonmedicinal	983.9	E864.3	—	E950.7	E962.1	E980.6
Povidone-iodine (anti-infective) NEC	976.0	E858.7	E946.0	E950.4	E962.0	E980.4
Practolol	972.0	E858.3	E942.0	E950.4	E962.0	E980.4
Pralidoxime (chloride)	977.2	E858.8	E947.2	E950.4	E962.0	E980.4
Pramoxine	968.5	E855.2	E938.5	E950.4	E962.0	E980.4
Prazosin	972.6	E858.3	E942.6	E950.4	E962.0	E980.4
Prednisolone	962.0	E858.0	E932.0	E950.4	E962.0	E980.4
ENT agent	976.6	E858.7	E946.6	E950.4	E962.0	E980.4
ophthalmic preparation	976.5	E858.7	E946.5	E950.4	E962.0	E980.4
topical NEC	976.0	E858.7	E946.0	E950.4	E962.0	E980.4
Prednisone	962.0	E858.0	E932.0	E950.4	E962.0	E980.4
Pregnanediol	962.2	E858.0	E932.2	E950.4	E962.0	E980.4
Pregneninolone	962.2	E858.0	E932.2	E950.4	E962.0	E980.4
Preludin	977.0	E858.8	E947.0	E950.4	E962.0	E980.4
Premarin	962.2	E858.0	E932.2	E950.4	E962.0	E980.4
Prenylamine	972.4	E858.3	E942.4	E950.4	E962.0	E980.4
Preparation H	976.8	E858.7	E946.8	E950.4	E962.0	E980.4
Preservatives	989.89	E866.8	—	E950.9	E962.1	E980.9
Pride of China	988.2	E865.3	—	E950.9	E962.1	E980.9
Prilocaine	968.9	E855.2	E938.9	E950.4	E962.0	E980.4
infiltration (subcutaneous)	968.5	E855.2	E938.5	E950.4	E962.0	E980.4
nerve block (peripheral) (plexus)	968.6	E855.2	E938.6	E950.4	E962.0	E980.4
Primaquine	961.4	E857	E931.4	E950.4	E962.0	E980.4
Primidone	966.3	E855.0	E936.3	E950.4	E962.0	E980.4
Primula (veris)	988.2	E865.4	—	E950.9	E962.1	E980.9
Prinadol	965.09	E850.2	E935.2	E950.0	E962.0	E980.0
Priscol, Priscoline	971.3	E855.6	E941.3	E950.4	E962.0	E980.4
Privet	988.2	E865.4	—	E950.9	E962.1	E980.9
Privine	971.2	E855.5	E941.2	E950.4	E962.0	E980.4
Pro-Banthine	971.1	E855.4	E941.1	E950.4	E962.0	E980.4
Probarbital	967.0	E851	E937.0	E950.1	E962.0	E980.1
Probenecid	974.7	E858.5	E944.7	E950.4	E962.0	E980.4
Procainamide (hydrochloride)	972.0	E858.3	E942.0	E950.4	E962.0	E980.4
Procaine (hydrochloride) (infiltration) (topical)	968.5	E855.2	E938.5	E950.4	E962.0	E980.4
nerve block (peripheral) (plexus)	968.6	E855.2	E938.6	E950.4	E962.0	E980.4
penicillin G	960.0	E856	E930.0	E950.4	E962.0	E980.4
spinal	968.7	E855.2	E938.7	E950.4	E962.0	E980.4
Procalmidol	969.5	E853.8	E939.5	E950.3	E962.0	E980.3
Procarbazine	963.1	E858.1	E933.1	E950.4	E962.0	E980.4
Prochlorperazine	969.1	E853.0	E939.1	E950.3	E962.0	E980.3
Procyclidine	966.4	E855.0	E936.4	E950.4	E962.0	E980.4
Producer gas	986	E868.8	—	E952.1	E962.2	E982.1
Profenamine	966.4	E855.0	E936.4	E950.4	E962.0	E980.4
Profenil	975.1	E858.6	E945.1	E950.4	E962.0	E980.4
Progesterones	962.2	E858.0	E932.2	E950.4	E962.0	E980.4
Progestin	962.2	E858.0	E932.2	E950.4	E962.0	E980.4
Progestogens (with estrogens)	962.2	E858.0	E932.2	E950.4	E962.0	E980.4
Progestone	962.2	E858.0	E932.2	E950.4	E962.0	E980.4
Proguanil	961.4	E857	E931.4	E950.4	E962.0	E980.4
Prolactin	962.4	E858.0	E932.4	E950.4	E962.0	E980.4
Proloid	962.7	E858.0	E932.7	E950.4	E962.0	E980.4
Proluton	962.2	E858.0	E932.2	E950.4	E962.0	E980.4
Promacetin	961.8	E857	E931.8	E950.4	E962.0	E980.4
Promazine	969.1	E853.0	E939.1	E950.3	E962.0	E980.3
Promedol	965.09	E850.2	E935.2	E950.0	E962.0	E980.0
Promethazine	967.8	E852.8	E937.8	E950.2	E962.0	E980.2
Promin	961.8	E857	E931.8	E950.4	E962.0	E980.4
Pronestyl (hydrochloride)	972.0	E858.3	E942.0	E950.4	E962.0	E980.4
Pronetalol, pronethalol	972.0	E858.3	E942.0	E950.4	E962.0	E980.4
Prontosil	961.0	E857	E931.0	E950.4	E962.0	E980.4
Propamidine isethionate	961.5	E857	E931.5	E950.4	E962.0	E980.4
Propanal (medicinal)	967.8	E852.8	E937.8	E950.2	E962.0	E980.2
Propane (gas) (distributed in mobile container)	987.0	E868.0	—	E951.1	E962.2	E981.1
distributed through pipes	987.0	E867	—	E951.0	E962.2	E981.0
incomplete combustion of — see Carbon monoxide, Propane						
Propanidid	968.3	E855.1	E938.3	E950.4	E962.0	E980.4
Propanol	980.3	E860.4	—	E950.9	E962.1	E980.9
Propantheline	971.1	E855.4	E941.1	E950.4	E962.0	E980.4
Proparacaine	968.5	E855.2	E938.5	E950.4	E962.0	E980.4
Propatyl nitrate	972.4	E858.3	E942.4	E950.4	E962.0	E980.4
Propicillin	960.0	E856	E930.0	E950.4	E962.0	E980.4
Propiolactone (vapor)	987.8	E869.8	—	E952.8	E962.2	E982.8
Propiomazine	967.8	E852.8	E937.8	E950.2	E962.0	E980.2
Propionaldehyde (medicinal)	967.8	E852.8	E937.8	E950.2	E962.0	E980.2
Propionate compound	976.0	E858.7	E946.0	E950.4	E962.0	E980.4
Propion gel	976.0	E858.7	E946.0	E950.4	E962.0	E980.4
Propitocaine	968.9	E855.2	E938.9	E950.4	E962.0	E980.4
infiltration (subcutaneous)	968.5	E855.2	E938.5	E950.4	E962.0	E980.4
nerve block (peripheral) (plexus)	968.6	E855.2	E938.6	E950.4	E962.0	E980.4
Propoxur	989.3	E863.2	—	E950.6	E962.1	E980.7
Propoxycaine	968.9	E855.2	E938.9	E950.4	E962.0	E980.4
infiltration (subcutaneous)	968.5	E855.2	E938.5	E950.4	E962.0	E980.4
nerve block (peripheral) (plexus)	968.6	E855.2	E938.6	E950.4	E962.0	E980.4
topical (surface)	968.5	E855.2	E938.5	E950.4	E962.0	E980.4
Propoxyphene (hydrochloride)	965.8	E850.8	E935.8	E950.0	E962.0	E980.0
Propranolol	972.0	E858.3	E942.0	E950.4	E962.0	E980.4
Propyl						
alcohol	980.3	E860.4	—	E950.9	E962.1	E980.9
carbinol	980.3	E860.4	—	E950.9	E962.1	E980.9
hexadrine	971.2	E855.5	E941.2	E950.4	E962.0	E980.4
iodone	977.8	E858.8	E947.8	E950.4	E962.0	E980.4
thiouracil	962.8	E858.0	E932.8	E950.4	E962.0	E980.4
Propylene	987.1	E869.8	—	E952.8	E962.2	E982.8
Propylparaben (ophthalmic)	976.5	E858.7	E946.5	E950.4	E962.0	E980.4
Proscillaridin	972.1	E858.3	E942.1	E950.4	E962.0	E980.4
Prostaglandins	975.0	E858.6	E945.0	E950.4	E962.0	E980.4
Prostigmin	971.0	E855.3	E941.0	E950.4	E962.0	E980.4
Protamine (sulfate)	964.5	E858.2	E934.5	E950.4	E962.0	E980.4
zinc insulin	962.3	E858.0	E932.3	E950.4	E962.0	E980.4
Protectants (topical)	976.3	E858.7	E946.3	E950.4	E962.0	E980.4
Protein hydrolysate	974.5	E858.5	E944.5	E950.4	E962.0	E980.4
Prothiaden — see Dothiepin hydrochloride						
Prothionamide	961.8	E857	E931.8	E950.4	E962.0	E980.4
Prothipendyl	969.5	E853.8	E939.5	E950.3	E962.0	E980.3
Protokylol	971.2	E855.5	E941.2	E950.4	E962.0	E980.4
Protopam	977.2	E858.8	E947.2	E950.4	E962.0	E980.4
Protoveratrine(s) (A) (B)	972.6	E858.3	E942.6	E950.4	E962.0	E980.4
Protriptyline	969.0	E854.0	E939.0	E950.3	E962.0	E980.3
Provera	962.2	E858.0	E932.2	E950.4	E962.0	E980.4
Provitamin A	963.5	E858.1	E933.5	E950.4	E962.0	E980.4
Proxymetacaine	968.5	E855.2	E938.5	E950.4	E962.0	E980.4
Proxyphylline	975.1	E858.6	E945.1	E950.4	E962.0	E980.4
Prozac — see Fluoxetine hydrochloride						
Prunus						
laurocerasus	988.2	E865.4	—	E950.9	E962.1	E980.9
virginiana	988.2	E865.4	—	E950.9	E962.1	E980.9
Prussic acid	989.0	E866.8	—	E950.9	E962.1	E980.9
vapor	987.7	E869.8	—	E952.8	E962.2	E982.8
Pseudoephedrine	971.2	E855.5	E941.2	E950.4	E962.0	E980.4
Psilocin	969.6	E854.1	E939.6	E950.3	E962.0	E980.3
Psilocybin	969.6	E854.1	E939.6	E950.3	E962.0	E980.3
PSP	977.8	E858.8	E947.8	E950.4	E962.0	E980.4
Psychedelic agents	969.6	E854.1	E939.6	E950.3	E962.0	E980.3
Psychodysleptics	969.6	E854.1	E939.6	E950.3	E962.0	E980.3
Psychostimulants	969.7	E854.2	E939.7	E950.3	E962.0	E980.3
Psychotherapeutic agents	969.9	E855.9	E939.9	E950.3	E962.0	E980.3
antidepressants	969.0	E854.0	E939.0	E950.3	E962.0	E980.3
specified NEC	969.8	E855.8	E939.8	E950.3	E962.0	E980.3
tranquilizers NEC	969.5	E853.9	E939.5	E950.3	E962.0	E980.3
Psychotomimetic agents	969.6	E854.1	E939.6	E950.3	E962.0	E980.3
Psychotropic agents	969.9	E854.8	E939.9	E950.3	E962.0	E980.3
specified NEC	969.8	E854.8	E939.8	E950.3	E962.0	E980.3
Psyllium	973.3	E858.4	E943.3	E950.4	E962.0	E980.4
Pteroylglutamic acid	964.1	E858.2	E934.1	E950.4	E962.0	E980.4
Pteroyltriglutamate	963.1	E858.1	E933.1	E950.4	E962.0	E980.4
PTFE	987.8	E869.8	—	E952.8	E962.2	E982.8
Pulsatilla	988.2	E865.4	—	E950.9	E962.1	E980.9
Purex (bleach)	983.9	E864.3	—	E950.7	E962.1	E980.6
Purine diuretics	974.1	E858.5	E944.1	E950.4	E962.0	E980.4

Purinethol — Table of Drugs and Chemicals

	Poisoning	External Cause (E-Code)				
		Accident	Therapeutic Use	Suicide Attempt	Assault	Undetermined
Purinethol	963.1	E858.1	E933.1	E950.4	E962.0	E980.4
PVP	964.8	E858.2	E934.8	E950.4	E962.0	E980.4
Pyrabital	965.7	E850.7	E935.7	E950.0	E962.0	E980.0
Pyramidon	965.5	E850.5	E935.5	E950.0	E962.0	E980.0
Pyrantel (pamoate)	961.6	E857	E931.6	E950.4	E962.0	E980.4
Pyrathiazine	963.0	E858.1	E933.0	E950.4	E962.0	E980.4
Pyrazinamide	961.8	E857	E931.8	E950.4	E962.0	E980.4
Pyrazinoic acid (amide)	961.8	E857	E931.8	E950.4	E962.0	E980.4
Pyrazole (derivatives)	965.5	E850.5	E935.5	E950.0	E962.0	E980.0
Pyrazolone (analgesics)	965.5	E850.5	E935.5	E950.0	E962.0	E980.0
Pyrethrins, pyrethrum	989.4	E863.4	—	E950.6	E962.1	E980.7
Pyribenzamine	963.0	E858.1	E933.0	E950.4	E962.0	E980.4
Pyridine (liquid) (vapor)	982.0	E862.4	—	E950.9	E962.1	E980.9
aldoxime chloride	977.2	E858.8	E947.2	E950.4	E962.0	E980.4
Pyridium	976.1	E858.7	E946.1	E950.4	E962.0	E980.4
Pyridostigmine	971.0	E855.3	E941.0	E950.4	E962.0	E980.4
Pyridoxine	963.5	E858.1	E933.5	E950.4	E962.0	E980.4
Pyrilamine	963.0	E858.1	E933.0	E950.4	E962.0	E980.4
Pyrimethamine	961.4	E857	E931.4	E950.4	E962.0	E980.4
Pyrogallic acid	983.0	E864.0	—	E950.7	E962.1	E980.6
Pyroxylin	976.3	E858.7	E946.3	E950.4	E962.0	E980.4
Pyrrobutamine	963.0	E858.1	E933.0	E950.4	E962.0	E980.4
Pyrrocaine	968.5	E855.2	E938.5	E950.4	E962.0	E980.4
Pyrvinium (pamoate)	961.6	E857	E931.6	E950.4	E962.0	E980.4
PZI	962.3	E858.0	E932.3	E950.4	E962.0	E980.4
Quaalude	967.4	E852.3	E937.4	E950.2	E962.0	E980.2
Quaternary ammonium derivatives	971.1	E855.4	E941.1	E950.4	E962.0	E980.4
Quicklime	983.2	E864.2	—	E950.7	E962.1	E980.6
Quinacrine	961.3	E857	E931.3	E950.4	E962.0	E980.4
Quinaglute	972.0	E858.3	E942.0	E950.4	E962.0	E980.4
Quinalbarbitone	967.0	E851	E937.0	E950.1	E962.0	E980.1
Quinestradiol	962.2	E858.0	E932.2	E950.4	E962.0	E980.4
Quinethazone	974.3	E858.5	E944.3	E950.4	E962.0	E980.4
Quinidine (gluconate) (polygalacturonate) (salts) (sulfate)	972.0	E858.3	E942.0	E950.4	E962.0	E980.4
Quinine	961.4	E857	E931.4	E950.4	E962.0	E980.4
Quiniobine	961.3	E857	E931.3	E950.4	E962.0	E980.4
Quinolines	961.3	E857	E931.3	E950.4	E962.0	E980.4
Quotane	968.5	E855.2	E938.5	E950.4	E962.0	E980.4
Rabies						
immune globulin (human)	964.6	E858.2	E934.6	E950.4	E962.0	E980.4
vaccine	979.1	E858.8	E949.1	E950.4	E962.0	E980.4
Racemoramide	965.09	E850.2	E935.2	E950.0	E962.0	E980.0
Racemorphan	965.09	E850.2	E935.2	E950.0	E962.0	E980.0
Radiator alcohol	980.1	E860.2	—	E950.9	E962.1	E980.9
Radio-opaque (drugs) (materials)	977.8	E858.8	E947.8	E950.4	E962.0	E980.4
Ranunculus	988.2	E865.4	—	E950.9	E962.1	E980.9
Rat poison	989.4	E863.7	—	E950.6	E962.1	E980.7
Rattlesnake (venom)	989.5	E905.0	—	E950.9	E962.1	E980.9
Raudixin	972.6	E858.3	E942.6	E950.4	E962.0	E980.4
Rautensin	972.6	E858.3	E942.6	E950.4	E962.0	E980.4
Rautina	972.6	E858.3	E942.6	E950.4	E962.0	E980.4
Rautotal	972.6	E858.3	E942.6	E950.4	E962.0	E980.4
Rauwiloid	972.6	E858.3	E942.6	E950.4	E962.0	E980.4
Rauwoldin	972.6	E858.3	E942.6	E950.4	E962.0	E980.4
Rauwolfia (alkaloids)	972.6	E858.3	E942.6	E950.4	E962.0	E980.4
Realgar	985.1	E866.3	—	E950.8	E962.1	E980.8
Red cells, packed	964.7	E858.2	E934.7	E950.4	E962.0	E980.4
Reducing agents, industrial NEC	983.9	E864.3	—	E950.7	E962.1	E980.6
Refrigerant gas (freon)	987.4	E869.2	—	E952.8	E962.2	E982.8
central nervous system	968.0	E855.1	E938.0	E950.4	E962.0	E980.4
not freon	987.9	E869.9	—	E952.9	E962.2	E982.9
Regroton	974.4	E858.5	E944.4	E950.4	E962.0	E980.4
Rela	968.0	E855.1	E938.0	E950.4	E962.0	E980.4
Relaxants, skeletal muscle (autonomic)	975.2	E858.6	E945.2	E950.4	E962.0	E980.4
Renese	974.3	E858.5	E944.3	E950.4	E962.0	E980.4
Renografin	977.8	E858.8	E947.8	E950.4	E962.0	E980.4
Replacement solutions	974.5	E858.5	E944.5	E950.4	E962.0	E980.4
Rescinnamine	972.6	E858.3	E942.6	E950.4	E962.0	E980.4
Reserpine	972.6	E858.3	E942.6	E950.4	E962.0	E980.4
Resorcin, resorcinol	976.4	E858.7	E946.4	E950.4	E962.0	E980.4
Respaire	975.5	E858.6	E945.5	E950.4	E962.0	E980.4
Respiratory agents NEC	975.8	E858.6	E945.8	E950.4	E962.0	E980.4
Retinoic acid	976.8	E858.7	E946.8	E950.4	E962.0	E980.4
Retinol	963.5	E858.1	E933.5	E950.4	E962.0	E980.4
Rh (D) immune globulin (human)	964.6	E858.2	E934.6	E950.4	E962.0	E980.4
Rhodine	965.1	E850.3	E935.3	E950.0	E962.0	E980.0
RhoGAM	964.6	E858.2	E934.6	E950.4	E962.0	E980.4
Riboflavin	963.5	E858.1	E933.5	E950.4	E962.0	E980.4
Ricin	989.89	E866.8	—	E950.9	E962.1	E980.9
Ricinus communis	988.2	E865.3	—	E950.9	E962.1	E980.9
Rickettsial vaccine NEC	979.6	E858.8	E949.6	E950.4	E962.0	E980.4
with viral and bacterial vaccine	979.7	E858.8	E949.7	E950.4	E962.0	E980.4
Rifampin	960.6	E856	E930.6	E950.4	E962.0	E980.4
Rimifon	961.8	E857	E931.8	E950.4	E962.0	E980.4
Ringer's injection (lactated)	974.5	E858.5	E944.5	E950.4	E962.0	E980.4
Ristocetin	960.8	E856	E930.8	E950.4	E962.0	E980.4
Ritalin	969.7	E854.2	E939.7	E950.3	E962.0	E980.3
Roach killers — see Pesticides						
Rocky Mountain spotted fever vaccine	979.6	E858.8	E949.6	E950.4	E962.0	E980.4
Rodenticides	989.4	E863.7	—	E950.6	E962.1	E980.7
Rohypnol	969.4	E853.2	E939.4	E950.3	E962.0	E980.3
Rolaids	973.0	E858.4	E943.0	E950.4	E962.0	E980.4
Rolitetracycline	960.4	E856	E930.4	E950.4	E962.0	E980.4
Romilar	975.4	E858.6	E945.4	E950.4	E962.0	E980.4
Rose water ointment	976.3	E858.7	E946.3	E950.4	E962.0	E980.4
Rosuvastatin calcium	972.1	E858.3	E942.2	E950.4	E962.0	E980.4
Rotenone	989.4	E863.7	—	E950.6	E962.1	E980.7
Rotoxamine	963.0	E858.1	E933.0	E950.4	E962.0	E980.4
Rough-on-rats	989.4	E863.7	—	E950.6	E962.1	E980.7
RU486	962.9	E858.0	E932.9	E950.4	E962.0	E980.4
Rubbing alcohol	980.2	E860.3	—	E950.9	E962.1	E980.9
Rubella virus vaccine	979.4	E858.8	E949.4	E950.4	E962.0	E980.4
Rubelogen	979.4	E858.8	E949.4	E950.4	E962.0	E980.4
Rubeovax	979.4	E858.8	E949.4	E950.4	E962.0	E980.4
Rubidomycin	960.7	E856	E930.7	E950.4	E962.0	E980.4
Rue	988.2	E865.4	—	E950.9	E962.1	E980.9
Ruta	988.2	E865.4	—	E950.9	E962.1	E980.9
Sabadilla (medicinal)	976.0	E858.7	E946.0	E950.4	E962.0	E980.4
pesticide	989.4	E863.4	—	E950.6	E962.1	E980.7
Sabin oral vaccine	979.5	E858.8	E949.5	E950.4	E962.0	E980.4
Saccharated iron oxide	964.0	E858.2	E934.0	E950.4	E962.0	E980.4
Saccharin	974.5	E858.5	E944.5	E950.4	E962.0	E980.4
Safflower oil	972.2	E858.3	E942.2	E950.4	E962.0	E980.4
Salbutamol sulfate	975.7	E858.6	E945.7	E950.4	E962.0	E980.4
Salicylamide	965.1	E850.3	E935.3	E950.0	E962.0	E980.0
Salicylate(s)	965.1	E850.3	E935.3	E950.0	E962.0	E980.0
methyl	976.3	E858.7	E946.3	E950.4	E962.0	E980.4
theobromine calcium	974.1	E858.5	E944.1	E950.4	E962.0	E980.4
Salicylazosulfapyridine	961.0	E857	E931.0	E950.4	E962.0	E980.4
Salicylhydroxamic acid	976.0	E858.7	E946.0	E950.4	E962.0	E980.4
Salicylic acid (keratolytic) NEC	976.4	E858.7	E946.4	E950.4	E962.0	E980.4
congeners	965.1	E850.3	E935.3	E950.0	E962.0	E980.0
salts	965.1	E850.3	E935.3	E950.0	E962.0	E980.0
Saliniazid	961.8	E857	E931.8	E950.4	E962.0	E980.4
Salol	976.3	E858.7	E946.3	E950.4	E962.0	E980.4
Salt (substitute) NEC	974.5	E858.5	E944.5	E950.4	E962.0	E980.4
Saluretics	974.3	E858.5	E944.3	E950.4	E962.0	E980.4
Saluron	974.3	E858.5	E944.3	E950.4	E962.0	E980.4
Salvarsan 606 (neosilver) (silver)	961.1	E857	E931.1	E950.4	E962.0	E980.4
Sambucus canadensis	988.2	E865.4	—	E950.9	E962.1	E980.9
berry	988.2	E865.3	—	E950.9	E962.1	E980.9
Sandril	972.6	E858.3	E942.6	E950.4	E962.0	E980.4
Sanguinaria canadensis	988.2	E865.4	—	E950.9	E962.1	E980.9
Saniflush (cleaner)	983.9	E861.3	—	E950.7	E962.1	E980.6
Santonin	961.6	E857	E931.6	E950.4	E962.0	E980.4
Santyl	976.8	E858.7	E946.8	E950.4	E962.0	E980.4
Sarkomycin	960.7	E856	E930.7	E950.4	E962.0	E980.4
Saroten	969.0	E854.0	E939.0	E950.3	E962.0	E980.3
Saturnine — see Lead						
Savin (oil)	976.4	E858.7	E946.4	E950.4	E962.0	E980.4
Scammony	973.1	E858.4	E943.1	E950.4	E962.0	E980.4
Scarlet red	976.8	E858.7	E946.8	E950.4	E962.0	E980.4
Scheele's green	985.1	E866.3	—	E950.8	E962.1	E980.8
insecticide	985.1	E863.4	—	E950.8	E962.1	E980.8
Schradan	989.3	E863.1	—	E950.6	E962.1	E980.7
Schweinfurt(h) green	985.1	E866.3	—	E950.8	E962.1	E980.8
insecticide	985.1	E863.4	—	E950.8	E962.1	E980.8
Scilla — see Squill						
Sclerosing agents	972.7	E858.3	E942.7	E950.4	E962.0	E980.4

Table of Drugs and Chemicals

Solvents, industrial

	Poisoning	External Cause (E-Code)				
		Accident	Therapeutic Use	Suicide Attempt	Assault	Undetermined
Scopolamine	971.1	E855.4	E941.1	E950.4	E962.0	E980.4
Scouring powder	989.89	E861.3	—	E950.9	E962.1	E980.9
Sea						
anemone (sting)	989.5	E905.6	—	E950.9	E962.1	E980.9
cucumber (sting)	989.5	E905.6	—	E950.9	E962.1	E980.9
snake (bite) (venom)	989.5	E905.0	—	E950.9	E962.1	E980.9
urchin spine (puncture)	989.5	E905.6	—	E950.9	E962.1	E980.9
Secbutabarbital	967.0	E851	E937.0	E950.1	E962.0	E980.1
Secbutabarbitone	967.0	E851	E937.0	E950.1	E962.0	E980.1
Secobarbital	967.0	E851	E937.0	E950.1	E962.0	E980.1
Seconal	967.0	E851	E937.0	E950.1	E962.0	E980.1
Secretin	977.8	E858.8	E947.8	E950.4	E962.0	E980.4
Sedatives, nonbarbiturate	967.9	E852.9	E937.9	E950.2	E962.0	E980.2
specified NEC	967.8	E852.8	E937.8	E950.2	E962.0	E980.2
Sedormid	967.8	E852.8	E937.8	E950.2	E962.0	E980.2
Seed (plant)	988.2	E865.3	—	E950.9	E962.1	E980.9
disinfectant or dressing	989.89	E866.5	—	E950.9	E962.1	E980.9
Selenium (fumes) NEC	985.8	E866.4	—	E950.9	E962.1	E980.9
disulfide or sulfide	976.4	E858.7	E946.4	E950.4	E962.0	E980.4
Selsun	976.4	E858.7	E946.4	E950.4	E962.0	E980.4
Senna	973.1	E858.4	E943.1	E950.4	E962.0	E980.4
Septisol	976.2	E858.7	E946.2	E950.4	E962.0	E980.4
Serax	969.4	E853.2	E939.4	E950.3	E962.0	E980.3
Serenesil	967.8	E852.8	E937.8	E950.2	E962.0	E980.2
Serenium (hydrochloride)	961.9	E857	E931.9	E950.4	E962.0	E980.4
Serepax — see Oxazepam						
Sernyl	968.3	E855.1	E938.3	E950.4	E962.0	E980.4
Serotonin	977.8	E858.8	E947.8	E950.4	E962.0	E980.4
Serpasil	972.6	E858.3	E942.6	E950.4	E962.0	E980.4
Sewer gas	987.8	E869.8	—	E952.8	E962.2	E982.8
Shampoo	989.6	E861.0	—	E950.9	E962.1	E980.9
Shellfish, nonbacterial or noxious	988.0	E865.1	—	E950.9	E962.1	E980.9
Silicones NEC	989.83	E866.8	E947.8	E950.9	E962.1	E980.9
Silvadene	976.0	E858.7	E946.0	E950.4	E962.0	E980.4
Silver (compound) (medicinal) NEC	976.0	E858.7	E946.0	E950.4	E962.0	E980.4
anti-infectives	976.0	E858.7	E946.0	E950.4	E962.0	E980.4
arsphenamine	961.1	E857	E931.1	E950.4	E962.0	E980.4
nitrate	976.0	E858.7	E946.0	E950.4	E962.0	E980.4
ophthalmic preparation	976.5	E858.7	E946.5	E950.4	E962.0	E980.4
toughened (keratolytic)	976.4	E858.7	E946.4	E950.4	E962.0	E980.4
nonmedicinal (dust)	985.8	E866.4	—	E950.9	E962.1	E980.9
protein (mild) (strong)	976.0	E858.7	E946.0	E950.4	E962.0	E980.4
salvarsan	961.1	E857	E931.1	E950.4	E962.0	E980.4
Simethicone	973.8	E858.4	E943.8	E950.4	E962.0	E980.4
Sinequan	969.0	E854.0	E939.0	E950.3	E962.0	E980.3
Singoserp	972.6	E858.3	E942.6	E950.4	E962.0	E980.4
Sintrom	964.2	E858.2	E934.2	E950.4	E962.0	E980.4
Sitosterols	972.2	E858.3	E942.2	E950.4	E962.0	E980.4
Skeletal muscle relaxants	975.2	E858.6	E945.2	E950.4	E962.0	E980.4
Skin						
agents (external)	976.9	E858.7	E946.9	E950.4	E962.0	E980.4
specified NEC	976.8	E858.7	E946.8	E950.4	E962.0	E980.4
test antigen	977.8	E858.8	E947.8	E950.4	E962.0	E980.4
Sleep-eze	963.0	E858.1	E933.0	E950.4	E962.0	E980.4
Sleeping draught (drug) (pill) (tablet)	967.9	E852.9	E937.9	E950.2	E962.0	E980.2
Smallpox vaccine	979.0	E858.8	E949.0	E950.4	E962.0	E980.4
Smelter fumes NEC	985.9	E866.4	—	E950.9	E962.1	E980.9
Smog	987.3	E869.1	—	E952.8	E962.2	E982.8
Smoke NEC	987.9	E869.9	—	E952.9	E962.2	E982.9
Smooth muscle relaxant	975.1	E858.6	E945.1	E950.4	E962.0	E980.4
Snail killer	989.4	E863.4	—	E950.6	E962.1	E980.7
Snake (bite) (venom)	989.5	E905.0	—	E950.9	E962.1	E980.9
Snuff	989.89	E866.8	—	E950.9	E962.1	E980.9
Soap (powder) (product)	989.6	E861.1	—	E950.9	E962.1	E980.9
bicarb	963.3	E858.1	E933.3	E950.4	E962.0	E980.4
chlorinated — see Sodium, hypochlorite						
medicinal, soft	976.2	E858.7	E946.2	E950.4	E962.0	E980.4
Soda (caustic)	983.2	E864.2	—	E950.7	E962.1	E980.6
Sodium						
acetosulfone	961.8	E857	E931.8	E950.4	E962.0	E980.4
acetrizoate	977.8	E858.8	E947.8	E950.4	E962.0	E980.4
amytal	967.0	E851	E937.0	E950.1	E962.0	E980.1
arsenate — see Arsenic						
bicarbonate	963.3	E858.1	E933.3	E950.4	E962.0	E980.4
bichromate	983.9	E864.3	—	E950.7	E962.1	E980.6
biphosphate	963.2	E858.1	E933.2	E950.4	E962.0	E980.4
bisulfate	983.9	E864.3	—	E950.7	E962.1	E980.6

	Poisoning	External Cause (E-Code)				
		Accident	Therapeutic Use	Suicide Attempt	Assault	Undetermined
Sodium — continued						
borate (cleanser)	989.6	E861.3	—	E950.9	E962.1	E980.9
bromide NEC	967.3	E852.2	E937.3	E950.2	E962.0	E980.2
cacodylate (nonmedicinal) NEC	978.8	E858.8	E948.8	E950.4	E962.0	E980.4
anti-infective	961.1	E857	E931.1	E950.4	E962.0	E980.4
herbicide	989.4	E863.5	—	E950.6	E962.1	E980.7
calcium edetate	963.8	E858.1	E933.8	E950.4	E962.0	E980.4
carbonate NEC	983.2	E864.2	—	E950.7	E962.1	E980.6
chlorate NEC	983.9	E864.3	—	E950.7	E962.1	E980.6
herbicide	983.9	E863.5	—	E950.7	E962.1	E980.6
chloride NEC	974.5	E858.5	E944.5	E950.4	E962.0	E980.4
chromate	983.9	E864.3	—	E950.7	E962.1	E980.6
citrate	963.3	E858.1	E933.3	E950.4	E962.0	E980.4
cyanide — see Cyanide(s)						
cyclamate	974.5	E858.5	E944.5	E950.4	E962.0	E980.4
diatrizoate	977.8	E858.8	E947.8	E950.4	E962.0	E980.4
dibunate	975.4	E858.6	E945.4	E950.4	E962.0	E980.4
dioctyl sulfosuccinate	973.2	E858.4	E943.2	E950.4	E962.0	E980.4
edetate	963.8	E858.1	E933.8	E950.4	E962.0	E980.4
ethacrynate	974.4	E858.5	E944.4	E950.4	E962.0	E980.4
fluoracetate (dust) (rodenticide)	989.4	E863.7	—	E950.6	E962.1	E980.7
fluoride — see Fluoride(s)						
free salt	974.5	E858.5	E944.5	E950.4	E962.0	E980.4
glucosulfone	961.8	E857	E931.8	E950.4	E962.0	E980.4
hydroxide	983.2	E864.2	—	E950.7	E962.1	E980.6
hypochlorite (bleach) NEC	983.9	E864.3	—	E950.7	E962.1	E980.6
disinfectant	983.9	E861.4	—	E950.7	E962.1	E980.6
medicinal (anti-infective) (external)	976.0	E858.7	E946.0	E950.4	E962.0	E980.4
vapor	987.8	E869.8	—	E952.8	E962.2	E982.8
hyposulfite	976.0	E858.7	E946.0	E950.4	E962.0	E980.4
indigotindisulfonate	977.8	E858.8	E947.8	E950.4	E962.0	E980.4
iodide	977.8	E858.8	E947.8	E950.4	E962.0	E980.4
iothalamate	977.8	E858.8	E947.8	E950.4	E962.0	E980.4
iron edetate	964.0	E858.2	E934.0	E950.4	E962.0	E980.4
lactate	963.3	E858.1	E933.3	E950.4	E962.0	E980.4
lauryl sulfate	976.2	E858.7	E946.2	E950.4	E962.0	E980.4
L-triiodothyronine	962.7	E858.0	E932.7	E950.4	E962.0	E980.4
metrizoate	977.8	E858.8	E947.8	E950.4	E962.0	E980.4
monofluoracetate (dust) (rodenticide)	989.4	E863.7	—	E950.6	E962.1	E980.7
morrhuate	972.7	E858.3	E942.7	E950.4	E962.0	E980.4
nafcillin	960.0	E856	E930.0	E950.4	E962.0	E980.4
nitrate (oxidizing agent)	983.9	E864.3	—	E950.7	E962.1	E980.6
nitrite (medicinal)	972.4	E858.3	E942.4	E950.4	E962.0	E980.4
nitroferricyanide	972.6	E858.3	E942.6	E950.4	E962.0	E980.4
nitroprusside	972.6	E858.3	E942.6	E950.4	E962.0	E980.4
para-aminohippurate	977.8	E858.8	E947.8	E950.4	E962.0	E980.4
perborate (nonmedicinal) NEC	989.89	E866.8	—	E950.9	E962.1	E980.9
medicinal	976.0	E858.7	E946.6	E950.4	E962.0	E980.4
soap	989.6	E861.1	—	E950.9	E962.1	E980.9
percarbonate — see Sodium, perborate						
phosphate	973.3	E858.4	E943.3	E950.4	E962.0	E980.4
polystyrene sulfonate	974.5	E858.5	E944.5	E950.4	E962.0	E980.4
propionate	976.0	E858.7	E946.0	E950.4	E962.0	E980.4
psylliate	972.7	E858.3	E942.7	E950.4	E962.0	E980.4
removing resins	974.5	E858.5	E944.5	E950.4	E962.0	E980.4
salicylate	965.1	E850.3	E935.3	E950.0	E962.0	E980.0
sulfate	973.3	E858.4	E943.3	E950.4	E962.0	E980.4
sulfoxone	961.8	E857	E931.8	E950.4	E962.0	E980.4
tetradecyl sulfate	972.7	E858.3	E942.7	E950.4	E962.0	E980.4
thiopental	968.3	E855.1	E938.3	E950.4	E962.0	E980.4
thiosalicylate	965.1	E850.3	E935.3	E950.0	E962.0	E980.0
thiosulfate	976.0	E858.7	E946.0	E950.4	E962.0	E980.4
tolbutamide	977.8	E858.8	E947.8	E950.4	E962.0	E980.4
tyropanoate	977.8	E858.8	E947.8	E950.4	E962.0	E980.4
valproate	966.3	E855.0	E936.3	E950.4	E962.0	E980.4
Solanine	977.8	E858.8	E947.8	E950.4	E962.0	E980.4
Solanum dulcamara	988.2	E865.4	—	E950.9	E962.1	E980.9
Solapsone	961.8	E857	E931.8	E950.4	E962.0	E980.4
Solasulfone	961.8	E857	E931.8	E950.4	E962.0	E980.4
Soldering fluid	983.1	E864.1	—	E950.7	E962.1	E980.6
Solid substance	989.9	E866.9	—	E950.9	E962.1	E980.9
specified NEC	989.9	E866.8	—	E950.9	E962.1	E980.9
Solvents, industrial	982.8	E862.9	—	E950.9	E962.1	E980.9
naphtha	981	E862.0	—	E950.9	E962.1	E980.9
petroleum	981	E862.0	—	E950.9	E962.1	E980.9
specified NEC	982.8	E862.4	—	E950.9	E962.1	E980.9

Soma — Table of Drugs and Chemicals

		External Cause (E-Code)				
	Poisoning	Accident	Therapeutic Use	Suicide Attempt	Assault	Undetermined
Soma	968.0	E855.1	E938.0	E950.4	E962.0	E980.4
Somatotropin	962.4	E858.0	E932.4	E950.4	E962.0	E980.4
Sominex	963.0	E858.1	E933.0	E950.4	E962.0	E980.4
Somnos	967.1	E852.0	E937.1	E950.2	E962.0	E980.2
Somonal	967.0	E851	E937.0	E950.1	E962.0	E980.1
Soneryl	967.0	E851	E937.0	E950.1	E962.0	E980.1
Soothing syrup	977.9	E858.9	E947.9	E950.5	E962.0	E980.5
Sopor	967.4	E852.3	E937.4	E950.2	E962.0	E980.2
Soporific drug	967.9	E852.9	E937.9	E950.2	E962.0	E980.2
specified type NEC	967.8	E852.8	E937.8	E950.2	E962.0	E980.2
Sorbitol NEC	977.4	E858.8	E947.4	E950.4	E962.0	E980.4
Sotradecol	972.7	E858.3	E942.7	E950.4	E962.0	E980.4
Spacoline	975.1	E858.6	E945.1	E950.4	E962.0	E980.4
Spanish fly	976.8	E858.7	E946.8	E950.4	E962.0	E980.4
Sparine	969.1	E853.0	E939.1	E950.3	E962.0	E980.3
Sparteine	975.0	E858.6	E945.0	E950.4	E962.0	E980.4
Spasmolytics	975.1	E858.6	E945.1	E950.4	E962.0	E980.4
anticholinergics	971.1	E855.4	E941.1	E950.4	E962.0	E980.4
Spectinomycin	960.8	E856	E930.8	E950.4	E962.0	E980.4
Speed	969.7	E854.2	E939.7	E950.3	E962.0	E980.3
Spermicides	976.8	E858.7	E946.8	E950.4	E962.0	E980.4
Spider (bite) (venom)	989.5	E905.1	—	E950.9	E962.1	E980.9
antivenin	979.9	E858.8	E949.9	E950.4	E962.0	E980.4
Spigelia (root)	961.6	E857	E931.6	E950.4	E962.0	E980.4
Spiperone	969.2	E853.1	E939.2	E950.3	E962.0	E980.3
Spiramycin	960.3	E856	E930.3	E950.4	E962.0	E980.4
Spirilene	969.5	E853.8	E939.5	E950.3	E962.0	E980.3
Spirit(s) (neutral) NEC	980.0	E860.1	—	E950.9	E962.1	E980.9
beverage	980.0	E860.0	—	E950.9	E962.1	E980.9
industrial	980.9	E860.9	—	E950.9	E962.1	E980.9
mineral	981	E862.0	—	E950.9	E962.1	E980.9
of salt — see Hydrochloric acid						
surgical	980.9	E860.9	—	E950.9	E962.1	E980.9
Spironolactone	974.4	E858.5	E944.4	E950.4	E962.0	E980.4
Sponge, absorbable (gelatin)	964.5	E858.2	E934.5	E950.4	E962.0	E980.4
Sporostacin	976.0	E858.7	E946.0	E950.4	E962.0	E980.4
Sprays (aerosol)	989.89	E866.8	—	E950.9	E962.1	E980.9
cosmetic	989.89	E866.7	—	E950.9	E962.1	E980.9
medicinal NEC	977.9	E858.9	E947.9	E950.5	E962.0	E980.5
pesticides — see Pesticides						
specified content — see substance specified						
Spurge flax	988.2	E865.4	—	E950.9	E962.1	E980.9
Spurges	988.2	E865.4	—	E950.9	E962.1	E980.9
Squill (expectorant) NEC	975.5	E858.6	E945.5	E950.4	E962.0	E980.4
rat poison	989.4	E863.7	—	E950.6	E962.1	E980.7
Squirting cucumber (cathartic)	973.1	E858.4	E943.1	E950.4	E962.0	E980.4
Stains	989.89	E866.8	—	E950.9	E962.1	E980.9
Stannous — see also Tin						
fluoride	976.7	E858.7	E946.7	E950.4	E962.0	E980.4
Stanolone	962.1	E858.0	E932.1	E950.4	E962.0	E980.4
Stanozolol	962.1	E858.0	E932.1	E950.4	E962.0	E980.4
Staphisagria or stavesacre (pediculicide)	976.0	E858.7	E946.0	E950.4	E962.0	E980.4
Stelazine	969.1	E853.0	E939.1	E950.3	E962.0	E980.3
Stemetil	969.1	E853.0	E939.1	E950.3	E962.0	E980.3
Sterculia (cathartic) (gum)	973.3	E858.4	E943.3	E950.4	E962.0	E980.4
Sternutator gas	987.8	E869.8	—	E952.8	E962.2	E982.8
Steroids NEC	962.0	E858.0	E932.0	E950.4	E962.0	E980.4
ENT agent	976.6	E858.7	E946.6	E950.4	E962.0	E980.4
ophthalmic preparation	976.5	E858.7	E946.5	E950.4	E962.0	E980.4
topical NEC	976.0	E858.7	E946.0	E950.4	E962.0	E980.4
Stibine	985.8	E866.4	—	E950.9	E962.1	E980.9
Stibophen	961.2	E857	E931.2	E950.4	E962.0	E980.4
Stilbamide, stilbamidine	961.5	E857	E931.5	E950.4	E962.0	E980.4
Stilbestrol	962.2	E858.0	E932.2	E950.4	E962.0	E980.4
Stimulants (central nervous system)	970.9	E854.3	E940.9	E950.4	E962.0	E980.4
analeptics	970.0	E854.3	E940.0	E950.4	E962.0	E980.4
opiate antagonist	970.1	E854.3	E940.1	E950.4	E962.0	E980.4
psychotherapeutic NEC	969.0	E854.0	E939.0	E950.3	E962.0	E980.3
specified NEC	970.8	E854.3	E940.8	E950.4	E962.0	E980.4
Storage batteries (acid) (cells)	983.1	E864.1	—	E950.7	E962.1	E980.6
Stovaine	968.9	E855.2	E938.9	E950.4	E962.0	E980.4
infiltration (subcutaneous)	968.5	E855.2	E938.5	E950.4	E962.0	E980.4
nerve block (peripheral) (plexus)	968.6	E855.2	E938.6	E950.4	E962.0	E980.4
spinal	968.7	E855.2	E938.7	E950.4	E962.0	E980.4
Stovaine — continued						
topical (surface)	968.5	E855.2	E938.5	E950.4	E962.0	E980.4
Stovarsal	961.1	E857	E931.1	E950.4	E962.0	E980.4
Stove gas — see Gas, utility						
Stoxil	976.5	E858.7	E946.5	E950.4	E962.0	E980.4
STP	969.6	E854.1	E939.6	E950.3	E962.0	E980.3
Stramonium (medicinal) NEC	971.1	E855.4	E941.1	E950.4	E962.0	E980.4
natural state	988.2	E865.4	—	E950.9	E962.1	E980.9
Streptodornase	964.4	E858.2	E934.4	E950.4	E962.0	E980.4
Streptoduocin	960.6	E856	E930.6	E950.4	E962.0	E980.4
Streptokinase	964.4	E858.2	E934.4	E950.4	E962.0	E980.4
Streptomycin	960.6	E856	E930.6	E950.4	E962.0	E980.4
Streptozocin	960.7	E856	E930.7	E950.4	E962.0	E980.4
Stripper (paint) (solvent)	982.8	E862.9	—	E950.9	E962.1	E980.9
Strobane	989.2	E863.0	—	E950.6	E962.1	E980.7
Strophanthin	972.1	E858.3	E942.1	E950.4	E962.0	E980.4
Strophanthus hispidus or kombe	988.2	E865.4	—	E950.9	E962.1	E980.9
Strychnine (rodenticide) (salts)	989.1	E863.7	—	E950.6	E962.1	E980.7
medicinal NEC	970.8	E854.3	E940.8	E950.4	E962.0	E980.4
Strychnos (ignatii) — see Strychnine						
Styramate	968.0	E855.1	E938.0	E950.4	E962.0	E980.4
Styrene	983.0	E864.0	—	E950.7	E962.1	E980.6
Succinimide (anticonvulsant)	966.2	E855.0	E936.2	E950.4	E962.0	E980.4
mercuric — see Mercury						
Succinylcholine	975.2	E858.6	E945.2	E950.4	E962.0	E980.4
Succinylsulfathiazole	961.0	E857	E931.0	E950.4	E962.0	E980.4
Sucrose	974.5	E858.5	E944.5	E950.4	E962.0	E980.4
Sulfacetamide	961.0	E857	E931.0	E950.4	E962.0	E980.4
ophthalmic preparation	976.5	E858.7	E946.5	E950.4	E962.0	E980.4
Sulfachlorpyridazine	961.0	E857	E931.0	E950.4	E962.0	E980.4
Sulfacytine	961.0	E857	E931.0	E950.4	E962.0	E980.4
Sulfadiazine	961.0	E857	E931.0	E950.4	E962.0	E980.4
silver (topical)	976.0	E858.7	E946.0	E950.4	E962.0	E980.4
Sulfadimethoxine	961.0	E857	E931.0	E950.4	E962.0	E980.4
Sulfadimidine	961.0	E857	E931.0	E950.4	E962.0	E980.4
Sulfaethidole	961.0	E857	E931.0	E950.4	E962.0	E980.4
Sulfafurazole	961.0	E857	E931.0	E950.4	E962.0	E980.4
Sulfaguanidine	961.0	E857	E931.0	E950.4	E962.0	E980.4
Sulfamerazine	961.0	E857	E931.0	E950.4	E962.0	E980.4
Sulfameter	961.0	E857	E931.0	E950.4	E962.0	E980.4
Sulfamethizole	961.0	E857	E931.0	E950.4	E962.0	E980.4
Sulfamethoxazole	961.0	E857	E931.0	E950.4	E962.0	E980.4
Sulfamethoxydiazine	961.0	E857	E931.0	E950.4	E962.0	E980.4
Sulfamethoxypyridazine	961.0	E857	E931.0	E950.4	E962.0	E980.4
Sulfamethylthiazole	961.0	E857	E931.0	E950.4	E962.0	E980.4
Sulfamylon	976.0	E858.7	E946.0	E950.4	E962.0	E980.4
Sulfan blue (diagnostic dye)	977.8	E858.8	E947.8	E950.4	E962.0	E980.4
Sulfanilamide	961.0	E857	E931.0	E950.4	E962.0	E980.4
Sulfanilylguanidine	961.0	E857	E931.0	E950.4	E962.0	E980.4
Sulfaphenazole	961.0	E857	E931.0	E950.4	E962.0	E980.4
Sulfaphenylthiazole	961.0	E857	E931.0	E950.4	E962.0	E980.4
Sulfaproxyline	961.0	E857	E931.0	E950.4	E962.0	E980.4
Sulfapyridine	961.0	E857	E931.0	E950.4	E962.0	E980.4
Sulfapyrimidine	961.0	E857	E931.0	E950.4	E962.0	E980.4
Sulfarsphenamine	961.1	E857	E931.1	E950.4	E962.0	E980.4
Sulfasalazine	961.0	E857	E931.0	E950.4	E962.0	E980.4
Sulfasomizole	961.0	E857	E931.0	E950.4	E962.0	E980.4
Sulfasuxidine	961.0	E857	E931.0	E950.4	E962.0	E980.4
Sulfinpyrazone	974.7	E858.5	E944.7	E950.4	E962.0	E980.4
Sulfisoxazole	961.0	E857	E931.0	E950.4	E962.0	E980.4
ophthalmic preparation	976.5	E858.7	E946.5	E950.4	E962.0	E980.4
Sulfomyxin	960.8	E856	E930.8	E950.4	E962.0	E980.4
Sulfonal	967.8	E852.8	E937.8	E950.2	E962.0	E980.2
Sulfonamides (mixtures)	961.0	E857	E931.0	E950.4	E962.0	E980.4
Sulfones	961.8	E857	E931.8	E950.4	E962.0	E980.4
Sulfonethylmethane	967.8	E852.8	E937.8	E950.2	E962.0	E980.2
Sulfonmethane	967.8	E852.8	E937.8	E950.2	E962.0	E980.2
Sulfonphthal, sulfonphthol	977.8	E858.8	E947.8	E950.4	E962.0	E980.4
Sulfonylurea derivatives, oral	962.3	E858.0	E932.3	E950.4	E962.0	E980.4
Sulfoxone	961.8	E857	E931.8	E950.4	E962.0	E980.4
Sulfur, sulfureted, sulfuric, sulfurous, sulfuryl (compounds) NEC	989.89	E866.8	—	E950.9	E962.1	E980.9
acid	983.1	E864.1	—	E950.7	E962.1	E980.6
dioxide	987.3	E869.1	—	E952.8	E962.2	E982.8

Table of Drugs and Chemicals

		External Cause (E-Code)							External Cause (E-Code)			
	Poisoning	Accident	Therapeutic Use	Suicide Attempt	Assault	Undetermined		Poisoning	Accident	Therapeutic Use	Suicide Attempt	Assault	Undetermined
Sulfur, sulfureted, sulfuric, sulfurous, sulfuryl (compounds) — continued							Tetanus — continued toxoid — continued with diphtheria toxoid — continued						
ether — see Ether(s)							with pertussis	978.6	E858.8	E948.6	E950.4	E962.0	E980.4
hydrogen	987.8	E869.8	—	E952.8	E962.2	E982.8	Tetrabenazine	969.5	E853.8	E939.5	E950.3	E962.0	E980.3
medicinal (keratolytic) (ointment) NEC	976.4	E858.7	E946.4	E950.4	E962.0	E980.4	Tetracaine (infiltration) (topical)	968.5	E855.2	E938.5	E950.4	E962.0	E980.4
pesticide (vapor)	989.4	E863.4	—	E950.6	E962.1	E980.7	nerve block (peripheral)						
vapor NEC	987.8	E869.8	—	E952.8	E962.2	E982.8	(plexus)	968.6	E855.2	E938.6	E950.4	E962.0	E980.4
Sulkowitch's reagent	977.8	E858.8	E947.8	E950.4	E962.0	E980.4	spinal	968.7	E855.2	E938.7	E950.4	E962.0	E980.4
Sulphadione	961.8	E857	E931.8	E950.4	E962.0	E980.4	Tetrachlorethylene — see Tetrachloroethylene						
Sulph — see also Sulf-													
Sulthiame, sultiame	966.3	E855.0	E936.3	E950.4	E962.0	E980.4	Tetrachlormethiazide	974.3	E858.5	E944.3	E950.4	E962.0	E980.4
Superinone	975.5	E858.6	E945.5	E950.4	E962.0	E980.4	Tetrachloroethane (liquid)						
Suramin	961.5	E857	E931.5	E950.4	E962.0	E980.4	(vapor)	982.3	E862.4	—	E950.9	E962.1	E980.9
Surfacaine	968.5	E855.2	E938.5	E950.4	E962.0	E980.4	paint or varnish	982.3	E861.6	—	E950.9	E962.1	E980.9
Surital	968.3	E855.1	E938.3	E950.4	E962.0	E980.4	Tetrachloroethylene (liquid)						
Sutilains	976.8	E858.7	E946.8	E950.4	E962.0	E980.4	(vapor)	982.3	E862.4	—	E950.9	E962.1	E980.9
Suxamethonium (bromide)							medicinal	961.6	E857	E931.6	E950.4	E962.0	E980.4
(chloride) (iodide)	975.2	E858.6	E945.2	E950.4	E962.0	E980.4	Tetrachloromethane — see Carbon, tetrachloride						
Suxethonium (bromide)	975.2	E858.6	E945.2	E950.4	E962.0	E980.4							
Sweet oil (birch)	976.3	E858.7	E946.3	E950.4	E962.0	E980.4	Tetracycline	960.4	E856	E930.4	E950.4	E962.0	E980.4
Sym-dichloroethyl ether	982.3	E862.4	—	E950.9	E962.1	E980.9	ophthalmic preparation	976.5	E858.7	E946.5	E950.4	E962.0	E980.4
Sympatholytics	971.3	E855.6	E941.3	E950.4	E962.0	E980.4	topical NEC	976.0	E858.7	E946.0	E950.4	E962.0	E980.4
Sympathomimetics	971.2	E855.5	E941.2	E950.4	E962.0	E980.4	Tetraethylammonium						
Synagis	979.6	E858.8	E949.6	E950.4	E962.0	E980.4	chloride	972.3	E858.3	E942.3	E950.4	E962.0	E980.4
Synalar	976.0	E858.7	E946.0	E950.4	E962.0	E980.4	Tetraethyl lead (antiknock						
Synthroid	962.7	E858.0	E932.7	E950.4	E962.0	E980.4	compound)	984.1	E862.1	—	E950.9	E962.1	E980.9
Syntocinon	975.0	E858.6	E945.0	E950.4	E962.0	E950.4	Tetraethyl pyrophosphate	989.3	E863.1	—	E950.6	E962.1	E980.7
Syrosingopine	972.6	E858.3	E942.6	E950.4	E962.0	E980.4	Tetraethylthiuram						
Systemic agents (primarily)	963.9	E858.1	E933.9	E950.4	E962.0	E980.4	disulfide	977.3	E858.8	E947.3	E950.4	E962.0	E980.4
specified NEC	963.8	E858.1	E933.8	E950.4	E962.0	E980.4	Tetrahydroaminoacridine	971.0	E855.3	E941.0	E950.4	E962.0	E980.4
Tablets — see also specified							Tetrahydrocannabinol	969.6	E854.1	E939.6	E950.3	E962.0	E980.3
substance	977.9	E858.9	E947.9	E950.5	E962.0	E980.5	Tetrahydronaphthalene	982.0	E862.4	—	E950.9	E962.1	E980.9
Tace	962.2	E858.0	E932.2	E950.4	E962.0	E980.4	Tetrahydrozoline	971.2	E855.5	E941.2	E950.4	E962.0	E980.4
Tacrine	971.0	E855.3	E941.0	E950.4	E962.0	E980.4	Tetralin	982.0	E862.4	—	E950.9	E962.1	E980.9
Talbutal	967.0	E851	E937.0	E950.1	E962.0	E980.1	Tetramethylthiuram (disulfide)						
Talc	976.3	E858.7	E946.3	E950.4	E962.0	E980.4	NEC	989.4	E863.6	—	E950.6	E962.1	E980.7
Talcum	976.3	E858.7	E946.3	E950.4	E962.0	E980.4	medicinal	976.2	E858.7	E946.2	E950.4	E962.0	E980.4
Tandearil, tanderil	965.5	E850.5	E935.5	E950.0	E962.0	E980.0	Tetronal	967.8	E852.8	E937.8	E950.2	E962.0	E980.2
Tannic acid	983.1	E864.1	—	E950.7	E962.1	E980.6	Tetryl	983.0	E864.0	—	E950.7	E962.1	E980.6
medicinal (astringent)	976.2	E858.7	E946.2	E950.4	E962.0	E980.4	Thalidomide	967.8	E852.8	E937.8	E950.2	E962.0	E980.2
Tannin — see Tannic acid							Thallium (compounds) (dust)						
Tansy	988.2	E865.4	—	E950.9	E962.1	E980.9	NEC	985.8	E866.4	—	E950.9	E962.1	E980.9
TAO	960.3	E856	E930.3	E950.4	E962.0	E980.4	pesticide (rodenticide)	985.8	E863.7	—	E950.6	E962.1	E980.7
Tapazole	962.8	E858.0	E932.8	E950.4	E962.0	E980.4	THC	969.6	E854.1	E939.6	E950.3	E962.0	E980.3
Tar NEC	983.0	E864.0	—	E950.7	E962.1	E980.6	Thebacon	965.09	E850.2	E935.2	E950.0	E962.0	E980.0
camphor — see Naphthalene							Thebaine	965.09	E850.2	E935.2	E950.0	E962.0	E980.0
fumes	987.8	E869.8	—	E952.8	E962.2	E982.8	Theobromine (calcium						
Taractan	969.3	E853.8	E939.3	E950.3	E962.0	E980.3	salicylate)	974.1	E858.5	E944.1	E950.4	E962.0	E980.4
Tarantula (venomous)	989.5	E905.1	—	E950.9	E962.1	E980.9	Theophylline (diuretic)	974.1	E858.5	E944.1	E950.4	E962.0	E980.4
Tartar emetic							ethylenediamine	975.7	E858.6	E945.7	E950.4	E962.0	E980.4
(anti-infective)	961.2	E857	E931.2	E950.4	E962.0	E980.4	Thiabendazole	961.6	E857	E931.6	E950.4	E962.0	E980.4
Tartaric acid	983.1	E864.1	—	E950.7	E962.1	E980.6	Thialbarbital,						
Tartrated antimony							thialbarbitone	968.3	E855.1	E938.3	E950.4	E962.0	E980.4
(anti-infective)	961.2	E857	E931.2	E950.4	E962.0	E980.4	Thiamine	963.5	E858.1	E933.5	E950.4	E962.0	E980.4
TCA — see Trichloroacetic acid							Thiamylal (sodium)	968.3	E855.1	E938.3	E950.4	E962.0	E980.4
TDI	983.0	E864.0	—	E950.7	E962.1	E980.6	Thiazesim	969.0	E854.0	E939.0	E950.3	E962.0	E980.3
vapor	987.8	E869.8	—	E952.8	E962.2	E982.8	Thiazides (diuretics)	974.3	E858.5	E944.3	E950.4	E962.0	E980.4
Tear gas	987.5	E869.3	—	E952.8	E962.2	E982.8	Thiethylperazine	963.0	E858.1	E933.0	E950.4	E962.0	E980.4
Teclothiazide	974.3	E858.5	E944.3	E950.4	E962.0	E980.4	Thimerosal (topical)	976.0	E858.7	E946.0	E950.4	E962.0	E980.4
Tegretol	966.3	E855.0	E936.3	E950.4	E962.0	E980.4	ophthalmic preparation	976.5	E858.7	E946.5	E950.4	E962.0	E980.4
Telepaque	977.8	E858.8	E947.8	E950.4	E962.0	E980.4	Thioacetazone	961.8	E857	E931.8	E950.4	E962.0	E980.4
Tellurium	985.8	E866.4	—	E950.9	E962.1	E980.9	Thiobarbiturates	968.3	E855.1	E938.3	E950.4	E962.0	E980.4
fumes	985.8	E866.4	—	E950.9	E962.1	E980.9	Thiobismol	961.2	E857	E931.2	E950.4	E962.0	E980.4
TEM	963.1	E858.1	E933.1	E950.4	E962.0	E980.4	Thiocarbamide	962.8	E858.0	E932.8	E950.4	E962.0	E980.4
Temazepan — see Benzodiazepines							Thiocarbarsone	961.1	E857	E931.1	E950.4	E962.0	E980.4
							Thiocarlide	961.8	E857	E931.8	E950.4	E962.0	E980.4
TEPA	963.1	E858.1	E933.1	E950.4	E962.0	E980.4	Thioguanine	963.1	E858.1	E933.1	E950.4	E962.0	E980.4
TEPP	989.3	E863.1	—	E950.6	E962.1	E980.7	Thiomercaptomerin	974.0	E858.5	E944.0	E950.4	E962.0	E980.4
Terbutaline	971.2	E855.5	E941.2	E950.4	E962.0	E980.4	Thiomerin	974.0	E858.5	E944.0	E950.4	E962.0	E980.4
Teroxalene	961.6	E857	E931.6	E950.4	E962.0	E980.4	Thiopental, thiopentone						
Terpin hydrate	975.5	E858.6	E945.5	E950.4	E962.0	E980.4	(sodium)	968.3	E855.1	E938.3	E950.4	E962.0	E980.4
Terramycin	960.4	E856	E930.4	E950.4	E962.0	E980.4	Thiopropazate	969.1	E853.0	E939.1	E950.3	E962.0	E980.3
Tessalon	975.4	E858.6	E945.4	E950.4	E962.0	E980.4	Thioproperazine	969.1	E853.0	E939.1	E950.3	E962.0	E980.3
Testosterone	962.1	E858.0	E932.1	E950.4	E962.0	E980.4	Thioridazine	969.1	E853.0	E939.1	E950.3	E962.0	E980.3
Tetanus (vaccine)	978.4	E858.8	E948.4	E950.4	E962.0	E980.4	Thio-TEPA, thiotepa	963.1	E858.1	E933.1	E950.4	E962.0	E980.4
antitoxin	979.9	E858.8	E949.9	E950.4	E962.0	E980.4	Thiothixene	969.3	E853.8	E939.3	E950.3	E962.0	E980.3
immune globulin (human)	964.6	E858.2	E934.6	E950.4	E962.0	E980.4	Thiouracil	962.8	E858.0	E932.8	E950.4	E962.0	E980.4
toxoid	978.4	E858.8	E948.4	E950.4	E962.0	E980.4	Thiourea	962.8	E858.0	E932.8	E950.4	E962.0	E980.4
with diphtheria toxoid	978.9	E858.8	E948.9	E950.4	E962.0	E980.4							

Table of Drugs and Chemicals

Substance	Poisoning	Accident	Therapeutic Use	Suicide Attempt	Assault	Undetermined
Thiphenamil	971.1	E855.4	E941.1	E950.4	E962.0	E980.4
Thiram NEC	989.4	E863.6	—	E950.6	E962.1	E980.7
medicinal	976.2	E858.7	E946.2	E950.4	E962.0	E980.4
Thonzylamine	963.0	E858.1	E933.0	E950.4	E962.0	E980.4
Thorazine	969.1	E853.0	E939.1	E950.3	E962.0	E980.3
Thornapple	988.2	E865.4	—	E950.9	E962.1	E980.9
Throat preparation (lozenges) NEC	976.6	E858.7	E946.6	E950.4	E962.0	E980.4
Thrombin	964.5	E858.2	E934.5	E950.4	E962.0	E980.4
Thrombolysin	964.4	E858.2	E934.4	E950.4	E962.0	E980.4
Thymol	983.0	E864.0	—	E950.7	E962.1	E980.6
Thymus extract	962.9	E858.0	E932.9	E950.4	E962.0	E980.4
Thyroglobulin	962.7	E858.0	E932.7	E950.4	E962.0	E980.4
Thyroid (derivatives) (extract)	962.7	E858.0	E932.7	E950.4	E962.0	E980.4
Thyrolar	962.7	E858.0	E932.7	E950.4	E962.0	E980.4
Thyrothrophin, thyrotropin	977.8	E858.8	E947.8	E950.4	E962.0	E980.4
Thyroxin(e)	962.7	E858.0	E932.7	E950.4	E962.0	E980.4
Tigan	963.0	E858.1	E933.0	E950.4	E962.0	E980.4
Tigloidine	968.0	E855.1	E938.0	E950.4	E962.0	E980.4
Tin (chloride) (dust) (oxide) NEC	985.8	E866.4	—	E950.9	E962.1	E980.9
anti-infectives	961.2	E857	E931.2	E950.4	E962.0	E980.4
Tinactin	976.0	E858.7	E946.0	E950.4	E962.0	E980.4
Tincture, iodine — see Iodine						
Tindal	969.1	E853.0	E939.1	E950.3	E962.0	E980.3
Titanium (compounds) (vapor)	985.8	E866.4	—	E950.9	E962.1	E980.9
ointment	976.3	E858.7	E946.3	E950.4	E962.0	E980.4
Titroid	962.7	E858.0	E932.7	E950.4	E962.0	E980.4
TMTD — see Tetramethylthiuram disulfide						
TNT	989.89	E866.8	—	E950.9	E962.1	E980.9
fumes	987.8	E869.8	—	E952.8	E962.2	E982.8
Toadstool	988.1	E865.5	—	E950.9	E962.1	E980.9
Tobacco NEC	989.84	E866.8	—	E950.9	E962.1	E980.9
Indian	988.2	E865.4	—	E950.9	E962.1	E980.9
smoke, second-hand	987.8	E869.4	—	—	—	—
Tocopherol	963.5	E858.1	E933.5	E950.4	E962.0	E980.4
Tocosamine	975.0	E858.6	E945.0	E950.4	E962.0	E980.4
Tofranil	969.0	E854.0	E939.0	E950.3	E962.0	E980.3
Toilet deodorizer	989.89	E866.8	—	E950.9	E962.1	E980.9
Tolazamide	962.3	E858.0	E932.3	E950.4	E962.0	E980.4
Tolazoline	971.3	E855.6	E941.3	E950.4	E962.0	E980.4
Tolbutamide	962.3	E858.0	E932.3	E950.4	E962.0	E980.4
sodium	977.8	E858.8	E947.8	E950.4	E962.0	E980.4
Tolmetin	965.69	E850.6	E935.6	E950.0	E962.0	E980.0
Tolnaftate	976.0	E858.7	E946.0	E950.4	E962.0	E980.4
Tolpropamine	976.1	E858.7	E946.1	E950.4	E962.0	E980.4
Tolserol	968.0	E855.1	E938.0	E950.4	E962.0	E980.4
Toluene (liquid) (vapor)	982.0	E862.4	—	E950.9	E962.1	E980.9
diisocyanate	983.0	E864.0	—	E950.7	E962.1	E980.6
Toluidine	983.0	E864.0	—	E950.7	E962.1	E980.6
vapor	987.8	E869.8	—	E952.8	E962.2	E982.8
Toluol (liquid) (vapor)	982.0	E862.4	—	E950.9	E962.1	E980.9
Tolylene-2, 4-diisocyanate	983.0	E864.0	—	E950.7	E962.1	E980.6
Tonics, cardiac	972.1	E858.3	E942.1	E950.4	E962.0	E980.4
Toxaphene (dust) (spray)	989.2	E863.0	—	E950.6	E962.1	E980.7
Toxoids NEC	978.8	E858.8	E948.8	E950.4	E962.0	E980.4
Tractor fuel NEC	981	E862.1	—	E950.9	E962.1	E980.9
Tragacanth	973.3	E858.4	E943.3	E950.4	E962.0	E980.4
Tramazoline	971.2	E855.5	E941.2	E950.4	E962.0	E980.4
Tranquilizers	969.5	E853.9	E939.5	E950.3	E962.0	E980.3
benzodiazepine-based	969.4	E853.2	E939.4	E950.3	E962.0	E980.3
butyrophenone-based	969.2	E853.1	E939.2	E950.3	E962.0	E980.3
major NEC	969.3	E853.8	E939.3	E950.3	E962.0	E980.3
phenothiazine-based	969.1	E853.0	E939.1	E950.3	E962.0	E980.3
specified NEC	969.5	E853.8	E939.5	E950.3	E962.0	E980.3
Trantoin	961.9	E857	E931.9	E950.4	E962.0	E980.4
Tranxene	969.4	E853.2	E939.4	E950.3	E962.0	E980.3
Tranylcypromine (sulfate)	969.0	E854.0	E939.0	E950.3	E962.0	E980.3
Trasentine	975.1	E858.6	E945.1	E950.4	E962.0	E980.4
Travert	974.5	E858.5	E944.5	E950.4	E962.0	E980.4
Trecator	961.8	E857	E931.8	E950.4	E962.0	E980.4
Tretinoin	976.8	E858.7	E946.8	E950.4	E962.0	E980.4
Triacetin	976.0	E858.7	E946.0	E950.4	E962.0	E980.4
Triacetyloleandomycin	960.3	E856	E930.3	E950.4	E962.0	E980.4
Triamcinolone	962.0	E858.0	E932.0	E950.4	E962.0	E980.4
ENT agent	976.6	E858.7	E946.6	E950.4	E962.0	E980.4
medicinal (keratolytic)	976.4	E858.7	E946.4	E950.4	E962.0	E980.4
Triamcinolone — continued ophthalmic preparation	976.5	E858.7	E946.5	E950.4	E962.0	E980.4
topical NEC	976.0	E858.7	E946.0	E950.4	E962.0	E980.4
Triamterene	974.4	E858.5	E944.4	E950.4	E962.0	E980.4
Triaziquone	963.1	E858.1	E933.1	E950.4	E962.0	E980.4
Tribromacetaldehyde	967.3	E852.2	E937.3	E950.2	E962.0	E980.2
Tribromoethanol	968.2	E855.1	E938.2	E950.4	E962.0	E980.4
Tribromomethane	967.3	E852.2	E937.3	E950.2	E962.0	E980.2
Trichlorethane	982.3	E862.4	—	E950.9	E962.1	E980.9
Trichlormethiazide	974.3	E858.5	E944.3	E950.4	E962.0	E980.4
Trichloroacetic acid	983.1	E864.1	—	E950.7	E962.1	E980.6
Trichloroethanol	967.1	E852.0	E937.1	E950.2	E962.0	E980.2
Trichloroethylene (liquid) (vapor)	982.3	E862.4	—	E950.9	E962.1	E980.9
anesthetic (gas)	968.2	E855.1	E938.2	E950.4	E962.0	E980.4
Trichloroethyl phosphate	967.1	E852.0	E937.1	E950.2	E962.0	E980.2
Trichlorofluoromethane NEC	987.4	E869.2	—	E952.8	E962.2	E982.8
Trichlorotriethylamine	963.1	E858.1	E933.1	E950.4	E962.0	E980.4
Trichomonacides NEC	961.5	E857	E931.5	E950.4	E962.0	E980.4
Trichomycin	960.1	E856	E930.1	E950.4	E962.0	E980.4
Triclofos	967.1	E852.0	E937.1	E950.2	E962.0	E980.2
Tricresyl phosphate	989.89	E866.8	—	E950.9	E962.1	E980.9
solvent	982.8	E862.4	—	E950.9	E962.1	E980.9
Tricyclamol	966.4	E855.0	E936.4	E950.4	E962.0	E980.4
Tridesilon	976.0	E858.7	E946.0	E950.4	E962.0	E980.4
Tridihexethyl	971.1	E855.4	E941.1	E950.4	E962.0	E980.4
Tridione	966.0	E855.0	E936.0	E950.4	E962.0	E980.4
Triethanolamine NEC	983.2	E864.2	—	E950.7	E962.1	E980.6
detergent	983.2	E861.0	—	E950.7	E962.1	E980.6
trinitrate	972.4	E858.3	E942.4	E950.4	E962.0	E980.4
Triethanomelamine	963.1	E858.1	E933.1	E950.4	E962.0	E980.4
Triethylene melamine	963.1	E858.1	E933.1	E950.4	E962.0	E980.4
Triethylenephosphoramide	963.1	E858.1	E933.1	E950.4	E962.0	E980.4
Triethylenethiophosphoramide	963.1	E858.1	E933.1	E950.4	E962.0	E980.4
Trifluoperazine	969.1	E853.0	E939.1	E950.3	E962.0	E980.3
Trifluperidol	969.2	E853.1	E939.2	E950.3	E962.0	E980.3
Triflupromazine	969.1	E853.0	E939.1	E950.3	E962.0	E980.3
Trihexyphenidyl	971.1	E855.4	E941.1	E950.4	E962.0	E980.4
Triiodothyronine	962.7	E858.0	E932.7	E950.4	E962.0	E980.4
Trilene	968.2	E855.1	E938.2	E950.4	E962.0	E980.4
Trimeprazine	963.0	E858.1	E933.0	E950.4	E962.0	E980.4
Trimetazidine	972.4	E858.3	E942.4	E950.4	E962.0	E980.4
Trimethadione	966.0	E855.0	E936.0	E950.4	E962.0	E980.4
Trimethaphan	972.3	E858.3	E942.3	E950.4	E962.0	E980.4
Trimethidinium	972.3	E858.3	E942.3	E950.4	E962.0	E980.4
Trimethobenzamide	963.0	E858.1	E933.0	E950.4	E962.0	E980.4
Trimethylcarbinol	980.8	E860.8	—	E950.9	E962.1	E980.9
Trimethylpsoralen	976.3	E858.7	E946.3	E950.4	E962.0	E980.4
Trimeton	963.0	E858.1	E933.0	E950.4	E962.0	E980.4
Trimipramine	969.0	E854.0	E939.0	E950.3	E962.0	E980.3
Trimustine	963.1	E858.1	E933.1	E950.4	E962.0	E980.4
Trinitrin	972.4	E858.3	E942.4	E950.4	E962.0	E980.4
Trinitrophenol	983.0	E864.0	—	E950.7	E962.1	E980.6
Trinitrotoluene	989.89	E866.8	—	E950.9	E962.1	E980.9
fumes	987.8	E869.8	—	E952.8	E962.2	E982.8
Trional	967.8	E852.8	E937.8	E950.2	E962.0	E980.2
Trioxide of arsenic — see Arsenic						
Trioxsalen	976.3	E858.7	E946.3	E950.4	E962.0	E980.4
Tripelennamine	963.0	E858.1	E933.0	E950.4	E962.0	E980.4
Triperidol	969.2	E853.1	E939.2	E950.3	E962.0	E980.3
Triprolidine	963.0	E858.1	E933.0	E950.4	E962.0	E980.4
Trisoralen	976.3	E858.7	E946.3	E950.4	E962.0	E980.4
Troleandomycin	960.3	E856	E930.3	E950.4	E962.0	E980.4
Trolnitrate (phosphate)	972.4	E858.3	E942.4	E950.4	E962.0	E980.4
Trometamol	963.3	E858.1	E933.3	E950.4	E962.0	E980.4
Tromethamine	963.3	E858.1	E933.3	E950.4	E962.0	E980.4
Tronothane	968.5	E855.2	E938.5	E950.4	E962.0	E980.4
Tropicamide	971.1	E855.4	E941.1	E950.4	E962.0	E980.4
Troxidone	966.0	E855.0	E936.0	E950.4	E962.0	E980.4
Tryparsamide	961.1	E857	E931.1	E950.4	E962.0	E980.4
Trypsin	963.4	E858.1	E933.4	E950.4	E962.0	E980.4
Tryptizol	969.0	E854.0	E939.0	E950.3	E962.0	E980.3
Tuaminoheptane	971.2	E855.5	E941.2	E950.4	E962.0	E980.4
Tuberculin (old)	977.8	E858.8	E947.8	E950.4	E962.0	E980.4
Tubocurare	975.2	E858.6	E945.2	E950.4	E962.0	E980.4
Tubocurarine	975.2	E858.6	E945.2	E950.4	E962.0	E980.4
Turkish green	969.6	E854.1	E939.6	E950.3	E962.0	E980.3
Turpentine (spirits of) (liquid) (vapor)	982.8	E862.4	—	E950.9	E962.1	E980.9

Table of Drugs and Chemicals

	Poisoning	External Cause (E-Code)				
		Accident	Therapeutic Use	Suicide Attempt	Assault	Undetermined
Tybamate	969.5	E853.8	E939.5	E950.3	E962.0	E980.3
Tyloxapol	975.5	E858.6	E945.5	E950.4	E962.0	E980.4
Tymazoline	971.2	E855.5	E941.2	E950.4	E962.0	E980.4
Typhoid vaccine	978.1	E858.8	E948.1	E950.4	E962.0	E980.4
Typhus vaccine	979.2	E858.8	E949.2	E950.4	E962.0	E980.4
Tyrothricin	976.0	E858.7	E946.0	E950.4	E962.0	E980.4
ENT agent	976.6	E858.7	E946.6	E950.4	E962.0	E980.4
ophthalmic preparation	976.5	E858.7	E946.5	E950.4	E962.0	E980.4
Undecenoic acid	976.0	E858.7	E946.0	E950.4	E962.0	E980.4
Undecylenic acid	976.0	E858.7	E946.0	E950.4	E962.0	E980.4
Unna's boot	976.3	E858.7	E946.3	E950.4	E962.0	E980.4
Uracil mustard	963.1	E858.1	E933.1	E950.4	E962.0	E980.4
Uramustine	963.1	E858.1	E933.1	E950.4	E962.0	E980.4
Urari	975.2	E858.6	E945.2	E950.4	E962.0	E980.4
Urea	974.4	E858.5	E944.4	E950.4	E962.0	E980.4
topical	976.8	E858.7	E946.8	E950.4	E962.0	E980.4
Urethan(e) (antineoplastic)	963.1	E858.1	E933.1	E950.4	E962.0	E980.4
Urginea (maritima) (scilla) — see Squill						
Uric acid metabolism agents NEC	974.7	E858.5	E944.7	E950.4	E962.0	E980.4
Urokinase	964.4	E858.2	E934.4	E950.4	E962.0	E980.4
Urokon	977.8	E858.8	E947.8	E950.4	E962.0	E980.4
Urotropin	961.9	E857	E931.9	E950.4	E962.0	E980.4
Urtica	988.2	E865.4	—	E950.9	E962.1	E980.9
Utility gas — see Gas, utility						
Vaccine NEC	979.9	E858.8	E949.9	E950.4	E962.0	E980.4
bacterial NEC	978.8	E858.8	E948.8	E950.4	E962.0	E980.4
with						
other bacterial component	978.9	E858.8	E948.9	E950.4	E962.0	E980.4
pertussis component	978.6	E858.8	E948.6	E950.4	E962.0	E980.4
viral-rickettsial component	979.7	E858.8	E949.7	E950.4	E962.0	E980.4
mixed NEC	978.9	E858.8	E948.9	E950.4	E962.0	E980.4
BCG	978.0	E858.8	E948.0	E950.4	E962.0	E980.4
cholera	978.2	E858.8	E948.2	E950.4	E962.0	E980.4
diphtheria	978.5	E858.8	E948.5	E950.4	E962.0	E980.4
influenza	979.6	E858.8	E949.6	E950.4	E962.0	E980.4
measles	979.4	E858.8	E949.4	E950.4	E962.0	E980.4
meningococcal	978.8	E858.8	E948.8	E950.4	E962.0	E980.4
mumps	979.6	E858.8	E949.6	E950.4	E962.0	E980.4
paratyphoid	978.1	E858.8	E948.1	E950.4	E962.0	E980.4
pertussis (with diphtheria toxoid) (with tetanus toxoid)	978.6	E858.8	E948.6	E950.4	E962.0	E980.4
plague	978.3	E858.8	E948.3	E950.4	E962.0	E980.4
poliomyelitis	979.5	E858.8	E949.5	E950.4	E962.0	E980.4
poliovirus	979.5	E858.8	E949.5	E950.4	E962.0	E980.4
rabies	979.1	E858.8	E949.1	E950.4	E962.0	E980.4
respiratory syncytial virus	979.6	E858.8	E949.6	E950.4	E962.0	E980.4
rickettsial NEC	979.6	E858.8	E949.6	E950.4	E962.0	E980.4
with						
bacterial component	979.7	E858.8	E949.7	E950.4	E962.0	E980.4
pertussis component	978.6	E858.8	E948.6	E950.4	E962.0	E980.4
viral component	979.7	E858.8	E949.7	E950.4	E962.0	E980.4
Rocky mountain spotted fever	979.6	E858.8	E949.6	E950.4	E962.0	E980.4
rotavirus	979.6	E858.8	E949.6	E950.4	E962.0	E980.4
rubella virus	979.4	E858.8	E949.4	E950.4	E962.0	E980.4
sabin oral	979.5	E858.8	E949.5	E950.4	E962.0	E980.4
smallpox	979.0	E858.8	E949.0	E950.4	E962.0	E980.4
tetanus	978.4	E858.8	E948.4	E950.4	E962.0	E980.4
typhoid	978.1	E858.8	E948.1	E950.4	E962.0	E980.4
typhus	979.2	E858.8	E949.2	E950.4	E962.0	E980.4
viral NEC	979.6	E858.8	E949.6	E950.4	E962.0	E980.4
with						
bacterial component	979.7	E858.8	E949.7	E950.4	E962.0	E980.4
pertussis component	978.6	E858.8	E948.6	E950.4	E962.0	E980.4
rickettsial component	979.7	E858.8	E949.7	E950.4	E962.0	E980.4
yellow fever	979.3	E858.8	E949.3	E950.4	E962.0	E980.4
Vaccinia immune globulin (human)	964.6	E858.2	E934.6	E950.4	E962.0	E980.4
Vaginal contraceptives	976.8	E858.7	E946.8	E950.4	E962.0	E980.4
Valethamate	971.1	E855.4	E941.1	E950.4	E962.0	E980.4
Valisone	976.0	E858.7	E946.0	E950.4	E962.0	E980.4
Valium	969.4	E853.2	E939.4	E950.3	E962.0	E980.3
Valmid	967.8	E852.8	E937.8	E950.2	E962.0	E980.2
Vanadium	985.8	E866.4	—	E950.9	E962.1	E980.9
Vancomycin	960.8	E856	E930.8	E950.4	E962.0	E980.4
Vapor — see also Gas	987.9	E869.9	—	E952.9	E962.2	E982.9
kiln (carbon monoxide)	986	E868.8	—	E952.1	E962.2	E982.1
Vapor — see also Gas — continued						
lead — see Lead						
specified source NEC (see also specific substance)	987.8	E869.8	—	E952.8	E962.2	E982.8
Varidase	964.4	E858.2	E934.4	E950.4	E962.0	E980.4
Varnish	989.89	E861.6	—	E950.9	E962.1	E980.9
cleaner	982.8	E862.9	—	E950.9	E962.1	E980.9
Vaseline	976.3	E858.7	E946.3	E950.4	E962.0	E980.4
Vasodilan	972.5	E858.3	E942.5	E950.4	E962.0	E980.4
Vasodilators NEC	972.5	E858.3	E942.5	E950.4	E962.0	E980.4
coronary	972.4	E858.3	E942.4	E950.4	E962.0	E980.4
Vasopressin	962.5	E858.0	E932.5	E950.4	E962.0	E980.4
Vasopressor drugs	962.5	E858.0	E932.5	E950.4	E962.0	E980.4
Venom, venomous (bite) (sting)	989.5	E905.9	—	E950.9	E962.1	E980.9
arthropod NEC	989.5	E905.5	—	E950.9	E962.1	E980.9
bee	989.5	E905.3	—	E950.9	E962.1	E980.9
centipede	989.5	E905.4	—	E950.9	E962.1	E980.9
hornet	989.5	E905.3	—	E950.9	E962.1	E980.9
lizard	989.5	E905.0	—	E950.9	E962.1	E980.9
marine animals or plants	989.5	E905.6	—	E950.9	E962.1	E980.9
millipede (tropical)	989.5	E905.4	—	E950.9	E962.1	E980.9
plant NEC	989.5	E905.7	—	E950.9	E962.1	E980.9
marine	989.5	E905.6	—	E950.9	E962.1	E980.9
scorpion	989.5	E905.2	—	E950.9	E962.1	E980.9
snake	989.5	E905.0	—	E950.9	E962.1	E980.9
specified NEC	989.5	E905.8	—	E950.9	E962.1	E980.9
spider	989.5	E905.1	—	E950.9	E962.1	E980.9
wasp	989.5	E905.3	—	E950.9	E962.1	E980.9
Ventolin — see Salbutamol sulfate						
Veramon	967.0	E851	E937.0	E950.1	E962.0	E980.1
Veratrum						
album	988.2	E865.4	—	E950.9	E962.1	E980.9
alkaloids	972.6	E858.3	E942.6	E950.4	E962.0	E980.4
viride	988.2	E865.4	—	E950.9	E962.1	E980.9
Verdigris — see also Copper	985.8	E866.4	—	E950.9	E962.1	E980.9
Veronal	967.0	E851	E937.0	E950.1	E962.0	E980.1
Veroxil	961.6	E857	E931.6	E950.4	E962.0	E980.4
Versidyne	965.7	E850.7	E935.7	E950.0	E962.0	E980.0
Viagra	972.5	E858.3	E942.5	E950.4	E962.0	E980.4
Vienna						
green	985.1	E866.3	—	E950.8	E962.1	E980.8
insecticide	985.1	E863.4	—	E950.6	E962.1	E980.7
red	989.89	E866.8	—	E950.9	E962.1	E980.9
pharmaceutical dye	977.4	E858.8	E947.4	E950.4	E962.0	E980.4
Vinbarbital, vinbarbitone	967.0	E851	E937.0	E950.1	E962.0	E980.1
Vinblastine	963.1	E858.1	E933.1	E950.4	E962.0	E980.4
Vincristine	963.1	E858.1	E933.1	E950.4	E962.0	E980.4
Vinesthene, vinethene	968.2	E855.1	E938.2	E950.4	E962.0	E980.4
Vinyl						
bital	967.0	E851	E937.0	E950.1	E962.0	E980.1
ether	968.2	E855.1	E938.2	E950.4	E962.0	E980.4
Vioform	961.3	E857	E931.3	E950.4	E962.0	E980.4
topical	976.0	E858.7	E946.0	E930.4	E962.0	E980.4
Viomycin	960.6	E856	E930.6	E950.4	E962.0	E980.4
Viosterol	963.5	E858.1	E933.5	E950.4	E962.0	E980.4
Viper (venom)	989.5	E905.0	—	E950.9	E962.1	E980.9
Viprynium (embonate)	961.6	E857	E931.6	E950.4	E962.0	E980.4
Virugon	961.7	E857	E931.7	E950.4	E962.0	E980.4
Visine	976.5	E858.7	E946.5	E950.4	E962.0	E980.4
Vitamins NEC	963.5	E858.1	E933.5	E950.4	E962.0	E980.4
B_{12}	964.1	E858.2	E934.1	E950.4	E962.0	E980.4
hematopoietic	964.1	E858.2	E934.1	E950.4	E962.0	E980.4
K	964.3	E858.2	E934.3	E950.4	E962.0	E980.4
Vleminckx's solution	976.4	E858.7	E946.4	E950.4	E962.0	E980.4
Voltaren — see Diclofenac sodium						
Warfarin (potassium) (sodium)	964.2	E858.2	E934.2	E950.4	E962.0	E980.4
rodenticide	989.4	E863.7	—	E950.6	E962.1	E980.7
Wasp (sting)	989.5	E905.3	—	E950.9	E962.1	E980.9
Water						
balance agents NEC	974.5	E858.5	E944.5	E950.4	E962.0	E980.4
gas	987.1	E868.1	—	E951.8	E962.2	E981.8
incomplete combustion of — see Carbon, monoxide, fuel, utility						
hemlock	988.2	E865.4	—	E950.9	E962.1	E980.9

Table of Drugs and Chemicals

	External Cause (E-Code)				
	Poisoning	Accident	Therapeutic Use	Suicide Attempt	Assault	Undetermined
Water — *continued*						
moccasin (venom)	989.5	E905.0	—	E950.9	E962.1	E980.9
Wax (paraffin) (petroleum)	981	E862.3	—	E950.9	E962.1	E980.9
automobile	989.89	E861.2	—	E950.9	E962.1	E980.9
floor	981	E862.0	—	E950.9	E962.1	E980.9
Weed killers NEC	989.4	E863.5	—	E950.6	E962.1	E980.7
Welldorm	967.1	E852.0	E937.1	E950.2	E962.0	E980.2
White						
arsenic — see Arsenic						
hellebore	988.2	E865.4	—	E950.9	E962.1	E980.9
lotion (keratolytic)	976.4	E858.7	E946.4	E950.4	E962.0	E980.4
spirit	981	E862.0	—	E950.9	E962.1	E980.9
Whitewashes	989.89	E861.6	—	E950.9	E962.1	E980.9
Whole blood	964.7	E858.2	E934.7	E950.4	E962.0	E980.4
Wild						
black cherry	988.2	E865.4	—	E950.9	E962.1	E980.9
poisonous plants NEC	988.2	E865.4	—	E950.9	E962.1	E980.9
Window cleaning fluid	989.89	E861.3	—	E950.9	E962.1	E980.9
Wintergreen (oil)	976.3	E858.7	E946.3	E950.4	E962.0	E980.4
Witch hazel	976.2	E858.7	E946.2	E950.4	E962.0	E980.4
Wood						
alcohol	980.1	E860.2	—	E950.9	E962.1	E980.9
spirit	980.1	E860.2	—	E950.9	E962.1	E980.9
Woorali	975.2	E858.6	E945.2	E950.4	E962.0	E980.4
Wormseed, American	961.6	E857	E931.6	E950.4	E962.0	E980.4
Xanthine diuretics	974.1	E858.5	E944.1	E950.4	E962.0	E980.4
Xanthocillin	960.0	E856	E930.0	E950.4	E962.0	E980.4
Xanthotoxin	976.3	E858.7	E946.3	E950.4	E962.0	E980.4
Xigris	964.2	E858.2	E934.2	E950.4	E962.0	E980.4
Xylene (liquid) (vapor)	982.0	E862.4	—	E950.9	E962.1	E980.9
Xylocaine (infiltration)						
(topical)	968.5	E855.2	E938.5	E950.4	E962.0	E980.4
nerve block (peripheral)						
(plexus)	968.6	E855.2	E938.6	E950.4	E962.0	E980.4
spinal	968.7	E855.2	E938.7	E950.4	E962.0	E980.4
Xylol (liquid) (vapor)	982.0	E862.4	—	E950.9	E962.1	E980.9
Xylometazoline	971.2	E855.5	E941.2	E950.4	E962.0	E980.4
Yellow						
fever vaccine	979.3	E858.8	E949.3	E950.4	E962.0	E980.4
jasmine	988.2	E865.4	—	E950.9	E962.1	E980.9
Yew	988.2	E865.4	—	E950.9	E962.1	E980.9
Zactane	965.7	E850.7	E935.7	E950.0	E962.0	E980.0
Zaroxolyn	974.3	E858.5	E944.3	E950.4	E962.0	E980.4
Zephiran (topical)	976.0	E858.7	E946.0	E950.4	E962.0	E980.4
ophthalmic preparation	976.5	E858.7	E946.5	E950.4	E962.0	E980.4
Zerone	980.1	E860.2	—	E950.9	E962.1	E980.9
Zinc (compounds) (fumes) (salts)						
(vapor) NEC	985.8	E866.4	—	E950.9	E962.1	E980.9
anti-infectives	976.0	E858.7	E946.0	E950.4	E962.0	E980.4
antivaricose	972.7	E858.3	E942.7	E950.4	E962.0	E980.4
bacitracin	976.0	E858.7	E946.0	E950.4	E962.0	E980.4
chloride	976.2	E858.7	E946.2	E950.4	E962.0	E980.4
gelatin	976.3	E858.7	E946.3	E950.4	E962.0	E980.4
oxide	976.3	E858.7	E946.3	E950.4	E962.0	E980.4
peroxide	976.0	E858.7	E946.0	E950.4	E962.0	E980.4
pesticides	985.8	E863.4	—	E950.6	E962.1	E980.7
phosphide (rodenticide)	985.8	E863.7	—	E950.6	E962.1	E980.7
stearate	976.3	E858.7	E946.3	E950.4	E962.0	E980.4
sulfate (antivaricose)	972.7	E858.3	E942.7	E950.4	E962.0	E980.4
ENT agent	976.6	E858.7	E946.6	E950.4	E962.0	E980.4
ophthalmic solution	976.5	E858.7	E946.5	E950.4	E962.0	E980.4
topical NEC	976.0	E858.7	E946.0	E950.4	E962.0	E980.4
undecylenate	976.0	E858.7	E946.0	E950.4	E962.0	E980.4
Zovant	964.2	E858.2	E934.2	E950.4	E962.0	E980.4
Zoxazolamine	968.0	E855.1	E938.0	E950.4	E962.0	E980.4
Zygadenus (venenosus)	988.2	E865.4	—	E950.9	E962.1	E980.9

SECTION 3

Alphabetic Index to External Causes of Injury and Poisoning (E Code)

This section contains the index to the codes which classify environmental events, circumstances, and other conditions as the cause of injury and other adverse effects. Where a code from the section Supplementary Classification of External Causes of Injury and Poisoning (E800-E999) is applicable, it is intended that the E code shall be used in addition to a code from the main body of the classification, Chapters 1 to 17.

The alphabetic index to the E codes is organized by main terms which describe the accident, circumstance, event, or specific agent which caused the injury or other adverse effect.

Note — Transport accidents (E800-E848) include accidents involving:

aircraft and spacecraft (E840-E845)

watercraft (E830-E838)

motor vehicle (E810-E825)

railway (E800-E807)

other road vehicles (E826-E829)

For definitions and examples related to transport accidents — see Volume 1 code categories E800-E848.

The fourth-digit subdivisions for use with categories E800-E848 to identify the injured person are found at the end of this section.

For identifying the place in which an accident or poisoning occurred (circumstances classifiable to categories E850-E869 and E880-E928) — see the listing in this section under "Accident, occurring."

See the Table of Drugs and Chemicals (Section 2 of this volume) for identifying the specific agent involved in drug overdose or a wrong substance given or taken in error, and for intoxication or poisoning by a drug or other chemical substance.

The specific adverse effect, reaction, or localized toxic effect to a correct drug or substance properly administered in therapeutic or prophylactic dosage should be classified according to the nature of the adverse effect (e.g., allergy, dermatitis, tachycardia) listed in Section 1 of this volume.

Abandonment

A

Abandonment
 causing exposure to weather conditions — *see* Exposure
 child, with intent to injure or kill E968.4
 helpless person, infant, newborn E904.0
  with intent to injure or kill E968.4
Abortion, criminal, injury to child E968.8
Abuse (alleged) (suspected)
 adult
  by
   child E967.4
   ex-partner E967.3
   ex-spouse E967.3
   father E967.0
   grandchild E967.7
   grandparent E967.6
   mother E967.2
   non-related caregiver E967.8
   other relative E967.7
   other specified person E967.1
   partner E967.3
   sibling E967.5
   spouse E967.3
   stepfather E967.0
   stepmother E967.2
   unspecified person E967.9
 child
  by
   boyfriend of parent or guardian E967.0
   child E967.4
   father E967.0
   female partner of parent or guardian E967.2
   girlfriend of parent or guardian E967.2
   grandchild E967.7
   grandparent E967.6
   male partner of parent or guardian E967.0
   mother E967.2
   non-related caregiver E967.8
   other relative E967.7
   other specified person(s) E967.1
   sibling E967.5
   stepfather E967.0
   stepmother E967.2
   unspecified person E967.9
Accident (to) E928.9
 aircraft (in transit) (powered) E841 ☑
  at landing, take-off E840 ☑
  due to, caused by cataclysm — *see* categories E908 ☑, E909 ☑
  late effect of E929.1
  unpowered (*see also* Collision, aircraft, unpowered) E842 ☑
  while alighting, boarding E843 ☑
 amphibious vehicle
  on
   land — *see* Accident, motor vehicle
   water — *see* Accident, watercraft
 animal-drawn vehicle NEC E827 ☑
 animal, ridden NEC E828 ☑
 balloon (*see also* Collision, aircraft, unpowered) E842 ☑
 caused by, due to
  abrasive wheel (metalworking) E919.3
  animal NEC E906.9
   being ridden (in sport or transport) E828 ☑
  avalanche NEC E909.2
  band saw E919.4
  bench saw E919.4
  bore, earth-drilling or mining (land) (seabed) E919.1
  bulldozer E919.7

Accident (to) — *continued*
 caused by, due to — *continued*
  cataclysmic
   earth surface movement or eruption E909.9
   storm E908.9
  chain
   hoist E919.2
    agricultural operations E919.0
    mining operations E919.1
   saw E920.1
  circular saw E919.4
  cold (excessive) (*see also* Cold, exposure to) E901.9
  combine E919.0
  conflagration — *see* Conflagration
  corrosive liquid, substance NEC E924.1
  cotton gin E919.8
  crane E919.2
   agricultural operations E919.0
   mining operations E919.1
  cutting or piercing instrument (*see also* Cut) E920.9
  dairy equipment E919.8
  derrick E919.2
   agricultural operations E919.0
   mining operations E919.1
  drill E920.1
   earth (land) (seabed) E919.1
   hand (powered) E920.1
    not powered E920.4
   metalworking E919.3
   woodworking E919.4
  earth(-)
   drilling machine E919.1
   moving machine E919.7
   scraping machine E919.7
  electric
   current (*see also* Electric shock) E925.9
   motor (*see also* Accident, machine, by type of machine)
    current (of) — *see* Electric shock
  elevator (building) (grain) E919.2
   agricultural operations E919.0
   mining operations E919.1
  environmental factors NEC E928.9
  excavating machine E919.7
  explosive material (*see also* Explosion) E923.9
  farm machine E919.0
  firearm missile — *see* Shooting
  fire, flames (*see also* Fire)
   conflagration — *see* Conflagration
  forging (metalworking) machine E919.3
  forklift (truck) E919.2
   agricultural operations E919.0
   mining operations E919.1
  gas turbine E919.5
  harvester E919.0
  hay derrick, mower, or rake E919.0
  heat (excessive) (*see also* Heat) E900.9
  hoist (*see also* Accident, caused by, due to, lift) E919.2
   chain — *see* Accident, caused by, due to, chain
   shaft E919.1
  hot
   liquid E924.0
    caustic or corrosive E924.1
   object (not producing fire or flames) E924.8
   substance E924.9
    caustic or corrosive E924.1
    liquid (metal) NEC E924.0
    specified type NEC E924.8
  human bite E928.3
  ignition — *see* Ignition
  internal combustion engine E919.5
  landslide NEC E909.2

Accident (to) — *continued*
 caused by, due to — *continued*
  lathe (metalworking) E919.3
   turnings E920.8
   woodworking E919.4
  lift, lifting (appliances) E919.2
   agricultural operations E919.0
   mining operations E919.1
   shaft E919.1
  lightning NEC E907
  machine, machinery (*see also* Accident, machine)
   drilling, metal E919.3
   manufacturing, for manufacture of
    beverages E919.8
    clothing E919.8
    foodstuffs E919.8
    paper E919.8
    textiles E919.8
   milling, metal E919.3
   moulding E919.4
   power press, metal E919.3
   printing E919.8
   rolling mill, metal E919.3
   sawing, metal E919.3
   specified type NEC E919.8
   spinning E919.8
   weaving E919.8
  natural factor NEC E928.9
  overhead plane E919.4
  plane E920.4
   overhead E919.4
  powered
   hand tool NEC E920.1
   saw E919.4
    hand E920.1
  printing machine E919.8
  pulley (block) E919.2
   agricultural operations E919.0
   mining operations E919.1
   transmission E919.6
  radial saw E919.4
  radiation — *see* Radiation
  reaper E919.0
  road scraper E919.7
   when in transport under its own power — *see* categories E810-E825 ☑
  roller coaster E919.8
  sander E919.4
  saw E920.4
   band E919.4
   bench E919.4
   chain E920.1
   circular E919.4
   hand E920.4
    powered E920.1
   powered, except hand E919.4
   radial E919.4
  sawing machine, metal E919.3
  shaft
   hoist E919.1
   lift E919.1
   transmission E919.6
  shears E920.4
   hand E920.4
    powered E920.1
   mechanical E919.3
  shovel E920.4
   steam E919.7
  spinning machine E919.8
  steam (*see also* Burning, steam)
   engine E919.5
   shovel E919.7
  thresher E919.0
  thunderbolt NEC E907
  tractor E919.0
   when in transport under its own power — *see* categories E810-E825 ☑
  transmission belt, cable, chain, gear, pinion, pulley, shaft E919.6
  turbine (gas) (water driven) E919.5
  under-cutter E919.1

Accident (to) — *continued*
 caused by, due to — *continued*
  weaving machine E919.8
  winch E919.2
   agricultural operations E919.0
   mining operations E919.1
 diving E883.0
  with insufficient air supply E913.2
 glider (hang) (*see also* Collision, aircraft, unpowered) E842 ☑
 hovercraft
  on
   land — *see* Accident, motor vehicle
   water — *see* Accident, watercraft
 ice yacht (*see also* Accident, vehicle NEC) E848
 in
  medical, surgical procedure
   as, or due to misadventure — *see* Misadventure
   causing an abnormal reaction or later complication without mention of misadventure — *see* Reaction, abnormal
 kite carrying a person (*see also* Collision, involving aircraft, unpowered) E842 ☑
 land yacht (*see also* Accident, vehicle NEC) E848
 late effect of — *see* Late effect
 launching pad E845 ☑
 machine, machinery (*see also* Accident, caused by, due to, by specific type of machine) E919.9
  agricultural including animal-powered E919.0
  earth-drilling E919.1
  earth moving or scraping E919.7
  excavating E919.7
  involving transport under own power on highway or transport vehicle — *see* categories E810-E825 ☑, E840-E845 ☑
  lifting (appliances) E919.2
  metalworking E919.3
  mining E919.1
  prime movers, except electric motors E919.5
   electric motors — *see* Accident, machine, by specific type of machine
  recreational E919.8
  specified type NEC E919.8
  transmission E919.6
  watercraft (deck) (engine room) (galley) (laundry) (loading) E836
  woodworking or forming E919.4
 motor vehicle (on public highway) (traffic) E819 ☑
  due to cataclysm — *see* categories E908 ☑, E909 ☑
  involving
   collision (*see also* Collision, motor vehicle) E812 ☑
   nontraffic, not on public highway — *see* categories E820-E825 ☑
   not involving collision — *see* categories E816-E819 ☑
  nonmotor vehicle NEC E829 ☑
   nonroad — *see* Accident, vehicle NEC
   road, except pedal cycle, animal-drawn vehicle, or animal being ridden E829 ☑
  nonroad vehicle NEC — *see* Accident, vehicle NEC
  not elsewhere classifiable involving
   cable car (not on rails) E847
    on rails E829 ☑
   coal car in mine E846

Index to External Causes

Accident (to) — *continued*
 not elsewhere classifiable involving — *continued*
  hand truck — *see* Accident, vehicle NEC
  logging car E846
  sled(ge), meaning snow or ice vehicle E848
  tram, mine or quarry E846
  truck
   mine or quarry E846
   self-propelled, industrial E846
   station baggage E846
  tub, mine or quarry E846
  vehicle NEC E848
   snow and ice E848
   used only on industrial premises E846
  wheelbarrow E848
 occurring (at) (in)
  apartment E849.0
  baseball field, diamond E849.4
  construction site, any E849.3
  dock E849.8
   yard E849.3
  dormitory E849.7
  factory (building) (premises) E849.3
  farm E849.1
   buildings E849.1
   house E849.0
  football field E849.4
  forest E849.8
  garage (place of work) E849.3
   private (home) E849.0
  gravel pit E849.2
  gymnasium E849.4
  highway E849.5
  home (private) (residential) E849.0
   institutional E849.7
  hospital E849.7
  hotel E849.6
  house (private) (residential) E849.0
   movie E849.6
   public E849.6
  institution, residential E849.7
  jail E849.7
  mine E849.2
  motel E849.6
  movie house E849.6
  office (building) E849.6
  orphanage E849.7
  park (public) E849.4
   mobile home E849.8
   trailer E849.8
  parking lot or place E849.8
  place
   industrial NEC E849.3
   parking E849.8
   public E849.8
    specified place NEC E849.5
   recreational NEC E849.4
   sport NEC E849.4
  playground (park) (school) E849.4
  prison E849.6
  public building NEC E849.6
  quarry E849.2
  railway
   line NEC E849.8
   yard E849.3
  residence
   home (private) E849.0
  resort (beach) (lake) (mountain) (seashore) (vacation) E849.4
  restaurant E849.6
  sand pit E849.2
  school (building) (private) (public) (state) E849.6
   reform E849.7
   riding E849.4
  seashore E849.8
   resort E849.4
  shop (place of work) E849.3
   commercial E849.6
  skating rink E849.4
  sports palace E849.4
  stadium E849.4

Accident (to) — *continued*
 occurring — *continued*
  store E849.6
  street E849.5
  swimming pool (public) E849.4
   private home or garden E849.0
  tennis court, public E849.4
  theatre, theater E849.6
  trailer court E849.8
  tunnel E849.8
   under construction E849.2
  warehouse E849.3
  yard
   dock E849.3
   industrial E849.3
   private (home) E849.0
   railway E849.3
 off-road type motor vehicle (not on public highway) NEC E821
  on public highway — *see* categories E810-E819 ☑
 pedal cycle E826 ☑
 railway E807 ☑
  due to cataclysm — *see* categories E908 ☑, E909 ☑
  involving
   avalanche E909.2
   burning by engine, locomotive, train (see also Explosion, railway engine) E803 ☑
   collision (see also Collision, railway) E800 ☑
   derailment (see also Derailment, railway) E802 ☑
   explosion (see also Explosion, railway engine) E803 ☑
   fall (see also Fall, from, railway rolling stock) E804 ☑
   fire (see also Explosion, railway engine) E803 ☑
   hitting by, being struck by object falling in, on, from, rolling stock, train, vehicle E806 ☑
    rolling stock, train, vehicle E805 ☑
   overturning, railway rolling stock, train, vehicle (see also Derailment, railway) E802 ☑
   running off rails, railway (see also Derailment, railway) E802 ☑
   specified circumstances NEC E806 ☑
   train or vehicle hit by
    avalanche E909.2
    falling object (earth, rock, tree) E806 ☑
    due to cataclysm — *see* categories E908 ☑, E909 ☑
    landslide E909.2
 roller skate E885.1
 scooter (nonmotorized) E885.0
 skateboard E885.2
 ski(ing) E885.3
  jump E884.9
  lift or tow (with chair or gondola) E847
 snowboard E885.4
 snow vehicle, motor driven (not on public highway) E820 ☑
  on public highway — *see* categories E810-E819 ☑
 spacecraft E845 ☑
 specified cause NEC E928.8
 street car E829 ☑
 traffic NEC E819 ☑
 vehicle NEC (with pedestrian) E848
  battery powered
   airport passenger vehicle E846
   truck (baggage) (mail) E846

Accident (to) — *continued*
 vehicle — *continued*
  powered commercial or industrial (with other vehicle or object within commercial or industrial premises) E846
  watercraft E838 ☑
   with
    drowning or submersion resulting from
     accident other than to watercraft E832 ☑
     accident to watercraft E830 ☑
    injury, except drowning or submersion, resulting from
     accident other than to watercraft — *see* categories E833-E838 ☑
     accident to watercraft E831 ☑
    due to, caused by cataclysm — *see* categories E908 ☑, E909 ☑
    machinery E836 ☑
Acid throwing E961
Acosta syndrome E902.0
Aeroneurosis E902.1
Aero-otitis media — *see* Effects of, air pressure
Aerosinusitis — *see* Effects of, air pressure
After-effect, late — *see* Late effect
Air
 blast
  in
   terrorism E979.2
   war operations E993
 embolism (traumatic) NEC E928.9
  in
   infusion or transfusion E874.1
   perfusion E874.2
 sickness E903
Alpine sickness E902.0
Altitude sickness — *see* Effects of, air pressure
Anaphylactic shock, anaphylaxis — *see also* Table of Drugs and Chemicals E947.9
 due to bite or sting (venomous) — *see* Bite, venomous
Andes disease E902.0
Apoplexy
 heat — *see* Heat
Arachnidism E905.1
Arson E968.0
Asphyxia, asphyxiation
 by
  chemical
   in
    terrorism E979.7
    war operations E997.2
  explosion — *see* Explosion
  food (bone) (regurgitated food) (seed) E911
  foreign object, except food E912
  fumes
   in
    terrorism (chemical weapons) E979.7
    war operations E997.2
  gas (see also Table of Drugs and Chemicals)
   in
    terrorism E979.7
    war operations E997.2
   legal
    execution E978
    intervention (tear) E972
   tear E972
  mechanical means (see also Suffocation) E913.9
 from
  conflagration — *see* Conflagration
  fire (see also Fire) E899
   in
    terrorism E979.3

Asphyxia, asphyxiation — *continued*
 from — *continued*
  fire (see also Fire) — *continued*
   in — *continued*
    war operations E990.9
  ignition — *see* Ignition
Aspiration
 foreign body — *see* Foreign body, aspiration
 mucus, not of newborn (with asphyxia, obstruction respiratory passage, suffocation) E912
 phlegm (with asphyxia, obstruction respiratory passage, suffocation) E912
 vomitus (with asphyxia, obstruction respiratory passage, suffocation) (see also Foreign body, aspiration, food) E911
Assassination (attempt) — *see also* Assault E968.9
Assault (homicidal) (by) (in) E968.9
 acid E961
  swallowed E962.1
 air gun E968.6
 BB gun E968.6
 bite NEC E968.8
  of human being E968.7
 bomb ((placed in) car or house) E965.8
  antipersonnel E965.5
  letter E965.7
  petrol E965.6
 brawl (hand) (fists) (foot) E960.0
 burning, burns (by fire) E968.0
  acid E961
   swallowed E962.1
  caustic, corrosive substance E961
   swallowed E962.1
  chemical from swallowing caustic, corrosive substance NEC E962.1
  hot liquid E968.3
  scalding E968.3
  vitriol E961
   swallowed E962.1
 caustic, corrosive substance E961
  swallowed E962.1
 cut, any part of body E966
 dagger E966
 drowning E964
 explosive(s) E965.9
  bomb (see also Assault, bomb) E965.8
  dynamite E965.8
 fight (hand) (fists) (foot) E960.0
  with weapon E968.9
   blunt or thrown E968.2
   cutting or piercing E966
   firearm — *see* Shooting, homicide
 fire E968.0
 firearm(s) — *see* Shooting, homicide
 garrotting E963
 gunshot (wound) — *see* Shooting, homicide
 hanging E963
 injury NEC E968.9
 knife E966
 late effect of E969
 ligature E963
 poisoning E962.9
  drugs or medicinals E962.0
  gas(es) or vapors, except drugs and medicinals E962.2
  solid or liquid substances, except drugs and medicinals E962.1
 puncture, any part of body E966
 pushing
  before moving object, train, vehicle E968.5
  from high place E968.1
 rape E960.1
 scalding E968.3
 shooting — *see* Shooting, homicide
 sodomy E960.1
 stab, any part of body E966

Assault

Assault — *continued*
- strangulation E963
- submersion E964
- suffocation E963
- transport vehicle E968.5
- violence NEC E968.9
- vitriol E961
  - swallowed E962.1
- weapon E968.9
  - blunt or thrown E968.2
  - cutting or piercing E966
  - firearm — *see* Shooting, homicide
- wound E968.9
  - cutting E966
  - gunshot — *see* Shooting, homicide
  - knife E966
  - piercing E966
  - puncture E966
  - stab E966

Attack by animal NEC E906.9

Avalanche E909.2
- falling on or hitting
  - motor vehicle (in motion) (on public highway) E909.2
  - railway train E909.2

Aviators' disease E902.1

B

Barotitis, barodontalgia, barosinusitis, barotrauma (otitic) (sinus) — *see* Effects of, air pressure

Battered
- baby or child (syndrome) — *see* Abuse, child; category E967 ☑
- person other than baby or child — *see* Assault

Bayonet wound — *see also* Cut, by bayonet E920.3
- in
  - legal intervention E974
  - terrorism E979.8
  - war operations E995

Bean in nose E912

Bed set on fire NEC E898.0

Beheading (by guillotine)
- homicide E966
- legal execution E978

Bending, injury in E927

Bends E902.0

Bite
- animal NEC E906.5
  - other specified (except arthropod) E906.3
  - venomous NEC E905.9
- arthropod (nonvenomous) NEC E906.4
  - venomous — *see* Sting
- black widow spider E905.1
- cat E906.3
- centipede E905.4
- cobra E905.0
- copperhead snake E905.0
- coral snake E905.0
- dog E906.0
- fer de lance E905.0
- gila monster E905.0
- human being
  - accidental E928.3
  - assault E968.7
- insect (nonvenomous) E906.4
  - venomous — *see* Sting
- krait E905.0
- late effect of — *see* Late effect
- lizard E906.2
  - venomous E905.0
- mamba E905.0
- marine animal
  - nonvenomous E906.3
    - snake E906.2
  - venomous E905.6
    - snake E905.0
- millipede E906.4
  - venomous E905.4
- moray eel E906.3
- rat E906.1
- rattlesnake E905.0
- rodent, except rat E906.3

Bite — *continued*
- serpent — *see* Bite, snake
- shark E906.3
- snake (venomous) E905.0
  - nonvenomous E906.2
  - sea E905.0
- spider E905.1
  - nonvenomous E906.4
- tarantula (venomous) E905.1
- venomous NEC E905.9
  - by specific animal — *see category* E905 ☑
- viper E905.0
- water moccasin E905.0

Blast (air)
- from nuclear explosion E996
- in
  - terrorism E979.2
    - from nuclear explosion E979.5
    - underwater E979.0
  - war operations E993
    - from nuclear explosion E996
    - underwater E992

Blizzard E908.3

Blow E928.9
- by law-enforcing agent, police (on duty) E975
  - with blunt object (baton) (nightstick) (stave) (truncheon) E973

Blowing up — *see also* Explosion E923.9

Brawl (hand) (fists) (foot) E960.0

Breakage (accidental)
- cable of cable car not on rails E847
- ladder (causing fall) E881.0
- part (any) of
  - animal-drawn vehicle E827 ☑
  - ladder (causing fall) E881.0
  - motor vehicle
    - in motion (on public highway) E818 ☑
    - not on public highway E825 ☑
  - nonmotor road vehicle, except animal-drawn vehicle or pedal cycle E829 ☑
  - off-road type motor vehicle (not on public highway) NEC E821 ☑
    - on public highway E818 ☑
  - pedal cycle E826 ☑
  - scaffolding (causing fall) E881.1
  - snow vehicle, motor-driven (not on public highway) E820 ☑
    - on public highway E818 ☑
  - vehicle NEC — *see* Accident, vehicle

Broken
- glass
  - fall on E888.0
  - injury by E920.8
- power line (causing electric shock) E925.1

Bumping against, into (accidentally)
- object (moving) E917.9
  - caused by crowd E917.1
    - with subsequent fall E917.6
  - furniture E917.3
    - with subsequent fall E917.7
  - in
    - running water E917.2
    - sports E917.0
      - with subsequent fall E917.5
  - stationary E917.4
    - with subsequent fall E917.8
- person(s) E917.9
  - with fall E886.9
    - in sports E886.0
  - as, or caused by, a crowd E917.1
    - with subsequent fall E917.6
  - in sports E917.0
    - with fall E886.0

Burning, burns (accidental) (by) (from) (on) E899
- acid (any kind) E924.1
  - swallowed — *see* Table of Drugs and Chemicals

Burning, burns — *continued*
- bedclothes (*see also* Fire, specified NEC) E898.0
- blowlamp (*see also* Fire, specified NEC) E898.1
- blowtorch (*see also* Fire, specified NEC) E898.1
- boat, ship, watercraft — *see* categories E830 ☑, E831 ☑, E837 ☑
- bonfire (controlled) E897
  - uncontrolled E892
- candle (*see also* Fire, specified NEC) E898.1
- caustic liquid, substance E924.1
  - swallowed — *see* Table of Drugs and Chemicals
- chemical E924.1
  - from swallowing caustic, corrosive substance — *see* Table of Drugs and Chemicals
  - in
    - terrorism E979.7
    - war operations E997.2
- cigar(s) or cigarette(s) (*see also* Fire, specified NEC) E898.1
- clothes, clothing, nightdress — *see* Ignition, clothes
  - with conflagration — *see* Conflagration
- conflagration — *see* Conflagration
- corrosive liquid, substance E924.1
  - swallowed — *see* Table of Drugs and Chemicals
- electric current (*see also* Electric shock) E925.9
- fire, flames (*see also* Fire) E899
- flare, Verey pistol E922.8
- heat
  - from appliance (electrical) E924.8
  - in local application, or packing during medical or surgical procedure E873.5
- homicide (attempt) (*see also* Assault, burning) E968.0
- hot
  - liquid E924.0
    - caustic or corrosive E924.1
  - object (not producing fire or flames) E924.8
  - substance E924.9
    - caustic or corrosive E924.1
    - liquid (metal) E924.0
    - specified type NEC E924.8
  - tap water E924.2
- ignition (*see also* Ignition)
  - clothes, clothing, nightdress (*see also* Ignition, clothes)
    - with conflagration — *see* Conflagration
  - highly inflammable material (benzine) (fat) (gasoline) (kerosene) (paraffin) (petrol) E894
- in
  - terrorism E979.3
    - from nuclear explosion E979.5
    - petrol bomb E979.3
  - war operations (from fire-producing device or conventional weapon) E990.9
    - from nuclear explosion E996
    - petrol bomb E990.0
- inflicted by other person
  - stated as
    - homicidal, intentional (*see also* Assault, burning) E968.0
    - undetermined whether accidental or intentional (*see also* Burn, stated as undetermined whether accidental or intentional) E988.1
- internal, from swallowed caustic, corrosive liquid, substance — *see* Table of Drugs and Chemicals
- lamp (*see also* Fire, specified NEC) E898.1

Burning, burns — *continued*
- late effect of NEC E929.4
- lighter (cigar) (cigarette) (*see also* Fire, specified NEC) E898.1
- lightning E907
- liquid (boiling) (hot) (molten) E924.0
  - caustic, corrosive (external) E924.1
    - swallowed — *see* Table of Drugs and Chemicals
- local application of externally applied substance in medical or surgical care E873.5
- machinery — *see* Accident, machine
- matches (*see also* Fire, specified NEC) E898.1
- medicament, externally applied E873.5
- metal, molten E924.0
- object (hot) E924.8
  - producing fire or flames — *see* Fire
- oven (electric) (gas) E924.8
- pipe (smoking) (*see also* Fire, specified NEC) E898.1
- radiation — *see* Radiation
- railway engine, locomotive, train (*see also* Explosion, railway engine) E803 ☑
- self-inflicted (unspecified whether accidental or intentional) E988.1
  - caustic or corrosive substance NEC E988.7
  - stated as intentional, purposeful E958.1
    - caustic or corrosive substance NEC E958.7
  - stated as undetermined whether accidental or intentional E988.1
    - caustic or corrosive substance NEC E988.7
- steam E924.0
  - pipe E924.8
- substance (hot) E924.9
  - boiling or molten E924.0
  - caustic, corrosive (external) E924.1
    - swallowed — *see* Table of Drugs and Chemicals
- suicidal (attempt) NEC E958.1
  - caustic substance E958.7
  - late effect of E959
- tanning bed E926.2
- therapeutic misadventure
  - overdose of radiation E873.2
- torch, welding (*see also* Fire, specified NEC) E898.1
- trash fire (*see also* Burning, bonfire) E897
- vapor E924.0
- vitriol E924.1
- x-rays E926.3
- in medical, surgical procedure — *see* Misadventure, failure, in dosage, radiation

Butted by animal E906.8

C

Cachexia, lead or saturnine E866.0
- from pesticide NEC (*see also* Table of Drugs and Chemicals) E863.4

Caisson disease E902.2

Capital punishment (any means) E978

Car sickness E903

Casualty (not due to war) NEC E928.9
- terrorism E979.8
- war (*see also* War operations) E995

Cat
- bite E906.3
- scratch E906.8

Cataclysmic (any injury)
- earth surface movement or eruption E909.9
  - specified type NEC E909.8
- storm or flood resulting from storm E908.9
  - specified type NEC E909.8

Catching fire — *see* Ignition

Index to External Causes

Caught
  between
    objects (moving) (stationary and moving) E918
      and machinery — see Accident, machine
  by cable car, not on rails E847
  in
    machinery (moving parts of) — see, Accident, machine
    object E918

Cave-in (causing asphyxia, suffocation (by pressure)) — see also Suffocation, due to, cave-in E913.3
  with injury other than asphyxia or suffocation E916
    with asphyxia or suffocation (see also Suffocation, due to, cave-in) E913.3
  struck or crushed by E916
    with asphyxia or suffocation (see also Suffocation, due to, cave-in) E913.3

Change(s) in air pressure — see also Effects of, air pressure
  sudden, in aircraft (ascent) (descent) (causing aeroneurosis or aviators' disease) E902.1

Chilblains E901.0
  due to manmade conditions E901.1

Choking (on) (any object except food or vomitus) E912
  apple E911
  bone E911
  food, any type (regurgitated) E911
  mucus or phlegm E912
  seed E911

Civil insurrection — see War operations

Cloudburst E908.8

Cold, exposure to (accidental) (excessive) (extreme) (place) E901.9
  causing chilblains or immersion foot E901.0
  due to
    manmade conditions E901.1
    specified cause NEC E901.8
    weather (conditions) E901.0
  late effect of NEC E929.5
  self-inflicted (undetermined whether accidental or intentional) E988.3
  suicidal E958.3
  suicide E958.3

Colic, lead, painter's, or saturnine — see category E866 ☑

Collapse
  building E916
    burning (uncontrolled fire) E891.8
      in terrorism E979.3
    private E890.8
  dam E909.3
  due to heat — see Heat
  machinery — see Accident, machine or vehicle
  man-made structure E909.3
  postoperative NEC E878.9
  structure
    burning (uncontrolled fire) NEC E891.8
      in terrorism E979.3

Collision (accidental)

Note — In the case of collisions between different types of vehicles, persons and objects, priority in classification is in the following order:

Aircraft
Watercraft
Motor vehicle
Railway vehicle
Pedal cycle
Animal-drawn vehicle
Animal being ridden
Streetcar or other nonmotor road vehicle
Other vehicle
Pedestrian or person using pedestrian conveyance
Object (except where falling from or set in motion by vehicle etc. listed above)

In the listing below, the combinations are listed only under the vehicle etc. having priority. For definitions, see Supplementary Classification of External Causes of Injury and Poisoning (E800-E999).

  aircraft (with object or vehicle) (fixed) (movable) (moving) E841 ☑
    with
      person (while landing, taking off) (without accident to aircraft) E844 ☑
      powered (in transit) (with unpowered aircraft) E841 ☑
      while landing, taking off E840 ☑
    unpowered E842 ☑
    while landing, taking off E840 ☑
  animal being ridden (in sport or transport) E828 ☑
    and
      animal (being ridden) (herded) (unattended) E828 ☑
      nonmotor road vehicle, except pedal cycle or animal-drawn vehicle E828 ☑
      object (fallen) (fixed) (movable) (moving) not falling from or set in motion by vehicle of higher priority E828 ☑
      pedestrian (conveyance or vehicle) E828 ☑
  animal-drawn vehicle E827 ☑
    and
      animal (being ridden) (herded) (unattended) E827 ☑
      nonmotor road vehicle, except pedal cycle E827 ☑
      object (fallen) (fixed) (movable) (moving) not falling from or set in motion by vehicle of higher priority E827 ☑
      pedestrian (conveyance or vehicle) E827 ☑
    streetcar E827 ☑
  motor vehicle (on public highway) (traffic accident) E812 ☑
    after leaving, running off, public highway (without antecedent collision) (without re-entry) E816 ☑
    with antecedent collision on public highway — see categories E810-E815 ☑
    with re-entrance collision with another motor vehicle E811 ☑
    and
      abutment (bridge) (overpass) E815 ☑

Collision — *continued*
  motor vehicle — *continued*
    and — *continued*
      animal (herded) (unattended) E815 ☑
      carrying person, property animal-drawn vehicle E813 ☑
      another motor vehicle (abandoned) (disabled) (parked) (stalled) (stopped) E812 ☑
        with, involving re-entrance (on same roadway) (across median strip) E811 ☑
      any object, person, or vehicle off the public highway resulting from a noncollision motor vehicle nontraffic accident E816 ☑
      avalanche, fallen or not moving E815 ☑
      falling E909.2
      boundary fence E815 ☑
      culvert E815 ☑
      fallen
        stone E815 ☑
        tree E815 ☑
      guard post or guard rail E815 ☑
      inter-highway divider E815 ☑
      landslide, fallen or not moving E815 ☑
      moving E909 ☑
      machinery (road) E815 ☑
      nonmotor road vehicle NEC E813 ☑
      object (any object, person, or vehicle off the public highway resulting from a noncollision motor vehicle nontraffic accident) E815 ☑
      off, normally not on, public highway resulting from a noncollision motor vehicle traffic accident E816 ☑
      pedal cycle E813 ☑
      pedestrian (conveyance) E814 ☑
      person (using pedestrian conveyance) E814 ☑
      post or pole (lamp) (light) (signal) (telephone) (utility) E815 ☑
      railway rolling stock, train, vehicle E810 ☑
      safety island E815 ☑
      street car E813 ☑
      traffic signal, sign, or marker (temporary) E815 ☑
      tree E815 ☑
      tricycle E813 ☑
      wall of cut made for road E815 ☑
    due to cataclysm — see categories E908 ☑, E909 ☑
    not on public highway, nontraffic accident E822 ☑
    and
      animal (carrying person, property) (herded) (unattended) E822 ☑
      animal-drawn vehicle E822 ☑
      another motor vehicle (moving), except off-road motor vehicle E822 ☑
      stationary E823 ☑
      avalanche, fallen, not moving E823 ☑
      moving E909.2
      landslide, fallen, not moving E823 ☑
      moving E909.2

Collision — *continued*
  motor vehicle — *continued*
    not on public highway, nontraffic accident — *continued*
    and — *continued*
      nonmotor vehicle (moving) E822 ☑
      stationary E823 ☑
      object (fallen) (normally) (fixed) (movable but not in motion) (stationary) E823 ☑
        moving, except when falling from, set in motion by, aircraft or cataclysm E822 ☑
      pedal cycle (moving) E822 ☑
      stationary E823 ☑
      pedestrian (conveyance) E822 ☑
      person (using pedestrian conveyance) E822 ☑
      railway rolling stock, train, vehicle (moving) E822 ☑
      stationary E823 ☑
      road vehicle (any) (moving) E822 ☑
      stationary E823 ☑
      tricycle (moving) E822 ☑
      stationary E823 ☑
    off-road type motor vehicle (not on public highway) E821 ☑
    and
      animal (being ridden) (-drawn vehicle) E821 ☑
      another off-road motor vehicle, except snow vehicle E821 ☑
      other motor vehicle, not on public highway E821 ☑
      other object or vehicle NEC, fixed or movable, not set in motion by aircraft, motor vehicle on highway, or snow vehicle, motor driven E821 ☑
      pedal cycle E821 ☑
      pedestrian (conveyance) E821 ☑
      railway train E821 ☑
    on public highway — see Collision, motor vehicle
  pedal cycle E826 ☑
    and
      animal (carrying person, property) (herded) (unherded) E826 ☑
      animal-drawn vehicle E826 ☑
      another pedal cycle E826 ☑
      nonmotor road vehicle E826 ☑
      object (fallen) (fixed) (movable) (moving) not falling from or set in motion by aircraft, motor vehicle, or railway train NEC E826 ☑
      pedestrian (conveyance) E826 ☑
      person (using pedestrian conveyance) E826 ☑
      street car E826 ☑
  pedestrian(s) (conveyance) E917.9
    with fall E886.9
      in sports E886.0
    and
      crowd, human stampede E917.1
        with subsequent fall E917.6
      furniture E917.3
        with subsequent fall E917.7
      machinery — see Accident, machine
      object (fallen) (moving) not falling from NEC, fixed or set in motion by any vehicle classifiable to E800-E848 ☑, E917.9

Collision

Collision — continued
  pedestrian(s) — continued
    and — continued
      object not falling from, fixed or set in motion by any vehicle classifiable to — continued
        with subsequent fall E917.6
        caused by a crowd E917.1
          with subsequent fall E917.6
        furniture E917.3
          with subsequent fall E917.7
        in
          running water E917.2
            with drowning or submersion — see Submersion
        sports E917.0
          with subsequent fall E917.5
        stationary E917.4
          with subsequent fall E917.8
        vehicle, nonmotor, nonroad E848
      in
        running water E917.2
          with drowning or submersion — see Submersion
        sports E917.0
          with fall E886.0
    person(s) (using pedestrian conveyance) (see also Collision, pedestrian) E917.9
  railway (rolling stock) (train) (vehicle) (with (subsequent) derailment, explosion, fall or fire) E800
    with antecedent derailment E802 ☑
    and
      animal (carrying person) (herded) (unattended) E801 ☑
      another railway train or vehicle E800 ☑
      buffers E801 ☑
      fallen tree on railway E801 ☑
      farm machinery, nonmotor (in transport) (stationary) E801 ☑
      gates E801 ☑
      nonmotor vehicle E801 ☑
      object (fallen) (fixed) (movable) (moving) not falling from, set in motion by, aircraft or motor vehicle NEC E801 ☑
      pedal cycle E801 ☑
      pedestrian (conveyance) E805 ☑
      person (using pedestrian conveyance) E805 ☑
      platform E801 ☑
      rock on railway E801 ☑
      street car E801 ☑
  snow vehicle, motor-driven (not on public highway) E820 ☑
    and
      animal (being ridden) (-drawn vehicle) E820 ☑
      another off-road motor vehicle E820 ☑
      other motor vehicle, not on public highway E820 ☑
      other object or vehicle NEC, fixed or movable, not set in motion by aircraft or motor vehicle on highway E820 ☑
      pedal cycle E820 ☑
      pedestrian (conveyance) E820 ☑
      railway train E820 ☑
    on public highway — see Collision, motor vehicle
  street car(s) E829 ☑

Collision — continued
  street car(s) — continued
    and
      animal, herded, not being ridden, unattended E829 ☑
      nonmotor road vehicle NEC E829 ☑
      object (fallen) (fixed) (movable) (moving) not falling from or set in motion by aircraft, animal-drawn vehicle, animal being ridden, motor vehicle, pedal cycle, or railway train E829 ☑
      pedestrian (conveyance) E829 ☑
      person (using pedestrian conveyance) E829 ☑
  vehicle
    animal-drawn — see Collision, animal-drawn vehicle
    motor — see Collision, motor vehicle
    nonmotor
      nonroad E848
      and
        another nonmotor, nonroad vehicle E848
        object (fallen) (fixed) (movable) (moving) not falling from or set in motion by aircraft, animal-drawn vehicle, animal being ridden, motor vehicle, nonmotor road vehicle, pedal cycle, railway train, or streetcar E848
      road, except animal being ridden, animal-drawn vehicle, or pedal cycle E829 ☑
      and
        animal, herded, not being ridden, unattended E829 ☑
        another nonmotor road vehicle, except animal being ridden, animal-drawn vehicle, or pedal cycle E829 ☑
        object (fallen) (fixed) (movable) (moving) not falling from or set in motion by, aircraft, animal-drawn vehicle, animal being ridden, motor vehicle, pedal cycle, or railway train E829 ☑
        pedestrian (conveyance) E829 ☑
        person (using pedestrian conveyance) E829 ☑
        vehicle, nonmotor, nonroad E829 ☑
  watercraft E838 ☑
    and
      person swimming or water skiing E838 ☑
    causing
      drowning, submersion E830 ☑
      injury except drowning, submersion E831 ☑
Combustion, spontaneous — see Ignition
Complication of medical or surgical procedure or treatment
  as an abnormal reaction — see Reaction, abnormal
  delayed, without mention of misadventure — see Reaction, abnormal
  due to misadventure — see Misadventure

Compression
  divers' squeeze E902.2
  trachea by
    food E911
    foreign body, except food E912
Conflagration
  building or structure, except private dwelling (barn) (church) (convalescent or residential home) (factory) (farm outbuilding) (hospital) (hotel) (institution) (educational) (domitory) (residential) (school) (shop) (store) (theater) E891.9
    with or causing (injury due to)
      accident or injury NEC E891.9
        specified circumstance NEC E891.8
      burns, burning E891.3
      carbon monoxide E891.2
      fumes E891.2
        polyvinylchloride (PVC) or similar material E891.1
      smoke E891.2
      causing explosion E891.0
    in terrorism E979.3
  not in building or structure E892
  private dwelling (apartment) (boarding house) (camping place) (caravan) (farmhouse) (home (private)) (house) (lodging house) (private garage) (rooming house) (tenement) E890.9
    with or causing (injury due to)
      accident or injury NEC E890.9
        specified circumstance NEC E890.8
      burns, burning E890.3
      carbon monoxide E890.2
      fumes E890.2
        polyvinylchloride (PVC) or similar material E890.1
      smoke E890.2
      causing explosion E890.0
Constriction, external
  caused by
    hair E928.4
    other object E928.5
Contact with
  dry ice E901.1
  liquid air, hydrogen, nitrogen E901.1
Cramp(s)
  Heat — see Heat
  swimmers (see also category E910) E910.2
    not in recreation or sport E910.3
Cranking (car) (truck) (bus) (engine), injury by E917.9
Crash
  aircraft (in transit) (powered) E841 ☑
    at landing, take-off E840 ☑
    in
      terrorism E979.1
      war operations E994
    on runway NEC E840 ☑
    stated as
      homicidal E968.8
      suicidal E958.6
      undetermined whether accidental or intentional E988.6
    unpowered E842 ☑
  glider E842 ☑
  motor vehicle (see also Accident, motor vehicle)
    homicidal E968.5
    suicidal E958.5
    undetermined whether accidental or intentional E988.5
Crushed (accidentally) E928.9
  between
    boat(s), ship(s), watercraft (and dock or pier) (without accident to watercraft) E838 ☑

Crushed — continued
  between — continued
    boat(s), ship(s), watercraft — continued
      after accident to, or collision, watercraft E831 ☑
    objects (moving) (stationary and moving) E918
  by
    avalanche NEC E909.2
    boat, ship, watercraft after accident to, collision, watercraft E831 ☑
    cave-in E916
      with asphyxiation or suffocation (see also Suffocation, due to, cave-in) E913.3
    crowd, human stampede E917.1
    falling
      aircraft (see also Accident, aircraft) E841 ☑
      in
        terrorism E979.1
        war operations E994
    earth, material E916
      with asphyxiation or suffocation (see also Suffocation, due to, cave-in) E913.3
    object E916
      on ship, watercraft E838 ☑
      while loading, unloading watercraft E838 ☑
    landslide NEC E909.2
    lifeboat after abandoning ship E831 ☑
    machinery — see Accident, machine
    railway rolling stock, train, vehicle (part of) E805 ☑
    street car E829 ☑
    vehicle NEC — see Accident, vehicle NEC
  in
    machinery — see Accident, machine
    object E918
    transport accident — see categories E800-E848
  late effect of NEC E929.9
Cut, cutting (any part of body) (accidental) E920.9
  by
    arrow E920.8
    axe E920.4
    bayonet (see also Bayonet wound) E920.3
    blender E920.2
    broken glass E920.8
      following fall E888.0
    can opener E920.4
      powered E920.2
    chisel E920.4
    circular saw E919.4
    cutting or piercing instrument (see also category) E920 ☑
      following fall E888.0
      late effect of E929.8
    dagger E920.3
    dart E920.8
    drill — see Accident, caused by drill
    edge of stiff paper E920.8
    electric
      beater E920.2
      fan E920.2
      knife E920.2
      mixer E920.2
    fork E920.4
    garden fork E920.4
    hand saw or tool (not powered) E920.4
      powered E920.1
    hedge clipper E920.4
      powered E920.1
    hoe E920.4

Index to External Causes

Cut, cutting — continued
  by — continued
    ice pick E920.4
    knife E920.3
      electric E920.2
    lathe turnings E920.8
    lawn mower E920.4
      powered E920.0
      riding E919.8
    machine — see Accident, machine
    meat
      grinder E919.8
      slicer E919.8
    nails E920.8
    needle E920.4
      hypodermic E920.5
    object, edged, pointed, sharp — see category E920 ☑
    following fall E888.0
    paper cutter E920.4
    piercing instrument (see also category) E920 ☑
    late effect of E929.8
    pitchfork E920.4
    powered
      can opener E920.2
      garden cultivator E920.1
        riding E919.8
      hand saw E920.1
      hand tool NEC E920.1
      hedge clipper E920.1
      household appliance or implement E920.2
      lawn mower (hand) E920.0
        riding E919.8
      rivet gun E920.1
      staple gun E920.1
    rake E920.4
    saw
      circular E919.4
      hand E920.4
    scissors E920.4
    screwdriver E920.4
    sewing machine (electric) (powered) E920.2
      not powered E920.4
    shears E920.4
    shovel E920.4
    spade E920.4
    splinters E920.8
    sword E920.3
    tin can lid E920.8
    wood slivers E920.8
  homicide (attempt) E966
  inflicted by other person
    stated as
      intentional, homicidal E966
      undetermined whether accidental or intentional E986
  late effect of NEC E929.8
  legal
    execution E978
    intervention E974
  self-inflicted (unspecified whether accidental or intentional) E986
    stated as intentional, purposeful E956
  stated as undetermined whether accidental or intentional E986
  suicidal (attempt) E956
  terrorism E979.8
  war operations E995
Cyclone E908.1

D

Death due to injury occurring one year or more previous — see Late effect
Decapitation (accidental circumstances) NEC E928.9
  homicidal E966
  legal execution (by guillotine) E978
Deprivation — see also Privation
  homicidal intent E968.4

Derailment (accidental)
  railway (rolling stock) (train) (vehicle) (with subsequent collision) E802 ☑
    with
      collision (antecedent) (see also Collision, railway) E800 ☑
      explosion (subsequent) (without antecedent collision) E802 ☑
        antecedent collision E803 ☑
      fall (without collision (antecedent)) E802 ☑
      fire (without collision (antecedent)) E802 ☑
  street car E829 ☑
Descent
  parachute (voluntary) (without accident to aircraft) E844 ☑
    due to accident to aircraft — see categories E840-E842 ☑
Desertion
  child, with intent to injure or kill E968.4
  helpless person, infant, newborn E904.0
    with intent to injure or kill E968.4
Destitution — see Privation
Disability, late effect or sequela of injury — see Late effect
Disease
  Andes E902.0
  aviators' E902.1
  caisson E902.2
  range E902.0
Divers' disease, palsy, paralysis, squeeze E902.0
Dog bite E906.0
Dragged by
  cable car (not on rails) E847
    on rails E829 ☑
  motor vehicle (on highway) E814 ☑
    not on highway, nontraffic accident E825 ☑
  street car E829 ☑
Drinking poison (accidental) — see Table of Drugs and Chemicals
Drowning — see Submersion
Dust in eye E914

E

Earth falling (on) (with asphyxia or suffocation (by pressure)) — see also Suffocation, due to, cave-in E913.3
  as, or due to, a cataclysm (involving any transport vehicle) — see categories E908 ☑, E909 ☑
  not due to cataclysmic action E913.3
    motor vehicle (in motion) (on public highway) E813 ☑
      not on public highway E825 ☑
    nonmotor road vehicle NEC E829 ☑
    pedal cycle E826 ☑
    railway rolling stock, train, vehicle E806 ☑
    street car E829 ☑
    struck or crushed by E916
      with asphyxiation or suffocation E913.3
      with injury other than asphyxia, suffocation E916
Earthquake (any injury) E909.0
Effect(s) (adverse) of
  air pressure E902.9
    at high altitude E902.9
      in aircraft E902.1
      residence or prolonged visit (causing conditions classifiable to E902.0) E902.0
    due to
      diving E902.2
      specified cause NEC E902.8
    in aircraft E902.1

Effect(s) (adverse) of — continued
  cold, excessive (exposure to) (see also Cold, exposure to) E901.9
  heat (excessive) (see also Heat) E900.9
  hot
    place — see Heat
    weather E900.0
  insulation — see Heat
  late — see Late effect of
  motion E903
  nuclear explosion or weapon
    in
      terrorism E979.5
      war operations (blast) (fireball) (heat) (radiation) (direct) (secondary) E996
  radiation — see Radiation
  terrorism, secondary E979.9
  travel E903
Electric shock, electrocution (accidental) (from exposed wire, faulty appliance, high voltage cable, live rail, open socket) (by) (in) E925.9
  appliance or wiring
    domestic E925.0
    factory E925.2
    farm (building) E925.8
      house E925.0
    home E925.0
    industrial (conductor) (control apparatus) (transformer) E925.2
    outdoors E925.8
    public building E925.8
    residential institution E925.8
    school E925.8
    specified place NEC E925.8
  caused by other person
    stated as
      intentional, homicidal E968.8
      undetermined whether accidental or intentional E988.4
  electric power generating plant, distribution station E925.1
  homicide (attempt) E968.8
  legal execution E978
  lightning E907
  machinery E925.9
    domestic E925.0
    factory E925.2
    farm E925.8
    home E925.0
  misadventure in medical or surgical procedure
    in electroshock therapy E873.4
  self-inflicted (undetermined whether accidental or intentional) E988.4
    stated as intentional E958.4
  stated as undetermined whether accidental or intentional E988.4
  suicidal (attempt) E958.4
  transmission line E925.1
Electrocution — see Electric shock
Embolism
  air (traumatic) NEC — see Air, embolism
Encephalitis
  lead or saturnine E866.0
    from pesticide NEC E863.4
Entanglement
  in
    bedclothes, causing suffocation E913.0
    wheel of pedal cycle E826 ☑
Entry of foreign body, material, any — see Foreign body
Execution, legal (any method) E978
Exhaustion
  cold — see Cold, exposure to
  due to excessive exertion E927
  heat — see Heat
Explosion (accidental) (in) (of) (on) E923.9
  acetylene E923.2
  aerosol can E921.8

Explosion

Explosion — continued
  aircraft (in transit) (powered) E841 ☑
    at landing, take-off E840 ☑
    in
      terrorism E979.1
      war operations E994
    unpowered E842 ☑
  air tank (compressed) (in machinery) E921.1
  anesthetic gas in operating theatre E923.2
  automobile tire NEC E921.8
    causing transport accident — see categories E810-E825 ☑
  blasting (cap) (materials) E923.1
  boiler (machinery), not on transport vehicle E921.0
    steamship — see Explosion, watercraft
  bomb E923.8
    in
      terrorism E979.2
      war operations E993
        after cessation of hostilities E998
        atom, hydrogen or nuclear E996
        injury by fragments from E991.9
          antipersonnel bomb E991.3
  butane E923.2
  caused by
    other person
      stated as
        intentional, homicidal — see Assault, explosive
        undetermined whether accidental or homicidal E985.5
  coal gas E923.2
  detonator E923.1
  dynamite E923.1
  explosive (material) NEC E923.9
    gas(es) E923.2
    missile E923.8
      in
        terrorism E979.2
        war operations E993
          injury by fragments from E991.9
            antipersonnel bomb E991.3
    used in blasting operations E923.1
  fire-damp E923.2
  fireworks E923.0
  gas E923.2
    cylinder (in machinery) E921.1
    pressure tank (in machinery) E921.1
  gasoline (fumes) (tank) not in moving motor vehicle E923.2
  grain store (military) (munitions) E923.8
  grenade E923.8
    in
      terrorism E979.2
      war operations E993
        injury by fragments from E991.9
  homicide (attempt) — see Assault, explosive
  hot water heater, tank (in machinery) E921.0
  in mine (of explosive gases) NEC E923.2
  late effect of NEC E929.8
  machinery (see also Accident, machine)
    pressure vessel — see Explosion, pressure vessel
  methane E923.2
  missile E923.8
    in
      terrorism E979.2
      war operations E993

Explosion — *continued*
  missile — *continued*
    in — *continued*
      war operations — *continued*
        injury by fragments from E991.9
  motor vehicle (part of)
    in motion (on public highway) E818 ☑
      not on public highway E825 ☑
  munitions (dump) (factory) E923.8
    in
      terrorism E979.2
      war operations E993
  of mine E923.8
    in
      terrorism
        at sea or in harbor E979.0
        land E979.2
        marine E979.0
      war operations
        after cessation of hostilities E998
        at sea or in harbor E992
        land E993
          after cessation of hostilities E998
          injury by fragments from E991.9
          marine E992
  own weapons
    in
      terrorism (*see also* Suicide) E979.2
      war operations E993
        injury by fragments from E991.9
          antipersonnel bomb E991.3
  pressure
    cooker E921.8
    gas tank (in machinery) E921.1
    vessel (in machinery) E921.9
      on transport vehicle — *see* categories E800-E848 ☑
      specified type NEC E921.8
  propane E923.2
  railway engine, locomotive, train (boiler) (with subsequent collision, derailment, fall) E803 ☑
    with
      collision (antecedent) (*see also* Collision, railway) E800 ☑
      derailment (antecedent) E802 ☑
      fire (without antecedent collision or derailment) E803 ☑
  secondary fire resulting from — *see* Fire
  self-inflicted (unspecified whether accidental or intentional) E985.5
    stated as intentional, purposeful E955.5
  shell (artillery) E923.8
    in
      terrorism E979.2
      war operations E993
        injury by fragments from E991.9
  stated as undetermined whether caused accidentally or purposely inflicted E985.5
  steam or water lines (in machinery) E921.0
  suicide (attempted) E955.5
  terrorism — *see* Terrorism, explosion
  torpedo E923.8
    in
      terrorism E979.0
      war operations E992
  transport accident — *see* categories E800-E848 ☑
  war operations — *see* War operations, explosion
  watercraft (boiler) E837 ☑

Explosion — *continued*
  watercraft — *continued*
    causing drowning, submersion (after jumping from watercraft) E830 ☑
Exposure (weather) (conditions) (rain) (wind) E904.3
  with homicidal intent E968.4
  excessive E904.3
    cold (*see also* Cold, exposure to) E901.9
      self-inflicted — *see* Cold, exposure to, self-inflicted
    heat (*see also* Heat) E900.9
  helpless person, infant, newborn due to abandonment or neglect E904.0
  noise E928.1
  prolonged in deep-freeze unit or refrigerator E901.1
  radiation — *see* Radiation
  resulting from transport accident — *see* categories E800-E848 ☑
  smoke from, due to
    fire — *see* Fire
    tobacco, second-hand E869.4
  vibration E928.2

F

Fallen on by
  animal (horse) (not being ridden) E906.8
    being ridden (in sport or transport) E828 ☑
Fall, falling (accidental) E888.9
  building E916
    burning E891.8
      private E890.8
  down
    escalator E880.0
    ladder E881.0
      in boat, ship, watercraft E833 ☑
    staircase E880.9
    stairs, steps — *see* Fall, from, stairs
  earth (with asphyxia or suffocation (by pressure)) (*see also* Earth, falling) E913.3
  from, off
    aircraft (at landing, take-off) (in-transit) (while alighting, boarding) E843 ☑
      resulting from accident to aircraft — *see* categories E840-E842 ☑
    animal (in sport or transport) E828 ☑
    animal-drawn vehicle E827 ☑
    balcony E882
    bed E884.4
    bicycle E826 ☑
    boat, ship, watercraft (into water) E832 ☑
      after accident to, collision, fire on E830 ☑
      and subsequently struck by (part of) boat E831 ☑
      and subsequently struck by (part of) while alighting, boat E831 ☑
      burning, crushed, sinking E830 ☑
      and subsequently struck by (part of) boat E831 ☑
    bridge E882
    building E882
      burning (uncontrolled fire) E891.8
        in terrorism E979.3
        private E890.8
    bunk in boat, ship, watercraft E834 ☑
      due to accident to watercraft E831 ☑
    cable car (not on rails) E847

Fall, falling — *continued*
  from, off — *continued*
    cable car — *continued*
      on rails E829 ☑
    car — *see* Fall from motor vehicle
    chair E884.2
    cliff E884.1
    commode E884.6
    curb (sidewalk) E880.1
    elevation aboard ship E834 ☑
      due to accident to ship E831 ☑
    embankment E884.9
    escalator E880.0
    fire escape E882
    flagpole E882
    furniture NEC E884.5
    gangplank (into water) (*see also* Fall, from, boat) E832 ☑
      to deck, dock E834 ☑
    hammock on ship E834 ☑
      due to accident to watercraft E831 ☑
    haystack E884.9
    high place NEC E884.9
      stated as undetermined whether accidental or intentional — *see* Jumping, from, high place
    horse (in sport or transport) E828 ☑
    in-line skates E885.1
    ladder E881.0
      in boat, ship, watercraft E833 ☑
      due to accident to watercraft E831 ☑
    machinery (*see also* Accident, machine)
      not in operation E884.9
    motor vehicle (in motion) (on public highway) E818 ☑
      not on public highway E825 ☑
      stationary, except while alighting, boarding, entering, leaving E884.9
      while alighting, boarding, entering, leaving E824 ☑
      stationary, except while alighting, boarding, entering, leaving E884.9
      while alighting, boarding, entering, leaving, except off-road type motor vehicle E817 ☑
      off-road type — *see* Fall, from, off-road type motor vehicle
    nonmotor road vehicle (while alighting, boarding) NEC E829 ☑
      stationary, except while alighting, boarding, entering, leaving E884.9
    off road type motor vehicle (not on public highway) NEC E821 ☑
      on public highway E818 ☑
      while alighting, boarding, entering, leaving E817 ☑
    snow vehicle — *see* Fall from snow vehicle, motor-driven
  one
    deck to another on ship E834 ☑
      due to accident to ship E831 ☑
    level to another NEC E884.9
      boat, ship, or watercraft E834 ☑
        due to accident to watercraft E831 ☑
  pedal cycle E826 ☑
  playground equipment E884.0

Fall, falling — *continued*
  from, off — *continued*
    railway rolling stock, train, vehicle (while alighting, boarding) E804 ☑
      with
        collision (*see also* Collision, railway) E800 ☑
        derailment (*see also* Derailment, railway) E802 ☑
        explosion (*see also* Explosion, railway engine) E803 ☑
    rigging (aboard ship) E834 ☑
      due to accident to watercraft E831 ☑
    roller skates E885.1
    scaffolding E881.1
    scooter (nonmotorized) E885.0
    sidewalk (curb) E880.1
      moving E885.9
    skateboard E885.2
    skis E885.3
    snowboard E885.4
    snow vehicle, motor-driven (not on public highway) E820 ☑
      on public highway E818 ☑
        while alighting, boarding, entering, leaving E817 ☑
    stairs, steps E880.9
      boat, ship, watercraft E833 ☑
        due to accident to watercraft E831 ☑
      motor bus, motor vehicle — *see* Fall, from, motor vehicle, while alighting, boarding
      street car E829 ☑
    stationary vehicle NEC E884.9
    stepladder E881.0
    street car (while boarding, alighting) E829 ☑
      stationary, except while boarding or alighting E884.9
    structure NEC E882
      burning (uncontrolled fire) E891.8
        in terrorism E979.3
    table E884.9
    toilet E884.6
    tower E882
    tree E884.9
    turret E882
    vehicle NEC (*see also* Accident, vehicle NEC)
      stationary E884.9
    viaduct E882
    wall E882
    wheelchair E884.3
    window E882
  in, on
    aircraft (at landing, take-off) (in-transit) E843 ☑
      resulting from accident to aircraft — *see* categories E840-E842 ☑
    boat, ship, watercraft E835 ☑
      due to accident to watercraft E831 ☑
    one level to another NEC E834 ☑
    on ladder, stairs E833 ☑
    cutting or piercing instrument or machine E888.0
    deck (of boat, ship, watercraft) E835 ☑
      due to accident to watercraft E831 ☑
    escalator E880.0
    gangplank E835 ☑
    glass, broken E888.0
    knife E888.0
    ladder E881.0
      in boat, ship, watercraft E833 ☑
        due to accident to watercraft E831 ☑

Index to External Causes

Fall, falling — *continued*
  in, on — *continued*
    object
      edged, pointed or sharp E888.0
      other E888.1
    pitchfork E888.0
    railway rolling stock, train, vehicle (while alighting, boarding) E804 ☑
      with
        collision (*see also* Collision, railway) E800 ☑
        derailment (*see also* Derailment, railway) E802 ☑
        explosion (*see also* Explosion, railway engine) E803 ☑
    scaffolding E881.1
    scissors E888.0
    staircase, stairs, steps (*see also* Fall, from, stairs) E880.9
    street car E829 ☑
    water transport (*see also* Fall, in, boat) E835 ☑
  into
    cavity E883.9
    dock E883.9
      from boat, ship, watercraft (*see also* Fall, from, boat) E832 ☑
    hold (of ship) E834 ☑
      due to accident to watercraft E831 ☑
    hole E883.9
    manhole E883.2
    moving part of machinery — *see* Accident, machine
    opening in surface NEC E883.9
    pit E883.9
    quarry E883.9
    shaft E883.9
    storm drain E883.2
    tank E883.9
    water (with drowning or submersion) E910.9
    well E883.1
  late effect of NEC E929.3
  object (*see also* Hit by, object, falling) E916
  other E888.8
  over
    animal E885.9
    cliff E884.1
    embankment E884.9
    small object E885.9
  overboard (*see also* Fall, from, boat) E832 ☑
  resulting in striking against object E888.1
    sharp E888.0
  rock E916
  same level NEC E888.9
    aircraft (any kind) E843 ☑
      resulting from accident to aircraft — *see* categories E840-E842 ☑
    boat, ship, watercraft E835 ☑
      due to accident to, collision, watercraft E831 ☑
    from
      collision, pushing, shoving, by or with other person(s) E886.9
        as, or caused by, a crowd E917.6
        in sports E886.0
      in-line skates E885.1
      roller skates E885.1
      scooter (nonmotorized) E885.0
      skateboard E885.2
      slipping stumbling, tripping E885
      snowboard E885.4
  snowslide E916
    as avalanche E909.2
  stone E916

Fall, falling — *continued*
  through
    hatch (on ship) E834 ☑
      due to accident to watercraft E831 ☑
    roof E882
    window E882
    timber E916
  while alighting from, boarding, entering, leaving
    aircraft (any kind) E843 ☑
    motor bus, motor vehicle — *see* Fall, from, motor vehicle, while alighting, boarding
    nonmotor road vehicle NEC E829 ☑
    railway train E804 ☑
    street car E829 ☑
Fell or jumped from high place, so stated — *see* Jumping, from, high place
Felo-de-se — *see also* Suicide E958.9
Fever
  heat — *see* Heat
  thermic — *see* Heat
Fight (hand) (fist) (foot) — *see also* Assault, fight E960.0
Fire (accidental) (caused by great heat from appliance (electrical), hot object or hot substance) (secondary, resulting from explosion) E899
  conflagration — *see* Conflagration
  controlled, normal (in brazier, fireplace, furnace, or stove) (charcoal) (coal) (coke) (electric) (gas) (wood)
    bonfire E897
    brazier, not in building or structure E897
    in building or structure, except private dwelling (barn) (church) (convalescent or residential home) (factory) (farm outbuilding) (hospital) (hotel) (institution (educational) (dormitory) (residential)) (private garage) (school) (shop) (store) (theatre) E896
    in private dwelling (apartment) (boarding house) (camping place) (caravan) (farmhouse) (home (private)) (house) (lodging house) (rooming house) (tenement) E895
    not in building or structure E897
    trash E897
  forest (uncontrolled) E892
  grass (uncontrolled) E892
  hay (uncontrolled) E892
  homicide (attempt) E968.0
    late effect of E969
  in, of, on, starting in E892
    aircraft (in transit) (powered) E841 ☑
      at landing, take-off E840 ☑
      stationary E892
      unpowered (balloon) (glider) E842 ☑
    balloon E842 ☑
    boat, ship, watercraft — *see* categories E830 ☑, E831 ☑, E837 ☑
    building or structure, except private dwelling (barn) (church) (convalescent or residential home) (factory) (farm outbuilding) (hospital) (hotel) (institution (educational) (dormitory) (residential)) (school) (shop) (store) (theatre) (*see also* Conflagration, building or structure, except private dwelling E891.9
    forest (uncontrolled) E892
    glider E842 ☑
    grass (uncontrolled) E892

Fire, hot object or hot substance — *continued*
  in, of, on, starting in — *continued*
    hay (uncontrolled) E892
    lumber (uncontrolled) E892
    machinery — *see* Accident, machine
    mine (uncontrolled) E892
    motor vehicle (in motion) (on public highway) E818 ☑
      not on public highway E825 ☑
      stationary E892
    prairie (uncontrolled) E892
    private dwelling (apartment) (boarding house) (camping place) (caravan) (farmhouse) (home (private)) (house) (lodging house) (private garage) (rooming house) (tenement) (*see also* Conflagration, private dwelling) E890.9
    railway rolling stock, train, vehicle (*see also* Explosion, railway engine) E803 ☑
      stationary E892
    room NEC E898.1
    street car (in motion) E829 ☑
      stationary E892
    terrorism (by fire-producing device) E979.3
    fittings or furniture (burning building) (uncontrolled fire) E979.3
    from nuclear explosion E979.5
    transport vehicle, stationary NEC E892
    tunnel (uncontrolled) E892
    war operations (by fire-producing device or conventional weapon) E990.9
      from nuclear explosion E996
      petrol bomb E990.0
  late effect of NEC E929.4
  lumber (uncontrolled) E892
  mine (uncontrolled) E892
  prairie (uncontrolled) E892
  self-inflicted (unspecified whether accidental or intentional) E988.1
    stated as intentional, purposeful E958.1
  specified NEC E898.1
  with
    conflagration — *see* Conflagration
    ignition (of)
      clothing — *see* Ignition, clothes
      highly inflammable material (benzine) (fat) (gasoline) (kerosene) (paraffin) (petrol) E894
  started by other person
    stated as
      with intent to injure or kill E968.0
      undetermined whether or not with intent to injure or kill E988.1
  suicide (attempted) E958.1
    late effect of E959
  tunnel (uncontrolled) E892
Fireball effects from nuclear explosion
  in
    terrorism E979.5
    war operations E996
Fireworks (explosion) E923.0
Flash burns from explosion — *see also* Explosion E923.9
Flood (any injury) (resulting from storm) E908.2
  caused by collapse of dam or man-made structure E909.3
Forced landing (aircraft) E840 ☑

Foreign body, object or material (entrance into) (accidental)
  air passage (causing injury) E915
    with asphyxia, obstruction, suffocation E912
      food or vomitus E911
    nose (with asphyxia, obstruction, suffocation) E912
      causing injury without asphyxia, obstruction, suffocation E915
  alimentary canal (causing injury) (with obstruction) E915
    with asphyxia, obstruction respiratory passage, suffocation E912
    food E911
    mouth E915
      with asphyxia, obstruction, suffocation E912
        food E911
    pharynx E915
      with asphyxia, obstruction, suffocation E912
        food E911
  aspiration (with asphyxia, obstruction respiratory passage, suffocation) E912
    causing injury without asphyxia, obstruction respiratory passage, suffocation E915
    food (regurgitated) (vomited) E911
      causing injury without asphyxia, obstruction respiratory passage, suffocation E915
  mucus (not of newborn) E912
  phlegm E912
  bladder (causing injury or obstruction) E915
  bronchus, bronchi — *see* Foreign body, air passages
  conjunctival sac E914
  digestive system — *see* Foreign body, alimentary canal
  ear (causing injury or obstruction) E915
  esophagus (causing injury or obstruction) (*see also* Foreign body, alimentary canal) E915
  eye (any part) E914
  eyelid E914
  hairball (stomach) (with obstruction) E915
  ingestion — *see* Foreign body, alimentary canal
  inhalation — *see* Foreign body, aspiration
  intestine (causing injury or obstruction) E915
  iris E914
  lacrimal apparatus E914
  larynx — *see* Foreign body, air passage
  late effect of NEC E929.8
  lung — *see* Foreign body, air passage
  mouth — *see* Foreign body, alimentary canal, mouth
  nasal passage — *see* Foreign body, air passage, nose
  nose — *see* Foreign body, air passage, nose
  ocular muscle E914
  operation wound (left in) — *see* Misadventure, foreign object
  orbit E914
  pharynx — *see* Foreign body, alimentary canal, pharynx
  rectum (causing injury or obstruction) E915
  stomach (hairball) (causing injury or obstruction) E915
  tear ducts or glands E914
  trachea — *see* Foreign body, air passage
  urethra (causing injury or obstruction) E915

Foreign body, object or material

Foreign body, object or material — *continued*
  vagina (causing injury or obstruction) E915
Found dead, injured
  from exposure (to) — *see* Exposure
  on
    public highway E819 ☑
    railway right of way E807 ☑
Fracture (circumstances unknown or unspecified) E887
  due to specified external means — *see* manner of accident
  late effect of NEC E929.3
  occurring in water transport NEC E835 ☑
Freezing — *see* Cold, exposure to
Frostbite E901.0
  due to manmade conditions E901.1
Frozen — *see* Cold, exposure to

G

Garrotting, homicidal (attempted) E963
Gored E906.8
Gunshot wound — *see also* Shooting E922.9

H

Hailstones, injury by E904.3
Hairball (stomach) (with obstruction) E915
Hanged himself — *see also* Hanging, self-inflicted E983.0
Hang gliding E842 ☑
Hanging (accidental) E913.8
  caused by other person
    in accidental circumstances E913.8
    stated as
      intentional, homicidal E963
      undetermined whether accidental or intentional E983.0
  homicide (attempt) E963
  in bed or cradle E913.0
  legal execution E978
  self-inflicted (unspecified whether accidental or intentional) E983.0
    in accidental circumstances E913.8
    stated as intentional, purposeful E953.0
    stated as undetermined whether accidental or intentional E983.0
  suicidal (attempt) E953.0
Heat (apoplexy) (collapse) (cramps) (effects of) (excessive) (exhaustion) (fever) (prostration) (stroke) E900.9
  due to
    manmade conditions (as listed in E900.1, except boat, ship, watercraft) E900.1
    weather (conditions) E900.0
  from
    electric heating appartus causing burning E924.8
    nuclear explosion
      in
        terrorism E979.5
        war operations E996
  generated in, boiler, engine, evaporator, fire room of boat, ship, watercraft E838 ☑
  inappropriate in local application or packing in medical or surgical procedure E873.5
  late effect of NEC E989
Hemorrhage
  delayed following medical or surgical treatment without mention of misadventure — *see* Reaction, abnormal
  during medical or surgical treatment as misadventure — *see* Misadventure, cut

High
  altitude, effects E902.9
  level of radioactivity, effects — *see* Radiation
  pressure effects (*see also* Effects of, air pressure)
    from rapid descent in water (causing caisson or divers' disease, palsy, or paralysis) E902.2
  temperature, effects — *see* Heat
Hit, hitting (accidental) by
  aircraft (propeller) (without accident to aircraft) E844 ☑
    unpowered E842 ☑
  avalanche E909.2
  being thrown against object in or part of
    motor vehicle (in motion) (on public highway) E818 ☑
      not on public highway E825 ☑
    nonmotor road vehicle NEC E829 ☑
    street car E829 ☑
  boat, ship, watercraft
    after fall from watercraft E838 ☑
    damaged, involved in accident E831 ☑
    while swimming, water skiing E838 ☑
  bullet (*see also* Shooting) E922.9
    from air gun E922.4
    in
      terrorism E979.4
      war operations E991.2
        rubber E991.0
  flare, Verey pistol (*see also* Shooting) E922.8
  hailstones E904.3
  landslide E909.2
  law-enforcing agent (on duty) E975
    with blunt object (baton) (night stick) (stave) (truncheon) E973
  machine — *see* Accident, machine
  missile
    firearm (*see also* Shooting) E922.9
    in
      terrorism — *see* Terrorism, missile
      war operations — *see* War operations, missile
  motor vehicle (on public highway) (traffic accident) E814 ☑
    not on public highway, nontraffic accident E822 ☑
  nonmotor road vehicle NEC E829 ☑
  object
    falling E916
      from, in, on
        aircraft E844 ☑
          due to accident to aircraft — *see* categories E840-E842 ☑
          unpowered E842 ☑
        boat, ship, watercraft E838 ☑
          due to accident to watercraft E831 ☑
        building E916
          burning (uncontrolled fire) E891.8
            in terrorism E979.3
            private E890.8
        cataclysmic
          earth surface movement or eruption E909.9
          storm E908.9
        cave-in E916
          with asphyxiation or suffocation (*see also* Suffocation, due to cave-in) E913.3
        earthquake E909.0
        motor vehicle (in motion) (on public highway) E818 ☑

Hit, hitting by — *continued*
  object — *continued*
    falling — *continued*
      from, in, on — *continued*
        motor vehicle — *continued*
          not on public highway E825 ☑
          stationary E916
        nonmotor road vehicle NEC E829
        pedal cycle E826 ☑
        railway rolling stock, train, vehicle E806 ☑
        street car E829 ☑
        structure, burning NEC E891.8
        vehicle, stationary E916
    moving NEC — *see* Striking against, object
    projected NEC — *see* Striking against, object
    set in motion by
      compressed air or gas, spring, striking, throwing — *see* Striking against, object
      explosion — *see* Explosion
    thrown into, on, or towards
      motor vehicle (in motion) (on public highway) E818 ☑
        not on public highway E825 ☑
      nonmotor road vehicle NEC E829 ☑
      pedal cycle E826 ☑
      street car E829 ☑
  off-road type motor vehicle (not on public highway) E821 ☑
    on public highway E814 ☑
  other person(s) E917.9
    with blunt or thrown object E917.9
      in sports E917.0
        with subsequent fall E917.5
    intentionally, homicidal E968.2
    as, or caused by, a crowd E917.1
      with subsequent fall E917.6
    in sports E917.0
  pedal cycle E826 ☑
  police (on duty) E975
    with blunt object (baton) (nightstick) (stave) (truncheon) E973
  railway, rolling stock, train, vehicle (part of) E805 ☑
  shot — *see* Shooting
  snow vehicle, motor-driven (not on public highway) E820 ☑
    on public highway E814 ☑
  street car E829 ☑
  vehicle NEC — *see* Accident, vehicle NEC
Homicide, homicidal (attempt) (justifiable) — *see also* Assault E968.9
Hot
  liquid, object, substance, accident caused by (*see also* Accident, caused by, hot, by type of substance)
  late effect of E929.8
  place, effects — *see* Heat
  weather, effects E900.0
Humidity, causing problem E904.3
Hunger E904.1
  resulting from
    abandonment or neglect E904.0
    transport accident — *see* categories E800-E848
Hurricane (any injury) E908.0
Hypobarism, hypobaropathy — *see* Effects of, air pressure
Hypothermia — *see* Cold, exposure to

I

Ictus
  caloris — *see* Heat

Ictus — *continued*
  solaris E900.0
Ignition (accidental)
  anesthetic gas in operating theatre E923.2
  bedclothes
    with
      conflagration — *see* Conflagration
      ignition (of)
        clothing — *see* Ignition, clothes
        highly inflammable material (benzine) (fat) (gasoline) (kerosene) (paraffin) (petrol) E894
  benzine E894
  clothes, clothing (from controlled fire) (in building) E893.9
    with conflagration — *see* Conflagration
    from
      bonfire E893.2
      highly inflammable material E894
      sources or material as listed in E893.8
      trash fire E893.2
      uncontrolled fire — *see* Conflagration
    in
      private dwelling E893.0
      specified building or structure, except private dwelling E893.1
    not in building or structure E893.2
  explosive material — *see* Explosion
  fat E894
  gasoline E894
  kerosene E894
  material
    explosive — *see* Explosion
    highly inflammable E894
      with conflagration — *see* Conflagration
      with explosion E923.2
  nightdress — *see* Ignition, clothes
  paraffin E894
  petrol E894
Immersion — *see* Submersion
Implantation of quills of porcupine E906.8
Inanition (from) E904.9
  hunger — *see* Lack of, food
  resulting from homicidal intent E968.4
  thirst — *see* Lack of, water
Inattention after, at birth E904.0
  homicidal, infanticidal intent E968.4
Infanticide — *see also* Assault
Ingestion
  foreign body (causing injury) (with obstruction) — *see* Foreign body, alimentary canal
  poisonous substance NEC — *see* Table of Drugs and Chemicals
Inhalation
  excessively cold substance, manmade E901.1
  foreign body — *see* Foreign body, aspiration
  liquid air, hydrogen, nitrogen E901.1
  mucus, not of newborn (with asphyxia, obstruction respiratory passage, suffocation) E912
  phlegm (with asphyxia, obstruction respiratory passage, suffocation) E912
  poisonous gas — *see* Table of Drugs and Chemicals
  smoke from, due to
    fire — *see* Fire
    tobacco, second-hand E869.4
  vomitus (with asphyxia, obstruction respiratory passage, suffocation) E911

Index to External Causes

Injury, injured (accidental(ly)) NEC E928.9
  by, caused by, from
    air rifle (BB gun) E922.4
    animal (not being ridden) NEC E906.9
      being ridden (in sport or transport) E828 ☑
    assault (see also Assault) E968.9
    avalanche E909.2
    bayonet (see also Bayonet wound) E920.3
    being thrown against some part of, or object in
      motor vehicle (in motion) (on public highway) E818 ☑
        not on public highway E825 ☑
      nonmotor road vehicle NEC E829 ☑
      off-road motor vehicle NEC E821 ☑
      railway train E806 ☑
      snow vehicle, motor-driven E820 ☑
      street car E829 ☑
    bending E927
    bite, human E928.3
    broken glass E920.8
    bullet — see Shooting
    cave-in (see also Suffocation, due to, cave-in) E913.3
      without asphyxiation or suffocation E916
    earth surface movement or eruption E909.9
      storm E908.9
    cloudburst E908.8
    cutting or piercing instrument (see also Cut) E920.9
    cyclone E908.1
    earthquake E909.0
    earth surface movement or eruption E909.9
    electric current (see also Electric shock) E925.9
    explosion (see also Explosion) E923.9
    fire — see Fire
    flare, Verey pistol E922.8
    flood E908.2
    foreign body — see Foreign body
    hailstones E904.3
    hurricane E908.0
    landslide E909.2
    law-enforcing agent, police, in course of legal intervention — see Legal intervention
    lightning E907
    live rail or live wire — see Electric shock
    machinery (see also Accident, machine)
      aircraft, without accident to aircraft E844 ☑
      boat, ship, watercraft (deck) (engine room) (galley) (laundry) (loading) E836 ☑
    missile
      explosive E923.8
      firearm — see Shooting
      in
        terrorism — see Terrorism, missile
        war operations — see War operations, missile
    moving part of motor vehicle (in motion) (on public highway) E818 ☑
      not on public highway, nontraffic accident E825 ☑
      while alighting, boarding, entering, leaving — see Fall, from, motor vehicle, while alighting, boarding

Injury, injured — continued
  by, caused by, from — continued
    nail E920.8
    needle (sewing) E920.4
      hypodermic E920.5
    noise E928.1
    object
      fallen on
        motor vehicle (in motion) (on public highway) E818 ☑
        not on public highway E825 ☑
      falling — see Hit by, object, falling
    paintball gun E922.5
    radiation — see Radiation
    railway rolling stock, train, vehicle (part of) E805 ☑
      door or window E806 ☑
    rotating propeller, aircraft E844 ☑
    rough landing of off-road type motor vehicle (after leaving ground or rough terrain) E821 ☑
    saber (see also Wound, saber) E920.3
    shot — see Shooting
    snow vehicle E820 ☑
    sound waves E928.1
    splinter or sliver, wood E920.8
    straining E927
    street car (door) E829 ☑
    suicide (attempt) E958.9
    sword E920.3
    terrorism — see Terrorism
    third rail — see Electric shock
    thunderbolt E907
    tidal wave E909.4
      caused by storm E908.0
    tornado E908.1
    torrential rain E908.2
    twisting E927
    vehicle NEC — see Accident, vehicle NEC
    vibration E928.2
    volcanic eruption E909.1
    weapon burst, in war operations E993
    weightlessness (in spacecraft, real or simulated) E928.0
    wood splinter or sliver E920.8
  due to
    civil insurrection — see War operations
      occurring after cessation of hostilities E998
    terrorism — see Terrorism
    war operations — see War operations
      occurring after cessation of hostilities E998
  homicidal (see also Assault) E968.9
  inflicted by
    in course of arrest (attempted), suppression of disturbance, maintenance of order, by law enforcing agents — see Legal intervention
    law-enforcing agent (on duty) — see Legal intervention
    other person
      stated as
        accidental E928.9
        homicidal, intentional — see Assault
        undetermined whether accidental or intentional — see Injury, stated as undetermined
    police (on duty) — see Legal intervention
  in, on
    civil insurrection — see War operations
    fight E960.0

Injury, injured — continued
  in, on — continued
    parachute descent (voluntary) (without accident to aircraft) E844 ☑
      with accident to aircraft — see categories E840-E842 ☑
    public highway E819
    railway right of way E807 ☑
    terrorism — see Terrorism
    war operations — see War operations
  late effect of E929.9
  purposely (inflicted) by other person(s) — see Assault
  self-inflicted (unspecified whether accidental or intentional) E988.9
    stated as
      accidental E928.9
      intentionally, purposely E958.9
  specified cause NEC E928.8
  stated as
    hanging E983.0
    knife E986
    late effect of E989
    puncture (any part of body) E986
    shooting — see Shooting, stated as undetermined whether accidental or intentional
    specified means NEC E988.8
    stab (any part of body) E986
    strangulation — see Suffocation, stated as undetermined whether accidental or intentional
    submersion E984
    suffocation — see Suffocation, stated as undetermined whether accidental or intentional
  undetermined whether accidentally or purposely inflicted (by) E988.9
    cut (any part of body) E986
    cutting or piercing instrument (classifiable to E920) E986
    drowning E984
    explosive(s) (missile) E985.5
    falling from high place E987.9
      manmade structure, except residential E987.1
      natural site E987.2
      residential premises E987.0
  to child due to criminal abortion E968.8

Insufficient nourishment — see also Lack of, food
  homicidal intent E968.4
Insulation, effects — see Heat
Interruption of respiration by
  food lodged in esophagus E911
  foreign body, except food, in esophagus E912
Intervention, legal — see Legal intervention
Intoxication, drug or poison — see Table of Drugs and Chemicals
Irradiation — see Radiation

J

Jammed (accidentally)
  between objects (moving) (stationary and moving) E918
  in object E918
Jumped or fell from high place, so stated — see Jumping, from high place, stated as
  in undetermined circumstances
Jumping
  before train, vehicle or other moving object (unspecified whether accidental or intentional) E988.0
    stated as
      intentional, purposeful E958.0
      suicidal (attempt) E958.0

Jumping — continued
  from
    aircraft
      by parachute (voluntarily) (without accident to aircraft) E844 ☑
      due to accident to aircraft — see categories E840-E842 ☑
    boat, ship, watercraft (into water)
      after accident to, fire on, watercraft E830 ☑
        and subsequently struck by (part of) boat E831 ☑
      burning, crushed, sinking E830 ☑
        and subsequently struck by (part of) boat E831 ☑
      voluntarily, without accident (to boat) with injury other than drowning or submersion E883.0
    building (see also Jumping, from, high place)
      burning (uncontrolled fire) E891.8
        in terrorism E979.3
        private E890.8
    cable car (not on rails) E847
      on rails E829 ☑
    high place
      in accidental circumstances or in sport — see categories E880-E884 ☑
      stated as
        with intent to injure self E957.9
          man-made structures NEC E957.1
          natural sites E957.2
          residential premises E957.0
        in undetermined circumstances E987.9
          man-made structures NEC E987.1
          natural sites E987.2
          residential premises E987.0
        suicidal (attempt) E957.9
          man-made structures NEC E957.1
          natural sites E957.1
          residential premises E957.0
    motor vehicle (in motion) (on public highway) — see Fall, from, motor vehicle
    nonmotor road vehicle NEC E829 ☑
    street car E829 ☑
    structure (see also Jumping, from, high place)
      burning NEC (uncontrolled fire) E891.8
        in terrorism E979.3
  into water
    with injury other than drowning or submersion E883.0
    drowning or submersion — see Submersion
    from, off, watercraft — see Jumping, from, boat

Justifiable homicide — see Assault

K

Kicked by
  animal E906.8
  person(s) (accidentally) E917.9
    with intent to injure or kill E960.0
    as, or caused by a crowd E917.1
      with subsequent fall E917.6
    in fight E960.0
    in sports E917.0
      with subsequent fall E917.5
Kicking against
  object (moving) E917.9

Kicking against

Kicking against — *continued*
  object — *continued*
    in sports E917.0
      with subsequent fall E917.5
    stationary E917.4
      with subsequent fall E917.8
  person — *see* Striking against, person
Killed, killing (accidentally) NEC — *see also* Injury E928.9
  in
    action — *see* War operations
    brawl, fight (hand) (fists) (foot) E960.0
      by weapon (*see also* Assault)
        cutting, piercing E966
        firearm — *see* Shooting, homicide
  self
    stated as
      accident E928.9
      suicide — *see* Suicide
    unspecified whether accidental or suicidal E988.9
Knocked down (accidentally) (by) NEC E928.9
  animal (not being ridden) E906.8
    being ridden (in sport or transport) E828 ☑
  blast from explosion (*see also* Explosion) E923.9
  crowd, human stampede E917.6
  late effect of — *see* Late effect
  person (accidentally) E917.9
    in brawl, fight E960.0
    in sports E917.5
  transport vehicle — *see* vehicle involved under Hit by
  while boxing E917.5

L

Laceration NEC E928.9
Lack of
  air (refrigerator or closed place), suffocation by E913.2
  care (helpless person) (infant) (newborn) E904.0
    homicidal intent E968.4
  food except as result of transport accident E904.1
    helpless person, infant, newborn due to
      abandonment or neglect E904.0
  water except as result of transport accident E904.2
    helpless person, infant, newborn due to
      abandonment or neglect E904.0
Landslide E909.2
  falling on, hitting
    motor vehicle (any) (in motion) (on or off public highway) E909.2
    railway rolling stock, train, vehicle E909.2
Late effect of
  accident NEC (accident classifiable to E928.9) E929.9
    specified NEC (accident classifiable to E910–E928.8) E929.8
  assault E969
  fall, accidental (accident classifiable to E880–E888) E929.3
  fire, accident caused by (accident classifiable to E890–E899) E929.4
  homicide, attempt (any means) E969
  injury due to terrorism E999.1
  injury undetermined whether accidentally or purposely inflicted (injury classifiable to E980–E988) E989
  legal intervention (injury classifiable to E970–E976) E977

Late effect of — *continued*
  medical or surgical procedure, test or therapy
    as, or resulting in, or from
      abnormal or delayed reaction or complication — *see* Reaction, abnormal
      misadventure — *see* Misadventure
  motor vehicle accident (accident classifiable to E810–E825) E929.0
  natural or environmental factor, accident due to (accident classifiable to E900–E909) E929.5
  poisoning, accidental (accident classifiable to E850–E858, E860–E869) E929.2
  suicide, attempt (any means) E959
  transport accident NEC (accident classifiable to E800–E807, E826–E838, E840–E848) E929.1
  war operations, injury due to (injury classifiable to E990–E998) E999.0
Launching pad accident E845 ☑
Legal
  execution, any method E978
  intervention (by) (injury from) E976
    baton E973
    bayonet E974
    blow E975
    blunt object (baton) (nightstick) (stave) (truncheon) E973
    cutting or piercing instrument E974
    dynamite E971
    execution, any method E973
    explosive(s) (shell) E971
    firearm(s) E970
    gas (asphyxiation) (poisoning) (tear) E972
    grenade E971
    late effect of E977
    machine gun E970
    manhandling E975
    mortar bomb E971
    nightstick E973
    revolver E970
    rifle E970
    specified means NEC E975
    stabbing E974
    stave E973
    truncheon E973
Lifting, injury in E927
Lightning (shock) (stroke) (struck by) E907
Liquid (noncorrosive) in eye E914
  corrosive E924.1
Loss of control
  motor vehicle (on public highway) (without antecedent collision) E816 ☑
    with
      antecedent collision on public highway — *see* Collision, motor vehicle
      involving any object, person or vehicle not on public highway E816 ☑
    not on public highway, non-traffic accident E825 ☑
      with antecedent collision — *see* Collision, motor vehicle, not on public highway
      on public highway — *see* Collision, motor vehicle
  off-road type motor vehicle (not on public highway) E821 ☑
    on public highway — *see* Loss of control, motor vehicle
  snow vehicle, motor-driven (not on public highway) E820 ☑
    on public highway — *see* Loss of control, motor vehicle

Lost at sea E832 ☑
  with accident to watercraft E830 ☑
  in war operations E995
Low
  pressure, effects — *see* Effects of, air pressure
  temperature, effects — *see* Cold, exposure to
Lying before train, vehicle or other moving object (unspecified whether accidental or intentional) E988.0
  stated as intentional, purposeful, suicidal (attempt) E958.0
Lynching — *see also* Assault E968.9

M

Malfunction, atomic power plant in water transport E838 ☑
Mangled (accidentally) NEC E928.9
Manhandling (in brawl, fight) E960.0
  legal intervention E975
Manslaughter (nonaccidental) — *see* Assault
Marble in nose E912
Mauled by animal E906.8
Medical procedure, complication of
  delayed or as an abnormal reaction without mention of misadventure — *see* Reaction, abnormal
  due to or as a result of misadventure — *see* Misadventure
Melting of fittings and furniture in burning
  in terrorism E979.3
Minamata disease E865.2
Misadventure(s) to patient(s) during surgical or medical care E876.9
  contaminated blood, fluid, drug or biological substance (presence of agents and toxins as listed in E875) E875.9
    administered (by) NEC E875.9
      infusion E875.0
      injection E875.1
      specified means NEC E875.2
      transfusion E875.0
      vaccination E875.1
  cut, cutting, puncture, perforation or hemorrhage (accidental) (inadvertent) (inappropriate) (during) E870.9
    aspiration of fluid or tissue (by puncture or catheterization, except heart) E870.5
      biopsy E870.8
      needle (aspirating) E870.5
    blood sampling E870.5
    catheterization E870.5
      heart E870.6
    dialysis (kidney) E870.2
    endoscopic examination E870.4
    enema E870.7
    infusion E870.1
    injection E870.3
    lumbar puncture E870.5
    needle biopsy E870.5
    paracentesis, abdominal E870.5
    perfusion E870.2
    specified procedure NEC E870.8
    surgical operation E870.0
    thoracentesis E870.5
    transfusion E870.1
    vaccination E870.3
  excessive amount of blood or other fluid during transfusion or infusion E873.0
  failure
    in dosage E873.9
      electroshock therapy E873.4
      inappropriate temperature (too hot or too cold) in local application and packing E873.5

Misadventure(s) to patient(s) during surgical or medical care — *continued*
  failure — *continued*
    in dosage — *continued*
      infusion
        excessive amount of fluid E873.0
        incorrect dilution of fluid E873.1
      insulin-shock therapy E873.4
      nonadministration of necessary drug or medicinal E873.6
      overdose (*see also* Overdose)
        radiation, in therapy E873.2
    radiation
      inadvertent exposure of patient (receiving radiation for test or therapy) E873.3
      not receiving radiation for test or therapy — *see* Radiation
      overdose E873.2
    specified procedure NEC E873.8
    transfusion
      excessive amount of blood E873.0
  mechanical, of instrument or apparatus (during procedure) E874.9
    aspiration of fluid or tissue (by puncture or catheterization, except of heart) E874.4
      biopsy E874.8
      needle (aspirating) E874.4
    blood sampling E874.4
    catheterization E874.4
      heart E874.5
    dialysis (kidney) E874.2
    endoscopic examination E874.3
    enema E874.8
    infusion E874.1
    injection E874.8
    lumbar puncture E874.4
    needle biopsy E874.4
    paracentesis, abdominal E874.4
    perfusion E874.2
    specified procedure NEC E874.8
    surgical operation E874.0
    thoracentesis E874.4
    transfusion E874.1
    vaccination E874.8
  sterile precautions (during procedure) E872.9
    aspiration of fluid or tissue (by puncture or catheterization, except of heart) E872.5
      biopsy E872.8
      needle (aspirating) E872.5
    blood sampling E872.5
    catheterization E872.5
      heart E872.6
    dialysis (kidney) E872.2
    endoscopic examination E872.4
    enema E872.8
    infusion E872.1
    injection E872.3
    lumbar puncture E872.5
    needle biopsy E872.5
    paracentesis, abdominal E872.5
    perfusion E872.2
    removal of catheter or packing E872.8
    specified procedure NEC E872.8
    surgical operation E872.0
    thoracentesis E872.5
    transfusion E872.1
    vaccination E872.3
  suture or ligature during surgical procedure E876.2
  to introduce or to remove tube or instrument E876.4

Index to External Causes

Misadventure(s) to patient(s) during surgical or medical care — *continued*
  failure — *continued*
    to introduce or to remove tube or instrument — *continued*
      foreign object left in body — *see* Misadventure, foreign object
  foreign object left in body (during procedure) E871.9
    aspiration of fluid or tissue (by puncture or catheterization, except heart) E871.5
    biopsy E871.8
      needle (aspirating) E871.5
    blood sampling E871.5
    catheterization E871.5
      heart E871.6
    dialysis (kidney) E871.2
    endoscopic examination E871.4
    enema E871.8
    infusion E871.1
    injection E871.3
    lumbar puncture E871.5
    needle biopsy E871.5
    paracentesis, abdominal E871.5
    perfusion E871.2
    removal of catheter or packing E871.7
    specified procedure NEC E871.8
    surgical operation E871.0
    thoracentesis E871.5
    transfusion E871.1
    vaccination E871.3
  hemorrhage — *see* Misadventure, cut
  inadvertent exposure of patient to radiation (being received for test or therapy) E873.3
  inappropriate
    operation performed E876.5
    temperature (too hot or too cold) in local application or packing E873.5
  infusion (*see also* Misadventure, by specific type, infusion)
    excessive amount of fluid E873.0
    incorrect dilution of fluid E873.1
    wrong fluid E876.1
  mismatched blood in transfusion E876.0
  nonadministration of necessary drug or medicinal E873.6
  overdose (*see also* Overdose)
    radiation, in therapy E873.2
  perforation — *see* Misadventure, cut
  performance of inappropriate operation E876.5
  puncture — *see* Misadventure, cut
  specified type NEC E876.8
    failure
      suture or ligature during surgical operation E876.2
      to introduce or to remove tube or instrument E876.4
        foreign object left in body E871.9
    infusion of wrong fluid E876.1
    performance of inappropriate operation E876.5
    transfusion of mismatched blood E876.0
    wrong
      fluid in infusion E876.1
      placement of endotracheal tube during anesthetic procedure E876.3
  transfusion (*see also* Misadventure, by specific type, transfusion)
    excessive amount of blood E873.0
    mismatched blood E876.0
  wrong
    drug given in error — *see* Table of Drugs and Chemicals
    fluid in infusion E876.1
    placement of endotracheal tube during anesthetic procedure E876.3

Motion (effects) E903
  sickness E903
Mountain sickness E902.0
Mucus aspiration or inhalation, not of newborn (with asphyxia, obstruction respiratory passage, suffocation) E912
Mudslide of cataclysmic nature E909.2
Murder (attempt) — *see also* Assault E968.9

N

Nail, injury by E920.8
Needlestick (sewing needle) E920.4
  hypodermic E920.5
Neglect — *see also* Privation
  criminal E968.4
  homicidal intent E968.4
Noise (causing injury) (pollution) E928.1

O

Object
  falling
    from, in, on, hitting
      aircraft E844 ☑
        due to accident to aircraft — *see* categories E840-E842 ☑
      machinery (*see also* Accident, machine)
        not in operation E916
      motor vehicle (in motion) (on public highway) E818 ☑
        not on public highway E825 ☑
        stationary E916
      nonmotor road vehicle NEC E829 ☑
      pedal cycle E826 ☑
      person E916
      railway rolling stock, train, vehicle E806 ☑
      street car E829 ☑
      watercraft E838 ☑
        due to accident to watercraft E831 ☑
  set in motion by
    accidental explosion of pressure vessel — *see* category E921 ☑
    firearm — *see* category E922 ☑
    machine(ry) — *see* Accident, machine
    transport vehicle — *see* categories E800-E848 ☑
  thrown from, in, on, towards
    aircraft E844 ☑
    cable car (not on rails) E847
      on rails E829 ☑
    motor vehicle (in motion) (on public highway) E818 ☑
      not on public highway E825 ☑
    nonmotor road vehicle NEC E829 ☑
    pedal cycle E826 ☑
    street car E829 ☑
    vehicle NEC — *see* Accident, vehicle NEC

Obstruction
  air passages, larynx, respiratory passages
    by
      external means NEC — *see* Suffocation
      food, any type (regurgitated) (vomited) E911
      material or object, except food E912

Obstruction — *continued*
  air passages, larynx, respiratory passages — *continued*
    by — *continued*
      mucus E912
      phlegm E912
      vomitus E911
  digestive tract, except mouth or pharynx
    by
      food, any type E915
      foreign body (any) E915
  esophagus
    without asphyxia or obstruction of respiratory passage E915
    food E911
    foreign body, except food E912
  mouth or pharynx
    by
      food, any type E911
      material or object, except food E912
  respiration — *see* Obstruction, air passages

Oil in eye E914
Overdose
  anesthetic (drug) — *see* Table of Drugs and Chemicals
  drug — *see* Table of Drugs and Chemicals
Overexertion (lifting) (pulling) (pushing) E927
Overexposure (accidental) (to)
  cold (*see also* Cold, exposure to) E901.9
    due to manmade conditions E901.1
  heat (*see also* Heat) E900.9
  radiation — *see* Radiation
  radioactivity — *see* Radiation
  sun, except sunburn E900.0
  weather — *see* Exposure
  wind — *see* Exposure
Overheated — *see also* Heat E900.9
Overlaid E913.0
Overturning (accidental)
  animal-drawn vehicle E827 ☑
  boat, ship, watercraft
    causing
      drowning, submersion E830 ☑
      injury except drowning, submersion E831 ☑
  machinery — *see* Accident, machine
  motor vehicle (*see also* Loss of control, motor vehicle) E816 ☑
    with antecedent collision on public highway — *see* Collision, motor vehicle
    not on public highway, nontraffic accident E825 ☑
      with antecedent collision — *see* Collision, motor vehicle, not on public highway
  nonmotor road vehicle NEC E829 ☑
  off-road type motor vehicle — *see* Loss of control, off-road type motor vehicle
  pedal cycle E826 ☑
  railway rolling stock, train, vehicle (*see also* Derailment, railway) E802 ☑
  street car E829 ☑
  vehicle NEC — *see* Accident, vehicle NEC

P

Palsy, divers' E902.2
Parachuting (voluntary) (without accident to aircraft) E844 ☑
  due to accident to aircraft — *see* categories E840-E842 ☑
Paralysis
  divers' E902.2
  lead or saturnine E866.0
    from pesticide NEC E863.4
Pecked by bird E906.8

Phlegm aspiration or inhalation (with asphyxia, obstruction respiratory passage, suffocation) E912
Piercing — *see also* Cut E920.9
Pinched
  between objects (moving) (stationary and moving) E918
  in object E918
Pinned under
  machine(ry) — *see* Accident, machine
Place of occurrence of accident — *see* Accident (to), occurring (at) (in)
Plumbism E866.0
  from insecticide NEC E863.4
Poisoning (accidental) (by) — *see also* Table of Drugs and Chemicals
  carbon monoxide
    generated by
      aircraft in transit E844 ☑
      motor vehicle
        in motion (on public highway) E818 ☑
        not on public highway E825 ☑
      watercraft (in transit) (not in transit) E838 ☑
  caused by injection of poisons or toxins into or through skin by plant thorns, spines, or other mechanism E905.7
  marine or sea plants E905.6
  fumes or smoke due to
    conflagration — *see* Conflagration
    explosion or fire — *see* Fire
    ignition — *see* Ignition
  gas
    in legal intervention E972
    legal execution, by E978
    on watercraft E838 ☑
    used as anesthetic — *see* Table of Drugs and Chemicals
  in
    terrorism (chemical weapons) E979.7
    war operations E997.2
      execution E978
      intervention
        by gas E972
  late effect of — *see* Late effect
  legal
Pressure, external, causing asphyxia, suffocation — *see also* Suffocation E913.9
Privation E904.9
  food (*see also* Lack of, food) E904.1
  helpless person, infant, newborn due to abandonment or neglect E904.0
  late effect of NEC E929.5
  resulting from transport accident — *see* categories E800-E848 ☑
  water (*see also* Lack of, water) E904.2
Projected objects, striking against or struck by — *see* Striking against, object
Prolonged stay in
  high altitude (causing conditions as listed in E902.0) E902.0
  weightless environment E928.0
Prostration
  heat — *see* Heat
Pulling, injury in E927
Puncture, puncturing — *see also* Cut E920.9
  by
    plant thorns or spines E920.8
      toxic reaction E905.7
        marine or sea plants E905.6
    sea-urchin spine E905.6
Pushing (injury in) (overexertion) E927
  by other person(s) (accidental) E917.9
    with fall E886.9
      in sports E886.0
    as, or caused by, a crowd, human stampede E917.1
      with subsequent fall E917.6

Pushing — continued
by other person(s) — continued
before moving vehicle or object
stated as
intentional, homicidal E968.5
undetemined whether accidental or intentional E988.8
from
high place
in accidental circum-stances — see categories E880-E884 ☑
stated as
intentional, homicidal E968.1
undetermined whether accidental or intentional E987.9
man-made structure, except residential E987.1
natural site E987.2
residential E987.0
motor vehicle (see also Fall, from, motor vehicle) E818 ☑
stated as
intentional, homicidal E968.5
undetermined whether accidental or intentional E988.8
in sports E917.0
with fall E886.0

R

Radiation (exposure to) E926.9
abnormal reaction to medical test or therapy E879.2
arc lamps E926.2
atomic power plant (malfunction) NEC E926.9
in water transport E838 ☑
electromagnetic, ionizing E926.3
gamma rays E926.3
in
terrorism (from or following nuclear explosion) (direct) (secondary) E979.5
laser E979.8
war operations (from or following nuclear explosion) (direct) (secondary) E996
laser(s) E997.0
water transport E838 ☑
inadvertent exposure of patient (receiving test or therapy) E873.3
infrared (heaters and lamps) E926.1
excessive heat E900.1
ionized, ionizing (particles, artificially accelerated) E926.8
electromagnetic E926.3
isotopes, radioactive — see Radiation, radioactive isotopes
laser(s) E926.4
in
terrorism E979.8
war operations E997.0
misadventure in medical care — see Misadventure, failure, in dosage, radiation
late effect of NEC E929.8
excessive heat from — see Heat
light sources (visible) (ultraviolet) E926.2
misadventure in medical or surgical procedure — see Misadventure, failure, in dosage, radiation
overdose (in medical or surgical procedure) E873.2
radar E926.0
radioactive isotopes E926.5
atomic power plant malfunction E926.5

Radiation — continued
radioactive isotopes — continued
atomic power plant malfunction — continued
in water transport E838 ☑
misadventure in medical or surgical treatment — see Misadventure, failure, in dosage, radiation
radiobiologicals — see Radiation, radioactive isotopes
radiofrequency E926.0
radiopharmaceuticals — see Radiation, radioactive isotopes
radium NEC E926.9
sun E926.2
excessive heat from E900.0
tanning bed E926.2
welding arc or torch E926.2
excessive heat from E900.1
x-rays (hard) (soft) E926.3
misadventure in medical or surgical treatment — see Misadventure, failure, in dosage, radiation

Rape E960.1

Reaction, abnormal to or following
(medical or surgical procedure) E879.9
amputation (of limbs) E878.5
anastomosis (arteriovenous) (blood vessel) (gastrojejunal) (skin) (tendon) (natural, artificial material, tissue) E878.2
external stoma, creation of E878.3
aspiration (of fluid) E879.4
tissue E879.8
biopsy E879.8
blood
sampling E879.7
transfusion
procedure E879.8
bypass — see Reaction, abnormal, anastomosis
catheterization
cardiac E879.0
urinary E879.6
colostomy E878.3
cystostomy E878.3
dialysis (kidney) E879.1
drugs or biologicals — see Table of Drugs and Chemicals
duodenostomy E878.3
electroshock therapy E879.3
formation of external stoma E878.3
gastrostomy E878.3
graft — see Reaction, abnormal, anastomosis
hypothermia E879.8
implant, implantation (of)
artificial
internal device (cardiac pacemaker) (electrodes in brain) (heart valve prosthesis) (orthopedic) E878.1
material or tissue (for anastomosis or bypass) E878.2
with creation of external stoma E878.3
natural tissues (for anastomosis or bypass) E878.2
with creation of external stoma E878.3
as transplantion — see Reaction, abnormal, transplant
infusion
procedure E879.8
injection
procedure E879.8
specific type of procedure) E879.9
insertion of gastric or duodenal sound E879.5
insulin-shock therapy E879.3
lumbar puncture E879.4
perfusion E879.1

Reaction, abnormal to or following — continued
procedures other than surgical operation (see also Reaction, abnormal, by)
specified procedure NEC E879.8
radiological procedure or therapy E879.2
removal of organ (partial) (total) NEC E878.6
with
anastomosis, bypass or graft E878.2
formation of external stoma E878.3
implant of artificial internal device E878.1
transplant(ation)
partial organ E878.4
whole organ E878.0
sampling
blood E879.7
fluid NEC E879.4
tissue E879.8
shock therapy E879.3
surgical operation (see also Reaction, abnormal, by specified type of operation) E878.9
restorative NEC E878.4
with
anastomosis, bypass or graft E878.2
fomation of external stoma E878.3
implant(ation) — see Reaction, abnormal, implant
transplant(ation) — see Reaction, abnormal, transplant
specified operation NEC E878.8
thoracentesis E879.4
transfusion
procedure E879.8
transplant, transplantation (heart) (kidney) (liver) E878.0
partial organ E878.4
ureterostomy E878.3
vaccination E879.8

Reduction in
atmospheric pressure (see also Effects of, air pressure)
while surfacing from
deep water diving causing caisson or divers' disease, palsy or paralysis E902.2
underground E902.8

Residual (effect) — see Late effect

Rock falling on or hitting (accidentally)
motor vehicle (in motion) (on public highway) E818 ☑
not on public highway E825 ☑
nonmotor road vehicle NEC E829 ☑
pedal cycle E826 ☑
person E916
railway rolling stock, train, vehicle E806 ☑

Running off, away
animal (being ridden) (in sport or transport) E828 ☑
not being ridden E906.8
animal-drawn vehicle E827 ☑
rails, railway (see also Derailment) E802 ☑
roadway
motor vehicle (without antecedent collision) E816 ☑
with
antecedent collision — see Collision motor vehicle
subsequent collision
involving any object, person or vehicle not on public highway E816 ☑

Running off, away — continued
roadway — continued
motor vehicle — continued
with — continued
subsequent collision — continued
on public highway E811 ☑
nontraffic accident E825 ☑
with antecedent collision — see Collision, motor vehicle, not on public highway
nonmotor road vehicle NEC E829 ☑
pedal cycle E826 ☑

Run over (accidentally) (by)
animal (not being ridden) E906.8
being ridden (in sport or transport) E828 ☑
animal-drawn vehicle E827 ☑
machinery — see Accident, machine
motor vehicle (on public highway) — see Hit by, motor vehicle
nonmotor road vehicle NEC E829 ☑
railway train E805 ☑
street car E829 ☑
vehicle NEC E848

S

Saturnism E866.0
from insecticide NEC E863.4

Scald, scalding (accidental) (by) (from) (in) E924.0
acid — see Scald, caustic
boiling tap water E924.2
caustic or corrosive liquid, substance E924.1
swallowed — see Table of Drugs and Chemicals
homicide (attempt) — see Assault, burning
inflicted by other person
stated as
intentional or homicidal E968.3
undetermined whether accidental or intentional E988.2
late effect of NEC E929.8
liquid (boiling) (hot) E924.0
local application of externally applied substance in medical or surgical care E873.5
molten metal E924.0
self-inflicted (unspecified whether accidental or intentional) E988.2
stated as intentional, purposeful E958.2
stated as undetermined whether accidental or intentional E988.2
steam E924.0
tap water (boiling) E924.2
transport accident — see categories E800-E848 ☑
vapor E924.0

Scratch, cat E906.8

Sea
sickness E903

Self-mutilation — see Suicide

Sequelae (of)
in
terrorism E999.1
war operations E999.0

Shock
anaphylactic (see also Table of Drugs and Chemicals) E947.9
due to
bite (venomous) — see Bite, venomous NEC
sting — see Sting
electric (see also Electric shock) E925.9
from electric appliance or current (see also Electric shock) E925.9

Shooting, shot (accidental(ly)) E922.9
air gun E922.4
BB gun E922.4

Index to External Causes

Shooting, shot — continued
- hand gun (pistol) (revolver) E922.0
- himself (see also Shooting, self-inflicted) E985.4
  - hand gun (pistol) (revolver) E985.0
  - military firearm, except hand gun E985.3
    - hand gun (pistol) (revolver) E985.0
  - rifle (hunting) E985.2
    - military E985.3
  - shotgun (automatic) E985.1
  - specified firearm NEC E985.4
  - Verey pistol E985.4
- homicide (attempt) E965.4
  - air gun E968.6
  - BB gun E968.6
  - hand gun (pistol) (revolver) E965.0
  - military firearm, except hand gun E965.3
    - hand gun (pistol) (revolver) E965.0
  - paintball gun E965.4
  - rifle (hunting) E965.2
    - military E965.3
  - shotgun (automatic) E965.1
  - specified firearm NEC E965.4
  - Verey pistol E965.4
- in
  - terrorism — see Terrorism, shooting
  - war operations — see War operations, shooting
- inflicted by other person
  - in accidental circumstances E922.9
    - hand gun (pistol) (revolver) E922.0
    - military firearm, except hand gun E922.3
      - hand gun (pistol) (revolver) E922.0
    - rifle (hunting) E922.2
      - military E922.3
    - shotgun (automatic) E922.1
    - specified firearm NEC E922.8
    - Verey pistol E922.8
  - stated as
    - intentional, homicidal E965.4
      - hand gun (pistol) (revolver) E965.0
      - military firearm, except hand gun E965.3
        - hand gun (pistol) (revolver) E965.0
      - paintball gun E965.4
      - rifle (hunting) E965.2
        - military E965.3
      - shotgun (automatic) E965.1
      - specified firearm E965.4
      - Verey pistol E965.4
    - undetermined whether accidental or intentional E985.4
      - air gun E985.6
      - BB gun E985.6
      - hand gun (pistol) (revolver) E985.0
      - military firearm, except hand gun E985.3
        - hand gun (pistol) (revolver) E985.0
      - paintball gun E985.7
      - rifle (hunting) E985.2
      - shotgun (automatic) E985.1
      - specified firearm NEC E985.4
      - Verey pistol E985.4
- legal
  - execution E978
  - intervention E970
- military firearm, except hand gun E922.3
  - hand gun (pistol) (revolver) E922.0
- paintball gun E922.5
- rifle (hunting) E922.2
  - military E922.3

Shooting, shot — continued
- self-inflicted (unspecified whether accidental or intentional) E985.4
  - air gun E985.6
  - BB gun E985.6
  - hand gun (pistol) (revolver) E985.0
  - military firearm, except hand gun E985.3
    - hand gun (pistol) (revolver) E985.0
  - paintball gun E985.7
  - rifle (hunting) E985.2
    - military E985.3
  - shotgun (automatic) E985.1
  - specified firearm NEC E985.4
  - stated as
    - accidental E922.9
      - hand gun (pistol) (revolver) E922.0
      - military firearm, except hand gun E922.3
        - hand gun (pistol) (revolver) E922.0
      - paintball gun E922.5
      - rifle (hunting) E922.2
        - military E922.3
      - shotgun (automatic) E922.1
      - specified firearm NEC E922.8
      - Verey pistol E922.8
    - intentional, purposeful E955.4
      - hand gun (pistol) (revolver) E955.0
      - military firearm, except hand gun E955.3
        - hand gun (pistol) (revolver) E955.0
      - paintball gun E955.7
      - rifle (hunting) E955.2
        - military E955.3
      - shotgun (automatic) E955.1
      - specified firearm NEC E955.4
      - Verey pistol E955.4
    - shotgun (automatic) E922.1
    - specified firearm NEC E922.8
    - stated as undetermined whether accidental or intentional E985.4
      - hand gun (pistol) (revolver) E985.0
      - military firearm, except hand gun E985.3
        - hand gun (pistol) (revolver) E985.0
      - paintball gun E985.7
      - rifle (hunting) E985.2
        - military E985.3
      - shotgun (automatic) E985.1
      - specified firearm NEC E985.4
      - Verey pistol E985.4
  - suicidal (attempt) E955.4
    - air gun E955.6
    - BB gun E955.6
    - hand gun (pistol) (revolver) E955.0
    - military firearm, except hand gun E955.3
      - hand gun (pistol) (revolver) E955.0
    - paintball gun E955.7
    - rifle (hunting) E955.2
      - military E955.3
    - shotgun (automatic) E955.1
    - specified firearm NEC E955.4
    - Verey pistol E955.4
  - Verey pistol E922.8
- **Shoving** (accidentally) by other person — see also Pushing by other person E917.9
- **Sickness**
  - air E903
  - alpine E902.0
  - car E903
  - motion E903
  - mountain E902.0
  - sea E903
  - travel E903
- **Sinking** (accidental)
  - boat, ship, watercraft (causing drowning, submersion) E830 ☑

Sinking — continued
- boat, ship, watercraft — continued
  - causing injury except drowning, submersion E831 ☑
- **Siriasis** E900.0
- **Skydiving** E844 ☑
- **Slashed wrists** — see also Cut, self-inflicted E986
- **Slipping** (accidental)
  - on
    - deck (of boat, ship, watercraft) (icy) (oily) (wet) E835 ☑
    - ice E885.9
    - ladder of ship E833 ☑
      - due to accident to watercraft E831 ☑
    - mud E885.9
    - oil E885.9
    - snow E885.9
    - stairs of ship E833 ☑
      - due to accident to watercraft E831 ☑
    - surface
      - slippery E885 ☑
      - wet E885 ☑
- **Sliver, wood, injury by** E920.8
- **Smothering, smothered** — see also Suffocation E913.9
- **Smouldering building or structure in terrorism** E979.3
- **Sodomy** (assault) E960.1
- **Solid substance in eye** (any part) or adnexa E914
- **Sound waves** (causing injury) E928.1
- **Splinter, injury by** E920.8
- **Stab, stabbing** E966
  - accidental — see Cut
- **Starvation** E904.1
  - helpless person, infant, newborn — see Lack of food
  - homicidal intent E968.4
  - late effect of NEC E929.5
  - resulting from accident connected with transport — see categories E800-E848 ☑
- **Stepped on**
  - by
    - animal (not being ridden) E906.8
      - being ridden (in sport or transport) E828 ☑
    - crowd E917.1
    - person E917.9
      - in sports E917.0
  - in sports E917.0
- **Stepping on**
  - object (moving) E917.9
    - in sports E917.0
    - with subsequent fall E917.5
    - stationary E917.4
      - with subsequent fall E917.8
  - person E917.9
    - as, or caused by a crowd E917.1
      - with subsequent fall E917.6
    - in sports E917.0
- **Sting** E905.9
  - ant E905.5
  - bee E905.3
  - caterpillar E905.5
  - coral E905.6
  - hornet E905.3
  - insect NEC E905.5
  - jellyfish E905.6
  - marine animal or plant E905.6
  - nematocysts E905.6
  - scorpion E905.2
  - sea anemone E905.6
  - sea cucumber E905.6
  - wasp E905.3
  - yellow jacket E905.3
- **Storm** E908.9
  - specified type NEC E908.8
- **Straining, injury in** E927
- **Strangling** — see Suffocation
- **Strangulation** — see Suffocation
- **Strenuous movements** (in recreational or other activities) E927

Striking against
- bottom (when jumping or diving into water) E883.0
- object (moving) E917.9
  - caused by crowd E917.1
    - with subsequent fall E917.6
  - furniture E917.3
    - with subsequent fall E917.7
  - in
    - running water E917.2
      - with drowning or submersion — see Submersion
    - sports E917.0
      - with subsequent fall E917.5
    - stationary E917.4
      - with subsequent fall E917.8
- person(s) E917.9
  - with fall E886.9
    - in sports E886.0
  - as, or caused by, a crowd E917.1
    - with subsequent fall E917.6
    - in sports E917.0
      - with fall E886.0
- **Stroke**
  - heat — see Heat
  - lightning E907
- **Struck by** — see also Hit by
  - bullet
    - in
      - terrorism E979.4
      - war operations E991.2
        - rubber E991.0
  - lightning E907
  - missile
    - in terrorism — see Terrorism, missile
  - object
    - falling
      - from, in, on
        - building
          - burning (uncontrolled fire)
            - in terrorism E979.3
  - thunderbolt E907
- **Stumbling over animal, carpet, curb, rug or (small) object (with fall)** E885.9
  - without fall — see Striking against, object
- **Submersion** (accidental) E910.8
  - boat, ship, watercraft (causing drowning, submersion) E830 ☑
    - causing injury except drowning, submersion E831 ☑
  - by other person
    - in accidental circumstances — see category E910
    - intentional, homicidal E964
    - stated as undetermined whether accidental or intentional E984
  - due to
    - accident
      - machinery — see Accident, machine
      - to boat, ship, watercraft E830 ☑
      - transport — see categories E800-E848 ☑
    - avalanche E909.2
    - cataclysmic
      - earth surface movement or eruption E909.9
      - storm E908.9
    - cloudburst E908.8
    - cyclone E908.1
    - fall
      - from
        - boat, ship, watercraft (not involved in accident) E832 ☑
        - burning, crushed E830 ☑
        - involved in accident, collision E830 ☑
        - gangplank (into water) E832 ☑
        - overboard NEC E832 ☑
    - flood E908.2

Submersion (accidental)

Submersion (accidental) — *continued*
due to — *continued*
  hurricane E908.0
  jumping into water E910.8
    from boat, ship, watercraft
      burning, crushed, sinking E830 ☑
      involved in accident, collision E830 ☑
      not involved in accident, for swim E910.2
    in recreational activity (without diving equipment) E910.2
      with or using diving equipment E910.1
    to rescue another person E910.3
  homicide (attempt) E964
  in
    bathtub E910.4
    specified activity, not sport, transport or recreational E910.3
    sport or recreational activity (without diving equipment) E910.2
      with or using diving equipment E910.1
    water skiing E910.0
    swimming pool NEC E910.8
  terrorism E979.8
  war operations E995
  water transport E832 ☑
    due to accident to boat, ship, watercraft E830 ☑
  landslide E909.2
    overturning boat, ship, watercraft E909.2
    sinking boat, ship, watercraft E909.2
    submersion boat, ship, watercraft E909.2
    tidal wave E909.4
      caused by storm E908.0
    torrential rain E908.2
  late effect of NEC E929.8
  quenching tank E910.8
  self-inflicted (unspecified whether accidental or intentional) E984
    in accidental circumstances — *see* category E910 ☑
    stated as intentional, purposeful E954
    stated as undetermined whether accidental or intentional E984
  suicidal (attempted) E954
  while
    attempting rescue of another person E910.3
    engaged in
      marine salvage E910.3
      underwater construction or repairs E910.3
    fishing, not from boat E910.2
    hunting, not from boat E910.2
    ice skating E910.2
    pearl diving E910.3
    placing fishing nets E910.3
    playing in water E910.2
    scuba diving E910.1
      nonrecreational E910.3
    skin diving E910.1
    snorkel diving E910.2
    spear fishing underwater E910.1
    surfboarding E910.2
    swimming (swimming pool) E910.2
    wading (in water) E910.2
    water skiing E910.0

Sucked
  into
    jet (aircraft) E844 ☑

Suffocation (accidental) (by external means) (by pressure) (mechanical) E913.9

Suffocation — *continued*
caused by other person
  in accidental circumstances — *see* category E913 ☑
  stated as
    intentional, homicidal E963
    undetermined whether accidental or intentional E983.8
      by, in
        hanging E983.0
        plastic bag E983.1
        specified means NEC E983.8
due to, by
  avalanche E909.2
  bedclothes E913.0
  bib E913.0
  blanket E913.0
  cave-in E913.3
    caused by cataclysmic earth surface movement or eruption E909.9
  conflagration — *see* Conflagration
  explosion — *see* Explosion
  falling earth, other substance E913.3
  fire — *see* Fire
  food, any type (ingestion) (inhalation) (regurgitated) (vomited) E911
  foreign body, except food (ingestion) (inhalation) E912
  ignition — *see* Ignition
  landslide E909.2
  machine(ry) — *see* Accident, machine
  material, object except food entering by nose or mouth, ingested, inhaled E912
  mucus (aspiration) (inhalation), not of newborn E912
  phlegm (aspiration) (inhalation) E912
  pillow E913.0
  plastic bag — *see* Suffocation, in, plastic bag
  sheet (plastic) E913.0
  specified means NEC E913.8
  vomitus (aspiration) (inhalation) E911
homicidal (attempt) E963
in
  airtight enclosed place E913.2
  baby carriage E913.0
  bed E913.0
  closed place E913.2
  cot, cradle E913.0
  perambulator E913.0
  plastic bag (in accidental circumstances) E913.1
    homicidal, purposely inflicted by other person E963
    self-inflicted (unspecified whether accidental or intentional) E983.1
      in accidental circumstances E913.1
    intentional, suicidal E953.1
    stated as undetermined whether accidentally or purposely inflicted E983.1
    suicidal, purposely self-inflicted E953.1
  refrigerator E913.2
self-inflicted (*see also* Suffocation, stated as undetermined whether accidental or intentional) E953.9
  in accidental circumstances — *see* category E913 ☑
  stated as intentional, purposeful — *see* Suicide, suffocation
stated as undetermined whether accidental or intentional E983.9
  by, in
    hanging E983.0

Suffocation — *continued*
stated as undetermined whether accidental or intentional — *continued*
  by, in — *continued*
    plastic bag E983.1
    specified means NEC E983.8
suicidal — *see* Suicide, suffocation

Suicide, suicidal (attempted) (by) E958.9
burning, burns E958.1
caustic substance E958.7
  poisoning E950.7
  swallowed E950.7
cold, extreme E958.3
cut (any part of body) E956
cutting or piercing instrument (classifiable to E920) E956
drowning E954
electrocution E958.4
explosive(s) (classifiable to E923) E955.5
fire E958.1
firearm (classifiable to E922) — *see* Shooting, suicidal
hanging E953.0
jumping
  before moving object, train, vehicle E958.0
  from high place — *see* Jumping, from, high place, stated as, suicidal
knife E956
late effect of E959
motor vehicle, crashing of E958.5
poisoning — *see* Table of Drugs and Chemicals
puncture (any part of body) E956
scald E958.2
shooting — *see* Shooting, suicidal
specified means NEC E958.8
stab (any part of body) E956
strangulation — *see* Suicide, suffocation
submersion E954
suffocation E953.9
  by, in
    hanging E953.0
    plastic bag E953.1
    specified means NEC E953.8
wound NEC E958.9

Sunburn E926.2
Sunstroke E900.0
Supersonic waves (causing injury) E928.1
Surgical procedure, complication of
delayed or as an abnormal reaction without mention of misadventure — *see* Reaction, abnormal
due to or as a result of misadventure — *see* Misadventure
Swallowed, swallowing
foreign body — *see* Foreign body, alimentary canal
poison — *see* Table of Drugs and Chemicals
substance
  caustic — *see* Table of Drugs and Chemicals
  corrosive — *see* Table of Drugs and Chemicals
  poisonous — *see* Table of Drugs and Chemicals
Swimmers cramp — *see also* category E910 E910.2
not in recreation or sport E910.3
Syndrome, battered
baby or child — *see* Abuse, child
wife — *see* Assault

T

Tackle in sport E886.0
Terrorism (injury) (by) (in) E979.8
air blast E979.2
aircraft burned, destroyed, exploded, shot down E979.1
used as a weapon E979.1

Terrorism — *continued*
anthrax E979.6
asphyxia from
  chemical (weapons) E979.7
  fire, conflagration (caused by fire-producing device) E979.3
    from nuclear explosion E979.5
  gas or fumes E979.7
bayonet E979.8
biological agents E979.6
blast (air) (effects) E979.2
  from nuclear explosion E979.5
  underwater E979.0
bomb (antipersonnel) (mortar) (explosion) (fragments) E979.2
bullet(s) (from carbine, machine gun, pistol, rifle, shotgun) E979.4
burn from
  chemical E979.7
  fire, conflagration (caused by fire-producing device) E979.3
    from nuclear explosion E979.5
  gas E979.7
burning aircraft E979.1
chemical E979.7
cholera E979.6
conflagration E979.3
crushed by falling aircraft E979.1
depth-charge E979.0
destruction of aircraft E979.1
disability, as sequelae one year or more after injury E999.1
drowning E979.8
effect
  of nuclear weapon (direct) (secondary) E979.5
  secondary NEC E979.9
  sequelae E999.1
explosion (artillery shell) (breech-block) (cannon block) E979.2
  aircraft E979.1
  bomb (antipersonnel) (mortar) E979.2
  nuclear (atom) (hydrogen) E979.5
  depth-charge E979.0
  grenade E979.2
  injury by fragments from E979.2
  land-mine E979.2
  marine weapon E979.0
  mine (land) E979.2
    at sea or in harbor E979.0
    marine E979.0
  missile (explosive) NEC E979.2
  munitions (dump) (factory) E979.2
  nuclear (weapon) E979.5
    other direct and secondary effects of E979.5
  sea-based artillery shell E979.0
  torpedo E979.0
exposure to ionizing radiation from nuclear explosion E979.5
falling aircraft E979.1
firearms E979.4
fireball effects from nuclear explosion E979.5
fire or fire-producing device E979.3
fragments from artillery shell, bomb NEC, grenade, guided missile, land-mine, rocket, shell, shrapnel E979.2
gas or fumes E979.7
grenade (explosion) (fragments) E979.2
guided missile (explosion) (fragments) E979.2
  nuclear E979.5
heat from nuclear explosion E979.5
hot substances E979.3
hydrogen cyanide E979.7
land-mine (explosion) (fragments) E979.2
laser(s) E979.8
late effect of E999.1
lewisite E979.7

Index to External Causes

Terrorism — *continued*
    lung irritant (chemical) (fumes) (gas) E979.7
    marine mine E979.0
    mine E979.2
        at sea E979.0
        in harbor E979.0
        land (explosion) (fragments) E979.2
        marine E979.0
    missile (explosion) (fragments) (guided) E979.2
        marine E979.0
        nuclear weapons E979.5
    mortar bomb (explosion) (fragments) E979.2
    mustard gas E979.7
    nerve gas E979.7
    nuclear weapons E979.5
    pellets (shotgun) E979.4
    petrol bomb E979.3
    phosgene E979.7
    piercing object E979.8
    poisoning (chemical) (fumes) (gas) E979.7
    radiation, ionizing from nuclear explosion E979.5
    rocket (explosion) (fragments) E979.2
    saber, sabre E979.8
    sarin E979.7
    screening smoke E979.7
    sequelae effect (of) E999.1
    shell (aircraft) (artillery) (cannon) (land-based) (explosion) (fragments) E979.2
        sea-based E979.0
    shooting E979.4
        bullet(s) E979.4
        pellet(s) (rifle) (shotgun) E979.4
    shrapnel E979.2
    smallpox E979.7
    stabbing object(s) E979.8
    submersion E979.8
    torpedo E979.0
    underwater blast E979.0
    vesicant (chemical) (fumes) (gas) E979.7
    weapon burst E979.2
Thermic fever E900.9
Thermoplegia E900.9
Thirst — *see also* Lack of water
    resulting from accident connected with transport — *see* categories E800–E848 ☑
Thrown (accidentally)
    against object in or part of vehicle
        by motion of vehicle
            aircraft E844 ☑
            boat, ship, watercraft E838 ☑
            motor vehicle (on public highway) E818 ☑
                not on public highway E825 ☑
                off-road type (not on public highway) E821 ☑
                on public highway E818 ☑
            snow vehicle E820 ☑
                on public highway E818 ☑
            nonmotor road vehicle NEC E829 ☑
            railway rolling stock, train, vehicle E806 ☑
            street car E829 ☑
    from
        animal (being ridden) (in sport or transport) E828 ☑
        high place, homicide (attempt) E968.1
        machinery — *see* Accident, machine
        vehicle NEC — *see* Accident, vehicle NEC
    off — *see* Thrown, from

Thrown — *continued*
    overboard (by motion of boat, ship, watercraft) E832 ☑
        by accident to boat, ship, watercraft E830 ☑
Thunderbolt NEC E907
Tidal wave (any injury) E909.4
    caused by storm E908.0
Took
    overdose of drug — *see* Table of Drugs and Chemicals
    poison — *see* Table of Drugs and Chemicals
Tornado (any injury) E908.1
Torrential rain (any injury) E908.2
Traffic accident NEC E819 ☑
Trampled by animal E906.8
    being ridden (in sport or transport) E828 ☑
Trapped (accidentally)
    between
        objects (moving) (stationary and moving) E918
    by
        door of
            elevator E918
            motor vehicle (on public highway) (while alighting, boarding) — *see* Fall, from, motor vehicle, while alighting
            railway train (underground) E806 ☑
            street car E829 ☑
            subway train E806 ☑
    in object E918
Travel (effects) E903
    sickness E903
Tree
    falling on or hitting E916
        motor vehicle (in motion) (on public highway) E818 ☑
            not on public highway E825 ☑
        nonmotor road vehicle NEC E829 ☑
        pedal cycle E826 ☑
        person E916
        railway rolling stock, train, vehicle E806 ☑
        street car E829 ☑
Trench foot E901.0
Tripping over animal, carpet, curb, rug, or small object (with fall) E885
    without fall — *see* Striking against, object
Tsunami E909.4
Twisting, injury in E927

V

Violence, nonaccidental — *see also* Assault E968.9
Volcanic eruption (any injury) E909.1
Vomitus in air passages (with asphyxia, obstruction or suffocation) E911

W

War operations (during hostilities) (injury) (by) (in) E995
    after cessation of hostilities, injury due to E998
    air blast E993
    aircraft burned, destroyed, exploded, shot down E994
    asphyxia from
        chemical E997.2
        fire, conflagration (caused by fire producing device or conventional weapon) E990.9
            from nuclear explosion E996
            petrol bomb E990.0
        fumes E997.2
        gas E997.2
    battle wound NEC E995

War operations — *continued*
    bayonet E995
    biological warfare agents E997.1
    blast (air) (effects) E993
        from nuclear explosion E996
        underwater E992
    bomb (mortar) (explosion) E993
        after cessation of hostilities E998
        fragments, injury by E991.9
        antipersonnel E991.3
    bullet(s) (from carbine, machine gun, pistol, rifle, shotgun) E991.2
        rubber E991.0
    burn from
        chemical E997.2
        fire, conflagration (caused by fire-producing device or conventional weapon) E990.9
            from nuclear explosion E996
            petrol bomb E990.0
        gas E997.2
    burning aircraft E994
    chemical E997.2
    chlorine E997.2
    conventional warfare, specified form NEC E995
    crushing by falling aircraft E994
    depth charge E992
    destruction of aircraft E994
    disability as sequela one year or more after injury E999.0
    drowning E995
    effect (direct) (secondary) nuclear weapon E996
    explosion (artillery shell) (breech block) (cannon shell) E993
        after cessation of hostilities of bomb, mine placed in war E998
        aircraft E994
        bomb (mortar) E993
            atom E996
            hydrogen E996
            injury by fragments from E991.9
                antipersonnel E991.3
            nuclear E996
        depth charge E992
        injury by fragments from E991.9
            antipersonnel E991.3
        marine weapon E992
        mine
            at sea or in harbor E992
            land E993
                injury by fragments from E991.9
            marine E992
        munitions (accidental) (being used in war) (dump) (factory) E993
        nuclear (weapon) E996
        own weapons (accidental) E993
            injury by fragments from E991.9
                antipersonnel E991.3
        sea-based artillery shell E992
        torpedo E992
    exposure to ionizing radiation from nuclear explosion E996
    falling aircraft E994
    fireball effects from nuclear explosion E996
    fire or fire-producing device E990.9
        petrol bomb E990.0
    fragments from
        antipersonnel bomb E991.3
        artillery shell, bomb NEC, grenade, guided missile, land mine, rocket, shell, shrapnel E991.9
    fumes E997.2
    gas E997.2
    grenade (explosion) E993
        fragments, injury by E991.9
    guided missile (explosion) E993
        fragments, injury by E991.9

War operations — *continued*
    guided missile — *continued*
        nuclear E996
    heat from nuclear explosion E996
    injury due to, but occurring after cessation of hostilities E998
    lacrimator (gas) (chemical) E997.2
    land mine (explosion) E993
        after cessation of hostilities E998
        fragments, injury by E991.9
    laser(s) E997.0
    late effect of E999.0
    lewisite E997.2
    lung irritant (chemical) (fumes) (gas) E997.2
    marine mine E992
    mine
        after cessation of hostilities E998
        at sea E992
        in harbor E992
        land (explosion) E993
            fragments, injury by E991.9
        marine E992
    missile (guided) (explosion) E993
        fragments, injury by E991.9
        marine E992
        nuclear E996
    mortar bomb (explosion) E993
        fragments, injury by E991.9
    mustard gas E997.2
    nerve gas E997.2
    phosgene E997.2
    poisoning (chemical) (fumes) (gas) E997.2
    radiation, ionizing from nuclear explosion E996
    rocket (explosion) E993
        fragments, injury by E991.9
    saber, sabre E995
    screening smoke E997.8
    shell (aircraft) (artillery) (cannon) (land based) (explosion) E993
        fragments, injury by E991.9
        sea-based E992
    shooting E991.2
        after cessation of hostilities E998
        bullet(s) E991.2
            rubber E991.0
        pellet(s) (rifle) E991.1
        shrapnel E991.9
        submersion E995
        torpedo E992
    unconventional warfare, except by nuclear weapon E997.9
        biological (warfare) E997.1
        gas, fumes, chemicals E997.2
        laser(s) E997.0
        specified type NEC E997.8
    underwater blast E992
    vesicant (chemical) (fumes) (gas) E997.2
    weapon burst E993
Washed
    away by flood — *see* Flood
    away by tidal wave — *see* Tidal wave
    off road by storm (transport vehicle) E908.9
    overboard E832 ☑
Weather exposure — *see also* Exposure
    cold E901.0
    hot E900.0
Weightlessness (causing injury) (effects of) (in spacecraft, real or simulated) E928.0
Wound (accidental) NEC — *see also* Injury E928.9
    battle (*see also* War operations) E995
    bayonet E920.3
    in
        legal intervention E974
        war operations E995
    gunshot — *see* Shooting
    incised — *see* Cut
    saber, sabre E920.3
        in war operations E995

Index to External Causes

Railway Accidents (E800-E807)

The following fourth-digit subdivisions are for use with categories E800-E807 to identify the injured person:

.0 **Railway employee**
Any person who by virtue of his employment in connection with a railway, whether by the railway company or not, is at increased risk of involvement in a railway accident, such as:
    catering staff on train
      postal staff on train
      driver
      railway fireman
      guard
      shunter
      porter
      sleeping car attendant

.1 **Passenger on railway**
Any authorized person traveling on a train, except a railway employee
    EXCLUDES intending passenger waiting at station (.8)
                  unauthorized rider on railway vehicle (.8)

.2 **Pedestrian** See definition (r), E-Codes-2

.3 **Pedal cyclist** See definition (p), E-Codes-2

.8 **Other specified person** Intending passenger waiting at station
Unauthorized rider on railway vehicle

.9 **Unspecified person**

Motor Vehicle Traffic and Nontraffic Accidents (E810-E825)

The following fourth-digit subdivisions are for use with categories E810-E819 and E820-E825 to identify the injured person:

.0 **Driver of motor vehicle other than motorcycle** See definition (1), E-Codes-2

.1 **Passenger in motor vehicle other than motorcycle** See definition (1), E-Codes-2

.2 **Motorcyclist** See definition (1), E-Codes-2

.3 **Passenger on motorcycle** See definition (1), E-Codes-2

.4 **Occupant of streetcar**

.5 **Rider of animal; occupant of animal-drawn vehicle**

.6 **Pedal cyclist** See definition (p), E-Codes-2

.7 **Pedestrian** See definition (r), E-Codes-2

.8 **Other specified person**
Occupant of vehicle other than above
Person in railway train involved in accident
Unauthorized rider of motor vehicle

.9 **Unspecified person**

Other Road Vehicle Accidents (E826-E829)
(animal-drawn vehicle, streetcar, pedal cycle, and other nonmotor road vehicle accidents)

The following fourth-digit subdivisions are for use with categories E826-E829 to identify the injured person:

.0 **Pedestrian** See definition (r), E-Codes-2

.1 **Pedal cyclist** (does not apply to codes E827, E828, E829) See definition (p), E-Codes-2

.2 **Rider of animal** (does not apply to code E829)

.3 **Occupant of animal-drawn vehicle** (does not apply to codes E828, E829)

.4 **Occupant of streetcar**

.8 **Other specified person**

.9 **Unspecified person**

Water Transport Accidents (E830-E838)

The following fourth-digit subdivisions are for use with categories E830-E838 to identify the injured person:

.0 **Occupant of small boat, unpowered**

.1 **Occupant of small boat, powered** See definition (t), E-Codes-2
    EXCLUDES water skier (.4)

.2 **Occupant of other watercraft — crew**
Persons:
  engaged in operation of watercraft
    providing passenger services [cabin attendants, ship's physician, catering personnel]
    working on ship during voyage in other capacity [musician in band, operators of shops and beauty parlors]

.3 **Occupant of other watercraft — other than crew**
Passenger
Occupant of lifeboat, other than crew, after abandoning ship

.4 **Water skier**

.5 **Swimmer**

.6 **Dockers, stevedores**
Longshoreman employed on the dock in loading and unloading ships

.8 **Other specified person**
Immigration and custom officials on board ship
Persons:
  accompanying passenger or member of crew visiting boat
Pilot (guiding ship into port)

.9 **Unspecified person**

Air and Space Transport Accidents (E840-E845)

The following fourth-digit subdivisions are for use with categories E840-E845 to identify the injured person:

.0 **Occupant of spacecraft**
  Crew
  Passenger (civilian)   in military aircraft [air force]
  (military)   [army] [national guard] [navy]
  Troops

.1 **Occupant of military aircraft, any**
    EXCLUDES occupants of aircraft operated under jurisdiction of police departments (.5) parachutist (.7)

.2 **Crew of commercial aircraft (powered) in surface to surface transport**

.3 **Other occupant of commercial aircraft (powered) in surface to surface transport**
Flight personnel:
  not part of crew
  on familiarization flight Passenger on aircraft

.4 **Occupant of commercial aircraft (powered) in surface to air transport**
Occupant [crew] [passenger] of aircraft (powered) engaged in activities, such as:
  air drops of emergency supplies
    air drops of parachutists, except from military craft
    crop dusting
    lowering of construction material [bridge or telephone pole]
    sky writing

.5 **Occupant of other powered aircraft**
Occupant [crew] [passenger] of aircraft (powered) engaged in activities, such as:
  aerial spraying (crops)(fire retardants)
    aerobatic flying
    aircraft racing
    rescue operation
    storm surveillance
    traffic suveillance
Occupant of private plane NOS

.6 **Occupant of unpowered aircraft, except parachutist**
Occupant of aircraft classifiable to E842

.7 **Parachutist (military)(other)**
Person making voluntary descent
  person making descent after accident to aircraft (.1-.6)

.8 **Ground crew, airline employee**
Persons employed at airfields (civil)(military) or launching pads, not occupants of aircraft

.9 **Other person**

1. INFECTIOUS AND PARASITIC DISEASES (001-139)

Note: Categories for "late effects" of infectious and parasitic diseases are to be found at 137-139.

INCLUDES diseases generally recognized as communicable or transmissible as well as a few diseases of unknown but possibly infectious origin

EXCLUDES acute respiratory infections (460-466)
carrier or suspected carrier of infectious organism (V02.0-V02.9)
certain localized infections
influenza (487.0-487.8)

INTESTINAL INFECTIOUS DISEASES (001-009)

EXCLUDES helminthiases (120.0-129)

4th 001 Cholera
DEF: An acute infectious enteritis caused by a potent enterotoxin elaborated by *Vibrio cholerae*; the vibrio produces a toxin in the intestinal tract that changes the permeability of the mucosa leading to diarrhea and dehydration.

- 001.0 Due to Vibrio cholerae
- 001.1 Due to Vibrio cholerae el tor
- 001.9 Cholera, unspecified

4th 002 Typhoid and paratyphoid fevers
DEF: Typhoid fever: an acute generalized illness caused by *Salmonella typhi*; notable clinical features are fever, headache, abdominal pain, cough, toxemia, leukopenia, abnormal pulse, rose spots on the skin, bacteremia, hyperplasia of intestinal lymph nodes, mesenteric lymphadenopathy, and Peyer's patches in the intestines.

DEF: Paratyphoid fever: a prolonged febrile illness, much like typhoid but usually less severe; caused by salmonella serotypes other than *S. typhi*, especially *S. enteritidis* serotypes paratyphi A and B and *S. choleraesuis*.

- 002.0 Typhoid fever
  Typhoid (fever) (infection) [any site]
- 002.1 Paratyphoid fever A
- 002.2 Paratyphoid fever B
- 002.3 Paratyphoid fever C
- 002.9 Paratyphoid fever, unspecified

4th 003 Other salmonella infections
INCLUDES infection or food poisoning by Salmonella [any serotype]

DEF: Infections caused by a genus of gram-negative, anaerobic bacteria of the family *Enterobacteriaceae*; affecting warm-blooded animals, like humans; major symptoms are enteric fevers, acute gastroenteritis and septicemia.

- 003.0 Salmonella gastroenteritis
  Salmonellosis
- 003.1 Salmonella septicemia
- 5th 003.2 Localized salmonella infections
  - 003.20 Localized salmonella infection, unspecified
  - 003.21 Salmonella meningitis
  - 003.22 Salmonella pneumonia
  - 003.23 Salmonella arthritis
  - 003.24 Salmonella osteomyelitis
  - 003.29 Other
- 003.8 Other specified salmonella infections
- 003.9 Salmonella infection, unspecified

4th 004 Shigellosis
INCLUDES bacillary dysentery

DEF: Acute infectious dysentery caused by the genus *Shigella*, of the family *Enterobacteriaceae*; affecting the colon causing the release of blood-stained stools with accompanying tenesmus, abdominal cramps and fever.

- 004.0 Shigella dysenteriae
  Infection by group A Shigella (Schmitz) (Shiga)
- 004.1 Shigella flexneri
  Infection by group B Shigella
- 004.2 Shigella boydii
  Infection by group C Shigella
- 004.3 Shigella sonnei
  Infection by group D Shigella
- 004.8 Other specified Shigella infections
- 004.9 Shigellosis, unspecified

4th 005 Other food poisoning (bacterial)
EXCLUDES salmonella infections (003.0-003.9)
toxic effect of:
  food contaminants (989.7)
  noxious foodstuffs (988.0-988.9)

DEF: Enteritis caused by ingesting contaminated foods and characterized by diarrhea, abdominal pain, vomiting; symptoms may be mild or life threatening.

- 005.0 Staphylococcal food poisoning
  Staphylococcal toxemia specified as due to food
- 005.1 Botulism
  Food poisoning due to Clostridium botulinum
- 005.2 Food poisoning due to Clostridium perfringens [C. welchii]
  Enteritis necroticans
- 005.3 Food poisoning due to other Clostridia
- 005.4 Food poisoning due to Vibrio parahaemolyticus
- 5th 005.8 Other bacterial food poisoning
  EXCLUDES salmonella food poisoning (003.0-003.9)
  - 005.81 Food poisoning due to Vibrio vulnificus
  - 005.89 Other bacterial food poisoning
    Food poisoning due to Bacillus cereus
- 005.9 Food poisoning, unspecified

4th 006 Amebiasis
INCLUDES infection due to Entamoeba histolytica
EXCLUDES amebiasis due to organisms other than Entamoeba histolytica (007.8)

DEF: Infection of the large intestine caused by *Entamoeba histolytica*; usually asymptomatic but symptoms may range from mild diarrhea to profound life-threatening dysentery. Extraintestinal complications include hepatic abscess, which may rupture into the lung, pericardium or abdomen, causing life-threatening infections.

- 006.0 Acute amebic dysentery without mention of abscess
  Acute amebiasis
- 006.1 Chronic intestinal amebiasis without mention of abscess
  Chronic: amebiasis   Chronic: amebic dysentery
- 006.2 Amebic nondysenteric colitis
  DEF: *Entamoeba histolytica* infection with inflamed colon but no dysentery.
- 006.3 Amebic liver abscess
  Hepatic amebiasis
- 006.4 Amebic lung abscess
  Amebic abscess of lung (and liver)
- 006.5 Amebic brain abscess
  Amebic abscess of brain (and liver) (and lung)
- 006.6 Amebic skin ulceration
  Cutaneous amebiasis
- 006.8 Amebic infection of other sites
  Amebic: Ameboma
    appendicitis
    balanitis
  EXCLUDES specific infections by free-living amebae (136.2)
- 006.9 Amebiasis, unspecified
  Amebiasis NOS

4th 007 Other protozoal intestinal diseases
INCLUDES protozoal: colitis   protozoal: dysentery
    diarrhea

- 007.0 Balantidiasis
  Infection by Balantidium coli
- 007.1 Giardiasis
  Infection by Giardia lamblia   Lambliasis

INFECTIOUS AND PARASITIC DISEASES

007.2 Coccidiosis
Infection by Isospora belli and Isospora hominis
Isosporiasis

007.3 Intestinal trichomoniasis
DEF: Colitis, diarrhea, or dysentery caused by the protozoa *Trichomonas*.

007.4 Cryptosporidiosis
AHA: 4Q, '97, 30
DEF: An intestinal infection by protozoan parasites causing intractable diarrhea in patients with AIDS and other immunosuppressed individuals.

007.5 Cyclosporiasis
AHA: 4Q, '00, 38
DEF: An infection of the small intestine by the protozoal organism, *Cyclospora caytenanesis*, spread to humans though ingestion of contaminated water or food. Symptoms include watery diarrhea with frequent explosive bowel movements, loss of appetite, loss of weight, bloating, increased gas, stomach cramps, nausea, vomiting, muscle aches, low grade fever, and fatigue.

007.8 Other specified protozoal intestinal diseases
Amebiasis due to organisms other than Entamoeba histolytica

007.9 Unspecified protozoal intestinal disease
Flagellate diarrhea
Protozoal dysentery NOS

√4th 008 Intestinal infections due to other organisms
INCLUDES: any condition classifiable to 009.0-009.3 with mention of the responsible organisms
EXCLUDES: food poisoning by these organisms (005.0-005.9)

√5th 008.0 Escherichia coli [E. coli]
AHA: 4Q, '92, 17

008.00 E. coli, unspecified
E. coli enteritis NOS

008.01 Enteropathogenic E. coli
DEF: E. coli causing inflammation of intestines.

008.02 Enterotoxigenic E. coli
DEF: A toxic reaction to E. coli of the intestinal mucosa, causing voluminous watery secretions.

008.03 Enteroinvasive E. coli
DEF: E. coli infection penetrating intestinal mucosa.

008.04 Enterohemorrhagic E. coli
DEF: E. coli infection penetrating the intestinal mucosa, producing microscopic ulceration and bleeding.

008.09 Other intestinal E. coli infections

008.1 Arizona group of paracolon bacilli

008.2 Aerobacter aerogenes
Enterobacter aeogenes

008.3 Proteus (mirabilis) (morganii)

√5th 008.4 Other specified bacteria
AHA: 4Q, '92, 18

008.41 Staphylococcus
Staphylococcal enterocolitis

008.42 Pseudomonas
AHA: 2Q, '89, 10

008.43 Campylobacter

008.44 Yersinia enterocolitica

008.45 Clostridium difficile
Pseudomembranous colitis
DEF: An overgrowth of a species of bacterium that is a part of the normal colon flora in human infants and sometimes in adults; produces a toxin that causes pseudomembranous enterocolitis; typically is seen in patients undergoing antibiotic therapy.

008.46 Other anaerobes
Anaerobic enteritis NOS
Bacteroides (fragilis)
Gram-negative anaerobes

008.47 Other gram-negative bacteria
Gram-negative enteritis NOS
EXCLUDES: gram-negative anaerobes (008.46)

008.49 Other
AHA: 2Q, '89, 10; 1Q, '88, 6

008.5 Bacterial enteritis, unspecified

√5th 008.6 Enteritis due to specified virus
AHA: 4Q, '92, 18

008.61 Rotavirus

008.62 Adenovirus

008.63 Norwalk virus
Norwalk-like agent

008.64 Other small round viruses [SRVs]
Small round virus NOS

008.65 Calicivirus
DEF: Enteritis due to a subgroup of *Picornaviruses*.

008.66 Astrovirus

008.67 Enterovirus NEC
Coxsackie virus   Echovirus
EXCLUDES: poliovirus (045.0-045.9)

008.69 Other viral enteritis
Torovirus
AHA: 1Q, '03, 10

008.8 Other organism, not elsewhere classified
Viral:
 enteritis NOS
 gastroenteritis
EXCLUDES: influenza with involvement of gastrointestinal tract (487.8)

√4th 009 Ill-defined intestinal infections
EXCLUDES: diarrheal disease or intestinal infection due to specified organism (001.0-008.8)
diarrhea following gastrointestinal surgery (564.4)
intestinal malabsorption (579.0-579.9)
ischemic enteritis (557.0-557.9)
other noninfectious gastroenteritis and colitis (558.1-558.9)
regional enteritis (555.0-555.9)
ulcerative colitis (556)

009.0 Infectious colitis, enteritis, and gastroenteritis
Colitis
Enteritis } septic
Gastroenteritis

Dysentery:
 NOS
 catarrhal
 hemorrhagic
AHA: 3Q, '99, 4

DEF: Colitis: An inflammation of mucous membranes of the colon.

DEF: Enteritis: An inflammation of mucous membranes of the small intestine.

DEF: Gastroenteritis: An inflammation of mucous membranes of stomach and intestines.

009.1 Colitis, enteritis, and gastroenteritis of presumed infectious origin
EXCLUDES: colitis NOS (558.9)
enteritis NOS (558.9)
gastroenteritis NOS (558.9)
AHA: 3Q, '99, 6

INFECTIOUS AND PARASITIC DISEASES

009.2   Infectious diarrhea
    Diarrhea:
      dysenteric
      epidemic
    Infectious diarrheal disease NOS

009.3   Diarrhea of presumed infectious origin
    EXCLUDES   diarrhea NOS (787.91)
    AHA: N-D, '87, 7

TUBERCULOSIS (010-018)

INCLUDES   infection by Mycobacterium tuberculosis (human) (bovine)

EXCLUDES   congenital tuberculosis (771.2)
      late effects of tuberculosis (137.0-137.4)

The following fifth-digit subclassification is for use with categories 010-018:

  0   unspecified
  1   bacteriological or histological examination not done
  2   bacteriological or histological examination unknown (at present)
  3   tubercle bacilli found (in sputum) by microscopy
  4   tubercle bacilli not found (in sputum) by microscopy, but found by bacterial culture
  5   tubercle bacilli not found by bacteriological examination, but tuberculosis confirmed histologically
  6   tubercle bacilli not found by bacteriological or histological examination but tuberculosis confirmed by other methods [inoculation of animals]

DEF: An infection by *Mycobacterium tuberculosis* causing the formation of small, rounded nodules, called tubercles, that can disseminate throughout the body via lymph and blood vessels. Localized tuberculosis is most often seen in the lungs.

010   Primary tuberculous infection
    DEF: Tuberculosis of the lungs occurring when the patient is first infected.

    010.0   Primary tuberculous infection
      EXCLUDES   nonspecific reaction to tuberculin skin test without active tuberculosis (795.5)
          positive PPD (795.5)
          positive tuberculin skin test without active tuberculosis (795.5)
      DEF: Hilar or paratracheal lymph node enlargement in pulmonary tuberculosis.

    010.1   Tuberculous pleurisy in primary progressive tuberculosis
      DEF: Inflammation and exudation in the lining of the tubercular lung.

    010.8   Other primary progressive tuberculosis
      EXCLUDES   tuberculous erythema nodosum (017.1)

    010.9   Primary tuberculous infection, unspecified

011   Pulmonary tuberculosis
    Use additional code to identify any associated silicosis (502)

    011.0   Tuberculosis of lung, infiltrative
    011.1   Tuberculosis of lung, nodular
    011.2   Tuberculosis of lung with cavitation
    011.3   Tuberculosis of bronchus
      EXCLUDES   isolated bronchial tuberculosis (012.2)
    011.4   Tuberculous fibrosis of lung
    011.5   Tuberculous bronchiectasis
    011.6   Tuberculous pneumonia [any form]
      DEF: Inflammatory pulmonary reaction to tuberculous cells.

    011.7   Tuberculous pneumothorax
      DEF: Spontaneous rupture of damaged tuberculous pulmonary tissue.

    011.8   Other specified pulmonary tuberculosis
    011.9   Pulmonary tuberculosis, unspecified
      Respiratory tuberculosis NOS
      Tuberculosis of lung NOS

012   Other respiratory tuberculosis
    EXCLUDES   respiratory tuberculosis, unspecified (011.9)

    012.0   Tuberculous pleurisy
      Tuberculosis of pleura
      Tuberculous empyema
      Tuberculous hydrothorax
      EXCLUDES   pleurisy with effusion without mention of cause (511.9)
          tuberculous pleurisy in primary progressive tuberculosis (010.1)
      DEF: Inflammation and exudation in the lining of the tubercular lung.

    012.1   Tuberculosis of intrathoracic lymph nodes
      Tuberculosis of lymph nodes:
        hilar
        mediastinal
        tracheobronchial
      Tuberculous tracheobronchial adenopathy
      EXCLUDES   that specified as primary (010.0-010.9)

    012.2   Isolated tracheal or bronchial tuberculosis
    012.3   Tuberculous laryngitis
      Tuberculosis of glottis

    012.8   Other specified respiratory tuberculosis
      Tuberculosis of: Tuberculosis of:
        mediastinum   nose (septum)
        nasopharynx   sinus [any nasal]

013   Tuberculosis of meninges and central nervous system

    013.0   Tuberculous meningitis
      Tuberculosis of meninges (cerebral) (spinal)
      Tuberculous:
        leptomeningitis
        meningoencephalitis
      EXCLUDES   tuberculoma of meninges (013.1)

    013.1   Tuberculoma of meninges
    013.2   Tuberculoma of brain
      Tuberculosis of brain (current disease)
    013.3   Tuberculous abscess of brain
    013.4   Tuberculoma of spinal cord
    013.5   Tuberculous abscess of spinal cord
    013.6   Tuberculous encephalitis or myelitis
    013.8   Other specified tuberculosis of central nervous system
    013.9   Unspecified tuberculosis of central nervous system
      Tuberculosis of central nervous system NOS

014   Tuberculosis of intestines, peritoneum, and mesenteric glands

    014.0   Tuberculous peritonitis
      Tuberculous ascites
      DEF: Tuberculous inflammation of the membrane lining the abdomen.

    014.8   Other
      Tuberculosis (of):
        anus
        intestine (large) (small)
        mesenteric glands
        rectum
        retroperitoneal (lymph nodes)
      Tuberculous enteritis

INFECTIOUS AND PARASITIC DISEASES

015 Tuberculosis of bones and joints
Use additional code to identify manifestation, as:
tuberculous:
arthropathy (711.4)
necrosis of bone (730.8)
osteitis (730.8)
osteomyelitis (730.8)
synovitis (727.01)
tenosynovitis (727.01)

015.0 Vertebral column
Pott's disease
Use additional code to identify manifestation, as:
curvature of spine [Pott's] (737.4)
kyphosis (737.4)
spondylitis (720.81)

015.1 Hip
015.2 Knee
015.5 Limb bones
Tuberculous dactylitis
015.6 Mastoid
Tuberculous mastoiditis
015.7 Other specified bone
015.8 Other specified joint
015.9 Tuberculosis of unspecified bones and joints

016 Tuberculosis of genitourinary system
016.0 Kidney
Renal tuberculosis
Use additional code to identify manifestation, as:
tuberculous:
nephropathy (583.81)
pyelitis (590.81)
pyelonephritis (590.81)

016.1 Bladder
016.2 Ureter
016.3 Other urinary organs
016.4 Epididymis ♂
016.5 Other male genital organs ♂
Use additional code to identify manifestation, as:
tuberculosis of:
prostate (601.4)
seminal vesicle (608.81)
testis (608.81)

016.6 Tuberculous oophoritis and salpingitis ♀
016.7 Other female genital organs ♀
Tuberculous:
cervicitis
endometritis

016.9 Genitourinary tuberculosis, unspecified

017 Tuberculosis of other organs
017.0 Skin and subcutaneous cellular tissue
Lupus:
exedens
vulgaris
Scrofuloderma
Tuberculosis:
colliquativa
Tuberculosis:
cutis
lichenoides
papulonecrotica
verrucosa cutis
EXCLUDES
lupus erythematosus (695.4)
disseminated (710.0)
lupus NOS (710.0)
nonspecific reaction to tuberculin skin test without active tuberculosis (795.5)
positive PPD (795.5)
positive tuberculin skin test without active tuberculosis (795.5)

017.1 Erythema nodosum with hypersensitivity reaction in tuberculosis
Bazin's disease
Erythema:
induratum
Erythema:
nodosum, tuberculous
Tuberculosis indurativa
EXCLUDES erythema nodosum NOS (695.2)
DEF: Tender, inflammatory, bilateral nodules appearing on the shins and thought to be an allergic reaction to tuberculotoxin.

017.2 Peripheral lymph nodes
Scrofula
Scrofulous abscess
Tuberculous adenitis
EXCLUDES tuberculosis of lymph nodes:
bronchial and mediastinal (012.1)
mesenteric and retroperitoneal (014.8)
tuberculous tracheobronchial adenopathy (012.1)
DEF: Scrofula: Old name for tuberculous cervical lymphadenitis.

017.3 Eye
Use additional code to identify manifestation, as:
tuberculous:
chorioretinitis, disseminated (363.13)
episcleritis (379.09)
interstitial keratitis (370.59)
iridocyclitis, chronic (364.11)
keratoconjunctivitis (phlyctenular) (370.31)

017.4 Ear
Tuberculosis of ear
Tuberculous otitis media
EXCLUDES tuberculous mastoiditis (015.6)

017.5 Thyroid gland
017.6 Adrenal glands
Addison's disease, tuberculous
017.7 Spleen
017.8 Esophagus
017.9 Other specified organs
Use additional code to identify manifestation, as:
tuberculosis of:
endocardium [any valve] (424.91)
myocardium (422.0)
pericardium (420.0)

018 Miliary tuberculosis
INCLUDES tuberculosis:
disseminated
generalized
miliary, whether of a single specified site, multiple sites, or unspecified site
polyserositis
DEF: A form of tuberculosis caused by caseous material carried through the bloodstream planting seedlike tubercles in various body organs.

018.0 Acute miliary tuberculosis
018.8 Other specified miliary tuberculosis
018.9 Miliary tuberculosis, unspecified

ZOONOTIC BACTERIAL DISEASES (020-027)

020 Plague
INCLUDES infection by Yersinia [Pasteurella] pestis

020.0 Bubonic
DEF: Most common acute and severe form of plague characterized by lymphadenopathy (buboes), chills, fever and headache.

020.1 Cellulocutaneous
DEF: Plague characterized by inflammation and necrosis of skin.

020.2 Septicemic
DEF: Plague characterized by massive infection in the bloodstream.

§ Requires fifth-digit. See beginning of section 010–018 for codes and definitions.

 Newborn Age: 0   Pediatric Age: 0-17   Maternity Age: 12-55   Adult Age: 15-124

Tabular List — **INFECTIOUS AND PARASITIC DISEASES** — 020.3–027.9

- **020.3 Primary pneumonic**
  DEF: Plague characterized by massive pulmonary infection.
- **020.4 Secondary pneumonic**
  DEF: Lung infection as a secondary complication of plague.
- **020.5 Pneumonic, unspecified**
- **020.8 Other specified types of plague**
  Abortive plague   Pestis minor
  Ambulatory plague
- **020.9 Plague, unspecified**

√4th **021 Tularemia**
INCLUDES:
  deerfly fever
  infection by Francisella [Pasteurella] tularensis
  rabbit fever

DEF: A febrile disease transmitted by the bites of deer flies, fleas and ticks, by inhalations of aerosolized *F. tulairensis* or by ingestion of contaminated food or water; patients quickly develop fever, chills, weakness, headache, backache and malaise.

- **021.0 Ulceroglandular tularemia**
  DEF: Lesions occur at the site *Francisella tularensis*; organism enters body, usually the fingers or hands.
- **021.1 Enteric tularemia**
  Tularemia: Tularemia:
    cryptogenic   typhoidal
    intestinal
- **021.2 Pulmonary tularemia**
  Bronchopneumonic tularemia
- **021.3 Oculoglandular tularemia**
  DEF: Painful conjunctival infection by *Francisella tularensis* organism with possible corneal, preauricular lymph, or lacrimal involvement.
- **021.8 Other specified tularemia**
  Tularemia:
    generalized or disseminated
    glandular
- **021.9 Unspecified tularemia**

√4th **022 Anthrax**
AHA: 4Q '02, 70

DEF: An infectious bacterial disease usually transmitted by contact with infected animals or their discharges or products; it is classified by primary routes of inoculation as cutaneous, gastrointestinal and by inhalation.

- **022.0 Cutaneous anthrax**
  Malignant pustule
- **022.1 Pulmonary anthrax**
  Respiratory anthrax   Wool-sorters' disease
- **022.2 Gastrointestinal anthrax**
- **022.3 Anthrax septicemia**
- **022.8 Other specified manifestations of anthrax**
- **022.9 Anthrax, unspecified**

√4th **023 Brucellosis**
INCLUDES:
  fever:
    Malta
    Mediterranean
    undulant

DEF: An infectious disease caused by gram-negative, *aerobic coccobacilli* organisms; it is transmitted to humans through contact with infected tissue or dairy products; fever, sweating, weakness and aching are symptoms of the disease.

- **023.0 Brucella melitensis**
  DEF: Infection from direct or indirect contact with infected sheep or goats.
- **023.1 Brucella abortus**
  DEF: Infection from direct or indirect contact with infected cattle.
- **023.2 Brucella suis**
  DEF: Infection from direct or indirect contact with infected swine.
- **023.3 Brucella canis**
  DEF: Infection from direct or indirect contact with infected dogs.
- **023.8 Other brucellosis**
  Infection by more than one organism
- **023.9 Brucellosis, unspecified**

024 Glanders
Infection by:
  Actinobacillus mallei
  Malleomyces mallei
  Pseudomonas mallei
Farcy
Malleus

DEF: Equine infection causing mucosal inflammation and skin ulcers in humans.

025 Melioidosis
Infection by:
  Malleomyces pseudomallei
  Pseudomonas pseudomallei
  Whitmore's bacillus
Pseudoglanders

DEF: Rare infection caused by *Pseudomonas pseudomallei*; clinical symptoms range from localized infection to fatal septicemia.

√4th **026 Rat-bite fever**
- **026.0 Spirillary fever**
  Rat-bite fever due to Spirillum minor [S. minus]
  Sodoku
- **026.1 Streptobacillary fever**
  Epidemic arthritic erythema
  Haverhill fever
  Rat-bite fever due to Streptobacillus moniliformis
- **026.9 Unspecified rat-bite fever**

√4th **027 Other zoonotic bacterial diseases**
- **027.0 Listeriosis**
  Infection } by Listeria monocytogenes
  Septicemia
  Use additional code to identify manifestation, as meningitis (320.7)
  EXCLUDES: congenital listeriosis (771.2)
- **027.1 Erysipelothrix infection**
  Erysipeloid (of Rosenbach)
  Infection } by Erysipelothrix insidiosa
  Septicemia   [E. rhusiopathiae]

  DEF: Usually associated with handling of fish, meat, or poultry; symptoms range from localized inflammation to septicemia.
- **027.2 Pasteurellosis**
  Pasteurella pseudotuberculosis infection
  Mesenteric adenitis   } by Pasteurella
  Septic infection (cat bite)   multocida [P.
   (dog bite)   septica]
  EXCLUDES: infection by:
    Francisella [Pasteurella] tularensis (021.0-021.9)
    Yersinia [Pasteurella] pestis (020.0-020.9)

  DEF: Swelling, abscesses, or septicemia from *Pasteurella multocida*, commonly transmitted to humans by a dog or cat scratch.
- **027.8 Other specified zoonotic bacterial diseases**
- **027.9 Unspecified zoonotic bacterial disease**

OTHER BACTERIAL DISEASES (030-041)

EXCLUDES bacterial venereal diseases (098.0-099.9)
bartonellosis (088.0)

✓4th 030 Leprosy
INCLUDES Hansen's disease
infection by Mycobacterium leprae

- **030.0 Lepromatous [type L]**
  Lepromatous leprosy (macular) (diffuse) (infiltrated) (nodular) (neuritic)
  DEF: Infectious disseminated leprosy bacilli with lesions and deformities.

- **030.1 Tuberculoid [type T]**
  Tuberculoid leprosy (macular) (maculoanesthetic) (major) (minor) (neuritic)
  DEF: Relatively benign, self-limiting leprosy with neuralgia and scales.

- **030.2 Indeterminate [group I]**
  Indeterminate [uncharacteristic] leprosy (macular) (neuritic)
  DEF: Uncharacteristic leprosy, frequently an early manifestation.

- **030.3 Borderline [group B]**
  Borderline or dimorphous leprosy (infiltrated) (neuritic)
  DEF: Transitional form of leprosy, neither lepromatous nor tuberculoid.

- **030.8 Other specified leprosy**
- **030.9 Leprosy, unspecified**

✓4th 031 Diseases due to other mycobacteria

- **031.0 Pulmonary**
  Battey disease
  Infection by Mycobacterium:
    avium
    intracellulare [Battey bacillus]
    kansasii

- **031.1 Cutaneous**
  Buruli ulcer
  Infection by Mycobacterium:
    marinum [M. balnei]
    ulcerans

- **031.2 Disseminated**
  Disseminated mycobacterium avium-intracellulare complex (DMAC)
  Mycobacterium avium-intracellulare complex (MAC) bacteremia
  AHA: 4Q, '97, 31
  DEF: Disseminated mycobacterium avium-intracellulare complex (DMAC): A serious systemic form of MAC commonly observed in patients in the late course of AIDS.
  DEF: Mycobacterium avium-intracellulare complex (MAC) bacterium: Human pulmonary disease, lymphadenitis in children and systemic disease in immunocompromised individuals caused by a slow growing, gram-positive, aerobic organism.

- **031.8 Other specified mycobacterial diseases**
- **031.9 Unspecified diseases due to mycobacteria**
  Atypical mycobacterium infection NOS

✓4th 032 Diphtheria
INCLUDES infection by Corynebacterium diphtheriae

- **032.0 Faucial diphtheria**
  Membranous angina, diphtheritic
  DEF: Diphtheria of the throat.

- **032.1 Nasopharyngeal diphtheria**
- **032.2 Anterior nasal diphtheria**
- **032.3 Laryngeal diphtheria**
  Laryngotracheitis, diphtheritic

- **✓5th 032.8 Other specified diphtheria**
  - 032.81 Conjunctival diphtheria
    Pseudomembranous diphtheritic conjunctivitis
  - 032.82 Diphtheritic myocarditis
  - 032.83 Diphtheritic peritonitis
  - 032.84 Diphtheritic cystitis
  - 032.85 Cutaneous diphtheria
  - 032.89 Other

- **032.9 Diphtheria, unspecified**

✓4th 033 Whooping cough
INCLUDES pertussis
Use additional code to identify any associated pneumonia (484.3)
DEF: An acute, highly contagious respiratory tract infection caused by *Bordetella pertussis* and *B. bronchiseptica*; characteristic paroxysmal cough.

- **033.0 Bordetella pertussis [B. pertussis]**
- **033.1 Bordetella parapertussis [B. parapertussis]**
- **033.8 Whooping cough due to other specified organism**
  Bordetella bronchiseptica [B. bronchiseptica]
- **033.9 Whooping cough, unspecified organism**

✓4th 034 Streptococcal sore throat and scarlet fever

- **034.0 Streptococcal sore throat**
  Septic: Streptococcal:
    angina   laryngitis
    sore throat   pharyngitis
  Streptococcal: tonsillitis
    angina

- **034.1 Scarlet fever**
  Scarlatina
  EXCLUDES parascarlatina (057.8)
  DEF: Streptococcal infection and fever with red rash spreading from trunk.

035 Erysipelas
EXCLUDES postpartum or puerperal erysipelas (670)
DEF: An acute superficial cellulitis involving the dermal lymphatics; it is often caused by group A streptococci.

✓4th 036 Meningococcal infection

- **036.0 Meningococcal meningitis**
  Cerebrospinal fever (meningococcal)
  Meningitis:
    cerebrospinal
    epidemic

- **036.1 Meningococcal encephalitis**
- **036.2 Meningococcemia**
  Meningococcal septicemia
- **036.3 Waterhouse-Friderichsen syndrome, meningococcal**
  Meningococcal hemorrhagic adrenalitis
  Meningococcic adrenal syndrome
  Waterhouse-Friderichsen syndrome NOS

- **✓5th 036.4 Meningococcal carditis**
  - 036.40 Meningococcal carditis, unspecified
  - 036.41 Meningococcal pericarditis
    DEF: Meningococcal infection of the outer membrane of the heart.
  - 036.42 Meningococcal endocarditis
    DEF: Meningococcal infection of the membranes lining the cavities of the heart.
  - 036.43 Meningococcal myocarditis
    DEF: Meningococcal infection of the muscle of the heart.

- **✓5th 036.8 Other specified meningococcal infections**
  - 036.81 Meningococcal optic neuritis
  - 036.82 Meningococcal arthropathy
  - 036.89 Other

- **036.9 Meningococcal infection, unspecified**
  Meningococcal infection NOS

N Newborn Age: 0   **P** Pediatric Age: 0-17   **M** Maternity Age: 12-55   **A** Adult Age: 15-124

INFECTIOUS AND PARASITIC DISEASES

037 Tetanus
EXCLUDES tetanus:
complicating:
abortion (634-638 with .0, 639.0)
ectopic or molar pregnancy (639.0)
neonatorum (771.3)
puerperal (670)

DEF: An acute, often fatal, infectious disease caused by the anaerobic, spore-forming bacillus *Clostridium tetani*; the bacillus most often enters the body through a contaminated wound, burns, surgical wounds, or cutaneous ulcers. Symptoms include lockjaw, spasms, seizures, and paralysis.

4th 038 Septicemia
Use additional code for systemic inflammatory response syndrome (SIRS) (995.91-995.92)

EXCLUDES
bacteremia (790.7)
during labor (659.3)
following ectopic or molar pregnancy (639.0)
following infusion, injection, transfusion, or vaccination (999.3)
postpartum, puerperal (670)
septicemia (sepsis) of newborn (771.81)
that complicating abortion (634-638 with .0, 639.0)

AHA: 2Q, '04, 16; 4Q, '88, 10; 3Q, '88, 12

DEF: A systemic disease associated with the presence and persistence of pathogenic microorganisms or their toxins in the blood.

038.0 Streptococcal septicemia
AHA: 4Q, '03, 79; 2Q, '96. 5

5th 038.1 Staphylococcal septicemia
AHA: 4Q, '97, 32

038.10 Staphylococcal septicemia, unspecified

038.11 Staphylococcus aureus septicemia
AHA: 1Q, '05, 7; 2Q, '00, 5; 4Q, '98, 42

038.19 Other staphylococcal septicemia
AHA: 2Q, '00, 5

038.2 Pneumococcal septicemia [Streptococcus pneumoniae septicemia]
AHA: 2Q, '96, 5; 1Q, '91, 13

038.3 Septicemia due to anaerobes
Septicemia due to bacteroides
EXCLUDES gas gangrene (040.0)
that due to anaerobic streptococci (038.0)

DEF: Infection of blood by microorganisms that thrive without oxygen.

5th 038.4 Septicemia due to other gram-negative organisms
DEF: Infection of blood by microorganisms categorized as gram-negative by Gram's method of staining for identification of bacteria.

038.40 Gram-negative organism, unspecified
Gram-negative septicemia NOS

038.41 Hemophilus influenzae [H. influenzae]

038.42 Escherichia coli [E. coli]
AHA: 4Q, '03, 73

038.43 Pseudomonas

038.44 Serratia

038.49 Other

038.8 Other specified septicemias
EXCLUDES septicemia (due to):
anthrax (022.3)
gonococcal (098.89)
herpetic (054.5)
meningococcal (036.2)
septicemic plague (020.2)

038.9 Unspecified septicemia
Septicemia NOS
EXCLUDES bacteremia NOS (790.7)
AHA: ▶2Q, '05, 18-19;◀ 2Q, '04, 16; 4Q, '03, 79; 2Q, '00, 3; 3Q, '99. 5. 9; 1Q, '98, 5; 3Q, '96, 16; 2Q, '96, 6

4th 039 Actinomycotic infections
INCLUDES
actinomycotic mycetoma
infection by Actinomycetales, such as species of Actinomyces, Actinomadura, Nocardia, Streptomyces
maduromycosis (actinomycotic)
schizomycetoma (actinomycotic)

DEF: Inflammatory lesions and abscesses at site of infection by *Actinomyces israelii*.

039.0 Cutaneous
Erythrasma   Trichomycosis axillaris

039.1 Pulmonary
Thoracic actinomycosis

039.2 Abdominal

039.3 Cervicofacial

039.4 Madura foot
EXCLUDES madura foot due to mycotic infection (117.4)

039.8 Of other specified sites

039.9 Of unspecified site
Actinomycosis NOS   Nocardiosis NOS
Maduromycosis NOS

4th 040 Other bacterial diseases
EXCLUDES
bacteremia NOS (790.7)
bacterial infection NOS (041.9)

040.0 Gas gangrene
Gas bacillus infection or gangrene
Infection by Clostridium:
histolyticum
oedematiens
perfringens [welchii]
septicum
sordellii
Malignant edema
Myonecrosis, clostridial
Myositis, clostridial
AHA: 1Q, '95, 11

040.1 Rhinoscleroma
DEF: Growths on the nose and nasopharynx caused by *Klebsiella rhinoscleromatis*.

040.2 Whipple's disease
Intestinal lipodystrophy

040.3 Necrobacillosis
DEF: Infection with *Fusobacterium necrophorum* causing abscess or necrosis.

5th 040.8 Other specified bacterial diseases
040.81 Tropical pyomyositis

040.82 Toxic shock syndrome
Use additional code to identify the organism
AHA: 4Q, '02, 44
DEF: Syndrome caused by staphylococcal exotoxin that may rapidly progress to severe and intractable shock; symptoms include characteristic sunburn-like rash with peeling of skin on palms and soles, sudden onset high fever, vomiting, diarrhea, malagia, and hypotension.

040.89 Other
AHA: N-D, '86, 7

4th 041 Bacterial infection in conditions classified elsewhere and of unspecified site
Note: This category is provided to be used as an additional code to identify the bacterial agent in diseases classified elsewhere. This category will also be used to classify bacterial infections of unspecified nature or site.

EXCLUDES
bacteremia NOS (790.7)
septicemia (038.0-038.9)

AHA: 2Q, '01, 12; J-A, '84, 19

INFECTIOUS AND PARASITIC DISEASES

041.0–046.9

Tabular List

- √5th **041.0 Streptococcus**
  - 041.00 Streptococcus, unspecified
  - 041.01 Group A
    - AHA: 1Q, '02, 3
  - 041.02 Group B
  - 041.03 Group C
  - 041.04 Group D [Enterococcus]
  - 041.05 Group G
  - 041.09 Other Streptococcus
- √5th **041.1 Staphylococcus**
  - 041.10 Staphylococcus, unspecified
  - 041.11 Staphylococcus aureus
    - AHA: 4Q, '03, 104, 106; 2Q, '01, 11; 4Q, '98, 42, 54;4Q, '97, 32
  - 041.19 Other Staphylococcus
- 041.2 Pneumococcus
- 041.3 Friedländer's bacillus
  - Infection by Klebsiella pneumoniae
- 041.4 Escherichia coli [E. coli]
- 041.5 Hemophilus influenzae [H. influenzae]
- 041.6 Proteus (mirabilis) (morganii)
- 041.7 Pseudomonas
  - AHA: 4Q, '02, 45
- √5th **041.8 Other specified bacterial infections**
  - 041.81 Mycoplasma
    - Eaton's agent
    - Pleuropneumonia-like organisms [PPLO]
  - 041.82 Bacteroides fragilis
    - DEF: Anaerobic gram-negative bacilli of the gastrointestinal tract; frequently implicated in intra-abdominal infection; commonly resistant to antibiotics.
  - 041.83 Clostridium perfringens
  - 041.84 Other anaerobes
    - Gram-negative anaerobes
    - EXCLUDES *Helicobacter pylori (041.86)*
  - 041.85 Other gram-negative organisms
    - Aerobacter aerogenes
    - Gram-negative bacteria NOS
    - Mima polymorpha
    - Serratia
    - EXCLUDES *gram-negative anaerobes (041.84)*
    - AHA: 1Q, 95, 18
  - 041.86 Helicobacter pylori [H. pylori]
    - AHA: 4Q, '95, 60
  - 041.89 Other specified bacteria
    - AHA: 2Q, '03, 7
- 041.9 Bacterial infection, unspecified
  - AHA: 2Q, '91, 9

HUMAN IMMUNODEFICIENCY VIRUS (HIV) INFECTION (042)

- 042 **Human immunodeficiency virus [HIV] disease**
  - Acquired immune deficiency syndrome
  - Acquired immunodeficiency syndrome
  - AIDS
  - AIDS-like syndrome
  - AIDS-related complex
  - ARC
  - HIV infection, symptomatic
  - Use additional code(s) to identify all manifestations of HIV.
  - Use additional code to identify HIV-2 infection (079.53)
  - EXCLUDES *asymptomatic HIV infection status (V08)*
    exposure to HIV virus (V01.79)
    nonspecific serologic evidence of HIV (795.71)
  - AHA: 1Q, '05, 7; 2Q, '04, 11; 1Q, '04, 5; 1Q, '03, 15; 1Q, '99, 14, 4Q, '97, 30, 31; 1Q, '93, 21; 2Q, '92, 11; 3Q, '90, 17; J-A, '87, 8

POLIOMYELITIS AND OTHER NON-ARTHROPOD-BORNE VIRAL DISEASES OF CENTRAL NERVOUS SYSTEM (045-049)

- √4th **045 Acute poliomyelitis**
  - EXCLUDES *late effects of acute poliomyelitis (138)*
  - The following fifth-digit subclassification is for use with category 045:
    - 0 poliovirus, unspecified type
    - 1 poliovirus type I
    - 2 poliovirus type II
    - 3 poliovirus type III
- √5th **045.0 Acute paralytic poliomyelitis specified as bulbar**
  - Infantile paralysis (acute) ⎫
  - Poliomyelitis (acute) ⎬ specified as bulbar
  - (anterior) ⎭
  - Polioencephalitis (acute) (bulbar)
  - Polioencephalomyelitis (acute) (anterior) (bulbar)
  - DEF: Acute paralytic infection occurring where the brain merges with the spinal cord; affecting breathing, swallowing, and heart rate.
- √5th **045.1 Acute poliomyelitis with other paralysis**
  - Paralysis:
    - acute atrophic, spinal
    - infantile, paralytic
  - Poliomyelitis (acute) ⎫
  - anterior ⎬ with paralysis except bulbar
  - epidemic ⎭
  - DEF: Paralytic infection affecting peripheral or spinal nerves.
- √5th **045.2 Acute nonparalytic poliomyelitis**
  - Poliomyelitis (acute) ⎫
  - anterior ⎬ specified as nonparalytic
  - epidemic ⎭
  - DEF: Nonparalytic infection causing pain, stiffness, and paresthesias.
- √5th **045.9 Acute poliomyelitis, unspecified**
  - Infantile paralysis ⎫
  - Poliomyelitis (acute) ⎬ unspecified whether paralytic or nonparalytic
  - anterior ⎪
  - epidemic ⎭
- √4th **046 Slow virus infection of central nervous system**
  - 046.0 Kuru
    - DEF: A chronic, progressive, fatal nervous system disorder; clinical symptoms include cerebellar ataxia, trembling, spasticity and progressive dementia.
  - 046.1 Jakob-Creutzfeldt disease
    - Subacute spongiform encephalopathy
    - DEF: Communicable, progressive spongiform encephalopathy thought to be caused by an infectious particle known as a "prion" (proteinaceous infection particle). This is a progressive, fatal disease manifested principally by mental deterioration.
  - 046.2 Subacute sclerosing panencephalitis
    - Dawson's inclusion body encephalitis
    - Van Bogaert's sclerosing leukoencephalitis
    - DEF: Progressive viral infection causing cerebral dysfunction, blindness, dementia, and death (SSPE).
  - 046.3 Progressive multifocal leukoencephalopathy
    - Multifocal leukoencephalopathy NOS
    - DEF: Infection affecting cerebral cortex in patients with weakened immune systems.
  - 046.8 Other specified slow virus infection of central nervous system
  - 046.9 Unspecified slow virus infection of central nervous system

INFECTIOUS AND PARASITIC DISEASES 047–053.79

√4th 047 Meningitis due to enterovirus
- INCLUDES meningitis:
  - abacterial
  - aseptic
  - viral
- EXCLUDES meningitis due to:
  - adenovirus (049.1)
  - arthropod-borne virus (060.0-066.9)
  - leptospira (100.81)
  - virus of:
    - herpes simplex (054.72)
    - herpes zoster (053.0)
    - lymphocytic choriomeningitis (049.0)
    - mumps (072.1)
    - poliomyelitis (045.0-045.9)
  - any other infection specifically classified elsewhere

AHA: J-F, '87, 6

- 047.0 Coxsackie virus
- 047.1 ECHO virus
  - Meningo-eruptive syndrome
- 047.8 Other specified viral meningitis
- 047.9 Unspecified viral meningitis
  - Viral meningitis NOS

048 Other enterovirus diseases of central nervous system
- Boston exanthem

√4th 049 Other non-arthropod-borne viral diseases of central nervous system
- EXCLUDES late effects of viral encephalitis (139.0)

- 049.0 Lymphocytic choriomeningitis
  - Lymphocytic:
    - meningitis (serous) (benign)
    - meningoencephalitis (serous) (benign)
- 049.1 Meningitis due to adenovirus
  - DEF: Inflammation of lining of brain caused by Arenaviruses and usually occurring in adults in fall and winter months.
- 049.8 Other specified non-arthropod-borne viral diseases of central nervous system
  - Encephalitis:
    - acute:
      - inclusion body
      - necrotizing
    - epidemic
    - lethargica
    - Rio Bravo
    - von Economo's disease
- 049.9 Unspecified non-arthropod-borne viral diseases of central nervous system
  - Viral encephalitis NOS

VIRAL DISEASES ACCOMPANIED BY EXANTHEM (050-057)
EXCLUDES arthropod-borne viral diseases (060.0-066.9)
Boston exanthem (048)

√4th 050 Smallpox
- 050.0 Variola major
  - Hemorrhagic (pustular) smallpox
  - Malignant smallpox
  - Purpura variolosa
  - DEF: Form of smallpox known for its high mortality; exists only in laboratories.
- 050.1 Alastrim
  - Variola minor
  - DEF: Mild form of smallpox known for its low mortality rate.
- 050.2 Modified smallpox
  - Varioloid
  - DEF: Mild form occurring in patients with history of infection or vaccination.
- 050.9 Smallpox, unspecified

√4th 051 Cowpox and paravaccinia
- 051.0 Cowpox
  - Vaccinia not from vaccination
  - EXCLUDES vaccinia (generalized) (from vaccination) (999.0)
  - DEF: A disease contracted by milking infected cows; vesicles usually appear on the fingers, may spread to hands and adjacent areas and usually disappear without scarring; other associated features of the disease may include local edema, lymphangitis and regional lymphadenitis with or without fever.
- 051.1 Pseudocowpox
  - Milkers' node
  - DEF: Hand lesions and mild fever in dairy workers caused by exposure to paravaccinia.
- 051.2 Contagious pustular dermatitis
  - Ecthyma contagiosum
  - Orf
  - DEF: Skin eruptions caused by exposure to poxvirus-infected sheep or goats.
- 051.9 Paravaccinia, unspecified

√4th 052 Chickenpox
DEF: Contagious infection by varicella-zoster virus causing rash with pustules and fever.
- 052.0 Postvaricella encephalitis
  - Postchickenpox encephalitis
- 052.1 Varicella (hemorrhagic) pneumonitis
- 052.2 Postvaricella myelitis
  - Postchickenpox myelitis
- 052.7 With other specified complications
  - AHA: 1Q, '02, 3
- 052.8 With unspecified complication
- 052.9 Varicella without mention of complication
  - Chickenpox NOS
  - Varicella NOS

√4th 053 Herpes zoster
- INCLUDES shingles, zona
- DEF: Self-limiting infection by varicella-zoster virus causing unilateral eruptions and neuralgia along affected nerves.
- 053.0 With meningitis
  - DEF: Varicella-zoster virus infection causing inflammation of the lining of the brain and/or spinal cord.
- √5th 053.1 With other nervous system complications
  - 053.10 With unspecified nervous system complication
  - 053.11 Geniculate herpes zoster
    - Herpetic geniculate ganglionitis
    - DEF: Unilateral eruptions and neuralgia along the facial nerve geniculum affecting face and outer and middle ear.
  - 053.12 Postherpetic trigeminal neuralgia
    - DEF: Severe oral or nasal pain following a herpes zoster infection.
  - 053.13 Postherpetic polyneuropathy
    - DEF: Multiple areas of pain following a herpes zoster infection.
  - 053.14 Herpes zoster myelitis
  - 053.19 Other
- √5th 053.2 With ophthalmic complications
  - 053.20 Herpes zoster dermatitis of eyelid
    - Herpes zoster ophthalmicus
  - 053.21 Herpes zoster keratoconjunctivitis
  - 053.22 Herpes zoster iridocyclitis
  - 053.29 Other
- √5th 053.7 With other specified complications
  - 053.71 Otitis externa due to herpes zoster
  - 053.79 Other

INFECTIOUS AND PARASITIC DISEASES

053.8 **With unspecified complication**
053.9 Herpes zoster without mention of complication
    Herpes zoster NOS

√4th **054 Herpes simplex**
    EXCLUDES congenital herpes simplex (771.2)

054.0 Eczema herpeticum
    Kaposi's varicelliform eruption
    DEF: Herpes simplex virus invading site of preexisting skin inflammation.

√5th 054.1 Genital herpes
    AHA: J-F, '87, 15, 16

    054.10 **Genital herpes, unspecified**
        Herpes progenitalis
    054.11 Herpetic vulvovaginitis ♀
    054.12 Herpetic ulceration of vulva ♀
    054.13 Herpetic infection of penis ♂
    054.19 Other

054.2 Herpetic gingivostomatitis
054.3 Herpetic meningoencephalitis
    Herpes encephalitis
    Simian B disease
    DEF: Inflammation of the brain and its lining; caused by infection of herpes simplex 1 in adults and simplex 2 in newborns.

√5th 054.4 With ophthalmic complications
    054.40 **With unspecified ophthalmic complication**
    054.41 Herpes simplex dermatitis of eyelid
    054.42 Dendritic keratitis
    054.43 Herpes simplex disciform keratitis
    054.44 Herpes simplex iridocyclitis
    054.49 Other

054.5 Herpetic septicemia
    AHA: 2Q, '00, 5

054.6 Herpetic whitlow
    Herpetic felon
    DEF: A primary infection of the terminal segment of a finger by herpes simplex; intense itching and pain start the disease, vesicles form, and tissue ultimately is destroyed.

√5th 054.7 With other specified complications
    054.71 Visceral herpes simplex
    054.72 Herpes simplex meningitis
    054.73 Herpes simplex otitis externa
    054.74 Herpes simplex myelitis
    054.79 Other

054.8 **With unspecified complication**
054.9 Herpes simplex without mention of complication

√4th **055 Measles**
    INCLUDES morbilli
                  rubeola

055.0 Postmeasles encephalitis
055.1 Postmeasles pneumonia
055.2 Postmeasles otitis media

√5th 055.7 With other specified complications
    055.71 Measles keratoconjunctivitis
        Measles keratitis
    055.79 Other

055.8 **With unspecified complication**
055.9 Measles without mention of complication

√4th **056 Rubella**
    INCLUDES German measles
    EXCLUDES congenital rubella (771.0)
    DEF: Acute but usually benign togavirus infection causing fever, sore throat, and rash; associated with complications to fetus as a result of maternal infection.

√5th 056.0 With neurological complications
    056.00 **With unspecified neurological complication**
    056.01 Encephalomyelitis due to rubella
        Encephalitis } due to rubella
        Meningoencephalitis
    056.09 Other

√5th 056.7 With other specified complications
    056.71 Arthritis due to rubella
    056.79 Other

056.8 **With unspecified complications**
056.9 Rubella without mention of complication

√4th **057 Other viral exanthemata**
    DEF: Skin eruptions or rashes and fever caused by viruses, including poxviruses.

057.0 Erythema infectiosum [fifth disease]
    DEF: A moderately contagious, benign, epidemic disease, usually seen in children, and of probable viral etiology; a red macular rash appears on the face and may spread to the limbs and trunk.

057.8 Other specified viral exanthemata
    Dukes (-Filatow) disease
    Exanthema subitum [sixth disease]
    Fourth disease
    Parascarlatina
    Pseudoscarlatina
    Roseola infantum

057.9 **Viral exanthem, unspecified**

ARTHROPOD-BORNE VIRAL DISEASES (060-066)
    Use additional code to identify any associated meningitis (321.2)
    EXCLUDES late effects of viral encephalitis (139.0)

√4th **060 Yellow fever**
    DEF: Fever and jaundice from infection by mosquito-borne virus of genus Flavivirus.

060.0 Sylvatic
    Yellow fever:
        jungle
        sylvan
    DEF: Yellow fever transmitted from animal to man, via mosquito.

060.1 Urban
    DEF: Yellow fever transmitted from man to man, via mosquito.

060.9 **Yellow fever, unspecified**

061 Dengue
    Breakbone fever
    EXCLUDES hemorrhagic fever caused by dengue virus (065.4)
    DEF: Acute, self-limiting infection by mosquito-borne virus characterized by fever and generalized aches

√4th **062 Mosquito-borne viral encephalitis**

062.0 Japanese encephalitis
    Japanese B encephalitis
    DEF: Flavivirus causing inflammation of the brain with a wide range of clinical manifestations

062.1 Western equine encephalitis
    DEF: Alphavirus WEE infection causing inflammation of the brain, found in areas west of the Mississippi; transmitted horse to mosquito to man.

062.2 Eastern equine encephalitis
    EXCLUDES Venezuelan equine encephalitis (066.2)
    DEF: Alphavirus EEE causing inflammation of the brain and spinal cord, found as far north as Canada and south into South America and Mexico; transmitted horse to mosquito to man.

INFECTIOUS AND PARASITIC DISEASES

062.3 St. Louis encephalitis
DEF: Epidemic form caused by Flavivirus and transmitted by mosquito, and characterized by fever, difficulty in speech, and headache.

062.4 Australian encephalitis
Australian arboencephalitis
Australian X disease
Murray Valley encephalitis
DEF: Flavivirus causing inflammation of the brain, occurring in Australia and New Guinea.

062.5 California virus encephalitis
Encephalitis:
 California
 La Crosse
Tahyna fever
DEF: Bunya virus causing inflammation of the brain.

062.8 Other specified mosquito-borne viral encephalitis
Encephalitis by Ilheus virus
EXCLUDES West Nile virus (066.40-066.49)

062.9 Mosquito-borne viral encephalitis, unspecified

063 Tick-borne viral encephalitis
INCLUDES diphasic meningoencephalitis

063.0 Russian spring-summer [taiga] encephalitis

063.1 Louping ill
DEF: Inflammation of brain caused by virus transmitted sheep to tick to man; incidence usually limited to British Isles.

063.2 Central European encephalitis
DEF: Inflammation of brain caused by virus transmitted by tick; limited to central Europe and presenting with two distinct phases.

063.8 Other specified tick-borne viral encephalitis
Langat encephalitis   Powassan encephalitis

063.9 Tick-borne viral encephalitis, unspecified

064 Viral encephalitis transmitted by other and unspecified arthropods
Arthropod-borne viral encephalitis, vector unknown
Negishi virus encephalitis
EXCLUDES viral encephalitis NOS (049.9)

065 Arthropod-borne hemorrhagic fever

065.0 Crimean hemorrhagic fever [CHF Congo virus]
Central Asian hemorrhagic fever

065.1 Omsk hemorrhagic fever

065.2 Kyasanur Forest disease

065.3 Other tick-borne hemorrhagic fever

065.4 Mosquito-borne hemorrhagic fever
Chikungunya hemorrhagic fever
Dengue hemorrhagic fever
EXCLUDES Chikungunya fever (066.3)
 dengue (061)
 yellow fever (060.0-060.9)

065.8 Other specified arthropod-borne hemorrhagic fever
Mite-borne hemorrhagic fever

065.9 Arthropod-borne hemorrhagic fever, unspecified
Arbovirus hemorrhagic fever NOS

066 Other arthropod-borne viral diseases

066.0 Phlebotomus fever
Changuinola fever   Sandfly fever
DEF: Sandfly-borne viral infection occurring in Asia, Middle East and South America.

066.1 Tick-borne fever
Nairobi sheep disease   Tick fever:
Tick fever: Kemerovo
 American mountain   Quaranfil
 Colorado

066.2 Venezuelan equine fever
Venezuelan equine encephalitis
DEF: Alphavirus VEE infection causing inflammation of the brain, usually limited to South America, Mexico, and Florida; transmitted horse to mosquito to man.

066.3 Other mosquito-borne fever
Fever (viral):   Fever (viral):
 Bunyamwera   Oropouche
 Bwamba   Pixuna
 Chikungunya   Rift valley
 Guama   Ross river
 Mayaro   Wesselsbron
 Mucambo   Zika
 O'Nyong-Nyong
EXCLUDES dengue (061)
 yellow fever (060.0-060.9)

066.4 West Nile fever
AHA: 4Q, '02, 44
DEF: Mosquito-borne fever causing fatal inflammation of the brain, the lining of the brain, or of the lining of the brain and spinal cord.

066.40 West Nile fever, unspecified
West Nile fever NOS
West Nile fever without complications
West Nile virus NOS

066.41 West Nile fever with encephalitis
West Nile encephalitis
West Nile encephalomyelitis
AHA: 4Q, '04, 51

066.42 West Nile fever with other neurologic manifestation
Use additional code to specify the neurologic manifestation
AHA: 4Q, '04, 51

066.49 West Nile fever with other complications
Use additional code to specify the other conditions

066.8 Other specified arthropod-borne viral diseases
Chandipura fever   Piry fever

066.9 Arthropod-borne viral disease, unspecified
Arbovirus infection NOS

OTHER DISEASES DUE TO VIRUSES AND CHLAMYDIAE (070-079)

070 Viral hepatitis
INCLUDES viral hepatitis (acute) (chronic)
EXCLUDES cytomegalic inclusion virus hepatitis (078.5)

The following fifth-digit subclassification is for use with categories 070.2 and 070.3:
 0 acute or unspecified, without mention of hepatitis delta
 1 acute or unspecified, with hepatitis delta
 2 chronic, without mention of hepatitis delta
 3 chronic, with hepatitis delta

DEF: Hepatitis A: HAV infection is self-limiting with flu like symptoms; transmission, fecal-oral.
DEF: Hepatitis B: HBV infection can be chronic and systemic; transmission, bodily fluids.
DEF: Hepatitis C: HCV infection can be chronic and systemic; transmission, blood transfusion and unidentified agents.
DEF: Hepatitis D (delta): HDV occurs only in the presence of hepatitis B virus.
DEF: Hepatitis E: HEV is epidemic form; transmission and nature under investigation.

070.0 Viral hepatitis A with hepatic coma

070.1 Viral hepatitis A without mention of hepatic coma
Infectious hepatitis

070.2 Viral hepatitis B with hepatic coma
AHA: 4Q, '91, 28

070.3 Viral hepatitis B without mention of hepatic coma
Serum hepatitis
AHA: 1Q, '93, 28; 4Q, '91, 28

070.4 Other specified viral hepatitis with hepatic coma
AHA: 4Q, '91, 28

070.41 Acute hepatitis C with hepatic coma

INFECTIOUS AND PARASITIC DISEASES
070.42–077.2

- **070.42** Hepatitis delta without mention of active hepatitis B disease with hepatic coma
  - Hepatitis delta with hepatitis B carrier state
- **070.43** Hepatitis E with hepatic coma
- **070.44** Chronic hepatitis C with hepatic coma
- **070.49** Other specified viral hepatitis with hepatic coma

√5th **070.5** Other specified viral hepatitis without mention of hepatic coma
AHA: 4Q, '91, 28

- **070.51** Acute hepatitis C without mention of hepatic coma
- **070.52** Hepatitis delta without mention of active hepatitits B disease or hepatic coma
- **070.53** Hepatitis E without mention of hepatic coma
- **070.54** Chronic hepatitis C without mention of hepatic coma
- **070.59** Other specified viral hepatitis without mention of hepatic coma

070.6 Unspecified viral hepatitis with hepatic coma
  EXCLUDES unspecified viral hepatitis C with hepatic coma (070.71)

√5th **070.7** Unspecified viral hepatitis C
- **070.70** Unspecified viral hepatitis C without hepatic coma
  - Unspecified viral hepatitis C NOS
  - AHA: 4Q, '04, 52
- **070.71** Unspecified viral hepatitis C with hepatic coma
  - AHA: 4Q, '04, 52

070.9 Unspecified viral hepatitis without mention of hepatic coma
  - Viral hepatitis NOS
  EXCLUDES unspecified viral hepatitis C without hepatic coma (070.70)

071 Rabies
  Hydrophobia   Lyssa
  DEF: Acute infectious disease of the CNS caused by a rhabdovirus; usually spread by virus-laden saliva from bites by infected animals; it progresses from fever, restlessness, and extreme excitability, to hydrophobia, seizures, confusion and death.

√4th **072** Mumps
  DEF: Acute infectious disease caused by paramyxovirus; usually seen in children less than 15 years of age; salivary glands are typically enlarged, and other organs, such as testes, pancreas and meninges, are often involved.

- **072.0** Mumps orchitis ♂
- **072.1** Mumps meningitis
- **072.2** Mumps encephalitis
  - Mumps meningoencephalitis
- **072.3** Mumps pancreatitis

√5th **072.7** Mumps with other specified complications
- **072.71** Mumps hepatitis
- **072.72** Mumps polyneuropathy
- **072.79** Other

072.8 Mumps with unspecified complication
072.9 Mumps without mention of complication
  Epidemic parotitis   Infectious parotitis

√4th **073** Ornithosis
  INCLUDES parrot fever
           psittacosis
  DEF: Chlamydia psittaci infection often transmitted from birds to humans.

- **073.0** With pneumonia
  - Lobular pneumonitis due to ornithosis
- **073.7** With other specified complications
- **073.8** With unspecified complication
- **073.9** Ornithosis, unspecified

√4th **074** Specific diseases due to Coxsackie virus
  EXCLUDES Coxsackie virus:
            infection NOS (079.2)
            meningitis (047.0)

- **074.0** Herpangina
  - Vesicular pharyngitis
  DEF: Acute infectious coxsackie virus infection causing throat lesions, fever, and vomiting; generally affects children in summer.

- **074.1** Epidemic pleurodynia
  - Bornholm disease   Epidemic:
  - Devil's grip   myalgia
                             myositis
  DEF: Paroxysmal pain in chest, accompanied by fever and usually limited to children and young adults; caused by coxsackie virus.

√5th **074.2** Coxsackie carditis
- **074.20** Coxsackie carditis, unspecified
- **074.21** Coxsackie pericarditis
  DEF: Coxsackie infection of the outer lining of the heart.
- **074.22** Coxsackie endocarditis
  DEF: Coxsackie infection within the heart's cavities.
- **074.23** Coxsackie myocarditis
  - Aseptic myocarditis of newborn
  DEF: Coxsackie infection of the muscle of the heart.

- **074.3** Hand, foot, and mouth disease
  - Vesicular stomatitis and exanthem
  DEF: Mild coxsackie infection causing lesions on hands, feet and oral mucosa; most commonly seen in preschool children.

- **074.8** Other specified diseases due to Coxsackie virus
  - Acute lymphonodular pharyngitis

075 Infectious mononucleosis
  - Glandular fever   Pfeiffer's disease
  - Monocytic angina
  AHA: 3Q, '01, 13; M-A, '87, 8
  DEF: Acute infection by Epstein-Barr virus causing fever, sore throat, enlarged lymph glands and spleen, and fatigue; usually seen in teens and young adults.

√4th **076** Trachoma
  EXCLUDES late effect of trachoma (139.1)
  DEF: A chronic infectious disease of the cornea and conjunctiva caused by a strain of the bacteria *Chlamydia trachomatis*; the infection can cause photophobia, pain, excessive tearing and sometimes blindness.

- **076.0** Initial stage
  - Trachoma dubium
- **076.1** Active stage
  - Granular conjunctivitis (trachomatous)
  - Trachomatous follicular conjunctivitis pannus
- **076.9** Trachoma, unspecified
  - Trachoma NOS

√4th **077** Other diseases of conjunctiva due to viruses and Chlamydiae
  EXCLUDES ophthalmic complications of viral diseases classified elsewhere

- **077.0** Inclusion conjunctivitis
  - Paratrachoma
  - Swimming pool conjunctivitis
  EXCLUDES inclusion blennorrhea (neonatal) (771.6)
  DEF: Pus in conjunctiva caused by *Chlamydiae trachomatis* infection.

- **077.1** Epidemic keratoconjunctivitis
  - Shipyard eye
  DEF: Highly contagious corneal or conjunctival infection caused by adenovirus type 8; symptoms include inflammation and corneal infiltrates.

- **077.2** Pharyngoconjunctival fever
  - Viral pharyngoconjunctivitis

N Newborn Age: 0 **P** Pediatric Age: 0-17 **M** Maternity Age: 12-55 **A** Adult Age: 15-124

INFECTIOUS AND PARASITIC DISEASES

077.3 Other adenoviral conjunctivitis
Acute adenoviral follicular conjunctivitis

077.4 Epidemic hemorrhagic conjunctivitis
Apollo:
  conjunctivitis
  disease
Conjunctivitis due to enterovirus type 70
Hemorrhagic conjunctivitis (acute) (epidemic)

077.8 Other viral conjunctivitis
Newcastle conjunctivitis

√5th **077.9 Unspecified diseases of conjunctiva due to viruses and Chlamydiae**

077.98 Due to Chlamydiae

077.99 Due to viruses
Viral conjunctivitis NOS

√4th **078 Other diseases due to viruses and Chlamydiae**
EXCLUDES: *viral infection NOS (079.0-079.9)*
viremia NOS (790.8)

078.0 Molluscum contagiosum
DEF: Benign poxvirus infection causing small bumps on the skin or conjunctiva; transmitted by close contact.

√5th **078.1 Viral warts**
Viral warts due to human papilloma virus
AHA: 2Q, '97, 9; 4Q, '93, 22
DEF: A keratotic papilloma of the epidermis caused by the human papilloma virus; the superficial vegetative lesions last for varying durations and eventually regress spontaneously.

078.10 Viral warts, unspecified
Condyloma NOS
Verruca:
  NOS
  Vulgaris
Warts (infectious)

078.11 Condyloma acuminatum
DEF: Clusters of mucosa or epidermal lesions on external genitalia; viral infection is sexually transmitted.

078.19 Other specified viral warts
Genital warts NOS   Verruca:
Verruca: plantaris
  plana

078.2 Sweating fever
Miliary fever   Sweating disease
DEF: A viral infection characterized by profuse sweating; various papular, vesicular and other eruptions cause the blockage of sweat glands.

078.3 Cat-scratch disease
Benign lymphoreticulosis (of inoculation)
Cat-scratch fever

078.4 Foot and mouth disease
Aphthous fever   Epizootic:
Epizootic: stomatitis
  aphthae
DEF: Ulcers on oral mucosa, legs, and feet after exposure to infected animal.

078.5 Cytomegaloviral disease
Cytomegalic inclusion disease
Salivary gland virus disease
Use additional code to identify manifestation, as:
  cytomegalic inclusion virus:
    hepatitis (573.1)
    pneumonia (484.1)
EXCLUDES: *congenital cytomegalovirus infection (771.1)*
AHA: 1Q, '03, 10; 3Q, '98, 4; 2Q, '93, 11; 1Q, '89, 9
DEF: A herpes virus inclusion associated with serious disease morbidity including fever, leukopenia, pneumonia, retinitis, hepatitis and organ transplant; often leads to syndromes such as hepatomegaly, splenomegaly and thrombocytopenia; a common post-transplant complication for organ transplant recipients.

078.6 Hemorrhagic nephrosonephritis
Hemorrhagic fever:
  epidemic
  Korean
  Russian
  with renal syndrome
DEF: Viral infection causing kidney dysfunction and bleeding disorders.

078.7 Arenaviral hemorrhagic fever
Hemorrhagic fever:
  Argentine
  Bolivian
  Junin virus
  Machupo virus

√5th **078.8 Other specified diseases due to viruses and Chlamydiae**
EXCLUDES: *epidemic diarrhea (009.2)*
lymphogranuloma venereum (099.1)

078.81 Epidemic vertigo

078.82 Epidemic vomiting syndrome
Winter vomiting disease

078.88 Other specified diseases due to Chlamydiae
AHA: 4Q, '96, 22

078.89 Other specified diseases due to viruses
Epidemic cervical myalgia
Marburg disease
Tanapox

√4th **079 Viral and chlamydial infection in conditions classified elsewhere and of unspecified site**
Note: This category is provided to be used as an additional code to identify the viral agent in diseases classifiable elsewhere. This category will also be used to classify virus infection of unspecified nature or site.

079.0 Adenovirus

079.1 ECHO virus
DEF: An "orphan" enteric RNA virus, certain serotypes of which are associated with human disease, especially aseptic meningitis.

079.2 Coxsackie virus
DEF: A heterogenous group of viruses associated with aseptic meningitis, myocarditis, pericarditis, and acute onset juvenile diabetes.

079.3 Rhinovirus
DEF: Rhinoviruses affect primarily the upper respiratory tract. Over 100 distinct types infect humans.

079.4 Human papillomavirus
AHA: 2Q, '97, 9; 4Q, '93, 22
DEF: Viral infection caused by the genus *Papillomavirus* causing cutaneous and genital warts, including verruca vulgaris and condyloma acuminatum; certain types are associated with cervical dysplasia, cancer and other genital malignancies.

√5th **079.5 Retrovirus**
EXCLUDES: *human immunodeficiency virus, type 1 [HIV-1] (042)*
human T-cell lymphotrophic virus, type III [HTLV-III] (042)
lymphadenopathy-associated virus [LAV] (042)
AHA: 4Q, '93, 22, 23
DEF: A large group of RNA viruses that carry reverse transcriptase and include the leukoviruses and lentiviruses.

079.50 Retrovirus, unspecified

079.51 Human T-cell lymphotrophic virus, type I [HTLV-I]

079.52 Human T-cell lymphotrophic virus, type II [HTLV-II]

INFECTIOUS AND PARASITIC DISEASES

079.53 Human immunodeficiency virus, type 2 [HIV-2]
079.59 Other specified retrovirus

079.6 Respiratory syncytial virus (RSV)
AHA: 4Q, '96, 27, 28
DEF: The major respiratory pathogen of young children, causing severe bronchitis and bronchopneumonia, and minor infection in adults.

√5th **079.8** Other specified viral and chlamydial infections
AHA: 1Q, '88, 12

079.81 Hantavirus
AHA: 4Q, '95, 60
DEF: An infection caused by the Muerto Canyon virus whose primary rodent reservoir is the deer mouse Peromyscus maniculatus; commonly characterized by fever, myalgias, headache, cough and rapid respiratory failure.

079.82 SARS-associated coronavirus
AHA: 4Q, '03, 46
DEF: A life-threatening respiratory disease described as severe acute respiratory syndrome (SARS); etiology coronavirus; most common presenting symptoms may range from mild to more severe forms of flu-like conditions; fever, chills, cough, headache, myalgia; diagnosis of SARS is based upon clinical, laboratory, and epidemiological criteria.x

079.88 Other specified chlamydial infection
079.89 Other specified viral infection

√5th **079.9** Unspecified viral and chlamydial infections
EXCLUDES viremia NOS (790.8)
AHA: 2Q, '91, 8

079.98 Unspecified chlamydial infection
Chlamydial infections NOS
079.99 Unspecified viral infection
Viral infections NOS

RICKETTSIOSES AND OTHER ARTHROPOD-BORNE DISEASES (080-088)
EXCLUDES arthropod-borne viral diseases (060.0-066.9)

080 Louse-borne [epidemic] typhus
Typhus (fever):   Typhus (fever):
   classical   exanthematic NOS
   epidemic   louse-borne
DEF: *Rickettsia prowazekii*; causes severe headache, rash, high fever.

√4th **081** Other typhus
081.0 Murine [endemic] typhus
Typhus (fever):   Typhus (fever):
   endemic   flea-borne
DEF: Milder typhus caused by *Rickettsia typhi (mooseri)*; transmitted by rat flea.

081.1 Brill's disease
Brill-Zinsser disease
Recrudescent typhus (fever)

081.2 Scrub typhus
Japanese river fever   Mite-borne typhus
Kedani fever   Tsutsugamushi
DEF: Typhus caused by *Rickettsia tsutsugamushi* transmitted by chigger.

081.9 Typhus, unspecified
Typhus (fever) NOS

√4th **082** Tick-borne rickettsioses
082.0 Spotted fevers
Rocky mountain spotted fever
Sao Paulo fever

082.1 Boutonneuse fever
African tick typhus   Marseilles fever
India tick typhus   Mediterranean tick fever
Kenya tick typhus

082.2 North Asian tick fever
Siberian tick typhus
082.3 Queensland tick typhus

√5th **082.4** Ehrlichiosis
AHA: 4Q, '00, 38

082.40 Ehrlichiosis, unspecified
082.41 Ehrlichiosis chaffeensis [E. chaffeensis]
DEF: A febrile illness caused by bacterial infection, also called human monocytic ehrlichiosis (HME). Causal organism is *Ehrlichia chaffeensis*, transmitted by the Lone Star tick, *Amblyomma americanum*. Symptoms include fever, chills, myalgia, nausea, vomiting, diarrhea, confusion, and severe headache occurring one week after a tick bite. Clinical findings are lymphadenopathy, rash, thrombocytopenia, leukopenia, and abnormal liver function tests.

082.49 Other ehrlichiosis

082.8 Other specified tick-borne rickettsioses
Lone star fever
AHA: 4Q, '99, 19

082.9 Tick-borne rickettsiosis, unspecified
Tick-borne typhus NOS

√4th **083** Other rickettsioses
083.0 Q fever
DEF: Infection of *Coxiella burnetii* usually acquired through airborne organisms.

083.1 Trench fever
Quintan fever   Wolhynian fever

083.2 Rickettsialpox
Vesicular rickettsiosis
DEF: Infection of *Rickettsia akari* usually acquired through a mite bite.

083.8 Other specified rickettsioses
083.9 Rickettsiosis, unspecified

√4th **084** Malaria
Note: Subcategories 084.0-084.6 exclude the listed conditions with mention of pernicious complications (084.8-084.9).
EXCLUDES congenital malaria (771.2)
DEF: Mosquito-borne disease causing high fever and prostration and cataloged by species of *Plasmodium: P. falciparum, P. malariae, P. ovale,* and *P. vivax.*

084.0 Falciparum malaria [malignant tertian]
Malaria (fever):
   by Plasmodium falciparum
   subtertian

084.1 Vivax malaria [benign tertian]
Malaria (fever) by Plasmodium vivax

084.2 Quartan malaria
Malaria (fever) by Plasmodium malariae
Malariae malaria

084.3 Ovale malaria
Malaria (fever) by Plasmodium ovale

084.4 Other malaria
Monkey malaria

084.5 Mixed malaria
Malaria (fever) by more than one parasite

084.6 Malaria, unspecified
Malaria (fever) NOS

084.7 Induced malaria
Therapeutically induced malaria
EXCLUDES accidental infection from syringe, blood transfusion, etc. (084.0-084.6, above, according to parasite species)
transmission from mother to child during delivery (771.2)

| Tabular List | INFECTIOUS AND PARASITIC DISEASES | 084.8–090.2 |

084.8 Blackwater fever
  Hemoglobinuric: Malarial hemoglobinuria
    fever (bilious)
    malaria
  DEF: Severe hemic and renal complication of *Plasmodium falciparum* infection.

084.9 Other pernicious complications of malaria
  Algid malaria
  Cerebral malaria
  Use additional code to identify complication, as:
    malarial:
      hepatitis (573.2)
      nephrosis (581.81)

√4th **085 Leishmaniasis**
  085.0 Visceral [kala-azar]
    Dumdum fever
    Infection by Leishmania:
      donovani
      infantum
    Leishmaniasis:
      dermal, post-kala-azar
      Mediterranean
      visceral (Indian)
  085.1 Cutaneous, urban
    Aleppo boil   Leishmaniasis, cutaneous:
    Baghdad boil   dry form
    Delhi boil   late
    Infection by Leishmania recurrent
      tropica (minor)   ulcerating
                         Oriental sore
  085.2 Cutaneous, Asian desert
    Infection by Leishmania tropica major
    Leishmaniasis, cutaneous:
      acute necrotizing
      rural
      wet form
      zoonotic form
  085.3 Cutaneous, Ethiopian
    Infection by Leishmania ethiopica
    Leishmaniasis, cutaneous:
      diffuse
      lepromatous
  085.4 Cutaneous, American
    Chiclero ulcer
    Infection by Leishmania mexicana
    Leishmaniasis tegumentaria diffusa
  085.5 Mucocutaneous (American)
    Espundia
    Infection by Leishmania braziliensis
    Uta
  085.9 Leishmaniasis, unspecified

√4th **086 Trypanosomiasis**
  Use additional code to identify manifestations, as:
    trypanosomiasis:
      encephalitis (323.2)
      meningitis (321.3)
  086.0 Chagas' disease with heart involvement
    American trypanosomiasis } with heart
    Infection by Trypanosoma }   involvement
      cruzi   }
    Any condition classifiable to 086.2 with heart involvement
  086.1 Chagas' disease with other organ involvement
    American   }
      trypanosomiasis   } with involvement of
    Infection by   }   organ other
      Trypanosoma cruzi   }   than heart
    Any condition classifiable to 086.2 with involvement of organ other than heart

086.2 Chagas' disease without mention of organ involvement
  American trypanosomiasis
  Infection by Trypanosoma cruzi
086.3 Gambian trypanosomiasis
  Gambian sleeping sickness
  Infection by Trypanosoma gambiense
086.4 Rhodesian trypanosomiasis
  Infection by Trypanosoma rhodesiense
  Rhodesian sleeping sickness
086.5 African trypanosomiasis, unspecified
  Sleeping sickness NOS
086.9 Trypanosomiasis, unspecified

√4th **087 Relapsing fever**
  INCLUDES recurrent fever
  DEF: Infection by *Borrelia*; symptoms are episodic and include fever and arthralgia.
  087.0 Louse-borne
  087.1 Tick-borne
  087.9 Relapsing fever, unspecified

√4th **088 Other arthropod-borne diseases**
  088.0 Bartonellosis
    Carrión's disease   Verruga peruana
    Oroya fever
  √5th **088.8 Other specified arthropod-borne diseases**
    088.81 Lyme disease
      Erythema chronicum migrans
      AHA: 4Q, '91, 15; 3Q, '90, 14; 2Q, '89, 10
      DEF: A recurrent multisystem disorder caused by the spirochete *Borrelia burgdorferi* with the carrier being the tick *Ixodes dammini*; the disease begins with lesions of erythema chronicum migrans; it is followed by arthritis of the large joints, myalgia, malaise, and neurological and cardiac manifestations.
    088.82 Babesiosis
      Babesiasis
      AHA: 4Q, '93, 23
      DEF: A tick-borne disease caused by infection of *Babesia*, characterized by fever, malaise, listlessness, severe anemia and hemoglobinuria.
    088.89 Other
  088.9 Arthropod-borne disease, unspecified

SYPHILIS AND OTHER VENEREAL DISEASES (090-099)
  EXCLUDES nonvenereal endemic syphilis (104.0)
            urogenital trichomoniasis (131.0)

√4th **090 Congenital syphilis**
  DEF: Infection by spirochete *Treponema pallidum* acquired in utero from the infected mother.
  090.0 Early congenital syphilis, symptomatic
    Congenital syphilitic: Congenital syphilitic:
      choroiditis   splenomegaly
      coryza (chronic)   Syphilitic (congenital):
      hepatomegaly   epiphysitis
      mucous patches   osteochondritis
      periostitis   pemphigus
    Any congenital syphilitic condition specified as early or manifest less than two years after birth
  090.1 Early congenital syphilis, latent
    Congenital syphilis without clinical manifestations, with positive serological reaction and negative spinal fluid test, less than two years after birth
  090.2 Early congenital syphilis, unspecified
    Congenital syphilis NOS, less than two years after birth

INFECTIOUS AND PARASITIC DISEASES

090.3 **Syphilitic interstitial keratitis**
Syphilitic keratitis:
parenchymatous
punctata profunda
EXCLUDES: interstitial keratitis NOS (370.50)

√5th **090.4** **Juvenile neurosyphilis**
Use additional code to identify any associated mental disorder
DEF: *Treponema pallidum* infection involving the nervous system.

090.40 **Juvenile neurosyphilis, unspecified**
Congenital neurosyphilis
Dementia paralytica juvenilis
Juvenile:
general paresis
tabes
taboparesis

090.41 **Congenital syphilitic encephalitis**
DEF: Congenital *Treponema pallidum* infection involving the brain.

090.42 **Congenital syphilitic meningitis**
DEF: Congenital *Treponema pallidum* infection involving the lining of the brain and/or spinal cord.

090.49 **Other**

090.5 **Other late congenital syphilis, symptomatic**
Gumma due to congenital syphilis
Hutchinson's teeth
Syphilitic saddle nose
Any congenital syphilitic condition specified as late or manifest two years or more after birth

090.6 **Late congenital syphilis, latent**
Congenital syphilis without clinical manifestations, with positive serological reaction and negative spinal fluid test, two years or more after birth

090.7 **Late congenital syphilis, unspecified**
Congenital syphilis NOS, two years or more after birth

090.9 **Congenital syphilis, unspecified**

√4th **091** **Early syphilis, symptomatic**
EXCLUDES: early cardiovascular syphilis (093.0-093.9)
early neurosyphilis (094.0-094.9)

091.0 **Genital syphilis (primary)**
Genital chancre
DEF: Genital lesion at the site of initial infection by *Treponema pallidum*.

091.1 **Primary anal syphilis**
DEF: Anal lesion at the site of initial infection by *Treponema pallidum*.

091.2 **Other primary syphilis**
Primary syphilis of: Primary syphilis of:
breast   lip
fingers   tonsils
DEF: Lesion at the site of initial infection by *Treponema pallidum*.

091.3 **Secondary syphilis of skin or mucous membranes**
Condyloma latum   Secondary syphilis of:
Secondary syphilis of: skin
anus   tonsils
mouth   vulva
pharynx
DEF: Transitory or chronic lesions following initial syphilis infection.

091.4 **Adenopathy due to secondary syphilis**
Syphilitic adenopathy (secondary)
Syphilitic lymphadenitis (secondary)

√5th **091.5** **Uveitis due to secondary syphilis**
091.50 **Syphilitic uveitis, unspecified**
091.51 **Syphilitic chorioretinitis (secondary)**
DEF: Inflammation of choroid and retina as a secondary infection.

091.52 **Syphilitic iridocyclitis (secondary)**
DEF: Inflammation of iris and ciliary body as a secondary infection.

√5th **091.6** **Secondary syphilis of viscera and bone**
091.61 **Secondary syphilitic periostitis**
DEF: Inflammation of outer layers of bone as a secondary infection.

091.62 **Secondary syphilitic hepatitis**
Secondary syphilis of liver

091.69 **Other viscera**

091.7 **Secondary syphilis, relapse**
Secondary syphilis, relapse (treated) (untreated)

√5th **091.8** **Other forms of secondary syphilis**
091.81 **Acute syphilitic meningitis (secondary)**
DEF: Sudden, severe inflammation of the lining of the brain and/or spinal cord as a secondary infection.

091.82 **Syphilitic alopecia**
DEF: Hair loss following initial syphilis infection.

091.89 **Other**

091.9 **Unspecified secondary syphilis**

√4th **092** **Early syphilis, latent**
INCLUDES: syphilis (acquired) without clinical manifestations, with positive serological reaction and negative spinal fluid test, less than two years after infection

092.0 **Early syphilis, latent, serological relapse after treatment**

092.9 **Early syphilis, latent, unspecified**

√4th **093** **Cardiovascular syphilis**
093.0 **Aneurysm of aorta, specified as syphilitic**
Dilatation of aorta, specified as syphilitic

093.1 **Syphilitic aortitis**
DEF: Inflammation of the aorta - the main artery leading from the heart.

√5th **093.2** **Syphilitic endocarditis**
DEF: Inflammation of the tissues lining the cavities of the heart.

093.20 **Valve, unspecified**
Syphilitic ostial coronary disease
093.21 **Mitral valve**
093.22 **Aortic valve**
Syphilitic aortic incompetence or stenosis
093.23 **Tricuspid valve**
093.24 **Pulmonary valve**

√5th **093.8** **Other specified cardiovascular syphilis**
093.81 **Syphilitic pericarditis**
DEF: Inflammation of the outer lining of the heart.

093.82 **Syphilitic myocarditis**
DEF: Inflammation of the muscle of the heart.

093.89 **Other**

093.9 **Cardiovascular syphilis, unspecified**

√4th **094** **Neurosyphilis**
Use additional code to identify any associated mental disorder

094.0 **Tabes dorsalis**
Locomotor ataxia (progressive)
Posterior spinal sclerosis (syphilitic)
Tabetic neurosyphilis
Use additional code to identify manifestation, as: neurogenic arthropathy [Charcot's joint disease] (713.5)
DEF: Progressive degeneration of nerves associated with long-term syphilis; causing pain, wasting away, incontinence, and ataxia.

N Newborn Age: 0   **P** Pediatric Age: 0-17   **M** Maternity Age: 12-55   **A** Adult Age: 15-124

INFECTIOUS AND PARASITIC DISEASES

094.1 General paresis
- Dementia paralytica
- General paralysis (of the insane) (progressive)
- Paretic neurosyphilis
- Taboparesis

DEF: Degeneration of brain associated with long-term syphilis, causing loss of brain function, progressive dementia, and paralysis.

094.2 Syphilitic meningitis
- Meningovascular syphilis
- EXCLUDES: acute syphilitic meningitis (secondary) (091.81)

DEF: Inflammation of the lining of the brain and/or spinal cord.

094.3 Asymptomatic neurosyphilis

094.8 Other specified neurosyphilis
- 094.81 Syphilitic encephalitis
- 094.82 Syphilitic Parkinsonism
  - DEF: Decreased motor function, tremors, and muscular rigidity.
- 094.83 Syphilitic disseminated retinochoroiditis
  - DEF: Inflammation of retina and choroid due to neurosyphilis.
- 094.84 Syphilitic optic atrophy
  - DEF: Degeneration of the eye and its nerves due to neurosyphilis.
- 094.85 Syphilitic retrobulbar neuritis
  - DEF: Inflammation of the posterior optic nerve due to neurosyphilis.
- 094.86 Syphilitic acoustic neuritis
  - DEF: Inflammation of acoustic nerve due to neurosyphilis.
- 094.87 Syphilitic ruptured cerebral aneurysm
- 094.89 **Other**

094.9 Neurosyphilis, unspecified
- Gumma (syphilitic) ⎫
- Syphilis (early) (late) ⎬ of central nervous system NOS
- Syphiloma ⎭

095 Other forms of late syphilis, with symptoms
- INCLUDES: gumma (syphilitic)
- syphilis, late, tertiary, or unspecified stage

- 095.0 Syphilitic episcleritis
- 095.1 Syphilis of lung
- 095.2 Syphilitic peritonitis
- 095.3 Syphilis of liver
- 095.4 Syphilis of kidney
- 095.5 Syphilis of bone
- 095.6 Syphilis of muscle
  - Syphilitic myositis
- 095.7 Syphilis of synovium, tendon, and bursa
  - Syphilitic: bursitis
  - Syphilitic: synovitis
- 095.8 **Other specified forms of late symptomatic syphilis**
  - EXCLUDES: cardiovascular syphilis (093.0-093.9)
  - neurosyphilis (094.0-094.9)
- 095.9 **Late symptomatic syphilis, unspecified**

096 Late syphilis, latent
- Syphilis (acquired) without clinical manifestations, with positive serological reaction and negative spinal fluid test, two years or more after infection

097 Other and unspecified syphilis
- 097.0 **Late syphilis, unspecified**
- 097.1 **Latent syphilis, unspecified**
  - Positive serological reaction for syphilis
- 097.9 **Syphilis, unspecified**
  - Syphilis (acquired) NOS
  - EXCLUDES: syphilis NOS causing death under two years of age (090.9)

098 Gonococcal infections
DEF: *Neisseria gonorrhoeae* infection generally acquired in utero or in sexual congress.

098.0 Acute, of lower genitourinary tract
- Gonococcal:
  - Bartholinitis (acute)
  - urethritis (acute)
  - vulvovaginitis (acute)
- Gonorrhea (acute):
  - NOS
  - genitourinary (tract) NOS

098.1 Acute, of upper genitourinary tract
- 098.10 **Gonococcal infection (acute) of upper genitourinary tract, site unspecified**
- 098.11 Gonococcal cystitis (acute)
  - Gonorrhea (acute) of bladder
- 098.12 Gonococcal prostatitis (acute) ♂
- 098.13 Gonococcal epididymo-orchitis (acute) ♂
  - Gonococcal orchitis (acute)
  - DEF: Acute inflammation of the testes.
- 098.14 Gonococcal seminal vesiculitis (acute) ♂
  - Gonorrhea (acute) of seminal vesicle
- 098.15 Gonococcal cervicitis (acute) ♀
  - Gonorrhea (acute) of cervix
- 098.16 Gonococcal endometritis (acute) ♀
  - Gonorrhea (acute) of uterus
- 098.17 Gonococcal salpingitis, specified as acute ♀
  - DEF: Acute inflammation of the fallopian tubes.
- 098.19 Other

098.2 Chronic, of lower genitourinary tract
- Gonococcal:
  - Bartholinitis
  - urethritis
  - vulvovaginitis
- Gonorrhea:
  - NOS
  - genitourinary (tract)
- specified as chronic or with duration of two months or more

Any condition classifiable to 098.0 specified as chronic or with duration of two months or more

098.3 Chronic, of upper genitourinary tract
- INCLUDES: any condition classifiable to 098.1 stated as chronic or with a duration of two months or more

- 098.30 **Chronic gonococcal infection of upper genitourinary tract, site unspecified**
- 098.31 Gonococcal cystitis, chronic
  - Any condition classifiable to 098.11, specified as chronic
  - Gonorrhea of bladder, chronic
- 098.32 Gonococcal prostatitis, chronic ♂
  - Any condition classifiable to 098.12, specified as chronic
- 098.33 Gonococcal epididymo-orchitis, chronic ♂
  - Any condition classifiable to 098.13, specified as chronic
  - Chronic gonococcal orchitis
  - DEF: Chronic inflammation of the testes.
- 098.34 Gonococcal seminal vesiculitis, chronic ♂
  - Any condition classifiable to 098.14, specified as chronic
  - Gonorrhea of seminal vesicle, chronic
- 098.35 Gonococcal cervicitis, chronic ♀
  - Any condition classifiable to 098.15, specified as chronic
  - Gonorrhea of cervix, chronic
- 098.36 Gonococcal endometritis, chronic ♀
  - Any condition classifiable to 098.16, specified as chronic
  - DEF: Chronic inflammation of the uterus.

Additional Digit Required | Unspecified Code | Other Specified Code | Manifestation Code | ▶◀ Revised Text | ● New Code | ▲ Revised Code Title

INFECTIOUS AND PARASITIC DISEASES

098.37 Gonococcal salpingitis (chronic) ♀
DEF: Chronic inflammation of the fallopian tubes.

098.39 Other

✓5th **098.4 Gonococcal infection of eye**
  098.40 Gonococcal conjunctivitis (neonatorum)
    Gonococcal ophthalmia (neonatorum)
    DEF: Inflammation and infection of conjunctiva present at birth.
  098.41 Gonococcal iridocyclitis
    DEF: Inflammation and infection of iris and ciliary body.
  098.42 Gonococcal endophthalmia
    DEF: Inflammation and infection of the contents of the eyeball.
  098.43 Gonococcal keratitis
    DEF: Inflammation and infection of the cornea.
  098.49 Other

✓5th **098.5 Gonococcal infection of joint**
  098.50 Gonococcal arthritis
    Gonococcal infection of joint NOS
  098.51 Gonococcal synovitis and tenosynovitis
  098.52 Gonococcal bursitis
    DEF: Inflammation of the sac-like cavities in a joint.
  098.53 Gonococcal spondylitis
  098.59 Other
    Gonococcal rheumatism

098.6 Gonococcal infection of pharynx

098.7 Gonococcal infection of anus and rectum
  Gonococcal proctitis

✓5th **098.8 Gonococcal infection of other specified sites**
  098.81 Gonococcal keratosis (blennorrhagica)
    DEF: Pustular skin lesions caused by *Neisseria gonorrhoeae*.
  098.82 Gonococcal meningitis
    DEF: Inflammation of the lining of the brain and/or spinal cord.
  098.83 Gonococcal pericarditis
    DEF: Inflammation of the outer lining of the heart.
  098.84 Gonococcal endocarditis
    DEF: Inflammation of the tissues lining the cavities of the heart.
  098.85 Other gonococcal heart disease
  098.86 Gonococcal peritonitis
    DEF: Inflammation of the membrane lining the abdomen.
  098.89 Other
    Gonococcemia

✓4th **099 Other venereal diseases**
  099.0 Chancroid
    Bubo (inguinal):   Chancre:
      chancroidal   Ducrey's
      due to Hemophilus   simple
        ducreyi   soft
    Ulcus molle (cutis) (skin)
    DEF: A sexually transmitted disease caused by *Haemophilus ducreyi*; it is identified by a painful primary ulcer at the site of inoculation (usually on the external genitalia) with related lymphadenitis.

  099.1 Lymphogranuloma venereum
    Climatic or tropical bubo
    (Durand-) Nicolas-Favre disease
    Esthiomene
    Lymphogranuloma inguinale
    DEF: Sexually transmitted infection of *Chlamydia trachomatis* causing skin lesions.

  099.2 Granuloma inguinale
    Donovanosis   Granuloma venereum
    Granuloma pudendi   Pudendal ulcer
      (ulcerating)
    DEF: Chronic, sexually transmitted infection of *Calymmatobacterium granulomatis*, resulting in progressive, anogenital skin ulcers.

  099.3 Reiter's disease
    Reiter's syndrome
    Use additional code for associated:
      arthropathy (711.1)
      conjunctivitis (372.33)
    DEF: A symptom complex of unknown etiology consisting of urethritis, conjunctivitis, arthritis and myocutaneous lesions. It occurs most commonly in young men and patients with HIV and may precede or follow AIDS. Also a form of reactive arthritis.

✓5th **099.4 Other nongonococcal urethritis [NGU]**
  099.40 Unspecified
    Nonspecific urethritis
  099.41 Chlamydia trachomatis
  099.49 Other specified organism

✓5th **099.5 Other venereal diseases due to Chlamydia trachomatis**
  EXCLUDES *Chlamydia trachomatis* infection of
            conjunctiva (076.0-076.9, 077.0, 077.9)
            Lymphogranuloma venereum (099.1)
  DEF: Venereal diseases caused by *Chlamydia trachomatis* at other sites besides the urethra (e.g., pharynx, anus and rectum, conjunctiva and peritoneum).

  099.50 Unspecified site
  099.51 Pharynx
  099.52 Anus and rectum
  099.53 Lower genitourinary sites
    EXCLUDES urethra (099.41)
    Use additional code to specify site of infection, such as:
      bladder (595.4)
      cervix (616.0)
      vagina and vulva (616.11)
  099.54 Other genitourinary sites
    Use additional code to specify site of infection, such as:
      pelvic inflammatory disease NOS (614.9)
      testis and epididymis (604.91)
  099.55 Unspecified genitourinary site
  099.56 Peritoneum
    Perihepatitis
  099.59 Other specified site

099.8 Other specified venereal diseases
099.9 Venereal disease, unspecified

OTHER SPIROCHETAL DISEASES (100-104)

✓4th **100 Leptospirosis**
DEF: An infection of any spirochete of the genus Leptospire in blood. This zoonosis is transmitted to humans most often by exposure with contaminated animal tissues or water and less often by contact with urine. Patients present with flulike symptoms, the most common being muscle aches involving the thighs and low back. Treatment is with hydration and antibiotics.

  100.0 Leptospirosis icterohemorrhagica
    Leptospiral or spirochetal jaundice (hemorrhagic)
    Weil's disease

✓5th **100.8 Other specified leptospiral infections**
  100.81 Leptospiral meningitis (aseptic)
  100.89 Other
    Fever: Infection by Leptospira:
      Fort Bragg   australis
      pretibial   bataviae
      swamp   pyrogenes

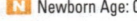

N Newborn Age: 0   P Pediatric Age: 0-17   M Maternity Age: 12-55   A Adult Age: 15-124

18 — Volume 1   2007 ICD•9•CM

INFECTIOUS AND PARASITIC DISEASES

100.9 *Leptospirosis, unspecified*

101 Vincent's angina
- Acute necrotizing ulcerative:
  - gingivitis
  - stomatitis
- Fusospirochetal pharyngitis
- Spirochetal stomatitis
- Trench mouth
- Vincent's:
  - gingivitis
  - infection [any site]

DEF: Painful ulceration with edema and hypermic patches of the oropharyngeal and throat membranes; it is caused by spreading of acute ulcerative gingivitis.

✓4th 102 Yaws
INCLUDES: frambesia, pian

DEF: An infectious, endemic, tropical disease caused by *Treponema pertenue*; it usually affects persons 15 years old or younger; a primary cutaneous lesion develops, then a granulomatous skin eruption, and occasionally lesions that destroy skin and bone.

- **102.0 Initial lesions**
  - Chancre of yaws
  - Frambesia, initial or primary
  - Initial frambesial ulcer
  - Mother yaw
- **102.1 Multiple papillomata and wet crab yaws**
  - Butter yaws
  - Frambesioma
  - Pianoma
  - Plantar or palmar papilloma of yaws
- **102.2 Other early skin lesions**
  - Cutaneous yaws, less than five years after infection
  - Early yaws (cutaneous) (macular) (papular) (maculopapular) (micropapular)
  - Frambeside of early yaws
- **102.3 Hyperkeratosis**
  - Ghoul hand
  - Hyperkeratosis, palmar or plantar (early) (late) due to yaws
  - Worm-eaten soles

  DEF: Overgrowth of the skin of the palms or bottoms of the feet, due to yaws.
- **102.4 Gummata and ulcers**
  - Gummatous frambeside
  - Nodular late yaws (ulcerated)

  DEF: Rubbery lesions and areas of dead skin caused by yaws.
- **102.5 Gangosa**
  - Rhinopharyngitis mutilans

  DEF: Massive, mutilating lesions of the nose and oral cavity caused by yaws.
- **102.6 Bone and joint lesions**
  - Goundou
  - Gumma, bone
  - Gummatous osteitis or periostitis
  } of yaws (late)
  - Hydrarthrosis
  - Osteitis
  - Periostitis (hypertrophic)
  } of yaws (early) (late)
- **102.7 Other manifestations**
  - Juxta-articular nodules of yaws
  - Mucosal yaws
- **102.8 Latent yaws**
  - Yaws without clinical manifestations, with positive serology
- **102.9** *Yaws, unspecified*

✓4th 103 Pinta

DEF: A chronic form of treponematosis, endemic in areas of tropical America; it is identified by the presence of red, violet, blue, coffee-colored or white spots on the skin.

- **103.0 Primary lesions**
  - Chancre (primary)
  - Papule (primary)
  - Pintid
  } of pinta [carate]
- **103.1 Intermediate lesions**
  - Erythematous plaques
  - Hyperchromic lesions
  - Hyperkeratosis
  } of pinta [carate]
- **103.2 Late lesions**
  - Cardiovascular lesions
  - Skin lesions:
    - achromic
    - cicatricial
    - dyschromic
  - Vitiligo
  } of pinta [carate]
- **103.3 Mixed lesions**
  - Achromic and hyperchromic skin lesions of pinta [carate]
- **103.9** *Pinta, unspecified*

✓4th 104 Other spirochetal infection
- **104.0 Nonvenereal endemic syphilis**
  - Bejel
  - Njovera

  DEF: *Treponema pallidum, T. pertenue,* or *T. carateum* infection transmitted non-sexually, causing lesions on mucosa and skin.
- **104.8 Other specified spirochetal infections**
  EXCLUDES: relapsing fever (087.0-087.9)
  syphilis (090.0-097.9)
- **104.9** *Spirochetal infection, unspecified*

MYCOSES (110-118)

Use additional code to identify manifestation as:
- arthropathy (711.6)
- meningitis (321.0-321.1)
- otitis externa (380.15)

EXCLUDES: infection by Actinomycetales, such as species of Actinomyces, Actinomadura, Nocardia, Streptomyces (039.0-039.9)

✓4th 110 Dermatophytosis
INCLUDES: infection by species of Epidermophyton, Microsporum, and Trichophyton
tinea, any type except those in 111

DEF: Superficial infection of the skin caused by a parasitic fungus.

- **110.0 Of scalp and beard**
  - Kerion
  - Sycosis, mycotic
  - Trichophytic tinea [black dot tinea], scalp
- **110.1 Of nail**
  - Dermatophytic onychia
  - Onychomycosis
  - Tinea unguium
- **110.2 Of hand**
  - Tinea manuum
- **110.3 Of groin and perianal area**
  - Dhobie itch
  - Eczema marginatum
  - Tinea cruris
- **110.4 Of foot**
  - Athlete's foot
  - Tinea pedis
- **110.5 Of the body**
  - Herpes circinatus
  - Tinea imbricata [Tokelau]
- **110.6 Deep seated dermatophytosis**
  - Granuloma trichophyticum
  - Majocchi's granuloma
- **110.8 Of other specified sites**
- **110.9** *Of unspecified site*
  - Favus NOS
  - Microsporic tinea NOS
  - Ringworm NOS

INFECTIOUS AND PARASITIC DISEASES

☑4th 111 Dermatomycosis, other and unspecified
- **111.0 Pityriasis versicolor**
  - Infection by Malassezia [Pityrosporum] furfur
  - Tinea flava
  - Tinea versicolor
- **111.1 Tinea nigra**
  - Infection by Cladosporium species
  - Keratomycosis nigricans
  - Microsporosis nigra
  - Pityriasis nigra
  - Tinea palmaris nigra
- **111.2 Tinea blanca**
  - Infection by Trichosporon (beigelii) cutaneum
  - White piedra
- **111.3 Black piedra**
  - Infection by Piedraia hortai
- **111.8 Other specified dermatomycoses**
- **111.9 Dermatomycosis, unspecified**

☑4th 112 Candidiasis
  - **INCLUDES** infection by Candida species
  - moniliasis
  - **EXCLUDES** neonatal monilial infection (771.7)
  - **DEF:** Fungal infection caused by *Candida*; usually seen in mucous membranes or skin.
- **112.0 Of mouth**
  - Thrush (oral)
- **112.1 Of vulva and vagina** ♀
  - Candidal vulvovaginitis   Monilial vulvovaginitis
- **112.2 Of other urogenital sites**
  - Candidal balanitis
  - AHA: 4Q, '03, 105; 4Q, '96, 33
- **112.3 Of skin and nails**
  - Candidal intertrigo   Candidal perionyxis
  - Candidal onychia   [paronychia]
- **112.4 Of lung**
  - Candidal pneumonia
  - AHA: 2Q, '98, 7
- **112.5 Disseminated**
  - Systemic candidiasis
  - AHA: 2Q, '00, 5; 2Q, '89, 10
- **☑5th 112.8 Of other specified sites**
  - **112.81 Candidal endocarditis**
  - **112.82 Candidal otitis externa**
    - Otomycosis in moniliasis
  - **112.83 Candidal meningitis**
  - **112.84 Candidal esophagitis**
    - AHA: 4Q, '92, 19
  - **112.85 Candidal enteritis**
    - AHA: 4Q, '92, 19
  - **112.89 Other**
    - AHA: 1Q, '92, 17; 3Q, '91, 20
- **112.9 Of unspecified site**

☑4th 114 Coccidioidomycosis
  - **INCLUDES** infection by Coccidioides (immitis)
  - Posada-Wernicke disease
  - AHA: 4Q, '93, 23
  - **DEF:** A fungal disease caused by inhalation of dust particles containing arthrospores of *Coccidioides immitis*; a self-limited respiratory infection; the primary form is known as San Joaquin fever, desert fever or valley fever.
- **114.0 Primary coccidioidomycosis (pulmonary)**
  - Acute pulmonary coccidioidomycosis
  - Coccidioidomycotic pneumonitis
  - Desert rheumatism
  - Pulmonary coccidioidomycosis
  - San Joaquin Valley fever
  - **DEF:** Acute, self-limiting *Coccidioides immitis* infection of the lung.
- **114.1 Primary extrapulmonary coccidioidomycosis**
  - Chancriform syndrome
  - Primary cutaneous coccidioidomycosis
  - **DEF:** Acute, self-limiting *Coccidioides immitis* infection in non-pulmonary site.
- **114.2 Coccidioidal meningitis**
  - **DEF:** *Coccidioides immitis* infection of the lining of the brain and/or spinal cord.
- **114.3 Other forms of progressive coccidioidomycosis**
  - Coccidioidal granuloma
  - Disseminated coccidioidomycosis
- **114.4 Chronic pulmonary coccidioidomycosis**
- **114.5 Pulmonary coccidioidomycosis, unspecified**
- **114.9 Coccidioidomycosis, unspecified**

☑4th 115 Histoplasmosis
  The following fifth-digit subclassification is for use with category 115:
  - 0 without mention of manifestation
  - 1 meningitis
  - 2 retinitis
  - 3 pericarditis
  - 4 endocarditis
  - 5 pneumonia
  - 9 other
- **☑5th 115.0 Infection by Histoplasma capsulatum**
  - American histoplasmosis
  - Darling's disease
  - Reticuloendothelial cytomycosis
  - Small form histoplasmosis
  - **DEF:** Infection resulting from inhalation of fungal spores, causing acute pneumonia, an influenza-like illness, or a disseminated disease of the reticuloendothelial system. In immunocompromised patients it can reactivate, affecting lungs, meninges, heart, peritoneum and adrenals.
- **☑5th 115.1 Infection by Histoplasma duboisii**
  - African histoplasmosis
  - Large form histoplasmosis
- **☑5th 115.9 Histoplasmosis, unspecified**
  - Histoplasmosis NOS

☑4th 116 Blastomycotic infection
- **116.0 Blastomycosis**
  - Blastomycotic dermatitis
  - Chicago disease
  - Cutaneous blastomycosis
  - Disseminated blastomycosis
  - Gilchrist's disease
  - Infection by Blastomyces [Ajellomyces] dermatitidis
  - North American blastomycosis
  - Primary pulmonary blastomycosis
- **116.1 Paracoccidioidomycosis**
  - Brazilian blastomycosis
  - Infection by Paracoccidioides [Blastomyces] brasiliensis
  - Lutz-Splendore-Almeida disease
  - Mucocutaneous-lymphangitic paracoccidioidomycosis
  - Pulmonary paracoccidioidomycosis
  - South American blastomycosis
  - Visceral paracoccidioidomycosis
- **116.2 Lobomycosis**
  - Infections by Loboa [Blastomyces] loboi
  - Keloidal blastomycosis
  - Lobo's disease

☑4th 117 Other mycoses
- **117.0 Rhinosporidiosis**
  - Infection by Rhinosporidium seeberi

117.1	**Sporotrichosis**	

- **117.1 Sporotrichosis**
  - Cutaneous sporotrichosis
  - Disseminated sporotrichosis
  - Infection by Sporothrix [Sporotrichum] schenckii
  - Lymphocutaneous sporotrichosis
  - Pulmonary sporotrichosis
  - Sporotrichosis of the bones
- **117.2 Chromoblastomycosis**
  - Chromomycosis
  - Infection by Cladosporidium carrionii, Fonsecaea compactum, Fonsecaea pedrosoi, Phialophora verrucosa
- **117.3 Aspergillosis**
  - Infection by Aspergillus species, mainly A. fumigatus, A. flavus group, A. terreus group
  - AHA: 4Q, '97, 40
- **117.4 Mycotic mycetomas**
  - Infection by various genera and species of Ascomycetes and Deuteromycetes, such as Acremonium [Cephalosporium] falciforme, Neotestudina rosatii, Madurella grisea, Madurella mycetomii, Pyrenochaeta romeroi, Zopfia [Leptosphaeria] senegalensis
  - Madura foot, mycotic
  - Maduromycosis, mycotic
  - EXCLUDES actinomycotic mycetomas (039.0-039.9)
- **117.5 Cryptococcosis**
  - Busse-Buschke's disease
  - European cryptococcosis
  - Infection by Cryptococcus neoformans
  - Pulmonary cryptococcosis
  - Systemic cryptococcosis
  - Torula
- **117.6 Allescheriosis [Petriellidosis]**
  - Infections by Allescheria [Petriellidium] boydii [Monosporium apiospermum]
  - EXCLUDES mycotic mycetoma (117.4)
- **117.7 Zygomycosis [Phycomycosis or Mucormycosis]**
  - Infection by species of Absidia, Basidiobolus, Conidiobolus, Cunninghamella, Entomophthora, Mucor, Rhizopus, Saksenaea
- **117.8 Infection by dematiacious fungi, [Phaehyphomycosis]**
  - Infection by dematiacious fungi, such as Cladosporium trichoides [bantianum], Dreschlera hawaiiensis, Phialophora gougerotii, Phialophora jeanselmi
- **117.9 Other and unspecified mycoses**
- **118 Opportunistic mycoses**
  - Infection of skin, subcutaneous tissues, and/or organs by a wide variety of fungi generally considered to be pathogenic to compromised hosts only (e.g., infection by species of Alternaria, Dreschlera, Fusarium)

HELMINTHIASES (120-129)

- **✓4th 120 Schistosomiasis [bilharziasis]**
  - DEF: Infection caused by *Schistosoma*, a genus of flukes or trematode parasites.
  - **120.0 Schistosoma haematobium**
    - Vesical schistosomiasis NOS
  - **120.1 Schistosoma mansoni**
    - Intestinal schistosomiasis NOS
  - **120.2 Schistosoma japonicum**
    - Asiatic schistosomiasis NOS
    - Katayama disease or fever
  - **120.3 Cutaneous**
    - Cercarial dermatitis
    - Infection by cercariae of Schistosoma
    - Schistosome dermatitis
    - Swimmers' itch
  - **120.8 Other specified schistosomiasis**
    - Infection by Schistosoma:
      - bovis
      - intercalatum
      - mattheii
      - spindale
    - Schistosomiasis chestermani
  - **120.9 Schistosomiasis, unspecified**
    - Blood flukes NOS
    - Hemic distomiasis
- **✓4th 121 Other trematode infections**
  - **121.0 Opisthorchiasis**
    - Infection by:
      - cat liver fluke
      - Opisthorchis (felineus) (tenuicollis) (viverrini)
  - **121.1 Clonorchiasis**
    - Biliary cirrhosis due to clonorchiasis
    - Chinese liver fluke disease
    - Hepatic distomiasis due to Clonorchis sinensis
    - Oriental liver fluke disease
  - **121.2 Paragonimiasis**
    - Infection by Paragonimus
    - Lung fluke disease (oriental)
    - Pulmonary distomiasis
  - **121.3 Fascioliasis**
    - Infection by Fasciola:
      - gigantica
      - hepatica
    - Liver flukes NOS
    - Sheep liver fluke infection
  - **121.4 Fasciolopsiasis**
    - Infection by Fasciolopsis (buski)
    - Intestinal distomiasis
  - **121.5 Metagonimiasis**
    - Infection by Metagonimus yokogawai
  - **121.6 Heterophyiasis**
    - Infection by:
      - Heterophyes heterophyes
      - Stellantchasmus falcatus
  - **121.8 Other specified trematode infections**
    - Infection by:
      - Dicrocoelium dendriticum
      - Echinostoma ilocanum
      - Gastrodiscoides hominis
  - **121.9 Trematode infection, unspecified**
    - Distomiasis NOS
    - Fluke disease NOS
- **✓4th 122 Echinococcosis**
  - INCLUDES echinococciasis
    - hydatid disease
    - hydatidosis
  - DEF: Infection caused by larval forms of tapeworms of the genus *Echinococcus*.
  - **122.0** Echinococcus granulosus infection of liver
  - **122.1** Echinococcus granulosus infection of lung
  - **122.2** Echinococcus granulosus infection of thyroid
  - **122.3** Echinococcus granulosus infection, other
  - **122.4** Echinococcus granulosus infection, unspecified
  - **122.5** Echinococcus multilocularis infection of liver
  - **122.6** Echinococcus multilocularis infection, other
  - **122.7** Echinococcus multilocularis infection, unspecified
  - **122.8** Echinococcosis, unspecified, of liver
  - **122.9** Echinococcosis, other and unspecified
- **✓4th 123 Other cestode infection**
  - **123.0 Taenia solium infection, intestinal form**
    - Pork tapeworm (adult) (infection)
  - **123.1 Cysticercosis**
    - Cysticerciasis
    - Infection by Cysticercus cellulosae [larval form of Taenia solium]
    - AHA: 2Q, '97, 8

INFECTIOUS AND PARASITIC DISEASES

123.2 **Taenia saginata infection**
  Beef tapeworm (infection)
  Infection by Taeniarhynchus saginatus

123.3 **Taeniasis, unspecified**

123.4 **Diphyllobothriasis, intestinal**
  Diphyllobothrium (adult) (latum) (pacificum) infection
  Fish tapeworm (infection)

123.5 **Sparganosis [larval diphyllobothriasis]**
  Infection by:
    Diphyllobothrium larvae
    Sparganum (mansoni) (proliferum)
    Spirometra larvae

123.6 **Hymenolepiasis**
  Dwarf tapeworm (infection)
  Hymenolepis (diminuta) (nana) infection
  Rat tapeworm (infection)

123.8 **Other specified cestode infection**
  Diplogonoporus (grandis) ⎫
  Dipylidium (caninum)   ⎬ infection
  Dog tapeworm (infection) ⎭

123.9 **Cestode infection, unspecified**
  Tapeworm (infection) NOS

124 **Trichinosis**
  Trichinella spiralis infection
  Trichinellosis
  Trichiniasis
  DEF: Infection by *Trichinella spiralis*, the smallest of the parasitic nematodes.

√4th 125 **Filarial infection and dracontiasis**

  125.0 **Bancroftian filariasis**
    Chyluria   ⎫
    Elephantiasis   ⎪
    Infection   ⎬ due to Wuchereria bancrofti
    Lymphadenitis   ⎪
    Lymphangitis   ⎭
    Wuchereriasis

  125.1 **Malayan filariasis**
    Brugia filariasis   ⎫
    Chyluria   ⎪
    Elephantiasis   ⎬ due to Brugia [Wuchereria]
    Infection   ⎪   malayi
    Lymphadenitis   ⎪
    Lymphangitis   ⎭

  125.2 **Loiasis**
    Eyeworm disease of Africa   Loa loa infection

  125.3 **Onchocerciasis**
    Onchocerca volvulus infection
    Onchocercais

  125.4 **Dipetalonemiasis**
    Infection by:
      Acanthocheilonema perstans
      Dipetalonema perstans

  125.5 **Mansonella ozzardi infection**
    Filariasis ozzardi

  125.6 **Other specified filariasis**
    Dirofilaria infection
    Infection by:
      Acanthocheilonema streptocerca
      Dipetalonema streptocerca

  125.7 **Dracontiasis**
    Guinea-worm infection
    Infection by Dracunculus medinensis

  125.9 **Unspecified filariasis**

√4th 126 **Ancylostomiasis and necatoriasis**
  INCLUDES cutaneous larva migrans due to Ancylostoma
    hookworm (disease) (infection)
    uncinariasis

  126.0 **Ancylostoma duodenale**
  126.1 **Necator americanus**
  126.2 **Ancylostoma braziliense**
  126.3 **Ancylostoma ceylanicum**
  126.8 **Other specified Ancylostoma**
  126.9 **Ancylostomiasis and necatoriasis, unspecified**
    Creeping eruption NOS
    Cutaneous larva migrans NOS

√4th 127 **Other intestinal helminthiases**

  127.0 **Ascariasis**
    Ascaridiasis
    Infection by Ascaris lumbricoides
    Roundworm infection

  127.1 **Anisakiasis**
    Infection by Anisakis larva

  127.2 **Strongyloidiasis**
    Infection by Strongyloides stercoralis
    EXCLUDES trichostrongyliasis (127.6)

  127.3 **Trichuriasis**
    Infection by Trichuris trichiuria
    Trichocephaliasis
    Whipworm (disease) (infection)

  127.4 **Enterobiasis**
    Infection by Enterobius vermicularis
    Oxyuriasis
    Oxyuris vermicularis infection
    Pinworm (disease) (infection)
    Threadworm infection

  127.5 **Capillariasis**
    Infection by Capillaria philippinensis
    EXCLUDES infection by *Capillaria hepatica* (128.8)

  127.6 **Trichostrongyliasis**
    Infection by Trichostrongylus species

  127.7 **Other specified intestinal helminthiasis**
    Infection by:
      Oesophagostomum apiostomum and related species
      Ternidens diminutus
      other specified intestinal helminth
    Physalopteriasis

  127.8 **Mixed intestinal helminthiasis**
    Infection by intestinal helminths classified to more than one of the categories 120.0-127.7
    Mixed helminthiasis NOS

  127.9 **Intestinal helminthiasis, unspecified**

√4th 128 **Other and unspecified helminthiases**

  128.0 **Toxocariasis**
    Larva migrans visceralis
    Toxocara (canis) (cati) infection
    Visceral larva migrans syndrome

  128.1 **Gnathostomiasis**
    Infection by Gnathostoma spinigerum and related species

  128.8 **Other specified helminthiasis**
    Infection by:
      Angiostrongylus cantonensis
      Capillaria hepatica
      other specified helminth

  128.9 **Helminth infection, unspecified**
    Helminthiasis NOS
    Worms NOS

129 **Intestinal parasitism, unspecified**

OTHER INFECTIOUS AND PARASITIC DISEASES (130–136)

√4th 130 **Toxoplasmosis**
  INCLUDES infection by toxoplasma gondii
    toxoplasmosis (acquired)
  EXCLUDES congenital toxoplasmosis (771.2)

  130.0 **Meningoencephalitis due to toxoplasmosis**
    Encephalitis due to acquired toxoplasmosis

  130.1 **Conjunctivitis due to toxoplasmosis**

  130.2 **Chorioretinitis due to toxoplasmosis**
    Focal retinochoroiditis due to acquired toxoplasmosis

N Newborn Age: 0   **P** Pediatric Age: 0-17   **M** Maternity Age: 12-55   **A** Adult Age: 15-124

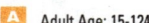

INFECTIOUS AND PARASITIC DISEASES 130.3–137.4

- **130.3** Myocarditis due to toxoplasmosis
- **130.4** Pneumonitis due to toxoplasmosis
- **130.5** Hepatitis due to toxoplasmosis
- **130.7** Toxoplasmosis of other specified sites
- **130.8** Multisystemic disseminated toxoplasmosis
  - Toxoplasmosis of multiple sites
- **130.9** Toxoplasmosis, unspecified

√4th **131 Trichomoniasis**
  - INCLUDES infection due to Trichomonas (vaginalis)

  √5th **131.0 Urogenital trichomoniasis**
  - **131.00** Urogenital trichomoniasis, unspecified
    - Fluor (vaginalis) } trichomonal or due
    - Leukorrhea (vaginalis) } to Trichomonas (vaginalis)
    - DEF: *Trichomonas vaginalis* infection of reproductive and urinary organs, transmitted through coitus.
  - **131.01** Trichomonal vulvovaginitis ♀
    - Vaginitis, trichomonal or due to Trichomonas (vaginalis)
    - DEF: *Trichomonas vaginalis* infection of vulva and vagina; often asymptomatic, transmitted through coitus.
  - **131.02** Trichomonal urethritis
    - DEF: *Trichomonas vaginalis* infection of the urethra.
  - **131.03** Trichomonal prostatitis ♂
    - DEF: *Trichomonas vaginalis* infection of the prostate.
  - **131.09** Other

  - **131.8 Other specified sites**
    - EXCLUDES intestinal (007.3)
  - **131.9 Trichomoniasis, unspecified**

√4th **132 Pediculosis and phthirus infestation**
  - **132.0** Pediculus capitis [head louse]
  - **132.1** Pediculus corporis [body louse]
  - **132.2** Phthirus pubis [pubic louse]
    - Pediculus pubis
  - **132.3** Mixed infestation
    - Infestation classifiable to more than one of the categories 132.0-132.2
  - **132.9** Pediculosis, unspecified

√4th **133 Acariasis**
  - **133.0** Scabies
    - Infestation by Sarcoptes scabiei
    - Norwegian scabies
    - Sarcoptic itch
  - **133.8** Other acariasis
    - Chiggers
    - Infestation by:
      - Demodex folliculorum
      - Trombicula
  - **133.9** Acariasis, unspecified
    - Infestation by mites NOS

√4th **134 Other infestation**
  - **134.0** Myiasis
    - Infestation by:
      - Dermatobia (hominis)
      - fly larvae
      - Gasterophilus (intestinalis)
      - maggots
      - Oestrus ovis
  - **134.1** Other arthropod infestation
    - Infestation by:
      - chigoe
      - sand flea
    - Tunga penetrans
    - Jigger disease
    - Tungiasis
    - Scarabiasis
  - **134.2** Hirudiniasis
    - Hirudiniasis (external) (internal)
    - Leeches (aquatic) (land)
  - **134.8** Other specified infestations
  - **134.9** Infestation, unspecified
    - Infestation (skin) NOS
    - Skin parasites NOS

- **135 Sarcoidosis**
  - Besnier-Boeck-Schaumann disease
  - Lupoid (miliary) of Boeck
  - Lupus pernio (Besnier)
  - Lymphogranulomatosis, benign (Schaumann's)
  - Sarcoid (any site):
    - NOS
    - Boeck
    - Darier-Roussy
  - Uveoparotid fever
  - DEF: A chronic, granulomatous reticulosis (abnormal increase in cells), affecting any organ or tissue; acute form has high rate of remission; chronic form is progressive.

√4th **136 Other and unspecified infectious and parasitic diseases**
  - **136.0** Ainhum
    - Dactylolysis spontanea
    - DEF: A disease affecting the toes, especially the fifth digit, and sometimes the fingers, especially seen in black adult males; it is characterized by a linear constriction around the affected digit leading to spontaneous amputation of the distal part of the digit.
  - **136.1** Behçet's syndrome
    - DEF: A chronic inflammatory disorder of unknown etiology involving the small blood vessels; it is characterized by recurrent aphthous ulceration of the oral and pharyngeal mucous membranes and the genitalia, skin lesions, severe uveitis, retinal vascularitis and optic atrophy.
  - **136.2** Specific infections by free-living amebae
    - Meningoencephalitis due to Naegleria
  - **136.3** Pneumocystosis
    - Pneumonia due to Pneumocystis carinii
    - ▶Pneumonia due to Pneumocystis jiroveci◀
    - AHA: 1Q, '05, 7; 1Q, '03, 15; N-D, '87, 5, 6
    - DEF: *Pneumocystis carinii* fungus causing pneumonia in immunocompromised patients; a leading cause of death among AIDS patients.
  - **136.4** Psorospermiasis
  - **136.5** Sarcosporidiosis
    - Infection by Sarcocystis lindemanni
    - DEF: Sarcocystis infection causing muscle cysts of intestinal inflammation.
  - **136.8** Other specified infectious and parasitic diseases
    - Candiru infestation
  - **136.9** Unspecified infectious and parasitic diseases
    - Infectious disease NOS
    - Parasitic disease NOS
    - AHA: 2Q, '91, 8

LATE EFFECTS OF INFECTIOUS AND PARASITIC DISEASES (137-139)

√4th **137 Late effects of tuberculosis**
  - Note: This category is to be used to indicate conditions classifiable to 010-018 as the cause of late effects, which are themselves classified elsewhere. The "late effects" include those specified as such, as sequelae, or as due to old or inactive tuberculosis, without evidence of active disease.
  - **137.0** Late effects of respiratory or unspecified tuberculosis
  - **137.1** Late effects of central nervous system tuberculosis
  - **137.2** Late effects of genitourinary tuberculosis
  - **137.3** Late effects of tuberculosis of bones and joints
  - **137.4** Late effects of tuberculosis of other specified organs

INFECTIOUS AND PARASITIC DISEASES

138 Late effects of acute poliomyelitis
> Note: This category is to be used to indicate conditions classifiable to 045 as the cause of late effects, which are themselves classified elsewhere. The "late effects" include conditions specified as such, or as sequelae, or as due to old or inactive poliomyelitis, without evidence of active disease.

✓4th **139 Late effects of other infectious and parasitic diseases**
> Note: This category is to be used to indicate conditions classifiable to categories 001-009, 020-041, 046-136 as the cause of late effects, which are themselves classified elsewhere. The "late effects" include conditions specified as such; they also include sequela of diseases classifiable to the above categories if there is evidence that the disease itself is no longer present.

139.0 Late effects of viral encephalitis
> Late effects of conditions classifiable to 049.8-049.9, 062-064

139.1 Late effects of trachoma
> Late effects of conditions classifiable to 076

139.8 Late effects of other and unspecified infectious and parasitic diseases
> AHA: 4Q, '91, 15; 3Q, '90, 14; M-A, '87, 8

2. NEOPLASMS (140-239)

Notes:

1. Content

This chapter contains the following broad groups:

140-195	Malignant neoplasms, stated or presumed to be primary, of specified sites, except of lymphatic and hematopoietic tissue
196-198	Malignant neoplasms, stated or presumed to be secondary, of specified sites
199	Malignant neoplasms, without specification of site
200-208	Malignant neoplasms, stated or presumed to be primary, of lymphatic and hematopoietic tissue
210-229	Benign neoplasms
230-234	Carcinoma in situ
235-238	Neoplasms of uncertain behavior [see Note at beginning of section]
239	Neoplasms of unspecified nature

2. Functional activity

All neoplasms are classified in this chapter, whether or not functionally active. An additional code from Chapter 3 may be used to identify such functional activity associated with any neoplasm, e.g.:

catecholamine-producing malignant pheochromocytoma of adrenal:

code 194.0, additional code 255.6

basophil adenoma of pituitary with Cushing's syndrome:

code 227.3, additional code 255.0

3. Morphology [Histology]

For those wishing to identify the histological type of neoplasms, a comprehensive coded nomenclature, which comprises the morphology rubrics of the ICD-Oncology, is given in Appendix A.

4. Malignant neoplasms overlapping site boundaries

Categories 140-195 are for the classification of primary malignant neoplasms according to their point of origin. A malignant neoplasm that overlaps two or more subcategories within a three-digit rubric and whose point of origin cannot be determined should be classified to the subcategory .8 "Other."

For example, "carcinoma involving tip and ventral surface of tongue" should be assigned to 141.8. On the other hand, "carcinoma of tip of tongue, extending to involve the ventral surface" should be coded to 141.2, as the point of origin, the tip, is known. Three subcategories (149.8, 159.8, 165.8) have been provided for malignant neoplasms that overlap the boundaries of three-digit rubrics within certain systems.

Overlapping malignant neoplasms that cannot be classified as indicated above should be assigned to the appropriate subdivision of category 195 (Malignant neoplasm of other and ill-defined sites).

AHA: 2Q, '90, 7

DEF: An abnormal growth, such as a tumor. Morphology determines behavior, i.e., whether it will remain intact (benign) or spread to adjacent tissue (malignant). The term mass is not synonymous with neoplasm, as it is often used to describe cysts and thickenings such as those occurring with hematoma or infection.

MALIGNANT NEOPLASM OF LIP, ORAL CAVITY, AND PHARYNX (140-149)

EXCLUDES carcinoma in situ (230.0)

✓4th **140 Malignant neoplasm of lip**

EXCLUDES skin of lip (173.0)

140.0 Upper lip, vermilion border
Upper lip:
NOS
external
Upper lip:
lipstick area

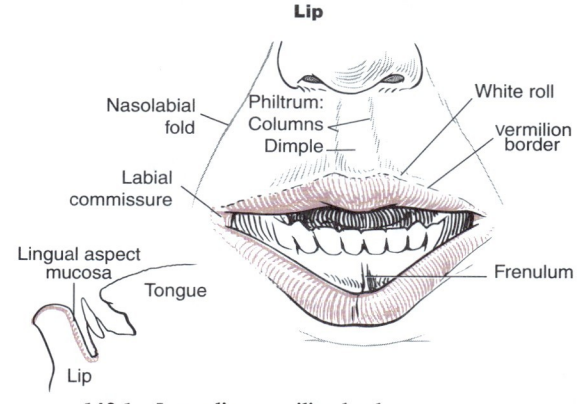

Lip

140.1 Lower lip, vermilion border
Lower lip:
NOS
external
Lower lip:
lipstick area

140.3 Upper lip, inner aspect
Upper lip:
buccal aspect
frenulum
Upper lip:
mucosa
oral aspect

140.4 Lower lip, inner aspect
Lower lip:
buccal aspect
frenulum
Lower lip:
mucosa
oral aspect

140.5 Lip, unspecified, inner aspect
Lip, not specified whether upper or lower:
buccal aspect
frenulum
mucosa
oral aspect

140.6 Commissure of lip
Labial commissure

140.8 Other sites of lip
Malignant neoplasm of contiguous or overlapping sites of lip whose point of origin cannot be determined

140.9 Lip, unspecified, vermilion border
Lip, not specified as upper or lower:
NOS
external
lipstick area

✓4th **141 Malignant neoplasm of tongue**

141.0 Base of tongue
Dorsal surface of base of tongue
Fixed part of tongue NOS

141.1 Dorsal surface of tongue
Anterior two-thirds of tongue, dorsal surface
Dorsal tongue NOS
Midline of tongue
EXCLUDES dorsal surface of base of tongue (141.0)

Tongue

141.2–146.4 NEOPLASMS — Tabular List

- **141.2** Tip and lateral border of tongue
- **141.3** Ventral surface of tongue
  Anterior two-thirds of tongue, ventral surface
  Frenulum linguae
- **141.4** Anterior two-thirds of tongue, part unspecified
  Mobile part of tongue NOS
- **141.5** Junctional zone
  Border of tongue at junction of fixed and mobile parts at insertion of anterior tonsillar pillar
- **141.6** Lingual tonsil
- **141.8** Other sites of tongue
  Malignant neoplasm of contiguous or overlapping sites of tongue whose point of origin cannot be determined
- **141.9** Tongue, unspecified
  Tongue NOS

✓4th **142** Malignant neoplasm of major salivary glands
  INCLUDES salivary ducts
  EXCLUDES malignant neoplasm of minor salivary glands:
    NOS (145.9)
    buccal mucosa (145.0)
    soft palate (145.3)
    tongue (141.0-141.9)
    tonsil, palatine (146.0)
- **142.0** Parotid gland
- **142.1** Submandibular gland
  Submaxillary gland
- **142.2** Sublingual gland
- **142.8** Other major salivary glands
  Malignant neoplasm of contiguous or overlapping sites of salivary glands and ducts whose point of origin cannot be determined
- **142.9** Salivary gland, unspecified
  Salivary gland (major) NOS

✓4th **143** Malignant neoplasm of gum
  INCLUDES alveolar (ridge) mucosa
    gingiva (alveolar) (marginal)
    interdental papillae
  EXCLUDES malignant odontogenic neoplasms (170.0-170.1)
- **143.0** Upper gum
- **143.1** Lower gum
- **143.8** Other sites of gum
  Malignant neoplasm of contiguous or overlapping sites of gum whose point of origin cannot be determined
- **143.9** Gum, unspecified

✓4th **144** Malignant neoplasm of floor of mouth
- **144.0** Anterior portion
  Anterior to the premolar-canine junction
- **144.1** Lateral portion

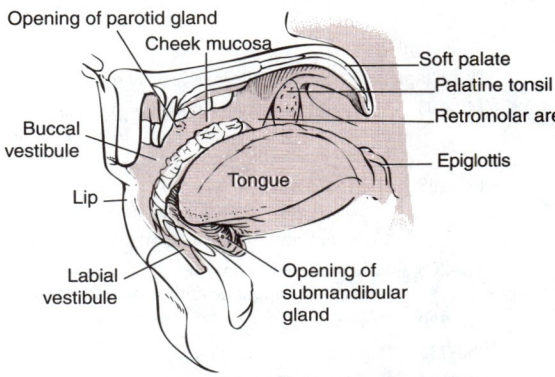

Mouth

- **144.8** Other sites of floor of mouth
  Malignant neoplasm of contiguous or overlapping sites of floor of mouth whose point of origin cannot be determined
- **144.9** Floor of mouth, part unspecified

✓4th **145** Malignant neoplasm of other and unspecified parts of mouth
  EXCLUDES mucosa of lips (140.0-140.9)
- **145.0** Cheek mucosa
  Buccal mucosa
  Cheek, inner aspect
- **145.1** Vestibule of mouth
  Buccal sulcus (upper) (lower)
  Labial sulcus (upper) (lower)
- **145.2** Hard palate
- **145.3** Soft palate
  EXCLUDES nasopharyngeal [posterior] [superior] surface of soft palate (147.3)
- **145.4** Uvula
- **145.5** Palate, unspecified
  Junction of hard and soft palate
  Roof of mouth
- **145.6** Retromolar area
- **145.8** Other specified parts of mouth
  Malignant neoplasm of contiguous or overlapping sites of mouth whose point of origin cannot be determined
- **145.9** Mouth, unspecified
  Buccal cavity NOS
  Minor salivary gland, unspecified site
  Oral cavity NOS

✓4th **146** Malignant neoplasm of oropharynx
- **146.0** Tonsil
  Tonsil: Tonsil:
    NOS   palatine
    faucial
  EXCLUDES lingual tonsil (141.6)
    pharyngeal tonsil (147.1)
  AHA: S-O, '87, 8
- **146.1** Tonsillar fossa
- **146.2** Tonsillar pillars (anterior) (posterior)
  Faucial pillar   Palatoglossal arch
  Glossopalatine fold   Palatopharyngeal arch
- **146.3** Vallecula
  Anterior and medial surface of the pharyngoepiglottic fold
- **146.4** Anterior aspect of epiglottis
  Epiglottis, free border [margin]
  Glossoepiglottic fold(s)
  EXCLUDES epiglottis:
    NOS (161.1)
    suprahyoid portion (161.1)

Main Salivary Glands

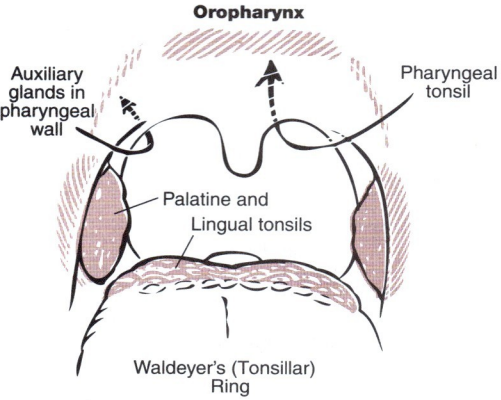

Oropharynx

146.5 Junctional region
Junction of the free margin of the epiglottis, the aryepiglottic fold, and the pharyngoepiglottic fold

146.6 Lateral wall of oropharynx

146.7 Posterior wall of oropharynx

146.8 Other specified sites of oropharynx
Branchial cleft
Malignant neoplasm of contiguous or overlapping sites of oropharynx whose point of origin cannot be determined

146.9 Oropharynx, unspecified
AHA: 2Q, '02, 6

√4ᵗʰ **147 Malignant neoplasm of nasopharynx**

147.0 Superior wall
Roof of nasopharynx

147.1 Posterior wall
Adenoid
Pharyngeal tonsil

147.2 Lateral wall
Fossa of Rosenmüller
Opening of auditory tube
Pharyngeal recess

147.3 Anterior wall
Floor of nasopharynx
Nasopharyngeal [posterior] [superior] surface of soft palate
Posterior margin of nasal septum and choanae

147.8 Other specified sites of nasopharynx
Malignant neoplasm of contiguous or overlapping sites of nasopharynx whose point of origin cannot be determined

147.9 Nasopharynx, unspecified
Nasopharyngeal wall NOS

√4ᵗʰ **148 Malignant neoplasm of hypopharynx**

148.0 Postcricoid region

148.1 Pyriform sinus
Pyriform fossa

Nasopharynx

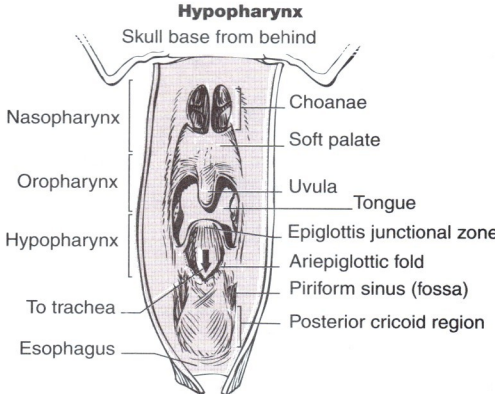

Hypopharynx

148.2 Aryepiglottic fold, hypopharyngeal aspect
Aryepiglottic fold or interarytenoid fold:
  NOS
  marginal zone
EXCLUDES aryepiglottic fold or interarytenoid fold, laryngeal aspect (161.1)

148.3 Posterior hypopharyngeal wall

148.8 Other specified sites of hypopharynx
Malignant neoplasm of contiguous or overlapping sites of hypopharynx whose point of origin cannot be determined

148.9 Hypopharynx, unspecified
Hypopharyngeal wall NOS
Hypopharynx NOS

√4ᵗʰ **149 Malignant neoplasm of other and ill-defined sites within the lip, oral cavity, and pharynx**

149.0 Pharynx, unspecified

149.1 Waldeyer's ring

149.8 Other
Malignant neoplasms of lip, oral cavity, and pharynx whose point of origin cannot be assigned to any one of the categories 140-148
EXCLUDES "book leaf" neoplasm [ventral surface of tongue and floor of mouth] (145.8)

149.9 Ill-defined

MALIGNANT NEOPLASM OF DIGESTIVE ORGANS AND PERITONEUM (150-159)
EXCLUDES carcinoma in situ (230.1-230.9)

√4ᵗʰ **150 Malignant neoplasm of esophagus**

150.0 Cervical esophagus

150.1 Thoracic esophagus

150.2 Abdominal esophagus
EXCLUDES adenocarcinoma (151.0)
  cardio-esophageal junction (151.0)

150.3 Upper third of esophagus
Proximal third of esophagus

150.4 Middle third of esophagus

150.5 Lower third of esophagus
Distal third of esophagus
EXCLUDES adenocarcinoma (151.0)
  cardio-esophageal junction (151.0)

150.8 Other specified part
Malignant neoplasm of contiguous or overlapping sites of esophagus whose point of origin cannot be determined

150.9 Esophagus, unspecified

√4ᵗʰ **151 Malignant neoplasm of stomach**
EXCLUDES ▶malignant stromal tumor of stomach (171.5)◀

151.0 Cardia
Cardiac orifice   Cardio-esophageal junction
EXCLUDES squamous cell carcinoma (150.2, 150.5)

NEOPLASMS

151.1 Pylorus
Prepylorus
Pyloric canal

151.2 Pyloric antrum
Antrum of stomach NOS

151.3 Fundus of stomach

151.4 Body of stomach

151.5 Lesser curvature, unspecified
Lesser curvature, not classifiable to 151.1-151.4

151.6 Greater curvature, unspecified
Greater curvature, not classifiable to 151.0-151.4

151.8 Other specified sites of stomach
Anterior wall, not classifiable to 151.0-151.4
Posterior wall, not classifiable to 151.0-151.4
Malignant neoplasm of contiguous or overlapping sites of stomach whose point of origin cannot be determined

151.9 Stomach, unspecified
Carcinoma ventriculi   Gastric cancer
AHA: 2Q, '01, 17

✓4th 152 Malignant neoplasm of small intestine, including duodenum
EXCLUDES ▸ malignant stromal tumor of small intestine (171.5) ◂

152.0 Duodenum

152.1 Jejunum

152.2 Ileum
EXCLUDES   ileocecal valve (153.4)

152.3 Meckel's diverticulum

152.8 Other specified sites of small intestine
Duodenojejunal junction
Malignant neoplasm of contiguous or overlapping sites of small intestine whose point of origin cannot be determined

152.9 Small intestine, unspecified

✓4th 153 Malignant neoplasm of colon

153.0 Hepatic flexure

153.1 Transverse colon

153.2 Descending colon
Left colon

153.3 Sigmoid colon
Sigmoid (flexure)
EXCLUDES   rectosigmoid junction (154.0)

153.4 Cecum
Ileocecal valve

153.5 Appendix

153.6 Ascending colon
Right colon

153.7 Splenic flexure

153.8 Other specified sites of large intestine
Malignant neoplasm of contiguous or overlapping sites of colon whose point of origin cannot be determined
EXCLUDES   ileocecal valve (153.4)
rectosigmoid junction (154.0)

153.9 Colon, unspecified
Large intestine NOS

✓4th 154 Malignant neoplasm of rectum, rectosigmoid junction, and anus

154.0 Rectosigmoid junction
Colon with rectum
Rectosigmoid (colon)

154.1 Rectum
Rectal ampulla

154.2 Anal canal
Anal sphincter
EXCLUDES   skin of anus (172.5, 173.5)
AHA: 1Q, '01, 8

154.3 Anus, unspecified
EXCLUDES   anus:
margin (172.5, 173.5)
skin (172.5, 173.5)
perianal skin (172.5, 173.5)

154.8 Other
Anorectum
Cloacogenic zone
Malignant neoplasm of contiguous or overlapping sites of rectum, rectosigmoid junction, and anus whose point of origin cannot be determined

✓4th 155 Malignant neoplasm of liver and intrahepatic bile ducts

155.0 Liver, primary
Carcinoma:
hepatocellular
liver cell
liver, specified as primary
Hepatoblastoma

155.1 Intrahepatic bile ducts
Canaliculi biliferi   Intrahepatic:
Interlobular: biliary passages
 bile ducts   canaliculi
 biliary canals   gall duct
EXCLUDES   hepatic duct (156.1)

155.2 Liver, not specified as primary or secondary

✓4th 156 Malignant neoplasm of gallbladder and extrahepatic bile ducts

156.0 Gallbladder

156.1 Extrahepatic bile ducts
Biliary duct or passage NOS
Common bile duct
Cystic duct
Hepatic duct
Sphincter of Oddi

156.2 Ampulla of Vater
DEF: Malignant neoplasm in the area of dilation at the juncture of the common bile and pancreatic ducts near the opening into the lumen of the duodenum.

156.8 Other specified sites of gallbladder and extrahepatic bile ducts
Malignant neoplasm of contiguous or overlapping sites of gallbladder and extrahepatic bile ducts whose point of origin cannot be determined

156.9 Biliary tract, part unspecified
Malignant neoplasm involving both intrahepatic and extrahepatic bile ducts

✓4th 157 Malignant neoplasm of pancreas

157.0 Head of pancreas
AHA: 2Q, '05, 9; 4Q, '00, 40

157.1 Body of pancreas

157.2 Tail of pancreas

157.3 Pancreatic duct
Duct of:
Santorini
Wirsung

NEOPLASMS

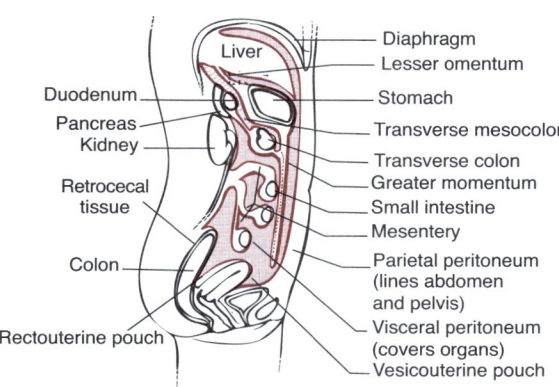
Retroperitoneum and Peritoneum

157.4 Islets of Langerhans
Islets of Langerhans, any part of pancreas
Use additional code to identify any functional activity

DEF: Malignant neoplasm within the structures of the pancreas that produce insulin, somatostatin and glucagon.

157.8 Other specified sites of pancreas
Ectopic pancreatic tissue
Malignant neoplasm of contiguous or overlapping sites of pancreas whose point of origin cannot be determined

157.9 Pancreas, part unspecified
AHA: 4Q, '89, 11

✓4th **158 Malignant neoplasm of retroperitoneum and peritoneum**

158.0 Retroperitoneum
Periadrenal tissue
Perinephric tissue
Perirenal tissue
Retrocecal tissue

158.8 Specified parts of peritoneum
Cul-de-sac (of Douglas)
Mesentery
Mesocolon
Omentum
Peritoneum:
  parietal
  pelvic
Rectouterine pouch
Malignant neoplasm of contiguous or overlapping sites of retroperitoneum and peritoneum whose point of origin cannot be determined

158.9 Peritoneum, unspecified

✓4th **159 Malignant neoplasm of other and ill-defined sites within the digestive organs and peritoneum**

159.0 Intestinal tract, part unspecified
Intestine NOS

159.1 Spleen, not elsewhere classified
Angiosarcoma } of spleen
Fibrosarcoma
EXCLUDES Hodgkin's disease (201.0-201.9)
          lymphosarcoma (200.1)
          reticulosarcoma (200.0)

159.8 Other sites of digestive system and intra-abdominal organs
Malignant neoplasm of digestive organs and peritoneum whose point of origin cannot be assigned to any one of the categories 150-158
EXCLUDES anus and rectum (154.8)
          cardio-esophageal junction (151.0)
          colon and rectum (154.0)

159.9 Ill-defined
Alimentary canal or tract NOS
Gastrointestinal tract NOS
EXCLUDES abdominal NOS (195.2)
          intra-abdominal NOS (195.2)

MALIGNANT NEOPLASM OF RESPIRATORY AND INTRATHORACIC ORGANS (160-165)
EXCLUDES carcinoma in situ (231.0-231.9)

✓4th **160 Malignant neoplasm of nasal cavities, middle ear, and accessory sinuses**

160.0 Nasal cavities
Cartilage of nose   Septum of nose
Conchae, nasal   Vestibule of nose
Internal nose
EXCLUDES nasal bone (170.0)
          nose NOS (195.0)
          olfactory bulb (192.0)
          posterior margin of septum and choanae (147.3)
          skin of nose (172.3, 173.3)
          turbinates (170.0)

160.1 Auditory tube, middle ear, and mastoid air cells
Antrum tympanicum   Tympanic cavity
Eustachian tube
EXCLUDES auditory canal (external) (172.2, 173.2)
          bone of ear (meatus) (170.0)
          cartilage of ear (171.0)
          ear (external) (skin) (172.2, 173.2)

160.2 Maxillary sinus
Antrum (Highmore) (maxillary)

160.3 Ethmoidal sinus

160.4 Frontal sinus

160.5 Sphenoidal sinus

160.8 Other
Malignant neoplasm of contiguous or overlapping sites of nasal cavities, middle ear, and accessory sinuses whose point of origin cannot be determined

160.9 Accessory sinus, unspecified

✓4th **161 Malignant neoplasm of larynx**

161.0 Glottis
Intrinsic larynx
Laryngeal commissure (anterior) (posterior)
True vocal cord
Vocal cord NOS

161.1 Supraglottis
Aryepiglottic fold or interarytenoid fold, laryngeal aspect
Epiglottis (suprahyoid portion) NOS
Extrinsic larynx
False vocal cords
Posterior (laryngeal) surface of epiglottis
Ventricular bands
EXCLUDES anterior aspect of epiglottis (146.4)
          aryepiglottic fold or interarytenoid fold:
            NOS (148.2)
            hypopharyngeal aspect (148.2)
            marginal zone (148.2)

161.2 Subglottis

161.3 Laryngeal cartilages
Cartilage: Cartilage:
  arytenoid   cuneiform
  cricoid   thyroid

161.8 Other specified sites of larynx
Malignant neoplasm of contiguous or overlapping sites of larynx whose point of origin cannot be determined

161.9 Larynx, unspecified

NEOPLASMS — Tabular List
162–170.7

✓4th 162 Malignant neoplasm of trachea, bronchus, and lung

- 162.0 Trachea
  - Cartilage } of trachea
  - Mucosa
- 162.2 Main bronchus
  - Carina
  - Hilus of lung
- 162.3 Upper lobe, bronchus or lung
  - AHA: 1Q, '04, 4
- 162.4 Middle lobe, bronchus or lung
- 162.5 Lower lobe, bronchus or lung
- 162.8 Other parts of bronchus or lung
  - Malignant neoplasm of contiguous or overlapping sites of bronchus or lung whose point of origin cannot be determined
- 162.9 Bronchus and lung, unspecified
  - AHA: 2Q, '97, 3; 4Q, '96, 48

✓4th 163 Malignant neoplasm of pleura

- 163.0 Parietal pleura
- 163.1 Visceral pleura
- 163.8 Other specified sites of pleura
  - Malignant neoplasm of contiguous or overlapping sites of pleura whose point of origin cannot be determined
- 163.9 Pleura, unspecified

✓4th 164 Malignant neoplasm of thymus, heart, and mediastinum

- 164.0 Thymus
- 164.1 Heart
  - Endocardium
  - Epicardium
  - Myocardium
  - Pericardium
  - **EXCLUDES** great vessels (171.4)
- 164.2 Anterior mediastinum
- 164.3 Posterior mediastinum
- 164.8 Other
  - Malignant neoplasm of contiguous or overlapping sites of thymus, heart, and mediastinum whose point of origin cannot be determined
- 164.9 Mediastinum, part unspecified

✓4th 165 Malignant neoplasm of other and ill-defined sites within the respiratory system and intrathoracic organs

- 165.0 Upper respiratory tract, part unspecified
- 165.8 Other
  - Malignant neoplasm of respiratory and intrathoracic organs whose point of origin cannot be assigned to any one of the categories 160-164
- 165.9 Ill-defined sites within the respiratory system
  - Respiratory tract NOS
  - **EXCLUDES** intrathoracic NOS (195.1)
  - thoracic NOS (195.1)

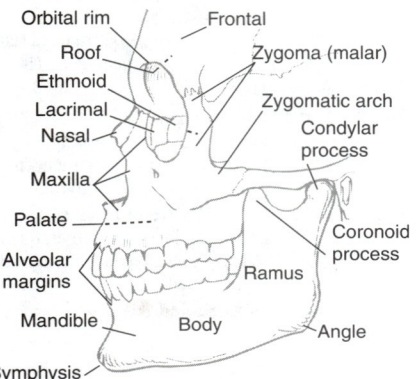

Skull

MALIGNANT NEOPLASM OF BONE, CONNECTIVE TISSUE, SKIN, AND BREAST (170-176)

EXCLUDES carcinoma in situ:
- breast (233.0)
- skin (232.0-232.9)

✓4th 170 Malignant neoplasm of bone and articular cartilage

INCLUDES cartilage (articular) (joint)
periosteum

EXCLUDES bone marrow NOS (202.9)
cartilage:
- ear (171.0)
- eyelid (171.0)
- larynx (161.3)
- nose (160.0)
synovia (171.0-171.9)

- 170.0 Bones of skull and face, except mandible
  - Bone: ethmoid, frontal, malar, nasal, occipital, orbital, parietal
  - Bone: sphenoid, temporal, zygomatic, Maxilla (superior), Turbinate, Upper jaw bone, Vomer
  - **EXCLUDES** carcinoma, any type except intraosseous or odontogenic:
    - maxilla, maxillary (sinus) (160.2)
    - upper jaw bone (143.0)
  - jaw bone (lower) (170.1)

- 170.1 Mandible
  - Inferior maxilla
  - Jaw bone NOS
  - Lower jaw bone
  - **EXCLUDES** carcinoma, any type except intraosseous or odontogenic:
    - jaw bone NOS (143.9)
    - lower (143.1)
    - upper jaw bone (170.0)

- 170.2 Vertebral column, excluding sacrum and coccyx
  - Spinal column   Vertebra
  - Spine
  - **EXCLUDES** sacrum and coccyx (170.6)

- 170.3 Ribs, sternum, and clavicle
  - Costal cartilage
  - Costovertebral joint
  - Xiphoid process

- 170.4 Scapula and long bones of upper limb
  - Acromion
  - Bones NOS of upper limb
  - Humerus
  - Radius
  - Ulna
  - AHA: 2Q, '99, 9

- 170.5 Short bones of upper limb
  - Carpal   Scaphoid (of hand)
  - Cuneiform, wrist   Semilunar or lunate
  - Metacarpal   Trapezium
  - Navicular, of hand   Trapezoid
  - Phalanges of hand   Unciform
  - Pisiform

- 170.6 Pelvic bones, sacrum, and coccyx
  - Coccygeal vertebra   Pubic bone
  - Ilium   Sacral vertebra
  - Ischium

- 170.7 Long bones of lower limb
  - Bones NOS of lower limb
  - Femur
  - Fibula
  - Tibia

NEOPLASMS

170.8 Short bones of lower limb
- Astragalus [talus]
- Calcaneus
- Cuboid
- Cuneiform, ankle
- Metatarsal
- Navicular (of ankle)
- Patella
- Phalanges of foot
- Tarsal

170.9 Bone and articular cartilage, site unspecified

✓4th 171 Malignant neoplasm of connective and other soft tissue

INCLUDES:
- blood vessel
- bursa
- fascia
- fat
- ligament, except uterine
- ▶malignant stromal tumors◀
- muscle
- peripheral, sympathetic, and parasympathetic nerves and ganglia
- synovia
- tendon (sheath)

EXCLUDES:
- cartilage (of):
  - articular (170.0-170.9)
  - larynx (161.3)
  - nose (160.0)
- connective tissue:
  - breast (174.0-175.9)
  - internal organs ▶(except stromal tumors)◀—code to malignant neoplasm of the site [e.g., leiomyosarcoma of stomach, 151.9]
- heart (164.1)
- uterine ligament (183.4)

171.0 Head, face, and neck
- Cartilage of: ear
- Cartilage of: eyelid

AHA: 2Q, '99, 6

171.2 Upper limb, including shoulder
- Arm
- Finger
- Forearm
- Hand

171.3 Lower limb, including hip
- Foot
- Leg
- Popliteal space
- Thigh
- Toe

171.4 Thorax
- Axilla
- Diaphragm
- Great vessels

EXCLUDES:
- heart (164.1)
- mediastinum (164.2-164.9)
- thymus (164.0)

171.5 Abdomen
- Abdominal wall
- Hypochondrium

EXCLUDES:
- peritoneum (158.8)
- retroperitoneum (158.0)

171.6 Pelvis
- Buttock
- Groin
- Inguinal region
- Perineum

EXCLUDES:
- pelvic peritoneum (158.8)
- retroperitoneum (158.0)
- uterine ligament, any (183.3-183.5)

171.7 Trunk, unspecified
- Back NOS
- Flank NOS

171.8 Other specified sites of connective and other soft tissue
- Malignant neoplasm of contiguous or overlapping sites of connective tissue whose point of origin cannot be determined

171.9 Connective and other soft tissue, site unspecified

✓4th 172 Malignant melanoma of skin

INCLUDES:
- melanocarcinoma
- melanoma (skin) NOS

EXCLUDES:
- skin of genital organs (184.0-184.9, 187.1-187.9)
- sites other than skin—code to malignant neoplasm of the site

DEF: Malignant neoplasm of melanocytes; most common in skin, may involve oral cavity, esophagus, anal canal, vagina, leptomeninges or conjunctiva.

172.0 Lip

EXCLUDES: vermilion border of lip (140.0-140.1, 140.9)

172.1 Eyelid, including canthus

172.2 Ear and external auditory canal
- Auricle (ear)
- Auricular canal, external
- External [acoustic] meatus
- Pinna

172.3 Other and unspecified parts of face
- Cheek (external)
- Chin
- Eyebrow
- Forehead
- Nose, external
- Temple

172.4 Scalp and neck

172.5 Trunk, except scrotum
- Axilla
- Breast
- Buttock
- Groin
- Perianal skin
- Perineum
- Umbilicus

EXCLUDES:
- anal canal (154.2)
- anus NOS (154.3)
- scrotum (187.7)

172.6 Upper limb, including shoulder
- Arm
- Finger
- Forearm
- Hand

172.7 Lower limb, including hip
- Ankle
- Foot
- Heel
- Knee
- Leg
- Popliteal area
- Thigh
- Toe

172.8 Other specified sites of skin
- Malignant melanoma of contiguous or overlapping sites of skin whose point of origin cannot be determined

172.9 Melanoma of skin, site unspecified

✓4th 173 Other malignant neoplasm of skin

INCLUDES:
- malignant neoplasm of:
  - sebaceous glands
  - sudoriferous, sudoriparous glands
  - sweat glands

EXCLUDES:
- Kaposi's sarcoma (176.0-176.9)
- malignant melanoma of skin (172.0-172.9)
- skin of genital organs (184.0-184.9, 187.1-187.9)

AHA: 1Q, '00, 18; 2Q, '96, 12

173.0 Skin of lip

EXCLUDES: vermilion border of lip (140.0-140.1, 140.9)

173.1 Eyelid, including canthus

EXCLUDES: cartilage of eyelid (171.0)

173.2 Skin of ear and external auditory canal
- Auricle (ear)
- Auricular canal, external
- External meatus
- Pinna

EXCLUDES: cartilage of ear (171.0)

173.3 Skin of other and unspecified parts of face
- Cheek, external
- Chin
- Eyebrow
- Forehead
- Nose, external
- Temple

AHA: 1Q, '00, 3

NEOPLASMS

173.4–182.8

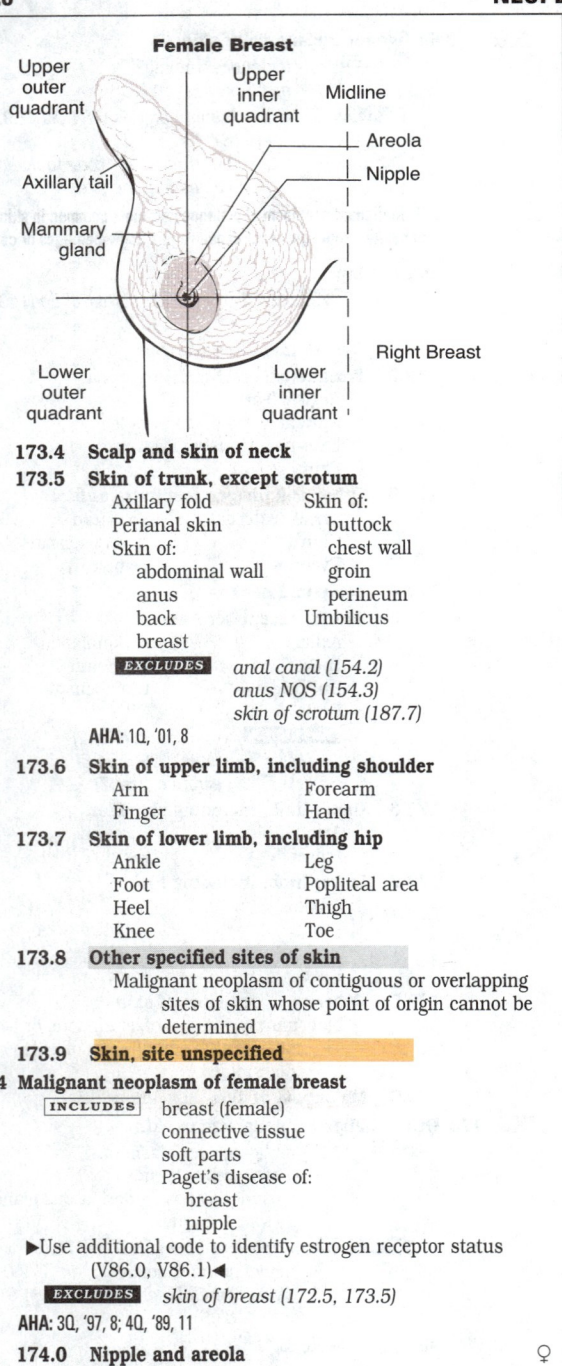

173.4 Scalp and skin of neck

173.5 Skin of trunk, except scrotum
Axillary fold
Perianal skin
Skin of:
  abdominal wall
  anus
  back
  breast
Skin of:
  buttock
  chest wall
  groin
  perineum
  Umbilicus
EXCLUDES: anal canal (154.2)
  anus NOS (154.3)
  skin of scrotum (187.7)
AHA: 1Q, '01, 8

173.6 Skin of upper limb, including shoulder
Arm
Finger
Forearm
Hand

173.7 Skin of lower limb, including hip
Ankle
Foot
Heel
Knee
Leg
Popliteal area
Thigh
Toe

173.8 Other specified sites of skin
Malignant neoplasm of contiguous or overlapping sites of skin whose point of origin cannot be determined

173.9 Skin, site unspecified

√4th **174 Malignant neoplasm of female breast**
INCLUDES: breast (female)
  connective tissue
  soft parts
  Paget's disease of:
    breast
    nipple
► Use additional code to identify estrogen receptor status (V86.0, V86.1) ◄
EXCLUDES: skin of breast (172.5, 173.5)
AHA: 3Q, '97, 8; 4Q, '89, 11

174.0 Nipple and areola ♀
174.1 Central portion ♀
174.2 Upper-inner quadrant ♀
174.3 Lower-inner quadrant ♀
174.4 Upper-outer quadrant ♀
AHA: 1Q, '04, 3
174.5 Lower-outer quadrant ♀
174.6 Axillary tail ♀
174.8 Other specified sites of female breast ♀
Ectopic sites
Inner breast
Lower breast
Malignant neoplasm of contiguous or overlapping sites of breast whose point of origin cannot be determined
Midline of breast
Outer breast
Upper breast

174.9 Breast (female), unspecified ♀
AHA: 3Q, '05, 11

√4th **175 Malignant neoplasm of male breast**
► Use additional code to identify estrogen receptor status (V86.0, V86.1) ◄
EXCLUDES: skin of breast (172.5, 173.5)

175.0 Nipple and areola ♂
175.9 Other and unspecified sites of male breast ♂
Ectopic breast tissue, male

√4th **176 Kaposi's sarcoma**
AHA: 4Q, '91, 24

176.0 Skin
176.1 Soft tissue
Blood vessel
Connective tissue
Fascia
Ligament
Lymphatic(s) NEC
Muscle
EXCLUDES: lymph glands and nodes (176.5)

176.2 Palate
176.3 Gastrointestinal sites
176.4 Lung
176.5 Lymph nodes
176.8 Other specified sites
Oral cavity NEC
176.9 Unspecified
Viscera NOS

MALIGNANT NEOPLASM OF GENITOURINARY ORGANS (179-189)
EXCLUDES: carcinoma in situ (233.1-233.9)

179 Malignant neoplasm of uterus, part unspecified ♀

√4th **180 Malignant neoplasm of cervix uteri**
INCLUDES: invasive malignancy [carcinoma]
EXCLUDES: carcinoma in situ (233.1)

180.0 Endocervix ♀
Cervical canal NOS   Endocervical gland
Endocervical canal
180.1 Exocervix ♀
180.8 Other specified sites of cervix ♀
Cervical stump
Squamocolumnar junction of cervix
Malignant neoplasm of contiguous or overlapping sites of cervix uteri whose point of origin cannot be determined
180.9 Cervix uteri, unspecified ♀

181 Malignant neoplasm of placenta
Choriocarcinoma NOS
Chorioepithelioma NOS
EXCLUDES: chorioadenoma (destruens) (236.1)
  hydatidiform mole (630)
    malignant (236.1)
  invasive mole (236.1)
  male choriocarcinoma NOS (186.0-186.9)

√4th **182 Malignant neoplasm of body of uterus**
EXCLUDES: carcinoma in situ (233.2)

182.0 Corpus uteri, except isthmus ♀
Cornu   Fundus
Endometrium   Myometrium
182.1 Isthmus ♀
Lower uterine segment
182.8 Other specified sites of body of uterus ♀
Malignant neoplasm of contiguous or overlapping sites of body of uterus whose point of origin cannot be determined
EXCLUDES: uterus NOS (179)

NEOPLASMS

183–190.6

✓4th **183 Malignant neoplasm of ovary and other uterine adnexa**
  EXCLUDES Douglas' cul-de-sac (158.8)
  183.0 Ovary ♀
    Use additional code to identify any functional activity
  183.2 Fallopian tube ♀
    Oviduct   Uterine tube
  183.3 Broad ligament ♀
    Mesovarium   Parovarian region
  183.4 Parametrium ♀
    Uterine ligament NOS Uterosacral ligament
  183.5 Round ligament ♀
    AHA: 3Q, '99, 5
  183.8 Other specified sites of uterine adnexa ♀
    Tubo-ovarian
    Utero-ovarian
    Malignant neoplasm of contiguous or overlapping sites of ovary and other uterine adnexa whose point of origin cannot be determined
  183.9 Uterine adnexa, unspecified ♀

✓4th **184 Malignant neoplasm of other and unspecified female genital organs**
  EXCLUDES carcinoma in situ (233.3)
  184.0 Vagina ♀
    Gartner's duct   Vaginal vault
  184.1 Labia majora ♀
    Greater vestibular [Bartholin's] gland
  184.2 Labia minora ♀
  184.3 Clitoris ♀
  184.4 Vulva, unspecified ♀
    External female genitalia NOS
    Pudendum
  184.8 Other specified sites of female genital organs ♀
    Malignant neoplasm of contiguous or overlapping sites of female genital organs whose point of origin cannot be determined
  184.9 Female genital organ, site unspecified ♀
    Female genitourinary tract NOS

185 Malignant neoplasm of prostate ♂
  EXCLUDES seminal vesicles (187.8)
  AHA: 3Q, '03, 13; 3Q, '99, 5; 3Q, '92, 7

✓4th **186 Malignant neoplasm of testis**
  Use additional code to identify any functional activity
  186.0 Undescended testis ♂
    Ectopic testis   Retained testis
  186.9 Other and unspecified testis ♂
    Testis: Testis:
      NOS   scrotal
      descended

✓4th **187 Malignant neoplasm of penis and other male genital organs**
  187.1 Prepuce ♂
    Foreskin
  187.2 Glans penis ♂
  187.3 Body of penis ♂
    Corpus cavernosum
  187.4 Penis, part unspecified ♂
    Skin of penis NOS
  187.5 Epididymis ♂
  187.6 Spermatic cord ♂
    Vas deferens
  187.7 Scrotum ♂
    Skin of scrotum
  187.8 Other specified sites of male genital organs ♂
    Seminal vesicle
    Tunica vaginalis
    Malignant neoplasm of contiguous or overlapping sites of penis and other male genital organs whose point of origin cannot be determined
  187.9 Male genital organ, site unspecified ♂
    Male genital organ or tract NOS

✓4th **188 Malignant neoplasm of bladder**
  EXCLUDES carcinoma in situ (233.7)
  188.0 Trigone of urinary bladder
  188.1 Dome of urinary bladder
  188.2 Lateral wall of urinary bladder
  188.3 Anterior wall of urinary bladder
  188.4 Posterior wall of urinary bladder
  188.5 Bladder neck
    Internal urethral orifice
  188.6 Ureteric orifice
  188.7 Urachus
  188.8 Other specified sites of bladder
    Malignant neoplasm of contiguous or overlapping sites of bladder whose point of origin cannot be determined
  188.9 Bladder, part unspecified
    Bladder wall NOS
    AHA: 1Q, '00, 5

✓4th **189 Malignant neoplasm of kidney and other and unspecified urinary organs**
  189.0 Kidney, except pelvis
    Kidney NOS   Kidney parenchyma
    AHA: ▶2Q, '05, 4;◀ 2Q, '04, 4
  189.1 Renal pelvis
    Renal calyces   Ureteropelvic junction
  189.2 Ureter
    EXCLUDES ureteric orifice of bladder (188.6)
  189.3 Urethra
    EXCLUDES urethral orifice of bladder (188.5)
  189.4 Paraurethral glands
  189.8 Other specified sites of urinary organs
    Malignant neoplasm of contiguous or overlapping sites of kidney and other urinary organs whose point of origin cannot be determined
  189.9 Urinary organ, site unspecified
    Urinary system NOS

MALIGNANT NEOPLASM OF OTHER AND UNSPECIFIED SITES (190-199)
  EXCLUDES carcinoma in situ (234.0-234.9)

✓4th **190 Malignant neoplasm of eye**
  EXCLUDES carcinoma in situ (234.0)
           eyelid (skin) (172.1, 173.1)
             cartilage (171.0)
           optic nerve (192.0)
           orbital bone (170.0)
  190.0 Eyeball, except conjunctiva, cornea, retina, and choroid
    Ciliary body   Sclera
    Crystalline lens Uveal tract
    Iris
  190.1 Orbit
    Connective tissue of orbit
    Extraocular muscle
    Retrobulbar
    EXCLUDES bone of orbit (170.0)
  190.2 Lacrimal gland
  190.3 Conjunctiva
  190.4 Cornea
  190.5 Retina
  190.6 Choroid

NEOPLASMS

190.7–196 — Tabular List

Brain — Midsagittal Section (between hemispheres)
Labels: Fourth ventricle, Cerebrum, Corpus callosum, Thalamus, Hypothalamus, Hypophysis, Pons, Medulla oblongata, Cerebellum

190.7 **Lacrimal duct**
Lacrimal sac   Nasolacrimal duct

190.8 **Other specified sites of eye**
Malignant neoplasm of contiguous or overlapping sites of eye whose point of origin cannot be determined

190.9 **Eye, part unspecified**

191 Malignant neoplasm of brain
EXCLUDES: cranial nerves (192.0)
retrobulbar area (190.1)

191.0 **Cerebrum, except lobes and ventricles**
Basal ganglia   Globus pallidus
Cerebral cortex   Hypothalamus
Corpus striatum   Thalamus

191.1 **Frontal lobe**
AHA: ►4Q, '05, 118◄

191.2 **Temporal lobe**
Hippocampus   Uncus

191.3 **Parietal lobe**

191.4 **Occipital lobe**

191.5 **Ventricles**
Choroid plexus   Floor of ventricle

191.6 **Cerebellum NOS**
Cerebellopontine angle

191.7 **Brain stem**
Cerebral peduncle   Midbrain
Medulla oblongata   Pons

191.8 **Other parts of brain**
Corpus callosum
Tapetum
Malignant neoplasm of contiguous or overlapping sites of brain whose point of origin cannot be determined

191.9 **Brain, unspecified**
Cranial fossa NOS

192 Malignant neoplasm of other and unspecified parts of nervous system
EXCLUDES: peripheral, sympathetic, and parasympathetic nerves and ganglia (171.0-171.9)

192.0 **Cranial nerves**
Olfactory bulb

192.1 **Cerebral meninges**
Dura (mater)   Meninges NOS
Falx (cerebelli) (cerebri)   Tentorium

192.2 **Spinal cord**
Cauda equina

192.3 **Spinal meninges**

192.8 **Other specified sites of nervous system**
Malignant neoplasm of contiguous or overlapping sites of other parts of nervous system whose point of origin cannot be determined

192.9 **Nervous system, part unspecified**
Nervous system (central) NOS
EXCLUDES: meninges NOS (192.1)

193 Malignant neoplasm of thyroid gland
Sipple's syndrome
Thyroglossal duct
Use additional code to identify any functional activity

194 Malignant neoplasm of other endocrine glands and related structures
Use additional code to identify any functional activity
EXCLUDES: islets of Langerhans (157.4)
ovary (183.0)
testis (186.0-186.9)
thymus (164.0)

194.0 **Adrenal gland**
Adrenal cortex   Suprarenal gland
Adrenal medulla

194.1 **Parathyroid gland**

194.3 **Pituitary gland and craniopharyngeal duct**
Craniobuccal pouch   Rathke's pouch
Hypophysis   Sella turcica
AHA: J-A, '85, 9

194.4 **Pineal gland**

194.5 **Carotid body**

194.6 **Aortic body and other paraganglia**
Coccygeal body   Para-aortic body
Glomus jugulare

194.8 **Other**
Pluriglandular involvement NOS
Note: If the sites of multiple involvements are known, they should be coded separately.

194.9 **Endocrine gland, site unspecified**

195 Malignant neoplasm of other and ill-defined sites
INCLUDES: malignant neoplasms of contiguous sites, not elsewhere classified, whose point of origin cannot be determined
EXCLUDES: malignant neoplasm:
lymphatic and hematopoietic tissue (200.0-208.9)
secondary sites (196.0-198.8)
unspecified site (199.0-199.1)

195.0 **Head, face, and neck**
Cheek NOS   Nose NOS
Jaw NOS   Supraclavicular region NOS
AHA: 4Q, '03, 107

195.1 **Thorax**
Axilla   Intrathoracic NOS
Chest (wall) NOS

195.2 **Abdomen**
Intra-abdominal NOS
AHA: 2Q, '97, 3

195.3 **Pelvis**
Groin
Inguinal region NOS
Presacral region
Sacrococcygeal region
Sites overlapping systems within pelvis, as:
rectovaginal (septum)
rectovesical (septum)

195.4 **Upper limb**

195.5 **Lower limb**

195.8 **Other specified sites**
Back NOS   Trunk NOS
Flank NOS

196 Secondary and unspecified malignant neoplasm of lymph nodes
EXCLUDES: any malignant neoplasm of lymph nodes, specified as primary (200.0-202.9)
Hodgkin's disease (201.0-201.9)
lymphosarcoma (200.1)
reticulosarcoma (200.0)
other forms of lymphoma (202.0-202.9)
AHA: 2Q, '92, 3; M-J, '85, 3

N Newborn Age: 0   P Pediatric Age: 0-17   M Maternity Age: 12-55   A Adult Age: 15-124

NEOPLASMS

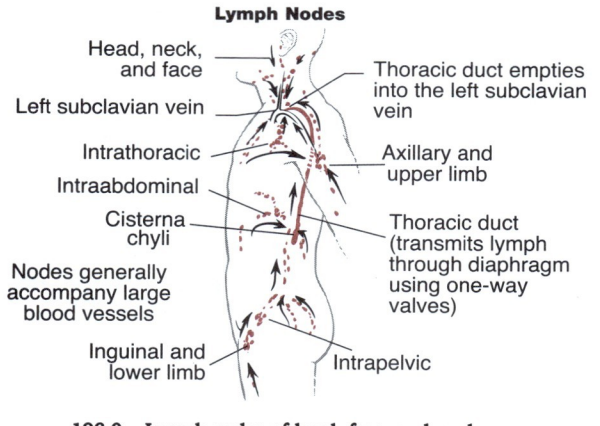

196.0 Lymph nodes of head, face, and neck
Cervical
Cervicofacial
Scalene
Supraclavicular

196.1 Intrathoracic lymph nodes
Bronchopulmonary
Intercostal
Mediastinal
Tracheobronchial

196.2 Intra-abdominal lymph nodes
Intestinal
Mesenteric
Retroperitoneal
AHA: 4Q, '03, 111

196.3 Lymph nodes of axilla and upper limb
Brachial
Epitrochlear
Infraclavicular
Pectoral

196.5 Lymph nodes of inguinal region and lower limb
Femoral
Groin
Popliteal
Tibial

196.6 Intrapelvic lymph nodes
Hypogastric
Iliac
Obturator
Parametrial

196.8 Lymph nodes of multiple sites

196.9 Site unspecified
Lymph nodes NOS

√4th **197 Secondary malignant neoplasm of respiratory and digestive systems**
EXCLUDES   lymph node metastasis (196.0-196.9)
AHA: M-J, '85, 3

197.0 Lung
Bronchus
AHA: 2Q, '99, 9

197.1 Mediastinum

197.2 Pleura
AHA: 4Q, '03, 110; 4Q, '89, 11

197.3 Other respiratory organs
Trachea

197.4 Small intestine, including duodenum

197.5 Large intestine and rectum

197.6 Retroperitoneum and peritoneum
AHA: 2Q, '04, 4; 4Q, '89, 11

197.7 Liver, specified as secondary
AHA: ▶2Q, '05, 9◀

197.8 Other digestive organs and spleen
AHA: 2Q, '97, 3; 2Q, '92, 3

√4th **198 Secondary malignant neoplasm of other specified sites**
EXCLUDES   lymph node metastasis (196.0-196.9)
AHA: M-J, '85, 3

198.0 Kidney

198.1 Other urinary organs

198.2 Skin
Skin of breast

198.3 Brain and spinal cord
AHA: 3Q, '99, 7

198.4 Other parts of nervous system
Meninges (cerebral) (spinal)
AHA: J-F, '87, 7

198.5 Bone and bone marrow
AHA: 4Q, '03, 110; 3Q, '99, 5; 2Q, '92, 3; 1Q, '91, 16; 4Q, '89, 10

198.6 Ovary   ♀

198.7 Adrenal gland
Suprarenal gland

√5th **198.8 Other specified sites**
198.81 Breast
EXCLUDES   skin of breast (198.2)
198.82 Genital organs
198.89 Other
EXCLUDES   retroperitoneal lymph nodes (196.2)
AHA: ▶2Q, '05, 4;◀ 2Q, '97, 4

√4th **199 Malignant neoplasm without specification of site**

199.0 Disseminated
Carcinomatosis ⎫
Generalized: ⎬ unspecified site
  cancer   ⎪   (primary)
  malignancy   ⎪   (secondary)
Multiple cancer ⎭
AHA: 4Q, '89, 10

199.1 Other
Cancer   ⎫ unspecified site
Carcinoma   ⎬   (primary)
Malignancy   ⎭   (secondary)

MALIGNANT NEOPLASM OF LYMPHATIC AND HEMATOPOIETIC TISSUE (200-208)

EXCLUDES   secondary neoplasm of:
  bone marrow (198.5)
  spleen (197.8)
  secondary and unspecified neoplasm of lymph nodes (196.0-196.9)

The following fifth-digit subclassification is for use with categories 200-202:
0 unspecified site, extranodal and solid organ sites
1 lymph nodes of head, face, and neck
2 intrathoracic lymph nodes
3 intra-abdominal lymph nodes
4 lymph nodes of axilla and upper limb
5 lymph nodes of inguinal region and lower limb
6 intrapelvic lymph nodes
7 spleen
8 lymph nodes of multiple sites

√4th **200 Lymphosarcoma and reticulosarcoma**
AHA: 2Q, '92, 3; N-D, '86, 5

√5th **200.0 Reticulosarcoma**
Lymphoma (malignant):
  histiocytic (diffuse):
    nodular
    pleomorphic cell type
    reticulum cell type
Reticulum cell sarcoma:
  NOS
  pleomorphic cell type
AHA: For Code 200.03: 3Q, '01, 12

DEF: Malignant lymphoma of primarily histiocytic cells; commonly originates in reticuloendothelium of lymph nodes.

200.1–202.9 NEOPLASMS Tabular List

§ ✓5th **200.1 Lymphosarcoma**
Lymphoblastoma (diffuse)
Lymphoma (malignant):
    lymphoblastic (diffuse)
    lymphocytic (cell type) (diffuse)
    lymphosarcoma type
Lymphosarcoma:
    NOS
    diffuse NOS
    lymphoblastic (diffuse)
    lymphocytic (diffuse)
    prolymphocytic

> **EXCLUDES** lymphosarcoma:
>   follicular or nodular (202.0)
>   mixed cell type (200.8)
>   lymphosarcoma cell leukemia (207.8)

DEF: Malignant lymphoma created from anaplastic lymphoid cells resembling lymphocytes or lymphoblasts.

§ ✓5th **200.2 Burkitt's tumor or lymphoma**
Malignant lymphoma, Burkitt's type
DEF: Large osteolytic lesion most common in jaw or as abdominal mass; usually found in central Africa but reported elsewhere.

§ ✓5th **200.8 Other named variants**
Lymphoma (malignant):
    lymphoplasmacytoid type
    mixed lymphocytic-histiocytic (diffuse)
Lymphosarcoma, mixed cell type (diffuse)
Reticulolymphosarcoma (diffuse)

✓4th **201 Hodgkin's disease**
AHA: 2Q, '92, 3; N-D, '86, 5
DEF: Painless, progressive enlargement of lymph nodes, spleen and general lymph tissue; symptoms include anorexia, lassitude, weight loss, fever, pruritis, night sweats, anemia.

§ ✓5th **201.0 Hodgkin's paragranuloma**
§ ✓5th **201.1 Hodgkin's granuloma**
AHA: 2Q, '99, 7
§ ✓5th **201.2 Hodgkin's sarcoma**
§ ✓5th **201.4 Lymphocytic-histiocytic predominance**
§ ✓5th **201.5 Nodular sclerosis**
Hodgkin's disease, nodular sclerosis:
    NOS
    cellular phase
§ ✓5th **201.6 Mixed cellularity**
§ ✓5th **201.7 Lymphocytic depletion**
Hodgkin's disease, lymphocytic depletion:
    NOS
    diffuse fibrosis
    reticular type
§ ✓5th **201.9 Hodgkin's disease, unspecified**
Hodgkin's: Malignant:
  disease NOS   lymphogranuloma
  lymphoma NOS   lymphogranulomatosis

✓4th **202 Other malignant neoplasms of lymphoid and histiocytic tissue**
AHA: 2Q, '92, 3; N-D, '86, 5

§ ✓5th **202.0 Nodular lymphoma**
Brill-Symmers disease
Lymphoma:
    follicular (giant)
    lymphocytic, nodular
Lymphosarcoma:
    follicular (giant)
    nodular
DEF: Lymphomatous cells clustered into nodules within the lymph node; usually occurs in older adults and may involve all nodes and possibly extranodal sites.

§ ✓5th **202.1 Mycosis fungoides**
AHA: 2Q, '92, 4
DEF: Type of cutaneous T-cell lymphoma; may evolve into generalized lymphoma; formerly thought to be of fungoid origin.

§ ✓5th **202.2 Sézary's disease**
AHA: 2Q, '99, 7
DEF: Type of cutaneous T-cell lymphoma with erythroderma, intense pruritus, peripheral lymphadenopathy, abnormal hyperchromatic mononuclear cells in skin, lymph nodes and peripheral blood.

§ ✓5th **202.3 Malignant histiocytosis**
Histiocytic medullary reticulosis
Malignant:
    reticuloendotheliosis
    reticulosis

§ ✓5th **202.4 Leukemic reticuloendotheliosis**
Hairy-cell leukemia
DEF: Chronic leukemia with large, mononuclear cells with "hairy" appearance in marrow, spleen, liver, blood.

§ ✓5th **202.5 Letterer-Siwe disease**
Acute:
    differentiated progressive histiocytosis
    histiocytosis X (progressive)
    infantile reticuloendotheliosis
    reticulosis of infancy

> **EXCLUDES** Hand-Schüller-Christian disease (277.89)
> histiocytosis (acute) (chronic) (277.89)
> histiocytosis X (chronic) (277.89)

DEF: A recessive reticuloendotheliosis of early childhood, with a hemorrhagic tendency, eczema-like skin eruption, hepato-splenomegaly, including lymph node enlargement, and progressive anemia; it is often a fatal disease with no established cause.

§ ✓5th **202.6 Malignant mast cell tumors**
Malignant: Mast cell sarcoma
  mastocytoma   Systemic tissue mast
  mastocytosis   cell disease

> **EXCLUDES** mast cell leukemia (207.8)

§ ✓5th **202.8 Other lymphomas**
Lymphoma (malignant):
    NOS
    diffuse

> **EXCLUDES** benign lymphoma (229.0)

AHA: 2Q, '92, 4

§ ✓5th **202.9 Other and unspecified malignant neoplasms of lymphoid and histiocytic tissue**
Follicular dendritic cell sarcoma
Interdigitating dendritic cell sarcoma
Langerhans cell sarcom
Malignant neoplasm of bone marrow NOS

---

§ Requires fifth-digit. See beginning of section 200–208 for codes and definitions.

N Newborn Age: 0   **P** Pediatric Age: 0-17   **M** Maternity Age: 12-55   **A** Adult Age: 15-124

Tabular List — NEOPLASMS

203 Multiple myeloma and immunoproliferative neoplasms

The following fifth-digit subclassification is for use with category 203:
- 0 without mention of remission
- 1 in remission

203.0 Multiple myeloma
Kahler's disease Myelomatosis
EXCLUDES solitary myeloma (238.6)
AHA: 1Q, '96, 16; 4Q, '91, 26

203.1 Plasma cell leukemia
Plasmacytic leukemia
AHA: 4Q, '90, 26; S-O, '86, 12

203.8 Other immunoproliferative neoplasms
AHA: 4Q, '90, 26; S-O, '86, 12

204 Lymphoid leukemia
INCLUDES leukemia:
- lymphatic
- lymphoblastic
- lymphocytic
- lymphogenous

AHA: 3Q, '93, 4

The following fifth-digit subclassification is for use with category 204:
- 0 without mention of remission
- 1 in remission

204.0 Acute
EXCLUDES acute exacerbation of chronic lymphoid leukemia (204.1)
AHA: 3Q, '99, 6

204.1 Chronic
204.2 Subacute
204.8 Other lymphoid leukemia
Aleukemic leukemia: Aleukemic leukemia:
- lymphatic   lymphoid
- lymphocytic

204.9 Unspecified lymphoid leukemia

205 Myeloid leukemia
INCLUDES leukemia:
- granulocytic
- myeloblastic
- myelocytic
- myelogenous
- myelomonocytic
- myelosclerotic
- myelosis

AHA: 3Q, '93, 3; 4Q, '91, 26; 4Q, '90, 3; M-J, '85, 18

The following fifth-digit subclassification is for use with category 205:
- 0 without mention of remission
- 1 in remission

205.0 Acute
Acute promyelocytic leukemia
EXCLUDES acute exacerbation of chronic myeloid leukemia (205.1)

205.1 Chronic
Eosinophilic leukemia
Neutrophilic leukemia
AHA: 1Q, 00, 6; J-A, '85, 13

205.2 Subacute
205.3 Myeloid sarcoma
Chloroma
Granulocytic sarcoma

205.8 Other myeloid leukemia
Aleukemic leukemia: Aleukemic leukemia:
- granulocytic   myeloid
- myelogenous   Aleukemic myelosis

205.9 Unspecified myeloid leukemia

206 Monocytic leukemia
INCLUDES leukemia:
- histiocytic
- monoblastic
- monocytoid

The following fifth-digit subclassification is for use with category 206:
- 0 without mention of remission
- 1 in remission

206.0 Acute
EXCLUDES acute exacerbation of chronic monocytic leukemia (206.1)

206.1 Chronic
206.2 Subacute
206.8 Other monocytic leukemia
Aleukemic: Aleukemic:
- monocytic leukemia   monocytoid leukemia

206.9 Unspecified monocytic leukemia

207 Other specified leukemia
EXCLUDES leukemic reticuloendotheliosis (202.4)
plasma cell leukemia (203.1)

The following fifth-digit subclassification is for use with category 207:
- 0 without mention of remission
- 1 in remission

207.0 Acute erythremia and erythroleukemia
Acute erythremic myelosis Erythremic myelosis
Di Guglielmo's disease

DEF: Erythremia: polycythemia vera.

DEF: Erythroleukemia: a malignant blood dyscrasia (a myeloproliferative disorder).

207.1 Chronic erythremia
Heilmeyer-Schöner disease

207.2 Megakaryocytic leukemia
Megakaryocytic myelosis Thrombocytic leukemia

207.8 Other specified leukemia
Lymphosarcoma cell leukemia

208 Leukemia of unspecified cell type

The following fifth-digit subclassification is for use with category 208:
- 0 without mention of remission
- 1 in remission

208.0 Acute
Acute leukemia NOS Stem cell leukemia
Blast cell leukemia
EXCLUDES acute exacerbation of chronic unspecified leukemia (208.1)

208.1 Chronic
Chronic leukemia NOS

208.2 Subacute
Subacute leukemia NOS

208.8 Other leukemia of unspecified cell type
208.9 Unspecified leukemia
Leukemia NOS

NEOPLASMS

BENIGN NEOPLASMS (210-229)

✓4th 210 Benign neoplasm of lip, oral cavity, and pharynx
EXCLUDES cyst (of):
  jaw (526.0-526.2, 526.89)
  oral soft tissue (528.4)
  radicular (522.8)

210.0 Lip
Frenulum labii
Lip (inner aspect) (mucosa) (vermilion border)
EXCLUDES labial commissure (210.4)
  skin of lip (216.0)

210.1 Tongue
Lingual tonsil

210.2 Major salivary glands
Gland:
  parotid
  sublingual
  submandibular
EXCLUDES benign neoplasms of minor salivary glands:
  NOS (210.4)
  buccal mucosa (210.4)
  lips (210.0)
  palate (hard) (soft) (210.4)
  tongue (210.1)
  tonsil, palatine (210.5)

210.3 Floor of mouth

210.4 Other and unspecified parts of mouth
Gingiva   Oral mucosa
Gum (upper) (lower)   Palate (hard) (soft)
Labial commissure   Uvula
Oral cavity NOS
EXCLUDES benign odontogenic neoplasms of bone (213.0-213.1)
  developmental odontogenic cysts (526.0)
  mucosa of lips (210.0)
  nasopharyngeal [posterior] [superior] surface of soft palate (210.7)

210.5 Tonsil
Tonsil (faucial) (palatine)
EXCLUDES lingual tonsil (210.1)
  pharyngeal tonsil (210.7)
  tonsillar:
    fossa (210.6)
    pillars (210.6)

210.6 Other parts of oropharynx
Branchial cleft or vestiges   Tonsillar:
Epiglottis, anterior aspect   fossa
Fauces NOS   pillars
Mesopharynx NOS   Vallecula
EXCLUDES epiglottis:
  NOS (212.1)
  suprahyoid portion (212.1)

210.7 Nasopharynx
Adenoid tissue   Pharyngeal tonsil
Lymphadenoid tissue   Posterior nasal septum

210.8 Hypopharynx
Arytenoid fold   Postcricoid region
Laryngopharynx   Pyriform fossa

210.9 Pharynx, unspecified
Throat NOS

✓4th 211 Benign neoplasm of other parts of digestive system
EXCLUDES ▶benign stromal tumors of digestive system (215.5)◄

211.0 Esophagus

211.1 Stomach
Body ⎫
Cardia ⎬ of stomach
Fundus ⎭
Cardiac orifice
Pylorus

211.2 Duodenum, jejunum, and ileum
Small intestine NOS
EXCLUDES ampulla of Vater (211.5)
  ileocecal valve (211.3)

211.3 Colon
Appendix   Ileocecal valve
Cecum   Large intestine NOS
EXCLUDES rectosigmoid junction (211.4)
AHA: 3Q, '05, 17; 2Q, '05, 16; 4Q, '01, 56

211.4 Rectum and anal canal
Anal canal or sphincter   Rectosigmoid junction
Anus NOS
EXCLUDES anus:
  margin (216.5)
  skin (216.5)
  perianal skin (216.5)

211.5 Liver and biliary passages
Ampulla of Vater   Gallbladder
Common bile duct   Hepatic duct
Cystic duct   Sphincter of Oddi

211.6 Pancreas, except islets of Langerhans

211.7 Islets of Langerhans
Islet cell tumor
Use additional code to identify any functional activity

211.8 Retroperitoneum and peritoneum
Mesentery   Omentum
Mesocolon   Retroperitoneal tissue

211.9 Other and unspecified site
Alimentary tract NOS
Digestive system NOS
Gastrointestinal tract NOS
Intestinal tract NOS
Intestine NOS
Spleen, not elsewhere classified

✓4th 212 Benign neoplasm of respiratory and intrathoracic organs

212.0 Nasal cavities, middle ear, and accessory sinuses
Cartilage of nose   Sinus:
Eustachian tube   ethomoidal
Nares   frontal
Septum of nose   maxillary
                       sphenoidal
EXCLUDES auditory canal (external) (216.2)
  bone of:
    ear (213.0)
    nose [turbinates] (213.0)
  cartilage of ear (215.0)
  ear (external) (skin) (216.2)
  nose NOS (229.8)
    skin (216.3)
  olfactory bulb (225.1)
  polyp of:
    accessory sinus (471.8)
    ear (385.30-385.35)
    nasal cavity (471.0)
  posterior margin of septum and choanae (210.7)

212.1 Larynx
Cartilage:
  arytenoid
  cricoid
  cuneiform
  thyroid
Epiglottis (suprahyoid portion) NOS
Glottis
Vocal cords (false) (true)
EXCLUDES epiglottis, anterior aspect (210.6)
  polyp of vocal cord or larynx (478.4)

212.2 Trachea

212.3 Bronchus and lung
Carina   Hilus of lung

212.4 Pleura

NEOPLASMS

- **212.5** Mediastinum
- **212.6** Thymus
- **212.7** Heart
  - EXCLUDES: great vessels (215.4)
- **212.8** Other specified sites
- **212.9** Site unspecified
  - Respiratory organ NOS
  - Upper respiratory tract NOS
  - EXCLUDES: intrathoracic NOS (229.8)
  - thoracic NOS (229.8)

✓4th 213 Benign neoplasm of bone and articular cartilage
INCLUDES: cartilage (articular) (joint)
periosteum

EXCLUDES: cartilage of:
- ear (215.0)
- eyelid (215.0)
- larynx (212.1)
- nose (212.0)
exostosis NOS (726.91)
synovia (215.0-215.9)

- **213.0** Bones of skull and face
  - EXCLUDES: lower jaw bone (213.1)
- **213.1** Lower jaw bone
- **213.2** Vertebral column, excluding sacrum and coccyx
- **213.3** Ribs, sternum, and clavicle
- **213.4** Scapula and long bones of upper limb
- **213.5** Short bones of upper limb
- **213.6** Pelvic bones, sacrum, and coccyx
- **213.7** Long bones of lower limb
- **213.8** Short bones of lower limb
- **213.9** Bone and articular cartilage, site unspecified

✓4th 214 Lipoma
INCLUDES:
- angiolipoma
- fibrolipoma
- hibernoma
- lipoma (fetal) (infiltrating) (intramuscular)
- myelolipoma
- myxolipoma

DEF: Benign tumor frequently composed of mature fat cells; may occasionally be composed of fetal fat cells.

- **214.0** Skin and subcutaneous tissue of face
- **214.1** Other skin and subcutaneous tissue
- **214.2** Intrathoracic organs
- **214.3** Intra-abdominal organs
- **214.4** Spermatic cord ♂
- **214.8** Other specified sites
  - AHA: 3Q, '94, 7
- **214.9** Lipoma, unspecified site

✓4th 215 Other benign neoplasm of connective and other soft tissue
INCLUDES:
- blood vessel
- bursa
- fascia
- ligament
- muscle
- peripheral, sympathetic, and parasympathetic nerves and ganglia
- synovia
- tendon (sheath)

EXCLUDES: cartilage:
- articular (213.0-213.9)
- larynx (212.1)
- nose (212.0)
connective tissue of:
- breast (217)
- internal organ, except lipoma and hemangioma—code to benign neoplasm of the site
lipoma (214.0-214.9)

- **215.0** Head, face, and neck
- **215.2** Upper limb, including shoulder
- **215.3** Lower limb, including hip
- **215.4** Thorax
  - EXCLUDES: heart (212.7)
  - mediastinum (212.5)
  - thymus (212.6)
- **215.5** Abdomen
  - Abdominal wall
  - ►Benign stromal tumors of abdomen◄
  - Hypochondrium
- **215.6** Pelvis
  - Buttock
  - Groin
  - Inguinal region
  - Perineum
  - EXCLUDES: uterine:
    - leiomyoma (218.0-218.9)
    - ligament, any (221.0)
- **215.7** Trunk, unspecified
  - Back NOS
  - Flank NOS
- **215.8** Other specified sites
- **215.9** Site unspecified

✓4th 216 Benign neoplasm of skin
INCLUDES:
- blue nevus
- dermatofibroma
- hydrocystoma
- pigmented nevus
- syringoadenoma
- syringoma

EXCLUDES: skin of genital organs (221.0-222.9)

AHA: 1Q, '00, 21

- **216.0** Skin of lip
  - EXCLUDES: vermilion border of lip (210.0)
- **216.1** Eyelid, including canthus
  - EXCLUDES: cartilage of eyelid (215.0)
- **216.2** Ear and external auditory canal
  - Auricle (ear)
  - Auricular canal, external
  - External meatus
  - Pinna
  - EXCLUDES: cartilage of ear (215.0)
- **216.3** Skin of other and unspecified parts of face
  - Cheek, external
  - Eyebrow
  - Nose, external
  - Temple
- **216.4** Scalp and skin of neck
  - AHA: 3Q, '91, 12
- **216.5** Skin of trunk, except scrotum
  - Axillary fold
  - Perianal skin
  - Skin of:
    - abdominal wall
    - anus
    - back
    - breast
  - Skin of:
    - buttock
    - chest wall
    - groin
    - perineum
    - Umbilicus
  - EXCLUDES: anal canal (211.4)
  - anus NOS (211.4)
  - skin of scrotum (222.4)
- **216.6** Skin of upper limb, including shoulder
- **216.7** Skin of lower limb, including hip
- **216.8** Other specified sites of skin
- **216.9** Skin, site unspecified

217 Benign neoplasm of breast
Breast (male) (female):
- connective tissue
- glandular tissue
Breast (male) (female):
- soft parts

EXCLUDES:
- adenofibrosis (610.2)
- benign cyst of breast (610.0)
- fibrocystic disease (610.1)
- skin of breast (216.5)

AHA: 1Q, '00, 4

NEOPLASMS

218 Uterine leiomyoma ✓4th
　INCLUDES　fibroid (bleeding) (uterine)
　　uterine:
　　　fibromyoma
　　　myoma

DEF: Benign tumor primarily derived from uterine smooth muscle tissue; may contain fibrous, fatty, or epithelial tissue; also called uterine fibroid or myoma.

- 218.0 Submucous leiomyoma of uterus ♀
- 218.1 Intramural leiomyoma of uterus ♀
　　Interstitial leiomyoma of uterus
- 218.2 Subserous leiomyoma of uterus ♀
- 218.9 **Leiomyoma of uterus, unspecified** ♀
　　AHA: 1Q, '03, 4

219 Other benign neoplasm of uterus ✓4th
- 219.0 Cervix uteri ♀
- 219.1 Corpus uteri ♀
　　Endometrium　　Myometrium
　　Fundus
- 219.8 Other specified parts of uterus ♀
- 219.9 **Uterus, part unspecified** ♀

220 Benign neoplasm of ovary ♀
　Use additional code to identify any functional activity (256.0-256.1)
　EXCLUDES　cyst:
　　　corpus albicans (620.2)
　　　corpus luteum (620.1)
　　　endometrial (617.1)
　　　follicular (atretic) (620.0)
　　　graafian follicle (620.0)
　　　ovarian NOS (620.2)
　　　retention (620.2)

221 Benign neoplasm of other female genital organs ✓4th
　INCLUDES　adenomatous polyp
　　　benign teratoma
　EXCLUDES　cyst:
　　　epoophoron (752.11)
　　　fimbrial (752.11)
　　　Gartner's duct (752.11)
　　　parovarian (752.11)

- 221.0 Fallopian tube and uterine ligaments ♀
　　Oviduct
　　Parametruim
　　Uterine ligament (broad) (round) (uterosacral)
　　Uterine tube
- 221.1 Vagina ♀
- 221.2 Vulva ♀
　　Clitoris
　　External female genitalia NOS
　　Greater vestibular [Bartholin's] gland
　　Labia (majora) (minora)
　　Pudendum
　　EXCLUDES　Bartholin's (duct) (gland) cyst (616.2)

Eyeball

- 221.8 Other specified sites of female genital organs ♀
- 221.9 **Female genital organ, site unspecified** ♀
　　Female genitourinary tract NOS

222 Benign neoplasm of male genital organs ✓4th
- 222.0 Testis ♂
　　Use additional code to identify any functional activity
- 222.1 Penis ♂
　　Corpus cavernosum　Prepuce
　　Glans penis
- 222.2 Prostate ♂
　　EXCLUDES　adenomatous hyperplasia of prostate (600.20-600.21)
　　　prostatic:
　　　　adenoma (600.20-600.21)
　　　　enlargement (600.00-600.01)
　　　　hypertrophy (600.00-600.01)
- 222.3 Epididymis ♂
- 222.4 Scrotum ♂
　　Skin of scrotum
- 222.8 Other specified sites of male genital organs ♂
　　Seminal vesicle
　　Spermatic cord
- 222.9 **Male genital organ, site unspecified** ♂
　　Male genitourinary tract NOS

223 Benign neoplasm of kidney and other urinary organs ✓4th
- 223.0 Kidney, except pelvis
　　Kidney NOS
　　EXCLUDES　renal:
　　　　calyces (223.1)
　　　　pelvis (223.1)
- 223.1 Renal pelvis
- 223.2 Ureter
　　EXCLUDES　ureteric orifice of bladder (223.3)
- 223.3 Bladder
- 223.8 Other specified sites of urinary organs ✓5th
　　- 223.81 Urethra
　　　EXCLUDES　urethral orifice of bladder (223.3)
　　- 223.89 Other
　　　Paraurethral glands
- 223.9 **Urinary organ, site unspecified**
　　Urinary system NOS

224 Benign neoplasm of eye ✓4th
　EXCLUDES　cartilage of eyelid (215.0)
　　　eyelid (skin) (216.1)
　　　optic nerve (225.1)
　　　orbital bone (213.0)
- 224.0 Eyeball, except conjunctiva, cornea, retina, and choroid
　　Ciliary body　　Sclera
　　Iris　　　　　Uveal tract
- 224.1 Orbit
　　EXCLUDES　bone of orbit (213.0)
- 224.2 Lacrimal gland
- 224.3 Conjunctiva
- 224.4 Cornea
- 224.5 Retina
　　EXCLUDES　hemangioma of retina (228.03)
- 224.6 Choroid
- 224.7 Lacrimal duct
　　Lacrimal sac
　　Nasolacrimal duct
- 224.8 Other specified parts of eye
- 224.9 **Eye, part unspecified**

N Newborn Age: 0　P Pediatric Age: 0-17　M Maternity Age: 12-55　A Adult Age: 15-124

NEOPLASMS

225 Benign neoplasm of brain and other parts of nervous system [4th]
  EXCLUDES
    hemangioma (228.02)
    neurofibromatosis (237.7)
    peripheral, sympathetic, and parasympathetic
      nerves and ganglia (215.0-215.9)
    retrobulbar (224.1)
  - **225.0** Brain
  - **225.1** Cranial nerves
      Acoustic neuroma
      AHA: 4Q, '04, 113
  - **225.2** Cerebral meninges
      Meninges NOS   Meningioma (cerebral)
  - **225.3** Spinal cord
      Cauda equina
  - **225.4** Spinal meninges
      Spinal meningioma
  - **225.8** Other specified sites of nervous system
  - **225.9** Nervous system, part unspecified
      Nervous system (central) NOS
      EXCLUDES meninges NOS (225.2)

226 Benign neoplasm of thyroid glands
  Use additional code to identify any functional activity

227 Benign neoplasm of other endocrine glands and related structures [4th]
  Use additional code to identify any functional activity
  EXCLUDES
    ovary (220)
    pancreas (211.6)
    testis (222.0)
  - **227.0** Adrenal gland
      Suprarenal gland
  - **227.1** Parathyroid gland
  - **227.3** Pituitary gland and craniopharyngeal duct (pouch)
      Craniobuccal pouch   Rathke's pouch
      Hypophysis   Sella turcica
  - **227.4** Pineal gland
      Pineal body
  - **227.5** Carotid body
  - **227.6** Aortic body and other paraganglia
      Coccygeal body   Para-aortic body
      Glomus jugulare
      AHA: N-D, '84, 17
  - **227.8** Other
  - **227.9** Endocrine gland, site unspecified

228 Hemangioma and lymphangioma, any site [4th]
  INCLUDES
    angioma (benign) (cavernous) (congenital) NOS
    cavernous nevus
    glomus tumor
    hemangioma (benign) (congenital)
  EXCLUDES
    benign neoplasm of spleen, except hemangioma
      and lymphangioma (211.9)
    glomus jugulare (227.6)
    nevus:
      NOS (216.0-216.9)
      blue or pigmented (216.0-216.9)
      vascular (757.32)
  AHA: 1Q, '00, 21
  - **228.0** Hemangioma, any site [5th]
      AHA: J-F, '85, 19
      DEF: A common benign tumor usually occurring in infancy; composed of newly formed blood vessels due to malformation of angioblastic tissue.
    - **228.00** Of unspecified site
    - **228.01** Of skin and subcutaneous tissue
    - **228.02** Of intracranial structures
    - **228.03** Of retina
    - **228.04** Of intra-abdominal structures
        Peritoneum   Retroperitoneal tissue
    - **228.09** Of other sites
        Systemic angiomatosis
        AHA: 3Q, '91, 20
  - **228.1** Lymphangioma, any site
      Congenital lymphangioma
      Lymphatic nevus

229 Benign neoplasm of other and unspecified sites [4th]
  - **229.0** Lymph nodes
      EXCLUDES lymphangioma (228.1)
  - **229.8** Other specified sites
      Intrathoracic NOS   Thoracic NOS
  - **229.9** Site unspecified

CARCINOMA IN SITU (230-234)

INCLUDES
  Bowen's disease
  erythroplasia
  Queyrat's erythroplasia
EXCLUDES leukoplakia—see Alphabetic Index

DEF: A neoplastic type; with tumor cells confined to epithelium of origin; without further invasion.

230 Carcinoma in situ of digestive organs [4th]
  - **230.0** Lip, oral cavity, and pharynx
      Gingiva   Oropharynx
      Hypopharynx   Salivary gland or duct
      Mouth [any part]   Tongue
      Nasopharynx
      EXCLUDES
        aryepiglottic fold or interarytenoid fold,
          laryngeal aspect (231.0)
        epiglottis:
          NOS (231.0)
          suprahyoid portion (231.0)
        skin of lip (232.0)
  - **230.1** Esophagus
  - **230.2** Stomach
      Body   }
      Cardia } of stomach
      Fundus }
      Cardiac orifice
      Pylorus
  - **230.3** Colon
      Appendix   Ileocecal valve
      Cecum   Large intestine NOS
      EXCLUDES rectosigmoid junction (230.4)
  - **230.4** Rectum
      Rectosigmoid junction
  - **230.5** Anal canal
      Anal sphincter
  - **230.6** Anus, unspecified
      EXCLUDES anus:
        margin (232.5)
        skin (232.5)
        perianal skin (232.5)
  - **230.7** Other and unspecified parts of intestine
      Duodenum   Jejunum
      Ileum   Small intestine NOS
      EXCLUDES ampulla of Vater (230.8)
  - **230.8** Liver and biliary system
      Ampulla of Vater   Gallbladder
      Common bile duct   Hepatic duct
      Cystic duct   Sphincter of Oddi
  - **230.9** Other and unspecified digestive organs
      Digestive organ NOS
      Gastrointestinal tract NOS
      Pancreas
      Spleen

231–236.2 NEOPLASMS Tabular List

✓4th 231 Carcinoma in situ of respiratory system
- **231.0 Larynx**
  - Cartilage:
    - arytenoid
    - cricoid
    - cuneiform
    - thyroid
  - Epiglottis:
    - NOS
    - posterior surface
    - suprahyoid portion
  - Vocal cords (false) (true)
  - EXCLUDES aryepiglottic fold or interarytenoid fold:
    - NOS (230.0)
    - hypopharyngeal aspect (230.0)
    - marginal zone (230.0)
- **231.1 Trachea**
- **231.2 Bronchus and lung**
  - Carina
  - Hilus of lung
- **231.8 Other specified parts of respiratory system**
  - Accessory sinuses
  - Middle ear
  - Nasal cavities
  - Pleura
  - EXCLUDES
    - ear (external) (skin) (232.2)
    - nose NOS (234.8)
    - skin (232.3)
- **231.9 Respiratory system, part unspecified**
  - Respiratory organ NOS

✓4th 232 Carcinoma in situ of skin
- INCLUDES pigment cells
- **232.0 Skin of lip**
  - EXCLUDES vermilion border of lip (230.0)
- **232.1 Eyelid, including canthus**
- **232.2 Ear and external auditory canal**
- **232.3 Skin of other and unspecified parts of face**
- **232.4 Scalp and skin of neck**
- **232.5 Skin of trunk, except scrotum**
  - Anus, margin
  - Axillary fold
  - Perianal skin
  - Skin of:
    - abdominal wall
    - anus
    - back
  - Skin of:
    - breast
    - buttock
    - chest wall
    - groin
    - perineum
    - Umbilicus
  - EXCLUDES
    - anal canal (230.5)
    - anus NOS (230.6)
    - skin of genital organs (233.3, 233.5-233.6)
- **232.6 Skin of upper limb, including shoulder**
- **232.7 Skin of lower limb, including hip**
- **232.8 Other specified sites of skin**
- **232.9 Skin, site unspecified**

✓4th 233 Carcinoma in situ of breast and genitourinary system
- **233.0 Breast**
  - EXCLUDES
    - Paget's disease (174.0-174.9)
    - skin of breast (232.5)
- **233.1 Cervix uteri** ♀
  - ▶Cervical intraepithelial glandular neoplasia◀
  - Cervical intraepithelial neoplasia III [CIN III]
  - Severe dysplasia of cervix
  - EXCLUDES
    - cervical intraepithelial neoplasia II [CIN II] (622.12)
    - cytologic evidence of malignancy without histologic confirmation ▶(795.06)◀
    - high grade squamous intraepithelial lesion (HGSIL) (795.04)
    - moderate dysplasia of cervix (622.12)
  - AHA: 3Q, '92, 7; 3Q, '92, 8; 1Q, '91, 11
- **233.2 Other and unspecified parts of uterus** ♀
- **233.3 Other and unspecified female genital organs** ♀
- **233.4 Prostate** ♂
- **233.5 Penis** ♂
- **233.6 Other and unspecified male genital organs** ♂
- **233.7 Bladder**
- **233.9 Other and unspecified urinary organs**

✓4th 234 Carcinoma in situ of other and unspecified sites
- **234.0 Eye**
  - EXCLUDES
    - cartilage of eyelid (234.8)
    - eyelid (skin) (232.1)
    - optic nerve (234.8)
    - orbital bone (234.8)
- **234.8 Other specified sites**
  - Endocrine gland [any]
- **234.9 Site unspecified**
  - Carcinoma in situ NOS

NEOPLASMS OF UNCERTAIN BEHAVIOR (235-238)

Note: Categories 235–238 classify by site certain histomorphologically well-defined neoplasms, the subsequent behavior of which cannot be predicted from the present appearance.

✓4th 235 Neoplasm of uncertain behavior of digestive and respiratory systems
- EXCLUDES ▶stromal tumors of uncertain behavior of digestive system (238.1)◀
- **235.0 Major salivary glands**
  - Gland:
    - parotid
    - sublingual
  - Gland:
    - submandibular
  - EXCLUDES minor salivary glands (235.1)
- **235.1 Lip, oral cavity, and pharynx**
  - Gingiva
  - Hypopharynx
  - Minor salivary glands
  - Mouth
  - Nasopharynx
  - Oropharynx
  - Tongue
  - EXCLUDES
    - aryepiglottic fold or interarytenoid fold, laryngeal aspect (235.6)
    - epiglottis:
      - NOS (235.6)
      - suprahyoid portion (235.6)
    - skin of lip (238.2)
- **235.2 Stomach, intestines, and rectum**
- **235.3 Liver and biliary passages**
  - Ampulla of Vater
  - Bile ducts [any]
  - Gallbladder
  - Liver
- **235.4 Retroperitoneum and peritoneum**
- **235.5 Other and unspecified digestive organs**
  - Anal:
    - canal
    - sphincter
  - Anus NOS
  - Esophagus
  - Pancreas
  - Spleen
  - EXCLUDES anus:
    - margin (238.2)
    - skin (238.2)
    - perianal skin (238.2)
- **235.6 Larynx**
  - EXCLUDES aryepiglottic fold or interarytenoid fold:
    - NOS (235.1)
    - hypopharyngeal aspect (235.1)
    - marginal zone (235.1)
- **235.7 Trachea, bronchus, and lung**
- **235.8 Pleura, thymus, and mediastinum**
- **235.9 Other and unspecified respiratory organs**
  - Accessory sinuses
  - Middle ear
  - Nasal cavities
  - Respiratory organ NOS
  - EXCLUDES
    - ear (external) (skin) (238.2)
    - nose (238.8)
    - skin (238.2)

✓4th 236 Neoplasm of uncertain behavior of genitourinary organs
- **236.0 Uterus** ♀
- **236.1 Placenta**
  - Chorioadenoma (destruens)
  - Invasive mole
  - Malignant hydatid(iform) mole
- **236.2 Ovary** ♀
  - Use additional code to identify any functional activity

	236.3	**Other and unspecified** female genital organs ♀
	236.4	**Testis** ♂
		Use additional code to identify any functional activity
	236.5	**Prostate** ♂
	236.6	**Other and unspecified** male genital organs ♂
	236.7	**Bladder**
✓5th	**236.9**	**Other and unspecified urinary organs**
	236.90	Urinary organ, unspecified
	236.91	Kidney and ureter
	236.99	Other

✓4th **237 Neoplasm of uncertain behavior of endocrine glands and nervous system**

- **237.0 Pituitary gland and craniopharyngeal duct**
  Use additional code to identify any functional activity
- **237.1 Pineal gland**
- **237.2 Adrenal gland**
  Suprarenal gland
  Use additional code to identify any functional activity
- **237.3 Paraganglia**
  Aortic body   Coccygeal body
  Carotid body   Glomus jugulare
  AHA: N-D, '84, 17
- **237.4 Other and unspecified endocrine glands**
  Parathyroid gland   Thyroid gland
- **237.5 Brain and spinal cord**
- **237.6 Meninges**
  Meninges: Meninges:
    NOS   spinal
    cerebral
- ✓5th **237.7 Neurofibromatosis**
  von Recklinghausen's disease
  DEF: An inherited condition with developmental changes in the nervous system, muscles, bones and skin; multiple soft tumors (neurofibromas) distributed over the entire body.
  - 237.70 Neurofibromatosis, unspecified
  - 237.71 Neurofibromatosis, type 1 [von Recklinghausen's disease]
  - 237.72 Neurofibromatosis, type 2 [acoustic neurofibromatosis]
    DEF: Inherited condition with cutaneous lesions, benign tumors of peripheral nerves and bilateral 8th nerve masses.
- **237.9 Other and unspecified parts of nervous system**
  Cranial nerves
  EXCLUDES peripheral, sympathetic, and parasympathetic nerves and ganglia (238.1)

✓4th **238 Neoplasm of uncertain behavior of other and unspecified sites and tissues**

- **238.0 Bone and articular cartilage**
  EXCLUDES cartilage:
    ear (238.1)
    eyelid (238.1)
    larynx (235.6)
    nose (235.9)
    synovia (238.1)
  AHA: 4Q, '04, 128
- **238.1 Connective and other soft tissue**
  Peripheral, sympathetic, and parasympathetic nerves and ganglia
  ▶Stromal tumors of digestive system◀
  EXCLUDES cartilage (of):
    articular (238.0)
    larynx (235.6)
    nose (235.9)
    connective tissue of breast (238.3)
- **238.2 Skin**
  EXCLUDES anus NOS (235.5)
    skin of genital organs (236.3, 236.6)
    vermilion border of lip (235.1)
- **238.3 Breast**
  EXCLUDES skin of breast (238.2)
- **238.4 Polycythemia vera**
  DEF: Abnormal proliferation of all bone marrow elements, increased red cell mass and total blood volume; unknown etiology, frequently associated with splenomegaly, leukocytosis, and thrombocythemia.
- **238.5 Histiocytic and mast cells**
  Mast cell tumor NOS
  Mastocytoma NOS
- **238.6 Plasma cells**
  Plasmacytoma NOS
  Solitary myeloma
- ✓5th **238.7 Other lymphatic and hematopoietic tissues**
  EXCLUDES ▶acute myelogenous leukemia (205.0)
    chronic myelomonocytic leukemia (205.1)◀
    myelofibrosis ▶(289.83)◀
    myelosclerosis NOS (289.89)
    myelosis:
      NOS (205.9)
      megakaryocytic (207.2)
  AHA: 3Q, '01, 13; 1Q, '97, 5; 2Q, '89, 8
  - ● 238.71 Essential thrombocythemia
    Essential hemorrhagic thrombocythemia
    Essential thrombocytosis
    Idiopathic (hemorrhagic) thrombocythemia
    Primary thrombocytosis
  - ● 238.72 Low grade myelodysplastic syndrome lesions
    Refractory anemia (RA)
    Refractory anemia with ringed sideroblasts (RARS)
    Refractory cytopenia with multilineage dysplasia (RCMD)
    Refractory cytopenia with multilineage dysplasia and ringed sideroblasts (RCMD-RS)
    DEF: Refractory anemia (RA): Form of bone marrow disorder (myelodysplastic syndrome) that interferes with red blood cell production in the bone marrow; malignancy unresponsive to hematinics; characteristic normal or hypercellular marrow with abnormal erythrocyte development and reticulocytopenia.
  - ● 238.73 High grade myelodysplastic syndrome lesions
    Refractory anemia with excess blasts-1 (RAEB-1)
    Refractory anemia with excess blasts-2 (RAEB-2)
  - ● 238.74 Myelodysplastic syndrome with 5q deletion
    5q minus syndrome NOS
    EXCLUDES constitutional 5q deletion (758.39)
      high grade myelodysplastic syndrome with 5q deletion (238.73)
  - ● 238.75 Myelodysplastic syndrome, unspecified

- **238.76 Myelofibrosis with myeloid metaplasia**
  Agnogenic myeloid metaplasia
  Idiopathic myelofibrosis (chronic)
  Myelosclerosis with myeloid metaplasia
  Primary myelofibrosis
  EXCLUDES
      myelofibrosis NOS (289.83)
      myelophthisic anemia (284.2)
      myelophthisis (284.2)
      secondary myelofibrosis (289.83)

- **238.79 Other lymphatic and hematopoietic tissues**
  Lymphoproliferative disease (chronic) NOS
  Megakaryocytic myelosclerosis
  Myeloproliferative disease (chronic) NOS
  Panmyelosis (acute)

238.8 Other specified sites
  Eye
  Heart
  EXCLUDES
      eyelid (skin) (238.2)
      cartilage (238.1)

238.9 Site unspecified

NEOPLASMS OF UNSPECIFIED NATURE (239)

✓4th 239 Neoplasms of unspecified nature
  Note: Category 239 classifies by site neoplasms of unspecified morphology and behavior. The term "mass," unless otherwise stated, is not to be regarded as a neoplastic growth.
  INCLUDES
      "growth" NOS
      neoplasm NOS
      new growth NOS
      tumor NOS

239.0 Digestive system
  EXCLUDES
      anus:
          margin (239.2)
          skin (239.2)
          perianal skin (239.2)

239.1 Respiratory system

239.2 Bone, soft tissue, and skin
  EXCLUDES
      anal canal (239.0)
      anus NOS (239.0)
      bone marrow (202.9)
      cartilage:
          larynx (239.1)
          nose (239.1)
      connective tissue of breast (239.3)
      skin of genital organs (239.5)
      vermilion border of lip (239.0)

239.3 Breast
  EXCLUDES
      skin of breast (239.2)

239.4 Bladder

239.5 Other genitourinary organs

239.6 Brain
  EXCLUDES
      cerebral meninges (239.7)
      cranial nerves (239.7)

239.7 Endocrine glands and other parts of nervous system
  EXCLUDES
      peripheral, sympathetic, and parasympathetic nerves and ganglia (239.2)

239.8 Other specified sites
  EXCLUDES
      eyelid (skin) (239.2)
      cartilage (239.2)
      great vessels (239.2)
      optic nerve (239.7)

239.9 Site unspecified

ENDOCRINE, NUTRITIONAL AND METABOLIC, IMMUNITY

Endocrine System
- Hypothalamus
- Pituitary (Hypophysis) gland
- Thyroid gland
- Thymus gland
- Pineal gland
- Parathyroid glands
- Adrenal (Suprarenal) glands
- Ovaries
- Pancreas
- Testes

3. ENDOCRINE, NUTRITIONAL AND METABOLIC DISEASES, AND IMMUNITY DISORDERS (240-279)

EXCLUDES endocrine and metabolic disturbances specific to the fetus and newborn (775.0-775.9)

Note: All neoplasms, whether functionally active or not, are classified in Chapter 2. Codes in Chapter 3 (i.e., 242.8, 246.0, 251-253, 255-259) may be used to identify such functional activity associated with any neoplasm, or by ectopic endocrine tissue.

DISORDERS OF THYROID GLAND (240-246)

240 Simple and unspecified goiter
DEF: An enlarged thyroid gland often caused by an inadequate dietary intake of iodine.

- **240.0 Goiter, specified as simple**
  Any condition classifiable to 240.9, specified as simple

- **240.9 Goiter, unspecified**
  Enlargement of thyroid
  Goiter or struma:
    NOS
    diffuse colloid
    endemic
  Goiter or struma:
    hyperplastic
    nontoxic (diffuse)
    parenchymatous
    sporadic
  EXCLUDES congenital (dyshormonogenic) goiter (246.1)

241 Nontoxic nodular goiter
EXCLUDES adenoma of thyroid (226)
cystadenoma of thyroid (226)

- **241.0 Nontoxic uninodular goiter**
  Thyroid nodule   Uninodular goiter (nontoxic)
  DEF: Enlarged thyroid, commonly due to decreased thyroid production, with single nodule; no clinical hypothyroidism.

- **241.1 Nontoxic multinodular goiter**
  Multinodular goiter (nontoxic)
  DEF: Enlarged thyroid, commonly due to decreased thyroid production with multiple nodules; no clinical hypothyroidism.

- **241.9 Unspecified nontoxic nodular goiter**
  Adenomatous goiter
  Nodular goiter (nontoxic) NOS
  Struma nodosa (simplex)

242 Thyrotoxicosis with or without goiter
EXCLUDES neonatal thyrotoxicosis (775.3)

The following fifth-digit subclassification is for use with category 242:
  0 without mention of thyrotoxic crisis or storm
  1 with mention of thyrotoxic crisis or storm

DEF: A condition caused by excess quantities of thyroid hormones being introduced into the tissues.

- **242.0 Toxic diffuse goiter**
  Basedow's disease
  Exophthalmic or toxic goiter NOS
  Graves' disease
  Primary thyroid hyperplasia
  DEF: Diffuse thyroid enlargement accompanied by hyperthyroidism, bulging eyes, and dermopathy.

- **242.1 Toxic uninodular goiter**
  Thyroid nodule   toxic or with
  Uninodular goiter hyperthyroidism
  DEF: Symptomatic hyperthyroidism with a single nodule on the enlarged thyroid gland. Abrupt onset of symptoms; including extreme nervousness, insomnia, weight loss, tremors, and psychosis or coma.

- **242.2 Toxic multinodular goiter**
  Secondary thyroid hyperplasia
  DEF: Symptomatic hyperthyroidism with multiple nodules on the enlarged thyroid gland. Abrupt onset of symptoms; including extreme nervousness, insomnia, weight loss, tremors, and psychosis or coma.

- **242.3 Toxic nodular goiter, unspecified**
  Adenomatous goiter
  Nodular goiter   toxic or with
  Struma nodosa   hyperthyroidism
  Any condition classifiable to 241.9 specified as toxic or with hyperthyroidism

- **242.4 Thyrotoxicosis from ectopic thyroid nodule**

- **242.8 Thyrotoxicosis of other specified origin**
  Overproduction of thyroid-stimulating hormone [TSH]
  Thyrotoxicosis:
    factitia from ingestion of excessive thyroid material
  Use additional E code to identify cause, if drug-induced

- **242.9 Thyrotoxicosis without mention of goiter or other cause**
  Hyperthyroidism NOS
  Thyrotoxicosis NOS

243 Congenital hypothyroidism
Congenital thyroid insufficiency
Cretinism (athyrotic) (endemic)
Use additional code to identify associated mental retardation
EXCLUDES congenital (dyshormonogenic) goiter (246.1)
DEF: Underproduction of thyroid hormone present from birth.

244 Acquired hypothyroidism
INCLUDES athyroidism (acquired)
hypothyroidism (acquired)
myxedema (adult) (juvenile)
thyroid (gland) insufficiency (acquired)

- **244.0 Postsurgical hypothyroidism**
  DEF: Underproduction of thyroid hormone due to surgical removal of all or part of the thyroid gland.

- **244.1 Other postablative hypothyroidism**
  Hypothyroidism following therapy, such as irradiation

- **244.2 Iodine hypothyroidism**
  Hypothyroidism resulting from administration or ingestion of iodide
  Use additional E code to identify drug

- **244.3 Other iatrogenic hypothyroidism**
  Hypothyroidism resulting from:
    P-aminosalicylic acid [PAS]
    Phenylbutazone
    Resorcinol
  Iatrogenic hypothyroidism NOS
  Use additional E code to identify drug

ENDOCRINE, NUTRITIONAL AND METABOLIC, IMMUNITY

244.8 Other specified acquired hypothyroidism
Secondary hypothyroidism NEC

AHA: J-A, '85, 9

244.9 Unspecified hypothyroidism
Hypothyroidism } primary or NOS
Myxedema

AHA: 3Q, '99, 19; 4Q, '96, 29

√4th 245 Thyroiditis

245.0 Acute thyroiditis
Abscess of thyroid
Thyroiditis:
  nonsuppurative, acute
  pyogenic
  suppurative
Use additional code to identify organism

DEF: Inflamed thyroid caused by infection, with abscess and liquid puris.

245.1 Subacute thyroiditis
Thyroiditis:
  de Quervain's
  giant cell
  granulomatous
  viral

DEF: Inflammation of the thyroid, characterized by fever and painful enlargement of the thyroid gland, with granulomas in the gland.

245.2 Chronic lymphocytic thyroiditis
Hashimoto's disease
Struma lymphomatosa
Thyroiditis:
  autoimmune
  lymphocytic (chronic)

DEF: Autoimmune disease of thyroid; lymphocytes infiltrate the gland and thyroid antibodies are produced; women more often affected.

245.3 Chronic fibrous thyroiditis
Struma fibrosa
Thyroiditis:
  invasive (fibrous)
  ligneous
  Riedel's

DEF: Persistent fibrosing inflammation of thyroid with adhesions to nearby structures; rare condition.

245.4 Iatrogenic thyroiditis
Use additional code to identify cause

DEF: Thyroiditis resulting from treatment or intervention by physician or in a patient intervention setting.

245.8 Other and unspecified chronic thyroiditis
Chronic thyroiditis: Chronic thyroiditis:
  NOS   nonspecific

245.9 Thyroiditis, unspecified
Thyroiditis NOS

√4th 246 Other disorders of thyroid

246.0 Disorders of thyrocalcitonin secretion
Hypersecretion of calcitonin or thyrocalcitonin

246.1 Dyshormonogenic goiter
Congenital (dyshormonogenic) goiter
Goiter due to enzyme defect in synthesis of thyroid hormone
Goitrous cretinism (sporadic)

246.2 Cyst of thyroid
EXCLUDES   cystadenoma of thyroid (226)

246.3 Hemorrhage and infarction of thyroid

246.8 Other specified disorders of thyroid
Abnormality of thyroid-binding globulin
Atrophy of thyroid
Hyper-TBG-nemia
Hypo-TBG-nemia

246.9 Unspecified disorder of thyroid

DISEASES OF OTHER ENDOCRINE GLANDS (250-259)

√4th 250 Diabetes mellitus
EXCLUDES   gestational diabetes (648.8)
           hyperglycemia NOS (790.6)
           neonatal diabetes mellitus (775.1)
           nonclinical diabetes (790.29)

The following fifth-digit subclassification is for use with category 250:

0 type II or unspecified type, not stated as uncontrolled
Fifth-digit 0 is for use for type II patients, even if the patient requires insulin
Use additional code, if applicable, for associated long-term (current) insulin use V58.67

1 type I [juvenile type], not stated as uncontrolled

2 type II or unspecified type, uncontrolled
Fifth-digit 2 is for use for type II patients, even if the patient requires insulin
Use additional code, if applicable, for associated long-term (current) insulin use V58.67

3 type I [juvenile type], uncontrolled

AHA: 4Q, '04, 56; 2Q, '04, 17; 2Q, '02, 13; 2Q,'01, 16; 2Q,'98, 15; 4Q, '97, 32; 2Q, '97, 14; 3Q, '96, 5; 4Q, '93, 19; 2Q, '92, 5; 3Q, '91, 3; 2Q, '90, 22; N-D, '85, 11

DEF: Diabetes mellitus: Inability to metabolize carbohydrates, proteins, and fats with insufficient secretion of insulin. Symptoms may be unremarkable, with long-term complications, involving kidneys, nerves, blood vessels, and eyes.

DEF: Uncontrolled diabetes: A nonspecific term indicating that the current treatment regimen does not keep the blood sugar level of a patient within acceptable levels.

√5th 250.0 Diabetes mellitus without mention of complication
Diabetes mellitus without mention of complication or manifestation classifiable to 250.1-250.9
Diabetes (mellitus) NOS

AHA: 4Q, '97, 32; 3Q, '91, 3, 12; N-D, '85, 11; For code 250.00: 1Q, '05, 15; 4Q, '04, 55; 4Q, '03, 105, 108; 2Q, '03, 16; 1Q, '02, 7, 11; For code: 250.01: 4Q, '04, 55; 4Q, '03, 110; 2Q, '03, 6; For code: 250.02: 1Q, '03, 5

√5th 250.1 Diabetes with ketoacidosis
Diabetic:
  acidosis } without mention of coma
  ketosis

AHA: 3Q, '91, 6; For code 250.11: 4Q, '03, 82

DEF: Diabetic hyperglycemic crisis causing ketone presence in body fluids.

√5th 250.2 Diabetes with hyperosmolarity
Hyperosmolar (nonketotic) coma

AHA: 4Q, '93, 19; 3Q, '91, 7

√5th 250.3 Diabetes with other coma
Diabetic coma (with ketoacidosis)
Diabetic hypoglycemic coma
Insulin coma NOS
EXCLUDES   diabetes with hyperosmolar coma (250.2)

AHA: 3Q, '91, 7,12

DEF: Coma (not hyperosmolar) caused by hyperglycemia or hypoglycemia as complication of diabetes.

√5th 250.4 Diabetes with renal manifestations
Use additional code to identify manifestation, as:
  chronic kidney disease (585.1-585.9)
  diabetic:
    nephropathy NOS (583.81)
    nephrosis (581.81)
    intercapillary glomerulosclerosis (581.81)
    Kimmelstiel-Wilson syndrome (581.81)

AHA: 3Q, '91, 8,12; S-O, '87, 9; S-O, '84, 3; For code: 250.40: 1Q, '03, 20

N Newborn Age: 0   **P** Pediatric Age: 0-17   **M** Maternity Age: 12-55   **A** Adult Age: 15-124

Tabular List — ENDOCRINE, NUTRITIONAL AND METABOLIC, IMMUNITY — 250.5–252.02

√5th **250.5 Diabetes with ophthalmic manifestations**
Use additional code to identify manifestation, as:
diabetic:
blindness (369.00-369.9)
cataract (366.41)
glaucoma (365.44)
macular edema (362.07)
retinal edema (362.07)
retinopathy (362.01-362.07)
AHA: ▶4Q, '05, 65;◀ ◀3Q, '91, 8; S-O, '85, 11;
For code 250.50: ▶4Q, '05, 67◀

√5th **250.6 Diabetes with neurological manifestations**
Use additional code to identify manifestation, as:
diabetic:
amyotrophy (358.1)
gastroparalysis (536.3)
gastroparesis (536.3)
mononeuropathy (354.0-355.9)
neurogenic arthropathy (713.5)
peripheral autonomic neuropathy (337.1)
polyneuropathy (357.2)
AHA: 2Q, '93, 6; 2Q, '92, 15; 3Q, '91, 9; N-D, '84, 9; **For code 250.60:** 4Q, '03, 105; **For code 250.61:** 2Q, '04, 7

√5th **250.7 Diabetes with peripheral circulatory disorders**
Use additional code to identify manifestation, as:
diabetic:
gangrene (785.4)
peripheral angiopathy (443.81)
DEF: Blood vessel damage or disease, usually in the feet, legs, or hands, as a complication of diabetes.
AHA 1Q, '96, 10; 3Q, '94, 5; 2Q, '94, 17; 3Q, '91, 10, 12; 3Q, '90, 15; **For code 250.70:** 1Q, '04, 14

√5th **250.8 Diabetes with other specified manifestations**
Diabetic hypoglycemia
Hypoglycemic shock
Use additional code to identify manifestation, as:
any associated ulceration (707.10-707.9)
diabetic bone changes (731.8)
Use additional E code to identify cause, if drug-induced
AHA: 4Q, '00, 44; 4Q, '97, 43; 2Q, '97, 16; 4Q, '93, 20; 3Q, '91, 10; **For code 250.80:** 1Q, '04, 14

√5th **250.9 Diabetes with unspecified complication**
AHA: 2Q, '92, 15; 3Q, '91, 7, 12

√4th **251 Other disorders of pancreatic internal secretion**

251.0 Hypoglycemic coma
Iatrogenic hyperinsulinism
Non-diabetic insulin coma
Use additional E code to identify cause, if drug-induced
EXCLUDES hypoglycemic coma in diabetes mellitus (250.3)
AHA: M-A, '85, 8
DEF: Coma induced by low blood sugar in non-diabetic patient.

251.1 Other specified hypoglycemia
Hyperinsulinism: Hyperplasia of pancreatic
NOS   islet beta cells NOS
ectopic
functional
EXCLUDES hypoglycemia:
in diabetes mellitus (250.8)
in infant of diabetic mother (775.0)
neonatal hypoglycemia (775.6)
hypoglycemic coma (251.0)
Use additional E code to identify cause, if drug-induced.
DEF: Excessive production of insulin by the pancreas; associated with obesity and insulin-producing tumors.
AHA: 1Q, '03, 10

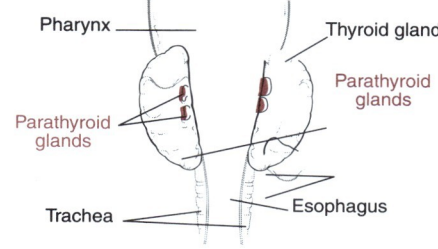
Dorsal View of Parathyroid Glands

251.2 Hypoglycemia, unspecified
Hypoglycemia:
NOS
reactive
spontaneous
EXCLUDES hypoglycemia:
with coma (251.0)
in diabetes mellitus (250.8)
leucine-induced (270.3)
AHA: M-A, '85, 8

251.3 Postsurgical hypoinsulinemia
Hypoinsulinemia following complete or partial pancreatectomy
Postpancreatectomy hyperglycemia
AHA: 3Q, '91, 6

251.4 Abnormality of secretion of glucagon
Hyperplasia of pancreatic islet alpha cells with glucagon excess
DEF: Production malfunction of a pancreatic hormone secreted by cells of the islets of Langerhans

251.5 Abnormality of secretion of gastrin
Hyperplasia of pancreatic alpha cells with gastrin excess
Zollinger-Ellison syndrome

251.8 Other specified disorders of pancreatic internal secretion
AHA: 2Q, '98, 15; 3Q, '91, 6

251.9 Unspecified disorder of pancreatic internal secretion
Islet cell hyperplasia NOS

√4th **252 Disorders of parathyroid gland**

√5th **252.0 Hyperparathyroidism**
EXCLUDES ectopic hyperparathyroidism (259.3)
DEF: Abnormally high secretion of parathyroid hormones causing bone deterioration, reduced renal function, kidney stones.

252.00 Hyperparathyroidism, unspecified

252.01 Primary hyperparathyroidism
Hyperplasia of parathyroid
DEF: Parathyroid dysfunction commonly caused by hyperplasia of two or more glands; characteristic hypercalcemia and increased parathyroid hormone levels.

252.02 Secondary hyperparathyroidism, non-renal
EXCLUDES secondary hyperparathyroidism (of renal origin) (588.81)
AHA: 4Q, '04, 57-59
DEF: Underlying disease of nonrenal origin decreases blood levels of calcium causing the parathyroid to release increased levels of parathyroid hormone; parathyroid hormone levels return to normal once underlying condition is treated and blood calcium levels are normal.

ENDOCRINE, NUTRITIONAL AND METABOLIC, IMMUNITY

252.08 **Other hyperparathyroidism**
Tertiary hyperparathyroidism
DEF: Tertiary hyperparathyroidism: chronic secondary hyperparathyroidism leads to adenomatous parathyroid causing irreversible abnormal production of parathyroid hormone (PTH); PTH remains high after the serum calcium levels are brought under control.

252.1 **Hypoparathyroidism**
Parathyroiditis (autoimmune)
Tetany:
  parathyroid
  parathyroprival
    EXCLUDES   *pseudohypoparathyroidism (275.4)*
                     pseudopseudohypoparathyroidism (275.4)
                     tetany NOS (781.7)
                     transitory neonatal hypoparathyroidism (775.4)
DEF: Abnormally low secretion of parathyroid hormones which causes decreased calcium and increased phosphorus in the blood. Resulting in muscle cramps, tetany, urinary frequency and cataracts.

252.8 **Other specified disorders of parathyroid gland**
Cyst   } of parathyroid gland
Hemorrhage

252.9 **Unspecified disorder of parathyroid gland**

√4th **253** **Disorders of the pituitary gland and its hypothalamic control**
    INCLUDES   the listed conditions whether the disorder is in the pituitary or the hypothalamus
    EXCLUDES   *Cushing's syndrome (255.0)*

253.0 **Acromegaly and gigantism**
Overproduction of growth hormone
DEF: Acromegaly: chronic, beginning in middle age; caused by hypersecretion of the pituitary growth hormone; produces enlarged parts of skeleton, especially the nose, ears, jaws, fingers and toes.
DEF: Gigantism: pituitary gigantism caused by excess growth of short flat bones; men may grow 78 to 80 inches tall.

253.1 **Other and unspecified anterior pituitary hyperfunction**
Forbes-Albright syndrome
    EXCLUDES   *overproduction of:*
                   ACTH (255.3)
                   thyroid-stimulating hormone [TSH] (242.8)
AHA: J-A, '85, 9
DEF: Spontaneous galactorrhea-amenorrhea syndrome unrelated to pregnancy; usually related to presence of pituitary tumor.

253.2 **Panhypopituitarism**
Cachexia, pituitary
Necrosis of pituitary (postpartum)
Pituitary insufficiency NOS
Sheehan's syndrome
Simmonds' disease
    EXCLUDES   *iatrogenic hypopituitarism (253.7)*
DEF: Damage to or absence of pituitary gland leading to impaired sexual function, weight loss, fatigue, bradycardia, hypotension, pallor, depression, and impaired growth in children; called Simmonds' disease if cachexia is prominent.

253.3 **Pituitary dwarfism**
Isolated deficiency of (human) growth hormone [HGH]
Lorain-Levi dwarfism
DEF: Dwarfism with infantile physical characteristics due to abnormally low secretion of growth hormone and gonadotropin deficiency.

253.4 **Other anterior pituitary disorders**
Isolated or partial deficiency of an anterior pituitary hormone, other than growth hormone
Prolactin deficiency
AHA: J-A, '85, 9

253.5 **Diabetes insipidus**
Vasopressin deficiency
    EXCLUDES   *nephrogenic diabetes insipidus (588.1)*
DEF: Metabolic disorder causing insufficient antidiuretic hormone release; symptoms include frequent urination, thirst, ravenous hunger, loss of weight, fatigue.

253.6 **Other disorders of neurohypophysis**
Syndrome of inappropriate secretion of antidiuretic hormone [ADH]
    EXCLUDES   *ectopic antidiuretic hormone secretion (259.3)*

253.7 **Iatrogenic pituitary disorders**
Hypopituitarism: Hypopituitarism:
  hormone-induced   postablative
  hypophysectomy-induced radiotherapy-induced
Use additional E code to identify cause
DEF: Pituitary dysfunction that results from drug therapy, radiation therapy, or surgery, causing mild to severe symptoms.

253.8 **Other disorders of the pituitary and other syndromes of diencephalohypophyseal origin**
Abscess of pituitary   Cyst of Rathke's pouch
Adiposogenital dystrophy Fröhlich's syndrome
    EXCLUDES   *craniopharyngioma (237.0)*

253.9 **Unspecified**
Dyspituitarism

√4th **254** **Diseases of thymus gland**
    EXCLUDES   *aplasia or dysplasia with immunodeficiency (279.2)*
                   hypoplasia with immunodeficiency (279.2)
                   myasthenia gravis (358.00-358.01)

254.0 **Persistent hyperplasia of thymus**
Hypertrophy of thymus
DEF: Continued abnormal growth of the twin lymphoid lobes that produce T lymphocytes.

254.1 **Abscess of thymus**

254.8 **Other specified diseases of thymus gland**
Atrophy } of thymus
Cyst
    EXCLUDES   *thymoma (212.6)*

254.9 **Unspecified disease of thymus gland**

√4th **255** **Disorders of adrenal glands**
    INCLUDES   the listed conditions whether the basic disorder is in the adrenals or is pituitary-induced

255.0 **Cushing's syndrome**
Adrenal hyperplasia due to excess ACTH
Cushing's syndrome:
  NOS
  iatrogenic
  idiopathic
  pituitary-dependent
Ectopic ACTH syndrome
Iatrogenic syndrome of excess cortisol
Overproduction of cortisol
Use additional E code to identify cause, if drug-induced
    EXCLUDES   *congenital adrenal hyperplasia (255.2)*
DEF: Due to adrenal cortisol oversecretion or glucocorticoid medications; may cause fatty tissue of the face, neck and body, osteoporosis and curvature of spine, hypertension, diabetes mellitus, female genitourinary problems, male impotence, degeneration of muscle tissues, weakness.

√5th **255.1** **Hyperaldosteronism**
AHA: 4Q, '03, 48
DEF: Oversecretion of aldosterone causing fluid retention, hypertension.

255.10 **Hyperaldosteronism, unspecified**
Aldosteronism NOS
▶Primary aldosteronism, unspecified◀
    EXCLUDES   *Conn's syndrome (255.12)*

ENDOCRINE, NUTRITIONAL AND METABOLIC, IMMUNITY

- **255.11** Glucocorticoid-remediable aldosteronism
  Familial aldosteronism type I
  EXCLUDES Conn's syndrome (255.12)
  DEF: A rare autosomal dominant familial form of primary aldosteronism in which the secretion of aldosterone is under the influence of adrenocorticotrophic hormone (ACTH) rather than the renin-angiotensin mechanism; characterized by moderate hypersecretion of aldosterone and suppressed plasma renin activity rapidly reversed by administration of glucosteroids; symptoms include hypertension and mild hypokalemia.

- **255.12** Conn's syndrome
  DEF: A type of primary aldosteronism caused by an adenoma of the glomerulosa cells in the adrenal cortex; presence of hypertension.

- **255.13** Bartter's syndrome
  DEF: A cluster of symptoms caused by a defect in the ability of the kidney to reabsorb potassium; signs include alkalosis (hypokalemic alkalosis), increased aldosterone, increased plasma renin, and normal blood pressure; symptoms include muscle cramping, weakness, constipation, frequency of urination, and failure to grow; also known as urinary potassium wasting or juxtaglomerular cell hyperplasia.

- **255.14** Other secondary aldosteronism

- **255.2** Adrenogenital disorders
  Achard-Thiers syndrome
  Adrenogenital syndromes, virilizing or feminizing, whether acquired or associated with congenital adrenal hyperplasia consequent on inborn enzyme defects in hormone synthesis
  Congenital adrenal hyperplasia
  Female adrenal pseudohermaphroditism
  Male:
    macrogenitosomia praecox
    sexual precocity with adrenal hyperplasia
  Virilization (female) (suprarenal)
  EXCLUDES adrenal hyperplasia due to excess ACTH (255.0)
  isosexual virilization (256.4)

- **255.3** Other corticoadrenal overactivity
  Acquired benign adrenal androgenic overactivity
  Overproduction of ACTH

- **255.4** Corticoadrenal insufficiency
  Addisonian crisis
  Addison's disease NOS
  Adrenal:
    atrophy (autoimmune)
    calcification
    crisis
    hemorrhage
    infarction
    insufficiency NOS
  EXCLUDES tuberculous Addison's disease (017.6)
  DEF: Underproduction of adrenal hormones causing low blood pressure.

- **255.5** Other adrenal hypofunction
  Adrenal medullary insufficiency
  EXCLUDES Waterhouse-Friderichsen syndrome (meningococcal) (036.3)

- **255.6** Medulloadrenal hyperfunction
  Catecholamine secretion by pheochromocytoma

- **255.8** Other specified disorders of adrenal glands
  Abnormality of cortisol-binding globulin

- **255.9** Unspecified disorder of adrenal glands

4th 256 Ovarian dysfunction
AHA: 4Q, '00, 51

- **256.0** Hyperestrogenism ♀
  DEF: Excess secretion of estrogen by the ovaries; characterized by ovaries containing multiple follicular cysts filled with serous fluid.

- **256.1** Other ovarian hyperfunction ♀
  Hypersecretion of ovarian androgens
  AHA: 3Q, '95, 15

- **256.2** Postablative ovarian failure ♀
  Ovarian failure: Ovarian failure:
    iatrogenic   postsurgical
    postirradiation
  Use additional code for states associated with artificial menopause (627.4)
  EXCLUDES acquired absence of ovary (V45.77)
  asymptomatic age-related (natural) postmenopausal status (V49.81)
  AHA: 2Q, '02, 12
  DEF: Failed ovarian function after medical or surgical intervention.

- **5th 256.3** Other ovarian failure
  Use additional code for states associated with natural menopause (627.2)
  EXCLUDES asymptomatic age-related (natural) postmenopausal status (V49.81)
  AHA: 4Q, '01, 41

  - **256.31** Premature menopause ♀
    DEF: Permanent cessation of ovarian function before the age of 40 occurring naturally of unknown cause.

  - **256.39** Other ovarian failure ♀
    Delayed menarche
    Ovarian hypofunction
    Primary ovarian failure NOS

- **256.4** Polycystic ovaries ♀
  Isosexual virilization   Stein-Leventhal syndrome
  DEF: Multiple serous filled cysts of ovary; symptoms of infertility, hirsutism, oligomenorrhea or amenorrhea.

- **256.8** Other ovarian dysfunction ♀
- **256.9** Unspecified ovarian dysfunction ♀

4th 257 Testicular dysfunction

- **257.0** Testicular hyperfunction ♂
  Hypersecretion of testicular hormones

- **257.1** Postablative testicular hypofunction ♂
  Testicular hypofunction: Testicular hypofunction:
    iatrogenic   postsurgical
    postirradiation

- **257.2** Other testicular hypofunction
  Defective biosynthesis of testicular androgen
  Eunuchoidism:
    NOS
    hypogonadotropic
  Failure:
    Leydig's cell, adult
    seminiferous tubule, adult
  Testicular hypogonadism
  EXCLUDES azoospermia (606.0)

- **257.8** Other testicular dysfunction
  EXCLUDES androgen insensitivity syndrome (259.5)

- **257.9** Unspecified testicular dysfunction ♂

4th 258 Polyglandular dysfunction and related disorders

- **258.0** Polyglandular activity in multiple endocrine adenomatosis
  Wermer's syndrome
  DEF: Wermer's syndrome: A rare hereditary condition characterized by the presence of adenomas or hyperplasia in more than one endocrine gland causing premature aging.

- **258.1** Other combinations of endocrine dysfunction
  Lloyd's syndrome
  Schmidt's syndrome

- **258.8** Other specified polyglandular dysfunction
- **258.9** Polyglandular dysfunction, unspecified

2007 ICD•9•CM

Volume 1 — 49

ENDOCRINE, NUTRITIONAL AND METABOLIC, IMMUNITY — Tabular List

259 Other endocrine disorders

259.0 Delay in sexual development and puberty, not elsewhere classified
Delayed puberty

259.1 Precocious sexual development and puberty, not elsewhere classified [P]
Sexual precocity:
 NOS
 constitutional
Sexual precocity:
 cryptogenic
 idiopathic

259.2 Carcinoid syndrome
Hormone secretion by carcinoid tumors
DEF: Presence of carcinoid tumors that spread to liver; characterized by cyanotic flushing of skin, diarrhea, bronchospasm, acquired tricuspid and pulmonary stenosis, sudden drops in blood pressure, edema, ascites.

259.3 Ectopic hormone secretion, not elsewhere classified
Ectopic:
 antidiuretic hormone secretion [ADH]
 hyperparathyroidism
EXCLUDES ectopic ACTH syndrome (255.0)
AHA: N-D, '85, 4

259.4 Dwarfism, not elsewhere classified
Dwarfism:
 NOS
 constitutional
EXCLUDES dwarfism:
  achondroplastic (756.4)
  intrauterine (759.7)
  nutritional (263.2)
  pituitary (253.3)
  renal (588.0)
  progeria (259.8)

259.5 Androgen insensitivity syndrome
Partial androgen insensitivity
Reifenstein syndrome
AHA: 4Q, '05, 53
DEF: X chromosome abnormality that prohibits the body from recognizing androgen; XY genotype with ambiguous genitalia; also called testicular feminization.

259.8 Other specified endocrine disorders
Pineal gland dysfunction Werner's syndrome
Progeria

259.9 Unspecified endocrine disorder
Disturbance: Infantilism NOS
 endocrine NOS
 hormone NOS

NUTRITIONAL DEFICIENCIES (260-269)
EXCLUDES deficiency anemias (280.0-281.9)

260 Kwashiorkor
Nutritional edema with dyspigmentation of skin and hair
DEF: Syndrome, particularly of children; excessive carbohydrate with inadequate protein intake, inhibited growth potential, anomalies in skin and hair pigmentation, edema and liver disease.

261 Nutritional marasmus
Nutritional atrophy   Severe malnutrition NOS
Severe calorie deficiency
DEF: Protein-calorie malabsorption or malnutrition of children; characterized by tissue wasting, dehydration, and subcutaneous fat depletion; may occur with infectious disease; also called infantile atrophy.

262 Other severe, protein-calorie malnutrition
Nutritional edema without mention of dyspigmentation of skin and hair
AHA: 4Q, '92, 24; J-A, '85, 12

263 Other and unspecified protein-calorie malnutrition
AHA: 4Q, '92, 24

263.0 Malnutrition of moderate degree
AHA: J-A, '85, 1
DEF: Malnutrition characterized by biochemical changes in electrolytes, lipids, blood plasma.

263.1 Malnutrition of mild degree
AHA: J-A, '85, 1

263.2 Arrested development following protein-calorie malnutrition
Nutritional dwarfism
Physical retardation due to malnutrition

263.8 Other protein-calorie malnutrition

263.9 Unspecified protein-calorie malnutrition
Dystrophy due to malnutrition
Malnutrition (calorie) NOS
EXCLUDES nutritional deficiency NOS (269.9)
AHA: 4Q, '03, 109; N-D, '84, 19

264 Vitamin A deficiency

264.0 With conjunctival xerosis
DEF: Vitamin A deficiency with conjunctival dryness.

264.1 With conjunctival xerosis and Bitot's spot
Bitot's spot in the young child
DEF: Vitamin A deficiency with conjunctival dryness, superficial spots of keratinized epithelium.

264.2 With corneal xerosis
DEF: Vitamin A deficiency with corneal dryness.

264.3 With corneal ulceration and xerosis
DEF: Vitamin A deficiency with corneal dryness, epithelial ulceration.

264.4 With keratomalacia
DEF: Vitamin A deficiency creating corneal dryness; progresses to corneal insensitivity, softness, necrosis; usually bilateral.

264.5 With night blindness
DEF: Vitamin A deficiency causing vision failure in dim light.

264.6 With xerophthalmic scars of cornea
DEF: Vitamin A deficiency with corneal scars from dryness.

264.7 Other ocular manifestations of vitamin A deficiency
Xerophthalmia due to vitamin A deficiency

264.8 Other manifestations of vitamin A deficiency
Follicular keratosis } due to vitamin A
Xeroderma   } deficiency

264.9 Unspecified vitamin A deficiency
Hypovitaminosis A NOS

265 Thiamine and niacin deficiency states

265.0 Beriberi
DEF: Inadequate vitamin B_1 (thiamine) intake, affects heart and peripheral nerves; individual may become edematous and develop cardiac disease due to the excess fluid; alcoholics and people with a diet of excessive polished rice prone to the disease.

265.1 Other and unspecified manifestations of thiamine deficiency
Other vitamin B_1 deficiency states

265.2 Pellagra
Deficiency: Deficiency:
 niacin (-tryptophan)   vitamin PP
 nicotinamide   Pellagra (alcoholic)
 nicotinic acid
DEF: Niacin deficiency causing dermatitis, inflammation of mucous membranes, diarrhea, and psychic disturbances.

266 Deficiency of B-complex components

266.0 Ariboflavinosis
Riboflavin [vitamin B_2] deficiency
AHA: S-O, '86, 10
DEF: Vitamin B_2 (riboflavin) deficiency marked by swollen lips and tongue fissures, corneal vascularization, scaling lesions, and anemia.

[N] Newborn Age: 0 [P] Pediatric Age: 0-17 [M] Maternity Age: 12-55 [A] Adult Age: 15-124

ENDOCRINE, NUTRITIONAL AND METABOLIC, IMMUNITY

266.1 Vitamin B_6 deficiency
Deficiency:
 pyridoxal
 pyridoxamine
Deficiency:
 pyridoxine
 Vitamin B_6 deficiency syndrome

EXCLUDES: vitamin B_6-responsive sideroblastic anemia (285.0)

DEF: Vitamin B_6 deficiency causing skin, lip, and tongue disturbances, peripheral neuropathy; and convulsions in infants.

266.2 Other B-complex deficiencies
Deficiency:
 cyanocobalamin
 folic acid
Deficiency:
 vitamin B_{12}

EXCLUDES: combined system disease with anemia (281.0-281.1)
deficiency anemias (281.0-281.9)
subacute degeneration of spinal cord with anemia (281.0-281.1)

266.9 Unspecified vitamin B deficiency

267 Ascorbic acid deficiency
Deficiency of vitamin C
Scurvy

EXCLUDES: scorbutic anemia (281.8)

DEF: Vitamin C deficiency causing swollen gums, myalgia, weight loss, and weakness.

268 Vitamin D deficiency

EXCLUDES: vitamin D-resistant:
osteomalacia (275.3)
rickets (275.3)

268.0 Rickets, active

EXCLUDES: celiac rickets (579.0)
renal rickets (588.0)

DEF: Inadequate vitamin D intake, usually in pediatrics, that affects bones most involved with muscular action; may cause nodules on ends and sides of bones; delayed closure of fontanels in infants; symptoms may include muscle soreness, and profuse sweating.

268.1 Rickets, late effect
Any condition specified as due to rickets and stated to be a late effect or sequela of rickets
Use additional code to identify the nature of late effect

DEF: Distorted or demineralized bones as a result of vitamin D deficiency.

268.2 Osteomalacia, unspecified
DEF: Softening of bones due to decrease in calcium; marked by pain, tenderness, muscular weakness, anorexia, and weight loss.

268.9 Unspecified vitamin D deficiency
Avitaminosis D

269 Other nutritional deficiencies

269.0 Deficiency of vitamin K

EXCLUDES: deficiency of coagulation factor due to vitamin K deficiency (286.7)
vitamin K deficiency of newborn (776.0)

269.1 Deficiency of other vitamins
Deficiency:
 vitamin E
Deficiency:
 vitamin P

269.2 Unspecified vitamin deficiency
Multiple vitamin deficiency NOS

269.3 Mineral deficiency, not elsewhere classified
Deficiency:
 calcium, dietary
Deficiency:
 iodine

EXCLUDES: deficiency:
calcium NOS (275.4)
potassium (276.8)
sodium (276.1)

269.8 Other nutritional deficiency

EXCLUDES: adult failure to thrive (783.7)
failure to thrive in childhood (783.41)
feeding problems (783.3)
newborn (779.3)

269.9 Unspecified nutritional deficiency

OTHER METABOLIC AND IMMUNITY DISORDERS (270-279)

Use additional code to identify any associated mental retardation

270 Disorders of amino-acid transport and metabolism

EXCLUDES: abnormal findings without manifest disease (790.0-796.9)
disorders of purine and pyrimidine metabolism (277.1-277.2)
gout (274.0-274.9)

270.0 Disturbances of amino-acid transport
Cystinosis
Cystinuria
Fanconi (-de Toni) (-Debré) syndrome
Glycinuria (renal)
Hartnup disease

270.1 Phenylketonuria [PKU]
Hyperphenylalaninemia

DEF: Inherited metabolic condition causing excess phenylpyruvic and other acids in urine; results in mental retardation, neurological manifestations, including spasticity and tremors, light pigmentation, eczema, and mousy odor.

270.2 Other disturbances of aromatic amino-acid metabolism
Albinism
Alkaptonuria
Alkaptonuric ochronosis
Disturbances of metabolism of tyrosine and tryptophan
Homogentisic acid defects
Hydroxykynureninuria
Hypertyrosinemia
Indicanuria
Kynureninase defects
Oasthouse urine disease
Ochronosis
Tyrosinosis
Tyrosinuria
Waardenburg syndrome

EXCLUDES: vitamin B_6-deficiency syndrome (266.1)

AHA: 3Q, '99, 20

270.3 Disturbances of branched-chain amino-acid metabolism
Disturbances of metabolism of leucine, isoleucine, and valine
Hypervalinemia
Intermittent branched-chain ketonuria
Leucine-induced hypoglycemia
Leucinosis
Maple syrup urine disease

AHA: 3Q, '00, 8

270.4 Disturbances of sulphur-bearing amino-acid metabolism
Cystathioninemia
Cystathioninuria
Disturbances of metabolism of methionine, homocystine, and cystathionine
Homocystinuria
Hypermethioninemia
Methioninemia

AHA: 1Q, '04, 6

270.5 Disturbances of histidine metabolism
Carnosinemia
Histidinemia
Hyperhistidinemia
Imidazole aminoaciduria

ENDOCRINE, NUTRITIONAL AND METABOLIC, IMMUNITY

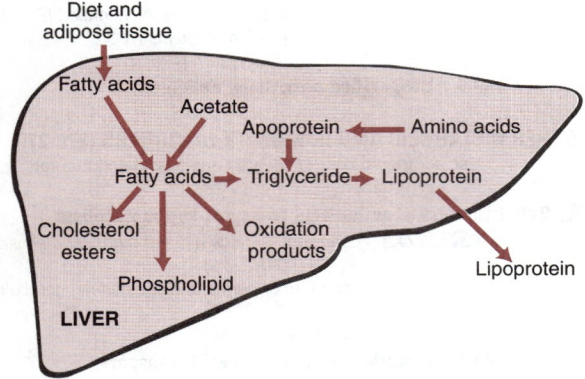

Lipid Metabolism

270.6 Disorders of urea cycle metabolism
Argininosuccinic aciduria
Citrullinemia
Disorders of metabolism of ornithine, citrulline, argininosuccinic acid, arginine, and ammonia
Hyperammonemia
Hyperornithinemia

270.7 Other disturbances of straight-chain amino-acid metabolism
Glucoglycinuria
Glycinemia (with methyl-malonic acidemia)
Hyperglycinemia
Hyperlysinemia
Other disturbances of metabolism of glycine, threonine, serine, glutamine, and lysine
Pipecolic acidemia
Saccharopinuria
AHA: 3Q, '00, 8

270.8 Other specified disorders of amino-acid metabolism
Alaninemia   Iminoacidopathy
Ethanolaminuria   Prolinemia
Glycoprolinuria   Prolinuria
Hydroxyprolinemia   Sarcosinemia
Hyperprolinemia

270.9 Unspecified disorder of amino-acid metabolism

✓4th **271 Disorders of carbohydrate transport and metabolism**
EXCLUDES   abnormality of secretion of glucagon (251.4)
           diabetes mellitus (250.0-250.9)
           hypoglycemia NOS (251.2)
           mucopolysaccharidosis (277.5)

271.0 Glycogenosis
Amylopectinosis
Glucose-6-phosphatase deficiency
Glycogen storage disease
McArdle's disease
Pompe's disease
von Gierke's disease
AHA: 1Q, '98, 5

DEF: Excess glycogen storage; rare inherited trait affects liver, kidneys; causes various symptoms depending on type, though often weakness, and muscle cramps.

271.1 Galactosemia
Galactose-1-phosphate uridyl transferase deficiency
Galactosuria

DEF: Any of three genetic disorders due to defective galactose metabolism; symptoms include failure to thrive in infancy, jaundice, liver and spleen damage, cataracts, and mental retardation.

271.2 Hereditary fructose intolerance
Essential benign fructosuria   Fructosemia

DEF: Chromosome recessive disorder of carbohydrate metabolism; in infants, occurs after dietary sugar introduced; characterized by enlarged spleen, yellowish cast to skin, and progressive inability to thrive.

271.3 Intestinal disaccharidase deficiencies and disaccharide malabsorption
Intolerance or malabsorption (congenital) (of):
  glucose-galactose
  lactose
  sucrose-isomaltose

271.4 Renal glycosuria
Renal diabetes

DEF: Persistent abnormal levels of glucose in urine, with normal blood glucose levels; caused by failure of the renal tubules to reabsorb glucose.

271.8 Other specified disorders of carbohydrate transport and metabolism
Essential benign pentosuria   Mannosidosis
Fucosidosis   Oxalosis
Glycolic aciduria   Xylosuria
Hyperoxaluria (primary)   Xylulosuria

271.9 Unspecified disorder of carbohydrate transport and metabolism

✓4th **272 Disorders of lipoid metabolism**
EXCLUDES   localized cerebral lipidoses (330.1)

272.0 Pure hypercholesterolemia
Familial hypercholesterolemia
Fredrickson Type IIa hyperlipoproteinemia
Hyperbetalipoproteinemia
Hyperlipidemia, Group A
Low-density-lipoid-type [LDL] hyperlipoproteinemia
AHA: 4Q, '05, 71

272.1 Pure hyperglyceridemia
Endogenous hyperglyceridemia
Fredrickson Type IV hyperlipoproteinemia
Hyperlipidemia, Group B
Hyperprebetalipoproteinemia
Hypertriglyceridemia, essential
Very-low-density-lipoid-type [VLDL] hyperlipoproteinemia

272.2 Mixed hyperlipidemia
Broad- or floating-betalipoproteinemia
Fredrickson Type IIb or III hyperlipoproteinemia
Hypercholesterolemia with endogenous hyperglyceridemia
Hyperbetalipoproteinemia with prebetalipoproteinemia
Tubo-eruptive xanthoma
Xanthoma tuberosum

DEF: Elevated levels of lipoprotein, a complex of fats and proteins, in blood due to inherited metabolic disorder.

272.3 Hyperchylomicronemia
Bürger-Grütz syndrome
Fredrickson type I or V hyperlipoproteinemia
Hyperlipidemia, Group D
Mixed hyperglyceridemia

272.4 Other and unspecified hyperlipidemia
Alpha-lipoproteinemia
Combined hyperlipidemia
Hyperlipidemia NOS
Hyperlipoproteinemia NOS
AHA: 1Q, '05, 17

DEF: Hyperlipoproteinemia: elevated levels of transient chylomicrons in the blood which are a form of lipoproteins which transport dietary cholesterol and triglycerides from the small intestine to the blood.

ENDOCRINE, NUTRITIONAL AND METABOLIC, IMMUNITY

272.5 Lipoprotein deficiencies
Abetalipoproteinemia
Bassen-Kornzweig syndrome
High-density lipoid deficiency (familial)
Hypoalphalipoproteinemia
Hypobetalipoproteinemia
DEF: Abnormally low levels of lipoprotein, a complex of fats and protein, in the blood.

272.6 Lipodystrophy
Barraquer-Simons disease
Progressive lipodystrophy
Use additional E code to identify cause, if iatrogenic
EXCLUDES intestinal lipodystrophy (040.2)
DEF: Disturbance of fat metabolism resulting in loss of fatty tissue in some areas of the body.

272.7 Lipidoses
Chemically-induced lipidosis
Disease:
  Anderson's
  Fabry's
  Gaucher's
  I cell [mucolipidosis I]
  lipoid storage NOS
  Niemann-Pick
  pseudo-Hurler's or mucolipidosis III
  triglyceride storage, Type I or II
  Wolman's or triglyceride storage, Type III
Mucolipidosis II
Primary familial xanthomatosis
EXCLUDES cerebral lipidoses (330.1)
Tay-Sachs disease (330.1)
DEF: Lysosomal storage diseases marked by an abnormal amount of lipids in reticuloendothelial cells.

272.8 Other disorders of lipoid metabolism
Hoffa's disease or liposynovitis prepatellaris
Launois-Bensaude's lipomatosis
Lipoid dermatoarthritis

272.9 Unspecified disorder of lipoid metabolism

273 Disorders of plasma protein metabolism
EXCLUDES agammaglobulinemia and hypogammaglobulinemia (279.0-279.2)
coagulation defects (286.0-286.9)
hereditary hemolytic anemias (282.0-282.9)

273.0 Polyclonal hypergammaglobulinemia
Hypergammaglobulinemic purpura:
  benign primary
  Waldenström's
DEF: Elevated blood levels of gamma globulins, frequently found in patients with chronic infectious diseases.

273.1 Monoclonal paraproteinemia
Benign monoclonal hypergammaglobulinemia [BMH]
Monoclonal gammopathy:
  NOS
  associated with lymphoplasmacytic dyscrasias
  benign
Paraproteinemia:
  benign (familial)
  secondary to malignant or inflammatory disease
DEF: Elevated blood levels of macroglobulins (plasma globulins of high weight); characterized by malignant neoplasms of bone marrow, spleen, liver, or lymph nodes; symptoms include weakness, fatigue, bleeding disorders, and vision problems.

273.2 Other paraproteinemias
Cryoglobulinemic: Mixed cryoglobulinemia
  purpura
  vasculitis

273.3 Macroglobulinemia
Macroglobulinemia (idiopathic) (primary)
Waldenström's macroglobulinemia

273.4 Alpha-1-antitrypsin deficiency
AAT deficiency
DEF: Disorder of plasma protein metabolism that results in a deficiency of Alpha-1-antitrypsin, an acute-phase reactive protein, released into the blood in response to infection or injury to protect tissue against the harmful effect of enzymes.

273.8 Other disorders of plasma protein metabolism
Abnormality of transport protein
Bisalbuminemia
AHA: 2Q, '98, 11

273.9 Unspecified disorder of plasma protein metabolism

274 Gout
EXCLUDES lead gout (984.0-984.9)
AHA: 2Q, '95, 4
DEF: Purine and pyrimidine metabolic disorders; manifested by hyperuricemia and recurrent acute inflammatory arthritis; monosodium urate or monohydrate crystals may be deposited in and around the joints, leading to joint destruction, and severe crippling.

274.0 Gouty arthropathy

274.1 Gouty nephropathy
  274.10 Gouty nephropathy, unspecified
    AHA: N-D, '85, 15
  274.11 Uric acid nephrolithiasis
    DEF: Sodium urate stones in the kidney.
  274.19 Other

274.8 Gout with other specified manifestations
  274.81 Gouty tophi of ear
    DEF: Chalky sodium urate deposit in the ear due to gout; produces chronic inflammation of external ear.
  274.82 Gouty tophi of other sites
    Gouty tophi of heart
  274.89 Other
    Use additional code to identify manifestations, as:
    gouty:
      iritis (364.11)
      neuritis (357.4)

274.9 Gout, unspecified

275 Disorders of mineral metabolism
EXCLUDES abnormal findings without manifest disease (790.0-796.9)

275.0 Disorders of iron metabolism
Bronzed diabetes
Hemochromatosis
Pigmentary cirrhosis (of liver)
EXCLUDES anemia:
  iron deficiency (280.0-280.9)
  sideroblastic (285.0)
AHA: 2Q, '97, 11

275.1 Disorders of copper metabolism
Hepatolenticular degeneration
Wilson's disease

275.2 Disorders of magnesium metabolism
Hypermagnesemia   Hypomagnesemia

275.3 Disorders of phosphorus metabolism
Familial hypophosphatemia
Hypophosphatasia
Vitamin D-resistant:
  osteomalacia
  rickets

275.4 Disorders of calcium metabolism
EXCLUDES parathyroid disorders (252.00-252.9)
vitamin D deficiency (268.0-268.9)
AHA: 4Q, '97, 33

  275.40 Unspecified disorder of calcium metabolism

ENDOCRINE, NUTRITIONAL AND METABOLIC, IMMUNITY

275.41 Hypocalcemia
DEF: Abnormally decreased blood calcium level; symptoms include hyperactive deep tendon reflexes, muscle, abdominal cramps, and carpopedal spasm.

275.42 Hypercalcemia
AHA: 4Q, '03, 110
DEF: Abnormally increased blood calcium level; symptoms include muscle weakness, fatigue, nausea, depression, and constipation.

275.49 Other disorders of calcium metabolism
Nephrocalcinosis
Pseudohypoparathyroidism
Pseudopseudohypoparathryoidism

DEF: Nephrocalcinosis: calcium phosphate deposits in the tubules of the kidney with resultant renal insufficiency.
DEF: Pseudohypoparathyroidism: inherited disorder with signs and symptoms of hypoparathyroidism; caused by inadequate response to parathyroid hormone, not hormonal deficiency. Symptoms include muscle cramps, tetany, urinary frequency, blurred vision due to cataracts, and dry scaly skin.
DEF: Pseudopseudohypoparathyroidism: clinical manifestations of hypoparathyroidism without affecting blood calcium levels.

275.8 Other specified disorders of mineral metabolism

275.9 Unspecified disorder of mineral metabolism

✓4th 276 Disorders of fluid, electrolyte, and acid-base balance
EXCLUDES: diabetes insipidus (253.5)
familial periodic paralysis (359.3)

276.0 Hyperosmolality and/or hypernatremia
Sodium [Na] excess   Sodium [Na] overload

276.1 Hyposmolality and/or hyponatremia
Sodium [Na] deficiency

276.2 Acidosis
Acidosis: Acidosis:
   NOS   metabolic
   lactic   respiratory
EXCLUDES: diabetic acidosis (250.1)
AHA: J-F, '87, 15
DEF: Disorder involves decrease of pH (hydrogen ion) concentration in blood and cellular tissues; caused by increase in acid and decrease in bicarbonate.

276.3 Alkalosis
Alkalosis: Alkalosis:
   NOS   respiratory
   metabolic
DEF: Accumulation of base (non-acid part of salt), or loss of acid without relative loss of base in body fluids; caused by increased arterial plasma bicarbonate concentration or loss of carbon dioxide due to hyperventilation.

276.4 Mixed acid-base balance disorder
Hypercapnia with mixed acid-base disorder

✓5th 276.5 Volume depletion
EXCLUDES: hypovolemic shock:
   postoperative (998.0)
   traumatic (958.4)
AHA: ►4Q, '05, 54; 2Q, '05, 9;◄ 1Q, '03, 5, 22; 3Q, '02, 21; 4Q, '97, 30; 2Q, '88, 9

276.50 Volume depletion, unspecified
DEF: ►Depletion of total body water (dehydration) and/or contraction of total intravascular plasma (hypovolemia).◄

276.51 Dehydration
DEF: ►Depletion of total body water; blood volume may be normal while fluid is pulled from other tissues.◄

276.52 Hypovolemia
Depletion of volume of plasma
DEF: ►Depletion of volume plasma; depletion of total blood volume.◄

276.6 Fluid overload
Fluid retention
EXCLUDES: ascites (789.5)
   localized edema (782.3)

276.7 Hyperpotassemia
Hyperkalemia   Potassium [K]:
Potassium [K]:   intoxication
   excess   overload
AHA: 1Q, '05, 9; 2Q,'01, 12
DEF: Elevated blood levels of potassium; symptoms include abnormal EKG readings, weakness; related to defective renal excretion.

276.8 Hypopotassemia
Hypokalemia   Potassium [K] deficiency
DEF: Decreased blood levels of potassium; symptoms include neuromuscular disorders.

276.9 Electrolyte and fluid disorders not elsewhere classified
Electrolyte imbalance   Hypochloremia
Hyperchloremia
EXCLUDES: electrolyte imbalance:
   associated with hyperemesis gravidarum (643.1)
   complicating labor and delivery (669.0)
   following abortion and ectopic or molar pregnancy (634-638 with .4, 639.4)
AHA: J-F, '87, 15

✓4th 277 Other and unspecified disorders of metabolism

✓5th 277.0 Cystic fibrosis
Fibrocystic disease of the pancreas
Mucoviscidosis
DEF: Generalized, genetic disorder of infants, children, and young adults marked by exocrine gland dysfunction; characterized by chronic pulmonary disease with excess mucus production, pancreatic deficiency, high levels of electrolytes in the sweat.
AHA: 4Q, '90, 16; 3Q, '90, 18

277.00 Without mention of meconium ileus
Cystic fibrosis NOS
AHA: 2Q, '03, 12

277.01 With meconium ileus N
Meconium:
   ileus (of newborn)
   obstruction of intestine in mucoviscidosis

277.02 With pulmonary manifestations
Cystic fibrosis with pulmonary exacerbation
Use additional code to identify any infectious organism present, such as: pseudomonas (041.7)
AHA: 4Q, '02, 45, 46

277.03 With gastrointestinal manifestations
EXCLUDES: with meconium ileus (277.01)
AHA: 4Q, '02, 45

277.09 With other manifestations

277.1 Disorders of porphyrin metabolism
Hematoporphyria   Porphyrinuria
Hematoporphyrinuria   Protocoproporphyria
Hereditary coproporphyria   Protoporphyria
Porphyria   Pyrroloporphyria

Tabular List — **ENDOCRINE, NUTRITIONAL AND METABOLIC, IMMUNITY** — 277.2–278.00

277.2 Other disorders of purine and pyrimidine metabolism
Hypoxanthine-guanine-phosphoribosyltransferase deficiency [HG-PRT deficiency]
Lesch-Nyhan syndrome
Xanthinuria
EXCLUDES: gout (274.0-274.9)
orotic aciduric anemia (281.4)

√5th **277.3 Amyloidosis**
AHA: 1Q, '96, 16
DEF: Conditions of diverse etiologies characterized by the accumulation of insoluble fibrillar proteins (amyloid) in various organs and tissues of the body, compromising vital functions.

● **277.30 Amyloidosis, unspecified**
Amyloidosis NOS

● **277.31 Familial Mediterranean fever**
Benign paroxysmal peritonitis
Hereditary amyloid nephropathy
Periodic familial polyserositis
Recurrent polyserositis

● **277.39 Other amyloidosis**
Hereditary cardiac amyloidosis
Inherited systemic amyloidosis
Neuropathic (Portuguese) (Swiss) amyloidosis
Secondary amyloidosis

277.4 Disorders of bilirubin excretion
Hyperbilirubinemia:
  congenital
  constitutional
Syndrome:
  Crigler-Najjar
Syndrome:
  Dubin-Johnson
  Gilbert's
  Rotor's
EXCLUDES: hyperbilirubinemias specific to the perinatal period (774.0-774.7)

277.5 Mucopolysaccharidosis
Gargoylism
Hunter's syndrome
Hurler's syndrome
Lipochondrodystrophy
Maroteaux-Lamy syndrome
Morquio-Brailsford disease
Osteochondrodystrophy
Sanfilippo's syndrome
Scheie's syndrome

DEF: Metabolism disorders evidenced by excretion of various mucopolysaccharides in urine and infiltration of these substances into connective tissue, with resulting various defects of bone, cartilage and connective tissue.

277.6 Other deficiencies of circulating enzymes
Hereditary angioedema

277.7 Dysmetabolic syndrome X
Use additional code for associated manifestation, such as:
  cardiovascular disease (414.00-414.07)
  obesity (278.00-278.01)
AHA: 4Q, '01, 42

DEF: A specific group of metabolic disorders that are related to the state of insulin resistance (decreased cellular response to insulin) without elevated blood sugars; often related to elevated cholesterol and triglycerides, obesity, cardiovascular disease, and high blood pressure.

√5th **277.8 Other specified disorders of metabolism**
AHA: 4Q, '03, 50; 2Q, '01, 18; S-O, '87, 9

277.81 Primary carnitine deficiency

277.82 Carnitine deficiency due to inborn errors of metabolism

277.83 Iatrogenic carnitine deficiency
Carnitine deficiency due to:
  hemodialysis
  valproic acid therapy

277.84 Other secondary carnitine deficiency

277.85 Disorders of fatty acid oxidation
Carnitine palmitoyltransferase deficiencies (CPT1, CPT2)
Glutaric aciduria type II (type IIA, IIB, IIC)
Long chain 3-hydroxyacyl CoA dehydrogenase deficiency (LCHAD)
Long chain/very long chain acyl CoA dehydrogenase deficiency (LCAD, VLCAD)
Medium chain acyl CoA dehydrogenase deficiency (MCAD)
Short chain acyl CoA dehydrogenase deficiency (SCAD)
EXCLUDES: primary carnitine deficiency (277.81)

277.86 Peroxisomal disorders
Adrenomyeloneuropathy
Neonatal adrenoleukodystrophy
Rhizomelic chrondrodysplasia punctata
X-linked adrenoleukodystrophy
Zellweger syndrome
EXCLUDES: infantile Refsum disease (356.3)

277.87 Disorders of mitochondrial metabolism
Kearns-Sayre syndrome
Mitochondrial Encephalopathy, Lactic Acidosis and Stroke-like episodes (MELAS syndrome)
Mitochondrial Neurogastrointestinal Encephalopathy syndrome (MNGIE)
Myoclonus with Epilepsy and with Ragged Red Fibers (MERRF syndrome)
Neuropathy, Ataxia and Retinitis Pigmentosa (NARP syndrome)
Use additional code for associated conditions
EXCLUDES: disorders of pyruvate metabolism (271.8)
Leber's optic atrophy (377.16)
Leigh's subacute necrotizing encephalopathy (330.8)
Reye's syndrome (331.81)
AHA: 4Q, '04, 62

277.89 Other specified disorders of metabolism
Hand-Schüller-Christian disease
Histiocytosis (acute) (chronic)
Histiocytosis X (chronic)
EXCLUDES: histiocytosis:
  acute differentiated progressive (202.5)
  X, acute (progressive) (202.5)

277.9 Unspecified disorder of metabolism
Enzymopathy NOS

√4th **278 Overweight, obesity and other hyperalimentation**
EXCLUDES: hyperalimentation NOS (783.6)
poisoning by vitamins NOS (963.5)
polyphagia (783.6)

√5th **278.0 Overweight and obesity**
Use additional code to identify Body Mass Index (BMI), if known ►(V85.0-V85.54)◄
EXCLUDES: adiposogenital dystrophy (253.8)
obesity of endocrine origin NOS (259.9)
AHA: 4Q, '05, 97

278.00 Obesity, unspecified
Obesity NOS
AHA: 4Q, '01, 42; 1Q, '99, 5, 6

Additional Digit Required — Unspecified Code — Other Specified Code — Manifestation Code — ►◄ Revised Text — ● New Code — ▲ Revised Code Title

2007 ICD•9•CM — October 2006 • Volume 1 — 55

278.01 Morbid obesity
  Severe obesity
  AHA: 3Q, '03, 6-8
  DEF: Increased weight beyond limits of skeletal and physical requirements (125 percent or more over ideal body weight), as a result of excess fat in subcutaneous connective tissues.
  DEF: ▶BMI (body mass index) between 30.0 and 39.9.◀

278.02 Overweight
  AHA: ▶4Q, '05, 55◀
  DEF: ▶BMI (body mass index) between 25 and 29.9.◀

278.1 Localized adiposity
  Fat pad

278.2 Hypervitaminosis A

278.3 Hypercarotinemia
  DEF: Elevated blood carotene level due to ingesting excess carotenoids or the inability to convert carotenoids to vitamin A.

278.4 Hypervitaminosis D
  DEF: Weakness, fatigue, loss of weight, and other symptoms resulting from ingesting excessive amounts of vitamin D.

278.8 Other hyperalimentation

✓4th **279 Disorders involving the immune mechanism**

✓5th **279.0 Deficiency of humoral immunity**
  DEF: Inadequate immune response to bacterial infections with potential reinfection by viruses due to lack of circulating immunoglobulins (acquired antibodies).

  279.00 Hypogammaglobulinemia, unspecified
    Agammaglobulinemia NOS
  279.01 Selective IgA immunodeficiency
  279.02 Selective IgM immunodeficiency
  279.03 Other selective immunoglobulin deficiencies
    Selective deficiency of IgG
  279.04 Congenital hypogammaglobulinemia
    Agammaglobulinemia:
      Bruton's type
      X-linked
  279.05 Immunodeficiency with increased IgM
    Immunodeficiency with hyper-IgM:
      autosomal recessive
      X-linked
  279.06 Common variable immunodeficiency
    Dysgammaglobulinemia (acquired) (congenital) (primary)
    Hypogammaglobulinemia:
      acquired primary
      congenital non-sex-linked
      sporadic
  279.09 Other
    Transient hypogammaglobulinemia of infancy

✓5th **279.1 Deficiency of cell-mediated immunity**

  279.10 Immunodeficiency with predominant T-cell defect, unspecified
    AHA: S-0, '87, 10

279.11 DiGeorge's syndrome
  Pharyngeal pouch syndrome
  Thymic hypoplasia
  DEF: Congenital disorder due to defective development of the third and fourth pharyngeal pouches; results in hypoplasia or aplasia of the thymus, parathyroid glands; related to congenital heart defects, anomalies of the great vessels, esophageal atresia, and abnormalities of facial structures.

279.12 Wiskott-Aldrich syndrome
  DEF: A disease characterized by chronic conditions, such as eczema, suppurative otitis media and anemia; it results from an X-linked recessive gene and is classified as an immune deficiency syndrome.

279.13 Nezelof's syndrome
  Cellular immunodeficiency with abnormal immunoglobulin deficiency
  DEF: Immune system disorder characterized by a pathological deficiency in cellular immunity and humoral antibodies resulting in inability to fight infectious diseases.

279.19 Other
  EXCLUDES ataxia-telangiectasia (334.8)

279.2 Combined immunity deficiency
  Agammaglobulinemia:
    autosomal recessive
    Swiss-type
    x-linked recessive
  Severe combined immunodeficiency [SCID]
  Thymic:
    alymophoplasia
    aplasia or dysplasia with immunodeficiency
  EXCLUDES thymic hypoplasia (279.11)
  DEF: Agammaglobulinemia: no immunoglobulins in the blood.
  DEF: Thymic alymphoplasia: severe combined immunodeficiency; result of failed lymphoid tissue development.

279.3 Unspecified immunity deficiency

279.4 Autoimmune disease, not elsewhere classified
  Autoimmune disease NOS
  EXCLUDES transplant failure or rejection (996.80-996.89)

279.8 Other specified disorders involving the immune mechanism
  Single complement [C1-C9] deficiency or dysfunction

279.9 Unspecified disorder of immune mechanism
  AHA: 3Q, '92, 13

| Tabular List | BLOOD AND BLOOD-FORMING ORGANS | 280–282.4 |

4. DISEASES OF THE BLOOD AND BLOOD-FORMING ORGANS (280–289)

EXCLUDES anemia complicating pregnancy or the puerperium (648.2)

✓4th 280 Iron deficiency anemias

INCLUDES anemia:
  asiderotic
  hypochromic-microcytic
  sideropenic

EXCLUDES familial microcytic anemia (282.49)

280.0 Secondary to blood loss (chronic)
  Normocytic anemia due to blood loss
  EXCLUDES acute posthemorrhagic anemia (285.1)
  AHA: 4Q, '93, 34

280.1 Secondary to inadequate dietary iron intake

280.8 Other specified iron deficiency anemias
  Paterson-Kelly syndrome
  Plummer-Vinson syndrome
  Sideropenic dysphagia

280.9 Iron deficiency anemia, unspecified
  Anemia:
    achlorhydric
    chlorotic
    idiopathic hypochromic
    iron [Fe] deficiency NOS

✓4th 281 Other deficiency anemias

281.0 Pernicious anemia
  Anemia:
    Addison's
    Biermer's
    congenital pernicious
  Congenital intrinsic factor [Castle's] deficiency
  EXCLUDES combined system disease without mention of anemia (266.2)
  subacute degeneration of spinal cord without mention of anemia (266.2)
  AHA: N-D, '84, 1; S-O, '84, 16
  DEF: Chronic progressive anemia due to Vitamin B$_{12}$ malabsorption; caused by lack of a secretion known as intrinsic factor, which is produced by the gastric mucosa of the stomach.

281.1 Other vitamin B$_{12}$ deficiency anemia
  Anemia:
    vegan's
    vitamin B$_{12}$ deficiency (dietary)
    due to selective vitamin B$_{12}$ malabsorption with proteinuria
  Syndrome:
    Imerslund's
    Imerslund-Gräsbeck
  EXCLUDES combined system disease without mention of anemia (266.2)
  subacute degeneration of spinal cord without mention of anemia (266.2)

281.2 Folate-deficiency anemia
  Congenital folate malabsorption
  Folate or folic acid deficiency anemia:
    NOS
    dietary
    drug-induced
  Goat's milk anemia
  Nutritional megaloblastic anemia (of infancy)
  Use additional E code to identify drug
  DEF: Macrocytic anemia resembles pernicious anemia but without absence of hydrochloric acid secretions; responsive to folic acid therapy.

281.3 Other specified megaloblastic anemias not elsewhere classified
  Combined B$_{12}$ and folate-deficiency anemia
  Refractory megaloblastic anemia
  DEF: Megaloblasts predominant in bone marrow with few normoblasts; rare familial type associated with proteinuria and genitourinary tract anomalies.

281.4 Protein-deficiency anemia
  Amino-acid-deficiency anemia

281.8 Anemia associated with other specified nutritional deficiency
  Scorbutic anemia

281.9 Unspecified deficiency anemia
  Anemia:
    dimorphic
    macrocytic
    megaloblastic NOS
    nutritional NOS
    simple chronic

✓4th 282 Hereditary hemolytic anemias

DEF: Escalated rate of erythrocyte destruction; similar to all anemias, occurs when imbalance exists between blood loss and blood production.

282.0 Hereditary spherocytosis
  Acholuric (familial) jaundice
  Congenital hemolytic anemia (spherocytic)
  Congenital spherocytosis
  Minkowski-Chauffard syndrome
  Spherocytosis (familial)
  EXCLUDES hemolytic anemia of newborn (773.0-773.5)
  DEF: Hereditary, chronic illness marked by abnormal red blood cell membrane; symptoms include enlarged spleen, jaundice; and anemia in severe cases.

282.1 Hereditary elliptocytosis
  Elliptocytosis (congenital)
  Ovalocytosis (congenital) (hereditary)
  DEF: Genetic hemolytic anemia characterized by malformed, elliptical erythrocytes; there is increased destruction of red cells with resulting anemia.

282.2 Anemias due to disorders of glutathione metabolism
  Anemia:
    6-phosphogluconic dehydrogenase deficiency
    enzyme deficiency, drug-induced
    erythrocytic glutathione deficiency
    glucose-6-phosphate dehydrogenase [G-6-PD] deficiency
    glutathione-reductase deficiency
    hemolytic nonspherocytic (hereditary), type I
  Disorder of pentose phosphate pathway
  Favism

282.3 Other hemolytic anemias due to enzyme deficiency
  Anemia:
    hemolytic nonspherocytic (hereditary), type II
    hexokinase deficiency
    pyruvate kinase [PK] deficiency
    triosephosphate isomerase deficiency

✓5th 282.4 Thalassemias
  EXCLUDES sickle-cell:
    disease (282.60-282.69)
    trait (282.5)
  AHA: 4Q, '03, 51
  DEF: A group of inherited hemolytic disorders characterized by decreased production of at least one of the four polypeptide globin chains which results in defective hemoglobin synthesis; symptoms include severe anemia, expanded marrow spaces, transfusional and absorptive iron overload, impaired growth rate, thickened cranial bones, and pathologic fractures.

282.41 **Sickle-cell thalassemia without crisis**
Sickle-cell thalassemia NOS
Thalassemia Hb-S disease without crisis

282.42 **Sickle-cell thalassemia with crisis**
Sickle-cell thalassemia with vaso-occlusive pain
Thalassemia Hb-S disease with crisis
Use additional code for type of crisis, such as:
acute chest syndrome (517.3)
splenic sequestration (289.52)

282.49 **Other thalassemia**
Cooley's anemia
Hb-Bart's disease
Hereditary leptocytosis
Mediterranean anemia (with other hemoglobinopathy)
Microdrepanocytosis
Thalassemia (alpha) (beta) (intermedia) (major) (minima) (minor) (mixed) (trait) (with other hemoglobinopathy)
Thalassemia NOS

282.5 **Sickle-cell trait**
Hb-AS genotype
Hemoglobin S [Hb-S] trait
Heterozygous:
hemoglobin S
Hb-S
> EXCLUDES that with other hemoglobinopathy (282.60-282.69)
> that with thalassemia (282.49)

DEF: Heterozygous genetic makeup characterized by one gene for normal hemoglobin and one for sickle-cell hemoglobin; clinical disease rarely present.

√5th **282.6** **Sickle-cell disease**
Sickle-cell anemia
> EXCLUDES sickle-cell thalassemia (282.41-282.42)
> sickle-cell trait (282.5)

DEF: Inherited blood disorder; sickle-shaped red blood cells are hard and pointed, clogging blood flow; anemia characterized by, periodic episodes of pain, acute abdominal discomfort, skin ulcerations of the legs, increased infections; occurs primarily in persons of African descent.

282.60 **Sickle-cell disease, unspecified**
Sickle-cell anemia NOS
AHA: 2Q, '97, 11

282.61 **Hb-SS disease without crisis**

282.62 **Hb-SS disease with crisis**
Hb-SS disease with vaso-occlusive pain
Sickle-cell crisis NOS
Use additional code for type of crisis, such as:
acute chest syndrome (517.3)
splenic sequestration (289.52)
AHA: 4Q, '03, 56; 2Q, '98, 8; 2Q, '91, 15

282.63 **Sickle-cell/Hb-C disease without crisis**
Hb-S/Hb-C disease without crisis

282.64 **Sickle-cell/Hb-C disease with crisis**
Hb-S/Hb-C disease with crisis
Sickle-cell/Hb-C disease with vaso-occlusive pain
Use additional code for type of crisis, such as:
acute chest syndrome (517.3)
splenic sequestration (289.52)
AHA: 4Q, '03, 51

282.68 **Other sickle-cell disease without crisis**
Hb-S/Hb-D
Hb-S/Hb-E
Sickle-cell/Hb-D
Sickle-cell/Hb-E
} disease without crisis
AHA: 4Q, '03, 51

282.69 **Other sickle-cell disease with crisis**
Hb-S/Hb-D
Hb-S/Hb-E
Sickle-cell/Hb-D
Sickle-cell/Hb-E
} disease with crisis
Other sickle-cell disease with vaso-occlusive pain
Use additional code for type of crisis, such as:
acute chest syndrome (517.3)
splenic sequestration (289.52)

282.7 **Other hemoglobinopathies**
Abnormal hemoglobin NOS
Congenital Heinz-body anemia
Disease:
hemoglobin C [Hb-C]
hemoglobin D [Hb-D]
hemoglobin E [Hb-E]
hemoglobin Zurich [Hb-Zurich]
Hemoglobinopathy NOS
Hereditary persistence of fetal hemoglobin [HPFH]
Unstable hemoglobin hemolytic disease
> EXCLUDES familial polycythemia (289.6)
> hemoglobin M [Hb-M] disease (289.7)
> high-oxygen-affinity hemoglobin (289.0)

DEF: Any disorder of hemoglobin due to alteration of molecular structure; may include overt anemia.

282.8 **Other specified hereditary hemolytic anemias**
Stomatocytosis

282.9 **Hereditary hemolytic anemia, unspecified**
Hereditary hemolytic anemia NOS

√4th **283** **Acquired hemolytic anemias**
AHA: N-D, '84, 1

DEF: Non-hereditary anemia characterized by premature destruction of red blood cells; caused by infectious organisms, poisons, and physical agents.

283.0 **Autoimmune hemolytic anemias**
Autoimmune hemolytic disease (cold type) (warm type)
Chronic cold hemagglutinin disease
Cold agglutinin disease or hemoglobinuria
Hemolytic anemia:
cold type (secondary) (symptomatic)
drug-induced
warm type (secondary) (symptomatic)
Use additional E code to identify cause, if drug-induced
> EXCLUDES Evans' syndrome (287.32)
> hemolytic disease of newborn (773.0-773.5)

√5th **283.1** **Non-autoimmune hemolytic anemias**
Use additional E code to identify cause
AHA: 4Q, '93, 25

DEF: Hemolytic anemia and thrombocytopenia with acute renal failure; relatively rare condition; 50 percent of patients require renal dialysis.

283.10 **Non-autoimmune hemolytic anemia, unspecified**

283.11 **Hemolytic-uremic syndrome**

283.19 **Other non-autoimmune hemolytic anemias**
Hemolytic anemia:
mechanical
microangiopathic
toxic

BLOOD AND BLOOD-FORMING ORGANS

283.2 Hemoglobinuria due to hemolysis from external causes
Acute intravascular hemolysis
Hemoglobinuria:
from exertion
march
paroxysmal (cold) (nocturnal)
due to other hemolysis
Marchiafava-Micheli syndrome
Use additional E code to identify cause

283.9 Acquired hemolytic anemia, unspecified
Acquired hemolytic anemia NOS
Chronic idiopathic hemolytic anemia

284 Aplastic anemia and other bone marrow failure syndromes
AHA: 1Q, '91, 14; N-D, '84, 1; S-O, '84, 16

DEF: Bone marrow failure to produce the normal amount of blood components; generally non-responsive to usual therapy.

284.0 Constitutional aplastic anemia
AHA: 1Q, '91, 14

284.01 Constitutional red blood cell aplasia
Aplasia, (pure) red cell:
congenital
of infants
primary
Blackfan-Diamond syndrome
Familial hypoplastic anemia

284.09 Other constitutional aplastic anemia
Fanconi's anemia
Pancytopenia with malformations

284.1 Pancytopenia
EXCLUDES pancytopenia (due to) (with):
aplastic anemia NOS (284.9)
bone marrow infiltration (284.2)
constitutional red blood cell aplasia (284.01)
drug induced (284.8)
hairy cell leukemia (202.4)
human immunodeficiency virus disease (042)
leukoerythroblastic anemia (284.2)
malformations (284.09)
myelodysplastic syndromes (238.72-238.75)
myeloproliferative disease (238.79)
other constitutional aplastic anemia (284.09)

284.2 Myelophthisis
Leukoerythroblastic anemia
Myelophthisic anemia
Code first the underlying disorder, such as:
malignant neoplasm of breast (174.0-174.9, 175.0-175.9)
tuberculosis (015.0-015.9)
EXCLUDES idiopathic myelofibrosis (238.76)
myelofibrosis NOS (289.83)
myelofibrosis with myeloid metaplasia (238.76)
primary myelofibrosis (238.76)
secondary myelofibrosis (289.83)

284.8 Other specified aplastic anemias
Aplastic anemia (due to):
chronic systemic disease
drugs
infection
radiation
toxic (paralytic)
Red cell aplasia (acquired) (adult) (pure) (with thymoma)
Use additional E code to identify cause
AHA: 3Q, '05, 11; 1Q, '97, 5; 1Q, '92, 15; 1Q, '91, 14

284.9 Aplastic anemia, unspecified
Anemia:
aplastic (idiopathic) NOS
aregenerative
hypoplastic NOS
nonregenerative
Medullary hypoplasia
EXCLUDES refractory anemia ▶(238.72)◀

285 Other and unspecified anemias
AHA: 1Q, '91, 14; N-D, '84, 1

285.0 Sideroblastic anemia
Anemia:
hypochromic with iron loading
sideroachrestic
sideroblastic:
acquired
congenital
hereditary
primary
secondary (drug-induced) (due to disease)
sex-linked hypochromic
vitamin B_6-responsive
Pyridoxine-responsive (hypochromic) anemia
Use additional E code to identify cause, if drug induced
EXCLUDES refractory sideroblastic anemia ▶(238.72)◀

DEF: Characterized by a disruption of final heme synthesis; results in iron overload of reticuloendothelial tissues.

285.1 Acute posthemorrhagic anemia
Anemia due to acute blood loss
EXCLUDES anemia due to chronic blood loss (280.0)
blood loss anemia NOS (280.0)
AHA: 2Q, '92, 15

285.2 Anemia of chronic disease
▶Anemia in chronic illness◀
AHA: 4Q, '00, 39

285.21 Anemia in chronic kidney disease
Anemia in end stage renal disease
Erythropoietin-resistant anemia (EPO resistant anemia)

285.22 Anemia in neoplastic disease

285.29 Anemia of other chronic disease
▶Anemia in other chronic illness◀

285.8 Other specified anemias
Anemia:
dyserythropoietic (congenital)
dyshematopoietic (congenital)
von Jaksch's
Infantile pseudoleukemia
AHA: 1Q, '91, 16

285.9 Anemia, unspecified
Anemia:
NOS
essential
normocytic, not due to blood loss
profound
progressive
secondary
Oligocythemia
EXCLUDES anemia (due to):
blood loss:
acute (285.1)
chronic or unspecified (280.0)
iron deficiency (280.0-280.9)
AHA: 1Q, '02, 14; 2Q, '92, 16; M-A, '85, 13; ND, '84, 1

BLOOD AND BLOOD-FORMING ORGANS

✓4ᵗʰ 286 Coagulation defects

286.0 Congenital factor VIII disorder
Antihemophilic globulin [AHG] deficiency
Factor VIII (functional) deficiency
Hemophilia:
  NOS
  A
  classical
  familial
  hereditary
Subhemophilia
  EXCLUDES factor VIII deficiency with vascular defect (286.4)

DEF: Hereditary, sex-linked, results in missing antihemophilic globulin (AHG) (factor VIII); causes abnormal coagulation characterized by increased tendency to bleeding, large bruises of skin, soft tissue; may also be bleeding in mouth, nose, gastrointestinal tract; after childhood, hemorrhages in joints, resulting in swelling and impaired function.

286.1 Congenital factor IX disorder
Christmas disease
Deficiency:
  factor IX (functional)
  plasma thromboplastin component [PTC]
Hemophilia B

DEF: Deficiency of plasma thromboplastin component (PTC) (factor IX) and plasma thromboplastin antecedent (PTA); PTC deficiency clinically indistinguishable from classical hemophilia; PTA deficiency found in both sexes.

286.2 Congenital factor XI deficiency
Hemophilia C
Plasma thromboplastin antecedent [PTA] deficiency
Rosenthal's disease

286.3 Congenital deficiency of other clotting factors
Congenital afibrinogenemia
Deficiency:
  AC globulin factor:
    I [fibrinogen]
    II [prothrombin]
    V [labile]
    VII [stable]
    X [Stuart-Prower]
    XII [Hageman]
    XIII [fibrin stabilizing]
  Laki-Lorand factor
  proaccelerin
Disease
  Owren's
  Stuart-Prower
Dysfibrinogenemia (congenital)
Dysprothrombinemia (constitutional)
Hypoproconvertinemia
Hypoprothrmbinemia (hereditary)
Parahemophilia

286.4 von Willebrand's disease
Angiohemophilia (A) (B)
Constitutional thrombopathy
Factor VIII deficiency with vascular defect
Pseudohemophilia type B
Vascular hemophilia
von Willebrand's (-Jürgens') disease
  EXCLUDES factor VIII deficiency:
    NOS (286.0)
    with functional defect (286.0)
    hereditary capillary fragility (287.8)

DEF: Abnormal blood coagulation caused by deficient blood Factor VII; congenital; symptoms include excess or prolonged bleeding, such as hemorrhage during menstruation, following birthing, or after surgical procedure.

286.5 Hemorrhagic disorder due to intrinsic circulating anticoagulants
Antithrombinemia
Antithromboplastinemia
Antithromboplastino-genemia
Hyperheparinemia
Increase in:
  anti-VIIIa
  anti-IXa
  anti-Xa
  anti-XIa
  antithrombin
Secondary hemophilia
Systemic lupus erythematosus [SLE] inhibitor

AHA: 3Q, '92, 15; 3Q, '90, 14

286.6 Defibrination syndrome
Afibrinogenemia, acquired
Consumption coagulopathy
Diffuse or disseminated intravascular coagulation [DIC syndrome]
Fibrinolytic hemorrhage, acquired
Hemorrhagic fibrinogenolysis
Pathologic fibrinolysis
Purpura:
  fibrinolytic
  fulminans
  EXCLUDES that complicating:
    abortion (634-638 with .1, 639.1)
    pregnancy or the puerperium (641.3, 666.3)
    disseminated intravascular coagulation in newborn (776.2)

AHA: 4Q, '93, 29

DEF: Characterized by destruction of circulating fibrinogen; often precipitated by other conditions, such as injury, causing release of thromboplastic particles in blood stream.

286.7 Acquired coagulation factor deficiency
Deficiency of coagulation factor due to:
  liver disease
  vitamin K deficiency
Hypoprothrombinemia, acquired
Use additional E code to identify cause, if drug induced
  EXCLUDES vitamin K deficiency of newborn (776.0)

AHA: 4Q, '93, 29

286.9 Other and unspecified coagulation defects
Defective coagulation NOS
Deficiency, coagulation factor NOS
Delay, coagulation
Disorder:
  coagulation
  hemostasis
  EXCLUDES abnormal coagulation profile (790.92)
    hemorrhagic disease of newborn (776.0)
    that complicating:
      abortion (634-638 with .1, 639.1)
      pregnancy or the puerperium (641.3, 666.3)

BLOOD AND BLOOD-FORMING ORGANS

✓4th 287 Purpura and other hemorrhagic conditions
  EXCLUDES: hemorrhagic thrombocythemia ▶(238.79)◀
  purpura fulminans (286.6)
  AHA: 1Q, '91, 14

- **287.0 Allergic purpura**
  Peliosis rheumatica
  Purpura:
    anaphylactoid
    autoimmune
    Henoch's
    nonthrombocytopenic:
      hemorrhagic
      idiopathic
  Purpura:
    rheumatica
    Schönlein-Henoch
    vascular
  Vasculitis, allergic
  EXCLUDES: hemorrhagic purpura (287.39)
  purpura annularis telangiectodes (709.1)
  DEF: Any hemorrhagic condition, thrombocytic or nonthrombocytopenic in origin, caused by a presumed allergic reaction.

- **287.1 Qualitative platelet defects**
  Thrombasthenia (hemorrhagic) (hereditary)
  Thrombocytasthenia
  Thrombocytopathy (dystrophic)
  Thrombopathy (Bernard-Soulier)
  EXCLUDES: von Willebrand's disease (286.4)

- **287.2 Other nonthrombocytopenic purpuras**
  Purpura:
    NOS
    senile
  Purpura:
    simplex

- **✓5th 287.3 Primary thrombocytopenia**
  EXCLUDES: thrombotic thrombocytopenic purpura (446.6)
  transient thrombocytopenia of newborn (776.1)
  AHA: 4Q, '05, 56
  DEF: Decrease in number of blood platelets in circulating blood and purpural skin hemorrhages.

  - **287.30 Primary thrombocytopenia, unspecified**
    Megakaryocytic hypoplasia
  - **287.31 Immune thrombocytopenic purpura**
    Idiopathic thrombocytopenic purpura
    Tidal platelet dysgenesis
    AHA: 4Q, '05, 57
    DEF: Tidal platelet dysgenesis: Platelet counts fluctuate from normal to very low within periods of 20 to 40 days and may involve autoimmune platelet destruction.
  - **287.32 Evans' syndrome**
    DEF: Combination of immunohemolytic anemia and autoimmune hemolytic anemia, sometimes with neutropenia.
  - **287.33 Congenital and hereditary thrombocytopenic purpura**
    Congenital and hereditary thrombocytopenia
    Thrombocytopenia with absent radii (TAR) syndrome
    EXCLUDES: Wiskott-Aldrich syndrome (279.12)
    DEF: Thrombocytopenia with absent radii (TAR) syndrome: autosomal recessive syndrome characterized by thrombocytopenia and bilateral radial aplasia; manifestations include skeletal, gastrointestinal, hematologic, and cardiac system abnormalities.
  - **287.39 Other primary thrombocytopenia**

- **287.4 Secondary thrombocytopenia**
  Posttransfusion purpura
  Thrombocytopenia (due to):
    dilutional
    drugs
    extracorporeal circulation of blood
    platelet alloimmunization
  Use additional E code to identify cause
  EXCLUDES: transient thrombocytopenia of newborn (776.1)
  AHA: 4Q, '99, 22; 4Q, '93, 29
  DEF: Reduced number of platelets in circulating blood as consequence of an underlying disease or condition.

- **287.5 Thrombocytopenia, unspecified**
- **287.8 Other specified hemorrhagic conditions**
  Capillary fragility (hereditary)
  Vascular pseudohemophilia
- **287.9 Unspecified hemorrhagic conditions**
  Hemorrhagic diathesis (familial)

✓4th 288 Diseases of white blood cells
  EXCLUDES: leukemia (204.0-208.9)
  AHA: 1Q, '91, 14

- ▲ **✓5th 288.0 Neutropenia**
  ▶Decreased absolute neutrophil count (ANC)
  Use additional code for any associated fever (780.6)◀
  EXCLUDES: ▶neutropenic splenomegaly (289.53)◀
  transitory neonatal neutropenia (776.7)
  AHA: 3Q, '05, 11; 3Q, '99, 6; 2Q, '99, 9; 3Q, '96, 16; 2Q, '96, 6
  DEF: Sudden, severe condition characterized by reduced number of white blood cells; results in sores in the throat, stomach or skin; symptoms include chills, fever; some drugs can bring on condition.

  - ● **288.00 Neutropenia, unspecified**
  - ● **288.01 Congenital neutropenia**
    Congenital agranulocytosis
    Infantile genetic agranulocytosis
    Kostmann's syndrome
  - ● **288.02 Cyclic neutropenia**
    Cyclic hematopoiesis
    Periodic neutropenia
  - ● **288.03 Drug induced neutropenia**
    Use additional E code to identify drug
  - ● **288.04 Neutropenia due to infection**
  - ● **288.09 Other neutropenia**
    Agranulocytosis
    Neutropenia:
      immune
      toxic

- **288.1 Functional disorders of polymorphonuclear neutrophils**
  Chronic (childhood) granulomatous disease
  Congenital dysphagocytosis
  Job's syndrome
  Lipochrome histiocytosis (familial)
  Progressive septic granulomatosis

- **288.2 Genetic anomalies of leukocytes**
  Anomaly (granulation) (granulocyte) or syndrome:
    Alder's (-Reilly)
    Chédiak-Steinbrinck (-Higashi)
    Jordan's
    May-Hegglin
    Pelger-Huet
  Hereditary:
    hypersegmentation
    hyposegmentation
    leukomelanopathy

BLOOD AND BLOOD-FORMING ORGANS

288.3 Eosinophilia
Eosinophilia:
   allergic
   hereditary
   idiopathic
Eosinophilia:
   secondary
Eosinophilic leukocytosis
> EXCLUDES Löffler's syndrome (518.3)
>   pulmonary eosinophilia (518.3)

AHA: 3Q, '00, 11

DEF: Elevated number of eosinophils in the blood; characteristic of allergic states and various parasitic infections.

● **288.4 Hemophagocytic syndromes**
Familial hemophagocytic lymphohistiocytosis
Familial hemophagocytic reticulosis
Hemophagocytic syndrome, infection-associated
Histiocytic syndromes
Macrophage activation syndrome

● √5ᵗʰ **288.5 Decreased white blood cell count**
> EXCLUDES neutropenia (288.01-288.09)

● **288.50 Leukocytopenia, unspecified**
Decreased leukocytes, unspecified
Decreased white blood cell count, unspecified
Leukopenia NOS

● **288.51 Lymphocytopenia**
Decreased lymphocytes

● **288.59 Other decreased white blood cell count**
Basophilic leukopenia
Eosinophilic leukopenia
Monocytopenia
Plasmacytopenia

● √5ᵗʰ **288.6 Elevated white blood cell count**
> EXCLUDES eosinophilia (288.3)

● **288.60 Leukocytosis, unspecified**
Elevated leukocytes, unspecified
Elevated white blood cell count, unspecified

● **288.61 Lymphocytosis (symptomatic)**
Elevated lymphocytes

● **288.62 Leukemoid reaction**
Basophilic leukemoid reaction
Lymphocytic leukemoid reaction
Monocytic leukemoid reaction
Myelocytic leukemoid reaction
Neutrophilic leukemoid reaction

● **288.63 Monocytosis (symptomatic)**
> EXCLUDES infectious mononucleosis (075)

● **288.64 Plasmacytosis**
● **288.65 Basophilia**
● **288.69 Other elevated white blood cell count**

288.8 Other specified disease of white blood cells
> EXCLUDES ▶ decreased white blood cell counts (288.50-288.59)
>   elevated white blood cell counts (288.60-288.69) ◀
>   immunity disorders (279.0-279.9)

AHA: M-A, '87, 12

288.9 Unspecified disease of white blood cells

√4ᵗʰ **289 Other diseases of blood and blood-forming organs**

289.0 Polycythemia, secondary
High-oxygen-affinity hemoglobin
Polycythemia:
   acquired
   benign
   due to:
      fall in plasma volume
      high altitude
   emotional
   erythropoietin
   hypoxemic
   nephrogenous
   relative
   spurious
   stress
> EXCLUDES polycythemia:
>   neonatal (776.4)
>   primary (238.4)
>   vera (238.4)

DEF: Elevated number of red blood cells in circulating blood as result of reduced oxygen supply to the tissues.

289.1 Chronic lymphadenitis
Chronic:
   adenitis   } any lymph node, except
   lymphadenitis } mesenteric
> EXCLUDES acute lymphadenitis (683)
>   mesenteric (289.2)
>   enlarged glands NOS (785.6)

DEF: Persistent inflammation of lymph node tissue; origin of infection is usually elsewhere.

289.2 Nonspecific mesenteric lymphadenitis
Mesenteric lymphadenitis (acute) (chronic)

DEF: Inflammation of the lymph nodes in peritoneal fold that encases abdominal organs; disease resembles acute appendicitis; unknown etiology.

289.3 Lymphadenitis, unspecified, except mesenteric

AHA: 2Q, '92, 8

289.4 Hypersplenism
"Big spleen" syndrome   Hypersplenia
Dyssplenism
> EXCLUDES primary splenic neutropenia
>   ▶(289.53)◀

DEF: An overactive spleen; it causes a deficiency of the peripheral blood components, an increase in bone marrow cells and sometimes a notable increase in the size of the spleen.

√5ᵗʰ **289.5 Other diseases of spleen**

289.50 Disease of spleen, unspecified
289.51 Chronic congestive splenomegaly
289.52 Splenic sequestration
Code first sickle-cell disease in crisis (282.42, 282.62, 282.64, 282.69)

AHA: 4Q, '03, 51

DEF: Blood is entrapped in the spleen due to vessel occlusion; most often associated with sickle-cell disease; spleen becomes enlarged and there is a sharp drop in hemoglobin.

● **289.53 Neutropenic splenomegaly**
289.59 Other
Lien migrans   Splenic:
Perisplenitis   fibrosis
Splenic: infarction
   abscess   rupture, nontraumatic
   atrophy   Splenitis
   cyst   Wandering spleen
> EXCLUDES bilharzial splenic fibrosis (120.0-120.9)
>   hepatolienal fibrosis (571.5)
>   splenomegaly NOS (789.2)

BLOOD AND BLOOD-FORMING ORGANS

289.6 Familial polycythemia
Familial:
  benign polycythemia
  erythrocytosis
DEF: Elevated number of red blood cells.

289.7 Methemoglobinemia
Congenital NADH [DPNH]-methemoglobin-reductase deficiency
Hemoglobin M [Hb-M] disease
Methemoglobinemia:
  NOS
  acquired (with sulfhemoglobinemia)
  hereditary
  toxic
Stokvis' disease
Sulfhemoglobinemia
Use additional E code to identify cause
DEF: Presence in the blood of methemoglobin, a chemically altered form of hemoglobin; causes cyanosis, headache, dizziness, ataxia dyspnea, tachycardia, nausea, stupor, coma, and, rarely, death.

289.8 Other specified diseases of blood and blood-forming organs
AHA: 4Q, '03, 56; 1Q, '02, 16; 2Q, '89, 8; M-A, '87, 12
DEF: Hypercoagulable states: a group of inherited or acquired abnormalities of specific proteins and anticoagulant factors; also called thromboembolic states or thrombotic disorders, these disorders result in the abnormal development of blood clots.

289.81 Primary hypercoagulable state
Activated protein C resistance
Antithrombin III deficiency
Factor V Leiden mutation
Lupus anticoagulant
Protein C deficiency
Protein S deficiency
Prothrombin gene mutation
DEF: Activated protein C resistance: decreased effectiveness of protein C to degrade factor V, necessary to inhibit clotting cascade; also called Factor V Leiden mutation.
DEF: Antithrombin III deficiency: deficiency in plasma antithrombin III one of six naturally occurring antithrombins that limit coagulation.
DEF: Factor V Leiden mutation: also called activated protein C resistance.
DEF: Lupus anticoagulant: deficiency in a circulating anticoagulant that inhibits the conversion of prothrombin into thrombin; autoimmune antibodies induce procoagulant surfaces in platelets; also called anti-phospholipid syndrome.
DEF: Protein C deficiency: deficiency of activated protein C which functions to bring the blood-clotting process into balance; same outcome as factor V Leiden mutation.
DEF: Protein S deficiency: similar to protein C deficiency; protein S is a vitamin K dependent cofactor in the activation of protein C.
DEF: Prothrombin gene mutation: increased levels of prothrombin, or factor II, a plasma protein that is converted to thrombin, which acts upon fibrinogen to form the fibrin.

289.82 Secondary hypercoagulable state

289.83 Myelofibrosis
Myelofibrosis NOS
Secondary myelofibrosis
Code first the underlying disorder, such as:
  malignant neoplasm of breast (174.0-174.9, 175.0-175.9)
EXCLUDES idiopathic myelofibrosis (238.76)
  leukoerythroblastic anemia (284.2)
  myelofibrosis with myeloid metaplasia (238.76)
  myelophthisic anemia (284.2)
  myelophthisis (284.2)
  primary myelofibrosis (238.76)

289.89 Other specified diseases of blood and blood-forming organs
Hypergammaglobulinemia
Pseudocholinesterase deficiency

289.9 Unspecified diseases of blood and blood-forming organs
Blood dyscrasia NOS
Erythroid hyperplasia
AHA: M-A, '85, 14

MENTAL DISORDERS

5. MENTAL DISORDERS (290-319)

PSYCHOSES (290-299)
EXCLUDES mental retardation (317-319)

ORGANIC PSYCHOTIC CONDITIONS (290-294)
INCLUDES psychotic organic brain syndrome
EXCLUDES nonpsychotic syndromes of organic etiology (310.0-310.9)
psychoses classifiable to 295-298 and without impairment of orientation, comprehension, calculation, learning capacity, and judgment, but associated with physical disease, injury, or condition affecting the brain [eg., following childbirth] (295.0-298.8)

✓4th 290 Dementias
Code first the associated neurological condition
EXCLUDES dementia due to alcohol (291.0-291.2)
dementia due to drugs (292.82)
dementia not classified as senile, presenile, or arteriosclerotic (294.10-294.11)
psychoses classifiable to 295-298 occurring in the senium without dementia or delirium (295.0-298.8)
senility with mental changes of nonpsychotic severity (310.1)
transient organic psychotic conditions (293.0-293.9)

290.0 Senile dementia, uncomplicated
Senile dementia:
  NOS
  simple type
EXCLUDES mild memory disturbances, not amounting to dementia, associated with senile brain disease (310.1)
senile dementia with:
  delirium or confusion (290.3)
  delusional [paranoid] features (290.20)
  depressive features (290.21)

AHA: 4Q, '99, 4

✓5th 290.1 Presenile dementia
Brain syndrome with presenile brain disease
EXCLUDES arteriosclerotic dementia (290.40-290.43)
dementia associated with other cerebral conditions (294.10-294.11)

AHA: N-D, '84, 20

290.10 Presenile dementia, uncomplicated
Presenile dementia:
  NOS
  simple type

290.11 Presenile dementia with delirium
Presenile dementia with acute confusional state
AHA: 1Q, '88, 3

290.12 Presenile dementia with delusional features
Presenile dementia, paranoid type

290.13 Presenile dementia with depressive features
Presenile dementia, depressed type

✓5th 290.2 Senile dementia with delusional or depressive features
EXCLUDES senile dementia:
  NOS (290.0)
  with delirium and/or confusion (290.3)

290.20 Senile dementia with delusional features
Senile dementia, paranoid type
Senile psychosis NOS

290.21 Senile dementia with depressive features

290.3 Senile dementia with delirium
Senile dementia with acute confusional state
EXCLUDES senile:
  dementia NOS (290.0)
  psychosis NOS (290.20)

✓5th 290.4 Vascular dementia
Multi-infarct dementia or psychosis
Use additional code to identify cerebral atherosclerosis (437.0)
EXCLUDES suspected cases with no clear evidence of arteriosclerosis (290.9)

AHA: 1Q, '88, 3

290.40 Vascular dementia, uncomplicated
Arteriosclerotic dementia:
  NOS
  simple type

290.41 Vascular dementia with delirium
Arteriosclerotic dementia with acute confusional state

290.42 Vascular dementia with delusions
Arteriosclerotic dementia, paranoid type

290.43 Vascular dementia with depressed mood
Arteriosclerotic dementia, depressed type

290.8 Other specified senile psychotic conditions
Presbyophrenic psychosis

290.9 Unspecified senile psychotic condition

✓4th 291 Alcohol induced mental disorders
EXCLUDES alcoholism without psychosis (303.0-303.9)
AHA: 1Q, '88, 3; S-O, '86, 3

291.0 Alcohol withdrawal delirium
Alcoholic delirium
Delirium tremens
EXCLUDES alcohol withdrawal (291.81)
AHA: 2Q, '91, 11

291.1 Alcohol induced persisting amnestic disorder
Alcoholic polyneuritic psychosis
Korsakoff's psychosis, alcoholic
Wernicke-Korsakoff syndrome (alcoholic)

DEF: Prominent and lasting reduced memory span, disordered time appreciation and confabulation, occurring in alcoholics, as sequel to acute alcoholic psychosis.

291.2 Alcohol induced persisting dementia
Alcoholic dementia NOS
Alcoholism associated with dementia NOS
Chronic alcoholic brain syndrome

Additional Digit Required · Unspecified Code · Other Specified Code · Manifestation Code · ▶◀ Revised Text · ● New Code · ▲ Revised Code Title

2007 ICD·9·CM Volume 1 — 65

MENTAL DISORDERS

291.3 **Alcohol induced psychotic disorder with hallucinations**
Alcoholic:
  hallucinosis (acute)
  psychosis with hallucinosis
  EXCLUDES alcohol withdrawal with delirium (291.0)
    schizophrenia (295.0-295.9) and paranoid states (297.0-297.9) taking the form of chronic hallucinosis with clear consciousness in an alcoholic

AHA: 2Q, '91, 11

DEF: Psychosis lasting less than six months with slight or no clouding of consciousness in which auditory hallucinations predominate.

291.4 **Idiosyncratic alcohol intoxication**
Pathologic:
  alcohol intoxication
  drunkenness
  EXCLUDES acute alcohol intoxication (305.0)
    in alcoholism (303.0)
    simple drunkenness (305.0)

DEF: Unique behavioral patterns, like belligerence, after intake of relatively small amounts of alcohol; behavior not due to excess consumption.

291.5 **Alcohol induced psychotic disorder with delusions**
Alcoholic: Alcoholic:
  paranoia   psychosis, paranoid type
  EXCLUDES nonalcoholic paranoid states (297.0-297.9)
    schizophrenia, paranoid type (295.3)

√5th **291.8** **Other specified alcohol induced mental disorders**
AHA: 3Q, '94, 13; J-A, '85, 10

  291.81 **Alcohol withdrawal**
  Alcohol:
    abstinence syndrome or symptoms
    withdrawal syndrome or symptoms
  EXCLUDES alcohol withdrawal:
    delirium (291.0)
    hallucinosis (291.3)
    delirium tremens (291.0)

  AHA: 4Q, '96, 28; 2Q, '91, 11

  291.82 **Alcohol induced sleep disorders**
  Alcohol induced circadian rhythm sleep disorders
  Alcohol induced hypersomnia
  Alcohol induced insomnia
  Alcohol induced parasomnia

  291.89 **Other**
  Alcohol induced anxiety disorder
  Alcohol induced mood disorder
  Alcohol induced sexual dysfunction

291.9 **Unspecified alcohol induced mental disorders**
Alcoholic:
  mania NOS
  psychosis NOS
Alcoholism (chronic) with psychosis
Alcohol related disorder NOS

√4th **292** **Drug induced mental disorders**
INCLUDES organic brain syndrome associated with consumption of drugs
Use additional code for any associated drug dependence (304.0-304.9)
Use additional E code to identify drug
AHA: 3Q, '04, 8; 2Q, '91, 11; S-O, '86, 3

  292.0 **Drug withdrawal**
  Drug:
    abstinence syndrome or symptoms
    withdrawal syndrome or symptoms
  AHA: 1Q, '97, 12; 1Q, '88, 3

√5th **292.1** **Drug induced psychotic disorders**
  292.11 **Drug induced psychotic disorder with delusions**
  Paranoid state induced by drugs

  292.12 **Drug induced psychotic disorder with hallucinations**
  Hallucinatory state induced by drugs
  EXCLUDES states following LSD or other hallucinogens, lasting only a few days or less ["bad trips"] (305.3)

292.2 **Pathological drug intoxication**
Drug reaction:
  NOS   }
  idiosyncratic } resulting in brief psychotic states
  pathologic   }
EXCLUDES expected brief psychotic reactions to hallucinogens ["bad trips"] (305.3)
  physiological side-effects of drugs (e.g., dystonias)

√5th **292.8** **Other specified drug induced mental disorders**
  292.81 **Drug induced delirium**
  AHA: 1Q, '88, 3

  292.82 **Drug induced persisting dementia**
  292.83 **Drug induced persisting amnestic disorder**
  292.84 **Drug induced mood disorder**
  Depressive state induced by drugs
  292.85 **Drug induced sleep disorders**
  Drug induced circadian rhythm sleep disorder
  Drug induced hypersomnia
  Drug induced insomnia
  Drug induced parasomnia

  292.89 **Other**
  Drug induced anxiety disorder
  Drug induced organic personality syndrome
  Drug induced sexual dysfunction
  Drug intoxication

292.9 **Unspecified drug induced mental disorder**
Drug related disorder NOS
Organic psychosis NOS due to or associated with drugs

√4th **293** **Transient mental disorders due to conditions classified elsewhere**
INCLUDES transient organic mental disorders not associated with alcohol or drugs
Code first the associated physical or neurological condition
EXCLUDES confusional state or delirium superimposed on senile dementia (290.3)
  dementia due to:
    alcohol (291.0-291.9)
    arteriosclerosis (290.40-290.43)
    drugs (292.82)
    senility (290.0)

  293.0 **Delirium due to conditions classified elsewhere**
  Acute:
    confusional state
    infective psychosis
    organic reaction
    posttraumatic organic psychosis
    psycho-organic syndrome
  Acute psychosis associated with endocrine, metabolic, or cerebrovascular disorder
  Epileptic:
    confusional state
    twilight state
  AHA: 1Q, '88, 3

MENTAL DISORDERS

293.1 Subacute delirium
Subacute:
confusional state
infective psychosis
organic reaction
posttraumatic organic psychosis
psycho-organic syndrome
psychosis associated with endocrine or metabolic disorder

293.8 Other specified transient mental disorders due to conditions classified elsewhere

293.81 Psychotic disorder with delusions in conditions classified elsewhere
Transient organic psychotic condition, paranoid type

293.82 Psychotic disorder with hallucinations in conditions classified elsewhere
Transient organic psychotic condition, hallucinatory type

293.83 Mood disorder in conditions classified elsewhere
Transient organic psychotic condition, depressive type

293.84 Anxiety disorder in conditions classified elsewhere
AHA: 4Q, '96, 29

293.89 Other
Catatonic disorder in conditions classified elsewhere

293.9 Unspecified transient mental disorder in conditions classified elsewhere
Organic psychosis:
infective NOS
posttraumatic NOS
transient NOS
Psycho-organic syndrome

294 Persistent mental disorders due to conditions classified elsewhere
INCLUDES organic psychotic brain syndromes (chronic), not elsewhere classified
AHA: M-A, '85, 12

294.0 Amnestic disorder in conditions classified elsewhere
Korsakoff's psychosis or syndrome (nonalcoholic)
Code first underlying condition
EXCLUDES alcoholic:
amnestic syndrome (291.1)
Korsakoff's psychosis (291.1)

294.1 Dementia in conditions classified elsewhere
Dementia of the Alzheimer's type
Code first any underlying physical condition, as:
dementia in:
Alzheimer's disease (331.0)
cerebral lipidoses (330.1)
dementia with Lewy bodies (331.82)
dementia with Parkinsonism (331.82)
epilepsy (345.0-345.9)
frontal dementia (331.19)
frontotemporal dementia (331.19)
general paresis [syphilis] (094.1)
hepatolenticular degeneration (275.1)
Huntington's chorea (333.4)
Jakob-Creutzfeldt disease (046.1)
multiple sclerosis (340)
Pick's disease of the brain (331.11)
polyarteritis nodosa (446.0)
syphilis (094.1)
EXCLUDES dementia:
arteriosclerotic (290.40-290.43)
presenile (290.10-290.13)
senile (290.0)
epileptic psychosis NOS (294.8)
AHA: 4Q, '00, 40; 1Q, '99, 14; N-D, '85, 5

294.10 Dementia in conditions classified elsewhere without behavioral disturbance
Dementia in conditions classified elsewhere NOS

294.11 Dementia in conditions classified elsewhere with behavioral disturbance
Aggressive behavior
Combative behavior
Violent behavior
Wandering off
AHA: 4Q, '00, 41

294.8 Other persistent mental disorders due to conditions classified elsewhere
Amnestic disorder NOS
Dementia NOS
Epileptic psychosis NOS
Mixed paranoid and affective organic psychotic states
Use additional code for associated epilepsy (345.0-345.9)
EXCLUDES mild memory disturbances, not amounting to dementia (310.1)
AHA: 3Q, '03, 14; 1Q, '88, 5

294.9 Unspecified persistent mental disorders due to conditions classified elsewhere
Cognitive disorder NOS
Organic psychosis (chronic)

OTHER PSYCHOSES (295-299)

Use additional code to identify any associated physical disease, injury, or condition affecting the brain with psychoses classifiable to 295-298

295 Schizophrenic disorders
INCLUDES schizophrenia of the types described in 295.0-295.9 occurring in children
EXCLUDES childhood type schizophrenia (299.9)
infantile autism (299.0)

The following fifth-digit subclassification is for use with category 295:
0 unspecified
1 subchronic
2 chronic
3 subchronic with acute exacerbation
4 chronic with acute exacerbation
5 in remission

DEF: Group of disorders with disturbances in thought (delusions, hallucinations), mood (blunted, flattened, inappropriate affect), sense of self, relationship to world; also bizarre, purposeless behavior, repetitious activity, or inactivity.

295.0 Simple type
Schizophrenia simplex
EXCLUDES latent schizophrenia (295.5)

295.1 Disorganized type
Hebephrenia   Hebephrenic type schizophrenia
DEF: Inappropriate behavior; results in extreme incoherence and disorganization of time, place and sense of social appropriateness; withdrawal from routine social interaction may occur.

295.2 Catatonic type
Catatonic (schizophrenia):   Schizophrenic:
agitation   catalepsy
excitation   catatonia
excited type   flexibilitas cerea
stupor
withdrawn type

DEF: Extreme changes in motor activity; one extreme is decreased response or reaction to the environment and the other is spontaneous activity.

MENTAL DISORDERS

295.3 Paranoid type
Paraphrenic schizophrenia
EXCLUDES involutional paranoid state (297.2)
paranoia (297.1)
paraphrenia (297.2)

DEF: Preoccupied with delusional suspicions and auditory hallucinations related to single theme; usually hostile, grandiose, overly religious, occasionally hypochondriacal.

295.4 Schizophreniform disorder
Oneirophrenia
Schizophreniform:
    attack
    psychosis, confusional type
EXCLUDES acute forms of schizophrenia of:
    catatonic type (295.2)
    hebephrenic type (295.1)
    paranoid type (295.3)
    simple type (295.0)
    undifferentiated type (295.8)

295.5 Latent schizophrenia
Latent schizophrenic reaction
Schizophrenia:
    borderline
    incipient
    prepsychotic
    prodromal
    pseudoneurotic
    pseudopsychopathic
EXCLUDES schizoid personality (301.20-301.22)

295.6 Residual type
Chronic undifferentiated schizophrenia
Restzustand (schizophrenic)
Schizophrenic residual state

295.7 Schizoaffective disorder
Cyclic schizophrenia
Mixed schizophrenic and affective psychosis
Schizo-affective psychosis
Schizophreniform psychosis, affective type

295.8 Other specified types of schizophrenia
Acute (undifferentiated) schizophrenia
Atypical schizophrenia
Cenesthopathic schizophrenia
EXCLUDES infantile autism (299.0)

295.9 Unspecified schizophrenia
Schizophrenia:
    NOS
    mixed NOS
    undifferentiated NOS
    undifferentiated type
Schizophrenic reaction NOS
Schizophreniform psychosis NOS
AHA: 3Q, '95, 6

296 Episodic mood disorders
INCLUDES episodic affective disorders
EXCLUDES neurotic depression (300.4)
reactive depressive psychosis (298.0)
reactive excitation (298.1)

The following fifth-digit subclassification is for use with categories 296.0-296.6:
0 unspecified
1 mild
2 moderate
3 severe, without mention of psychotic behavior
4 severe, specified as with psychotic behavior
5 in partial or unspecified remission
6 in full remission

AHA: M-A, '85, 14

296.0 Bipolar I disorder, single manic episode
Hypomania (mild) NOS
Hypomanic psychosis
Mania (monopolar) NOS
Manic-depressive psychosis
    or reaction:
    hypomanic
    manic
} single episode or unspecified

EXCLUDES circular type, if there was a previous attack of depression (296.4)

DEF: Mood disorder identified by hyperactivity; may show extreme agitation or exaggerated excitability; speech and thought processes may be accelerated.

296.1 Manic disorder, recurrent episode
Any condition classifiable to 296.0, stated to be recurrent
EXCLUDES circular type, if there was a previous attack of depression (296.4)

296.2 Major depressive disorder, single episode
Depressive psychosis
Endogenous depression
Involutional melancholia
Manic-depressive psychosis
    or reaction,
    depressed type
Monopolar depression
Psychotic depression
} single episode or unspecified

EXCLUDES circular type, if previous attack was of manic type (296.5)
depression NOS (311)
reactive depression (neurotic) (300.4)
psychotic (298.0)

DEF: Mood disorder that produces depression; may exhibit as sadness, low self-esteem, or guilt feelings; other manifestations may be withdrawal from friends and family; interrupted normal sleep.

296.3 Major depressive disorder, recurrent episode
Any condition classifiable to 296.2, stated to be recurrent
EXCLUDES circular type, if previous attack was of manic type (296.5)
depression NOS (311)
reactive depression (neurotic) (300.4)
psychotic (298.0)

296.4 Bipolar I disorder, most recent episode (or current) manic
Bipolar disorder, now manic
Manic-depressive psychosis, circular type but currently manic
EXCLUDES brief compensatory or rebound mood swings (296.99)

296.5 Bipolar I disorder, most recent episode (or current) depressed
Bipolar disorder, now depressed
Manic-depressive psychosis, circular type but currently depressed
EXCLUDES brief compensatory or rebound mood swings (296.99)

296.6 Bipolar I disorder, most recent episode (or current) mixed
Manic-depressive psychosis, circular type, mixed

296.7 Bipolar I disorder, most recent episode (or current) unspecified
Atypical bipolar affective disorder NOS
Manic-depressive psychosis, circular type, current condition not specified as either manic or depressive

DEF: Manic-depressive disorder referred to as bipolar because of the mood range from manic to depressive.

---

§ Requires fifth-digit. See category 295 for codes and definitions.

N Newborn Age: 0   **P** Pediatric Age: 0-17   **M** Maternity Age: 12-55   **A** Adult Age: 15-124

MENTAL DISORDERS

✓5th 296.8 Other and unspecified bipolar disorders
- **296.80 Bipolar disorder, unspecified**
  - Bipolar disorder NOSx
  - Manic-depressive:
    - reaction NOS
    - syndrome NOS
- **296.81 Atypical manic disorder**
- **296.82 Atypical depressive disorder**
- **296.89 Other**
  - Bipolar II disorder
  - Manic-depressive psychosis, mixed type

✓5th 296.9 Other and unspecified episodic mood disorder
- EXCLUDES: psychogenic affective psychoses (298.0-298.8)
- **296.90 Unspecified episodic mood disorder**
  - Affective psychosis NOS
  - Melancholia NOS
  - Mood disorder NOS
  - AHA: M-A, '85, 14
- **296.99 Other specified episodic mood disorder**
  - Mood swings:
    - brief compensatory
    - rebound

✓4th 297 Delusional disorders
- INCLUDES: paranoid disorders
- EXCLUDES:
  - acute paranoid reaction (298.3)
  - alcoholic jealousy or paranoid state (291.5)
  - paranoid schizophrenia (295.3)
- **297.0 Paranoid state, simple**
- **297.1 Delusional disorder**
  - Chronic paranoid psychosis
  - Sander's disease
  - Systematized delusions
  - EXCLUDES: paranoid personality disorder (301.0)
- **297.2 Paraphrenia**
  - Involutional paranoid state Paraphrenia (involutional)
  - Late paraphrenia
  - DEF: Paranoid schizophrenic disorder that persists over a prolonged period but does not distort personality despite persistent delusions.
- **297.3 Shared psychotic disorder**
  - Folie à deux
  - Induced psychosis or paranoid disorder
  - DEF: Mental disorder two people share; first person with the delusional disorder convinces second person because of a close relationship and shared experiences to accept the delusions.
- **297.8 Other specified paranoid states**
  - Paranoia querulans Sensitiver Beziehungswahn
  - EXCLUDES:
    - acute paranoid reaction or state (298.3)
    - senile paranoid state (290.20)
- **297.9 Unspecified paranoid state**
  - Paranoid:
    - disorder NOS
    - psychosis NOS
  - Paranoid:
    - reaction NOS
    - state NOS
  - AHA: J-A, '85, 9

✓4th 298 Other nonorganic psychoses
- INCLUDES: psychotic conditions due to or provoked by:
  - emotional stress
  - environmental factors as major part of etiology
- **298.0 Depressive type psychosis**
  - Psychogenic depressive psychosis
  - Psychotic reactive depression
  - Reactive depressive psychosis
  - EXCLUDES:
    - manic-depressive psychosis, depressed type (296.2-296.3)
    - neurotic depression (300.4)
    - reactive depression NOS (300.4)

- **298.1 Excitative type psychosis**
  - Acute hysterical psychosis Reactive excitation
  - Psychogenic excitation
  - EXCLUDES: manic-depressive psychosis, manic type (296.0-296.1)
  - DEF: Affective disorder similar to manic-depressive psychosis, in the manic phase, seemingly brought on by stress.
- **298.2 Reactive confusion**
  - Psychogenic confusion
  - Psychogenic twilight state
  - EXCLUDES: acute confusional state (293.0)
  - DEF: Confusion, disorientation, cloudiness in consciousness; brought on by severe emotional upheaval.
- **298.3 Acute paranoid reaction**
  - Acute psychogenic paranoid psychosis
  - Bouffée délirante
  - EXCLUDES: paranoid states (297.0-297.9)
- **298.4 Psychogenic paranoid psychosis**
  - Protracted reactive paranoid psychosis
- **298.8 Other and unspecified reactive psychosis**
  - Brief psychotic disorder
  - Brief reactive psychosis NOS
  - Hysterical psychosis
  - Psychogenic psychosis NOS
  - Psychogenic stupor
  - EXCLUDES: acute hysterical psychosis (298.1)
- **298.9 Unspecified psychosis**
  - Atypical psychosis
  - Psychosis NOS
  - Psychotic disorder NOS

✓4th 299 Pervasive developmental disorders
- EXCLUDES: adult type psychoses occurring in childhood, as:
  - affective disorders (296.0-296.9)
  - manic-depressive disorders (296.0-296.9)
  - schizophrenia (295.0-295.9)

The following fifth-digit subclassification is for use with category 299:
- 0 current or active state
- 1 residual state

✓5th 299.0 Autistic disorder
- Childhood autism
- Infantile psychosis
- Kanner's syndrome
- EXCLUDES:
  - disintegrative psychosis (299.1)
  - Heller's syndrome (299.1)
  - schizophrenic syndrome of childhood (299.9)
- DEF: Severe mental disorder of children, results in impaired social behavior; abnormal development of communicative skills, appears to be unaware of the need for emotional support and offers little emotional response to family members.

✓5th 299.1 Childhood disintegrative disorder
- Heller's syndrome
- Use additional code to identify any associated neurological disorder
- EXCLUDES:
  - infantile autism (299.0)
  - schizophrenic syndrome of childhood (299.9)
- DEF: Mental disease of children identified by impaired development of reciprocal social skills, verbal and nonverbal communication skills, imaginative play.

✓5th 299.8 Other specified pervasive developmental disorders
- Asperger's disorder
- Atypical childhood psychosis
- Borderline psychosis of childhood
- EXCLUDES: simple stereotypes without psychotic disturbance (307.3)

MENTAL DISORDERS — Tabular List

§ ✓5ᵗʰ **299.9 Unspecified pervasive developmental disorder**
    Child psychosis NOS
    Schizophrenia, childhood type NOS
    Schizophrenic syndrome of childhood NOS
    EXCLUDES schizophrenia of adult type occurring in childhood (295.0-295.9)

NEUROTIC DISORDERS, PERSONALITY DISORDERS, AND OTHER NONPSYCHOTIC MENTAL DISORDERS (300-316)

✓4ᵗʰ **300 Anxiety, dissociative and somatoform disorders**

✓5ᵗʰ **300.0 Anxiety states**
    EXCLUDES anxiety in:
        acute stress reaction (308.0)
        transient adjustment reaction (309.24)
        neurasthenia (300.5)
        psychophysiological disorders (306.0-306.9)
        separation anxiety (309.21)
    DEF: Mental disorder characterized by anxiety and avoidance behavior not particularly related to any specific situation or stimulus; symptoms include emotional instability, apprehension, fatigue.

    300.00 Anxiety state, unspecified
        Anxiety: Anxiety:
            neurosis   state (neurotic)
            reaction   Atypical anxiety disorder
    AHA: 1Q, '02, 6

    300.01 Panic disorder without agoraphobia
        Panic: Panic:
            attack   state
        EXCLUDES panic disorder with agoraphobia (300.21)
    DEF: Neurotic disorder characterized by recurrent panic or anxiety, apprehension, fear or terror; symptoms include shortness of breath, palpitations, dizziness, faintness or shakiness; fear of dying may persist or fear of other morbid consequences.

    300.02 Generalized anxiety disorder
    300.09 Other

✓5ᵗʰ **300.1 Dissociative, conversion and factitious disorders**
    EXCLUDES
        adjustment reaction (309.0-309.9)
        anorexia nervosa (307.1)
        gross stress reaction (308.0-308.9)
        hysterical personality (301.50-301.59)
        psychophysiologic disorders (306.0-306.9)

    300.10 Hysteria, unspecified
    300.11 Conversion disorder
        Astasia-abasia, hysterical
        Conversion hysteria or reaction
        Hysterical
            blindness
            deafness
            paralysis
    AHA: N-D, '85, 15
    DEF: Mental disorder that impairs physical functions with no physiological basis; sensory motor symptoms include seizures, paralysis, temporary blindness; increase in stress or avoidance of unpleasant responsibilities may precipitate.

    300.12 Dissociative amnesia
        Hysterical amnesia

    300.13 Dissociative fugue
        Hysterical fugue
    DEF: Dissociative hysteria; identified by loss of memory, flight from familiar surroundings; conscious activity is not associated with perception of surroundings, no later memory of episode.

    300.14 Dissociative identity disorder
        Dissociative identity disorder

    300.15 Dissociative disorder or reaction, unspecified
    DEF: Hysterical neurotic episode; sudden but temporary changes in perceived identity, memory, consciousness, segregated memory patterns exist separate from dominant personality.

    300.16 Factitious disorder with predominantly psychological signs and symptoms
        Compensation neurosis
        Ganser's syndrome, hysterical
    DEF: A disorder characterized by the purposeful assumption of mental illness symptoms; the symptoms are not real, possibly representing what the patient imagines mental illness to be like, and are acted out more often when another person is present.

    300.19 Other and unspecified factitious illness
        Factitious disorder (with combined psychological and physical signs and symptoms) (with predominantly physical signs and symptoms) NOS
        EXCLUDES multiple operations or hospital addiction syndrome (301.51)

✓5ᵗʰ **300.2 Phobic disorders**
    EXCLUDES anxiety state not associated with a specific situation or object (300.00-300.09)
        obsessional phobias (300.3)

    300.20 Phobia, unspecified
        Anxiety-hysteria NOS
        Phobia NOS

    300.21 Agoraphobia with panic disorder
        Fear of:
            open spaces
            streets   } with panic attacks
            travel
        Panic disorder with agoraphobia
        EXCLUDES agoraphobia without panic disorder (300.22)
            panic disorder without agoraphobia (300.01)

    300.22 Agoraphobia without mention of panic attacks
        Any condition classifiable to 300.21 without mention of panic attacks

    300.23 Social phobia
        Fear of:
            eating in public
            public speaking
            washing in public

    300.29 Other isolated or specific phobias
        Acrophobia
        Animal phobias
        Claustrophobia
        Fear of crowds

§ Requires fifth-digit. See category 299 for codes and definitions.

 Newborn Age: 0   Pediatric Age: 0-17   M Maternity Age: 12-55   Adult Age: 15-124

MENTAL DISORDERS

300.3 Obsessive-compulsive disorders
Anancastic neurosis   Obsessional phobia [any]
Compulsive neurosis
EXCLUDES obsessive-compulsive symptoms occurring in:
endogenous depression (296.2-296.3)
organic states (eg., encephalitis)
schizophrenia (295.0-295.9)

300.4 Dysthymic disorder
Anxiety depression
Depression with anxiety
Depressive reaction
Neurotic depressive state
Reactive depression
EXCLUDES adjustment reaction with depressive symptoms (309.0-309.1)
depression NOS (311)
manic-depressive psychosis, depressed type (296.2-296.3)
reactive depressive psychosis (298.0)
DEF: Depression without psychosis; less severe depression related to personal change or unexpected circumstances; also referred to as "reactional depression."

300.5 Neurasthenia
Fatigue neurosis
Nervous debility
Psychogenic:
  asthenia
  general fatigue
Use additional code to identify any associated physical disorder
EXCLUDES anxiety state (300.00-300.09)
neurotic depression (300.4)
psychophysiological disorders (306.0-306.9)
specific nonpsychotic mental disorders following organic brain damage (310.0-310.9)
DEF: Physical and mental symptoms caused primarily by what is known as mental exhaustion; symptoms include chronic weakness, fatigue.

300.6 Depersonalization disorder
Derealization (neurotic)
Neurotic state with depersonalization episode
EXCLUDES depersonalization associated with:
anxiety (300.00-300.09)
depression (300.4)
manic-depressive disorder or psychosis (296.0-296.9)
schizophrenia (295.0-295.9)
DEF: Dissociative disorder characterized by feelings of strangeness about self or body image; symptoms include dizziness, anxiety, fear of insanity, loss of reality of surroundings.

300.7 Hypochondriasis
Body dysmorphic disorder
EXCLUDES hypochondriasis in:
hysteria (300.10-300.19)
manic-depressive psychosis, depressed type (296.2-296.3)
neurasthenia (300.5)
obsessional disorder (300.3)
schizophrenia (295.0-295.9)

√5th 300.8 Somatoform disorders
  300.81 Somatization disorder
    Briquet's disorder
    Severe somatoform disorder
  300.82 Undifferentiated somatoform disorder
    Atypical somatoform disorder
    Somatoform disorder NOS
    AHA: 4Q, '96, 29
    DEF: Disorders in which patients have symptoms that suggest an organic disease but no evidence of physical disorder after repeated testing.
  300.89 Other somatoform disorders
    Occupational neurosis, including writers' cramp
    Psychasthenia
    Psychasthenic neurosis

  300.9 Unspecified nonpsychotic mental disorder
    Psychoneurosis NOS

√4th 301 Personality disorders
INCLUDES character neurosis
Use additional code to identify any associated neurosis or psychosis, or physical condition
EXCLUDES nonpsychotic personality disorder associated with organic brain syndromes (310.0-310.9)

  301.0 Paranoid personality disorder
    Fanatic personality
    Paranoid personality (disorder)
    Paranoid traits
    EXCLUDES acute paranoid reaction (298.3)
    alcoholic paranoia (291.5)
    paranoid schizophrenia (295.3)
    paranoid states (297.0-297.9)
    AHA: J-A, '85, 9

  √5th 301.1 Affective personality disorder
    EXCLUDES affective psychotic disorders (296.0-296.9)
    neurasthenia (300.5)
    neurotic depression (300.4)
    301.10 Affective personality disorder, unspecified
    301.11 Chronic hypomanic personality disorder
      Chronic hypomanic disorder
      Hypomanic personality
    301.12 Chronic depressive personality disorder
      Chronic depressive disorder
      Depressive character or personality
    301.13 Cyclothymic disorder
      Cycloid personality
      Cyclothymia
      Cyclothymic personality

  √5th 301.2 Schizoid personality disorder
    EXCLUDES schizophrenia (295.0-295.9)
    301.20 Schizoid personality disorder, unspecified
    301.21 Introverted personality
    301.22 Schizotypal personality disorder

  301.3 Explosive personality disorder
    Aggressive:
      personality
      reaction
    Aggressiveness
    Emotional instability (excessive)
    Pathological emotionality
    Quarrelsomeness
    EXCLUDES dyssocial personality (301.7)
    hysterical neurosis (300.10-300.19)

301.4 Obsessive-compulsive personality disorder
Anancastic personality
Obsessional personality
EXCLUDES obsessive-compulsive disorder (300.3)
phobic state (300.20-300.29)

✓5th 301.5 Histrionic personality disorder
EXCLUDES hysterical neurosis (300.10-300.19)

DEF: Extreme emotional behavior, often theatrical; often concerned about own appeal; may demand attention, exhibit seductive behavior.

301.50 Histrionic personality disorder, unspecified
Hysterical personality NOS

301.51 Chronic factitious illness with physical symptoms
Hospital addiction syndrome
Multiple operations syndrome
Munchausen syndrome

301.59 Other histrionic personality disorder
Personality:
emotionally unstable
labile
psychoinfantile

301.6 Dependent personality disorder
Asthenic personality
Inadequate personality
Passive personality
EXCLUDES neurasthenia (300.5)
passive-aggressive personality (301.84)

DEF: Overwhelming feeling of helplessness; fears of abandonment may persist; difficulty in making personal decisions without confirmation by others; low self-esteem due to irrational sensitivity to criticism.

301.7 Antisocial personality disorder
Amoral personality
Asocial personality
Dyssocial personality
Personality disorder with predominantly sociopathic or asocial manifestation
EXCLUDES disturbance of conduct without specifiable personality disorder (312.0-312.9)
explosive personality (301.3)

AHA: S-O, '84, 16

DEF: Continuous antisocial behavior that violates rights of others; social traits include extreme aggression, total disregard for traditional social rules.

✓5th 301.8 Other personality disorders
301.81 Narcissistic personality disorder
DEF: Grandiose fantasy or behavior, lack of social empathy, hypersensitive to the lack of others' judgment, exploits others; also sense of entitlement to have expectations met, need for continual admiration.

301.82 Avoidant personality disorder
DEF: Personality disorder marked by feelings of social inferiority; sensitivity to criticism, emotionally restrained due to fear of rejection.

301.83 Borderline personality disorder
DEF: Personality disorder characterized by unstable moods, self-image, and interpersonal relationships; uncontrolled anger, impulsive and self-destructive acts, fears of abandonment, feelings of emptiness and boredom, recurrent suicide threats or self-mutilation.

301.84 Passive-aggressive personality
DEF: Pattern of procrastination and refusal to meet standards; introduce own obstacles to success and exploit failure.

301.89 Other
Personality:
eccentric
"haltlose" type
immature
masochistic
psychoneurotic
EXCLUDES psychoinfantile personality (301.59)

301.9 Unspecified personality disorder
Pathological personality NOS
Personality disorder NOS
Psychopathic:
constitutional state
personality (disorder)

✓4th 302 Sexual and gender identity disorders
EXCLUDES sexual disorder manifest in:
organic brain syndrome (290.0-294.9, 310.0-310.9)
psychosis (295.0-298.9)

302.0 Ego-dystonic sexual orientation
Ego-dystonic lesbianism
Sexual orientation conflict disorder
EXCLUDES homosexual pedophilia (302.2)

302.1 Zoophilia
Bestiality
DEF: A sociodeviant disorder marked by engaging in sexual intercourse with animals.

302.2 Pedophilia
DEF: A sociodeviant condition of adults characterized by sexual activity with children.

302.3 Transvestic fetishism
EXCLUDES trans-sexualism (302.5)
DEF: The desire to dress in clothing of opposite sex.

302.4 Exhibitionism
DEF: Sexual deviant behavior; exposure of genitals to strangers; behavior prompted by intense sexual urges and fantasies.

✓5th 302.5 Trans-sexualism
EXCLUDES transvestism (302.3)
DEF: Gender identity disturbance; overwhelming desire to change anatomic sex, due to belief that individual is a member of the opposite sex.

302.50 With unspecified sexual history
302.51 With asexual history
302.52 With homosexual history
302.53 With heterosexual history

302.6 Gender identity disorder in children
Feminism in boys
Gender identity disorder NOS
EXCLUDES gender identity disorder in adult (302.85)
trans-sexualism (302.50-302.53)
transvestism (302.3)

✓5th 302.7 Psychosexual dysfunction
EXCLUDES impotence of organic origin (607.84)
normal transient symptoms from ruptured hymen
transient or occasional failures of erection due to fatigue, anxiety, alcohol, or drugs

302.70 Psychosexual dysfunction, unspecified
Sexual dysfunction NOS

302.71 Hypoactive sexual desire disorder
EXCLUDES decreased sexual desire NOS (799.81)

MENTAL DISORDERS

302.72 With inhibited sexual excitement
Female sexual arousal disorder
Frigidity
Impotence
Male erectile disorder

302.73 Female orgasmic disorder ♀
302.74 Male orgasmic disorder ♂
302.75 Premature ejaculation ♂
302.76 Dyspareunia, psychogenic ♀
Dyspareunia, psychogenic
DEF: Difficult or painful sex due to psychosomatic state.

302.79 With other specified psychosexual dysfunctions
Sexual aversion disorder

√5th **302.8 Other specified psychosexual disorders**

302.81 Fetishism
DEF: Psychosexual disorder noted for intense sexual urges and arousal precipitated by fantasies; use of inanimate objects, such as clothing, to stimulate sexual arousal, orgasm.

302.82 Voyeurism
DEF: Psychosexual disorder characterized by uncontrollable impulse to observe others, without their knowledge, who are nude or engaged in sexual activity.

302.83 Sexual masochism
DEF: Psychosexual disorder noted for need to achieve sexual gratification through humiliating or hurtful acts inflicted on self.

302.84 Sexual sadism
DEF: Psychosexual disorder noted for need to achieve sexual gratification through humiliating or hurtful acts inflicted on someone else.

302.85 Gender identity disorder in adolescents or adults
EXCLUDES   gender identity disorder NOS (302.6)
gender identity disorder in children (302.6)

302.89 Other
Frotteurism
Nymphomania
Satyriasis

302.9 Unspecified psychosexual disorder
Paraphilia NOS
Pathologic sexuality NOS
Sexual deviation NOS
Sexual disorder NOS

√4th **303 Alcohol dependence syndrome**
Use additional code to identify any associated condition, as:
alcoholic psychoses (291.0-291.9)
drug dependence (304.0-304.9)
physical complications of alcohol, such as:
cerebral degeneration (331.7)
cirrhosis of liver (571.2)
epilepsy (345.0-345.9)
gastritis (535.3)
hepatitis (571.1)
liver damage NOS (571.3)
EXCLUDES   drunkenness NOS (305.0)

The following fifth-digit subclassification is for use with category 303:
0 unspecified
1 continuous
2 episodic
3 in remission

AHA: 3Q, '95, 6; 2Q, '91, 9; 4Q, '88, 8; S-O, '86, 3

√5th **303.0 Acute alcoholic intoxication**
Acute drunkenness in alcoholism

√5th **303.9 Other and unspecified alcohol dependence**
Chronic alcoholism
Dipsomania
AHA: 2Q, '02, 4; 2Q, '89, 9

√4th **304 Drug dependence**
EXCLUDES   nondependent abuse of drugs (305.1-305.9)

The following fifth-digit subclassification is for use with category 304:
0 unspecified
1 continuous
2 episodic
3 in remission

AHA: 2Q, '91, 10; 4Q, '88, 8; S-O, '86, 3

√5th **304.0 Opioid type dependence**
Heroin
Meperidine
Methadone
Morphine
Opium
Opium alkaloids and their derivatives
Synthetics with morphine-like effects

√5th **304.1 Sedative, hypnotic or anxiolytic dependence**
Barbiturates
Nonbarbiturate sedatives and tranquilizers with a similar effect:
chlordiazepoxide
diazepam
glutethimide
meprobamate
methaqualone

√5th **304.2 Cocaine dependence**
Coca leaves and derivatives

√5th **304.3 Cannabis dependence**
Hashish
Hemp
Marihuana

√5th **304.4 Amphetamine and other psychostimulant dependence**
Methylphenidate
Phenmetrazine

√5th **304.5 Hallucinogen dependence**
Dimethyltryptamine [DMT]
Lysergic acid diethylamide [LSD] and derivatives
Mescaline
Psilocybin

√5th **304.6 Other specified drug dependence**
Absinthe addiction
Glue sniffing
Inhalant dependence
Phencyclidine dependence
EXCLUDES   tobacco dependence (305.1)

√5th **304.7 Combinations of opioid type drug with any other**
AHA: M-A, '86, 12

√5th **304.8 Combinations of drug dependence excluding opioid type drug**
AHA: M-A, '86, 12

√5th **304.9 Unspecified drug dependence**
Drug addiction NOS   Drug dependence NOS
AHA: For code 304.90: 4Q, '03, 103

MENTAL DISORDERS

✓4th 305 Nondependent abuse of drugs

Note: Includes cases where a person, for whom no other diagnosis is possible, has come under medical care because of the maladaptive effect of a drug on which he is not dependent and that he has taken on his own initiative to the detriment of his health or social functioning.

EXCLUDES
- alcohol dependence syndrome (303.0-303.9)
- drug dependence (304.0-304.9)
- drug withdrawal syndrome (292.0)
- poisoning by drugs or medicinal substances (960.0-979.9)

The following fifth-digit subclassification is for use with codes 305.0, 305.2-305.9:
- 0 unspecified
- 1 continuous
- 2 episodic
- 3 in remission

AHA: 2Q, '91, 10; 4Q, '88, 8; S-O, '86, 3

✓5th 305.0 Alcohol abuse
Drunkenness NOS
Excessive drinking of alcohol NOS
"Hangover" (alcohol)
Inebriety NOS

EXCLUDES
- acute alcohol intoxication in alcoholism (303.0)
- alcoholic psychoses (291.0-291.9)

AHA: 3Q, '96, 16

305.1 Tobacco use disorder
Tobacco dependence

EXCLUDES
- history of tobacco use (V15.82)
- ▶smoking complicating pregnancy (649.0)
- tobacco use disorder complicating pregnancy (649.0)◀

AHA: 2Q, '96, 10; N-D, '84, 12

✓5th 305.2 Cannabis abuse

✓5th 305.3 Hallucinogen abuse
Acute intoxication from hallucinogens ["bad trips"]
LSD reaction

✓5th 305.4 Sedative, hypnotic or anxiolytic abuse

✓5th 305.5 Opioid abuse

✓5th 305.6 Cocaine abuse
AHA: 1Q, '93, 25; For code 305.60: 1Q, '05, 6

✓5th 305.7 Amphetamine or related acting sympathomimetic abuse
AHA: For code 305.70: 2Q, '03, 10-11

✓5th 305.8 Antidepressant type abuse

✓5th 305.9 Other, mixed, or unspecified drug abuse
Caffeine intoxication
Inhalant abuse
"Laxative habit"
Misuse of drugs NOS
Nonprescribed use of drugs or patent medicinals
Phencyclidine abuse

AHA: 3Q, '99, 20

✓4th 306 Physiological malfunction arising from mental factors

INCLUDES psychogenic:
- physical symptoms ⎫ not involving
- physiological ⎬ tissue
- manifestations ⎭ damage

EXCLUDES
- hysteria (300.11-300.19)
- physical symptoms secondary to a psychiatric disorder classified elsewhere
- psychic factors associated with physical conditions involving tissue damage classified elsewhere (316)
- specific nonpsychotic mental disorders following organic brain damage (310.0-310.9)

DEF: Functional disturbances or interruptions due to mental or psychological causes; no tissue damage sustained in these conditions.

306.0 Musculoskeletal
Psychogenic paralysis
Psychogenic torticollis

EXCLUDES
- Gilles de la Tourette's syndrome (307.23)
- paralysis as hysterical or conversion reaction (300.11)
- tics (307.20-307.22)

306.1 Respiratory
Psychogenic:
- air hunger
- cough
- hiccough
- hyperventilation
- yawning

EXCLUDES psychogenic asthma (316 and 493.9)

306.2 Cardiovascular
Cardiac neurosis
Cardiovascular neurosis
Neurocirculatory asthenia
Psychogenic cardiovascular disorder

EXCLUDES psychogenic paroxysmal tachycardia (316 and 427.2)

AHA: J-A, '85, 14

DEF: Neurocirculatory asthenia: functional nervous and circulatory irregularities with palpitations, dyspnea, fatigue, rapid pulse, precordial pain, fear of effort, discomfort during exercise, anxiety; also called DaCosta's syndrome, Effort syndrome, Irritable or Soldier's Heart.

306.3 Skin
Psychogenic pruritus

EXCLUDES psychogenic:
- alopecia (316 and 704.00)
- dermatitis (316 and 692.9)
- eczema (316 and 691.8 or 692.9)
- urticaria (316 and 708.0-708.9)

306.4 Gastrointestinal
Aerophagy
Cyclical vomiting, psychogenic
Diarrhea, psychogenic
Nervous gastritis
Psychogenic dyspepsia
EXCLUDES
cyclical vomiting NOS (536.2)
globus hystericus (300.11)
mucous colitis (316 and 564.9)
psychogenic:
cardiospasm (316 and 530.0)
duodenal ulcer (316 and 532.0-532.9)
gastric ulcer (316 and 531.0-531.9)
peptic ulcer NOS (316 and 533.0-533.9)
vomiting NOS (307.54)

AHA: 2Q, '89, 11

DEF: Aerophagy: excess swallowing of air, usually unconscious; related to anxiety; results in distended abdomen or belching, often interpreted by the patient as a physical disorder.

√5ᵗʰ **306.5 Genitourinary**
EXCLUDES
enuresis, psychogenic (307.6)
frigidity (302.72)
impotence (302.72)
psychogenic dyspareunia (302.76)

306.50 Psychogenic genitourinary malfunction, unspecified

306.51 Psychogenic vaginismus ♀
Functional vaginismus
DEF: Psychogenic response resulting in painful contractions of vaginal canal muscles; can be severe enough to prevent sexual intercourse.

306.52 Psychogenic dysmenorrhea ♀
306.53 Psychogenic dysuria
306.59 Other

AHA: M-A, '87, 11

306.6 Endocrine
306.7 Organs of special sense
EXCLUDES
hysterical blindness or deafness (300.11)
psychophysical visual disturbances (368.16)

306.8 Other specified psychophysiological malfunction
Bruxism
Teeth grinding

306.9 Unspecified psychophysiological malfunction
Psychophysiologic disorder NOS
Psychosomatic disorder NOS

√4ᵗʰ **307 Special symptoms or syndromes, not elsewhere classified**
Note: This category is intended for use if the psychopathology is manifested by a single specific symptom or group of symptoms which is not part of an organic illness or other mental disorder classifiable elsewhere.
EXCLUDES
those due to mental disorders classified elsewhere
those of organic origin

307.0 Stuttering
EXCLUDES
dysphasia (784.5)
lisping or lalling (307.9)
retarded development of speech (315.31-315.39)

307.1 Anorexia nervosa
EXCLUDES
eating disturbance NOS (307.50)
feeding problem (783.3)
of nonorganic origin (307.59)
loss of appetite (783.0)
of nonorganic origin (307.59)

AHA: 4Q, '89, 11

√5ᵗʰ **307.2 Tics**
EXCLUDES
nail-biting or thumb-sucking (307.9)
stereotypes occurring in isolation (307.3)
tics of organic origin (333.3)

DEF: Involuntary muscle response usually confined to the face, shoulders.

307.20 Tic disorder, unspecified
Tic disorder NOS
307.21 Transient tic disorder
307.22 Chronic motor or vocal tic disorder
307.23 Tourette's disorder
Motor-verbal tic disorder
DEF: Syndrome of facial and vocal tics in childhood; progresses to spontaneous or involuntary jerking, obscene utterances, other uncontrollable actions considered inappropriate.

307.3 Stereotypic movement disorder
Body-rocking
Head banging
Spasmus nutans
Stereotypes NOS
EXCLUDES
tics (307.20-307.23)
of organic origin (333.3)

√5ᵗʰ **307.4 Specific disorders of sleep of nonorganic origin**
EXCLUDES
narcolepsy (347.00-347.11)
organic hypersomnia (327.10-327.19)
organic insomnia (327.00-327.09)
those of unspecified cause (780.50-780.59)

307.40 Nonorganic sleep disorder, unspecified
307.41 Transient disorder of initiating or maintaining sleep
Adjustment insomnia
Hyposomnia } associated with inter-
Insomnia } mittent emotional
Sleeplessness } reactions or conflicts

307.42 Persistent disorder of initiating or maintaining sleep
Hyposomnia, insomnia, or sleeplessness associated with:
anxiety
conditioned arousal
depression (major) (minor)
psychosis
Idiopathic insomnia
Paradoxical insomnia
Primary insomnia
Psychophysiological insomnia

307.43 Transient disorder of initiating or maintaining wakefulness
Hypersomnia associated with acute or intermittent emotional reactions or conflicts

307.44 Persistent disorder of initiating or maintaining wakefulness
Hypersomnia associated with depression (major) (minor)
Insufficient sleep syndrome
Primary hypersomnia
EXCLUDES sleep deprivation (V69.4)

307.45 Circadian rhythm sleep disorder of nonorganic origin

MENTAL DISORDERS

307.46 Sleep arousal disorder
Night terror disorder
Night terrors
Sleep terror disorder
Sleepwalking
Somnambulism

DEF: Sleepwalking marked by extreme terror, panic, screaming, confusion; no recall of event upon arousal; term may refer to simply the act of sleepwalking.

307.47 Other dysfunctions of sleep stages or arousal from sleep
Nightmare disorder
Nightmares:
  NOS
  REM-sleep type
Sleep drunkenness

307.48 Repetitive intrusions of sleep
Repetitive intrusion of sleep with:
  atypical polysomnographic features
  environmental disturbances
  repeated REM-sleep interruptions

307.49 Other
"Short-sleeper"
Subjective insomnia complaint

√5th 307.5 Other and unspecified disorders of eating
EXCLUDES anorexia:
  nervosa (307.1)
  of unspecified cause (783.0)
overeating, of unspecified cause (783.6)
vomiting:
  NOS (787.0)
  cyclical (536.2)
  psychogenic (306.4)

307.50 Eating disorder, unspecified
Eating disorder NOS

307.51 Bulimia nervosa
Overeating of nonorganic origin

DEF: Mental disorder commonly characterized by binge eating followed by self-induced vomiting; perceptions of being fat; and fear the inability to stop eating voluntarily.

307.52 Pica
Perverted appetite of nonorganic origin

DEF: Compulsive eating disorder characterized by craving for substances, other than food; such as paint chips or dirt.

307.53 Rumination disorder
Regurgitation, of nonorganic origin, of food with reswallowing
EXCLUDES obsessional rumination (300.3)

307.54 Psychogenic vomiting

307.59 Other
Feeding disorder of infancy or early childhood of nonorganic origin
Infantile feeding disturbances } of nonorganic origin
Loss of appetite

307.6 Enuresis
Enuresis (primary) (secondary) of nonorganic origin
EXCLUDES enuresis of unspecified cause (788.3)

DEF: Involuntary urination past age of normal control; also called bedwetting; no trace to biological problem; focus on psychological issues.

307.7 Encopresis
Encopresis (continuous) (discontinuous) of nonorganic origin
EXCLUDES encopresis of unspecified cause (787.6)

DEF: Inability to control bowel movements; cause traced to psychological, not biological, problems.

√5th 307.8 Pain disorders related to psychological factors
307.80 Psychogenic pain, site unspecified
307.81 Tension headache
EXCLUDES headache:
  NOS (784.0)
  migraine (346.0-346.9)

AHA: N-D, '85, 16

307.89 Other
Code first to ►type or◄ site of pain
EXCLUDES pain disorder exclusively attributed to psychological factors (307.80)
psychogenic pain (307.80)

307.9 Other and unspecified special symptoms or syndromes, not elsewhere classified
Communication disorder NOS
Hair plucking
Lalling
Lisping
Masturbation
Nail-biting
Thumb-sucking

√4th 308 Acute reaction to stress
INCLUDES catastrophic stress
combat fatigue
gross stress reaction (acute)
transient disorders in response to exceptional physical or mental stress which usually subside within hours or days
EXCLUDES adjustment reaction or disorder (309.0-309.9)
chronic stress reaction (309.1-309.9)

308.0 Predominant disturbance of emotions
Anxiety
Emotional crisis } as acute reaction to exceptional [gross] stress
Panic state

308.1 Predominant disturbance of consciousness
Fugues as acute reaction to exceptional [gross] stress

308.2 Predominant psychomotor disturbance
Agitation states } as acute reaction to exceptional [gross] stress
Stupor

308.3 Other acute reactions to stress
Acute situational disturbance
Acute stress disorder
EXCLUDES prolonged posttraumatic emotional disturbance (309.81)

308.4 Mixed disorders as reaction to stress
308.9 Unspecified acute reaction to stress

√4th 309 Adjustment reaction
INCLUDES adjustment disorders
reaction (adjustment) to chronic stress
EXCLUDES acute reaction to major stress (308.0-308.9)
neurotic disorders (300.0-300.9)

309.0 Adjustment disorder with depressed mood
Grief reaction
EXCLUDES affective psychoses (296.0-296.9)
neurotic depression (300.4)
prolonged depressive reaction (309.1)
psychogenic depressive psychosis (298.0)

309.1 Prolonged depressive reaction
EXCLUDES affective psychoses (296.0-296.9)
brief depressive reaction (309.0)
neurotic depression (300.4)
psychogenic depressive psychosis (298.0)

MENTAL DISORDERS

√5th 309.2 With predominant disturbance of other emotions

309.21 Separation anxiety disorder

DEF: Abnormal apprehension by a child when physically separated from support environment; byproduct of abnormal symbiotic child-parent relationship.

309.22 Emancipation disorder of adolescence and early adult life

DEF: Adjustment reaction of late adolescence; conflict over independence from parental supervision; symptoms include difficulty in making decisions, increased reliance on parental advice, deliberate adoption of values in opposition of parents.

309.23 Specific academic or work inhibition

309.24 Adjustment disorder with anxiety

309.28 Adjustment disorder with mixed anxiety and depressed mood

Adjustment reaction with anxiety and depression

309.29 Other

Culture shock

309.3 Adjustment disorder with disturbance of conduct

Conduct disturbance } as adjustment reaction
Destructiveness

EXCLUDES: destructiveness in child (312.9)
disturbance of conduct NOS (312.9)
dyssocial behavior without manifest psychiatric disorder (V71.01-V71.02)
personality disorder with predominantly sociopathic or asocial manifestations (301.7)

309.4 Adjustment disorder with mixed disturbance of emotions and conduct

√5th 309.8 Other specified adjustment reactions

309.81 Posttraumatic stress disorder

Chronic posttraumatic stress disorder
Concentration camp syndrome
Posttraumatic stress disorder NOS
▶Post-traumatic stress disorder (PTSD)◀

EXCLUDES: acute stress disorder (308.3)
posttraumatic brain syndrome:
nonpsychotic (310.2)
psychotic (293.0-293.9)

DEF: Preoccupation with traumatic events beyond normal experience; events such as rape, personal assault, combat, natural disasters, accidents, torture precipitate disorder; also recurring flashbacks of trauma; symptoms include difficulty remembering, sleeping, or concentrating, and guilt feelings for surviving.

309.82 Adjustment reaction with physical symptoms

309.83 Adjustment reaction with withdrawal

Elective mutism as adjustment reaction
Hospitalism (in children) NOS

309.89 Other

309.9 Unspecified adjustment reaction

Adaptation reaction NOS
Adjustment reaction NOS

√4th 310 Specific nonpsychotic mental disorders due to brain damage

EXCLUDES: neuroses, personality disorders, or other nonpsychotic conditions occurring in a form similar to that seen with functional disorders but in association with a physical condition (300.0-300.9, 301.0-301.9)

310.0 Frontal lobe syndrome

Lobotomy syndrome
Postleucotomy syndrome [state]

EXCLUDES: postcontusion syndrome (310.2)

310.1 Personality change due to conditions classified elsewhere

Cognitive or personality change of other type, of nonpsychotic severity
Organic psychosyndrome of nonpsychotic severity
Presbyophrenia NOS
Senility with mental changes of nonpsychotic severity

EXCLUDES: memory loss of unknown cause (780.93)

AHA: 2Q, '05, 6

DEF: Personality disorder caused by organic factors, such as brain lesions, head trauma, or cerebrovascular accident (CVA).

310.2 Postconcussion syndrome

Postcontusion syndrome or encephalopathy
Posttraumatic brain syndrome, nonpsychotic
Status postcommotio cerebri

EXCLUDES: frontal lobe syndrome (310.0)
postencephalitic syndrome (310.8)
any organic psychotic conditions following head injury (293.0-294.0)

AHA: 4Q, '90, 24

DEF: Nonpsychotic disorder due to brain trauma, causes symptoms unrelated to any disease process; symptoms include amnesia, serial headaches, rapid heartbeat, fatigue, disrupted sleep patterns, inability to concentrate.

310.8 Other specified nonpsychotic mental disorders following organic brain damage

Mild memory disturbance
Postencephalitic syndrome
Other focal (partial) organic psychosyndromes

310.9 Unspecified nonpsychotic mental disorder following organic brain damage

AHA: 4Q, '03, 103

311 Depressive disorder, not elsewhere classified

Depressive disorder NOS   Depression NOS
Depressive state NOS

EXCLUDES: acute reaction to major stress with depressive symptoms (308.0)
affective personality disorder (301.10-301.13)
affective psychoses (296.0-296.9)
brief depressive reaction (309.0)
depressive states associated with stressful events (309.0-309.1)
disturbance of emotions specific to childhood and adolescence, with misery and unhappiness (313.1)
mixed adjustment reaction with depressive symptoms (309.4)
neurotic depression (300.4)
prolonged depressive adjustment reaction (309.1)
psychogenic depressive psychosis (298.0)

AHA: 4Q, '03, 75

MENTAL DISORDERS

312 Disturbance of conduct, not elsewhere classified ✓4th
  EXCLUDES
  adjustment reaction with disturbance of conduct (309.3)
  drug dependence (304.0-304.9)
  dyssocial behavior without manifest psychiatric disorder (V71.01-V71.02)
  personality disorder with predominantly sociopathic or asocial manifestations (301.7)
  sexual deviations (302.0-302.9)

The following fifth-digit subclassification is for use with categories 312.0-312.2:
  0 unspecified
  1 mild
  2 moderate
  3 severe

312.0 Undersocialized conduct disorder, aggressive type ✓5th
  Aggressive outburst
  Anger reaction
  Unsocialized aggressive disorder
  DEF: Mental condition identified by behaviors disrespectful of others' rights and of age-appropriate social norms or rules; symptoms include bullying, vandalism, verbal and physical abusiveness, lying, stealing, defiance.

312.1 Undersocialized conduct disorder, unaggressive type ✓5th
  Childhood truancy, unsocialized
  Solitary stealing
  Tantrums

312.2 Socialized conduct disorder ✓5th
  Childhood truancy, socialized   Group delinquency
  EXCLUDES gang activity without manifest psychiatric disorder (V71.01)

312.3 Disorders of impulse control, not elsewhere classified ✓5th
  312.30 Impulse control disorder, unspecified
  312.31 Pathological gambling
  312.32 Kleptomania
  312.33 Pyromania
  312.34 Intermittent explosive disorder
  312.35 Isolated explosive disorder
  312.39 Other
    Trichotillomania

312.4 Mixed disturbance of conduct and emotions
  Neurotic delinquency
  EXCLUDES compulsive conduct disorder (312.3)

312.8 Other specified disturbances of conduct, not elsewhere classified ✓5th
  312.81 Conduct disorder, childhood onset type
  312.82 Conduct disorder, adolescent onset type
  312.89 Other conduct disorder
    Conduct disorder of unspecified onset

312.9 Unspecified disturbance of conduct
  Delinquency (juvenile)
  Disruptive behavior disorder NOS

313 Disturbance of emotions specific to childhood and adolescence ✓4th
  EXCLUDES
  adjustment reaction (309.0-309.9)
  emotional disorder of neurotic type (300.0-300.9)
  masturbation, nail-biting, thumbsucking, and other isolated symptoms (307.0-307.9)

313.0 Overanxious disorder
  Anxiety and fearfulness ⎫ of childhood and
  Overanxious disorder   ⎭ adolescence
  EXCLUDES
  abnormal separation anxiety (309.21)
  anxiety states (300.00-300.09)
  hospitalism in children (309.83)
  phobic state (300.20-300.29)

313.1 Misery and unhappiness disorder
  EXCLUDES depressive neurosis (300.4)

313.2 Sensitivity, shyness, and social withdrawal disorder ✓5th
  EXCLUDES
  infantile autism (299.0)
  schizoid personality (301.20-301.22)
  schizophrenia (295.0-295.9)
  313.21 Shyness disorder of childhood
    Sensitivity reaction of childhood or adolescence
  313.22 Introverted disorder of childhood
    Social withdrawal   ⎫ of childhood or
    Withdrawal reaction ⎭ adolescence
  313.23 Selective mutism
    EXCLUDES elective mutism as adjustment reaction (309.83)

313.3 Relationship problems
  Sibling jealousy
  EXCLUDES relationship problems associated with aggression, destruction, or other forms of conduct disturbance (312.0-312.9)

313.8 Other or mixed emotional disturbances of childhood or adolescence ✓5th
  313.81 Oppositional defiant disorder
    DEF: Mental disorder of children noted for pervasive opposition, defiance of authority.
  313.82 Identity disorder
    Identity problem
    DEF: Distress of adolescents caused by inability to form acceptable self-identity; uncertainty about career choice, sexual orientation, moral values.
  313.83 Academic underachievement disorder
  313.89 Other P
    Reactive attachment disorder of infancy or early childhood

313.9 Unspecified emotional disturbance of childhood or adolescence P
  Mental disorder of infancy, childhood or adolescence NOS

314 Hyperkinetic syndrome of childhood ✓4th
  EXCLUDES hyperkinesis as symptom of underlying disorder—code the underlying disorder
  DEF: A behavioral disorder usually diagnosed at an early age; characterized by the inability to focus attention for a normal period of time.

314.0 Attention deficit disorder ✓5th
  Adult   Child
  314.00 Without mention of hyperactivity
    Predominantly inattentive type
    AHA: 1Q, '97, 8
  314.01 With hyperactivity
    Combined type
    Overactivity NOS
    Predominantly hyperactive/impulsive type
    Simple disturbance of attention with overactivity
    AHA: 1Q, '97, 8

314.1 Hyperkinesis with developmental delay
  Developmental disorder of hyperkinesis
  Use additional code to identify any associated neurological disorder

314.2 Hyperkinetic conduct disorder
  Hyperkinetic conduct disorder without developmental delay
  EXCLUDES hyperkinesis with significant delays in specific skills (314.1)

MENTAL DISORDERS

Tabular List

314.8 Other specified manifestations of hyperkinetic syndrome

314.9 Unspecified hyperkinetic syndrome
Hyperkinetic reaction of childhood or adolescence NOS
Hyperkinetic syndrome NOS

√4th 315 Specific delays in development
EXCLUDES: that due to a neurological disorder (320.0-389.9)

√5th 315.0 Specific reading disorder

315.00 Reading disorder, unspecified

315.01 Alexia
DEF: Lack of ability to understand written language; manifestation of aphasia.

315.02 Developmental dyslexia
DEF: Serious impairment of reading skills unexplained in relation to general intelligence and teaching processes; it can be inherited or congenital.

315.09 Other
Specific spelling difficulty

315.1 Mathematics disorder
Dyscalculia

315.2 Other specific learning difficulties
Disorder of written expression
EXCLUDES: specific arithmetical disorder (315.1)
specific reading disorder (315.00-315.09)

√5th 315.3 Developmental speech or language disorder

315.31 Expressive language disorder
Developmental aphasia
Word deafness
EXCLUDES: acquired aphasia (784.3)
elective mutism (309.83, 313.0, 313.23)

315.32 Mixed receptive-expressive language disorder
AHA: ▶2Q, '05, 5;◀ 4Q, '96, 30

315.39 Other
Developmental articulation disorder
Dyslalia
Phonological disorder
EXCLUDES: lisping and lalling (307.9)
stammering and stuttering (307.0)

315.4 Developmental coordination disorder
Clumsiness syndrome
Dyspraxia syndrome
Specific motor development disorder

315.5 Mixed development disorder
AHA: 2Q, '02, 11

315.8 Other specified delays in development

315.9 Unspecified delay in development
Developmental disorder NOS
Learning disorder NOS

316 Psychic factors associated with diseases classified elsewhere
Psychologic factors in physical conditions classified elsewhere
Use additional code to identify the associated physical condition, as:
psychogenic:
asthma (493.9)
dermatitis (692.9)
duodenal ulcer (532.0-532.9)
eczema (691.8, 692.9)
gastric ulcer (531.0-531.9)
mucous colitis (564.9)
paroxysmal tachycardia (427.2)
ulcerative colitis (556)
urticaria (708.0-708.9)
psychosocial dwarfism (259.4)
EXCLUDES: physical symptoms and physiological malfunctions, not involving tissue damage, of mental origin (306.0-306.9)

MENTAL RETARDATION (317-319)

Use additional code(s) to identify any associated psychiatric or physical condition(s)

317 Mild mental retardation
High-grade defect
IQ 50-70
Mild mental subnormality

√4th 318 Other specified mental retardation

318.0 Moderate mental retardation
IQ 35-49
Moderate mental subnormality

318.1 Severe mental retardation
IQ 20-34
Severe mental subnormality

318.2 Profound mental retardation
IQ under 20
Profound mental subnormality

319 Unspecified mental retardation
Mental deficiency NOS
Mental subnormality NOS

6. NERVOUS SYSTEM AND SENSE ORGANS (320-389)

INFLAMMATORY DISEASES OF THE CENTRAL NERVOUS SYSTEM (320-326)

✓4th 320 Bacterial meningitis

INCLUDES:
- arachnoiditis ⎫
- leptomeningitis ⎪
- meningitis ⎬ bacterial
- meningoencephalitis ⎪
- meningomyelitis ⎪
- pachymeningitis ⎭

AHA: J-F, '87, 6

DEF: Bacterial infection causing inflammation of the lining of the brain and/or spinal cord.

320.0 Hemophilus meningitis
Meningitis due to Hemophilus influenzae [H. influenzae]

320.1 Pneumococcal meningitis

320.2 Streptococcal meningitis

320.3 Staphylococcal meningitis

320.7 Meningitis in other bacterial diseases classified elsewhere
Code first underlying disease, as:
- actinomycosis (039.8)
- listeriosis (027.0)
- typhoid fever (002.0)
- whooping cough (033.0-033.9)

EXCLUDES: meningitis (in):
- epidemic (036.0)
- gonococcal (098.82)
- meningococcal (036.0)
- salmonellosis (003.21)
- syphilis:
  - NOS (094.2)
  - congenital (090.42)
  - meningovascular (094.2)
  - secondary (091.81)
- tuberculous (013.0)

✓5th 320.8 Meningitis due to other specified bacteria

320.81 Anaerobic meningitis
- Bacteroides (fragilis)
- Gram-negative anaerobes

320.82 Meningitis due to gram-negative bacteria, not elsewhere classified
- Aerobacter aerogenes
- Escherichia coli [E. coli]
- Friedländer bacillus
- Klebsiella pneumoniae
- Proteus morganii
- Pseudomonas

EXCLUDES: gram-negative anaerobes (320.81)

320.89 Meningitis due to other specified bacteria
- Bacillus pyocyaneus

320.9 Meningitis due to unspecified bacterium
Meningitis:
- bacterial NOS
- purulent NOS
- pyogenic NOS
- suppurative NOS

✓4th 321 Meningitis due to other organisms

INCLUDES:
- arachnoiditis ⎫
- leptomeningitis ⎬ due to organisms
- meningitis ⎪ other than
- pachymeningitis ⎭ bacteria

AHA: J-F, '87, 6

DEF: Infection causing inflammation of the lining of the brain and/or spinal cord, due to organisms other than bacteria.

321.0 Cryptococcal meningitis
Code first underlying disease (117.5)

321.1 Meningitis in other fungal diseases
Code first underlying disease (110.0-118)

EXCLUDES: meningitis in:
- candidiasis (112.83)
- coccidioidomycosis (114.2)
- histoplasmosis (115.01, 115.11, 115.91)

321.2 Meningitis due to viruses not elsewhere classified
Code first underlying disease, as:
- meningitis due to arbovirus (060.0-066.9)

EXCLUDES: meningitis (due to):
- abacterial (047.0-047.9)
- adenovirus (049.1)
- aseptic NOS (047.9)
- Coxsackie (virus)(047.0)
- ECHO virus (047.1)
- enterovirus (047.0-047.9)
- herpes simplex virus (054.72)
- herpes zoster virus (053.0)
- lymphocytic choriomeningitis virus (049.0)
- mumps (072.1)
- viral NOS (047.9)
- meningo-eruptive syndrome (047.1)

AHA: 4Q, '04, 51

321.3 Meningitis due to trypanosomiasis
Code first underlying disease (086.0-086.9)

321.4 Meningitis in sarcoidosis
Code first underlying disease (135)

321.8 Meningitis due to other nonbacterial organisms classified elsewhere
Code first underlying disease

EXCLUDES: leptospiral meningitis (100.81)

✓4th 322 Meningitis of unspecified cause

INCLUDES:
- arachnoiditis ⎫
- leptomeningitis ⎬ with no organism
- meningitis ⎪ specified as
- pachymeningitis ⎭ cause

AHA: J-F, '87, 6

DEF: Infection causing inflammation of the lining of the brain and/or spinal cord, due to unspecified cause.

322.0 Nonpyogenic meningitis
Meningitis with clear cerebrospinal fluid

322.1 Eosinophilic meningitis

322.2 Chronic meningitis

322.9 Meningitis, unspecified

✓4th 323 Encephalitis, myelitis, and encephalomyelitis

INCLUDES:
- acute disseminated encephalomyelitis
- meningoencephalitis, except bacterial
- meningomyelitis, except bacterial
- ▶myelitis:◀
  - ascending
  - transverse

EXCLUDES: ▶acute transverse myelitis NOS (341.20)
acute transverse myelitis in conditions classified elsewhere (341.21)◀
bacterial:
- meningoencephalitis (320.0-320.9)
- meningomyelitis (320.0-320.9)
▶idiopathic transverse myelitis (341.22)◀

DEF: Encephalitis: inflammation of brain tissues.
DEF: Myelitis: inflammation of the spinal cord.
DEF: Encephalomyelitis: inflammation of brain and spinal cord.

NERVOUS SYSTEM AND SENSE ORGANS

323.0 Encephalitis, myelitis, and encephalomyelitis in viral diseases classified elsewhere
Code first underlying disease, as:
- cat-scratch disease (078.3)
- infectious mononucleosis (075)
- ornithosis (073.7)

323.01 Encephalitis and encephalomyelitis in viral diseases classified elsewhere
EXCLUDES encephalitis (in):
- arthropod-borne viral (062.0-064)
- herpes simplex (054.3)
- mumps (072.2)
- other viral diseases of central nervous system (049.8-049.9)
- poliomyelitis (045.0-045.9)
- rubella (056.01)
- slow virus infections of central nervous system (046.0-046.9)
- viral NOS (049.9)
- West Nile (066.41)

323.02 Myelitis in viral diseases classified elsewhere
EXCLUDES myelitis (in):
- herpes simplex (054.74)
- herpes zoster (053.14)
- poliomyelitis (045.0-045.9)
- rubella (056.01)
- other viral diseases of central nervous system (049.8-049.9)

323.1 Encephalitis, myelitis, and encephalomyelitis in rickettsial diseases classified elsewhere
Code first underlying disease (080-083.9)
DEF: Inflammation of the brain caused by rickettsial disease carried by louse, tick, or mite.

323.2 Encephalitis, myelitis, and encephalomyelitis in protozoal diseases classified elsewhere
Code first underlying disease, as:
- malaria (084.0-084.9)
- trypanosomiasis (086.0-086.9)

DEF: Inflammation of the brain caused by protozoal disease carried by mosquitoes and flies.

323.4 Other encephalitis, myelitis, and encephalomyelitis due to infection classified elsewhere
Code first underlying disease

323.41 Other encephalitis and encephalomyelitis due to infection classified elsewhere
EXCLUDES encephalitis (in):
- meningococcal (036.1)
- syphilis:
  - NOS (094.81)
  - congenital (090.41)
- toxoplasmosis (130.0)
- tuberculosis (013.6)
- meningoencephalitis due to free-living ameba [Naegleria] (136.2)

323.42 Other myelitis due to infection classified elsewhere
EXCLUDES myelitis (in):
- syphilis (094.89)
- tuberculosis (013.6)

323.5 Encephalitis, myelitis, and encephalomyelitis following immunization procedures
Use additional E code to identify vaccine

323.51 Encephalitis and encephalomyelitis following immunization procedures
Encephalitis postimmunization or postvaccinal
Encephalomyelitis postimmunization or postvaccinal

323.52 Myelitis following immunization procedures
Myelitis postimmunization or postvaccinal

323.6 Postinfectious encephalitis, myelitis, and encephalomyelitis
Code first underlying disease
DEF: Infection, inflammation of brain several weeks following the outbreak of a systemic infection.

323.61 Infectious acute disseminated encephalomyelitis [ADEM]
Acute necrotizing hemorrhagic encephalopathy
EXCLUDES noninfectious acute disseminated encephalomyelitis (ADEM) (323.81)

323.62 Other postinfectious encephalitis and encephalomyelitis
EXCLUDES encephalitis:
- postchickenpox (052.0)
- postmeasles (055.0)

323.63 Postinfectious myelitis
EXCLUDES
- postchickenpox myelitis (052.2)
- herpes simplex myelitis (054.74)
- herpes zoster myelitis (053.14)

323.7 Toxic encephalitis, myelitis, and encephalomyelitis
Code first underlying cause, as:
- carbon tetrachloride (982.1)
- hydroxyquinoline derivatives (961.3)
- lead (984.0-984.9)
- mercury (985.0)
- thallium (985.8)

AHA: 2Q, '97, 8

323.71 Toxic encephalitis and encephalomyelitis
323.72 Toxic myelitis

323.8 Other causes of encephalitis, myelitis, and encephalomyelitis

323.81 Other causes of encephalitis and encephalomyelitis
Noninfectious acute disseminated encephalomyelitis (ADEM)

323.82 Other causes of myelitis
Transverse myelitis NOS

323.9 Unspecified cause of encephalitis, myelitis, and encephalomyelitis

324 Intracranial and intraspinal abscess

324.0 Intracranial abscess
Abscess (embolic):
- cerebellar
- cerebral

Abscess (embolic) of brain [any part]:
- epidural
- extradural
- otogenic
- subdural

EXCLUDES tuberculous (013.3)

324.1 Intraspinal abscess
Abscess (embolic) of spinal cord [any part]:
- epidural
- extradural
- subdural

EXCLUDES tuberculous (013.5)

NERVOUS SYSTEM AND SENSE ORGANS

324.9 Of unspecified site
  Extradural or subdural abscess NOS

325 Phlebitis and thrombophlebitis of intracranial venous sinuses

  Embolism ⎫
  Endophlebitis ⎪ of cavernous, lateral, or
  Phlebitis, septic or suppurative ⎬ other intracranial
  Thrombophlebitis ⎪ or unspecified
  Thrombosis ⎭ intracranial venous sinus

  EXCLUDES that specified as:
    complicating pregnancy, childbirth, or the puerperium (671.5)
    of nonpyogenic origin (437.6)

  DEF: Inflammation and formation of blood clot in a vein within the brain or its lining.

326 Late effects of intracranial abscess or pyogenic infection
  Note: This category is to be used to indicate conditions whose primary classification is to 320-325 [excluding 320.7, 321.0-321.8, ▶323.01-323.42,◀ 323.6-323.7] as the cause of late effects, themselves classifiable elsewhere. The "late effects" include conditions specified as such, or as sequelae, which may occur at any time after the resolution of the causal condition.
  Use additional code to identify condition, as:
    hydrocephalus (331.4)
    paralysis (342.0-342.9, 344.0-344.9)

▶ORGANIC SLEEP DISORDERS (327)◀

√4th 327 Organic sleep disorders
  AHA: 4Q, '05, 59-64

√5th 327.0 Organic disorders of initiating and maintaining sleep [Organic insomnia]
  EXCLUDES insomnia NOS (780.52)
    insomnia not due to a substance or known physiological condition (307.41-307.42)
    insomnia with sleep apnea NOS (780.51)

  327.00 Organic insomnia, unspecified
  327.01 Insomnia due to medical condition classified elsewhere
    Code first underlying condition
    EXCLUDES insomnia due to mental disorder (327.02)
  327.02 Insomnia due to mental disorder
    Code first mental disorder
    EXCLUDES alcohol induced insomnia (291.82)
      drug induced insomnia (292.85)
  327.09 Other organic insomnia

√5th 327.1 Organic disorder of excessive somnolence [Organic hypersomnia]
  EXCLUDES hypersomnia NOS (780.54)
    hypersomnia not due to a substance or known physiological condition (307.43-307.44)
    hypersomnia with sleep apnea NOS (780.53)

  327.10 Organic hypersomnia, unspecified
  327.11 Idiopathic hypersomnia with long sleep time
  327.12 Idiopathic hypersomnia without long sleep time
  327.13 Recurrent hypersomnia
    Kleine-Levin syndrome
    Menstrual related hypersomnia

  327.14 Hypersomnia due to medical condition classified elsewhere
    Code first underlying condition
    EXCLUDES hypersomnia due to mental disorder (327.15)
  327.15 Hypersomnia due to mental disorder
    Code first mental disorder
    EXCLUDES alcohol induced hypersomnia (291.82)
      drug induced hypersomnia (292.85)
  327.19 Other organic hypersomnia

√5th 327.2 Organic sleep apnea
  EXCLUDES Cheyne-Stokes breathing (786.04)
    hypersomnia with sleep apnea NOS (780.53)
    insomnia with sleep apnea NOS (780.51)
    sleep apnea in newborn (770.81-770.82)
    sleep apnea NOS (780.57)

  327.20 Organic sleep apnea, unspecified
  327.21 Primary central sleep apnea
  327.22 High altitude periodic breathing
  327.23 Obstructive sleep apnea (adult) (pediatric)
  327.24 Idiopathic sleep related nonobstructive alveolar hypoventilation
    Sleep related hypoxia
  327.25 Congenital central alveolar hypoventilation syndrome
  327.26 Sleep related hypoventilation/hypoxemia in conditions classifiable elsewhere
    Code first underlying condition
  327.27 Central sleep apnea in conditions classified elsewhere
    Code first underlying condition
  327.29 Other organic sleep apnea

√5th 327.3 Circadian rhythm sleep disorder
  Organic disorder of sleep wake cycle
  Organic disorder of sleep wake schedule
  EXCLUDES alcohol induced circadian rhythm sleep disorder (291.82)
    circadian rhythm sleep disorder of nonorganic origin (307.45)
    disruption of 24 hour sleep wake cycle NOS (780.55)
    drug induced circadian rhythm sleep disorder (292.85)

  327.30 Circadian rhythm sleep disorder, unspecified
  327.31 Circadian rhythm sleep disorder, delayed sleep phase type
  327.32 Circadian rhythm sleep disorder, advanced sleep phase type
  327.33 Circadian rhythm sleep disorder, irregular sleep-wake type
  327.34 Circadian rhythm sleep disorder, free-running type
  327.35 Circadian rhythm sleep disorder, jet lag type
  327.36 Circadian rhythm sleep disorder, shift work type
  327.37 Circadian rhythm sleep disorder in conditions classified elsewhere
    Code first underlying condition
  327.39 Other circadian rhythm sleep disorder

NERVOUS SYSTEM AND SENSE ORGANS

√5th 327.4 Organic parasomnia
> EXCLUDES alcohol induced parasomnia (291.82)
> drug induced parasomnia (292.85)
> parasomnia not due to a known physiological condition (307.47)

- **327.40** Organic parasomnia, unspecified
- **327.41** Confusional arousals
- **327.42** REM sleep behavior disorder
- **327.43** Recurrent isolated sleep paralysis
- **327.44** *Parasomnia in conditions classified elsewhere*
  Code first underlying condition
- **327.49** *Other organic parasomnia*

√5th 327.5 Organic sleep related movement disorders
> EXCLUDES ▶ restless legs syndrome (333.94) ◀
> sleep related movement disorder NOS (780.58)

- **327.51** Periodic limb movement disorder
  Periodic limb movement sleep disorder
- **327.52** Sleep related leg cramps
- **327.53** Sleep related bruxism
- **327.59** *Other organic sleep related movement disorders*

327.8 Other organic sleep disorders

HEREDITARY AND DEGENERATIVE DISEASES OF THE CENTRAL NERVOUS SYSTEM (330-337)

> EXCLUDES hepatolenticular degeneration (275.1)
> multiple sclerosis (340)
> other demyelinating diseases of central nervous system (341.0-341.9)

√4th 330 Cerebral degenerations usually manifest in childhood
Use additional code to identify associated mental retardation

- **330.0 Leukodystrophy**
  Krabbe's disease
  Leukodystrophy NOS
  globoid cell
  metachromatic
  sudanophilic
  Pelizaeus-Merzbacher disease
  Sulfatide lipidosis

  DEF: Hereditary disease of arylsulfatase or cerebroside sulfatase; characterized by a diffuse loss of myelin in CNS; infantile form causes blindness, motor disturbances, rigidity, mental deterioration and, occasionally, convulsions.

- **330.1 Cerebral lipidoses**
  Amaurotic (familial) idiocy
  Disease:
    Batten
    Jansky-Bielschowsky
    Kufs'
  Disease:
    Spielmeyer-Vogt
    Tay-Sachs
    Gangliosidosis

  DEF: Genetic disorder causing abnormal lipid accumulation in the reticuloendothelial cells of the brain.

- **330.2** *Cerebral degeneration in generalized lipidoses*
  Code first underlying disease, as:
    Fabry's disease (272.7)
    Gaucher's disease (272.7)
    Niemann-Pick disease (272.7)
    sphingolipidosis (272.7)

- **330.3** *Cerebral degeneration of childhood in other diseases classified elsewhere*
  Code first underlying disease, as:
    Hunter's disease (277.5)
    mucopolysaccharidosis (277.5)

- **330.8 Other specified cerebral degenerations in childhood**
  Alpers' disease or gray-matter degeneration
  Infantile necrotizing encephalomyelopathy
  Leigh's disease
  Subacute necrotizing encephalopathy or encephalomyelopathy

  AHA: N-D, '85, 5

- **330.9 Unspecified cerebral degeneration in childhood**

√4th 331 Other cerebral degenerations

- **331.0 Alzheimer's disease**
  AHA: 4Q, '00, 41; 4Q, '99, 7; N-D, '84, 20

  DEF: Diffuse atrophy of cerebral cortex; causing a progressive decline in intellectual and physical functions, including memory loss, personality changes and profound dementia.

- **√5th 331.1 Frontotemporal dementia**
  Use additional code for associated behavioral disturbance (294.10-294.11)

  AHA: 4Q, '03, 57

  DEF: Rare, progressive degenerative brain disease, similar to Alzheimer's; cortical atrophy affects the frontal and temporal lobes.

  - **331.11 Pick's disease**
    DEF: A less common form of progressive frontotemporal dementia with asymmetrical atrophy of the frontal and temporal regions of the cerebral cortex including abnormal rounded brain cells called Pick cells together with the presence of abnormal staining of protein (called tau) within the cells, called Pick bodies; symptoms include prominent apathy, deterioration of social skills, behavioral changes such as disinhibition and restlessness, echolalia, impairment of language, memory, and intellect, increased carelessness, poor personal hygiene, and decreased attention span.

  - **331.19** *Other frontotemporal dementia*
    Frontal dementia

- **331.2 Senile degeneration of brain**
  > EXCLUDES senility NOS (797)

- **331.3 Communicating hydrocephalus**
  > EXCLUDES congenital hydrocephalus (741.0, 742.3)

  AHA: S-O, '85, 12

  DEF: Subarachnoid hemorrhage and meningitis causing excess buildup of cerebrospinal fluid in cavities due to nonabsorption of fluid back through fluid pathways.

- **331.4 Obstructive hydrocephalus**
  Acquired hydrocephalus NOS
  > EXCLUDES congenital hydrocephalus (741.0, 742.3)

  AHA: 4Q, '03, 106; 1Q, '99, 9

  DEF: Obstruction of cerebrospinal fluid passage from brain into spinal canal.

- **331.7** *Cerebral degeneration in diseases classified elsewhere*
  Code first underlying disease, as:
    alcoholism (303.0-303.9)
    beriberi (265.0)
    cerebrovascular disease (430-438)
    congenital hydrocephalus (741.0, 742.3)
    neoplastic disease (140.0-239.9)
    myxedema (244.0-244.9)
    vitamin B_{12} deficiency (266.2)
  > EXCLUDES cerebral degeneration in:
  >   Jakob-Creutzfeldt disease (046.1)
  >   progressive multifocal leukoencephalopathy (046.3)
  >   subacute spongiform encephalopathy (046.1)

NERVOUS SYSTEM AND SENSE ORGANS

331.8 Other cerebral degeneration

331.81 Reye's syndrome

DEF: Rare childhood illness, often developed after a bout of viral upper respiratory infection; characterized by vomiting, elevated serum transaminase, changes in liver and other viscera; symptoms may be followed by an encephalopathic phase with brain swelling, disturbances of consciousness and seizures; can be fatal.

331.82 Dementia with Lewy bodies
Dementia with Parkinsonism
Lewy body dementia
Lewy body disease
Use additional code for associated behavioral disturbance (294.10-294.11)

AHA: 4Q, '03, 57

DEF: A cerebral dementia with neurophysiologic changes including increased hippocampal volume, hypoperfusion in the occipital lobes, and beta amyloid deposits with neurofibrillarity tangles, atrophy of cortex and brainstem, hallmark neuropsychologic characteristics are fluctuating cognition with pronounced variation in attention and alertness; recurrent hallucinations; and parkinsonism.

331.83 Mild cognitive impairment, so stated

EXCLUDES altered mental status (780.97)
cerebral degeneration (331.0-331.9)
change in mental status (780.97)
cognitive deficits following (late effects of) cerebral hemorrhage or infarction (438.0)
cognitive impairment due to intracranial or head injury (850-854, 959.01)
cognitive impairment due to late effect of intracranial injury (907.0)
dementia (290.0-290.43, 294.8)
mild memory disturbance (310.8)
neurologic neglect syndrome (781.8)
personality change, nonpsychotic (310.1)

331.89 Other
Cerebral ataxia

331.9 Cerebral degeneration, unspecified

332 Parkinson's disease
EXCLUDES dementia with Parkinsonism (331.82)

332.0 Paralysis agitans
Parkinsonism or Parkinson's disease:
NOS
idiopathic
primary

AHA: M-A, '87, 7

DEF: Form of parkinsonism; progressive, occurs in senior years; characterized by masklike facial expression; condition affects ability to stand erect, walk smoothly; weakened muscles, also tremble and involuntarily movement.

332.1 Secondary Parkinsonism
Neuroleptic-induced Parkinsonism
Parkinsonism due to drugs
Use additional E code to identify drug, if drug-induced

EXCLUDES Parkinsonism (in):
Huntington's disease (333.4)
progressive supranuclear palsy (333.0)
Shy-Drager syndrome (333.0)
syphilitic (094.82)

333 Other extrapyramidal disease and abnormal movement disorders

INCLUDES other forms of extrapyramidal, basal ganglia, or striatopallidal disease

EXCLUDES abnormal movements of head NOS (781.0)
sleep related movement disorders (327.51-327.59)

333.0 Other degenerative diseases of the basal ganglia
Atrophy or degeneration:
olivopontocerebellar [Déjérine-Thomas syndrome]
pigmentary pallidal [Hallervorden-Spatz disease]
striatonigral
Parkinsonian syndrome associated with:
idiopathic orthostatic hypotension
symptomatic orthostatic hypotension
Progressive supranuclear ophthalmoplegia
Shy-Drager syndrome

AHA: 3Q, '96, 8

333.1 Essential and other specified forms of tremor
Benign essential tremor
Familial tremor
Medication-induced postural tremor
Use additional E code to identify drug, if drug-induced

EXCLUDES tremor NOS (781.0)

333.2 Myoclonus
Familial essential myoclonus
Progressive myoclonic epilepsy
Unverricht-Lundborg disease
Use additional E code to identify drug, if drug-induced

AHA: 3Q, '97, 4; M-A, '87, 12

DEF: Spontaneous movements or contractions of muscles.

333.3 Tics of organic origin
Use additional E code to identify drug, if drug-induced

EXCLUDES Gilles de la Tourette's syndrome (307.23)
habit spasm (307.22)
tic NOS (307.20)

333.4 Huntington's chorea

DEF: Genetic disease; characterized by chronic progressive mental deterioration; dementia and death within 15 years of onset.

333.5 Other choreas
Hemiballism(us)
Paroxysmal choreo-athetosis
Use additional E code to identify drug, if drug-induced

EXCLUDES Sydenham's or rheumatic chorea (392.0-392.9)

333.6 Genetic torsion dystonia
Dystonia:
deformans progressiva
musculorum deformans
(Schwalbe-) Ziehen-Oppenheim disease

DEF: Sustained muscular contractions, causing twisting and repetitive movements that result in abnormal postures of trunk and limbs; etiology unknown.

333.7 Acquired torsion dystonia

333.71 Athetoid cerebral palsy
Double athetosis (syndrome)
Vogt's disease

EXCLUDES infantile cerebral palsy (343.0-343.9)

NERVOUS SYSTEM AND SENSE ORGANS

- **333.72** **Acute dystonia due to drugs**
  Acute dystonic reaction due to drugs
  Neuroleptic induced acute dystonia
  Use additional E code to identify drug
  > EXCLUDES: blepharospasm due to drugs (333.85)
  > orofacial dyskinesia due to drugs (333.85)
  > secondary Parkinsonism (332.1)
  > subacute dyskinesia due to drugs (333.85)
  > tardive dyskinesia (333.85)

- **333.79** **Other acquired torsion dystonia**

- √5th **333.8** **Fragments of torsion dystonia**
  Use additional E code to identify drug, if drug-induced

  - **333.81** **Blepharospasm**
    > EXCLUDES: blepharospasm due to drugs (333.85)
    DEF: Uncontrolled winking or blinking due to orbicularis oculi muscle spasm.

  - **333.82** **Orofacial dyskinesia**
    > EXCLUDES: orofacial dyskinesia due to drugs (333.85)
    DEF: Uncontrolled movement of mouth or facial muscles.

  - **333.83** **Spasmodic torticollis**
    > EXCLUDES: torticollis:
    > NOS (723.5)
    > hysterical (300.11)
    > psychogenic (306.0)
    DEF: Uncontrolled movement of head due to spasms of neck muscle.

  - **333.84** **Organic writers' cramp**
    > EXCLUDES: pychogenic (300.89)

  - **333.85** **Subacute dyskinesia due to drugs**
    Blepharospasm due to drugs
    Orofacial dyskinesia due to drugs
    Tardive dyskinesia
    Use additional E code to identify drug
    > EXCLUDES: acute dystonia due to drugs (333.72)
    > acute dystonic reaction due to drugs (333.72)
    > secondary Parkinsonism (332.1)

  - **333.89** **Other**

- √5th **333.9** **Other and unspecified extrapyramidal diseases and abnormal movement disorders**

  - **333.90** **Unspecified extrapyramidal disease and abnormal movement disorder**
    Medication-induced movement disorders NOS
    Use additional E code to identify drug, if drug-induced

  - **333.91** **Stiff-man syndrome**

  - **333.92** **Neuroleptic malignant syndrome**
    Use additional E code to identify drug
    > EXCLUDES: neuroleptic induced Parkinsonism (332.1)
    AHA: 4Q, '94, 37

  - **333.93** **Benign shuddering attacks**
    AHA: 4Q, '94, 37

  - **333.94** **Restless legs syndrome [RLS]**

  - **333.99** **Other**
    Neuroleptic-induced acute akathisia
    Use additional E code to identify drug, if drug-induced
    AHA: 4Q, '04, 95; 2Q, '04, 12; 4Q, '94, 37

- √4th **334** **Spinocerebellar disease**
  > EXCLUDES: olivopontocerebellar degeneration (333.0)
  > peroneal muscular atrophy (356.1)

  - **334.0** **Friedreich's ataxia**
    DEF: Genetic recessive disease of children; sclerosis of dorsal, lateral spinal cord columns; characterized by ataxia, speech impairment, swaying and irregular movements, with muscle paralysis, especially of lower limbs.

  - **334.1** **Hereditary spastic paraplegia**

  - **334.2** **Primary cerebellar degeneration**
    Cerebellar ataxia:
      Marie's
      Sanger-Brown
      Dyssynergia cerebellaris myoclonica
    Primary cerebellar degeneration:
      NOS
      hereditary
      sporadic
    AHA: M-A, '87, 9

  - **334.3** **Other cerebellar ataxia**
    Cerebellar ataxia NOS
    Use additional E code to identify drug, if drug-induced

  - **334.4** **Cerebellar ataxia in diseases classified elsewhere**
    Code first underlying disease, as:
      alcoholism (303.0-303.9)
      myxedema (244.0-244.9)
      neoplastic disease (140.0-239.9)

  - **334.8** **Other spinocerebellar diseases**
    Ataxia-telangiectasia [Louis-Bar syndrome]
    Corticostriatal-spinal degeneration

  - **334.9** **Spinocerebellar disease, unspecified**

- √4th **335** **Anterior horn cell disease**

  - **335.0** **Werdnig-Hoffmann disease**
    Infantile spinal muscular atrophy
    Progressive muscular atrophy of infancy
    DEF: Spinal muscle atrophy manifested in prenatal period or shortly after birth; symptoms include hypotonia, atrophy of skeletal muscle; death occurs in infancy.

  - √5th **335.1** **Spinal muscular atrophy**

    - **335.10** **Spinal muscular atrophy, unspecified**

    - **335.11** **Kugelberg-Welander disease**
      Spinal muscular atrophy:
        familial
        juvenile
      DEF: Hereditary; juvenile muscle atrophy; appears during first two decades of life; due to lesions of anterior horns of spinal cord; includes wasting, diminution of lower body muscles and twitching.

    - **335.19** **Other**
      Adult spinal muscular atrophy

  - √5th **335.2** **Motor neuron disease**

    - **335.20** **Amyotrophic lateral sclerosis**
      Motor neuron disease (bulbar) (mixed type)
      AHA: 4Q, '95, 81

    - **335.21** **Progressive muscular atrophy**
      Duchenne-Aran muscular atrophy
      Progressive muscular atrophy (pure)

    - **335.22** **Progressive bulbar palsy**

    - **335.23** **Pseudobulbar palsy**

    - **335.24** **Primary lateral sclerosis**

    - **335.29** **Other**

  - **335.8** **Other anterior horn cell diseases**

  - **335.9** **Anterior horn cell disease, unspecified**

NERVOUS SYSTEM AND SENSE ORGANS

√4th 336 Other diseases of spinal cord

336.0 Syringomyelia and syringobulbia
AHA: 1Q, '89, 10

336.1 Vascular myelopathies
Acute infarction of spinal cord (embolic) (nonembolic)
Arterial thrombosis of spinal cord
Edema of spinal cord
Hematomyelia
Subacute necrotic myelopathy

336.2 Subacute combined degeneration of spinal cord in diseases classified elsewhere
Code first underlying disease, as:
pernicious anemia (281.0)
other vitamin B_{12} deficiency anemia (281.1)
vitamin B_{12} deficiency (266.2)

336.3 Myelopathy in other diseases classified elsewhere
Code first underlying disease, as:
myelopathy in neoplastic disease (140.0-239.9)
EXCLUDES myelopathy in:
intervertebral disc disorder (722.70-722.73)
spondylosis (721.1, 721.41-721.42, 721.91)
AHA: 3Q, '99, 5

336.8 Other myelopathy
Myelopathy: drug-induced
Myelopathy: radiation-induced
Use additonal E code to identify cause

336.9 Unspecified disease of spinal cord
Cord compression NOS   Myelopathy NOS
EXCLUDES myelitis ▶(323.02, 323.1, 323.2, 323.42, 323.52, 323.63, 323.72, 323.82, 323.9)◀
spinal (canal) stenosis (723.0, 724.00-724.09)

√4th 337 Disorders of the autonomic nervous system
INCLUDES disorders of peripheral autonomic, sympathetic, parasympathetic, or vegetative system
EXCLUDES familial dysautonomia [Riley-Day syndrome] (742.8)

337.0 Idiopathic peripheral autonomic neuropathy
Carotid sinus syncope or syndrome
Cervical sympathetic dystrophy or paralysis

337.1 Peripheral autonomic neuropathy in disorders classified elsewhere
Code first underlying disease, as:
amyloidosis ▶(277.30-277.39)◀
diabetes (250.6)
AHA: 2Q, '93, 6; 3Q, '91, 9; N-D, '84, 9

√5th 337.2 Reflex sympathetic dystrophy
AHA: 4Q, '93, 24

DEF: Disturbance of the sympathetic nervous system evidenced by sweating, pain, pallor and edema following injury to nerves or blood vessels.

337.20 Reflex sympathetic dystrophy, unspecified
337.21 Reflex sympathetic dystrophy of the upper limb
337.22 Reflex sympathetic dystrophy of the lower limb
337.29 Reflex sympathetic dystrophy of other specified site

337.3 Autonomic dysreflexia
Use additional code to identify the cause, such as:
decubitus ulcer (707.00-707.09)
fecal impaction (560.39)
urinary tract infection (599.0)
AHA: 4Q, '98, 37

DEF: Noxious stimuli evokes paroxysmal hypertension, bradycardia, excess sweating, headache, pilomotor responses, facial flushing, and nasal congestion due to uncontrolled parasympathetic nerve response; usually occurs in patients with spinal cord injury above major sympathetic outflow tract (T_6).

337.9 Unspecified disorder of autonomic nervous system

▶**PAIN (338)**◀

√4th 338 Pain, not elsewhere classified
Use additional code to identify:
pain associated with psychological factors (307.89)
EXCLUDES generalized pain (780.96)
localized pain, unspecified type—code to pain by site
pain disorder exclusively attributed to psychological factors (307.80)

338.0 Central pain syndrome
Déjérine-Roussy syndrome
Myelopathic pain syndrome
Thalamic pain syndrome (hyperesthetic)

√5th 338.1 Acute pain
338.11 Acute pain due to trauma
338.12 Acute post-thoracotomy pain
Post-thoracotomy pain NOS
338.18 Other acute postoperative pain
Postoperative pain NOS
338.19 Other acute pain
EXCLUDES neoplasm related acute pain (338.3)

√5th 338.2 Chronic pain
EXCLUDES causalgia (355.9)
lower limb (355.71)
upper limb (354.4)
chronic pain syndrome (338.4)
myofascial pain syndrome (729.1)
neoplasm related chronic pain (338.3)
reflex sympathetic dystrophy (337.20-337.29)

338.21 Chronic pain due to trauma
338.22 Chronic post-thoracotomy pain
338.28 Other chronic postoperative pain
338.29 Other chronic pain

338.3 Neoplasm related pain (acute) (chronic)
Cancer associated pain
Pain due to malignancy (primary) (secondary)
Tumor associated pain

338.4 Chronic pain syndrome
Chronic pain associated with significant psychosocial dysfunction

OTHER DISORDERS OF THE CENTRAL NERVOUS SYSTEM (340-349)

340 Multiple sclerosis
Disseminated or multiple sclerosis:
NOS
brain stem
cord
generalized

341 Other demyelinating diseases of central nervous system

341.0 Neuromyelitis optica

341.1 Schilder's disease
Baló's concentric sclerosis
Encephalitis periaxialis:
concentrica [Baló's]
diffusa [Schilder's]

DEF: Chronic leukoencephalopathy of children and adolescents; symptoms include blindness, deafness, bilateral spasticity and progressive mental deterioration.

341.2 Acute (transverse) myelitis
EXCLUDES acute (transverse) myelitis (in) (due to):
following immunization procedures (323.52)
infection classified elsewhere (323.42)
postinfectious (323.63)
protozoal diseases classified elsewhere (323.2)
rickettsial diseases classified elsewhere (323.1)
toxic (323.72)
viral diseases classified elsewhere (323.02)
transverse myelitis NOS (323.82)

341.20 Acute (transverse) myelitis NOS

341.21 Acute (transverse) myelitis in conditions classified elsewhere
Code first underlying condition

341.22 Idiopathic transverse myelitis

341.8 Other demyelinating diseases of central nervous system
Central demyelination of corpus callosum
Central pontine myelinosis
Marchiafava (-Bignami) disease
AHA: N-D, '87, 6

341.9 Demyelinating disease of central nervous system, unspecified

342 Hemiplegia and hemiparesis
Note: This category is to be used when hemiplegia (complete) (incomplete) is reported without further specification, or is stated to be old or long-standing but of unspecified cause. The category is also for use in multiple coding to identify these types of hemiplegia resulting from any cause.

EXCLUDES congenital (343.1)
hemiplegia due to late effect of cerebrovascular accident (438.20-438.22)
infantile NOS (343.4)

The following fifth-digits are for use with codes 342.0-342.9:
0 affecting unspecified side
1 affecting dominant side
2 affecting nondominant side

AHA: 4Q, '94, 38

342.0 Flaccid hemiplegia
342.1 Spastic hemiplegia
342.8 Other specified hemiplegia
342.9 Hemiplegia, unspecified
AHA: 4Q, '98, 87

343 Infantile cerebral palsy
INCLUDES cerebral:
palsy NOS
spastic infantile paralysis
congenital spastic paralysis (cerebral)
Little's disease
paralysis (spastic) due to birth injury:
intracranial
spinal

EXCLUDES athetoid cerebral palsy (333.71)
hereditary cerebral paralysis, such as:
hereditary spastic paraplegia (334.1)
Vogt's disease (333.71)
spastic paralysis specified as noncongenital or noninfantile (344.0-344.9)

343.0 Diplegic
Congenital diplegia   Congenital paraplegia
DEF: Paralysis affecting both sides of the body simultaneously.

343.1 Hemiplegic
Congenital hemiplegia
EXCLUDES infantile hemiplegia NOS (343.4)

343.2 Quadriplegic
Tetraplegic

343.3 Monoplegic

343.4 Infantile hemiplegia
Infantile hemiplegia (postnatal) NOS

343.8 Other specified infantile cerebral palsy

343.9 Infantile cerebral palsy, unspecified
Cerebral palsy NOS
AHA: 4Q, '05, 89

344 Other paralytic syndromes
Note: This category is to be used when the listed conditions are reported without further specification or are stated to be old or long-standing but of unspecified cause. The category is also for use in multiple coding to identify these conditions resulting from any cause.

INCLUDES paralysis (complete) (incomplete), except as classifiable to 342 and 343
EXCLUDES congenital or infantile cerebral palsy (343.0-343.9)
hemiplegia (342.0-342.9)
congenital or infantile (343.1, 343.4)

344.0 Quadriplegia and quadriparesis

344.00 Quadriplegia unspecified
AHA: 4Q, '03, 103; 4Q, '98, 38

344.01 C_1-C_4 complete
344.02 C_1-C_4 incomplete
344.03 C_5-C_7 complete
344.04 C_5-C_7 incomplete
344.09 Other
AHA: 1Q, '01, 12; 4Q, '98, 39

344.1 Paraplegia
Paralysis of both lower limbs
Paraplegia (lower)
AHA: 4Q, '03, 110; M-A, '87, 10

344.2 Diplegia of upper limbs
Diplegia (upper)   Paralysis of both upper limbs

344.3 Monoplegia of lower limb
Paralysis of lower limb
EXCLUDES monoplegia of lower limb due to late effect of cerebrovascular accident (438.40-438.42)

344.30 Affecting unspecified side
344.31 Affecting dominant side
344.32 Affecting nondominant side

NERVOUS SYSTEM AND SENSE ORGANS

344.4 **Monoplegia of upper limb**
Paralysis of upper limb
> EXCLUDES: monoplegia of upper limb due to late effect of cerebrovascular accident (438.30-438.32)

- 344.40 Affecting unspecified side
- 344.41 Affecting dominant side
- 344.42 Affecting nondominant side

344.5 **Unspecified monoplegia**

344.6 **Cauda equina syndrome**
DEF: Dull pain and paresthesias in sacrum, perineum and bladder due to compression of spinal nerve roots; pain radiates down buttocks, back of thigh, calf of leg and into foot with prickling, burning sensations.

- 344.60 Without mention of neurogenic bladder
- 344.61 With neurogenic bladder
  - Acontractile bladder
  - Autonomic hyperreflexia
  - Cord bladder
  - Detrusor hyperreflexia of bladder

AHA: M-J, '87, 12; M-A, '87, 10

344.8 **Other specified paralytic syndromes**
- 344.81 Locked-in state
  AHA: 4Q, '93, 24
  DEF: State of consciousness where patients are paralyzed and unable to respond to environmental stimuli; patients have eye movements, and stimuli can enter the brain but patients cannot respond to stimuli.
- 344.89 Other specified paralytic syndrome
  AHA: 2Q, '99, 4

344.9 **Paralysis, unspecified**

345 **Epilepsy and recurrent seizures**
> EXCLUDES: progressive myoclonic epilepsy (333.2)

The following fifth-digit subclassification is for use with categories 345.0, .1, .4–.9:
- 0 without mention of intractable epilepsy
- 1 with intractable epilepsy

AHA: 1Q, '93, 24; 2Q, '92, 8 4Q, '92, 23

DEF: Brain disorder characterized by electrical-like disturbances; may include occasional impairment or loss of consciousness, abnormal motor phenomena and psychic or sensory disturbances.

345.0 **Generalized nonconvulsive epilepsy**
- Absences:
  - atonic
  - typical
- Minor epilepsy
- Petit mal
- Pykno-epilepsy
- Seizures:
  - akinetic
  - atonic

AHA: For code 345.00: 1Q, '04, 18

345.1 **Generalized convulsive epilepsy**
- Epileptic seizures:
  - clonic
  - myoclonic
  - tonic
- Epileptic seizures:
  - tonic-clonic
  - Grand mal
  - Major epilepsy

> EXCLUDES: convulsions:
> NOS (780.39)
> infantile (780.39)
> newborn (779.0)
> infantile spasms (345.6)

AHA: 3Q, '97, 4

DEF: Convulsive seizures with tension of limbs (tonic) or rhythmic contractions (clonic).

345.2 **Petit mal status**
Epileptic absence status
DEF: Minor myoclonic spasms and sudden momentary loss of consciousness in epilepsy.

345.3 **Grand mal status**
Status epilepticus NOS
> EXCLUDES: epilepsia partialis continua (345.7)
> status:
> psychomotor (345.7)
> temporal lobe (345.7)

AHA: 3Q, '05, 12

DEF: Sudden loss of consciousness followed by generalized convulsions in epilepsy.

345.4 **Localization-related (focal) (partial) epilepsy and epileptic syndromes with complex partial seizures**
Epilepsy:
- limbic system
- partial:
  - secondarily generalized
  - ▶with impairment of consciousness◀
  - with memory and ideational disturbances
- psychomotor
- psychosensory
- temporal lobe
Epileptic automatism

345.5 **Localization-related (focal) (partial) epilepsy and epileptic syndromes with simple partial seizures**
Epilepsy:
- Bravais-Jacksonian NOS
- focal (motor) NOS
- Jacksonian NOS
- motor partial
- partial NOS:
  - ▶without impairment of consciousness◀
- sensory-induced
- somatomotor
- somatosensory
- visceral
- visual

345.6 **Infantile spasms**
- Hypsarrhythmia
- Lightning spasms
- Salaam attacks

> EXCLUDES: salaam tic (781.0)

AHA: N-D, '84, 12

345.7 **Epilepsia partialis continua**
Kojevnikov's epilepsy
DEF: Continuous muscle contractions and relaxation; result of abnormal neural discharge.

345.8 **Other forms of epilepsy and recurrent seizures**
Epilepsy:
- cursive [running]
Epilepsy:
- gelastic

345.9 **Epilepsy, unspecified**
Epileptic convulsions, fits, or seizures NOS
▶Recurrent seizures NOS
Seizure disorder NOS◀

> EXCLUDES: ▶convulsion (convulsive) disorder (780.39)◀
> convulsive seizure or fit NOS
> ▶(780.39)◀
> ▶recurrent convulsions (780.39)◀

AHA: N-D, '87, 12

346 **Migraine**
DEF: Benign vascular headache of extreme pain; commonly associated with irritability, nausea, vomiting and often photophobia; premonitory visual hallucination of a crescent in the visual field (scotoma).

The following fifth-digit subclassification is for use with category 346:
- 0 without mention of intractable migraine
- 1 with intractable migraine, so stated

346.0 **Classical migraine**
Migraine preceded or accompanied by transient focal neurological phenomena
Migraine with aura

NERVOUS SYSTEM AND SENSE ORGANS

346.1 ✓5th **Common migraine**
  Atypical migraine
  Sick headache

346.2 ✓5th **Variants of migraine**
  Cluster headache
  Histamine cephalgia
  Horton's neuralgia
  Migraine:
    abdominal
    basilar
  Migraine:
    lower half
    retinal
  Neuralgia:
    ciliary
    migrainous

346.8 ✓5th **Other forms of migraine**
  Migraine:
    hemiplegic
  Migraine:
    ophthalmoplegic

346.9 ✓5th **Migraine, unspecified**
  AHA: N-D, '85, 16

347 ✓4th **Cataplexy and narcolepsy**
  DEF: Cataplexy: sudden onset of muscle weakness with loss of tone and strength; caused by aggressive or spontaneous emotions.
  DEF: Narcolepsy: brief, recurrent, uncontrollable episodes of sound sleep.

347.0 ✓5th **Narcolepsy**
  347.00 Without cataplexy
    Narcolepsy NOS
  347.01 With cataplexy

347.1 ✓5th **Narcolepsy in conditions classified elsewhere**
  Code first underlying condition
  347.10 Without cataplexy
  347.11 With cataplexy

348 ✓4th **Other conditions of brain**

348.0 Cerebral cysts
  Arachnoid cyst
  Porencephalic cyst
  Porencephaly, acquired
  Pseudoporencephaly
  EXCLUDES porencephaly (congenital) (742.4)

348.1 Anoxic brain damage
  EXCLUDES that occurring in:
    abortion (634-638 with .7, 639.8)
    ectopic or molar pregnancy (639.8)
    labor or delivery (668.2, 669.4)
  that of newborn (767.0, 768.0-768.9, 772.1-772.2)
  Use additional E code to identify cause
  DEF: Brain injury due to lack of oxygen, other than birth trauma.

348.2 Benign intracranial hypertension
  Pseudotumor cerebri
  EXCLUDES hypertensive encephalopathy (437.2)
  DEF: Elevated pressure in brain due to fluid retention in brain cavities.

348.3 ✓5th **Encephalopathy, not elsewhere classified**
  AHA: 4Q, '03, 58; 3Q, '97, 4
  348.30 Encephalopathy, unspecified
  348.31 Metabolic encephalopathy
    Septic encephalopathy
    EXCLUDES ▶toxic metabolic encephalopathy (349.82)◀

348.39 Other encephalopathy
  EXCLUDES encephalopathy:
    alcoholic (291.2)
    hepatic (572.2)
    hypertensive (437.2)
    toxic (349.82)

348.4 Compression of brain
  Compression } brain (stem)
  Herniation
  Posterior fossa compression syndrome
  AHA: 4Q, '94, 37
  DEF: Elevated pressure in brain due to blood clot, tumor, fracture, abscess, other condition.

348.5 Cerebral edema
  DEF: Elevated pressure in the brain due to fluid retention in brain tissues.

348.8 Other conditions of brain
  Cerebral:
    calcification
  Cerebral:
    fungus
  AHA: S-O, '87, 9

348.9 Unspecified condition of brain

349 ✓4th **Other and unspecified disorders of the nervous system**

349.0 Reaction to spinal or lumbar puncture
  Headache following lumbar puncture
  AHA: 2Q, '99, 9; 3Q, '90, 18

349.1 Nervous system complications from surgically implanted device
  EXCLUDES immediate postoperative complications (997.00-997.09)
  mechanical complications of nervous system device (996.2)

349.2 Disorders of meninges, not elsewhere classified
  Adhesions, meningeal (cerebral) (spinal)
  Cyst, spinal meninges
  Meningocele, acquired
  Pseudomeningocele, acquired
  AHA: 2Q, '98, 18; 3Q, '94, 4

349.8 ✓5th **Other specified disorders of nervous system**
  349.81 Cerebrospinal fluid rhinorrhea
    EXCLUDES cerebrospinal fluid otorrhea (388.61)
    DEF: Cerebrospinal fluid discharging from the nose; caused by fracture of frontal bone with tearing of dura mater and arachnoid.
  349.82 Toxic encephalopathy
    ▶Toxic metabolic encephalopathy◀
    Use additional E code, if desired, to identify cause
    AHA 4Q, '93, 29
    DEF: Brain tissue degeneration due to toxic substance.
  349.89 Other

349.9 Unspecified disorders of nervous system
  Disorder of nervous system (central) NOS

Cranial Nerves
- Olfactory bulb (I)
- Optic nerve (II)
- Oculomotor nerve (III)
- Trochlear nerve (IV)
- Trigeminal nerve (V)
- Abducens nerve (VI)
- Pons
- Facial nerve (VII)
- Vestibulocochlear nerve (VIII)
- Glossopharyngeal nerve (IX)
- Vagus nerve (X)
- Accessory nerve (XI)
- Hypoglossal nerve (XII)

N Newborn Age: 0 P Pediatric Age: 0-17 M Maternity Age: 12-55 A Adult Age: 15-124

NERVOUS SYSTEM AND SENSE ORGANS

DISORDERS OF THE PERIPHERAL NERVOUS SYSTEM (350-359)

EXCLUDES diseases of:
    acoustic [8th] nerve (388.5)
    oculomotor [3rd, 4th, 6th] nerves (378.0-378.9)
    optic [2nd] nerve (377.0-377.9)
    peripheral autonomic nerves (337.0-337.9)
    neuralgia
    neuritis } NOS or "rheumatic" (729.2)
    radiculitis
    peripheral neuritis in pregnancy (646.4)

✓4th 350 Trigeminal nerve disorders
INCLUDES disorders of 5th cranial nerve

350.1 Trigeminal neuralgia
    Tic douloureux   Trigeminal neuralgia NOS
    Trifacial neuralgia
    EXCLUDES postherpetic (053.12)

350.2 Atypical face pain

350.8 Other specified trigeminal nerve disorders

350.9 Trigeminal nerve disorder, unspecified

✓4th 351 Facial nerve disorders
INCLUDES disorders of 7th cranial nerve
EXCLUDES that in newborn (767.5)

351.0 Bell's palsy
    Facial palsy
    DEF: Unilateral paralysis of face due to lesion on facial nerve; produces facial distortion.

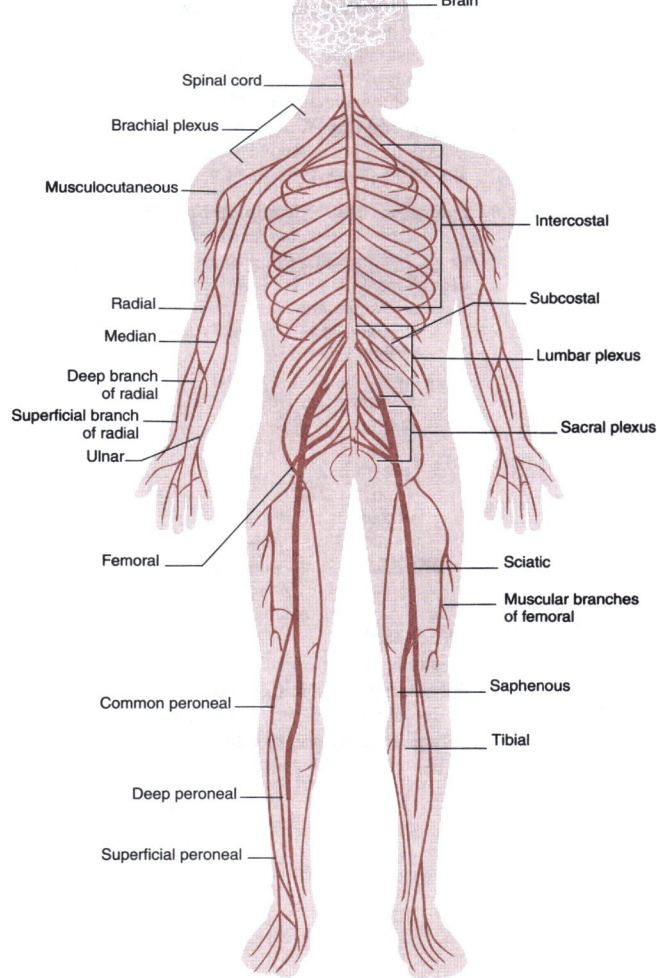
Peripheral Nervous System

351.1 Geniculate ganglionitis
    Geniculate ganglionitis NOS
    EXCLUDES herpetic (053.11)
    DEF: Inflammation of tissue at bend in facial nerve.

351.8 Other facial nerve disorders
    Facial myokymia   Melkersson's syndrome
    AHA: 3Q, '02, 13

351.9 Facial nerve disorder, unspecified

✓4th 352 Disorders of other cranial nerves

352.0 Disorders of olfactory [1st] nerve

352.1 Glossopharyngeal neuralgia
    AHA: 2Q, '02, 8
    DEF: Pain between throat and ear along petrosal and jugular ganglia.

352.2 Other disorders of glossopharyngeal [9th] nerve

352.3 Disorders of pneumogastric [10th] nerve
    Disorders of vagal nerve
    EXCLUDES paralysis of vocal cords or larynx (478.30-478.34)
    DEF: Nerve disorder affecting ear, tongue, pharynx, larynx, esophagus, viscera and thorax.

352.4 Disorders of accessory [11th] nerve
    DEF: Nerve disorder affecting palate, pharynx, larynx, thoracic viscera, sternocleidomastoid and trapezius muscles.

352.5 Disorders of hypoglossal [12th] nerve
    DEF: Nerve disorder affecting tongue muscles.

352.6 Multiple cranial nerve palsies
    Collet-Sicard syndrome   Polyneuritis cranialis

352.9 Unspecified disorder of cranial nerves

✓4th 353 Nerve root and plexus disorders
EXCLUDES conditions due to:
    intervertebral disc disorders (722.0-722.9)
    spondylosis (720.0-721.9)
    vertebrogenic disorders (723.0-724.9)

353.0 Brachial plexus lesions
    Cervical rib syndrome
    Costoclavicular syndrome
    Scalenus anticus syndrome
    Thoracic outlet syndrome
    EXCLUDES brachial neuritis or radiculitis NOS (723.4)
    that in newborn (767.6)
    DEF: Acquired disorder in tissue along nerves in shoulder; causes corresponding motor and sensory dysfunction.

353.1 Lumbosacral plexus lesions
    DEF: Acquired disorder in tissue along nerves in lower back; causes corresponding motor and sensory dysfunction.

353.2 Cervical root lesions, not elsewhere classified

353.3 Thoracic root lesions, not elsewhere classified

353.4 Lumbosacral root lesions, not elsewhere classified

353.5 Neuralgic amyotrophy
    Parsonage-Aldren-Turner syndrome

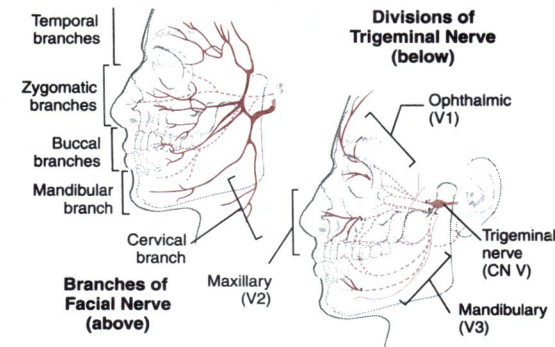
Trigeminal and Facial Nerve Branches

✓4th / ✓5th Additional Digit Required   Unspecified Code   Other Specified Code   Manifestation Code   ▶◀ Revised Text   ● New Code   ▲ Revised Code Title

NERVOUS SYSTEM AND SENSE ORGANS

353.6 Phantom limb (syndrome)
DEF: Abnormal tingling or a burning sensation, transient aches, and intermittent or continuous pain perceived as originating in the absent limb.

353.8 Other nerve root and plexus disorders

353.9 Unspecified nerve root and plexus disorder

354 Mononeuritis of upper limb and mononeuritis multiplex
DEF: Inflammation of a single nerve; known as mononeuritis multiplex when several nerves in unrelated body areas are affected.

354.0 Carpal tunnel syndrome
Median nerve entrapment   Partial thenar atrophy
DEF: Compression of median nerve by tendons; causes pain, tingling, numbness and burning sensation in hand.

354.1 Other lesion of median nerve
Median nerve neuritis

354.2 Lesion of ulnar nerve
Cubital tunnel syndrome
Tardy ulnar nerve palsy

354.3 Lesion of radial nerve
Acute radial nerve palsy
AHA: N-D, '87, 6

354.4 Causalgia of upper limb
EXCLUDES causalgia:
    NOS (355.9)
    lower limb (355.71)
DEF: Peripheral nerve damage, upper limb; usually due to injury; causes burning sensation and trophic skin changes.

354.5 Mononeuritis multiplex
Combinations of single conditions classifiable to 354 or 355

354.8 Other mononeuritis of upper limb

354.9 Mononeuritis of upper limb, unspecified

355 Mononeuritis of lower limb

355.0 Lesion of sciatic nerve
EXCLUDES sciatica NOS (724.3)
AHA: 2Q, '89, 12
DEF: Acquired disorder of sciatic nerve; causes motor and sensory dysfunction in back, buttock and leg.

355.1 Meralgia paresthetica
Lateral cutaneous femoral nerve of thigh compression or syndrome
DEF: Inguinal ligament entraps lateral femoral cutaneous nerve; causes tingling, pain and numbness along outer thigh.

355.2 Other lesion of femoral nerve

355.3 Lesion of lateral popliteal nerve
Lesion of common peroneal nerve

355.4 Lesion of medial popliteal nerve

355.5 Tarsal tunnel syndrome
DEF: Compressed, entrapped posterior tibial nerve; causes tingling, pain and numbness in sole of foot.

355.6 Lesion of plantar nerve
Morton's metatarsalgia, neuralgia, or neuroma

355.7 Other mononeuritis of lower limb
355.71 Causalgia of lower limb
EXCLUDES causalgia:
    NOS (355.9)
    upper limb (354.4)
DEF: Dysfunction of lower limb peripheral nerve, usually due to injury; causes burning pain and trophic skin changes.

355.79 Other mononeuritis of lower limb

355.8 Mononeuritis of lower limb, unspecified

355.9 Mononeuritis of unspecified site
Causalgia NOS
EXCLUDES causalgia:
    lower limb (355.71)
    upper limb (354.4)

356 Hereditary and idiopathic peripheral neuropathy

356.0 Hereditary peripheral neuropathy
Déjérine-Sottas disease

356.1 Peroneal muscular atrophy
Charcôt-Marie-Tooth disease
Neuropathic muscular atrophy
DEF: Genetic disorder, in muscles innervated by peroneal nerves; symptoms include muscle wasting in lower limbs and locomotor difficulties.

356.2 Hereditary sensory neuropathy
DEF: Inherited disorder in dorsal root ganglia, optic nerve, and cerebellum, causing sensory losses, shooting pains, and foot ulcers.

356.3 Refsum's disease
Heredopathia atactica polyneuritiformis
DEF: Genetic disorder of lipid metabolism; causes persistent, painful inflammation of nerves and retinitis pigmentosa.

356.4 Idiopathic progressive polyneuropathy

356.8 Other specified idiopathic peripheral neuropathy
Supranuclear paralysis

356.9 Unspecified

357 Inflammatory and toxic neuropathy

357.0 Acute infective polyneuritis
Guillain-Barré syndrome Postinfectious polyneuritis
AHA: 2Q, '98, 12
DEF: Guillain-Barré syndrome: acute demyelinatry polyneuropathy preceded by viral illness (i.e., herpes, cytomegalovirus [CMV], Epstein-Barr virus [EBV]) or a bacterial illness; areflexic motor paralysis with mild sensory disturbance and acellular rise in spinal fluid protein.

357.1 Polyneuropathy in collagen vascular disease
Code first underlying disease, as:
    disseminated lupus erythematosus (710.0)
    polyarteritis nodosa (446.0)
    rheumatoid arthritis (714.0)

357.2 Polyneuropathy in diabetes
Code first underlying disease (250.6)
AHA: 4Q, '03, 105; 2Q, '92, 15; 3Q, '91, 9

357.3 Polyneuropathy in malignant disease
Code first underlying disease (140.0-208.9)

357.4 Polyneuropathy in other diseases classified elsewhere
Code first underlying disease, as:
    amyloidosis ▶(277.30-277.39)◀
    beriberi (265.0)
    ▶chronic uremia (585.9)◀
    deficiency of B vitamins (266.0-266.9)
    diphtheria (032.0-032.9)
    hypoglycemia (251.2)
    pellagra (265.2)
    porphyria (277.1)
    sarcoidosis (135)
    uremia ▶NOS (586)◀
EXCLUDES polyneuropathy in:
    herpes zoster (053.13)
    mumps (072.72)
AHA: 2Q, '98, 15

357.5 Alcoholic polyneuropathy

357.6 Polyneuropathy due to drugs
Use additional E code to identify drug

357.7 Polyneuropathy due to other toxic agents
Use additional E code to identify toxic agent

NERVOUS SYSTEM AND SENSE ORGANS

√5ᵗʰ 357.8 Other
AHA: 4Q, '02, 47; 2Q, '98, 12

357.81 Chronic inflammatory demyelinating polyneuritis
DEF: Chronic inflammatory demyelinating polyneuritis: inflammation of peripheral nerves resulting in destruction of myelin sheath; associated with diabetes mellitus, dysproteinemias, renal failure and malnutrition; symptoms include tingling, numbness, burning pain, diminished tendon reflexes, weakness, and atrophy in lower extremities.

357.82 Critical illness polyneuropathy
Acute motor neuropathy
AHA: 4Q, '03, 111
DEF: An acute axonal neuropathy, both sensory and motor, that is associated with Systemic Inflammatory Response Syndrome (SIRS).

357.89 Other inflammatory and toxic neuropathy

357.9 Unspecified

√4ᵗʰ 358 Myoneural disorders

√5ᵗʰ 358.0 Myasthenia gravis
AHA: 4Q, '03, 59
DEF: Autoimmune disorder of acetylcholine at neuromuscular junction; causing fatigue of voluntary muscles.

358.00 Myasthenia gravis without (acute) exacerbation
Myasthenia gravis NOS

358.01 Myasthenia gravis with (acute) exacerbation
Myasthenia gravis in crisis
AHA: 1Q, '05, 4; 4Q, '04, 139

358.1 Myasthenic syndromes in diseases classified elsewhere
Amyotrophy } from stated cause classified elsewhere
Eaton-Lambert syndrome
Code first underlying disease, as:
  botulism (005.1)
  diabetes mellitus (250.6)
  hypothyroidism (244.0-244.9)
  malignant neoplasm (140.0-208.9)
  pernicious anemia (281.0)
  thyrotoxicosis (242.0-242.9)

358.2 Toxic myoneural disorders
Use additional E code to identify toxic agent

358.8 Other specified myoneural disorders

358.9 Myoneural disorders, unspecified
AHA: 2Q, '02, 16

√4ᵗʰ 359 Muscular dystrophies and other myopathies
EXCLUDES   idiopathic polymyositis (710.4)

359.0 Congenital hereditary muscular dystrophy
Benign congenital myopathy
Central core disease
Centronuclear myopathy
Myotubular myopathy
Nemaline body disease
EXCLUDES   arthrogryposis multiplex congenita (754.89)
DEF: Genetic disorder; causing progressive or nonprogressive muscle weakness.

359.1 Hereditary progressive muscular dystrophy
Muscular dystrophy: Muscular dystrophy:
  NOS   Gower's
  distal   Landouzy-Déjérine
  Duchenne   limb-girdle
  Erb's   ocular
  fascioscapulohumeral   oculopharyngeal
DEF: Genetic degenerative, muscle disease; causes progressive weakness, wasting of muscle with no nerve involvement.

359.2 Myotonic disorders
Dystrophia myotonica   Paramyotonia congenita
Eulenburg's disease   Steinert's disease
Myotonia congenita   Thomsen's disease
DEF: Impaired movement due to spasmatic, rigid muscles.

359.3 Familial periodic paralysis
Hypokalemic familial periodic paralysis
DEF: Genetic disorder; characterized by rapidly progressive flaccid paralysis; attacks often occur after exercise or exposure to cold or dietary changes.

359.4 Toxic myopathy
Use additional E code to identify toxic agent
AHA: 1Q, '88, 5
DEF: Muscle disorder caused by toxic agent.

359.5 Myopathy in endocrine diseases classified elsewhere
Code first underlying disease, as:
  Addison's disease (255.4)
  Cushing's syndrome (255.0)
  hypopituitarism (253.2)
  myxedema (244.0-244.9)
  thyrotoxicosis (242.0-242.9)
DEF: Muscle disorder secondary to dysfunction in hormone secretion.

359.6 Symptomatic inflammatory myopathy in diseases classified elsewhere
Code first underlying disease, as:
  amyloidosis ▶(277.30-277.39)◀
  disseminated lupus erythematosus (710.0)
  malignant neoplasm (140.0-208.9)
  polyarteritis nodosa (446.0)
  rheumatoid arthritis (714.0)
  sarcoidosis (135)
  scleroderma (710.1)
  Sjögren's disease (710.2)

√5ᵗʰ 359.8 Other myopathies
AHA: 4Q, '02, 47; 3Q, '90, 17

359.81 Critical illness myopathy
Acute necrotizing myopathy
Acute quadriplegic myopathy
Intensive care (ICU) myopathy
Myopathy of critical illness

359.89 Other myopathies

359.9 Myopathy, unspecified

DISORDERS OF THE EYE AND ADNEXA (360-379)

√4ᵗʰ 360 Disorders of the globe
INCLUDES   disorders affecting multiple structures of eye

√5ᵗʰ 360.0 Purulent endophthalmitis
EXCLUDES ▶ bleb associated endophthalmitis (379.63)◀

360.00 Purulent endophthalmitis, unspecified
360.01 Acute endophthalmitis
360.02 Panophthalmitis
360.03 Chronic endophthalmitis
360.04 Vitreous abscess

√5ᵗʰ 360.1 Other endophthalmitis
EXCLUDES ▶ bleb associated endophthalmitis (379.63)◀

360.11 Sympathetic uveitis
DEF: Inflammation of vascular layer of uninjured eye; follows injury to other eye.

360.12 Panuveitis
DEF: Inflammation of entire vascular layer of eye, including choroid, iris and ciliary body.

360.13 Parasitic endophthalmitis NOS
DEF: Parasitic infection causing inflammation of the entire eye.

360.14–360.9 NERVOUS SYSTEM AND SENSE ORGANS

360.14 **Ophthalmia nodosa**
DEF: Conjunctival inflammation caused by embedded hairs.

360.19 **Other**
Phacoanaphylactic endophthalmitis

√5th 360.2 **Degenerative disorders of globe**
AHA: 3Q, '91, 3

360.20 **Degenerative disorder of globe, unspecified**

360.21 **Progressive high (degenerative) myopia**
Malignant myopia
DEF: Severe, progressive nearsightedness in adults, complicated by serious disease of the choroid; leads to retinal detachment and blindness.

360.23 **Siderosis**
DEF: Iron pigment deposits within tissue of eyeball; caused by high iron content of blood.

360.24 **Other metallosis**
Chalcosis
DEF: Metal deposits, other than iron, within eyeball tissues.

360.29 **Other**
EXCLUDES: xerophthalmia (264.7)

√5th 360.3 **Hypotony of eye**
360.30 **Hypotony, unspecified**
DEF: Low osmotic pressure causing lack of tone, tension and strength.

360.31 **Primary hypotony**
360.32 **Ocular fistula causing hypotony**
DEF: Low intraocular pressure due to leak through abnormal passage.

360.33 **Hypotony associated with other ocular disorders**
360.34 **Flat anterior chamber**
DEF: Low pressure behind cornea, causing compression.

√5th 360.4 **Degenerated conditions of globe**
360.40 **Degenerated globe or eye, unspecified**
360.41 **Blind hypotensive eye**
Atrophy of globe
Phthisis bulbi
DEF: Vision loss due to extremely low intraocular pressure.

360.42 **Blind hypertensive eye**
Absolute glaucoma
DEF: Vision loss due to painful, high intraocular pressure.

360.43 **Hemophthalmos, except current injury**
EXCLUDES: traumatic (871.0-871.9, 921.0-921.9)
DEF: Pool of blood within eyeball, not from current injury.

360.44 **Leucocoria**
DEF: Whitish mass or reflex in the pupil behind lens; also called cat's eye reflex; often indicative of retinoblastoma.

√5th 360.5 **Retained (old) intraocular foreign body, magnetic**
EXCLUDES: current penetrating injury with magnetic foreign body (871.5)
retained (old) foreign body of orbit (376.6)

360.50 **Foreign body, magnetic, intraocular, unspecified**
360.51 Foreign body, magnetic, in anterior chamber
360.52 Foreign body, magnetic, in iris or ciliary body
360.53 Foreign body, magnetic, in lens
360.54 Foreign body, magnetic, in vitreous
360.55 Foreign body, magnetic, in posterior wall
360.59 **Foreign body, magnetic, in other or multiple sites**

√5th 360.6 **Retained (old) intraocular foreign body, nonmagnetic**
Retained (old) foreign body:
  NOS
  nonmagnetic
EXCLUDES: current penetrating injury with (nonmagnetic) foreign body (871.6)
retained (old) foreign body in orbit (376.6)

360.60 **Foreign body, intraocular, unspecified**
360.61 Foreign body in anterior chamber
360.62 Foreign body in iris or ciliary body
360.63 Foreign body in lens
360.64 Foreign body in vitreous
360.65 Foreign body in posterior wall
360.69 **Foreign body in other or multiple sites**

√5th 360.8 **Other disorders of globe**
360.81 Luxation of globe
DEF: Displacement of eyeball.

360.89 **Other**

360.9 **Unspecified disorder of globe**

NERVOUS SYSTEM AND SENSE ORGANS

✓4th 361 Retinal detachments and defects
DEF: Light-sensitive layer at back of eye, separates from blood supply; disrupting vision.

✓5th 361.0 Retinal detachment with retinal defect
Rhegmatogenous retinal detachment
EXCLUDES: detachment of retinal pigment epithelium (362.42-362.43)
retinal detachment (serous) (without defect) (361.2)

- 361.00 Retinal detachment with retinal defect, unspecified
- 361.01 Recent detachment, partial, with single defect
- 361.02 Recent detachment, partial, with multiple defects
- 361.03 Recent detachment, partial, with giant tear
- 361.04 Recent detachment, partial, with retinal dialysis
  Dialysis (juvenile) of retina (with detachment)
- 361.05 Recent detachment, total or subtotal
- 361.06 Old detachment, partial
  Delimited old retinal detachment
- 361.07 Old detachment, total or subtotal

✓5th 361.1 Retinoschisis and retinal cysts
EXCLUDES: juvenile retinoschisis (362.73)
microcystoid degeneration of retina (362.62)
parasitic cyst of retina (360.13)

- 361.10 Retinoschisis, unspecified
  DEF: Separation of retina due to degenerative process of aging; should not be confused with acute retinal detachment.
- 361.11 Flat retinoschisis
  DEF: Slow, progressive split of retinal sensory layers.
- 361.12 Bullous retinoschisis
  DEF: Fluid retention between split retinal sensory layers.
- 361.13 Primary retinal cysts
- 361.14 Secondary retinal cysts
- 361.19 Other
  Pseudocyst of retina

361.2 Serous retinal detachment
Retinal detachment without retinal defect
EXCLUDES: central serous retinopathy (362.41)
retinal pigment epithelium detachment (362.42-362.43)

✓5th 361.3 Retinal defects without detachment
EXCLUDES: chorioretinal scars after surgery for detachment (363.30-363.35)
peripheral retinal degeneration without defect (362.60-362.66)

- 361.30 Retinal defect, unspecified
  Retinal break(s) NOS
- 361.31 Round hole of retina without detachment
- 361.32 Horseshoe tear of retina without detachment
  Operculum of retina without mention of detachment
- 361.33 Multiple defects of retina without detachment

✓5th 361.8 Other forms of retinal detachment
- 361.81 Traction detachment of retina
  Traction detachment with vitreoretinal organization
- 361.89 Other
  AHA: 3Q, '99, 12

361.9 Unspecified retinal detachment
AHA: N-D, '87, 10

✓4th 362 Other retinal disorders
EXCLUDES: chorioretinal scars (363.30-363.35)
chorioretinitis (363.0-363.2)

✓5th 362.0 Diabetic retinopathy
Code first diabetes (250.5)
AHA: ▶4Q, '05, 65;◄ 3Q, '91, 8
DEF: Retinal changes in diabetes of long duration; causes hemorrhages, microaneurysms, waxy deposits and proliferative noninflammatory degenerative disease of retina.

- 362.01 Background diabetic retinopathy
  Diabetic retinal microaneurysms
  Diabetic retinopathy NOS
- 362.02 Proliferative diabetic retinopathy
  AHA: 3Q, '96, 5
  DEF: ▶Occurrence of the ischemic effects of vessel blockages result in neovascularization; new blood vessels begin to form to compensate for restricted blood flow; multiple areas of the retina and inner vitreous may be affected.◄
- 362.03 Nonproliferative diabetic retinopathy NOS
- 362.04 Mild nonproliferative diabetic retinopathy
  DEF: ▶Early stages of degenerative condition of the retina due to diabetes; microaneurysm formation; small balloon-like swelling of the retinal vessels.◄
- 362.05 Moderate nonproliferative diabetic retinopathy
  DEF: ▶Stage of degenerative condition of the retina due to diabetes with pronounced microaneurysms; vessel blockages can occur.◄
- 362.06 Severe nonproliferative diabetic retinopathy
  AHA: ▶4Q, '05, 67◄
  DEF: ▶Stage of degenerative condition of the retina due to diabetes in which vascular breakdown in the retina results in multiple vascular blockages, or "beadings," intraretinal hemorrhages can be numerous.◄
- 362.07 Diabetic macular edema
  Note: Code 362.07 must be used with a code for diabetic retinopathy (362.01-362.06)
  Diabetic retinal edema
  DEF: ▶Leakage from retinal blood vessels causes swelling of the macula and impaired vision; exudates or plaques may develop in the posterior pole of the retina due to the breakdown of retinal vasculature.◄

✓5th 362.1 Other background retinopathy and retinal vascular changes
- 362.10 Background retinopathy, unspecified
- 362.11 Hypertensive retinopathy
  AHA: 3Q, '90, 3
  DEF: Retinal irregularities caused by systemic hypertension.
- 362.12 Exudative retinopathy
  Coats' syndrome
  AHA: 3Q, '99, 12

362.13 Changes in vascular appearance
Vascular sheathing of retina
Use additional code for any associated atherosclerosis (440.8)

362.14 Retinal microaneurysms NOS
DEF: Microscopic dilation of retinal vessels in nondiabetic.

362.15 Retinal telangiectasia
DEF: Dilation of blood vessels of the retina.

362.16 Retinal neovascularization NOS
Neovascularization: choroidal
Neovascularization: subretinal
DEF: New and abnormal vascular growth in the retina.

362.17 Other intraretinal microvascular abnormalities
Retinal sclerosis   Retinal varices

362.18 Retinal vasculitis
Eales' disease
Retinal: arteritis
Retinal: endarteritis
Retinal: perivasculitis
Retinal: phlebitis
DEF: Inflammation of retinal blood vessels.

✓5th 362.2 Other proliferative retinopathy

362.21 Retrolental fibroplasia
DEF: Fibrous tissue in vitreous, from retina to lens, causing blindness; associated with premature infants requiring high amounts of oxygen.

362.29 Other nondiabetic proliferative retinopathy
AHA: 3Q, '96, 5

✓5th 362.3 Retinal vascular occlusion
DEF: Obstructed blood flow to and from retina.

362.30 Retinal vascular occlusion, unspecified
362.31 Central retinal artery occlusion
362.32 Arterial branch occlusion
362.33 Partial arterial occlusion
Hollenhorst plaque
Retinal microembolism

362.34 Transient arterial occlusion
Amaurosis fugax
AHA: 1Q, '00, 16

362.35 Central retinal vein occlusion
AHA: 2Q, '93, 6

362.36 Venous tributary (branch) occlusion
362.37 Venous engorgement
Occlusion: incipient } of retinal vein
Occlusion: partial

✓5th 362.4 Separation of retinal layers
EXCLUDES retinal detachment (serous) (361.2)
rhegmatogenous (361.00-361.07)

362.40 Retinal layer separation, unspecified
362.41 Central serous retinopathy
DEF: Serous-filled blister causing detachment of retina from pigment epithelium.

362.42 Serous detachment of retinal pigment epithelium
Exudative detachment of retinal pigment epithelium
DEF: Blister of fatty fluid causing detachment of retina from pigment epithelium.

362.43 Hemorrhagic detachment of retinal pigment epithelium
DEF: Blood-filled blister causing detachment of retina from pigment epithelium.

✓5th 362.5 Degeneration of macula and posterior pole
EXCLUDES degeneration of optic disc (377.21-377.24)
hereditary retinal degeneration [dystrophy] (362.70-362.77)

362.50 Macular degeneration (senile), unspecified
362.51 Nonexudative senile macular degeneration
Senile macular degeneration:
atrophic
dry

362.52 Exudative senile macular degeneration
Kuhnt-Junius degeneration
Senile macular degeneration:
disciform
wet
DEF: Leakage in macular blood vessels with loss of visual acuity.

362.53 Cystoid macular degeneration
Cystoid macular edema
DEF: Retinal swelling and cyst formation in macula.

362.54 Macular cyst, hole, or pseudohole
362.55 Toxic maculopathy
Use additional E code to identify drug, if drug induced

362.56 Macular puckering
Preretinal fibrosis

362.57 Drusen (degenerative)
DEF: White, hyaline deposits on Bruch's membrane (lamina basalis choroideae).

✓5th 362.6 Peripheral retinal degenerations
EXCLUDES hereditary retinal degeneration [dystrophy] (362.70-362.77)
retinal degeneration with retinal defect (361.00-361.07)

362.60 Peripheral retinal degeneration, unspecified
362.61 Paving stone degeneration
DEF: Degeneration of peripheral retina; causes thinning through which choroid is visible.

362.62 Microcystoid degeneration
Blessig's cysts   Iwanoff's cysts

362.63 Lattice degeneration
Palisade degeneration of retina
DEF: Degeneration of retina; often bilateral, usually benign; characterized by lines intersecting at irregular intervals in peripheral retina; retinal thinning and retinal holes may occur.

362.64 Senile reticular degeneration
DEF: Net-like appearance of retina; sign of degeneration.

362.65 Secondary pigmentary degeneration
Pseudoretinitis pigmentosa

362.66 Secondary vitreoretinal degenerations

✓5th 362.7 Hereditary retinal dystrophies
DEF: Genetically induced progressive changes in retina.

362.70 Hereditary retinal dystrophy, unspecified
362.71 Retinal dystrophy in systemic or cerebroretinal lipidoses
Code first underlying disease, as:
cerebroretinal lipidoses (330.1)
systemic lipidoses (272.7)

362.72 Retinal dystrophy in other systemic disorders and syndromes
Code first underlying disease, as:
Bassen-Kornzweig syndrome (272.5)
Refsum's disease (356.3)

362.73 Vitreoretinal dystrophies
Juvenile retinoschisis

362.74 Pigmentary retinal dystrophy
Retinal dystrophy, albipunctate
Retinitis pigmentosa

- **362.75 Other dystrophies primarily involving the sensory retina**
  - Progressive cone(-rod) dystrophy
  - Stargardt's disease
- **362.76 Dystrophies primarily involving the retinal pigment epithelium**
  - Fundus flavimaculatus
  - Vitelliform dystrophy
- **362.77 Dystrophies primarily involving Bruch's membrane**
  - Dystrophy:
    - hyaline
    - pseudoinflammatory foveal
  - Hereditary drusen

362.8 Other retinal disorders
EXCLUDES chorioretinal inflammations (363.0-363.2)
chorioretinal scars (363.30-363.35)

- **362.81 Retinal hemorrhage**
  - Hemorrhage:
    - preretinal
    - retinal (deep) (superficial)
    - subretinal
  - AHA: 4Q, '96, 43
- **362.82 Retinal exudates and deposits**
- **362.83 Retinal edema**
  - Retinal:
    - cotton wool spots
    - edema (localized) (macular) (peripheral)
  - DEF: Retinal swelling due to fluid accumulation.
- **362.84 Retinal ischemia**
  - DEF: Reduced retinal blood supply.
- **362.85 Retinal nerve fiber bundle defects**
- **362.89 Other retinal disorders**

362.9 Unspecified retinal disorder

363 Chorioretinal inflammations, scars, and other disorders of choroid

363.0 Focal chorioretinitis and focal retinochoroiditis
EXCLUDES focal chorioretinitis or retinochoroiditis in:
histoplasmosis (115.02, 115.12, 115.92)
toxoplasmosis (130.2)
congenital infection (771.2)

- **363.00 Focal chorioretinitis, unspecified**
  - Focal:
    - choroiditis or chorioretinitis NOS
    - retinitis or retinochoroiditis NOS
- **363.01 Focal choroiditis and chorioretinitis, juxtapapillary**
- **363.03 Focal choroiditis and chorioretinitis of other posterior pole**
- **363.04 Focal choroiditis and chorioretinitis, peripheral**
- **363.05 Focal retinitis and retinochoroiditis, juxtapapillary**
  - Neuroretinitis
- **363.06 Focal retinitis and retinochoroiditis, macular or paramacular**
- **363.07 Focal retinitis and retinochoroiditis of other posterior pole**
- **363.08 Focal retinitis and retinochoroiditis, peripheral**

363.1 Disseminated chorioretinitis and disseminated retinochoroiditis
EXCLUDES disseminated choroiditis or chorioretinitis in secondary syphilis (091.51)
neurosyphilitic disseminated retinitis or retinochoroiditis (094.83)
retinal (peri)vasculitis (362.18)

- **363.10 Disseminated chorioretinitis, unspecified**
  - Disseminated:
    - choroiditis or chorioretinitis NOS
    - retinitis or retinochoroiditis NOS
- **363.11 Disseminated choroiditis and chorioretinitis, posterior pole**
- **363.12 Disseminated choroiditis and chorioretinitis, peripheral**
- **363.13 Disseminated choroiditis and chorioretinitis, generalized**
  - Code first any underlying disease, as:
    - tuberculosis (017.3)
- **363.14 Disseminated retinitis and retinochoroiditis, metastatic**
- **363.15 Disseminated retinitis and retinochoroiditis, pigment epitheliopathy**
  - Acute posterior multifocal placoid pigment epitheliopathy
  - DEF: Widespread inflammation of retina and choroid; characterized by pigmented epithelium involvement.

363.2 Other and unspecified forms of chorioretinitis and retinochoroiditis
EXCLUDES panophthalmitis (360.02)
sympathetic uveitis (360.11)
uveitis NOS (364.3)

- **363.20 Chorioretinitis, unspecified**
  - Choroiditis NOS   Uveitis, posterior NOS
  - Retinitis NOS
- **363.21 Pars planitis**
  - Posterior cyclitis
  - DEF: Inflammation of peripheral retina and ciliary body; characterized by bands of white cells.
- **363.22 Harada's disease**
  - DEF: Retinal detachment and bilateral widespread exudative choroiditis; symptoms include headache, vomiting, increased lymphocytes in cerebrospinal fluid; and temporary or permanent deafness may occur.

363.3 Chorioretinal scars
Scar (postinflammatory) (postsurgical) (posttraumatic):
choroid
retina

- **363.30 Chorioretinal scar, unspecified**
- **363.31 Solar retinopathy**
  - DEF: Retinal scarring caused by solar radiation.
- **363.32 Other macular scars**
- **363.33 Other scars of posterior pole**
- **363.34 Peripheral scars**
- **363.35 Disseminated scars**

363.4 Choroidal degenerations
- **363.40 Choroidal degeneration, unspecified**
  - Choroidal sclerosis NOS
- **363.41 Senile atrophy of choroid**
  - DEF: Wasting away of choroid; due to aging.
- **363.42 Diffuse secondary atrophy of choroid**
  - DEF: Wasting away of choroid in systemic disease.
- **363.43 Angioid streaks of choroid**
  - DEF: Degeneration of choroid; characterized by dark brown steaks radiating from optic disk; occurs with pseudoxanthoma, elasticum or Paget's disease.

363.5 Hereditary choroidal dystrophies
Hereditary choroidal atrophy:
partial [choriocapillaris]
total [all vessels]

- **363.50 Hereditary choroidal dystrophy or atrophy, unspecified**
- **363.51 Circumpapillary dystrophy of choroid, partial**
- **363.52 Circumpapillary dystrophy of choroid, total**
  - Helicoid dystrophy of choroid

363.53 Central dystrophy of choroid, partial
Dystrophy, choroidal: central areolar
Dystrophy, choroidal: circinate

363.54 Central choroidal atrophy, total
Dystrophy, choroidal: central gyrate
Dystrophy, choroidal: serpiginous

363.55 Choroideremia
DEF: Hereditary choroid degeneration, occurs in first decade; characterized by constricted visual field and ultimately blindness in males; less debilitating in females.

363.56 Other diffuse or generalized dystrophy, partial
Diffuse choroidal sclerosis

363.57 Other diffuse or generalized dystrophy, total
Generalized gyrate atrophy, choroid

363.6 Choroidal hemorrhage and rupture
- 363.61 Choroidal hemorrhage, unspecified
- 363.62 Expulsive choroidal hemorrhage
- 363.63 Choroidal rupture

363.7 Choroidal detachment
- 363.70 Choroidal detachment, unspecified
- 363.71 Serous choroidal detachment
  DEF: Detachment of choroid from sclera; due to blister of serous fluid.
- 363.72 Hemorrhagic choroidal detachment
  DEF: Detachment of choroid from sclera; due to blood-filled blister.

363.8 Other disorders of choroid
363.9 Unspecified disorder of choroid

364 Disorders of iris and ciliary body

364.0 Acute and subacute iridocyclitis
Anterior uveitis
Cyclitis
Iridocyclitis } acute, subacute

EXCLUDES: gonococcal (098.41)
herpes simplex (054.44)
herpes zoster (053.22)

- 364.00 Acute and subacute iridocyclitis, unspecified
- 364.01 Primary iridocyclitis
- 364.02 Recurrent iridocyclitis
- 364.03 Secondary iridocyclitis, infectious
- 364.04 Secondary iridocyclitis, noninfectious
  Aqueous: cells, fibrin
  Aqueous: flare
- 364.05 Hypopyon
  DEF: Accumulation of white blood cells between cornea and lens.

364.1 Chronic iridocyclitis
EXCLUDES: posterior cyclitis (363.21)
- 364.10 Chronic iridocyclitis, unspecified
- 364.11 Chronic iridocyclitis in diseases classified elsewhere
  Code first underlying disease, as:
  sarcoidosis (135)
  tuberculosis (017.3)
  EXCLUDES: syphilitic iridocyclitis (091.52)
  DEF: Persistent inflammation of iris and ciliary body; due to underlying disease or condition.

364.2 Certain types of iridocyclitis
EXCLUDES: posterior cyclitis (363.21)
sympathetic uveitis (360.11)
- 364.21 Fuchs' heterochromic cyclitis
  DEF: Chronic cyclitis characterized by differences in the color of the two irises; the lighter iris appears in the inflamed eye.
- 364.22 Glaucomatocyclitic crises
  DEF: One-sided form of secondary open angle glaucoma; recurrent, uncommon and of short duration; causes high intraocular pressure, rarely damage.
- 364.23 Lens-induced iridocyclitis
  DEF: Inflammation of iris; due to immune reaction to proteins in lens following trauma or other lens abnormality.
- 364.24 Vogt-Koyanagi syndrome
  DEF: Uveomeningitis with exudative iridocyclitis and choroiditis; causes depigmentation of hair and skin, detached retina; tinnitus and loss of hearing may occur.

364.3 Unspecified iridocyclitis
Uveitis NOS

364.4 Vascular disorders of iris and ciliary body
- 364.41 Hyphema
  Hemorrhage of iris or ciliary body
  DEF: Hemorrhage in anterior chamber; also called hyphemia or "blood shot" eyes.
- 364.42 Rubeosis iridis
  Neovascularization of iris or ciliary body
  DEF: Blood vessel and connective tissue formation on surface of iris; symptomatic of diabetic retinopathy, central retinal vein occlusion and retinal detachment.

364.5 Degenerations of iris and ciliary body
- 364.51 Essential or progressive iris atrophy
- 364.52 Iridoschisis
  DEF: Splitting of iris into two layers.
- 364.53 Pigmentary iris degeneration
  Acquired heterochromia
  Pigment dispersion syndrome } of iris
- 364.54 Degeneration of pupillary margin
  Atrophy of sphincter
  Ectropion of pigment epithelium } of iris
- 364.55 Miotic cysts of pupillary margin
  DEF: Serous-filled sacs in pupillary margin of iris.
- 364.56 Degenerative changes of chamber angle
- 364.57 Degenerative changes of ciliary body
- 364.59 Other iris atrophy
  Iris atrophy (generalized) (sector shaped)

364.6 Cysts of iris, ciliary body, and anterior chamber
EXCLUDES: miotic pupillary cyst (364.55)
parasitic cyst (360.13)
- 364.60 Idiopathic cysts
  DEF: Fluid-filled sacs in iris or ciliary body; unknown etiology.
- 364.61 Implantation cysts
  Epithelial down-growth, anterior chamber
  Implantation cysts (surgical) (traumatic)
- 364.62 Exudative cysts of iris or anterior chamber
- 364.63 Primary cyst of pars plana
  DEF: Fluid-filled sacs of outermost ciliary ring.
- 364.64 Exudative cyst of pars plana
  DEF: Protein, fatty-filled sacs of outermost ciliary ring; due to fluid lead from blood vessels.

364.7 Adhesions and disruptions of iris and ciliary body
EXCLUDES: flat anterior chamber (360.34)
- 364.70 Adhesions of iris, unspecified
  Synechiae (iris) NOS
- 364.71 Posterior synechiae
  DEF: Adhesion binding iris to lens.
- 364.72 Anterior synechiae
  DEF: Adhesion binding the iris to cornea.

NERVOUS SYSTEM AND SENSE ORGANS

364.73 Goniosynechiae
Peripheral anterior synechiae
DEF: Adhesion binding the iris to cornea at the angle of the anterior chamber.

364.74 Pupillary membranes
Iris bombé
Pupillary: occlusion
Pupillary: seclusion
DEF: Membrane traversing the pupil and blocking vision.

364.75 Pupillary abnormalities
Deformed pupil   Rupture of sphincter, pupil
Ectopic pupil

364.76 Iridodialysis
DEF: Separation of the iris from the ciliary body base; due to trauma or surgical accident.

364.77 Recession of chamber angle
DEF: Receding of anterior chamber angle of the eye; restricts vision.

364.8 Other disorders of iris and ciliary body
Prolapse of iris NOS
EXCLUDES   prolapse of iris in recent wound (871.1)

364.9 Unspecified disorder of iris and ciliary body

365 Glaucoma
EXCLUDES   blind hypertensive eye [absolute glaucoma] (360.42)
congenital glaucoma (743.20-743.22)
DEF: Rise in intraocular pressure which restricts blood flow; multiple causes.

365.0 Borderline glaucoma [glaucoma suspect]
AHA: 1Q, '90, 8

365.00 Preglaucoma, unspecified

365.01 Open angle with borderline findings
Open angle with:
  borderline intraocular pressure
  cupping of optic discs
DEF: Minor block of aqueous outflow from eye.

365.02 Anatomical narrow angle
365.03 Steroid responders
365.04 Ocular hypertension
DEF: High fluid pressure within eye; no apparent cause.

365.1 Open-angle glaucoma

365.10 Open-angle glaucoma, unspecified
Wide-angle glaucoma NOS

365.11 Primary open angle glaucoma
Chronic simple glaucoma
DEF: High intraocular pressure, despite free flow of aqueous.

365.12 Low tension glaucoma
365.13 Pigmentary glaucoma
DEF: High intraocular pressure; due to iris pigment granules blocking aqueous flow.

365.14 Glaucoma of childhood
Infantile or juvenile glaucoma

365.15 Residual stage of open angle glaucoma

365.2 Primary angle-closure glaucoma

365.20 Primary angle-closure glaucoma, unspecified

365.21 Intermittent angle-closure glaucoma
Angle-closure glaucoma:
  interval
  subacute
DEF: Recurring attacks of high intraocular pressure; due to blocked aqueous flow.

365.22 Acute angle-closure glaucoma
DEF: Sudden, severe rise in intraocular pressure due to blockage in aqueous drainage.

365.23 Chronic angle-closure glaucoma
AHA: 2Q, '98, 16

365.24 Residual stage of angle-closure glaucoma

365.3 Corticosteroid-induced glaucoma
DEF: Elevated intraocular pressure; due to long-term corticosteroid therapy.

365.31 Glaucomatous stage
365.32 Residual stage

365.4 Glaucoma associated with congenital anomalies, dystrophies, and systemic syndromes

365.41 Glaucoma associated with chamber angle anomalies
Code first associated disorder, as:
  Axenfeld's anomaly (743.44)
  Rieger's anomaly or syndrome (743.44)

365.42 Glaucoma associated with anomalies of iris
Code first associated disorder, as:
  aniridia (743.45)
  essential iris atrophy (364.51)

365.43 Glaucoma associated with other anterior segment anomalies
Code first associated disorder, as:
  microcornea (743.41)

365.44 Glaucoma associated with systemic syndromes
Code first associated disease, as:
  neurofibromatosis (237.7)
  Sturge-Weber (-Dimitri) syndrome (759.6)

365.5 Glaucoma associated with disorders of the lens

365.51 Phacolytic glaucoma
Use additional code for associated hypermature cataract (366.18)
DEF: Elevated intraocular pressure; due to lens protein blocking aqueous flow.

365.52 Pseudoexfoliation glaucoma
Use additional code for associated pseudoexfoliation of capsule (366.11)
DEF: Glaucoma characterized by small grayish particles deposited on the lens.

365.59 Glaucoma associated with other lens disorders
Use additional code for associated disorder, as:
  dislocation of lens (379.33-379.34)
  spherophakia (743.36)

365.6 Glaucoma associated with other ocular disorders

365.60 Glaucoma associated with unspecified ocular disorder

365.61 Glaucoma associated with pupillary block
Use additional code for associated disorder, as:
  seclusion of pupil [iris bombé] (364.74)
DEF: Acute, open-angle glaucoma caused by mature cataract; aqueous flow is blocked by lens material and macrophages.

365.62 Glaucoma associated with ocular inflammations
Use additional code for associated disorder, as:
  glaucomatocyclitic crises (364.22)
  iridocyclitis (364.0-364.3)

365.63 Glaucoma associated with vascular disorders
Use additional code for associated disorder, as:
  central retinal vein occlusion (362.35)
  hyphema (364.41)

NERVOUS SYSTEM AND SENSE ORGANS

365.64 Glaucoma associated with tumors or cysts
Use additional code for associated disorder, as:
benign neoplasm (224.0-224.9)
epithelial down-growth (364.61)
malignant neoplasm (190.0-190.9)

365.65 Glaucoma associated with ocular trauma
Use additional code for associated condition, as:
contusion of globe (921.3)
recession of chamber angle (364.77)

365.8 Other specified forms of glaucoma
365.81 Hypersecretion glaucoma
365.82 Glaucoma with increased episcleral venous pressure
365.83 Aqueous misdirection
Malignant glaucoma
AHA: 4Q, '02, 48
DEF: A form of glaucoma that occurs when aqueous humor flows into the posterior chamber of the eye (vitreous) rather than through the normal recycling channels into the anterior chamber.

365.89 Other specified glaucoma
AHA: 2Q, '98, 16

365.9 Unspecified glaucoma
AHA: 3Q, '03, 14; 2Q, '01, 16

366 Cataract
EXCLUDES congenital cataract (743.30-743.34)
DEF: A variety of conditions that create a cloudy, or calcified lens that obstructs vision.

366.0 Infantile, juvenile, and presenile cataract
366.00 Nonsenile cataract, unspecified
366.01 Anterior subcapsular polar cataract
DEF: Defect within the front, center lens surface.
366.02 Posterior subcapsular polar cataract
DEF: Defect within the rear, center lens surface.
366.03 Cortical, lamellar, or zonular cataract
DEF: Opacities radiating from center to edge of lens; appear as thin, concentric layers of lens.
366.04 Nuclear cataract
366.09 Other and combined forms of nonsenile cataract

366.1 Senile cataract
AHA: 3Q, '91, 9; S-O, '85, 10
366.10 Senile cataract, unspecified
AHA: 1Q, '03, 5
366.11 Pseudoexfoliation of lens capsule
366.12 Incipient cataract
Cataract: Cataract:
coronary   punctate
immature NOS   Water clefts
DEF: Minor disorders of lens not affecting vision; due to aging.

Aqueous Misdirection Syndrome

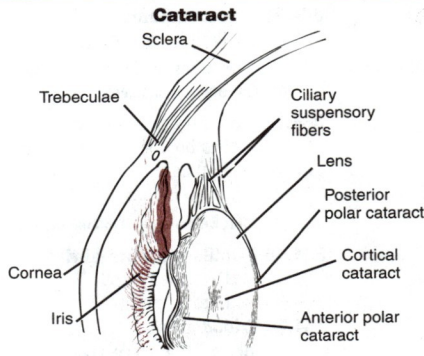
Cataract

366.13 Anterior subcapsular polar senile cataract
366.14 Posterior subcapsular polar senile cataract
366.15 Cortical senile cataract
366.16 Nuclear sclerosis
Cataracta brunescens
Nuclear cataract
366.17 Total or mature cataract
366.18 Hypermature cataract
Morgagni cataract
366.19 Other and combined forms of senile cataract

366.2 Traumatic cataract
366.20 Traumatic cataract, unspecified
366.21 Localized traumatic opacities
Vossius' ring
366.22 Total traumatic cataract
366.23 Partially resolved traumatic cataract

366.3 Cataract secondary to ocular disorders
366.30 Cataracta complicata, unspecified
366.31 Glaucomatous flecks (subcapsular)
Code first underlying glaucoma (365.0-365.9)
366.32 Cataract in inflammatory disorders
Code first underlying condition, as:
chronic choroiditis (363.0-363.2)
366.33 Cataract with neovascularization
Code first underlying condition, as:
chronic iridocyclitis (364.10)
366.34 Cataract in degenerative disorders
Sunflower cataract
Code first underlying condition, as:
chalcosis (360.24)
degenerative myopia (360.21)
pigmentary retinal dystrophy (362.74)

366.4 Cataract associated with other disorders
366.41 Diabetic cataract
Code first diabetes (250.5)
AHA: 3Q, '91, 9; S-O, '85, 11
366.42 Tetanic cataract
Code first underlying disease, as:
calcinosis (275.4)
hypoparathyroidism (252.1)
366.43 Myotonic cataract
Code first underlying disorder (359.2)
366.44 Cataract associated with other syndromes
Code first underlying condition, as:
craniofacial dysostosis (756.0)
galactosemia (271.1)
366.45 Toxic cataract
Drug-induced cataract
Use additional E code to identify drug or other toxic substance
366.46 Cataract associated with radiation and other physical influences
Use additional E code to identify cause

NERVOUS SYSTEM AND SENSE ORGANS

366.5 After-cataract
- **366.50** After-cataract, unspecified
  - Secondary cataract NOS
- **366.51** Soemmering's ring
  - DEF: A donut-shaped lens remnant and a capsule behind the pupil as a result of cataract surgery or trauma.
- **366.52** Other after-cataract, not obscuring vision
- **366.53** After-cataract, obscuring vision

366.8 Other cataract
- Calcification of lens

366.9 Unspecified cataract

367 Disorders of refraction and accommodation

367.0 Hypermetropia
- Far-sightedness
- Hyperopia
- DEF: Refraction error, called also hyperopia, focal point is posterior to retina; abnormally short anteroposterior diameter or subnormal refractive power; causes farsightedness.

367.1 Myopia
- Near-sightedness
- DEF: Refraction error, focal point is anterior to retina; causes near-sightedness.

367.2 Astigmatism
- **367.20** Astigmatism, unspecified
- **367.21** Regular astigmatism
- **367.22** Irregular astigmatism

367.3 Anisometropia and aniseikonia
- **367.31** Anisometropia
  - DEF: Eyes with refractive powers that differ by at least one diopter.
- **367.32** Aniseikonia
  - DEF: Eyes with unequal retinal imaging; usually due to refractive error.

367.4 Presbyopia
- DEF: Loss of crystalline lens elasticity; causes errors of accommodation; due to aging.

367.5 Disorders of accommodation
- **367.51** Paresis of accommodation
  - Cycloplegia
  - DEF: Partial paralysis of ciliary muscle; causing focus problems.
- **367.52** Total or complete internal ophthalmoplegia
  - DEF: Total paralysis of ciliary muscle; large pupil incapable of focus.
- **367.53** Spasm of accommodation
  - DEF: Abnormal contraction of ciliary muscle; causes focus problems.

367.8 Other disorders of refraction and accommodation
- **367.81** Transient refractive change
- **367.89** Other
  - Drug-induced } disorders of refraction
  - Toxic } & accommodation

367.9 Unspecified disorder of refraction and accommodation

368 Visual disturbances
- EXCLUDES: electrophysiological disturbances (794.11-794.14)

368.0 Amblyopia ex anopsia
- DEF: Vision impaired due to disuse; esotropia often cause.
- **368.00** Amblyopia, unspecified
- **368.01** Strabismic amblyopia
  - Suppression amblyopia
- **368.02** Deprivation amblyopia
  - DEF: Decreased vision associated with suppressed retinal image of one eye.
- **368.03** Refractive amblyopia

368.1 Subjective visual disturbances
- **368.10** Subjective visual disturbance, unspecified
- **368.11** Sudden visual loss
- **368.12** Transient visual loss
  - Concentric fading   Scintillating scotoma
- **368.13** Visual discomfort
  - Asthenopia   Photophobia
  - Eye strain
- **368.14** Visual distortions of shape and size
  - Macropsia   Micropsia
  - Metamorphopsia
- **368.15** Other visual distortions and entoptic phenomena
  - Photopsia   Refractive:
  - Refractive: polyopia
  - diplopia   Visual halos
- **368.16** Psychophysical visual disturbances
  - Visual: Visual:
  - agnosia   hallucinations
  - disorientation syndrome

368.2 Diplopia
- Double vision

368.3 Other disorders of binocular vision
- **368.30** Binocular vision disorder, unspecified
- **368.31** Suppression of binocular vision
- **368.32** Simultaneous visual perception without fusion
- **368.33** Fusion with defective stereopsis
  - DEF: Faulty depth perception though normal ability to focus.
- **368.34** Abnormal retinal correspondence

368.4 Visual field defects
- **368.40** Visual field defect, unspecified
- **368.41** Scotoma involving central area
  - Scotoma: Scotoma:
  - central   paracentral
  - centrocecal
  - DEF: Vision loss (blind spot) in central five degrees of visual field.
- **368.42** Scotoma of blind spot area
  - Enlarged: Paracecal scotoma
  - angioscotoma
  - blind spot
- **368.43** Sector or arcuate defects
  - Scotoma:
  - arcuate
  - Bjerrum
  - Seidel
  - DEF: Arc-shaped blind spot caused by retinal nerve damage.
- **368.44** Other localized visual field defect
  - Scotoma: Visual field defect:
  - NOS   nasal step
  - ring   peripheral
- **368.45** Generalized contraction or constriction
- **368.46** Homonymous bilateral field defects
  - Hemianopsia (altitudinal) (homonymous)
  - Quadrant anopia
  - DEF: Disorders found in the corresponding vertical halves of the visual fields of both eyes.
- **368.47** Heteronymous bilateral field defects
  - Hemianopsia: Hemianopsia:
  - binasal   bitemporal
  - DEF: Disorders in the opposite halves of the visual fields of both eyes.

368.5 Color vision deficiencies
- Color blindness
- **368.51** Protan defect
  - Protanomaly   Protanopia
  - DEF: Mild difficulty distinguishing green and red hues with shortened spectrum; sex-linked affecting one percent of males.

368.52 Deutan defect
Deuteranomaly   Deuteranopia
DEF: Male-only disorder; difficulty in distinguishing green and red, no shortened spectrum.

368.53 Tritan defect
Tritanomaly   Tritanopia
DEF: Difficulty in distinguishing blue and yellow; occurs often due to drugs, retinal detachment and central nervous system diseases.

368.54 Achromatopsia
Monochromatism (cone) (rod)
DEF: Complete color blindness; caused by disease, injury to retina, optic nerve or pathway.

368.55 Acquired color vision deficiencies
368.59 Other color vision deficiencies

✓5th **368.6 Night blindness**
Nyctalopia
DEF: Nyctalopia: disorder of vision in dim light or night blindness.

368.60 Night blindness, unspecified
368.61 Congenital night blindness
Hereditary night blindness
Oguchi's disease
368.62 Acquired night blindness
EXCLUDES   that due to vitamin A deficiency (264.5)
368.63 Abnormal dark adaptation curve
Abnormal threshold } of cones or rods
Delayed adaptation
368.69 Other night blindness

368.8 Other specified visual disturbances
Blurred vision NOS
AHA: 4Q, '02, 56

368.9 Unspecified visual disturbance
AHA: 1Q, '04, 15

✓4th **369 Blindness and low vision**
Note: Visual impairment refers to a functional limitation of the eye (e.g., limited visual acuity or visual field). It should be distinguished from visual disability, indicating a limitation of the abilities of the individual (e.g., limited reading skills, vocational skills), and from visual handicap, indicating a limitation of personal and socioeconomic independence (e.g., limited mobility, limited employability).

The levels of impairment defined in the table on this page are based on the recommendations of the WHO Study Group on Prevention of Blindness (Geneva, November 6–10, 1972; WHO Technical Report Series 518), and of the International Council of Ophthalmology (1976).

Note that definitions of blindness vary in different settings.

For international reporting WHO defines blindness as profound impairment. This definition can be applied to blindness of one eye (369.1, 369.6) and to blindness of the individual (369.0).

For determination of benefits in the U.S.A., the definition of legal blindness as severe impairment is often used. This definition applies to blindness of the individual only.

EXCLUDES   correctable impaired vision due to refractive errors (367.0-367.9)

✓5th **369.0 Profound impairment, both eyes**
369.00 Impairment level not further specified
Blindness:
NOS according to WHO definition
both eyes
369.01 Better eye: total impairment; lesser eye: total impairment

Classification		LEVELS OF VISUAL IMPAIRMENT	Additional descriptors which may be encountered
"legal"	WHO	Visual acuity and/or visual field limitation (whichever is worse)	
LEGAL BLINDNESS (U.S.A.) both eyes	(NEAR-) NORMAL VISION	RANGE OF NORMAL VISION 20/10 20/13 20/16 20/20 20/25 2.0 1.6 1.25 1.0 0.8	
		NEAR-NORMAL VISION 20/30 20/40 20/50 20/60 0.7 0.6 0.5 0.4 0.3	
	LOW VISION	MODERATE VISUAL IMPAIRMENT 20/70 20/80 20/100 20/125 20/160 0.25 0.20 0.16 0.12	Moderate low vision
		SEVERE VISUAL IMPAIRMENT 20/200 20/250 20/320 20/400 0.10 0.08 0.06 0.05 Visual field: 20 degrees or less	Severe low vision, "Legal" blindness
	BLINDNESS (WHO) one or both eyes	PROFOUND VISUAL IMPAIRMENT 20/500 20/630 20/800 20/1000 0.04 0.03 0.025 0.02 Count fingers at: less than 3m (10 ft.) Visual field: 10 degrees or less	Profound low vision, Moderate blindness
		NEAR-TOTAL VISUAL IMPAIRMENT Visual acuity: less than 0.02 (20/1000) Count fingers at: 1m (3 ft.) or less Hand movements: 5m (15 ft.) or less Light projection, light perception Visual field: 5 degrees or less	Severe blindness, Near-total blindness
		TOTAL VISUAL IMPAIRMENT No light perception (NLP)	Total blindness

Visual acuity refers to best achievable acuity with correction.
Non-listed Snellen fractions may be classified by converting to the nearest decimal equivalent, e.g. 10/200 = 0.05, 6/30 = 0.20.
CF (count fingers) without designation of distance, may be classified to profound impairment.
HM (hand motion) without designation of distance, may be classified to near-total impairment.
Visual field measurements refer to the largest field diameter for a 1/100 white test object.

369.02 Better eye: near-total impairment; lesser eye: not further specified
369.03 Better eye: near-total impairment; lesser eye: total impairment
369.04 Better eye: near-total impairment; lesser eye: near-total impairment
369.05 Better eye: profound impairment; lesser eye: not further specified
369.06 Better eye: profound impairment; lesser eye: total impairment
369.07 Better eye: profound impairment; lesser eye: near-total impairment
369.08 Better eye: profound impairment; lesser eye: profound impairment

✓5th **369.1 Moderate or severe impairment, better eye, profound impairment lesser eye**
369.10 Impairment level not further specified
Blindness, one eye, low vision other eye
369.11 Better eye: severe impairment; lesser eye: blind, not further specified
369.12 Better eye: severe impairment; lesser eye: total impairment
369.13 Better eye: severe impairment; lesser eye: near-total impairment
369.14 Better eye: severe impairment; lesser eye: profound impairment

NERVOUS SYSTEM AND SENSE ORGANS

369.15 Better eye: moderate impairment; lesser eye: blind, not further specified
369.16 Better eye: moderate impairment; lesser eye: total impairment
369.17 Better eye: moderate impairment; lesser eye: near-total impairment
369.18 Better eye: moderate impairment; lesser eye: profound impairment

369.2 Moderate or severe impairment, both eyes
   369.20 Impairment level not further specified
      Low vision, both eyes NOS
   369.21 Better eye: severe impairment; lesser eye: not further specified
   369.22 Better eye: severe impairment; lesser eye: severe impairment
   369.23 Better eye: moderate impairment; lesser eye: not further specified
   369.24 Better eye: moderate impairment; lesser eye: severe impairment
   369.25 Better eye: moderate impairment; lesser eye: moderate impairment

369.3 Unqualified visual loss, both eyes
   EXCLUDES blindness NOS:
      legal [U.S.A. definition] (369.4)
      WHO definition (369.00)

369.4 Legal blindness, as defined in U.S.A.
   Blindness NOS according to U.S.A. definition
   EXCLUDES legal blindness with specification of impairment level (369.01-369.08, 369.11-369.14, 369.21-369.22)

369.6 Profound impairment, one eye
   369.60 Impairment level not further specified
      Blindness, one eye
   369.61 One eye: total impairment; other eye: not specified
   369.62 One eye: total impairment; other eye: near-normal vision
   369.63 One eye: total impairment; other eye: normal vision
   369.64 One eye: near-total impairment; other eye: not specified
   369.65 One eye: near-total impairment; other eye: near-normal vision
   369.66 One eye: near-total impairment; other eye: normal vision
   369.67 One eye: profound impairment; other eye: not specified
   369.68 One eye: profound impairment; other eye: near-normal vision
   369.69 One eye: profound impairment; other eye: normal vision

369.7 Moderate or severe impairment, one eye
   369.70 Impairment level not further specified
      Low vision, one eye
   369.71 One eye: severe impairment; other eye: not specified
   369.72 One eye: severe impairment; other eye: near-normal vision
   369.73 One eye: severe impairment; other eye: normal vision
   369.74 One eye: moderate impairment; other eye: not specified
   369.75 One eye: moderate impairment; other eye: near-normal vision
   369.76 One eye: moderate impairment; other eye: normal vision

369.8 Unqualified visual loss, one eye
369.9 Unspecified visual loss
   AHA: 4Q, '02, 114; 3Q, '02, 20

370 Keratitis
   370.0 Corneal ulcer
      EXCLUDES that due to vitamin A deficiency (264.3)
      370.00 Corneal ulcer, unspecified
      370.01 Marginal corneal ulcer
      370.02 Ring corneal ulcer
      370.03 Central corneal ulcer
      370.04 Hypopyon ulcer
         Serpiginous ulcer
         DEF: Corneal ulcer with an accumulation of pus in the eye's anterior chamber.
      370.05 Mycotic corneal ulcer
         DEF: Fungal infection causing corneal tissue loss.
      370.06 Perforated corneal ulcer
         DEF: Tissue loss through all layers of cornea.
      370.07 Mooren's ulcer
         DEF: Tissue loss, with chronic inflammation, at junction of cornea and sclera; seen in elderly.

   370.2 Superficial keratitis without conjunctivitis
      EXCLUDES dendritic [herpes simplex] keratitis (054.42)
      370.20 Superficial keratitis, unspecified
      370.21 Punctate keratitis
         Thygeson's superficial punctate keratitis
         DEF: Formation of cellular and fibrinous deposits (keratic precipitates) on posterior surface; deposits develop after injury or iridocyclitis.
      370.22 Macular keratitis
         Keratitis: Keratitis:
          areolar   stellate
          nummular striate
      370.23 Filamentary keratitis
         DEF: Keratitis characterized by twisted filaments of mucoid material on the cornea's surface.
      370.24 Photokeratitis
         Snow blindness
         Welders' keratitis
         AHA: 3Q, '96, 6
         DEF: Painful, inflamed cornea; due to extended exposure to ultraviolet light.

   370.3 Certain types of keratoconjunctivitis
      370.31 Phlyctenular keratoconjunctivitis
         Phlyctenulosis
         Use additional code for any associated tuberculosis (017.3)
         DEF: Miniature blister on conjunctiva or cornea; associated with tuberculosis and malnutrition disorders.
      370.32 Limbar and corneal involvement in vernal conjunctivitis
         Use additional code for vernal conjunctivitis (372.13)
         DEF: Corneal itching and inflammation in conjunctivitis; often limited to lining of eyelids.
      370.33 Keratoconjunctivitis sicca, not specified as Sjögren's
         EXCLUDES Sjögren's syndrome (710.2)
         DEF: Inflammation of conjunctiva and cornea; characterized by "horny" looking tissue and excess blood in these areas; decreased flow of lacrimal (tear) is a contributing factor.
      370.34 Exposure keratoconjunctivitis
         AHA: 3Q, '96, 6
         DEF: Incomplete closure of eyelid causing dry, inflamed eye.
      370.35 Neurotrophic keratoconjunctivitis

NERVOUS SYSTEM AND SENSE ORGANS

✓5th 370.4 Other and unspecified keratoconjunctivitis
- **370.40 Keratoconjunctivitis, unspecified**
  Superficial keratitis with conjunctivitis NOS
- **370.44 Keratitis or keratoconjunctivitis in exanthema**
  Code first underlying condition (050.0-052.9)
  EXCLUDES: herpes simplex (054.43)
  herpes zoster (053.21)
  measles (055.71)
- **370.49 Other**
  EXCLUDES: epidemic keratoconjunctivitis (077.1)

✓5th 370.5 Interstitial and deep keratitis
- **370.50 Interstitial keratitis, unspecified**
- **370.52 Diffuse interstitial keratitis**
  Cogan's syndrome
  DEF: Inflammation of cornea; with deposits in middle corneal layers; may obscure vision.
- **370.54 Sclerosing keratitis**
  DEF: Chronic corneal inflammation leading to opaque scarring.
- **370.55 Corneal abscess**
  DEF: Pocket of pus and inflammation on the cornea.
- **370.59 Other**
  EXCLUDES: disciform herpes simplex keratitis (054.43)
  syphilitic keratitis (090.3)

✓5th 370.6 Corneal neovascularization
- **370.60 Corneal neovascularization, unspecified**
- **370.61 Localized vascularization of cornea**
  DEF: Limited infiltration of cornea by new blood vessels.
- **370.62 Pannus (corneal)**
  AHA: 3Q, '02, 20
  DEF: Buildup of superficial vascularization and granulated tissue under epithelium of cornea.
- **370.63 Deep vascularization of cornea**
  DEF: Deep infiltration of cornea by new blood vessels.
- **370.64 Ghost vessels (corneal)**

370.8 Other forms of keratitis
AHA: 3Q, '94, 5

370.9 Unspecified keratitis

✓4th 371 Corneal opacity and other disorders of cornea
- **✓5th 371.0 Corneal scars and opacities**
  EXCLUDES: that due to vitamin A deficiency (264.6)
  - **371.00 Corneal opacity, unspecified**
    Corneal scar NOS
  - **371.01 Minor opacity of cornea**
    Corneal nebula
  - **371.02 Peripheral opacity of cornea**
    Corneal macula not interfering with central vision
  - **371.03 Central opacity of cornea**
    Corneal:
      leucoma } interfering with central
      macula } vision
  - **371.04 Adherent leucoma**
    DEF: Dense, opaque corneal growth adhering to the iris; also spelled as leukoma.
  - **371.05 Phthisical cornea**
    Code first underlying tuberculosis (017.3)

- **✓5th 371.1 Corneal pigmentations and deposits**
  - **371.10 Corneal deposit, unspecified**
  - **371.11 Anterior pigmentations**
    Stähli's lines
  - **371.12 Stromal pigmentations**
    Hematocornea
  - **371.13 Posterior pigmentations**
    Krukenberg spindle
  - **371.14 Kayser-Fleischer ring**
    DEF: Copper deposits forming ring at outer edge of cornea; seen in Wilson's disease and other liver disorders.
  - **371.15 Other deposits associated with metabolic disorders**
  - **371.16 Argentous deposits**
    DEF: Silver deposits in cornea.

- **✓5th 371.2 Corneal edema**
  - **371.20 Corneal edema, unspecified**
  - **371.21 Idiopathic corneal edema**
    DEF: Corneal swelling and fluid retention of unknown cause.
  - **371.22 Secondary corneal edema**
    DEF: Corneal swelling and fluid retention caused by an underlying disease, injury, or condition.
  - **371.23 Bullous keratopathy**
    DEF: Corneal degeneration; characterized by recurring, rupturing epithelial "blisters;" ruptured blebs expose corneal nerves, cause great pain; occurs in glaucoma, iridocyclitis and Fuchs' epithelial dystrophy.
  - **371.24 Corneal edema due to wearing of contact lenses**

- **✓5th 371.3 Changes of corneal membranes**
  - **371.30 Corneal membrane change, unspecified**
  - **371.31 Folds and rupture of Bowman's membrane**
  - **371.32 Folds in Descemet's membrane**
  - **371.33 Rupture in Descemet's membrane**

- **✓5th 371.4 Corneal degenerations**
  - **371.40 Corneal degeneration, unspecified**
  - **371.41 Senile corneal changes**
    Arcus senilis   Hassall-Henle bodies
  - **371.42 Recurrent erosion of cornea**
    EXCLUDES: Mooren's ulcer (370.07)
  - **371.43 Band-shaped keratopathy**
    DEF: Horizontal bands of superficial corneal calcium deposits.
  - **371.44 Other calcerous degenerations of cornea**
  - **371.45 Keratomalacia NOS**
    EXCLUDES: that due to vitamin A deficiency (264.4)
    DEF: Destruction of the cornea by keratinization of the epithelium with ulceration and perforation of the cornea; seen in cases of vitamin A deficiency.
  - **371.46 Nodular degeneration of cornea**
    Salzmann's nodular dystrophy
  - **371.48 Peripheral degenerations of cornea**
    Marginal degeneration of cornea [Terrien's]
  - **371.49 Other**
    Discrete colliquative keratopathy

- **✓5th 371.5 Hereditary corneal dystrophies**
  DEF: Genetic disorder; leads to opacities, edema or lesions of cornea.
  - **371.50 Corneal dystrophy, unspecified**
  - **371.51 Juvenile epithelial corneal dystrophy**
  - **371.52 Other anterior corneal dystrophies**
    Corneal dystrophy:
      microscopic cystic
      ring-like
  - **371.53 Granular corneal dystrophy**
  - **371.54 Lattice corneal dystrophy**
  - **371.55 Macular corneal dystrophy**

NERVOUS SYSTEM AND SENSE ORGANS

371.56 **Other stromal corneal dystrophies**
Crystalline corneal dystrophy

371.57 **Endothelial corneal dystrophy**
Combined corneal dystrophy
Cornea guttata
Fuchs' endothelial dystrophy

371.58 **Other posterior corneal dystrophies**
Polymorphous corneal dystrophy

√5th 371.6 **Keratoconus**
DEF: Bilateral bulging protrusion of anterior cornea; often due to noninflammatory thinning.

371.60 Keratoconus, unspecified
371.61 **Keratoconus, stable condition**
371.62 **Keratoconus, acute hydrops**

√5th 371.7 **Other corneal deformities**
371.70 Corneal deformity, unspecified
371.71 **Corneal ectasia**
DEF: Bulging protrusion of thinned, scarred cornea.

371.72 **Descemetocele**
DEF: Protrusion of Descemet's membrane into cornea.

371.73 **Corneal staphyloma**
DEF: Protrusion of cornea into adjacent tissue.

√5th 371.8 **Other corneal disorders**
371.81 **Corneal anesthesia and hypoesthesia**
DEF: Decreased or absent sensitivity of cornea.

371.82 **Corneal disorder due to contact lens**
EXCLUDES *corneal edema due to contact lens (371.24)*
DEF: Contact lens wear causing cornea disorder, excluding swelling.

371.89 **Other**
AHA: 3Q, '99, 12

371.9 Unspecified corneal disorder

√4th 372 **Disorders of conjunctiva**
EXCLUDES *keratoconjunctivitis (370.3-370.4)*

√5th 372.0 **Acute conjunctivitis**
372.00 Acute conjunctivitis, unspecified
372.01 **Serous conjunctivitis, except viral**
EXCLUDES *viral conjunctivitis NOS (077.9)*

372.02 **Acute follicular conjunctivitis**
Conjunctival folliculosis NOS
EXCLUDES *conjunctivitis:*
adenoviral (acute follicular) (077.3)
epidemic hemorrhagic (077.4)
inclusion (077.0)
Newcastle (077.8)
epidemic keratoconjunctivitis (077.1)
pharyngoconjunctival fever (077.2)
DEF: Severe conjunctival inflammation with dense infiltrations of lymphoid tissues of inner eyelids; may be traced to a viral or chlamydial etiology.

372.03 Other mucopurulent conjunctivitis
Catarrhal conjunctivitis
EXCLUDES *blennorrhea neonatorum (gonococcal) (098.40)*
neonatal conjunctivitis (771.6)
ophthalmia neonatorum NOS (771.6)

372.04 **Pseudomembranous conjunctivitis**
Membranous conjunctivitis
EXCLUDES *diphtheritic conjunctivitis (032.81)*
DEF: Severe inflammation of conjunctiva; false membrane develops on inner surface of eyelid; membrane can be removed without harming epithelium, due to bacterial infections, toxic and allergic factors, and viral infections.

372.05 **Acute atopic conjunctivitis**
DEF: Sudden, severe conjunctivitis due to allergens.

√5th 372.1 **Chronic conjunctivitis**
372.10 Chronic conjunctivitis, unspecified
372.11 **Simple chronic conjunctivitis**
372.12 **Chronic follicular conjunctivitis**
DEF: Persistent inflammation of conjunctiva; with infiltration of lymphoid tissue of inner eyelids.

372.13 **Vernal conjunctivitis**
AHA: 3Q, '96, 8

372.14 Other chronic allergic conjunctivitis
AHA: 3Q, '96, 8

372.15 *Parasitic conjunctivitis*
Code first underlying disease, as:
filariasis (125.0-125.9)
mucocutaneous leishmaniasis (085.5)

√5th 372.2 **Blepharoconjunctivitis**
372.20 Blepharoconjunctivitis, unspecified
372.21 **Angular blepharoconjunctivitis**
DEF: Inflammation at junction of upper and lower eyelids; may block lacrimal secretions.

372.22 **Contact blepharoconjunctivitis**

√5th 372.3 **Other and unspecified conjunctivitis**
372.30 Conjunctivitis, unspecified
372.31 Rosacea conjunctivitis
Code first underlying rosacea dermatitis (695.3)

372.33 *Conjunctivitis in mucocutaneous disease*
Code first underlying disease, as:
erythema multiforme (695.1)
Reiter's disease (099.3)
EXCLUDES *ocular pemphigoid (694.61)*

372.39 **Other**

√5th 372.4 **Pterygium**
EXCLUDES *pseudopterygium (372.52)*
DEF: Wedge-shaped, conjunctival thickening that advances from the inner corner of the eye toward the cornea.

372.40 Pterygium, unspecified
372.41 **Peripheral pterygium, stationary**
372.42 **Peripheral pterygium, progressive**
372.43 **Central pterygium**
372.44 **Double pterygium**
372.45 **Recurrent pterygium**

√5th 372.5 **Conjunctival degenerations and deposits**
372.50 Conjunctival degeneration, unspecified
372.51 **Pinguecula**
DEF: Proliferative spot on the bulbar conjunctiva located near the sclerocorneal junction, usually on the nasal side; it is seen in elderly people.

372.52 **Pseudopterygium**
DEF: Conjunctival scar joined to the cornea; it looks like a pterygium but is not attached to the tissue.

372.53–374.14 NERVOUS SYSTEM AND SENSE ORGANS

372.53 Conjunctival xerosis
EXCLUDES: conjunctival xerosis due to vitamin A deficiency (264.0, 264.1, 264.7)
DEF: Dry conjunctiva due to vitamin A deficiency; related to Bitot's spots; may develop into xerophthalmia and keratomalacia.

372.54 Conjunctival concretions
DEF: Calculus or deposit on conjunctiva.

372.55 Conjunctival pigmentations
Conjunctival argyrosis
DEF: Color deposits in conjunctiva.

372.56 Conjunctival deposits

✓5th **372.6 Conjunctival scars**
372.61 Granuloma of conjunctiva
372.62 Localized adhesions and strands of conjunctiva
DEF: Abnormal fibrous connections in conjunctiva.
372.63 Symblepharon
Extensive adhesions of conjunctiva
DEF: Adhesion of the eyelids to the eyeball.
372.64 Scarring of conjunctiva
Contraction of eye socket (after enucleation)

✓5th **372.7 Conjunctival vascular disorders and cysts**
372.71 Hyperemia of conjunctiva
DEF: Conjunctival blood vessel congestion causing eye redness.
372.72 Conjunctival hemorrhage
Hyposphagma
Subconjunctival hemorrhage
372.73 Conjunctival edema
Chemosis of conjunctiva
Subconjunctival edema
DEF: Fluid retention and swelling in conjunctival tissue.
372.74 Vascular abnormalities of conjunctiva
Aneurysm(ata) of conjunctiva
372.75 Conjunctival cysts
DEF: Abnormal sacs of fluid in conjunctiva.

✓5th **372.8 Other disorders of conjunctiva**
372.81 Conjunctivochalasis
AHA: 4Q, '00, 41
DEF: Bilateral condition of redundant conjunctival tissue between globe and lower eyelid margin; may cover lower punctum, interferring with normal tearing.
372.89 Other disorders of conjunctiva

372.9 Unspecified disorder of conjunctiva

✓4th **373 Inflammation of eyelids**
✓5th **373.0 Blepharitis**
EXCLUDES: blepharoconjunctivitis (372.20-372.22)
373.00 Blepharitis, unspecified
373.01 Ulcerative blepharitis
373.02 Squamous blepharitis

✓5th **373.1 Hordeolum and other deep inflammation of eyelid**
DEF: Purulent, localized, staphylococcal infection in sebaceous glands of eyelids.
373.11 Hordeolum externum
Hordeolum NOS
Stye
DEF: Infection of oil gland in eyelash follicles.
373.12 Hordeolum internum
Infection of meibomian gland
DEF: Infection of oil gland of eyelid margin.
373.13 Abscess of eyelid
Furuncle of eyelid
DEF: Inflamed pocket of pus on eyelid.

373.2 Chalazion
Meibomian (gland) cyst
EXCLUDES: infected meibomian gland (373.12)
DEF: Chronic inflammation of the meibomian gland, causing an eyelid mass.

✓5th **373.3 Noninfectious dermatoses of eyelid**
373.31 Eczematous dermatitis of eyelid
373.32 Contact and allergic dermatitis of eyelid
373.33 Xeroderma of eyelid
373.34 Discoid lupus erythematosus of eyelid

373.4 Infective dermatitis of eyelid of types resulting in deformity
Code first underlying disease, as:
leprosy (030.0-030.9)
lupus vulgaris (tuberculous) (017.0)
yaws (102.0-102.9)

373.5 Other infective dermatitis of eyelid
Code first underlying disease, as:
actinomycosis (039.3)
impetigo (684)
mycotic dermatitis (110.0-111.9)
vaccinia (051.0)
postvaccination (999.0)
EXCLUDES: herpes:
simplex (054.41)
zoster (053.20)

373.6 Parasitic infestation of eyelid
Code first underlying disease, as:
leishmaniasis (085.0-085.9)
loiasis (125.2)
onchocerciasis (125.3)
pediculosis (132.0)

373.8 Other inflammations of eyelids
373.9 Unspecified inflammation of eyelid

✓4th **374 Other disorders of eyelids**
✓5th **374.0 Entropion and trichiasis of eyelid**
DEF: Entropion: turning inward of eyelid edge toward eyeball.
DEF: Trichiasis: ingrowing eyelashes marked by irritation with possible distortion of sight.
374.00 Entropion, unspecified A
374.01 Senile entropion
374.02 Mechanical entropion
374.03 Spastic entropion
374.04 Cicatricial entropion
374.05 Trichiasis without entropion

✓5th **374.1 Ectropion**
DEF: Turning outward (eversion) of eyelid edge; exposes palpebral conjunctiva; dryness, irritation result.
374.10 Ectropion, unspecified A
374.11 Senile ectropion
374.12 Mechanical ectropion
374.13 Spastic ectropion
374.14 Cicatricial ectropion

Entropion and Ectropion

NERVOUS SYSTEM AND SENSE ORGANS

374.2 Lagophthalmos (5th)
DEF: Incomplete closure of eyes; causes dry eye and other complications.
- 374.20 Lagophthalmos, unspecified
- 374.21 Paralytic lagophthalmos
- 374.22 Mechanical lagophthalmos
- 374.23 Cicatricial lagophthalmos

374.3 Ptosis of eyelid (5th)
- 374.30 Ptosis of eyelid, unspecified
  - AHA: 2Q, '96, 11
- 374.31 Paralytic ptosis
  - DEF: Drooping of upper eyelid due to nerve disorder.
- 374.32 Myogenic ptosis
  - DEF: Drooping of upper eyelid due to muscle disorder.
- 374.33 Mechanical ptosis
  - DEF: Outside force causes drooping of upper eyelid.
- 374.34 Blepharochalasis
  - Pseudoptosis
  - DEF: Loss of elasticity, thickened or indurated skin of eyelids associated with recurrent episodes of idiopathic edema causing intracellular tissue atrophy.

374.4 Other disorders affecting eyelid function (5th)
  EXCLUDES: blepharoclonus (333.81)
  blepharospasm (333.81)
  facial nerve palsy (351.0)
  third nerve palsy or paralysis (378.51-378.52)
  tic (psychogenic) (307.20-307.23)
  organic (333.3)
- 374.41 Lid retraction or lag
- 374.43 Abnormal innervation syndrome
  - Jaw-blinking
  - Paradoxical facial movements
- 374.44 Sensory disorders
- 374.45 Other sensorimotor disorders
  - Deficient blink reflex
- 374.46 Blepharophimosis
  - Ankyloblepharon
  - DEF: Narrowing of palpebral fissure horizontally; caused by laterally displaced inner canthi; either acquired or congenital.

374.5 Degenerative disorders of eyelid and periocular area (5th)
- 374.50 Degenerative disorder of eyelid, unspecified
- 374.51 Xanthelasma
  - Xanthoma (planum) (tuberosum) of eyelid
  - Code first underlying condition (272.0-272.9)
  - DEF: Fatty tumors of eyelid linked to high fat content of blood.
- 374.52 Hyperpigmentation of eyelid
  - Chloasma   Dyspigmentation
  - DEF: Excess pigment of eyelid.
- 374.53 Hypopigmentation of eyelid
  - Vitiligo of eyelid
  - DEF: Lack of color pigment of the eyelid.
- 374.54 Hypertrichosis of eyelid
  - DEF: Excess eyelash growth.
- 374.55 Hypotrichosis of eyelid
  - Madarosis of eyelid
  - DEF: Less than normal, or absent, eyelashes.
- 374.56 Other degenerative disorders of skin affecting eyelid

374.8 Other disorders of eyelid (5th)
- 374.81 Hemorrhage of eyelid
  - EXCLUDES: black eye (921.0)
- 374.82 Edema of eyelid
  - Hyperemia of eyelid
  - DEF: Swelling and fluid retention in eyelid.
- 374.83 Elephantiasis of eyelid
  - DEF: Filarial disease causing dermatitis and enlarged eyelid.
- 374.84 Cysts of eyelids
  - Sebaceous cyst of eyelid
- 374.85 Vascular anomalies of eyelid
- 374.86 Retained foreign body of eyelid
- 374.87 Dermatochalasis
  - DEF: Acquired form of connective tissue disorder associated with decreased elastic tissue and abnormal elastin formation resulting in loss of elasticity of the skin of the eyelid, generally associated with aging.
- 374.89 Other disorders of eyelid

374.9 Unspecified disorder of eyelid

375 Disorders of lacrimal system (4th)

375.0 Dacryoadenitis (5th)
- 375.00 Dacryoadenitis, unspecified
- 375.01 Acute dacryoadenitis
  - DEF: Severe, sudden inflammation of lacrimal gland.
- 375.02 Chronic dacryoadenitis
  - DEF: Persistent inflammation of lacrimal gland.
- 375.03 Chronic enlargement of lacrimal gland

375.1 Other disorders of lacrimal gland (5th)
- 375.11 Dacryops
  - DEF: Overproduction and constant flow of tears; may cause distended lacrimal duct.
- 375.12 Other lacrimal cysts and cystic degeneration
- 375.13 Primary lacrimal atrophy
- 375.14 Secondary lacrimal atrophy
  - DEF: Wasting away of lacrimal gland due to another disease.
- 375.15 Tear film insufficiency, unspecified
  - Dry eye syndrome
  - AHA: 3Q, '96, 6
  - DEF: Eye dryness and irritation due to insufficient tear production.
- 375.16 Dislocation of lacrimal gland

375.2 Epiphora (5th)
DEF: Abnormal development of tears due to stricture of lacrimal passages.
- 375.20 Epiphora, unspecified as to cause
- 375.21 Epiphora due to excess lacrimation
  - DEF: Tear overflow due to overproduction.
- 375.22 Epiphora due to insufficient drainage
  - DEF: Tear overflow due to blocked drainage.

375.3 Acute and unspecified inflammation of lacrimal passages (5th)
  EXCLUDES: neonatal dacryocystitis (771.6)
- 375.30 Dacryocystitis, unspecified
- 375.31 Acute canaliculitis, lacrimal

Lacrimal System

375.32 Acute dacryocystitis
  Acute peridacryocystitis
375.33 Phlegmonous dacryocystitis
  DEF: Infection of tear sac with pockets of pus.

375.4 Chronic inflammation of lacrimal passages
375.41 Chronic canaliculitis
375.42 Chronic dacryocystitis
375.43 Lacrimal mucocele

375.5 Stenosis and insufficiency of lacrimal passages
375.51 Eversion of lacrimal punctum
  DEF: Abnormal turning outward of tear duct.
375.52 Stenosis of lacrimal punctum
  DEF: Abnormal narrowing of tear duct.
375.53 Stenosis of lacrimal canaliculi
375.54 Stenosis of lacrimal sac
  DEF: Abnormal narrowing of tear sac.
375.55 Obstruction of nasolacrimal duct, neonatal
  EXCLUDES congenital anomaly of nasolacrimal duct (743.65)
  DEF: Acquired, abnormal obstruction of lacrimal system, from eye to nose; in an infant.
375.56 Stenosis of nasolacrimal duct, acquired
375.57 Dacryolith
  DEF: Concretion or stone in lacrimal system.

375.6 Other changes of lacrimal passages
375.61 Lacrimal fistula
  DEF: Abnormal communication from lacrimal system.
375.69 Other

375.8 Other disorders of lacrimal system
375.81 Granuloma of lacrimal passages
  DEF: Abnormal nodules within lacrimal system.
375.89 Other

375.9 Unspecified disorder of lacrimal system

376 Disorders of the orbit

376.0 Acute inflammation of orbit
376.00 Acute inflammation of orbit, unspecified
376.01 Orbital cellulitis
  Abscess of orbit
  DEF: Infection of tissue between orbital bone and eyeball.
376.02 Orbital periostitis
  DEF: Inflammation of connective tissue covering orbital bone.
376.03 Orbital osteomyelitis
  DEF: Inflammation of orbital bone.
376.04 Tenonitis

376.1 Chronic inflammatory disorders of orbit
376.10 Chronic inflammation of orbit, unspecified
376.11 Orbital granuloma
  Pseudotumor (inflammatory) of orbit
  DEF: Abnormal nodule between orbital bone and eyeball.
376.12 Orbital myositis
  DEF: Painful inflammation of eye muscles.
376.13 *Parasitic infestation of orbit*
  Code first underlying disease, as:
  hydatid infestation of orbit (122.3, 122.6, 122.9)
  myiasis of orbit (134.0)

376.2 Endocrine exophthalmos
  Code first underlying thyroid disorder (242.0-242.9)
376.21 *Thyrotoxic exophthalmos*
  DEF: Bulging eyes due to hyperthyroidism.
376.22 *Exophthalmic ophthalmoplegia*
  DEF: Inability to rotate eye due to bulging eyes.

376.3 Other exophthalmic conditions
376.30 Exophthalmos, unspecified
  DEF: Abnormal protrusion of eyeball.
376.31 Constant exophthalmos
  DEF: Continuous, abnormal protrusion or bulging of eyeball.
376.32 Orbital hemorrhage
  DEF: Bleeding behind the eyeball, causing forward bulge.
376.33 Orbital edema or congestion
  DEF: Fluid retention behind eyeball, causing forward bulge.
376.34 Intermittent exophthalmos
376.35 Pulsating exophthalmos
  DEF: Bulge or protrusion; associated with a carotid-cavernous fistula.
376.36 Lateral displacement of globe
  DEF: Abnormal displacement of the eyeball away from nose, toward temple.

376.4 Deformity of orbit
376.40 Deformity of orbit, unspecified
376.41 Hypertelorism of orbit
  DEF: Abnormal increase in interorbital distance; associated with congenital facial deformities; may be accompanied by mental deficiency.
376.42 Exostosis of orbit
  DEF: Abnormal bony growth of orbit.
376.43 Local deformities due to bone disease
  DEF: Acquired abnormalities of orbit; due to bone disease.
376.44 Orbital deformities associated with craniofacial deformities
376.45 Atrophy of orbit
  DEF: Wasting away of bone tissue of orbit.
376.46 Enlargement of orbit
376.47 Deformity due to trauma or surgery

376.5 Enophthalmos
  DEF: Recession of eyeball deep into eye socket.
376.50 Enophthalmos, unspecified as to cause
376.51 Enophthalmos due to atrophy of orbital tissue
376.52 Enophthalmos due to trauma or surgery

376.6 Retained (old) foreign body following penetrating wound of orbit
  Retrobulbar foreign body

376.8 Other orbital disorders
376.81 Orbital cysts
  Encephalocele of orbit
  AHA: 3Q, '99, 13
376.82 Myopathy of extraocular muscles
  DEF: Disease in the muscles that control eyeball movement.
376.89 Other

376.9 Unspecified disorder of orbit

377 Disorders of optic nerve and visual pathways

377.0 Papilledema
377.00 Papilledema, unspecified
377.01 Papilledema associated with increased intracranial pressure
377.02 Papilledema associated with decreased ocular pressure
377.03 Papilledema associated with retinal disorder
377.04 Foster-Kennedy syndrome
  DEF: Retrobulbar optic neuritis, central scotoma and optic atrophy; caused by tumors in frontal lobe of brain that press downward.

NERVOUS SYSTEM AND SENSE ORGANS

377.1 Optic atrophy
- 377.10 Optic atrophy, unspecified
- 377.11 Primary optic atrophy
  - EXCLUDES: neurosyphilitic optic atrophy (094.84)
- 377.12 Postinflammatory optic atrophy
  - DEF: Adverse effect of inflammation causing wasting away of eye.
- 377.13 Optic atrophy associated with retinal dystrophies
  - DEF: Progressive changes in retinal tissue due to metabolic disorder causing wasting away of eye.
- 377.14 Glaucomatous atrophy [cupping] of optic disc
- 377.15 Partial optic atrophy
  - Temporal pallor of optic disc
- 377.16 Hereditary optic atrophy
  - Optic atrophy:
    - dominant hereditary
    - Leber's

377.2 Other disorders of optic disc
- 377.21 Drusen of optic disc
- 377.22 Crater-like holes of optic disc
- 377.23 Coloboma of optic disc
  - DEF: Ocular malformation caused by the failure of fetal fissure of optic stalk to close.
- 377.24 Pseudopapilledema

377.3 Optic neuritis
  - EXCLUDES: meningococcal optic neuritis (036.81)
- 377.30 Optic neuritis, unspecified
- 377.31 Optic papillitis
  - DEF: Swelling and inflammation of optic disc.
- 377.32 Retrobulbar neuritis (acute)
  - EXCLUDES: syphilitic retrobulbar neuritis (094.85)
  - DEF: Inflammation of optic nerve immediately behind the eyeball.
- 377.33 Nutritional optic neuropathy
  - DEF: Malnutrition causing optic nerve disorder.
- 377.34 Toxic optic neuropathy
  - Toxic amblyopia
  - DEF: Toxic substance causing optic nerve disorder.
- 377.39 Other
  - EXCLUDES: ischemic optic neuropathy (377.41)

377.4 Other disorders of optic nerve
- 377.41 Ischemic optic neuropathy
  - DEF: Decreased blood flow affecting optic nerve.
- 377.42 Hemorrhage in optic nerve sheaths
  - DEF: Bleeding in meningeal lining of optic nerve.
- 377.43 Optic nerve hypoplasia
- 377.49 Other
  - Compression of optic nerve

377.5 Disorders of optic chiasm
- 377.51 Associated with pituitary neoplasms and disorders
  - DEF: Abnormal pituitary growth causing disruption in nerve chain from retina to brain.
- 377.52 Associated with other neoplasms
  - DEF: Abnormal growth, other than pituitary, causing disruption in nerve chain from retina to brain.
- 377.53 Associated with vascular disorders
  - DEF: Vascular disorder causing disruption in nerve chain from retina to brain.
- 377.54 Associated with inflammatory disorders
  - DEF: Inflammatory disease causing disruption in nerve chain from retina to brain.

377.6 Disorders of other visual pathways
- 377.61 Associated with neoplasms
- 377.62 Associated with vascular disorders
- 377.63 Associated with inflammatory disorders

377.7 Disorders of visual cortex
  - EXCLUDES: visual:
    - agnosia (368.16)
    - hallucinations (368.16)
    - halos (368.15)
- 377.71 Associated with neoplasms
- 377.72 Associated with vascular disorders
- 377.73 Associated with inflammatory disorders
- 377.75 Cortical blindness
  - DEF: Blindness due to brain disorder, rather than eye disorder.

377.9 Unspecified disorder of optic nerve and visual pathways

378 Strabismus and other disorders of binocular eye movements
  - EXCLUDES: nystagmus and other irregular eye movements (379.50-379.59)
  - DEF: Misalignment of the eyes due to imbalance in extraocular muscles.

378.0 Esotropia
  - Convergent concomitant strabismus
  - EXCLUDES: intermittent esotropia (378.20-378.22)
  - DEF: Visual axis deviation created by one eye fixing upon an image and the other eye deviating inward.
- 378.00 Esotropia, unspecified
- 378.01 Monocular esotropia
- 378.02 Monocular esotropia with A pattern
- 378.03 Monocular esotropia with V pattern
- 378.04 Monocular esotropia with other noncomitancies
  - Monocular esotropia with X or Y pattern
- 378.05 Alternating esotropia
- 378.06 Alternating esotropia with A pattern
- 378.07 Alternating esotropia with V pattern
- 378.08 Alternating esotropia with other noncomitancies
  - Alternating esotropia with X or Y pattern

378.1 Exotropia
  - Divergent concomitant strabismus
  - EXCLUDES: intermittent exotropia (378.20, 378.23-378.24)
  - DEF: Visual axis deviation created by one eye fixing upon an image and the other eye deviating outward.
- 378.10 Exotropia, unspecified
- 378.11 Monocular exotropia
- 378.12 Monocular exotropia with A pattern
- 378.13 Monocular exotropia with V pattern

Eye Musculature

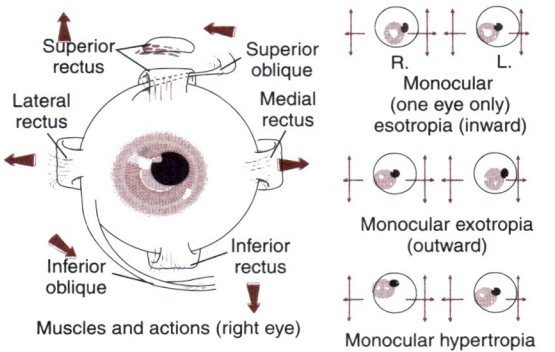

Muscles and actions (right eye)

Monocular (one eye only) esotropia (inward)

Monocular exotropia (outward)

Monocular hypertropia (upward)

2007 ICD·9·CM

NERVOUS SYSTEM AND SENSE ORGANS

378.14 Monocular exotropia with other noncomitancies
Monocular exotropia with X or Y pattern

378.15 Alternating exotropia
378.16 Alternating exotropia with A pattern
378.17 Alternating exotropia with V pattern
378.18 Alternating exotropia with other noncomitancies
Alternating exotropia with X or Y pattern

√5th **378.2** Intermittent heterotropia
EXCLUDES vertical heterotropia (intermittent) (378.31)
DEF: Deviation of eyes seen only at intervals; it is also called strabismus.

378.20 Intermittent heterotropia, unspecified
Intermittent:
esotropia NOS
exotropia NOS

378.21 Intermittent esotropia, monocular
378.22 Intermittent esotropia, alternating
378.23 Intermittent exotropia, monocular
378.24 Intermittent exotropia, alternating

√5th **378.3** Other and unspecified heterotropia
378.30 Heterotropia, unspecified
378.31 Hypertropia
Vertical heterotropia (constant) (intermittent)
378.32 Hypotropia
378.33 Cyclotropia
378.34 Monofixation syndrome
Microtropia
378.35 Accommodative component in esotropia

√5th **378.4** Heterophoria
DEF: Deviation occurring only when the other eye is covered.

378.40 Heterophoria, unspecified
378.41 Esophoria
378.42 Exophoria
378.43 Vertical heterophoria
378.44 Cyclophoria
378.45 Alternating hyperphoria

√5th **378.5** Paralytic strabismus
DEF: Deviation of the eye due to nerve paralysis affecting muscle.

378.50 Paralytic strabismus, unspecified
378.51 Third or oculomotor nerve palsy, partial
AHA: 3Q, '91, 9

378.52 Third or oculomotor nerve palsy, total
AHA: 2Q, '89, 12

378.53 Fourth or trochlear nerve palsy
AHA: 2Q, '01, 21

378.54 Sixth or abducens nerve palsy
AHA: 2Q, '89, 12

378.55 External ophthalmoplegia
378.56 Total ophthalmoplegia

√5th **378.6** Mechanical strabismus
DEF: Deviation of the eye due to an outside force on extraocular muscle.

378.60 Mechanical strabismus, unspecified
378.61 Brown's (tendon) sheath syndrome
DEF: Congenital or acquired shortening of the anterior sheath of the superior oblique muscle; the eye is unable to move upward and inward; it is usually unilateral.

378.62 Mechanical strabismus from other musculofascial disorders
378.63 Limited duction associated with other conditions

√5th **378.7** Other specified strabismus
378.71 Duane's syndrome
DEF: Congenital; affects one eye; due to abnormal fibrous bands attached to rectus muscle; inability to abduct affected eye with retraction of globe.

378.72 Progressive external ophthalmoplegia
DEF: Paralysis progressing from one eye muscle to another.

378.73 Strabismus in other neuromuscular disorders

√5th **378.8** Other disorders of binocular eye movements
EXCLUDES nystagmus (379.50-379.56)

378.81 Palsy of conjugate gaze
DEF: Muscle dysfunction impairing parallel movement of the eye.

378.82 Spasm of conjugate gaze
DEF: Muscle contractions impairing parallel movement of eye.

378.83 Convergence insufficiency or palsy
378.84 Convergence excess or spasm
378.85 Anomalies of divergence
378.86 Internuclear ophthalmoplegia
DEF: Eye movement anomaly due to brainstem lesion.

378.87 Other dissociated deviation of eye movements
Skew deviation

378.9 Unspecified disorder of eye movements
Ophthalmoplegia NOS Strabismus NOS
AHA: 2Q, '01, 21

√4th **379** Other disorders of eye
√5th **379.0** Scleritis and episcleritis
EXCLUDES syphilitic episcleritis (095.0)

379.00 Scleritis, unspecified
Episcleritis NOS

379.01 Episcleritis periodica fugax
DEF: Hyperemia (engorgement) of the sclera and overlying conjunctiva characterized by a sudden onset and short duration.

379.02 Nodular episcleritis
DEF: Inflammation of the outermost layer of the sclera, with formation of nodules.

379.03 Anterior scleritis
379.04 Scleromalacia perforans
DEF: Scleral thinning, softening and degeneration; seen with rheumatoid arthritis.

379.05 Scleritis with corneal involvement
Scleroperikeratitis

379.06 Brawny scleritis
DEF: Severe inflammation of the sclera; with thickened corneal margins.

379.07 Posterior scleritis
Sclerotenonitis

379.09 Other
Scleral abscess

√5th **379.1** Other disorders of sclera
EXCLUDES blue sclera (743.47)

379.11 Scleral ectasia
Scleral staphyloma NOS
DEF: Protrusion of the contents of the eyeball where the sclera has thinned.

379.12 Staphyloma posticum
DEF: Ring-shaped protrusion or bulging of sclera and uveal tissue at posterior pole of eye.

379.13 Equatorial staphyloma
DEF: Ring-shaped protrusion or bulging of sclera and uveal tissue midway between front and back of eye.

N Newborn Age: 0   P Pediatric Age: 0-17   M Maternity Age: 12-55   A Adult Age: 15-124

110 — Volume 1   2007 ICD•9•CM

NERVOUS SYSTEM AND SENSE ORGANS

379.14 Anterior staphyloma, localized
379.15 Ring staphyloma
379.16 Other degenerative disorders of sclera
379.19 Other

✓5th **379.2 Disorders of vitreous body**
DEF: Disorder of clear gel that fills space between retina and lens.

379.21 Vitreous degeneration
  Vitreous: cavitation
  Vitreous: liquefaction
  detachment
379.22 Crystalline deposits in vitreous
  Asteroid hyalitis
  Synchysis scintillans
379.23 Vitreous hemorrhage
  AHA: 3Q, '91, 15
379.24 Other vitreous opacities
  Vitreous floaters
379.25 Vitreous membranes and strands
379.26 Vitreous prolapse
  DEF: Slipping of vitreous from normal position.
379.29 Other disorders of vitreous
  EXCLUDES vitreous abscess (360.04)
  AHA: 1Q, '99, 11

✓5th **379.3 Aphakia and other disorders of lens**
  EXCLUDES after-cataract (366.50-366.53)
379.31 Aphakia
  EXCLUDES cataract extraction status (V45.61)
  DEF: Absence of eye's crystalline lens.
379.32 Subluxation of lens
379.33 Anterior dislocation of lens
  DEF: Lens displaced toward iris.
379.34 Posterior dislocation of lens
  DEF: Lens displaced backward toward vitreous.
379.39 Other disorders of lens

✓5th **379.4 Anomalies of pupillary function**
379.40 Abnormal pupillary function, unspecified
379.41 Anisocoria
  DEF: Unequal pupil diameter.
379.42 Miosis (persistent), not due to miotics
  DEF: Abnormal contraction of pupil less than 2 millimeters.
379.43 Mydriasis (persistent), not due to mydriatics
  DEF: Morbid dilation of pupil.
379.45 Argyll Robertson pupil, atypical
  Argyll Robertson phenomenon or pupil, nonsyphilitic
  EXCLUDES Argyll Robertson pupil (syphilitic) (094.89)
  DEF: Failure of pupil to respond to light; affects both eyes; may be caused by diseases such as syphilis of the central nervous system or miosis.
379.46 Tonic pupillary reaction
  Adie's pupil or syndrome
379.49 Other
  Hippus
  Pupillary paralysis

✓5th **379.5 Nystagmus and other irregular eye movements**
379.50 Nystagmus, unspecified
  AHA: 4Q, '02, 68; 2Q, '01, 21
  DEF: Involuntary, rapid, rhythmic movement of eyeball; vertical, horizontal, rotatory or mixed; cause may be congenital, acquired, physiological, neurological, myopathic, or due to ocular diseases.

379.51 Congenital nystagmus
379.52 Latent nystagmus
379.53 Visual deprivation nystagmus
379.54 Nystagmus associated with disorders of the vestibular system
379.55 Dissociated nystagmus
379.56 Other forms of nystagmus
379.57 Deficiencies of saccadic eye movements
  Abnormal optokinetic response
  DEF: Saccadic eye movements; small, rapid, involuntary movements by both eyes simultaneously, due to changing point of fixation on visualized object.
379.58 Deficiencies of smooth pursuit movements
379.59 Other irregularities of eye movements
  Opsoclonus

● ✓5th **379.6 Inflammation (infection) of postprocedural bleb**
  Postprocedural blebitis
● 379.60 Inflammation (infection) of postprocedural bleb, unspecified
● 379.61 Inflammation (infection) of postprocedural bleb, stage 1
● 379.62 Inflammation (infection) of postprocedural bleb, stage 2
● 379.63 Inflammation (infection) of postprocedural bleb, stage 3
  Bleb associated endophthalmitis

379.8 Other specified disorders of eye and adnexa
✓5th **379.9 Unspecified disorder of eye and adnexa**
379.90 Disorder of eye, unspecified
379.91 Pain in or around eye
379.92 Swelling or mass of eye
379.93 Redness or discharge of eye
379.99 Other ill-defined disorders of eye
  EXCLUDES blurred vision NOS (368.8)

DISEASES OF THE EAR AND MASTOID PROCESS (380-389)

✓4th **380 Disorders of external ear**
✓5th **380.0 Perichondritis and chondritis of pinna**
  Chondritis of auricle
  Perichondritis of auricle
380.00 Perichondritis of pinna, unspecified
380.01 Acute perichondritis of pinna
380.02 Chronic perichondritis of pinna
380.03 Chondritis of pinna
  AHA: 4Q, '04, 76
  DEF: Infection that has progressed into the cartilage; presents as indurated and edematous skin over the pinna; vascular compromise occurs with tissue necrosis and deformity.

✓5th **380.1 Infective otitis externa**
380.10 Infective otitis externa, unspecified
  Otitis externa (acute):   Otitis externa (acute):
    NOS   hemorrhagica
    circumscribed   infective NOS
    diffuse

Ear and Mastoid Process

✓4th Additional Digit Required | Unspecified Code | Other Specified Code | Manifestation Code | ▶◀ Revised Text | ● New Code | ▲ Revised Code Title

NERVOUS SYSTEM AND SENSE ORGANS — Tabular List

380.11 Acute infection of pinna
EXCLUDES furuncular otitis externa (680.0)

380.12 Acute swimmers' ear
Beach ear
Tank ear
DEF: Otitis externa due to swimming.

380.13 Other acute infections of external ear
Code first underlying disease, as:
erysipelas (035)
impetigo (684)
seborrheic dermatitis (690.10-690.18)
EXCLUDES herpes simplex (054.73)
herpes zoster (053.71)

380.14 Malignant otitis externa
DEF: Severe necrotic otitis externa; due to bacteria.

380.15 Chronic mycotic otitis externa
Code first underlying disease, as:
aspergillosis (117.3)
otomycosis NOS (111.9)
EXCLUDES candidal otitis externa (112.82)

380.16 Other chronic infective otitis externa
Chronic infective otitis externa NOS

√5th 380.2 Other otitis externa
380.21 Cholesteatoma of external ear
Keratosis obturans of external ear (canal)
EXCLUDES cholesteatoma NOS (385.30-385.35)
postmastoidectomy (383.32)
DEF: Cystlike mass filled with debris, including cholesterol; rare, congenital condition.

380.22 Other acute otitis externa
Acute otitis externa: Acute otitis externa:
  actinic   eczematoid
  chemical   reactive
  contact

380.23 Other chronic otitis externa
Chronic otitis externa NOS

√5th 380.3 Noninfectious disorders of pinna
380.30 Disorder of pinna, unspecified
380.31 Hematoma of auricle or pinna
380.32 Acquired deformities of auricle or pinna
EXCLUDES cauliflower ear (738.7)
AHA: 3Q, '03, 12

380.39 Other
EXCLUDES gouty tophi of ear (274.81)

380.4 Impacted cerumen
Wax in ear

√5th 380.5 Acquired stenosis of external ear canal
Collapse of external ear canal
380.50 Acquired stenosis of external ear canal, unspecified as to cause
380.51 Secondary to trauma
DEF: Narrowing of external ear canal; due to trauma.
380.52 Secondary to surgery
DEF: Postsurgical narrowing of external ear canal.
380.53 Secondary to inflammation
DEF: Narrowing, external ear canal; due to chronic inflammation.

√5th 380.8 Other disorders of external ear
380.81 Exostosis of external ear canal
380.89 Other

380.9 Unspecified disorder of external ear

√4th 381 Nonsuppurative otitis media and Eustachian tube disorders
√5th 381.0 Acute nonsuppurative otitis media
Acute tubotympanic catarrh
Otitis media, acute or subacute:
  catarrhal   transudative
  exudative   with effusion
EXCLUDES otitic barotrauma (993.0)

381.00 Acute nonsuppurative otitis media, unspecified
381.01 Acute serous otitis media
Acute or subacute secretory otitis media
DEF: Sudden, severe infection of middle ear.
381.02 Acute mucoid otitis media
Acute or subacute seromucinous otitis media
Blue drum syndrome
DEF: Sudden, severe infection of middle ear, with mucous.
381.03 Acute sanguinous otitis media
DEF: Sudden, severe infection of middle ear, with blood.
381.04 Acute allergic serous otitis media
381.05 Acute allergic mucoid otitis media
381.06 Acute allergic sanguinous otitis media

√5th 381.1 Chronic serous otitis media
Chronic tubotympanic catarrh
381.10 Chronic serous otitis media, simple or unspecified
DEF: Persistent infection of middle ear, without pus.
381.19 Other
Serosanguinous chronic otitis media

√5th 381.2 Chronic mucoid otitis media
Glue ear
EXCLUDES adhesive middle ear disease (385.10-385.19)
DEF: Chronic condition; characterized by viscous fluid in middle ear; due to obstructed Eustachian tube.

381.20 Chronic mucoid otitis media, simple or unspecified
381.29 Other
Mucosanguinous chronic otitis media

381.3 Other and unspecified chronic nonsuppurative otitis media
Otitis media, chronic: Otitis media, chronic:
  allergic   seromucinous
  exudative   transudative
  secretory   with effusion

381.4 Nonsuppurative otitis media, not specified as acute or chronic
Otitis media: Otitis media:
  allergic   seromucinous
  catarrhal   serous
  exudative   transudative
  mucoid   with effusion
  secretory

√5th 381.5 Eustachian salpingitis
381.50 Eustachian salpingitis, unspecified
381.51 Acute Eustachian salpingitis
DEF: Sudden, severe inflammation of Eustachian tube.
381.52 Chronic Eustachian salpingitis
DEF: Persistent inflammation of Eustachian tube.

NERVOUS SYSTEM AND SENSE ORGANS

381.6 ☑5ᵗʰ **Obstruction of Eustachian tube**
  Stenosis } of Eustachian tube
  Stricture

  381.60 Obstruction of Eustachian tube, unspecified
  381.61 Osseous obstruction of Eustachian tube
    Obstruction of Eustachian tube from cholesteatoma, polyp, or other osseous lesion
  381.62 Intrinsic cartilagenous obstruction of Eustachian tube
    DEF: Blockage of Eustachian tube; due to cartilage overgrowth.
  381.63 Extrinsic cartilagenous obstruction of Eustachian tube
    Compression of Eustachian tube

381.7 Patulous Eustachian tube
  DEF: Distended, oversized Eustachian tube.

☑5ᵗʰ **381.8 Other disorders of Eustachian tube**
  381.81 Dysfunction of Eustachian tube
  381.89 Other

381.9 Unspecified Eustachian tube disorder

☑4ᵗʰ **382 Suppurative and unspecified otitis media**
☑5ᵗʰ **382.0 Acute suppurative otitis media**
  Otitis media, acute: Otitis media, acute:
    necrotizing NOS   purulent

  382.00 Acute suppurative otitis media without spontaneous rupture of ear drum
    DEF: Sudden, severe inflammation of middle ear, with pus.
  382.01 Acute suppurative otitis media with spontaneous rupture of ear drum
    DEF: Sudden, severe inflammation of middle ear, with pressure tearing ear drum tissue.
  382.02 *Acute suppurative otitis media in diseases classified elsewhere*
    Code first underlying disease, as:
      influenza (487.8)
      scarlet fever (034.1)
    EXCLUDES postmeasles otitis (055.2)

382.1 Chronic tubotympanic suppurative otitis media
  Benign chronic suppurative
    otitis media   } (with anterior perforation of ear drum)
  Chronic tubotympanic disease
  DEF: Inflammation of tympanic cavity and auditory tube; with pus formation.

382.2 Chronic atticoantral suppurative otitis media
  Chronic atticoantral
    disease   } (with posterior or superior marginal perforation of ear drum)
  Persistent mucosal disease
  DEF: Inflammation of upper tympanic membrane and mastoid antrum; with pus formation.

382.3 Unspecified chronic suppurative otitis media
  Chronic purulent otitis media
    EXCLUDES tuberculous otitis media (017.4)

382.4 Unspecified suppurative otitis media
  Purulent otitis media NOS

382.9 Unspecified otitis media
  Otitis media: Otitis media:
    NOS   chronic NOS
    acute NOS
  AHA: N-D, '84, 16

☑4ᵗʰ **383 Mastoiditis and related conditions**
☑5ᵗʰ **383.0 Acute mastoiditis**
  Abscess of mastoid   Empyema of mastoid
  383.00 Acute mastoiditis without complications
    DEF: Sudden, severe inflammation of mastoid air cells.
  383.01 Subperiosteal abscess of mastoid
    DEF: Pocket of pus within mastoid bone.
  383.02 Acute mastoiditis with other complications
    Gradenigo's syndrome

383.1 Chronic mastoiditis
  Caries of mastoid
  Fistula of mastoid
    EXCLUDES tuberculous mastoiditis (015.6)
  DEF: Persistent inflammation of mastoid air cells.

☑5ᵗʰ **383.2 Petrositis**
  Coalescing osteitis }
  Inflammation   } of petrous bone
  Osteomyelitis   }

  383.20 **Petrositis, unspecified**
  383.21 Acute petrositis
    DEF: Sudden, severe inflammation of dense bone behind ear.
  383.22 Chronic petrositis
    DEF: Persistent inflammation of dense bone behind ear.

☑5ᵗʰ **383.3 Complications following mastoidectomy**
  383.30 **Postmastoidectomy complication, unspecified**
  383.31 Mucosal cyst of postmastoidectomy cavity
    DEF: Mucous-lined cyst cavity following removal of mastoid bone.
  383.32 Recurrent cholesteatoma of postmastoidectomy cavity
    DEF: Cystlike mass of cell debris in cavity following removal of mastoid bone.
  383.33 Granulations of postmastoidectomy cavity
    Chronic inflammation of postmastoidectomy cavity
    DEF: Granular tissue in cavity following removal of mastoid bone.

☑5ᵗʰ **383.8 Other disorders of mastoid**
  383.81 Postauricular fistula
    DEF: Abnormal passage behind mastoid cavity.
  383.89 Other

383.9 Unspecified mastoiditis

☑4ᵗʰ **384 Other disorders of tympanic membrane**
☑5ᵗʰ **384.0 Acute myringitis without mention of otitis media**
  384.00 **Acute myringitis, unspecified**
    Acute tympanitis NOS
    DEF: Sudden, severe inflammation of ear drum.
  384.01 Bullous myringitis
    Myringitis bullosa hemorrhagica
    DEF: Type of viral otitis media characterized by the appearance of serous or hemorrhagic blebs on the tympanic membrane.
  384.09 Other

2007 ICD•9•CM — Volume 1 — 113

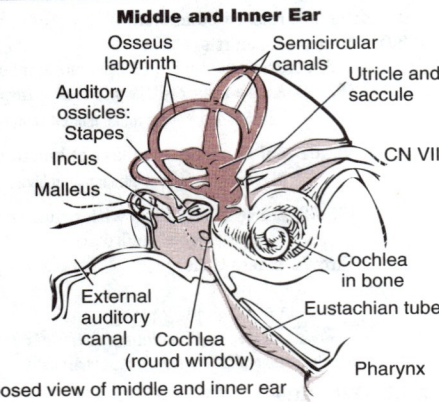

Middle and Inner Ear — Exposed view of middle and inner ear

Cholesteatoma

384.1 Chronic myringitis without mention of otitis media
Chronic tympanitis
DEF: Persistent inflammation of ear drum; with no evidence of middle ear infection.

√5th **384.2 Perforation of tympanic membrane**
Perforation of ear drum: NOS
persistent posttraumatic
Perforation of ear drum: postinflammatory
EXCLUDES: otitis media with perforation of tympanic membrane (382.00-382.9)
traumatic perforation [current injury] (872.61)

384.20 Perforation of tympanic membrane, unspecified
384.21 Central perforation of tympanic membrane
384.22 Attic perforation of tympanic membrane
Pars flaccida
384.23 Other marginal perforation of tympanic membrane
384.24 Multiple perforations of tympanic membrane
384.25 Total perforation of tympanic membrane

√5th **384.8 Other specified disorders of tympanic membrane**
384.81 Atrophic flaccid tympanic membrane
Healed perforation of ear drum
384.82 Atrophic nonflaccid tympanic membrane

384.9 Unspecified disorder of tympanic membrane

√4th **385 Other disorders of middle ear and mastoid**
EXCLUDES: mastoiditis (383.0-383.9)

√5th **385.0 Tympanosclerosis**
385.00 Tympanosclerosis, unspecified as to involvement
385.01 Tympanosclerosis involving tympanic membrane only
DEF: Tough, fibrous tissue impeding functions of ear drum.
385.02 Tympanosclerosis involving tympanic membrane and ear ossicles
DEF: Tough, fibrous tissue impeding functions of middle ear bones (stapes, malleus, incus).
385.03 Tympanosclerosis involving tympanic membrane, ear ossicles, and middle ear
DEF: Tough, fibrous tissue impeding functions of ear drum, middle ear bones and middle ear canal.
385.09 Tympanosclerosis involving other combination of structures

√5th **385.1 Adhesive middle ear disease**
Adhesive otitis
Otitis media: chronic adhesive
Otitis media: fibrotic
EXCLUDES: glue ear (381.20-381.29)
DEF: Adhesions of middle ear structures.

385.10 Adhesive middle ear disease, unspecified as to involvement
385.11 Adhesions of drum head to incus
385.12 Adhesions of drum head to stapes
385.13 Adhesions of drum head to promontorium
385.19 Other adhesions and combinations

√5th **385.2 Other acquired abnormality of ear ossicles**
385.21 Impaired mobility of malleus
Ankylosis of malleus
385.22 Impaired mobility of other ear ossicles
Ankylosis of ear ossicles, except malleus
385.23 Discontinuity or dislocation of ear ossicles
DEF: Disruption in auditory chain; created by malleus, incus and stapes.
385.24 Partial loss or necrosis of ear ossicles
DEF: Tissue loss in malleus, incus and stapes.

√5th **385.3 Cholesteatoma of middle ear and mastoid**
Cholesterosis
Epidermosis
Keratosis
Polyp
} of (middle) ear

EXCLUDES: cholesteatoma:
external ear canal (380.21)
recurrent of postmastoidectomy cavity (383.32)
DEF: Cystlike mass of middle ear and mastoid antrum filled with debris, including cholesterol.

385.30 Cholesteatoma, unspecified
385.31 Cholesteatoma of attic
385.32 Cholesteatoma of middle ear
385.33 Cholesteatoma of middle ear and mastoid
AHA: 3Q, '00, 10
DEF: Cystlike mass of cell debris in middle ear and mastoid air cells behind ear.
385.35 Diffuse cholesteatosis

√5th **385.8 Other disorders of middle ear and mastoid**
385.82 Cholesterin granuloma
DEF: Granuloma formed of fibrotic tissue; contains cholesterol crystals surrounded by foreign-body cells; found in the middle ear and mastoid area.
385.83 Retained foreign body of middle ear
AHA: 3Q, '94, 7; N-D, '87, 9
385.89 Other

385.9 Unspecified disorder of middle ear and mastoid

√4th **386 Vertiginous syndromes and other disorders of vestibular system**
EXCLUDES: vertigo NOS (780.4)
AHA: M-A, '85, 12

NERVOUS SYSTEM AND SENSE ORGANS

386.0 Ménière's disease
Endolymphatic hydrops
Lermoyez's syndrome
Ménière's syndrome or vertigo
DEF: Distended membranous labyrinth of middle ear from endolymphatic hydrops; causes ischemia, failure of nerve function; hearing and balance dysfunction; symptoms include fluctuating deafness, ringing in ears and dizziness.

- 386.00 Ménière's disease, unspecified
  Ménière's disease (active)
- 386.01 Active Ménière's disease, cochleovestibular
- 386.02 Active Ménière's disease, cochlear
- 386.03 Active Ménière's disease, vestibular
- 386.04 Inactive Ménière's disease
  Ménière's disease in remission

386.1 Other and unspecified peripheral vertigo
EXCLUDES epidemic vertigo (078.81)
- 386.10 Peripheral vertigo, unspecified
- 386.11 Benign paroxysmal positional vertigo
  Benign paroxysmal positional nystagmus
- 386.12 Vestibular neuronitis
  Acute (and recurrent) peripheral vestibulopathy
  DEF: Transient benign vertigo, unknown cause; characterized by response to caloric stimulation on one side, nystagmus with rhythmic movement of eyes; normal auditory function present; occurs in young adults.
- 386.19 Other
  Aural vertigo
  Otogenic vertigo

386.2 Vertigo of central origin
Central positional nystagmus
Malignant positional vertigo

386.3 Labyrinthitis
- 386.30 Labyrinthitis, unspecified
- 386.31 Serous labyrinthitis
  Diffuse labyrinthitis
  DEF: Inflammation of labyrinth; with fluid buildup.
- 386.32 Circumscribed labyrinthitis
  Focal labyrinthitis
- 386.33 Suppurative labyrinthitis
  Purulent labyrinthitis
  DEF: Inflammation of labyrinth; with pus.
- 386.34 Toxic labyrinthitis
  DEF: Inflammation of labyrinth; due to toxic reaction.
- 386.35 Viral labyrinthitis

386.4 Labyrinthine fistula
- 386.40 Labyrinthine fistula, unspecified
- 386.41 Round window fistula
- 386.42 Oval window fistula
- 386.43 Semicircular canal fistula
- 386.48 Labyrinthine fistula of combined sites

386.5 Labyrinthine dysfunction
- 386.50 Labyrinthine dysfunction, unspecified
- 386.51 Hyperactive labyrinth, unilateral
  DEF: Oversensitivity of labyrinth to auditory signals; affecting one ear.
- 386.52 Hyperactive labyrinth, bilateral
  DEF: Oversensitivity of labyrinth to auditory signals; affecting both ears.
- 386.53 Hypoactive labyrinth, unilateral
  DEF: Reduced sensitivity of labyrinth to auditory signals; affecting one ear.
- 386.54 Hypoactive labyrinth, bilateral
  DEF: Reduced sensitivity of labyrinth to auditory signals; affecting both ears.
- 386.55 Loss of labyrinthine reactivity, unilateral
  DEF: Reduced reaction of labyrinth to auditory signals; affecting one ear.
- 386.56 Loss of labyrinthine reactivity, bilateral
  DEF: Reduced reaction of labyrinth to auditory signals; affecting both ears.
- 386.58 Other forms and combinations

386.8 Other disorders of labyrinth
386.9 Unspecified vertiginous syndromes and labyrinthine disorders

387 Otosclerosis
INCLUDES otospongiosis
DEF: Synonym for otospongiosis, spongy bone formation in the labyrinth bones of the ear; it causes progressive hearing impairment.

- 387.0 Otosclerosis involving oval window, nonobliterative
  DEF: Tough, fibrous tissue impeding functions of oval window.
- 387.1 Otosclerosis involving oval window, obliterative
  DEF: Tough, fibrous tissue blocking oval window.
- 387.2 Cochlear otosclerosis
  Otosclerosis involving: Otosclerosis involving:
  otic capsule   round window
  DEF: Tough, fibrous tissue impeding functions of cochlea.
- 387.8 Other otosclerosis
- 387.9 Otosclerosis, unspecified

388 Other disorders of ear
388.0 Degenerative and vascular disorders of ear
- 388.00 Degenerative and vascular disorders, unspecified
- 388.01 Presbyacusis
  DEF: Progressive, bilateral perceptive hearing loss caused by advancing age; it is also known as presbycusis.
- 388.02 Transient ischemic deafness
  DEF: Restricted blood flow to auditory organs causing temporary hearing loss.

388.1 Noise effects on inner ear
- 388.10 Noise effects on inner ear, unspecified
- 388.11 Acoustic trauma (explosive) to ear
  Otitic blast injury
- 388.12 Noise-induced hearing loss

388.2 Sudden hearing loss, unspecified
388.3 Tinnitus
DEF: Abnormal noises in ear; may be heard by others beside the affected individual; noises include ringing, clicking, roaring and buzzing.
- 388.30 Tinnitus, unspecified
- 388.31 Subjective tinnitus
- 388.32 Objective tinnitus

388.4 Other abnormal auditory perception
- 388.40 Abnormal auditory perception, unspecified
- 388.41 Diplacusis
  DEF: Perception of a single auditory sound as two sounds at two different levels of intensity.
- 388.42 Hyperacusis
  DEF: Exceptionally acute sense of hearing caused by such conditions as Bell's palsy; this term may also refer to painful sensitivity to sounds.
- 388.43 Impairment of auditory discrimination
  DEF: Impaired ability to distinguish tone of sound.
- 388.44 Recruitment
  DEF: Perception of abnormally increased loudness caused by a slight increase in sound intensity; it is a term used in audiology.

388.5 Disorders of acoustic nerve
Acoustic neuritis
Degeneration } of acoustic or eighth nerve
Disorder

EXCLUDES: acoustic neuroma (225.1)
syphilitic acoustic neuritis (094.86)

AHA: M-A, '87, 8

√5th 388.6 Otorrhea
- **388.60** Otorrhea, unspecified
Discharging ear NOS
- **388.61** Cerebrospinal fluid otorrhea
EXCLUDES: cerebrospinal fluid rhinorrhea (349.81)
DEF: Spinal fluid leakage from ear.
- **388.69** Other
Otorrhagia

√5th 388.7 Otalgia
- **388.70** Otalgia, unspecified
Earache NOS
- **388.71** Otogenic pain
- **388.72** Referred pain

388.8 Other disorders of ear

388.9 Unspecified disorder of ear

√4th 389 Hearing loss

√5th 389.0 Conductive hearing loss
Conductive deafness
AHA: 4Q, '89, 5
DEF: Dysfunction in sound-conducting structures of external or middle ear causing hearing loss.
- **389.00** Conductive hearing loss, unspecified
- **389.01** Conductive hearing loss, external ear
- **389.02** Conductive hearing loss, tympanic membrane
- **389.03** Conductive hearing loss, middle ear
- **389.04** Conductive hearing loss, inner ear
- **389.08** Conductive hearing loss of combined types

√5th 389.1 Sensorineural hearing loss
Perceptive hearing loss or deafness
EXCLUDES: abnormal auditory perception (388.40-388.44)
psychogenic deafness (306.7)
AHA: 4Q, '89, 5
DEF: Nerve conduction causing hearing loss.
- **389.10** Sensorineural hearing loss, unspecified
AHA: 1Q, '93, 29
- **389.11** Sensory hearing loss, bilateral
- **389.12** Neural hearing loss, bilateral
- **389.14** Central hearing loss, bilateral
- **389.15** Sensorineural hearing loss, unilateral
- **389.16** Sensorineural hearing loss, asymmetrical
- **389.18** Sensorineural hearing loss of combined types, bilateral

389.2 Mixed conductive and sensorineural hearing loss
Deafness or hearing loss of type classifiable to 389.0 with type classifiable to 389.1

389.7 Deaf mutism, not elsewhere classifiable
Deaf, nonspeaking

389.8 Other specified forms of hearing loss

389.9 Unspecified hearing loss
Deafness NOS
AHA: 1Q, '04, 15

7. DISEASES OF THE CIRCULATORY SYSTEM (390-459)

ACUTE RHEUMATIC FEVER (390-392)

DEF: Febrile disease occurs mainly in children or young adults following throat infection by group A streptococci; symptoms include fever, joint pain, lesions of heart, blood vessels and joint connective tissue, abdominal pain, skin changes, and chorea.

390 Rheumatic fever without mention of heart involvement
Arthritis, rheumatic, acute or subacute
Rheumatic fever (active) (acute)
Rheumatism, articular, acute or subacute
EXCLUDES that with heart involvement (391.0-391.9)

391 Rheumatic fever with heart involvement
EXCLUDES chronic heart diseases of rheumatic origin (393.0-398.9) unless rheumatic fever is also present or there is evidence of recrudescence or activity of the rheumatic process

391.0 Acute rheumatic pericarditis
Rheumatic:
  fever (active) (acute) with pericarditis
  pericarditis (acute)
Any condition classifiable to 390 with pericarditis
EXCLUDES that not specified as rheumatic (420.0-420.9)

DEF: Sudden, severe inflammation of heart lining due to rheumatic fever.

391.1 Acute rheumatic endocarditis
Rheumatic:
  endocarditis, acute
  fever (active) (acute) with endocarditis or valvulitis
  valvulitis acute
Any condition classifiable to 390 with endocarditis or valvulitis

DEF: Sudden, severe inflammation of heart cavities due to rheumatic fever.

391.2 Acute rheumatic myocarditis
Rheumatic fever (active) (acute) with myocarditis
Any condition classifiable to 390 with myocarditis

DEF: Sudden, severe inflammation of heart muscles due to rheumatic fever.

391.8 Other acute rheumatic heart disease
Rheumatic:
  fever (active) (acute) with other or multiple types of heart involvement
  pancarditis, acute
Any condition classifiable to 390 with other or multiple types of heart involvement

391.9 Acute rheumatic heart disease, unspecified
Rheumatic:
  carditis, acute
  fever (active) (acute) with unspecified type of heart involvement
  heart disease, active or acute
Any condition classifiable to 390 with unspecified type of heart involvement

392 Rheumatic chorea
INCLUDES Sydenham's chorea
EXCLUDES chorea:
  NOS (333.5)
  Huntington's (333.4)

DEF: Childhood disease linked with rheumatic fever and streptococcal infections; symptoms include spasmodic, involuntary movements of limbs or facial muscles, psychic symptoms, and irritability.

392.0 With heart involvement
Rheumatic chorea with heart involvement of any type classifiable to 391

392.9 Without mention of heart involvement

CHRONIC RHEUMATIC HEART DISEASE (393-398)

393 Chronic rheumatic pericarditis
Adherent pericardium, rheumatic
Chronic rheumatic:
  mediastinopericarditis
  myopericarditis
EXCLUDES pericarditis NOS or not specified as rheumatic (423.0-423.9)

DEF: Persistent inflammation of heart lining due to rheumatic heart disease.

394 Diseases of mitral valve
EXCLUDES that with aortic valve involvement (396.0-396.9)

394.0 Mitral stenosis
Mitral (valve):
  obstruction (rheumatic)
  stenosis NOS

DEF: Narrowing, of mitral valve between left atrium and left ventricle due to rheumatic heart disease.

394.1 Rheumatic mitral insufficiency
Rheumatic mitral: Rheumatic mitral:
  incompetence   regurgitation
EXCLUDES that not specified as rheumatic (424.0)
AHA: ▶2Q, '05, 14◀

DEF: Malfunction of mitral valve between left atrium and left ventricle due to rheumatic heart disease.

394.2 Mitral stenosis with insufficiency
Mitral stenosis with incompetence or regurgitation

DEF: A narrowing or stricture of the mitral valve situated between the left atrium and left ventricle. The stenosis interferes with blood flow from the atrium into the ventricle. If the valve does not completely close, it becomes insufficient (inadequate) and cannot prevent regurgitation (abnormal backward flow) into the atrium when the left ventricle contracts. This abnormal function is also called incompetence.

394.9 Other and unspecified mitral valve diseases
Mitral (valve):   Mitral (valve):
  disease (chronic)   failure

395 Diseases of aortic valve
EXCLUDES that not specified as rheumatic (424.1)
that with mitral valve involvement (396.0-396.9)

395.0 Rheumatic aortic stenosis
Rheumatic aortic (valve) obstruction
AHA: 4Q, '88, 8

DEF: Narrowing of the aortic valve; results in backflow into ventricle due to rheumatic heart disease.

395.1 Rheumatic aortic insufficiency
Rheumatic aortic: Rheumatic aortic:
  incompetence   regurgitation

DEF: Malfunction of the aortic valve; results in backflow into left ventricle due to rheumatic heart disease.

395.2 Rheumatic aortic stenosis with insufficiency
Rheumatic aortic stenosis with incompetence or regurgitation

DEF: Malfunction and narrowing, of the aortic valve; results in backflow into left ventricle due to rheumatic heart disease.

395.9 Other and unspecified rheumatic aortic diseases
Rheumatic aortic (valve) disease

396 Diseases of mitral and aortic valves
INCLUDES involvement of both mitral and aortic valves, whether specified as rheumatic or not
AHA: N-D, '87, 8

396.0 Mitral valve stenosis and aortic valve stenosis
Atypical aortic (valve) stenosis
Mitral and aortic (valve) obstruction (rheumatic)

396.1 Mitral valve stenosis and aortic valve insufficiency

396.2 Mitral valve insufficiency and aortic valve stenosis
AHA: 2Q, '00, 16

CIRCULATORY SYSTEM

396.3 Mitral valve insufficiency and aortic valve insufficiency
Mitral and aortic (valve): incompetence
Mitral and aortic (valve): regurgitation

396.8 Multiple involvement of mitral and aortic valves
Stenosis and insufficiency of mitral or aortic valve with stenosis or insufficiency, or both, of the other valve

396.9 Mitral and aortic valve diseases, unspecified

√4th **397** Diseases of other endocardial structures

397.0 Diseases of tricuspid valve
Tricuspid (valve) (rheumatic):
  disease
  insufficiency
  obstruction
  regurgitation
  stenosis
AHA: 2Q, '00, 16

DEF: Malfunction of the valve between right atrium and right ventricle due to rheumatic heart disease.

397.1 Rheumatic diseases of pulmonary valve
EXCLUDES that not specified as rheumatic (424.3)

397.9 Rheumatic diseases of endocardium, valve unspecified
Rheumatic:
  endocarditis (chronic)
  valvulitis (chronic)
EXCLUDES that not specified as rheumatic (424.90-424.99)

√4th **398** Other rheumatic heart disease

398.0 Rheumatic myocarditis
Rheumatic degeneration of myocardium
EXCLUDES myocarditis not specified as rheumatic (429.0)

DEF: Chronic inflammation of heart muscle due to rheumatic heart disease.

√5th **398.9** Other and unspecified rheumatic heart diseases

398.90 Rheumatic heart disease, unspecified
Rheumatic: Rheumatic:
  carditis   heart disease NOS
EXCLUDES carditis not specified as rheumatic (429.89)
heart disease NOS not specified as rheumatic (429.9)

398.91 Rheumatic heart failure (congestive)
Rheumatic left ventricular failure
AHA: ▶2Q, '05, 14;◀ 1Q, '95, 6; 3Q, '88, 3

DEF: Decreased cardiac output, edema and hypertension due to rheumatic heart disease.

398.99 Other

HYPERTENSIVE DISEASE (401-405)

EXCLUDES that complicating pregnancy, childbirth, or the puerperium (642.0-642.9)
that involving coronary vessels (410.00-414.9)
AHA: 3Q, '90, 3; 2Q, '89, 12; S-O, '87, 9; J-A, '84, 11

√4th **401** Essential hypertension
INCLUDES high blood pressure
  hyperpiesia
  hyperpiesis
  hypertension (arterial) (essential) (primary) (systemic)
  hypertensive vascular:
    degeneration
    disease
EXCLUDES elevated blood pressure without diagnosis of hypertension (796.2)
pulmonary hypertension (416.0-416.9)
that involving vessels of:
  brain (430-438)
  eye (362.11)
AHA: 2Q, '92, 5

DEF: Hypertension that occurs without apparent organic cause; idiopathic.

401.0 Malignant
AHA: M-J, '85, 19

DEF: Severe high arterial blood pressure; results in necrosis in kidney, retina, etc.; hemorrhages occur and death commonly due to uremia or rupture of cerebral vessel.

401.1 Benign
DEF: Mildly elevated arterial blood pressure.

401.9 Unspecified
AHA: ▶4Q, '05, 71; 3Q, '05, 8;◀ 4Q, '04, 78; 4Q, '03, 105, 108, 111; 3Q, '03, 14; 2Q, '03, 16; 4Q, '97, 37

√4th **402** Hypertensive heart disease
INCLUDES hypertensive:
  cardiomegaly
  cardiopathy
  cardiovascular disease
  heart (disease) (failure)
any condition classifiable to 429.0-429.3, 429.8, 429.9 due to hypertension
Use additional code to specify type of heart failure (428.0-428.43), if known
AHA: 4Q, '02, 49; 2Q, '93, 9; N-D, '84, 18

√5th **402.0** Malignant
  402.00 Without heart failure
  402.01 With heart failure

√5th **402.1** Benign
  402.10 Without heart failure
  402.11 With heart failure

√5th **402.9** Unspecified
  402.90 Without heart failure
  402.91 With heart failure
AHA: 4Q, '02, 52; 1Q, '93, 19; 2Q, '89, 12

Sections of Heart Muscle

Tabular List — CIRCULATORY SYSTEM — 403–410.1

▲ ✓4th 403 Hypertensive chronic kidney disease

INCLUDES
arteriolar nephritis
arteriosclerosis of:
  kidney
  renal arterioles
arteriosclerotic nephritis (chronic) (interstitial)
hypertensive:
  nephropathy
  renal failure
  uremia (chronic)
nephrosclerosis
renal sclerosis with hypertension
any condition classifiable to 585, 586, or 587
  with any condition classifiable to 401

EXCLUDES
acute renal failure (584.5-584.9)
renal disease stated as not due to hypertension
renovascular hypertension (405.0-405.9 with fifth-digit 1)

The following fifth-digit subclassification is for use with category 403:

▲ 0 with chronic kidney disease stage I through stage IV, or unspecified
  ▶Use additional code to identify the stage of chronic kidney disease (585.1-585.4, 585.9)◀

▲ 1 with chronic kidney disease stage V or end stage renal disease
  ▶Use additional code to identify the stage of chronic kidney disease (585.5, 585.6)◀

AHA: 4Q, '05, 68; 4Q, '92, 22; 2Q, '92, 5

✓5th 403.0 Malignant
✓5th 403.1 Benign
✓5th 403.9 **Unspecified**
  AHA: For code 403.91: 4Q, '05, 69; 1Q, '04, 14; 1Q, '03, 20; 2Q, '01, 11; 3Q, '91, 8

▲ ✓4th 404 Hypertensive heart and chronic kidney disease

INCLUDES
disease:
  cardiorenal
  cardiovascular renal
any condition classifiable to 402 with any condition classifiable to 403

Use additional code to specify type of heart failure (428.0-428.43), if known

The following fifth-digit subclassification is for use with category 404:

▲ 0 without heart failure and with chronic kidney disease stage I through stage IV, or unspecified
  ▶Use additional code to identify the stage of chronic kidney disease (585.1-585.4, 585.9)◀

▲ 1 with heart failure and with chronic kidney disease stage I through stage IV, or unspecified
  ▶Use additional code to identify the stage of chronic kidney disease (585.1-585.4, 585.9)◀

▲ 2 without heart failure and with chronic kidney disease stage V or end stage renal disease
  ▶Use additional code to identify the stage of chronic kidney disease (585.5, 585.6)◀

▲ 3 with heart failure and chronic kidney disease stage V or end stage renal disease
  ▶Use additional code to identify the stage of chronic kidney disease (585.5-585.6)◀

AHA: 4Q, '05, 68; 4Q, '02, 49; 3Q, '90, 3; J-A, '84, 14

✓5th 404.0 Malignant
✓5th 404.1 Benign
✓5th 404.9 **Unspecified**

✓4th 405 Secondary hypertension
AHA: 3Q, '90, 3; S-O, '87, 9, 11; J-A, '84, 14

DEF: High arterial blood pressure due to or with a variety of primary diseases, such as renal disorders, CNS disorders, endocrine, and vascular diseases.

✓5th 405.0 Malignant
  405.01 Renovascular
  405.09 Other
✓5th 405.1 Benign
  405.11 Renovascular
  405.19 Other
✓5th 405.9 Unspecified
  405.91 **Renovascular**
  405.99 **Other**
  AHA: 3Q, '00, 4

ISCHEMIC HEART DISEASE (410-414)

INCLUDES that with mention of hypertension
Use additional code to identify presence of hypertension (401.0-405.9)

AHA: 3Q, '91, 10; J-A, '84, 5

✓4th 410 Acute myocardial infarction

INCLUDES
cardiac infarction
coronary (artery):
  embolism
  occlusion
  rupture
  thrombosis
infarction of heart, myocardium, or ventricle
rupture of heart, myocardium, or ventricle
ST elevation (STEMI) and non-ST elevation (NSTEMI) myocardial infarction
any condition classifiable to 414.1-414.9 specified as acute or with a stated duration of 8 weeks or less

The following fifth-digit subclassification is for use with category 410:

0 **episode of care unspecified**
  Use when the source document does not contain sufficient information for the assignment of fifth digit 1 or 2.

1 initial episode of care
  Use fifth-digit 1 to designate the first episode of care (regardless of facility site) for a newly diagnosed myocardial infarction. The fifth-digit 1 is assigned regardless of the number of times a patient may be transferred during the initial episode of care.

2 subsequent episode of care
  Use fifth-digit 2 to designate an episode of care following the initial episode when the patient is admitted for further observation, evaluation or treatment for a myocardial infarction that has received initial treatment, but is still less than 8 weeks old.

AHA: 4Q, '05, 69; 3Q, '01, 21; 3Q, '98, 15; 4Q, '97, 37; 3Q, '95, 9; 4Q, '92, 24; 1Q, '92,10; 3Q, '91, 18; 1Q, '91, 14; 3Q, '89, 3

DEF: A sudden insufficiency of blood supply to an area of the heart muscle; usually due to a coronary artery occlusion.

✓5th 410.0 Of anterolateral wall
  ST elevation myocardial infarction (STEMI) of anterolateral wall

✓5th 410.1 **Of other anterior wall**
  Infarction:
    anterior (wall) ⎫
      NOS   ⎬ (with contiguous portion of intraventricular septum)
    anteroapical ⎪
    anteroseptal ⎭
  ST elevation myocardial infarction (STEMI) of other anterior wall

AHA: For code 410.11: 3Q, '03, 10

CIRCULATORY SYSTEM

Acute Myocardial Infarction

Arteries of the Heart

§ ✓5ᵗʰ **410.2 Of inferolateral wall**
ST elevation myocardial infarction (STEMI) of inferolateral wall

§ ✓5ᵗʰ **410.3 Of inferoposterior wall**
ST elevation myocardial infarction (STEMI) of inferoposterior wall

§ ✓5ᵗʰ **410.4 Of other inferior wall**
Infarction:
diaphragmatic wall NOS } (with contiguous portion of intraventricular septum)
inferior (wall) NOS
ST elevation myocardial infarction (STEMI) of other inferior wall
AHA: 1Q, '00, 7, 26; 4Q, '99, 9; 3Q, '97, 10; **For code 410.41:** 2Q, '01, 8, 9

§ ✓5ᵗʰ **410.5 Of other lateral wall**
Infarction:
apical-lateral
basal-lateral
high lateral
posterolateral
ST elevation myocardial infarction (STEMI) of other lateral wall

§ ✓5ᵗʰ **410.6 True posterior wall infarction**
Infarction:
posterobasal
strictly posterior
ST elevation myocardial infarction (STEMI) of true posterior wall

§ ✓5ᵗʰ **410.7 Subendocardial infarction**
Non-ST elevation myocardial infarction (NSTEMI)
Nontransmural infarction
AHA: 1Q, '00, 7; **For code 410.71:** ▶4Q, '05, 71; 2Q, '05, 19◀

§ ✓5ᵗʰ **410.8 Of other specified sites**
Infarction of:
atrium
papillary muscle
septum alone
ST elevation myocardial infarction (STEMI) of other specified sites

§ ✓5ᵗʰ **410.9 Unspecified site**
Acute myocardial infarction NOS
Coronary occlusion NOS
Myocardial infarction NOS
AHA: 1Q, '96, 17; 1Q, '92, 9; **For code 410.91:** ▶2Q, '05, 18;◀ 3Q, '02, 5

✓4ᵗʰ **411 Other acute and subacute forms of ischemic heart disease**
AHA: 4Q, '94, 55; 3Q, '91, 24

411.0 Postmyocardial infarction syndrome
Dressler's syndrome
DEF: Complication developing several days/weeks after myocardial infarction; symptoms include fever, leukocytosis, chest pain, evidence of pericarditis, pleurisy, and pneumonitis; tendency to recur.

411.1 Intermediate coronary syndrome
Impending infarction   Preinfarction syndrome
Preinfarction angina   Unstable angina
EXCLUDES: angina (pectoris) (413.9)
decubitus (413.0)
AHA: ▶4Q, '05, 105;◀ 2Q, '04, 3; 1Q, '03, 12; 3Q, '01, 15; 2Q, '01, 7, 9; 4Q, '98, 86; 2Q, '96, 10; 3Q, '91, 24; 1Q, '91, 14; 3Q, '90, 6; 4Q, '89, 10
DEF: A condition representing an intermediate stage between angina of effort and acute myocardial infarction. It is often documented by the physician as "unstable angina."

✓5ᵗʰ **411.8 Other**
AHA: 3Q, '91, 18; 3Q, '89, 4

411.81 Acute coronary occlusion without myocardial infarction
Acute coronary (artery):
embolism
obstruction } without or not resulting in myocardial infarction
occlusion
thrombosis
EXCLUDES: obstruction without infarction due to atherosclerosis (414.00-414.0)
occlusion without infarction due to atherosclerosis (414.00-414.07)
AHA: 3Q, '91, 24; 1Q, '91, 14
DEF: Interrupted blood flow to a portion of the heart; without tissue death.

411.89 Other
Coronary insufficiency (acute)
Subendocardial ischemia
AHA: 3Q, '01, 14; 1Q, '92, 9

412 Old myocardial infarction
Healed myocardial infarction
Past myocardial infarction diagnosed on ECG [EKG] or other special investigation, but currently presenting no symptoms
AHA: 2Q, '03, 10; 2Q, '01, 9; 3Q, '98, 15; 2Q, '91, 22; 3Q, '90, 7

✓4ᵗʰ **413 Angina pectoris**
DEF: Severe constricting pain in the chest, often radiating from the precordium to the left shoulder and down the arm, due to ischemia of the heart muscle; usually caused by coronary disease; pain is often precipitated by effort or excitement.

413.0 Angina decubitus
Nocturnal angina
DEF: Angina occurring only in the recumbent position.

413.1 Prinzmetal angina
Variant angina pectoris
DEF: Angina occurring when patient is recumbent; associated with ST-segment elevations.

§ Requires fifth-digit. See category 410 for codes and definitions.

CIRCULATORY SYSTEM

413.9 **Other and unspecified angina pectoris**
    Angina:
        NOS
        cardiac
        of effort
    Anginal syndrome
    Status anginosus
    Stenocardia
    Syncope anginosa
    EXCLUDES *preinfarction angina (411.1)*
    AHA: 3Q, '02, 4; 3Q, '91, 16; 3Q, '90, 6

414 Other forms of chronic ischemic heart disease
    EXCLUDES *arteriosclerotic cardiovascular disease [ASCVD] (429.2)*
        cardiovascular:
            arteriosclerosis or sclerosis (429.2)
            degeneration or disease (429.2)

  414.0 Coronary atherosclerosis
    Arteriosclerotic heart disease [ASHD]
    Atherosclerotic heart disease
    Coronary (artery):
        arteriosclerosis
        arteritis or endarteritis
        atheroma
        sclerosis
        stricture
    EXCLUDES *embolism of graft (996.72)*
        occlusion NOS of graft (996.72)
        thrombus of graft (996.72)
    AHA: 2Q, '97, 13; 2Q, '95, 17; 4Q, '94, 49; 2Q, '94, 13; 1Q, '94, 6; 3Q, '90, 7
    DEF: A chronic condition marked by thickening and loss of elasticity of the coronary artery; caused by deposits of plaque containing cholesterol, lipoid material and lipophages.

    414.00 Of unspecified type of vessel, native or graft
      AHA: 1Q, '04, 24; 2Q, '03, 16; 3Q, '01, 15; 4Q, '99, 4; 3Q, '97, 15; 4Q, '96, 31

    414.01 Of native coronary artery
      AHA: ▶4Q, '05, 71;◀ 2Q, '04, 3; 4Q, '03, 108; 3Q, '03, 9, 14; 3Q, '02, 4-9; 3Q, '01, 15; 2Q, '01, 8, 9; 3Q, '97, 15; 2Q, '96, 10; 4Q, '96, 31
      DEF: Plaque deposits in natural heart vessels.

    414.02 Of autologous vein bypass graft
      DEF: Plaque deposit in grafted vein originating within patient.

    414.03 Of nonautologous biological bypass graft
      DEF: Plaque deposits in grafted vessel originating outside patient.

    414.04 Of artery bypass graft
      Internal mammary artery
      AHA: 4Q, '96, 31
      DEF: Plaque deposits in grafted artery originating within patient.

    414.05 Of unspecified type of bypass graft
      Bypass graft NOS
      AHA: 3Q, '97, 15; 4Q, '96, 31

    414.06 Of native coronary artery of transplanted heart
      AHA: 4Q, '03, 60

    414.07 Of bypass graft (artery) (vein) of transplanted heart

  414.1 Aneurysm and dissection of heart
    AHA: 4Q, '02, 54

    414.10 Aneurysm of heart (wall)
      Aneurysm (arteriovenous):
        mural
        ventricular

    414.11 Aneurysm of coronary vessels
      Aneurysm (arteriovenous) of coronary vessels
      AHA: 3Q, '03, 10; 1Q, '99, 17
      DEF: Dilatation of all three-vessel wall layers forming a sac filled with blood.

Anatomy

Blood Flow

    414.12 Dissection of coronary artery
      DEF: A tear in the intimal arterial wall of a coronary artery resulting in the sudden intrusion of blood within the layers of the wall.

    414.19 Other aneurysm of heart
      Arteriovenous fistula, acquired, of heart

  414.8 Other specified forms of chronic ischemic heart disease
    Chronic coronary insufficiency
    Ischemia, myocardial (chronic)
    Any condition classifiable to 410 specified as chronic, or presenting with symptoms after 8 weeks from date of infarction
    EXCLUDES *coronary insufficiency (acute) (411.89)*
    AHA: 3Q, '01, 15; 1Q, '92, 10; 3Q, '90, 7, 15; 2Q, '90, 19

  414.9 Chronic ischemic heart disease, unspecified
    Ischemic heart disease NOS

DISEASES OF PULMONARY CIRCULATION (415-417)

415 Acute pulmonary heart disease

  415.0 Acute cor pulmonale
    EXCLUDES *cor pulmonale NOS (416.9)*
    DEF: A heart-lung disease marked by dilation and failure of the right side of heart; due to pulmonary embolism; ventilatory function is impaired and pulmonary hypertension results within hours.

  415.1 Pulmonary embolism and infarction
    Pulmonary (artery) (vein):
      apoplexy
      embolism
      infarction (hemorrhagic)
      thrombosis
    EXCLUDES *that complicating:*
      abortion (634-638 with .6, 639.6)
      ectopic or molar pregnancy (639.6)
      pregnancy, childbirth, or the puerperium (673.0-673.8)
    AHA: 4Q, '90, 25
    DEF: Embolism: closure of the pulmonary artery or branch; due to thrombosis (blood clot).
    DEF: Infarction: necrosis of lung tissue; due to obstructed arterial blood supply, most often by pulmonary embolism.

415.11–422.91 — **CIRCULATORY SYSTEM** — Tabular List

- **415.11 Iatrogenic pulmonary embolism and infarction**
  AHA: 4Q, '95, 58
- **415.19 Other**

√4ᵗʰ 416 Chronic pulmonary heart disease

- **416.0 Primary pulmonary hypertension**
  Idiopathic pulmonary arteriosclerosis
  Pulmonary hypertension (essential) (idiopathic) (primary)
  DEF: A rare increase in pulmonary circulation, often resulting in right ventricular failure or fatal syncope.
- **416.1 Kyphoscoliotic heart disease**
  DEF: High blood pressure within the lungs as a result of curvature of the spine.
- **416.8 Other chronic pulmonary heart diseases**
  Pulmonary hypertension, secondary
- **416.9 Chronic pulmonary heart disease, unspecified**
  Chronic cardiopulmonary disease
  Cor pulmonale (chronic) NOS

√4ᵗʰ 417 Other diseases of pulmonary circulation

- **417.0 Arteriovenous fistula of pulmonary vessels**
  EXCLUDES congenital arteriovenous fistula (747.3)
  DEF: Abnormal communication between blood vessels within lung.
- **417.1 Aneurysm of pulmonary artery**
  EXCLUDES congenital aneurysm (747.3)
- **417.8 Other specified diseases of pulmonary circulation**
  Pulmonary: arteritis
  Pulmonary: endarteritis
  Rupture } of pulmonary vessel
  Stricture
- **417.9 Unspecified disease of pulmonary circulation**

OTHER FORMS OF HEART DISEASE (420-429)

√4ᵗʰ 420 Acute pericarditis

INCLUDES acute:
  mediastinopericarditis
  myopericarditis
  pericardial effusion
  pleuropericarditis
  pneumopericarditis
EXCLUDES acute rheumatic pericarditis (391.0)
  postmyocardial infarction syndrome [Dressler's] (411.0)
DEF: Inflammation of the pericardium (heart sac); pericardial friction rub results from this inflammation and is heard as a scratchy or leathery sound.

- **420.0 Acute pericarditis in diseases classified elsewhere**
  Code first underlying disease, as:
    actinomycosis (039.8)
    amebiasis (006.8)
    ►chronic uremia (585.9)◄
    nocardiosis (039.8)
    tuberculosis (017.9)
    uremia ►NOS (586)◄
  EXCLUDES pericarditis (acute) (in):
    Coxsackie (virus) (074.21)
    gonococcal (098.83)
    histoplasmosis (115.0-115.9 with fifth-digit 3)
    meningococcal infection (036.41)
    syphilitic (093.81)

- √5ᵗʰ **420.9 Other and unspecified acute pericarditis**
  - **420.90 Acute pericarditis, unspecified**
    Pericarditis (acute):   Pericarditis (acute):
      NOS   sicca
      infective NOS
    AHA: 2Q, '89, 12
  - **420.91 Acute idiopathic pericarditis**
    Pericarditis, acute: Pericarditis, acute:
      benign   viral
      nonspecific
  - **420.99 Other**
    Pericarditis (acute):
      pneumococcal
      purulent
      staphylococcal
      streptococcal
      suppurative
    Pneumopyopericardium
    Pyopericardium
    EXCLUDES pericarditis in diseases classified elsewhere (420.0)

√4ᵗʰ 421 Acute and subacute endocarditis

DEF: Bacterial inflammation of the endocardium (intracardiac area); major symptoms include fever, fatigue, heart murmurs, splenomegaly, embolic episodes and areas of infarction.

- **421.0 Acute and subacute bacterial endocarditis**
  Endocarditis (acute)   Endocarditis (acute)
    (chronic) (subacute):   (chronic) (subacute):
    bacterial   ulcerative
    infective NOS   vegetative
    lenta   Infective aneurysm
    malignant   Subacute bacterial
    purulent   endocarditis [SBE]
    septic
  Use additional code to identify infectious organism [e.g., Streptococcus 041.0, Staphylococcus 041.1]
  AHA: 1Q, '99, 12; 1Q, '91, 15

- **421.1 Acute and subacute infective endocarditis in diseases classified elsewhere**
  Code first underlying disease, as:
    blastomycosis (116.0)
    Q fever (083.0)
    typhoid (fever) (002.0)
  EXCLUDES endocarditis (in):
    Coxsackie (virus) (074.22)
    gonococcal (098.84)
    histoplasmosis (115.0-115.9 with fifth-digit 4)
    meningococcal infection (036.42)
    monilial (112.81)

- **421.9 Acute endocarditis, unspecified**
  Endocarditis
  Myoendocarditis } acute or subacute
  Periendocarditis
  EXCLUDES acute rheumatic endocarditis (391.1)

√4ᵗʰ 422 Acute myocarditis

EXCLUDES acute rheumatic myocarditis (391.2)
DEF: Acute inflammation of the muscular walls of the heart (myocardium).

- **422.0 Acute myocarditis in diseases classified elsewhere**
  Code first underlying disease, as:
    myocarditis (acute):
      influenzal (487.8)
      tuberculous (017.9)
  EXCLUDES myocarditis (acute) (due to):
    aseptic, of newborn (074.23)
    Coxsackie (virus) (074.23)
    diphtheritic (032.82)
    meningococcal infection (036.43)
    syphilitic (093.82)
    toxoplasmosis (130.3)

- √5ᵗʰ **422.9 Other and unspecified acute myocarditis**
  - **422.90 Acute myocarditis, unspecified**
    Acute or subacute (interstitial) myocarditis
  - **422.91 Idiopathic myocarditis**
    Myocarditis (acute or subacute):
      Fiedler's
      giant cell
      isolated (diffuse) (granulomatous)
      nonspecific granulomatous

422.92 Septic myocarditis
Myocarditis, acute or subacute:
pneumococcal
staphylococcal
Use additional code to identify infectious organism [e.g., Staphylococcus 041.1]
EXCLUDES myocarditis, acute or subacute:
in bacterial diseases classified elsewhere (422.0)
streptococcal (391.2)

422.93 Toxic myocarditis
DEF: Inflammation of the heart muscle due to an adverse reaction to certain drugs or chemicals reaching the heart through the bloodstream.

422.99 Other

√4ᵗʰ **423 Other diseases of pericardium**
EXCLUDES that specified as rheumatic (393)

423.0 Hemopericardium
DEF: Blood in the pericardial sac (pericardium).

423.1 Adhesive pericarditis
Adherent pericardium   Pericarditis:
Fibrosis of pericardium   adhesive
Milk spots   obliterative
                                Soldiers' patches
DEF: Two layers of serous pericardium adhere to each other by fibrous adhesions.

423.2 Constrictive pericarditis
Concato's disease
Pick's disease of heart (and liver)
DEF: Inflammation identified by a rigid, thickened and sometimes calcified pericardium; ventricles of the heart cannot be adequately filled and congestive heart failure may result.

423.8 Other specified diseases of pericardium
Calcification } of pericardium
Fistula
AHA: 2Q, '89, 12

423.9 Unspecified disease of pericardium

√4ᵗʰ **424 Other diseases of endocardium**
EXCLUDES bacterial endocarditis (421.0-421.9)
rheumatic endocarditis (391.1, 394.0-397.9)
syphilitic endocarditis (093.20-093.24)

424.0 Mitral valve disorders
Mitral (valve):
incompetence
insufficiency } NOS of specified cause, except rheumatic
regurgitation

EXCLUDES mitral (valve):
disease (394.9)
failure (394.9)
stenosis (394.0)
the listed conditions:
specified as rheumatic (394.1)
unspecified as to cause but with mention of:
diseases of aortic valve (396.0-396.9)
mitral stenosis or obstruction (394.2)
AHA: 2Q, '00, 16; 3Q, '98, 11; N-D, '87, 8; N-D, '84, 8

424.1 Aortic valve disorders
Aortic (valve):
incompetence
insufficiency } NOS of specified cause, except rheumatic
regurgitation
stenosis

EXCLUDES hypertrophic subaortic stenosis (425.1)
that specified as rheumatic (395.0-395.9)
that of unspecified cause but with mention of diseases of mitral valve (396.0-396.9)
AHA: 4Q, '88, 8; N-D, '87, 8

424.2 Tricuspid valve disorders, specified as nonrheumatic
Tricuspid valve:
incompetence
insufficiency } of specified cause, except rheumatic
regurgitation
stenosis

EXCLUDES rheumatic or of unspecified cause (397.0)

424.3 Pulmonary valve disorders
Pulmonic: Pulmonic:
incompetence NOS   regurgitation NOS
insufficiency NOS   stenosis NOS

EXCLUDES that specified as rheumatic (397.1)

√5ᵗʰ **424.9 Endocarditis, valve unspecified**

424.90 Endocarditis, valve unspecified, unspecified cause
Endocarditis (chronic):
NOS
nonbacterial thrombotic
Valvular:
incompetence
insufficiency
regurgitation } of unspecified valve, unspecified cause
stenosis
Valvulitis (chronic)

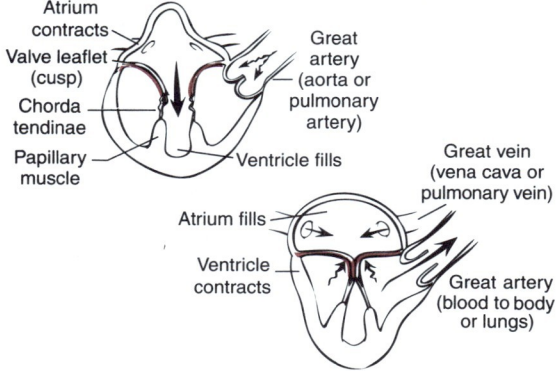

Normal Heart Valve Function

Heart Valve Disorders

Valve stenosis
(trouble opening)

Incompetent valve
(trouble closing)
causes regurgitation
(backflow of blood)

Insufficient valve
(unable to close completely)
Shortened, fused chorda tendinae
Ventricular hypertrophy

CIRCULATORY SYSTEM

Nerve Conduction of the Heart

424.91 Endocarditis in diseases classified elsewhere
Code first underlying disease as:
atypical verrucous endocarditis [Libman-Sacks] (710.0)
disseminated lupus erythematosus (710.0)
tuberculosis (017.9)
EXCLUDES: syphilitic (093.20-093.24)

424.99 Other
Any condition classifiable to 424.90 with specified cause, except rheumatic
EXCLUDES: endocardial fibroelastosis (425.3)
that specified as rheumatic (397.9)

√4th **425 Cardiomyopathy**
INCLUDES: myocardiopathy
AHA: J-A, '85, 15

425.0 Endomyocardial fibrosis

425.1 Hypertrophic obstructive cardiomyopathy
Hypertrophic subaortic stenosis (idiopathic)
DEF: Cardiomyopathy marked by left ventricle hypertrophy, enlarged septum; results in obstructed blood flow.

425.2 Obscure cardiomyopathy of Africa
Becker's disease
Idiopathic mural endomyocardial disease

425.3 Endocardial fibroelastosis
Elastomyofibrosis
DEF: A condition marked by left ventricle hypertrophy and conversion of the endocardium into a thick fibroelastic coat; capacity of the ventricle may be reduced, but is often increased.

425.4 Other primary cardiomyopathies
Cardiomyopathy: Cardiomyopathy:
NOS   idiopathic
congestive   nonobstructive
constrictive   obstructive
familial   restrictive
hypertrophic   Cardiovascular collagenosis
AHA: 2Q, '05, 14; 1Q, '00, 22; 4Q, '97, 55; 2Q, '90, 19

425.5 Alcoholic cardiomyopathy
AHA: S-O, '85, 15
DEF: Heart disease as result of excess alcohol consumption.

425.7 Nutritional and metabolic cardiomyopathy
Code first underlying disease, as:
amyloidosis ►(277.30-277.39)◄
beriberi (265.0)
cardiac glycogenosis (271.0)
mucopolysaccharidosis (277.5)
thyrotoxicosis (242.0-242.9)
EXCLUDES: gouty tophi of heart (274.82)

425.8 Cardiomyopathy in other diseases classified elsewhere
Code first underlying disease, as:
Friedreich's ataxia (334.0)
myotonia atrophica (359.2)
progressive muscular dystrophy (359.1)
sarcoidosis (135)
EXCLUDES: cardiomyopathy in Chagas' disease (086.0)
AHA: 2Q, '93, 9

425.9 Secondary cardiomyopathy, unspecified

√4th **426 Conduction disorders**
DEF: Disruption or disturbance in the electrical impulses that regulate heartbeats.

426.0 Atrioventricular block, complete
Third degree atrioventricular block

√5th **426.1 Atrioventricular block, other and unspecified**

426.10 Atrioventricular block, unspecified
Atrioventricular [AV] block (incomplete) (partial)

426.11 First degree atrioventricular block
Incomplete atrioventricular block, first degree
Prolonged P-R interval NOS

426.12 Mobitz (type) II atrioventricular block
Incomplete atrioventricular block:
Mobitz (type) II
second degree, Mobitz (type) II
DEF: Impaired conduction of excitatory impulse from cardiac atrium to ventricle through AV node.

426.13 Other second degree atrioventricular block
Incomplete atrioventricular block:
Mobitz (type) I [Wenckebach's]
second degree:
NOS
Mobitz (type) I
with 2:1 atrioventricular response [block]
Wenckebach's phenomenon
DEF: Wenckebach's phenomenon: impulses generated at constant rate to sinus node, P-R interval lengthens; results in cycle of ventricular inadequacy and shortened P-R interval; second-degree A-V block commonly called "Mobitz type 1."

426.2 Left bundle branch hemiblock
Block:
left anterior fascicular
left posterior fascicular

426.3 Other left bundle branch block
Left bundle branch block:
NOS
anterior fascicular with posterior fascicular
complete
main stem

426.4 Right bundle branch block
AHA: 3Q, '00, 3

√5th **426.5 Bundle branch block, other and unspecified**

426.50 Bundle branch block, unspecified

426.51 Right bundle branch block and left posterior fascicular block

426.52 Right bundle branch block and left anterior fascicular block

426.53 Other bilateral bundle branch block
Bifascicular block NOS
Bilateral bundle branch block NOS
Right bundle branch with left bundle branch block (incomplete) (main stem)

426.54 Trifascicular block

CIRCULATORY SYSTEM

426.6 Other heart block
　　Intraventricular block:　　Sinoatrial block
　　　NOS　　　　　　　　　Sinoauricular block
　　　diffuse
　　　myofibrillar

426.7 Anomalous atrioventricular excitation
　　Atrioventricular conduction:
　　　accelerated
　　　accessory
　　　pre-excitation
　　Ventricular pre-excitation
　　Wolff-Parkinson-White syndrome
　　DEF: Wolff-Parkinson-White: normal conduction pathway is bypassed; results in short P-R interval on EKG; tendency to supraventricular tachycardia.

426.8 Other specified conduction disorders
　426.81 Lown-Ganong-Levine syndrome
　　Syndrome of short P-R interval, normal QRS complexes, and supraventricular tachycardias
　426.82 Long QT syndrome
　　AHA: ▶4Q, '05, 72◀
　　DEF: ▶Condition characterized by recurrent syncope, malignant arrhythmias, and sudden death; characteristic prolonged Q-T interval on electrocardiogram.◀
　426.89 Other
　　Dissociation:
　　　atrioventricular [AV]
　　　interference
　　　isorhythmic
　　Nonparoxysmal AV nodal tachycardia

426.9 Conduction disorder, unspecified
　Heart block NOS　　Stokes-Adams syndrome

427 Cardiac dysrhythmias
　EXCLUDES　that complicating:
　　abortion (634-638 with .7, 639.8)
　　ectopic or molar pregnancy (639.8)
　　labor or delivery (668.1, 669.4)
　AHA: J-A, '85, 15
　DEF: Disruption or disturbance in the rhythm of heartbeats.

427.0 Paroxysmal supraventricular tachycardia
　Paroxysmal tachycardia:　Paroxysmal tachycardia:
　　atrial [PAT]　　　　　　　junctional
　　atrioventricular [AV]　　nodal
　DEF: Rapid atrial rhythm.

427.1 Paroxysmal ventricular tachycardia
　Ventricular tachycardia (paroxysmal)
　AHA: 3Q, '95, 9; M-A, '86, 11
　DEF: Rapid ventricular rhythm.

427.2 Paroxysmal tachycardia, unspecified
　Bouveret-Hoffmann syndrome
　Paroxysmal tachycardia:
　　NOS
　　essential

427.3 Atrial fibrillation and flutter
　427.31 Atrial fibrillation
　　AHA:▶3Q, '05, 8;◀ 4Q, '04, 78, 121; 3Q, '04, 7; 4Q, '03, 95, 105; 1Q, '03, 8; 2Q, '99, 17; 3Q, '95, 8
　　DEF: Irregular, rapid atrial contractions.
　427.32 Atrial flutter
　　AHA: 4Q, '03, 94
　　DEF: Regular, rapid atrial contractions.

427.4 Ventricular fibrillation and flutter
　427.41 Ventricular fibrillation
　　AHA: 3Q, '02, 5
　　DEF: Irregular, rapid ventricular contractions.
　427.42 Ventricular flutter
　　DEF: Regular, rapid, ventricular contractions.

427.5 Cardiac arrest
　Cardiorespiratory arrest
　AHA: 3Q,'02, 5; 2Q, '00, 12; 3Q, '95, 8; 2Q, '88, 8

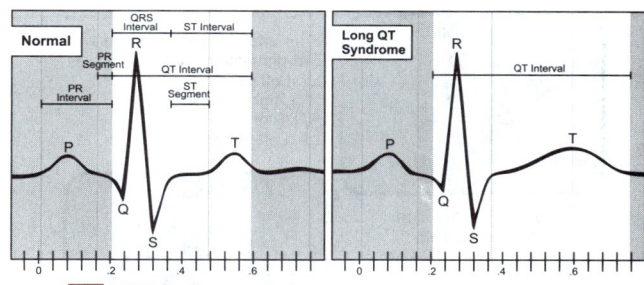
▶Normal and Long QT Electrocardiogram◀

427.6 Premature beats
　427.60 Premature beats, unspecified
　　Ectopic beats　　Premature contractions
　　Extrasystoles　　　or systoles NOS
　　Extrasystolic arrhythmia
　427.61 Supraventricular premature beats
　　Atrial premature beats, contractions, or systoles
　427.69 Other
　　Ventricular premature beats, contractions, or systoles
　　AHA: 4Q, '93, 42

427.8 Other specified cardiac dysrhythmias
　427.81 Sinoatrial node dysfunction
　　Sinus bradycardia:　　Syndrome:
　　　persistent　　　　　　　sick sinus
　　　severe　　　　　　　　tachycardia-bradycardia
　　EXCLUDES　sinus bradycardia NOS (427.89)
　　AHA: 3Q, '00, 8
　　DEF: Complex cardiac arrhythmia; appears as severe sinus bradycardia, sinus bradycardia with tachycardia, or sinus bradycardia with atrioventricular block.
　427.89 Other
　　Rhythm disorder:　　Rhythm disorder:
　　　coronary sinus　　　　nodal
　　　ectopic　　　　　　　Wandering (atrial) pacemaker
　　EXCLUDES　carotid sinus syncope (337.0)
　　　　　　　neonatal bradycardia (779.81)
　　　　　　　neonatal tachycardia (779.82)
　　　　　　　reflex bradycardia (337.0)
　　　　　　　tachycardia NOS (785.0)

427.9 Cardiac dysrhythmia, unspecified
　Arrhythmia (cardiac) NOS
　AHA: 2Q, '89, 10

428 Heart failure
　Code, if applicable, heart failure due to hypertension first (402.0-402.9, with fifth-digit 1 or 404.0-404.9 with fifth-digit 1 or 3)
　EXCLUDES　following cardiac surgery (429.4)
　　　　　　　rheumatic (398.91)
　　　　　　　that complicating:
　　　　　　　　abortion (634-638 with .7, 639.8)
　　　　　　　　ectopic or molar pregnancy (639.8)
　　　　　　　　labor or delivery (668.1, 669.4)
　AHA: 4Q, '02, 49; 3Q, '98, 5; 2Q, '90, 16; 2Q, '90, 19; 2Q, '89, 10; 3Q, '88, 3

428.0 Congestive heart failure, unspecified
　Congestive heart disease
　Right heart failure (secondary to left heart failure)
　EXCLUDES　fluid overload NOS (276.6)
　AHA:▶4Q, '05, 120; 3Q, '05, 8;◀1Q, '05, 5, 9; 4Q, '04, 140; 3Q, '04, 7; 4Q, '03, 109; 1Q, '03, 9; 4Q, '02, 52; 2Q, '01, 13; 4Q, '00, 48; 2Q, '00, 16; 1Q, '00, 22; 4Q, '99, 4; 1Q, '99, 11; 4Q, '97, 55; 3Q, '97, 10; 3Q, '96, 9; 3Q, '91, 18; 3Q, '91, 19; 2Q, '89, 12
　DEF: Mechanical inadequacy; caused by inability of heart to pump and circulate blood; results in fluid collection in lungs, hypertension, congestion and edema of tissue.

CIRCULATORY SYSTEM

Echocardiography of Heart Failure

Four-chamber echocardiograms, two-dimensional views.
LV: Left ventricle
RV: Right ventricle
RA: Right atrium
LA: Left atrium

Systolic dysfunction with dilated LV

Diastolic dysfunction with LV hypertrophy

428.1 Left heart failure
Acute edema of lung } with heart disease NOS
Acute pulmonary edema } or heart failure

Cardiac asthma
Left ventricular failure

DEF: Mechanical inadequacy of left ventricle; causing fluid in lungs.

√5th 428.2 Systolic heart failure
EXCLUDES combined systolic and diastolic heart failure (428.40-428.43)

DEF: Heart failure due to a defect in expulsion of blood caused by an abnormality in systolic function, or ventricular contractile dysfunction.

- **428.20** Unspecified
- **428.21** Acute
- **428.22** Chronic
  - AHA: ▶4Q, '05, 120◀
- **428.23** Acute on chronic
  - AHA: 1Q, '03, 9

√5th 428.3 Diastolic heart failure
EXCLUDES combined systolic and diastolic heart failure (428.40-428.43)

DEF: Heart failure due to resistance to ventricular filling caused by an abnormality in the diastolic function.

- **428.30** Unspecified
  - AHA: 4Q, '02, 52
- **428.31** Acute
- **428.32** Chronic
- **428.33** Acute on chronic

√5th 428.4 Combined systolic and diastolic heart failure
- **428.40** Unspecified
- **428.41** Acute
  - AHA: 4Q, '04, 140
- **428.42** Chronic
- **428.43** Acute on chronic
  - AHA: 4Q, '02, 52

428.9 Heart failure, unspecified
Cardiac failure NOS   Myocardial failure NOS
Heart failure NOS   Weak heart
AHA: 2Q, '89, 10; N-D, '85, 14

√4th 429 Ill-defined descriptions and complications of heart disease

429.0 Myocarditis, unspecified
Myocarditis:
  NOS
  chronic (interstitial)   } (with mention of
  fibroid   arteriosclerosis)
  senile

Use additional code to identify presence of arteriosclerosis

EXCLUDES
  acute or subacute (422.0-422.9)
  rheumatic (398.0)
  acute (391.2)
  that due to hypertension (402.0-402.9)

429.1 Myocardial degeneration
Degeneration of heart or myocardium:
  fatty
  mural   } (with mention of
  muscular   arteriosclerosis)
Myocardial:
  degeneration
  disease

Use additional code to identify presence of arteriosclerosis

EXCLUDES that due to hypertension (402.0-402.9)

429.2 Cardiovascular disease, unspecified
Arteriosclerotic cardiovascular disease [ASCVD]
Cardiovascular arteriosclerosis
Cardiovascular:
  degeneration
  disease   } (with mention of
  sclerosis   arteriosclerosis)

Use additional code to identify presence of arteriosclerosis

EXCLUDES that due to hypertension (402.0-402.9)

429.3 Cardiomegaly
Cardiac: Ventricular dilatation
  dilatation
  hypertrophy

EXCLUDES that due to hypertension (402.0-402.9)

429.4 Functional disturbances following cardiac surgery
Cardiac insufficiency } following cardiac surgery
Heart failure   } or due to prosthesis

Postcardiotomy syndrome
Postvalvulotomy syndrome

EXCLUDES cardiac failure in the immediate postoperative period (997.1)

AHA: 2Q, '02, 12; N-D, '85, 6

429.5 Rupture of chordae tendineae
DEF: Torn tissue, between heart valves and papillary muscles.

429.6 Rupture of papillary muscle
DEF: Torn muscle, between chordae tendineae and heart wall.

√5th 429.7 Certain sequelae of myocardial infarction, not elsewhere classified
Use additional code to identify the associated myocardial infarction:
  with onset of 8 weeks or less (410.00-410.92)
  with onset of more than 8 weeks (414.8)

EXCLUDES
  congenital defects of heart (745, 746)
  coronary aneurysm (414.11)
  disorders of papillary muscle (429.6, 429.81)
  postmyocardial infarction syndrome (411.0)
  rupture of chordae tendineae (429.5)

AHA: 3Q, '89, 5

- **429.71** Acquired cardiac septal defect   **A**
  EXCLUDES acute septal infarction (410.00-410.92)
  DEF: Abnormal communication, between opposite heart chambers; due to defect of septum; not present at birth.

- **429.79** Other   **A**
  Mural thrombus (atrial) (ventricular), acquired, following myocardial infarction
  AHA: 1Q, '92, 10

√5th 429.8 Other ill-defined heart diseases
- **429.81** Other disorders of papillary muscle
  Papillary muscle: Papillary muscle:
    atrophy   incompetence
    degeneration   incoordination
    dysfunction   scarring

CIRCULATORY SYSTEM

429.82 Hyperkinetic heart disease
DEF: Condition of unknown origin in young adults; marked by increased cardiac output at rest, increased rate of ventricular ejection; may lead to heart failure.

● **429.83 Takotsubo syndrome**
Broken heart syndrome
Reversible left ventricular dysfunction following sudden emotional stress
Stress induced cardiomyopathy
Transient left ventricular apical ballooning syndrome

429.89 Other
Carditis
EXCLUDES: *that due to hypertension (402.0-402.9)*
AHA: 3Q, '05, 14; 1Q, '92, 10

429.9 Heart disease, unspecified
Heart disease (organic) NOS   Morbus cordis NOS
EXCLUDES: *that due to hypertension (402.0-402.9)*
AHA: 1Q, '93, 19

CEREBROVASCULAR DISEASE (430-438)

INCLUDES: with mention of hypertension (conditions classifiable to 401-405)
Use additional code to identify presence of hypertension
EXCLUDES: *any condition classifiable to 430-434, 436, 437 occurring during pregnancy, childbirth, or the puerperium, or specified as puerperal (674.0)*
iatrogenic cerebrovascular infarction or hemorrhage (997.02)
AHA: 1Q, '93, 27; 3Q, '91, 10; 3Q, '90, 3; 2Q, '89, 8; M-A, '85, 6

430 Subarachnoid hemorrhage
Meningeal hemorrhage
Ruptured:
  berry aneurysm
  (congenital) cerebral aneurysm NOS
EXCLUDES: *syphilitic ruptured cerebral aneurysm (094.87)*
AHA: 4Q, '04, 77
DEF: Bleeding in space between brain and lining.

431 Intracerebral hemorrhage
Hemorrhage (of):
  basilar
  bulbar
  cerebellar
  cerebral
  cerebromeningeal
  cortical
Hemorrhage (of):
  internal capsule
  intrapontine
  pontine
  subcortical
  ventricular
Rupture of blood vessel in brain
DEF: Bleeding within the brain.
AHA: 4Q, '04, 77

✓4th **432 Other and unspecified intracranial hemorrhage**
AHA: 4Q, '04, 77

432.0 Nontraumatic extradural hemorrhage
Nontraumatic epidural hemorrhage
DEF: Bleeding, nontraumatic, between skull and brain lining.

432.1 Subdural hemorrhage
Subdural hematoma, nontraumatic
DEF: Bleeding, between outermost and other layers of brain lining.

432.9 Unspecified intracranial hemorrhage
Intracranial hemorrhage NOS

✓4th **433 Occlusion and stenosis of precerebral arteries**
INCLUDES: embolism, narrowing, obstruction, thrombosis } of basilar, carotid, and vertebral arteries
EXCLUDES: *insufficiency NOS of precerebral arteries (435.0-435.9)*

The following fifth-digit subclassification is for use with category 433:
  0 without mention of cerebral infarction
  1 with cerebral infarction
AHA: 2Q, '95, 14; 3Q, '90, 16
DEF: Blockage, stricture, arteries branching into brain.

✓5th **433.0 Basilar artery**
✓5th **433.1 Carotid artery**
  AHA: 1Q, '00, 16; For code 433.10: 1Q, '02, 7, 10
✓5th **433.2 Vertebral artery**
✓5th **433.3 Multiple and bilateral**
  AHA: 2Q, '02, 19
✓5th **433.8 Other specified precerebral artery**
✓5th **433.9 Unspecified precerebral artery**
  Precerebral artery NOS

✓4th **434 Occlusion of cerebral arteries**
The following fifth-digit subclassification is for use with category 434:
  0 without mention of cerebral infarction
  1 with cerebral infarction
AHA: 2Q, '95, 14

✓5th **434.0 Cerebral thrombosis**
  Thrombosis of cerebral arteries
  AHA: For code 434.01: 4Q, '04, 77
✓5th **434.1 Cerebral embolism**
  AHA: 3Q, '97, 11; For code 434.11: 4Q, '04, 77
✓5th **434.9 Cerebral artery occlusion, unspecified**
  AHA: 4Q, '98, 87; For code 434.91: 4Q, '04, 77-78

✓4th **435 Transient cerebral ischemia**
INCLUDES: cerebrovascular insufficiency (acute) with transient focal neurological signs and symptoms
insufficiency of basilar, carotid, and vertebral arteries
spasm of cerebral arteries
EXCLUDES: *acute cerebrovascular insufficiency NOS (437.1) that due to any condition classifiable to 433 (433.0-433.9)*
DEF: Temporary restriction of blood flow, to arteries branching into brain.

435.0 Basilar artery syndrome

CIRCULATORY SYSTEM — Tabular List

435.1 Vertebral artery syndrome

435.2 Subclavian steal syndrome
DEF: Cerebrovascular insufficiency, due to occluded subclavian artery; symptoms include pain in mastoid and posterior head regions, flaccid paralysis of arm and diminished or absent radial pulse on affected side.

435.3 Vertebrobasilar artery syndrome
AHA: 4Q, '95, 60
DEF: Transient ischemic attack; due to brainstem dysfunction; symptoms include confusion, vertigo, binocular blindness, diplopia, unilateral or bilateral weakness and paresthesis of extremities.

435.8 Other specified transient cerebral ischemias

435.9 Unspecified transient cerebral ischemia
Impending cerebrovascular accident
Intermittent cerebral ischemia
Transient ischemic attack [TIA]
AHA: N-D, '85, 12

436 Acute, but ill-defined, cerebrovascular disease
Apoplexy, apoplectic:
  NOS
  attack
  cerebral
Apoplexy, apoplectic:
  seizure
  Cerebral seizure

EXCLUDES any condition classifiable to categories 430-435
  cerebrovascular accident (434.91)
  CVA (ischemic) (434.91)
    embolic (434.11)
    hemorrhagic (430, 431, 432.0-432.9)
    thrombotic (434.01)
  postoperative cerebrovascular accident (997.02)
  stroke (ischemic) (434.91)
    embolic (434.11)
    hemorrhagic (430, 431, 432.0-432.9)
    thrombotic (434.01)
AHA: ▶4Q, '04, 77;◀ 4Q, '99, 3

437 Other and ill-defined cerebrovascular disease

437.0 Cerebral atherosclerosis
Atheroma of cerebral arteries
Cerebral arteriosclerosis

437.1 Other generalized ischemic cerebrovascular disease
Acute cerebrovascular insufficiency NOS
Cerebral ischemia (chronic)

437.2 Hypertensive encephalopathy
AHA: J-A, '84, 14
DEF: Cerebral manifestations (such as visual disturbances and headache) due to high blood pressure.

437.3 Cerebral aneurysm, nonruptured
Internal carotid artery, intracranial portion
Internal carotid artery NOS
EXCLUDES congenital cerebral aneurysm, nonruptured (747.81)
  internal carotid artery, extracranial portion (442.81)

437.4 Cerebral arteritis
AHA: 4Q, '99, 21
DEF: Inflammation of a cerebral artery or arteries.

437.5 Moyamoya disease
DEF: Cerebrovascular ischemia; vessels occlude and rupture causing tiny hemorrhages at base of brain; predominantly affects Japanese.

437.6 Nonpyogenic thrombosis of intracranial venous sinus
EXCLUDES pyogenic (325)

437.7 Transient global amnesia
AHA: 4Q, '92, 20
DEF: Episode of short-term memory loss, not often recurrent; pathogenesis unknown; with no signs or symptoms of neurological disorder.

437.8 Other

437.9 Unspecified
Cerebrovascular disease or lesion NOS

438 Late effects of cerebrovascular disease
Note: This category is to be used to indicate conditions in 430-437 as the cause of late effects. The "late effects" include conditions specified as such, as sequelae, which may occur at any time after the onset of the causal condition.
AHA: 4Q, '99, 4, 6, 7; 4Q, '98, 39, 88; 4Q, '97, 35, 37; 4Q, '92, 21;N-D,'86, 12; M-A, '86, 7

438.0 Cognitive deficits

438.1 Speech and language deficits
  438.10 Speech and language deficit, unspecified
  438.11 Aphasia
    AHA: 4Q, '03, 105; 4Q, '97, 36
    DEF: Impairment or absence of the ability to communicate by speech, writing or signs or to comprehend the spoken or written language due to disease or injury to the brain. Total aphasia is the loss of function of both sensory and motor areas of the brain.
  438.12 Dysphasia
    AHA: 4Q, '99, 3, 9
    DEF: Impaired speech; marked by inability to sequence language.
  438.19 Other speech and language deficits

438.2 Hemiplegia/hemiparesis
DEF: Paralysis of one side of the body.
  438.20 Hemiplegia affecting unspecified side
    AHA: 4Q, '03, 105; 4Q, '99, 3, 9
  438.21 Hemiplegia affecting dominant side
  438.22 Hemiplegia affecting nondominant side
    AHA: 4Q, '03, 105; 1Q, '02, 16

438.3 Monoplegia of upper limb
DEF: Paralysis of one limb or one muscle group.
  438.30 Monoplegia of upper limb affecting unspecified side
  438.31 Monoplegia of upper limb affecting dominant side
  438.32 Monoplegia of upper limb affecting nondominant side

438.4 Monoplegia of lower limb
  438.40 Monoplegia of lower limb affecting unspecified side
  438.41 Monoplegia of lower limb affecting dominant side
  438.42 Monoplegia of lower limb affecting nondominant side

438.5 Other paralytic syndrome
Use additional code to identify type of paralytic syndrome, such as:
  locked-in state (344.81)
  quadriplegia (344.00-344.09)
EXCLUDES late effects of cerebrovascular accident with:
  hemiplegia/hemiparesis (438.20-438.22)
  monoplegia of lower limb (438.40-438.42)
  monoplegia of upper limb (438.30-438.32)
  438.50 Other paralytic syndrome affecting unspecified side
  438.51 Other paralytic syndrome affecting dominant side
  438.52 Other paralytic syndrome affecting nondominant side
  438.53 Other paralytic syndrome, bilateral
    AHA: 4Q, '98, 39

438.6 Alterations of sensations
Use additional code to identify the altered sensation

438.7 Disturbances of vision
Use additional code to identify the visual disturbance
AHA: 4Q, '02, 56

CIRCULATORY SYSTEM

Map of Major Arteries

(Anatomical diagram showing major arteries of the body, including: Facial, Internal carotid, External carotid, Right and left common carotid, Vertebral, Brachiocephalic, Thyrocervical trunk, Subclavian, Internal mammary, Pulmonary, Subclavian, Aorta (Thoracic/Abdominal), Axillary, Brachial, Intercostal, Celiac trunk, Splenic, Renal, Superior mesenteric, Ovarian/testicular, Inferior mesenteric, Common iliac, Radial, Internal iliac, Ulnar, External iliac, Digital, Deep femoral, Femoral, Popliteal, Posterior tibial, Anterior tibial, Peroneal, Dorsalis pedis, Plantar, Digital)

Branches of Abdominal Aorta: Common hepatic, Hepatic, Celiac trunk, Left gastric, Short gastric, Cystic, Right gastric, Splenic, Gastroepiploic, Superior mesenteric, Colic, Ileocolic, Inferior mesenteric, Superior rectal, Left colic

---

√5th 438.8 Other late effects of cerebrovascular disease

438.81 Apraxia
DEF: Inability to activate learned movements; no known sensory or motor impairment.

438.82 Dysphagia
DEF: Inability or difficulty in swallowing.

438.83 Facial weakness
Facial droop

438.84 Ataxia
AHA: 4Q, '02, 56

438.85 Vertigo

438.89 Other late effects of cerebrovascular disease
Use additional code to identify the late effect
AHA: 1Q, '05, 13; 4Q, '98, 39

438.9 Unspecified late effects of cerebrovascular disease

DISEASES OF ARTERIES, ARTERIOLES, AND CAPILLARIES (440-448)

√4th 440 Atherosclerosis

INCLUDES:
arteriolosclerosis
arteriosclerosis (obliterans) (senile)
arteriosclerotic vascular disease
atheroma
degeneration:
  arterial   vascular
  arteriovascular
endarteritis deformans or obliterans
senile:
  arteritis   endarteritis

EXCLUDES:
atheroembolism (445.01-445.89)
atherosclerosis of bypass graft of the extremities (440.30-440.32)

DEF: Stricture and reduced elasticity of an artery; due to plaque deposits.

440.0 Of aorta
AHA: 2Q, '93, 7; 2Q, '93, 8; 4Q, '88, 8

√4th Additional Digit Required
√5th
Unspecified Code   Other Specified Code   Manifestation Code   ►◄ Revised Text   ● New Code   ▲ Revised Code Title

2007 ICD•9•CM

CIRCULATORY SYSTEM

440.1–442.83

440.1 Of renal artery
  EXCLUDES: atherosclerosis of renal arterioles (403.00-403.91)

✓5th 440.2 Of native arteries of the extremities
  EXCLUDES: atherosclerosis of bypass graft of the extremities (440.30-440.32)
  AHA: 4Q, '94, 49; 4Q, '93, 27; 4Q, '92, 25; 3Q, '90, 15; M-A, '87, 6

  440.20 Atherosclerosis of the extremities, unspecified

  440.21 Atherosclerosis of the extremities with intermittent claudication
    DEF: Atherosclerosis; marked by pain, tension and weakness after walking; no symptoms while at rest.

  440.22 Atherosclerosis of the extremities with rest pain
    INCLUDES: any condition classifiable to 440.21
    DEF: Atherosclerosis, marked by pain, tension and weakness while at rest.

  440.23 Atherosclerosis of the extremities with ulceration
    INCLUDES: any condition classifiable to 440.21 and 440.22
    Use additional code for any associated ulceration (707.10-707.9)
    AHA: 4Q, '00, 44

  440.24 Atherosclerosis of the extremities with gangrene
    INCLUDES: any condition classifiable to 440.21, 440.22, and 440.23 with ischemic gangrene 785.4
    ▶Use additional code for any associated ulceration (707.10-707.9)◀
    EXCLUDES: gas gangrene (040.0)
    AHA: 4Q, '03, 109; 3Q, '03, 14; 4Q, '95, 54; 1Q, '95, 11

  440.29 Other

✓5th 440.3 Of bypass graft of extremities
  EXCLUDES: atherosclerosis of native arteries of the extremities (440.21-440.24)
  embolism [occlusion NOS] [thrombus] of graft (996.74)
  AHA: 4Q, '94, 49

  440.30 Of unspecified graft
  440.31 Of autologous vein bypass graft
  440.32 Of nonautologous biological bypass graft

440.8 Of other specified arteries
  EXCLUDES: basilar (433.0)
    carotid (433.1)
    cerebral (437.0)
    coronary (414.00-414.07)
    mesenteric (557.1)
    precerebral (433.0-433.9)
    pulmonary (416.0)
    vertebral (433.2)

440.9 Generalized and unspecified atherosclerosis
  Arteriosclerotic vascular disease NOS
  EXCLUDES: arteriosclerotic cardiovascular disease [ASCVD] (429.2)

✓4th 441 Aortic aneurysm and dissection
  EXCLUDES: syphilitic aortic aneurysm (093.0)
    traumatic aortic aneurysm (901.0, 902.0)

✓5th 441.0 Dissection of aorta
  AHA: 4Q, '89, 10
  DEF: Dissection or splitting of wall of the aorta; due to blood entering through intimal tear or interstitial hemorrhage.

  441.00 Unspecified site

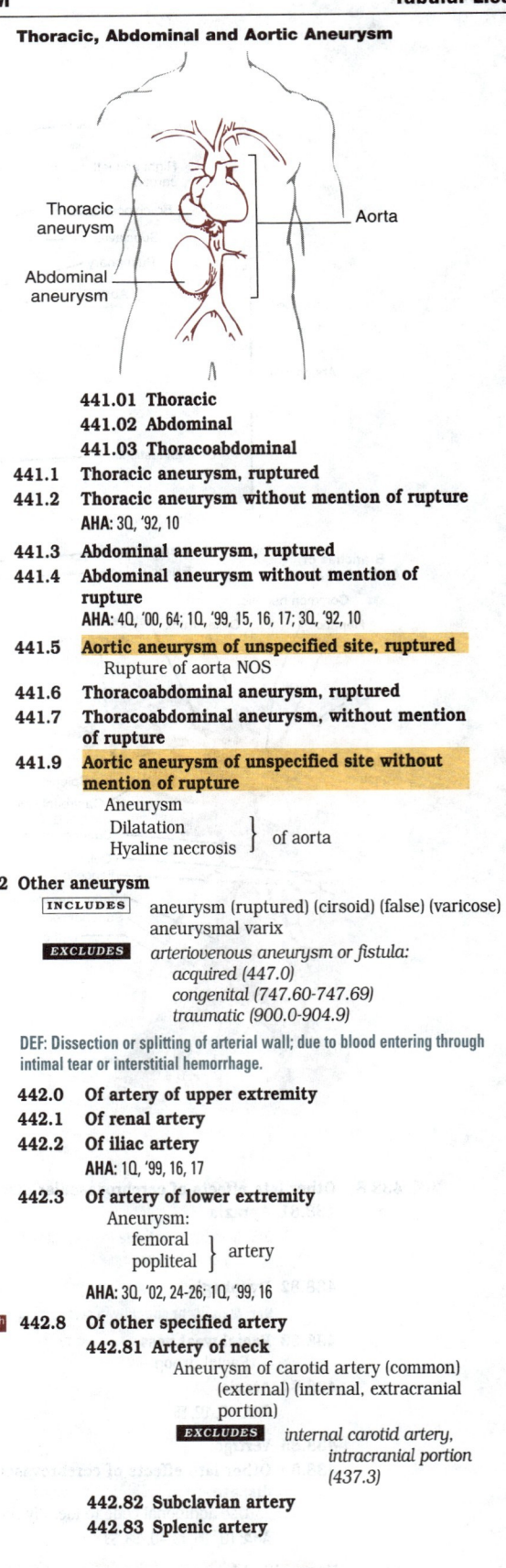

Thoracic, Abdominal and Aortic Aneurysm

  441.01 Thoracic
  441.02 Abdominal
  441.03 Thoracoabdominal
441.1 Thoracic aneurysm, ruptured
441.2 Thoracic aneurysm without mention of rupture
  AHA: 3Q, '92, 10
441.3 Abdominal aneurysm, ruptured
441.4 Abdominal aneurysm without mention of rupture
  AHA: 4Q, '00, 64; 1Q, '99, 15, 16, 17; 3Q, '92, 10
441.5 Aortic aneurysm of unspecified site, ruptured
  Rupture of aorta NOS
441.6 Thoracoabdominal aneurysm, ruptured
441.7 Thoracoabdominal aneurysm, without mention of rupture
441.9 Aortic aneurysm of unspecified site without mention of rupture
  Aneurysm
  Dilatation   } of aorta
  Hyaline necrosis

✓4th 442 Other aneurysm
  INCLUDES: aneurysm (ruptured) (cirsoid) (false) (varicose) aneurysmal varix
  EXCLUDES: arteriovenous aneurysm or fistula:
    acquired (447.0)
    congenital (747.60-747.69)
    traumatic (900.0-904.9)
  DEF: Dissection or splitting of arterial wall; due to blood entering through intimal tear or interstitial hemorrhage.

  442.0 Of artery of upper extremity
  442.1 Of renal artery
  442.2 Of iliac artery
    AHA: 1Q, '99, 16, 17
  442.3 Of artery of lower extremity
    Aneurysm:
      femoral   } artery
      popliteal
    AHA: 3Q, '02, 24-26; 1Q, '99, 16

✓5th 442.8 Of other specified artery
  442.81 Artery of neck
    Aneurysm of carotid artery (common) (external) (internal, extracranial portion)
    EXCLUDES: internal carotid artery, intracranial portion (437.3)
  442.82 Subclavian artery
  442.83 Splenic artery

CIRCULATORY SYSTEM

442.84 Other visceral artery
Aneurysm:
celiac
gastroduodenal
gastroepiploic
hepatic
pancreaticoduodenal
} artery

442.89 Other
Aneurysm:
mediastinal } artery
EXCLUDES
cerebral (nonruptured) (437.3)
congenital (747.81)
ruptured (430)
coronary (414.11)
heart (414.10)
pulmonary (417.1)

442.9 Of unspecified site

443 Other peripheral vascular disease

443.0 Raynaud's syndrome
Raynaud's:
disease
phenomenon (secondary)
Use additional code to identify gangrene (785.4)
DEF: Constriction of the arteries, due to cold or stress; bilateral ischemic attacks of fingers, toes, nose or ears; symptoms include pallor, paresthesia and pain; more common in females.

443.1 Thromboangiitis obliterans [Buerger's disease]
Presenile gangrene
DEF: Inflammatory disease of extremity blood vessels, mainly the lower; occurs primarily in young men and leads to tissue ischemia and gangrene.

443.2 Other arterial dissection
EXCLUDES
dissection of aorta (441.00-441.03)
dissection of coronary arteries (414.12)
AHA: 4Q, '02, 54

- 443.21 Dissection of carotid artery
- 443.22 Dissection of iliac artery
- 443.23 Dissection of renal artery
- 443.24 Dissection of vertebral artery
- 443.29 Dissection of other artery

443.8 Other specified peripheral vascular diseases

- 443.81 Peripheral angiopathy in diseases classified elsewhere
Code first underlying disease, as:
diabetes mellitus (250.7)
AHA: 1Q, '04, 14; 3Q, '91, 10

- 443.82 Erythromelalgia
AHA: ▶4Q, '05, 73◀
DEF: ▶Rare syndrome of paroxysmal vasodilation; maldistribution of blood flow causes redness, pain, increased skin temperature, and burning sensations in various parts of the body.◀

- 443.89 Other
Acrocyanosis   Erythrocyanosis
Acroparesthesia:
simple [Schultze's type]
vasomotor [Nothnagel's type]
EXCLUDES
chilblains (991.5)
frostbite (991.0-991.3)
immersion foot (991.4)

443.9 Peripheral vascular disease, unspecified
Intermittent claudication NOS
Peripheral:
angiopathy NOS
vascular disease NOS
Spasm of artery
EXCLUDES
atherosclerosis of the arteries of the extremities (440.20-440.22)
spasm of cerebral artery (435.0-435.9)
AHA: 4Q, '92, 25; 3Q, '91, 10

Arterial Diseases and Disorders

444 Arterial embolism and thrombosis
INCLUDES
infarction:
embolic
thrombotic
occlusion
EXCLUDES
atheroembolism (445.01-445.89)
that complicating:
abortion (634-638 with .6, 639.6)
ectopic or molar pregnancy (639.6)
pregnancy, childbirth, or the pueperium (673.0-673.8)
AHA: 2Q, '92, 11; 4Q, '90, 27

444.0 Of abdominal aorta
Aortic bifurcation syndrome   Leriche's syndrome
Aortoiliac obstruction   Saddle embolus
AHA: 2Q, '93, 7; 4Q, '90, 27

444.1 Of thoracic aorta
Embolism or thrombosis of aorta (thoracic)

444.2 Of arteries of the extremities
AHA: M-A, '87, 6

- 444.21 Upper extremity
- 444.22 Lower extremity
Arterial embolism or thrombosis:
femoral
peripheral NOS
popliteal
EXCLUDES
iliofemoral (444.81)
AHA: 3Q, '03, 10; 1Q, '03, 17; 3Q, '90, 16

444.8 Of other specified artery

- 444.81 Iliac artery
AHA: 1Q, '03, 16

- 444.89 Other
EXCLUDES
basilar (433.0)
carotid (433.1)
cerebral (434.0-434.9)
coronary (410.00-410.92)
mesenteric (557.0)
ophthalmic (362.30-362.34)
precerebral (433.0-433.9)
pulmonary (415.19)
renal (593.81)
retinal (362.30-362.34)
vertebral (433.2)

444.9 Of unspecified artery

445 Atheroembolism
INCLUDES
atherothrombotic microembolism
cholesterol embolism
AHA: 4Q, '02, 57

445.0 Of extremities
- 445.01 Upper extremity
- 445.02 Lower extremity

445.8–448.9 — **CIRCULATORY SYSTEM** — Tabular List

445.8 Of other sites [5th]
445.81 Kidney
▶Use additional code for any associated acute renal failure or chronic kidney disease (584, 585)◀
445.89 Other site

446 Polyarteritis nodosa and allied conditions [4th]
446.0 Polyarteritis nodosa
Disseminated necrotizing periarteritis
Necrotizing angiitis
Panarteritis (nodosa)
Periarteritis (nodosa)

DEF: Inflammation of small and mid-size arteries; symptoms related to involved arteries in kidneys, muscles, gastrointestinal tract and heart; results in tissue death.

446.1 Acute febrile mucocutaneous lymph node syndrome [MCLS]
Kawasaki disease

DEF: Acute febrile disease of children; marked by erythema of conjunctiva and mucous membranes of upper respiratory tract, skin eruptions and edema.

446.2 Hypersensitivity angiitis [5th]
EXCLUDES antiglomerular basement membrane disease without pulmonary hemorrhage (583.89)

446.20 Hypersensitivity angiitis, unspecified
446.21 Goodpasture's syndrome
Antiglomerular basement membrane antibody-mediated nephritis with pulmonary hemorrhage
Use additional code to identify renal disease (583.81)

DEF: Glomerulonephritis associated with hematuria, progresses rapidly; results in death from renal failure.

446.29 Other specified hypersensitivity angiitis
AHA: 1Q, '95, 3

446.3 Lethal midline granuloma
Malignant granuloma of face

DEF: Granulomatous lesion; in nose or paranasal sinuses; often fatal; occurs chiefly in males.

AHA: 3Q, '00, 11

446.4 Wegener's granulomatosis
Necrotizing respiratory granulomatosis
Wegener's syndrome

DEF: A disease occurring mainly in men; marked by necrotizing granulomas and ulceration of the upper respiratory tract; underlying condition is a vasculitis affecting small vessels and is possibly due to an immune disorder.

AHA: 3Q, '00, 11

446.5 Giant cell arteritis
Bagratuni's syndrome
Horton's disease
Cranial arteritis
Temporal arteritis

DEF: Inflammation of arteries; due to giant cells affecting carotid artery branches, resulting in occlusion; symptoms include fever, headache and neurological problems; occurs in elderly.

446.6 Thrombotic microangiopathy
Moschcowitz's syndrome
Thrombotic thrombocytopenic purpura

DEF: Blockage of small blood vessels; due to hyaline deposits; symptoms include purpura, CNS disorders; results in protracted disease or rapid death.

446.7 Takayasu's disease
Aortic arch arteritis   Pulseless disease

DEF: Progressive obliterative arteritis of brachiocephalic trunk, left subclavian, and left common carotid arteries above aortic arch; results in ischemia in brain, heart and arm; pulses impalpable in head, neck and arms; more common in young adult females.

447 Other disorders of arteries and arterioles [4th]
447.0 Arteriovenous fistula, acquired
Arteriovenous aneurysm, acquired

EXCLUDES cerebrovascular (437.3)
coronary (414.19)
pulmonary (417.0)
surgically created arteriovenous shunt or fistula:
   complication (996.1, 996.61-996.62)
   status or presence (V45.1)
traumatic (900.0-904.9)

DEF: Communication between an artery and vein caused by error in healing.

447.1 Stricture of artery
AHA: 2Q, '93, 8; M-A, '87, 6

447.2 Rupture of artery
Erosion
Fistula, except arteriovenous } of artery
Ulcer

EXCLUDES traumatic rupture of artery (900.0-904.9)

447.3 Hyperplasia of renal artery
Fibromuscular hyperplasia of renal artery

DEF: Overgrowth of cells in muscular lining of renal artery.

447.4 Celiac artery compression syndrome
Celiac axis syndrome   Marable's syndrome

447.5 Necrosis of artery
447.6 Arteritis, unspecified
Aortitis NOS   Endarteritis NOS

EXCLUDES arteritis, endarteritis:
   aortic arch (446.7)
   cerebral (437.4)
   coronary (414.00-414.07)
   deformans (440.0-440.9)
   obliterans (440.0-440.9)
   pulmonary (417.8)
   senile (440.0-440.9)
polyarteritis NOS (446.0)
syphilitic aortitis (093.1)

AHA: 1Q, '95, 3

447.8 Other specified disorders of arteries and arterioles
Fibromuscular hyperplasia of arteries, except renal

447.9 Unspecified disorders of arteries and arterioles

448 Disease of capillaries [4th]
448.0 Hereditary hemorrhagic telangiectasia
Rendu-Osler-Weber disease

DEF: Genetic disease with onset after puberty; results in multiple telangiectases, dilated venules on skin and mucous membranes; recurrent bleeding may occur.

448.1 Nevus, non-neoplastic
Nevus:
   araneus
   senile
Nevus:
   spider
   stellar

EXCLUDES neoplastic (216.0-216.9)
port wine (757.32)
strawberry (757.32)

DEF: Enlarged or malformed blood vessels of skin; results in reddish swelling, skin patch, or birthmark.

448.9 Other and unspecified capillary diseases
Capillary:
   hemorrhage
   hyperpermeability
Capillary:
   thrombosis

EXCLUDES capillary fragility (hereditary) (287.8)

CIRCULATORY SYSTEM

Map of Major Veins

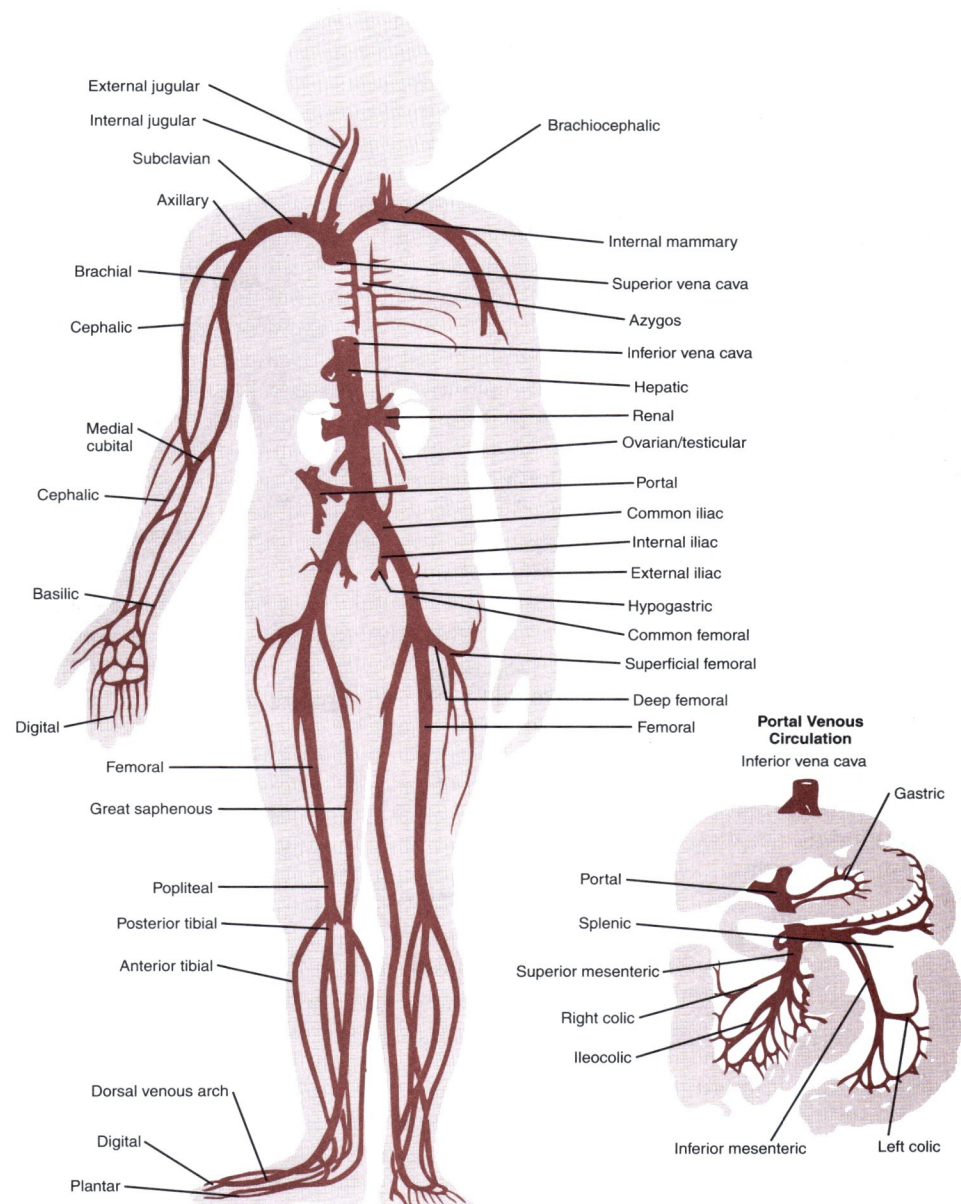

DISEASES OF VEINS AND LYMPHATICS, AND OTHER DISEASES OF CIRCULATORY SYSTEM (451-459)

✓4th 451 Phlebitis and thrombophlebitis

INCLUDES
- endophlebitis
- inflammation, vein
- periphlebitis
- suppurative phlebitis

Use additional E code to identify drug, if drug-induced

EXCLUDES that complicating:
- abortion (634-638 with .7, 639.8)
- ectopic or molar pregnancy (639.8)
- pregnancy, childbirth, or the puerperium (671.0-671.9)

that due to or following:
- implant or catheter device (996.61-996.62)
- infusion, perfusion, or transfusion (999.2)

AHA: 1Q, '92, 16

DEF: Inflammation of a vein (phlebitis) with formation of a thrombus (thrombophlebitis).

451.0 Of superficial vessels of lower extremities
AHA: 3Q, '91, 16

Saphenous vein (greater) (lesser)

✓5th 451.1 Of deep vessels of lower extremities
AHA: 3Q, '91, 16

451.11 Femoral vein (deep) (superficial)

451.19 Other
Femoropopliteal vein   Tibial vein
Popliteal vein

451.2 Of lower extremities, unspecified
AHA: 4Q, '04, 80

✓5th 451.8 Of other sites
EXCLUDES intracranial venous sinus (325)
nonpyogenic (437.6)
portal (vein) (572.1)

451.81 Iliac vein

CIRCULATORY SYSTEM — Tabular List

451.82–455.8

- **451.82** Of superficial veins of upper extremities
  - Antecubital vein
  - Cephalic vein
  - Basilic vein
- **451.83** Of deep veins of upper extremities
  - Brachial vein
  - Ulnar vein
  - Radial vein
- **451.84** Of upper extremities, unspecified
- **451.89** Other
  - Axillary vein
  - Jugular vein
  - Subclavian vein
  - Thrombophlebitis of breast (Mondor's disease)
- **451.9** Of unspecified site

452 Portal vein thrombosis
  Portal (vein) obstruction
  EXCLUDES hepatic vein thrombosis (453.0)
            phlebitis of portal vein (572.1)
  DEF: Formation of a blood clot in main vein of liver.

√4th 453 Other venous embolism and thrombosis
  EXCLUDES that complicating:
            abortion (634-638 with .7, 639.8)
            ectopic or molar pregnancy (639.8)
            pregnancy, childbirth, or the puerperium (671.0-671.9)
            that with inflammation, phlebitis, and thrombophlebitis (451.0-451.9)
  AHA: 1Q, '92, 16

- **453.0** Budd-Chiari syndrome
  Hepatic vein thrombosis
  DEF: Thrombosis or other obstruction of hepatic vein; symptoms include enlarged liver, extensive collateral vessels, intractable ascites and severe portal hypertension.

- **453.1** Thrombophlebitis migrans
  DEF: Slow, advancing thrombophlebitis; appearing first in one vein then another.

- **453.2** Of vena cava
- **453.3** Of renal vein
- **√5th 453.4** Venous embolism and thrombosis of deep vessels of lower extremity
  - **453.40** Venous embolism and thrombosis of unspecified deep vessels of lower extremity
    - Deep vein thrombosis NOS
    - DVT NOS
  - **453.41** Venous embolism and thrombosis of deep vessels of proximal lower extremity
    - Femoral
    - Thigh
    - Iliac
    - Upper leg NOS
    - Popliteal
    AHA: 4Q, '04, 79
  - **453.42** Venous embolism and thrombosis of deep vessels of distal lower extremity
    - Calf
    - Peroneal
    - Lower leg NOS
    - Tibial

- **453.8** Of other specified veins
  EXCLUDES cerebral (434.0-434.9)
            coronary (410.00-410.92)
            intracranial venous sinus (325)
              nonpyogenic (437.6)
            mesenteric (557.0)
            portal (452)
            precerebral (433.0-433.9)
            pulmonary (415.19)
  AHA: 3Q, '91, 16; M-A, '87, 6

- **453.9** Of unspecified site
  Embolism of vein
  Thrombosis (vein)

√4th 454 Varicose veins of lower extremities
  EXCLUDES that complicating pregnancy, childbirth, or the puerperium (671.0)
  AHA: 2Q, '91, 20
  DEF: Dilated leg veins; due to incompetent vein valves that allow reversed blood flow and cause tissue erosion or weakness of wall; may be painful.

- **454.0** With ulcer [A]
  Varicose ulcer (lower extremity, any part)
  Varicose veins with ulcer of lower extremity [any part] or of unspecified site
  Any condition classifiable to 454.9 with ulcer or specified as ulcerated
  AHA: 4Q, '99, 18

- **454.1** With inflammation [A]
  Stasis dermatitis
  Varicose veins with inflammation of lower extremity [any part] or of unspecified site
  Any condition classifiable to 454.9 with inflammation or specified as inflamed

- **454.2** With ulcer and inflammation [A]
  Varicose veins with ulcer and inflammation of lower extremity [any part] or of unspecified site
  Any condition classifiable to 454.9 with ulcer and inflammation

- **454.8** With other complications
  Edema
  Pain
  Swelling
  AHA: 4Q, '02, 58

- **454.9** Asymptomatic varicose veins [A]
  Phlebectasia
  Varicose veins } of lower extremity [any part] or of unspecified site
  Varix
  Varicose veins NOS
  AHA: 4Q, '02, 58

√4th 455 Hemorrhoids
  INCLUDES hemorrhoids (anus) (rectum)
            piles
            varicose veins, anus or rectum
  EXCLUDES that complicating pregnancy, childbirth, or the puerperium (671.8)
  DEF: Varicose condition of external hemorrhoidal veins causing painful swellings at the anus.

- **455.0** Internal hemorrhoids without mention of complication
  AHA: ▶3Q, '05, 17◀
- **455.1** Internal thrombosed hemorrhoids
- **455.2** Internal hemorrhoids with other complication
  Internal hemorrhoids:
    bleeding
    prolapsed
  Internal hemorrhoids:
    strangulated
    ulcerated
  AHA: ▶3Q, '05, 17;◀ 1Q, '03, 8
- **455.3** External hemorrhoids without mention of complication
  AHA: ▶3Q, '05, 17◀
- **455.4** External thrombosed hemorrhoids
- **455.5** External hemorrhoids with other complication
  External hemorrhoids:
    bleeding
    prolapsed
  External hemorrhoids:
    strangulated
    ulcerated
  AHA: ▶3Q, '05, 17;◀ 1Q, '03, 8
- **455.6** Unspecified hemorrhoids without mention of complication
  Hemorrhoids NOS
- **455.7** Unspecified thrombosed hemorrhoids
  Thrombosed hemorrhoids, unspecified whether internal or external
- **455.8** Unspecified hemorrhoids with other complication
  Hemorrhoids, unspecified whether internal or external:
    bleeding
    prolapsed
    strangulated
    ulcerated

[N] Newborn Age: 0   [P] Pediatric Age: 0-17   [M] Maternity Age: 12-55   [A] Adult Age: 15-124

Tabular List
CIRCULATORY SYSTEM
455.9–459.0

455.9 Residual hemorrhoidal skin tags
Skin tags, anus or rectum

√4ᵗʰ **456 Varicose veins of other sites**

456.0 Esophageal varices with bleeding
DEF: Distended, tortuous, veins of lower esophagus, usually due to portal hypertension.

456.1 Esophageal varices without mention of bleeding

√5ᵗʰ **456.2 Esophageal varices in diseases classified elsewhere**
Code first underlying disease, as:
cirrhosis of liver (571.0-571.9)
portal hypertension (572.3)

456.20 With bleeding
AHA: N-D, '85, 14

456.21 Without mention of bleeding
AHA: ▶3Q, '05, 15;◀ 2Q, '02, 4

456.3 Sublingual varices
DEF: Distended, tortuous veins beneath tongue.

456.4 Scrotal varices ♂
Varicocele

456.5 Pelvic varices
Varices of broad ligament

456.6 Vulval varices ♀
Varices of perineum
EXCLUDES that complicating pregnancy, childbirth, or the puerperium (671.1)

456.8 Varices of other sites
Varicose veins of nasal septum (with ulcer)
EXCLUDES placental varices (656.7)
retinal varices (362.17)
varicose ulcer of unspecified site (454.0)
varicose veins of unspecified site (454.9)

AHA: 2Q, '02, 4

√4ᵗʰ **457 Noninfectious disorders of lymphatic channels**

457.0 Postmastectomy lymphedema syndrome ▲
Elephantiasis
Obliteration of lymphatic vessel } due to mastectomy

DEF: Reduced lymphatic circulation following mastectomy; symptoms include swelling of the arm on the operative side.

AHA: 2Q, '02, 12

457.1 Other lymphedema
Elephantiasis   Lymphedema:
 (nonfilarial) NOS   praecox
Lymphangiectasis   secondary
Lymphedema: Obliteration, lymphatic vessel
 acquired (chronic)
EXCLUDES elephantiasis (nonfilarial):
congenital (757.0)
eyelid (374.83)
vulva (624.8)

AHA: 3Q, '04, 5

DEF: Fluid retention due to reduced lymphatic circulation; due to other than mastectomy.

457.2 Lymphangitis
Lymphangitis: Lymphangitis:
 NOS   subacute
 chronic
EXCLUDES acute lymphangitis (682.0-682.9)

457.8 Other noninfectious disorders of lymphatic channels
Chylocele (nonfilarial) Lymph node or vessel:
Chylous: fistula
 ascites   infarction
 cyst   rupture
EXCLUDES chylocele:
filarial (125.0-125.9)
tunica vaginalis (nonfilarial) (608.84)

AHA: 1Q, '04, 5; 3Q, '03, 17

457.9 Unspecified noninfectious disorder of lymphatic channels

√4ᵗʰ **458 Hypotension**
INCLUDES hypopiesis
EXCLUDES cardiovascular collapse (785.50)
maternal hypotension syndrome (669.2)
shock (785.50-785.59)
Shy-Drager syndrome (333.0)

458.0 Orthostatic hypotension
Hypotension: Hypotension:
 orthostatic (chronic) postural
AHA: 3Q, '00, 8; 3Q, '91, 9

DEF: Low blood pressure; occurs when standing.

458.1 Chronic hypotension
Permanent idiopathic hypotension
DEF: Persistent low blood pressure.

√5ᵗʰ **458.2 Iatrogenic hypotension**
AHA: 4Q, '03, 60; 3Q, '02, 12; 4Q, '95, 57
DEF: Abnormally low blood pressure; due to medical treatment.

458.21 Hypotension of hemodialysis
Intra-dialytic hypotension
AHA: 4Q, '03, 61

458.29 Other iatrogenic hypotension
Postoperative hypotension

458.8 Other specified hypotension
AHA: 4Q, '97, 37

458.9 Hypotension, unspecified
Hypotension (arterial) NOS

√4ᵗʰ **459 Other disorders of circulatory system**

459.0 Hemorrhage, unspecified
Rupture of blood vessel NOS
Spontaneous hemorrhage NEC
EXCLUDES hemorrhage:
gastrointestinal NOS (578.9)
in newborn NOS (772.9)
secondary or recurrent following trauma (958.2)
traumatic rupture of blood vessel (900.0-904.9)

AHA: 4Q, '90, 26

CIRCULATORY SYSTEM

459.1 **Postphlebitic syndrome**
Chronic venous hypertension due to deep vein thrombosis
> EXCLUDES: chronic venous hypertension without deep vein thrombosis (459.30-459.39)

AHA: 4Q, '02, 58; 2Q, '91, 20

DEF: Various conditions following deep vein thrombosis; including edema, pain, stasis dermatitis, cellulitis, varicose veins and ulceration of the lower leg.

459.10 **Postphlebitic syndrome without complications**
Asymptomatic postphlebitic syndrome
Postphlebitic syndrome NOS

459.11 **Postphlebitic syndrome with ulcer**

459.12 **Postphlebitic syndrome with inflammation**

459.13 **Postphlebitic syndrome with ulcer and inflammation**

459.19 **Postphlebitic syndrome with other complication**

459.2 **Compression of vein**
Stricture of vein
Vena cava syndrome (inferior) (superior)

459.3 **Chronic venous hypertension (idiopathic)**
Stasis edema
> EXCLUDES: chronic venous hypertension due to deep vein thrombosis (459.10-459.19)
> varicose veins (454.0-454.9)

AHA: 4Q, '02, 59

459.30 **Chronic venous hypertension without complications**
Asymptomatic chronic venous hypertension
Chronic venous hypertension NOS

459.31 **Chronic venous hypertension with ulcer**

AHA: 4Q, '02, 43

459.32 **Chronic venous hypertension with inflammation**

459.33 **Chronic venous hypertension with ulcer and inflammation**

459.39 **Chronic venous hypertension with other complication**

459.8 **Other specified disorders of circulatory system**

459.81 **Venous (peripheral) insufficiency, unspecified**
Chronic venous insufficiency NOS
Use additional code for any associated ulceration (707.10-707.9)

AHA: 3Q, '04, 5; 2Q, '91, 20; M-A, '87, 6

DEF: Insufficient drainage, venous blood, any part of body, results in edema or dermatosis.

459.89 **Other**
Collateral circulation (venous), any site
Phlebosclerosis
Venofibrosis

459.9 **Unspecified circulatory system disorder**

RESPIRATORY SYSTEM

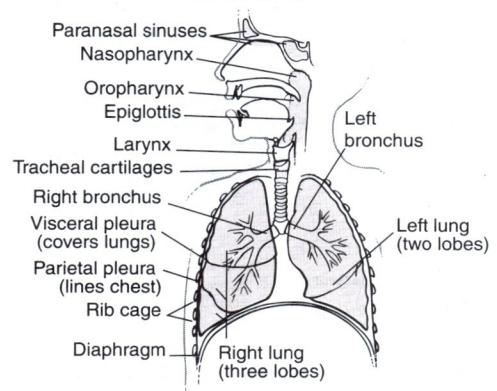

8. DISEASES OF THE RESPIRATORY SYSTEM (460-519)

Use additional code to identify infectious organism

ACUTE RESPIRATORY INFECTIONS (460-466)

EXCLUDES pneumonia and influenza (480.0-487.8)

460 Acute nasopharyngitis [common cold]
- Coryza (acute)
- Nasal catarrh, acute
- Nasopharyngitis:
  - NOS
  - acute
- Nasopharyngitis: infective NOS
- Rhinitis:
  - acute
  - infective

EXCLUDES nasopharyngitis, chronic (472.2)
- pharyngitis:
  - acute or unspecified (462)
  - chronic (472.1)
- rhinitis:
  - allergic (477.0-477.9)
  - chronic or unspecified (472.0)
- sore throat:
  - acute or unspecified (462)
  - chronic (472.1)

AHA: 1Q, '88, 12

DEF: Acute inflammation of mucous membranes; extends from nares to pharynx.

✓4th 461 Acute sinusitis

INCLUDES
- abscess
- empyema
- infection
- inflammation
- suppuration

acute, of sinus (accessory) (nasal)

EXCLUDES chronic or unspecified sinusitis (473.0-473.9)

- **461.0 Maxillary**
  - Acute antritis
- **461.1 Frontal**
- **461.2 Ethmoidal**
- **461.3 Sphenoidal**
- **461.8 Other acute sinusitis**
  - Acute pansinusitis
- **461.9 Acute sinusitis, unspecified**
  - Acute sinusitis NOS

462 Acute pharyngitis
- Acute sore throat NOS
- Pharyngitis (acute):
  - NOS
  - gangrenous
  - infective
  - phlegmonous
  - pneumococcal
- Pharyngitis (acute):
  - staphylococcal
  - suppurative
  - ulcerative
- Sore throat (viral) NOS
- Viral pharyngitis

EXCLUDES abscess:
- peritonsillar [quinsy] (475)
- pharyngeal NOS (478.29)
- retropharyngeal (478.24)
- chronic pharyngitis (472.1)
- infectious mononucleosis (075)
- that specified as (due to):
  - Coxsackie (virus) (074.0)
  - gonococcus (098.6)
  - herpes simplex (054.79)
  - influenza (487.1)
  - septic (034.0)
  - streptococcal (034.0)

AHA: 4Q, '99, 26; S-O, '85, 8

463 Acute tonsillitis
- Tonsillitis (acute):
  - NOS
  - follicular
  - gangrenous
  - infective
  - pneumococcal
- Tonsillitis (acute):
  - septic
  - staphylococcal
  - suppurative
  - ulcerative
  - viral

EXCLUDES
- chronic tonsillitis (474.0)
- hypertrophy of tonsils (474.1)
- peritonsillar abscess [quinsy] (475)
- sore throat:
  - acute or NOS (462)
  - septic (034.0)
- streptococcal tonsillitis (034.0)

AHA: N-D, '84, 16

✓4th 464 Acute laryngitis and tracheitis

EXCLUDES
- that associated with influenza (487.1)
- that due to Streptococcus (034.0)

✓5th 464.0 Acute laryngitis
- Laryngitis (acute):
  - NOS
  - edematous
  - Hemophilus influenzae [H. influenzae]
  - pneumococcal
  - septic
  - suppurative
  - ulcerative

EXCLUDES
- chronic laryngitis (476.0-476.1)
- influenzal laryngitis (487.1)

AHA: 4Q, '01, 42

- **464.00 Without mention of obstruction**
- **464.01 With obstruction**

✓5th 464.1 Acute tracheitis
- Tracheitis (acute):
  - NOS
  - catarrhal
- Tracheitis (acute):
  - viral

EXCLUDES chronic tracheitis (491.8)

- **464.10 Without mention of obstruction**
- **464.11 With obstruction**

✓5th 464.2 Acute laryngotracheitis
- Laryngotracheitis (acute)
- Tracheitis (acute) with laryngitis (acute)

EXCLUDES chronic laryngotracheitis (476.1)

- **464.20 Without mention of obstruction**
- **464.21 With obstruction**

RESPIRATORY SYSTEM

464.3 Acute epiglottitis
Viral epiglottitis
EXCLUDES: epiglottitis, chronic (476.1)
- 464.30 Without mention of obstruction
- 464.31 With obstruction

464.4 Croup
Croup syndrome
DEF: Acute laryngeal obstruction due to allergy, foreign body or infection; symptoms include barking cough, hoarseness and harsh, persistent high-pitched respiratory sound.

464.5 Supraglottitis, unspecified
AHA: 4Q, '01, 42
DEF: A rapidly advancing generalized upper respiratory infection of the lingual tonsillar area, epiglottic folds, false vocal cords, and the epiglottis; seen most commonly in children, but can affect people of any age.
- 464.50 Without mention of obstruction
  AHA: 4Q, '01, 43
- 464.51 With obstruction

465 Acute upper respiratory infections of multiple or unspecified sites
EXCLUDES: upper respiratory infection due to:
influenza (487.1)
Streptococcus (034.0)
- 465.0 Acute laryngopharyngitis
  DEF: Acute infection of the vocal cords and pharynx.
- 465.8 Other multiple sites
  Multiple URI
- 465.9 Unspecified site
  Acute URI NOS
  Upper respiratory infection (acute)

466 Acute bronchitis and bronchiolitis
INCLUDES: that with:
bronchospasm
obstruction
- 466.0 Acute bronchitis
  Bronchitis, acute or subacute:
  fibrinous
  membranous
  pneumococcal
  purulent
  septic
  Bronchitis, acute or subacute:
  viral
  with tracheitis
  Croupous bronchitis
  Tracheobronchitis, acute
  EXCLUDES: acute bronchitis with chronic obstructive pulmonary disease (491.22)
  AHA: 4Q, '04, 137; 1Q, '04, 3; 4Q, '02, 46; 4Q, '96, 28; 4Q, '91, 24; 1Q, '88, 12
  DEF: Acute inflammation of main branches of bronchial tree due to infectious or irritant agents; symptoms include cough with a varied production of sputum, fever, substernal soreness, and lung rales.
- 466.1 Acute bronchiolitis
  Bronchiolitis (acute)   Capillary pneumonia
  DEF: Acute inflammation of finer subdivisions of bronchial tree due to infectious or irritant agents; symptoms include cough with a varied production of sputum, fever, substernal soreness, and lung rales.
  - 466.11 Acute bronchiolitis due to respiratory syncytial virus (RSV)
    AHA: 1Q, '05, 10; 4Q, '96, 27
  - 466.19 Acute bronchiolitis due to other infectious organisms
    Use additional code to identify organism

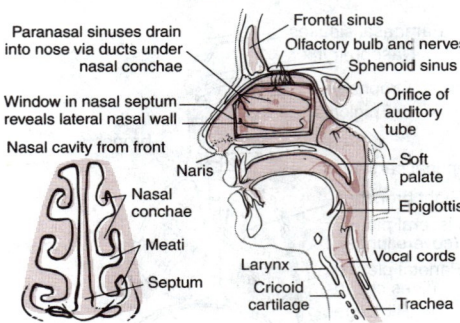

Upper Respiratory System

OTHER DISEASES OF THE UPPER RESPIRATORY TRACT (470-478)

470 Deviated nasal septum
Deflected septum (nasal) (acquired)
EXCLUDES: congenital (754.0)

471 Nasal polyps
EXCLUDES: adenomatous polyps (212.0)
- 471.0 Polyp of nasal cavity
  Polyp:
  choanal
  nasopharyngeal
- 471.1 Polypoid sinus degeneration
  Woakes' syndrome or ethmoiditis
- 471.8 Other polyp of sinus
  Polyp of sinus: Polyp of sinus:
  accessory   maxillary
  ethmoidal   sphenoidal
- 471.9 Unspecified nasal polyp
  Nasal polyp NOS

472 Chronic pharyngitis and nasopharyngitis
- 472.0 Chronic rhinitis
  Ozena   Rhinitis:
  Rhinitis: hypertrophic
  NOS   obstructive
  atrophic   purulent
  granulomatous   ulcerative
  EXCLUDES: allergic rhinitis (477.0-477.9)
  DEF: Persistent inflammation of mucous membranes of nose.
- 472.1 Chronic pharyngitis
  Chronic sore throat   Pharyngitis:
  Pharyngitis: granular (chronic)
  atrophic   hypertrophic
- 472.2 Chronic nasopharyngitis
  EXCLUDES: acute or unspecified nasopharyngitis (460)
  DEF: Persistent inflammation of mucous membranes extending from nares to pharynx.

Paranasal Sinuses

N Newborn Age: 0 | P Pediatric Age: 0-17 | M Maternity Age: 12-55 | A Adult Age: 15-124

138 — Volume 1   2007 ICD•9•CM

RESPIRATORY SYSTEM

✓4th 473 Chronic sinusitis
    INCLUDES: abscess, empyema, infection, suppuration (chronic) of sinus (accessory) (nasal)
    EXCLUDES: acute sinusitis (461.0-461.9)

- **473.0 Maxillary**
  Antritis (chronic)
- **473.1 Frontal**
- **473.2 Ethmoidal**
  EXCLUDES: Woakes' ethmoiditis (471.1)
- **473.3 Sphenoidal**
- **473.8 Other chronic sinusitis**
  Pansinusitis (chronic)
- **473.9 Unspecified sinusitis (chronic)**
  Sinusitis (chronic) NOS

✓4th 474 Chronic disease of tonsils and adenoids

- **✓5th 474.0 Chronic tonsillitis and adenoiditis**
  EXCLUDES: acute or unspecified tonsillitis (463)
  AHA: 4Q, '97, 38
  - 474.00 Chronic tonsillitis
  - 474.01 Chronic adenoiditis
  - 474.02 Chronic tonsillitis and adenoiditis
- **✓5th 474.1 Hypertrophy of tonsils and adenoids**
  Enlargement, Hyperplasia, Hypertrophy of tonsils or adenoids
  EXCLUDES: that with:
    adenoiditis (474.01)
    adenoiditis and tonsillitis (474.02)
    tonsillitis (474.00)
  - 474.10 Tonsils with adenoid
    AHA: 2Q, '05, 16
  - 474.11 Tonsils alone
  - 474.12 Adenoids alone
- **474.2 Adenoid vegetations**
  DEF: Fungus-like growth of lymph tissue between the nares and pharynx.
- **474.8 Other chronic disease of tonsils and adenoids**
  Amygdalolith   Tonsillar tag
  Calculus, tonsil   Ulcer, tonsil
  Cicatrix of tonsil (and adenoid)
- **474.9 Unspecified chronic disease of tonsils and adenoids**
  Disease (chronic) of tonsils (and adenoids)

475 Peritonsillar abscess
Abscess of tonsil   Quinsy
Peritonsillar cellulitis
EXCLUDES: tonsillitis:
  acute or NOS (463)
  chronic (474.0)

✓4th 476 Chronic laryngitis and laryngotracheitis
- **476.0 Chronic laryngitis**
  Laryngitis: catarrhal, hypertrophic
  Laryngitis: sicca
- **476.1 Chronic laryngotracheitis**
  Laryngitis, chronic, with tracheitis (chronic)
  Tracheitis, chronic, with laryngitis
  EXCLUDES: chronic tracheitis (491.8)
    laryngitis and tracheitis, acute or unspecified (464.00-464.51)

✓4th 477 Allergic rhinitis
  INCLUDES: allergic rhinitis (nonseasonal) (seasonal)
  hay fever
  spasmodic rhinorrhea
  EXCLUDES: allergic rhinitis with asthma (bronchial) (493.0)
DEF: True immunoglobulin E (IgE)-mediated allergic reaction of nasal mucosa; seasonal (typical hay fever) or perennial (year-round allergens: dust, food, dander).

- **477.0 Due to pollen**
  Pollinosis
- **477.1 Due to food**
  AHA: 4Q, '00, 42
- **477.2 Due to animal (cat) (dog) hair and dander**
- **477.8 Due to other allergen**
- **477.9 Cause unspecified**
  AHA: 2Q, '97, 9

✓4th 478 Other diseases of upper respiratory tract
- **478.0 Hypertrophy of nasal turbinates**
  DEF: Overgrowth, enlargement of shell-shaped bones, in nasal cavity.
- **✓5th 478.1 Other diseases of nasal cavity and sinuses**
  EXCLUDES: varicose ulcer of nasal septum (456.8)
  - 478.11 Nasal mucositis (ulcerative)
    Use additional E code to identify adverse effects of therapy, such as:
    antineoplastic and immunosuppressive drugs (E930.7, E933.1)
    radiation therapy (E879.2)
  - 478.19 Other diseases of nasal cavity and sinuses
    Abscess, Necrosis, Ulcer of nose (septum)
    Cyst or mucocele of sinus (nasal)
    Rhinolith
- **✓5th 478.2 Other diseases of pharynx, not elsewhere classified**
  - 478.20 Unspecified disease of pharynx
  - 478.21 Cellulitis of pharynx or nasopharynx
  - 478.22 Parapharyngeal abscess
  - 478.24 Retropharyngeal abscess
    DEF: Purulent infection, behind pharynx and front of precerebral fascia.
  - 478.25 Edema of pharynx or nasopharynx
  - 478.26 Cyst of pharynx or nasopharynx
  - 478.29 Other
    Abscess of pharynx or nasopharynx
    EXCLUDES: ulcerative pharyngitis (462)
- **✓5th 478.3 Paralysis of vocal cords or larynx**
  DEF: Loss of motor ability of vocal cords or larynx; due to nerve or muscle damage.
  - 478.30 Paralysis, unspecified
    Laryngoplegia   Paralysis of glottis
  - 478.31 Unilateral, partial
  - 478.32 Unilateral, complete
  - 478.33 Bilateral, partial
  - 478.34 Bilateral, complete
- **478.4 Polyp of vocal cord or larynx**
  EXCLUDES: adenomatous polyps (212.1)
- **478.5 Other diseases of vocal cords**
  Abscess, Cellulitis, Granuloma, Leukoplakia of vocal cords
  Chorditis (fibrinous) (nodosa) (tuberosa)
  Singers' nodes
- **478.6 Edema of larynx**
  Edema (of): glottis, subglottic
  Edema (of): supraglottic

RESPIRATORY SYSTEM

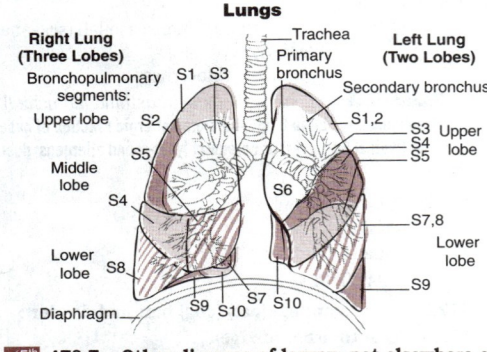

✓5th 478.7 Other diseases of larynx, not elsewhere classified
  - 478.70 Unspecified disease of larynx
  - 478.71 Cellulitis and perichondritis of larynx
    - DEF: Inflammation of deep soft tissues or lining of bone of the larynx.
  - 478.74 Stenosis of larynx
  - 478.75 Laryngeal spasm
    - Laryngismus (stridulus)
    - DEF: Involuntary muscle contraction of the larynx.
  - 478.79 Other
    - Abscess
    - Necrosis
    - Obstruction } of larynx
    - Pachyderma
    - Ulcer
    - EXCLUDES ulcerative laryngitis (464.00-464.01)
    - AHA: 3Q, '91, 20

478.8 Upper respiratory tract hypersensitivity reaction, site unspecified
  - EXCLUDES hypersensitivity reaction of lower respiratory tract, as:
    - extrinsic allergic alveolitis (495.0-495.9)
    - pneumoconiosis (500-505)

478.9 Other and unspecified diseases of upper respiratory tract
  - Abscess
  - Cicatrix } of trachea

PNEUMONIA AND INFLUENZA (480-487)
  - EXCLUDES pneumonia:
    - allergic or eosinophilic (518.3)
    - aspiration:
      - NOS (507.0)
      - newborn (770.18)
      - solids and liquids (507.0-507.8)
    - congenital (770.0)
    - lipoid (507.1)
    - passive (514)
    - rheumatic (390)

✓4th 480 Viral pneumonia
  - 480.0 Pneumonia due to adenovirus
  - 480.1 Pneumonia due to respiratory syncytial virus
    - AHA: 4Q, '96, 28; 1Q, '88, 12
  - 480.2 Pneumonia due to parainfluenza virus
  - 480.3 Pneumonia due to SARS-associated coronavirus
    - AHA: 4Q, '03, 46-47
    - DEF: A severe adult respiratory syndrome caused by the coronavirus, specified as inflammation of the lungs with consolidation.
  - 480.8 Pneumonia due to other virus not elsewhere classified
    - EXCLUDES congenital rubella pneumonitis (771.0)
      - influenza with pneumonia, any form (487.0)
      - pneumonia complicating viral diseases classified elsewhere (484.1-484.8)
  - 480.9 Viral pneumonia, unspecified
    - AHA: 3Q, '98, 5

481 Pneumococcal pneumonia [Streptococcus pneumoniae pneumonia]
  - Lobar pneumonia, organism unspecified
  - AHA: 2Q, '98, 7; 4Q, '92, 19; 1Q, '92, 18; 1Q, '91, 13; 1Q, '88, 13; M-A, '85, 6

✓4th 482 Other bacterial pneumonia
  - AHA: 4Q, '93, 39
  - 482.0 Pneumonia due to Klebsiella pneumoniae
  - 482.1 Pneumonia due to Pseudomonas
  - 482.2 Pneumonia due to Hemophilus influenzae [H. influenzae]
    - AHA: ▶2Q, '05, 19◀
  - ✓5th 482.3 Pneumonia due to Streptococcus
    - EXCLUDES Streptococcus pneumoniae (481)
    - AHA: 1Q, '88, 13
    - 482.30 Streptococcus, unspecified
    - 482.31 Group A
    - 482.32 Group B
    - 482.39 Other Streptococcus
  - ✓5th 482.4 Pneumonia due to Staphylococcus
    - AHA: 3Q, '91, 16
    - 482.40 Pneumonia due to Staphylococcus, unspecified
    - 482.41 Pneumonia due to Staphylococcus aureus
    - 482.49 Other Staphylococcus pneumonia
  - ✓5th 482.8 Pneumonia due to other specified bacteria
    - EXCLUDES pneumonia, complicating infectious disease classified elsewhere (484.1-484.8)
    - AHA: 3Q, '88, 11
    - 482.81 Anaerobes
      - Bacteroides (melaninogenicus)
      - Gram-negative anaerobes
    - 482.82 Escherichia coli [E. coli]
    - 482.83 Other gram-negative bacteria
      - Gram-negative pneumonia NOS
      - Proteus
      - Serratia marcescens
      - EXCLUDES gram-negative anaerobes (482.81)
        - Legionnaires' disease (482.84)
      - AHA: 2Q, '98, 5; 3Q, '94, 9
    - 482.84 Legionnaires' disease
      - AHA: 4Q, '97, 38
      - DEF: Severe and often fatal infection by *Legionella pneumophilia*; symptoms include high fever, gastrointestinal pain, headache, myalgia, dry cough, and pneumonia; transmitted airborne via air conditioning systems, humidifiers, water faucets, shower heads; not person-to-person contact.
    - 482.89 Other specified bacteria
      - AHA: 2Q, '97, 6
  - 482.9 Bacterial pneumonia unspecified
    - AHA: 2Q, '98, 6; 2Q, '97, 6; 1Q, '94, 17

N Newborn Age: 0 **P** Pediatric Age: 0-17 **M** Maternity Age: 12-55 **A** Adult Age: 15-124

RESPIRATORY SYSTEM

✓4th **483 Pneumonia due to other specified organism**
AHA: N-D, '87, 5

483.0 Mycoplasma pneumoniae
Eaton's agent
Pleuropneumonia-like organism [PPLO]

483.1 Chlamydia
AHA: 4Q, '96, 31

483.8 Other specified organism

✓4th **484 Pneumonia in infectious diseases classified elsewhere**
EXCLUDES influenza with pneumonia, any form (487.0)

484.1 Pneumonia in cytomegalic inclusion disease
Code first underlying disease, as (078.5)

484.3 Pneumonia in whooping cough
Code first underlying disease, as (033.0-033.9)

484.5 Pneumonia in anthrax
Code first underlying disease (022.1)

484.6 Pneumonia in aspergillosis
Code first underlying disease (117.3)
AHA: 4Q, '97, 40

484.7 Pneumonia in other systemic mycoses
Code first underlying disease
EXCLUDES pneumonia in:
candidiasis (112.4)
coccidioidomycosis (114.0)
histoplasmosis (115.0-115.9 with fifth-digit 5)

484.8 Pneumonia in other infectious diseases classified elsewhere
Code first underlying disease, as:
Q fever (083.0)
typhoid fever (002.0)
EXCLUDES pneumonia in:
actinomycosis (039.1)
measles (055.1)
nocardiosis (039.1)
ornithosis (073.0)
Pneumocystis carinii (136.3)
salmonellosis (003.22)
toxoplasmosis (130.4)
tuberculosis (011.6)
tularemia (021.2)
varicella (052.1)

485 Bronchopneumonia, organism unspecified
Bronchopneumonia: Pneumonia:
 hemorrhagic   lobular
 terminal   segmental
Pleurobronchopneumonia
EXCLUDES bronchiolitis (acute) (466.11-466.19)
chronic (491.8)
lipoid pneumonia (507.1)

486 Pneumonia, organism unspecified
EXCLUDES hypostatic or passive pneumonia (514)
influenza with pneumonia, any form (487.0)
inhalation or aspiration pneumonia due to foreign materials (507.0-507.8)
pneumonitis due to fumes and vapors (506.0)
AHA: 4Q, '99, 6; 3Q, '99, 9; 3Q, '98, 7; 2Q, '98, 4, 5; 1Q, '98, 8; 3Q, '97, 9; 3Q, '94, 10; 3Q, '88, 11

✓4th **487 Influenza**
EXCLUDES Hemophilus influenzae [H. influenzae]:
infection NOS (041.5)
laryngitis (464.00-464.01)
meningitis (320.0)

487.0 With pneumonia
Influenza with pneumonia, any form
Influenzal:
 bronchopneumonia
 pneumonia
Use additional code to identify the type of pneumonia (480.0-480.9, 481, 482.0-482.9, 483.0-483.8, 485)

487.1 With other respiratory manifestations
Influenza NOS   Influenzal:
Influenzal: pharyngitis
 laryngitis   respiratory infection
                          (upper) (acute)
AHA: ▶2Q, '05, 18;◀ 4Q, '99, 26

487.8 With other manifestations
Encephalopathy due to influenza
Influenza with involvement of gastrointestinal tract
EXCLUDES "intestinal flu" [viral gastroenteritis] (008.8)

CHRONIC OBSTRUCTIVE PULMONARY DISEASE AND ALLIED CONDITIONS (490-496)
AHA: 3Q, '88, 5

490 Bronchitis, not specified as acute or chronic
Bronchitis NOS:
 catarrhal
 with tracheitis NOS
Tracheobronchitis NOS
EXCLUDES bronchitis:
allergic NOS (493.9)
asthmatic NOS (493.9)
due to fumes and vapors (506.0)

✓4th **491 Chronic bronchitis**
EXCLUDES chronic obstructive asthma (493.2)

491.0 Simple chronic bronchitis
Catarrhal bronchitis, chronic
Smokers' cough

491.1 Mucopurulent chronic bronchitis
Bronchitis (chronic) (recurrent):
 fetid
 mucopurulent
 purulent
AHA: 3Q, '88, 12

DEF: Chronic bronchial infection characterized by both mucus and pus secretions in the bronchial tree; recurs after asymptomatic periods; signs are coughing, expectoration and secondary changes in the lung.

✓5th **491.2 Obstructive chronic bronchitis**
Bronchitis:
 emphysematous
 obstructive (chronic) (diffuse)
Bronchitis with:
 chronic airway obstruction
 emphysema
EXCLUDES asthmatic bronchitis (acute) NOS (493.9)
chronic obstructive asthma (493.2)
AHA: 3Q, '97, 9; 4Q, '91, 25; 2Q, '91, 21

491.20 Without exacerbation
Emphysema with chronic bronchitis
AHA: 3Q, '97, 9

RESPIRATORY SYSTEM

Interrelationship Between Chronic Airway Obstruction, Chronic Bronchitis and Emphysema

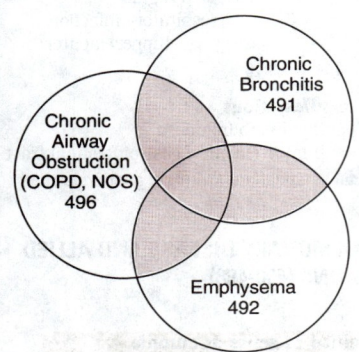

Shaded area: Obstructive Chronic Bronchitis (Chronic Bronchitis with COPD) 491.20-491.21

491.21 With (acute) exacerbation
Acute exacerbation of chronic obstructive pulmonary disease [COPD]
Decompensated chronic obstructive pulmonary disease [COPD]
Decompensated chronic obstructive pulmonary disease [COPD] with exacerbation
EXCLUDES chronic obstructive asthma with acute exacerbation (493.22)
AHA: 1Q, '04, 3; 3Q, '02, 18, 19; 4Q, '01, 43; 2Q, '96, 10

491.22 With acute bronchitis
AHA: 4Q, '04, 82

491.8 Other chronic bronchitis
Chronic: Chronic:
  tracheitis   tracheobronchitis

491.9 Unspecified chronic bronchitis

☑4th **492 Emphysema**
AHA: 2Q, '91, 21

492.0 Emphysematous bleb
Giant bullous emphysema
Ruptured emphysematous bleb
Tension pneumatocele
Vanishing lung
AHA: 2Q, '93, 3

DEF: Formation of vesicle or bulla in emphysematous lung, more than one millimeter; contains serum or blood.

492.8 Other emphysema
Emphysema (lung or pulmonary):
  NOS
  centriacinar
  centrilobular
  obstructive
  panacinar
  panlobular
Emphysema (lung or pulmonary):
  unilateral
  vesicular
  MacLeod's syndrome
  Swyer-James syndrome
  Unilateral hyperlucent lung
EXCLUDES emphysema:
  with chronic bronchitis (491.20-491.22)
  compensatory (518.2)
  due to fumes and vapors (506.4)
  interstitial (518.1)
    newborn (770.2)
  mediastinal (518.1)
  surgical (subcutaneous) (998.81)
  traumatic (958.7)
AHA: 1Q, '05, 4; 4Q, '93, 41; J-A, '84, 17

☑4th **493 Asthma**
EXCLUDES wheezing NOS (786.07)
The following fifth-digit subclassification is for use with codes 493.0-493.2, 493.9:
  0 unspecified
  1 with status asthmaticus
  2 with (acute) exacerbation

AHA: 4Q, '04, 137; 4Q, '03, 62; 4Q, '01, 43; 4Q, '00, 42; 1Q, '91, 13; 3Q, '88, 9; J-A, '85, 8; N-D, '84, 17

DEF: Status asthmaticus: Severe, intractable episode of asthma unresponsive to normal therapeutic measures.

☑5th **493.0 Extrinsic asthma**
Asthma: Asthma:
  allergic with   hay
    stated cause   platinum
  atopic   Hay fever with asthma
  childhood
EXCLUDES asthma:
  allergic NOS (493.9)
  detergent (507.8)
  miners' (500)
  wood (495.8)

DEF: Transient stricture of airway diameters of bronchi; due to environmental factor; also called allergic (bronchial) asthma.

☑5th **493.1 Intrinsic asthma**
Late-onset asthma
AHA: 3Q, '88, 9; M-A, '85, 7

DEF: Transient stricture, of airway diameters of bronchi; due to pathophysiological disturbances.

☑5th **493.2 Chronic obstructive asthma**
Asthma with chronic obstructive pulmonary disease [COPD]
Chronic asthmatic bronchitis
EXCLUDES acute bronchitis (466.0)
chronic obstructive bronchitis (491.20-491.22)
AHA: 4Q, '03, 108; 2Q, '91, 21; 2Q, '90, 20

DEF: Persistent narrowing of airway diameters in the bronchial tree, restricting airflow and causing constant labored breathing.

☑5th **493.8 Other forms of asthma**
AHA: 4Q, '03, 62

493.81 Exercise induced bronchospasm
493.82 Cough variant asthma

☑5th **493.9 Asthma, unspecified**
Asthma (bronchial) (allergic NOS)
Bronchitis:
  allergic
  asthmatic
AHA: 4Q, '97, 40; For code 493.90: 4Q, '04, 137; 4Q, '03, 108; 4Q, '99, 25; 1Q, '97, 7; For code 493.91: 1Q, '05, 5; For code 493.92: 1Q, '03, 9

☑4th **494 Bronchiectasis**
Bronchiectasis (fusiform) (postinfectious) (recurrent)
Bronchiolectasis
EXCLUDES congenital (748.61)
tuberculous bronchiectasis (current disease) (011.5)
AHA: 4Q, '00, 42

DEF: Dilation of bronchi; due to infection or chronic conditions; causes decreased lung capacity and recurrent infections of lungs.

494.0 Bronchiectasis without acute exacerbation
494.1 Bronchiectasis with acute exacerbation

RESPIRATORY SYSTEM

√4th 495 Extrinsic allergic alveolitis
  INCLUDES: allergic alveolitis and pneumonitis due to inhaled organic dust particles of fungal, thermophilic actinomycete, or other origin
  DEF: Pneumonitis due to particles inhaled into lung, often at workplace; symptoms include cough, chills, fever, increased heart and respiratory rates; develops within hours of exposure.

  495.0 Farmers' lung
  495.1 Bagassosis
  495.2 Bird-fanciers' lung
      Budgerigar-fanciers' disease or lung
      Pigeon-fanciers' disease or lung
  495.3 Suberosis
      Cork-handlers' disease or lung
  495.4 Malt workers' lung
      Alveolitis due to Aspergillus clavatus
  495.5 Mushroom workers' lung
  495.6 Maple bark-strippers' lung
      Alveolitis due to Cryptostroma corticale
  495.7 "Ventilation" pneumonitis
      Allergic alveolitis due to fungal, thermophilic actinomycete, and other organisms growing in ventilation [air conditioning] systems
  495.8 **Other specified allergic alveolitis and pneumonitis**
      Cheese-washers' lung
      Coffee workers' lung
      Fish-meal workers' lung
      Furriers' lung
      Grain-handlers' disease or lung
      Pituitary snuff-takers' disease
      Sequoiosis or red-cedar asthma
      Wood asthma
  495.9 **Unspecified allergic alveolitis and pneumonitis**
      Alveolitis, allergic (extrinsic)
      Hypersensitivity pneumonitis

496 Chronic airway obstruction, not elsewhere classified
  Note: This code is not to be used with any code from categories 491-493
  Chronic:
    nonspecific lung disease
    obstructive lung disease
    obstructive pulmonary disease [COPD] NOS
  EXCLUDES: chronic obstructive lung disease [COPD] specified (as) (with):
    allergic alveolitis (495.0-495.9)
    asthma (493.20-493.22)
    bronchiectasis (494.0-494.1)
    bronchitis (491.20-491.22)
      with emphysema (491.20-491.22)
      ▶decompensated (491.21)◀
    emphysema (492.0-492.8)
  AHA: 4Q, '03, 109; 2Q, '00, 15; 2Q, '92, 16; 2Q, '91, 21; 3Q, '88, 56

PNEUMOCONIOSES AND OTHER LUNG DISEASES DUE TO EXTERNAL AGENTS (500-508)

DEF: Permanent deposits of particulate matter, within lungs; due to occupational or environmental exposure; results in chronic induration and fibrosis. (See specific listings in 500-508 code range)

500 Coal workers' pneumoconiosis A
    Anthracosilicosis   Coal workers' lung
    Anthracosis   Miner's asthma
    Black lung disease

501 Asbestosis A

502 Pneumoconiosis due to other silica or silicates
    Pneumoconiosis due to talc
    Silicotic fibrosis (massive) of lung
    Silicosis (simple) (complicated)

503 Pneumoconiosis due to other inorganic dust
    Aluminosis (of lung)   Graphite fibrosis (of lung)
    Baritosis   Siderosis
    Bauxite fibrosis (of lung) Stannosis
    Berylliosis

504 Pneumonopathy due to inhalation of other dust
    Byssinosis   Flax-dressers' disease
    Cannabinosis
    EXCLUDES: allergic alveolitis (495.0-495.9)
      asbestosis (501)
      bagassosis (495.1)
      farmers' lung (495.0)

505 Pneumoconiosis, unspecified

√4th 506 Respiratory conditions due to chemical fumes and vapors
  Use additional E code to identify cause

  506.0 **Bronchitis and pneumonitis due to fumes and vapors**
      Chemical bronchitis (acute)
  506.1 **Acute pulmonary edema due to fumes and vapors**
      Chemical pulmonary edema (acute)
      EXCLUDES: acute pulmonary edema NOS (518.4)
        chronic or unspecified pulmonary edema (514)
      AHA: 3Q, '88, 4
  506.2 **Upper respiratory inflammation due to fumes and vapors**
      AHA: 3Q, '05, 10
  506.3 **Other acute and subacute respiratory conditions due to fumes and vapors**
  506.4 **Chronic respiratory conditions due to fumes and vapors**
      Emphysema (diffuse) (chronic) ⎫
      Obliterative bronchiolitis (chronic) (subacute) ⎬ due to inhalation of chemical fumes and vapors
      Pulmonary fibrosis (chronic) ⎭
  506.9 **Unspecified respiratory conditions due to fumes and vapors**
      Silo-fillers' disease

√4th 507 Pneumonitis due to solids and liquids
  EXCLUDES: fetal aspiration pneumonitis (770.18)
  AHA: 3Q, '91, 16

  507.0 **Due to inhalation of food or vomitus**
      Aspiration pneumonia (due to):   Aspiration pneumonia (due to):
        NOS   milk
        food (regurgitated)   saliva
        gastric secretions   vomitus
      AHA: 1Q, '89, 10
  507.1 **Due to inhalation of oils and essences**
      Lipoid pneumonia (exogenous)
      EXCLUDES: endogenous lipoid pneumonia (516.8)
  507.8 **Due to other solids and liquids**
      Detergent asthma

√4th 508 Respiratory conditions due to other and unspecified external agents
  Use additional E code to identify cause

  508.0 **Acute pulmonary manifestations due to radiation**
      Radiation pneumonitis
      AHA: 2Q, '88, 4
  508.1 **Chronic and other pulmonary manifestations due to radiation**
      Fibrosis of lung following radiation
  508.8 **Respiratory conditions due to other specified external agents**
  508.9 **Respiratory conditions due to unspecified external agent**

OTHER DISEASES OF RESPIRATORY SYSTEM (510-519)

√4th 510 Empyema
  Use additional code to identify infectious organism (041.0-041.9)
  EXCLUDES: abscess of lung (513.0)
  DEF: Purulent infection, within pleural space.

RESPIRATORY SYSTEM

510.0 With fistula
Fistula:
- bronchocutaneous
- bronchopleural
- hepatopleural

Fistula:
- mediastinal
- pleural
- thoracic

Any condition classifiable to 510.9 with fistula

DEF: Purulent infection of respiratory cavity; with communication from cavity to another structure.

510.9 Without mention of fistula
Abscess:
- pleura
- thorax

Empyema (chest) (lung) (pleura)

Fibrinopurulent pleurisy

Pleurisy:
- purulent

Pleurisy:
- septic
- seropurulent
- suppurative

Pyopneumothorax

Pyothorax

AHA: 3Q, '94, 6

✓4th 511 Pleurisy

EXCLUDES malignant pleural effusion (197.2)
pleurisy with mention of tuberculosis, current disease (012.0)

DEF: Inflammation of serous membrane of lungs and lining of thoracic cavity; causes exudation in cavity or membrane surface.

511.0 Without mention of effusion or current tuberculosis
- Adhesion, lung or pleura
- Calcification of pleura
- Pleurisy (acute) (sterile):
  - diaphragmatic
  - fibrinous
  - interlobar

Pleurisy:
- NOS
- pneumococcal
- staphylococcal
- streptococcal

Thickening of pleura

AHA: 3Q, '94, 5

511.1 With effusion, with mention of a bacterial cause other than tuberculosis
Pleurisy with effusion (exudative) (serous):
- pneumococcal
- staphylococcal
- streptococcal
- other specified nontuberculous bacterial cause

511.8 Other specified forms of effusion, except tuberculous
- Encysted pleurisy
- Hemopneumothorax
- Hemothorax
- Hydropneumothorax
- Hydrothorax

EXCLUDES traumatic (860.2-860.5, 862.29, 862.39)

AHA: 1Q, '97, 10

511.9 Unspecified pleural effusion
- Pleural effusion NOS
- Pleurisy:
  - exudative
  - serofibrinous

Pleurisy:
- serous
- with effusion NOS

AHA: 2Q, '03, 7; 3Q, '91, 19; 4Q, '89, 11

✓4th 512 Pneumothorax

DEF: Collapsed lung; due to gas or air in pleural space.

512.0 Spontaneous tension pneumothorax
AHA: 3Q, '94, 5
DEF: Leaking air from lung into lining causing collapse.

512.1 Iatrogenic pneumothorax
Postoperative pneumothorax
AHA: 4Q, '94, 40
DEF: Air trapped in the lining of the lung following surgery.

512.8 Other spontaneous pneumothorax
Pneumothorax:
- NOS
- acute

Pneumothorax:
- chronic

EXCLUDES pneumothorax:
congenital (770.2)
traumatic (860.0-860.1, 860.4-860.5)
tuberculous, current disease (011.7)

AHA: 2Q, '93, 3

✓4th 513 Abscess of lung and mediastinum

513.0 Abscess of lung
- Abscess (multiple) of lung
- Gangrenous or necrotic pneumonia
- Pulmonary gangrene or necrosis

AHA: 2Q, '98, 7

513.1 Abscess of mediastinum

514 Pulmonary congestion and hypostasis
Hypostatic:
- bronchopneumonia
- pneumonia

Passive pneumonia
Pulmonary congestion (chronic) (passive)

Pulmonary edema:
- NOS
- chronic

EXCLUDES acute pulmonary edema:
NOS (518.4)
with mention of heart disease or failure (428.1)
▶hypostatic pneumonia due to or specified as a specific type of pneumonia—code to the type of pneumonia (480.0-480.9, 481, 482.0-482.49, 483.0-483.8, 485, 486, 487.0)◀

AHA: 2Q, '98, 6; 3Q, '88, 5

DEF: Excessive retention of interstitial fluid in the lungs and pulmonary vessels; due to poor circulation.

515 Postinflammatory pulmonary fibrosis
- Cirrhosis of lung
- Fibrosis of lung (atrophic) (confluent) (massive) (perialveolar) (peribronchial) } chronic or unspecified
- Induration of lung

DEF: Fibrosis and scarring of the lungs due to inflammatory reaction.

✓4th 516 Other alveolar and parietoalveolar pneumonopathy

516.0 Pulmonary alveolar proteinosis
DEF: Reduced ventilation; due to proteinaceous deposits on alveoli; symptoms include dyspnea, cough, chest pain, weakness, weight loss, and hemoptysis.

516.1 Idiopathic pulmonary hemosiderosis
Essential brown induration of lung
Code first underlying disease (275.0)
DEF: Fibrosis of alveolar walls; marked by abnormal amounts hemosiderin in lungs; primarily affects children; symptoms include anemia, fluid in lungs, and blood in sputum; etiology unknown.

516.2 Pulmonary alveolar microlithiasis
DEF: Small calculi in pulmonary alveoli resembling sand-like particles on x-ray.

516.3 Idiopathic fibrosing alveolitis
- Alveolar capillary block
- Diffuse (idiopathic) (interstitial) pulmonary fibrosis
- Hamman-Rich syndrome

516.8 Other specified alveolar and parietoalveolar pneumonopathies
- Endogenous lipoid pneumonia
- Interstitial pneumonia (desquamative) (lymphoid)

EXCLUDES lipoid pneumonia, exogenous or unspecified (507.1)

AHA: 1Q, '92, 12

516.9 Unspecified alveolar and parietoalveolar pneumonopathy

N Newborn Age: 0   **P** Pediatric Age: 0-17   **M** Maternity Age: 12-55   **A** Adult Age: 15-124

RESPIRATORY SYSTEM

517 Lung involvement in conditions classified elsewhere
EXCLUDES rheumatoid lung (714.81)

517.1 Rheumatic pneumonia
Code first underlying disease (390)

517.2 Lung involvement in systemic sclerosis
Code first underlying disease (710.1)

517.3 Acute chest syndrome
Code first sickle-cell disease in crisis (282.42, 282.62, 282.64, 282.69)
AHA: 4Q, '03, 51, 56

517.8 Lung involvement in other diseases classified elsewhere
Code first underlying disease, as:
  amyloidosis ▶(277.30-277.39)◀
  polymyositis (710.4)
  sarcoidosis (135)
  Sjögren's disease (710.2)
  systemic lupus erythematosus (710.0)
EXCLUDES syphilis (095.1)
AHA: 2Q, '03, 7

518 Other diseases of lung

518.0 Pulmonary collapse
Atelectasis   Middle lobe syndrome
Collapse of lung
EXCLUDES atelectasis:
  congenital (partial) (770.5)
  primary (770.4)
  tuberculous, current disease (011.8)
AHA: 4Q, '90, 25

518.1 Interstitial emphysema
Mediastinal emphysema
EXCLUDES surgical (subcutaneous) emphysema (998.81)
  that in fetus or newborn (770.2)
  traumatic emphysema (958.7)
DEF: Escaped air from the alveoli trapped in the interstices of the lung; trauma or cough may cause the disease.

518.2 Compensatory emphysema
DEF: Distention of all or part of the lung caused by disease processes or surgical intervention that decreased volume in another part of the lung; overcompensation reaction to the loss of capacity in another part of the lung.

518.3 Pulmonary eosinophilia
Eosinophilic asthma   Pneumonia:
Löffler's syndrome   eosinophilic
Pneumonia: Tropical eosinophilia
  allergic
DEF: Infiltration, into pulmonary parenchyma of eosinophilia; results in cough, fever, and dyspnea.

518.4 Acute edema of lung, unspecified
Acute pulmonary edema NOS
Pulmonary edema, postoperative
EXCLUDES pulmonary edema:
  acute, with mention of heart disease or failure (428.1)
  chronic or unspecified (514)
  due to external agents (506.0-508.9)
DEF: Severe, sudden fluid retention within lung tissues.

518.5 Pulmonary insufficiency following trauma and surgery
Adult respiratory distress syndrome
Pulmonary insufficiency following:
  shock
  surgery
  trauma
Shock lung
EXCLUDES adult respiratory distress syndrome associated with other conditions (518.82)
  pneumonia:
    aspiration (507.0)
    hypostatic (514)
  respiratory failure in other conditions (518.81, 518.83-518.84)
AHA: 4Q, '04, 139; 3Q, '88, 3; 3Q, '88, 7; S-O, '87, 1

518.6 Allergic bronchopulmonary aspergillosis
AHA: 4Q, '97, 39
DEF: Noninvasive hypersensitive reaction; due to allergic reaction to *Aspergillus fumigatus* (mold).

518.7 Transfusion related acute lung injury [TRALI]

518.8 Other diseases of lung

518.81 Acute respiratory failure
Respiratory failure NOS
EXCLUDES acute and chronic respiratory failure (518.84)
  acute respiratory distress (518.82)
  chronic respiratory failure (518.83)
  respiratory arrest (799.1)
  respiratory failure, newborn (770.84)
AHA: 4Q, '05, 96; 2Q, '05, 19; 1Q, '05, 3-8; 4Q, '04, 139; 1Q, '03, 15; 4Q, '98, 41; 3Q, '91, 14; 2Q, '91, 3; 4Q, '90, 25; 2Q, '90, 20; 3Q, '88, 7; 3Q, '88, 10; S-O, '87, 1

518.82 Other pulmonary insufficiency, not elsewhere classified
Acute respiratory distress
Acute respiratory insufficiency
Adult respiratory distress syndrome NEC
EXCLUDES adult respiratory distress syndrome associated with trauma and surgery (518.5)
  pulmonary insufficiency following trauma and surgery (518.5)
  respiratory distress:
    NOS (786.09)
    newborn (770.89)
    syndrome, newborn (769)
  shock lung (518.5)
AHA: 4Q, '03, 105; 2Q, '91, 21; 3Q, '88, 7

518.83 Chronic respiratory failure
AHA: 4Q, '05, 96; 4Q, '03, 103, 111

518.84 Acute and chronic respiratory failure
Acute on chronic respiratory failure

518.89 Other diseases of lung, not elsewhere classified
Broncholithiasis   Lung disease NOS
Calcification of lung   Pulmolithiasis
AHA: 3Q, '90, 18; 4Q, '88, 6

DEF: Broncholithiasis: calculi in lumen of transbronchial tree.

DEF: Pulmolithiasis: calculi in lung.

RESPIRATORY SYSTEM

√4th 519 Other diseases of respiratory system

√5th 519.0 Tracheostomy complications

519.00 Tracheostomy complication, unspecified

519.01 Infection of tracheostomy
Use additional code to identify type of infection, such as:
abscess or cellulitis of neck (682.1)
septicemia (038.0-038.9)
Use additional code to identify organism (041.00-041.9)

AHA: 4Q, '98, 41

519.02 Mechanical complication of tracheostomy
Tracheal stenosis due to tracheostomy

519.09 Other tracheostomy complications
Hemorrhage due to tracheostomy
Tracheoesophageal fistula due to tracheostomy

√5th 519.1 Other diseases of trachea and bronchus, not elsewhere classified

AHA: 3Q, '02, 18; 3Q, '88, 6

- **519.11 Acute bronchospasm**
Bronchospasm NOS
  EXCLUDES *acute bronchitis with bronchospasm (466.0)*
  asthma (493.00-493.92)
  exercise induced bronchospasm (493.81)

- **519.19 Other diseases of trachea and bronchus**
Calcification
Stenosis   } of bronchus or trachea
Ulcer

519.2 Mediastinitis
DEF: Inflammation of tissue between organs behind sternum.

519.3 Other diseases of mediastinum, not elsewhere classified
Fibrosis
Hernia   } of mediastinum
Retraction

519.4 Disorders of diaphragm
Diaphragmitis   Relaxation of diaphragm
Paralysis of diaphragm
  EXCLUDES *congenital defect of diaphragm (756.6)*
  diaphragmatic hernia (551-553 with .3)
  congenital (756.6)

519.8 Other diseases of respiratory system, not elsewhere classified
AHA: 4Q, '89, 12

519.9 Unspecified disease of respiratory system
Respiratory disease (chronic) NOS

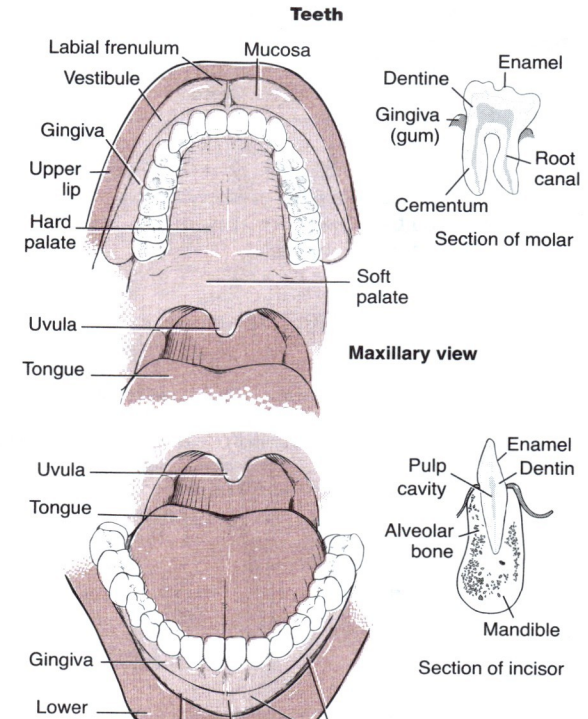

9. DISEASES OF THE DIGESTIVE SYSTEM (520-579)

DISEASES OF ORAL CAVITY, SALIVARY GLANDS, AND JAWS (520-529)

✓4th 520 Disorders of tooth development and eruption

520.0 Anodontia
Absence of teeth (complete) (congenital) (partial)
Hypodontia
Oligodontia
EXCLUDES: acquired absence of teeth (525.10-525.19)

520.1 Supernumerary teeth
Distomolar   Paramolar
Fourth molar   Supplemental teeth
Mesiodens
EXCLUDES: supernumerary roots (520.2)

520.2 Abnormalities of size and form
Concrescence ⎫
Fusion   ⎬ of teeth
Gemination   ⎭

Dens evaginatus   Microdontia
Dens in dente   Peg-shaped [conical] teeth
Dens invaginatus   Supernumerary roots
Enamel pearls   Taurodontism
Macrodontia   Tuberculum paramolare
EXCLUDES: that due to congenital syphilis (090.5)
tuberculum Carabelli, which is regarded as a normal variation

520.3 Mottled teeth
Dental fluorosis
Mottling of enamel
Nonfluoride enamel opacities

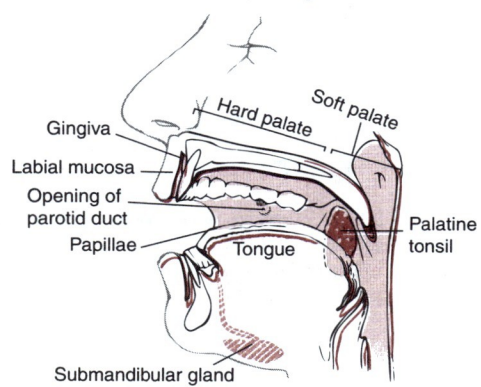

520.4 Disturbances of tooth formation
Aplasia and hypoplasia of cementum
Dilaceration of tooth
Enamel hypoplasia (neonatal) (postnatal) (prenatal)
Horner's teeth
Hypocalcification of teeth
Regional odontodysplasia
Turner's tooth
EXCLUDES: Hutchinson's teeth and mulberry molars in congenital syphilis (090.5)
mottled teeth (520.3)

520.5 Hereditary disturbances in tooth structure, not elsewhere classified
Amelogenesis   ⎫
Dentinogenesis ⎬ imperfecta
Odontogenesis ⎭

Dentinal dysplasia   Shell teeth

520.6 Disturbances in tooth eruption
Teeth: Tooth eruption:
  embedded   late
  impacted   obstructed
  natal   premature
  neonatal
  ▶prenatal◀
  primary [deciduous]:
    persistent
    shedding, premature
EXCLUDES: exfoliation of teeth (attributable to disease of surrounding tissues) (525.0-525.19)

AHA: 2Q, '05, 15

520.7 Teething syndrome

520.8 Other specified disorders of tooth development and eruption
Color changes during tooth formation
Pre-eruptive color changes
EXCLUDES: posteruptive color changes (521.7)

520.9 Unspecified disorder of tooth development and eruption

DIGESTIVE SYSTEM

521 Diseases of hard tissues of teeth [4th]

521.0 Dental caries [5th]
AHA: 4Q, '01, 44

- **521.00** Dental caries, unspecified
- **521.01** Dental caries limited to enamel
  - Initial caries
  - White spot lesion
- **521.02** Dental caries extending into dentine
- **521.03** Dental caries extending into pulp
- **521.04** Arrested dental caries
- **521.05** Odontoclasia
  - Infantile melanodontia
  - Melanodontoclasia
  - EXCLUDES: internal and external resorption of teeth (521.40-521.49)
  - DEF: A pathological dental condition described as stained areas, loss of tooth substance, and hypoplasia linked to nutritional deficiencies during tooth development and to cariogenic oral conditions; synonyms are melanodontoclasia and infantile melanodontia.
- **521.06** Dental caries pit and fissure
  - ▶Primary dental caries, pit and fissure origin◀
- **521.07** Dental caries of smooth surface
  - ▶Primary dental caries, smooth surface origin◀
- **521.08** Dental caries of root surface
  - ▶Primary dental caries, root surface◀
- **521.09** Other dental caries
  - AHA: 3Q, '02, 14

521.1 Excessive attrition (approximal wear) (occlusal wear) [5th]
- **521.10** Excessive attrition, unspecified
- **521.11** Excessive attrition, limited to enamel
- **521.12** Excessive attrition, extending into dentine
- **521.13** Excessive attrition, extending into pulp
- **521.14** Excessive attrition, localized
- **521.15** Excessive attrition, generalized

521.2 Abrasion [5th]
Abrasion:
- dentifrice
- habitual
- occupational   } of teeth
- ritual
- traditional
- Wedge defect NOS

- **521.20** Abrasion, unspecified
- **521.21** Abrasion, limited to enamel
- **521.22** Abrasion, extending into dentine
- **521.23** Abrasion, extending into pulp
- **521.24** Abrasion, localized
- **521.25** Abrasion, generalized

521.3 Erosion [5th]
Erosion of teeth:
- NOS
- due to:
  - medicine
  - persistent vomiting

Erosion of teeth:
- idiopathic
- occupational

- **521.30** Erosion, unspecified
- **521.31** Erosion, limited to enamel
- **521.32** Erosion, extending into dentine
- **521.33** Erosion, extending into pulp
- **521.34** Erosion, localized
- **521.35** Erosion, generalized

521.4 Pathological resorption [5th]
DEF: Loss of dentin and cementum due to disease process.

- **521.40** Pathological resorption, unspecified
- **521.41** Pathological resorption, internal
- **521.42** Pathological resorption, external
- **521.49** Other pathological resorption
  - Internal granuloma of pulp

521.5 Hypercementosis
Cementation hyperplasia
DEF: Excess deposits of cementum, on tooth root.

521.6 Ankylosis of teeth
DEF: Adhesion of tooth to surrounding bone.

521.7 Intrinsic posteruptive color changes
Staining [discoloration] of teeth:
- NOS
- due to:
  - drugs
  - metals
  - pulpal bleeding

EXCLUDES: accretions [deposits] on teeth (523.6)
extrinsic color changes (523.6)
pre-eruptive color changes (520.8)

521.8 Other specified diseases of hard tissues of teeth [5th]
- **521.81** Cracked tooth
  - EXCLUDES: asymptomatic craze lines in enamel—omit code
  - broken tooth due to trauma (873.63, 873.73)
  - fractured tooth due to trauma (873.63, 873.73)
- **521.89** Other specified diseases of hard tissues of teeth
  - Irradiated enamel
  - Sensitive dentin

521.9 Unspecified disease of hard tissues of teeth

522 Diseases of pulp and periapical tissues [4th]

522.0 Pulpitis
Pulpal:
- abscess
- polyp

Pulpitis:
- acute
- chronic (hyperplastic) (ulcerative)
- suppurative

522.1 Necrosis of the pulp
Pulp gangrene
DEF: Death of pulp tissue.

522.2 Pulp degeneration
Denticles
Pulp calcifications
Pulp stones

522.3 Abnormal hard tissue formation in pulp
Secondary or irregular dentin

522.4 Acute apical periodontitis of pulpal origin
DEF: Severe inflammation of periodontal ligament due to pulpal inflammation or necrosis.

522.5 Periapical abscess without sinus
Abscess:
- dental
- dentoalveolar

EXCLUDES: periapical abscess with sinus (522.7)

522.6 Chronic apical periodontitis
Apical or periapical granuloma
Apical periodontitis NOS

522.7 Periapical abscess with sinus
Fistula:
- alveolar process
- dental

522.8 Radicular cyst
Cyst:
- apical (periodontal)
- periapical
- radiculodental
- residual radicular

EXCLUDES: lateral developmental or lateral periodontal cyst (526.0)

DEF: Cyst in tissue around tooth apex due to chronic infection of granuloma around root.

522.9 Other and unspecified diseases of pulp and periapical tissues

DIGESTIVE SYSTEM

523 Gingival and periodontal diseases [4th]

523.0 Acute gingivitis [5th]
EXCLUDES acute necrotizing ulcerative gingivitis (101)
herpetic gingivostomatitis (054.2)

- **523.00 Acute gingivitis, plaque induced**
  Acute gingivitis NOS
- **523.01 Acute gingivitis, non-plaque induced**

523.1 Chronic gingivitis [5th]
Gingivitis (chronic): desquamative, hyperplastic
Gingivitis (chronic): simple marginal, ulcerative
EXCLUDES herpetic gingivostomatitis (054.2)

- **523.10 Chronic gingivitis, plaque induced**
  Chronic gingivitis NOS
  Gingivitis NOS
- **523.11 Chronic gingivitis, non-plaque induced**

523.2 Gingival recession [5th]
Gingival recession (postinfective) (postoperative)

- **523.20 Gingival recession, unspecified**
- **523.21 Gingival recession, minimal**
- **523.22 Gingival recession, moderate**
- **523.23 Gingival recession, severe**
- **523.24 Gingival recession, localized**
- **523.25 Gingival recession, generalized**

▲ 523.3 Aggressive and acute periodontitis [5th]
Acute:
  pericementitis
  pericoronitis
EXCLUDES acute apical periodontitis (522.4)
periapical abscess (522.5, 522.7)
DEF: Severe inflammation, of tissues supporting teeth.

- **523.30 Aggressive periodontitis, unspecified**
- **523.31 Aggressive periodontitis, localized**
  Periodontal abscess
- **523.32 Aggressive periodontitis, generalized**
- **523.33 Acute periodontitis**

523.4 Chronic periodontitis [5th]
Chronic pericoronitis
Pericementitis (chronic)
Periodontitis:
  complex
  simplex
  NOS
EXCLUDES chronic apical periodontitis (522.6)

- **523.40 Chronic periodontitis, unspecified**
- **523.41 Chronic periodontitis, localized**
- **523.42 Chronic periodontitis, generalized**

523.5 Periodontosis

523.6 Accretions on teeth
Dental calculus:
  subgingival
  supragingival
Deposits on teeth:
  betel
  materia alba
Deposits on teeth:
  soft
  tartar
  tobacco
Extrinsic discoloration of teeth
EXCLUDES intrinsic discoloration of teeth (521.7)
DEF: Foreign material on tooth surface, usually plaque or calculus.

523.8 Other specified periodontal diseases
Giant cell:
  epulis
  peripheral granuloma
Gingival:
  cysts
  enlargement NOS
  fibromatosis
Gingival polyp
Periodontal lesions due to traumatic occlusion
Peripheral giant cell granuloma
EXCLUDES leukoplakia of gingiva (528.6)

523.9 Unspecified gingival and periodontal disease
AHA: 3Q, '02, 14

524 Dentofacial anomalies, including malocclusion [4th]

524.0 Major anomalies of jaw size [5th]
EXCLUDES hemifacial atrophy or hypertrophy (754.0)
unilateral condylar hyperplasia or hypoplasia of mandible (526.89)

- **524.00 Unspecified anomaly**
  DEF: Unspecified deformity of jaw size.
- **524.01 Maxillary hyperplasia**
  DEF: Overgrowth or overdevelopment of upper jaw bone.
- **524.02 Mandibular hyperplasia**
  DEF: Overgrowth or overdevelopment of lower jaw bone.
- **524.03 Maxillary hypoplasia**
  DEF: Incomplete or underdeveloped, upper jaw bone.
- **524.04 Mandibular hypoplasia**
  DEF: Incomplete or underdeveloped, lower jaw bone.
- **524.05 Macrogenia**
  DEF: Enlarged, jaw, especially chin; affects bone, soft tissue, or both.
- **524.06 Microgenia**
  DEF: Underdeveloped mandible, characterized by an extremely small chin.
- **524.07 Excessive tuberosity of jaw**
  ►Entire maxillary tuberosity◄
- **524.09 Other specified anomaly**

524.1 Anomalies of relationship of jaw to cranial base [5th]
- **524.10 Unspecified anomaly**
  Prognathism   Retrognathism
  DEF: Prognathism: protrusion of lower jaw.
  DEF: Retrognathism: jaw is located posteriorly to a normally positioned jaw; backward position of mandible.
- **524.11 Maxillary asymmetry**
  DEF: Absence of symmetry of maxilla.
- **524.12 Other jaw asymmetry**
- **524.19 Other specified anomaly**

524.2 Anomalies of dental arch relationship [5th]
►Anomaly of dental arch◄
EXCLUDES hemifacial atrophy or hypertrophy (754.0)
soft tissue impingement (524.81-524.82)
unilateral condylar hyperplasia or hypoplasia of mandible (526.89)

- **524.20 Unspecified anomaly of dental arch relationship**
- ▲ **524.21 Malocclusion, Angle's class I**
  Neutro-occlusion
- ▲ **524.22 Malocclusion, Angle's class II**
  Disto-occlusion Division I
  Disto-occlusion Division II

Angle's Classification of Malocclusion

Normal occlusion

Class I Malocclusion

Class II Malocclusion

Class III Malocclusion

DIGESTIVE SYSTEM — Tabular List

- **524.23** Malocclusion, Angle's class III
  - Mesio-occlusion
- **524.24** Open anterior occlusal relationship
  - ▶Anterior open bite◀
- **524.25** Open posterior occlusal relationship
  - ▶Posterior open bite◀
- **524.26** Excessive horizontal overlap
  - ▶Excessive horizontal overjet◀
- **524.27** Reverse articulation
  - Anterior articulation
  - ▶Crossbite◀
  - Posterior articulation
- **524.28** Anomalies of interarch distance
  - Excessive interarch distance
  - Inadequate interarch distance
- **524.29** Other anomalies of dental arch relationship
  - ▶Other anomalies of dental arch◀

√5th **524.3** Anomalies of tooth position of fully erupted teeth
  - EXCLUDES: impacted or embedded teeth with abnormal position of such teeth or adjacent teeth (520.6)
- **524.30** Unspecified anomaly of tooth position
  - Diastema of teeth NOS
  - Displacement of teeth NOS
  - Transposition of teeth NOS
- **524.31** Crowding of teeth
- **524.32** Excessive spacing of teeth
- **524.33** Horizontal displacement of teeth
  - ▶Tipped teeth◀
  - Tipping of teeth
- **524.34** Vertical displacement of teeth
  - ▶Extruded tooth◀
  - Infraeruption of teeth
  - ▶Intruded tooth◀
  - Supraeruption of teeth
- **524.35** Rotation of tooth/teeth
- **524.36** Insufficient interocclusal distance of teeth (ridge)
  - ▶Lack of adequate intermaxillary vertical dimension◀
- **524.37** Excessive interocclusal distance of teeth
  - ▶Excessive intermaxillary vertical dimension◀
  - Loss of occlusal vertical dimension
- **524.39** Other anomalies of tooth position

524.4 Malocclusion, unspecified
  - DEF: Malposition of top and bottom teeth; interferes with chewing.

√5th **524.5** Dentofacial functional abnormalities
- **524.50** Dentofacial functional abnormality, unspecified
- **524.51** Abnormal jaw closure
- **524.52** Limited mandibular range of motion
- **524.53** Deviation in opening and closing of the mandible
- **524.54** Insufficient anterior guidance
  - ▶Insufficient anterior occlusal guidance◀
- **524.55** Centric occlusion maximum intercuspation discrepancy
  - ▶Centric occlusion of teeth discrepancy◀
- **524.56** Non-working side interference
  - ▶Balancing side interference◀
- **524.57** Lack of posterior occlusal support
- **524.59** Other dentofacial functional abnormalities
  - Abnormal swallowing
  - Mouth breathing
  - Sleep postures
  - Tongue, lip, or finger habits

√5th **524.6** Temporomandibular joint disorders
  - EXCLUDES: current temporomandibular joint:
    - dislocation (830.0-830.1)
    - strain (848.1)
- **524.60** Temporomandibular joint disorders, unspecified
  - Temporomandibular joint-pain-dysfunction syndrome [TMJ]
- **524.61** Adhesions and ankylosis (bony or fibrous)
  - DEF: Stiffening or union of temporomandibular joint due to bony or fibrous union across joint.
- **524.62** Arthralgia of temporomandibular joint
  - DEF: Pain in temporomandibular joint; not inflammatory in nature.
- **524.63** Articular disc disorder (reducing or non-reducing)
- **524.64** Temporomandibular joint sounds on opening and/or closing the jaw
- **524.69** Other specified temporomandibular joint disorders

√5th **524.7** Dental alveolar anomalies
- **524.70** Unspecified alveolar anomaly
- **524.71** Alveolar maxillary hyperplasia
  - DEF: Excessive tissue formation in the dental alveoli of upper jaw.
- **524.72** Alveolar mandibular hyperplasia
  - DEF: Excessive tissue formation in the dental alveoli of lower jaw.
- **524.73** Alveolar maxillary hypoplasia
  - DEF: Incomplete or underdeveloped, alveolar tissue of upper jaw.
- **524.74** Alveolar mandibular hypoplasia
  - DEF: Incomplete or underdeveloped, alveolar tissue of lower jaw.
- **524.75** Vertical displacement of alveolus and teeth
  - Extrusion of alveolus and teeth
- **524.76** Occlusal plane deviation
- **524.79** Other specified alveolar anomaly

√5th **524.8** Other specified dentofacial anomalies
- **524.81** Anterior soft tissue impingement
- **524.82** Posterior soft tissue impingement
- **524.89** Other specified dentofacial anomalies

524.9 Unspecified dentofacial anomalies

√4th **525** Other diseases and conditions of the teeth and supporting structures
- **525.0** Exfoliation of teeth due to systemic causes
  - DEF: Deterioration of teeth and surrounding structures due to systemic disease.

√5th **525.1** Loss of teeth due to trauma, extraction, or periodontal disease
  - Code first class of edentulism (525.40-525.44, 525.50-525.54)
  - AHA: 4Q, '05, 74; 4Q, '01, 44
- **525.10** Acquired absence of teeth, unspecified
  - Tooth extraction status, NOS
- **525.11** Loss of teeth due to trauma
- **525.12** Loss of teeth due to periodontal disease
- **525.13** Loss of teeth due to caries
- **525.19** Other loss of teeth

√5th **525.2** Atrophy of edentulous alveolar ridge
- **525.20** Unspecified atrophy of edentulous alveolar ridge
  - Atrophy of the mandible NOS
  - Atrophy of the maxilla NOS
- **525.21** Minimal atrophy of the mandible
- **525.22** Moderate atrophy of the mandible

- 525.23 Severe atrophy of the mandible
- 525.24 Minimal atrophy of the maxilla
- 525.25 Moderate atrophy of the maxilla
- 525.26 Severe atrophy of the maxilla
- 525.3 **Retained dental root**
- √5ᵗʰ 525.4 **Complete edentulism**
  Use additional code to identify cause of edentulism (525.10-525.19)
  AHA: ▶4Q, '05, 74◀
  - 525.40 **Complete edentulism, unspecified**
    Edentulism NOS
  - 525.41 Complete edentulism, class I
  - 525.42 Complete edentulism, class II
  - 525.43 Complete edentulism, class III
  - 525.44 Complete edentulism, class IV
- √5ᵗʰ 525.5 **Partial edentulism**
  Use additional code to identify cause of edentulism (525.10-525.19)
  AHA: ▶4Q, '05, 74◀
  - 525.50 **Partial edentulism, unspecified**
  - 525.51 Partial edentulism, class I
  - 525.52 Partial edentulism, class II
  - 525.53 Partial edentulism, class III
  - 525.54 Partial edentulism, class IV
- ● √5ᵗʰ 525.6 **Unsatisfactory restoration of tooth**
  Defective bridge, crown, fillings
  Defective dental restoration
  EXCLUDES dental restoration status (V45.84)
  unsatisfactory endodontic treatment (526.61-526.69)
  - ● 525.60 **Unspecified unsatisfactory restoration of tooth**
    Unspecified defective dental restoration
  - ● 525.61 **Open restoration margins**
    Dental restoration failure of marginal integrity
    Open margin on tooth restoration
  - ● 525.62 **Unrepairable overhanging of dental restorative materials**
    Overhanging of tooth restoration
  - ● 525.63 **Fractured dental restorative material without loss of material**
    EXCLUDES cracked tooth (521.81)
    fractured tooth (873.63, 873.73)
  - ● 525.64 **Fractured dental restorative material with loss of material**
    EXCLUDES cracked tooth (521.81)
    fractured tooth (873.63, 873.73)
  - ● 525.65 **Contour of existing restoration of tooth biologically incompatible with oral health**
    Dental restoration failure of periodontal anatomical integrity
    Unacceptable contours of existing restoration
    Unacceptable morphology of existing restoration
  - ● 525.66 **Allergy to existing dental restorative material**
    Use additional code to identify the specific type of allergy
  - ● 525.67 **Poor aesthetics of existing restoration**
    Dental restoration aesthetically inadequate or displeasing
  - ● 525.69 **Other unsatisfactory restoration of existing tooth**
- 525.8 **Other specified disorders of the teeth and supporting structures**
  Enlargement of alveolar ridge NOS
  Irregular alveolar process
- 525.9 **Unspecified disorder of the teeth and supporting structures**

√4ᵗʰ 526 **Diseases of the jaws**
- 526.0 **Developmental odontogenic cysts**
  Cyst: dentigerous, eruption, follicular, lateral developmental
  Cyst: lateral periodontal, primordial, Keratocyst
  EXCLUDES radicular cyst (522.8)
- 526.1 **Fissural cysts of jaw**
  Cyst: globulomaxillary, incisor canal, median anterior maxillary
  Cyst: median palatal, nasopalatine, palatine of papilla
  EXCLUDES cysts of oral soft tissues (528.4)
- 526.2 **Other cysts of jaws**
  Cyst of jaw: NOS, aneurysmal
  Cyst of jaw: hemorrhagic, traumatic
- 526.3 **Central giant cell (reparative) granuloma**
  EXCLUDES peripheral giant cell granuloma (523.8)
- 526.4 **Inflammatory conditions**
  Abscess
  Osteitis
  Osteomyelitis (neonatal)
  Periostitis
  } of jaw (acute) (chronic) (suppurative)
  Sequestrum of jaw bone
  EXCLUDES alveolar osteitis (526.5)
- 526.5 **Alveolitis of jaw**
  Alveolar osteitis   Dry socket
  DEF: Inflammation, of alveoli or tooth socket.
- ● √5ᵗʰ 526.6 **Periradicular pathology associated with previous endodontic treatment**
  - ● 526.61 Perforation of root canal space
  - ● 526.62 Endodontic overfill
  - ● 526.63 Endodontic underfill
  - ● 526.69 **Other periradicular pathology associated with previous endodontic treatment**
- √5ᵗʰ 526.8 **Other specified diseases of the jaws**
  - 526.81 **Exostosis of jaw**
    Torus mandibularis   Torus palatinus
    DEF: Spur or bony outgrowth on the jaw.
  - 526.89 **Other**
    Cherubism
    Fibrous dysplasia
    Latent bone cyst
    Osteoradionecrosis
    } of jaw(s)
    Unilateral condylar hyperplasia or hypoplasia of mandible
- 526.9 **Unspecified disease of the jaws**

√4ᵗʰ 527 **Diseases of the salivary glands**
- 527.0 **Atrophy**
  DEF: Wasting away, necrosis of salivary gland tissue.
- 527.1 **Hypertrophy**
  DEF: Overgrowth or overdeveloped salivary gland tissue.
- 527.2 **Sialoadenitis**
  Parotitis: NOS, allergic, toxic
  Sialoangitis
  Sialodochitis
  EXCLUDES epidemic or infectious parotitis (072.0-072.9)
  uveoparotid fever (135)
  DEF: Inflammation of salivary gland.

DIGESTIVE SYSTEM — Tabular List

527.3 **Abscess**

527.4 **Fistula**
> EXCLUDES: congenital fistula of salivary gland (750.24)

527.5 **Sialolithiasis**
Calculus } of salivary gland or duct
Stone
Sialodocholithiasis

527.6 **Mucocele**
Mucous:
  extravasation cyst of salivary gland
  retention cyst of salivary gland
Ranula
DEF: Dilated salivary gland cavity filled with mucous.

527.7 **Disturbance of salivary secretion**
Hyposecretion   Sialorrhea
Ptyalism   Xerostomia

527.8 **Other specified diseases of the salivary glands**
Benign lymphoepithelial lesion of salivary gland
Sialectasia
Sialosis
Stenosis } of salivary duct
Stricture

527.9 **Unspecified disease of the salivary glands**

√4th **528 Diseases of the oral soft tissues, excluding lesions specific for gingiva and tongue**

▲ √5th **528.0 Stomatitis and mucositis (ulcerative)**
> EXCLUDES: ▶cellulitis and abscess of mouth (528.3)
> diphtheritic stomatitis (032.0)
> epizootic stomatitis (078.4)
> gingivitis (523.0-523.1)
> oral thrush (112.0)
> Stevens-Johnson syndrome (695.1)◀
> stomatitis:
>   acute necrotizing ulcerative (101)
>   aphthous (528.2)
>   gangrenous (528.1)
>   herpetic (054.2)
>   Vincent's (101)

AHA: 2Q, '99, 9

DEF: Stomatitis: Inflammation of oral mucosa; labial and buccal mucosa, tongue, palate, floor of the mouth, and gingivae.

• **528.00 Stomatitis and mucositis, unspecified**
Mucositis NOS
Ulcerative mucositis NOS
Ulcerative stomatitis NOS
Vesicular stomatitis NOS

• **528.01 Mucositis (ulcerative) due to antineoplastic therapy**
Use additional E code to identify adverse effects of therapy, such as:
antineoplastic and immunosuppressive drugs (E930.7, E933.1)
radiation therapy (E879.2)

• **528.02 Mucositis (ulcerative) due to other drugs**
Use additional E code to identify drug

• **528.09 Other stomatitis and mucositis (ulcerative)**

528.1 Cancrum oris
Gangrenous stomatitis   Noma
DEF: A severely gangrenous lesion of mouth due to fusospirochetal infection; destroys buccal, labial and facial tissues; can be fatal; found primarily in debilitated and malnourished children.

528.2 Oral aphthae
Aphthous stomatitis   Recurrent aphthous ulcer
Canker sore   Stomatitis herpetiformis
Periadenitis mucosa
  necrotica recurrens
> EXCLUDES: herpetic stomatitis (054.2)

DEF: Small oval or round ulcers of the mouth marked by a grayish exudate and a red halo effect.

528.3 Cellulitis and abscess
Cellulitis of mouth (floor)   Oral fistula
Ludwig's angina
> EXCLUDES: abscess of tongue (529.0)
> cellulitis or abscess of lip (528.5)
> fistula (of):
>   dental (522.7)
>   lip (528.5)
>   gingivitis ▶(523.00-523.11)◀

528.4 Cysts
Dermoid cyst
Epidermoid cyst
Epstein's pearl
Lymphoepithelial cyst } of mouth
Nasoalveolar cyst
Nasolabial cyst
> EXCLUDES: cyst:
>   gingiva (523.8)
>   tongue (529.8)

528.5 Diseases of lips
Abscess
Cellulitis } of lip(s)
Fistula
Hypertrophy
Cheilitis: Cheilodynia
  NOS   Cheilosis
  angular
> EXCLUDES: actinic cheilitis (692.79)
> congenital fistula of lip (750.25)
> leukoplakia of lips (528.6)

AHA: S-O, '86, 10

528.6 Leukoplakia of oral mucosa, including tongue
Leukokeratosis of   Leukoplakia of:
  oral mucosa   lips
Leukoplakia of: tongue
  gingiva
> EXCLUDES: carcinoma in situ (230.0, 232.0)
> leukokeratosis nicotina palati (528.79)

DEF: Thickened white patches of epithelium on mucous membranes of mouth.

√5th **528.7 Other disturbances of oral epithelium, including tongue**
> EXCLUDES: carcinoma in situ (230.0, 232.0)
> leukokeratosis NOS (702)

528.71 Minimal keratinized residual ridge mucosa
▶Minimal keratinization of alveolar ridge mucosa◀

528.72 Excessive keratinized residual ridge mucosa
▶Excessive keratinization of alveolar ridge mucosa◀

528.79 Other disturbances of oral epithelium, including tongue
Erythroplakia of mouth or tongue
Focal epithelial hyperplasia of mouth or tongue
Leukoedema of mouth or tongue
Leukokeratosis nicotina palate
▶Other oral epithelium disturbances◀

528.8 Oral submucosal fibrosis, including of tongue

528.9 Other and unspecified diseases of the oral soft tissues
Cheek and lip biting   Melanoplakia
Denture sore mouth   Papillary hyperplasia of palate
Denture stomatitis
Eosinophilic granuloma
Irritative hyperplasia } of oral mucosa
Pyogenic granuloma
Ulcer (traumatic)

DIGESTIVE SYSTEM

✓4th 529 Diseases and other conditions of the tongue

529.0 Glossitis
Abscess }
Ulceration (traumatic) } of tongue

EXCLUDES glossitis:
benign migratory (529.1)
Hunter's (529.4)
median rhomboid (529.2)
Moeller's (529.4)

529.1 Geographic tongue
Benign migratory glossitis
Glossitis areata exfoliativa

DEF: Chronic glossitis; marked by filiform papillae atrophy and inflammation; no known etiology.

529.2 Median rhomboid glossitis
DEF: A noninflammatory, congenital disease characterized by rhomboid-like lesions at the middle third of the tongue's dorsal surface.

529.3 Hypertrophy of tongue papillae
Black hairy tongue   Hypertrophy of foliate papillae
Coated tongue   Lingua villosa nigra

529.4 Atrophy of tongue papillae
Bald tongue   Glossitis:
Glazed tongue   Moeller's
Glossitis: Glossodynia exfoliativa
    Hunter's   Smooth atrophic tongue

529.5 Plicated tongue
Fissured }
Furrowed } tongue
Scrotal   }

EXCLUDES fissure of tongue, congenital (750.13)

DEF: Cracks, fissures or furrows, on dorsal surface of tongue.

529.6 Glossodynia
Glossopyrosis   Painful tongue

EXCLUDES glossodynia exfoliativa (529.4)

529.8 Other specified conditions of the tongue
Atrophy   }
Crenated   }
Enlargement } (of) tongue
Hypertrophy }

Glossocele
Glossoptosis

EXCLUDES erythroplasia of tongue (528.79)
leukoplakia of tongue (528.6)
macroglossia (congenital) (750.15)
microglossia (congenital) (750.16)
oral submucosal fibrosis (528.8)

529.9 Unspecified condition of the tongue

DISEASES OF ESOPHAGUS, STOMACH, AND DUODENUM
▶(530-538)◀

✓4th 530 Diseases of esophagus
EXCLUDES esophageal varices (456.0-456.2)

530.0 Achalasia and cardiospasm
Achalasia (of cardia)   Megaesophagus
Aperistalsis of esophagus

EXCLUDES congenital cardiospasm (750.7)

DEF: Failure of smooth muscle fibers to relax, at gastrointestinal junctures; such as esophagogastric sphincter when swallowing.

✓5th 530.1 Esophagitis
Abscess of esophagus   Esophagitis:
Esophagitis: peptic
    NOS   postoperative
    chemical   regurgitant
Use additional E code to identify cause, if induced by chemical

EXCLUDES tuberculous esophagitis (017.8)

AHA: 4Q, '93, 27; 1Q, '92, 17; 3Q, '91, 20

530.10 Esophagitis, unspecified
AHA: 3Q, '05, 17

530.11 Reflux esophagitis
AHA: 4Q, '95, 82

DEF: Inflammation of lower esophagus; due to regurgitated gastric acid from malfunctioning lower esophageal sphincter; causes heartburn and substernal pain.

530.12 Acute esophagitis
AHA: 4Q, '01, 45

DEF: An acute inflammation of the mucous lining or submucosal coat of the esophagus.

530.19 Other esophagitis
AHA: 3Q, '01, 10

✓5th 530.2 Ulcer of esophagus
Ulcer of esophagus
    fungal
    peptic
Ulcer of esophagus due to ingestion of:
    aspirin
    chemicals
    medicines
Use additional E code to identify cause, if induced by chemical or drug

AHA: 4Q, '03, 63

530.20 Ulcer of esophagus without bleeding
Ulcer of esophagus NOS

530.21 Ulcer of esophagus with bleeding
EXCLUDES bleeding esophageal varices (456.0, 456.20)

530.3 Stricture and stenosis of esophagus
Compression of esophagus
Obstruction of esophagus

EXCLUDES congenital stricture of esophagus (750.3)

AHA: 2Q, '01, 4; 2Q, '97, 3; 1Q, '88, 13

530.4 Perforation of esophagus
Rupture of esophagus

EXCLUDES traumatic perforation of esophagus (862.22, 862.32, 874.4-874.5)

530.5 Dyskinesia of esophagus
Corkscrew esophagus   Esophagospasm
Curling esophagus   Spasm of esophagus

EXCLUDES cardiospasm (530.0)

AHA: 1Q, '88, 13; N-D, '84, 19

DEF: Difficulty performing voluntary esophageal movements.

Esophagus

✓4th / ✓5th Additional Digit Required   Unspecified Code   Other Specified Code   Manifestation Code   ▶◀ Revised Text   ● New Code   ▲ Revised Code Title

2007 ICD•9•CM   October 2006 • Volume 1 — 153

530.6 Diverticulum of esophagus, acquired
Diverticulum, acquired:
 epiphrenic
 pharyngoesophageal
 pulsion
 subdiaphragmatic
 traction
 Zenker's (hypopharyngeal)
Esophageal pouch, acquired
Esophagocele, acquired

EXCLUDES: congenital diverticulum of esophagus (750.4)

AHA: J-F, '85, 3

530.7 Gastroesophageal laceration-hemorrhage syndrome
Mallory-Weiss syndrome

DEF: Laceration of distal esophagus and proximal stomach due to vomiting, hiccups or other sustained activity.

√5th **530.8 Other specified disorders of esophagus**

530.81 Esophageal reflux
Gastroesophageal reflux
EXCLUDES: reflux esophagitis (530.11)
AHA: 2Q, '01, 4; 1Q, '95, 7; 4Q, '92, 27

DEF: Regurgitation of the gastric contents into esophagus and possibly pharynx; where aspiration may occur between the vocal cords and down into the trachea.

530.82 Esophageal hemorrhage
EXCLUDES: hemorrhage due to esophageal varices (456.0-456.2)
AHA: 1Q, '05, 17

530.83 Esophageal leukoplakia

530.84 Tracheoesophageal fistula
EXCLUDES: congenital tracheoesophageal fistula (750.3)

530.85 Barrett's esophagus
AHA: 4Q, '03, 63

DEF: A metaplastic disorder in which specialized columnar epithelial cells replace the normal squamous epithelial cells; an acquired condition secondary to chronic gastroesophageal reflux damage to the mucosa; associated with increased risk of developing adenocarcinoma.

530.86 Infection of esophagostomy
Use additional code to specify infection

530.87 Mechanical complication of esophagostomy
Malfunction of esophagostomy

530.89 Other
EXCLUDES: Paterson-Kelly syndrome (280.8)

530.9 Unspecified disorder of esophagus

√4th **531 Gastric ulcer**
INCLUDES: ulcer (peptic):
 prepyloric
 pylorus
 stomach
Use additional E code to identify drug, if drug-induced
EXCLUDES: peptic ulcer NOS (533.0-533.9)

The following fifth-digit subclassification is for use with category 531:
 0 without mention of obstruction
 1 with obstruction

AHA: 1Q, '91, 15; 4Q, '90, 27

DEF: Destruction of tissue in lumen of stomach due to action of gastric acid and pepsin on gastric mucosa decreasing resistance to ulcers.

√5th **531.0 Acute with hemorrhage**
AHA: N-D, '84, 15

√5th **531.1 Acute with perforation**

√5th **531.2 Acute with hemorrhage and perforation**

√5th **531.3 Acute without mention of hemorrhage or perforation**

√5th **531.4 Chronic or unspecified with hemorrhage**
AHA: 4Q, '90, 22

√5th **531.5 Chronic or unspecified with perforation**

√5th **531.6 Chronic or unspecified with hemorrhage and perforation**

√5th **531.7 Chronic without mention of hemorrhage or perforation**

√5th **531.9 Unspecified as acute or chronic, without mention of hemorrhage or perforation**

√4th **532 Duodenal ulcer**
INCLUDES: erosion (acute) of duodenum
 ulcer (peptic):
  duodenum
  postpyloric
Use additional E code to identify drug, if drug-induced
EXCLUDES: peptic ulcer NOS (533.0-533.9)

The following fifth-digit subclassification is for use with category 532:
 0 without mention of obstruction
 1 with obstruction

AHA: 4Q, '90, 27; 1Q, '91, 15

DEF: Ulcers in duodenum due to action of gastric acid and pepsin on mucosa decreasing resistance to ulcers.

√5th **532.0 Acute with hemorrhage**
AHA: 4Q, '90, 22

√5th **532.1 Acute with perforation**

√5th **532.2 Acute with hemorrhage and perforation**

√5th **532.3 Acute without mention of hemorrhage or perforation**

√5th **532.4 Chronic or unspecified with hemorrhage**

√5th **532.5 Chronic or unspecified with perforation**

√5th **532.6 Chronic or unspecified with hemorrhage and perforation**

√5th **532.7 Chronic without mention of hemorrhage or perforation**

√5th **532.9 Unspecified as acute or chronic, without mention of hemorrhage or perforation**

DIGESTIVE SYSTEM

533 Peptic ulcer, site unspecified
INCLUDES gastroduodenal ulcer NOS
peptic ulcer NOS
stress ulcer NOS

Use additional E code to identify drug, if drug-induced

EXCLUDES peptic ulcer:
duodenal (532.0-532.9)
gastric (531.0-531.9)

The following fifth-digit subclassification is for use with category 533:
- 0 without mention of obstruction
- 1 with obstruction

AHA: 1Q, '91, 15; 4Q, '90, 27

- **533.0** Acute with hemorrhage
- **533.1** Acute with perforation
- **533.2** Acute with hemorrhage and perforation
- **533.3** Acute without mention of hemorrhage and perforation
- **533.4** Chronic or unspecified with hemorrhage
- **533.5** Chronic or unspecified with perforation
- **533.6** Chronic or unspecified with hemorrhage and perforation
- **533.7** Chronic without mention of hemorrhage or perforation
  AHA: 2Q, '89, 16
- **533.9** Unspecified as acute or chronic, without mention of hemorrhage or perforation

534 Gastrojejunal ulcer
INCLUDES ulcer (peptic) or erosion:
anastomotic
gastrocolic
gastrointestinal
gastrojejunal
jejunal
marginal
stomal

EXCLUDES primary ulcer of small intestine (569.82)

The following fifth-digit subclassification is for use with category 534:
- 0 without mention of obstruction
- 1 with obstruction

AHA: 1Q, '91, 15; 4Q, '90, 27

- **534.0** Acute with hemorrhage
- **534.1** Acute with perforation
- **534.2** Acute with hemorrhage and perforation
- **534.3** Acute without mention of hemorrhage or perforation
- **534.4** Chronic or unspecified with hemorrhage
- **534.5** Chronic or unspecified with perforation
- **534.6** Chronic or unspecified with hemorrhage and perforation
- **534.7** Chronic without mention of hemorrhage or perforation
- **534.9** Unspecified as acute or chronic, without mention of hemorrhage or perforation

535 Gastritis and duodenitis

The following fifth-digit subclassification is for use with category 535:
- 0 without mention of hemorrhage
- 1 with hemorrhage

AHA: 2Q, '92, 9; 4Q, '91, 25

- **535.0** Acute gastritis
  AHA: 2Q, '92, 8; N-D, '86, 9
- **535.1** Atrophic gastritis
  Gastritis: Gastritis:
  atrophic-hyperplastic   chronic (atrophic)
  AHA: 1Q, '94, 18
  DEF: Inflammation of stomach, with mucous membrane atrophy and peptic gland destruction.
- **535.2** Gastric mucosal hypertrophy
  Hypertrophic gastritis
- **535.3** Alcoholic gastritis
- **535.4** Other specified gastritis
  Gastritis: Gastritis:
  allergic   superficial
  bile induced   toxic
  irritant
  AHA: 4Q, '90, 27
- **535.5** Unspecified gastritis and gastroduodenitis
  AHA: For code 535.50: 3Q, '05, 17; 4Q, '99, 25
- **535.6** Duodenitis
  AHA: For code 535.60: 3Q, '05, 17
  DEF: Inflammation of intestine, between pylorus and jejunum.

536 Disorders of function of stomach
EXCLUDES functional disorders of stomach specified as psychogenic (306.4)

- **536.0** Achlorhydria
  DEF: Absence of gastric acid due to gastric mucosa atrophy; unresponsive to histamines; also known as gastric anacidity.
- **536.1** Acute dilatation of stomach
  Acute distention of stomach
- **536.2** Persistent vomiting
  Habit vomiting
  Persistent vomiting [not of pregnancy]
  Uncontrollable vomiting
  EXCLUDES excessive vomiting in pregnancy (643.0-643.9)
  vomiting NOS (787.0)
- **536.3** Gastroparesis
  Gastroparalysis
  AHA: 2Q, '04, 7; 2Q, '01, 4; 4Q, '94, 42
  DEF: Slight degree of paralysis within muscular coat of stomach.
- **536.4** Gastrostomy complications
  AHA: 4Q, '98, 42
  - **536.40** Gastrostomy complication, unspecified
  - **536.41** Infection of gastrostomy
    Use additional code to specify type of infection, such as:
    abscess or cellulitis of abdomen (682.2)
    septicemia (038.0-038.9)
    Use additional code to identify organism (041.00-041.9)
    AHA: 4Q, '98, 42
  - **536.42** Mechanical complication of gastrostomy
  - **536.49** Other gastrostomy complications
    AHA: 4Q, '98, 42
- **536.8** Dyspepsia and other specified disorders of function of stomach
  Achylia gastrica   Hyperchlorhydria
  Hourglass contraction   Hypochlorhydria
    of stomach   Indigestion
  Hyperacidity   ▶ Tachygastria ◀
  EXCLUDES achlorhydria (536.0)
  heartburn (787.1)
  AHA: 2Q, '93, 6; 2Q, '89, 16; N-D, '84, 9
- **536.9** Unspecified functional disorder of stomach
  Functional gastrointestinal:
  disorder
  disturbance
  irritation

DIGESTIVE SYSTEM

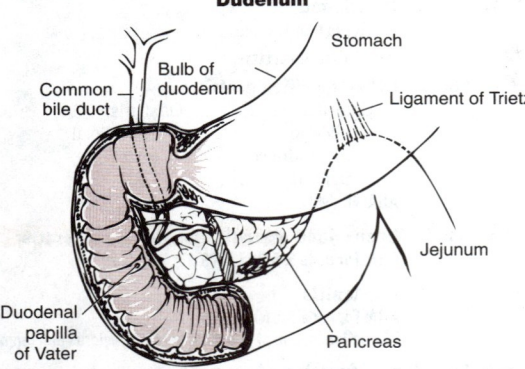

- **537 Other disorders of stomach and duodenum** [✓4th]
  - **537.0 Acquired hypertrophic pyloric stenosis**
    - Constriction ⎫
    - Obstruction ⎬ of pylorus, acquired or adult
    - Stricture ⎭
    - EXCLUDES congenital or infantile pyloric stenosis (750.5)
    - AHA: 2Q, '01, 4; J-F, '85, 14
  - **537.1 Gastric diverticulum**
    - EXCLUDES congenital diverticulum of stomach (750.7)
    - AHA: J-F, '85, 4
    - DEF: Herniated sac or pouch, within stomach or duodenum.
  - **537.2 Chronic duodenal ileus**
    - DEF: Persistent obstruction between pylorus and jejunum.
  - **537.3 Other obstruction of duodenum**
    - Cicatrix ⎫
    - Stenosis ⎬ of duodenum
    - Stricture ⎪
    - Volvulus ⎭
    - EXCLUDES congenital obstruction of duodenum (751.1)
  - **537.4 Fistula of stomach or duodenum**
    - Gastrocolic fistula   Gastrojejunocolic fistula
  - **537.5 Gastroptosis**
    - DEF: Downward displacement of stomach.
  - **537.6 Hourglass stricture or stenosis of stomach**
    - Cascade stomach
    - EXCLUDES congenital hourglass stomach (750.7)
    - hourglass contraction of stomach (536.8)
  - **537.8 Other specified disorders of stomach and duodenum** [✓5th]
    - AHA: 4Q, '91, 25
    - **537.81 Pylorospasm**
      - EXCLUDES congenital pylorospasm (750.5)
      - DEF: Spasm of the pyloric sphincter.
    - **537.82 Angiodysplasia of stomach and duodenum (without mention of hemorrhage)**
      - AHA: 3Q, '96, 10; 4Q, '90, 4
    - **537.83 Angiodysplasia of stomach and duodenum with hemorrhage**
      - DEF: Bleeding of stomach and duodenum due to vascular abnormalities.
    - **537.84 Dieulafoy lesion (hemorrhagic) of stomach and duodenum**
      - AHA: 4Q, '02, 60
      - DEF: An abnormally large and convoluted submucosal artery protruding through a defect in the mucosa in the stomach or intestines that can erode the epithelium causing hemorrhaging; also called Dieulafoy's vascular malformation.
    - **537.89 Other**
      - Gastric or duodenal:
        - prolapse
        - rupture
      - Intestinal metaplasia of gastric mucosa
      - Passive congestion of stomach
      - EXCLUDES diverticula of duodenum (562.00-562.01)
      - gastrointestinal hemorrhage (578.0-578.9)
      - AHA: 3Q, '05, 15; N-D, '84, 7
  - **537.9 Unspecified disorder of stomach and duodenum**
- **538 Gastrointestinal mucositis (ulcerative)**
  - Use additional E code to identify adverse effects of therapy, such as:
    - antineoplastic and immunosuppressive drugs (E930.7, E933.1)
    - radiation therapy (E879.2)
  - EXCLUDES mucositis (ulcerative) of mouth and oral soft tissue (528.00- 528.09)

APPENDICITIS (540-543)

- **540 Acute appendicitis** [✓4th]
  - AHA: N-D, '84, 19
  - DEF: Inflammation of vermiform appendix due to fecal obstruction, neoplasm or foreign body of appendiceal lumen; causes infection, edema and infarction of appendiceal wall; may result in mural necrosis, and perforation.
  - **540.0 With generalized peritonitis**
    - Appendicitis (acute):   with:
      - fulminating   perforation
      - gangrenous   peritonitis (generalized)
      - obstructive   rupture
    - Cecitis (acute)
    - Rupture of appendix
    - EXCLUDES acute appendicitis with peritoneal abscess (540.1)
  - **540.1 With peritoneal abscess**
    - With generalized peritonitis   Abscess of appendix
    - AHA: N-D, '84, 19
  - **540.9 Without mention of peritonitis**
    - Acute:
      - appendicitis:
        - fulminating ⎫
        - gangrenous ⎬ without mention of
        - inflamed   ⎪ perforation, peritonitis,
        - obstructive ⎪ or rupture
        - cecitis   ⎭
    - AHA: 1Q, '01, 15; 4Q, '97, 52
- **541 Appendicitis, unqualified**
  - AHA: 2Q, '90, 26
- **542 Other appendicitis**
  - Appendicitis: Appendicitis:
    - chronic   relapsing
    - recurrent   subacute
  - EXCLUDES hyperplasia (lymphoid) of appendix (543.0)
  - AHA: 1Q, '01, 15

N Newborn Age: 0   P Pediatric Age: 0-17   M Maternity Age: 12-55   A Adult Age: 15-124

Tabular List — DIGESTIVE SYSTEM 543–551.9

✓4th 543 Other diseases of appendix

543.0 Hyperplasia of appendix (lymphoid)
DEF: Proliferation of cells in appendix tissue.

543.9 Other and unspecified diseases of appendix
Appendicular or appendiceal:
  colic
  concretion
  fistula
Diverticulum ⎫
Fecalith   ⎪
Intussusception ⎬ of appendix
Mucocele   ⎪
Stercolith   ⎭

HERNIA OF ABDOMINAL CAVITY (550-553)
INCLUDES hernia:
  acquired
  congenital, except diaphragmatic or hiatal

✓4th 550 Inguinal hernia
INCLUDES
  bubonocele
  inguinal hernia (direct) (double) (indirect) (oblique) (sliding)
  scrotal hernia

The following fifth-digit subclassification is for use with category 550:

  0 unilateral or unspecified (not specified as recurrent)
    Unilateral NOS
  1 unilateral or unspecified, recurrent
  2 bilateral (not specified as recurrent)
    Bilateral NOS
  3 bilateral, recurrent

AHA: N-D, '85, 12
DEF: Hernia: protrusion of an abdominal organ or tissue through inguinal canal.
DEF: Indirect inguinal hernia: (external or oblique) leaves abdomen through deep inguinal ring, passes through inguinal canal lateral to the inferior epigastric artery.
DEF: Direct inguinal hernia: (internal) emerges between inferior epigastric artery and rectus muscle edge.

✓5th 550.0 Inguinal hernia, with gangrene
Inguinal hernia with gangrene (and obstruction)

✓5th 550.1 Inguinal hernia, with obstruction, without mention of gangrene
Inguinal hernia with mention of incarceration, irreducibility, or strangulation

Inguinal Hernia

Hernias of Abdominal Cavity

✓5th 550.9 Inguinal hernia, without mention of obstruction or gangrene
Inguinal hernia NOS
AHA: For code 550.91: 3Q, '03, 10; 1Q, '03, 4

✓4th 551 Other hernia of abdominal cavity, with gangrene
INCLUDES that with gangrene (and obstruction)

✓5th 551.0 Femoral hernia with gangrene
  551.00 Unilateral or unspecified (not specified as recurrent)
    Femoral hernia NOS with gangrene
  551.01 Unilateral or unspecified, recurrent
  551.02 Bilateral (not specified as recurrent)
  551.03 Bilateral, recurrent

551.1 Umbilical hernia with gangrene
Parumbilical hernia specified as gangrenous

✓5th 551.2 Ventral hernia with gangrene
  551.20 Ventral, unspecified, with gangrene
  551.21 Incisional, with gangrene
    Hernia:
      postoperative ⎫ specified as
      recurrent, ventral ⎭ gangrenous
  551.29 Other
    Epigastric hernia specified as gangrenous

551.3 Diaphragmatic hernia with gangrene
Hernia:
  hiatal (esophageal) ⎫
    (sliding)   ⎬ specified as
  paraesophageal   ⎪ gangrenous
  Thoracic stomach   ⎭
EXCLUDES congenital diaphragmatic hernia (756.6)

551.8 Hernia of other specified sites, with gangrene
Any condition classifiable to 553.8 if specified as gangrenous

551.9 Hernia of unspecified site, with gangrene
Any condition classifiable to 553.9 if specified as gangrenous

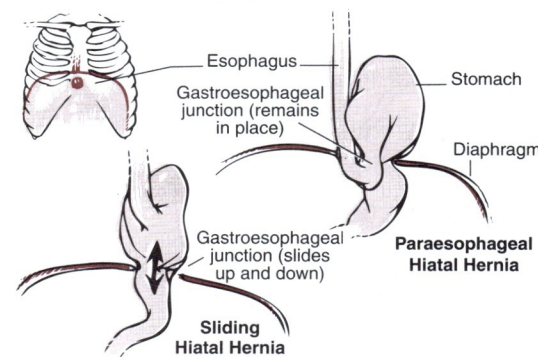
Diaphragmatic Hernia

✓4th / ✓5th Additional Digit Required | Unspecified Code | Other Specified Code | Manifestation Code | ►◄ Revised Text | ● New Code | ▲ Revised Code Title

2007 ICD•9•CM   Volume 1 — 157

DIGESTIVE SYSTEM

Femoral Hernia

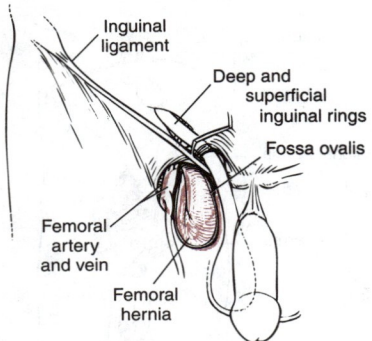

✓4th **552 Other hernia of abdominal cavity, with obstruction, but without mention of gangrene**
  EXCLUDES that with mention of gangrene (551.0-551.9)

✓5th **552.0 Femoral hernia with obstruction**
  Femoral hernia specified as incarcerated, irreducible, strangulated, or causing obstruction

  552.00 Unilateral or unspecified (not specified as recurrent)
  552.01 Unilateral or unspecified, recurrent
  552.02 Bilateral (not specified as recurrent)
  552.03 Bilateral, recurrent

552.1 Umbilical hernia with obstruction
  Parumbilical hernia specified as incarcerated, irreducible, strangulated, or causing obstruction

✓5th **552.2 Ventral hernia with obstruction**
  Ventral hernia specified as incarcerated, irreducible, strangulated, or causing obstruction

  552.20 Ventral, unspecified, with obstruction
  552.21 Incisional, with obstruction
    Hernia:
      postoperative
      recurrent,
      ventral
    } specified as incarcerated, irreducible, strangulated, or causing obstruction
    AHA: 3Q, '03, 11

  552.29 Other
    Epigastric hernia specified as incarcerated, irreducible, strangulated, or causing obstruction

552.3 Diaphragmatic hernia with obstruction
  Hernia:
    hiatal (esophageal) (sliding)
    paraesophageal
    Thoracic stomach
    } specified as incarcerated, irreducible, strangulated, or causing obstruction
  EXCLUDES congenital diaphragmatic hernia (756.6)

Large Intestine

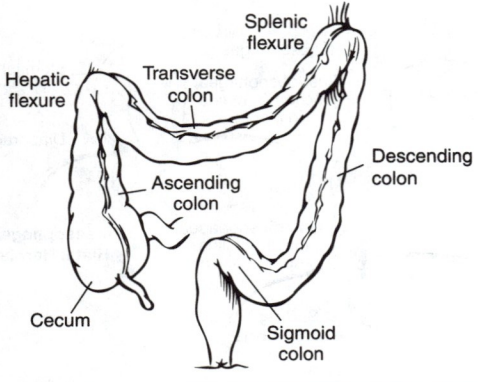

552.8 Hernia of other specified sites, with obstruction
  Any condition classifiable to 553.8 if specified as incarcerated, irreducible, strangulated, or causing obstruction
  EXCLUDES hernia due to adhesion with obstruction (560.81)
  AHA: 1Q, '04, 10

552.9 Hernia of unspecified site, with obstruction
  Any condition classifiable to 553.9 if specified as incarcerated, irreducible, strangulated, or causing obstruction

✓4th **553 Other hernia of abdominal cavity without mention of obstruction or gangrene**
  EXCLUDES the listed conditions with mention of:
    gangrene (and obstruction) (551.0-551.9)
    obstruction (552.0-552.9)

✓5th **553.0 Femoral hernia**
  553.00 Unilateral or unspecified (not specified as recurrent)
    Femoral hernia NOS
  553.01 Unilateral or unspecified, recurrent
  553.02 Bilateral (not specified as recurrent)
  553.03 Bilateral, recurrent

553.1 Umbilical hernia
  Parumbilical hernia

✓5th **553.2 Ventral hernia**
  553.20 Ventral, unspecified
    AHA: 3Q, '03, 6
  553.21 Incisional
    Hernia: Hernia:
      postoperative   recurrent, ventral
    AHA: 3Q, '03, 6
  553.29 Other
    Hernia: Hernia:
      epigastric   spigelian

553.3 Diaphragmatic hernia
  Hernia:
    hiatal (esophageal) (sliding)
    paraesophageal
  Thoracic stomach
  EXCLUDES congenital:
    diaphragmatic hernia (756.6)
    hiatal hernia (750.6)
    esophagocele (530.6)
  AHA: 2Q, '01, 6; 1Q, '00, 6

553.8 Hernia of other specified sites
  Hernia: Hernia:
    ischiatic   retroperitoneal
    ischiorectal   sciatic
    lumbar   Other abdominal
    obturator   hernia of specified
    pudendal   site
  EXCLUDES vaginal enterocele (618.6)

553.9 Hernia of unspecified site
  Enterocele   Hernia:
  Epiplocele   intestinal
  Hernia: intra-abdominal
    NOS   Rupture (nontraumatic)
    interstitial   Sarcoepiplocele

NONINFECTIOUS ENTERITIS AND COLITIS (555-558)

✓4th 555 Regional enteritis
INCLUDES Crohn's disease
Granulomatous enteritis
EXCLUDES ulcerative colitis (556)
DEF: Inflammation of intestine; classified to site.

555.0 Small intestine
Ileitis: Regional enteritis or
  regional Crohn's disease of:
  segmental duodenum
  terminal ileum
    jejunum

555.1 Large intestine
Colitis: Regional enteritis or
  granulmatous Crohn's disease of:
  regional colon
  transmural large bowel
    rectum
AHA: 3Q, '99, 8

555.2 Small intestine with large intestine
Regional ileocolitis
AHA: 1Q, '03, 18

555.9 Unspecified site
Crohn's disease NOS   Regional enteritis NOS
AHA: ▶2Q, '05, 11;◀ 3Q, '99, 8; 4Q, '97, 42; 2Q, '97, 3

✓4th 556 Ulcerative colitis
AHA: 3Q, '99, 8
DEF: Chronic inflammation of mucosal lining of intestinal tract; may be single area or entire colon.

556.0 Ulcerative (chronic) enterocolitis
556.1 Ulcerative (chronic) ileocolitis
556.2 Ulcerative (chronic) proctitis
556.3 Ulcerative (chronic) proctosigmoiditis
556.4 Pseudopolyposis of colon
556.5 Left-sided ulcerative (chronic) colitis
556.6 Universal ulcerative (chronic) colitis
Pancolitis
556.8 Other ulcerative colitis
556.9 Ulcerative colitis, unspecified
Ulcerative enteritis NOS
AHA: 1Q, '03, 10

✓4th 557 Vascular insufficiency of intestine
EXCLUDES necrotizing enterocolitis of the newborn (777.5)
DEF: Inadequacy of intestinal vessels.

557.0 Acute vascular insufficiency of intestine
Acute:
  hemorrhagic enterocolitis
  ischemic colitis, enteritis, or enterocolitis
  massive necrosis of intestine
Bowel infarction
Embolism of mesenteric artery
Fulminant enterocolitis
Hemorrhagic necrosis of intestine
Infarction of appendices epiploicae
Intestinal gangrene
Intestinal infarction (acute) (agnogenic)
  (hemorrhagic) (nonocclusive)
Mesenteric infarction (embolic) (thrombotic)
Necrosis of intestine
Terminal hemorrhagic enteropathy
Thrombosis of mesenteric artery
AHA: 4Q, '01, 53

557.1 Chronic vascular insufficiency of intestine
Angina, abdominal
Chronic ischemic colitis, enteritis, or enterocolitis
Ischemic stricture of intestine
Mesenteric:
  angina
  artery syndrome (superior)
  vascular insufficiency
AHA: 3Q, '96, 9; 4Q, '90, 4; N-D, '86, 11; N-D, '84, 7

557.9 Unspecified vascular insufficiency of intestine
Alimentary pain due to vascular insufficiency
Ischemic colitis, enteritis, or enterocolitis NOS

✓4th 558 Other and unspecified noninfectious gastroenteritis and colitis
EXCLUDES infectious:
  colitis, enteritis, or gastroenteritis (009.0-009.1)
  diarrhea (009.2-009.3)

558.1 Gastroenteritis and colitis due to radiation
Radiation enterocolitis

558.2 Toxic gastroenteritis and colitis
Use additional E code, if desired, to identify cause

558.3 Allergic gastroenteritis and colitis
Use additional code to identify type of food allergy
  (V15.01-V15.05)
AHA: 1Q, '03, 12; 4Q, '00, 42
DEF: True immunoglobulin E (IgE)-mediated allergic reaction of the lining of the stomach, intestines, or colon to food proteins; causes nausea, vomiting, diarrhea, and abdominal cramping.

558.9 Other and unspecified noninfectious gastroenteritis and colitis
Colitis
Enteritis
Gastroenteritis   } NOS, dietetic, or
Ileitis   noninfectious
Jejunitis
Sigmoiditis
AHA: 3Q, '99, 4, 6; N-D, '87, 7

OTHER DISEASES OF INTESTINES AND PERITONEUM (560-569)

✓4th 560 Intestinal obstruction without mention of hernia
EXCLUDES duodenum (537.2-537.3)
  inguinal hernia with obstruction (550.1)
  intestinal obstruction complicating hernia
    (552.0-552.9)
  mesenteric:
    embolism (557.0)
    infarction (557.0)
    thrombosis (557.0)
  neonatal intestinal obstruction (277.01, 777.1-777.2, 777.4)

560.0 Intussusception
Intussusception (colon) (intestine) (rectum)
Invagination of intestine or colon
EXCLUDES intussusception of appendix (543.9)
AHA: 4Q, '98, 82
DEF: Prolapse of a bowel section into adjacent section; occurs primarily in children; symptoms include paroxysmal pain, vomiting, presence of lower abdominal tumor and blood, and mucous passage from rectum.

560.1 Paralytic ileus
Adynamic ileus
Ileus (of intestine) (of bowel) (of colon)
Paralysis of intestine or colon
EXCLUDES gallstone ileus (560.31)
AHA: J-F, '87, 13
DEF: Obstruction of ileus due to inhibited bowel motility.

560.2 Volvulus
Knotting
Strangulation } of intestine, bowel, or colon
Torsion
Twist
DEF: Entanglement of bowel; causes obstruction; may compromise bowel circulation.

DIGESTIVE SYSTEM

560.3–564.6

Volvulus, Diverticulitis

- √5th **560.3 Impaction of intestine**
  - **560.30 Impaction of intestine, unspecified**
    - Impaction of colon
  - **560.31 Gallstone ileus**
    - Obstruction of intestine by gallstone
  - **560.39 Other**
    - Concretion of intestine   Fecal impaction
    - Enterolith
    - AHA: 4Q, '98, 38

- √5th **560.8 Other specified intestinal obstruction**
  - **560.81 Intestinal or peritoneal adhesions with obstruction (postoperative) (postinfection)**
    - EXCLUDES adhesions without obstruction (568.0)
    - AHA: 4Q, '95, 55; 3Q, '95, 6; N-D, '87, 9
    - DEF: Obstruction of peritoneum or intestine due to abnormal union of tissues.
  - **560.89 Other**
    - Acute pseudo-obstruction of intestine
    - Mural thickening causing obstruction
    - EXCLUDES ischemic stricture of intestine (557.1)
    - AHA: 2Q, '97, 3; 1Q, '88, 6

- **560.9 Unspecified intestinal obstruction**
  - Enterostenosis
  - Obstruction
  - Occlusion   } of intestine or colon
  - Stenosis
  - Stricture
  - EXCLUDES congenital stricture or stenosis of intestine (751.1-751.2)

- √4th **562 Diverticula of intestine**
  - Use additional code to identify any associated: peritonitis (567.0-567.9)
  - EXCLUDES congenital diverticulum of colon (751.5)
  - diverticulum of appendix (543.9)
  - Meckel's diverticulum (751.0)
  - AHA: 4Q, '91, 25; J-F, '85, 1

- √5th **562.0 Small intestine**
  - **562.00 Diverticulosis of small intestine (without mention of hemorrhage)**
    - Diverticulosis:
      - duodenum
      - ileum   } without mention of diverticulitis
      - jejunum
    - DEF: Saclike herniations of mucous lining of small intestine.
  - **562.01 Diverticulitis of small intestine (without mention of hemorrhage)**
    - Diverticulitis (with diverticulosis):
      - duodenum
      - ileum
      - jejunum
      - small intestine
    - DEF: Inflamed saclike herniations of mucous lining of small intestine.
  - **562.02 Diverticulosis of small intestine with hemorrhage**
  - **562.03 Diverticulitis of small intestine with hemorrhage**

- √5th **562.1 Colon**
  - **562.10 Diverticulosis of colon (without mention of hemorrhage)**
    - Diverticulosis:
      - NOS
      - intestine (large)   } without mention of diverticulitis
      - Diverticular disease (colon)
    - AHA: ▶3Q, '05, 17;◄ 3Q, '02, 15; 4Q, '90, 21; J-F, '85, 5
    - DEF: Saclike herniations of mucous lining of large intestine
  - **562.11 Diverticulitis of colon (without mention of hemorrhage)**
    - Diverticulitis (with diverticulosis):
      - NOS   intestine (large)
      - colon
    - AHA: 1Q, '96, 14; J-F, '85, 5
    - DEF: Inflamed saclike herniations of mucosal lining of large intestine.
  - **562.12 Diverticulosis of colon with hemorrhage**
  - **562.13 Diverticulitis of colon with hemorrhage**

- √4th **564 Functional digestive disorders, not elsewhere classified**
  - EXCLUDES functional disorders of stomach (536.0-536.9)
  - those specified as psychogenic (306.4)

- √5th **564.0 Constipation**
  - AHA: 4Q, '01, 45
  - **564.00 Constipation, unspecified**
  - **564.01 Slow transit constipation**
    - DEF: Delay in the transit of fecal material through the colon secondary to smooth muscle dysfunction or decreased peristaltic contractions along the colon: also called colonic inertia or delayed transit.
  - **564.02 Outlet dysfunction constipation**
    - DEF: Failure to relax the paradoxical contractions of the striated pelvic floor muscles during the attempted defecation.
  - **564.09 Other constipation**

- **564.1 Irritable bowel syndrome**
  - Irritable colon   Spastic colon
  - AHA: 1Q, '88, 6
  - DEF: Functional gastrointestinal disorder (FGID); symptoms following meals include diarrhea, constipation, abdominal pain; other symptoms include bloating, gas, distended abdomen, nausea, vomiting, appetite loss, emotional distress, and depression.

- **564.2 Postgastric surgery syndromes**
  - Dumping syndrome   Postgastrectomy syndrome
  - Jejunal syndrome   Postvagotomy syndrome
  - EXCLUDES malnutrition following gastrointestinal surgery (579.3)
  - postgastrojejunostomy ulcer (534.0-534.9)
  - AHA: 1Q, '95, 11

- **564.3 Vomiting following gastrointestinal surgery**
  - Vomiting (bilious) following gastrointestinal surgery

- **564.4 Other postoperative functional disorders**
  - Diarrhea following gastrointestinal surgery
  - EXCLUDES colostomy and enterostomy complications (569.60-569.69)

- **564.5 Functional diarrhea**
  - EXCLUDES diarrhea:
    - NOS (787.91)
    - psychogenic (306.4)
  - DEF: Diarrhea with no detectable organic cause.

- **564.6 Anal spasm**
  - Proctalgia fugax

N Newborn Age: 0   P Pediatric Age: 0-17   M Maternity Age: 12-55   A Adult Age: 15-124

DIGESTIVE SYSTEM

Rectum and Anus

Anal Fistula and Abscess

564.7 Megacolon, other than Hirschsprung's
Dilatation of colon
EXCLUDES megacolon:
congenital [Hirschsprung's] (751.3)
toxic (556)
DEF: Enlarged colon; congenital or acquired; can occur acutely or become chronic.

√5th 564.8 Other specified functional disorders of intestine
EXCLUDES malabsorption (579.0-579.9)
AHA: 1Q, '88, 6

564.81 Neurogenic bowel
AHA: 1Q, '01, 12; 4Q, '98, 45
DEF: Disorder of bowel due to spinal cord lesion above conus medullaris; symptoms include precipitous micturition, nocturia, catheter intolerance, headache, sweating, nasal obstruction and spastic contractions.

564.89 Other functional disorders of intestine
Atony of colon
DEF: Absence of normal bowel tone or strength.

564.9 Unspecified functional disorder of intestine

√4th 565 Anal fissure and fistula

565.0 Anal fissure
Tear of anus, nontraumatic
EXCLUDES traumatic (863.89, 863.99)
DEF: Ulceration of cleft at anal mucosa; causes pain, itching, bleeding, infection, and sphincter spasm; may occur with hemorrhoids.

565.1 Anal fistula
Fistula: Fistula:
  anorectal   rectum to skin
  rectal
EXCLUDES fistula of rectum to internal organs—
see Alphabetic Index
ischiorectal fistula (566)
rectovaginal fistula (619.1)
DEF: Abnormal opening on cutaneous surface near anus; may lack connection with rectum.

566 Abscess of anal and rectal regions
Abscess: Cellulitis:
  ischiorectal   anal
  perianal   perirectal
  perirectal   rectal
                Ischiorectal fistula

√4th 567 Peritonitis and retroperitoneal infections
EXCLUDES peritonitis:
benign paroxysmal ▶(277.31)◀
pelvic, female (614.5, 614.7)
periodic familial ▶(277.31)◀
puerperal (670)
with or following:
abortion (634-638 with .0, 639.0)
appendicitis (540.0-540.1)
ectopic or molar pregnancy (639.0)
DEF: Inflammation of the peritoneal cavity.

567.0 Peritonitis in infectious diseases classified elsewhere
Code first underlying disease
EXCLUDES peritonitis:
gonococcal (098.86)
syphilitic (095.2)
tuberculous (014.0)

567.1 Pneumococcal peritonitis

√5th 567.2 Other suppurative peritonitis
AHA: 4Q, '05, 74; 2Q, '01, 11, 12; 3Q, '99, 9; 2Q, '98, 19

567.21 Peritonitis (acute) generalized
Pelvic peritonitis, male

567.22 Peritoneal abscess
Abscess (of):   Abscess (of):
  abdominopelvic   retrocecal
  mesenteric   subdiaphragmatic
  omentum   subhepatic
  peritoneum   subphrenic

567.23 Spontaneous bacterial peritonitis
EXCLUDES ▶ bacterial peritonitis NOS (567.29)◀

567.29 Other suppurative peritonitis
Subphrenic peritonitis

√5th 567.3 Retroperitoneal infections
AHA: 4Q, '05, 74

567.31 Psoas muscle abscess
DEF: Infection that extends into or around the psoas muscle that connects the lumbar vertebrae to the femur.

567.38 Other retroperitoneal abscess
AHA: 4Q, '05, 77

567.39 Other retroperitoneal infections

√5th 567.8 Other specified peritonitis
AHA: 4Q, '05, 74

567.81 Choleperitonitis
Peritonitis due to bile
DEF: Inflammation or infection due to presence of bile in the peritoneum resulting from rupture of the bile passages or gallbladder.

Psoas Muscle Abscess

567.82 Sclerosing mesenteritis
- Fat necrosis of peritoneum
- (Idiopathic) sclerosing mesenteric fibrosis
- Mesenteric lipodystrophy
- Mesenteric panniculitis
- Retractile mesenteritis

AHA: ▶4Q, '05, 77◀

DEF: ▶Inflammatory processes involving the mesenteric fat; progresses to fibrosis and necrosis of tissue.◀

567.89 Other specified peritonitis
- Chronic proliferative peritonitis
- Mesenteric saponification
- Peritonitis due to urine

567.9 Unspecified peritonitis
- Peritonitis: NOS
- Peritonitis: of unspecified cause

AHA: 1Q, '04, 10

568 Other disorders of peritoneum

568.0 Peritoneal adhesions (postoperative) (postinfection)
- Adhesions (of):
  - abdominal (wall)
  - diaphragm
  - intestine
  - male pelvis
- Adhesions (of):
  - mesenteric
  - omentum
  - stomach
- Adhesive bands

EXCLUDES adhesions:
  pelvic, female (614.6)
  with obstruction:
    duodenum (537.3)
    intestine (560.81)

AHA: 3Q, '03, 7, 11; 4Q, '95, 55; 3Q, '95, 7; S-O, '85, 11

DEF: Abnormal union of tissues in peritoneum.

568.8 Other specified disorders of peritoneum

568.81 Hemoperitoneum (nontraumatic)

568.82 Peritoneal effusion (chronic)

EXCLUDES ascites NOS (789.5)

DEF: Persistent leakage of fluid within peritoneal cavity.

568.89 Other
- Peritoneal: cyst
- Peritoneal: granuloma

568.9 Unspecified disorder of peritoneum

569 Other disorders of intestine

569.0 Anal and rectal polyp
- Anal and rectal polyp NOS

EXCLUDES adenomatous anal and rectal polyp (211.4)

569.1 Rectal prolapse
- Procidentia:
  - anus (sphincter)
  - rectum (sphincter)
- Proctoptosis
- Prolapse:
  - anal canal
  - rectal mucosa

EXCLUDES prolapsed hemorrhoids (455.2, 455.5)

569.2 Stenosis of rectum and anus
- Stricture of anus (sphincter)

569.3 Hemorrhage of rectum and anus

EXCLUDES gastrointestinal bleeding NOS (578.9)
  melena (578.1)

AHA: ▶3Q, '05, 17◀

569.4 Other specified disorders of rectum and anus

569.41 Ulcer of anus and rectum
- Solitary ulcer } of anus (sphincter) or
- Stercoral ulcer }   rectum (sphincter)

569.42 Anal or rectal pain

AHA: 1Q, '03, 8; 1Q, '96, 13

569.49 Other
- Granuloma } of rectum (sphincter)
- Rupture }
- Hypertrophy of anal papillae
- Proctitis NOS

EXCLUDES fistula of rectum to:
  internal organs—see Alphabetic Index
  skin (565.1)
  hemorrhoids (455.0-455.9)
  incontinence of sphincter ani (787.6)

569.5 Abscess of intestine

EXCLUDES appendiceal abscess (540.1)

569.6 Colostomy and enterostomy complications

AHA: 4Q, '95, 58

DEF: Complication in a surgically created opening, from intestine to surface skin.

569.60 Colostomy and enterostomy complication, unspecified

569.61 Infection of colostomy or enterostomy
- Use additional code to identify organism (041.00-041.9)
- Use additional code to specify type of infection, such as:
  - abscess or cellulitis of abdomen (682.2)
  - septicemia (038.0-038.9)

569.62 Mechanical complication of colostomy and enterostomy
- Malfunction of colostomy and enterostomy

AHA: ▶2Q, '05, 11;◀ 1Q, '03, 10; 4Q, '98, 44

569.69 Other complication
- Fistula
- Hernia
- Prolapse

AHA: 3Q, '98, 16

569.8 Other specified disorders of intestine

AHA: 4Q, '91, 25

569.81 Fistula of intestine, excluding rectum and anus
- Fistula:
  - abdominal wall
  - enterocolic
- Fistula:
  - enteroenteric
  - ileorectal

EXCLUDES fistula of intestine to internal organs—see Alphabetic Index
  persistent postoperative fistula (998.6)

AHA: 3Q, '99, 8

569.82 Ulceration of intestine
- Primary ulcer of intestine
- Ulceration of colon

EXCLUDES that with perforation (569.83)

569.83 Perforation of intestine

569.84 Angiodysplasia of intestine (without mention of hemorrhage)

AHA: 3Q, '96, 10; 4Q, '90, 4; 4Q, '90, 21

DEF: Small vascular abnormalities of the intestinal tract without bleeding problems.

569.85 Angiodysplasia of intestine with hemorrhage

AHA: 3Q, '96, 9

DEF: Small vascular abnormalities of the intestinal tract with bleeding problems.

569.86 Dieulafoy lesion (hemorrhagic) of intestine

AHA: 4Q, '02, 60-61

Tabular List — DIGESTIVE SYSTEM

569.89 Other
Enteroptosis
Granuloma } of intestine
Prolapse

Pericolitis
Perisigmoiditis
Visceroptosis

EXCLUDES gangrene of intestine, mesentery, or omentum (557.0)
hemorrhage of intestine NOS (578.9)
obstruction of intestine (560.0-560.9)

AHA: 3Q, '96, 9

569.9 Unspecified disorder of intestine

OTHER DISEASES OF DIGESTIVE SYSTEM (570-579)

570 Acute and subacute necrosis of liver
Acute hepatic failure
Acute or subacute hepatitis, not specified as infective
Necrosis of liver (acute) (diffuse) (massive) (subacute)
Parenchymatous degeneration of liver
Yellow atrophy (liver) (acute) (subacute)

EXCLUDES icterus gravis of newborn (773.0-773.2)
serum hepatitis (070.2-070.3)
that with:
    abortion (634-638 with .7, 639.8)
    ectopic or molar pregnancy (639.8)
    pregnancy, childbirth, or the puerperium (646.7)
viral hepatitis (070.0-070.9)

AHA: 2Q, '05, 9; 1Q, '00, 22

√4ᵗʰ 571 Chronic liver disease and cirrhosis

571.0 Alcoholic fatty liver A
571.1 Acute alcoholic hepatitis A
Acute alcoholic liver disease
AHA: 2Q, '02, 4

571.2 Alcoholic cirrhosis of liver A
Florid cirrhosis   Laennec's cirrhosis (alcoholic)
AHA: 2Q, '02, 4; 1Q, '02, 3; N-D, '85, 14
DEF: Fibrosis and dysfunction, of liver; due to alcoholic liver disease.

571.3 Alcoholic liver damage, unspecified A

√5ᵗʰ 571.4 Chronic hepatitis
EXCLUDES viral hepatitis (acute) (chronic) (070.0-070.9)

571.40 Chronic hepatitis, unspecified
571.41 Chronic persistent hepatitis
571.49 Other
Chronic hepatitis: Recurrent hepatitis
    active
    aggressive
AHA: 3Q, '99, 19; N-D, '85, 14

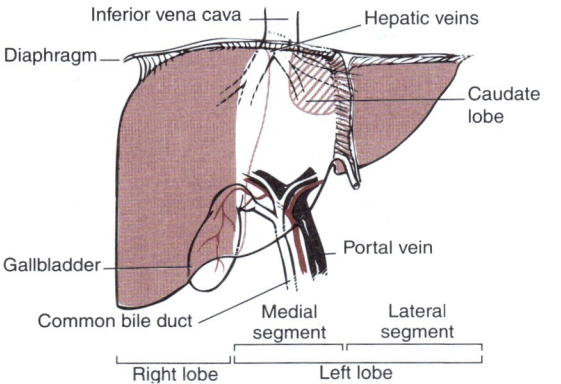
Liver

571.5 Cirrhosis of liver without mention of alcohol
Cirrhosis of liver: Cirrhosis of liver:
    NOS   postnecrotic
    cryptogenic   Healed yellow atrophy
    macronodular   (liver)
    micronodular   Portal cirrhosis
    posthepatitic
DEF: Fibrosis and dysfunction of liver; not alcohol related.

571.6 Biliary cirrhosis
Chronic nonsuppurative destructive cholangitis
Cirrhosis:
    cholangitic
    cholestatic

571.8 Other chronic nonalcoholic liver disease
Chronic yellow atrophy (liver)
Fatty liver, without mention of alcohol
AHA: 2Q, '96, 12

571.9 Unspecified chronic liver disease without mention of alcohol

√4ᵗʰ 572 Liver abscess and sequelae of chronic liver disease
572.0 Abscess of liver
EXCLUDES amebic liver abscess (006.3)

572.1 Portal pyemia
Phlebitis of portal vein   Pylephlebitis
Portal thrombophlebitis   Pylethrombophlebitis
DEF: Inflammation of portal vein or branches; may be due to intestinal disease; symptoms include fever, chills, jaundice, sweating, and abscess in various body parts.

572.2 Hepatic coma
Hepatic encephalopathy   Portal-systemic
Hepatocerebral intoxication   encephalopathy
AHA: 2Q, '05, 9; 1Q, '02, 3; 3Q, '95, 14

572.3 Portal hypertension
AHA: 3Q, '05, 15
DEF: Abnormally high blood pressure in the portal vein.

572.4 Hepatorenal syndrome
EXCLUDES that following delivery (674.8)
AHA: 3Q, '93, 15
DEF: Hepatic and renal failure characterized by cirrhosis with ascites or obstructive jaundice, oliguria, and low sodium concentration.

572.8 Other sequelae of chronic liver disease

√4ᵗʰ 573 Other disorders of liver
EXCLUDES amyloid or lardaceous degeneration of liver ▶(277.39)◀
congenital cystic disease of liver (751.62)
glycogen infiltration of liver (271.0)
hepatomegaly NOS (789.1)
portal vein obstruction (452)

573.0 Chronic passive congestion of liver
DEF: Blood accumulation in liver tissue.

573.1 Hepatitis in viral diseases classified elsewhere
Code first underlying disease as:
    Coxsackie virus disease (074.8)
    cytomegalic inclusion virus disease (078.5)
    infectious mononucleosis (075)
EXCLUDES hepatitis (in):
    mumps (072.71)
    viral (070.0-070.9)
    yellow fever (060.0-060.9)

573.2 Hepatitis in other infectious diseases classified elsewhere
Code first underlying disease, as:
    malaria (084.9)
EXCLUDES hepatitis in:
    late syphilis (095.3)
    secondary syphilis (091.62)
    toxoplasmosis (130.5)

573.3 Hepatitis, unspecified
Toxic (noninfectious) hepatitis
Use additional E code to identify cause
AHA: 3Q, '98, 3, 4; 4Q, '90, 26

573.4–575.6 DIGESTIVE SYSTEM — Tabular List

- **573.4** Hepatic infarction
- **573.8** Other specified disorders of liver
  - Hepatoptosis
- **573.9** Unspecified disorder of liver

√4th **574 Cholelithiasis**

The following fifth-digit subclassification is for use with category 574:
- 0 without mention of obstruction
- 1 with obstruction

√5th **574.0 Calculus of gallbladder with acute cholecystitis**
Biliary calculus
Calculus of cystic duct } with acute cholecystitis
Cholelithiasis
Any condition classifiable to 574.2 with acute cholecystitis
AHA: 4Q, '96, 32

√5th **574.1 Calculus of gallbladder with other cholecystitis**
Biliary calculus
Calculus of cystic duct } with cholecystitis
Cholelithiasis
Cholecystitis with cholelithiasis NOS
Any condition classifiable to 574.2 with cholecystitis (chronic)
AHA: 3Q, '99, 9; 4Q, '96, 32, 69; 2Q, '96, 13; For code 574.10: 1Q, '03, 5

√5th **574.2 Calculus of gallbladder without mention of cholecystitis**
Biliary:
  calculus NOS
  colic NOS
Calculus of cystic duct
Cholelithiasis NOS
Colic (recurrent) of gallbladder
Gallstone (impacted)
AHA: For code 574.20: 1Q, '88, 14

√5th **574.3 Calculus of bile duct with acute cholecystitis**
Calculus of bile duct [any] } with acute cholecystitis
Choledocholithiasis
Any condition classifiable to 574.5 with acute cholecystitis

√5th **574.4 Calculus of bile duct with other cholecystitis**
Calculus of bile duct [any] } with cholecystitis
Choledocholithiasis   (chronic)
Any condition classifiable to 574.5 with cholecystitis (chronic)

√5th **574.5 Calculus of bile duct without mention of cholecystitis**
Calculus of:
  bile duct [any]
  common duct
  hepatic duct
Choledocholithiasis
Hepatic:
  colic (recurrent)
  lithiasis
AHA: 3Q, '94, 11

√5th **574.6 Calculus of gallbladder and bile duct with acute cholecystitis**
Any condition classifiable to 574.0 and 574.3
AHA: 4Q, '96, 32

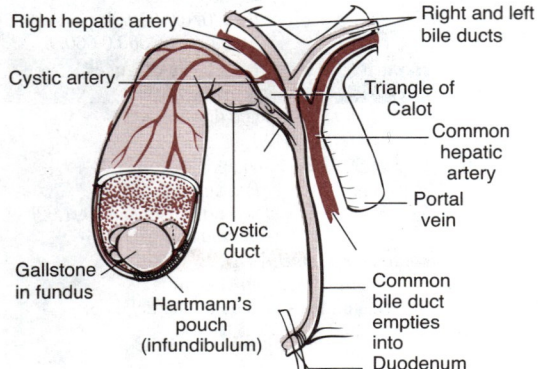
Gallbladder and Bile Ducts

√5th **574.7 Calculus of gallbladder and bile duct with other cholecystitis**
Any condition classifiable to 574.1 and 574.4
AHA: 4Q, '96, 32

√5th **574.8 Calculus of gallbladder and bile duct with acute and chronic cholecystitis**
Any condition classifiable to 574.6 and 574.7
AHA: 4Q, '96, 32

√5th **574.9 Calculus of gallbladder and bile duct without cholecystitis**
Any condition classifiable to 574.2 and 574.5
AHA: 4Q, '96, 32

√4th **575 Other disorders of gallbladder**

575.0 Acute cholecystitis
Abscess of gallbladder
Angiocholecystitis
Cholecystitis:
  emphysematous (acute)
  gangrenous   } without mention of calculus
  suppurative
Empyema of gallbladder
Gangrene of gallbladder

EXCLUDES that with:
  acute and chronic cholecystitis (575.12)
  choledocholithiasis (574.3)
  choledocholithiasis and cholelithiasis (574.6)
  cholelithiasis (574.0)
AHA: 3Q, '91, 17

√5th **575.1 Other cholecystitis**
Cholecystitis:
  NOS   } without mention of calculus
  chronic

EXCLUDES that with:
  choledocholithiasis (574.4)
  choledocholithiasis and cholelithiasis (574.8)
  cholelithiasis (574.1)
AHA: 4Q, '96, 32

- **575.10 Cholecystitis, unspecified**
  Cholecystitis NOS
- **575.11** Chronic cholecystitis
- **575.12** Acute and chronic cholecystitis
  AHA: 4Q, '97, 52; 4Q, '96, 32

575.2 Obstruction of gallbladder
Occlusion
Stenosis   } of cystic duct or gallbladder without mention of calculus
Stricture

EXCLUDES that with calculus (574.0-574.2 with fifth-digit 1)

575.3 Hydrops of gallbladder
Mucocele of gallbladder
AHA: 2Q, '89, 13
DEF: Serous fluid accumulation in bladder.

575.4 Perforation of gallbladder
Rupture of cystic duct or gallbladder

575.5 Fistula of gallbladder
Fistula: Fistula:
  cholecystoduodenal   cholecystoenteric

575.6 Cholesterolosis of gallbladder
Strawberry gallbladder
AHA: 4Q, '90, 17
DEF: Cholesterol deposits in gallbladder tissue.

DIGESTIVE SYSTEM

575.8 Other specified disorders of gallbladder
Adhesions
Atrophy
Cyst   } (of) cystic duct or gallbladder
Hypertrophy
Nonfunctioning
Ulcer

Biliary dyskinesia
  EXCLUDES Hartmann's pouch of intestine (V44.3)
            nonvisualization of gallbladder (793.3)
AHA: 4Q, '90, 26; 2Q, '89, 13

575.9 Unspecified disorder of gallbladder

√4th **576 Other disorders of biliary tract**
  EXCLUDES that involving the:
            cystic duct (575.0-575.9)
            gallbladder (575.0-575.9)

576.0 Postcholecystectomy syndrome
AHA: 1Q, '88, 10
DEF: Jaundice or abdominal pain following cholecystectomy.

576.1 Cholangitis
Cholangitis: Cholangitis:
  NOS   recurrent
  acute   sclerosing
  ascending   secondary
  chronic   stenosing
  primary   suppurative
AHA: 2Q, '99, 13

576.2 Obstruction of bile duct
Occlusion } of bile duct, except cystic
Stenosis   } duct, without mention
Stricture } of calculus
  EXCLUDES congenital (751.61)
            that with calculus (574.3-574.5 with fifth-digit 1)
AHA: 3Q, '03, 17-18; 1Q, '01, 8; 2Q, '99, 13

576.3 Perforation of bile duct
Rupture of bile duct, except cystic duct

576.4 Fistula of bile duct
Choledochoduodenal fistula

576.5 Spasm of sphincter of Oddi

576.8 Other specified disorders of biliary tract
Adhesions
Atrophy
Cyst   } of bile duct [any]
Hypertrophy
Stasis
Ulcer
  EXCLUDES congenital choledochal cyst (751.69)
AHA: 3Q, '03, 17; 2Q, '99, 14

576.9 Unspecified disorder of biliary tract

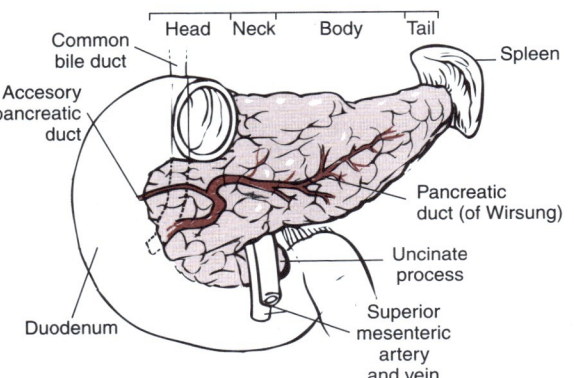

√4th **577 Diseases of pancreas**

577.0 Acute pancreatitis
Abscess of pancreas   Pancreatitis:
Necrosis of pancreas: acute (recurrent)
  acute   apoplectic
  infective   hemorrhagic
Pancreatitis: subacute
  NOS   suppurative
  EXCLUDES mumps pancreatitis (072.3)
AHA: 3Q, '99, 9; 2Q, '98, 19; 2Q, '96, 13; 2Q, '89, 9

577.1 Chronic pancreatitis
Chronic pancreatitis: Pancreatitis:
  NOS   painless
  infectious   recurrent
  interstitial   relapsing
AHA: 1Q, '01, 8; 2Q, '96, 13; 3Q, '94, 11

577.2 Cyst and pseudocyst of pancreas

577.8 Other specified diseases of pancreas
Atrophy
Calculus   } of pancreas
Cirrhosis
Fibrosis

Pancreatic: Pancreatic:
  infantilism   necrosis:
  necrosis: fat
    NOS   Pancreatolithiasis
    aseptic
  EXCLUDES fibrocystic disease of pancreas (277.00-277.09)
            islet cell tumor of pancreas (211.7)
            pancreatic steatorrhea (579.4)
AHA: 1Q, '01, 8

577.9 Unspecified disease of pancreas

√4th **578 Gastrointestinal hemorrhage**
  EXCLUDES that with mention of:
            angiodysplasia of stomach and duodenum (537.83)
            angiodysplasia of intestine (569.85)
            diverticulitis, intestine:
              large (562.13)
              small (562.03)
            diverticulosis, intestine:
              large (562.12)
              small (562.02)
            gastritis and duodenitis (535.0-535.6)
            ulcer:
              duodenal, gastric, gastrojejuunal or peptic (531.00-534.91)
AHA: 2Q, '92, 9; 4Q, '90, 20

578.0 Hematemesis
Vomiting of blood
AHA: 2Q, '02, 4

578.1 Blood in stool
Melena
  EXCLUDES melena of the newborn (772.4, 777.3)
            occult blood (792.1)
AHA: 2Q, '92, 8

578.9 Hemorrhage of gastrointestinal tract, unspecified
Gastric hemorrhage
Intestinal hemorrhage
AHA: ▶3Q, '05, 17;◀ N-D, '86, 9

579 Intestinal malabsorption

579.0 Celiac disease
Celiac: Gee (-Herter) disease
  crisis Gluten enteropathy
  infantilism Idiopathic steatorrhea
  rickets Nontropical sprue

DEF: Malabsorption syndrome due to gluten consumption; symptoms include fetid, bulky, frothy, oily stools; distended abdomen, gas, weight loss, asthenia, electrolyte depletion and vitamin B, D and K deficiency.

579.1 Tropical sprue
Sprue: Tropical steatorrhea
  NOS
  tropical

DEF: Diarrhea, occurs in tropics; may be due to enteric infection and malnutrition.

579.2 Blind loop syndrome
Postoperative blind loop syndrome

DEF: Obstruction or impaired passage in small intestine due to alterations, from strictures or surgery; causes stasis, abnormal bacterial flora, diarrhea, weight loss, multiple vitamin deficiency, and megaloblastic anemia.

579.3 Other and unspecified postsurgical nonabsorption
Hypoglycemia ⎫ following gastrointestinal
Malnutrition ⎭   surgery

AHA: 4Q, '03, 104

579.4 Pancreatic steatorrhea
DEF: Excess fat in feces due to absence of pancreatic juice in intestine.

579.8 Other specified intestinal malabsorption
Enteropathy: Steatorrhea (chronic)
  exudative
  protein-losing

AHA: 1Q, '88, 6

579.9 Unspecified intestinal malabsorption
Malabsorption syndrome NOS

AHA: 4Q, '04, 59

GENITOURINARY SYSTEM

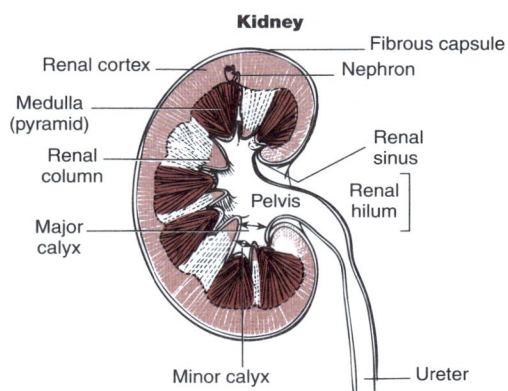

10. DISEASES OF THE GENITOURINARY SYSTEM (580-629)

NEPHRITIS, NEPHROTIC SYNDROME, AND NEPHROSIS (580-589)

EXCLUDES ▶hypertensive chronic kidney disease (403.00-403.91, 404.00-404.93)◀

580 Acute glomerulonephritis
   INCLUDES acute nephritis
   DEF: Acute, severe inflammation in tuft of capillaries that filter the kidneys.

- **580.0 With lesion of proliferative glomerulonephritis**
  - Acute (diffuse) proliferative glomerulonephritis
  - Acute poststreptococcal glomerulonephritis
- **580.4 With lesion of rapidly progressive glomerulonephritis**
  - Acute nephritis with lesion of necrotizing glomerulitis
  - DEF: Acute glomerulonephritis; progresses to ESRD with diffuse epithelial proliferation.
- **580.8 With other specified pathological lesion in kidney**
  - **580.81 Acute glomerulonephritis in diseases classified elsewhere**
    - Code first underlying disease, as:
      - infectious hepatitis (070.0-070.9)
      - mumps (072.79)
      - subacute bacterial endocarditis (421.0)
      - typhoid fever (002.0)
  - **580.89 Other**
    - Glomerulonephritis, acute, with lesion of:
      - exudative nephritis
      - interstitial (diffuse) (focal) nephritis
- **580.9 Acute glomerulonephritis with unspecified pathological lesion in kidney**
  - Glomerulonephritis:
    - NOS
    - hemorrhagic
  - Nephritis
  - Nephropathy
  } specified as acute

581 Nephrotic syndrome
   DEF: Disease process marked by symptoms such as; extensive edema, notable proteinuria, hypoalbuminemia, and susceptibility to intercurrent infections.

- **581.0 With lesion of proliferative glomerulonephritis**
- **581.1 With lesion of membranous glomerulonephritis**
  - Epimembranous nephritis
  - Idiopathic membranous glomerular disease
  - Nephrotic syndrome with lesion of:
    - focal glomerulosclerosis
    - sclerosing membranous glomerulonephritis
    - segmental hyalinosis
- **581.2 With lesion of membranoproliferative glomerulonephritis**
  - Nephrotic syndrome with lesion (of):
    - endothelial
    - hypocomplementemic persistent
    - lobular
    - mesangiocapillary
    - mixed membranous and proliferative
    } glomerulonephritis
  - DEF: Glomerulonephritis combined with clinical features of nephrotic syndrome; characterized by uneven thickening of glomerular capillary walls and mesangial cell increase; slowly progresses to ESRD.
- **581.3 With lesion of minimal change glomerulonephritis**
  - Foot process disease
  - Lipoid nephrosis
  - Minimal change:
    - glomerular disease
    - glomerulitis
    - nephrotic syndrome
- **581.8 With other specified pathological lesion in kidney**
  - **581.81 Nephrotic syndrome in diseases classified elsewhere**
    - Code first underlying disease, as:
      - amyloidosis ▶(277.30-277.39)◀
      - diabetes mellitus (250.4)
      - malaria (084.9)
      - polyarteritis (446.0)
      - systemic lupus erythematosus (710.0)
    - **EXCLUDES** nephrosis in epidemic hemorrhagic fever (078.6)
    - AHA: 3Q, '91, 8,12; S-O, '85, 3
  - **581.89 Other**
    - Glomerulonephritis with edema and lesion of:
      - exudative nephritis
      - interstitial (diffuse) (focal) nephritis
- **581.9 Nephrotic syndrome with unspecified pathological lesion in kidney**
  - Glomerulonephritis with edema NOS
  - Nephritis:
    - nephrotic NOS
    - with edema NOS
  - Nephrosis NOS
  - Renal disease with edema NOS

582 Chronic glomerulonephritis
   INCLUDES chronic nephritis
   DEF: Slow progressive type of nephritis characterized by inflammation of the capillary loops in the glomeruli of the kidney, which leads to renal failure.

- **582.0 With lesion of proliferative glomerulonephritis**
  - Chronic (diffuse) proliferative glomerulonephritis
- **582.1 With lesion of membranous glomerulonephritis**
  - Chronic glomerulonephritis:
    - membranous
    - sclerosing
  - Focal glomerulosclerosis
  - Segmental hyalinosis
  - AHA: S-O, '84, 16

582.2 **With lesion of membranoproliferative glomerulonephritis**
Chronic glomerulonephritis:
  endothelial
  hypocomplementemic persistent
  lobular
  membranoproliferative
  mesangiocapillary
  mixed membranous and proliferative
DEF: Chronic glomerulonephritis with mesangial cell proliferation.

582.4 **With lesion of rapidly progressive glomerulonephritis**
Chronic nephritis with lesion of necrotizing glomerulitis
DEF: Chronic glomerulonephritis rapidly progresses to ESRD; marked by diffuse epithelial proliferation.

√5th **582.8** **With other specified pathological lesion in kidney**
582.81 Chronic glomerulonephritis in diseases classified elsewhere
Code first underlying disease, as:
  amyloidosis ►(277.30-277.39)◄
  systemic lupus erythematosus (710.0)
582.89 Other
Chronic glomerulonephritis with lesion of:
  exudative nephritis
  interstitial (diffuse) (focal) nephritis

582.9 **Chronic glomerulonephritis with unspecified pathological lesion in kidney**
Glomerulonephritis:
  NOS
  hemorrhagic   } specified as chronic
Nephritis
Nephropathy
AHA: 2Q, '01, 12

√4th **583 Nephritis and nephropathy, not specified as acute or chronic**
INCLUDES "renal disease" so stated, not specified as acute or chronic but with stated pathology or cause

583.0 **With lesion of proliferative glomerulonephritis**
Proliferative:
  glomerulonephritis   Proliferative:
  (diffuse) NOS   nephritis NOS
                          nephropathy NOS

583.1 **With lesion of membranous glomerulonephritis**
Membranous:
  glomerulonephritis NOS
  nephritis NOS
Membranous nephropathy:
  NOS
DEF: Kidney inflammation or dysfunction with deposits on glomerular capillary basement membranes.

583.2 **With lesion of membranoproliferative glomerulonephritis**
Membranoproliferative:
  glomerulonephritis NOS
  nephritis NOS
  nephropathy NOS
Nephritis NOS, with lesion of:
  hypocomplementemic
    persistent
  lobular
  mesangiocapillary   } glomerulonephritis
  mixed membranous
    and proliferative
DEF: Kidney inflammation or dysfunction with mesangial cell proliferation.

583.4 **With lesion of rapidly progressive glomerulonephritis**
Necrotizing or rapidly progressive:
  glomerulitis NOS
  glomerulonephritis NOS
  nephritis NOS
  nephropathy NOS
Nephritis, unspecified, with lesion of necrotizing glomerulitis
DEF: Kidney inflammation or dysfunction; rapidly progresses to ESRD marked by diffuse epithelial proliferation.

583.6 **With lesion of renal cortical necrosis**
Nephritis NOS   } with (renal) cortical
Nephropathy NOS   }   necrosis
Renal cortical necrosis NOS

583.7 **With lesion of renal medullary necrosis**
Nephritis NOS   } with (renal) medullary
Nephropathy NOS   }   [papillary] necrosis

√5th **583.8** **With other specified pathological lesion in kidney**
583.81 Nephritis and nephropathy, not specified as acute or chronic, in diseases classified elsewhere
Code first underlying disease, as:
  amyloidosis ►(277.30-277.39)◄
  diabetes mellitus (250.4)
  gonococcal infection (098.19)
  Goodpasture's syndrome (446.21)
  systemic lupus erythematosus (710.0)
  tuberculosis (016.0)
EXCLUDES gouty nephropathy (274.10)
         syphilitic nephritis (095.4)
AHA: 2Q, '03, 7; 3Q, '91, 8; S-O, '85, 3

583.89 Other
Glomerulitis   } with lesion of:
Glomerulonephritis }   exudative
Nephritis   }   nephritis
Nephropathy   }   interstitial
Renal disease   }   nephritis

583.9 **With unspecified pathological lesion in kidney**
Glomerulitis NOS   Nephritis NOS
Glomerulonephritis NOS   Nephropathy NOS
EXCLUDES nephropathy complicating pregnancy, labor, or the puerperium (642.0-642.9, 646.2)
         renal disease NOS with no stated cause (593.9)

√4th **584 Acute renal failure**
EXCLUDES following labor and delivery (669.3)
         posttraumatic (958.5)
         that complicating:
           abortion (634-638 with .3, 639.3)
           ectopic or molar pregnancy (639.3)
AHA: 1Q, '93, 18; 2Q, '92, 5; 4Q, '92, 22
DEF: State resulting from increasing urea and related substances from the blood (azotemia), often with urine output of less than 500 ml per day.

584.5 **With lesion of tubular necrosis**
Lower nephron nephrosis
Renal failure with (acute) tubular necrosis
Tubular necrosis:
  NOS
  acute
DEF: Acute decline in kidney efficiency with destruction of tubules.

584.6 **With lesion of renal cortical necrosis**
DEF: Acute decline in kidney efficiency with destruction of renal tissues that filter blood.

584.7 **With lesion of renal medullary [papillary] necrosis**
Necrotizing renal papillitis
DEF: Acute decline in kidney efficiency with destruction of renal tissues that collect urine.

GENITOURINARY SYSTEM

584.8 With other specified pathological lesion in kidney
AHA: N-D, '85, 1

584.9 Acute renal failure, unspecified
AHA: 2Q, '05, 18; 2Q, '03, 7; 1Q, '03, 22; 3Q, '02, 21, 28; 2Q, '01, 14; 1Q, '00, 22; 3Q, '96, 9; 4Q, '88, 1

585 Chronic kidney disease [CKD]
Chronic uremia
►Code first hypertensive chronic kidney disease, if applicable, (403.00-403.91, 404.00-404.94)◄
Use additional code to identify kidney transplant status, if applicable (V42.0)
Use additional code to identify manifestation as:
uremic:
neuropathy (357.4)
pericarditis (420.0)
AHA: 4Q, '05, 68, 77; 1Q, '04, 5; 4Q, '03, 61, 111; 2Q, '03, 7; 2Q, '01, 12, 13; 1Q, '01, 3; 4Q, '98, 55; 3Q, '98, 6, 7; 2Q, '98, 20; 3Q, '96, 9; 1Q, '93, 18; 3Q, '91, 8; 4Q, '89, 1; N-D, '85, 15; S-O, '84, 3

585.1 Chronic kidney disease, Stage I
DEF: Some kidney damage; normal or slightly increased GFR (> 90).

585.2 Chronic kidney disease, Stage II (mild)
DEF: Kidney damage with mild decrease in GFR (60–89).

585.3 Chronic kidney disease, Stage III (moderate)
AHA: 4Q, '05, 69
DEF: Kidney damage with moderate decrease in GFR (30–59).

585.4 Chronic kidney disease, Stage IV (severe)
DEF: Kidney damage with severe decrease in GFR (15–29).

585.5 Chronic kidney disease, Stage V
EXCLUDES ►chronic kidney disease, stage V requiring chronic dialysis (585.6)◄
DEF: Kidney failure with GFR value of less than 15.

585.6 End stage renal disease
►Chronic kidney disease requiring chronic dialysis◄
AHA: 4Q, '05, 79
DEF: Federal government indicator of a stage V CKD patient undergoing treatment by dialysis or transplantation.

585.9 Chronic kidney disease, unspecified
Chronic renal disease
Chronic renal failure NOS
Chronic renal insufficiency
AHA: 4Q, '05, 79

586 Renal failure, unspecified
Uremia NOS
EXCLUDES following labor and delivery (669.3)
posttraumatic renal failure (958.5)
that complicating:
abortion (634-638 with .3, 639.3)
ectopic or molar pregnancy (639.3)
uremia:
extrarenal (788.9)
prerenal (788.9)
with any condition classifiable to 401 (403.0-403.9 with fifth-digit 1)
AHA: 3Q, '98, 6; 1Q, '93, 18

DEF: Renal failure: kidney functions cease; malfunction may be due to inability to excrete metabolized substances or retain level of electrolytes.
DEF: Uremia: excess urea, creatinine and other nitrogenous products of protein and amino acid metabolism in blood due to reduced excretory function in bilateral kidney disease; also called azotemia.

587 Renal sclerosis, unspecified
Atrophy of kidney
Contracted kidney
Renal:
cirrhosis
fibrosis
EXCLUDES nephrosclerosis (arteriolar) (arteriosclerotic) (403.00-403.92)
with hypertension (403.00-403.91)

Genitourinary System

588 Disorders resulting from impaired renal function

588.0 Renal osteodystrophy
Azotemic osteodystrophy
Phosphate-losing tubular disorders
Renal:
dwarfism
infantilism
rickets
DEF: Bone disorder that results in various bone diseases such as osteomalacia, osteoporosis or osteosclerosis; caused by impaired renal function, an abnormal level of phosphorus in the blood and impaired stimulation of the parathyroid.

588.1 Nephrogenic diabetes insipidus
EXCLUDES diabetes insipidus NOS (253.5)
DEF: Type of diabetes due to renal tubules inability to reabsorb water; not responsive to vasopressin; may develop into chronic renal insufficiency.

588.8 Other specified disorders resulting from impaired renal function
EXCLUDES secondary hypertension (405.0-405.9)

588.81 Secondary hyperparathyroidism (of renal origin)
Secondary hyperparathyroidism NOS
AHA: 4Q, '04, 58-59
DEF: Parathyroid dysfunction caused by chronic renal failure; phosphate clearance is impaired, phosphate is released from bone, vitamin D is not produced, intestinal calcium absorption is low, and blood levels of calcium are lowered causing excessive production of parathyroid hormone.

588.89 Other specified disorders resulting from impaired renal function
Hypokalemic nephropathy

588.9 Unspecified disorder resulting from impaired renal function

589 Small kidney of unknown cause
589.0 Unilateral small kidney
589.1 Bilateral small kidneys
589.9 Small kidney, unspecified

OTHER DISEASES OF URINARY SYSTEM (590-599)

590 Infections of kidney
Use additional code to identify organism, such as Escherichia coli [E. coli] (041.4)

590.0 Chronic pyelonephritis
Chronic pyelitis
Chronic pyonephrosis
Code, if applicable, any causal condition first

590.00 Without lesion of renal medullary necrosis
590.01 With lesion of renal medullary necrosis

590.1 Acute pyelonephritis
Acute pyelitis   Acute pyonephrosis

590.10 Without lesion of renal medullary necrosis
590.11 With lesion of renal medullary necrosis

GENITOURINARY SYSTEM

590.2 Renal and perinephric abscess
Abscess:
  kidney
  nephritic
Abscess:
  perirenal
  Carbuncle of kidney

590.3 Pyeloureteritis cystica
Infection of renal pelvis and ureter
Ureteritis cystica
DEF: Inflammation and formation of submucosal cysts in the kidney, pelvis, and ureter.

√5th **590.8 Other pyelonephritis or pyonephrosis, not specified as acute or chronic**

590.80 Pyelonephritis, unspecified
Pyelitis NOS   Pyelonephritis NOS
AHA: 1Q, '98, 10; 4Q, '97, 40

590.81 Pyelitis or pyelonephritis in diseases classified elsewhere
Code first underlying disease, as:
  tuberculosis (016.0)

590.9 Infection of kidney, unspecified
EXCLUDES urinary tract infection NOS (599.0)

591 Hydronephrosis
Hydrocalycosis   Hydroureteronephrosis
Hydronephrosis
EXCLUDES congenital hydronephrosis (753.29)
          hydroureter (593.5)
AHA: 2Q, '98, 9
DEF: Distention of kidney and pelvis, with urine build-up due to ureteral obstruction; pyonephrosis may result.

√4th **592 Calculus of kidney and ureter**
EXCLUDES nephrocalcinosis (275.4)

592.0 Calculus of kidney
Nephrolithiasis NOS   Staghorn calculus
Renal calculus or stone   Stone in kidney
EXCLUDES uric acid nephrolithiasis (274.11)
AHA: 1Q, '00, 4

592.1 Calculus of ureter
Ureteric stone   Ureterolithiasis
AHA: 2Q, '98, 9; 1Q, '98, 10; 1Q, '91, 11

592.9 Urinary calculus, unspecified
AHA: 1Q, '98, 10; 4Q, '97, 40

√4th **593 Other disorders of kidney and ureter**

593.0 Nephroptosis
Floating kidney   Mobile kidney

593.1 Hypertrophy of kidney

593.2 Cyst of kidney, acquired
Cyst (multiple) (solitary) of kidney, not congenital
Peripelvic (lymphatic) cyst
EXCLUDES calyceal or pyelogenic cyst of kidney (591)
          congenital cyst of kidney (753.1)
          polycystic (disease of) kidney (753.1)
AHA: 4Q, '90, 3
DEF: Abnormal, fluid-filled sac in the kidney, not present at birth.

593.3 Stricture or kinking of ureter
Angulation } of ureter (post-operative)
Constriction
Stricture of pelviureteric junction
AHA: 2Q, '98, 9
DEF: Stricture or knot in tube connecting kidney to bladder.

593.4 Other ureteric obstruction
Idiopathic retroperitoneal fibrosis
Occlusion NOS of ureter
EXCLUDES that due to calculus (592.1)
AHA: 2Q, '97, 4

593.5 Hydroureter
EXCLUDES congenital hydroureter (753.22)
          hydroureteronephrosis (591)

593.6 Postural proteinuria
Benign postural proteinuria
Orthostatic proteinuria
EXCLUDES proteinuria NOS (791.0)
DEF: Excessive amounts of serum protein in the urine caused by the body position, e.g., orthostatic and lordotic.

√5th **593.7 Vesicoureteral reflux**
AHA: 4Q, '94, 42
DEF: Backflow of urine, from bladder into ureter due to obstructed bladder neck.

593.70 Unspecified or without reflux nephropathy
593.71 With reflux nephropathy, unilateral
593.72 With reflux nephropathy, bilateral
593.73 With reflux nephropathy NOS

√5th **593.8 Other specified disorders of kidney and ureter**

593.81 Vascular disorders of kidney
Renal (artery):   Renal (artery):
  embolism   thrombosis
  hemorrhage   Renal infarction

593.82 Ureteral fistula
Intestinoureteral fistula
EXCLUDES fistula between ureter and female genital tract (619.0)
DEF: Abnormal communication, between tube connecting kidney to bladder and another structure.

593.89 Other
Adhesions, kidney   Polyp of ureter
  or ureter   Pyelectasia
Periureteritis   Ureterocele
EXCLUDES tuberculosis of ureter (016.2)
          ureteritis cystica (590.3)

593.9 Unspecified disorder of kidney and ureter
Acute renal disease
Acute renal insufficiency
Renal disease NOS
Salt-losing nephritis or syndrome
EXCLUDES chronic renal insufficiency (585.9)
          cystic kidney disease (753.1)
          nephropathy, so stated (583.0-583.9)
          renal disease:
            arising in pregnancy or the puerperium (642.1-642.2, 642.4-642.7, 646.2)
            not specified as acute or chronic, but with stated pathology or cause (583.0-583.9)
AHA: ►4Q, '05, 79;◄ 1Q, '93, 17

√4th **594 Calculus of lower urinary tract**

594.0 Calculus in diverticulum of bladder
DEF: Stone or mineral deposit in abnormal sac on the bladder wall.

594.1 Other calculus in bladder
Urinary bladder stone
EXCLUDES staghorn calculus (592.0)
DEF: Stone or mineral deposit in bladder.

594.2 Calculus in urethra
DEF: Stone or mineral deposit in tube that empties urine from bladder.

594.8 Other lower urinary tract calculus
AHA: J-F, '85, 16

594.9 Calculus of lower urinary tract, unspecified
EXCLUDES calculus of urinary tract NOS (592.9)

√4th **595 Cystitis**
EXCLUDES prostatocystitis (601.3)
Use additional code to identify organism, such as Escherichia coli [E. coli] (041.4)

595.0 Acute cystitis
EXCLUDES trigonitis (595.3)
AHA: 2Q, '99, 15
DEF: Acute inflammation of bladder.

GENITOURINARY SYSTEM

Tabular List

595.1 Chronic interstitial cystitis
Hunner's ulcer   Submucous cystitis
Panmural fibrosis of bladder
DEF: Inflamed lesion affecting bladder wall; symptoms include urinary frequency, pain on bladder filling, nocturia, and distended bladder.

595.2 Other chronic cystitis
Chronic cystitis NOS   Subacute cystitis
EXCLUDES trigonitis (595.3)
DEF: Persistent inflammation of bladder.

595.3 Trigonitis
Follicular cystitis   Urethrotrigonitis
Trigonitis (acute) (chronic)
DEF: Inflammation of the triangular area of the bladder called the trigonum vesicae.

595.4 Cystitis in diseases classified elsewhere
Code first underlying disease, as:
actinomycosis (039.8)
amebiasis (006.8)
bilharziasis (120.0-120.9)
Echinococcus infestation (122.3, 122.6)
EXCLUDES cystitis:
diphtheritic (032.84)
gonococcal (098.11, 098.31)
monilial (112.2)
trichomonal (131.09)
tuberculous (016.1)

√5th 595.8 Other specified types of cystitis

595.81 Cystitis cystica
DEF: Inflammation of the bladder characterized by formation of multiple cysts.

595.82 Irradiation cystitis
Use additional E code to identify cause
DEF: Inflammation of the bladder due to effects of radiation.

595.89 Other
Abscess of bladder   Cystitis:
Cystitis: emphysematous
bullous   glandularis

595.9 Cystitis, unspecified

√4th 596 Other disorders of bladder
Use additional code to identify urinary incontinence (625.6, 788.30-788.39)
AHA: M-A, '87, 10

596.0 Bladder neck obstruction
Contracture (acquired)   of bladder neck or
Obstruction (acquired)   vesicourethral
Stenosis (acquired)   orifice
EXCLUDES congenital (753.6)
AHA: 3Q '02, 28; 2Q, '01, 14; N-D, '86, 10
DEF: Bladder outlet and vesicourethral obstruction; occurs more often in males as a consequence of benign prostatic hypertrophy or prostatic cancer; may also occur in either sex due to strictures, following radiation, cystoscopy, catheterization, injury, infection, blood clots, bladder cancer, impaction or disease compressing bladder neck.

596.1 Intestinovesical fistula
Fistula: Fistula:
enterovesical   vesicoenteric
vesicocolic   vesicorectal
DEF: Abnormal communication, between intestine and bladder.

596.2 Vesical fistula, not elsewhere classified
Fistula: Fistula:
bladder NOS   vesicocutaneous
urethrovesical   vesicoperineal
EXCLUDES fistula between bladder and female genital tract (619.0)
DEF: Abnormal communication between bladder and another structure.

596.3 Diverticulum of bladder
Diverticulitis   } of bladder
Diverticulum (acquired) (false)
EXCLUDES that with calculus in diverticulum of bladder (594.0)
DEF: Abnormal pouch in bladder wall.

596.4 Atony of bladder
High compliance bladder
Hypotonicity   } of bladder
EXCLUDES neurogenic bladder (596.54)
DEF: Distended, bladder with loss of expulsive force; linked to CNS disease.

√5th 596.5 Other functional disorders of bladder
EXCLUDES cauda equina syndrome with neurogenic bladder (344.61)

596.51 Hypertonicity of bladder
Hyperactivity   Overactive bladder
DEF: Abnormal tension of muscular wall of bladder; may appear after surgery of voluntary nerve.

596.52 Low bladder compliance
DEF: Low bladder capacity; causes increased pressure and frequent urination.

596.53 Paralysis of bladder
DEF: Impaired bladder motor function due to nerve or muscle damage.

596.54 Neurogenic bladder NOS
AHA: 1Q, '01, 12
DEF: Unspecified dysfunctional bladder due to lesion of central, peripheral nervous system; may result in incontinence, residual urine retention, urinary infection, stones and renal failure.

596.55 Detrusor sphincter dyssynergia
DEF: Instability of the urinary bladder sphincter muscle associated with urinary incontinence.

596.59 Other functional disorder of bladder
Detrusor instability
DEF: Detrusor instability: instability of bladder; marked by uninhibited contractions often leading to incontinence.

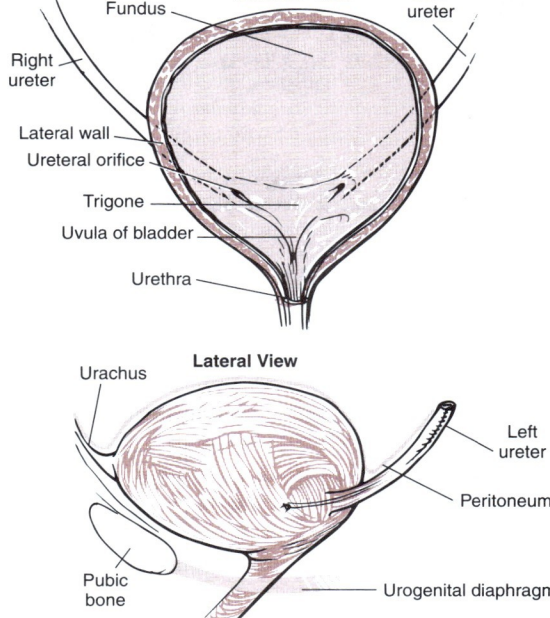

Bladder — Anterior View / Lateral View

2007 ICD•9•CM   Volume 1 — 171

GENITOURINARY SYSTEM

596.6 Rupture of bladder, nontraumatic

596.7 Hemorrhage into bladder wall
Hyperemia of bladder
EXCLUDES *acute hemorrhagic cystitis (595.0)*

596.8 Other specified disorders of bladder
Bladder:
 calcified
 contracted
Bladder:
 hemorrhage
 hypertrophy
EXCLUDES *cystocele, female (618.01-618.02, 618.09, 618.2-618.4)*
hernia or prolapse of bladder, female (618.01-618.02, 618.09, 618.2-618.4)
AHA: J-F, '85, 8

596.9 Unspecified disorder of bladder
AHA: J-F, '85, 8

✓4th **597** Urethritis, not sexually transmitted, and urethral syndrome
EXCLUDES *nonspecific urethritis, so stated (099.4)*

597.0 Urethral abscess
Abscess:
 periurethral
 urethral (gland)
Abscess of:
 bulbourethral gland
Abscess of:
 Cowper's gland
 Littré's gland
Periurethral cellulitis
EXCLUDES *urethral caruncle (599.3)*
DEF: Pocket of pus in tube that empties urine from the bladder.

✓5th **597.8** Other urethritis
 597.80 Urethritis, unspecified
 597.81 Urethral syndrome NOS
 597.89 Other
 Adenitis, Skene's glands
 Cowperitis
 Meatitis, urethral
 Ulcer, urethra (meatus)
 Verumontanitis
 EXCLUDES *trichomonal (131.02)*

✓4th **598** Urethral stricture
Use additional code to identify urinary incontinence (625.6, 788.30-788.39)
INCLUDES pinhole meatus
stricture of urinary meatus
EXCLUDES *congenital stricture of urethra and urinary meatus (753.6)*
DEF: Narrowing of tube that empties urine from bladder.

✓5th **598.0** Urethral stricture due to infection
 598.00 Due to unspecified infection
 598.01 Due to infective diseases classified elsewhere
 Code first underlying disease, as:
 gonococcal infection (098.2)
 schistosomiasis (120.0-120.9)
 syphilis (095.8)

598.1 Traumatic urethral stricture
Stricture of urethra:
 late effect of injury
Stricture of urethra:
 postobstetric
EXCLUDES *postoperative following surgery on genitourinary tract (598.2)*

598.2 Postoperative urethral stricture
Postcatheterization stricture of urethra
AHA: 3Q, '97, 6

598.8 Other specified causes of urethral stricture
AHA: N-D, '84, 9

598.9 Urethral stricture, unspecified

✓4th **599** Other disorders of urethra and urinary tract

599.0 Urinary tract infection, site not specified
EXCLUDES *candidiasis of urinary tract (112.2)*
urinary tract infection of newborn (771.82)
Use additional code to identify organism, such as Escherichia coli [E. coli] (041.4)
AHA: 3Q, '05, 12; 2Q, '04, 13; 4Q, '03, 79; 4Q, '99, 6; 2Q, '99, 15; 1Q, '98, 5; 2Q, '96, 7; 4Q, '96, 33; 2Q, '95, 7; 1Q, '92, 13

599.1 Urethral fistula
Fistula:
 urethroperineal
 urethrorectal
Urinary fistula NOS
EXCLUDES *fistula:*
 urethroscrotal (608.89)
 urethrovaginal (619.0)
 urethrovesicovaginal (619.0)
AHA: 3Q, '97, 6

599.2 Urethral diverticulum
DEF: Abnormal pouch in urethral wall.

599.3 Urethral caruncle
Polyp of urethra

599.4 Urethral false passage
DEF: Abnormal opening in urethra due to surgery, trauma or disease.

599.5 Prolapsed urethral mucosa
Prolapse of urethra   Urethrocele
EXCLUDES *urethrocele, female (618.03, 618.09, 618.2-618.4)*

✓5th **599.6** Urinary obstruction
Use additional code to identify urinary incontinence (625.6, 788.30-788.39)
EXCLUDES *obstructive nephropathy NOS (593.89)*
AHA: 4Q, '05, 80

 599.60 Urinary obstruction, unspecified
 Obstructive uropathy NOS
 Urinary (tract) obstruction NOS

 599.69 Urinary obstruction, not elsewhere classified
 ▶Code, if applicable, any causal condition first, such as:
 hyperplasia of prostate (600.0-600.9 with fifth-digit 1)◀

599.7 Hematuria
Hematuria (benign) (essential)
EXCLUDES *hemoglobinuria (791.2)*
AHA: 1Q, '00, 5; 3Q, '95, 8
DEF: Blood in urine.

✓5th **599.8** Other specified disorders of urethra and urinary tract
Use additional code to identify urinary incontinence (625.6, 788.30-788.39)
EXCLUDES *symptoms and other conditions classifiable to 788.0-788.2, 788.4-788.9, 791.0-791.9*

 599.81 Urethral hypermobility
 DEF: Hyperactive urethra.

 599.82 Intrinsic (urethral) spincter deficiency [ISD]
 AHA: 2Q, '96, 15
 DEF: Malfunctioning urethral sphincter.

 599.83 Urethral instability
 DEF: Inconsistent functioning of urethra.

 599.84 Other specified disorders of urethra
 Rupture of urethra (nontraumatic)
 Urethral:
 cyst
 granuloma
 DEF: Rupture of urethra; due to herniation or breaking down of tissue; not due to trauma.
 DEF: Urethral cyst: abnormal sac in urethra; usually fluid filled.
 DEF: Granuloma: inflammatory cells forming small nodules in urethra.

GENITOURINARY SYSTEM

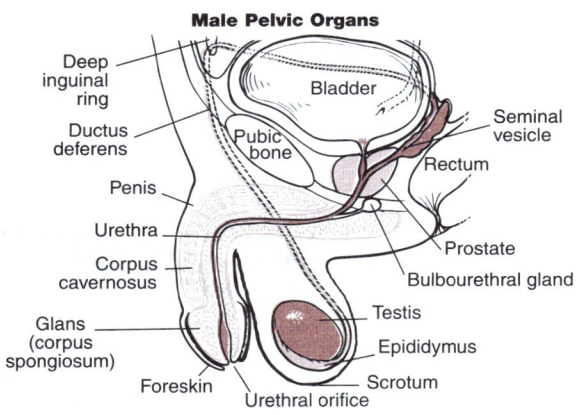

599.89 Other specified disorders of urinary tract

599.9 Unspecified disorder of urethra and urinary tract

DISEASES OF MALE GENITAL ORGANS (600-608)

600 Hyperplasia of prostate
  INCLUDES ▶enlarged prostate◀
  AHA: 3Q, '05, 20; 4Q, '00, 43; 3Q, '94, 12; 3Q, '92, 7; N-D, '86, 10
  DEF: Fibrostromal proliferation in periurethral glands, causes blood in urine; etiology unknown.

  600.0 Hypertrophy (benign) of prostate
    Benign prostatic hypertrophy
    Enlargement of prostate
    Smooth enlarged prostate
    Soft enlarged prostate
    AHA: 4Q, '03, 63; 1Q, '03, 6; 3Q '02, 28; 2Q, '01, 14

    600.00 Hypertrophy (benign) of prostate without urinary obstruction and other lower urinary tract symptoms [LUTS]

    600.01 Hypertrophy (benign) of prostate with urinary obstruction and other lower urinary tract symptoms [LUTS]
      Hypertrophy (benign) of prostate with urinary retention
      ▶Use additional code to identify symptoms:
        incomplete bladder emptying (788.21)
        nocturia (788.43)
        straining on urination (788.65)
        urinary frequency (788.41)
        urinary hesitancy (788.64)
        urinary incontinence (788.30-788.39)
        urinary obstruction (599.69)
        urinary retention (788.20)
        urinary urgency (788.63)
        weak urinary stream (788.62)◀
      AHA: 4Q, '03, 64

  600.1 Nodular prostate
    Hard, firm prostate   Multinodular prostate
    EXCLUDES malignant neoplasm of prostate (185)
    AHA: 4Q, '03, 63
    DEF: Hard, firm nodule in prostate.

    600.10 Nodular prostate without urinary obstruction
      Nodular prostate NOS

    600.11 Nodular prostate with urinary obstruction
      Nodular prostate with urinary retention

  600.2 Benign localized hyperplasia of prostate
    Adenofibromatous hypertrophy of prostate
    Adenoma of prostate
    Fibroadenoma of prostate
    Fibroma of prostate
    Myoma of prostate
    Polyp of prostate
    EXCLUDES benign neoplasms of prostate (222.2)
              hypertrophy of prostate (600.00-600.01)
              malignant neoplasm of prostate (185)
    AHA: 4Q, '03, 63
    DEF: Benign localized hyperplasia is a clearly defined epithelial tumor. Other terms used for this condition are adenofibromatous hypertrophy of prostate, adenoma of prostate, fibroadenoma of prostate, fibroma of prostate, myoma of prostate, and polyp of prostate.

    600.20 Benign localized hyperplasia of prostate without urinary obstruction and other lower urinary tract symptoms [LUTS]
      Benign localized hyperplasia of prostate NOS

    600.21 Benign localized hyperplasia of prostate with urinary obstruction and other lower urinary tract symptoms [LUTS]
      Benign localized hyperplasia of prostate with urinary retention
      ▶Use additional code to identify symptoms:
        incomplete bladder emptying (788.21)
        nocturia (788.43)
        straining on urination (788.65)
        urinary frequency (788.41)
        urinary hesitancy (788.64)
        urinary incontinence (788.30-788.39)
        urinary obstruction (599.69)
        urinary retention (788.20)
        urinary urgency (788.63)
        weak urinary stream (788.62)◀

  600.3 Cyst of prostate
    DEF: Sacs of fluid, which differentiate this from either nodular or adenomatous tumors.

  600.9 Hyperplasia of prostate, unspecified
    Median bar
    Prostatic obstruction NOS
    AHA: 4Q, '03, 63

    600.90 Hyperplasia of prostate, unspecified, without urinary obstruction and other lower urinary tract symptoms [LUTS]
      Hyperplasia of prostate NOS

    600.91 Hyperplasia of prostate, unspecified with urinary obstruction and other lower urinary tract symptoms [LUTS]
      Hyperplasia of prostate, unspecified, with urinary retention
      ▶Use additional code to identify symptoms:
        incomplete bladder emptying (788.21)
        nocturia (788.43)
        straining on urination (788.65)
        urinary frequency (788.41)
        urinary hesitancy (788.64)
        urinary incontinence (788.30-788.39)
        urinary obstruction (599.69)
        urinary retention (788.20)
        urinary urgency (788.63)
        weak urinary stream (788.62)◀

601 Inflammatory diseases of prostate
  Use additional code to identify organism, such as Staphylococcus (041.1), or Streptococcus (041.0)

  601.0 Acute prostatitis
  601.1 Chronic prostatitis
  601.2 Abscess of prostate
  601.3 Prostatocystitis

GENITOURINARY SYSTEM
Tabular List

601.4 Prostatitis in diseases classified elsewhere A ♂
Code first underlying disease, as:
actinomycosis (039.8)
blastomycosis (116.0)
syphilis (095.8)
tuberculosis (016.5)
EXCLUDES prostatitis:
gonococcal (098.12, 098.32)
monilial (112.2)
trichomonal (131.03)

601.8 Other specified inflammatory diseases of prostate A ♂
Prostatitis: Prostatitis:
cavitary   granulomatous
diverticular

601.9 Prostatitis, unspecified A ♂
Prostatitis NOS

√4th **602 Other disorders of prostate**

602.0 Calculus of prostate A ♂
Prostatic stone
DEF: Stone or mineral deposit in prostate.

602.1 Congestion or hemorrhage of prostate A ♂
DEF: Bleeding or fluid collection in prostate.

602.2 Atrophy of prostate A ♂

602.3 Dysplasia of prostate ♂
Prostatic intraepithelial neoplasia I (PIN I)
Prostatic intraepithelial neoplasia II (PIN II)
EXCLUDES prostatic intraepithelial neoplasia III (PIN III) (233.4)
AHA: 4Q, '01, 46
DEF: Abnormality of shape and size of the intraepithelial tissues of the prostate; pre-malignant condition characterized by stalks and absence of a basilar cell layer; synonyms are intraductal dysplasia, large acinar atypical hyperplasia, atypical primary hyperplasia, hyperplasia with malignant changes, marked atypia, or duct-acinar dysplasia.

602.8 Other specified disorders of prostate A ♂
Fistula
Infarction } of prostate
Periprostatic adhesions

602.9 Unspecified disorder of prostate A ♂

√4th **603 Hydrocele**
INCLUDES hydrocele of spermatic cord, testis, or tunica vaginalis
EXCLUDES congenital (778.6)
DEF: Circumscribed collection of fluid in tunica vaginalis, spermatic cord or testis.

603.0 Encysted hydrocele

603.1 Infected hydrocele
Use additional code to identify organism

603.8 Other specified types of hydrocele

603.9 Hydrocele, unspecified

Common Inguinal Canal Anomalies

√4th **604 Orchitis and epididymitis**
Use additional code to identify organism, such as Escherichia coli [E. coli] (041.4), Staphylococcus (041.1), or Streptococcus (041.0)

604.0 Orchitis, epididymitis, and epidymo-orchitis, with abscess ♂
Abscess of epididymis or testis

√5th **604.9 Other orchitis, epididymitis, and epididymo-orchitis, without mention of abscess**

604.90 Orchitis and epididymitis, unspecified ♂

604.91 Orchitis and epididymitis in diseases classified elsewhere ♂
Code first underlying disease, as:
diphtheria (032.89)
filariasis (125.0-125.9)
syphilis (095.8)
EXCLUDES orchitis:
gonococcal (098.13, 098.33)
mumps (072.0)
tuberculous (016.5)
tuberculous epididymitis (016.4)

604.99 Other ♂

605 Redundant prepuce and phimosis ♂
Adherent prepuce   Phimosis (congenital)
Paraphimosis   Tight foreskin
DEF: Constriction of preputial orifice causing inability of the prepuce to be drawn back over the glans; it may be congenital or caused by infection.

√4th **606 Infertility, male**
AHA: 2Q, '96, 9

606.0 Azoospermia A ♂
Absolute infertility
Infertility due to:
germinal (cell) aplasia
spermatogenic arrest (complete)
DEF: Absence of spermatozoa in the semen or inability to produce spermatozoa.

606.1 Oligospermia A ♂
Infertility due to:
germinal cell desquamation
hypospermatogenesis
incomplete spermatogenic arrest
DEF: Insufficient number of sperm in semen.

606.8 Infertility due to extratesticular causes A ♂
Infertility due to: Infertility due to:
drug therapy   radiation
infection   systemic disease
obstruction of efferent
ducts

606.9 Male infertility, unspecified A ♂

√4th **607 Disorders of penis**
EXCLUDES phimosis (605)

607.0 Leukoplakia of penis ♂
Kraurosis of penis
EXCLUDES carcinoma in situ of penis (233.5)
erythroplasia of Queyrat (233.5)
DEF: White, thickened patches on glans penis.

607.1 Balanoposthitis ♂
Balanitis
Use additional code to identify organism
DEF: Inflammation of glans penis and prepuce.

607.2 Other inflammatory disorders of penis ♂
Abscess
Boil   } of corpus cavernosum or penis
Carbuncle
Cellulitis
Cavernitis (penis)
Use additional code to identify organism
EXCLUDES herpetic infection (054.13)

607.3 Priapism ♂
Painful erection
DEF: Prolonged penile erection without sexual stimulation.

GENITOURINARY SYSTEM

607.8 Other specified disorders of penis [5th]
- **607.81** Balanitis xerotica obliterans ♂
  - Induratio penis plastica
  - DEF: Inflammation of the glans penis, caused by stricture of the opening of the prepuce.
- **607.82** Vascular disorders of penis ♂
  - Embolism
  - Hematoma (nontraumatic)
  - Hemorrhage
  - Thrombosis
  } of corpus cavernosum or penis
- **607.83** Edema of penis ♂
  - DEF: Fluid retention within penile tissues.
- **607.84** Impotence of organic origin ♂ [A]
  - EXCLUDES nonorganic (302.72)
  - AHA: 3Q, '91, 11
  - DEF: Physiological cause interfering with erection.
- **607.85** Peyronie's disease ♂
  - AHA: 4Q, '03, 64
  - DEF: A severe curvature of the erect penis due to fibrosis of the cavernous sheaths.
- **607.89** Other ♂
  - Atrophy
  - Fibrosis
  - Hypertrophy
  - Ulcer (chronic)
  } of corpus cavernosum or penis

607.9 Unspecified disorder of penis ♂

608 Other disorders of male genital organs [4th]
- **608.0** Seminal vesiculitis ♂
  - Abscess
  - Cellulitis
  } of seminal vesicle
  - Vesiculitis (seminal)
  - Use additional code to identify organism
  - EXCLUDES gonococcal infection (098.14, 098.34)
  - DEF: Inflammation of seminal vesicle.
- **608.1** Spermatocele ♂
  - DEF: Cystic enlargement of the epididymis or the testis; the cysts contain spermatozoa.
- **608.2** Torsion of testis [5th]
  - DEF: Twisted or rotated testis; may compromise blood flow.
  - **608.20** Torsion of testis, unspecified ♂
  - **608.21** Extravaginal torsion of spermatic cord ♂
  - **608.22** Intravaginal torsion of spermatic cord ♂
  - **608.23** Torsion of appendix testis ♂
  - **608.24** Torsion of appendix epididymis ♂
- **608.3** Atrophy of testis ♂
- **608.4** Other inflammatory disorders of male genital organs ♂
  - Abscess
  - Boil
  - Carbuncle
  - Cellulitis
  } of scrotum, spermatic cord, testis [except abscess], tunica vaginalis, or vas deferens
  - Vasitis
  - Use additional code to identify organism
  - EXCLUDES abscess of testis (604.0)

Torsion of Testis

Torsion of testis

Testes after correction showing bilateral fixation

608.8 Other specified disorders of male genital organs [5th]
- **608.81** Disorders of male genital organs in diseases classified elsewhere ♂
  - Code first underlying disease, as:
    - filariasis (125.0-125.9)
    - tuberculosis (016.5)
- **608.82** Hematospermia ♂
  - AHA: 4Q, '01, 46
  - DEF: Presence of blood in the ejaculate; relatively common, affecting men of any age after puberty; cause is often difficult to determine since the semen originates in several organs, often the result of a viral bacterial infection and inflammation.
- **608.83** Vascular disorders ♂
  - Hematoma (non-traumatic)
  - Hemorrhage
  - Thrombosis
  } of seminal vesicle, spermatic cord, testis, scrotum, tunica vaginalis, or vas deferens
  - Hematocele NOS, male
  - AHA: 4Q, '03, 110
- **608.84** Chylocele of tunica vaginalis ♂
  - DEF: Chylous effusion into tunica vaginalis; due to infusion of lymphatic fluids.
- **608.85** Stricture ♂
  - Stricture of:
    - spermatic cord
    - tunica vaginalis
  - Stricture of:
    - vas deferens
- **608.86** Edema ♂
- **608.87** Retrograde ejaculation ♂
  - AHA: 4Q, '01, 46
  - DEF: Condition where the semen travels to the bladder rather than out through the urethra due to damaged nerves causing the bladder neck to remain open during ejaculation.
- **608.89** Other ♂
  - Atrophy
  - Fibrosis
  - Hypertrophy
  - Ulcer
  } of seminal vesicle, spermatic cord, testis, scrotum, tunica vaginalis, or vas deferens
  - EXCLUDES atrophy of testis (608.3)

608.9 Unspecified disorder of male genital organs ♂

DISORDERS OF BREAST (610-611)

610 Benign mammary dysplasias [4th]
- **610.0** Solitary cyst of breast
  - Cyst (solitary) of breast
- **610.1** Diffuse cystic mastopathy [A]
  - Chronic cystic mastitis
  - Cystic breast
  - Fibrocystic disease of breast
  - DEF: Extensive formation of nodular cysts in breast tissue; symptoms include tenderness, change in size and hyperplasia of ductal epithelium.
- **610.2** Fibroadenosis of breast
  - Fibroadenosis of breast:
    - NOS
    - chronic
    - cystic
  - Fibroadenosis of breast:
    - diffuse
    - periodic
    - segmental
  - DEF: Non-neoplastic nodular condition of breast.
- **610.3** Fibrosclerosis of breast
  - DEF: Fibrous tissue in breast.

GENITOURINARY SYSTEM — Tabular List

610.4 Mammary duct ectasia
Comedomastitis
Duct ectasia
Mastitis:
 periductal
 plasma cell
DEF: Atrophy of duct epithelium; causes distended collecting ducts of mammary gland; drying up of breast secretion, intraductal inflammation and periductal and interstitial chronic inflammatory reaction.

610.8 Other specified benign mammary dysplasias
Mazoplasia   Sebaceous cyst of breast

610.9 Benign mammary dysplasia, unspecified

√4ᵗʰ **611 Other disorders of breast**
 EXCLUDES that associated with lactation or the puerperium (675.0-676.9)

611.0 Inflammatory disease of breast
Abscess (acute) (chronic) (nonpuerperal) of:
 areola
 breast
 Mammillary fistula
Mastitis (acute) (subacute) (nonpuerperal):
 NOS
 infective
 retromammary
 submammary
 EXCLUDES carbuncle of breast (680.2)
 chronic cystic mastitis (610.1)
 neonatal infective mastitis (771.5)
 thrombophlebitis of breast [Mondor's disease] (451.89)

611.1 Hypertrophy of breast
Gynecomastia
Hypertrophy of breast: NOS
Hypertrophy of breast: massive pubertal

611.2 Fissure of nipple

611.3 Fat necrosis of breast
Fat necrosis (segmental) of breast
DEF: Splitting of neutral fats in adipose tissue cells as a result of trauma; a firm circumscribed mass is then formed in the breast.

611.4 Atrophy of breast

611.5 Galactocele
DEF: Milk-filled cyst in breast; due to blocked duct.

611.6 Galactorrhea not associated with childbirth
DEF: Flow of milk not associated with childbirth or pregnancy.

√5ᵗʰ **611.7 Signs and symptoms in breast**
 611.71 Mastodynia
  Pain in breast
 611.72 Lump or mass in breast
  AHA: 2Q, '03, 4-5
 611.79 Other
  Induration of breast   Nipple discharge
  Inversion of nipple   Retraction of nipple

611.8 Other specified disorders of breast
Hematoma (nontraumatic)
Infarction
} of breast
Occlusion of breast duct
Subinvolution of breast (postlactational) (postpartum)

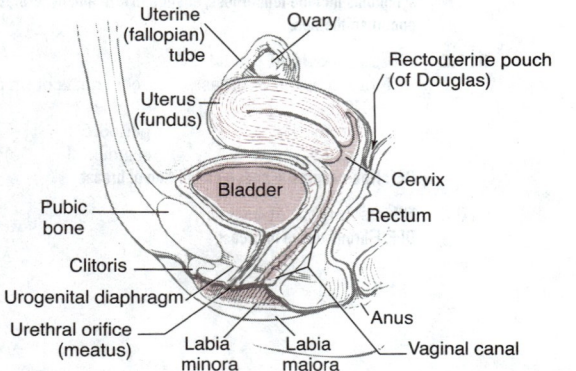
Female Genitourinary System

611.9 Unspecified breast disorder

INFLAMMATORY DISEASE OF FEMALE PELVIC ORGANS (614-616)
Use additional code to identify organism, such as Staphylococcus (041.1), or Streptococcus (041.0)
 EXCLUDES that associated with pregnancy, abortion, childbirth, or the puerperium (630-676.9)

√4ᵗʰ **614 Inflammatory disease of ovary, fallopian tube, pelvic cellular tissue, and peritoneum**
 EXCLUDES endometritis (615.0-615.9)
  major infection following delivery (670)
  that complicating:
   abortion (634-638 with .0, 639.0)
   ectopic or molar pregnancy (639.0)
   pregnancy or labor (646.6)

614.0 Acute salpingitis and oophoritis ♀
Any condition classifiable to 614.2, specified as acute or subacute
DEF: Acute inflammation, of ovary and fallopian tube.

614.1 Chronic salpingitis and oophoritis ♀
Hydrosalpinx
Salpingitis:
 follicularis
 isthmica nodosa
Any condition classifiable to 614.2, specified as chronic
DEF: Persistent inflammation of ovary and fallopian tube.

614.2 Salpingitis and oophoritis not specified as acute, subacute, or chronic ♀
Abscess (of):
 fallopian tube
 ovary
 tubo-ovarian
Oophoritis
Perioophoritis
Pyosalpinx
Perisalpingitis
Salpingitis
Salpingo-oophoritis
Tubo-ovarian inflammatory disease
 EXCLUDES gonococcal infection (chronic) (098.37)
  acute (098.17)
  tuberculous (016.6)
AHA: 2Q, '91, 5

614.3 Acute parametritis and pelvic cellulitis ♀
Acute inflammatory pelvic disease
Any condition classifiable to 614.4, specified as acute
DEF: Parametritis: inflammation of the parametrium; pelvic cellulitis is a synonym for parametritis.

614.4 Chronic or unspecified parametritis and pelvic cellulitis ♀
Abscess (of):
 broad ligament
 parametrium
 pelvis, female
 pouch of Douglas
} chronic or NOS
Chronic inflammatory pelvic disease
Pelvic cellulitis, female
 EXCLUDES tuberculous (016.7)

614.5 Acute or unspecified pelvic peritonitis, female ♀
AHA: ▶4Q, '05, 74◄

614.6 Pelvic peritoneal adhesions, female (postoperative) (postinfection) ♀
Adhesions:
 peritubal
 tubo-ovarian
Use additional code to identify any associated infertility (628.2)
AHA: 3Q, '03, 6; 1Q, '03, 4; 3Q, '95, 7; 3Q, '94, 12
DEF: Fibrous scarring abnormally joining structures within abdomen.

614.7 Other chronic pelvic peritonitis, female ♀
 EXCLUDES tuberculous (016.7)

614.8 Other specified inflammatory disease of female pelvic organs and tissues ♀

N Newborn Age: 0 **P** Pediatric Age: 0-17 **M** Maternity Age: 12-55 **A** Adult Age: 15-124

Tabular List — GENITOURINARY SYSTEM   614.9–617.3

614.9 *Unspecified inflammatory disease of female pelvic organs and tissues* ♀
  Pelvic infection or inflammation, female NOS
  Pelvic inflammatory disease [PID]

√4th 615 Inflammatory diseases of uterus, except cervix
  EXCLUDES *following delivery (670)*
    hyperplastic endometritis (621.30-621.33)
    that complicating:
      abortion (634-638 with .0, 639.0)
      ectopic or molar pregnancy (639.0)
      pregnancy or labor (646.6)

  615.0 Acute ♀
    Any condition classifiable to 615.9, specified as acute or subacute

  615.1 Chronic ♀
    Any condition classifiable to 615.9, specified as chronic

  615.9 *Unspecified inflammatory disease of uterus* ♀
    Endometritis   Myometritis
    Endomyometritis   Perimetritis
    Intrauterine infection   Pyometra
    Metritis   Uterine abscess

√4th 616 Inflammatory disease of cervix, vagina, and vulva
  EXCLUDES *that complicating:*
    abortion (634-638 with .0, 639.0)
    ectopic or molar pregnancy (639.0)
    pregnancy, childbirth, or the puerperium (646.6)

  616.0 Cervicitis and endocervicitis ♀
    Cervicitis   } with or without mention of
    Endocervicitis}   erosion or ectropion
    Nabothian (gland) cyst or follicle
    EXCLUDES *erosion or ectropion without mention of cervicitis (622.0)*

  √5th 616.1 Vaginitis and vulvovaginitis
    DEF: Inflammation or infection of vagina or external female genitalia.

    616.10 *Vaginitis and vulvovaginitis, unspecified* ♀
      Vaginitis:
        NOS
        postirradiation
      Vulvitis NOS
      Vulvovaginitis NOS
      Use additional code to identify organism, such as Escherichia coli [E. coli] (041.4), Staphylococcus (041.1), or Streptococcus (041.0)
      EXCLUDES *noninfective leukorrhea (623.5)*
        postmenopausal or senile vaginitis (627.3)

    616.11 *Vaginitis and vulvovaginitis in diseases classified elsewhere* ♀
      Code first underlying disease, as:
        pinworm vaginitis (127.4)
      EXCLUDES *herpetic vulvovaginitis (054.11)*
        monilial vulvovaginitis (112.1)
        trichomonal vaginitis or vulvovaginitis (131.01)

  616.2 Cyst of Bartholin's gland ♀
    Bartholin's duct cyst
    DEF: Fluid-filled sac within gland of vaginal orifice.

  616.3 Abscess of Bartholin's gland ♀
    Vulvovaginal gland abscess

  616.4 Other abscess of vulva ♀
    Abscess   }
    Carbuncle } of vulva
    Furuncle   }

  √5th 616.5 Ulceration of vulva

    616.50 *Ulceration of vulva, unspecified* ♀
      Ulcer NOS of vulva

    616.51 *Ulceration of vulva in diseases classified elsewhere* ♀
      Code first underlying disease, as:
        Behçet's syndrome (136.1)
        tuberculosis (016.7)
      EXCLUDES *vulvar ulcer (in):*
        gonococcal (098.0)
        herpes simplex (054.12)
        syphilitic (091.0)

  616.8 Other specified inflammatory diseases of cervix, vagina, and vulva ♀
    EXCLUDES *noninflammatory diseases of:*
      cervix (622.0-622.9)
      vagina (623.0-623.9)
      vulva (624.0-6249)

    • **616.81 Mucositis (ulcerative) of cervix, vagina, and vulva** ♀
      Use additional E code to identify adverse effects of therapy, such as: antineoplastic and immunosuppressive drugs (E930.7, E933.1)
      radiation therapy (E879.2)

    • **616.89 Other inflammatory disease of cervix, vagina and vulva** ♀
      Caruncle, vagina or labium
      Ulcer, vagina

  616.9 *Unspecified inflammatory disease of cervix, vagina, and vulva* ♀

OTHER DISORDERS OF FEMALE GENITAL TRACT (617-629)

√4th 617 Endometriosis

  617.0 Endometriosis of uterus ♀
    Adenomyosis   Endometriosis:
    Endometriosis: internal
      cervix   myometrium
    EXCLUDES *stromal endometriosis (236.0)*
    AHA: 3Q, '92, 7
    DEF: Aberrant uterine mucosal tissue; creating products of menses and inflamed uterine tissues.

  617.1 Endometriosis of ovary ♀
    Chocolate cyst of ovary
    Endometrial cystoma of ovary
    DEF: Aberrant uterine tissue; creating products of menses and inflamed ovarian tissues.

  617.2 Endometriosis of fallopian tube ♀
    DEF: Aberrant uterine tissue; creating products of menses and inflamed tissues of fallopian tubes.

  617.3 Endometriosis of pelvic peritoneum ♀
    Endometriosis: Endometriosis:
      broad ligament   parametrium
      cul-de-sac (Douglas')   round ligament
    DEF: Aberrant uterine tissue; creating products of menses and inflamed peritoneum tissues.

Common Sites of Endometriosis

Common sites of endometriosis, in descending order of frequency:
(1) ovary
(2) cul de sac
(3) uterosacral ligaments
(4) broad ligaments
(5) fallopian tube
(6) uterovesical fold
(7) round ligament
(8) vermiform appedix
(9) vagina
(10) rectovaginal septum

GENITOURINARY SYSTEM

617.4 Endometriosis of rectovaginal septum and vagina ♀
DEF: Aberrant uterine tissue; creating products of menses and inflamed tissues in and behind vagina.

617.5 Endometriosis of intestine ♀
Endometriosis:
  appendix
  colon
Endometriosis:
  rectum
DEF: Aberrant uterine tissue; creating products of menses and inflamed intestinal tissues.

617.6 Endometriosis in scar of skin ♀

617.8 Endometriosis of other specified sites ♀
Endometriosis:
  bladder
  lung
Endometriosis:
  umbilicus
  vulva

617.9 Endometriosis, site unspecified ♀

✓4th **618 Genital prolapse**
Use additional code to identify urinary incontinence (625.6, 788.31, 788.33-788.39)
EXCLUDES that complicating pregnancy, labor, or delivery (654.4)

✓5th **618.0 Prolapse of vaginal walls without mention of uterine prolapse**
EXCLUDES that with uterine prolapse (618.2-618.4)
  enterocele (618.6)
  vaginal vault prolapse following hysterectomy (618.5)

  618.00 Unspecified prolapse of vaginal walls ♀
  Vaginal prolapse NOS

  618.01 Cystocele, midline ♀
  Cystocele NOS
  DEF: Defect in the pubocervical fascia, the supportive layer of the bladder, causing bladder drop and herniated into the vagina along the midline.

  618.02 Cystocele, lateral ♀
  Paravaginal
  DEF: Loss of support of the lateral attachment of the vagina at the arcus tendinous results in bladder drop; bladder herniates into the vagina laterally; also called paravaginal defect.

  618.03 Urethrocele ♀
  618.04 Rectocele ♀
  Proctocele
  618.05 Perineocele ♀
  618.09 Other prolapse of vaginal walls without mention of uterine prolapse ♀
  Cystourethrocele

618.1 Uterine prolapse without vaginal wall prolapse ♀
Descensus uteri
Uterine prolapse:
  NOS
  complete
Uterine prolapse:
  first degree
  second degree
  third degree
EXCLUDES that with mention of cystocele, urethrocele, or rectocele (618.2-618.4)

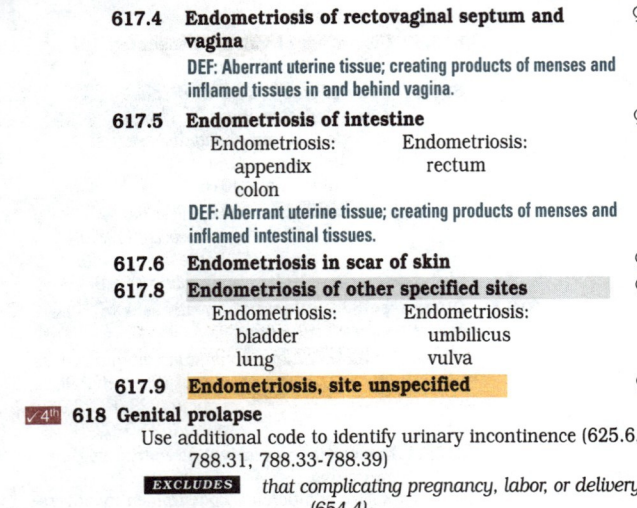

Vaginal Midline Cystocele

Vaginal Lateral Cystocele

618.2 Uterovaginal prolapse, incomplete ♀
DEF: Downward displacement of uterus downward into vagina.

618.3 Uterovaginal prolapse, complete ♀
DEF: Downward displacement of uterus exposed within external genitalia.

618.4 Uterovaginal prolapse, unspecified ♀

618.5 Prolapse of vaginal vault after hysterectomy ♀

618.6 Vaginal enterocele, congenital or acquired ♀
Pelvic enterocele, congenital or acquired
DEF: Vaginal vault hernia formed by the loop of the small intestine protruding into the rectal vaginal pouch; can also accompany uterine prolapse or follow hysterectomy.

618.7 Old laceration of muscles of pelvic floor ♀

✓5th **618.8 Other specified genital prolapse**
  618.81 Incompetence or weakening of pubocervical tissue ♀
  618.82 Incompetence or weakening of rectovaginal tissue ♀
  618.83 Pelvic muscle wasting ♀
  Disuse atrophy of pelvic muscles and anal sphincter
  618.84 Cervical stump prolapse ♀
  618.89 Other specified genital prolapse ♀
  Incompetence or weakening of pelvic fundus
  Relaxation of vaginal outlet or pelvis

618.9 Unspecified genital prolapse ♀

✓4th **619 Fistula involving female genital tract**
EXCLUDES vesicorectal and intestinovesical fistula (596.1)

619.0 Urinary-genital tract fistula, female ♀
Fistula:
  cervicovesical
  ureterovaginal
  urethrovaginal
  urethrovesicovaginal
Fistula:
  ureteroureteric
  uterovesical
  vesicervicovaginal
  vesicovaginal

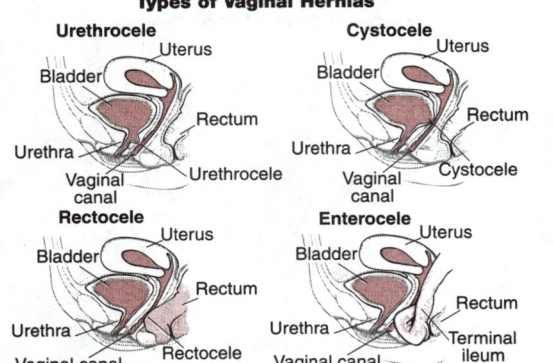

Types of Vaginal Hernias

GENITOURINARY SYSTEM

619.1 Digestive-genital tract fistula, female ♀
Fistula:
  intestinouterine
  intestinovaginal
  rectovaginal
Fistula:
  rectovulval
  sigmoidovaginal
  uterorectal

619.2 Genital tract-skin fistula, female ♀
Fistula:
  uterus to abdominal wall
  vaginoperineal

619.8 Other specified fistulas involving female genital tract ♀
Fistula:
  cervix
  cul-de-sac (Douglas')
Fistula:
  uterus
  vagina
DEF: Abnormal communication between female reproductive tract and skin.

619.9 Unspecified fistula involving female genital tract ♀

✓4th **620 Noninflammatory disorders of ovary, fallopian tube, and broad ligament**
EXCLUDES hydrosalpinx (614.1)

620.0 Follicular cyst of ovary ♀
Cyst of graafian follicle
DEF: Fluid-filled, encapsulated cyst due to occluded follicle duct that secretes hormones into ovaries.

620.1 Corpus luteum cyst or hematoma ♀
Corpus luteum hemorrhage or rupture
Lutein cyst
DEF: Fluid-filled cyst due to serous developing from corpus luteum or clotted blood.

620.2 Other and unspecified ovarian cyst ♀
Cyst:
  NOS
  corpus albicans
  retention NOS
  serous
  theca-lutein
} of ovary
Simple cystoma of ovary
EXCLUDES cystadenoma (benign) (serous) (220)
  developmental cysts (752.0)
  neoplastic cysts (220)
  polycystic ovaries (256.4)
  Stein-Leventhal syndrome (256.4)

620.3 Acquired atrophy of ovary and fallopian tube ♀
Senile involution of ovary

620.4 Prolapse or hernia of ovary and fallopian tube ♀
Displacement of ovary and fallopian tube
Salpingocele

620.5 Torsion of ovary, ovarian pedicle, or fallopian tube ♀
Torsion:
  accessory tube
Torsion:
  hydatid of Morgagni

620.6 Broad ligament laceration syndrome ♀
Masters-Allen syndrome

620.7 Hematoma of broad ligament ♀
Hematocele, broad ligament
DEF: Blood within peritoneal fold that supports uterus.

Uterus and Ovaries

620.8 Other noninflammatory disorders of ovary, fallopian tube, and broad ligament ♀
Cyst
Polyp
} of broad ligament or fallopian tube
Infarction
Rupture
} of ovary or fallopian tube
Hematosalpinx
EXCLUDES hematosalpinx in ectopic pregnancy (639.2)
  peritubal adhesions (614.6)
  torsion of ovary, ovarian pedicle, or fallopian tube (620.5)

620.9 Unspecified noninflammatory disorder of ovary, fallopian tube, and broad ligament ♀

✓4th **621 Disorders of uterus, not elsewhere classified**

621.0 Polyp of corpus uteri ♀
Polyp:
  endometrium
Polyp:
  uterus NOS
EXCLUDES cervical polyp NOS (622.7)

621.1 Chronic subinvolution of uterus ♀
EXCLUDES puerperal (674.8)
AHA: 1Q, '91, 11
DEF: Abnormal size of uterus after delivery; the uterus does not return to its normal size after the birth of a child.

621.2 Hypertrophy of uterus ♀
Bulky or enlarged uterus
EXCLUDES puerperal (674.8)

✓5th **621.3 Endometrial hyperplasia**
Hyperplasia (adenomatous) (cystic) (glandular) of endometrium
DEF: Abnormal cystic overgrowth of endometrial tissue.

621.30 Endometrial hyperplasia, unspecified ♀
Endometrial hyperplasia NOS

621.31 Simple endometrial hyperplasia without atypia ♀

621.32 Complex endometrial hyperplasia without atypia ♀

621.33 Endometrial hyperplasia with atypia ♀

621.4 Hematometra ♀
Hemometra
EXCLUDES that in congenital anomaly (752.2-752.3)
DEF: Accumulated blood in uterus.

621.5 Intrauterine synechiae ♀
Adhesions of uterus
Band(s) of uterus

621.6 Malposition of uterus ♀
Anteversion
Retroflexion
Retroversion
} of uterus
EXCLUDES malposition complicating pregnancy, labor, or delivery (654.3-654.4)
  prolapse of uterus (618.1-618.4)

621.7 Chronic inversion of uterus ♀
EXCLUDES current obstetrical trauma (665.2)
  prolapse of uterus (618.1-618.4)

621.8 Other specified disorders of uterus, not elsewhere classified ♀
Atrophy, acquired
Cyst
Fibrosis NOS
Old laceration (postpartum)
Ulcer
} of uterus
EXCLUDES bilharzial fibrosis (120.0-120.9)
  endometriosis (617.0)
  fistulas (619.0-619.8)
  inflammatory diseases (615.0-615.9)

621.9 Unspecified disorder of uterus ♀

GENITOURINARY SYSTEM

✓4th 622 Noninflammatory disorders of cervix
EXCLUDES abnormality of cervix complicating pregnancy, labor, or delivery (654.5-654.6)
fistula (619.0-619.8)

622.0 Erosion and ectropion of cervix ♀
Eversion } of cervix
Ulcer
EXCLUDES that in chronic cervicitis (616.0)
DEF: Ulceration or turning outward of uterine cervix.

✓5th 622.1 Dysplasia of cervix (uteri)
EXCLUDES abnormal results from cervical cytologic examination without histologic confirmation (795.00-795.09)
carcinoma in situ of cervix (233.1)
cervical intraepithelial neoplasia III [CIN III] (233.1)

AHA: 1Q, '91, 11
DEF: Abnormal cell structures in portal between uterus and vagina.

622.10 Dysplasia of cervix, unspecified ♀
Anaplasia of cervix
Cervical atypism
Cervical dysplasia NOS

622.11 Mild dysplasia of cervix ♀
Cervical intraepithelial neoplasia I [CIN I]

622.12 Moderate dysplasia of cervix ♀
Cervical intraepithelial neoplasia II [CIN II]
EXCLUDES carcinoma in situ of cervix (233.1)
cervical intraepithelial neoplasia III [CIN III] (233.1)
severe dysplasia (233.1)

622.2 Leukoplakia of cervix (uteri) ♀
DEF: Abnormal cell structures in portal between uterus and vagina.
EXCLUDES carcinoma in situ of cervix (233.1)
DEF: Thickened, white patches on portal between uterus and vagina.

622.3 Old laceration of cervix ♀
Adhesions
Band(s) } of cervix
Cicatrix (postpartum)
EXCLUDES current obstetrical trauma (665.3)
DEF: Scarring or other evidence of old wound on cervix.

622.4 Stricture and stenosis of cervix ♀
Atresia (acquired)
Contracture } of cervix
Occlusion
Pinpoint os uteri
EXCLUDES congenital (752.49)
that complicating labor (654.6)

622.5 Incompetence of cervix ♀
EXCLUDES complicating pregnancy (654.5)
that affecting fetus or newborn (761.0)
DEF: Inadequate functioning of cervix; marked by abnormal widening during pregnancy; causing miscarriage.

622.6 Hypertrophic elongation of cervix ♀
DEF: Overgrowth of cervix tissues extending down into vagina.

622.7 Mucous polyp of cervix ♀
Polyp NOS of cervix
EXCLUDES adenomatous polyp of cervix (219.0)

622.8 Other specified noninflammatory disorders of cervix ♀
Atrophy (senile)
Cyst
Fibrosis } of cervix
Hemorrhage
EXCLUDES endometriosis (617.0)
fistula (619.0-619.8)
inflammatory diseases (616.0)

622.9 Unspecified noninflammatory disorder of cervix ♀

✓4th 623 Noninflammatory disorders of vagina
EXCLUDES abnormality of vagina complicating pregnancy, labor, or delivery (654.7)
congenital absence of vagina (752.49)
congenital diaphragm or bands (752.49)
fistulas involving vagina (619.0-619.8)

623.0 Dysplasia of vagina ♀
EXCLUDES carcinoma in situ of vagina (233.3)

623.1 Leukoplakia of vagina ♀
DEF: Thickened white patches on vaginal canal.

623.2 Stricture or atresia of vagina ♀
Adhesions (postoperative) (postradiation) of vagina
Occlusion of vagina
Stenosis, vagina
Use additional E code to identify any external cause
EXCLUDES congenital atresia or stricture (752.49)

623.3 Tight hymenal ring ♀
Rigid hymen
Tight hymenal ring } acquired or congenital
Tight introitus
EXCLUDES imperforate hymen (752.42)

623.4 Old vaginal laceration ♀
EXCLUDES old laceration involving muscles of pelvic floor (618.7)
DEF: Scarring or other evidence of old wound on vagina.

623.5 Leukorrhea, not specified as infective ♀
Leukorrhea NOS of vagina
Vaginal discharge NOS
EXCLUDES trichomonal (131.00)
DEF: Viscid whitish discharge, from vagina.

623.6 Vaginal hematoma ♀
EXCLUDES current obstetrical trauma (665.7)

623.7 Polyp of vagina ♀

623.8 Other specified noninflammatory disorders of vagina ♀
Cyst } of vagina
Hemorrhage

623.9 Unspecified noninflammatory disorder of vagina ♀

✓4th 624 Noninflammatory disorders of vulva and perineum
EXCLUDES abnormality of vulva and perineum complicating pregnancy, labor, or delivery (654.8)
condyloma acuminatum (078.1)
fistulas involving:
  perineum — see Alphabetic Index
  vulva (619.0-619.8)
vulval varices (456.6)
vulvar involvement in skin conditions (690-709.9)

624.0 Dystrophy of vulva ♀
Kraurosis } of vulva
Leukoplakia
EXCLUDES carcinoma in situ of vulva (233.3)

624.1 Atrophy of vulva ♀

624.2 Hypertrophy of clitoris ♀
EXCLUDES that in endocrine disorders (255.2, 256.1)

624.3 Hypertrophy of labia ♀
Hypertrophy of vulva NOS
DEF: Overgrowth of fleshy folds on either side of vagina.

624.4 Old laceration or scarring of vulva ♀
DEF: Scarring or other evidence of old wound on external female genitalia.

624.5 Hematoma of vulva ♀
EXCLUDES that complicating delivery (664.5)
DEF: Blood in tissue of external genitalia.

624.6 Polyp of labia and vulva ♀

GENITOURINARY SYSTEM

624.8 Other specified noninflammatory disorders of vulva and perineum ♀
Cyst
Edema   } of vulva
Stricture
AHA: 1Q, '03, 13; 1Q, '95, 8

624.9 Unspecified noninflammatory disorder of vulva and perineum ♀

✓4th **625 Pain and other symptoms associated with female genital organs**

625.0 Dyspareunia ♀
EXCLUDES   psychogenic dyspareunia (302.76)
DEF: Difficult or painful sexual intercourse.

625.1 Vaginismus ♀
Colpospasm   Vulvismus
EXCLUDES   psychogenic vaginismus (306.51)
DEF: Vaginal spasms; due to involuntary contraction of musculature; prevents intercourse.

625.2 Mittelschmerz ♀
Intermenstrual pain   Ovulation pain
DEF: Pain occurring between menstrual periods.

625.3 Dysmenorrhea ♀
Painful menstruation
EXCLUDES   psychogenic dysmenorrhea (306.52)
AHA: 2Q, '94, 12

625.4 Premenstrual tension syndromes ♀
Menstrual:
  migraine
  molimen
Premenstrual dysphoric disorder
Premenstrual syndrome
Premenstrual tension NOS
AHA: 4Q, '03, 116

625.5 Pelvic congestion syndrome ♀
Congestion-fibrosis syndrome   Taylor's syndrome
DEF: Excessive accumulated of blood in vessels of pelvis; may occur after orgasm; causes abnormal menstruation, lower back pain and vaginal discharge.

625.6 Stress incontinence, female ♀
EXCLUDES   mixed incontinence (788.33)
            stress incontinence, male (788.32)
DEF: Involuntary leakage of urine due to insufficient sphincter control; occurs upon sneezing, laughing, coughing, sudden movement or lifting.

625.8 Other specified symptoms associated with female genital organs ♀
AHA: N-D, '85, 16

625.9 Unspecified symptom associated with female genital organs ♀

✓4th **626 Disorders of menstruation and other abnormal bleeding from female genital tract**
EXCLUDES   menopausal and premenopausal bleeding (627.0)
            pain and other symptoms associated with menstrual cycle (625.2-625.4)
            postmenopausal bleeding (627.1)

626.0 Absence of menstruation ♀
Amenorrhea (primary) (secondary)

626.1 Scanty or infrequent menstruation ♀
Hypomenorrhea   Oligomenorrhea

626.2 Excessive or frequent menstruation ♀
Heavy periods   Menorrhagia
Menometrorrhagia   Plymenorrhea
EXCLUDES   premenopausal (627.0)
            that in puberty (626.3)

626.3 Puberty bleeding ♀
Excessive bleeding associated with onset of menstrual periods
Pubertal menorrhagia

626.4 Irregular menstrual cycle ♀
Irregular: Irregular:
  bleeding NOS   periods
  menstruation

626.5 Ovulation bleeding ♀
Regular intermenstrual bleeding

626.6 Metrorrhagia ♀
Bleeding unrelated to menstrual cycle
Irregular intermenstrual bleeding

626.7 Postcoital bleeding ♀
DEF: Bleeding from vagina after sexual intercourse.

626.8 Other ♀
Dysfunctional or functional uterine hemorrhage NOS
Menstruation:
  retained
  suppression of

626.9 Unspecified ♀

✓4th **627 Menopausal and postmenopausal disorders**
EXCLUDES   asymptomatic age-related (natural) postmenopausal status (V49.81)

627.0 Premenopausal menorrhagia ♀
Excessive bleeding associated with onset of menopause
Menorrhagia:
  climacteric
  menopausal
  preclimacteric

627.1 Postmenopausal bleeding ♀

627.2 Symptomatic menopausal or female climacteric states ♀
Symptoms, such as flushing, sleeplessness, headache, lack of concentration, associated with the menopause

627.3 Postmenopausal atrophic vaginitis ♀
Senile (atrophic) vaginitis

627.4 Symptomatic states associated with artificial menopause ♀
Postartificial menopause syndromes
Any condition classifiable to 627.1, 627.2, or 627.3 which follows induced menopause
DEF: Conditions arising after hysterectomy.

627.8 Other specified menopausal and postmenopausal disorders ♀
EXCLUDES   premature menopause NOS (256.31)

627.9 Unspecified menopausal and postmenopausal disorder ♀

✓4th **628 Infertility, female**
INCLUDES   primary and secondary sterility
AHA: 2Q, '96, 9; 1Q, '95, 7
DEF: Infertility: inability to conceive for at least one year with regular intercourse.
DEF: Primary infertility: occurring in patients who have never conceived.
DEF: Secondary infertility; occurring in patients who have previously conceived.

628.0 Associated with anovulation ♀
Anovulatory cycle
Use additional code for any associated Stein-Leventhal syndrome (256.4)

628.1 Of pituitary-hypothalamic origin ♀
Code first underlying cause, as:
  adiposogenital dystrophy (253.8)
  anterior pituitary disorder (253.0-253.4)

628.2 Of tubal origin ♀
Infertility associated with congenital anomaly of tube
Tubal:
  block
  occlusion
  stenosis
Use additional code for any associated peritubal adhesions (614.6)

628.3 Of uterine origin ♀
Infertility associated with congenital anomaly of uterus
Nonimplantation
Use additional code for any associated tuberculous endometritis (016.7)

628.4 Of cervical or vaginal origin ♀
Infertility associated with:
anomaly of cervical mucus
congenital structural anomaly
dysmucorrhea

628.8 Of other specified origin ♀
628.9 Of unspecified origin ♀

√4th **629 Other disorders of female genital organs**

629.0 Hematocele, female, not elsewhere classified ♀
EXCLUDES hematocele or hematoma:
broad ligament (620.7)
fallopian tube (620.8)
that associated with ectopic pregnancy (633.00-633.91)
uterus (621.4)
vagina (623.6)
vulva (624.5)

629.1 Hydrocele, canal of Nuck ♀
Cyst of canal of Nuck (acquired)
EXCLUDES congenital (752.41)

√5th **629.2 Female genital mutilation status**
Female circumcision status
▶Female genital cutting◀
AHA: 4Q, '04, 88

629.20 Female genital mutilation status, unspecified ♀
▶Female genital cutting status, unspecified◀
Female genital mutilation status NOS

629.21 Female genital mutilation Type I status ♀
Clitorectomy status
▶Female genital cutting Type I status◀
DEF: Female genital mutilation involving clitorectomy, with part or all of the clitoris removed.

629.22 Female genital mutilation Type II status ♀
Clitorectomy with excision of labia minora status
▶Female genital cutting Type II status◀
AHA: 4Q, '04, 90
DEF: Female genital mutilation involving clitoris and the labia minora amputation.

629.23 Female genital mutilation Type III status ♀
▶Female genital cutting Type III status◀
Infibulation status
AHA: 4Q, '04, 90
DEF: Female genital mutilation involving removal, most or all of the labia minora excised, labia majora incised which is then made into a hood of skin over the urethral and vaginal opening.

• **629.29 Other female genital mutilation status** ♀
Female genital cutting Type IV status
Female genital mutilation Type IV status
Other female genital cutting status

√5th **629.8 Other specified disorders of female genital organs**

• **629.81 Habitual aborter without current pregnancy** ♀
EXCLUDES habitual aborter with current pregnancy (646.3)

• **629.89 Other specified disorders of female genital organs**

629.9 Unspecified disorder of female genital organs ♀

11. COMPLICATIONS OF PREGNANCY, CHILDBIRTH AND THE PUERPERIUM (630-677)

ECTOPIC AND MOLAR PREGNANCY (630-633)

Use additional code from category 639 to identify any complications

630 Hydatidiform mole
Trophoblastic disease NOS   Vesicularmole
EXCLUDES: chorioadenoma (destruens) (236.1)
chorionepithelioma (181)
malignant hydatidiform mole (236.1)
DEF: Abnormal product of pregnancy; marked by mass of cysts resembling bunch of grapes due to chorionic villi proliferation, and dissolution; must be surgically removed.

631 Other abnormal product of conception
Blighted ovum
Mole:
  NOS
  carneous
Mole:
  fleshy
  stone

632 Missed abortion
Early fetal death before completion of 22 weeks' gestation with retention of dead fetus
Retained products of conception, not following spontaneous or induced abortion or delivery
EXCLUDES: failed induced abortion (638.0-638.9)
fetal death (intrauterine) (late) (656.4)
missed delivery (656.4)
that with abnormal product of conception (630, 631)
AHA: 1Q, '01, 5

633 Ectopic pregnancy
INCLUDES: ruptured ectopic pregnancy
AHA: 4Q, '02, 61
DEF: Fertilized egg develops outside uterus.

633.0 Abdominal pregnancy
Intraperitoneal pregnancy
633.00 Abdominal pregnancy without intrauterine pregnancy
633.01 Abdominal pregnancy with intrauterine pregnancy

633.1 Tubal pregnancy
Fallopian pregnancy
Rupture of (fallopian) tube due to pregnancy
Tubal abortion
AHA: 2Q, '90, 27
633.10 Tubal pregnancy without intrauterine pregnancy
633.11 Tubal pregnancy with intrauterine pregnancy

633.2 Ovarian pregnancy
633.20 Ovarian pregnancy without intrauterine pregnancy
633.21 Ovarian pregnancy with intrauterine pregnancy

633.8 Other ectopic pregnancy
Pregnancy:
  cervical
  combined
  cornual
Pregnancy:
  intraligamentous
  mesometric
  mural
633.80 Other ectopic pregnancy without intrauterine pregnancy
633.81 Other ectopic pregnancy with intrauterine pregnancy

633.9 Unspecified ectopic pregnancy
633.90 Unspecified ectopic pregnancy without intrauterine pregnancy
633.91 Unspecified ectopic pregnancy with intrauterine pregnancy

Ectopic Pregnancy Sites

OTHER PREGNANCY WITH ABORTIVE OUTCOME (634-639)

The following fourth-digit subdivisions are for use with categories 634-638:

.0 Complicated by genital tract and pelvic infection
Endometritis
Salpingo-oophoritis
Sepsis NOS
Septicemia NOS
Any condition classifiable to 639.0, with condition classifiable to 634-638
EXCLUDES: urinary tract infection (634-638 with .7)

.1 Complicated by delayed or excessive hemorrhage
Afibrinogenemia
Defibrination syndrome
Intravascular hemolysis
Any condition classifiable to 639.1, with condition classifiable to 634-638

.2 Complicated by damage to pelvic organs and tissues
Laceration, perforation, or tear of:
  bladder
  uterus
Any condition classifiable to 639.2, with condition classifiable to 634-638

.3 Complicated by renal failure
Oliguria
Uremia
Any condition classifiable to 639.3, with condition classifiable to 634-638

.4 Complicated by metabolic disorder
Electrolyte imbalance with conditions classifiable to 634-638

.5 Complicated by shock
Circulatory collapse
Shock (postoperative) (septic)
Any condition classifiable to 639.5, with condition classifiable to 634-638

.6 Complicated by embolism
Embolism:
  NOS
  amniotic fluid
  pulmonary
Any condition classifiable to 639.6, with condition classifiable to 634-638

.7 With other specified complications
Cardiac arrest or failure
Urinary tract infection
Any condition classifiable to 639.8, with condition classifiable to 634-638

.8 With unspecified complication

.9 Without mention of complication

COMPLICATIONS OF PREGNANCY, CHILDBIRTH AND THE PUERPERIUM

§ ✓4th 634 Spontaneous abortion

INCLUDES: miscarriage
spontaneous abortion

Requires fifth-digit to identify stage:
0 unspecified
1 incomplete
2 complete

AHA: 2Q, '91, 16

DEF: Spontaneous premature expulsion of the products of conception from the uterus.

- ✓5th 634.0 Complicated by genital tract and pelvic infection ♀
- ✓5th 634.1 Complicated by delayed or excessive hemorrhage ♀
  AHA: For code 634.11: 1Q, '03, 6
- ✓5th 634.2 Complicated by damage to pelvic organs or tissues ♀
- ✓5th 634.3 Complicated by renal failure ♀
- ✓5th 634.4 Complicated by metabolic disorder ♀
- ✓5th 634.5 Complicated by shock ♀
- ✓5th 634.6 Complicated by embolism ♀
- ✓5th 634.7 With other specified complications ♀
- ✓5th 634.8 With unspecified complication ♀
- ✓5th 634.9 Without mention of complication ♀

§ ✓4th 635 Legally induced abortion

INCLUDES: abortion or termination of pregnancy:
elective
legal
therapeutic

EXCLUDES: menstrual extraction or regulation (V25.3)

Requires fifth-digit to identify stage:
0 unspecified
1 incomplete
2 complete

AHA: 2Q, '94, 14

DEF: Intentional expulsion of products of conception from uterus performed by medical professionals inside boundaries of law.

- ✓5th 635.0 Complicated by genital tract and pelvic infection ♀
- ✓5th 635.1 Complicated by delayed or excessive hemorrhage ♀
- ✓5th 635.2 Complicated by damage to pelvic organs or tissues ♀
- ✓5th 635.3 Complicated by renal failure ♀
- ✓5th 635.4 Complicated by metabolic disorder ♀
- ✓5th 635.5 Complicated by shock ♀
- ✓5th 635.6 Complicated by embolism ♀
- ✓5th 635.7 With other specified complications ♀
- ✓5th 635.8 With unspecified complication ♀
- ✓5th 635.9 Without mention of complication ♀

§ ✓4th 636 Illegally induced abortion

INCLUDES: abortion:
criminal
illegal
abortion:
self-induced

Requires fifth-digit to identify stage:
0 unspecified
1 incomplete
2 complete

DEF: Intentional expulsion of products of conception from uterus; outside boundaries of law.

- ✓5th 636.0 Complicated by genital tract and pelvic infection ♀
- ✓5th 636.1 Complicated by delayed or excessive hemorrhage ♀
- ✓5th 636.2 Complicated by damage to pelvic organs or tissues ♀
- ✓5th 636.3 Complicated by renal failure ♀
- ✓5th 636.4 Complicated by metabolic disorder ♀
- ✓5th 636.5 Complicated by shock ♀
- ✓5th 636.6 Complicated by embolism ♀
- ✓5th 636.7 With other specified complications ♀
- ✓5th 636.8 With unspecified complication ♀
- ✓5th 636.9 Without mention of complication ♀

§ ✓4th 637 Unspecified abortion

INCLUDES: abortion NOS
retained products of conception following abortion, not classifiable elsewhere

Requires fifth-digit to identify stage:
0 unspecified
1 incomplete
2 complete

- ✓5th 637.0 Complicated by genital tract and pelvic infection ♀
- ✓5th 637.1 Complicated by delayed or excessive hemorrhage ♀
- ✓5th 637.2 Complicated by damage to pelvic organs or tissues ♀
- ✓5th 637.3 Complicated by renal failure ♀
- ✓5th 637.4 Complicated by metabolic disorder ♀
- ✓5th 637.5 Complicated by shock ♀
- ✓5th 637.6 Complicated by embolism ♀
- ✓5th 637.7 With other specified complications ♀
- ✓5th 637.8 With unspecified complication ♀
- ✓5th 637.9 Without mention of complication ♀

§ ✓4th 638 Failed attempted abortion

INCLUDES: failure of attempted induction of (legal) abortion

EXCLUDES: incomplete abortion (634.0-637.9)

DEF: Continued pregnancy despite an attempted legal abortion.

- 638.0 Complicated by genital tract and pelvic infection ♀
- 638.1 Complicated by delayed or excessive hemorrhage ♀
- 638.2 Complicated by damage to pelvic organs or tissues ♀
- 638.3 Complicated by renal failure ♀
- 638.4 Complicated by metabolic disorder ♀
- 638.5 Complicated by shock ♀
- 638.6 Complicated by embolism ♀
- 638.7 With other specified complications ♀
- 638.8 With unspecified complication ♀
- 638.9 Without mention of complication ♀

✓4th 639 Complications following abortion and ectopic and molar pregnancies

Note: This category is provided for use when it is required to classify separately the complications classifiable to the fourth-digit level in categories 634-638; for example:

a) when the complication itself was responsible for an episode of medical care, the abortion, ectopic or molar pregnancy itself having been dealt with at a previous episode

b) when these conditions are immediate complications of ectopic or molar pregnancies classifiable to 630-633 where they cannot be identified at fourth-digit level.

§ See beginning of section 634–639 for fourth-digit definitions.

Tabular List — **COMPLICATIONS OF PREGNANCY, CHILDBIRTH AND THE PUERPERIUM** — 639.0–641.1

639.0 Genital tract and pelvic infection M ♀
- Endometritis
- Parametritis
- Pelvic peritonitis
- Salpingitis
- Salpingo-oophoritis
- Sepsis NOS
- Septicemia NOS

} following conditions classifiable to 630-638

EXCLUDES urinary tract infection (639.8)

639.1 Delayed or excessive hemorrhage M ♀
- Afibrinogenemia
- Defibrination syndrome
- Intravascular hemolysis

} following conditions classifiable to 630-638

639.2 Damage to pelvic organs and tissues M ♀
- Laceration, perforation, or tear of:
  - bladder
  - bowel
  - broad ligament
  - cervix
  - periurethral tissue
  - uterus
  - vagina

} following conditions classifiable to 630-638

639.3 Renal failure M ♀
- Oliguria
- Renal:
  - failure (acute)
  - shutdown
  - tubular necrosis
- Uremia

} following conditions classifiable to 630-638

639.4 Metabolic disorders M ♀
- Electrolyte imbalance following conditions classifiable to 630-638

639.5 Shock M ♀
- Circulatory collapse
- Shock (postoperative) (septic)

} following conditions classifiable to 630-638

639.6 Embolism M ♀
- Embolism:
  - NOS
  - air
  - amniotic fluid
  - blood-clot
  - fat
  - pulmonary
  - pyemic
  - septic
  - soap

} following conditions classifiable to 630-638

639.8 Other specified complications following abortion or ectopic and molar pregnancy M ♀
- Acute yellow atrophy or necrosis of liver
- Cardiac arrest or failure
- Cerebral anoxia
- Urinary tract infection

} following conditions classifiable to 630-638

639.9 Unspecified complication following abortion or ectopic and molar pregnancy M ♀
- Complication(s) not further specified following conditions classifiable to 630-638

COMPLICATIONS MAINLY RELATED TO PREGNANCY ▶(640-649)◀

INCLUDES the listed conditions even if they arose or were present during labor, delivery, or the puerperium

AHA: 2Q, '90, 11

The following fifth-digit subclassification is for use with categories ▶640-649◀ to denote the current episode of care. Valid fifth-digits are in [brackets] under each code.

0 unspecified as to episode of care or not applicable

1 delivered, with or without mention of antepartum condition
- Antepartum condition with delivery
- Delivery NOS (with mention of antepartum complication during current episode of care)
- Intrapartum obstetric condition (with mention of antepartum complication during current episode of care)
- Pregnancy, delivered (with mention of antepartum complication during current episode of care)

2 delivered, with mention of postpartum complication
- Delivery with mention of puerperal complication during current episode of care

3 antepartum condition or complication
- Antepartum obstetric condition, not delivered during the current episode of care

4 postpartum condition or complication
- Postpartum or puerperal obstetric condition or complication following delivery that occurred:
  - during previous episode of care
  - outside hospital, with subsequent admission for observation or care

AHA: 2Q, '90, 11

√4th **640 Hemorrhage in early pregnancy**
INCLUDES hemorrhage before completion of 22 weeks' gestation

√5th **640.0 Threatened abortion** M ♀
[0,1,3]
DEF: Bloody discharge during pregnancy; cervix may be dilated and pregnancy is threatened, but the pregnancy is not terminated.

√5th **640.8 Other specified hemorrhage in early pregnancy** M ♀
[0,1,3]

√5th **640.9 Unspecified hemorrhage in early pregnancy** M ♀
[0,1,3]

√4th **641 Antepartum hemorrhage, abruptio placentae, and placenta previa**

√5th **641.0 Placenta previa without hemorrhage** M ♀
[0,1,3]
- Low implantation of placenta
- Placenta previa noted:
  - during pregnancy
  - before labor (and delivered by cesarean delivery)

} without hemorrhage

DEF: Placenta implanted in lower segment of uterus; commonly causes hemorrhage in the last trimester of pregnancy.

√5th **641.1 Hemorrhage from placenta previa** M ♀
[0,1,3]
- Low-lying placenta
- Placenta previa:
  - incomplete
  - marginal
  - partial
  - total

} NOS or with hemorrhage (intrapartum)

EXCLUDES hemorrhage from vasa previa (663.5)

COMPLICATIONS OF PREGNANCY, CHILDBIRTH AND THE PUERPERIUM

Placenta Previa: Low (marginal) implantation, Partial placenta previa, Total placenta previa

§ √5ᵗʰ **641.2 Premature separation of placenta**
[0,1,3]
Ablatio placentae
Abruptio placentae
Accidental antepartum hemorrhage
Couvelaire uterus
Detachment of placenta (premature)
Premature separation of normally implanted placenta

DEF: Abruptio placentae: premature detachment of the placenta, characterized by shock, oliguria and decreased fibrinogen.

§ √5ᵗʰ **641.3 Antepartum hemorrhage associated with coagulation defects**
[0,1,3]
Antepartum or intrapartum hemorrhage associated with:
afibrinogenemia
hyperfibrinolysis
hypofibrinogenemia

EXCLUDES ▶coagulation defects not associated with antepartum hemorrhage (649.3)◀

DEF: Uterine hemorrhage prior to delivery.

§ √5ᵗʰ **641.8 Other antepartum hemorrhage**
[0,1,3]
Antepartum or intrapartum hemorrhage associated with:
trauma
uterine leiomyoma

§ √5ᵗʰ **641.9 Unspecified antepartum hemorrhage**
[0,1,3]
Hemorrhage: Hemorrhage:
 antepartum NOS   of pregnancy NOS
 intrapartum NOS

√4ᵗʰ **642 Hypertension complicating pregnancy, childbirth, and the puerperium**

§ √5ᵗʰ **642.0 Benign essential hypertension complicating pregnancy, childbirth, and the puerperium**
[0-4]
Hypertension: specified as complicating,
 benign essential   or as a reason for
 chronic NOS   obstetric care during
 essential   pregnancy, childbirth

Abruptio Placentae: (concealed bleeding), (apparent hemorrhage), (concealed hemorrhage)

§ √5ᵗʰ **642.1 Hypertension secondary to renal disease, complicating pregnancy, childbirth, and the puerperium**
[0-4]
Hypertension secondary to renal disease, specified as complicating, or as a reason for obstetric care during pregnancy, childbirth or the puerperium

§ √5ᵗʰ **642.2 Other pre-existing hypertension complicating pregnancy, childbirth, and the puerperium**
[0-4]
Hypertensive: specified as
 ▶chronic kidney◀   complicating, or
  disease   as a reason for
 heart and ▶chronic   obstetric care
  kidney◀ disease   during pregnancy,
 heart disease   childbirth, or the
Malignant hypertension   puerperium

§ √5ᵗʰ **642.3 Transient hypertension of pregnancy**
[0-4]
Gestational hypertension
Transient hypertension, so described, in pregnancy, childbirth or the puerperium

AHA: 3Q, '90, 4

§ √5ᵗʰ **642.4 Mild or unspecified pre-eclampsia**
[0-4]
Hypertension in pregnancy, childbirth or the puerperium, not specified as pre-existing, with either albuminuria or edema, or both; mild or unspecified
Pre-eclampsia: Toxemia (pre-eclamptic):
 NOS   NOS
 mild   mild

EXCLUDES albuminuria in pregnancy, without mention of hypertension (646.2)
edema in pregnancy, without mention of hypertension (646.1)

§ √5ᵗʰ **642.5 Severe pre-eclampsia**
[0-4]
Hypertension in pregnancy, childbirth or the puerperium, not specified as pre-existing, with either albuminuria or edema, or both; specified as severe
Pre-eclampsia, severe
Toxemia (pre-eclamptic), severe

AHA: N-D, '85, 3

§ √5ᵗʰ **642.6 Eclampsia**
[0-4]
Toxemia: Toxemia:
 eclamptic   with convulsions

§ √5ᵗʰ **642.7 Pre-eclampsia or eclampsia superimposed on pre-existing hypertension**
[0-4]
Conditions classifiable to 642.4-642.6, with conditions classifiable to 642.0-642.2

§ √5ᵗʰ **642.9 Unspecified hypertension complicating pregnancy, childbirth, or the puerperium**
[0-4]
Hypertension NOS, without mention of albuminuria or edema, complicating pregnancy, childbirth or the puerperium

√4ᵗʰ **643 Excessive vomiting in pregnancy**

INCLUDES hyperemesis
vomiting:
 persistent   } arising during pregnancy
 vicious

hyperemesis gravidarum

§ √5ᵗʰ **643.0 Mild hyperemesis gravidarum**
[0,1,3]
Hyperemesis gravidarum, mild or unspecified, starting before the end of the 22nd week of gestation

DEF: Detrimental vomiting and nausea.

---

§ Requires fifth digit. Valid digits are in [brackets] under each code. See beginning of section 640–649 for codes and definitions.

N Newborn Age: 0   **P** Pediatric Age: 0-17   **M** Maternity Age: 12-55   **A** Adult Age: 15-124

COMPLICATIONS OF PREGNANCY, CHILDBIRTH AND THE PUERPERIUM

643.1–647.5

§ ✓5th **643.1** **Hyperemesis gravidarum with metabolic disturbance** [M] ♀
[0,1,3]
Hyperemesis gravidarum, starting before the end of the 22nd week of gestation, with metabolic disturbance, such as:
carbohydrate depletion
dehydration
electrolyte imbalance

§ ✓5th **643.2** **Late vomiting of pregnancy** [M] ♀
[0,1,3]
Excessive vomiting starting after 22 completed weeks of gestation

§ ✓5th **643.8** **Other vomiting complicating pregnancy** [M] ♀
[0,1,3]
Vomiting due to organic disease or other cause, specified as complicating pregnancy, or as a reason for obstetric care during pregnancy
Use additional code to specify cause

§ ✓5th **643.9** **Unspecified vomiting of pregnancy** [M] ♀
[0,1,3]
Vomiting as a reason for care during pregnancy, length of gestation unspecified

✓4th **644** **Early or threatened labor**

§ ✓5th **644.0** **Threatened premature labor** [M] ♀
[0,3]
Premature labor after 22 weeks, but before 37 completed weeks of gestation without delivery
EXCLUDES that occurring before 22 completed weeks of gestation (640.0)

§ ✓5th **644.1** **Other threatened labor** [M] ♀
[0,3]
False labor:
  NOS
  after 37 completed weeks of gestation } without delivery
  Threatened labor NOS

§ ✓5th **644.2** **Early onset of delivery** [M] ♀
[0,1]
Onset (spontaneous) of delivery
Premature labor with onset of delivery } before 37 completed weeks of gestation

AHA: 2Q, '91, 16

✓4th **645** **Late pregnancy**
AHA: 4Q, '00, 43; 4Q, '91, 26

§ ✓5th **645.1** **Post term pregnancy** [M] ♀
[0,1,3]
Pregnancy over 40 completed weeks to 42 completed weeks gestation

§ ✓5th **645.2** **Prolonged pregnancy** [M] ♀
[0,1,3]
Pregnancy which has advanced beyond 42 completed weeks of gestation

✓4th **646** **Other complications of pregnancy, not elsewhere classified**
Use additional code(s) to further specify complication
AHA: 4Q, '95, 59

§ ✓5th **646.0** **Papyraceous fetus** [M] ♀
[0,1,3]
Fetus that dies in the second trimester of pregnancy and is retained in the uterus, with subsequent atrophy and mummification; commonly occurs in twin pregnancy, nonviable fetus becomes compressed by growth of living twin and exhibits parchment-like skin.

§ ✓5th **646.1** **Edema or excessive weight gain in pregnancy, without mention of hypertension** [M] ♀
[0-4]
Gestational edema   Maternal obesity syndrome
EXCLUDES that with mention of hypertension (642.0-642.9)

§ ✓5th **646.2** **Unspecified renal disease in pregnancy, without mention of hypertension** [M] ♀
[0-4]
Albuminuria
Nephropathy NOS } in pregnancy or the puerperium, without mention of hypertension
Renal disease NOS
Uremia

Gestational proteinuria
EXCLUDES that with mention of hypertension (642.0-642.9)

§ ✓5th **646.3** **Habitual aborter** [M] ♀
[0,1,3]
EXCLUDES with current abortion (634.0-634.9)
without current pregnancy (629.9)
DEF: Three or more consecutive spontaneous abortions.

§ ✓5th **646.4** **Peripheral neuritis in pregnancy** [M] ♀
[0-4]

§ ✓5th **646.5** **Asymptomatic bacteriuria in pregnancy** [M] ♀
[0-4]

§ ✓5th **646.6** **Infections of genitourinary tract in pregnancy** [M] ♀
[0-4]
Conditions classifiable to 590, 595, 597, 599.0, 616 complicating pregnancy, childbirth or the puerperium
Conditions classifiable to (614.0-614.5, 614.7-614.9, 615) complicating pregnancy or labor
EXCLUDES major puerperal infection (670)
AHA: For code 646.63: 4Q, '04, 90

§ ✓5th **646.7** **Liver disorders in pregnancy** [M] ♀
[0,1,3]
Acute yellow atrophy of liver (obstetric) (true)
Icterus gravis } of pregnancy
Necrosis of liver
EXCLUDES hepatorenal syndrome following delivery (674.8)
viral hepatitis (647.6)

§ ✓5th **646.8** **Other specified complications of pregnancy** [M] ♀
[0-4]
Fatigue during pregnancy
Herpes gestationis
Insufficient weight gain of pregnancy
AHA: 3Q, '98, 16, J-F, '85, 15

§ ✓5th **646.9** **Unspecified complication of pregnancy** [M] ♀
[0,1,3]

✓4th **647** **Infectious and parasitic conditions in the mother classifiable elsewhere, but complicating pregnancy, childbirth, or the puerperium**
INCLUDES the listed conditions when complicating the pregnant state, aggravated by the pregnancy, or when a main reason for obstetric care
EXCLUDES those conditions in the mother known or suspected to have affected the fetus (655.0-655.9)
Use additional code(s) to further specify complication

§ ✓5th **647.0** **Syphilis** [M] ♀
[0-4] Conditions classifiable to 090-097

§ ✓5th **647.1** **Gonorrhea** [M] ♀
[0-4] Conditions classifiable to 098

§ ✓5th **647.2** **Other venereal diseases** [M] ♀
[0-4] Conditions classifiable to 099

§ ✓5th **647.3** **Tuberculosis** [M] ♀
[0-4] Conditions classifiable to 010-018

§ ✓5th **647.4** **Malaria** [M] ♀
[0-4] Conditions classifiable to 084

§ ✓5th **647.5** **Rubella** [M] ♀
[0-4] Conditions classifiable to 056

§ Requires fifth digit. Valid digits are in [brackets] under each code. See beginning of section 640–649 for codes and definitions.

Additional Digit Required   Unspecified Code   Other Specified Code   Manifestation Code   ▶◀ Revised Text   ● New Code   ▲ Revised Code Title

2007 ICD•9•CM   Volume 1 — 187

COMPLICATIONS OF PREGNANCY, CHILDBIRTH AND THE PUERPERIUM

§ √5th **647.6** Other viral diseases
[0-4] Conditions classifiable to 042 and 050-079, except 056
AHA: J-F, '85, 15

§ √5th **647.8** Other specified infectious and parasitic diseases
[0-4]

§ √5th **647.9** Unspecified infection or infestation
[0-4]

√4th **648** Other current conditions in the mother classifiable elsewhere, but complicating pregnancy, childbirth, or the puerperium
> INCLUDES the listed conditions when complicating the pregnant state, aggravated by the pregnancy, or when a main reason for obstetric care
>
> EXCLUDES those conditions in the mother known or suspected to have affected the fetus (655.0-665.9)

Use additional code(s) to identify the condition

§ √5th **648.0** Diabetes mellitus
[0-4] Conditions classifiable to 250
> EXCLUDES gestational diabetes (648.8)

AHA: 3Q, '91, 5, 11

§ √5th **648.1** Thyroid dysfunction
[0-4] Conditions classifiable to 240-246

§ √5th **648.2** Anemia
[0-4] Conditions classifiable to 280-285
AHA: For Code 648.22: 1Q, '02, 14

§ √5th **648.3** Drug dependence
[0-4] Conditions classifiable to 304
AHA: 2Q, '98, 13; 4Q, '88, 8

§ √5th **648.4** Mental disorders
[0-4] Conditions classifiable to 290-303, ▶305.0, 305.2-305.9, 306-316, 317-319◄
AHA: 2Q, '98, 13; 4Q, '95, 63

§ √5th **648.5** Congenital cardiovascular disorders
[0-4] Conditions classifiable to 745-747

§ √5th **648.6** Other cardiovascular diseases
[0-4] Conditions classifiable to 390-398, 410-429
> EXCLUDES cerebrovascular disorders in the puerperium (674.0)
> peripartum cardiomyopathy (674.5)
> venous complications (671.0-671.9)

AHA: 3Q, '98, 11

§ √5th **648.7** Bone and joint disorders of back, pelvis, and lower limbs
[0-4] Conditions classifiable to 720-724, and those classifiable to 711-719 or 725-738, specified as affecting the lower limbs

§ √5th **648.8** Abnormal glucose tolerance
[0-4] Conditions classifiable to 790.21-790.29
Gestational diabetes
Use additional code, if applicable, for associated long-term (current) insulin use (V58.67)
AHA: 3Q, '91, 5; For code 648.83: 4Q, '04, 56
DEF: Glucose intolerance arising in pregnancy, resolving at end of pregnancy.

§ √5th **648.9** Other current conditions classifiable elsewhere
[0-4] Conditions classifiable to 440-459
Nutritional deficiencies [conditions classifiable to 260-269]
AHA: 4Q, '04, 88; N-D, '87, 10; For code 648.91: 1Q, '02, 14; For code 648.93: 4Q, '04, 90

√4th **649** Other conditions or status of the mother complicating pregnancy, childbirth, or the puerperium

§ √5th **649.0** Tobacco use disorder complicating pregnancy, childbirth, or the puerperium
[0-4] Smoking complicating pregnancy, childbirth, or the puerperium

§ √5th **649.1** Obesity complicating pregnancy, childbirth, or the puerperium
[0-4] Use additional code to identify the obesity (278.00, 278.01)

§ √5th **649.2** Bariatric surgery status complicating pregnancy, childbirth, or the puerperium
[0-4] Gastric banding status complicating pregnancy, childbirth, or the puerperium
Gastric bypass status for obesity complicating pregnancy, childbirth, or the puerperium
Obesity surgery status complicating pregnancy, childbirth, or the puerperium

§ √5th **649.3** Coagulation defects complicating pregnancy, childbirth, or the puerperium
[0-4] Conditions classifiable to 286
Use additional code to identify the specific coagulation defect (286.0-286.9)
> EXCLUDES coagulation defects causing antepartum hemorrhage (641.3)
> postpartum coagulation defects (666.3)

§ √5th **649.4** Epilepsy complicating pregnancy, childbirth, or the puerperium
[0-4] Conditions classifiable to 345
Use additional code to identify the specific type of epilepsy (345.00-345.91)
> EXCLUDES eclampsia (642.6)

§ √5th **649.5** Spotting complicating pregnancy
[0,1,3]
> EXCLUDES antepartum hemorrhage (641.0 641.9)
> hemorrhage in early pregnancy (640.0-640.9)

§ √5th **649.6** Uterine size date discrepancy
[0-4]

NORMAL DELIVERY, AND OTHER INDICATIONS FOR CARE IN PREGNANCY, LABOR, AND DELIVERY (650-659)

The following fifth-digit subclassification is for use with categories 651-659 to denote the current episode of care. Valid fifth-digits are in [brackets] under each code.
0 unspecified as to episode of care or not applicable
1 delivered, with or without mention of antepartum condition
2 delivered, with mention of postpartum complication
3 antepartum condition or complication
4 postpartum condition or complication

650 Normal delivery
Delivery requiring minimal or no assistance, with or without episiotomy, without fetal manipulation [e.g., rotation version] or instrumentation [forceps] of spontaneous, cephalic, vaginal, full-term, single, live-born infant. This code is for use as a single diagnosis code and is not to be used with any other code in the range 630-676.
> EXCLUDES breech delivery (assisted) (spontaneous) NOS (652.2)
> delivery by vacuum extractor, forceps, cesarean section, or breech extraction, without specified complication (669.5-669.7)

Use additional code to indicate outcome of delivery (V27.0)
AHA: 2Q, '02, 10; 3Q, '01, 12; 3Q, '00, 5; 4Q, '95, 28, 59

√4th **651** Multiple gestation

§ √5th **651.0** Twin pregnancy
[0,1,3]

§ Requires fifth digit. Valid digits are in [brackets] under each code. See beginning of section 640–649 for codes and definitions.

COMPLICATIONS OF PREGNANCY, CHILDBIRTH AND THE PUERPERIUM 651.1–654.1

Malposition and Malpresentation

Cephalopelvic Disproportion

§ ✓5th **651.1 Triplet pregnancy** M ♀
[0,1,3]

§ ✓5th **651.2 Quadruplet pregnancy** M ♀
[0,1,3]

§ ✓5th **651.3 Twin pregnancy with fetal loss and retention of one fetus** M ♀
[0,1,3]
    Vanishing twin syndrome (651.33)

§ ✓5th **651.4 Triplet pregnancy with fetal loss and retention of one or more fetus(es)** M ♀
[0,1,3]

§ ✓5th **651.5 Quadruplet pregnancy with fetal loss and retention of one or more fetus(es)** M ♀
[0,1,3]

§ ✓5th **651.6 Other multiple pregnancy with fetal loss and retention of one or more fetus(es)** M ♀
[0,1,3]

§ ✓5th **651.7 Multiple gestation following (elective) fetal reduction** M ♀
[0,1,3]
    Fetal reduction of multiple fetuses reduced to single fetus
    AHA: For code 651.71: ▶4Q, '05, 81◀

§ ✓5th **651.8 Other specified multiple gestation** M ♀
[0,1,3]

§ ✓5th **651.9 Unspecified multiple gestation** M ♀
[0,1,3]

✓4th **652 Malposition and malpresentation of fetus**
    Code first any associated obstructed labor (660.0)

§ ✓5th **652.0 Unstable lie** M ♀
[0,1,3]
    DEF: Changing fetal position.

§ ✓5th **652.1 Breech or other malpresentation successfully converted to cephalic presentation** M ♀
[0,1,3]
    Cephalic version NOS

§ ✓5th **652.2 Breech presentation without mention of version** M ♀
[0,1,3]
    Breech delivery (assisted) (spontaneous) NOS   Complete breech
    Buttocks presentation   Frank breech
    EXCLUDES footling presentation (652.8)
               incomplete breech (652.8)
    DEF: Fetal presentation of buttocks or feet at birth canal.

§ ✓5th **652.3 Transverse or oblique presentation** M ♀
[0,1,3]
    Oblique lie   Transverse lie
    EXCLUDES transverse arrest of fetal head (660.3)
    DEF: Delivery of fetus, shoulder first.

§ ✓5th **652.4 Face or brow presentation** M ♀
[0,1,3]
    Mentum presentation

§ ✓5th **652.5 High head at term** M ♀
[0,1,3]
    Failure of head to enter pelvic brim

§ ✓5th **652.6 Multiple gestation with malpresentation of one fetus or more** M ♀
[0,1,3]

§ ✓5th **652.7 Prolapsed arm** M ♀
[0,1,3]

§ ✓5th **652.8 Other specified malposition or malpresentation** M ♀
[0,1,3]
    Compound presentation

§ ✓5th **652.9 Unspecified malposition or malpresentation** M ♀
[0,1,3]

✓4th **653 Disproportion**
    Code first any associated obstructed labor (660.1)

§ ✓5th **653.0 Major abnormality of bony pelvis, not further specified** M ♀
[0,1,3]
    Pelvic deformity NOS

§ ✓5th **653.1 Generally contracted pelvis** M ♀
[0,1,3]
    Contracted pelvis NOS

§ ✓5th **653.2 Inlet contraction of pelvis** M ♀
[0,1,3]
    Inlet contraction (pelvis)

§ ✓5th **653.3 Outlet contraction of pelvis** M ♀
[0,1,3]
    Outlet contraction (pelvis)

§ ✓5th **653.4 Fetopelvic disproportion** M ♀
[0,1,3]
    Cephalopelvic disproportion NOS
    Disproportion of mixed maternal and fetal origin, with normally formed fetus

§ ✓5th **653.5 Unusually large fetus causing disproportion** M ♀
[0,1,3]
    Disproportion of fetal origin with normally formed fetus
    Fetal disproportion NOS
    EXCLUDES that when the reason for medical care was concern for the fetus (656.6)

§ ✓5th **653.6 Hydrocephalic fetus causing disproportion** M ♀
[0,1,3]
    EXCLUDES that when the reason for medical care was concern for the fetus (655.0)

§ ✓5th **653.7 Other fetal abnormality causing disproportion** M ♀
[0,1,3]
    Conjoined twins   Fetal:
    Fetal: myelomeningocele
      ascites   sacral teratoma
      hydrops   tumor

§ ✓5th **653.8 Disproportion of other origin** M ♀
[0,1,3]
    EXCLUDES shoulder (girdle) dystocia (660.4)

§ ✓5th **653.9 Unspecified disproportion** M ♀
[0,1,3]

✓4th **654 Abnormality of organs and soft tissues of pelvis**
    INCLUDES the listed conditions during pregnancy, childbirth or the puerperium
    Code first any associated obstructed labor (660.2)

§ ✓5th **654.0 Congenital abnormalities of uterus** M ♀
[0-4]
    Double uterus   Uterus bicornis

§ ✓5th **654.1 Tumors of body of uterus** M ♀
[0-4]
    Uterine fibroids

---

§ Requires fifth digit. Valid digits are in [brackets] under each code. See beginning of section 640–649 for codes and definitions.

COMPLICATIONS OF PREGNANCY, CHILDBIRTH AND THE PUERPERIUM

§ ✓5th **654.2 Previous cesarean delivery** Ⓜ♀
[0,1,3]   Uterine scar from previous cesarean delivery
          AHA: 1Q, '92, 8

§ ✓5th **654.3 Retroverted and incarcerated gravid uterus** Ⓜ♀
[0-4]   DEF: Retroverted: tilted back uterus; no change in angle of longitudinal axis.
        DEF: Incarcerated: immobile, fixed uterus.

§ ✓5th **654.4 Other abnormalities in shape or position of gravid uterus and of neighboring structures** Ⓜ♀
[0-4]
          Cystocele   Prolapse of gravid uterus
          Pelvic floor repair   Rectocele
          Pendulous abdomen   Rigid pelvic floor

§ ✓5th **654.5 Cervical incompetence** Ⓜ♀
[0-4]   Presence of Shirodkar suture with or without mention of cervical incompetence
        DEF: Abnormal cervix; tendency to dilate in second trimester; causes premature fetal expulsion.
        DEF: Shirodkar suture: purse-string suture used to artificially close incompetent cervix.

§ ✓5th **654.6 Other congenital or acquired abnormality of cervix** Ⓜ♀
[0-4]
          Cicatricial cervix   Rigid cervix (uteri)
          Polyp of cervix   Stenosis or stricture of cervix
          Previous surgery to cervix   Tumor of cervix

§ ✓5th **654.7 Congenital or acquired abnormality of vagina** Ⓜ♀
[0-4]
          Previous surgery to vagina   Stricture of vagina
          Septate vagina   Tumor of vagina
          Stenosis of vagina (acquired) (congenital)

§ ✓5th **654.8 Congenital or acquired abnormality of vulva** Ⓜ♀
[0-4]
          Fibrosis of perineum   Rigid perineum
          Persistent hymen   Tumor of vulva
          Previous surgery to perineum or vulva
          EXCLUDES   varicose veins of vulva (671.1)
          AHA: 1Q, '03, 14

§ ✓5th **654.9 Other and unspecified** Ⓜ♀
[0-4]   Uterine scar NEC

✓4th **655 Known or suspected fetal abnormality affecting management of mother**
          INCLUDES   the listed conditions in the fetus as a reason for observation or obstetrical care of the mother, or for termination of pregnancy
          AHA: 3Q, '90, 4

§ ✓5th **655.0 Central nervous system malformation in fetus** Ⓜ♀
[0,1,3]   Fetal or suspected fetal:
            anencephaly
            hydrocephalus
            spina bifida (with myelomeningocele)

§ ✓5th **655.1 Chromosomal abnormality in fetus** Ⓜ♀
[0,1,3]

§ ✓5th **655.2 Hereditary disease in family possibly affecting fetus** Ⓜ♀
[0,1,3]

§ ✓5th **655.3 Suspected damage to fetus from viral disease in the mother** Ⓜ♀
[0,1,3]   Suspected damage to fetus from maternal rubella

§ ✓5th **655.4 Suspected damage to fetus from other disease in the mother** Ⓜ♀
[0,1,3]   Suspected damage to fetus from maternal:
            alcohol addiction
            listeriosis
            toxoplasmosis

§ ✓5th **655.5 Suspected damage to fetus from drugs** Ⓜ♀
[0,1,3]

§ ✓5th **655.6 Suspected damage to fetus from radiation** Ⓜ♀
[0,1,3]

§ ✓5th **655.7 Decreased fetal movements** Ⓜ♀
[0,1,3]   AHA: 4Q, '97, 41

§ ✓5th **655.8 Other known or suspected fetal abnormality, not elsewhere classified** Ⓜ♀
[0,1,3]   Suspected damage to fetus from:
            environmental toxins
            intrauterine contraceptive device

§ ✓5th **655.9 Unspecified** Ⓜ♀
[0,1,3]

✓4th **656 Other fetal and placental problems affecting management of mother**

§ ✓5th **656.0 Fetal-maternal hemorrhage** Ⓜ♀
[0,1,3]   Leakage (microscopic) of fetal blood into maternal circulation

§ ✓5th **656.1 Rhesus isoimmunization** Ⓜ♀
[0,1,3]   Anti-D [Rh] antibodies
          Rh incompatibility
          DEF: Antibodies developing against Rh factor; mother with Rh negative develops antibodies against Rh positive fetus.

§ ✓5th **656.2 Isoimmunization from other and unspecified blood-group incompatibility** Ⓜ♀
[0,1,3]   ABO isoimmunization

§ ✓5th **656.3 Fetal distress** Ⓜ♀
[0,1,3]   Fetal metabolic acidemia
          EXCLUDES   abnormal fetal acid-base balance (656.8)
                     abnormality in fetal heart rate or rhythm (659.7)
                     fetal bradycardia (659.7)
                     fetal tachycardia (659.7)
                     meconium in liquor (656.8)
          AHA: N-D, '86, 4
          DEF: Life-threatening disorder; fetal anoxia, hemolytic disease and other miscellaneous diseases cause fetal distress.

§ ✓5th **656.4 Intrauterine death** Ⓜ♀
[0,1,3]   Fetal death:
            NOS
            after completion of 22 weeks' gestation
            late
          Missed delivery
          EXCLUDES   missed abortion (632)

§ ✓5th **656.5 Poor fetal growth** Ⓜ♀
[0,1,3]   "Light-for-dates"   "Small-for-dates"
          "Placental insufficiency"

§ ✓5th **656.6 Excessive fetal growth** Ⓜ♀
[0,1,3]   "Large-for-dates"

§ ✓5th **656.7 Other placental conditions** Ⓜ♀
[0,1,3]   Abnormal placenta   Placental infarct
          EXCLUDES   placental polyp (674.4)
                     placentitis (658.4)

§ ✓5th **656.8 Other specified fetal and placental problems** Ⓜ♀
[0,1,3]   Abnormal acid-base balance
          Intrauterine acidosis
          Lithopedian
          Meconium in liquor
          DEF: Lithopedion: Calcified fetus; not expelled by mother.

§ ✓5th **656.9 Unspecified fetal and placental problem** Ⓜ♀
[0,1,3]

✓4th **657 Polyhydramnios** Ⓜ♀
[0,1,3]
§ ✓5th   Use 0 as fourth-digit for this category
         Hydramnios
         AHA: 4Q, '91, 26
         DEF: Excess amniotic fluid.

---

§ Requires fifth digit. Valid digits are in [brackets] under each code. See beginning of section 640–649 for codes and definitions.

Ⓝ Newborn Age: 0   Ⓟ Pediatric Age: 0-17   Ⓜ Maternity Age: 12-55   Ⓐ Adult Age: 15-124

COMPLICATIONS OF PREGNANCY, CHILDBIRTH AND THE PUERPERIUM

658 Other problems associated with amniotic cavity and membranes
EXCLUDES: amniotic fluid embolism (673.1)

- **658.0** Oligohydramnios [0,1,3]
  Oligohydramnios without mention of rupture of membranes
  DEF: Deficient amount of amniotic fluid.

- **658.1** Premature rupture of membranes [0,1,3]
  Rupture of amniotic sac less than 24 hours prior to the onset of labor
  AHA: For code 658.13: 1Q, '01, 5; 4Q, '98, 77

- **658.2** Delayed delivery after spontaneous or unspecified rupture of membranes [0,1,3]
  Prolonged rupture of membranes NOS
  Rupture of amniotic sac 24 hours or more prior to the onset of labor

- **658.3** Delayed delivery after artificial rupture of membranes [0,1,3]

- **658.4** Infection of amniotic cavity [0,1,3]
  Amnionitis   Membranitis
  Chorioamnionitis   Placentitis

- **658.8** Other [0,1,3]
  Amnion nodosum   Amniotic cyst

- **658.9** Unspecified [0,1,3]

659 Other indications for care or intervention related to labor and delivery, not elsewhere classified

- **659.0** Failed mechanical induction [0,1,3]
  Failure of induction of labor by surgical or other instrumental methods

- **659.1** Failed medical or unspecified induction [0,1,3]
  Failed induction NOS
  Failure of induction of labor by medical methods, such as oxytocic drugs

- **659.2** Maternal pyrexia during labor, unspecified [0,1,3]
  DEF: Fever during labor.

- **659.3** Generalized infection during labor [0,1,3]
  Septicemia during labor

- **659.4** Grand multiparity [0,1,3]
  EXCLUDES: supervision only, in pregnancy (V23.3)
  without current pregnancy (V61.5)
  DEF: Having borne six or more children previously.

- **659.5** Elderly primigravida [0,1,3]
  First pregnancy in a woman who will be 35 years of age or older at expected date of delivery
  EXCLUDES: supervision only, in pregnancy (V23.81)
  AHA: 3Q, '01, 12

- **659.6** Elderly multigravida [0,1,3]
  Second or more pregnancy in a woman who will be 35 years of age or older at expected date of delivery
  EXCLUDES: elderly primigravida 659.5
  supervision only, in pregnancy (V23.82)
  AHA: 3Q, '01, 12

- **659.7** Abnormality in fetal heart rate or rhythm [0,1,3]
  Depressed fetal heart tones
  Fetal:
    bradycardia
    tachycardia
  Fetal heart rate decelerations
  Non-reassuring fetal heart rate or rhythm
  AHA: 4Q, '98, 48

- **659.8** Other specified indications for care or intervention related to labor and delivery [0,1,3]
  Pregnancy in a female less than 16 years old at expected date of delivery
  Very young maternal age
  AHA: 3Q, '01, 12

- **659.9** Unspecified indication for care or intervention related to labor and delivery [0,1,3]

COMPLICATIONS OCCURRING MAINLY IN THE COURSE OF LABOR AND DELIVERY (660-669)

The following fifth-digit subclassification is for use with categories 660-669 to denote the current episode of care. Valid fifth-digits are in [brackets] under each code.
0 unspecified as to episode of care or not applicable
1 delivered, with or without mention of antepartum condition
2 delivered, with mention of postpartum complication
3 antepartum condition or complication
4 postpartum condition or complication

660 Obstructed labor
AHA: 3Q, '95, 10

- **660.0** Obstruction caused by malposition of fetus at onset of labor [0,1,3]
  Any condition classifiable to 652, causing obstruction during labor
  Use additional code from 652.0-652.9 to identify condition

- **660.1** Obstruction by bony pelvis [0,1,3]
  Any condition classifiable to 653, causing obstruction during labor
  Use additional code from 653.0-653.9 to identify condition

- **660.2** Obstruction by abnormal pelvic soft tissues [0,1,3]
  Prolapse of anterior lip of cervix
  Any condition classifiable to 654, causing obstruction during labor
  Use additional code from 654.0-654.9 to identify condition

- **660.3** Deep transverse arrest and persistent occipitoposterior position [0,1,3]

- **660.4** Shoulder (girdle) dystocia [0,1,3]
  Impacted shoulders
  DEF: Obstructed labor due to impacted fetal shoulders.

- **660.5** Locked twins [0,1,3]

- **660.6** Failed trial of labor, unspecified [0,1,3]
  Failed trial of labor, without mention of condition or suspected condition

- **660.7** Failed forceps or vacuum extractor, unspecified [0,1,3]
  Application of ventouse or forceps, without mention of condition

- **660.8** Other causes of obstructed labor [0,1,3]
  Use additional code to identify condition
  AHA: 4Q, '04, 88

- **660.9** Unspecified obstructed labor [0,1,3]
  Dystocia: Dystocia:
    NOS   maternal NOS
    fetal NOS

---

§ Requires fifth digit. Valid digits are in [brackets] under each code. See beginning of section 640–649 for codes and definitions.

2007 ICD•9•CM

COMPLICATIONS OF PREGNANCY, CHILDBIRTH AND THE PUERPERIUM

661–665.1

√4th 661 Abnormality of forces of labor

§ √5th **661.0 Primary uterine inertia** M♀
[0,1,3]
Failure of cervical dilation
Hypotonic uterine dysfunction, primary
Prolonged latent phase of labor
DEF: Lack of efficient contractions during labor causing prolonged labor.

§ √5th **661.1 Secondary uterine inertia** M♀
[0,1,3]
Arrested active phase of labor
Hypotonic uterine dysfunction, secondary

§ √5th **661.2 Other and unspecified uterine inertia** M♀
[0,1,3]
Desultory labor   Poor contractions
Irregular labor   Slow slope active phase of labor

§ √5th **661.3 Precipitate labor** M♀
[0,1,3] **DEF:** Rapid labor and delivery.

§ √5th **661.4 Hypertonic, incoordinate, or prolonged** M♀
[0,1,3] **uterine contractions**
Cervical spasm
Contraction ring (dystocia)
Dyscoordinate labor
Hourglass contraction of uterus
Hypertonic uterine dysfunction
Incoordinate uterine action
Retraction ring (Bandl's) (pathological)
Tetanic contractions
Uterine dystocia NOS
Uterine spasm

§ √5th **661.9 Unspecified abnormality of labor** M♀
[0,1,3]

√4th 662 Long labor

§ √5th **662.0 Prolonged first stage** M♀
[0,1,3]

§ √5th **662.1 Prolonged labor, unspecified** M♀
[0,1,3]

§ √5th **662.2 Prolonged second stage** M♀
[0,1,3]

§ √5th **662.3 Delayed delivery of second twin, triplet, etc.** M♀
[0,1,3]

√4th 663 Umbilical cord complications

§ √5th **663.0 Prolapse of cord** M♀
[0,1,3]
Presentation of cord
DEF: Abnormal presentation of fetus; marked by protruding umbilical cord during labor; can cause fetal death.

§ √5th **663.1 Cord around neck, with compression** M♀
[0,1,3]
Cord tightly around neck

Perineal Lacerations

First degree
Second degree
Anus
Third degree
Fourth degree

§ √5th **663.2 Other and unspecified cord entanglement,** M♀
[0,1,3] **with compression**
Entanglement of cords of twins in mono-amniotic sac
Knot in cord (with compression)

§ √5th **663.3 Other and unspecified cord entanglement,** M♀
[0,1,3] **without mention of compression**
AHA: For code 663.31: 2Q, '03, 9

§ √5th **663.4 Short cord** M♀
[0,1,3]

§ √5th **663.5 Vasa previa** M♀
[0,1,3] **DEF:** Abnormal presentation of fetus marked by blood vessels of umbilical cord in front of fetal head.

§ √5th **663.6 Vascular lesions of cord** M♀
[0,1,3]
Bruising of cord   Thrombosis of vessels of
Hematoma of cord   cord

§ √5th **663.8 Other umbilical cord complications** M♀
[0,1,3]
Velamentous insertion of umbilical cord

§ √5th **663.9 Unspecified umbilical cord complication** M♀
[0,1,3]

√4th 664 Trauma to perineum and vulva during delivery
INCLUDES damage from instruments
that from extension of episiotomy
AHA: 1Q, '92, 11; N-D, '84, 10

§ √5th **664.0 First-degree perineal laceration** M♀
[0,1,4]
Perineal laceration, rupture, or tear involving:
fourchette   skin
hymen   vagina
labia   vulva

§ √5th **664.1 Second-degree perineal laceration** M♀
[0,1,4]
Perineal laceration, rupture, or tear (following episiotomy) involving:
pelvic floor
perineal muscles
vaginal muscles
EXCLUDES that involving anal sphincter (664.2)

§ √5th **664.2 Third-degree perineal laceration** M♀
[0,1,4]
Perineal laceration, rupture, or tear (following episiotomy) involving:
anal sphincter
rectovaginal septum
sphincter NOS
EXCLUDES that with anal or rectal mucosal laceration (664.3)

§ √5th **664.3 Fourth-degree perineal laceration** M♀
[0,1,4]
Perineal laceration, rupture, or tear as classifiable to 664.2 and involving also:
anal mucosa
rectal mucosa

§ √5th **664.4 Unspecified perineal laceration** M♀
[0,1,4]
Central laceration
AHA: 1Q, '92, 8

§ √5th **664.5 Vulval and perineal hematoma** M♀
[0,1,4] **AHA:** N-D, '84, 10

§ √5th **664.8 Other specified trauma to perineum and vulva** M♀
[0,1,4]

§ √5th **664.9 Unspecified trauma to perineum and vulva** M♀
[0,1,4]

√4th 665 Other obstetrical trauma
INCLUDES damage from instruments

§ √5th **665.0 Rupture of uterus before onset of labor** M♀
[0,1,3]

§ √5th **665.1 Rupture of uterus during labor** M♀
[0,1]
Rupture of uterus NOS

§ Requires fifth digit. Valid digits are in [brackets] under each code. See beginning of section 640–649 for codes and definitions.

N Newborn Age: 0   **P** Pediatric Age: 0-17   **M** Maternity Age: 12-55   **A** Adult Age: 15-124

COMPLICATIONS OF PREGNANCY, CHILDBIRTH AND THE PUERPERIUM

665.2–669.9

§ √5th **665.2** Inversion of uterus Ⓜ ♀
[0,2,4]

§ √5th **665.3** Laceration of cervix Ⓜ ♀
[0,1,4]

§ √5th **665.4** High vaginal laceration Ⓜ ♀
[0,1,4]
Laceration of vaginal wall or sulcus without mention of perineal laceration

§ √5th **665.5** Other injury to pelvic organs Ⓜ ♀
[0,1,4]
Injury to:
  bladder
  urethra
AHA: M-A, '87, 10

§ √5th **665.6** Damage to pelvic joints and ligaments Ⓜ ♀
[0,1,4]
Avulsion of inner symphyseal cartilage
Damage to coccyx
Separation of symphysis (pubis)
AHA: N-D, '84, 12

§ √5th **665.7** Pelvic hematoma Ⓜ ♀
[0,1,2,4]
Hematoma of vagina

§ √5th **665.8** Other specified obstetrical trauma Ⓜ ♀
[0-4]

§ √5th **665.9** Unspecified obstetrical trauma Ⓜ ♀
[0-4]

√4th **666** Postpartum hemorrhage
AHA: 1Q, '88, 14

§ √5th **666.0** Third-stage hemorrhage Ⓜ ♀
[0,2,4]
Hemorrhage associated with retained, trapped, or adherent placenta
Retained placenta NOS

§ √5th **666.1** Other immediate postpartum hemorrhage Ⓜ ♀
[0,2,4]
Atony of uterus ►with hemorrhage◄
Hemorrhage within the first 24 hours following delivery of placenta
Postpartum hemorrhage (atonic) NOS
EXCLUDES ► atony of uterus without hemorrhage (669.8)◄

§ √5th **666.2** Delayed and secondary postpartum hemorrhage Ⓜ ♀
[0,2,4]
Hemorrhage:
  after the first 24 hours following delivery
  associated with retained portions of placenta or membranes
Postpartum hemorrhage specified as delayed or secondary
Retained products of conception NOS, following delivery

§ √5th **666.3** Postpartum coagulation defects Ⓜ ♀
[0,2,4]
Postpartum: Postpartum:
  afibrinogenemia   fibrinolysis

√4th **667** Retained placenta or membranes, without hemorrhage
Requires fifth-digit; valid digits are in [brackets] under each code. See beginning of section 660-669 for definitions.
AHA: 1Q, '88, 14
DEF: Postpartum condition resulting from failure to expel placental membrane tissues due to failed contractions of uterine wall.

§ √5th **667.0** Retained placenta without hemorrhage Ⓜ ♀
[0,2,4]
Placenta accreta
Retained placenta: } without hemorrhage
  NOS
  total

§ √5th **667.1** Retained portions of placenta or membranes, without hemorrhage Ⓜ ♀
[0,2,4]
Retained products of conception following delivery, without hemorrhage

√4th **668** Complications of the administration of anesthetic or other sedation in labor and delivery
INCLUDES complications arising from the administration of a general or local anesthetic, analgesic, or other sedation in labor and delivery
EXCLUDES reaction to spinal or lumbar puncture (349.0)
spinal headache (349.0)
Use additional code(s) to further specify complication

§ √5th **668.0** Pulmonary complications Ⓜ ♀
[0-4]
Inhalation [aspiration] of stomach contents or secretions } following anesthesia or other sedation in labor or delivery
Mendelson's syndrome
Pressure collapse of lung

§ √5th **668.1** Cardiac complications Ⓜ ♀
[0-4]
Cardiac arrest or failure following anesthesia or other sedation in labor and delivery

§ √5th **668.2** Central nervous system complications Ⓜ ♀
[0-4]
Cerebral anoxia following anesthesia or other sedation in labor and delivery

§ √5th **668.8** Other complications of anesthesia or other sedation in labor and delivery Ⓜ ♀
[0-4]
AHA: 2Q, '99, 9

§ √5th **668.9** Unspecified complication of anesthesia and other sedation Ⓜ ♀
[0-4]

√4th **669** Other complications of labor and delivery, not elsewhere classified

§ √5th **669.0** Maternal distress Ⓜ ♀
[0-4]
Metabolic disturbance in labor and delivery

§ √5th **669.1** Shock during or following labor and delivery Ⓜ ♀
[0-4]
Obstetric shock

§ √5th **669.2** Maternal hypotension syndrome Ⓜ ♀
[0-4]
DEF: Low arterial blood pressure, in mother, during labor and delivery.

§ √5th **669.3** Acute renal failure following labor and delivery Ⓜ ♀
[0,2,4]

§ √5th **669.4** Other complications of obstetrical surgery and procedures Ⓜ ♀
[0-4]
Cardiac: } following cesarean or other obstetrical surgery or procedure, including delivery NOS
  arrest
  failure
Cerebral anoxia
EXCLUDES complications of obstetrical surgical wounds (674.1-674.3)

§ √5th **669.5** Forceps or vacuum extractor delivery without mention of indication Ⓜ ♀
[0,1]
Delivery by ventouse, without mention of indication

§ √5th **669.6** Breech extraction, without mention of indication Ⓜ ♀
[0,1]
EXCLUDES breech delivery NOS (652.2)

§ √5th **669.7** Cesarean delivery, without mention of indication Ⓜ ♀
[0,1]
AHA: For code 669.71: 1Q, '01, 11

§ √5th **669.8** Other complications of labor and delivery Ⓜ ♀
[0-4]

§ √5th **669.9** Unspecified complication of labor and delivery Ⓜ ♀
[0-4]

§ Requires fifth digit. Valid digits are in [brackets] under each code. See beginning of section 640–649 for codes and definitions.

√4th / √5th Additional Digit Required   Unspecified Code   Other Specified Code   Manifestation Code   ►◄ Revised Text   ● New Code   ▲ Revised Code Title

2007 ICD•9•CM

COMPLICATIONS OF PREGNANCY, CHILDBIRTH AND THE PUERPERIUM

670–674.2 | **Tabular List**

COMPLICATIONS OF THE PUERPERIUM (670-677)

Note: Categories 671 and 673-676 include the listed conditions even if they occur during pregnancy or childbirth.

The following fifth-digit subclassification is for use with categories 670-676 to denote the current episode of care. Valid fifth-digits are in [brackets] under each code.

- 0 unspecified as to episode of care or not applicable
- 1 delivered, with or without mention of antepartum condition
- 2 delivered, with mention of postpartum complication
- 3 antepartum condition or complication
- 4 postpartum condition or complication

✓4th 670 Major puerperal infection
[0,2,4]
§ ✓5th Use 0 as fourth-digit for this category
Puerperal:
 endometritis
 fever (septic)
 pelvic:
  cellulitis
  sepsis
  peritonitis
  pyemia
  salpingitis
  septicemia

EXCLUDES infection following abortion (639.0)
minor genital tract infection following delivery (646.6)
puerperal pyrexia NOS (672)
puerperal fever NOS (672)
puerperal pyrexia of unknown origin (672)
urinary tract infection following delivery (646.6)

AHA: 4Q, '91, 26; 2Q, '91, 7

DEF: Infection and inflammation, following childbirth.

✓4th 671 Venous complications in pregnancy and the puerperium

§ ✓5th **671.0 Varicose veins of legs**
[0-4] Varicose veins NOS
DEF: Distended, tortuous veins on legs associated with pregnancy.

§ ✓5th **671.1 Varicose veins of vulva and perineum**
[0-4] DEF: Distended, tortuous veins on external female genitalia associated with pregnancy.

§ ✓5th **671.2 Superficial thrombophlebitis**
[0-4] Thrombophlebitis (superficial)

§ ✓5th **671.3 Deep phlebothrombosis, antepartum**
[0,1,3] Deep-vein thrombosis, antepartum

§ ✓5th **671.4 Deep phlebothrombosis, postpartum**
[0,2,4] Deep-vein thrombosis, postpartum
Pelvic thrombophlebitis, postpartum
Phlegmasia alba dolens (puerperal)

§ ✓5th **671.5 Other phlebitis and thrombosis**
[0-4] Cerebral venous thrombosis
Thrombosis of intracranial venous sinus

§ ✓5th **671.8 Other venous complications**
[0-4] Hemorrhoids

§ ✓5th **671.9 Unspecified venous complication**
[0-4] Phlebitis NOS   Thrombosis NOS

✓4th 672 Pyrexia of unknown origin during the puerperium
[0,2,4]
§ ✓5th Use 0 as fourth-digit for this category
Postpartum fever NOS   Puerperal pyrexia NOS
Puerperal fever NOS

AHA: 4Q, '91, 26

DEF: Fever of unknown origin experienced by the mother after childbirth.

✓4th 673 Obstetrical pulmonary embolism
Requires fifth-digit; valid digits are in [brackets] under each code. See beginning of section 670-676 for definitions.
INCLUDES pulmonary emboli in pregnancy, childbirth or the puerperium, or specified as puerperal
EXCLUDES embolism following abortion (639.6)

§ ✓5th **673.0 Obstetrical air embolism**
[0-4] DEF: Sudden blocking of pulmonary artery with air or nitrogen bubbles during puerperium..

§ ✓5th **673.1 Amniotic fluid embolism**
[0-4] DEF: Sudden onset of pulmonary artery blockage from amniotic fluid entering the mother's circulation near the end of pregnancy due to strong uterine contractions.

§ ✓5th **673.2 Obstetrical blood-clot embolism**
[0-4] Puerperal pulmonary embolism NOS
AHA: For code 673.24: 1Q, '05, 6
DEF: Blood clot blocking artery in the lung; associated with pregnancy.

§ ✓5th **673.3 Obstetrical pyemic and septic embolism**
[0-4]

§ ✓5th **673.8 Other pulmonary embolism**
[0-4] Fat embolism

✓4th 674 Other and unspecified complications of the puerperium, not elsewhere classified

§ ✓5th **674.0 Cerebrovascular disorders in the puerperium**
[0-4] Any condition classifiable to 430-434, 436-437 occurring during pregnancy, childbirth or the puerperium, or specified as puerperal
EXCLUDES intracranial venous sinus thrombosis (671.5)

§ ✓5th **674.1 Disruption of cesarean wound**
[0,2,4] Dehiscence or disruption of uterine wound
EXCLUDES uterine rupture before onset of labor (665.0)
uterine rupture during labor (665.1)

§ ✓5th **674.2 Disruption of perineal wound**
[0,2,4] Breakdown of perineum   Disruption of wound of:
Disruption of wound of: perineal laceration
 episiotomy   Secondary perineal tear

AHA: For code 674.24: 1Q, '97, 9

Lactation Process: Ejection Reflex Arc

---

§ Requires fifth digit. Valid digits are in [brackets] under each code. See beginning of section 640-649 for codes and definitions.

N Newborn Age: 0   P Pediatric Age: 0-17   M Maternity Age: 12-55   A Adult Age: 15-124

COMPLICATIONS OF PREGNANCY, CHILDBIRTH AND THE PUERPERIUM

674.3 Other complications of obstetrical surgical wounds [0,2,4]
Hematoma
Hemorrhage } of cesarean section or perineal wound
Infection

EXCLUDES: damage from instruments in delivery (664.0-665.9)

AHA: 2Q, '91, 7

674.4 Placental polyp
[0,2,4]

674.5 Peripartum cardiomyopathy
[0-4]
Postpartum cardiomyopathy

AHA: 4Q, '03, 65

DEF: Any structural or functional abnormality of the ventricular myocardium, non-inflammatory disease of obscure or unknown etiology with onset during the postpartum period.

674.8 Other
[0,2,4]
Hepatorenal syndrome, following delivery
Postpartum:
   subinvolution of uterus
   uterine hypertrophy

AHA: 3Q, '98, 16

674.9 Unspecified
[0,2,4]
Sudden death of unknown cause during the puerperium

675 Infections of the breast and nipple associated with childbirth

INCLUDES: the listed conditions during pregnancy, childbirth or the puerperium

675.0 Infections of nipple
[0-4]
Abscess of nipple

675.1 Abscess of breast
[0-4]
Abscess: Mastitis:
  mammary   purulent
  subareolar   retromammary
  submammary submammary

675.2 Nonpurulent mastitis
[0-4]
Lymphangitis of breast Mastitis:
Mastitis: interstitial
  NOS   parenchymatous

675.8 Other specified infections of the breast and nipple
[0-4]

675.9 Unspecified infection of the breast and nipple
[0-4]

676 Other disorders of the breast associated with childbirth and disorders of lactation

INCLUDES: the listed conditions during pregnancy, the puerperium, or lactation

676.0 Retracted nipple
[0-4]

676.1 Cracked nipple
[0-4]
Fissure of nipple

676.2 Engorgement of breasts
[0-4]
DEF: Abnormal accumulation of milk in ducts of breast.

676.3 Other and unspecified disorder of breast
[0-4]

676.4 Failure of lactation
[0-4]
Agalactia
DEF: Abrupt ceasing of milk secretion by breast.

676.5 Suppressed lactation
[0-4]

676.6 Galactorrhea
[0-4]
EXCLUDES: galactorrhea not associated with childbirth (611.6)

DEF: Excessive or persistent milk secretion by breast; may be in absence of nursing.

676.8 Other disorders of lactation
[0-4]
Galactocele
DEF: Galactocele: obstructed mammary gland, creating retention cyst, results in milk-filled cysts enlarging mammary gland.

676.9 Unspecified disorder of lactation
[0-4]

677 Late effect of complication of pregnancy, childbirth, and the puerperium

Note: This category is to be used to indicate conditions in 632-648.9 and 651-676.9 as the cause of the late effect, themselves classifiable elsewhere. The "late effects" include conditions specified as such, or as sequelae, which may occur at any time after puerperium.
Code first any sequelae

AHA: 1Q, '97, 9; 4Q, '94, 42

SKIN AND SUBCUTANEOUS TISSUE 680–682.1

12. DISEASES OF THE SKIN AND SUBCUTANEOUS TISSUE (680-709)

INFECTIONS OF SKIN AND SUBCUTANEOUS TISSUE (680-686)

EXCLUDES certain infections of skin classified under "Infectious and Parasitic Diseases," such as:
- erysipelas (035)
- erysipeloid of Rosenbach (027.1)
- herpes:
  - simplex (054.0-054.9)
  - zoster (053.0-053.9)
- molluscum contagiosum (078.0)
- viral warts (078.1)

680 Carbuncle and furuncle

INCLUDES boil
furunculosis

DEF: Carbuncle: necrotic boils in skin and subcutaneous tissue of neck or back mainly due to staphylococcal infection.

DEF: Furuncle: circumscribed inflammation of corium and subcutaneous tissue due to staphylococcal infection.

680.0 Face
Ear [any part]
Face [any part, except eye]
Nose (septum)
Temple (region)
EXCLUDES eyelid (373.13)
lacrimal apparatus (375.31)
orbit (376.01)

680.1 Neck

680.2 Trunk
Abdominal wall
Back [any part, except buttocks]
Breast
Chest wall
Flank
Groin
Pectoral region
Perineum
Umbilicus
EXCLUDES buttocks (680.5)
external genital organs:
female (616.4)
male (607.2, 608.4)

680.3 Upper arm and forearm
Arm [any part, except hand]
Axilla
Shoulder

680.4 Hand
Finger [any]
Thumb
Wrist

680.5 Buttock
Anus
Gluteal region

680.6 Leg, except foot
Ankle
Hip
Knee
Thigh

Skin and Subcutaneous Layer

680.7 Foot
Heel
Toe

680.8 Other specified sites
Head [any part, except face]
Scalp
EXCLUDES external genital organs:
female (616.4)
male (607.2, 608.4)

680.9 Unspecified site
Boil NOS
Carbuncle NOS
Furuncle NOS

681 Cellulitis and abscess of finger and toe
INCLUDES that with lymphangitis
Use additional code to identify organism, such as Staphylococcus (041.1)
AHA: 2Q, '91, 5; J-F, '87, 12

DEF: Acute suppurative inflammation and edema in subcutaneous tissue or muscle of finger or toe.

681.0 Finger
681.00 Cellulitis and abscess, unspecified
681.01 Felon
Pulp abscess
Whitlow
EXCLUDES herpetic whitlow (054.6)

DEF: Painful abscess of fingertips caused by infection in the closed space of terminal phalanx.

681.02 Onychia and paronychia of finger
Panaritium } of finger
Perionychia

DEF: Onychia: inflammation of nail matrix; causes nail loss.

DEF: Paronychia: inflammation of tissue folds around nail.

681.1 Toe
681.10 Cellulitis and abscess, unspecified
AHA: 1Q, '05, 14
681.11 Onychia and paronychia of toe
Panaritium } of toe
Perionychia

681.9 Cellulitis and abscess of unspecified digit
Infection of nail NOS

682 Other cellulitis and abscess
INCLUDES abscess (acute) } (with lymphangitis)
cellulitis (diffuse) } except of finger
lymphangitis, acute } or toe
Use additional code to identify organism, such as Staphylococcus (041.1)
EXCLUDES lymphangitis (chronic) (subacute) (457.2)
AHA: 2Q, '91, 5; J-F, '87, 12; S-O, '85, 10

DEF: Cellulitis: Acute suppurative inflammation of deep subcutaneous tissue and sometimes muscle due to infection of wound, burn or other lesion.

682.0 Face
Cheek, external
Chin
Forehead
Nose, external
Submandibular
Temple (region)
EXCLUDES ear [any part] (380.10-380.16)
eyelid (373.13)
lacrimal apparatus (375.31)
lip (528.5)
mouth (528.3)
nose (internal) (478.1)
orbit (376.01)

682.1 Neck

682.2 Trunk
  Abdominal wall
  Back [any part, except buttock]
  Chest wall
  Flank
  Groin
  Pectoral region
  Perineum
  Umbilicus, except newborn
  EXCLUDES anal and rectal regions (566)
        breast:
          NOS (611.0)
          puerperal (675.1)
        external genital organs:
          female (616.3-616.4)
          male (604.0, 607.2, 608.4)
        umbilicus, newborn (771.4)
  AHA: 4Q, '98, 42

682.3 Upper arm and forearm
  Arm [any part, except hand]
  Axilla
  Shoulder
  EXCLUDES hand (682.4)
  AHA: 2Q, '03, 7

682.4 Hand, except fingers and thumb
  Wrist
  EXCLUDES finger and thumb (681.00-681.02)

682.5 Buttock
  Gluteal region
  EXCLUDES anal and rectal regions (566)

682.6 Leg, except foot
  Ankle
  Hip
  Knee
  Thigh
  AHA: 3Q, '04, 5; 4Q, '03, 108

682.7 Foot, except toes
  Heel
  EXCLUDES toe (681.10-681.11)

682.8 Other specified sites
  Head [except face]
  Scalp
  EXCLUDES face (682.0)

682.9 Unspecified site
  Abscess NOS
  Cellulitis NOS
  Lymphangitis, acute NOS
  EXCLUDES lymphangitis NOS (457.2)

683 Acute lymphadenitis
  Abscess (acute)
  Adenitis, acute   } lymph gland or node,
  Lymphadenitis, acute   except mesenteric
  Use additional code to identify organism, such as
    Staphylococcus (041.1)
  EXCLUDES enlarged glands NOS (785.6)
        lymphadenitis:
          chronic or subacute, except mesenteric
            (289.1)
          mesenteric (acute) (chronic) (subacute) (289.2)
          unspecified (289.3)
  DEF: Acute inflammation of lymph nodes due to primary infection located elsewhere in the body.

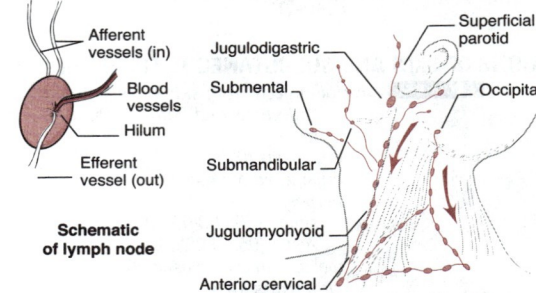

684 Impetigo
  Impetiginization of other dermatoses
  Impetigo (contagiosa) [any site] [any organism]:
    bullous
    circinate
    neonatorum
    simplex
  Pemphigus neonatorum
  EXCLUDES impetigo herpetiformis (694.3)
  DEF: Infectious skin disease commonly occurring in children; caused by group A streptococci or *Staphylococcus aureus*; skin lesions usually appear on the face and consist of subcorneal vesicles and bullae that burst and form yellow crusts.

√4th **685 Pilonidal cyst**
  INCLUDES fistula   } coccygeal or pilonidal
        sinus
  DEF: Hair-containing cyst or sinus in the tissues of the sacrococcygeal area; often drains through opening at the postanal dimple.

  685.0 With abscess
  685.1 Without mention of abscess

√4th **686 Other local infections of skin and subcutaneous tissue**
  Use additional code to identify any infectious organism (041.0-041.8)

√5th **686.0 Pyoderma**
    Dermatitis: Dermatitis:
      purulent   suppurative
      septic
    DEF: Nonspecific purulent skin disease related most to furuncles, pustules, or possibly carbuncles.

    686.00 Pyoderma, unspecified
    686.01 Pyoderma gangrenosum
      AHA: 4Q, '97, 42
      DEF: Persistent debilitating skin disease, characterized by irregular, boggy, blue-red ulcerations, with central healing and undermined edges.

    686.09 Other pyoderma

SKIN AND SUBCUTANEOUS TISSUE

686.1 **Pyogenic granuloma**
Granuloma:
  septic
  suppurative
  telangiectaticum
  EXCLUDES pyogenic granuloma of oral mucosa (528.9)

DEF: Solitary polypoid capillary hemangioma often associated with local irritation, trauma, and superimposed inflammation; located on the skin and gingival or oral mucosa.

686.8 **Other specified local infections of skin and subcutaneous tissue**
Bacterid (pustular)
Dermatitis vegetans
Ecthyma
Perlèche
  EXCLUDES dermatitis infectiosa eczematoides (690.8)
  panniculitis (729.30-729.39)

686.9 **Unspecified local infection of skin and subcutaneous tissue**
Fistula of skin NOS
Skin infection NOS
  EXCLUDES fistula to skin from internal organs — see Alphabetic Index

OTHER INFLAMMATORY CONDITIONS OF SKIN AND SUBCUTANEOUS TISSUE (690-698)
  EXCLUDES panniculitis (729.30-729.39)

√4ᵗʰ **690 Erythematosquamous dermatosis**
  EXCLUDES eczematous dermatitis of eyelid (373.31)
  parakeratosis variegata (696.2)
  psoriasis (696.0-696.1)
  seborrheic keratosis (702.11-702.19)

DEF: Dry material desquamated from the scalp, associated with disease.

√5ᵗʰ **690.1** **Seborrheic dermatitis**
AHA: 4Q, '95, 58

  690.10 **Seborrheic dermatitis, unspecified**
  Seborrheic dermatitis NOS

  690.11 **Seborrhea capitis**   P
  Cradle cap

  690.12 **Seborrheic infantile dermatitis**   P

  690.18 **Other seborrheic dermatitis**

690.8 **Other erythematosquamous dermatosis**

√4ᵗʰ **691 Atopic dermatitis and related conditions**

DEF: Atopic dermatitis: chronic, pruritic, inflammatory skin disorder found on the face and antecubital and popliteal fossae; noted in persons with a hereditary predisposition to pruritus, and often accompanied by allergic rhinitis, hay fever, asthma, and extreme itching; also called allergic dermatitis, allergic or atopic eczema, or disseminated neurodermatitis.

691.0 **Diaper or napkin rash**
Ammonia dermatitis
Diaper or napkin:
  dermatitis
  erythema
  rash
Psoriasiform napkin eruption

691.8 **Other atopic dermatitis and related conditions**
Atopic dermatitis
Besnier's prurigo
Eczema:
  atopic
  flexural
  intrinsic (allergic)
Neurodermatitis:
  atopic
  diffuse (of Brocq)

√4ᵗʰ **692 Contact dermatitis and other eczema**
  INCLUDES dermatitis:
    NOS
    contact
    occupational
    venenata
  eczema (acute) (chronic):
    NOS
    allergic
    erythematous
    occupational
  EXCLUDES allergy NOS (995.3)
    contact dermatitis of eyelids (373.32)
    dermatitis due to substances taken internally (693.0-693.9)
    eczema of external ear (380.22)
    perioral dermatitis (695.3)
    urticarial reactions (708.0-708.9, 995.1)

DEF: Contact dermatitis: acute or chronic dermatitis caused by initial irritant effect of a substance, or by prior sensitization to a substance coming once again in contact with skin.

692.0 **Due to detergents**
692.1 **Due to oils and greases**
692.2 **Due to solvents**
Dermatitis due to solvents of:
  chlorocompound
  cyclohexane
  ester   } group
  glycol
  hydrocarbon
  ketone

692.3 **Due to drugs and medicines in contact with skin**
Dermatitis (allergic)   Dermatitis (allergic)
  (contact) due to: (contact) due to:
  arnica   neomycin
  fungicides   pediculocides
  iodine   phenols
  keratolytics   scabicides
  mercurials   any drug applied to skin
Dermatitis medicamentosa due to drug applied to skin
Use additional E code to identify drug
  EXCLUDES allergy NOS due to drugs ▶(995.27)◀
    dermatitis due to ingested drugs (693.0)
    dermatitis medicamentosa NOS (693.0)

692.4 **Due to other chemical products**
Dermatitis due to:
  acids
  adhesive plaster
  alkalis
  caustics
  dichromate
  insecticide
  nylon
  plastic
  rubber
AHA: 2Q, '89, 16

692.5 **Due to food in contact with skin**
Dermatitis, contact,   Dermatitis, contact,
  due to: due to:
  cereals   fruit
  fish   meat
  flour   milk
  EXCLUDES dermatitis due to:
    dyes (692.89)
    ingested foods (693.1)
    preservatives (692.89)

692.6 Due to plants [except food]
Dermatitis due to:
  lacquer tree [Rhus verniciflua]
  poison:
    ivy [Rhus toxicodendron]
    oak [Rhus diversiloba]
    sumac [Rhus venenata]
    vine [Rhus radicans]
  primrose [Primula]
  ragweed [Senecio jacobae]
  other plants in contact with the skin
> EXCLUDES allergy NOS due to pollen (477.0)
> nettle rash (708.8)

√5th 692.7 Due to solar radiation
> EXCLUDES sunburn due to other ultraviolet radiation exposure (692.82)

692.70 Unspecified dermatitis due to sun

692.71 Sunburn
  First degree sunburn
  Sunburn NOS
AHA: 4Q, '01, 47

692.72 Acute dermatitis due to solar radiation
  Acute solar skin damage NOS
  Berlogue dermatitis
  Photoallergic response
  Phototoxic response
  Polymorphus light eruption
> EXCLUDES sunburn (692.71, 692.76-692.77)

Use additional E code to identify drug, if drug induced

DEF: Berloque dermatitis: phytophotodermatitis due to sun exposure after use of a product containing bergamot oil; causes red patches, which may turn brown.

DEF: Photoallergic response: dermatitis due to hypersensitivity to the sun; causes papulovesicular, eczematous or exudative eruptions.

DEF: Phototoxic response: chemically induced sensitivity to sun causes burn-like reaction, occasionally vesiculation and subsequent hyperpigmentation.

DEF: Polymorphous light eruption: inflammatory skin eruptions due to sunlight exposure; eruptions differ in size and shape.

DEF: Acute solar skin damage (NOS): rapid, unspecified injury to skin from sun.

692.73 Actinic reticuloid and actinic granuloma

DEF: Actinic reticuloid: dermatosis aggravated by light, causes chronic eczema-like eruption on exposed skin which extends to other unexposed surfaces; occurs in the eldery.

DEF: Actinic granuloma: inflammatory response of skin to sun causing small nodule of microphages.

692.74 Other chronic dermatitis due to solar radiation
  Solar elastosis
  Chronic solar skin damage NOS
> EXCLUDES actinic [solar] keratosis (702.0)

DEF: Solar elastosis: premature aging of skin of light-skinned people; causes inelasticity, thinning or thickening, wrinkling, dryness, scaling and hyperpigmentation.

DEF: Chronic solar skin damage (NOS): chronic skin impairment due to exposure to the sun, not otherwise specified.

692.75 Disseminated superficial actinic porokeratosis [DSAP]
AHA: 4Q, '00, 43

DEF: Autosomal dominant skin condition occurring in skin that has been overexposed to the sun. Primarily affects women over the age of 16; characterized by numerous superficial annular, keratotic, brownish-red spots or thickenings with depressed centers and sharp, ridged borders. High risk that condition will evolve into squamous cell carcinoma.

692.76 Sunburn of second degree
AHA: 4Q, '01, 47

692.77 Sunburn of third degree
AHA: 4Q, '01, 47

692.79 Other dermatitis due to solar radiation
  Hydroa aestivale
  Photodermatitis   } (due to sun)
  Photosensitiveness
  Solar skin damage NOS

√5th 692.8 Due to other specified agents

692.81 Dermatitis due to cosmetics

692.82 Dermatitis due to other radiation
  Infrared rays
  Light
  Radiation NOS
  Tanning bed
  Ultraviolet rays
  X-rays
> EXCLUDES solar radiation (692.70-692.79)

AHA: 4Q, '01, 47; 3Q, '00, 5

692.83 Dermatitis due to metals
  Jewelry

692.84 Due to animal (cat) (dog) dander
  Due to animal (cat) (dog) hair

692.89 Other
Dermatitis due to:
  cold weather
  dyes
  hot weather
  preservatives
> EXCLUDES allergy (NOS) (rhinitis) due to animal hair or dander (477.2)
> allergy to dust (477.8)
> sunburn (692.71, 692.76-692.77)

692.9 Unspecified cause
Dermatitis:
  NOS
  contact NOS
  venenata NOS
Eczema NOS

√4th 693 Dermatitis due to substances taken internally
> EXCLUDES adverse effect NOS of drugs and medicines ▶(995.20)◀
> allergy NOS (995.3)
> contact dermatitis (692.0-692.9)
> urticarial reactions (708.0-708.9, 995.1)

DEF: Inflammation of skin due to ingested substance.

693.0 Due to drugs and medicines
  Dermatitis medicamentosa NOS
  Use additional E code to identify drug
> EXCLUDES that due to drugs in contact with skin (692.3)

693.1 Due to food

693.8 Due to other specified substances taken internally

693.9 Due to unspecified substance taken internally
> EXCLUDES dermatitis NOS (692.9)

SKIN AND SUBCUTANEOUS TISSUE

✓4th 694 Bullous dermatoses

694.0 Dermatitis herpetiformis
Dermatosis herpetiformis   Hydroa herpetiformis
Duhring's disease
EXCLUDES herpes gestationis (646.8)
dermatitis herpetiformis:
juvenile (694.2)
senile (694.5)

DEF: Chronic, relapsing multisystem disease manifested most in the cutaneous system; seen as an extremely pruritic eruption of various combinations of lesions that frequently heal leaving hyperpigmentation or hypopigmentation and occasionally scarring; usually associated with an asymptomatic gluten-sensitive enteropathy, and immunogenic factors are believed to play a role in its origin.

694.1 Subcorneal pustular dermatosis
Sneddon-Wilkinson disease or syndrome

DEF: Chronic relapses of sterile pustular blebs beneath the horny skin layer of the trunk and skin folds; resembles dermatitis herpetiformis.

694.2 Juvenile dermatitis herpetiformis
Juvenile pemphigoid

694.3 Impetigo herpetiformis

DEF: Rare dermatosis associated with pregnancy; marked by itching pustules in third trimester, hypocalcemia, tetany, fever and lethargy; may result in maternal or fetal death.

694.4 Pemphigus
Pemphigus:
NOS
erythematosus
foliaceus
malignant
vegetans
vulgaris
EXCLUDES pemphigus neonatorum (684)

DEF: Chronic, relapsing, sometimes fatal skin diseases; causes vesicles, bullae; autoantibodies against intracellular connections cause acantholysis.

694.5 Pemphigoid
Benign pemphigus NOS
Bullous pemphigoid
Herpes circinatus bullosus
Senile dermatitis herpetiformis

✓5th 694.6 Benign mucous membrane pemphigoid
Cicatricial pemphigoid
Mucosynechial atrophic bullous dermatitis

694.60 Without mention of ocular involvement

694.61 With ocular involvement
Ocular pemphigus

694.8 Other specified bullous dermatoses
EXCLUDES herpes gestationis (646.8)

694.9 Unspecified bullous dermatoses

✓4th 695 Erythematous conditions

695.0 Toxic erythema
Erythema venenatum

695.1 Erythema multiforme
Erythema iris   Scalded skin syndrome
Herpes iris   Stevens-Johnson syndrome
Lyell's syndrome   Toxic epidermal necrolysis

DEF: Symptom complex with a varied skin eruption pattern of macular, bullous, papular, nodose, or vesicular lesions on the neck, face, and legs; gastritis and rheumatic pains are also noticeable, first-seen symptoms; complex is secondary to a number of factors, including infections, ingestants, physical agents, malignancy and pregnancy.

695.2 Erythema nodosum
EXCLUDES tuberculous erythema nodosum (017.1)

DEF: Panniculitis (an inflammatory reaction of the subcutaneous fat) of women, usually seen as a hypersensitivity reaction to various infections, drugs, sarcoidosis, and specific enteropathies; the acute stage is often associated with other symptoms, including fever, malaise, and arthralgia; the lesions are pink to blue in color, appear in crops as tender nodules and are found on the front of the legs below the knees.

695.3 Rosacea
Acne:
erythematosa
rosacea
Perioral dermatitis
Rhinophyma

DEF: Chronic skin disease, usually of the face, characterized by persistent erythema and sometimes by telangiectasis with acute episodes of edema, engorgement papules, and pustules.

695.4 Lupus erythematosus
Lupus:
erythematodes (discoid)
erythematosus (discoid), not disseminated
EXCLUDES lupus (vulgaris) NOS (017.0)
systemic [disseminated] lupus erythematosus (710.0)

DEF: Group of connective tissue disorders occurring as various cutaneous diseases of unknown origin; it primarily affects women between the ages of 20 and 40.

✓5th 695.8 Other specified erythematous conditions

695.81 Ritter's disease
Dermatitis exfoliativa neonatorum

DEF: Infectious skin disease of infants and young children marked by eruptions ranging from a localized bullous type to widespread development of easily ruptured fine vesicles and bullae; results in exfoliation of large planes of skin and leaves raw areas; also called staphylococcal scalded skin syndrome.

695.89 Other
Erythema intertrigo
Intertrigo
Pityriasis rubra (Hebra)
EXCLUDES mycotic intertrigo (111.0-111.9)

AHA:: S-O, '86, 10

695.9 Unspecified erythematous condition
Erythema NOS
Erythroderma (secondary)

✓4th 696 Psoriasis and similar disorders

696.0 Psoriatic arthropathy

DEF: Psoriasis associated with inflammatory arthritis; often involves interphalengeal joints.

696.1 Other psoriasis
Acrodermatitis continua
Dermatitis repens
Psoriasis:
NOS
any type, except arthropathic
EXCLUDES psoriatic arthropathy (696.0)

696.2 Parapsoriasis
Parakeratosis variegata
Parapsoriasis lichenoides chronica
Pityriasis lichenoides et varioliformis

DEF: Erythrodermas similar to lichen, planus and psoriasis; symptoms include redness and itching; resistant to treatment.

SKIN AND SUBCUTANEOUS TISSUE

696.3 Pityriasis rosea
Pityriasis circinata (et maculata)
DEF: Common, self-limited rash of unknown etiology marked by a solitary erythematous, salmon or fawn-colored herald plaque on the trunk, arms or thighs; followed by development of papular or macular lesions that tend to peel and form a scaly collarette.

696.4 Pityriasis rubra pilaris
Devergie's disease   Lichen ruber acuminatus
EXCLUDES pityriasis rubra (Hebra) (695.89)
DEF: Inflammatory disease of hair follicles; marked by firm, red lesions topped by horny plugs; may form patches; occurs on fingers elbows, knees.

696.5 Other and unspecified pityriasis
Pityriasis:
  NOS
  alba
  streptogenes
EXCLUDES pityriasis:
  simplex (690.18)
  versicolor (111.0)

696.8 Other

✓4th 697 Lichen
EXCLUDES lichen:
  obtusus corneus (698.3)
  pilaris (congenital) (757.39)
  ruber acuminatus (696.4)
  sclerosus et atrophicus (701.0)
  scrofulosus (017.0)
  simplex chronicus (698.3)
  spinulosus (congenital) (757.39)
  urticatus (698.2)

697.0 Lichen planus
Lichen:
  planopilaris
  ruber planus
DEF: Inflammatory, pruritic skin disease; marked by angular, flat-top, violet-colored papules; may be acute and widespread or chronic and localized.

697.1 Lichen nitidus
Pinkus' disease
DEF: Chronic, inflammatory, usually asymptomatic skin disorder, characterized by numerous glistening, flat-topped, discrete, smooth, skin-colored micropapules most often on penis, lower abdomen, inner thighs, wrists, forearms, breasts and buttocks.

697.8 Other lichen, not elsewhere classified
Lichen:
  ruber moniliforme
  striata

697.9 Lichen, unspecified

✓4th 698 Pruritus and related conditions
EXCLUDES pruritus specified as psychogenic (306.3)
DEF: Pruritus: Intense, persistent itching due to irritation of sensory nerve endings from organic or psychogenic causes.

698.0 Pruritus ani
Perianal itch

698.1 Pruritus of genital organs

698.2 Prurigo
Lichen urticatus
Prurigo:
  NOS
  Hebra's
  mitis
  simplex
Urticaria papulosa (Hebra)
EXCLUDES prurigo nodularis (698.3)

698.3 Lichenification and lichen simplex chronicus
Hyde's disease
Neurodermatitis (circumscripta) (local)
Prurigo nodularis
EXCLUDES neurodermatitis, diffuse (of Brocq) (691.8)
DEF: Lichenification: thickening of skin due to prolonged rubbing or scratching.
DEF: Lichen simplex chronicus: eczematous dermatitis, of face, neck, extremities, scrotum, vulva, and perianal region due to repeated itching, rubbing and scratching; spontaneous or evolves with other dermatoses.

698.4 Dermatitis factitia [artefacta]
Dermatitis ficta
Neurotic excoriation
Use additional code to identify any associated mental disorder
DEF: Various types of self-inflicted skin lesions characterized in appearance as an erythema to a gangrene.

698.8 Other specified pruritic conditions
Pruritu
  hiemalis
  senilis
Winter itch

698.9 Unspecified pruritic disorder
Itch NOS
Pruritus NOS

OTHER DISEASES OF SKIN AND SUBCUTANEOUS TISSUE (700-709)
EXCLUDES conditions confined to eyelids (373.0-374.9)
congenital conditions of skin, hair, and nails (757.0-757.9)

700 Corns and callosities
Callus
Clavus
DEF: Corns: conical or horny thickening of skin on toes, due to friction, pressure from shoes and hosiery; pain and inflammation may develop.
DEF: Callosities: localized overgrowth (hyperplasia) of the horny epidermal layer due to pressure or friction.

✓4th 701 Other hypertrophic and atrophic conditions of skin
EXCLUDES dermatomyositis (710.3)
hereditary edema of legs (757.0)
scleroderma (generalized) (710.1)

701.0 Circumscribed scleroderma
Addison's keloid
Dermatosclerosis, localized
Lichen sclerosus et atrophicus
Morphea
Scleroderma, circumscribed or localized
DEF: Thickened, hardened, skin and subcutaneous tissue; may involve musculoskeletal system.

701.1 Keratoderma, acquired
Acquired:
  ichthyosis
  keratoderma palmaris et plantaris
Elastosis perforans serpiginosa
Hyperkeratosis:
  NOS
  follicularis in cutem penetrans
  palmoplantaris climacterica
Keratoderma:
  climactericum
  tylodes, progressive
Keratosis (blennorrhagica)
EXCLUDES Darier's disease [keratosis follicularis] (congenital) (757.39)
keratosis:
  arsenical (692.4)
  gonococcal (098.81)

AHA: 4Q, '94, 48

SKIN AND SUBCUTANEOUS TISSUE

701.2 Acquired acanthosis nigricans
Keratosis nigricans
DEF: Diffuse velvety hyperplasia of the spinous skin layer of the axilla and other body folds marked by gray, brown, or black pigmentation; in adult form it is often associated with an internal carcinoma (malignant acanthosis nigricans) in a benign, nevoid form it is relatively generalized; benign juvenile form with obesity is sometimes caused by an endocrine disturbance.

701.3 Striae atrophicae
Atrophic spots of skin
Atrophoderma maculatum
Atrophy blanche (of Milian)
Degenerative colloid atrophy
Senile degenerative atrophy
Striae distensae
DEF: Bands of atrophic, depressed, wrinkled skin associated with stretching of skin from pregnancy, obesity, or rapid growth during puberty.

701.4 Keloid scar
Cheloid
Hypertrophic scar
Keloid
DEF: Overgrowth of scar tissue due to excess amounts of collagen during connective tissue repair; occurs mainly on upper trunk, face.

701.5 Other abnormal granulation tissue
Excessive granulation

701.8 Other specified hypertrophic and atrophic conditions of skin
Acrodermatitis atrophicans chronica
Atrophia cutis senilis
Atrophoderma neuriticum
Confluent and reticulate papillomatosis
Cutis laxa senilis
Elastosis senilis
Folliculitis ulerythematosa reticulata
Gougerot-Carteaud syndrome or disease

701.9 Unspecified hypertrophic and atrophic conditions of skin
Atrophoderma
Skin tag

√4ᵗʰ **702 Other dermatoses**
EXCLUDES   carcinoma in situ (232.0-232.9)

702.0 Actinic keratosis
AHA: 1Q, '92, 18
DEF: Wart-like growth, red or skin-colored; may form a cutaneous horn.

√5ᵗʰ **702.1 Seborrheic keratosis**
DEF: Common, benign, lightly pigmented, warty growth composed of basaloid cells.

702.11 Inflamed seborrheic keratosis
AHA: 4Q, '94, 48

702.19 Other seborrheic keratosis
Seborrheic keratosis NOS

702.8 Other specified dermatoses

√4ᵗʰ **703 Diseases of nail**
EXCLUDES   congenital anomalies (757.5)
onychia and paronychia (681.02, 681.11)

703.0 Ingrowing nail
Ingrowing nail with infection
Unguis incarnatus
EXCLUDES   infection, nail NOS (681.9)

703.8 Other specified diseases of nail
Dystrophia unguium
Hypertrophy of nail
Koilonychia
Leukonychia (punctata) (striata)
Onychauxis
Onychogryposis
Onycholysis

703.9 Unspecified disease of nail

√4ᵗʰ **704 Diseases of hair and hair follicles**
EXCLUDES   congenital anomalies (757.4)

√5ᵗʰ **704.0 Alopecia**
EXCLUDES   madarosis (374.55)
syphilitic alopecia (091.82)
DEF: Lack of hair, especially on scalp; often called baldness; may be partial or total; occurs at any age.

704.00 Alopecia, unspecified
Baldness
Loss of hair

704.01 Alopecia areata
Ophiasis
DEF: Alopecia areata: usually reversible, inflammatory, patchy hair loss found in beard or scalp.
DEF: Ophiasis: alopecia areata of children; marked by band around temporal and occipital scalp margins.

704.02 Telogen effluvium
DEF: Shedding of hair from premature telogen development in follicles due to stress, including shock, childbirth, surgery, drugs or weight loss.

704.09 Other
Folliculitis decalvans
Hypotrichosis:
NOS
postinfectional NOS
Pseudopelade

704.1 Hirsutism
Hypertrichosis:
NOS
lanuginosa, acquired
Polytrichia
EXCLUDES   hypertrichosis of eyelid (374.54)
DEF: Excess hair growth; often in unexpected places and amounts.

704.2 Abnormalities of the hair
Atrophic hair
Clastothrix
Fragilitas crinium
Trichiasis:
NOS
cicatrical
Trichorrhexis (nodosa)
EXCLUDES   trichiasis of eyelid (374.05)

704.3 Variations in hair color
Canities (premature)
Grayness, hair (premature)
Heterochromia of hair
Poliosis:
NOS
circumscripta, acquired

704.8 Other specified diseases of hair and hair follicles
Folliculitis: Sycosis:
  NOS   NOS
  abscedens et suffodiens   barbae [not parasitic]
  pustular   lupoid
Perifolliculitis: vulgaris
  NOS
  capitis abscedens et suffodiens
  scalp

704.9 Unspecified disease of hair and hair follicles

√4ᵗʰ **705 Disorders of sweat glands**

705.0 Anhidrosis
Hypohidrosis   Oligohidrosis
DEF: Lack or deficiency of ability to sweat.

705.1 Prickly heat
Heat rash   Sudamina
Miliaria rubra (tropicalis)

SKIN AND SUBCUTANEOUS TISSUE

✓5th 705.2 Focal hyperhidrosis
EXCLUDES generalized (secondary) hyperhidrosis (780.8)

705.21 Primary focal hyperhidrosis
Focal hyperhidrosis NOS
Hyperhidrosis NOS
Hyperhidrosis of:
  axilla
  face
  palms
  soles

AHA: 4Q, '04, 91

DEF: A rare condition that is a disorder of the sweat glands resulting in excessive production of sweat; occurs in the absence of any underlying or causative condition and is almost always focal, confined to one or more specific areas of the body.

705.22 Secondary focal hyperhidrosis
Frey's syndrome

AHA: 4Q, '04, 91

DEF: Secondary focal hyperhidrosis: a symptom of an underlying disease process resulting in excessive sweating beyond what the body requires to maintain thermal control, confined to one or more specific areas of the body.

DEF: Frey's syndrome: an auriculotemporal syndrome due to lesion on the parotid gland; characteristic redness and excessive sweating on the cheek in connection with eating.

✓5th 705.8 Other specified disorders of sweat glands

705.81 Dyshidrosis
Cheiropompholyx
Pompholyx

DEF: Vesicular eruption, on hands, feet causing itching and burning.

705.82 Fox-Fordyce disease
DEF: Chronic, usually pruritic disease chiefly of women evidenced by small follicular papular eruptions, especially in the axillary and pubic areas; develops from the closure and rupture of the affected apocrine glands' intraepidermal portion of the ducts.

705.83 Hidradenitis
Hidradenitis suppurativa
DEF: Inflamed sweat glands.

705.89 Other
Bromhidrosis
Chromhidrosis
Granulosis rubra nasi
Urhidrosis
EXCLUDES generalized hyperhidrosis (780.8)
hidrocystoma (216.0-216.9)

DEF: Bromhidrosis: foul-smelling axillary sweat due to decomposed bacteria.
DEF: Chromhidrosis: secretion of colored sweat.
DEF: Granulosis rubra nasi: idiopathic condition of children; causes redness, sweating around nose, face and chin; tends to end by puberty.
DEF: Urhidrosis: urinous substance, such as uric acid, in sweat; occurs in uremia.

705.9 Unspecified disorder of sweat glands
Disorder of sweat glands NOS

✓4th 706 Diseases of sebaceous glands

706.0 Acne varioliformis
Acne: Acne:
  frontalis   necrotica

DEF: Rare form of acne characterized by persistent brown papulopustules usually on the brow and temporoparietal part of the scalp.

Four Stages of Decubitus Ulcers

First Stage Nonblanchable erythema

Second Stage Partial thickness skin loss involving epidermis, dermis, or both

Third Stage Full thickness skin loss extending through subcutaneous tissue

Fourth Stage Full thickness skin loss extending to muscle and bone

706.1 Other acne
Acne:
  NOS
  conglobata
  cystic
  pustular
  vulgaris
Blackhead
Comedo
EXCLUDES acne rosacea (695.3)

706.2 Sebaceous cyst
Atheroma, skin
Keratin cyst
Wen

DEF: Benign epidermal cyst, contains sebum and keratin; presents as firm, circumscribed nodule.

706.3 Seborrhea
EXCLUDES seborrhea:
  capitis (690.11)
  sicca (690.18)
seborrheic:
  dermatitis (690.10)
  keratosis (702.11-702.19)

DEF: Seborrheic dermatitis marked by excessive secretion of sebum; the sebum forms an oily coating, crusts, or scales on the skin; it is also called hypersteatosis.

706.8 Other specified diseases of sebaceous glands
Asteatosis (cutis)   Xerosis cutis

706.9 Unspecified disease of sebaceous glands

✓4th 707 Chronic ulcer of skin
INCLUDES non-infected sinus of skin
non-healing ulcer
EXCLUDES specific infections classified under "Infectious and Parasitic Diseases" (001.0-136.9)
varicose ulcer (454.0, 454.2)

AHA: 4Q, '04, 92

✓5th 707.0 Decubitus ulcer
Bed sore
Decubitus ulcer [any site]
Plaster ulcer
Pressure ulcer

AHA: 1Q, '04, 14; 4Q, '03, 110; 4Q, '99, 20; 1Q, '96, 15; 3Q, '90, 15; N-D, '87, 9

707.00 Unspecified site
707.01 Elbow
707.02 Upper back
Shoulder blades
707.03 Lower back
Sacrum

AHA: 1Q, '05, 16

707.04 Hip

N Newborn Age: 0   **P** Pediatric Age: 0-17   **M** Maternity Age: 12-55   **A** Adult Age: 15-124

SKIN AND SUBCUTANEOUS TISSUE

Cutaneous Lesions
Surface Lesions: Fissure, Polyp growth, Ulcer
Solid Lesions: Flat macule, Slightly elevated wheal, Solid papule
Sac Lesions: Cyst, Clear fluid vesicle, Pustule

- **707.05** Buttock
- **707.06** Ankle
- **707.07** Heel
  - AHA: 1Q, '05, 16
- **707.09** Other site
  - Head

√5th **707.1** Ulcer of lower limbs, except decubitus
  Ulcer, chronic:
   neurogenic } of lower limb
   trophic
  Code, if applicable, any casual condition first:
   atherosclerosis of the extremities with ulceration (440.23)
   chronic venous hypertension with ulcer (459.31)
   chronic venous hypertension with ulcer and inflammation (459.33)
   diabetes mellitus (250.80-250.83)
   postphlebitic syndrome with ulcer (459.11)
   postphlebitic syndrome with ulcer and inflammation (459.13)
  AHA: 4Q, '00, 44; 4Q, '99, 15

- **707.10** Ulcer of lower limb, unspecified
  - AHA: 3Q, '04, 5; 4Q, '02, 43
- **707.11** Ulcer of thigh
- **707.12** Ulcer of calf
- **707.13** Ulcer of ankle
- **707.14** Ulcer of heel and midfoot
  - Plantar surface of midfoot
- **707.15** Ulcer of other part of foot
  - Toes
- **707.19** Ulcer of other part of lower limb

707.8 Chronic ulcer of other specified sites
  Ulcer, chronic:
   neurogenic } of other specified sites
   trophic

707.9 Chronic ulcer of unspecified site
  Chronic ulcer NOS
  Trophic ulcer NOS
  Tropical ulcer NOS
  Ulcer of skin NOS

√4th **708** Urticaria
  EXCLUDES edema:
   angioneurotic (995.1)
   Quincke's (995.1)
   hereditary angioedema (277.6)
   urticaria:
    giant (995.1)
    papulosa (Hebra) (698.2)
    pigmentosa (juvenile) (congenital) (757.33)
  DEF: Skin disorder marked by raised edematous patches of skin or mucous membrane with intense itching; also called hives.

- **708.0** Allergic urticaria
- **708.1** Idiopathic urticaria
- **708.2** Urticaria due to cold and heat
  - Thermal urticaria
- **708.3** Dermatographic urticaria
  - Dermatographia   Factitial urticaria
- **708.4** Vibratory urticaria
- **708.5** Cholinergic urticaria
- **708.8** Other specified urticaria
  - Nettle rash
  - Urticaria:
    chronic
    recurrent periodic
- **708.9** Urticaria, unspecified
  - Hives NOS

√4th **709** Other disorders of skin and subcutaneous tissue

√5th **709.0** Dyschromia
  EXCLUDES albinism (270.2)
   pigmented nevus (216.0-216.9)
   that of eyelid (374.52-374.53)
  DEF: Pigment disorder of skin or hair.

- **709.00** Dyschromia, unspecified
- **709.01** Vitiligo
  - DEF: Persistent, progressive development of nonpigmented white patches on otherwise normal skin.
- **709.09** Other

709.1 Vascular disorders of skin
  Angioma serpiginosum
  Purpura (primary) annularis telangiectodes

709.2 Scar conditions and fibrosis of skin
  Adherent scar (skin)
  Cicatrix
  Disfigurement (due to scar)
  Fibrosis, skin NOS
  Scar NOS
  EXCLUDES keloid scar (701.4)
  AHA: N-D, '84, 19

709.3 Degenerative skin disorders
  Calcinosis: Degeneration, skin
   circumscripta   Deposits, skin
   cutis   Senile dermatosis NOS
  Colloid milium   Subcutaneous calcification

709.4 Foreign body granuloma of skin and subcutaneous tissue
  EXCLUDES residual foreign body without granuloma of skin and subcutaneous tissue (729.6)
   that of muscle (728.82)

709.8 Other specified disorders of skin
  Epithelial hyperplasia Vesicular eruption
  Menstrual dermatosis
  AHA: N-D, '87, 6
  DEF: Epithelial hyperplasia: increased number of epitheleal cells.
  DEF: Vesicular eruption: liquid-filled structures appearing through skin.

709.9 Unspecified disorder of skin and subcutaneous tissue
  Dermatosis NOS

13. DISEASES OF THE MUSCULOSKELETAL SYSTEM AND CONNECTIVE TISSUE (710-739)

The following fifth-digit subclassification is for use with categories 711-712, 715-716, 718-719, and 730:

- 0 site unspecified
- 1 shoulder region
  - Acromioclavicular joint(s)
  - Clavicle
  - Glenohumeral joint(s)
  - Scapula
  - Sternoclavicular joint(s)
- 2 upper arm
  - Elbow joint
  - Humerus
- 3 forearm
  - Radius
  - Wrist joint
  - Ulna
- 4 hand
  - Carpus
  - Phalanges [fingers]
  - Metacarpus
- 5 pelvic region and thigh
  - Buttock
  - Hip (joint)
  - Femur
- 6 lower leg
  - Fibula
  - Patella
  - Knee joint
  - Tibia
- 7 ankle and foot
  - Ankle joint
  - Phalanges, foot
  - Digits [toes]
  - Tarsus
  - Metatarsus
  - Other joints in foot
- 8 other specified sites
  - Head
  - Skull
  - Neck
  - Trunk
  - Ribs
  - Vertebral column
- 9 multiple sites

ARTHROPATHIES AND RELATED DISORDERS (710-719)

EXCLUDES disorders of spine (720.0-724.9)

710 Diffuse diseases of connective tissue

INCLUDES all collagen diseases whose effects are not mainly confined to a single system

EXCLUDES those affecting mainly the cardiovascular system, i.e., polyarteritis nodosa and allied conditions (446.0-446.7)

710.0 Systemic lupus erythematosus
Disseminated lupus erythematosus
Libman-Sacks disease
Use additional code to identify manifestation, as:
  endocarditis (424.91)
  nephritis (583.81)
    chronic (582.81)
  nephrotic syndrome (581.81)
EXCLUDES lupus erythematosus (discoid) NOS (695.4)

AHA: 2Q, '03, 7-8; 2Q, '97, 8

DEF: A chronic multisystemic inflammatory disease affecting connective tissue; marked by anemia, leukopenia, muscle and joint pains, fever, rash of a butterfly pattern around cheeks and forehead area; of unknown etiology.

710.1 Systemic sclerosis
Acrosclerosis
Progressive systemic sclerosis
CRST syndrome
Scleroderma
EXCLUDES circumscribed scleroderma (701.0)
Use additional code to identify manifestation, as:
  lung involvement (517.2)
  myopathy (359.6)

AHA: 1Q, '88, 6

DEF: Systemic disease, involving excess fibrotic collagen build-up; symptoms include thickened skin; fibrotic degenerative changes in various organs; and vascular abnormalities; condition occurs more often in females.

710.2 Sicca syndrome
Keratoconjunctivitis sicca
Sjögren's disease

DEF: Autoimmune disease; associated with keratoconjunctivitis, laryngopharyngitis, rhinitis, dry mouth, enlarged parotid gland, and chronic polyarthritis.

710.3 Dermatomyositis
Poikilodermatomyositis
Polymyositis with skin involvement

DEF: Polymyositis associated with flat-top purple papules on knuckles; marked by upper eyelid rash, edema of eyelids and orbit area, red rash on forehead, neck, shoulders, trunk and arms; symptoms include fever, weight loss aching muscles; visceral cancer (in individuals older than 40).

710.4 Polymyositis
DEF: Chronic, progressive, inflammatory skeletal muscle disease; causes weakness of limb girdles, neck, pharynx; may precede or follow scleroderma, Sjogren's disease, systemic lupus erythematosus, arthritis, or malignancy.

710.5 Eosinophilia myalgia syndrome
Toxic oil syndrome
Use additional E code to identify drug, if drug induced

AHA: 4Q, '92, 21

DEF: Eosinophilia myalgia syndrome (EMS): inflammatory, multisystem fibrosis; associated with ingesting elementary L-tryptophan; symptoms include myalgia, weak limbs and bulbar muscles, distal sensory loss, areflexia, arthralgia, cough, fever, fatigue, skin rashes, myopathy, and eosinophil counts greater than 1000/microliter.

DEF: Toxic oil syndrome: syndrome similar to EMS due to ingesting contaminated cooking oil.

710.8 Other specified diffuse diseases of connective tissue
Multifocal fibrosclerosis (idiopathic) NEC
Systemic fibrosclerosing syndrome

AHA: M-A, '87, 12

710.9 Unspecified diffuse connective tissue disease
Collagen disease NOS

MUSCULOSKELETAL SYSTEM AND CONNECTIVE TISSUE

✓4th 711 Arthropathy associated with infections

INCLUDES: arthritis, arthropathy, polyarthritis, polyarthropathy — associated with conditions classifiable below

EXCLUDES: rheumatic fever (390)

The following fifth-digit subclassification is for use with category 711; valid digits are in [brackets] under each code. See list at beginning of chapter for definitions.

0 site unspecified
1 shoulder region
2 upper arm
3 forearm
4 hand
5 pelvic region and thigh
6 lower leg
7 ankle and foot
8 other specified sites
9 multiple sites

AHA: 1Q, '92, 17

§ ✓5th 711.0 Pyogenic arthritis
[0-9]
Arthritis or polyarthritis (due to):
coliform [Escherichia coli]
Hemophilus influenzae [H. influenzae]
pneumococcal
Pseudomonas
staphylococcal
streptococcal
Pyarthrosis
Use additional code to identify infectious organism (041.0-041.8)

AHA: 1Q, '92, 16; 1Q, '91, 15

DEF: Infectious arthritis caused by various bacteria; marked by inflamed synovial membranes, and purulent effusion in joints.

§ ✓5th 711.1 Arthropathy associated with Reiter's disease and nonspecific urethritis
[0-9]
Code first underlying disease as:
nonspecific urethritis (099.4)
Reiter's disease (099.3)

DEF: Reiter's disease: joint disease marked by diarrhea, urethritis, conjunctivitis, keratosis and arthritis; of unknown etiology; affects young males.

DEF: Urethritis: inflamed urethra.

§ ✓5th 711.2 Arthropathy in Behçet's syndrome
[0-9]
Code first underlying disease (136.1)

DEF: Behçet's syndrome: chronic inflammatory disorder, of unknown etiology; affects small blood vessels; causes ulcers of oral and pharyngeal mucous membranes and genitalia, skin lesions, retinal vasculitis, optic atrophy and severe uveitis.

§ ✓5th 711.3 Postdysenteric arthropathy
[0-9]
Code first underlying disease as:
dysentery (009.0)
enteritis, infectious (008.0-009.3)
paratyphoid fever (002.1-002.9)
typhoid fever (002.0)

EXCLUDES: salmonella arthritis (003.23)

§ ✓5th 711.4 Arthropathy associated with other bacterial diseases
[0-9]
Code first underlying disease as:
diseases classifiable to 010-040, 090-099, except as in 711.1, 711.3, and 713.5
leprosy (030.0-030.9)
tuberculosis (015.0-015.9)

EXCLUDES: gonococcal arthritis (098.50)
meningococcal arthritis (036.82)

§ ✓5th 711.5 Arthropathy associated with other viral diseases
[0-9]
Code first underlying disease as:
diseases classifiable to 045-049, 050-079, 480, 487
O'nyong nyong (066.3)

EXCLUDES: that due to rubella (056.71)

§ ✓5th 711.6 Arthropathy associated with mycoses
[0-9]
Code first underlying disease (110.0-118)

§ ✓5th 711.7 Arthropathy associated with helminthiasis
[0-9]
Code first underlying disease as:
filariasis (125.0-125.9)

§ ✓5th 711.8 Arthropathy associated with other infectious and parasitic diseases
[0-9]
Code first underlying disease as:
diseases classifiable to 080-088, 100-104, 130-136

EXCLUDES: arthropathy associated with sarcoidosis (713.7)

AHA: 4Q, '91, 15; 3Q, '90, 14

§ ✓5th 711.9 Unspecified infective arthritis
[0-9]
Infective arthritis or polyarthritis (acute) (chronic) (subacute) NOS

✓4th 712 Crystal arthropathies

INCLUDES: crystal-induced arthritis and synovitis
EXCLUDES: gouty arthropathy (274.0)

DEF: Joint disease due to urate crystal deposit in joints or synovial membranes.

The following fifth-digit subclassification is for use with category 712; valid digits are in [brackets] under each code. See list at beginning of chapter for definitions.

0 site unspecified
1 shoulder region
2 upper arm
3 forearm
4 hand
5 pelvic region and thigh
6 lower leg
7 ankle and foot
8 other specified sites
9 multiple sites

§ ✓5th 712.1 Chondrocalcinosis due to dicalcium phosphate crystals
[0-9]
Chondrocalcinosis due to dicalcium phosphate crystals (with other crystals)
Code first underlying disease (275.4)

§ ✓5th 712.2 Chondrocalcinosis due to pyrophosphate crystals
[0-9]
Code first underlying disease (275.4)

§ ✓5th 712.3 Chondrocalcinosis, unspecified
[0-9]
Code first underlying disease (275.4)

§ ✓5th 712.8 Other specified crystal arthropathies
[0-9]

§ ✓5th 712.9 Unspecified crystal arthropathy
[0-9]

✓4th 713 Arthropathy associated with other disorders classified elsewhere

INCLUDES: arthritis, arthropathy, polyarthritis, polyarthropathy — associated with conditions classifiable below

---

§ Requires fifth digit. Valid digits are in [brackets] under each code. See beginning of section 710-739 for codes and definitions.

N Newborn Age: 0   P Pediatric Age: 0-17   M Maternity Age: 12-55   A Adult Age: 15-124

MUSCULOSKELETAL SYSTEM AND CONNECTIVE TISSUE

713.0 Arthropathy associated with other endocrine and metabolic disorders
Code first underlying disease as:
acromegaly (253.0)
hemochromatosis (275.0)
hyperparathyroidism (252.00-252.08)
hypogammaglobulinemia (279.00-279.09)
hypothyroidism (243-244.9)
lipoid metabolism disorder (272.0-272.9)
ochronosis (270.2)
EXCLUDES arthropathy associated with:
amyloidosis (713.7)
crystal deposition disorders, except gout (712.1-712.9)
diabetic neuropathy (713.5)
gouty arthropathy (274.0)

713.1 Arthropathy associated with gastrointestinal conditions other than infections
Code first underlying disease as:
regional enteritis (555.0-555.9)
ulcerative colitis (556)

713.2 Arthropathy associated with hematological disorders
Code first underlying disease as:
hemoglobinopathy (282.4-282.7)
hemophilia (286.0-286.2)
leukemia (204.0-208.9)
malignant reticulosis (202.3)
multiple myelomatosis (203.0)
EXCLUDES arthropathy associated with Henoch-Schönlein purpura (713.6)

713.3 Arthropathy associated with dermatological disorders
Code first underlying disease as:
erythema multiforme (695.1)
erythema nodosum (695.2)
EXCLUDES psoriatic arthropathy (696.0)

713.4 Arthropathy associated with respiratory disorders
Code first underlying disease as:
diseases classifiable to 490-519
EXCLUDES arthropathy associated with respiratory infections (711.0, 711.4-711.8)

713.5 Arthropathy associated with neurological disorders
Charcôt's arthropathy } associated with diseases classifiable elsewhere
Neuropathic arthritis
Code first underlying disease as:
neuropathic joint disease [Charcôt's joints]:
NOS (094.0)
diabetic (250.6)
syringomyelic (336.0)
tabetic [syphilitic] (094.0)

713.6 Arthropathy associated with hypersensitivity reaction
Code first underlying disease as:
Henoch (-Schönlein) purpura (287.0)
serum sickness (999.5)
EXCLUDES allergic arthritis NOS (716.2)

713.7 Other general diseases with articular involvement
Code first underlying disease as:
amyloidosis ▶(277.30-277.39)◀
familial Mediterranean fever ▶(277.31)◀
sarcoidosis (135)
AHA: 2Q, '97, 12

713.8 Arthropathy associated with other conditions classifiable elsewhere
Code first underlying disease as:
conditions classifiable elsewhere except as in 711.1-711.8, 712, and 713.0-713.7

√4ᵗʰ 714 Rheumatoid arthritis and other inflammatory polyarthropathies
EXCLUDES rheumatic fever (390)
rheumatoid arthritis of spine NOS (720.0)
AHA: 2Q, '95, 3

714.0 Rheumatoid arthritis
Arthritis or polyarthritis:
atrophic
rheumatic (chronic)
Use additional code to identify manifestation, as:
myopathy (359.6)
polyneuropathy (357.1)
EXCLUDES juvenile rheumatoid arthritis NOS (714.30)
AHA: 1Q, '90, 5
DEF: Chronic systemic disease principally of joints, manifested by inflammatory changes in articular structures and synovial membranes, atrophy, and loss in bone density.

714.1 Felty's syndrome
Rheumatoid arthritis with splenoadenomegaly and leukopenia
DEF: Syndrome marked by rheumatoid arthritis, splenomegaly, leukopenia, pigmented spots on lower extremity skin, anemia, and thrombocytopenia.

714.2 Other rheumatoid arthritis with visceral or systemic involvement
Rheumatoid carditis

√5ᵗʰ 714.3 Juvenile chronic polyarthritis
DEF: Rheumatoid arthritis of more than one joint; lasts longer than six weeks in age 17 or younger; symptoms include fever, erythematous rash, weight loss, lymphadenopathy, hepatosplenomegaly and pericarditis.

714.30 Polyarticular juvenile rheumatoid arthritis, chronic or unspecified
Juvenile rheumatoid arthritis NOS
Still's disease

714.31 Polyarticular juvenile rheumatoid arthritis, acute

714.32 Pauciarticular juvenile rheumatoid arthritis

714.33 Monoarticular juvenile rheumatoid arthritis

714.4 Chronic postrheumatic arthropathy
Chronic rheumatoid nodular fibrositis
Jaccoud's syndrome
DEF: Persistent joint disorder; follows previous rheumatic infection.

√5ᵗʰ 714.8 Other specified inflammatory polyarthropathies
714.81 Rheumatoid lung
Caplan's syndrome
Diffuse interstitial rheumatoid disease of lung
Fibrosing alveolitis, rheumatoid
DEF: Lung disorders associated with rheumatoid arthritis.

714.89 Other

714.9 Unspecified inflammatory polyarthropathy
Inflammatory polyarthropathy or polyarthritis NOS
EXCLUDES polyarthropathy NOS (716.5)

MUSCULOSKELETAL SYSTEM AND CONNECTIVE TISSUE

715 Osteoarthrosis and allied disorders
Note: Localized, in the subcategories below, includes bilateral involvement of the same site.

INCLUDES arthritis or polyarthritis:
   degenerative
   hypertrophic
   degenerative joint disease
   osteoarthritis

EXCLUDES Marie-Strümpell spondylitis (720.0)
   osteoarthrosis [osteoarthritis] of spine (721.0-721.9)

The following fifth-digit subclassification is for use with category 715; valid digits are in [brackets] under each code. See list at beginning of chapter for definitions.
   0 site unspecified
   1 shoulder region
   2 upper arm
   3 forearm
   4 hand
   5 pelvic region and thigh
   6 lower leg
   7 ankle and foot
   8 other specified sites
   9 multiple sites

§ 715.0 Osteoarthrosis, generalized
[0,4,9]
   Degenerative joint disease, involving multiple joints
   Primary generalized hypertrophic osteoarthrosis
   DEF: Chronic noninflammatory arthritis; marked by degenerated articular cartilage and enlarged bone; symptoms include pain and stiffness with activity; occurs among elderly.

§ 715.1 Osteoarthrosis, localized, primary
[0-8]
   Localized osteoarthropathy, idiopathic

§ 715.2 Osteoarthrosis, localized, secondary
[0-8]
   Coxae malum senilis

§ 715.3 Osteoarthrosis, localized, not specified whether primary or secondary
[0-8]
   Otto's pelvis
   AHA: For code 715.35: 3Q, '04, 12; 2Q, '04, 15;
   For code 715.36: 4Q, '03, 118; 2Q, '95, 5

§ 715.8 Osteoarthrosis involving, or with mention of more than one site, but not specified as generalized
[0,9]

§ 715.9 Osteoarthrosis, unspecified whether generalized or localized
[0-8]
   AHA: For code 715.90: 2Q, '97, 12

716 Other and unspecified arthropathies
EXCLUDES cricoarytenoid arthropathy (478.79)

The following fifth-digit subclassification is for use with category 716; valid digits are in [brackets] under each code. See list at beginning of chapter for definitions.
   0 site unspecified
   1 shoulder region
   2 upper arm
   3 forearm
   4 hand
   5 pelvic region and thigh
   6 lower leg
   7 ankle and foot
   8 other specified sites
   9 multiple sites

AHA: 2Q, '95, 3

§ 716.0 Kaschin-Beck disease
[0-9]
   Endemic polyarthritis
   DEF: Chronic degenerative disease of spine and peripheral joints; occurs in eastern Siberian, northern Chinese, and Korean youth; may a mycotoxicosis caused by eating cereals infected with fungus.

§ 716.1 Traumatic arthropathy
[0-9]
   AHA: For Code 716.11: 1Q, '02, 9

§ 716.2 Allergic arthritis
[0-9]
   EXCLUDES arthritis associated with Henoch-Schönlein purpura or serum sickness (713.6)

§ 716.3 Climacteric arthritis ♀
[0-9]
   Menopausal arthritis
   DEF: Ovarian hormone deficiency; causes pain in small joints, shoulders, elbows or knees; affects females at menopause; also called arthropathia ovaripriva.

§ 716.4 Transient arthropathy
[0-9]
   EXCLUDES palindromic rheumatism (719.3)

§ 716.5 Unspecified polyarthropathy or polyarthritis
[0-9]

§ 716.6 Unspecified monoarthritis
[0-8]
   Coxitis

§ 716.8 Other specified arthropathy
[0-9]

§ 716.9 Arthropathy, unspecified
[0-9]
   Arthritis } (acute) (chronic) (subacute)
   Arthropathy
   Articular rheumatism (chronic)
   Inflammation of joint NOS

717 Internal derangement of knee
INCLUDES degeneration
   rupture, old } of articular cartilage or meniscus of knee
   tear, old

EXCLUDES acute derangement of knee (836.0-836.6)
   ankylosis (718.5)
   contracture (718.4)
   current injury (836.0-836.6)
   deformity (736.4-736.6)
   recurrent dislocation (718.3)

717.0 Old bucket handle tear of medial meniscus
   Old bucket handle tear of unspecified cartilage

717.1 Derangement of anterior horn of medial meniscus

717.2 Derangement of posterior horn of medial meniscus

717.3 Other and unspecified derangement of medial meniscus
   Degeneration of internal semilunar cartilage

Disruption and Tears of Meniscus

Bucket-handle

Flap-type

Radial
Peripheral

Horizontal cleavage

Vertical

Congenital discoid meniscus

§ Requires fifth digit. Valid digits are in [brackets] under each code. See beginning of section 710-739 for codes and definitions.

MUSCULOSKELETAL SYSTEM AND CONNECTIVE TISSUE

Internal Derangements of Knee

√5th 717.4 Derangement of lateral meniscus
- 717.40 Derangement of lateral meniscus, unspecified
- 717.41 Bucket handle tear of lateral meniscus
- 717.42 Derangement of anterior horn of lateral meniscus
- 717.43 Derangement of posterior horn of lateral meniscus
- 717.49 Other

717.5 Derangement of meniscus, not elsewhere classified
  Congenital discoid meniscus
  Cyst of semilunar cartilage
  Derangement of semilunar cartilage NOS

717.6 Loose body in knee
  Joint mice, knee
  Rice bodies, knee (joint)
  DEF: The presence in the joint synovial area of a small, frequently calcified, loose body created from synovial membrane, organized fibrin fragments of articular cartilage or arthritis osteophytes.

717.7 Chondromalacia of patella
  Chondromalacia patellae
  Degeneration [softening] of articular cartilage of patella
  AHA: M-A, '85, 14; N-D, '84, 9
  DEF: Softened patella cartilage.

√5th 717.8 Other internal derangement of knee
- 717.81 Old disruption of lateral collateral ligament
- 717.82 Old disruption of medial collateral ligament
- 717.83 Old disruption of anterior cruciate ligament
- 717.84 Old disruption of posterior cruciate ligament
- 717.85 Old disruption of other ligaments of knee
  Capsular ligament of knee
- 717.89 Other
  Old disruption of ligaments of knee NOS

717.9 Unspecified internal derangement of knee
  Derangement NOS of knee

√4th 718 Other derangement of joint
  EXCLUDES current injury (830.0-848.9)
  jaw (524.60-524.69)

The following fifth-digit subclassification is for use with category 718; valid digits are in [brackets] under each code. See list at beginning of chapter for definitions.
- 0 site unspecified
- 1 shoulder region
- 2 upper arm
- 3 forearm
- 4 hand
- 5 pelvic region and thigh
- 6 lower leg
- 7 ankle and foot
- 8 other specified sites
- 9 multiple sites

§ √5th 718.0 Articular cartilage disorder
[0-5,7-9]
  Meniscus: disorder, rupture, old
  Meniscus: tear, old
  Old rupture of ligament(s) of joint NOS
  EXCLUDES articular cartilage disorder:
    in ochronosis (270.2)
    knee (717.0-717.9)
  chondrocalcinosis (275.4)
  metastatic calcification (275.4)

§ √5th 718.1 Loose body in joint
[0-5,7-9]
  Joint mice
  EXCLUDES knee (717.6)
  AHA: For code 718.17: 2Q, '01, 15
  DEF: Calcified loose bodies in synovial fluid; due to arthritic osteophytes.

§ √5th 718.2 Pathological dislocation
[0-9]
  Dislocation or displacement of joint, not recurrent and not current injury
  Spontaneous dislocation (joint)

§ √5th 718.3 Recurrent dislocation of joint
[0-9] **AHA:** N-D, '87, 7

§ √5th 718.4 Contracture of joint
[0-9] **AHA:** 4Q, '98, 40

§ √5th 718.5 Ankylosis of joint
[0-9]
  Ankylosis of joint (fibrous) (osseous)
  EXCLUDES spine (724.9)
    stiffness of joint without mention of ankylosis (719.5)
  DEF: Immobility and solidification, of joint; due to disease, injury or surgical procedure.

§ √5th 718.6 Unspecified intrapelvic protrusion of acetabulum
[0,5]
  Protrusio acetabuli, unspecified
  DEF: Sinking of the floor of acetabulum; causing femoral head to protrude, limits hip movement; of unknown etiology.

§ √5th 718.7 Developmental dislocation of joint
[0-9]
  EXCLUDES congenital dislocation of joint (754.0-755.8)
    traumatic dislocation of joint (830-839)
  AHA: 4Q, '01, 48

§ √5th 718.8 Other joint derangement, not elsewhere classified
[0-9]
  Flail joint (paralytic)
  Instability of joint
  EXCLUDES deformities classifiable to 736 (736.0-736.9)
  AHA: For code 718.81: 2Q, '00, 14

---

§ Requires fifth digit. Valid digits are in [brackets] under each code. See beginning of section 710–739 for codes and definitions.

MUSCULOSKELETAL SYSTEM AND CONNECTIVE TISSUE

Joint Derangements and Disorders

§ ⎷5th 718.9 Unspecified derangement of joint
[0-5,7-9]   EXCLUDES   knee (717.5)

⎷4th 719 Other and unspecified disorders of joint
EXCLUDES   jaw (524.60-524.69)

The following fifth-digit subclassification is for use with codes 719.0-719.6, 719.8-719.9; valid digits are in [brackets] under each code. See list at beginning of chapter for definitions.

0 site unspecified
1 shoulder region
2 upper arm
3 forearm
4 hand
5 pelvic region and thigh
6 lower leg
7 ankle and foot
8 other specified sites
9 multiple sites

§ ⎷5th 719.0 Effusion of joint
[0-9]   Hydrarthrosis
Swelling of joint, with or without pain
EXCLUDES   intermittent hydrarthrosis (719.3)

§ ⎷5th 719.1 Hemarthrosis
[0-9]   EXCLUDES   current injury (840.0-848.9)

§ ⎷5th 719.2 Villonodular synovitis
[0-9]   DEF: Overgrowth of synovial tissue, especially at knee joint; due to macrophage infiltration of giant cells in synovial villi and fibrous nodules.

§ ⎷5th 719.3 Palindromic rheumatism
[0-9]   Hench-Rosenberg syndrome
Intermittent hydrarthrosis
DEF: Recurrent episodes of afebrile arthritis and periarthritis marked by their complete disappearance after a few days or hours; causes swelling, redness, and disability usually affecting only one joint; no known cause; affects adults of either sex.

§ ⎷5th 719.4 Pain in joint
[0-9]   Arthralgia
AHA: For code 719.46: 1Q, '01, 3

§ ⎷5th 719.5 Stiffness of joint, not elsewhere classified
[0-9]

§ ⎷5th 719.6 Other symptoms referable to joint
[0-9]   Joint crepitus   Snapping hip
AHA: 1Q, '94, 15

719.7 Difficulty in walking
EXCLUDES   abnormality of gait (781.2)
AHA: 2Q, '04, 15; 4Q, '03, 66

§ ⎷5th 719.8 Other specified disorders of joint
[0-9]   Calcification of joint   Fistula of joint
EXCLUDES   temporomandibular joint-pain-dysfunction syndrome [Costen's syndrome] (524.60)

§ ⎷5th 719.9 Unspecified disorder of joint
[0-9]

DORSOPATHIES (720-724)

EXCLUDES   curvature of spine (737.0-737.9)
osteochondrosis of spine (juvenile) (732.0)
adult (732.8)

⎷4th 720 Ankylosing spondylitis and other inflammatory spondylopathies

720.0 Ankylosing spondylitis
Rheumatoid arthritis of spine NOS
Spondylitis:
   Marie-Strümpell
   rheumatoid
DEF: Rheumatoid arthritis of spine and sacroiliac joints; fusion and deformity in spine follows; affects mainly males; cause unknown.

720.1 Spinal enthesopathy
Disorder of peripheral ligamentous or muscular attachments of spine
Romanus lesion
DEF: Tendinous or muscular vertebral bone attachment abnormality.

720.2 Sacroiliitis, not elsewhere classified
Inflammation of sacroiliac joint NOS
DEF: Pain due to inflammation in joint, at juncture of sacrum and hip.

⎷5th 720.8 Other inflammatory spondylopathies
720.81 Inflammatory spondylopathies in diseases classified elsewhere
Code first underlying disease as:
   tuberculosis (015.0)
720.89 Other

720.9 Unspecified inflammatory spondylopathy
Spondylitis NOS

⎷4th 721 Spondylosis and allied disorders
AHA: 2Q, '89, 14

DEF: Degenerative changes in spinal joint.

721.0 Cervical spondylosis without myelopathy
Cervical or cervicodorsal: Cervical or cervicodorsal:
   arthritis   spondylarthritis
   osteoarthritis

721.1 Cervical spondylosis with myelopathy
Anterior spinal artery compression syndrome
Spondylogenic compression of cervical spinal cord
Vertebral artery compression syndrome

Normal Anatomy of Vertebral Disc

§ Requires fifth digit. Valid digits are in [brackets] under each code. See beginning of section 710-739 for codes and definitions.

N Newborn Age: 0   P Pediatric Age: 0-17   M Maternity Age: 12-55   A Adult Age: 15-1244

Tabular List — **MUSCULOSKELETAL SYSTEM AND CONNECTIVE TISSUE** — 721.2–723.0

721.2 Thoracic spondylosis without myelopathy
Thoracic:
    arthritis
    osteoarthritis
Thoracic:
    spondylarthritis

721.3 Lumbosacral spondylosis without myelopathy
Lumbar or lumbosacral:
    arthritis
    osteoarthritis
Lumbar or lumbosacral:
    spondylarthritis
AHA: 4Q, '02, 107

√5th **721.4 Thoracic or lumbar spondylosis with myelopathy**
  721.41 Thoracic region
    Spondylogenic compression of thoracic spinal cord
  721.42 Lumbar region
    Spondylogenic compression of lumbar spinal cord

721.5 Kissing spine
  Baastrup's syndrome
  DEF: Compression of spinous processes of adjacent vertebrae; due to mutual contact.

721.6 Ankylosing vertebral hyperostosis

721.7 Traumatic spondylopathy
  Kümmell's disease or spondylitis

721.8 Other allied disorders of spine

√5th **721.9 Spondylosis of unspecified site**
  721.90 Without mention of myelopathy
    Spinal:
        arthritis (deformans) (degenerative) (hypertrophic)
        osteoarthritis NOS
    Spondylarthrosis NOS
  721.91 With myelopathy
    Spondylogenic compression of spinal cord NOS

√4th **722 Intervertebral disc disorders**
  AHA: 1Q, '88. 10

722.0 Displacement of cervical intervertebral disc without myelopathy
  Neuritis (brachial) or radiculitis due to displacement or rupture of cervical intervertebral disc
  Any condition classifiable to 722.2 of the cervical or cervicothoracic intervertebral disc

√5th **722.1 Displacement of thoracic or lumbar intervertebral disc without myelopathy**
  722.10 Lumbar intervertebral disc without myelopathy
    Lumbago or sciatica due to displacement of intervertebral disc
    Neuritis or radiculitis due to displacement or rupture of lumbar intervertebral disc
    Any condition classifiable to 722.2 of the lumbar or lumbosacral intervertebral disc
  AHA: 3Q, '03, 12; 1Q, '03, 7; 4Q, '02, 107

  722.11 Thoracic intervertebral disc without myelopathy
    Any condition classifiable to 722.2 of thoracic intervertebral disc

722.2 Displacement of intervertebral disc, site unspecified, without myelopathy
  Discogenic syndrome NOS
  Herniation of nucleus pulposus NOS
  Intervertebral disc NOS:
      extrusion
      prolapse
      protrusion
      rupture
  Neuritis or radiculitis due to displacement or rupture of intervertebral disc

√5th **722.3 Schmorl's nodes**
  DEF: Irregular bone defect in the margin of the vertebral body; causes herniation into end plate of vertebral body.
  722.30 Unspecified region
  722.31 Thoracic region
  722.32 Lumbar region
  722.39 Other

722.4 Degeneration of cervical intervertebral disc
  Degeneration of cervicothoracic intervertebral disc

√5th **722.5 Degeneration of thoracic or lumbar intervertebral disc**
  722.51 Thoracic or thoracolumbar intervertebral disc
  722.52 Lumbar or lumbosacral intervertebral disc
  AHA: 4Q, '04, 133

722.6 Degeneration of intervertebral disc, site unspecified
  Degenerative disc disease NOS
  Narrowing of intervertebral disc or space NOS

√5th **722.7 Intervertebral disc disorder with myelopathy**
  722.70 Unspecified region
  722.71 Cervical region
  722.72 Thoracic region
  722.73 Lumbar region

√5th **722.8 Postlaminectomy syndrome**
  AHA: J-F, '87, 7
  DEF: Spinal disorder due to spinal laminectomy surgery.
  722.80 Unspecified region
  722.81 Cervical region
  722.82 Thoracic region
  722.83 Lumbar region
  AHA: 2Q, '97, 15

√5th **722.9 Other and unspecified disc disorder**
  Calcification of intervertebral cartilage or disc
  Discitis
  722.90 Unspecified region
    AHA: N-D, '84, 19
  722.91 Cervical region
  722.92 Thoracic region
  722.93 Lumbar region

√4th **723 Other disorders of cervical region**
  EXCLUDES conditions due to:
              intervertebral disc disorders (722.0-722.9)
              spondylosis (721.0-721.9)
  AHA: 3Q, '94, 14; 2Q, '89, 14

723.0 Spinal stenosis in cervical region
  AHA: 4Q, '03, 101

Derangement of Vertebral Disc
(Nucleus pulposus Herniates through Annulus; Spinal cord; Spinal nerve; Spinal stenosis; Schmorl's nodule; Osteophyte; Folded or thickened ligamentum flavum; Collapsed disk; Laminectomy and/or diskectomy decompresses spinal canal)

√4th Additional Digit Required | Unspecified Code | Other Specified Code | Manifestation Code | ▶◀ Revised Text | ● New Code | ▲ Revised Code Title
2007 ICD•9•CM — Volume 1 — 213

MUSCULOSKELETAL SYSTEM AND CONNECTIVE TISSUE — Tabular List

723.1–726.31

Spinal Stenosis in Cervical Region — Spinal cord in fluid-filled Dural sac, Posterior longitudinal ligament, Vertebral body

Old displacement/dislocation of C1 on C2 — Spinal cord, Spinal canal

Torticollis

723.1 Cervicalgia
Pain in neck
DEF: Pain in cervical spine or neck region.

723.2 Cervicocranial syndrome
Barré-Liéou syndrome
Posterior cervical sympathetic syndrome
DEF: Neurologic disorder of upper cervical spine and nerve roots.

723.3 Cervicobrachial syndrome (diffuse)
AHA: N-D, '85, 12
DEF: Complex of symptoms due to scalenus anterior muscle compressing the brachial plexus; pain radiates from shoulder to arm or back of neck.

723.4 Brachial neuritis or radiculitis NOS
Cervical radiculitis
Radicular syndrome of upper limbs

723.5 Torticollis, unspecified
Contracture of neck
EXCLUDES:
 congenital (754.1)
 due to birth injury (767.8)
 hysterical (300.11)
 ocular torticollis (781.93)
 psychogenic (306.0)
 spasmodic (333.83)
 traumatic, current (847.0)
AHA: 2Q, '01, 21; 1Q, '95, 7
DEF: Abnormally positioned neck relative to head; due to cervical muscle or fascia contractions; also called wryneck.

723.6 Panniculitis specified as affecting neck
DEF: Inflammation of the panniculus adiposus (subcutaneous fat) in the neck.

723.7 Ossification of posterior longitudinal ligament in cervical region

723.8 Other syndromes affecting cervical region
Cervical syndrome NEC
Klippel's disease
Occipital neuralgia
AHA: 1Q, '00, 7

723.9 Unspecified musculoskeletal disorders and symptoms referable to neck
Cervical (region) disorder NOS

√4th **724 Other and unspecified disorders of back**
EXCLUDES: collapsed vertebra (code to cause, e.g., osteoporosis, 733.00-733.09)
 conditions due to:
  intervertebral disc disorders (722.0-722.9)
  spondylosis (721.0-721.9)
AHA: 2Q, '89, 14

√5th **724.0 Spinal stenosis, other than cervical**
 724.00 Spinal stenosis, unspecified region
 724.01 Thoracic region
 724.02 Lumbar region
  AHA: 4Q, '99, 13
 724.09 Other

724.1 Pain in thoracic spine

724.2 Lumbago
Low back pain Lumbalgia
Low back syndrome
AHA: N-D, '85, 12

724.3 Sciatica
Neuralgia or neuritis of sciatic nerve
EXCLUDES: specified lesion of sciatic nerve (355.0)
AHA: 2Q, '89, 12

724.4 Thoracic or lumbosacral neuritis or radiculitis, unspecified
Radicular syndrome of lower limbs
AHA: 2Q, '99, 3

724.5 Backache, unspecified
Vertebrogenic (pain) syndrome NOS

724.6 Disorders of sacrum
Ankylosis | lumbosacral or sacroiliac (joint)
Instability |

√5th **724.7 Disorders of coccyx**
 724.70 Unspecified disorder of coccyx
 724.71 Hypermobility of coccyx
 724.79 Other
  Coccygodynia

724.8 Other symptoms referable to back
Ossification of posterior longitudinal ligament NOS
Panniculitis specified as sacral or affecting back

724.9 Other unspecified back disorders
Ankylosis of spine NOS
Compression of spinal nerve root NEC
Spinal disorder NOS
EXCLUDES: sacroiliitis (720.2)

RHEUMATISM, EXCLUDING THE BACK (725-729)
INCLUDES: disorders of muscles and tendons and their attachments, and of other soft tissues

725 Polymyalgia rheumatica
DEF: Joint and muscle pain, pelvis, and shoulder girdle stiffness, high sedimentation rate and temporal arteritis; occurs in elderly.

√4th **726 Peripheral enthesopathies and allied syndromes**
Note: Enthesopathies are disorders of peripheral ligamentous or muscular attachments.
EXCLUDES: spinal enthesopathy (720.1)

726.0 Adhesive capsulitis of shoulder

√5th **726.1 Rotator cuff syndrome of shoulder and allied disorders**
 726.10 Disorders of bursae and tendons in shoulder region, unspecified
  Rotator cuff syndrome NOS
  Supraspinatus syndrome NOS
  AHA: 2Q, '01, 11
 726.11 Calcifying tendinitis of shoulder
 726.12 Bicipital tenosynovitis
 726.19 Other specified disorders
  EXCLUDES: complete rupture of rotator cuff, nontraumatic (727.61)

726.2 Other affections of shoulder region, not elsewhere classified
Periarthritis of shoulder Scapulohumeral fibrositis

√5th **726.3 Enthesopathy of elbow region**
 726.30 Enthesopathy of elbow, unspecified
 726.31 Medial epicondylitis

N Newborn Age: 0 P Pediatric Age: 0-17 M Maternity Age: 12-55 A Adult Age: 15-1244

Bunion

Ganglia

726.32 Lateral epicondylitis
Epicondylitis NOS   Tennis elbow
Golfers' elbow

726.33 Olecranon bursitis
Bursitis of elbow

726.39 Other

726.4 Enthesopathy of wrist and carpus
Bursitis of hand or wrist
Periarthritis of wrist

726.5 Enthesopathy of hip region
Bursitis of hip   Psoas tendinitis
Gluteal tendinitis   Trochanteric tendinitis
Iliac crest spur

✓5th **726.6 Enthesopathy of knee**

726.60 Enthesopathy of knee, unspecified
Bursitis of knee NOS

726.61 Pes anserinus tendinitis or bursitis
DEF: Inflamed tendons of sartorius, gracilis and semitendinosus muscles of medial aspect of knee.

726.62 Tibial collateral ligament bursitis
Pellegrini-Stieda syndrome

726.63 Fibular collateral ligament bursitis

726.64 Patellar tendinitis

726.65 Prepatellar bursitis

726.69 Other
Bursitis: Bursitis:
  infrapatellar   subpatellar

✓5th **726.7 Enthesopathy of ankle and tarsus**

726.70 Enthesopathy of ankle and tarsus, unspecified
Metatarsalgia NOS
EXCLUDES Morton's metatarsalgia (355.6)

726.71 Achilles bursitis or tendinitis

726.72 Tibialis tendinitis
Tibialis (anterior) (posterior) tendinitis

726.73 Calcaneal spur
DEF: Overgrowth of calcaneous bone; causes pain on walking; due to chronic avulsion injury of plantar fascia from calcaneus.

726.79 Other
Peroneal tendinitis

726.8 Other peripheral enthesopathies

✓5th **726.9 Unspecified enthesopathy**

726.90 Enthesopathy of unspecified site
Capsulitis NOS
Periarthritis NOS
Tendinitis NOS

726.91 Exostosis of unspecified site
Bone spur NOS
AHA: 2Q, '01, 15

✓4th **727 Other disorders of synovium, tendon, and bursa**

✓5th **727.0 Synovitis and tenosynovitis**

727.00 Synovitis and tenosynovitis, unspecified
Synovitis NOS
Tenosynovitis NOS

727.01 Synovitis and tenosynovitis in diseases classified elsewhere
Code first underlying disease as:
  tuberculosis (015.0-015.9)
EXCLUDES crystal-induced (275.4)
          gonococcal (098.51)
          gouty (274.0)
          syphilitic (095.7)

727.02 Giant cell tumor of tendon sheath

727.03 Trigger finger (acquired)
DEF: Stenosing tenosynovitis or nodule in flexor tendon; cessation of flexion or extension movement in finger, followed by snapping into place.

727.04 Radial styloid tenosynovitis
de Quervain's disease

727.05 Other tenosynovitis of hand and wrist

727.06 Tenosynovitis of foot and ankle

727.09 Other

727.1 Bunion
DEF: Enlarged first metatarsal head due to inflamed bursa; results in laterally displaced great toe.

727.2 Specific bursitides often of occupational origin
Beat: Miners':
  elbow   elbow
  hand   knee
  knee
Chronic crepitant synovitis of wrist

727.3 Other bursitis
Bursitis NOS
EXCLUDES bursitis:
          gonococcal (098.52)
          subacromial (726.19)
          subcoracoid (726.19)
          subdeltoid (726.19)
          syphilitic (095.7)
          "frozen shoulder" (726.0)

✓5th **727.4 Ganglion and cyst of synovium, tendon, and bursa**

727.40 Synovial cyst, unspecified
EXCLUDES that of popliteal space (727.51)
AHA: 2Q, '97, 6

727.41 Ganglion of joint

727.42 Ganglion of tendon sheath

727.43 Ganglion, unspecified

727.49 Other
Cyst of bursa

✓5th **727.5 Rupture of synovium**

727.50 Rupture of synovium, unspecified

727.51–728.88 MUSCULOSKELETAL SYSTEM AND CONNECTIVE TISSUE

727.51 Synovial cyst of popliteal space
Baker's cyst (knee)

727.59 Other

√5th **727.6** Rupture of tendon, nontraumatic

727.60 Nontraumatic rupture of unspecified tendon

727.61 Complete rupture of rotator cuff

727.62 Tendons of biceps (long head)

727.63 Extensor tendons of hand and wrist

727.64 Flexor tendons of hand and wrist

727.65 Quadriceps tendon

727.66 Patellar tendon

727.67 Achilles tendon

727.68 Other tendons of foot and ankle

727.69 Other

√5th **727.8** Other disorders of synovium, tendon, and bursa

727.81 Contracture of tendon (sheath)
Short Achilles tendon (acquired)

727.82 Calcium deposits in tendon and bursa
Calcification of tendon NOS
Calcific tendinitis NOS
EXCLUDES peripheral ligamentous or muscular attachments (726.0-726.9)

727.83 Plica syndrome
Plica knee
AHA: 4Q, '00, 44
DEF: A fold in the synovial tissue that begins to form before birth, creating a septum between two pockets of synovial tissue; two most common plicae are the medial patellar plica and the suprapatellar plica. Plica syndrome, or plica knee, refers to symptomatic plica. Experienced by females more commonly than males.

727.89 Other
Abscess of bursa or tendon
EXCLUDES xanthomatosis localized to tendons (272.7)
AHA: 2Q, '89, 15

727.9 Unspecified disorder of synovium, tendon, and bursa

√4th **728** Disorders of muscle, ligament, and fascia
EXCLUDES enthesopathies (726.0-726.9)
muscular dystrophies (359.0-359.1)
myoneural disorders (358.00-358.9)
myopathies (359.2-359.9)
old disruption of ligaments of knee (717.81-717.89)

728.0 Infective myositis
Myositis:
  purulent
  suppurative
EXCLUDES myositis:
  epidemic (074.1)
  interstitial (728.81)
  syphilitic (095.6)
  tropical (040.81)
DEF: Inflamed connective septal tissue of muscle.

√5th **728.1** Muscular calcification and ossification

728.10 Calcification and ossification, unspecified
Massive calcification (paraplegic)

728.11 Progressive myositis ossificans
DEF: Progressive myositic disease; marked by bony tissue formed by voluntary muscle; occurs among very young.

728.12 Traumatic myositis ossificans
Myositis ossificans (circumscripta)

728.13 Postoperative heterotopic calcification
DEF: Abnormal formation of calcium deposits in muscular tissue after surgery, marked by a corresponding loss of muscle tone and tension.

728.19 Other
Polymyositis ossificans

728.2 Muscular wasting and disuse atrophy, not elsewhere classified
Amyotrophia NOS   Myofibrosis
EXCLUDES neuralgic amyotrophy (353.5)
pelvic muscle wasting and disuse atrophy (618.83)
progressive muscular atrophy (335.0-335.9)

728.3 Other specific muscle disorders
Arthrogryposis
Immobility syndrome (paraplegic)
EXCLUDES arthrogryposis multiplex congenita (754.89)
stiff-man syndrome (333.91)

728.4 Laxity of ligament

728.5 Hypermobility syndrome

728.6 Contracture of palmar fascia **A**
Dupuytren's contracture
DEF: Dupuytren's contracture: flexion deformity of finger, due to shortened, thickened fibrosing of palmar fascia; cause unknown; associated with long-standing epilepsy; occurs more often in males.

√5th **728.7** Other fibromatoses

728.71 Plantar fascial fibromatosis
Contracture of plantar fascia
Plantar fasciitis (traumatic)
DEF: Plantar fascia fibromatosis; causes nodular swelling and pain; not associated with contractures.

728.79 Other
Garrod's or knuckle pads
Nodular fasciitis
Pseudosarcomatous fibromatosis (proliferative) (subcutaneous)
DEF: Knuckle pads: pea-size nodules on dorsal surface of interphalangeal joints; new growth of fibrous tissue with thickened dermis and epidermis.

√5th **728.8** Other disorders of muscle, ligament, and fascia

728.81 Interstitial myositis
DEF: Inflammation of septal connective parts of muscle tissue.

728.82 Foreign body granuloma of muscle
Talc granuloma of muscle

728.83 Rupture of muscle, nontraumatic

728.84 Diastasis of muscle
Diastasis recti (abdomen)
EXCLUDES diastasis recti complicating pregnancy, labor, and delivery (665.8)
DEF: Muscle separation, such as recti abdominis after repeated pregnancies.

728.85 Spasm of muscle

728.86 Necrotizing fasciitis
Use additional code to identify:
  infectious organism (041.00-041.89)
  gangrene (785.4), if applicable
AHA: 4Q, '95, 54
DEF: Fulminating infection begins with extensive cellulitis, spreads to superficial and deep fascia; causes thrombosis of subcutaneous vessels, and gangrene of underlying tissue.

728.87 Muscle weakness (generalized)
EXCLUDES generalized weakness (780.79)
AHA: 1Q, '05, 13; 4Q, '03, 66

728.88 Rhabdomyolysis
AHA: 4Q, '03, 66
DEF: A disintegration or destruction of muscle; an acute disease characterized by the excretion of myoglobin into the urine.

MUSCULOSKELETAL SYSTEM AND CONNECTIVE TISSUE

728.89 **Other**
Eosinophilic fasciitis
Use additional E code to identify drug, if drug induced
AHA: 3Q, '02, 28; 2Q, '01, 14, 15

DEF: Eosinophilic fasciitis: inflammation of fascia of extremities associated with eosinophilia, edema, and swelling; occurs alone or as part of myalgia syndrome.

728.9 **Unspecified disorder of muscle, ligament, and fascia**
AHA: 4Q, '88, 11

729 **Other disorders of soft tissues**
EXCLUDES:
acroparesthesia (443.89)
carpal tunnel syndrome (354.0)
disorders of the back (720.0-724.9)
entrapment syndromes (354.0-355.9)
palindromic rheumatism (719.3)
periarthritis (726.0-726.9)
psychogenic rheumatism (306.0)

729.0 **Rheumatism, unspecified and fibrositis**
DEF: General term describes diseases of muscle, tendon, nerve, joint, or bone; symptoms include pain and stiffness.

729.1 **Myalgia and myositis, unspecified**
Fibromyositis NOS
DEF: Myalgia: muscle pain.
DEF: Myositis: inflamed voluntary muscle.
DEF: Fibromyositis: inflamed fibromuscular tissue.

729.2 **Neuralgia, neuritis, and radiculitis, unspecified**
EXCLUDES:
brachial radiculitis (723.4)
cervical radiculitis (723.4)
lumbosacral radiculitis (724.4)
mononeuritis (354.0-355.9)
radiculitis due to intervertebral disc involvement (722.0-722.2, 722.7)
sciatica (724.3)

DEF: Neuralgia: paroxysmal pain along nerve symptoms include brief pain and tenderness at point nerve exits.
DEF: Neuritis: inflamed nerve, symptoms include paresthesia, paralysis and loss of reflexes at nerve site.
DEF: Radiculitis: inflamed nerve root.

729.3 **Panniculitis, unspecified**
DEF: Inflammatory reaction of subcutaneous fat; causes nodules; often develops in abdominal region.

729.30 **Panniculitis, unspecified site**
Weber-Christian disease
DEF: Febrile, nodular, nonsuppurative, relapsing inflammation of subcutaneous fat.

729.31 Hypertrophy of fat pad, knee
Hypertrophy of infrapatellar fat pad

729.39 Other site
EXCLUDES:
panniculitis specified as (affecting):
back (724.8)
neck (723.6)
sacral (724.8)

729.4 **Fasciitis, unspecified**
EXCLUDES:
necrotizing fasciitis (728.86)
nodular fasciitis (728.79)
AHA: 2Q, '94, 13

729.5 Pain in limb

729.6 Residual foreign body in soft tissue
EXCLUDES:
foreign body granuloma:
muscle (728.82)
skin and subcutaneous tissue (709.4)

729.7 Nontraumatic compartment syndrome
EXCLUDES:
compartment syndrome NOS (958.90)
traumatic compartment syndrome (958.90-958.99)

729.71 Nontraumatic compartment syndrome of upper extremity
Nontraumatic compartment syndrome of shoulder, arm, forearm, wrist, hand and fingers

729.72 Nontraumatic compartment syndrome of lower extremity
Nontraumatic compartment syndrome of hip, buttock, thigh, leg, foot and toes

729.73 Nontraumatic compartment syndrome of abdomen

729.79 Nontraumatic compartment syndrome of other sites

729.8 Other musculoskeletal symptoms referable to limbs
729.81 Swelling of limb
AHA: 4Q, '88, 6

729.82 Cramp

729.89 Other
EXCLUDES:
abnormality of gait (781.2)
tetany (781.7)
transient paralysis of limb (781.4)
AHA: 4Q, '88, 12

729.9 **Other and unspecified disorders of soft tissue**
Polyalgia

OSTEOPATHIES, CHONDROPATHIES, AND ACQUIRED MUSCULOSKELETAL DEFORMITIES (730-739)

730 Osteomyelitis, periostitis, and other infections involving bone
EXCLUDES:
jaw (526.4-526.5)
petrous bone (383.2)

Use additional code to identify organism, such as Staphylococcus (041.1)

The following fifth-digit subclassification is for use with category 730; valid digits are in [brackets] under each code. See list at beginning of chapter for definitions.
0 site unspecified
1 shoulder region
2 upper arm
3 forearm
4 hand
5 pelvic region and thigh
6 lower leg
7 ankle and foot
8 other specified sites
9 multiple sites

AHA: 4Q, '97, 43

DEF: Osteomyelitis: bacterial inflammation of bone tissue and marrow.
DEF: Periostitis: inflammation of specialized connective tissue; causes swelling of bone and aching pain.

§ **730.0** **Acute osteomyelitis**
[0-9] Abscess of any bone except accessory sinus, jaw, or mastoid
Acute or subacute osteomyelitis, with or without mention of periostitis
▶Use additional code to identify major osseous defect, if applicable (731.3)◀
AHA: For code 730.06: 1Q, '02, 4; For code 730.07: 1Q, '04, 14

---

§ Requires fifth digit. Valid digits are in [brackets] under each code. See beginning of section 710-739 for codes and definitions.

MUSCULOSKELETAL SYSTEM AND CONNECTIVE TISSUE

730.1 Chronic osteomyelitis
[0-9]
- Brodie's abscess
- Chronic or old osteomyelitis, with or without mention of periostitis
- Sequestrum of bone
- Sclerosing osteomyelitis of Garré

▶Use additional code to identify major osseous defect, if applicable (731.3)◀

EXCLUDES: aseptic necrosis of bone (733.40-733.49)

AHA: For code 730.17: 3Q, '00, 4

730.2 Unspecified osteomyelitis
[0-9]
- Osteitis or osteomyelitis NOS, with or without mention of periostitis

▶Use additional code to identify major osseous defect, if applicable (731.3)◀

730.3 Periostitis without mention of osteomyelitis
[0-9]
- Abscess of periosteum } without mention of osteomyelitis
- Periostosis

EXCLUDES: that in secondary syphilis (091.61)

730.7 Osteopathy resulting from poliomyelitis
[0-9]
Code first underlying disease (045.0-045.9)

730.8 Other infections involving bone in diseases classified elsewhere
[0-9]
Code first underlying disease as:
- tuberculosis (015.0-015.9)
- typhoid fever (002.0)

EXCLUDES: syphilis of bone NOS (095.5)

AHA: 2Q, '97, 16; 3Q, '91, 10

730.9 Unspecified infection of bone
[0-9]

731 Osteitis deformans and osteopathies associated with other disorders classified elsewhere

DEF: Osteitis deformans: Bone disease marked by episodes of increased bone loss, excessive repair attempts follow; causes weakened, deformed bones with increased mass, bowed long bones, deformed flat bones, pain and pathological fractures; may be fatal if associated with congestive heart failure, giant cell tumors or bone sarcoma; also called Paget's disease.

731.0 Osteitis deformans without mention of bone tumor
Paget's disease of bone

731.1 Osteitis deformans in diseases classified elsewhere
Code first underlying disease as:
- malignant neoplasm of bone (170.0-170.9)

731.2 Hypertrophic pulmonary osteoarthropathy
Bamberger-Marie disease

DEF: Clubbing, of fingers and toes; related to enlarged ends of long bones; due to chronic lung and heart disease.

731.3 Major osseous defects
Code first underlying disease, if known, such as:
- aseptic necrosis (733.40-733.49)
- malignant neoplasm of bone (170.0-170.9)
- osteomyelitis (730.00-730.29)
- osteoporosis (733.00-733.09)
- peri-prosthetic osteolysis (996.45)

731.8 Other bone involvement in diseases classified elsewhere
Code first underlying disease as:
- diabetes mellitus (250.8)

Use additional code to specify bone condition, such as:
- acute osteomyelitis (730.00-730.09)

AHA: 1Q, '04, 14; 4Q, '97, 43; 2Q, '97, 16

732 Osteochondropathies

DEF: Conditions related to both bone and cartilage, or conditions in which cartilage is converted to bone (enchondral ossification).

732.0 Juvenile osteochondrosis of spine
Juvenile osteochondrosis (of):
- marginal or vertebral epiphysis (of Scheuermann)
- spine NOS

Vertebral epiphysitis

EXCLUDES: adolescent postural kyphosis (737.0)

732.1 Juvenile osteochondrosis of hip and pelvis
- Coxa plana
- Ischiopubic synchondrosis (of van Neck)
- Osteochondrosis (juvenile) of:
  - acetabulum
  - head of femur (of Legg-Calvé-Perthes)
  - iliac crest (of Buchanan)
  - symphysis pubis (of Pierson)
- Pseudocoxalgia

732.2 Nontraumatic slipped upper femoral epiphysis
Slipped upper femoral epiphysis NOS

732.3 Juvenile osteochondrosis of upper extremity
Osteochondrosis (juvenile) of:
- capitulum of humerus (of Panner)
- carpal lunate (of Kienbock)
- hand NOS
- head of humerus (of Haas)
- heads of metacarpals (of Mauclaire)
- lower ulna (of Burns)
- radial head (of Brailsford)
- upper extremity NOS

732.4 Juvenile osteochondrosis of lower extremity, excluding foot
Osteochondrosis (juvenile) of:
- lower extremity NOS
- primary patellar center (of Köhler)
- proximal tibia (of Blount)
- secondary patellar center (of Sinding-Larsen)
- tibial tubercle (of Osgood-Schlatter)

Tibia vara

732.5 Juvenile osteochondrosis of foot
- Calcaneal apophysitis
- Epiphysitis, os calcis
- Osteochondrosis (juvenile) of:
  - astragalus (of Diaz)
  - calcaneum (of Sever)
  - foot NOS
  - metatarsal:
    - second (of Freiberg)
    - fifth (of Iselin)
  - os tibiale externum (of Haglund)
  - tarsal navicular (of Köhler)

732.6 Other juvenile osteochondrosis
- Apophysitis
- Epiphysitis } specified as juvenile, of other
- Osteochondritis   site, or site NOS
- Osteochondrosis

732.7 Osteochondritis dissecans

732.8 Other specified forms of osteochondropathy
Adult osteochondrosis of spine

732.9 Unspecified osteochondropathy
- Apophysitis   } NOS
- Epiphysitis   } not specified as adult or juve-
- Osteochondritis   nile, of unspecified site
- Osteochondrosis

---

§ Requires fifth digit. Valid digits are in [brackets] under each code. See beginning of section 710–739 for codes and definitions.

N Newborn Age: 0   P Pediatric Age: 0-17   M Maternity Age: 12-55   A Adult Age: 15-124

MUSCULOSKELETAL SYSTEM AND CONNECTIVE TISSUE

✓4th 733 Other disorders of bone and cartilage

EXCLUDES
- bone spur (726.91)
- cartilage of, or loose body in, joint (717.0-717.9, 718.0-718.9)
- giant cell granuloma of jaw (526.3)
- osteitis fibrosa cystica generalisata (252.01)
- osteomalacia (268.2)
- polyostotic fibrous dysplasia of bone (756.54)
- prognathism, retrognathism (524.1)
- xanthomatosis localized to bone (272.7)

✓5th 733.0 Osteoporosis
▶Use additional code to identify major osseous defect, if applicable (731.3)◀

DEF: Bone mass reduction that ultimately results in fractures after minimal trauma; dorsal kyphosis or loss of height often occur.

733.00 Osteoporosis, unspecified
Wedging of vertebra NOS
AHA: 3Q, '01, 19; 2Q, '98, 12

733.01 Senile osteoporosis
Postmenopausal osteoporosis

733.02 Idiopathic osteoporosis

733.03 Disuse osteoporosis

733.09 Other
Drug-induced osteoporosis
Use additional E code to identify drug
AHA: 4Q, '03, 108

✓5th 733.1 Pathologic fracture
Spontaneous fracture
EXCLUDES
- stress fracture (733.93-733.95)
- traumatic fracture (800-829)

AHA: 4Q, '93, 25; N-D, '86, 10; N-D, '85, 16

DEF: Fracture due to bone structure weakening by pathological processes (e.g., osteoporosis, neoplasms and osteomalacia).

733.10 Pathologic fracture, unspecified site

733.11 Pathologic fracture of humerus

733.12 Pathologic fracture of distal radius and ulna
Wrist NOS

733.13 Pathologic fracture of vertebrae
Collapse of vertebra NOS
AHA: 3Q, '99, 5

733.14 Pathologic fracture of neck of femur
Femur NOS   Hip NOS
AHA: 1Q, '01, 1; 1Q, '96, 16

733.15 Pathologic fracture of other specified part of femur
AHA: 2Q, '98, 12

733.16 Pathologic fracture of tibia or fibula
Ankle NOS

733.19 Pathologic fracture of other specified site

✓5th 733.2 Cyst of bone

733.20 Cyst of bone (localized), unspecified

733.21 Solitary bone cyst
Unicameral bone cyst

733.22 Aneurysmal bone cyst
DEF: Solitary bone lesion, bulges into periosteum; marked by calcified rim.

733.29 Other
Fibrous dysplasia (monostotic)
EXCLUDES
- cyst of jaw (526.0-526.2, 526.89)
- osteitis fibrosa cystica (252.01)
- polyostotic fibrousdyplasia of bone (756.54)

733.3 Hyperostosis of skull
Hyperostosis interna frontalis
Leontiasis ossium
DEF: Abnormal bone growth on inner aspect of cranial bones.

✓5th 733.4 Aseptic necrosis of bone
▶Use additional code to identify major osseous defect, if applicable (731.3)◀
EXCLUDES osteochondropathies (732.0-732.9)

DEF: Infarction of bone tissue due to a nonfectious etiology, such as a fracture, ischemic disorder or administration of immunosuppressive drugs; leads to degenerative joint disease or nonunion of fractures.

733.40 Aseptic necrosis of bone, site unspecified

733.41 Head of humerus

733.42 Head and neck of femur
Femur NOS
EXCLUDES Legg-Calvé-Perthes disease (732.1)

733.43 Medial femoral condyle

733.44 Talus

733.49 Other

733.5 Osteitis condensans
Piriform sclerosis of ilium
DEF: Idiopathic condition marked by low back pain; associated with oval or triangular sclerotic, opaque bone next to sacroiliac joints in the ileum.

733.6 Tietze's disease
Costochondral junction syndrome
Costochondritis
DEF: Painful, idiopathic, nonsuppurative, swollen costal cartilage sometimes confused with cardiac symptoms because the anterior chest pain resembles that of coronary artery disease.

733.7 Algoneurodystrophy
Disuse atrophy of bone
Sudeck's atrophy
DEF: Painful, idiopathic.

✓5th 733.8 Malunion and nonunion of fracture
AHA: 2Q, '94, 5

733.81 Malunion of fracture

733.82 Nonunion of fracture
Pseudoarthrosis (bone)

✓5th 733.9 Other and unspecified disorders of bone and cartilage

733.90 Disorder of bone and cartilage, unspecified

733.91 Arrest of bone development or growth
Epiphyseal arrest

733.92 Chondromalacia
Chondromalacia:
  NOS
  localized, except patella
  systemic
  tibial plateau
EXCLUDES chondromalacia of patella (717.7)
DEF: Articular cartilage softening.

733.93 Stress fracture of tibia or fibula
Stress reaction of tibia or fibula
AHA: 4Q, '01, 48

733.94 Stress fracture of the metatarsals
Stress reaction of metatarsals
AHA: 4Q, '01, 48

733.95 Stress fracture of other bone
Stress reaction of other bone
AHA: 4Q, '01, 48

733.99 Other
Diaphysitis
Hypertrophy of bone
Relapsing polychondritis
AHA: J-F, '87, 14

Acquired Deformities of Toe

Acquired Deformities of Forearm

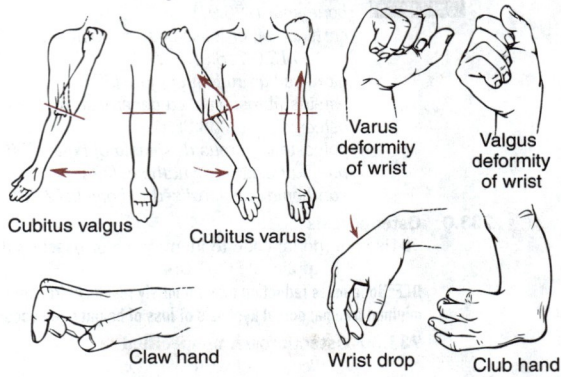

734 Flat foot
Pes planus (acquired)
Talipes planus (acquired)
EXCLUDES congenital (754.61)
rigid flat foot (754.61)
spastic (everted) flat foot (754.61)

735 Acquired deformities of toe
EXCLUDES congenital (754.60-754.69, 755.65-755.66)

735.0 Hallux valgus (acquired)
DEF: Angled displacement of the great toe, causing it to ride over or under other toes.

735.1 Hallux varus (acquired)
DEF: Angled displacement of the great toe toward the body midline, away from the other toes.

735.2 Hallux rigidus
DEF: Limited flexion movement at metatarsophalangeal joint of great toe; due to degenerative joint disease.

735.3 Hallux malleus
DEF: Extended proximal phalanx, flexed distal phalanges, of great toe; foot resembles claw or hammer.

735.4 Other hammer toe (acquired)

735.5 Claw toe (acquired)
DEF: Hyperextended proximal phalanges, flexed middle and distal phalanges.

735.8 Other acquired deformities of toe

735.9 Unspecified acquired deformity of toe

736 Other acquired deformities of limbs
EXCLUDES congenital (754.3-755.9)

736.0 Acquired deformities of forearm, excluding fingers

736.00 Unspecified deformity
Deformity of elbow, forearm, hand, or wrist (acquired) NOS

736.01 Cubitus valgus (acquired)
DEF: Deviation of the elbow away from the body midline upon extension; it occurs when the palm is turning outward.

736.02 Cubitus varus (acquired)
DEF: Elbow joint displacement angled laterally; when the forearm is extended, it is deviated toward the midline of the body; also called "gun stock" deformity.

736.03 Valgus deformity of wrist (acquired)
DEF: Abnormal angulation away from the body midline.

736.04 Varus deformity of wrist (acquired)
DEF: Abnormal angulation toward the body midline.

736.05 Wrist drop (acquired)
DEF: Inability to extend the hand at the wrist due to extensor muscle paralysis.

736.06 Claw hand (acquired)
DEF: Flexion and atrophy of the hand and fingers; found in ulnar nerve lesions, syringomyelia, and leprosy.

736.07 Club hand, acquired
DEF: Twisting of the hand out of shape or position; caused by the congenital absence of the ulna or radius.

736.09 Other

736.1 Mallet finger
DEF: Permanently flexed distal phalanx.

736.2 Other acquired deformities of finger

736.20 Unspecified deformity
Deformity of finger (acquired) NOS

736.21 Boutonniere deformity
DEF: A deformity of the finger caused by flexion of the proximal interphalangeal joint and hyperextension of the distal joint; also called buttonhole deformity.

736.22 Swan-neck deformity
DEF: Flexed distal and hyperextended proximal interphalangeal joint.

736.29 Other
EXCLUDES trigger finger (727.03)
AHA: 2Q, '05, 7; 2Q, '89, 13

736.3 Acquired deformities of hip

736.30 Unspecified deformity
Deformity of hip (acquired) NOS

736.31 Coxa valga (acquired)
DEF: Increase of at least 140 degrees in the angle formed by the axis of the head and the neck of the femur, and the axis of its shaft.

736.32 Coxa vara (acquired)
DEF: The bending downward of the neck of the femur: causing difficulty in movement; a right angle or less may be formed by the axis of the head and neck of the femur, and the axis of its shaft.

736.39 Other
AHA: 2Q, '91, 18

Acquired Deformities of Lower Limb

MUSCULOSKELETAL SYSTEM AND CONNECTIVE TISSUE

Scoliosis and Kyphoscoliosis

Scoliosis

Kyphoscoliosis

Acquired Deformities of Hip

Genu valga (knock-knee) — Normal angle — Coxa valga — Coxa vara — Genu vara (bowleg)

- **736.4** Genu valgum or varum (acquired)
  - **736.41** Genu valgum (acquired)
    DEF: Abnormally close together and an abnormally large space between the ankles; also called "knock-knees."
  - **736.42** Genu varum (acquired)
    DEF: Abnormally separated knees and the inward bowing of the legs; it is also called "bowlegs."
- **736.5** Genu recurvatum (acquired)
  DEF: Hyperextended knees; also called "backknee."
- **736.6** Other acquired deformities of knee
  Deformity of knee (acquired) NOS
- **736.7** Other acquired deformities of ankle and foot
  EXCLUDES deformities of toe (acquired) (735.0-735.9)
  pes planus (acquired) (734)
  - **736.70** Unspecified deformity of ankle and foot, acquired
  - **736.71** Acquired equinovarus deformity
    Clubfoot, acquired
    EXCLUDES clubfoot not specified as acquired (754.5-754.7)
  - **736.72** Equinus deformity of foot, acquired
    DEF: A plantar flexion deformity that forces people to walk on their toes.
  - **736.73** Cavus deformity of foot
    EXCLUDES that with claw foot (736.74)
    DEF: Abnormally high longitudinal arch of the foot.
  - **736.74** Claw foot, acquired
    DEF: High foot arch with hyperextended toes at metatarsophalangeal joint and flexed toes at distal joints; also called "main en griffe."
  - **736.75** Cavovarus deformity of foot, acquired
    DEF: Inward turning of the heel from the midline of the leg and an abnormally high longitudinal arch.
  - **736.76** Other calcaneus deformity
  - **736.79** Other
    Acquired:
    pes
    talipes } not elsewhere classified
- **736.8** Acquired deformities of other parts of limbs
  - **736.81** Unequal leg length (acquired)
  - **736.89** Other
    Deformity (acquired):
    arm or leg, not elsewhere classified
    shoulder
- **736.9** Acquired deformity of limb, site unspecified
- **737** Curvature of spine
  EXCLUDES congenital (754.2)
  - **737.0** Adolescent postural kyphosis
    EXCLUDES osteochondrosis of spine (juvenile) (732.0)
    adult (732.8)

- **737.1** Kyphosis (acquired)
  - **737.10** Kyphosis (acquired) (postural)
  - **737.11** Kyphosis due to radiation
  - **737.12** Kyphosis, postlaminectomy
    AHA: J-F, '87, 7
  - **737.19** Other
    EXCLUDES that associated with conditions classifiable elsewhere (737.41)
- **737.2** Lordosis (acquired)
  DEF: Swayback appearance created by an abnormally increased spinal curvature; it is also referred to as "hollow back" or "saddle back."
  - **737.20** Lordosis (acquired) (postural)
  - **737.21** Lordosis, postlaminectomy
  - **737.22** Other postsurgical lordosis
  - **737.29** Other
    EXCLUDES that associated with conditions classifiable elsewhere (737.42)
- **737.3** Kyphoscoliosis and scoliosis
  DEF: Kyphoscoliosis: backward and lateral curvature of the spinal column; it is found in vertebral osteochondrosis.
  DEF: Scoliosis: an abnormal deviation of the spine to the left or right of the midline
  - **737.30** Scoliosis [and kyphoscoliosis], idiopathic
    AHA: 3Q, '03, 19
  - **737.31** Resolving infantile idiopathic scoliosis
  - **737.32** Progressive infantile idiopathic scoliosis
    AHA: 3Q, '02, 12
  - **737.33** Scoliosis due to radiation
  - **737.34** Thoracogenic scoliosis

Kyphosis and Lordosis

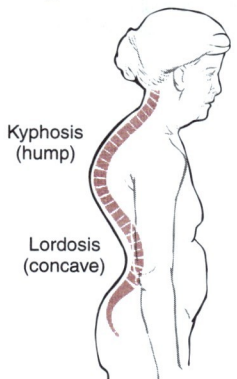

Kyphosis (hump)
Lordosis (concave)

MUSCULOSKELETAL SYSTEM AND CONNECTIVE TISSUE

737.39 Other

> EXCLUDES: that associated with conditions classifiable elsewhere (737.43)
> that in kyphoscoliotic heart disease (416.1)

AHA: 2Q, '02, 16

✓5th 737.4 Curvature of spine associated with other conditions
Code first associated condition as:
Charcôt-Marie-Tooth disease (356.1)
mucopolysaccharidosis (277.5)
neurofibromatosis (237.7)
osteitis deformans (731.0)
osteitis fibrosa cystica (252.01)
osteoporosis (733.00-733.09)
poliomyelitis (138)
tuberculosis [Pott's curvature] (015.0)

737.40 Curvature of spine, unspecified
737.41 Kyphosis
737.42 Lordosis
737.43 Scoliosis

737.8 Other curvatures of spine

737.9 Unspecified curvature of spine
Curvature of spine (acquired) (idiopathic) NOS
Hunchback, acquired
> EXCLUDES: deformity of spine NOS (738.5)

✓4th 738 Other acquired deformity
> EXCLUDES: congenital (754.0-756.9, 758.0-759.9)
> dentofacial anomalies (524.0-524.9)

738.0 Acquired deformity of nose
Deformity of nose (acquired)
Overdevelopment of nasal bones
> EXCLUDES: deflected or deviated nasal septum (470)

✓5th 738.1 Other acquired deformity of head
738.10 Unspecified deformity
738.11 Zygomatic hyperplasia
DEF: Abnormal enlargement of the zygoma (processus zygomaticus temporalis).

738.12 Zygomatic hypoplasia
DEF: Underdevelopment of the zygoma (processus zygomaticus temporalis).

738.19 Other specified deformity
AHA: 2Q, '03, 13

738.2 Acquired deformity of neck

738.3 Acquired deformity of chest and rib
Deformity: Pectus:
  chest (acquired)   carinatum, acquired
  rib (acquired)   excavatum, acquired

738.4 Acquired spondylolisthesis
Degenerative spondylolisthesis
Spondylolysis, acquired
> EXCLUDES: congenital (756.12)

DEF: Vertebra displaced forward over another; due to bilateral defect in vertebral arch, eroded articular surface of posterior facts and elongated pedicle between fifth lumbar vertebra and sacrum.

738.5 Other acquired deformity of back or spine
Deformity of spine NOS
> EXCLUDES: curvature of spine (737.0-737.9)

738.6 Acquired deformity of pelvis
Pelvic obliquity
> EXCLUDES: intrapelvic protrusion of acetabulum (718.6)
> that in relation to labor and delivery (653.0-653.4, 653.8-653.9)

DEF: Pelvic obliquity: slanting or inclination of the pelvis at an angle between 55 and 60 degrees between the plane of the pelvis and the horizontal plane.

738.7 Cauliflower ear
DEF: Abnormal external ear; due to injury, subsequent perichondritis.

738.8 Acquired deformity of other specified site
Deformity of clavicle
AHA: 2Q, '01, 15

738.9 Acquired deformity of unspecified site

✓4th 739 Nonallopathic lesions, not elsewhere classified
> INCLUDES: segmental dysfunction
> somatic dysfunction

DEF: Disability, loss of function or abnormality of a body part that is neither classifiable to a particular system nor brought about therapeutically to counteract another disease.

739.0 Head region
Occipitocervical region

739.1 Cervical region
Cervicothoracic region

739.2 Thoracic region
Thoracolumbar region

739.3 Lumbar region
Lumbosacral region

739.4 Sacral region
Sacrococcygeal region Sacroiliac region

739.5 Pelvic region
Hip region
Pubic region

739.6 Lower extremities

739.7 Upper extremities
Acromioclavicular region
Sternoclavicular region

739.8 Rib cage
Costochondral region Sternochondral region
Costovertebral region

739.9 Abdomen and other
AHA: 2Q, '89, 14

14. CONGENITAL ANOMALIES (740-759)

✓4th 740 Anencephalus and similar anomalies

740.0 Anencephalus
- Acrania
- Amyelencephalus
- Hemicephaly
- Hemianencephaly

DEF: Fetus without cerebrum, cerebellum and flat bones of skull.

740.1 Craniorachischisis

DEF: Congenital slit in cranium and vertebral column.

740.2 Iniencephaly

DEF: Spinal cord passes through enlarged occipital bone (foramen magnum); absent vertebral bone layer and spinal processes; resulting in both reduction in number and proper fusion of the vertebrae.

✓4th 741 Spina bifida

EXCLUDES: spina bifida occulta (756.17)

The following fifth-digit subclassification is for use with category 741:
- 0 unspecified region
- 1 cervical region
- 2 dorsal [thoracic] region
- 3 lumbar region

AHA: 3Q, '94, 7

DEF: Lack of closure of spinal cord's bony encasement; marked by cord protrusion into lumbosacral area; evident by elevated alpha-fetoprotein of amniotic fluid.

✓5th 741.0 With hydrocephalus
- Arnold-Chiari syndrome, type II
- Any condition classifiable to 741.9 with any condition classifiable to 742.3
- Chiari malformation, type II

AHA: 4Q, '97, 51; 4Q, '94, 37; S-O, '87, 10

✓5th 741.9 Without mention of hydrocephalus
- Hydromeningocele (spinal)
- Hydromyelocele
- Meningocele (spinal)
- Meningomyelocele
- Myelocele
- Myelocystocele
- Rachischisis
- Spina bifida (aperta)
- Syringomyelocele

✓4th 742 Other congenital anomalies of nervous system

EXCLUDES: congenital central alveolar hypoventilation syndrome (327.25)

742.0 Encephalocele
- Encephalocystocele
- Encephalomyelocele
- Hydroencephalocele
- Hydromeningocele, cranial
- Meningocele, cerebral
- Meningoencephalocele

AHA: 4Q, '94, 37

DEF: Brain tissue protrudes through skull defect.

742.1 Microcephalus
- Hydromicrocephaly
- Micrencephaly

DEF: Extremely small head or brain.

742.2 Reduction deformities of brain
- Absence
- Agenesis
- Aplasia
- Hypoplasia
} of part of brain

- Agyria
- Arhinencephaly
- Holoprosencephaly
- Microgyria

AHA: 3Q, '03, 15; 4Q, '94, 37

742.3 Congenital hydrocephalus
- Aqueduct of Sylvius:
  - anomaly
  - obstruction, congenital
  - stenosis
- Atresia of foramina of Magendie and Luschka
- Hydrocephalus in newborn

EXCLUDES: hydrocephalus:
- acquired (331.3-331.4)
- due to congenital toxoplasmosis (771.2)
- with any condition classifiable to 741.9 (741.0)

AHA: ▶4Q, '05, 83◀

DEF: Fluid accumulation within the skull; involves subarachnoid (external) or ventricular (internal) brain spaces.

742.4 Other specified anomalies of brain
- Congenital cerebral cyst
- Macroencephaly
- Macrogyria
- Megalencephaly
- Multiple anomalies of brain NOS
- Porencephaly
- Ulegyria

AHA: 1Q, '99, 9; 3Q, '92, 12

✓5th 742.5 Other specified anomalies of spinal cord

742.51 Diastematomyelia

DEF: Congenital anomaly often associated with spina bifida; the spinal cord is separated into halves by bony tissue resembling a "spike" (spicule), each half surrounded by a dural sac.

742.53 Hydromyelia
- Hydrorhachis

DEF: Dilated central spinal cord canal; characterized by increased fluid accumulation.

742.59 Other
- Amyelia
- Atelomyelia
- Congenital anomaly of spinal meninges
- Defective development of cauda equina
- Hypoplasia of spinal cord
- Myelatelia
- Myelodysplasia

AHA: 2Q, '91, 14; 1Q, '89, 10

742.8 Other specified anomalies of nervous system
- Agenesis of nerve
- Displacement of brachial plexus
- Familial dysautonomia
- Jaw-winking syndrome
- Marcus-Gunn syndrome
- Riley-Day syndrome

EXCLUDES   neurofibromatosis (237.7)

742.9 Unspecified anomaly of brain, spinal cord, and nervous system

Anomaly
Congenital: of:
  disease   brain
  lesion   nervous system
  Deformity   spinal cord

743 Congenital anomalies of eye

743.0 Anophthalmos
DEF: Complete absence of the eyes or the presence of vestigial eyes.

743.00 Clinical anophthalmos, unspecified
- Agenesis   } of eye
- Congenital absence
- Anophthalmos NOS

743.03 Cystic eyeball, congenital

743.06 Cryptophthalmos
DEF: Eyelids continue over eyeball, results in apparent absence of eyelids.

743.1 Microphthalmos
- Dysplasia   } of eye
- Hypoplasia
- Rudimentary eye

DEF: Abnormally small eyeballs, may be opacities of cornea and lens, scarring of choroid and retina.

743.10 Microphthalmos, unspecified
743.11 Simple microphthalmos
743.12 Microphthalmos associated with other anomalies of eye and adnexa

743.2 Buphthalmos
Glaucoma: Hydrophthalmos
  congenital
  newborn

EXCLUDES   glaucoma of childhood (365.14)
traumatic glaucoma due to birth injury (767.8)

DEF: Distended, enlarged fibrous coats of eye; due to intraocular pressure of congenital glaucoma.

743.20 Buphthalmos, unspecified
743.21 Simple buphthalmos
743.22 Buphthalmos associated with other ocular anomalies
- Keratoglobus, congenital } associated with buphthalmos
- Megalocornea

743.3 Congenital cataract and lens anomalies
EXCLUDES   infantile cataract (366.00-366.09)
DEF: Opaque eye lens.

743.30 Congenital cataract, unspecified

743.31 Capsular and subcapsular cataract
743.32 Cortical and zonular cataract
743.33 Nuclear cataract
743.34 Total and subtotal cataract, congenital
743.35 Congenital aphakia
- Congenital absence of lens

743.36 Anomalies of lens shape
- Microphakia   Spherophakia

743.37 Congenital ectopic lens
743.39 Other

743.4 Coloboma and other anomalies of anterior segment
DEF: Coloboma: ocular tissue defect associated with defect of ocular fetal intraocular fissure; may cause small pit on optic disk, major defects of iris, ciliary body, choroid, and retina.

743.41 Anomalies of corneal size and shape
- Microcornea
EXCLUDES   that associated with buphthalmos (743.22)

743.42 Corneal opacities, interfering with vision, congenital
743.43 Other corneal opacities, congenital
743.44 Specified anomalies of anterior chamber, chamber angle, and related structures
- Anomaly: Anomaly:
  Axenfeld's   Rieger's
  Peters'

743.45 Aniridia
AHA: 3Q, '02, 20
DEF: Incompletely formed or absent iris; affects both eyes; dominant trait; also called congenital hyperplasia of iris.

743.46 Other specified anomalies of iris and ciliary body
- Anisocoria, congenital   Coloboma of iris
- Atresia of pupil   Corectopia

743.47 Specified anomalies of sclera
743.48 Multiple and combined anomalies of anterior segment
743.49 Other

743.5 Congenital anomalies of posterior segment
743.51 Vitreous anomalies
- Congenital vitreous opacity

743.52 Fundus coloboma
DEF: Absent retinal and choroidal tissue; occurs in lower fundus; a bright white ectatic zone of exposed sclera extends into and changes the optic disk.

743.53 Chorioretinal degeneration, congenital
743.54 Congenital folds and cysts of posterior segment
743.55 Congenital macular changes
743.56 Other retinal changes, congenital
AHA: 3Q, '99, 12

743.57 Specified anomalies of optic disc
- Coloboma of optic disc (congenital)

743.58 Vascular anomalies
- Congenital retinal aneurysm

743.59 Other

743.6 Congenital anomalies of eyelids, lacrimal system, and orbit
743.61 Congenital ptosis
DEF: Drooping of eyelid.

743.62 Congenital deformities of eyelids
- Ablepharon   Congenital:
- Absence of eyelid   ectropion
- Accessory eyelid   entropion

AHA: 1Q, '00, 22

CONGENITAL ANOMALIES

743.63 Other specified congenital anomalies of eyelid
Absence, agenesis, of cilia

743.64 Specified congenital anomalies of lacrimal gland

743.65 Specified congenital anomalies of lacrimal passages
Absence, agenesis of:
    lacrimal apparatus
    punctum lacrimale
    Accessory lacrimal canal

743.66 Specified congenital anomalies of orbit

743.69 Other
Accessory eye muscles

743.8 Other specified anomalies of eye
    EXCLUDES   congenital nystagmus (379.51)
        ocular albinism (270.2)
        ▶optic nerve hypoplasia (377.43)◀
        retinitis pigmentosa (362.74)

743.9 Unspecified anomaly of eye
Congenital:
    anomaly NOS } of eye [any part]
    deformity NOS

✓4th 744 Congenital anomalies of ear, face, and neck
EXCLUDES   anomaly of:
    cervical spine (754.2, 756.10-756.19)
    larynx (748.2-748.3)
    nose (748.0-748.1)
    parathyroid gland (759.2)
    thyroid gland (759.2)
    cleft lip (749.10-749.25)

✓5th 744.0 Anomalies of ear causing impairment of hearing
    EXCLUDES   congenital deafness without mention of cause (389.0-389.9)

744.00 Unspecified anomaly of ear with impairment of hearing

744.01 Absence of external ear
Absence of:
    auditory canal (external)
    auricle (ear) (with stenosis or atresia of auditory canal)

744.02 Other anomalies of external ear with impairment of hearing
Atresia or stricture of auditory canal (external)

744.03 Anomaly of middle ear, except ossicles
Atresia or stricture of osseous meatus (ear)

744.04 Anomalies of ear ossicles
Fusion of ear ossicles

744.05 Anomalies of inner ear
Congenital anomaly of:
    membranous labyrinth
    organ of Corti

744.09 Other
Absence of ear, congenital

744.1 Accessory auricle
Accessory tragus   Supernumerary:
Polyotia   ear
Preauricular appendage lobule
DEF: Redundant tissue or structures of ear.

✓5th 744.2 Other specified anomalies of ear
    EXCLUDES   that with impairment of hearing (744.00-744.09)

744.21 Absence of ear lobe, congenital

744.22 Macrotia
DEF: Abnormally large pinna of ear.

744.23 Microtia
DEF: Hypoplasia of pinna; associated with absent or closed auditory canal.

744.24 Specified anomalies of Eustachian tube
Absence of Eustachian tube

744.29 Other
Bat ear   Prominence of auricle
Darwin's tubercle Ridge ear
Pointed ear
    EXCLUDES   preauricular sinus (744.46)

744.3 Unspecified anomaly of ear
Congenital:
    anomaly NOS } of ear, not elsewhere
    deformity NOS   classified

✓5th 744.4 Branchial cleft cyst or fistula; preauricular sinus

744.41 Branchial cleft sinus or fistula
Branchial:
    sinus (external) (internal)
    vestige
DEF: Cyst due to failed closure of embryonic branchial cleft.

744.42 Branchial cleft cyst

744.43 Cervical auricle

744.46 Preauricular sinus or fistula

744.47 Preauricular cyst

744.49 Other
Fistula (of):   Fistula (of):
  auricle, congenital cervicoaural

744.5 Webbing of neck
Pterygium colli
DEF: Thick, triangular skinfold, stretches from lateral side of neck across shoulder; associated with Turner's and Noonan's syndromes.

✓5th 744.8 Other specified anomalies of face and neck

744.81 Macrocheilia
Hypertrophy of lip, congenital
DEF: Abnormally large lips.

744.82 Microcheilia
DEF: Abnormally small lips.

744.83 Macrostomia
DEF: Bilateral or unilateral anomaly, of mouth due to malformed maxillary and mandibular processes; results in mouth extending toward ear.

744.84 Microstomia
DEF: Abnormally small mouth.

744.89 Other
    EXCLUDES   congenital fistula of lip (750.25)
        musculoskeletal anomalies (754.0-754.1, 756.0)

744.9 Unspecified anomalies of face and neck
Congenital:
    anomaly NOS } of face [any part] or
    deformity NOS neck [any part]

✓4th 745 Bulbus cordis anomalies and anomalies of cardiac septal closure

745.0 Common truncus
Absent septum   } between aorta and
Communication   pulmonary artery
  (abnormal)

Aortic septal defect
Common aortopulmonary trunk
Persistent truncus arteriosus

Heart Defects

Atrial septal defect
Ventricular septal defect
Aortic stenosis
Patent ductus arteriosus
Pulmonary stenosis
Transposition of the great vessels
Tetralogy of Fallot

745.1 Transposition of great vessels

    745.10 Complete transposition of great vessels
        Transposition of great vessels:
          NOS
          classical

    745.11 Double outlet right ventricle
        Dextratransposition of aorta
        Incomplete transposition of great vessels
        Origin of both great vessels from right ventricle
        Taussig-Bing syndrome or defect

    745.12 Corrected transposition of great vessels
    745.19 Other

745.2 Tetralogy of Fallot
    Fallot's pentalogy
    Ventricular septal defect with pulmonary stenosis or atresia, dextraposition of aorta, and hypertrophy of right ventricle
    EXCLUDES Fallot's triad (746.09)
    DEF: Obstructed cardiac outflow causes pulmonary stenosis, interventricular septal defect and right ventricular hypertrophy.

745.3 Common ventricle
    Cor triloculare biatriatum
    Single ventricle

745.4 Ventricular septal defect
    Eisenmenger's defect or complex
    Gerbo dedefect
    Interventricular septal defect
    Left ventricular-right atrial communication
    Roger's disease
    EXCLUDES common atrioventricular canal type (745.69)
               single ventricle (745.3)

745.5 Ostium secundum type atrial septal defect
    Defect: Patent or persistent:
      atrium secundum   foramen ovale
      fossa ovalis   ostium secundum
    Lutembacher's syndrome
    DEF: Opening in atrial septum due to failure of the septum secundum and the endocardial cushions to fuse; there is a rim of septum surrounding the defect.

745.6 Endocardial cushion defects
    DEF: Atrial and/or ventricular septal defects causing abnormal fusion of cushions in atrioventricular canal.

    745.60 Endocardial cushion defect, unspecified type
        DEF: Septal defect due to imperfect fusion of endocardial cushions.

    745.61 Ostium primum defect
        Persistent ostium primum
        DEF: Opening in low, posterior septum primum; causes cleft in basal portion of atrial septum; associated with cleft mitral valve.

    745.69 Other
        Absence of atrial septum
        Atrioventricular canal type ventricular septal defect
        Common atrioventricular canal
        Common atrium

745.7 Cor biloculare
    Absence of atrial and ventricular septa
    DEF: Atrial and ventricular septal defect; marked by heart with two cardiac chambers (one atrium, one ventricle), and one atrioventricular valve.

745.8 Other

745.9 Unspecified defect of septal closure
    Septal defect NOS

746 Other congenital anomalies of heart
    EXCLUDES endocardial fibroelastosis (425.3)

746.0 Anomalies of pulmonary valve
    EXCLUDES infundibular or subvalvular pulmonic stenosis (746.83)
               tetralogy of Fallot (745.2)

    746.00 Pulmonary valve anomaly, unspecified
    746.01 Atresia, congenital
        Congenital absence of pulmonary valve
    746.02 Stenosis, congenital
        DEF: Stenosis of opening between pulmonary artery and right ventricle; causes obstructed blood outflow from right ventricle.
    746.09 Other
        Congenital insufficiency of pulmonary valve
        Fallot's triad or trilogy

746.1 Tricuspid atresia and stenosis, congenital
    Absence of tricuspid valve

746.2 Ebstein's anomaly
    DEF: Malformation of the tricuspid valve characterized by septal and posterior leaflets attaching to the wall of the right ventricle; causing the right ventricle to fuse with the atrium producing a large right atrium and a small ventricle; causes a malfunction of the right ventricle with accompanying complications such as heart failure and abnormal cardiac rhythm.

746.3 Congenital stenosis of aortic valve
    Congenital aortic stenosis
    EXCLUDES congenital:
              subaortic stenosis (746.81)
              supravalvular aortic stenosis (747.22)
    AHA: 4Q, '88, 8
    DEF: Stenosis of orifice of aortic valve; obstructs blood outflow from left ventricle.

746.4 Congenital insufficiency of aortic valve
    Bicuspid aortic valve
    Congenital aortic insufficiency
    DEF: Impaired functioning of aortic valve due to incomplete closure; causes backflow (regurgitation) of blood from aorta to left ventricle.

746.5 Congenital mitral stenosis
    Fused commissure   ⎫
    Parachute deformity   ⎬ of mitral valve
    Supernumerary cusps   ⎭
    DEF: Stenosis of left atrioventricular orifice.

746.6 Congenital mitral insufficiency
    DEF: Impaired functioning of mitral valve due to incomplete closure; causes backflow of blood from left ventricle to left atrium.

746.7 Hypoplastic left heart syndrome
    Atresia, or marked hypoplasia, of aortic orifice or valve, with hypoplasia of ascending aorta and defective development of left ventricle (with mitral valve atresia)

CONGENITAL ANOMALIES

746.8 Other specified anomalies of heart
    746.81 Subaortic stenosis
        DEF: Stenosis, of left ventricular outflow tract due to fibrous tissue ring or septal hypertrophy below aortic valve.
    746.82 Cor triatriatum
        DEF: Transverse septum divides left atrium due to failed resorption of embryonic common pulmonary vein; results in three atrial chambers.
    746.83 Infundibular pulmonic stenosis
        Subvalvular pulmonic stenosis
        DEF: Stenosis of right ventricle outflow tract within infundibulum due to fibrous diaphragm below valve or long, narrow fibromuscular channel.
    746.84 Obstructive anomalies of heart, not elsewhere classified
        Uhl's disease
    746.85 Coronary artery anomaly
        Anomalous origin or communication of coronary artery
        Arteriovenous malformation of coronary artery
        Coronary artery:
            absence
            arising from aorta or pulmonary trunk
            single
        AHA: N-D, '85, 3
    746.86 Congenital heart block
        Complete or incomplete atrioventricular [AV] block
        DEF: Impaired conduction of electrical impulses; due to maldeveloped junctional tissue.
    746.87 Malposition of heart and cardiac apex
        Abdominal heart   Levocardia (isolated)
        Dextrocardia   Mesocardia
        Ectopia cordis
        EXCLUDES   dextrocardia with complete transposition of viscera (759.3)
    746.89 Other
        Atresia } of cardiac vein
        Hypoplasia
        Congenital:
            cardiomegaly
            diverticulum, left ventricle
            pericardial defect
        AHA: 3Q, '00, 3; 1Q, '99, 11; J-F, '85, 3

746.9 Unspecified anomaly of heart
    Congenital:
        anomaly of heart NOS
        heart disease NOS

747 Other congenital anomalies of circulatory system
    747.0 Patent ductus arteriosus
        Patent ductus Botalli   Persistent ductus arteriosus
        DEF: Open lumen in ductus arteriosus causes arterial blood recirculation in lungs; inhibits blood supply to aorta; symptoms such as shortness of breath more noticeable upon activity.
    747.1 Coarctation of aorta
        DEF: Localized deformity of aortic media seen as a severe constriction of the vessel lumen; major symptom is high blood pressure in the arms and low pressure in the legs; a CVA, rupture of the aorta, bacterial endocarditis or congestive heart failure can follow if left untreated.
        747.10 Coarctation of aorta (preductal) (postductal)
            Hypoplasia of aortic arch
            AHA: 1Q, '99, 11; 4Q, '88, 8
        747.11 Interruption of aortic arch

747.2 Other anomalies of aorta
    747.20 Anomaly of aorta, unspecified
    747.21 Anomalies of aortic arch
        Anomalous origin, right subclavian artery
        Dextraposition of aorta
        Double aortic arch
        Kommerell's diverticulum
        Overriding aorta
        Persistent:
            convolutions, aortic arch
            right aortic arch
        Vascular ring
        EXCLUDES   hypoplasia of aortic arch (747.10)
        AHA: 1Q, '03, 15
    747.22 Atresia and stenosis of aorta
        Absence
        Aplasia   } of aorta
        Hypoplasia
        Stricture
        Supra (valvular)-aortic stenosis
        EXCLUDES   congenital aortic (valvular) stenosis or stricture, so stated (746.3)
                            hypoplasia of aorta in hypoplastic left heart syndrome (746.7)
    747.29 Other
        Aneurysm of sinus of Valsalva
        Congenital:
            aneurysm   } of aorta
            dilation

747.3 Anomalies of pulmonary artery
    Agenesis
    Anomaly
    Atresia   } of pulmonary artery
    Coarctation
    Hypoplasia
    Stenosis
    Pulmonary arteriovenous aneurysm
    AHA: 1Q, '94, 15; 4Q, '88, 8

747.4 Anomalies of great veins
    747.40 Anomaly of great veins, unspecified
        Anomaly NOS of:
            pulmonary veins
            vena cava
    747.41 Total anomalous pulmonary venous connection
        Total anomalous pulmonary venous return [TAPVR]:
            subdiaphragmatic
            supradiaphragmatic
    747.42 Partial anomalous pulmonary venous connection
        Partial anomalous pulmonary venous return
    747.49 Other anomalies of great veins
        Absence
        Congenital   } of vena cava (inferior) (superior)
            stenosis
        Persistent:
            left posterior cardinal vein
            left superior vena cava
        Scimitar syndrome
        Transposition of pulmonary veins NOS

747.5 Absence or hypoplasia of umbilical artery
    Single umbilical artery

CONGENITAL ANOMALIES

✓5th 747.6 Other anomalies of peripheral vascular system
Absence ⎫
Anomaly ⎬ of artery or vein, not elsewhere classified
Atresia ⎭
Arteriovenous aneurysm (peripheral)
Arteriovenous malformation of the peripheral vascular system
Congenital:
   aneurysm (peripheral)
Congenital:
   phlebectasia
   stricture, artery
   varix
Multiple renal arteries

EXCLUDES anomalies of:
   cerebral vessels (747.81)
   pulmonary artery (747.3)
   congenital retinal aneurysm (743.58)
   hemangioma (228.00-228.09)
   lymphangioma (228.1)

747.60 Anomaly of the peripheral vascular system, unspecified site
747.61 Gastrointestinal vessel anomaly
   AHA: 3Q '96, 10
747.62 Renal vessel anomaly
747.63 Upper limb vessel anomaly
747.64 Lower limb vessel anomaly
747.69 Anomalies of other specified sites of peripheral vascular system

✓5th 747.8 Other specified anomalies of circulatory system
747.81 Anomalies of cerebrovascular system
Arteriovenous malformation of brain
Cerebral arteriovenous aneurysm, congenital
Congenital anomalies of cerebral vessels
EXCLUDES ruptured cerebral (arteriovenous) aneurysm (430)

747.82 Spinal vessel anomaly
Arteriovenous malformation of spinal vessel
AHA: 3Q, '95, 5

747.83 Persistent fetal circulation [N]
Persistent pulmonary hypertension
Primary pulmonary hypertension of newborn
AHA: 4Q, '02, 62

DEF: A return to fetal-type circulation due to constriction of pulmonary arterioles and opening of the ductus arteriosus and foramen ovale, right-to-left shunting occurs, oxygenation of the blood does not occur, and the lungs remain constricted after birth; PFC is seen in term or post-term infants causes include asphyxiation, meconium aspiration syndrome, acidosis, sepsis, and developmental immaturity.

747.89 Other
Aneurysm, congenital, specified site not elsewhere classified
EXCLUDES congenital aneurysm:
   coronary (746.85)
   peripheral (747.6)
   pulmonary (747.3)
   retinal (743.58)
AHA: 4Q, '02, 63

747.9 Unspecified anomaly of circulatory system

✓4th 748 Congenital anomalies of respiratory system
EXCLUDES congenital central alveolar hypoventilation syndrome (327.25)
congenital defect of diaphragm (756.6)

748.0 Choanal atresia
Atresia ⎫
Congenital stenosis ⎬ of nares (anterior) (posterior)

DEF: Occluded posterior nares (choana), bony or membranous due to failure of embryonic bucconasal membrane to rupture.

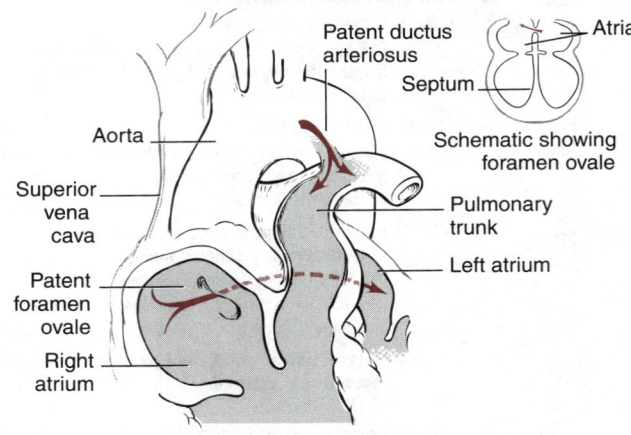
Persistent Fetal Circulation

748.1 Other anomalies of nose
Absent nose
Accessory nose
Cleft nose
Congenital:
   deformity of nose
Congenital:
   notching of tip of nose
   perforation of wall of nasal sinus
Deformity of wall of nasal sinus
EXCLUDES congenital deviation of nasal septum (754.0)

748.2 Web of larynx
Web of larynx:
   NOS
   glottic
Web of larynx:
   subglottic

DEF: Malformed larynx; marked by thin, translucent, or thick, fibrotic spread between vocal folds; affects speech.

748.3 Other anomalies of larynx, trachea, and bronchus
Absence or agenesis of:
   bronchus
   larynx
   trachea
Anomaly(of):
   cricoid cartilage
   epiglottis
   thyroid cartilage
   tracheal cartilage
Atresia (of):
   epiglottis
   glottis
   larynx
   trachea
Cleft thyroid, cartilage, congenital
Congenital:
   dilation, trachea
   stenosis:
     larynx
     trachea
   tracheocele
Diverticulum:
   bronchus
   trachea
Fissure of epiglottis
Laryngocele
Posterior cleft of cricoid cartilage (congenital)
Rudimentary tracheal bronchus
Stridor, laryngeal, congenital

AHA: 1Q, '99, 14

748.4 Congenital cystic lung
Disease, lung:
   cystic, congenital
   polycystic, congenital
Honeycomb lung, congenital
EXCLUDES acquired or unspecified cystic lung (518.89)

DEF: Enlarged air spaces of lung parenchyma.

748.5 Agenesis, hypoplasia, and dysplasia of lung
Absence of lung (fissures) (lobe)
Aplasia of lung
Hypoplasia of lung (lobe)
Sequestration of lung

✓5th 748.6 Other anomalies of lung
748.60 Anomaly of lung, unspecified
748.61 Congenital bronchiectasis
748.69 Other
Accessory lung (lobe)
Azygos lobe (fissure), lung

[N] Newborn Age: 0   [P] Pediatric Age: 0-17   [M] Maternity Age: 12-55   [A] Adult Age: 15-124

Cleft Lip and Palate

Unilateral cleft lip — No cleft palate

Cleft lip with cleft alveolar ridge — No cleft palate

Unilateral cleft lip and cleft palate — Alveolar ridge — Cleft palate

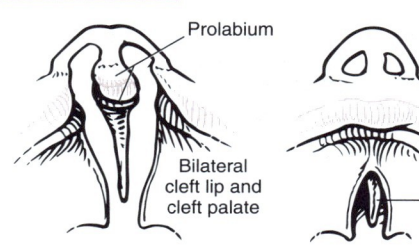
Prolabium — Bilateral cleft lip and cleft palate — Isolated cleft palate

748.8 Other specified anomalies of respiratory system
Abnormal communication between pericardial and pleural sacs
Anomaly, pleural folds
Atresia of nasopharynx
Congenital cyst of mediastinum

748.9 Unspecified anomaly of respiratory system
Anomaly of respiratory system NOS

749 Cleft palate and cleft lip

749.0 Cleft palate
- 749.00 Cleft palate, unspecified
- 749.01 Unilateral, complete
- 749.02 Unilateral, incomplete
  Cleft uvula
- 749.03 Bilateral, complete
- 749.04 Bilateral, incomplete

749.1 Cleft lip
Cheiloschisis   Harelip
Congenital fissure of lip   Labium leporinum
- 749.10 Cleft lip, unspecified
- 749.11 Unilateral, complete
- 749.12 Unilateral, incomplete
- 749.13 Bilateral, complete
- 749.14 Bilateral, incomplete

749.2 Cleft palate with cleft lip
Cheilopalatoschisis
- 749.20 Cleft palate with cleft lip, unspecified
- 749.21 Unilateral, complete
- 749.22 Unilateral, incomplete
- 749.23 Bilateral, complete
  AHA: 1Q, '96, 14
- 749.24 Bilateral, incomplete
- 749.25 Other combinations

750 Other congenital anomalies of upper alimentary tract
EXCLUDES dentofacial anomalies (524.0-524.9)

750.0 Tongue tie
Ankyloglossia
DEF: Restricted tongue movement due to lingual frenum extending toward tip of tongue. Tongue may be fused to mouth floor affecting speech.

750.1 Other anomalies of tongue
- 750.10 Anomaly of tongue, unspecified
- 750.11 Aglossia
  DEF: Absence of tongue.
- 750.12 Congenital adhesions of tongue
- 750.13 Fissure of tongue
  Bifid tongue   Double tongue
- 750.15 Macroglossia
  Congenital hypertrophy of tongue
- 750.16 Microglossia
  Hypoplasia of tongue
- 750.19 Other

750.2 Other specified anomalies of mouth and pharynx
- 750.21 Absence of salivary gland
- 750.22 Accessory salivary gland
- 750.23 Atresia, salivary duct
  Imperforate salivary duct
- 750.24 Congenital fistula of salivary gland
- 750.25 Congenital fistula of lip
  Congenital (mucus) lip pits
- 750.26 Other specified anomalies of mouth
  Absence of uvula
- 750.27 Diverticulum of pharynx
  Pharyngeal pouch
- 750.29 Other specified anomalies of pharynx
  Imperforate pharynx

750.3 Tracheoesophageal fistula, esophageal atresia and stenosis
Absent esophagus
Atresia of esophagus
Congenital:
  esophageal ring
  stenosis of esophagus
  stricture of esophagus
Congenital fistula:
  esophagobronchial
  esophagotracheal
Imperforate esophagus
Webbed esophagus

750.4 Other specified anomalies of esophagus
Dilatation, congenital
Displacement, congenital
Diverticulum
Duplication
Giant
} (of) esophagus

Esophageal pouch
EXCLUDES congenital hiatus hernia (750.6)
AHA: J-F, '85, 3

750.5 Congenital hypertrophic pyloric stenosis
Congenital or infantile:
  constriction
  hypertrophy
  spasm
  stenosis
  stricture
} of pylorus

DEF: Obstructed pylorus due to overgrowth of pyloric muscle.

750.6 Congenital hiatus hernia
Displacement of cardia through esophageal hiatus
EXCLUDES congenital diaphragmatic hernia (756.6)

750.7 Other specified anomalies of stomach
Congenital:
  cardiospasm
  hourglass stomach
Displacement of stomach
Diverticulum of stomach, congenital
Duplication of stomach
Megalogastria
Microgastria
Transposition of stomach

750.8 Other specified anomalies of upper alimentary tract

CONGENITAL ANOMALIES — Tabular List

750.9 **Unspecified anomaly of upper alimentary tract**
Congenital:
anomaly NOS } of upper alimentary tract
deformity NOS } [any part, except tongue]

✓4th **751 Other congenital anomalies of digestive system**

751.0 Meckel's diverticulum
Meckel's diverticulum (displaced) (hypertrophic)
Persistent:
omphalomesenteric duct
vitelline duct
AHA: 1Q, '04, 10

DEF: Malformed sacs or appendages of ileum of small intestine; can cause strangulation, volvulus and intussusception.

751.1 Atresia and stenosis of small intestine [P]
Atresia of: Atresia of:
  duodenum   intestine NOS
  ileum
Congenital:
  absence
  obstruction } of small intestine or
  stenosis   } intestine NOS
  stricture
Imperforate jejunum

751.2 Atresia and stenosis of large intestine, rectum, and anal canal [P]
Absence:
  anus (congenital)
  appendix, congenital
  large intestine, congenital
  rectum
Atresia of:
  anus
  colon
  rectum
Congenital or infantile:
  obstruction of large intestine
  occlusion of anus
  stricture of anus
Imperforate:
  anus
  rectum
Stricture of rectum, congenital
AHA: 2Q, '98, 16

751.3 Hirschsprung's disease and other congenital functional disorders of colon
Aganglionosis
Congenital dilation of colon
Congenital megacolon
Macrocolon

DEF: Hirschsprung's disease: enlarged or dilated colon (megacolon), with absence of ganglion cells in the narrowed wall distally; causes inability to defecate.

751.4 Anomalies of intestinal fixation
Congenital adhesions: Rotation of cecum or colon:
  omental, anomalous   failure of
  peritoneal   incomplete
  Jackson's membrane   insufficient
  Malrotation of colon   Universal mesentery

751.5 Other anomalies of intestine
Congenital diverticulum, colon
Dolichocolon
Duplication of:
  anus
  appendix
  cecum
  intestine
Ectopic anus
Megaloappendix
Megaloduodenum
Microcolon
Persistent cloaca
Transposition of:
  appendix
  colon
  intestine
AHA: 3Q, '02, 11; 3Q, '01, 8

✓5th **751.6 Anomalies of gallbladder, bile ducts, and liver**

751.60 Unspecified anomaly of gallbladder, bile ducts, and liver

751.61 Biliary atresia [P]
Congenital:
  absence
  hypoplasia   } of bile duct (common)
  obstruction } or passage
  stricture
AHA: S-O, '87, 8

751.62 Congenital cystic disease of liver
Congenital polycystic disease of liver
Fibrocystic disease of liver

751.69 Other anomalies of gallbladder, bile ducts, and liver
Absence of:
  gallbladder, congenital
  liver (lobe)
Accessory:
  hepatic ducts
  liver
Congenital:
  choledochal cyst
  hepatomegaly
Duplication of:
  biliary duct
  cystic duct
  gallbladder
  liver
Floating:
  gallbladder
  liver
Intrahepatic gallbladder
AHA: S-O, '87, 8

751.7 Anomalies of pancreas
Absence
Accessory
Agenesis   } (of) pancreas
Annular
Hypoplasia
Ectopic pancreatic tissue
Pancreatic heterotopia
EXCLUDES diabetes mellitus:
  congenital (250.0-250.9)
  neonatal (775.1)
fibrocystic disease of pancreas (277.00-277.09)

751.8 Other specified anomalies of digestive system
Absence (complete) (partial) of alimentary tract NOS
Duplication   } of digestive organs NOS
Malposition, congenital
EXCLUDES congenital diaphragmatic hernia (756.6)
congenital hiatus hernia (750.6)

CONGENITAL ANOMALIES

751.9 Unspecified anomaly of digestive system
Congenital:
  anomaly NOS
  deformity NOS } of digestive system NOS

752 Congenital anomalies of genital organs
  EXCLUDES syndromes associated with anomalies in the number and form of chromosomes (758.0-758.9)
  testicular feminization syndrome (259.5)

752.0 Anomalies of ovaries ♀
  Absence, congenital
  Accessory
  Ectopic
  Streak } (of) ovary

752.1 Anomalies of fallopian tubes and broad ligaments
  752.10 Unspecified anomaly of fallopian tubes and broad ligaments ♀
  752.11 Embryonic cyst of fallopian tubes and broad ligaments ♀
    Cyst: Cyst:
      epoophoron   parovarian
      fimbrial
    AHA: S-O, '85, 13
  752.19 Other ♀
    Absence
    Accessory
    Atresia } (of) fallopian tube or broad ligament

752.2 Doubling of uterus ♀
  Didelphic uterus
  Doubling of uterus [any degree] (associated with doubling of cervix and vagina)

752.3 Other anomalies of uterus ♀
  Absence, congenital
  Agenesis
  Aplasia
  Bicornuate } (of) uterus
  Uterus unicornis
  Uterus with only one functioning horn

752.4 Anomalies of cervix, vagina, and external female genitalia
  752.40 Unspecified anomaly of cervix, vagina, and external female genitalia ♀
  752.41 Embryonic cyst of cervix, vagina, and external female genitalia ♀
    Cyst of:
      canal of Nuck, congenital
      Gartner's duct
      vagina, embryonal
      vulva, congenital
    DEF: Embryonic fluid-filled cysts, of cervix, vagina or external female genitalia.
  752.42 Imperforate hymen ♀
    DEF: Complete closure of membranous fold around external opening of vagina.
  752.49 Other anomalies of cervix, vagina, and external female genitalia ♀
    Absence
    Agenesis } of cervix, clitoris, vagina, or vulva
    Congenital stenosis or stricture of:
      cervical canal
      vagina
    EXCLUDES double vagina associated with total duplication (752.2)

752.5 Undescended and retractile testicle
  AHA: 4Q, '96, 33
  752.51 Undescended testis ♂
    Cryptorchism
    Ectopic testis
  752.52 Retractile testis ♂

Hypospadias and Epispadias

Hypospadias (ventral view) — Glans penis, Glandular hypospadias, Penile hypospadias, Scrotal hypospadias, Scrotum, Scrotal raphe, Penile raphe

Epispadias (dorsal view) — Normal external urethral orifice, Glans penis, Foreskin (retracted), Epispadias

752.6 Hypospadias and epispadias and other penile anomalies
  AHA: 4Q, '96, 34, 35
  752.61 Hypospadias ♂
    AHA: 3Q, '97, 6
    DEF: Abnormal opening of urethra on the ventral surface of the penis or perineum; also a rare defect of vagina.
    AHA: 4Q, '03, 67-68
  752.62 Epispadias ♂
    Anaspadias
    DEF: Epispadias: urethra opening on dorsal surface of penis; in females appears as a slit in the upper wall of urethra.
  752.63 Congenital chordee ♂
    DEF: Ventral bowing of penis due to fibrous band along corpus spongiosum; occurs with hypospadias.
  752.64 Micropenis ♂
  752.65 Hidden penis ♂
  752.69 Other penile anomalies ♂

752.7 Indeterminate sex and pseudohermaphroditism
  Gynandrism   Pseudohermaphroditism
  Hermaphroditism   (male) (female)
  Ovotestis   Pure gonadal dysgenesis
  EXCLUDES pseudohermaphroditism:
    female, with adrenocortical disorder (255.2)
    male, with gonadal disorder (257.8)
    with specified chromosomal anomaly (758.0-758.9)
    testicular feminization syndrome (259.5)
  DEF: Pseudohermaphroditism: presence of gonads of one sex and external genitalia of other sex.

752.8 Other specified anomalies of genital organs
  EXCLUDES congenital hydrocele (778.6)
    penile anomalies (752.61-752.69)
    phimosis or paraphimosis (605)
  752.81 Scrotal transposition ♂
    AHA: 4Q, '03, 67-68
  752.89 Other specified anomalies of genital organs
    Absence of: Fusion of testes
      prostate   Hypoplasia of testis
      spermatic cord   Monorchism
      vas deferens   Polyorchism
    Anorchism
    Aplasia (congenital) of:
      prostate
      round ligament
      testicle
    Atresia of:
      ejaculatory duct
      vas deferens

CONGENITAL ANOMALIES

752.9 Unspecified anomaly of genital organs
  Congenital:
    anomaly NOS } of genital organ, not
    deformity NOS } elsewhere classified

✓4ᵗʰ 753 Congenital anomalies of urinary system

753.0 Renal agenesis and dysgenesis
  Atrophy of kidney:
    congenital
    infantile
  Congenital absence of kidney(s)
  Hypoplasia of kidney(s)

✓5ᵗʰ 753.1 Cystic kidney disease
  EXCLUDES acquired cyst of kidney (593.2)
  AHA: 4Q, '90, 3

753.10 Cystic kidney disease, unspecified
753.11 Congenital single renal cyst
753.12 Polycystic kidney, unspecified type
753.13 Polycystic kidney, autosomal dominant
  DEF: Slow progressive disease characterized by bilateral cysts causing increased kidney size and impaired function.

753.14 Polycystic kidney, autosomal recessive
  DEF: Rare disease characterized by multiple cysts involving kidneys and liver, producing renal and hepatic failure in childhood or adolescence.

753.15 Renal dysplasia
753.16 Medullary cystic kidney
  Nephronopthisis
  DEF: Diffuse kidney disease results in uremia onset prior to age 20.

753.17 Medullary sponge kidney
  DEF: Dilated collecting tubules; usually asymptomatic but calcinosis in tubules may cause renal insufficiency.

753.19 Other specified cystic kidney disease
  Multicystic kidney

✓5ᵗʰ 753.2 Obstructive defects of renal pelvis and ureter
  AHA: 4Q, '96, 35

753.20 Unspecified obstructive defect of renal pelvis and ureter
753.21 Congenital obstruction of ureteropelvic junction
  DEF: Stricture at junction of ureter and renal pelvis.

753.22 Congenital obstruction of ureterovesical junction
  Adynamic ureter
  Congenital hydroureter
  DEF: Stricture at junction of ureter and bladder.

753.23 Congenital ureterocele
753.29 Other

753.3 Other specified anomalies of kidney
  Accessory kidney   Fusion of kidneys
  Congenital: Giant kidney
    calculus of kidney   Horseshoe kidney
    displaced kidney   Hyperplasia of kidney
  Discoid kidney   Lobulation of kidney
  Double kidney with   Malrotation of kidney
    double pelvis   Trifid kidney (pelvis)
  Ectopic kidney

753.4 Other specified anomalies of ureter
  Absent ureter   Double ureter
  Accessory ureter   Ectopic ureter
  Deviation of ureter   Implantation, anomalous
  Displaced ureteric orifice   of ureter

753.5 Exstrophy of urinary bladder
  Ectopia vesicae
  Extroversion of bladder
  DEF: Absence of lower abdominal and anterior bladder walls with posterior bladder wall protrusion.

753.6 Atresia and stenosis of urethra and bladder neck
  Congenital obstruction:
    bladder neck
    urethra
  Congenital stricture of:
    urethra (valvular)
    urinary meatus
    vesicourethral orifice
  Imperforate urinary meatus
  Impervious urethra
  Urethral valve formation

753.7 Anomalies of urachus
  Cyst
  Fistula } (of) urachussinus
  Patent
  Persistent umbilical sinus

753.8 Other specified anomalies of bladder and urethra
  Absence, congenital of: Congenital urethrorectal
    bladder   fistula
    urethra   Congenital prolapse of:
  Accessory: bladder (mucosa)
    bladder   urethra
    urethra   Double:
  Congenital: urethra
    diverticulum of bladder   urinary meatus
    hernia of bladder

753.9 Unspecified anomaly of urinary system
  Congenital:
    anomaly NOS } of urinary system [any part,
    deformity NOS } except urachus]

✓4ᵗʰ 754 Certain congenital musculoskeletal deformities
  INCLUDES nonteratogenic deformities which are considered to be due to intrauterine malposition and pressure

754.0 Of skull, face, and jaw
  Asymmetry of face   Dolichocephaly
  Compression facies   Plagiocephaly
  Depressions in skull   Potter's facies
  Deviation of nasal   Squashed or bent nose,
    septum, congenital   congenital
  EXCLUDES dentofacial anomalies (524.0-524.9)
            syphilitic saddle nose (090.5)

754.1 Of sternocleidomastoid muscle
  Congenital sternomastoid torticollis
  Congenital wryneck
  Contracture of sternocleidomastoid (muscle)
  Sternomastoid tumor

754.2 Of spine
  Congenital postural:
    lordosis
    scoliosis

✓5ᵗʰ 754.3 Congenital dislocation of hip

754.30 Congenital dislocation of hip, unilateral
  Congenital dislocation of hip NOS
754.31 Congenital dislocation of hip, bilateral
754.32 Congenital subluxation of hip, unilateral
  Congenital flexion deformity, hip or thigh
  Predislocation status of hip at birth
  Preluxation of hip, congenital
754.33 Congenital subluxation of hip, bilateral
754.35 Congenital dislocation of one hip with subluxation of other hip

✓5ᵗʰ 754.4 Congenital genu recurvatum and bowing of long bones of leg

754.40 Genu recurvatum
  DEF: Backward curving of knee joint.
754.41 Congenital dislocation of knee (with genu recurvatum)
  DEF: Elevated, outward rotation of heel; also called clubfoot.

N Newborn Age: 0   P Pediatric Age: 0-17   M Maternity Age: 12-55   A Adult Age: 15-124

CONGENITAL ANOMALIES

754.42 Congenital bowing of femur
754.43 Congenital bowing of tibia and fibula
754.44 Congenital bowing of unspecified long bones of leg

✓5th 754.5 Varus deformities of feet
  EXCLUDES acquired (736.71, 736.75, 736.79)
  754.50 Talipes varus
    Congenital varus deformity of foot, unspecified
    Pes varus
    DEF: Inverted foot marked by outer sole resting on ground.
  754.51 Talipes equinovarus
    Equinovarus (congenital)
  754.52 Metatarsus primus varus
    DEF: Malformed first metatarsal bone, with bone angled toward body.
  754.53 Metatarsus varus
  754.59 Other
    Talipes calcaneovarus

✓5th 754.6 Valgus deformities of feet
  EXCLUDES valgus deformity of foot (acquired) (736.79)
  754.60 Talipes valgus
    Congenital valgus deformity of foot, unspecified
  754.61 Congenital pes planus
    Congenital rocker bottom flat foot
    Flat foot, congenital
    EXCLUDES pes planus (acquired) (734)
  754.62 Talipes calcaneovalgus
  754.69 Other
    Talipes: equinovalgus   Talipes: planovalgus

✓5th 754.7 Other deformities of feet
  EXCLUDES acquired (736.70-736.79)
  754.70 Talipes, unspecified
    Congenital deformity of foot NOS
  754.71 Talipes cavus
    Cavus foot (congenital)
  754.79 Other
    Asymmetric talipes   Talipes:
    Talipes: equinus
    calcaneus

✓5th 754.8 Other specified nonteratogenic anomalies
  754.81 Pectus excavatum
    Congenital funnel chest
  754.82 Pectus carinatum
    Congenital pigeon chest [breast]
  754.89 Other
    Club hand (congenital)
    Congenital:
      deformity of chest wall
      dislocation of elbow
    Generalized flexion contractures of lower limb joints, congenital
    Spade-like hand (congenital)

✓4th 755 Other congenital anomalies of limbs
  EXCLUDES those deformities classifiable to 754.0-754.8

✓5th 755.0 Polydactyly
  755.00 Polydactyly, unspecified digits
    Supernumerary digits
  755.01 Of fingers
    Accessory fingers
  755.02 Of toes
    Accessory toes

✓5th 755.1 Syndactyly
  Symphalangy   Webbing of digits
  755.10 Of multiple and unspecified sites
  755.11 Of fingers without fusion of bone

  755.12 Of fingers with fusion of bone
  755.13 Of toes without fusion of bone
  755.14 Of toes with fusion of bone

✓5th 755.2 Reduction deformities of upper limb
  755.20 Unspecified reduction deformity of upper limb
    Ectromelia NOS } of upper limb
    Hemimelia NOS
    Shortening of arm, congenital
  755.21 Transverse deficiency of upper limb
    Amelia of upper limb
    Congenital absence of:
      fingers, all (complete or partial)
      forearm, including hand and fingers
      upper limb, complete
    Congenital amputation of upper limb
    Transverse hemimelia of upper limb
  755.22 Longitudinal deficiency of upper limb, not elsewhere classified
    Phocomelia NOS of upper limb
    Rudimentary arm
  755.23 Longitudinal deficiency, combined, involving humerus, radius, and ulna (complete or incomplete)
    Congenital absence of arm and forearm (complete or incomplete) with or without metacarpal deficiency and/or phalangeal deficiency, incomplete
    Phocomelia, complete, of upper limb
  755.24 Longitudinal deficiency, humeral, complete or partial (with or without distal deficiencies, incomplete)
    Congenital absence of humerus (with or without absence of some [but not all] distal elements)
    Proximal phocomelia of upper limb
  755.25 Longitudinal deficiency, radioulnar, complete or partial (with or without distal deficiencies, incomplete)
    Congenital absence of radius and ulna (with or without absence of some [but not all] distal elements)
    Distal phocomelia of upper limb
  755.26 Longitudinal deficiency, radial, complete or partial (with or without distal deficiencies, incomplete)
    Agenesis of radius
    Congenital absence of radius (with or without absence of some [but not all] distal elements)
  755.27 Longitudinal deficiency, ulnar, complete or partial (with or without distal deficiencies, incomplete)
    Agenesis of ulna
    Congenital absence of ulna (with or without absence of some [but not all] distal elements)
  755.28 Longitudinal deficiency, carpals or metacarpals, complete or partial (with or without incomplete phalangeal deficiency)
  755.29 Longitudinal deficiency, phalanges, complete or partial
    Absence of finger, congenital
    Aphalangia of upper limb, terminal, complete or partial
    EXCLUDES terminal deficiency of all five digits (755.21)
    transverse deficiency of phalanges (755.21)

CONGENITAL ANOMALIES — Tabular List

755.3 Reduction deformities of lower limb [5th]

755.30 Unspecified reduction deformity of lower limb
- Ectromelia NOS } of lower limb
- Hemimelia NOS
- Shortening of leg, congenital

755.31 Transverse deficiency of lower limb
- Amelia of lower limb
- Congenital absence of:
  - foot
  - leg, including foot and toes
  - lower limb, complete
  - toes, all, complete
- Transverse hemimelia of lower limb

755.32 Longitudinal deficiency of lower limb, not elsewhere classified
- Phocomelia NOS of lower limb

755.33 Longitudinal deficiency, combined, involving femur, tibia, and fibula (complete or incomplete)
- Congenital absence of thigh and (lower) leg (complete or incomplete) with or without metacarpal deficiency and/or phalangeal deficiency, incomplete
- Phocomelia, complete, of lower limb

755.34 Longitudinal deficiency, femoral, complete or partial (with or without distal deficiencies, incomplete)
- Congenital absence of femur (with or without absence of some [but not all] distal elements)
- Proximal phocomelia of lower limb

755.35 Longitudinal deficiency, tibiofibular, complete or partial (with or without distal deficiencies, incomplete)
- Congenital absence of tibia and fibula (with or without absence of some [but not all] distal elements)
- Distal phocomelia of lower limb

755.36 Longitudinal deficiency, tibia, complete or partial (with or without distal deficiencies, incomplete)
- Agenesis of tibia
- Congenital absence of tibia (with or without absence of some [but not all] distal elements)

755.37 Longitudinal deficiency, fibular, complete or partial (with or without distal deficiencies, incomplete)
- Agenesis of fibula
- Congenital absence of fibula (with or without absence of some [but not all] distal elements)

755.38 Longitudinal deficiency, tarsals or metatarsals, complete or partial (with or without incomplete phalangeal deficiency)

755.39 Longitudinal deficiency, phalanges, complete or partial
- Absence of toe, congenital
- Aphalangia of lower limb, terminal, complete or partial
- **EXCLUDES** *terminal deficiency of all five digits (755.31)*
  transverse deficiency of phalanges (755.31)

755.4 Reduction deformities, unspecified limb
- Absence, congenital (complete or partial) of limb NOS
- Amelia
- Ectromelia } of unspecified limb
- Hemimelia
- Phocomelia

755.5 Other anomalies of upper limb, including shoulder girdle [5th]

755.50 Unspecified anomaly of upper limb

755.51 Congenital deformity of clavicle

755.52 Congenital elevation of scapula
- Sprengel's deformity

755.53 Radioulnar synostosis

755.54 Madelung's deformity
- **DEF:** Distal ulnar overgrowth or radial shortening; also called carpus curvus.

755.55 Acrocephalosyndactyly
- Apert's syndrome
- **DEF:** Premature cranial suture fusion (craniostenosis); marked by cone-shaped or pointed (acrocephaly) head and webbing of the fingers (syndactyly); it is very similar to craniofacial dysostosis.

755.56 Accessory carpal bones

755.57 Macrodactylia (fingers)
- **DEF:** Abnormally large fingers, toes.

755.58 Cleft hand, congenital
- Lobster-claw hand
- **DEF:** Extended separation between fingers into metacarpus; also may refer to large fingers and absent middle fingers of hand.

755.59 Other
- Cleidocranial dysostosis
- Cubitus:
  - valgus, congenital
  - varus, congenital
- **EXCLUDES** *club hand (congenital) (754.89)*
  congenital dislocation of elbow (754.89)

755.6 Other anomalies of lower limb, including pelvic girdle [5th]

755.60 Unspecified anomaly of lower limb

755.61 Coxa valga, congenital
- **DEF:** Abnormally wide angle between the neck and shaft of the femur.

755.62 Coxa vara, congenital
- **DEF:** Diminished angle between neck and shaft of femur.

755.63 Other congenital deformity of hip (joint)
- Congenital anteversion of femur (neck)
- **EXCLUDES** *congenital dislocation of hip (754.30-754.35)*
- **AHA:** 1Q, '94, 15; S-O, '84, 15

755.64 Congenital deformity of knee (joint)
- Congenital:
  - absence of patella
  - genu valgum [knock-knee]
  - genu varum [bowleg]
- Rudimentary patella

755.65 Macrodactylia of toes
- **DEF:** Abnormally large toes.

755.66 Other anomalies of toes
- Congenital: hallux valgus, hallux varus
- Congenital: hammer toe

755.67 Anomalies of foot, not elsewhere classified
- Astragaloscaphoid synostosis
- Calcaneonavicular bar
- Coalition of calcaneus
- Talonavicular synostosis
- Tarsal coalitions

CONGENITAL ANOMALIES

755.69 Other
Congenital:
angulation of tibia
deformity (of):
ankle (joint)
sacroiliac (joint)
fusion of sacroiliac joint

755.8 Other specified anomalies of unspecified limb

755.9 Unspecified anomaly of unspecified limb
Congenital:
anomaly NOS } of unspecified limb
deformity NOS
EXCLUDES reduction deformity of unspecified limb (755.4)

756 Other congenital musculoskeletal anomalies
EXCLUDES those deformities classifiable to 754.0-754.8

756.0 Anomalies of skull and face bones
Absence of skull bones
Acrocephaly
Congenital deformity of forehead
Craniosynostosis
Crouzon's disease
Hypertelorism
Imperfect fusion of skull
Oxycephaly
Platybasia
Premature closure of cranial sutures
Tower skull
Trigonocephaly
EXCLUDES acrocephalosyndactyly [Apert's syndrome] (755.55)
dentofacial anomalies (524.0-524.9)
skull defects associated with brain anomalies, such as:
anencephalus (740.0)
encephalocele (742.0)
hydrocephalus (742.3)
microcephalus (742.1)
AHA: 3Q, '98, 9; 3Q, '96, 15

756.1 Anomalies of spine

756.10 Anomaly of spine, unspecified

756.11 Spondylolysis, lumbosacral region
Prespondylolisthesis (lumbosacral)
DEF: Bilateral or unilateral defect through the pars interarticularis of a vertebra causes spondylolisthesis.

756.12 Spondylolisthesis
DEF: Downward slipping of lumbar vertebra over next vertebra; usually related to pelvic deformity.

756.13 Absence of vertebra, congenital

756.14 Hemivertebra
DEF: Incomplete development of one side of a vertebra.

756.15 Fusion of spine [vertebra], congenital

756.16 Klippel-Feil syndrome
DEF: Short, wide neck; limits range of motion due to abnormal number of cervical vertebra or fused hemivertebrae.

756.17 Spina bifida occulta
EXCLUDES spina bifida (aperta) (741.0-741.9)
DEF: Spina bifida marked by a bony spinal canal defect without a protrusion of the cord or meninges; it is diagnosed by radiography and has no symptoms.

756.19 Other
Platyspondylia
Supernumerary vertebra

756.2 Cervical rib
Supernumerary rib in the cervical region
DEF: Costa cervicalis: extra rib attached to cervical vertebra.

756.3 Other anomalies of ribs and sternum
Congenital absence of:
rib
sternum
Congenital:
fissure of sternum
fusion of ribs
Sternum bifidum
EXCLUDES nonteratogenic deformity of chest wall (754.81-754.89)

756.4 Chondrodystrophy
Achondroplasia
Chondrodystrophia (fetalis)
Dyschondroplasia
Enchondromatosis
Ollier's disease
EXCLUDES lipochondrodystrophy [Hurler's syndrome] (277.5)
Morquio's disease (277.5)
AHA: 2Q, '02, 16; S-O, '87, 10
DEF: Abnormal development of cartilage.

756.5 Osteodystrophies

756.50 Osteodystrophy, unspecified

756.51 Osteogenesis imperfecta
Fragilitas ossium
Osteopsathyrosis
DEF: A collagen disorder commonly characterized by brittle, osteoporotic, easily fractured bones, hypermobility of joints, blue sclerae, and a tendency to hemorrhage.

756.52 Osteopetrosis
DEF: Abnormally dense bone, optic atrophy, hepatosplenomegaly, deafness; sclerosing depletes bone marrow and nerve foramina of skull; often fatal.

756.53 Osteopoikilosis
DEF: Multiple sclerotic foci on ends of long bones, stippling in round, flat bones; identified by x-ray.

756.54 Polyostotic fibrous dysplasia of bone
DEF: Fibrous tissue displaces bone results in segmented ragged-edge café-au-lait spots; occurs in girls of early puberty.

756.55 Chondroectodermal dysplasia
Ellis-van Creveld syndrome
DEF: Inadequate enchondral bone formation; impaired development of hair and teeth, polydactyly, and cardiac septum defects.

756.56 Multiple epiphyseal dysplasia

756.59 Other
Albright (-McCune)-Sternberg syndrome

756.6 Anomalies of diaphragm
Absence of diaphragm
Congenital hernia:
diaphragmatic
Congenital hernia:
foramen of Morgagni
Eventration of diaphragm
EXCLUDES congenital hiatus hernia (750.6)

756.7 Anomalies of abdominal wall

756.70 Anomaly of abdominal wall, unspecified

756.71 Prune belly syndrome
Eagle-Barrett syndrome
Prolapse of bladder mucosa
AHA: 4Q, '97, 44
DEF: Prune belly syndrome: absence of lower rectus abdominis muscle and lower and medial oblique muscles; results in dilated bladder and ureters, dysplastic kidneys and hydronephrosis; more common in male infants with undescended testicles.

CONGENITAL ANOMALIES

756.79 Other congenital anomalies of abdominal wall
Exomphalos   Omphalocele
Gastroschisis
EXCLUDES: umbilical hernia (551-553 with .1)

DEF: Exomphalos: umbilical hernia prominent navel.

DEF: Gastroschisis: fissure of abdominal wall, results in protruding small or large intestine.

DEF: Omphalocele: hernia of umbilicus due to impaired abdominal wall; results in membrane-covered intestine protruding through peritoneum and amnion.

756.8 Other specified anomalies of muscle, tendon, fascia, and connective tissue

756.81 Absence of muscle and tendon
Absence of muscle (pectoral)

756.82 Accessory muscle

756.83 Ehlers-Danlos syndrome
DEF: Danlos syndrome: connective tissue disorder causes hyperextended skin and joints; results in fragile blood vessels with bleeding, poor wound healing and subcutaneous pseudotumors.

756.89 Other
Amyotrophia congenita
Congenital shortening of tendon
AHA: 3Q, '99, 16

756.9 Other and unspecified anomalies of musculoskeletal system
Congenital:
  anomaly NOS   } of musculoskeletal system,
  deformity NOS } not elsewhere classified

757 Congenital anomalies of the integument
INCLUDES: anomalies of skin, subcutaneous tissue, hair, nails, and breast
EXCLUDES: hemangioma (228.00-228.09)
pigmented nevus (216.0-216.9)

757.0 Hereditary edema of legs
Congenital lymphedema   Milroy's disease
Hereditary trophedema

757.1 Ichthyosis congenita
Congenital ichthyosis
Harlequin fetus
Ichthyosiform erythroderma
DEF: Overproduction of skin cells causes scaling of skin; may result in stillborn fetus or death soon after birth.

757.2 Dermatoglyphic anomalies
Abnormal palmar creases
DEF: Abnormal skin-line patterns of fingers, palms, toes and soles; initial finding of possible chromosomal abnormalities.

757.3 Other specified anomalies of skin

757.31 Congenital ectodermal dysplasia
DEF: Tissues and structures originate in embryonic ectoderm; includes anhidrotic and hidrotic ectodermal dysplasia and EEC syndrome.

757.32 Vascular hamartomas
Birthmarks   Strawberry nevus
Port-wine stain
DEF: Benign tumor of blood vessels; due to malformed angioblastic tissues.

757.33 Congenital pigmentary anomalies of skin
Congenital poikiloderma
Urticaria pigmentosa
Xeroderma pigmentosum
EXCLUDES: albinism (270.2)

757.39 Other
Accessory skin tags, congenital
Congenital scar
Epidermolysis bullosa
Keratoderma (congenital)
EXCLUDES: pilonidal cyst (685.0-685.1)

757.4 Specified anomalies of hair
Congenital: Congenital:
  alopecia   hypertrichosis
  atrichosis   monilethrix
  beaded hair   Persistent lanugo

757.5 Specified anomalies of nails
Anonychia   Congenital:
Congenital: leukonychia
  clubnail   onychauxis
  koilonychia   pachyonychia

757.6 Specified anomalies of breast
Absent
Accessory   } breast or nipple
Supernumerary

Hypoplasia of breast
EXCLUDES: absence of pectoral muscle (756.81)

757.8 Other specified anomalies of the integument

757.9 Unspecified anomaly of the integument
Congenital:
  anomaly NOS   } of integument
  deformity NOS

758 Chromosomal anomalies
INCLUDES: syndromes associated with anomalies in the number and form of chromosomes
Use additional codes for conditions associated with the chromosomal anomalies

758.0 Down's syndrome
Mongolism   Trisomy:
Translocation Down's   21 or 22
  syndrome   G

758.1 Patau's syndrome
Trisomy: Trisomy:
  13   D_1
DEF: Trisomy of 13th chromosome; characteristic failure to thrive, severe mental impairment, seizures, abnormal eyes, low-set ears and sloped forehead.

758.2 Edwards' syndrome
Trisomy: Trisomy:
  18   E_3
DEF: Trisomy of 18th chromosome; characteristic mental and physical impairments; mainly affects females.

758.3 Autosomal deletion syndromes

758.31 Cri-du-chat syndrome
Deletion 5p
DEF: Hereditary congenital syndrome caused by a microdeletion of short arm of chromosome 5; characterized by catlike cry in newborn, microencephaly, severe mental deficiency, and hypertelorism.

758.32 Velo-cardio-facial syndrome
Deletion 22q11.2
DEF: Microdeletion syndrome affecting multiple organs; characteristic cleft palate, heart defects, elongated face with almond-shaped eyes, wide nose, small ears, weak immune systems, weak musculature, hypothyroidism, short stature, and scoliosis; deletion at q11.2 on the long arm of the chromosome 22.

758.33 Other microdeletions
Miller-Dieker syndrome
Smith-Magenis syndrome
DEF: Miller-Dieker syndrome: deletion from the short arm of chromosome 17; characteristic mental retardation, speech and motor development delays, neurological complications, and multiple abnormalities affecting the kidneys, heart, gastrointestinal tract, and other organ; death in infancy or early childhood.

DEF: Smith-Magenis syndrome: deletion in a certain area of chromosome 17 that results in craniofacial changes, speech delay, hoarse voice, hearing loss in many, and behavioral problems, such as self-destructive head banging, wrist biting, and tearing at nails.

N Newborn Age: 0   **P** Pediatric Age: 0-17   **M** Maternity Age: 12-55   **A** Adult Age: 15-124

Tabular List   **CONGENITAL ANOMALIES**

         758.39 Other autosomal deletions
- **758.4 Balanced autosomal translocation in normal individual**
- **758.5 Other conditions due to autosomal anomalies**
  - Accessory autosomes NEC
- **758.6 Gonadal dysgenesis**
  - Ovarian dysgenesis   XO syndrome
  - Turner's syndrome
  - **EXCLUDES**   pure gonadal dysgenesis (752.7)
  - **DEF:** Impaired embryonic development of seminiferous tubes; results in small testes, azoospermia, infertility and enlarged mammary glands.
- **758.7 Klinefelter's syndrome** ♂
  - XXY syndrome
- ✓5th **758.8 Other conditions due to chromosome anomalies**
  - **758.81 Other conditions due to sex chromosome anomalies**
  - **758.89 Other**
- **758.9 Conditions due to anomaly of unspecified chromosome**

✓4th **759 Other and unspecified congenital anomalies**
- **759.0 Anomalies of spleen**
  - Aberrant ⎫
  - Absent   ⎬ spleen
  - Accessory ⎭
  - Congenital splenomegaly
  - Ectopic spleen
  - Lobulation of spleen
- **759.1 Anomalies of adrenal gland**
  - Aberrant ⎫
  - Absent   ⎬ adrenal gland
  - Accessory ⎭
  - **EXCLUDES**   adrenogenital disorders (255.2)
  -                  congenital disorders of steroid metabolism (255.2)
- **759.2 Anomalies of other endocrine glands**
  - Absent parathyroid gland
  - Accessory thyroid gland
  - Persistent thyroglossal or thyrolingual duct
  - Thyroglossal (duct) cyst
  - **EXCLUDES**   congenital:
  -                  goiter (246.1)
  -                  hypothyroidism (243)
- **759.3 Situs inversus**
  - Situs inversus or transversus:
    - abdominalis
    - thoracis
  - Transposition of viscera:
    - abdominal
    - thoracic
  - **EXCLUDES**   dextrocardia without mention of complete transposition (746.87)
  - **DEF:** Laterally transposed thoracic and abdominal viscera.
- **759.4 Conjoined twins**
  - Craniopagus   Thoracopagus
  - Dicephalus   Xiphopagus
  - Pygopagus
- **759.5 Tuberous sclerosis**
  - Bourneville's disease   Epiloia
  - **DEF:** Hamartomas of brain, retina and viscera, impaired mental ability, seizures and adenoma sebaceum.
- **759.6 Other hamartoses, not elsewhere classified**
  - Syndrome: Syndrome:
  -    Peutz-Jeghers   von Hippel-Lindau
  -    Sturge-Weber (-Dimitri)
  - **EXCLUDES**   neurofibromatosis (237.7)
  - **AHA:** 3Q, '92, 12
  - **DEF:** Peutz-Jeghers: hereditary syndrome characterized by hamartomas of small intestine.
  - **DEF:** Sturge-Weber: congenital syndrome characterized by unilateral port-wine stain over trigeminal nerve, underlying meninges and cerebral cortex.
  - **DEF:** von Hipple-Lindau: hereditary syndrome of congenital angiomatosis of the retina and cerebellum.
- **759.7 Multiple congenital anomalies, so described**
  - Congenital:
    - anomaly, multiple NOS
    - deformity, multiple NOS
- ✓5th **759.8 Other specified anomalies**
  - **AHA:** S-O, '87, 9; S-O, '85, 11
  - **759.81 Prader-Willi syndrome**
  - **759.82 Marfan syndrome**
    - **AHA:** 3Q, '93, 11
  - **759.83 Fragile X syndrome**
    - **AHA:** 4Q, '94, 41
  - **759.89 Other**
    - Congenital malformation syndromes affecting multiple systems, not elsewhere classified
    - Laurence-Moon-Biedl syndrome
    - **AHA:** ▶2Q, '05, 17;◀ 2Q, '04, 12; 1Q, '01, 3; 3Q, '99, 17, 18; 3Q, '98, 8
- **759.9 Congenital anomaly, unspecified**

Tabular List — CONDITIONS IN THE PERINATAL PERIOD — 760–761.7

15. CERTAIN CONDITIONS ORIGINATING IN THE PERINATAL PERIOD (760-779)

INCLUDES conditions which have their origin in the perinatal period, before birth through the first 28 days after birth, even though death or morbidity occurs later

Use additional code(s) to further specify condition

MATERNAL CAUSES OF PERINATAL MORBIDITY AND MORTALITY (760-763)

AHA: 2Q, '89, 14; 3Q, '90, 5

√4th 760 Fetus or newborn affected by maternal conditions which may be unrelated to present pregnancy

INCLUDES the listed maternal conditions only when specified as a cause of mortality or morbidity of the fetus or newborn

EXCLUDES maternal endocrine and metabolic disorders affecting fetus or newborn (775.0-775.9)

AHA: 1Q, '94, 8; 2Q, '92, 12; N-D, '84, 11

- **760.0 Maternal hypertensive disorders**
  Fetus or newborn affected by maternal conditions classifiable to 642

- **760.1 Maternal renal and urinary tract diseases**
  Fetus or newborn affected by maternal conditions classifiable to 580-599

- **760.2 Maternal infections**
  Fetus or newborn affected by maternal infectious disease classifiable to 001-136 and 487, but fetus or newborn not manifesting that disease
  EXCLUDES congenital infectious diseases (771.0-771.8)
  maternal genital tract and other localized infections (760.8)

- **760.3 Other chronic maternal circulatory and respiratory diseases**
  Fetus or newborn affected by chronic maternal conditions classifiable to 390-459, 490-519, 745-748

- **760.4 Maternal nutritional disorders**
  Fetus or newborn affected by:
  maternal disorders classifiable to 260-269
  maternal malnutrition NOS
  EXCLUDES fetal malnutrition (764.10-764.29)

- **760.5 Maternal injury**
  Fetus or newborn affected by maternal conditions classifiable to 800-995

- **760.6 Surgical operation on mother**
  EXCLUDES cesarean section for present delivery (763.4)
  damage to placenta from amniocentesis, cesarean section, or surgical induction (762.1)
  previous surgery to uterus or pelvic organs (763.89)

- **√5th 760.7 Noxious influences affecting fetus or newborn via placenta or breast milk**
  Fetus or newborn affected by noxious substance transmitted via placenta or breast milk
  EXCLUDES anesthetic and analgesic drugs administered during labor and delivery (763.5)
  drug withdrawal syndrome in newborn (779.5)

  AHA: 3Q, '91, 21

  - **760.70 Unspecified noxious substance**
    Fetus or newborn affected by:
    Drug NEC
  - **760.71 Alcohol**
    Fetal alcohol syndrome
  - **760.72 Narcotics**
  - **760.73 Hallucinogenic agents**
  - **760.74 Anti-infectives**
    Antibiotics
    Antifungals
  - **760.75 Cocaine**
    AHA: 3Q, '94, 6; 2Q, '92, 12; 4Q, '91, 26
  - **760.76 Diethylstilbestrol [DES]**
    AHA: 4Q, '94, 45
  - **760.77 Anticonvulsants** N
    Carbamazepine
    Phenobarbital
    Phenytoin
    Valproic acid
    AHA: ▶4Q, '05, 82◀
  - **760.78 Antimetabolic agents** N
    Methotrexate
    Retinoic acid
    Statins
    AHA: ▶4Q, '05, 82-83◀
  - **760.79 Other**
    Fetus or newborn affected by:
    immune sera ⎫
    medicinal agents ⎬ transmitted via placenta
    NEC ⎬ or breast milk
    toxic substance NEC ⎭

- **760.8 Other specified maternal conditions affecting fetus or newborn**
  Maternal genital tract and other localized infection affecting fetus or newborn, but fetus or newborn not manifesting that disease
  EXCLUDES maternal urinary tract infection affecting fetus or newborn (760.1)

- **760.9 Unspecified maternal condition affecting fetus or newborn**

√4th 761 Fetus or newborn affected by maternal complications of pregnancy

INCLUDES the listed maternal conditions only when specified as a cause of mortality or morbidity of the fetus or newborn

- **761.0 Incompetent cervix**
  DEF: Inadequate functioning of uterine cervix.

- **761.1 Premature rupture of membranes**

- **761.2 Oligohydramnios**
  EXCLUDES that due to premature rupture of membranes (761.1)
  DEF: Deficient amniotic fluid.

- **761.3 Polyhydramnios**
  Hydramnios (acute) (chronic)
  DEF: Excess amniotic fluid.

- **761.4 Ectopic pregnancy**
  Pregnancy:
  abdominal
  intraperitoneal
  tubal

- **761.5 Multiple pregnancy**
  Triplet (pregnancy)
  Twin (pregnancy)

- **761.6 Maternal death**

- **761.7 Malpresentation before labor**
  Breech presentation ⎫
  External version ⎬
  Oblique lie ⎬ before labor
  Transverse lie ⎬
  Unstable lie ⎭

761.8 Other specified maternal complications of pregnancy affecting fetus or newborn
    Spontaneous abortion, fetus

761.9 Unspecified maternal complication of pregnancy affecting fetus or newborn

✓4th 762 Fetus or newborn affected by complications of placenta, cord, and membranes
    INCLUDES the listed maternal conditions only when specified as a cause of mortality or morbidity in the fetus or newborn
    AHA: 1Q, '94, 8

762.0 Placenta previa N
    DEF: Placenta developed in lower segment of uterus; causes hemorrhaging in last trimester.

762.1 Other forms of placental separation and hemorrhage N
    Abruptio placentae
    Antepartum hemorrhage
    Damage to placenta from amniocentesis, cesarean section, or surgical induction
    Maternal blood loss
    Premature separation of placenta
    Rupture of marginal sinus

762.2 Other and unspecified morphological and functional abnormalities of placenta N
    Placental:
        dysfunction
        infarction
        insufficiency

762.3 Placental transfusion syndromes N
    Placental and cord abnormality resulting in twin-to-twin or other transplacental transfusion
    Use additional code to indicate resultant condition in fetus or newborn:
        fetal blood loss (772.0)
        polycythemia neonatorum (776.4)

762.4 Prolapsed cord N
    Cord presentation

762.5 Other compression of umbilical cord N
    Cord around neck
    Entanglement of cord
    Knot in cord
    Torsion of cord
    AHA: 2Q, '03, 9

762.6 Other and unspecified conditions of umbilical cord N
    Short cord
    Thrombosis
    Varices   } of umbilical cord
    Velamentous insertion
    Vasa previa
    EXCLUDES infection of umbilical cord (771.4)
              single umbilical artery (747.5)

762.7 Chorioamnionitis N
    Amnionitis
    Membranitis
    Placentitis
    DEF: Inflamed fetal membrane.

762.8 Other specified abnormalities of chorion and amnion N

762.9 Unspecified abnormality of chorion and amnion N

✓4th 763 Fetus or newborn affected by other complications of labor and delivery
    INCLUDES the listed conditions only when specified as a cause of mortality or morbidity in the fetus or newborn
    AHA: 1Q, '94, 8

763.0 Breech delivery and extraction N

763.1 Other malpresentation, malposition, and disproportion during labor and delivery N
    Fetus or newborn affected by:
        abnormality of bony pelvis
        contracted pelvis
        persistent occipitoposterior position
        shoulder presentation
        transverse lie
        conditions classifiable to 652, 653, and 660

763.2 Forceps delivery N
    Fetus or newborn affected by forceps extraction

763.3 Delivery by vacuum extractor N

763.4 Cesarean delivery N
    EXCLUDES placental separation or hemorrhage from cesarean section (762.1)

763.5 Maternal anesthesia and analgesia N
    Reactions and intoxications from maternal opiates and tranquilizers during labor and delivery
    EXCLUDES drug withdrawal syndrome in newborn (779.5)

763.6 Precipitate delivery N
    Rapid second stage

763.7 Abnormal uterine contractions N
    Fetus or newborn affected by:
        contraction ring
        hypertonic labor
        hypotonic uterine dysfunction
        uterine inertia or dysfunction
        conditions classifiable to 661, except 661.3

✓5th 763.8 Other specified complications of labor and delivery affecting fetus or newborn
    AHA: 4Q, '98, 46

763.81 Abnormality in fetal heart rate or rhythm before the onset of labor N

763.82 Abnormality in fetal heart rate or rhythm during labor N
    AHA: 4Q, '98, 46

763.83 Abnormality in fetal heart rate or rhythm, unspecified as to time of onset N

763.84 Meconium passage during delivery N
    EXCLUDES meconium aspiration (770.11, 770.12)
              meconium staining (779.84)
    AHA: ▶4Q, '05, 83◀
    DEF: ▶Fetal intestinal activity that increases in response to a distressed state during delivery; anal sphincter relaxes, and meconium is passed into the amniotic fluid.◀

763.89 Other specified complications of labor and delivery affecting fetus or newborn N
    Fetus or newborn affected by:
        abnormality of maternal soft tissues
        destructive operation on live fetus to facilitate delivery
        induction of labor (medical)
        previous surgery to uterus or pelvic organs
        other conditions classifiable to 650-669
        other procedures used in labor and delivery

Tabular List — **CONDITIONS IN THE PERINATAL PERIOD** — 763.9–767.19

763.9 Unspecified complication of labor and delivery affecting fetus or newborn N

OTHER CONDITIONS ORIGINATING IN THE PERINATAL PERIOD (764-779)

The following fifth-digit subclassification is for use with category 764 and codes 765.0 and 765.1 to denote birthweight:

- 0 unspecified [weight]
- 1 less than 500 grams
- 2 500-749 grams
- 3 750-999 grams
- 4 1,000-1,249 grams
- 5 1,250-1,499 grams
- 6 1,500-1,749 grams
- 7 1,750-1,999 grams
- 8 2,000-2,499 grams
- 9 2,500 grams and over

√4th **764 Slow fetal growth and fetal malnutrition**
AHA: 3Q, '04, 4; 4Q, '02, 63; 1Q,'94, 8; 2Q, '91, 19; 2Q, '89, 15

√5th **764.0 "Light-for-dates" without mention of fetal malnutrition** N
Infants underweight for gestational age
"Small-for-dates"

√5th **764.1 "Light-for-dates" with signs of fetal malnutrition** N
Infants "light-for-dates" classifiable to 764.0, who in addition show signs of fetal malnutrition, such as dry peeling skin and loss of subcutaneous tissue

√5th **764.2 Fetal malnutrition without mention of "light-for-dates"** N
Infants, not underweight for gestational age, showing signs of fetal malnutrition, such as dry peeling skin and loss of subcutaneous tissue
Intrauterine malnutrition

√5th **764.9 Fetal growth retardation, unspecified** N
Intrauterine growth retardation
AHA: For code 764.97: 1Q, '97, 6

√4th **765 Disorders relating to short gestation and low birthweight**
INCLUDES the listed conditions, without further specification, as causes of mortality, morbidity, or additional care, in fetus or newborn
AHA: 1Q, '97, 6; 1Q, '94, 8; 2Q, '91, 19; 2Q, '89, 15

√5th **765.0 Extreme immaturity** N
Note: Usually implies a birthweight of less than 1000 grams.
Use additional code for weeks of gestation (765.20-765.29)
AHA: 3Q, '04, 4; 4Q, '02, 63; For code 765.03: 4Q, '01, 51

√5th **765.1 Other preterm infants** N
Note: Usually implies a birthweight of 1000-2499 grams.
Prematurity NOS
Prematurity or small size, not classifiable to 765.0 or as "light-for-dates" in 764
Use additional code for weeks of gestation (765.20-765.29)
AHA: 3Q, '04, 4; 4Q, '02, 63; For code 765.10: 1Q, '94, 14; For code 765.17: 1Q, '97, 6; For code 765.18: 4Q, '02, 64

√5th **765.2 Weeks of gestation**
AHA: 3Q, '04, 4; 4Q, '02, 63

765.20 Unspecified weeks of gestation N
765.21 Less than 24 completed weeks of gestation N
765.22 24 completed weeks of gestation N
765.23 25-26 completed weeks of gestation N
765.24 27-28 completed weeks of gestation N
765.25 29-30 completed weeks of gestation N
765.26 31-32 completed weeks of gestation N
765.27 33-34 completed weeks of gestation N
765.28 35-36 completed weeks of gestation N
AHA: 4Q, '02, 64
765.29 37 or more completed weeks of gestation N

√4th **766 Disorders relating to long gestation and high birthweight**
INCLUDES the listed conditions, without further specification, as causes of mortality, morbidity, or additional care, in fetus or newborn

766.0 Exceptionally large baby N
Note: Usually implies a birthweight of 4500 grams or more.

766.1 Other "heavy-for-dates" infants N
Other fetus or infant "heavy-" or "large-for-dates" regardless of period of gestation

√5th **766.2 Late infant, not "heavy-for-dates"**
AHA: 4Q, '03, 69

766.21 Post-term infant N
Infant with gestation period over 40 completed weeks to 42 completed weeks
766.22 Prolonged gestation of infant N
Infant with gestation period over 42 completed weeks
Postmaturity NOS

√4th **767 Birth trauma**

767.0 Subdural and cerebral hemorrhage N
Subdural and cerebral hemorrhage, whether described as due to birth trauma or to intrapartum anoxia or hypoxia
Subdural hematoma (localized)
Tentorial tear
Use additional code to identify cause
EXCLUDES intraventricular hemorrhage (772.10-772.14)
subarachnoid hemorrhage (772.2)

√5th **767.1 Injuries to scalp**
AHA: 4Q, '03, 69

767.11 Epicranial subaponeurotic hemorrhage (massive) N
Subgaleal hemorrhage
DEF: A hemorrhage that occurs within the space between the galea aponeurotica, or epicranial aponeurosis, which is a thin tendinous structure that is attached to the skull laterally and provides an insertion site for the occipitalis posteriorly and the frontalis muscle anteriorly, and the periosteum of the skull.

767.19 Other injuries to scalp
Caput succedaneum
Cephalhematoma
Chignon (from vacuum extraction)

CONDITIONS IN THE PERINATAL PERIOD

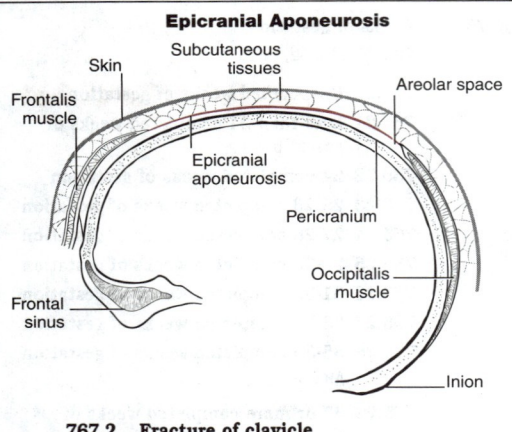

767.2 Fracture of clavicle

767.3 Other injuries to skeleton
Fracture of: long bones
Fracture of: skull
EXCLUDES congenital dislocation of hip (754.30-754.35)
fracture of spine, congenital (767.4)

767.4 Injury to spine and spinal cord
Dislocation
Fracture
Laceration
Rupture
} of spine or spinal cord due to birth trauma

767.5 Facial nerve injury
Facial palsy

767.6 Injury to brachial plexus
Palsy or paralysis:
brachial
Erb (-Duchenne)
Klumpke (-Déjérine)

767.7 Other cranial and peripheral nerve injuries
Phrenic nerve paralysis

767.8 Other specified birth trauma
Eye damage
Hematoma of:
liver (subcapsular)
testes
vulva
Rupture of:
liver
spleen
Scalpel wound
Traumatic glaucoma
EXCLUDES hemorrhage classifiable to 772.0-772.9

767.9 Birth trauma, unspecified
Birth injury NOS

768 Intrauterine hypoxia and birth asphyxia
Use only when associated with newborn morbidity classifiable elsewhere
EXCLUDES ▶acidemia NOS of newborn (775.81)
acidosis NOS of newborn (775.81)
cerebral ischemia NOS (779.2)
hypoxia NOS of newborn (770.88)
mixed metabolic and respiratory acidosis of newborn (775.81)
respiratory arrest of newborn (770.87)◀
AHA: 4Q, '92, 20
DEF: Oxygen intake insufficiency due to interrupted placental circulation or premature separation of placenta.

768.0 Fetal death from asphyxia or anoxia before onset of labor or at unspecified time

768.1 Fetal death from asphyxia or anoxia during labor

768.2 Fetal distress before onset of labor, in liveborn infant
Fetal metabolic acidemia before onset of labor, in liveborn infant

768.3 Fetal distress first noted during labor and delivery, in liveborn infant
Fetal metabolic acidemia first noted during labor ▶and delivery,◀ in liveborn infant

768.4 Fetal distress, unspecified as to time of onset, in liveborn infant
Fetal metabolic acidemia unspecified as to time of onset, in liveborn infant
AHA: N-D, '86, 10

768.5 Severe birth asphyxia
Birth asphyxia with neurologic involvement
EXCLUDES ▶hypoxic-ischemic encephalopathy [HIE] (768.7)◀
AHA: N-D, '86, 3

768.6 Mild or moderate birth asphyxia
Other specified birth asphyxia (without mention of neurologic involvement)
EXCLUDES ▶hypoxic-ischemic encephalopathy [HIE] (768.7)◀
AHA: N-D, '86, 3

768.7 Hypoxic-ischemic encephalopathy [HIE]

768.9 Unspecified birth asphyxia in liveborn infant
Anoxia
Asphyxia
} NOS, in liveborn infant

769 Respiratory distress syndrome
Cardiorespiratory distress syndrome of newborn
Hyaline membrane disease (pulmonary)
Idiopathic respiratory distress syndrome [IRDS or RDS] of newborn
Pulmonary hypoperfusion syndrome
EXCLUDES transient tachypnea of newborn (770.6)
AHA: 1Q, '89, 10; N-D, '86, 6
DEF: Severe chest contractions upon air intake and expiratory grunting; infant appears blue due to oxygen deficiency and has rapid respiratory rate; formerly called hyaline membrane disease.

770 Other respiratory conditions of fetus and newborn

770.0 Congenital pneumonia
Infective pneumonia acquired prenatally
EXCLUDES pneumonia from infection acquired after birth (480.0-486)
AHA: 1Q, '05, 10

770.1 Fetal and newborn aspiration
EXCLUDES aspiration of postnatal stomach contents (770.85, 770.86)
meconium passage during delivery (763.84)
meconium staining (779.84)
AHA: 4Q, '05, 83

770.10 Fetal and newborn aspiration, unspecified

770.11 Meconium aspiration without respiratory symptoms
Meconium aspiration NOS

CONDITIONS IN THE PERINATAL PERIOD

770.12 Meccanium aspiration with respiratory symptoms [N]
- Meconium aspiration pneumonia
- Meconium aspiration pneumonitis
- Meconium aspiration syndrome NOS
- Use additional code to identify any secondary pulmonary hypertension (416.8), if applicable

DEF: Meconium aspiration syndrome: aspiration of fetal intestinal material during or prior to delivery, usually a complication of placental insufficiency, causing pneumonitis and bronchial obstruction (inflammatory reaction of lungs).

770.13 Aspiration of clear amniotic fluid without respiratory symptoms [N]
- Aspiration of clear amniotic fluid NOS

770.14 Aspiration of clear amniotic fluid with respiratory symptoms [N]
- Aspiration of clear amniotic fluid with pneumonia
- Aspiration of clear amniotic fluid with pneumonitis
- Use additional code to identify any secondary pulmonary hypertension (416.8), if applicable

770.15 Aspiration of blood without respiratory symptoms [N]
- Aspiration of blood NOS

770.16 Aspiration of blood with respiratory symptoms [N]
- Aspiration of blood with pneumonia
- Aspiration of blood with pneumonitis
- Use additional code to identify any secondary pulmonary hypertension (416.8), if applicable

770.17 Other fetal and newborn aspiration without respiratory symptoms [N]

770.18 Other fetal and newborn aspiration with respiratory symptoms [N]
- Other aspiration pneumonia
- Other aspiration pneumonitis
- Use additional code to identify any secondary pulmonary hypertension (416.8), if applicable

770.2 Interstitial emphysema and related conditions [N]
- Pneumomediastinum
- Pneumopericardium
- Pneumothorax
} originating in the perinatal period

770.3 Pulmonary hemorrhage [N]
- Hemorrhage:
  - alveolar (lung)
  - intra-alveolar (lung)
  - massive pulmonary
} originating in the perinatal period

770.4 Primary atelectasis [N]
- Pulmonary immaturity NOS

DEF: Alveoli fail to expand causing insufficient air intake by newborn.

770.5 Other and unspecified atelectasis [N]
- Atelectasis:
  - NOS
  - partial
  - secondary
  - Pulmonary collapse
} originating in the perinatal period

770.6 Transitory tachypnea of newborn [N]
- Idiopathic tachypnea of newborn
- Wet lung syndrome
- EXCLUDES respiratory distress syndrome (769)

AHA: 4Q, '95, 4; 1Q, '94, 12; 3Q, '93, 7; 1Q, '89, 10; N-D, '86, 6

DEF: Quick, shallow breathing of newborn; short-term problem.

770.7 Chronic respiratory disease arising in the perinatal period
- Bronchopulmonary dysplasia
- Interstitial pulmonary fibrosis of prematurity
- Wilson-Mikity syndrome

AHA: 2Q, '91, 19; N-D, '86, 11

√5th 770.8 Other respiratory problems after birth
- EXCLUDES ▶mixed metabolic and respiratory acidosis of newborn (775.81)◀

AHA: 4Q, '02, 65; 2Q, '98, 10; 2Q, '96, 10

770.81 Primary apnea of newborn
- Apneic spells of newborn NOS
- Essential apnea of newborn
- Sleep apnea of newborn

DEF: Cessation of breathing when a neonate makes no respiratory effort for 15 seconds, resulting in cyanosis and bradycardia.

770.82 Other apnea of newborn [N]
- Obstructive apnea of newborn

770.83 Cyanotic attacks of newborn [N]

770.84 Respiratory failure of newborn [N]
- EXCLUDES respiratory distress syndrome (769)

770.85 Aspiration of postnatal stomach contents without respiratory symptoms [N]
- Aspiration of postnatal stomach contents NOS

AHA: 4Q, '05, 83

770.86 Aspiration of postnatal stomach contents with respiratory symptoms [N]
- Aspiration of postnatal stomach contents with pneumonia
- Aspiration of postnatal stomach contents with pneumonitis
- Use additional code to identify any secondary pulmonary hypertension (416.8), if applicable

AHA: 4Q, '05, 83

● **770.87 Respiratory arrest of newborn** [N]
● **770.88 Hypoxemia of newborn** [N]
- Hypoxia NOS of newborn

770.89 Other respiratory problems after birth [N]

770.9 Unspecified respiratory condition of fetus and newborn [N]

√4th 771 Infections specific to the perinatal period
- INCLUDES infections acquired before or during birth or via the umbilicus or during the first 28 days after birth
- EXCLUDES congenital pneumonia (770.0)
  - congenital syphilis (090.0-090.9)
  - maternal infectious disease as a cause of mortality or morbidity in fetus or newborn, but fetus or newborn not manifesting the disease (760.2)
  - ophthalmia neonatorum due to gonococcus (098.40)
  - other infections not specifically classified to this category

AHA: N-D, '85, 4

771.0 Congenital rubella [N]
- Congenital rubella pneumonitis

771.1 Congenital cytomegalovirus infection [N]
- Congenital cytomegalic inclusion disease

771.2 Other congenital infections
Congenital:
  herpes simplex
  listeriosis
  malaria
  toxoplasmosis
  tuberculosis

771.3 Tetanus neonatorum
Tetanus omphalitis
EXCLUDES hypocalcemic tetany (775.4)
DEF: Severe infection of central nervous system; due to exotoxin of tetanus bacillus from navel infection prompted by nonsterile technique during umbilical ligation.

771.4 Omphalitis of the newborn
Infection:
  navel cord
  umbilical stump
EXCLUDES tetanus omphalitis (771.3)
DEF: Inflamed umbilicus.

771.5 Neonatal infective mastitis
EXCLUDES noninfective neonatal mastitis (778.7)

771.6 Neonatal conjunctivitis and dacryocystitis
Ophthalmia neonatorum NOS
EXCLUDES ophthalmia neonatorum due to gonococcus (098.40)

771.7 Neonatal Candida infection
Neonatal moniliasis
Thrush in newborn

√5th **771.8 Other infection specific to the perinatal period**
Use additional code to identify organism (041.00-041.9)
AHA: 4Q, '02, 66

  771.81 Septicemia [sepsis] of newborn
  771.82 Urinary tract infection of newborn
  771.83 Bacteremia of newborn
  771.89 Other infections specific to the perinatal period
    Intra-amniotic infection of fetus NOS
    Infection of newborn NOS

√4th **772 Fetal and neonatal hemorrhage**
EXCLUDES hematological disorders of fetus and newborn (776.0-776.9)

  772.0 Fetal blood loss
  Fetal blood loss from:
    cut end of co-twin's cord
    placenta
    ruptured cord
    vasa previa
  Fetal exsanguination
  Fetal hemorrhage into:
    co-twin
    mother's circulation

√5th **772.1 Intraventricular hemorrhage**
  Intraventricular hemorrhage from any perinatal cause
  AHA: 4Q, '01, 49; 3Q, '92, 8; 4Q, '88, 8

  772.10 Unspecified grade
  772.11 Grade I
    Bleeding into germinal matrix
  772.12 Grade II
    Bleeding into ventricle
  772.13 Grade III
    Bleeding with enlargement of ventricle
    AHA: 4Q, '01, 51
  772.14 Grade IV
    Bleeding into cerebral cortex

772.2 Subarachnoid hemorrhage
Subarachnoid hemorrhage from any perinatal cause
EXCLUDES subdural and cerebral hemorrhage (767.0)

772.3 Umbilical hemorrhage after birth
Slipped umbilical ligature

772.4 Gastrointestinal hemorrhage
EXCLUDES swallowed maternal blood (777.3)

772.5 Adrenal hemorrhage

772.6 Cutaneous hemorrhage
Bruising
Ecchymoses
Petechiae   } in fetus or newborn
Superficial hematoma

772.8 Other specified hemorrhage of fetus or newborn
EXCLUDES hemorrhagic disease of newborn (776.0)
  pulmonary hemorrhage (770.3)

772.9 Unspecified hemorrhage of newborn

√4th **773 Hemolytic disease of fetus or newborn, due to isoimmunization**
DEF: Hemolytic anemia of fetus or newborn due to maternal antibody formation against fetal erythrocytes; infant blood contains nonmaternal antigen.

  773.0 Hemolytic disease due to Rh isoimmunization
  Anemia
  Erythroblastosis
    (fetalis)
  Hemolytic disease   } due to RH:
    (fetus) (newborn)   antibodies
  Jaundice   isoimmunization
                               maternal/fetal
                               incompatibility
  Rh hemolytic disease
  Rh isoimmunization

  773.1 Hemolytic disease due to ABO isoimmunization
  ABO hemolytic disease
  ABO isoimmunization
  Anemia
  Erythroblastosis
    (fetalis)   } due to ABO:
  Hemolytic disease   antibodies
    (fetus) (newborn)   isoimmunization
  Jaundice   maternal/fetal
                                 incompatibility
  AHA: 3Q, '92, 8
  DEF: Incompatible Rh fetal-maternal blood grouping; prematurely destroys red blood cells; detected by Coombs test.

  773.2 Hemolytic disease due to other and unspecified isoimmunization
  Erythroblastosis (fetalis) (neonatorum) NOS
  Hemolytic disease (fetus) (newborn) NOS
  Jaundice or anemia due to other and unspecified blood-group incompatibility
  AHA: 1Q, '94, 13

  773.3 Hydrops fetalis due to isoimmunization
  Use additional code to identify type of isoimmunization (773.0-773.2)
  DEF: Massive edema of entire body and severe anemia; may result in fetal death or stillbirth.

  773.4 Kernicterus due to isoimmunization
  Use additional code to identify type of isoimmunization (773.0-773.2)
  DEF: Complication of erythroblastosis fetalis associated with severe neural symptoms, high blood bilirubin levels and nerve cell destruction; results in bilirubin-pigmented gray matter of central nervous system.

  773.5 Late anemia due to isoimmunization

Tabular List — **CONDITIONS IN THE PERINATAL PERIOD** — 774–776.2

√4th **774 Other perinatal jaundice**

- **774.0 Perinatal jaundice from hereditary hemolytic anemias** N
  - *Code first underlying disease (282.0-282.9)*
- **774.1 Perinatal jaundice from other excessive hemolysis** N
  - Fetal or neonatal jaundice from:
    - bruising
    - drugs or toxins transmitted from mother
    - infection
    - polycythemia
    - swallowed maternal blood
  - Use additional code to identify cause
  - EXCLUDES jaundice due to isoimmunization (773.0-773.2)
- **774.2 Neonatal jaundice associated with preterm delivery** N
  - Hyperbilirubinemia of prematurity
  - Jaundice due to delayed conjugation associated with preterm delivery
  - AHA: 3Q, '91, 21
- √5th **774.3 Neonatal jaundice due to delayed conjugation from other causes**
  - **774.30 Neonatal jaundice due to delayed conjugation, cause unspecified** N
    - DEF: Jaundice of newborn with abnormal bilirubin metabolism; causes excess accumulated unconjugated bilirubin in blood.
  - **774.31 Neonatal jaundice due to delayed conjugation in diseases classified elsewhere** N
    - *Code first underlying diseases as:*
      - *congenital hypothyroidism (243)*
      - *Crigler-Najjar syndrome (277.4)*
      - *Gilbert's syndrome (277.4)*
  - **774.39 Other** N
    - Jaundice due to delayed conjugation from causes, such as:
      - breast milk inhibitors
      - delayed development of conjugating system
- **774.4 Perinatal jaundice due to hepatocellular damage** N
  - Fetal or neonatal hepatitis
  - Giant cell hepatitis
  - Inspissated bile syndrome
- **774.5 Perinatal jaundice from other causes** N
  - *Code first underlying cause as:*
    - *congenital obstruction of bile duct (751.61)*
    - *galactosemia (271.1)*
    - *Mucoviscidosis (277.00-277.09)*
- **774.6 Unspecified fetal and neonatal jaundice** N
  - Icterus neonatorum
  - Neonatal hyperbilirubinemia (transient)
  - Physiologic jaundice NOS in newborn
  - EXCLUDES that in preterm infants (774.2)
  - AHA: 1Q, '94, 13; 2Q, '89, 15
- **774.7 Kernicterus not due to isoimmunization** N
  - Bilirubin encephalopathy
  - Kernicterus of newborn NOS
  - EXCLUDES kernicterus due to isoimmunization (773.4)

√4th **775 Endocrine and metabolic disturbances specific to the fetus and newborn**

INCLUDES transitory endocrine and metabolic disturbances caused by the infant's response to maternal endocrine and metabolic factors, its removal from them, or its adjustment to extrauterine existence

- **775.0 Syndrome of "infant of a diabetic mother"** N
  - Maternal diabetes mellitus affecting fetus or newborn (with hypoglycemia)
  - AHA: 1Q, '04, 7-8; 3Q, '91, 5
- **775.1 Neonatal diabetes mellitus** N
  - Diabetes mellitus syndrome in newborn infant
  - AHA: 3Q, '91, 6
- **775.2 Neonatal myasthenia gravis** N
- **775.3 Neonatal thyrotoxicosis** N
  - Neonatal hyperthyroidism (transient)
- **775.4 Hypocalcemia and hypomagnesemia of newborn** N
  - Cow's milk hypocalcemia
  - Hypocalcemic tetany, neonatal
  - Neonatal hypoparathyroidism
  - Phosphate-loading hypocalcemia
- **775.5 Other transitory neonatal electrolyte disturbances** N
  - Dehydration, neonatal
  - AHA: 1Q, '05, 9
- **775.6 Neonatal hypoglycemia** N
  - EXCLUDES infant of mother with diabetes mellitus (775.0)
  - AHA: 1Q, '94, 8
- ▲ **775.7 Late metabolic acidosis of newborn** N
- ● **775.8 Other neonatal endocrine and metabolic disturbances**
  - **775.81 Other acidosis of newborn** N
    - Acidemia NOS of newborn
    - Acidosis of newborn NOS
    - Mixed metabolic and respiratory acidosis of newborn
  - ● **775.89 Other neonatal endocrine and metabolic disturbances** N
    - Amino-acid metabolic disorders described as transitory
- **775.9 Unspecified endocrine and metabolic disturbances specific to the fetus and newborn** N

√4th **776 Hematological disorders of fetus and newborn**

INCLUDES disorders specific to the fetus or newborn

- **776.0 Hemorrhagic disease of newborn** N
  - Hemorrhagic diathesis of newborn
  - Vitamin K deficiency of newborn
  - EXCLUDES fetal or neonatal hemorrhage (772.0-772.9)
- **776.1 Transient neonatal thrombocytopenia** N
  - Neonatal thrombocytopenia due to:
    - exchange transfusion
    - idiopathic maternal thrombocytopenia
    - isoimmunization
  - DEF: Temporary decrease in blood platelets of newborn.
- **776.2 Disseminated intravascular coagulation in newborn** N
  - DEF: Disseminated intravascular coagulation of newborn: clotting disorder due to excess thromboplastic agents in blood as a result of disease or trauma; causes blood clotting within vessels and reduces available elements necessary for blood coagulation.

776.3 Other transient neonatal disorders of coagulation [N]
  Transient coagulation defect, newborn

776.4 Polycythemia neonatorum [N]
  Plethora of newborn
  Polycythemia due to:
    donor twin transfusion
    maternal-fetal transfusion
  DEF: Abnormal increase of total red blood cells of newborn.

776.5 Congenital anemia [N]
  Anemia following fetal blood loss
  EXCLUDES anemia due to isoimmunization (773.0-773.2, 773.5)
            hereditary hemolytic anemias (282.0-282.9)

776.6 Anemia of prematurity [N]

776.7 Transient neonatal neutropenia [N]
  Isoimmune neutropenia
  Maternal transfer neutropenia
  EXCLUDES congenital neutropenia (nontransient) ▶(288.01)◀
  DEF: Decreased neutrophilic leukocytes in blood of newborn.

776.8 Other specified transient hematological disorders [N]

776.9 Unspecified hematological disorder specific to fetus or newborn [N]

✓4ᵗʰ **777** Perinatal disorders of digestive system
  INCLUDES disorders specific to the fetus and newborn
  EXCLUDES intestinal obstruction classifiable to 560.0-560.9

777.1 Meconium obstruction [N]
  Congenital fecaliths
  Delayed passage of meconium
  Meconium ileus NOS
  Meconium plug syndrome
  EXCLUDES meconium ileus in cystic fibrosis (277.01)
  DEF: Meconium blocked digestive tract of newborn.

777.2 Intestinal obstruction due to inspissated milk [N]

777.3 Hematemesis and melena due to swallowed maternal blood [N]
  Swallowed blood syndrome in newborn
  EXCLUDES that not due to swallowed maternal blood (772.4)

777.4 Transitory ileus of newborn [N]
  EXCLUDES Hirschsprung's disease (751.3)

777.5 Necrotizing enterocolitis in fetus or newborn [N]
  Pseudomembranous enterocolitis in newborn
  DEF: Acute inflammation of small intestine due to pseudomembranous plaque over ulceration; may be due to aggressive antibiotic therapy.

777.6 Perinatal intestinal perforation [N]
  Meconium peritonitis

777.8 Other specified perinatal disorders of digestive system [N]

777.9 Unspecified perinatal disorder of digestive system [N]

✓4ᵗʰ **778** Conditions involving the integument and temperature regulation of fetus and newborn

778.0 Hydrops fetalis not due to isoimmunization [N]
  Idiopathic hydrops
  EXCLUDES hydrops fetalis due to isoimmunization (773.3)
  DEF: Edema of entire body, unrelated to immune response.

778.1 Sclerema neonatorum [N]
  Subcutaneous fat necrosis
  DEF: Diffuse, rapidly progressing white, waxy, nonpitting hardening of tissue, usually of legs and feet, life-threatening; found in preterm or debilitated infants; unknown etiology.

778.2 Cold injury syndrome of newborn [N]

778.3 Other hypothermia of newborn [N]

778.4 Other disturbances of temperature regulation of newborn [N]
  Dehydration fever in newborn
  Environmentally-induced pyrexia
  Hyperthermia in newborn
  Transitory fever of newborn

778.5 Other and unspecified edema of newborn [N]
  Edema neonatorum

778.6 Congenital hydrocele [N]
  Congenital hydrocele of tunica vaginalis

778.7 Breast engorgement in newborn [N]
  Noninfective mastitis of newborn
  EXCLUDES infective mastitis of newborn (771.5)

778.8 Other specified conditions involving the integument of fetus and newborn [N]
  Urticaria neonatorum
  EXCLUDES impetigo neonatorum (684)
            pemphigus neonatorum (684)

778.9 Unspecified condition involving the integument and temperature regulation of fetus and newborn [N]

✓4ᵗʰ **779** Other and ill-defined conditions originating in the perinatal period

779.0 Convulsions in newborn [N]
  Fits }
  Seizures } in newborn
  AHA: N-D, '94, 11

779.1 Other and unspecified cerebral irritability in newborn [N]

779.2 Cerebral depression, coma, and other abnormal cerebral signs [N]
  ▶Cerebral ischemia NOS of newborn◀
  CNS dysfunction in newborn NOS
  EXCLUDES ▶ cerebral ischemia due to birth trauma (767.0)
            intrauterine cerebral ischemia (768.2-768.9)
            intraventricular hemorrhage (772.10-772.14)◀

779.3 Feeding problems in newborn [N]
  Regurgitation of food
  Slow feeding   } in newborn
  Vomiting
  AHA: 2Q, '89, 15

779.4 Drug reactions and intoxications specific to newborn [N]
  Gray syndrome from chloramphenicol administration in newborn
  EXCLUDES fetal alcohol syndrome (760.71)
            reactions and intoxications from maternal opiates and tranquilizers (763.5)

779.5 Drug withdrawal syndrome in newborn [N]
  Drug withdrawal syndrome in infant of dependent mother
  EXCLUDES fetal alcohol syndrome (760.71)
  AHA: 3Q, '94, 6

779.6 Termination of pregnancy (fetus) N
Fetal death due to:
  induced abortion
  termination of pregnancy
EXCLUDES spontaneous abortion (fetus) (761.8)

779.7 Periventricular leukomalacia
AHA: 4Q, '01, 50, 51

DEF: Necrosis of white matter adjacent to lateral ventricles with the formation of cysts; cause of PVL has not been firmly established, but thought to be related to inadequate blood flow in certain areas of the brain.

√5ᵗʰ **779.8 Other specified conditions originating in the perinatal period**
AHA: 4Q, '02, 67; 1Q, '94, 15

779.81 Neonatal bradycardia N
EXCLUDES abnormality in fetal heart rate or rhythm complicating labor and delivery (763.81-763.83)
bradycardia due to birth asphyxia (768.5-768.9)

779.82 Neonatal tachycardia N
EXCLUDES abnormality in fetal heart rate or rhythm complicating labor and delivery (763.81-763.83)

779.83 Delayed separation of umbilical cord N
AHA: 4Q, '03, 71

779.84 Meconium staining N
EXCLUDES meconium aspiration (770.11, 770.12)
meconium passage during delivery (763.84)
AHA: 4Q, '05, 83, 88

779.85 Cardiac arrest of newborn N

779.89 Other specified conditions originating in the perinatal period N
Use addtional code to specify condition
AHA: 1Q, '05, 9

779.9 Unspecified condition originating in the perinatal period N
Congenital debility NOS
Stillbirth NEC

16. SYMPTOMS, SIGNS, AND ILL-DEFINED CONDITIONS (780-799)

This section includes symptoms, signs, abnormal results of laboratory or other investigative procedures, and ill-defined conditions regarding which no diagnosis classifiable elsewhere is recorded.

Signs and symptoms that point rather definitely to a given diagnosis are assigned to some category in the preceding part of the classification. In general, categories 780-796 include the more ill-defined conditions and symptoms that point with perhaps equal suspicion to two or more diseases or to two or more systems of the body, and without the necessary study of the case to make a final diagnosis. Practically all categories in this group could be designated as "not otherwise specified," or as "unknown etiology," or as "transient." The Alphabetic Index should be consulted to determine which symptoms and signs are to be allocated here and which to more specific sections of the classification; the residual subcategories numbered .9 are provided for other relevant symptoms which cannot be allocated elsewhere in the classification.

The conditions and signs or symptoms included in categories 780-796 consist of: (a) cases for which no more specific diagnosis can be made even after all facts bearing on the case have been investigated; (b) signs or symptoms existing at the time of initial encounter that proved to be transient and whose causes could not be determined; (c) provisional diagnoses in a patient who failed to return for further investigation or care; (d) cases referred elsewhere for investigation or treatment before the diagnosis was made; (e) cases in which a more precise diagnosis was not available for any other reason; (f) certain symptoms which represent important problems in medical care and which it might be desired to classify in addition to a known cause.

SYMPTOMS (780-789)
AHA: 1Q, '91, 12; 2Q, '90, 3; 2Q, '90, 5; 2Q, '90, 15; M-A, '85, 3

780 General symptoms

780.0 Alteration of consciousness
EXCLUDES coma:
  diabetic (250.2-250.3)
  hepatic (572.2)
  originating in the perinatal period (779.2)
AHA: 4Q, '92, 20

780.01 Coma
AHA: 3Q, '96, 16
DEF: State of unconsciousness from which the patient cannot be awakened.

780.02 Transient alteration of awareness
DEF: Temporary, recurring spells of reduced consciousness.

780.03 Persistent vegetative state
DEF: Persistent wakefulness without consciousness due to nonfunctioning cerebral cortex.

780.09 Other
  Drowsiness   Stupor
  Semicoma   Unconsciousness
  Somnolence

780.1 Hallucinations
  Hallucinations: Hallucinations:
    NOS   olfactory
    auditory   tactile
    gustatory
EXCLUDES those associated with mental disorders, as functional psychoses (295.0-298.9)
  organic brain syndromes (290.0-294.9, 310.0-310.9)
  visual hallucinations (368.16)
DEF: Perception of external stimulus in absence of stimulus; inability to distinguish between real and imagined.

780.2 Syncope and collapse
  Blackout   (Near) (Pre) syncope
  Fainting   Vasovagal attack
EXCLUDES carotid sinus syncope (337.0)
  heat syncope (992.1)
  neurocirculatory asthenia (306.2)
  orthostatic hypotension (458.0)
  shock NOS (785.50)
AHA: 1Q, '02, 6; 3Q, '00, 12; 3Q, '95, 14; N-D, '85, 12
DEF: Sudden unconsciousness due to reduced blood flow to brain.

780.3 Convulsions
EXCLUDES convulsions:
  epileptic (345.10-345.91)
  in newborn (779.0)
AHA: 2Q, '97, 8; 1Q, '97, 12; 3Q, '94, 9; 1Q, '93, 24; 4Q, '92, 23; N-D, '87, 12
DEF: Sudden, involuntary contractions of the muscles.

780.31 Febrile convulsions (simple), unspecified
  Febrile seizure ▶NOS◀
AHA: 4Q, '97, 45

780.32 Complex febrile convulsions
  Febrile seizure:
    atypical
    complex
    complicated
EXCLUDES status epilepticus (345.3)

780.39 Other convulsions
  Convulsive disorder NOS
  Fit NOS
  ▶Recurrent convulsions NOS◀
  Seizure NOS
AHA: 4Q, '04, 51; 1Q, '03, 7; 2Q, '99, 17; 4Q, '98, 39

780.4 Dizziness and giddiness
  Light-headedness
  Vertigo NOS
EXCLUDES Ménière's disease and other specified vertiginous syndromes (386.0-386.9)
AHA: 2Q, '03, 11; 3Q, '00, 12; 2Q, '97, 9; 2Q, '91, 17
DEF: Whirling sensations in head with feeling of falling.

780.5 Sleep disturbances
EXCLUDES circadian rhythm sleep disorders (327.30-327.39)
  organic hypersomnia (327.10-327.19)
  organic insomnia (327.00-327.09)
  organic sleep apnea (327.20-327.29)
  organic sleep related movement disorders (327.51-327.59)
  parasomnias (327.40-327.49)
  that of nonorganic origin (307.40-307.49)
AHA: 4Q, '05, 59

780.50 Sleep disturbance, unspecified

780.51 Insomnia with sleep apnea, unspecified
DEF: Transient cessation of breathing disturbing sleep.

780.52 Insomnia, unspecified
DEF: Inability to maintain adequate sleep cycle.

780.53 Hypersomnia with sleep apnea, unspecified
AHA: 1Q, '93, 28; N-D, '85, 4
DEF: Autonomic response inhibited during sleep; causes insufficient oxygen intake, acidosis and pulmonary hypertension.

780.54 Hypersomnia, unspecified
DEF: Prolonged sleep cycle.

780.55 Disruptions of 24 hour sleep wake cycle, unspecified

780.56 Dysfunctions associated with sleep stages or arousal from sleep

780.57 Unspecified sleep apnea
AHA: 1Q, '01, 6 ; 1Q, '97, 5; 1Q, '93, 28

780.58 Sleep related movement disorder, unspecified
EXCLUDES ▶ restless legs syndrome (333.94)◀
AHA: 4Q, '04, 95

780.59 Other

780.6 Fever
Chills with fever
Fever NOS
Fever of unknown origin (FUO)
Hyperpyrexia NOS
Pyrexia
Pyrexia of unknown origin
▶Code first underlying condition when associated fever is present, such as with:
leukemia (codes from categories 204-208)
neutropenia (288.00-288.09)
sickle-cell disease (282.60-282.69)◀
EXCLUDES pyrexia of unknown origin (during):
in newborn (778.4)
labor (659.2)
the puerperium (672)
AHA: 3Q, '05, 16; 3Q, '00, 13; 4Q, '99, 26; 2Q, '91, 8
DEF: Elevated body temperature; no known cause.

√5ᵗʰ **780.7** Malaise and fatigue
EXCLUDES debility, unspecified (799.3)
fatigue (during):
combat (308.0-308.9)
heat (992.6)
pregnancy (646.8)
neurasthenia (300.5)
senile asthenia (797)
AHA: 4Q, '88, 12; M-A, '87, 8
DEF: Indefinite feeling of debility or lack of good health.

780.71 Chronic fatigue syndrome
AHA: 4Q, '98, 48
DEF: Persistent fatigue, symptoms include weak muscles, sore throat, lymphadenitis, headache, depression and mild fever; no known cause; also called chronic mononucleosis, benign myalgic encephalomyelitis, Iceland disease and neurosthenia.

780.79 Other malaise and fatigue
Asthenia NOS
Lethargy
Postviral (asthenic) syndrome
Tiredness
AHA: 4Q, '04, 78; 1Q, '00, 6; 4Q, '99, 26
DEF: Asthenia: any weakness, lack of strength or loss of energy, especially neuromuscular.
DEF: Lethargy: listlessness, drowsiness, stupor and apathy.
DEF: Postviral (asthenic) syndrome: listlessness, drowsiness, stupor and apathy; follows acute viral infection.
DEF: Tiredness: general exhaustion or fatigue.

780.8 Generalized hyperhidrosis
Diaphoresis
Excessive sweating
Secondary hyperhidrosis
EXCLUDES focal (localized) (primary) (secondary) hyperhidrosis (705.21-705.22)
Frey's syndrome (705.22)
DEF: Excessive sweating, appears as droplets on skin; generalized.

√5ᵗʰ **780.9** Other general symptoms
EXCLUDES hypothermia:
NOS (accidental) (991.6)
due to anesthesia (995.89)
of newborn (778.2-778.3)
memory disturbance as part of a pattern of mental disorder
AHA: 4Q, '02, 67; 4Q, '99, 10; 3Q, '93, 11; N-D, '85, 12

780.91 Fussy infant (baby) P
780.92 Excessive crying of infant (baby) N
EXCLUDES excessive crying of child, adolescent or adult (780.95)

780.93 Memory loss
Amnesia (retrograde)
Memory loss NOS
EXCLUDES mild memory disturbance due to organic brain damage (310.1)
transient global amnesia (437.7)
AHA: 4Q, '03, 71

780.94 Early satiety
AHA: 4Q, '03, 72
DEF: The premature feeling of being full; mechanism of satiety is mutlifactorial.

780.95 Excessive crying of child, adolescent, or adult
EXCLUDES excessive crying of infant (baby) (780.92)
AHA: 4Q, '05, 89

780.96 Generalized pain
Pain NOS

780.97 Altered mental status
Change in mental status
EXCLUDES altered level of consciousness (780.01-780.09)
altered mental status due to known condition—code to condition
delirium NOS (780.09)

780.99 Other general symptoms
Chill(s) NOS
Hypothermia, not associated with low environmental temperature
AHA: 4Q, '03, 103

√4ᵗʰ **781** Symptoms involving nervous and musculoskeletal systems
EXCLUDES depression NOS (311)
disorders specifically relating to:
back (724.0-724.9)
hearing (388.0-389.9)
joint (718.0-719.9)
limb (729.0-729.9)
neck (723.0-723.9)
vision (368.0-369.9)
pain in limb (729.5)

781.0 Abnormal involuntary movements
Abnormal head movements
Fasciculation
Spasms NOS
Tremor NOS
EXCLUDES abnormal reflex (796.1)
chorea NOS (333.5)
infantile spasms (345.60-345.61)
spastic paralysis (342.1, 343.0-344.9)
specified movement disorders classifiable to 333 (333.0-333.9)
that of nonorganic origin (307.2-307.3)

781.1 Disturbances of sensation of smell and taste
Anosmia
Parageusia
Parosmia
DEF: Anosmia: loss of sense of smell due to organic factors, including loss of olfactory nerve conductivity, cerebral disease, nasal fossae formation and peripheral olfactory nerve diseases; can also be psychological disorder.
DEF: Parageusia: distorted sense of taste, or bad taste in mouth.
DEF: Parosmia: distorted sense of smell.

SYMPTOMS, SIGNS, AND ILL-DEFINED CONDITIONS

781.2 **Abnormality of gait**
Gait:
  ataxic
  paralytic
Gait:
  spastic
  staggering

EXCLUDES ataxia:
  NOS (781.3)
  locomotor (progressive) (094.0)
difficulty in walking (719.7)

AHA: 2Q, '05, 6; 2Q, '04, 15

DEF: Abnormal, asymmetric gait.

781.3 **Lack of coordination**
Ataxia NOS   Muscular incoordination

EXCLUDES ataxic gait (781.2)
cerebellar ataxia (334.0-334.9)
difficulty in walking (719.7)
vertigo NOS (780.4)

AHA: 4Q, '04, 51; 3Q, '97, 12

781.4 **Transient paralysis of limb**
Monoplegia, transient NOS

EXCLUDES paralysis (342.0-344.9)

781.5 **Clubbing of fingers**
DEF: Enlarged soft tissue of distal fingers.

781.6 **Meningismus**
Dupré's syndrome   Meningism

AHA: 3Q, '00, 13; J-F, '87, 7

DEF: Condition with signs and symptoms that resemble meningeal irritation; it is associated with febrile illness and dehydration with no evidence of infection.

781.7 **Tetany**
Carpopedal spasm

EXCLUDES tetanus neonatorum (771.3)
tetany:
  hysterical (300.11)
  newborn (hypocalcemic) (775.4)
  parathyroid (252.1)
  psychogenic (306.0)

DEF: Nerve and muscle hyperexcitability; symptoms include muscle spasms, twitching, cramps, laryngospasm with inspiratory stridor, hyperreflexia and choreiform movements.

781.8 **Neurologic neglect syndrome**
Asomatognosia   Left-sided neglect
Hemi-akinesia   Sensory extinction
Hemi-inattention   Sensory neglect
Hemispatial neglect Visuospatial neglect

AHA: 4Q, '94, 37

√5th **781.9** **Other symptoms involving nervous and musculoskeletal systems**
AHA: 4Q, '00, 45

781.91 **Loss of height**
EXCLUDES osteoporosis (733.00-733.09)

781.92 **Abnormal posture**

781.93 **Ocular torticollis**
AHA: 4Q, '02, 68

DEF: Abnormal head posture as a result of a contracted state of cervical muscles to correct a visual disturbance; either double vision or a visual field defect.

781.94 **Facial weakness**
Facial droop

EXCLUDES facial weakness due to late effect of cerebrovascular accident (438.83)

AHA: 4Q, '03, 72

781.99 **Other symptoms involving nervous and musculoskeletal systems**

√4th **782** **Symptoms involving skin and other integumentary tissue**
EXCLUDES symptoms relating to breast (611.71-611.79)

782.0 **Disturbance of skin sensation**
Anesthesia of skin   Hypoesthesia
Burning or prickling   Numbness
  sensation   Paresthesia
Hyperesthesia   Tingling

782.1 **Rash and other nonspecific skin eruption**
Exanthem
EXCLUDES vesicular eruption (709.8)

782.2 **Localized superficial swelling, mass, or lump**
Subcutaneous nodules
EXCLUDES localized adiposity (278.1)

782.3 **Edema**
Anasarca   Localized edema NOS
Dropsy
EXCLUDES ascites (789.5)
edema of:
  newborn NOS (778.5)
  pregnancy (642.0-642.9, 646.1)
fluid retention (276.6)
hydrops fetalis (773.3, 778.0)
hydrothorax (511.8)
nutritional edema (260, 262)

AHA: 2Q, '00, 18

DEF: Edema: excess fluid in intercellular body tissue.
DEF: Anasarca: massive edema in all body tissues.
DEF: Dropsy: serous fluid accumulated in body cavity or cellular tissue.
DEF: Localized edema: edema in specific body areas.

782.4 **Jaundice, unspecified, not of newborn**
Cholemia NOS   Icterus NOS
EXCLUDES jaundice in newborn (774.0-774.7)
due to isoimmunization (773.0-773.2, 773.4)

DEF: Bilirubin deposits of skin, causing yellow cast.

782.5 **Cyanosis**
EXCLUDES newborn (770.83)

DEF: Deficient oxygen of blood; causes blue cast to skin.

√5th **782.6** **Pallor and flushing**
782.61 **Pallor**
782.62 **Flushing**
Excessive blushing

782.7 **Spontaneous ecchymoses**
Petechiae
EXCLUDES ecchymosis in fetus or newborn (772.6)
purpura (287.0-287.9)

DEF: Hemorrhagic spots of skin; resemble freckles.

782.8 **Changes in skin texture**
Induration } of skin
Thickening

782.9 **Other symptoms involving skin and integumentary tissues**

√4th **783** **Symptoms concerning nutrition, metabolism, and development**

783.0 **Anorexia**
Loss of appetite
EXCLUDES anorexia nervosa (307.1)
loss of appetite of nonorganic origin (307.59)

783.1 **Abnormal weight gain**
EXCLUDES excessive weight gain in pregnancy (646.1)
obesity (278.00)
  morbid (278.01)

Additional Digit Required

SYMPTOMS, SIGNS, AND ILL-DEFINED CONDITIONS — Tabular List

783.2 **Abnormal loss of weight and underweight**
Use additional code to identify Body Mass Index (BMI), if known ▶(V85.0-V85.54)◀
AHA: 4Q, '00, 45

783.21 **Loss of weight**
AHA: 4Q, '05, 96

783.22 **Underweight**
AHA: 4Q, '05, 96

783.3 **Feeding difficulties and mismanagement**
Feeding problem (elderly) (infant)
EXCLUDES: feeding disturbance or problems:
 in newborn (779.3)
 of nonorganic origin (307.50-307.59)
AHA: 3Q, '97, 12

783.4 **Lack of expected normal physiological development in childhood**
EXCLUDES: delay in sexual development and puberty (259.0)
 gonadal dysgenesis (758.6)
 pituitary dwarfism (253.3)
 slow fetal growth and fetal malnutrition (764.00-764.99)
 specific delays in mental development (315.0-315.9)
AHA: 4Q, '00, 45; 3Q, '97, 4

783.40 **Lack of normal physiological development, unspecified**
Inadequate development
Lack of development

783.41 **Failure to thrive** [P]
Failure to gain weight
AHA: 1Q, '03, 12
DEF: Organic failure to thrive: acute or chronic illness that interferes with nutritional intake, absorption, metabolism excretion and energy requirements. Nonorganic FTT is symptom of neglect or abuse.

783.42 **Delayed milestones** [P]
Late talker   Late walker

783.43 **Short stature**
Growth failure   Lack of growth
Growth retardation Physical retardation
DEF: Constitutional short stature: stature inconsistent with chronological age. Genetic short stature is when skeletal maturation matches chronological age.

783.5 **Polydipsia**
Excessive thirst

783.6 **Polyphagia**
Excessive eating   Hyperalimentation NOS
EXCLUDES: disorders of eating of nonorganic origin (307.50-307.59)

783.7 **Adult failure to thrive** [A]

783.9 **Other symptoms concerning nutrition, metabolism, and development**
Hypometabolism
EXCLUDES: abnormal basal metabolic rate (794.7)
 dehydration (276.51)
 other disorders of fluid, electrolyte, and acid-base balance (276.0-276.9)
AHA: 2Q, '04, 3

784 **Symptoms involving head and neck**
EXCLUDES: encephalopathy NOS (348.30)
 specific symptoms involving neck classifiable to 723 (723.0-723.9)

784.0 **Headache**
Facial pain   Pain in head NOS
EXCLUDES: atypical face pain (350.2)
 migraine (346.0-346.9)
 tension headache (307.81)
AHA: 3Q, '00, 13; 1Q, '90, 4; 3Q, '92, 14

784.1 **Throat pain**
EXCLUDES: dysphagia (787.2)
 neck pain (723.1)
 sore throat (462)
 chronic (472.1)

784.2 **Swelling, mass, or lump in head and neck**
Space-occupying lesion, intracranial NOS
AHA: 1Q, '03, 8

784.3 **Aphasia**
EXCLUDES: ▶aphasia due to late effects of cerebrovascular disease (438.11)◀
 developmental aphasia (315.31)
AHA: 4Q, '04, 78; 4Q, '98, 87; 3Q, '97, 12
DEF: Inability to communicate through speech, written word, or sign language.

784.4 **Voice disturbance**

784.40 **Voice disturbance, unspecified**

784.41 **Aphonia**
Loss of voice

784.49 **Other**
Change in voice   Hypernasality
Dysphonia   Hyponasality
Hoarseness

784.5 **Other speech disturbance**
Dysarthria   Slurred speech
Dysphasia
EXCLUDES: stammering and stuttering (307.0)
 that of nonorganic origin (307.0, 307.9)

784.6 **Other symbolic dysfunction**
EXCLUDES: developmental learning delays (315.0-315.9)

784.60 **Symbolic dysfunction, unspecified**

784.61 **Alexia and dyslexia**
Alexia (with agraphia)
DEF: Alexia: inability to understand written word due to central brain lesion.
DEF: Dyslexia: ability to recognize letters but inability to read, spell, and write words; genetic.

784.69 **Other**
Acalculia   Agraphia NOS
Agnosia   Apraxia

784.7 **Epistaxis**
Hemorrhage from nose   Nosebleed
AHA: 3Q, '04, 7

784.8 **Hemorrhage from throat**
EXCLUDES: hemoptysis (786.3)

784.9 **Other symptoms involving head and neck**

784.91 **Postnasal drip**

784.99 **Other symptoms involving head and neck**
Choking sensation   Mouth breathing
Halitosis   Sneezing

785 **Symptoms involving cardiovascular system**
EXCLUDES: heart failure NOS (428.9)

785.0 **Tachycardia, unspecified**
Rapid heart beat
EXCLUDES: neonatal tachycardia (779.82)
 paroxysmal tachycardia (427.0-427.2)
AHA: 2Q, '03, 11
DEF: Excessively rapid heart rate.

785.1 **Palpitations**
Awareness of heart beat
EXCLUDES: specified dysrhythmias (427.0-427.9)

785.2 **Undiagnosed cardiac murmurs**
Heart murmurs NOS
AHA: 4Q, '92, 16

[N] Newborn Age: 0   [P] Pediatric Age: 0-17   [M] Maternity Age: 12-55   [A] Adult Age: 15-124

SYMPTOMS, SIGNS, AND ILL-DEFINED CONDITIONS

785.3 **Other abnormal heart sounds**
Cardiac dullness, increased or decreased
Friction fremitus, cardiac
Precordial friction

785.4 **Gangrene**
Gangrene:
  NOS
  spreading cutaneous
Gangrenous cellulitis
Phagedena
Code first any associated underlying condition

> **EXCLUDES** gangrene of certain sites — see Alphabetic Index
> gangrene with atherosclerosis of the extremities (440.24)
> gas gangrene (040.0)

AHA: 1Q, '04, 14; 3Q, '91, 12; 3Q, '90, 15; M-A, '86, 12
DEF: Gangrene: necrosis of skin tissue due to bacterial infection, diabetes, embolus and vascular supply loss.
DEF: Gangrenous cellulitis: group A streptococcal infection; begins with severe cellulitis, spreads to superficial and deep fascia; produces gangrene of underlying tissues.

√5th 785.5 **Shock without mention of trauma**

785.50 **Shock, unspecified**
Failure of peripheral circulation
AHA: 2Q, '96, 10
DEF: Peripheral circulatory failure due to heart insufficiencies.

785.51 **Cardiogenic shock**
AHA: ▶3Q, '05, 14◀
DEF: Shock syndrome: associated with myocardial infarction, cardiac tamponade and massive pulmonary embolism; symptoms include mental confusion, reduced blood pressure, tachycardia, pallor and cold, clammy skin.

785.52 **Septic shock**
Shock:
  endotoxic
  gram-negative
Code first:
  systemic inflammatory response syndrome due to infectious process with organ dysfunction (995.92)
AHA: ▶2Q, '05, 18-19;◀ 4Q, '03, 73, 79

785.59 **Other**
Shock:
  hypovolemic

> **EXCLUDES** shock (due to):
> anesthetic (995.4)
> anaphylactic (995.0)
> due to serum (999.4)
> electric (994.8)
> following abortion (639.5)
> lightning (994.0)
> obstetrical (669.1)
> postoperative (998.0)
> traumatic (958.4)

AHA: 2Q, '00, 3

785.6 **Enlargement of lymph nodes**
Lymphadenopathy   "Swollen glands"

> **EXCLUDES** lymphadenitis (chronic) (289.1-289.3)
> acute (683)

785.9 **Other symptoms involving cardiovascular system**
Bruit (arterial)   Weak pulse

√4th 786 **Symptoms involving respiratory system and other chest symptoms**

√5th 786.0 **Dyspnea and respiratory abnormalities**

786.00 **Respiratory abnormality, unspecified**

786.01 **Hyperventilation**

> **EXCLUDES** hyperventilation, psychogenic (306.1)

DEF: Rapid breathing causes carbon dioxide loss from blood.

786.02 **Orthopnea**
DEF: Difficulty breathing except in upright position.

786.03 **Apnea**

> **EXCLUDES** apnea of newborn (770.81, 770.82)
> sleep apnea (780.51, 780.53, 780.57)

AHA: 4Q, '98, 50
DEF: Cessation of breathing.

786.04 **Cheyne-Stokes respiration**
AHA: 4Q, '98, 50
DEF: Rhythmic increase of depth and frequency of breathing with apnea; occurs in frontal lobe and diencephalic dysfunction.

786.05 **Shortness of breath**
AHA: 4Q, '99, 25; 1Q, '99, 6; 4Q, '98, 50
DEF: Inability to take in sufficient oxygen.

786.06 **Tachypnea**

> **EXCLUDES** transitory tachypnea of newborn (770.6)

AHA: 4Q, '98, 50
DEF: Abnormal rapid respiratory rate; called hyperventilation.

786.07 **Wheezing**

> **EXCLUDES** asthma (493.00-493.92)

AHA: 4Q, '98, 50
DEF: Stenosis of respiratory passageway; causes whistling sound; due to asthma, coryza, croup, emphysema, hay fever, edema, and pleural effusion.

786.09 **Other**

> **EXCLUDES** respiratory distress:
> following trauma and surgery (518.5)
> newborn (770.89)
> syndrome (newborn) (769)
> adult (518.5)
> respiratory failure (518.81, 518.83-518.84)
> newborn (770.84)

AHA: ▶4Q, '05, 90;◀ 2Q, '98, 10; 1Q, '97, 7; 1Q, '90, 9

786.1 **Stridor**

> **EXCLUDES** congenital laryngeal stridor (748.3)

DEF: Obstructed airway causes harsh sound.

786.2 **Cough**

> **EXCLUDES** cough:
> psychogenic (306.1)
> smokers' (491.0)
> with hemorrhage (786.3)

AHA: 4Q, '99, 26

786.3 **Hemoptysis**
Cough with hemorrhage
Pulmonary hemorrhage NOS

> **EXCLUDES** pulmonary hemorrhage of newborn (770.3)

AHA: 4Q, '90, 26
DEF: Coughing up blood or blood-stained sputum.

786.4 **Abnormal sputum**
Abnormal:
  amount
  color   (of) sputum
  odor
Excessive

√5th 786.5 **Chest pain**

786.50 **Chest pain, unspecified**
AHA: 1Q, '03, 6; 1Q, '02, 4; 4Q, '99, 25

786.51 **Precordial pain**
DEF: Chest pain over heart and lower thorax.

SYMPTOMS, SIGNS, AND ILL-DEFINED CONDITIONS

786.52 Painful respiration
Pain:
  anterior chest wall
  pleuritic
Pleurodynia
EXCLUDES epidemic pleurodynia (074.1)
AHA: N-D, '84, 17

786.59 Other
Discomfort
Pressure } in chest
Tightness
EXCLUDES pain in breast (611.71)
AHA: 1Q, '02, 6

786.6 Swelling, mass, or lump in chest
EXCLUDES lump in breast (611.72)

786.7 Abnormal chest sounds
Abnormal percussion, chest   Rales
Friction sounds, chest   Tympany, chest
EXCLUDES wheezing (786.07)

786.8 Hiccough
EXCLUDES psychogenic hiccough (306.1)

786.9 Other symptoms involving respiratory system and chest
Breath-holding spell

787 Symptoms involving digestive system
EXCLUDES constipation (564.00-564.09)
  pylorospasm (537.81)
    congenital (750.5)

787.0 Nausea and vomiting
Emesis
EXCLUDES hematemesis NOS (578.0)
vomiting:
  bilious, following gastrointestinal surgery (564.3)
  cyclical (536.2)
    psychogenic (306.4)
  excessive, in pregnancy (643.0-643.9)
  habit (536.2)
  of newborn (779.3)
  psychogenic NOS (307.54)
AHA: M-A, '85, 11

787.01 Nausea with vomiting
AHA: 1Q, '03, 5

787.02 Nausea alone
AHA: 3Q, '00, 12; 2Q, '97, 9

787.03 Vomiting alone

787.1 Heartburn
Pyrosis   Waterbrash
EXCLUDES dyspepsia or indigestion (536.8)
AHA: 2Q, '01, 6

787.2 Dysphagia
Difficulty in swallowing
AHA: 4Q, '03, 103, 109; 2Q, '01, 4

787.3 Flatulence, eructation, and gas pain
Abdominal distention (gaseous)
Bloating
Tympanites (abdominal) (intestinal)
EXCLUDES aerophagy (306.4)
DEF: Flatulence: excess air or gas in intestine or stomach.
DEF: Eructation: belching, expelling gas through mouth.
DEF: Gas pain: gaseous pressure affecting gastrointestinal system.

787.4 Visible peristalsis
Hyperperistalsis
DEF: Increase in involuntary movements of intestines.

787.5 Abnormal bowel sounds
Absent bowel sounds
Hyperactive bowel sounds

787.6 Incontinence of feces
Encopresis NOS
Incontinence of sphincter ani
EXCLUDES that of nonorganic origin (307.7)
AHA: 1Q, '97, 9

787.7 Abnormal feces
Bulky stools
EXCLUDES abnormal stool content (792.1)
melena:
  NOS (578.1)
  newborn (772.4, 777.3)

787.9 Other symptoms involving digestive system
EXCLUDES gastrointestinal hemorrhage (578.0-578.9)
  intestinal obstruction (560.0-560.9)
  specific functional digestive disorders:
    esophagus (530.0-530.9)
    stomach and duodenum (536.0-536.9)
    those not elsewhere classified (564.00-564.9)

787.91 Diarrhea
Diarrhea NOS
AHA: 4Q, '95, 54

787.99 Other
Change in bowel habits   Tenesmus (rectal)
DEF: Tenesmus: painful, ineffective straining at the rectum with limited passage of fecal matter.

788 Symptoms involving urinary system
EXCLUDES hematuria (599.7)
  nonspecific findings on examination of the urine (791.0-791.9)
  small kidney of unknown cause (589.0-589.9)
  uremia NOS (586)
  ▶urinary obstruction (599.60, 599.69)◀

788.0 Renal colic
Colic (recurrent) of: Colic (recurrent) of:
  kidney   ureter
AHA: 3Q, '04, 8
DEF: Kidney pain.

788.1 Dysuria
Painful urination   Strangury

788.2 Retention of urine
▶Code, if applicable, any causal condition first, such as:
  hyperplasia of prostate (600.0-600.9 with fifth-digit 1)◀
DEF: Accumulation of urine in the bladder due to inability to void.

788.20 Retention of urine, unspecified
AHA: 2Q, '04, 18; 3Q, '03, 12-13; 1Q, '03, 6; 3Q, '96, 10

788.21 Incomplete bladder emptying

788.29 Other specified retention of urine

788.3 Urinary incontinence
Code, if applicable, any causal condition first, such as:
  congenital ureterocele (753.23)
  genital prolapse (618.00-618.9)
  ▶hyperplasia of prostate (600.0-600.9 with fifth-digit 1)◀
EXCLUDES that of nonorganic origin (307.6)
AHA: 4Q, '92, 22

788.30 Urinary incontinence, unspecified
Enuresis NOS

788.31 Urge incontinence
AHA: 1Q, '00, 19
DEF: Inability to control urination, upon urge to urinate.

788.32 Stress incontinence, male ♂
EXCLUDES stress incontinence, female (625.6)
DEF: Inability to control urination associated with weak sphincter in males.

SYMPTOMS, SIGNS, AND ILL-DEFINED CONDITIONS

788.33 Mixed incontinence, (male) (female)
Urge and stress
DEF: Urge, stress incontinence: involuntary discharge of urine due to anatomic displacement.

788.34 Incontinence without sensory awareness
DEF: Involuntary discharge of urine without sensory warning.

788.35 Post-void dribbling
DEF: Involuntary discharge of residual urine after voiding.

788.36 Nocturnal enuresis
DEF: Involuntary discharge of urine during the night.

788.37 Continuous leakage
DEF: Continuous, involuntary urine seepage.

788.38 Overflow incontinence
DEF: Leakage caused by pressure of retained urine in the bladder after the bladder has fully contracted due to weakened bladder muscles or an obstruction of the urethra.

788.39 Other urinary incontinence

√5th **788.4** Frequency of urination and polyuria
▶Code, if applicable, any causal condition first, such as:
hyperplasia of prostate (600.0-600.9 with fifth-digit 1)◀

788.41 Urinary frequency
Frequency of micturition

788.42 Polyuria
DEF: Excessive urination.

788.43 Nocturia
DEF: Urination affecting sleep patterns.

788.5 Oliguria and anuria
Deficient secretion of urine
Suppression of urinary secretion
EXCLUDES that complicating:
abortion (634-638 with .3, 639.3)
ectopic or molar pregnancy (639.3)
pregnancy, childbirth, or the puerperium (642.0-642.9, 646.2)
DEF: Oliguria: diminished urinary secretion related to fluid intake.
DEF: Anuria: lack of urinary secretion due to renal failure or obstructed urinary tract.

√5th **788.6** Other abnormality of urination
▶Code, if applicable, any causal condition first, such as:
hyperplasia of prostate (600.0-600.9 with fifth-digit 1)◀

788.61 Splitting of urinary stream
Intermittent urinary stream

788.62 Slowing of urinary stream
Weak stream

788.63 Urgency of urination
EXCLUDES urge incontinence (788.31, 788.33)
AHA: 4Q, '03, 74
DEF: Feeling of intense need to urinate; abrupt sensation of imminent urination.

● **788.64** Urinary hesitancy
● **788.65** Straining on urination
788.69 Other

788.7 Urethral discharge
Penile discharge   Urethrorrhea

788.8 Extravasation of urine
DEF: Leaking or infiltration of urine into tissues.

788.9 Other symptoms involving urinary system
Extrarenal uremia   Vesical:
Vesical: tenesmus
    pain
AHA: 1Q, '05, 12; 4Q, '88, 1

√4th **789** Other symptoms involving abdomen and pelvis
EXCLUDES symptoms referable to genital organs:
female (625.0-625.9)
male (607.0-608.9)
psychogenic (302.70-302.79)

The following fifth-digit subclassification is to be used for codes 789.0, 789.3, 789.4, 789.6:
0 unspecified site
1 right upper quadrant
2 left upper quadrant
3 right lower quadrant
4 left lower quadrant
5 periumbilic
6 epigastric
7 generalized
9 other specified site
Multiple sites

√5th **789.0** Abdominal pain
Colic: Cramps, abdominal
    NOS
    infantile
EXCLUDES renal colic (788.0)
AHA: 1Q, '95, 3; For code 789.06: 1Q, '02, 5

789.1 Hepatomegaly
Enlargement of liver

789.2 Splenomegaly
Enlargement of spleen

√5th **789.3** Abdominal or pelvic swelling, mass, or lump
Diffuse or generalized swelling or mass:
abdominal NOS   umbilical
EXCLUDES abdominal distention (gaseous) (787.3)
ascites (789.5)

√5th **789.4** Abdominal rigidity

789.5 Ascites
Fluid in peritoneal cavity
AHA: 2Q, '05, 8; 4Q, '89, 11
DEF: Serous fluid effusion and accumulation in abdominal cavity.

√5th **789.6** Abdominal tenderness
Rebound tenderness

789.9 Other symptoms involving abdomen and pelvis
Umbilical: Umbilical:
    bleeding   discharge

NONSPECIFIC ABNORMAL FINDINGS (790-796)
AHA: 2Q, '90, 16

√4th **790** Nonspecific findings on examination of blood
EXCLUDES abnormality of:
platelets (287.0-287.9)
thrombocytes (287.0-287.9)
white blood cells ▶(288.00-288.9)◀

√5th **790.0** Abnormality of red blood cells
EXCLUDES anemia:
congenital (776.5)
newborn, due to isoimmunization (773.0-773.2, 773.5)
of premature infant (776.6)
other specified types (280.0-285.9)
hemoglobin disorders (282.5-282.7)
polycythemia:
familial (289.6)
neonatorum (776.4)
secondary (289.0)
vera (238.4)
AHA: 4Q, '00, 46

790.01 Precipitous drop in hematocrit
Drop in hematocrit

790.09 Other abnormality of red blood cells
Abnormal red cell morphology NOS
Abnormal red cell volume NOS
Anisocytosis
Poikilocytosis

790.1 Elevated sedimentation rate

SYMPTOMS, SIGNS, AND ILL-DEFINED CONDITIONS
Tabular List

790.2 Abnormal glucose [5th]
- EXCLUDES:
  - diabetes mellitus (250.00-250.93)
  - dysmetabolic syndrome X (277.7)
  - gestational diabetes (648.8)
  - glycosuria (791.5)
  - hypoglycemia (251.2)
  - that complicating pregnancy, childbirth, or puerperium (648.8)
- AHA: 4Q, '03, 74; 3Q, '91, 5

790.21 Impaired fasting glucose
- Elevated fasting glucose

790.22 Impaired glucose tolerance test (oral)
- Elevated glucose tolerance test

790.29 Other abnormal glucose
- Abnormal glucose NOS
- Abnormal non-fasting glucose
- ▶Hyperglycemia NOS◀
- Pre-diabetes NOS
- AHA: 2Q, '05, 21

790.3 Excessive blood level of alcohol
- Elevated blood-alcohol
- AHA: S-O, '86, 3

790.4 Nonspecific elevation of levels of transaminase or lactic acid dehydrogenase [LDH]

790.5 Other nonspecific abnormal serum enzyme levels
- Abnormal serum level of:
  - acid phosphatase
  - alkaline phosphatase
  - amylase
  - lipase
- EXCLUDES: deficiency of circulating enzymes (277.6)

790.6 Other abnormal blood chemistry
- Abnormal blood level of: Abnormal blood level of:
  - cobalt   lithium
  - copper   magnesium
  - iron   mineral
  - ▶lead◀   zinc
- EXCLUDES:
  - abnormality of electrolyte or acid-base balance (276.0-276.9)
  - hypoglycemia NOS (251.2)
  - ▶lead poisoning (984.0-984.9)◀
  - specific finding indicating abnormality of:
    - amino-acid transport and metabolism (270.0-270.9)
    - carbohydrate transport and metabolism (271.0-271.9)
    - lipid metabolism (272.0-272.9)
  - uremia NOS (586)
- AHA: 4Q, '88, 1

790.7 Bacteremia
- EXCLUDES:
  - bacteremia of newborn (771.83)
  - septicemia (038)
- Use additional code to identify organism (041)
- AHA: 2Q, '03, 7; 4Q, '93, 29; 3Q, '88, 12
- DEF: Laboratory finding of bacteria in the blood in the absence of two or more signs of sepsis; transient in nature, progresses to septicemia with severe infectious process.

790.8 Viremia, unspecified
- AHA: 4Q, '88, 10
- DEF: Presence of a virus in the blood stream.

790.9 Other nonspecific findings on examination of blood [5th]
- AHA: 4Q, '93, 29

790.91 Abnormal arterial blood gases

790.92 Abnormal coagulation profile
- Abnormal or prolonged:
  - bleeding time
  - coagulation time
  - partial thromboplastin time [PTT]
  - prothrombintime [PT]
- EXCLUDES: coagulation (hemorrhagic) disorders (286.0-286.9)

790.93 Elevated prostate specific antigen, [PSA] A ♂

790.94 Euthyroid sick syndrome
- AHA: 4Q, '97, 45
- DEF: Transient alteration of thyroid hormone metabolism due to nonthyroid illness or stress.

790.95 Elevated C-reactive protein [CRP]
- DEF: Inflammation in an arterial wall results in elevated C-reactive protein (CRP) in the blood; CRP is a recognized risk factor in cardiovascular disease.

790.99 Other
- AHA: 2Q, '03, 14

791 Nonspecific findings on examination of urine [4th]
- EXCLUDES:
  - hematuria NOS (599.7)
  - specific findings indicating abnormality of:
    - amino-acid transport and metabolism (270.0-270.9)
    - carbohydrate transport and metabolism (271.0-271.9)

791.0 Proteinuria
- Albuminuria
- Bence-Jones proteinuria
- EXCLUDES:
  - postural proteinuria (593.6)
  - that arising during pregnancy or the puerperium (642.0-642.9, 646.2)
- AHA: 3Q, '91, 8
- DEF: Excess protein in urine.

791.1 Chyluria
- EXCLUDES: filarial (125.0-125.9)
- DEF: Excess chyle in urine.

791.2 Hemoglobinuria
- DEF: Free hemoglobin in blood due to rapid hemolysis of red blood cells.

791.3 Myoglobinuria
- DEF: Myoglobin (oxygen-transporting pigment) in urine.

791.4 Biliuria
- DEF: Bile pigments in urine.

791.5 Glycosuria
- EXCLUDES: renal glycosuria (271.4)
- DEF: Sugar in urine.

791.6 Acetonuria
- Ketonuria
- DEF: Excess acetone in urine.

791.7 Other cells and casts in urine

791.9 Other nonspecific findings on examination of urine
- Crystalluria
- Elevated urine levels of:
  - 17-ketosteroids
  - catecholamines
  - indolacetic acid
- Elevated urine levels of:
  - vanillylmandelic acid [VMA]
- Melanuria
- AHA: 1Q, '05, 12

N Newborn Age: 0   P Pediatric Age: 0-17   M Maternity Age: 12-55   A Adult Age: 15-124

SYMPTOMS, SIGNS, AND ILL-DEFINED CONDITIONS

✓4th 792 Nonspecific abnormal findings in other body substances
  EXCLUDES: that in chromosomal analysis (795.2)

- **792.0 Cerebrospinal fluid**
- **792.1 Stool contents**
  - Abnormal stool color
  - Fat in stool
  - Mucus in stool
  - Occult stool
  - Pus in stool
  - EXCLUDES: blood in stool [melena] (578.1)
    newborn (772.4, 777.3)
  - AHA: 2Q, '92, 9
- **792.2 Semen** ♂
  - Abnormal spermatozoa
  - EXCLUDES: azoospermia (606.0)
    oligospermia (606.1)
- **792.3 Amniotic fluid** M ♀
  - AHA: N-D, '86, 4
  - DEF: Nonspecific abnormal findings in amniotic fluid.
- **792.4 Saliva**
  - EXCLUDES: that in chromosomal analysis (795.2)
- **792.5 Cloudy (hemodialysis) (peritoneal) dialysis effluent**
- **792.9 Other nonspecific abnormal findings in body substances**
  - Peritoneal fluid
  - Pleural fluid
  - Synovial fluid
  - Vaginal fluids

✓4th 793 Nonspecific abnormal findings on radiological and other examination of body structure
  INCLUDES: nonspecific abnormal findings of:
    thermography
    ultrasound examination [echogram]
    x-ray examination
  EXCLUDES: abnormal results of function studies and radioisotope scans (794.0-794.9)

- **793.0 Skull and head**
  - EXCLUDES: nonspecific abnormal echoencephalogram (794.01)
- **793.1 Lung field**
  - Coin lesion
  - Shadow } (of) lung
  - DEF: Coin lesion of lung: coin-shaped, solitary pulmonary nodule.
- **793.2 Other intrathoracic organ**
  - Abnormal:
    - echocardiogram
    - heart shadow
  - Abnormal:
    - ultrasound cardiogram
    - Mediastinal shift
- **793.3 Biliary tract**
  - Nonvisualization of gallbladder
- **793.4 Gastrointestinal tract**
- **793.5 Genitourinary organs**
  - Filling defect:
    - bladder
    - kidney
  - Filling defect:
    - ureter
  - AHA: 4Q, '00, 46
- **793.6 Abdominal area, including retroperitoneum**
- **793.7 Musculoskeletal system**
- **✓5th 793.8 Breast**
  - AHA: 4Q, '01, 51
  - **793.80 Abnormal mammogram, unspecified**
  - **793.81 Mammographic microcalcification**
    - EXCLUDES: ▶mammographic calcification (793.89)
      mammographic calculus (793.89)◄
    - DEF: Calcium and cellular debris deposits in the breast that can't be felt but are detected on a mammogram; can be a sign of cancer, benign conditions, or changes in the breast tissue as a result of inflammation, injury, or obstructed duct.
  - **793.89 Other abnormal findings on radiological examination of breast**
    - ▶Mammographic calcification
    - Mammographic calculus◄

- **✓5th 793.9 Other**
  - EXCLUDES: abnormal finding by radioisotope localization of placenta (794.9)
  - ● **793.91 Image test inconclusive due to excess body fat**
    - Use additional code to identify Body Mass Index (BMI), if known (V85.0-V85.54)
  - ● **793.99 Other nonspecific abnormal findings on radiological and other examinations of body structure**
    - Abnormal:
      - placental finding by x-ray or ultrasound method
      - radiological findings in skin and subcutaneous tissue

✓4th 794 Nonspecific abnormal results of function studies
  INCLUDES: radioisotope:
    scans
    uptake studies
    scintiphotography

- **✓5th 794.0 Brain and central nervous system**
  - **794.00 Abnormal function study, unspecified**
  - **794.01 Abnormal echoencephalogram**
  - **794.02 Abnormal electroencephalogram [EEG]**
  - **794.09 Other**
    - Abnormal brain scan
- **✓5th 794.1 Peripheral nervous system and special senses**
  - **794.10 Abnormal response to nerve stimulation, unspecified**
  - **794.11 Abnormal retinal function studies**
    - Abnormal electroretinogram [ERG]
  - **794.12 Abnormal electro-oculogram [EOG]**
  - **794.13 Abnormal visually evoked potential**
  - **794.14 Abnormal oculomotor studies**
  - **794.15 Abnormal auditory function studies**
    - AHA: 1Q, '04, 15-16
  - **794.16 Abnormal vestibular function studies**
  - **794.17 Abnormal electromyogram [EMG]**
    - EXCLUDES: that of eye (794.14)
  - **794.19 Other**
- **794.2 Pulmonary**
  - Abnormal lung scan
  - Reduced: ventilatory capacity
  - Reduced: vital capacity
- **✓5th 794.3 Cardiovascular**
  - **794.30 Abnormal function study, unspecified**
  - **794.31 Abnormal electrocardiogram [ECG] [EKG]**
    - EXCLUDES: long QT syndrome (426.82)
  - **794.39 Other**
    - Abnormal:
      - ballistocardiogram
      - phonocardiogram
    - Abnormal:
      - vectorcardiogram
- **794.4 Kidney**
  - Abnormal renal function test
- **794.5 Thyroid**
  - Abnormal thyroid: scan
  - Abnormal thyroid: uptake
- **794.6 Other endocrine function study**
- **794.7 Basal metabolism**
  - Abnormal basal metabolic rate [BMR]
- **794.8 Liver**
  - Abnormal liver scan
- **794.9 Other**
  - Bladder
  - Pancreas
  - Placenta
  - Spleen

SYMPTOMS, SIGNS, AND ILL-DEFINED CONDITIONS

795 Other and nonspecific abnormal cytological, histological, immunological and DNA test findings
EXCLUDES nonspecific abnormalities of red blood cells (790.01-790.09)

795.0 Abnormal Papanicolaou smear of cervix and cervical HPV
Abnormal thin preparation smear of cervix
Abnormal cervical cytology

EXCLUDES
- carcinoma in-situ of cervix (233.1)
- cervical intraepithelial neoplasia I (CIN I) (622.11)
- cervical intraepithelial neoplasia II (CIN II) (622.12)
- cervical intraepithelial neoplasia III (CIN III) (233.1)
- dysplasia (histologically confirmed) of cervix (uteri) NOS (622.10)
- mild dysplasia (histologically confirmed) (622.11)
- moderate dysplasia (histologically confirmed) (622.12)
- severe dysplasia (histologically confirmed) (233.1)

AHA: 4Q, '02, 69

795.00 Abnormal glandular Papanicolaou smear of cervix
Atypical endocervical cells NOS
Atypical endometrial cells NOS
Atypical glandular cells NOS

795.01 Papanicolaou smear of cervix with atypical squamous cells of undetermined significance [ASC-US]

795.02 Papanicolaou smear of cervix with atypical squamous cells cannot exclude high grade squamous intraepithelial lesion [ASC-H]

795.03 Papanicolaou smear of cervix with low grade squamous intraepithelial lesion [LGSIL]

795.04 Papanicolaou smear of cervix with high grade squamous intraepithelial lesion [HGSIL]

795.05 Cervical high risk human papillomavirus [HPV] DNA test positive

795.06 Papanicolaou smear of cervix with cytologic evidence of malignancy

795.08 Unsatisfactory smear
Inadequate sample

795.09 Other abnormal Papanicolaou smear of cervix and cervical HPV
Cervical low risk human papillomavirus HPV) DNA test positive
Use additional code for associated human papillomavirus (079.4)

EXCLUDES encounter for Papanicolaou cervical smear to confirm findings of recent normal smear following initial abnormal smear (V72.32)

795.1 Nonspecific abnormal Papanicolaou smear of other site

795.2 Nonspecific abnormal findings on chromosomal analysis
Abnormal karyotype

795.3 Nonspecific positive culture findings
Positive culture findings in:
- nose
- sputum
- throat
- wound

EXCLUDES that of:
- blood (790.7-790.8)
- urine (791.9)

795.31 Nonspecific positive findings for anthrax
Positive findings by nasal swab
AHA: 4Q, '02, 70

795.39 Other nonspecific positive culture findings

795.4 Other nonspecific abnormal histological findings

795.5 Nonspecific reaction to tuberculin skin test without active tuberculosis
Abnormal result of Mantoux test
PPD positive
Tuberculin (skin test):
- positive
- reactor

795.6 False positive serological test for syphilis
False positive Wassermann reaction

795.7 Other nonspecific immunological findings
EXCLUDES
- ▶abnormal tumor markers (795.81-795.89)
- elevated prostate specific antigen [PSA] (790.93)
- elevated tumor associated antigens (795.81-795.89)◀
- isoimmunization, in pregnancy (656.1-656.2)
- affecting fetus or newborn (773.0-773.2)

AHA: 2Q, '93, 6

795.71 Nonspecific serologic evidence of human immunodeficiency virus [HIV]
Inclusive human immunodeficiency [HIV] test (adult) (infant)

Note: This code is ONLY to be used when a test finding is reported as nonspecific. Asymptomatic positive findings are coded to V08. If any HIV infection symptom or condition is present, see code 042. Negative findings are not coded.

EXCLUDES
- acquired immunodeficiency syndrome [AIDS] (042)
- asymptomatic human immunodeficiency virus, [HIV] infection status (V08)
- HIV infection, symptomatic (042)
- human immunodeficiency virus [HIV] disease (042)
- positive (status) NOS (V08)

AHA: 2Q, '04, 11; 1Q, '93, 21; 1Q, '93, 22; 2Q, '92, 11; J-A, '87, 24

795.79 Other and unspecified nonspecific immunological findings
Raised antibody titer
Raised level of immunoglobulins

795.8 Abnormal tumor markers
Elevated tumor associated antigens [TAA]
Elevated tumor specific antigens [TSA]
EXCLUDES elevated prostate specific antigen [PSA] (790.93)

795.81 Elevated carcinoembryonic antigen [CEA]

795.82 Elevated cancer antigen 125 [CA 125]

795.89 Other abnormal tumor markers

796 Other nonspecific abnormal findings

796.0 Nonspecific abnormal toxicological findings
Abnormal levels of heavy metals or drugs in blood, urine, or other tissue
EXCLUDES excessive blood level of alcohol (790.3)
AHA: 1Q, '97, 16

SYMPTOMS, SIGNS, AND ILL-DEFINED CONDITIONS

796.1 Abnormal reflex

796.2 Elevated blood pressure reading without diagnosis of hypertension
> Note: This category is to be used to record an episode of elevated blood pressure in a patient in whom no formal diagnosis of hypertension has been made, or as an incidental finding.

AHA: 2Q, '03, 11; 3Q, '90, 4; J-A, '84, 12

796.3 Nonspecific low blood pressure reading

796.4 Other abnormal clinical findings
AHA: 1Q, '97, 16

796.5 Abnormal finding on antenatal screening
AHA: 4Q, '97, 46

796.6 Abnormal findings on neonatal screening
EXCLUDES: nonspecific serologic evidence of human immunodeficiency virus [HIV] (795.71)
AHA: 4Q, '04, 99

796.9 Other

ILL-DEFINED AND UNKNOWN CAUSES OF MORBIDITY AND MORTALITY (797-799)

797 Senility without mention of psychosis
Old age   Senile:
Senescence   debility
Senile asthenia exhaustion
EXCLUDES: senile psychoses (290.0-290.9)

798 Sudden death, cause unknown

798.0 Sudden infant death syndrome
Cot death   Sudden death of nonspecific
Crib death   cause in infancy
DEF: Sudden Infant Death Syndrome (SIDS): death of infant under age one due to nonspecific cause.

798.1 Instantaneous death

798.2 Death occurring in less than 24 hours from onset of symptoms, not otherwise explained
Death known not to be violent or instantaneous, for which no cause could be discovered
Died without sign of disease

798.9 Unattended death
Death in circumstances where the body of the deceased was found and no cause could be discovered
Found dead

799 Other ill-defined and unknown causes of morbidity and mortality
DEF: Weakened organ functions due to complex chronic medical conditions.

799.0 Asphyxia and hypoxemia
EXCLUDES: asphyxia and hypoxemia (due to):
carbon monoxide (986)
hypercapnia (786.09)
inhalation of food or foreign body (932-934.9)
newborn (768.0-768.9)
traumatic (994.7)

799.01 Asphyxia
AHA: 4Q, '05, 90
DEF: Lack of oxygen in inspired air, causing a deficiency of oxygen in tissues (hypoxia) and elevated levels of arterial carbon dioxide (hypercapnia).

799.02 Hypoxemia
AHA: 4Q, '05, 90
DEF: Deficient oxygenation of the blood.

799.1 Respiratory arrest
Cardiorespiratory failure
EXCLUDES: cardiac arrest (427.5)
failure of peripheral circulation (785.50)
respiratory distress:
NOS (786.09)
acute (518.82)
following trauma and surgery (518.5)
newborn (770.89)
syndrome (newborn) (769)
adult (following trauma and surgery) (518.5)
other (518.82)
respiratory failure (518.81, 518.83-518.84)
newborn (770.84)
respiratory insufficiency (786.09)
acute (518.82)

799.2 Nervousness
"Nerves"

799.3 Debility, unspecified
EXCLUDES: asthenia (780.79)
nervous debility (300.5)
neurasthenia (300.5)
senile asthenia (797)

799.4 Cachexia
Wasting disease
▶Code first underlying condition, if known◀
AHA: 3Q, '90, 17
DEF: General ill health and poor nutrition.

799.8 Other ill-defined conditions

799.81 Decreased libido
Decreased sexual desire
EXCLUDES: psychosexual dysfunction with inhibited sexual desire (302.71)
AHA: 4Q, '03, 75

799.89 Other ill-defined conditions
DEF: General ill health and poor nutrition.

799.9 Other unknown and unspecified cause
Undiagnosed disease, not specified as to site or system involved
Unknown cause of morbidity or mortality
AHA: 1Q, '98,.4; 1Q, '90, 20

17. INJURY AND POISONING (800-999)

Use E code(s) to identify the cause and intent of the injury or poisoning (E800-E999)

Note:

1. The principle of multiple coding of injuries should be followed wherever possible. Combination categories for multiple injuries are provided for use when there is insufficient detail as to the nature of the individual conditions, or for primary tabulation purposes when it is more convenient to record a single code; otherwise, the component injuries should be coded separately.

    Where multiple sites of injury are specified in the titles, the word "with" indicates involvement of both sites, and the word "and" indicates involvement of either or both sites. The word "finger" thumb.

2. Categories for "late effect" of injuries are to be found at 905-909.

FRACTURES (800-829)

EXCLUDES   malunion (733.81)
nonunion (733.82)
pathological or spontaneous fracture (733.10-733.19)
stress fractures (733.93-733.95)

The terms "condyle," "coronoid process," "ramus," and "symphysis" indicate the portion of the bone fractured, not the name of the bone involved.

The descriptions "closed" and "open" used in the fourth-digit subdivisions include the following terms:

closed (with or without delayed healing):
- comminuted
- depressed
- elevated
- fissured
- fracture NOS
- greenstick
- impacted
- linear
- simple
- slipped epiphysis
- spiral

open (with or without delayed healing):
- compound
- infected
- missile
- puncture
- with foreign body

A fracture not indicated as closed or open should be classified as closed.

AHA: 4Q, '90, 26; 3Q, '90, 5; 3Q, '90, 13; 2Q, '90, 7; 2Q, '89, 15, S-O, '85, 3

FRACTURE OF SKULL (800-804)

The following fifth-digit subclassification is for use with the appropriate codes in categories 800, 801, 803, and 804:

0 unspecified state of consciousness
1 with no loss of consciousness
2 with brief [less than one hour] loss of consciousness
3 with moderate [1-24 hours] loss of consciousness
4 with prolonged [more than 24 hours] loss of consciousness and return to pre-existing conscious level
5 with prolonged [more than 24 hours] loss of consciousness, without return to pre-existing conscious level
   Use fifth-digit 5 to designate when a patient is unconscious and dies before regaining consciousness, regardless of the duration of the loss of consciousness
6 with loss of consciousness of unspecified duration
9 with concussion, unspecified

- **800** Fracture of vault of skull
  - **INCLUDES**   frontal bone
    parietal bone

  AHA: 4Q, '96, 36

  DEF: Fracture of bone that forms skull dome and protects brain.

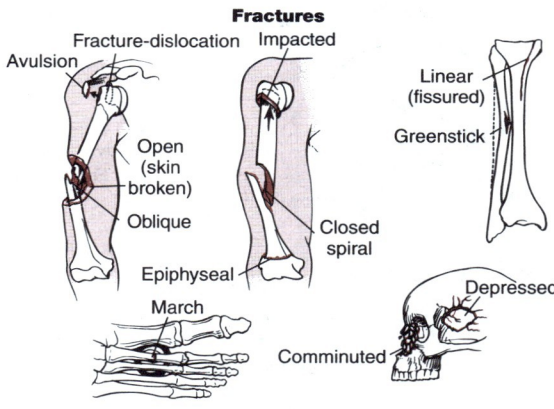

- 800.0 Closed without mention of intracranial injury
- 800.1 Closed with cerebral laceration and contusion
- 800.2 Closed with subarachnoid, subdural, and extradural hemorrhage
- 800.3 Closed with other and unspecified intracranial hemorrhage
- 800.4 Closed with intracranial injury of other and unspecified nature
- 800.5 Open without mention of intracranial injury
- 800.6 Open with cerebral laceration and contusion
- 800.7 Open with subarachnoid, subdural, and extradural hemorrhage
- 800.8 Open with other and unspecified intracranial hemorrhage
- 800.9 Open with intracranial injury of other and unspecified nature

- **801** Fracture of base of skull
  - **INCLUDES**   fossa:
    anterior
    middle
    posterior
    occiput bone
    orbital roof
    sinus:
    ethmoid
    frontal
    sphenoid bone
    temporal bone

  AHA: 4Q, '96, 36

  DEF: Fracture of bone that forms skull floor.

- 801.0 Closed without mention of intracranial injury
- 801.1 Closed with cerebral laceration and contusion
- 801.2 Closed with subarachnoid, subdural, and extradural hemorrhage
  AHA: 4Q, '96, 36
- 801.3 Closed with other and unspecified intracranial hemorrhage
- 801.4 Closed with intracranial injury of other and unspecified nature
- 801.5 Open without mention of intracranial injury
- 801.6 Open with cerebral laceration and contusion
- 801.7 Open with subarachnoid, subdural, and extradural hemorrhage
- 801.8 Open with other and unspecified intracranial hemorrhage
- 801.9 Open with intracranial injury of other and unspecified nature

- **802** Fracture of face bones
  AHA: 4Q, '96, 36

  - 802.0 Nasal bones, closed

INJURY AND POISONING

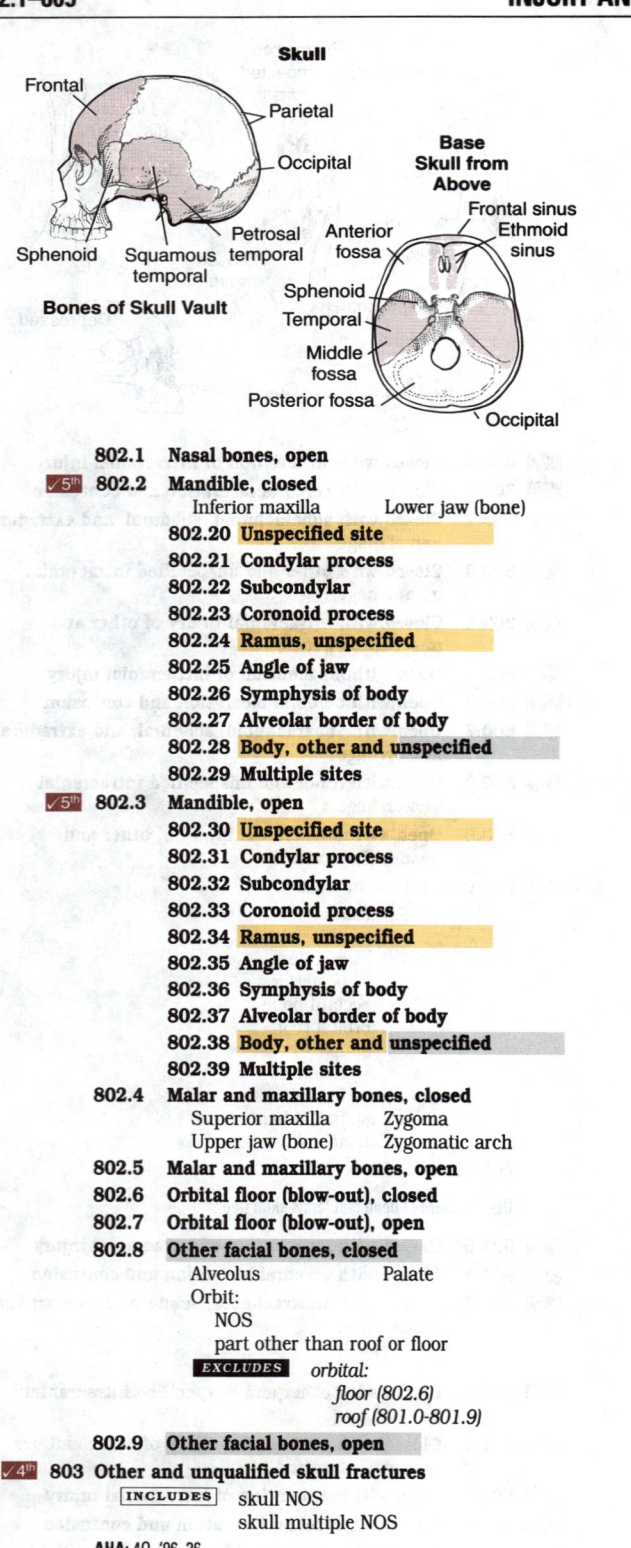

802.1 Nasal bones, open
√5th 802.2 Mandible, closed
    Inferior maxilla   Lower jaw (bone)
    802.20 Unspecified site
    802.21 Condylar process
    802.22 Subcondylar
    802.23 Coronoid process
    802.24 Ramus, unspecified
    802.25 Angle of jaw
    802.26 Symphysis of body
    802.27 Alveolar border of body
    802.28 Body, other and unspecified
    802.29 Multiple sites
√5th 802.3 Mandible, open
    802.30 Unspecified site
    802.31 Condylar process
    802.32 Subcondylar
    802.33 Coronoid process
    802.34 Ramus, unspecified
    802.35 Angle of jaw
    802.36 Symphysis of body
    802.37 Alveolar border of body
    802.38 Body, other and unspecified
    802.39 Multiple sites
802.4 Malar and maxillary bones, closed
    Superior maxilla   Zygoma
    Upper jaw (bone)   Zygomatic arch
802.5 Malar and maxillary bones, open
802.6 Orbital floor (blow-out), closed
802.7 Orbital floor (blow-out), open
802.8 Other facial bones, closed
    Alveolus   Palate
    Orbit:
      NOS
      part other than roof or floor
    EXCLUDES orbital:
        floor (802.6)
        roof (801.0-801.9)
802.9 Other facial bones, open
√4th 803 Other and unqualified skull fractures
    INCLUDES skull NOS
        skull multiple NOS
    AHA: 4Q, '96, 36
§ √5th 803.0 Closed without mention of intracranial injury
§ √5th 803.1 Closed with cerebral laceration and contusion
§ √5th 803.2 Closed with subarachnoid, subdural, and extradural hemorrhage
§ √5th 803.3 Closed with other and unspecified intracranial hemorrhage
§ √5th 803.4 Closed with intracranial injury of other and unspecified nature
§ √5th 803.5 Open without mention of intracranial injury
§ √5th 803.6 Open with cerebral laceration and contusion
§ √5th 803.7 Open with subarachnoid, subdural, and extradural hemorrhage
§ √5th 803.8 Open with other and unspecified intracranial hemorrhage
§ √5th 803.9 Open with intracranial injury of other and unspecified nature
√4th 804 Multiple fractures involving skull or face with other bones
    AHA: 4Q, '96, 36
§ √5th 804.0 Closed without mention of intracranial injury
§ √5th 804.1 Closed with cerebral laceration and contusion
§ √5th 804.2 Closed with subarachnoid, subdural, and extradural hemorrhage
§ √5th 804.3 Closed with other and unspecified intracranial hemorrhage
§ √5th 804.4 Closed with intracranial injury of other and unspecified nature
§ √5th 804.5 Open without mention of intracranial injury
§ √5th 804.6 Open with cerebral laceration and contusion
§ √5th 804.7 Open with subarachnoid, subdural, and extradural hemorrage
§ √5th 804.8 Open with other and unspecified intracranial hemorrhage
§ √5th 804.9 Open with intracranial injury of other and unspecified nature

FRACTURE OF NECK AND TRUNK (805-809)

√4th 805 Fracture of vertebral column without mention of spinal cord injury
    INCLUDES   neural arch
        spine
        spinous process
        transverse process
        vertebra

The following fifth-digit subclassification is for use with codes 805.0-805.1:
    0 cervical vertebra, unspecified level
    1 first cervical vertebra
    2 second cervical vertebra
    3 third cervical vertebra
    4 fourth cervical vertebra
    5 fifth cervical vertebra
    6 sixth cervical vertebra
    7 seventh cervical vertebra
    8 multiple cervical vertebrae

§ Requires fifth-digit. See beginning of section 800-804 for codes and definitions.

N Newborn Age: 0   P Pediatric Age: 0-17   M Maternity Age: 12-55   A Adult Age: 15-124

Tabular List — INJURY AND POISONING

§5th 805.0 Cervical, closed
  Atlas   Axis
§5th 805.1 Cervical, open
   805.2 Dorsal [thoracic], closed
   805.3 Dorsal [thoracic], open
   805.4 Lumbar, closed
     AHA: 4Q, '99, 12
   805.5 Lumbar, open
   805.6 Sacrum and coccyx, closed
   805.7 Sacrum and coccyx, open
   805.8 Unspecified, closed
   805.9 Unspecified, open

§4th 806 **Fracture of vertebral column with spinal cord injury**
   INCLUDES   any condition classifiable to 805 with:
        complete or incomplete transverse lesion (of cord)
        hematomyelia
        injury to:
          cauda equina
          nerve
        paralysis
        paraplegia
        quadriplegia
        spinal concussion

§5th 806.0 Cervical, closed
   806.00 C_1-C_4 level with unspecified spinal cord injury
     Cervical region NOS with spinal cord injury NOS
   806.01 C_1-C_4 level with complete lesion of cord
   806.02 C_1-C_4 level with anterior cord syndrome
   806.03 C_1-C_4 level with central cord syndrome
   806.04 C_1-C_4 level with other specified spinal cord injury
     C_1-C_4 level with:
       incomplete spinal cord lesion NOS
       posterior cord syndrome
   806.05 C_5-C_7 level with unspecified spinal cord injury
   806.06 C_5-C_7 level with complete lesion of cord
   806.07 C_5-C_7 level with anterior cord syndrome
   806.08 C_5-C_7 level with central cord syndrome
   806.09 C_5-C_7 level with other specified spinal cord injury
     C_5-C_7 level with:
       incomplete spinal cord lesion NOS
       posterior cord syndrome

§5th 806.1 Cervical, open
   806.10 C_1-C_4 level with unspecified spinal cord injury
   806.11 C_1-C_4 level with complete lesion of cord
   806.12 C_1-C_4 level with anterior cord syndrome
   806.13 C_1-C_4 level with central cord syndrome
   806.14 C_1-C_4 level with other specified spinal cord injury
     C_1-C_4 level with:
       incomplete spinal cord lesion NOS
       posterior cord syndrome

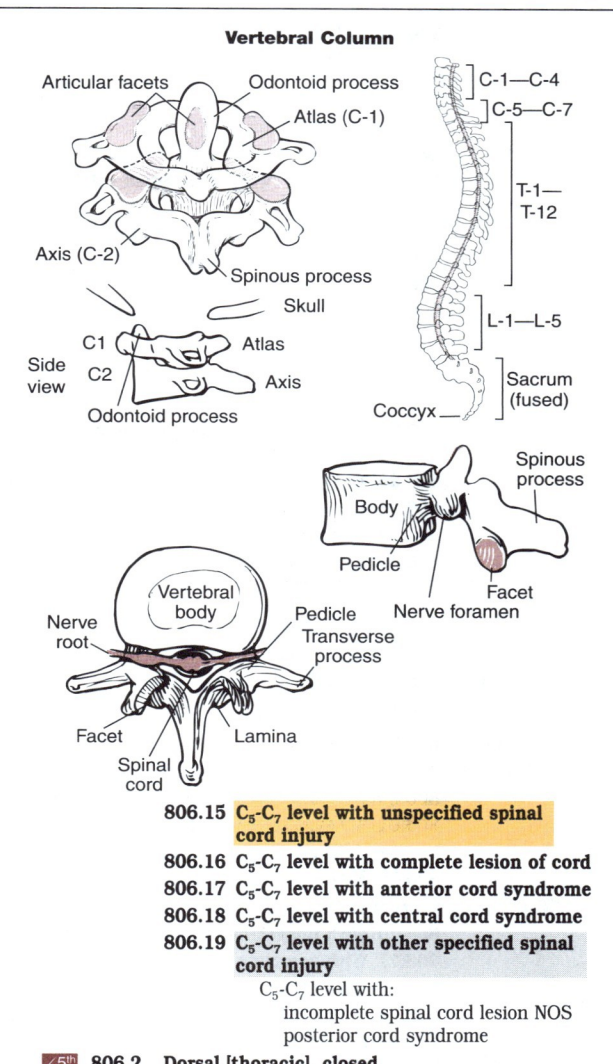

   806.15 C_5-C_7 level with unspecified spinal cord injury
   806.16 C_5-C_7 level with complete lesion of cord
   806.17 C_5-C_7 level with anterior cord syndrome
   806.18 C_5-C_7 level with central cord syndrome
   806.19 C_5-C_7 level with other specified spinal cord injury
     C_5-C_7 level with:
       incomplete spinal cord lesion NOS
       posterior cord syndrome

§5th 806.2 Dorsal [thoracic], closed
   806.20 T_1-T_6 level with unspecified spinal cord injury
     Thoracic region NOS with spinal cord injury NOS
   806.21 T_1-T_6 level with complete lesion of cord
   806.22 T_1-T_6 level with anterior cord syndrome
   806.23 T_1-T_6 level with central cord syndrome
   806.24 T_1-T_6 level with other specified spinal cord injury
     T_1-T_6 level with:
       incomplete spinal cord lesion NOS
       posterior cord syndrome
   806.25 T_7-T_{12} level with unspecified spinal cord injury
   806.26 T_7-T_{12} level with complete lesion of cord
   806.27 T_7-T_{12} level with anterior cord syndrome
   806.28 T_7-T_{12} level with central cord syndrome

INJURY AND POISONING

806.29 T$_7$-T$_{12}$ level with other specified spinal cord injury
  T$_7$-T$_{12}$ level with:
    incomplete spinal cord lesion NOS
    posterior cord syndrome

√5th **806.3** Dorsal [thoracic], open
  806.30 T$_1$-T$_6$ level with unspecified spinal cord injury
  806.31 T$_1$-T$_6$ level with complete lesion of cord
  806.32 T$_1$-T$_6$ level with anterior cord syndrome
  806.33 T$_1$-T$_6$ level with central cord syndrome
  806.34 T$_1$-T$_6$ level with other specified spinal cord injury
    T$_1$-T$_6$ level with:
      incomplete spinal cord lesion NOS
      posterior cord syndrome
  806.35 T$_7$-T$_{12}$ level with unspecified spinal cord injury
  806.36 T$_7$-T$_{12}$ level with complete lesion of cord
  806.37 T$_7$-T$_{12}$ level with anterior cord syndrome
  806.38 T$_7$-T$_{12}$ level with central cord syndrome
  806.39 T$_7$-T$_{12}$ level with other specified spinal cord injury
    T$_7$-T$_{12}$ level with:
      incomplete spinal cord lesion NOS
      posterior cord syndrome

806.4 Lumbar, closed
  AHA: 4Q, '99, 11, 13

806.5 Lumbar, open

√5th **806.6** Sacrum and coccyx, closed
  806.60 With unspecified spinal cord injury
  806.61 With complete cauda equina lesion
  806.62 With other cauda equina injury
  806.69 With other spinal cord injury

√5th **806.7** Sacrum and coccyx, open
  806.70 With unspecified spinal cord injury
  806.71 With complete cauda equina lesion
  806.72 With other cauda equina injury
  806.79 With other spinal cord injury

806.8 Unspecified, closed
806.9 Unspecified, open

√4th **807** Fracture of rib(s), sternum, larynx, and trachea
  The following fifth-digit subclassification is for use with codes 807.0-807.1:
    0 rib(s), unspecified
    1 one rib
    2 two ribs
    3 three ribs
    4 four ribs
    5 five ribs
    6 six ribs
    7 seven ribs
    8 eight or more ribs
    9 multiple ribs, unspecified

√5th **807.0** Rib(s), closed
√5th **807.1** Rib(s), open
807.2 Sternum, closed
  DEF: Break in flat bone (breast bone) in anterior thorax.
807.3 Sternum, open
  DEF: Break, with open wound, in flat bone in mid anterior thorax.
807.4 Flail chest
807.5 Larynx and trachea, closed
  Hyoid bone   Trachea
  Thyroid cartilage
807.6 Larynx and trachea, open

√4th **808** Fracture of pelvis
  808.0 Acetabulum, closed
  808.1 Acetabulum, open
  808.2 Pubis, closed
  808.3 Pubis, open
  √5th **808.4** Other specified part, closed
    808.41 Ilium
    808.42 Ischium
    808.43 Multiple pelvic fractures with disruption of pelvic circle
    808.49 Other
      Innominate bone   Pelvic rim
  √5th **808.5** Other specified part, open
    808.51 Ilium
    808.52 Ischium
    808.53 Multiple pelvic fractures with disruption of pelvic circle
    808.59 Other
  808.8 Unspecified, closed
  808.9 Unspecified, open

√4th **809** Ill-defined fractures of bones of trunk
  INCLUDES bones of trunk with other bones except those of skull and face
    multiple bones of trunk
  EXCLUDES multiple fractures of:
    pelvic bones alone (808.0-808.9)
    ribs alone (807.0-807.1, 807.4)
    ribs or sternum with limb bones (819.0-819.1, 828.0-828.1)
    skull or face with other bones (804.0-804.9)

809.0 Fracture of bones of trunk, closed
809.1 Fracture of bones of trunk, open

FRACTURE OF UPPER LIMB (810-819)

√4th **810** Fracture of clavicle
  INCLUDES collar bone
    interligamentous part of clavicle
  The following fifth-digit subclassification is for use with category 810:
    0 unspecified part
      Clavicle NOS
    1 sternal end of clavicle
    2 shaft of clavicle
    3 acromial end of clavicle

√5th **810.0** Closed
√5th **810.1** Open

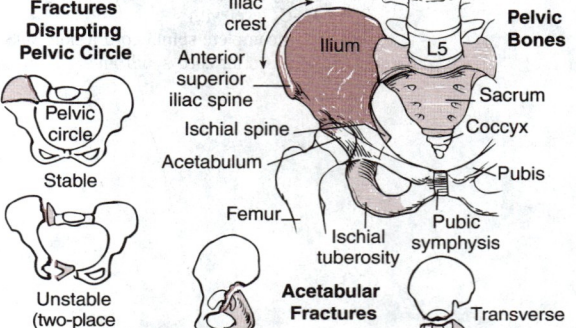

Pelvis and Pelvic Fractures
Fractures Disrupting Pelvic Circle — Pelvic circle — Stable — Unstable (two-place fracture)
Iliac crest — Ilium — L5 — Anterior superior iliac spine — Sacrum — Ischial spine — Coccyx — Acetabulum — Pubis — Femur — Ischial tuberosity — Pubic symphysis — Pelvic Bones
Acetabular Fractures — Posterior pillar — Transverse

INJURY AND POISONING

811 Fracture of scapula
INCLUDES shoulder blade

The following fifth-digit subclassification is for use with category 811:
- 0 unspecified part
- 1 acromial process
    - Acromion (process)
- 2 coracoid process
- 3 glenoid cavity and neck of scapula
- 9 other

- 811.0 Closed
- 811.1 Open

812 Fracture of humerus

- 812.0 Upper end, closed
    - 812.00 Upper end, unspecified part
        - Proximal end   Shoulder
    - 812.01 Surgical neck
        - Neck of humerus NOS
    - 812.02 Anatomical neck
    - 812.03 Greater tuberosity
    - 812.09 Other
        - Head   Upper epiphysis
        - Lesser tuberosity

- 812.1 Upper end, open
    - 812.10 Upper end, unspecified part
    - 812.11 Surgical neck
    - 812.12 Anatomical neck
    - 812.13 Greater tuberosity
    - 812.19 Other

- 812.2 Shaft or unspecified part, closed
    - 812.20 Unspecified part of humerus
        - Humerus NOS   Upper arm NOS
    - 812.21 Shaft of humerus
        - AHA: ▶4Q, '05, 129;◀ 3Q, '99, 14

- 812.3 Shaft or unspecified part, open
    - 812.30 Unspecified part of humerus
    - 812.31 Shaft of humerus

- 812.4 Lower end, closed
    - Distal end of humerus
    - Elbow
    - 812.40 Lower end, unspecified part
    - 812.41 Supracondylar fracture of humerus
    - 812.42 Lateral condyle
        - External condyle
    - 812.43 Medial condyle
        - Internal epicondyle
    - 812.44 Condyle(s), unspecified
        - Articular process NOS
        - Lower epiphysis NOS
    - 812.49 Other
        - Multiple fractures of lower end
        - Trochlea

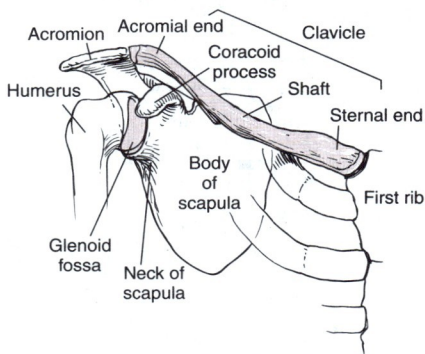

Right Clavicle and Scapula, Anterior View

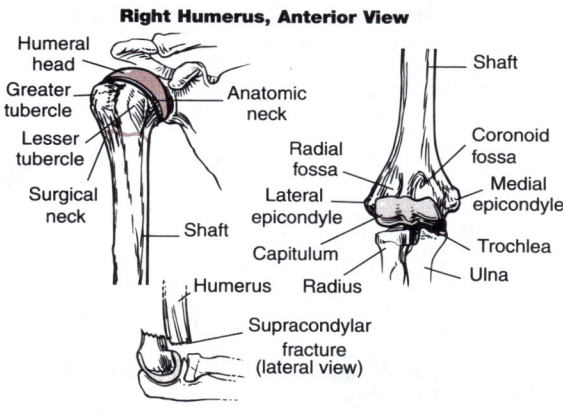

Right Humerus, Anterior View

- 812.5 Lower end, open
    - 812.50 Lower end, unspecified part
    - 812.51 Supracondylar fracture of humerus
    - 812.52 Lateral condyle
    - 812.53 Medial condyle
    - 812.54 Condyle(s), unspecified
    - 812.59 Other

813 Fracture of radius and ulna

- 813.0 Upper end, closed
    - Proximal end
    - 813.00 Upper end of forearm, unspecified
    - 813.01 Olecranon process of ulna
    - 813.02 Coronoid process of ulna
    - 813.03 Monteggia's fracture
        - DEF: Fracture near the head of the ulnar shaft, causing dislocation of the radial head.
    - 813.04 Other and unspecified fractures of proximal end of ulna (alone)
        - Multiple fractures of ulna, upper end
    - 813.05 Head of radius
    - 813.06 Neck of radius
    - 813.07 Other and unspecified fractures of proximal end of radius (alone)
        - Multiple fractures of radius, upper end
    - 813.08 Radius with ulna, upper end [any part]

- 813.1 Upper end, open
    - 813.10 Upper end of forearm, unspecified
    - 813.11 Olecranon process of ulna
    - 813.12 Coronoid process of ulna
    - 813.13 Monteggia's fracture
    - 813.14 Other and unspecified fractures of proximal end of ulna (alone)
    - 813.15 Head of radius
    - 813.16 Neck of radius
    - 813.17 Other and unspecified fractures of proximal end of radius (alone)
    - 813.18 Radius with ulna, upper end [any part]

- 813.2 Shaft, closed
    - 813.20 Shaft, unspecified
    - 813.21 Radius (alone)
    - 813.22 Ulna (alone)
    - 813.23 Radius with ulna

- 813.3 Shaft, open
    - 813.30 Shaft, unspecified
    - 813.31 Radius (alone)
    - 813.32 Ulna (alone)
    - 813.33 Radius with ulna

- 813.4 Lower end, closed
    - Distal end
    - 813.40 Lower end of forearm, unspecified

INJURY AND POISONING

Right Radius and Ulna, Anterior View

813.41 Colles' fracture
Smith's fracture
DEF: Break of lower end of radius; associated with backward movement of the radius lower section.

813.42 Other fractures of distal end of radius (alone)
Dupuytren's fracture, radius
Radius, lower end
DEF: Dupuytren's fracture: fracture and dislocation of the forearm; the fracture is of the radius above the wrist, and the dislocation is of the ulna at the lower end.

813.43 Distal end of ulna (alone)
Ulna: Ulna:
 head   lower epiphysis
 lower end styloid process

813.44 Radius with ulna, lower end

813.45 Torus fracture of radius
AHA: 4Q, '02, 70

√5th **813.5 Lower end, open**
813.50 Lower end of forearm, unspecified
813.51 Colles' fracture
813.52 Other fractures of distal end of radius (alone)
813.53 Distal end of ulna (alone)
813.54 Radius with ulna, lower end

√5th **813.8 Unspecified part, closed**
813.80 Forearm, unspecified
813.81 Radius (alone)
AHA: 2Q, '98, 19
813.82 Ulna (alone)
813.83 Radius with ulna

√5th **813.9 Unspecified part, open**
813.90 Forearm, unspecified
813.91 Radius (alone)
813.92 Ulna (alone)
813.93 Radius with ulna

√4th **814 Fracture of carpal bone(s)**
The following fifth-digit subclassification is for use with category 814:
0 carpal bone, unspecified
  Wrist NOS
1 navicular [scaphoid] of wrist
2 lunate [semilunar] bone of wrist
3 triquetral [cuneiform] bone of wrist
4 pisiform
5 trapezium bone [larger multangular]
6 trapezoid bone [smaller multangular]
7 capitate bone [os magnum]
8 hamate [unciform] bone
9 other

√5th 814.0 Closed
√5th 814.1 Open

√4th **815 Fracture of metacarpal bone(s)**
INCLUDES: hand [except finger]
          metacarpus
The following fifth-digit subclassification is for use with category 815:
0 metacarpal bone(s), site unspecified
1 base of thumb [first] metacarpal
  Bennett's fracture
2 base of other metacarpal bone(s)
3 shaft of metacarpal bone(s)
4 neck of metacarpal bone(s)
9 multiple sites of metacarpus

√5th 815.0 Closed
√5th 815.1 Open

√4th **816 Fracture of one or more phalanges of hand**
INCLUDES: finger(s) thumb
The following fifth-digit subclassification is for use with category 816:
0 phalanx or phalanges, unspecified
1 middle or proximal phalanx or phalanges
2 distal phalanx or phalanges
3 multiple sites

√5th 816.0 Closed
√5th 816.1 Open
AHA: For code 816.12: 4Q, '03, 77

√4th **817 Multiple fractures of hand bones**
INCLUDES: metacarpal bone(s) with phalanx or phalanges of same hand
817.0 Closed
817.1 Open

√4th **818 Ill-defined fractures of upper limb**
INCLUDES: arm NOS
          multiple bones of same upper limb
EXCLUDES: multiple fractures of:
            metacarpal bone(s) with phalanx or phalanges (817.0-817.1)
            phalanges of hand alone (816.0-816.1)
            radius with ulna (813.0-813.9)
818.0 Closed
818.1 Open

√4th **819 Multiple fractures involving both upper limbs, and upper limb with rib(s) and sternum**
INCLUDES: arm(s) with rib(s) or sternum
          both arms [any bones]
819.0 Closed
819.1 Open

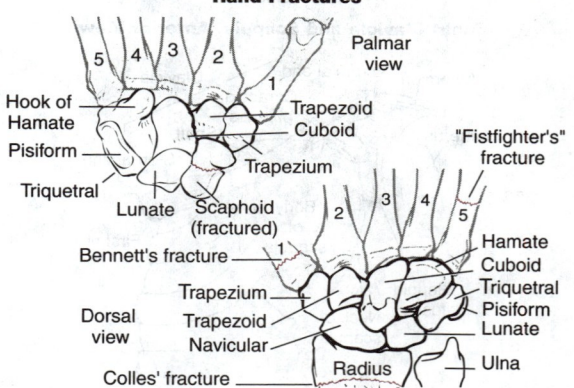
Hand Fractures

FRACTURE OF LOWER LIMB (820-829)

✓4th 820 Fracture of neck of femur
  ✓5th 820.0 Transcervical fracture, closed
    820.00 Intracapsular section, unspecified
    820.01 Epiphysis (separation) (upper)
      Transepiphyseal
    820.02 Midcervical section
      Transcervical NOS
      AHA: 3Q, '03, 12
    820.03 Base of neck
      Cervicotrochanteric section
    820.09 Other
      Head of femur   Subcapital
  ✓5th 820.1 Transcervical fracture, open
    820.10 Intracapsular section, unspecified
    820.11 Epiphysis (separation) (upper)
    820.12 Midcervical section
    820.13 Base of neck
    820.19 Other
  ✓5th 820.2 Pertrochanteric fracture, closed
    820.20 Trochanteric section, unspecified
      Trochanter: NOS   Trochanter: lesser
      greater
    820.21 Intertrochanteric section
    820.22 Subtrochanteric section
  ✓5th 820.3 Pertrochanteric fracture, open
    820.30 Trochanteric section, unspecified
    820.31 Intertrochanteric section
    820.32 Subtrochanteric section
  820.8 Unspecified part of neck of femur, closed
    Hip NOS   Neck of femur NOS
  820.9 Unspecified part of neck of femur, open

✓4th 821 Fracture of other and unspecified parts of femur
  ✓5th 821.0 Shaft or unspecified part, closed
    821.00 Unspecified part of femur
      Thigh   Upper leg
      EXCLUDES   hip NOS (820.8)
    821.01 Shaft
      AHA: 1Q, '99, 5
  ✓5th 821.1 Shaft or unspecified part, open
    821.10 Unspecified part of femur
    821.11 Shaft
  ✓5th 821.2 Lower end, closed
    Distal end
    821.20 Lower end, unspecified part
    821.21 Condyle, femoral
    821.22 Epiphysis, lower (separation)
    821.23 Supracondylar fracture of femur
      Multiple fractures of lower end
    821.29 Other
      Multiple fractures of lower end
  ✓5th 821.3 Lower end, open
    821.30 Lower end, unspecified part
    821.31 Condyle, femoral
    821.32 Epiphysis, lower (separation)
    821.33 Supracondylar fracture of femur
    821.39 Other

✓4th 822 Fracture of patella
  822.0 Closed
  822.1 Open

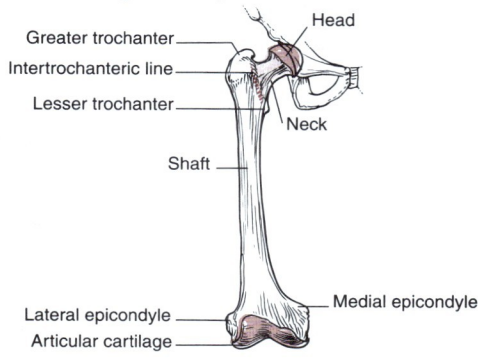

Right Femur, Anterior View

✓4th 823 Fracture of tibia and fibula
  EXCLUDES   Dupuytren's fracture (824.4-824.5)
    ankle (824.4-824.5)
    radius (813.42, 813.52)
    Pott's fracture (824.4-824.5)
    that involving ankle (824.0-824.9)

The following fifth-digit subclassification is for use with category 823:
  0 tibia alone
  1 fibula alone
  2 fibula with tibia

  ✓5th 823.0 Upper end, closed
    Head   Tibia:
    Proximal end   condyles
       tuberosity
  ✓5th 823.1 Upper end, open
  ✓5th 823.2 Shaft, closed
  ✓5th 823.3 Shaft, open
  ✓5th 823.4 Torus fracture
    DEF: A bone deformity in children, occurring commonly in the tibia and fibula, in which the bone bends and buckles but does not fracture.
    AHA: 4Q, '02, 70
  ✓5th 823.8 Unspecified part, closed
    Lower leg NOS
    AHA: For code 823.82: 1Q, '97, 8
  ✓5th 823.9 Unspecified part, open

✓4th 824 Fracture of ankle
  824.0 Medial malleolus, closed
    Tibia involving: Tibia involving:
      ankle   malleolus
    AHA: 1Q, '04, 9
  824.1 Medial malleolus, open
  824.2 Lateral malleolus, closed
    Fibula involving: Fibula involving:
      ankle   malleolus
    AHA: 2Q, '02, 3

Torus Fracture

INJURY AND POISONING

824.3 Lateral malleolus, open
824.4 Bimalleolar, closed
 Dupuytren's fracture, fibula   Pott's fracture
 DEF: Bimalleolar, closed: Breaking of both nodules (malleoli) on either side of ankle joint, without an open wound.
 DEF: Dupuytren's fracture (Pott's fracture): The breaking of the farthest end of the lower leg bone (fibula), with injury to the farthest end joint of the other lower leg bone (tibia).
824.5 Bimalleolar, open
824.6 Trimalleolar, closed
 Lateral and medial malleolus with anterior or posterior lip of tibia
824.7 Trimalleolar, open
824.8 Unspecified, closed
 Ankle NOS
 AHA: 3Q, '00, 12
824.9 Unspecified, open

√4th **825** Fracture of one or more tarsal and metatarsal bones
 825.0 Fracture of calcaneus, closed
  Heel bone   Os calcis
 825.1 Fracture of calcaneus, open
 √5th **825.2** Fracture of other tarsal and metatarsal bones, closed
  825.20 Unspecified bone(s) of foot [except toes]
   Instep
  825.21 Astragalus
   Talus
  825.22 Navicular [scaphoid], foot
  825.23 Cuboid
  825.24 Cuneiform, foot
  825.25 Metatarsal bone(s)
  825.29 Other
   Tarsal with metatarsal bone(s) only
   EXCLUDES calcaneus (825.0)
 √5th **825.3** Fracture of other tarsal and metatarsal bones, open
  825.30 Unspecified bone(s) of foot [except toes]
  825.31 Astragalus
  825.32 Navicular [scaphoid], foot
  825.33 Cuboid
  825.34 Cuneiform, foot
  825.35 Metatarsal bone(s)
  825.39 Other

√4th **826** Fracture of one or more phalanges of foot
 INCLUDES toe(s)
 826.0 Closed
 826.1 Open

√4th **827** Other, multiple, and ill-defined fractures of lower limb
 INCLUDES leg NOS
  multiple bones of same lower limb
 EXCLUDES multiple fractures of:
  ankle bones alone (824.4-824.9)
  phalanges of foot alone (826.0-826.1)
  tarsal with metatarsal bones (825.29, 825.39)
  tibia with fibula (823.0-823.9 with fifth-digit 2)
 827.0 Closed
 827.1 Open

√4th **828** Multiple fractures involving both lower limbs, lower with upper limb, and lower limb(s) with rib(s) and sternum
 INCLUDES arm(s) with leg(s) [any bones]
  both legs [any bones]
  leg(s) with rib(s) or sternum
 828.0 Closed
 828.1 Open

√4th **829** Fracture of unspecified bones
 829.0 Unspecified bone, closed
 829.1 Unspecified bone, open

DISLOCATION (830-839)

 INCLUDES displacement
  subluxation
 EXCLUDES congenital dislocation (754.0-755.8)
  pathological dislocation (718.2)
  recurrent dislocation (718.3)

The descriptions "closed" and "open," used in the fourth-digit subdivisions, include the following terms:
 closed: open:
  complete   compound
  dislocation NOS   infected
  partial   with foreign body
  simple
  uncomplicated

A dislocation not indicated as closed or open should be classified as closed.

AHA: 3Q, '90, 12

√4th **830** Dislocation of jaw
 INCLUDES jaw (cartilage) (meniscus)
  mandible
  maxilla (inferior)
  temporomandibular (joint)
 830.0 Closed dislocation
 830.1 Open dislocation

INJURY AND POISONING

✓4th 831 Dislocation of shoulder

> EXCLUDES   sternoclavicular joint (839.61, 839.71)
> sternum (839.61, 839.71)

The following fifth-digit subclassification is for use with category 831:

- 0 shoulder, unspecified
  Humerus NOS
- 1 anterior dislocation of humerus
- 2 posterior dislocation of humerus
- 3 inferior dislocation of humerus
- 4 acromioclavicular (joint)
  Clavicle
- 9 other
  Scapula

- ✓5th 831.0 Closed dislocation
- ✓5th 831.1 Open dislocation

✓4th 832 Dislocation of elbow

The following fifth-digit subclassification is for use with category 832:

- 0 elbow unspecified
- 1 anterior dislocation of elbow
- 2 posterior dislocation of elbow
- 3 medial dislocation of elbow
- 4 lateral dislocation of elbow
- 9 other

- ✓5th 832.0 Closed dislocation
- ✓5th 832.1 Open dislocation

✓4th 833 Dislocation of wrist

The following fifth-digit subclassification is for use with category 833:

- 0 wrist, unspecified part
  Carpal (bone)
  Radius, distal end
- 1 radioulnar (joint), distal
- 2 radiocarpal (joint)
- 3 midcarpal (joint)
- 4 carpometacarpal (joint)
- 5 metacarpal (bone), proximal end
- 9 other
  Ulna, distal end

- ✓5th 833.0 Closed dislocation
- ✓5th 833.1 Open dislocation

✓4th 834 Dislocation of finger

> INCLUDES   finger(s)
> phalanx of hand
> thumb

The following fifth-digit subclassification is for use with category 834:

- 0 finger, unspecified part
- 1 metacarpophalangeal (joint)
  Metacarpal (bone), distal end
- 2 interphalangeal (joint), hand

- ✓5th 834.0 Closed dislocation
- ✓5th 834.1 Open dislocation

✓4th 835 Dislocation of hip

The following fifth-digit subclassification is for use with category 835:

- 0 dislocation of hip, unspecified
- 1 posterior dislocation
- 2 obturator dislocation
- 3 other anterior dislocation

- ✓5th 835.0 Closed dislocation
- ✓5th 835.1 Open dislocation

✓4th 836 Dislocation of knee

> EXCLUDES   dislocation of knee:
> old or pathological (718.2)
> recurrent (718.3)
> internal derangement of knee joint (717.0-717.5, 717.8-717.9)
> old tear of cartilage or meniscus of knee (717.0-717.5, 717.8-717.9)

- 836.0 Tear of medial cartilage or meniscus of knee, current
  Bucket handle tear:
  NOS } current injury
  medial meniscus
- 836.1 Tear of lateral cartilage or meniscus of knee, current
- 836.2 Other tear of cartilage or meniscus of knee, current
  Tear of:
  cartilage (semilunar) } current injury, not specified as medial or lateral
  meniscus
- 836.3 Dislocation of patella, closed
- 836.4 Dislocation of patella, open
- ✓5th 836.5 Other dislocation of knee, closed
  - 836.50 Dislocation of knee, unspecified
  - 836.51 Anterior dislocation of tibia, proximal end
    Posterior dislocation of femur, distal end
  - 836.52 Posterior dislocation of tibia, proximal end
    Anterior dislocation of femur, distal end
  - 836.53 Medial dislocation of tibia, proximal end
  - 836.54 Lateral dislocation of tibia, proximal end
  - 836.59 Other
- ✓5th 836.6 Other dislocation of knee, open
  - 836.60 Dislocation of knee, unspecified
  - 836.61 Anterior dislocation of tibia, proximal end
  - 836.62 Posterior dislocation of tibia, proximal end
  - 836.63 Medial dislocation of tibia, proximal end
  - 836.64 Lateral dislocation of tibia, proximal end
  - 836.69 Other

✓4th 837 Dislocation of ankle

> INCLUDES   astragalus
> fibula, distal end
> navicular, foot
> scaphoid, foot
> tibia, distal end

- 837.0 Closed dislocation
- 837.1 Open dislocation

✓4th 838 Dislocation of foot

The following fifth-digit subclassification is for use with category 838:

- 0 foot, unspecified
- 1 tarsal (bone), joint unspecified
- 2 midtarsal (joint)
- 3 tarsometatarsal (joint)
- 4 metatarsal (bone), joint unspecified
- 5 metatarsophalangeal (joint)
- 6 interphalangeal (joint), foot
- 9 other
  Phalanx of foot
  Toe(s)

- ✓5th 838.0 Closed dislocation
- ✓5th 838.1 Open dislocation

✓4th 839 Other, multiple, and ill-defined dislocations

- ✓5th 839.0 Cervical vertebra, closed
  Cervical spine   Neck
  - 839.00 Cervical vertebra, unspecified
  - 839.01 First cervical vertebra

INJURY AND POISONING

839.02 Second cervical vertebra
839.03 Third cervical vertebra
839.04 Fourth cervical vertebra
839.05 Fifth cervical vertebra
839.06 Sixth cervical vertebra
839.07 Seventh cervical vertebra
839.08 Multiple cervical vertebrae

√5th 839.1 Cervical vertebra, open
839.10 Cervical vertebra, unspecified
839.11 First cervical vertebra
839.12 Second cervical vertebra
839.13 Third cervical vertebra
839.14 Fourth cervical vertebra
839.15 Fifth cervical vertebra
839.16 Sixth cervical vertebra
839.17 Seventh cervical vertebra
839.18 Multiple cervical vertebrae

√5th 839.2 Thoracic and lumbar vertebra, closed
839.20 Lumbar vertebra
839.21 Thoracic vertebra
Dorsal [thoracic] vertebra

√5th 839.3 Thoracic and lumbar vertebra, open
839.30 Lumbar vertebra
839.31 Thoracic vertebra

√5th 839.4 Other vertebra, closed
839.40 Vertebra, unspecified site
Spine NOS
839.41 Coccyx
839.42 Sacrum
Sacroiliac (joint)
839.49 Other

√5th 839.5 Other vertebra, open
839.50 Vertebra, unspecified site
839.51 Coccyx
839.52 Sacrum
839.59 Other

√5th 839.6 Other location, closed
839.61 Sternum
Sternoclavicular joint
839.69 Other
Pelvis

√5th 839.7 Other location, open
839.71 Sternum
839.79 Other

839.8 Multiple and ill-defined, closed
Arm
Back
Hand
Multiple locations, except fingers or toes alone
Other ill-defined locations
Unspecified location

839.9 Multiple and ill-defined, open

SPRAINS AND STRAINS OF JOINTS AND ADJACENT MUSCLES (840-848)

INCLUDES: avulsion, hemarthrosis, laceration, rupture, sprain, strain, tear of: joint capsule, ligament, muscle, tendon

EXCLUDES: laceration of tendon in open wounds (880-884 and 890-894 with .2)

√4th 840 Sprains and strains of shoulder and upper arm
840.0 Acromioclavicular (joint) (ligament)
840.1 Coracoclavicular (ligament)
840.2 Coracohumeral (ligament)
840.3 Infraspinatus (muscle) (tendon)
840.4 Rotator cuff (capsule)
EXCLUDES: complete rupture of rotator cuff, nontraumatic (727.61)
840.5 Subscapularis (muscle)
840.6 Supraspinatus (muscle) (tendon)
840.7 Superior glenoid labrum lesion
SLAP lesion
AHA: 4Q, '01, 52
DEF: Detachment injury of the superior aspect of the glenoid labrum which is the ring of fibrocartilage attached to the rim of the glenoid cavity of the scapula.
840.8 Other specified sites of shoulder and upper arm
840.9 Unspecified site of shoulder and upper arm
Arm NOS
Shoulder NOS

√4th 841 Sprains and strains of elbow and forearm
841.0 Radial collateral ligament
841.1 Ulnar collateral ligament
841.2 Radiohumeral (joint)
841.3 Ulnohumeral (joint)
841.8 Other specified sites of elbow and forearm
841.9 Unspecified site of elbow and forearm
Elbow NOS

√4th 842 Sprains and strains of wrist and hand
√5th 842.0 Wrist
842.00 Unspecified site
842.01 Carpal (joint)
842.02 Radiocarpal (joint) (ligament)
842.09 Other
Radioulnar joint, distal
√5th 842.1 Hand
842.10 Unspecified site
842.11 Carpometacarpal (joint)
842.12 Metacarpophalangeal (joint)
842.13 Interphalangeal (joint)
842.19 Other
Midcarpal (joint)

√4th 843 Sprains and strains of hip and thigh
843.0 Iliofemoral (ligament)
843.1 Ischiocapsular (ligament)
843.8 Other specified sites of hip and thigh
843.9 Unspecified site of hip and thigh
Hip NOS
Thigh NOS

√4th 844 Sprains and strains of knee and leg
844.0 Lateral collateral ligament of knee
844.1 Medial collateral ligament of knee
844.2 Cruciate ligament of knee
844.3 Tibiofibular (joint) (ligament), superior
844.8 Other specified sites of knee and leg
844.9 Unspecified site of knee and leg
Knee NOS   Leg NOS

√4th 845 Sprains and strains of ankle and foot
√5th 845.0 Ankle
845.00 Unspecified site
AHA: 2Q, '02, 3
845.01 Deltoid (ligament), ankle
Internal collateral (ligament), ankle
845.02 Calcaneofibular (ligament)
845.03 Tibiofibular (ligament), distal
AHA: 1Q, '04, 9
845.09 Other
Achilles tendon

 Pediatric Age: 0-17   Maternity Age: 12-55   Adult Age: 15-124

INJURY AND POISONING

✓5th **845.1 Foot**
- 845.10 Unspecified site
- 845.11 Tarsometatarsal (joint) (ligament)
- 845.12 Metatarsophalangeal (joint)
- 845.13 Interphalangeal (joint), toe
- 845.19 Other

✓4th **846 Sprains and strains of sacroiliac region**
- 846.0 Lumbosacral (joint) (ligament)
- 846.1 Sacroiliac ligament
- 846.2 Sacrospinatus (ligament)
- 846.3 Sacrotuberous (ligament)
- 846.8 Other specified sites of sacroiliac region
- 846.9 Unspecified site of sacroiliac region

✓4th **847 Sprains and strains of other and unspecified parts of back**
  EXCLUDES lumbosacral (846.0)
- 847.0 Neck
    - Anterior longitudinal (ligament), cervical
    - Atlanto-axial (joints)
    - Atlanto-occipital (joints)
    - Whiplash injury
    - EXCLUDES neck injury NOS (959.0)
      thyroid region (848.2)
- 847.1 Thoracic
- 847.2 Lumbar
- 847.3 Sacrum
    - Sacrococcygeal (ligament)
- 847.4 Coccyx
- 847.9 Unspecified site of back
    - Back NOS

✓4th **848 Other and ill-defined sprains and strains**
- 848.0 Septal cartilage of nose
- 848.1 Jaw
    - Temporomandibular (joint) (ligament)
- 848.2 Thyroid region
    - Cricoarytenoid (joint) (ligament)
    - Cricothyroid (joint) (ligament)
    - Thyroid cartilage
- 848.3 Ribs
    - Chondrocostal (joint)
    - Costal cartilage
    } without mention of injury to sternum

✓5th **848.4 Sternum**
- 848.40 Unspecified site
- 848.41 Sternoclavicular (joint) (ligament)
- 848.42 Chondrosternal (joint)
- 848.49 Other
    - Xiphoid cartilage
- 848.5 Pelvis
    - Symphysis pubis
    - EXCLUDES that in childbirth (665.6)
- 848.8 Other specified sites of sprains and strains
- 848.9 Unspecified site of sprain and strain

INTRACRANIAL INJURY, EXCLUDING THOSE WITH SKULL FRACTURE (850-854)

EXCLUDES intracranial injury with skull fracture (800-801 and 803-804, except .0 and .5)
open wound of head without intracranial injury (870.0-873.9)
skull fracture alone (800-801 and 803-804 with .0, .5)

The description "with open intracranial wound," used in the fourth-digit subdivisions, those specified as open or with mention of infection or foreign body.

The following fifth-digit subclassification is for use with categories 851-854:

- 0 unspecified state of consciousness
- 1 with no loss of consciousness
- 2 with brief [less than one hour] loss of consciousness
- 3 with moderate [1-24 hours] loss of consciousness
- 4 with prolonged [more than 24 hours] loss of consciousness and return to pre-existing conscious level
- 5 with prolonged [more than 24 hours] loss of consciousness, without return to pre-existing conscious level
    - Use fifth-digit 5 to designate when a patient is unconscious and dies before regaining consciousness, regardless of the duration of the loss of consciousness
- 6 with loss of consciousness of unspecified duration
- 9 with concussion, unspecified

AHA: 1Q, '93, 22

✓4th **850 Concussion**
  INCLUDES commotio cerebri
  EXCLUDES concussion with:
    cerebral laceration or contusion (851.0-851.9)
    cerebral hemorrhage (852-853)
    head injury NOS (959.01)

AHA: 2Q, '96, 6; 4Q, '90, 24

- 850.0 With no loss of consciousness
    - Concussion with mental confusion or disorientation, without loss of consciousness

✓5th 850.1 With brief loss of consciousness
    - Loss of consciousness for less than one hour
    - AHA: 4Q, '03, 76; 1Q, '99, 10; 2Q, '92, 5

    - 850.11 With loss of consciousness of 30 minutes or less
    - 850.12 With loss of consciousness from 31 to 59 minutes

- 850.2 With moderate loss of consciousness
    - Loss of consciousness for 1-24 hours
- 850.3 With prolonged loss of consciousness and return to pre-existing conscious level
    - Loss of consciousness for more than 24 hours with complete recovery
- 850.4 With prolonged loss of consciousness, without return to pre-existing conscious level
- 850.5 With loss of consciousness of unspecified duration
- 850.9 Concussion, unspecified

✓4th **851 Cerebral laceration and contusion**
AHA: 4Q, '96, 36; 1Q, '93, 22; 4Q, '90, 24

✓5th 851.0 Cortex (cerebral) contusion without mention of open intracranial wound

✓5th 851.1 Cortex (cerebral) contusion with open intracranial wound
AHA: 1Q, '92, 9

851.2–861.0   INJURY AND POISONING   Tabular List

§ ✓5th 851.2 Cortex (cerebral) laceration without mention of open intracranial wound

§ ✓5th 851.3 Cortex (cerebral) laceration with open intracranial wound

§ ✓5th 851.4 Cerebellar or brain stem contusion without mention of open intracranial wound

§ ✓5th 851.5 Cerebellar or brain stem contusion with open intracranial wound

§ ✓5th 851.6 Cerebellar or brain stem laceration without mention of open intracranial wound

§ ✓5th 851.7 Cerebellar or brain stem laceration with open intracranial wound

§ ✓5th 851.8 **Other and unspecified cerebral laceration and contusion, without mention of open intracranial wound**
- Brain (membrane) NOS
- AHA: 4Q, '96, 37

§ ✓5th 851.9 **Other and unspecified cerebral laceration and contusion, with open intracranial wound**

✓4th 852 Subarachnoid, subdural, and extradural hemorrhage, following injury
- EXCLUDES cerebral contusion or laceration (with hemorrhage) (851.0-851.9)
- DEF: Bleeding from lining of brain; due to injury.

§ ✓5th 852.0 Subarachnoid hemorrhage following injury without mention of open intracranial wound
- Middle meningeal hemorrhage following injury

§ ✓5th 852.1 Subarachnoid hemorrhage following injury with open intracranial wound

§ ✓5th 852.2 Subdural hemorrhage following injury without mention of open intracranial wound
- AHA: 4Q, '96, 43

§ ✓5th 852.3 Subdural hemorrhage following injury with open intracranial wound

§ ✓5th 852.4 Extradural hemorrhage following injury without mention of open intracranial wound
- Epidural hematoma following injury

§ ✓5th 852.5 Extradural hemorrhage following injury with open intracranial wound

✓4th 853 Other and unspecified intracranial hemorrhage following injury

§ ✓5th 853.0 **Without mention of open intracranial wound**
- Cerebral compression due to injury
- Intracranial hematoma following injury
- Traumatic cerebral hemorrhage
- AHA: 3Q, '90, 14

§ ✓5th 853.1 **With open intracranial wound**

✓4th 854 Intracranial injury of other and unspecified nature
- INCLUDES brain injury NOS
  - cavernous sinus
  - intracranial injury
- EXCLUDES any condition classifiable to 850-853
  - head injury NOS (959.01)
- AHA: 1Q, '99, 10; 2Q, '92, 6

§ ✓5th 854.0 **Without mention of open intracranial wound**
- AHA: For code 854.00: ▶2Q, '05, 6◀

§ ✓5th 854.1 **With open intracranial wound**

INTERNAL INJURY OF THORAX, ABDOMEN, AND PELVIS (860-869)

INCLUDES blast injuries
- blunt trauma
- bruise
- concussion injuries (except cerebral)
- crushing
- hematoma
- laceration
- puncture
- tear
- traumatic rupture

} of internal organs

EXCLUDES concussion NOS (850.0-850.9)
- flail chest (807.4)
- foreign body entering through orifice (930.0-939.9)
- injury to blood vessels (901.0-902.9)

The description "with open wound," used in the fourth-digit subdivisions, those with mention of infection or foreign body.

✓4th 860 Traumatic pneumothorax and hemothorax
- AHA: 2Q, '93, 4
- DEF: Traumatic pneumothorax: air or gas leaking into pleural space of lung due to trauma.
- DEF: Traumatic hemothorax: blood buildup in pleural space of lung due to trauma.

860.0 Pneumothorax without mention of open wound into thorax
860.1 Pneumothorax with open wound into thorax
860.2 Hemothorax without mention of open wound into thorax
860.3 Hemothorax with open wound into thorax
860.4 Pneumohemothorax without mention of open wound into thorax
860.5 Pneumohemothorax with open wound into thorax

✓4th 861 Injury to heart and lung
- EXCLUDES injury to blood vessels of thorax (901.0-901.9)

✓5th 861.0 Heart, without mention of open wound into thorax
- AHA: 1Q, '92, 9

§ Requires fifth-digit. See beginning of section 850–854 for codes and definitions.

N Newborn Age: 0   P Pediatric Age: 0-17   M Maternity Age: 12-55   A Adult Age: 15-124

Tabular List — **INJURY AND POISONING** — 861.00–864.1

- 861.00 **Unspecified injury**
- 861.01 Contusion
  - Cardiac contusion
  - Myocardial contusion
  - DEF: Bruising within the pericardium with no mention of open wound.
- 861.02 Laceration without penetration of heart chambers
  - DEF: Tearing injury of heart tissue, without penetration of chambers; no open wound.
- 861.03 Laceration with penetration of heart chambers

√5th 861.1 Heart, with open wound into thorax
- 861.10 **Unspecified injury**
- 861.11 Contusion
- 861.12 Laceration without penetration of heart chambers
- 861.13 Laceration with penetration of heart chambers

√5th 861.2 Lung, without mention of open wound into thorax
- 861.20 **Unspecified injury**
- 861.21 Contusion
  - DEF: Bruising of lung without mention of open wound.
- 861.22 Laceration

√5th 861.3 Lung, with open wound into thorax
- 861.30 **Unspecified injury**
- 861.31 Contusion
- 861.32 Laceration

√4th 862 Injury to other and unspecified intrathoracic organs
  - EXCLUDES injury to blood vessels of thorax (901.0-901.9)
- 862.0 Diaphragm, without mention of open wound into cavity
- 862.1 Diaphragm, with open wound into cavity

√5th 862.2 Other specified intrathoracic organs, without mention of open wound into cavity
- 862.21 Bronchus
- 862.22 Esophagus
- 862.29 Other
  - Pleura   Thymus gland

√5th 862.3 Other specified intrathoracic organs, with open wound into cavity
- 862.31 Bronchus
- 862.32 Esophagus
- 862.39 Other

- 862.8 Multiple and unspecified intrathoracic organs, without mention of open wound into cavity
  - Crushed chest
  - Multiple intrathoracic organs
- 862.9 Multiple and unspecified intrathoracic organs, with open wound into cavity

√4th 863 Injury to gastrointestinal tract
  - EXCLUDES anal sphincter laceration during delivery (664.2)
    bile duct (868.0-868.1 with fifth-digit 2)
    gallbladder (868.0-868.1 with fifth-digit 2)
- 863.0 Stomach, without mention of open wound into cavity
- 863.1 Stomach, with open wound into cavity

√5th 863.2 Small intestine, without mention of open wound into cavity
- 863.20 **Small intestine, unspecified site**
- 863.21 Duodenum
- 863.29 Other

√5th 863.3 Small intestine, with open wound into cavity
- 863.30 **Small intestine, unspecified site**
- 863.31 Duodenum
- 863.39 Other

√5th 863.4 Colon or rectum, without mention of open wound into cavity
- 863.40 **Colon, unspecified site**
- 863.41 Ascending [right] colon
- 863.42 Transverse colon
- 863.43 Descending [left] colon
- 863.44 Sigmoid colon
- 863.45 Rectum
- 863.46 Multiple sites in colon and rectum
- 863.49 Other

√5th 863.5 Colon or rectum, with open wound into cavity
- 863.50 **Colon, unspecified site**
- 863.51 Ascending [right] colon
- 863.52 Transverse colon
- 863.53 Descending [left] colon
- 863.54 Sigmoid colon
- 863.55 Rectum
- 863.56 Multiple sites in colon and rectum
- 863.59 Other

√5th 863.8 Other and unspecified gastrointestinal sites, without mention of open wound into cavity
- 863.80 **Gastrointestinal tract, unspecified site**
- 863.81 Pancreas, head
- 863.82 Pancreas, body
- 863.83 Pancreas, tail
- 863.84 Pancreas, multiple and unspecified sites
- 863.85 Appendix
- 863.89 Other
  - Intestine NOS

√5th 863.9 Other and unspecified gastrointestinal sites, with open wound into cavity
- 863.90 **Gastrointestinal tract, unspecified site**
- 863.91 Pancreas, head
- 863.92 Pancreas, body
- 863.93 Pancreas, tail
- 863.94 Pancreas, multiple and unspecified sites
- 863.95 Appendix
- 863.99 Other

√4th 864 Injury to liver

The following fifth-digit subclassification is for use with category 864:
- 0 **unspecified injury**
- 1 hematoma and contusion
- 2 laceration, minor
  - Laceration involving capsule only, or without significant involvement of hepatic parenchyma [i.e., less than 1 cm deep]
- 3 laceration, moderate
  - Laceration involving parenchyma but without major disruption of parenchyma [i.e., less than 10 cm long and less than 3 cm deep]
- 4 laceration, major
  - Laceration with significant disruption of hepatic parenchyma [i.e., 10 cm long and 3 cm deep]
  - Multiple moderate lacerations, with or without hematoma
  - Stellate lacerations of liver
- 5 **laceration, unspecified**
- 9 other

√5th 864.0 Without mention of open wound into cavity
√5th 864.1 With open wound into cavity

Additional Digit Required | Unspecified Code | Other Specified Code | Manifestation Code | ▶◀ Revised Text | ● New Code | ▲ Revised Code Title

865–872.01 INJURY AND POISONING Tabular List

☑4th 865 Injury to spleen

The following fifth-digit subclassification is for use with category 865:

- 0 unspecified injury
- 1 hematoma without rupture of capsule
- 2 capsular tears, without major disruption of parenchyma
- 3 laceration extending into parenchyma
- 4 massive parenchymal disruption
- 9 other

☑5th 865.0 Without mention of open wound into cavity
☑5th 865.1 With open wound into cavity

☑4th 866 Injury to kidney

The following fifth-digit subclassification is for use with category 866:

- 0 unspecified injury
- 1 hematoma without rupture of capsule
- 2 laceration
- 3 complete disruption of kidney parenchyma

☑5th 866.0 Without mention of open wound into cavity
☑5th 866.1 With open wound into cavity

☑4th 867 Injury to pelvic organs

EXCLUDES injury during delivery (664.0-665.9)

867.0 Bladder and urethra, without mention of open wound into cavity
AHA: N-D, '85, 15

867.1 Bladder and urethra, with open wound into cavity
867.2 Ureter, without mention of open wound into cavity
867.3 Ureter, with open wound into cavity
867.4 Uterus, without mention of open wound into cavity ♀
867.5 Uterus, with open wound into cavity ♀
867.6 Other specified pelvic organs, without mention of open wound into cavity
   Fallopian tube   Seminal vesicle
   Ovary   Vas deferens
   Prostate
867.7 Other specified pelvic organs, with open wound into cavity
867.8 Unspecified pelvic organ, without mention of open wound into cavity
867.9 Unspecified pelvic organ, with open wound into cavity

☑4th 868 Injury to other intra-abdominal organs

The following fifth-digit subclassification is for use with category 868:

- 0 unspecified intra-abdominal organ
- 1 adrenal gland
- 2 bile duct and gallbladder
- 3 peritoneum
- 4 retroperitoneum
- 9 other and multiple intra-abdominal organs

☑5th 868.0 Without mention of open wound into cavity
☑5th 868.1 With open wound into cavity

☑4th 869 Internal injury to unspecified or ill-defined organs

INCLUDES internal injury NOS
multiple internal injury NOS

869.0 Without mention of open wound into cavity
869.1 With open wound into cavity
AHA: 2Q, '89, 15

OPEN WOUND (870-897)

INCLUDES
animal bite
avulsion
cut
laceration
puncture wound
traumatic amputation

EXCLUDES
burn (940.0-949.5)
crushing (925-929.9)
puncture of internal organs (860.0-869.1)
superficial injury (910.0-919.9)
that incidental to:
   dislocation (830.0-839.9)
   fracture (800.0-829.1)
   internal injury (860.0-869.1)
   intracranial injury (851.0-854.1)

Note: The description "complicated" used in the fourth-digit subdivisions includes those with mention of delayed healing, delayed treatment, foreign body, or infection. Use additional code to identify infection

AHA: 4Q, '01, 52

OPEN WOUND OF HEAD, NECK, AND TRUNK (870-879)

☑4th 870 Open wound of ocular adnexa

870.0 Laceration of skin of eyelid and periocular area
870.1 Laceration of eyelid, full-thickness, not involving lacrimal passages
870.2 Laceration of eyelid involving lacrimal passages
870.3 Penetrating wound of orbit, without mention of foreign body
870.4 Penetrating wound of orbit with foreign body
   EXCLUDES retained (old) foreign body in orbit (376.6)
870.8 Other specified open wounds of ocular adnexa
870.9 Unspecified open wound of ocular adnexa

☑4th 871 Open wound of eyeball

EXCLUDES 2nd cranial nerve [optic] injury (950.0-950.9)
3rd cranial nerve [oculomotor] injury (951.0)

871.0 Ocular laceration without prolapse of intraocular tissue
AHA: 3Q, '96, 7

DEF: Tear in ocular tissue without displacing structures.

871.1 Ocular laceration with prolapse or exposure of intraocular tissue
871.2 Rupture of eye with partial loss of intraocular tissue
DEF: Forcible tearing of eyeball, with tissue loss.

871.3 Avulsion of eye
   Traumatic enucleation
DEF: Traumatic extraction of eyeball from socket.

871.4 Unspecified laceration of eye
871.5 Penetration of eyeball with magnetic foreign body
   EXCLUDES retained (old) magnetic foreign body in globe (360.50-360.59)
871.6 Penetration of eyeball with (nonmagnetic) foreign body
   EXCLUDES retained (old) (nonmagnetic) foreign body in globe (360.60-360.69)
871.7 Unspecified ocular penetration
871.9 Unspecified open wound of eyeball

☑4th 872 Open wound of ear

☑5th 872.0 External ear, without mention of complication
872.00 External ear, unspecified site
872.01 Auricle, ear
   Pinna
DEF: Open wound of fleshy, outer ear.

N Newborn Age: 0   P Pediatric Age: 0-17   M Maternity Age: 12-55   A Adult Age: 15-124

274 — Volume 1   2007 ICD•9•CM

| Tabular List | INJURY AND POISONING | 872.02–877.1 |

872.02 **Auditory canal**
DEF: Open wound of passage from external ear to eardrum.

√5th 872.1 **External ear, complicated**
872.10 External ear, unspecified site
872.11 Auricle, ear
872.12 Auditory canal

√5th 872.6 **Other specified parts of ear, without mention of complication**
872.61 Ear drum
Drumhead   Tympanic membrane
872.62 Ossicles
872.63 Eustachian tube
DEF: Open wound of channel between nasopharynx and tympanic cavity.
872.64 Cochlea
DEF: Open wound of snail shell shaped tube of inner ear.
872.69 Other and multiple sites

√5th 872.7 **Other specified parts of ear, complicated**
872.71 Ear drum
872.72 Ossicles
872.73 Eustachian tube
872.74 Cochlea
872.79 Other and multiple sites

872.8 **Ear, part unspecified, without mention of complication**
Ear NOS

872.9 **Ear, part unspecified, complicated**

√4th 873 **Other open wound of head**
873.0 Scalp, without mention of complication
873.1 Scalp, complicated

√5th 873.2 **Nose, without mention of complication**
873.20 Nose, unspecified site
873.21 Nasal septum
DEF: Open wound between nasal passages.
873.22 Nasal cavity
DEF: Open wound of nostrils.
873.23 Nasal sinus
DEF: Open wound of mucous-lined respiratory cavities.
873.29 Multiple sites

√5th 873.3 **Nose, complicated**
873.30 Nose, unspecified site
873.31 Nasal septum
873.32 Nasal cavity
873.33 Nasal sinus
873.39 Multiple sites

√5th 873.4 **Face, without mention of complication**
873.40 Face, unspecified site
873.41 Cheek
873.42 Forehead
Eyebrow
AHA: 4Q, '96, 43
873.43 Lip
873.44 Jaw
873.49 Other and multiple sites

√5th 873.5 **Face, complicated**
873.50 Face, unspecified site
873.51 Cheek
873.52 Forehead
873.53 Lip
873.54 Jaw
873.59 Other and multiple sites

√5th 873.6 **Internal structures of mouth, without mention of complication**
873.60 Mouth, unspecified site
873.61 Buccal mucosa
DEF: Open wound of inside of cheek.
873.62 Gum (alveolar process)
873.63 Tooth (broken) (fractured) (due to trauma)
EXCLUDES ▶ cracked tooth (521.81)◀
AHA: 1Q, '04, 17
873.64 Tongue and floor of mouth
873.65 Palate
DEF: Open wound of roof of mouth.
873.69 Other and multiple sites

√5th 873.7 **Internal structures of mouth, complicated**
873.70 Mouth, unspecified site
873.71 Buccal mucosa
873.72 Gum (alveolar process)
873.73 Tooth (broken) (fractured) (due to trauma)
EXCLUDES ▶ cracked tooth (521.81)◀
AHA: 1Q, '04, 17
873.74 Tongue and floor of mouth
873.75 Palate
873.79 Other and multiple sites

873.8 **Other and unspecified open wound of head without mention of complication**
Head NOS

873.9 **Other and unspecified open wound of head, complicated**

√4th 874 **Open wound of neck**
√5th 874.0 **Larynx and trachea, without mention of complication**
874.00 Larynx with trachea
874.01 Larynx
874.02 Trachea

√5th 874.1 **Larynx and trachea, complicated**
874.10 Larynx with trachea
874.11 Larynx
874.12 Trachea

874.2 Thyroid gland, without mention of complication
874.3 Thyroid gland, complicated
874.4 Pharynx, without mention of complication
Cervical esophagus
874.5 Pharynx, complicated
874.8 **Other and unspecified parts, without mention of complication**
Nape of neck   Throat NOS
Supraclavicular region
874.9 Other and unspecified parts, complicated

√4th 875 **Open wound of chest (wall)**
EXCLUDES open wound into thoracic cavity (860.0-862.9)
traumatic pneumothorax and hemothorax (860.1, 860.3, 860.5)
AHA: 3Q, '93, 17
875.0 Without mention of complication
875.1 Complicated

√4th 876 **Open wound of back**
INCLUDES loin
lumbar region
EXCLUDES open wound into thoracic cavity (860.0-862.9)
traumatic pneumothorax and hemothorax (860.1, 860.3, 860.5)
876.0 Without mention of complication
876.1 Complicated

√4th 877 **Open wound of buttock**
INCLUDES sacroiliac region
877.0 Without mention of complication
877.1 Complicated

INJURY AND POISONING

878–893.0

✓4th 878 Open wound of genital organs (external), including traumatic amputation
  EXCLUDES: injury during delivery (664.0-665.9)
  internal genital organs (867.0-867.9)
- 878.0 Penis, without mention of complication ♂
- 878.1 Penis, complicated ♂
- 878.2 Scrotum and testes, without mention of complication ♂
- 878.3 Scrotum and testes, complicated ♂
- 878.4 Vulva, without mention of complication ♀
  Labium (majus) (minus)
- 878.5 Vulva, complicated ♀
- 878.6 Vagina, without mention of complication ♀
- 878.7 Vagina, complicated ♀
- 878.8 Other and unspecified parts, without mention of complication
- 878.9 Other and unspecified parts, complicated

✓4th 879 Open wound of other and unspecified sites, except limbs
- 879.0 Breast, without mention of complication
- 879.1 Breast, complicated
- 879.2 Abdominal wall, anterior, without mention of complication
  Abdominal wall NOS   Pubic region
  Epigastric region   Umbilical region
  Hypogastric region
  AHA: 2Q, '91, 22
- 879.3 Abdominal wall, anterior, complicated
- 879.4 Abdominal wall, lateral, without mention of complication
  Flank   Iliac (region)
  Groin   Inguinal region
  Hypochondrium
- 879.5 Abdominal wall, lateral, complicated
- 879.6 Other and unspecified parts of trunk, without mention of complication
  Pelvic region   Trunk NOS
  Perineum
- 879.7 Other and unspecified parts of trunk, complicated
- 879.8 Open wound(s) (multiple) of unspecified site(s) without mention of complication
  Multiple open wounds NOS   Open wound NOS
- 879.9 Open wound(s) (multiple) of unspecified site(s), complicated

OPEN WOUND OF UPPER LIMB (880-887)
AHA: N-D, '85, 5

✓4th 880 Open wound of shoulder and upper arm
The following fifth-digit subclassification is for use with category 880:
  0 shoulder region
  1 scapular region
  2 axillary region
  3 upper arm
  9 multiple sites

- ✓5th 880.0 Without mention of complication
- ✓5th 880.1 Complicated
- ✓5th 880.2 With tendon involvement

✓4th 881 Open wound of elbow, forearm, and wrist
The following fifth-digit subclassification is for use with category 881:
  0 forearm
  1 elbow
  2 wrist

- ✓5th 881.0 Without mention of complication
- ✓5th 881.1 Complicated
- ✓5th 881.2 With tendon involvement

✓4th 882 Open wound of hand except finger(s) alone
- 882.0 Without mention of complication
- 882.1 Complicated
- 882.2 With tendon involvement

✓4th 883 Open wound of finger(s)
  INCLUDES: fingernail
  thumb (nail)
- 883.0 Without mention of complication
- 883.1 Complicated
- 883.2 With tendon involvement

✓4th 884 Multiple and unspecified open wound of upper limb
  INCLUDES: arm NOS
  multiple sites of one upper limb
  upper limb NOS
- 884.0 Without mention of complication
- 884.1 Complicated
- 884.2 With tendon involvement

✓4th 885 Traumatic amputation of thumb (complete) (partial)
  INCLUDES: thumb(s) (with finger(s) of either hand)
- 885.0 Without mention of complication
  AHA: 1Q, '03, 7
- 885.1 Complicated

✓4th 886 Traumatic amputation of other finger(s) (complete) (partial)
  INCLUDES: finger(s) of one or both hands, without mention of thumb(s)
- 886.0 Without mention of complication
- 886.1 Complicated

✓4th 887 Traumatic amputation of arm and hand (complete) (partial)
- 887.0 Unilateral, below elbow, without mention of complication
- 887.1 Unilateral, below elbow, complicated
- 887.2 Unilateral, at or above elbow, without mention of complication
- 887.3 Unilateral, at or above elbow, complicated
- 887.4 Unilateral, level not specified, without mention of complication
- 887.5 Unilateral, level not specified, complicated
- 887.6 Bilateral [any level], without mention of complication
  One hand and other arm
- 887.7 Bilateral [any level], complicated

OPEN WOUND OF LOWER LIMB (890-897)
AHA: N-D, '85, 5

✓4th 890 Open wound of hip and thigh
- 890.0 Without mention of complication
- 890.1 Complicated
- 890.2 With tendon involvement

✓4th 891 Open wound of knee, leg [except thigh], and ankle
  INCLUDES: leg NOS
  multiple sites of leg, except thigh
  EXCLUDES: that of thigh (890.0-890.2)
  with multiple sites of lower limb (894.0-894.2)
- 891.0 Without mention of complication
- 891.1 Complicated
- 891.2 With tendon involvement

✓4th 892 Open wound of foot except toe(s) alone
  INCLUDES: heel
- 892.0 Without mention of complication
- 892.1 Complicated
- 892.2 With tendon involvement

✓4th 893 Open wound of toe(s)
  INCLUDES: toenail
- 893.0 Without mention of complication

| Tabular List | INJURY AND POISONING | 893.1–902.9 |

- 893.1 Complicated
- 893.2 With tendon involvement

✓4th 894 Multiple and unspecified open wound of lower limb
  INCLUDES: lower limb NOS
  multiple sites of one lower limb, with thigh
- 894.0 Without mention of complication
- 894.1 Complicated
- 894.2 With tendon involvement

✓4th 895 Traumatic amputation of toe(s) (complete) (partial)
  INCLUDES: toe(s) of one or both feet
- 895.0 Without mention of complication
- 895.1 Complicated

✓4th 896 Traumatic amputation of foot (complete) (partial)
- 896.0 Unilateral, without mention of complication
- 896.1 Unilateral, complicated
- 896.2 Bilateral, without mention of complication
  EXCLUDES: one foot and other leg (897.6-897.7)
- 896.3 Bilateral, complicated

✓4th 897 Traumatic amputation of leg(s) (complete) (partial)
- 897.0 Unilateral, below knee, without mention of complication
- 897.1 Unilateral, below knee, complicated
- 897.2 Unilateral, at or above knee, without mention of complication
- 897.3 Unilateral, at or above knee, complicated
- 897.4 Unilateral, level not specified, without mention of complication
- 897.5 Unilateral, level not specified, complicated
- 897.6 Bilateral [any level], without mention of complication
  One foot and other leg
- 897.7 Bilateral [any level], complicated
  AHA: 3Q, '90, 5

INJURY TO BLOOD VESSELS (900-904)

INCLUDES:
- arterial hematoma
- avulsion
- cut
- laceration
- rupture
- traumatic aneurysm or fistula (arteriovenous)

of blood vessel, secondary to other injuries e.g., fracture or open wound

EXCLUDES: accidental puncture or laceration during medical procedure (998.2)
intracranial hemorrhage following injury (851.0-854.1)

AHA: 3Q, '90, 5

✓4th 900 Injury to blood vessels of head and neck
- ✓5th 900.0 Carotid artery
  - 900.00 Carotid artery, unspecified
  - 900.01 Common carotid artery
  - 900.02 External carotid artery
  - 900.03 Internal carotid artery
- 900.1 Internal jugular vein
- ✓5th 900.8 Other specified blood vessels of head and neck
  - 900.81 External jugular vein
    Jugular vein NOS
  - 900.82 Multiple blood vessels of head and neck
  - 900.89 Other
- 900.9 Unspecified blood vessel of head and neck

✓4th 901 Injury to blood vessels of thorax
  EXCLUDES: traumatic hemothorax (860.2-860.5)
- 901.0 Thoracic aorta
- 901.1 Innominate and subclavian arteries
- 901.2 Superior vena cava
- 901.3 Innominate and subclavian veins
- ✓5th 901.4 Pulmonary blood vessels
  - 901.40 Pulmonary vessel(s), unspecified
  - 901.41 Pulmonary artery
  - 901.42 Pulmonary vein
- ✓5th 901.8 Other specified blood vessels of thorax
  - 901.81 Intercostal artery or vein
  - 901.82 Internal mammary artery or vein
  - 901.83 Multiple blood vessels of thorax
  - 901.89 Other
    Azygos vein
    Hemiazygos vein
- 901.9 Unspecified blood vessel of thorax

✓4th 902 Injury to blood vessels of abdomen and pelvis
- 902.0 Abdominal aorta
- ✓5th 902.1 Inferior vena cava
  - 902.10 Inferior vena cava, unspecified
  - 902.11 Hepatic veins
  - 902.19 Other
- ✓5th 902.2 Celiac and mesenteric arteries
  - 902.20 Celiac and mesenteric arteries, unspecified
  - 902.21 Gastric artery
  - 902.22 Hepatic artery
  - 902.23 Splenic artery
  - 902.24 Other specified branches of celiac axis
  - 902.25 Superior mesenteric artery (trunk)
  - 902.26 Primary branches of superior mesenteric artery
    Ileocolic artery
  - 902.27 Inferior mesenteric artery
  - 902.29 Other
- ✓5th 902.3 Portal and splenic veins
  - 902.31 Superior mesenteric vein and primary subdivisions
    Ileocolic vein
  - 902.32 Inferior mesenteric vein
  - 902.33 Portal vein
  - 902.34 Splenic vein
  - 902.39 Other
    Cystic vein   Gastric vein
- ✓5th 902.4 Renal blood vessels
  - 902.40 Renal vessel(s), unspecified
  - 902.41 Renal artery
  - 902.42 Renal vein
  - 902.49 Other
    Suprarenal arteries
- ✓5th 902.5 Iliac blood vessels
  - 902.50 Iliac vessel(s), unspecified
  - 902.51 Hypogastric artery
  - 902.52 Hypogastric vein
  - 902.53 Iliac artery
  - 902.54 Iliac vein
  - 902.55 Uterine artery ♀
  - 902.56 Uterine vein ♀
  - 902.59 Other
- ✓5th 902.8 Other specified blood vessels of abdomen and pelvis
  - 902.81 Ovarian artery ♀
  - 902.82 Ovarian vein ♀
  - 902.87 Multiple blood vessels of abdomen and pelvis
  - 902.89 Other
- 902.9 Unspecified blood vessel of abdomen and pelvis

INJURY AND POISONING

✓4th 903 Injury to blood vessels of upper extremity
- **✓5th 903.0 Axillary blood vessels**
  - 903.00 Axillary vessel(s), unspecified
  - 903.01 Axillary artery
  - 903.02 Axillary vein
- 903.1 Brachial blood vessels
- 903.2 Radial blood vessels
- 903.3 Ulnar blood vessels
- 903.4 Palmar artery
- 903.5 Digital blood vessels
- 903.8 Other specified blood vessels of upper extremity
  - Multiple blood vessels of upper extremity
- 903.9 Unspecified blood vessel of upper extremity

✓4th 904 Injury to blood vessels of lower extremity and unspecified sites
- 904.0 Common femoral artery
  - Femoral artery above profunda origin
- 904.1 Superficial femoral artery
- 904.2 Femoral veins
- 904.3 Saphenous veins
  - Saphenous vein (greater) (lesser)
- **✓5th 904.4 Popliteal blood vessels**
  - 904.40 Popliteal vessel(s), unspecified
  - 904.41 Popliteal artery
  - 904.42 Popliteal vein
- **✓5th 904.5 Tibial blood vessels**
  - 904.50 Tibial vessel(s), unspecified
  - 904.51 Anterior tibial artery
  - 904.52 Anterior tibial vein
  - 904.53 Posterior tibial artery
  - 904.54 Posterior tibial vein
- 904.6 Deep plantar blood vessels
- 904.7 Other specified blood vessels of lower extremity
  - Multiple blood vessels of lower extremity
- 904.8 Unspecified blood vessel of lower extremity
- 904.9 Unspecified site
  - Injury to blood vessel NOS

LATE EFFECTS OF INJURIES, POISONINGS, TOXIC EFFECTS, AND OTHER EXTERNAL CAUSES (905-909)

Note: These categories are to be used to indicate conditions classifiable to 800-999 as the cause of late effects, which are themselves classified elsewhere. The "late effects" include those specified as such, or as sequelae, which may occur at any time after the acute injury.

✓4th 905 Late effects of musculoskeletal and connective tissue injuries
AHA: 1Q, '95, 10; 2Q, '94, 3
- 905.0 Late effect of fracture of skull and face bones
  - Late effect of injury classifiable to 800-804
  - AHA: 3Q, '97, 12
- 905.1 Late effect of fracture of spine and trunk without mention of spinal cord lesion
  - Late effect of injury classifiable to 805, 807-809
- 905.2 Late effect of fracture of upper extremities
  - Late effect of injury classifiable to 810-819
- 905.3 Late effect of fracture of neck of femur
  - Late effect of injury classifiable to 820
- 905.4 Late effect of fracture of lower extremities
  - Late effect of injury classifiable to 821-827
- 905.5 Late effect of fracture of multiple and unspecified bones
  - Late effect of injury classifiable to 828-829
- 905.6 Late effect of dislocation
  - Late effect of injury classifiable to 830-839
- 905.7 Late effect of sprain and strain without mention of tendon injury
  - Late effect of injury classifiable to 840-848, except tendon injury
- 905.8 Late effect of tendon injury
  - Late effect of tendon injury due to:
    open wound [injury classifiable to 880-884 with .2, 890-894 with .2]
    sprain and strain [injury classifiable to 840-848]
  - AHA: 2Q, '89, 13; 2Q, '89, 15
- 905.9 Late effect of traumatic amputation
  - Late effect of injury classifiable to 885-887, 895-897
  - **EXCLUDES** late amputation stump complication (997.60-997.69)

✓4th 906 Late effects of injuries to skin and subcutaneous tissues
- 906.0 Late effect of open wound of head, neck, and trunk
  - Late effect of injury classifiable to 870-879
- 906.1 Late effect of open wound of extremities without mention of tendon injury
  - Late effect of injury classifiable to 880-884, 890-894 except .2
- 906.2 Late effect of superficial injury
  - Late effect of injury classifiable to 910-919
- 906.3 Late effect of contusion
  - Late effect of injury classifiable to 920-924
- 906.4 Late effect of crushing
  - Late effect of injury classifiable to 925-929
- 906.5 Late effect of burn of eye, face, head, and neck
  - Late effect of injury classifiable to 940-941
  - AHA: 4Q, '04, 76
- 906.6 Late effect of burn of wrist and hand
  - Late effect of injury classifiable to 944
  - AHA: 4Q, '94, 22
- 906.7 Late effect of burn of other extremities
  - Late effect of injury classifiable to 943 or 945
  - AHA: 4Q, '94, 22
- 906.8 Late effect of burns of other specified sites
  - Late effect of injury classifiable to 942, 946-947
  - AHA: 4Q, '94, 22
- 906.9 Late effect of burn of unspecified site
  - Late effect of injury classifiable to 948-949
  - AHA: 4Q, '94, 22

✓4th 907 Late effects of injuries to the nervous system
- 907.0 Late effect of intracranial injury without mention of skull fracture
  - Late effect of injury classifiable to 850-854
  - AHA: 4Q, '03, 103; 3Q, '90, 14
- 907.1 Late effect of injury to cranial nerve
  - Late effect of injury classifiable to 950-951
- 907.2 Late effect of spinal cord injury
  - Late effect of injury classifiable to 806, 952
  - AHA: 4Q, '03, 103; 4Q, '98, 38
- 907.3 Late effect of injury to nerve root(s), spinal plexus(es), and other nerves of trunk
  - Late effect of injury classifiable to 953-954
- 907.4 Late effect of injury to peripheral nerve of shoulder girdle and upper limb
  - Late effect of injury classifiable to 955
- 907.5 Late effect of injury to peripheral nerve of pelvic girdle and lower limb
  - Late effect of injury classifiable to 956
- 907.9 Late effect of injury to other and unspecified nerve
  - Late effect of injury classifiable to 957

✓4th 908 Late effects of other and unspecified injuries
- 908.0 Late effect of internal injury to chest
  - Late effect of injury classifiable to 860-862

Tabular List — INJURY AND POISONING — 908.1–912.9

908.1 Late effect of internal injury to intra-abdominal organs
  Late effect of injury classifiable to 863-866, 868

908.2 Late effect of internal injury to other internal organs
  Late effect of injury classifiable to 867 or 869

908.3 Late effect of injury to blood vessel of head, neck, and extremities
  Late effect of injury classifiable to 900, 903-904

908.4 Late effect of injury to blood vessel of thorax, abdomen, and pelvis
  Late effect of injury classifiable to 901-902

908.5 Late effect of foreign body in orifice
  Late effect of injury classifiable to 930-939

908.6 Late effect of certain complications of trauma
  Late effect of complications classifiable to 958

908.9 Late effect of unspecified injury
  Late effect of injury classifiable to 959
  AHA: 3Q, '00, 4

√4th 909 Late effects of other and unspecified external causes

909.0 Late effect of poisoning due to drug, medicinal or biological substance
  Late effect of conditions classifiable to 960-979
  EXCLUDES late effect of adverse effect of drug, medicinal or biological substance (909.5)
  AHA: 4Q, '03, 103

909.1 Late effect of toxic effects of nonmedical substances
  Late effect of conditions classifiable to 980-989

909.2 Late effect of radiation
  Late effect of conditions classifiable to 990

909.3 Late effect of complications of surgical and medical care
  Late effect of conditions classifiable to 996-999
  AHA: 1Q, '93, 29

909.4 Late effect of certain other external causes
  Late effect of conditions classifiable to 991-994

909.5 Late effect of adverse effect of drug, medical or biological substance
  EXCLUDES late effect of poisoning due to drug, medical or biological substance (909.0)
  AHA: 4Q, '94, 48

909.9 Late effect of other and unspecified external causes

SUPERFICIAL INJURY (910-919)

EXCLUDES burn (blisters) (940.0-949.5)
  contusion (920-924.9)
  foreign body:
    granuloma (728.82)
    inadvertently left in operative wound (998.4)
    residual in soft tissue (729.6)
  insect bite, venomous (989.5)
  open wound with incidental foreign body (870.0-897.7)

AHA: 2Q, '89, 15

√4th 910 Superficial injury of face, neck, and scalp except eye
INCLUDES cheek
  ear
  gum
  lip
  nose
  throat
EXCLUDES eye and adnexa (918.0-918.9)

910.0 Abrasion or friction burn without mention of infection
910.1 Abrasion or friction burn, infected
910.2 Blister without mention of infection
910.3 Blister, infected
910.4 Insect bite, nonvenomous, without mention of infection
910.5 Insect bite, nonvenomous, infected
910.6 Superficial foreign body (splinter) without major open wound and without mention of infection
910.7 Superficial foreign body (splinter) without major open wound, infected
910.8 Other and unspecified superficial injury of face, neck, and scalp without mention of infection
910.9 Other and unspecified superficial injury of face, neck, and scalp, infected

√4th 911 Superficial injury of trunk
INCLUDES abdominal wall
  anus
  back
  breast
  buttock
  mchest wall
  flank
  groin
  interscapular region
  labium (majus) (minus)
  penis
  perineum
  scrotum
  testis
  vagina
  vulva
EXCLUDES hip (916.0-916.9)
  scapular region (912.0-912.9)

911.0 Abrasion or friction burn without mention of infection
  AHA: 3Q, '01, 10
911.1 Abrasion or friction burn, infected
911.2 Blister without mention of infection
911.3 Blister, infected
911.4 Insect bite, nonvenomous, without mention of infection
911.5 Insect bite, nonvenomous, infected
911.6 Superficial foreign body (splinter) without major open wound and without mention of infection
911.7 Superficial foreign body (splinter) without major open wound, infected
911.8 Other and unspecified superficial injury of trunk without mention of infection
911.9 Other and unspecified superficial injury of trunk, infected

√4th 912 Superficial injury of shoulder and upper arm
INCLUDES axilla
  scapular region

912.0 Abrasion or friction burn without mention of infection
912.1 Abrasion or friction burn, infected
912.2 Blister without mention of infection
912.3 Blister, infected
912.4 Insect bite, nonvenomous, without mention of infection
912.5 Insect bite, nonvenomous, infected
912.6 Superficial foreign body (splinter) without major open wound and without mention of infection
912.7 Superficial foreign body (splinter) without major open wound, infected
912.8 Other and unspecified superficial injury of shoulder and upper arm without mention of infection
912.9 Other and unspecified superficial injury of shoulder and upper arm, infected

INJURY AND POISONING
Tabular List

✓4th 913 Superficial injury of elbow, forearm, and wrist
- 913.0 Abrasion or friction burn without mention of infection
- 913.1 Abrasion or friction burn, infected
- 913.2 Blister without mention of infection
- 913.3 Blister, infected
- 913.4 Insect bite, nonvenomous, without mention of infection
- 913.5 Insect bite, nonvenomous, infected
- 913.6 Superficial foreign body (splinter) without major open wound and without mention of infection
- 913.7 Superficial foreign body (splinter) without major open wound, infected
- 913.8 Other and unspecified superficial injury of elbow, forearm, and wrist without mention of infection
- 913.9 Other and unspecified superficial injury of elbow, forearm, and wrist, infected

✓4th 914 Superficial injury of hand(s) except finger(s) alone
- 914.0 Abrasion or friction burn without mention of infection
- 914.1 Abrasion or friction burn, infected
- 914.2 Blister without mention of infection
- 914.3 Blister, infected
- 914.4 Insect bite, nonvenomous, without mention of infection
- 914.5 Insect bite, nonvenomous, infected
- 914.6 Superficial foreign body (splinter) without major open wound and without mention of infection
- 914.7 Superficial foreign body (splinter) without major open wound, infected
- 914.8 Other and unspecified superficial injury of hand without mention of infection
- 914.9 Other and unspecified superficial injury of hand, infected

✓4th 915 Superficial injury of finger(s)
  INCLUDES fingernail
            thumb (nail)
- 915.0 Abrasion or friction burn without mention of infection
- 915.1 Abrasion or friction burn, infected
- 915.2 Blister without mention of infection
- 915.3 Blister, infected
- 915.4 Insect bite, nonvenomous, without mention of infection
- 915.5 Insect bite, nonvenomous, infected
- 915.6 Superficial foreign body (splinter) without major open wound and without mention of infection
- 915.7 Superficial foreign body (splinter) without major open wound, infected
- 915.8 Other and unspecified superficial injury of fingers without mention of infection
  AHA: 3Q, '01, 10
- 915.9 Other and unspecified superficial injury of fingers, infected

✓4th 916 Superficial injury of hip, thigh, leg, and ankle
- 916.0 Abrasion or friction burn without mention of infection
- 916.1 Abrasion or friction burn, infected
- 916.2 Blister without mention of infection
- 916.3 Blister, infected
- 916.4 Insect bite, nonvenomous, without mention of infection
- 916.5 Insect bite, nonvenomous, infected
- 916.6 Superficial foreign body (splinter) without major open wound and without mention of infection
- 916.7 Superficial foreign body (splinter) without major open wound, infected
- 916.8 Other and unspecified superficial injury of hip, thigh, leg, and ankle without mention of infection
- 916.9 Other and unspecified superficial injury of hip, thigh, leg, and ankle, infected

✓4th 917 Superficial injury of foot and toe(s)
  INCLUDES heel
            toenail
- 917.0 Abrasion or friction burn without mention of infection
- 917.1 Abrasion or friction burn, infected
- 917.2 Blister without mention of infection
- 917.3 Blister, infected
- 917.4 Insect bite, nonvenomous, without mention of infection
- 917.5 Insect bite, nonvenomous, infected
- 917.6 Superficial foreign body (splinter) without major open wound and without mention of infection
- 917.7 Superficial foreign body (splinter) without major open wound, infected
- 917.8 Other and unspecified superficial injury of foot and toes without mention of infection
  AHA: 1Q, '03, 13
- 917.9 Other and unspecified superficial injury of foot and toes, infected
  AHA: 1Q, '03, 13

✓4th 918 Superficial injury of eye and adnexa
  EXCLUDES burn (940.0-940.9)
            foreign body on external eye (930.0-930.9)
- 918.0 Eyelids and periocular area
    Abrasion   Superficial foreign body
    Insect bite   (splinter)
- 918.1 Cornea
    Corneal abrasion   Superficial laceration
    EXCLUDES corneal injury due to contact lens (371.82)
- 918.2 Conjunctiva
- 918.9 Other and unspecified superficial injuries of eye
    Eye (ball) NOS

✓4th 919 Superficial injury of other, multiple, and unspecified sites
  EXCLUDES multiple sites classifiable to the same three-digit category (910.0-918.9)
- 919.0 Abrasion or friction burn without mention of infection
- 919.1 Abrasion or friction burn, infected
- 919.2 Blister without mention of infection
- 919.3 Blister, infected
- 919.4 Insect bite, nonvenomous, without mention of infection
- 919.5 Insect bite, nonvenomous, infected
- 919.6 Superficial foreign body (splinter) without major open wound and without mention of infection
- 919.7 Superficial foreign body (splinter) without major open wound, infected
- 919.8 Other and unspecified superficial injury without mention of infection
- 919.9 Other and unspecified superficial injury, infected

Tabular List — INJURY AND POISONING — 920–927.9

CONTUSION WITH INTACT SKIN SURFACE (920-924)

INCLUDES: bruise, hematoma } without fracture or open wound

EXCLUDES:
- concussion (850.0-850.9)
- hemarthrosis (840.0-848.9)
- internal organs (860.0-869.1)
- that incidental to:
  - crushing injury (925-929.9)
  - dislocation (830.0-839.9)
  - fracture (800.0-829.1)
  - internal injury (860.0-869.1)
  - intracranial injury (850.0-854.1)
  - nerve injury (950.0-957.9)
  - open wound (870.0-897.7)

920 Contusion of face, scalp, and neck except eye(s)
- Cheek
- Ear (auricle)
- Gum
- Lip
- Mandibular joint area
- Nose
- Throat

✓4th **921 Contusion of eye and adnexa**
- 921.0 Black eye, not otherwise specified
- 921.1 Contusion of eyelids and periocular area
- 921.2 Contusion of orbital tissues
- 921.3 Contusion of eyeball
  - AHA: J-A, '85, 16
- 921.9 Unspecified contusion of eye
  - Injury of eye NOS

✓4th **922 Contusion of trunk**
- 922.0 Breast
- 922.1 Chest wall
- 922.2 Abdominal wall
  - Flank
  - Groin
- ✓5th 922.3 Back
  - AHA: 4Q, '96, 39
  - 922.31 Back
    - EXCLUDES: interscapular region (922.33)
  - 922.32 Buttock
    - AHA: 3Q, '99, 14
  - 922.33 Interscapular region
- 922.4 Genital organs
  - Labium (majus) (minus)
  - Penis
  - Perineum
  - Scrotum
  - Vulva
  - Vagina
  - Testis
- 922.8 Multiple sites of trunk
- 922.9 Unspecified part
  - Trunk NOS

✓4th **923 Contusion of upper limb**
- ✓5th 923.0 Shoulder and upper arm
  - 923.00 Shoulder region
  - 923.01 Scapular region
  - 923.02 Axillary region
  - 923.03 Upper arm
  - 923.09 Multiple sites
- ✓5th 923.1 Elbow and forearm
  - 923.10 Forearm
  - 923.11 Elbow
- ✓5th 923.2 Wrist and hand(s), except finger(s) alone
  - 923.20 Hand(s)
  - 923.21 Wrist
- 923.3 Finger
  - Fingernail
  - Thumb (nail)
- 923.8 Multiple sites of upper limb
- 923.9 Unspecified part of upper limb
  - Arm NOS

✓4th **924 Contusion of lower limb and of other and unspecified sites**
- ✓5th 924.0 Hip and thigh
  - 924.00 Thigh
  - 924.01 Hip
- ✓5th 924.1 Knee and lower leg
  - 924.10 Lower leg
  - 924.11 Knee
- ✓5th 924.2 Ankle and foot, excluding toe(s)
  - 924.20 Foot
    - Heel
  - 924.21 Ankle
- 924.3 Toe
  - Toenail
- 924.4 Multiple sites of lower limb
- 924.5 Unspecified part of lower limb
  - Leg NOS
- 924.8 Multiple sites, not elsewhere classified
  - AHA: 1Q, '03, 7
- 924.9 Unspecified site

CRUSHING INJURY (925-929)

Use additional code to identify any associated injuries, such as:
- fractures (800-829)
- internal injuries (860.0-869.1)
- intracranial injuries (850.0-854.1)

AHA: 4Q, '03, 77; 2Q, '93, 7

✓4th **925 Crushing injury of face, scalp, and neck**
- Cheek
- Ear
- Larynx
- Pharynx
- Throat
- 925.1 Crushing injury of face and scalp
  - Cheek
  - Ear
- 925.2 Crushing injury of neck
  - Larynx
  - Pharynx
  - Throat

✓4th **926 Crushing injury of trunk**
- 926.0 External genitalia
  - Labium (majus) (minus)
  - Penis
  - Scrotum
  - Testis
  - Vulva
- ✓5th 926.1 Other specified sites
  - 926.11 Back
  - 926.12 Buttock
  - 926.19 Other
    - Breast
- 926.8 Multiple sites of trunk
- 926.9 Unspecified site
  - Trunk NOS

✓4th **927 Crushing injury of upper limb**
- ✓5th 927.0 Shoulder and upper arm
  - 927.00 Shoulder region
  - 927.01 Scapular region
  - 927.02 Axillary region
  - 927.03 Upper arm
  - 927.09 Multiple sites
- ✓5th 927.1 Elbow and forearm
  - 927.10 Forearm
  - 927.11 Elbow
- ✓5th 927.2 Wrist and hand(s), except finger(s) alone
  - 927.20 Hand(s)
  - 927.21 Wrist
- 927.3 Finger(s)
  - AHA: 4Q, '03, 77
- 927.8 Multiple sites of upper limb
- 927.9 Unspecified site
  - Arm NOS

INJURY AND POISONING

928–941.0

✓4th 928 Crushing injury of lower limb
- **✓5th 928.0 Hip and thigh**
  - 928.00 Thigh
  - 928.01 Hip
- **✓5th 928.1 Knee and lower leg**
  - 928.10 Lower leg
  - 928.11 Knee
- **✓5th 928.2 Ankle and foot, excluding toe(s) alone**
  - 928.20 Foot
    - Heel
  - 928.21 Ankle
- 928.3 Toe(s)
- 928.8 Multiple sites of lower limb
- 928.9 Unspecified site
  - Leg NOS

✓4th 929 Crushing injury of multiple and unspecified sites
- 929.0 Multiple sites, not elsewhere classified
- 929.9 Unspecified site

EFFECTS OF FOREIGN BODY ENTERING THROUGH ORIFICE (930-939)

EXCLUDES foreign body:
- granuloma (728.82)
- inadvertently left in operative wound (998.4, 998.7)
- in open wound (800-839, 851-897)
- residual in soft tissues (729.6)
- superficial without major open wound (910-919 with .6 or .7)

✓4th 930 Foreign body on external eye

EXCLUDES foreign body in penetrating wound of:
- eyeball (871.5-871.6)
  - retained (old) (360.5-360.6)
- ocular adnexa (870.4)
  - retained (old) (376.6)

- 930.0 Corneal foreign body
- 930.1 Foreign body in conjunctival sac
- 930.2 Foreign body in lacrimal punctum
- 930.8 Other and combined sites
- 930.9 Unspecified site
  - External eye NOS

931 Foreign body in ear
- Auditory canal
- Auricle

932 Foreign body in nose
- Nasal sinus
- Nostril

✓4th 933 Foreign body in pharynx and larynx
- 933.0 Pharynx
  - Nasopharynx
  - Throat NOS
- 933.1 Larynx
  - Asphyxia due to foreign body
  - Choking due to:
    - food (regurgitated)
    - phlegm

✓4th 934 Foreign body in trachea, bronchus, and lung
- 934.0 Trachea
- 934.1 Main bronchus
  - AHA: 3Q, '02, 18
- 934.8 Other specified parts
  - Bronchioles
  - Lung
- 934.9 Respiratory tree, unspecified
  - Inhalation of liquid or vomitus, lower respiratory tract NOS

✓4th 935 Foreign body in mouth, esophagus, and stomach
- 935.0 Mouth
- 935.1 Esophagus
  - AHA: 1Q, '88, 13
- 935.2 Stomach

936 Foreign body in intestine and colon

937 Foreign body in anus and rectum
- Rectosigmoid (junction)

938 Foreign body in digestive system, unspecified
- Alimentary tract NOS
- Swallowed foreign body

✓4th 939 Foreign body in genitourinary tract
- 939.0 Bladder and urethra
- 939.1 Uterus, any part ♀
  - EXCLUDES intrauterine contraceptive device:
    - complications from (996.32, 996.65)
    - presence of (V45.51)
- 939.2 Vulva and vagina ♀
- 939.3 Penis ♂
- 939.9 Unspecified site

BURNS (940-949)

INCLUDES burns from:
- electrical heating appliance
- electricity
- flame
- hot object
- lightning
- radiation
- chemical burns (external) (internal)
- scalds

EXCLUDES friction burns (910-919 with .0, .1)
sunburn (692.71, 692.76-692.77)

AHA: 4Q, '94, 22; 2Q, '90, 7; 4Q, '88, 3; M-A, '86, 9

✓4th 940 Burn confined to eye and adnexa
- 940.0 Chemical burn of eyelids and periocular area
- 940.1 Other burns of eyelids and periocular area
- 940.2 Alkaline chemical burn of cornea and conjunctival sac
- 940.3 Acid chemical burn of cornea and conjunctival sac
- 940.4 Other burn of cornea and conjunctival sac
- 940.5 Burn with resulting rupture and destruction of eyeball
- 940.9 Unspecified burn of eye and adnexa

✓4th 941 Burn of face, head, and neck

EXCLUDES mouth (947.0)

The following fifth-digit subclassification is for use with category 941:
- 0 face and head, unspecified site
- 1 ear [any part]
- 2 eye (with other parts of face, head, and neck)
- 3 lip(s)
- 4 chin
- 5 nose (septum)
- 6 scalp [any part]
  - Temple (region)
- 7 forehead and cheek
- 8 neck
- 9 multiple sites [except with eye] of face, head, and neck

AHA: 4Q, '94, 22; M-A, '86, 9

✓5th 941.0 Unspecified degree

Burns
Degrees of Burns

First (redness) | Second (blistering) | Third (fill thickness) | Deep Third (deep necrosis) — Eschar

INJURY AND POISONING

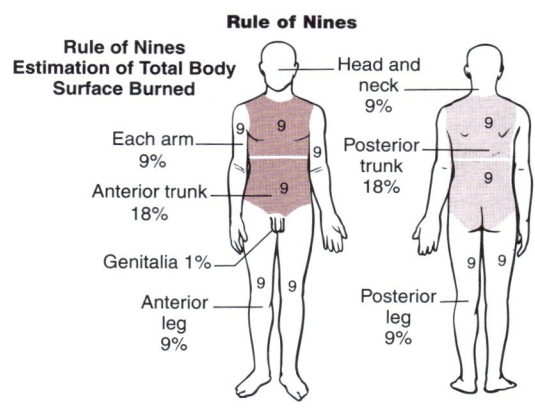

Rule of Nines
Estimation of Total Body Surface Burned
- Head and neck 9%
- Each arm 9%
- Anterior trunk 18%
- Posterior trunk 18%
- Genitalia 1%
- Anterior leg 9%
- Posterior leg 9%

✓5ᵗʰ **941.1** Erythema [first degree]
  AHA: For code 941.19: ▶3Q, '05, 10◀

✓5ᵗʰ **941.2** Blisters, epidermal loss [second degree]

✓5ᵗʰ **941.3** Full-thickness skin loss [third degree NOS]

✓5ᵗʰ **941.4** Deep necrosis of underlying tissues [deep third degree] without mention of loss of a body part

✓5ᵗʰ **941.5** Deep necrosis of underlying tissues [deep third degree] with loss of a body part

✓4ᵗʰ **942** Burn of trunk
  EXCLUDES scapular region (943.0-943.5 with fifth-digit 6)

  The following fifth-digit subclassification is for use with category 942:
  0 trunk, unspecified site
  1 breast
  2 chest wall, excluding breast and nipple
  3 abdominal wall
    Flank   Groin
  4 back [any part]
    Buttock   Interscapular region
  5 genitalia
    Labium (majus) (minus)   Scrotum
    Penis   Testis
    Perineum   Vulva
  9 other and multiple sites of trunk

  AHA: 4Q, '94, 22; M-A, '86, 9

✓5ᵗʰ **942.0** Unspecified degree
✓5ᵗʰ **942.1** Erythema [first degree]
✓5ᵗʰ **942.2** Blisters, epidermal loss [second degree]
✓5ᵗʰ **942.3** Full-thickness skin loss [third degree NOS]
✓5ᵗʰ **942.4** Deep necrosis of underlying tissues [deep third degree] without mention of loss of a body part
✓5ᵗʰ **942.5** Deep necrosis of underlying tissues [deep third degree] with loss of a body part

✓4ᵗʰ **943** Burn of upper limb, except wrist and hand

  The following fifth-digit subclassification is for use with category 943:
  0 upper limb, unspecified site
  1 forearm
  2 elbow
  3 upper arm
  4 axilla
  5 shoulder
  6 scapular region
  9 multiple sites of upper limb, except wrist and hand

  AHA: 4Q, '94, 22; M-A, '86, 9

✓5ᵗʰ **943.0** Unspecified degree
✓5ᵗʰ **943.1** Erythema [first degree]
✓5ᵗʰ **943.2** Blisters, epidermal loss [second degree]
✓5ᵗʰ **943.3** Full-thickness skin loss [third degree NOS]
✓5ᵗʰ **943.4** Deep necrosis of underlying tissues [deep third degree] without mention of loss of a body part

✓5ᵗʰ **943.5** Deep necrosis of underlying tissues [deep third degree] with loss of a body part

✓4ᵗʰ **944** Burn of wrist(s) and hand(s)

  The following fifth-digit subclassification is for use with category 944:
  0 hand, unspecified site
  1 single digit [finger (nail)] other than thumb
  2 thumb (nail)
  3 two or more digits, not including thumb
  4 two or more digits including thumb
  5 palm
  6 back of hand
  7 wrist
  8 multiple sites of wrist(s) and hand(s)

✓5ᵗʰ **944.0** Unspecified degree
✓5ᵗʰ **944.1** Erythema [first degree]
✓5ᵗʰ **944.2** Blisters, epidermal loss [second degree]
✓5ᵗʰ **944.3** Full-thickness skin loss [third degree NOS]
✓5ᵗʰ **944.4** Deep necrosis of underlying tissues [deep third degree] without mention of loss of a body part
✓5ᵗʰ **944.5** Deep necrosis of underlying tissues [deep third degree] with loss of a body part

✓4ᵗʰ **945** Burn of lower limb(s)

  The following fifth-digit subclassification is for use with category 945:
  0 lower limb [leg], unspecified site
  1 toe(s) (nail)
  2 foot
  3 ankle
  4 lower leg
  5 knee
  6 thigh [any part]
  9 multiple sites of lower limb(s)

  AHA: 4Q, '94, 22; M-A, '86, 9

✓5ᵗʰ **945.0** Unspecified degree
✓5ᵗʰ **945.1** Erythema [first degree]
✓5ᵗʰ **945.2** Blisters, epidermal loss [second degree]
✓5ᵗʰ **945.3** Full-thickness skin loss [third degree NOS]
✓5ᵗʰ **945.4** Deep necrosis of underlying tissues [deep third degree] without mention of loss of a body part
✓5ᵗʰ **945.5** Deep necrosis of underlying tissues [deep third degree] with loss of a body part

✓4ᵗʰ **946** Burns of multiple specified sites
  INCLUDES burns of sites classifiable to more than one three-digit category in 940-945
  EXCLUDES multiple burns NOS (949.0-949.5)
  AHA: 4Q, '94, 22; M-A, '86, 9

946.0 Unspecified degree
946.1 Erythema [first degree]
946.2 Blisters, epidermal loss [second degree]
946.3 Full-thickness skin loss [third degree NOS]
946.4 Deep necrosis of underlying tissues [deep third degree] without mention of loss of a body part
946.5 Deep necrosis of underlying tissues [deep third degree] with loss of a body part

✓4ᵗʰ **947** Burn of internal organs
  INCLUDES burns from chemical agents (ingested)
  AHA: 4Q, '94, 22; M-A, '86, 9

  947.0 Mouth and pharynx
    Gum   Tongue
  947.1 Larynx, trachea, and lung
  947.2 Esophagus
  947.3 Gastrointestinal tract
    Colon   Small intestine
    Rectum   Stomach

INJURY AND POISONING

947.4 Vagina and uterus ♀
947.8 Other specified sites
947.9 Unspecified site

✓4th **948 Burns classified according to extent of body surface involved**

Note: This category is to be used when the site of the burn is unspecified, or with categories 940-947 when the site is specified.

EXCLUDES sunburn (692.71, 692.76-692.77)

The following fifth-digit subclassification is for use with category 948 to indicate the percent of body surface with third degree burn; valid digits are in [brackets] under each code:

0 less than 10 percent or unspecified
1 10-19%
2 20-29%
3 30-39%
4 40-49%
5 50-59%
6 60-69%
7 70-79%
8 80-89%
9 90% or more of body surface

AHA: 4Q, '94, 22; 4Q, '88, 3; M-A, '86, 9; N-D, '84, 13

✓5th 948.0 Burn [any degree] involving less than 10 percent of body surface
[0]

✓5th 948.1 10-19 percent of body surface
[0-1]

✓5th 948.2 20-29 percent of body surface
[0-2]

✓5th 948.3 30-39 percent of body surface
[0-3]

✓5th 948.4 40-49 percent of body surface
[0-4]

✓5th 948.5 50-59 percent of body surface
[0-5]

✓5th 948.6 60-69 percent of body surface
[0-6]

✓5th 948.7 70-79 percent of body surface
[0-7]

✓5th 948.8 80-89 percent of body surface
[0-8]

✓5th 948.9 90 percent or more of body surface
[0-9]

✓4th **949 Burn, unspecified**

INCLUDES burn NOS multiple burns NOS
EXCLUDES burn of unspecified site but with statement of the extent of body surface involved (948.0-948.9)

AHA: 4Q, '94, 22; M-A, '86, 9

949.0 Unspecified degree
949.1 Erythema [first degree]
949.2 Blisters, epidermal loss [second degree]
949.3 Full-thickness skin loss [third degree NOS]
949.4 Deep necrosis of underlying tissues [deep third degree] without mention of loss of a body part
949.5 Deep necrosis of underlying tissues [deep third degree] with loss of a body part

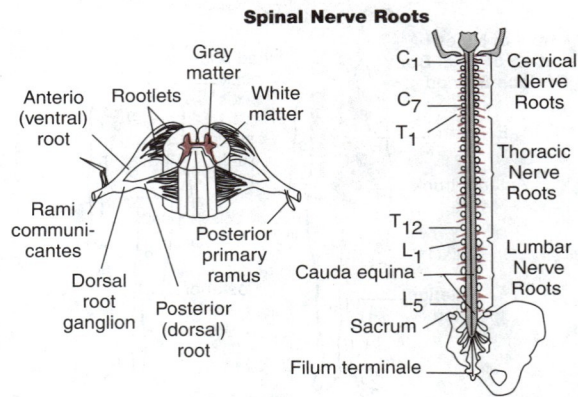

INJURY TO NERVES AND SPINAL CORD (950-957)

INCLUDES division of nerve
lesion in continuity
traumatic neuroma   (with open wound)
traumatic transient paralysis

EXCLUDES accidental puncture or laceration during medical procedure (998.2)

✓4th **950 Injury to optic nerve and pathways**
950.0 Optic nerve injury
Second cranial nerve
950.1 Injury to optic chiasm
950.2 Injury to optic pathways
950.3 Injury to visual cortex
950.9 Unspecified
Traumatic blindness NOS

✓4th **951 Injury to other cranial nerve(s)**
951.0 Injury to oculomotor nerve
Third cranial nerve
951.1 Injury to trochlear nerve
Fourth cranial nerve
951.2 Injury to trigeminal nerve
Fifth cranial nerve
951.3 Injury to abducens nerve
Sixth cranial nerve
951.4 Injury to facial nerve
Seventh cranial nerve
951.5 Injury to acoustic nerve
Auditory nerve   Traumatic deafness NOS
Eighth cranial nerve
951.6 Injury to accessory nerve
Eleventh cranial nerve
951.7 Injury to hypoglossal nerve
Twelfth cranial nerve
951.8 Injury to other specified cranial nerves
Glossopharyngeal [9th cranial] nerve
Olfactory [1st cranial] nerve
Pneumogastric [10th cranial] nerve
Traumatic anosmia NOS
Vagus [10th cranial] nerve
951.9 Injury to unspecified cranial nerve

✓4th **952 Spinal cord injury without evidence of spinal bone injury**
✓5th 952.0 Cervical
952.00 C_1-C_4 level with unspecified spinal cord injury
Spinal cord injury, cervical region NOS
952.01 C_1-C_4 level with complete lesion of spinal cord
952.02 C_1-C_4 level with anterior cord syndrome
952.03 C_1-C_4 level with central cord syndrome

INJURY AND POISONING

- 952.04 C_1-C_4 level with other specified spinal cord injury
  - Incomplete spinal cord lesion at C_1-C_4 level:
    - NOS
    - with posterior cord syndrome
- 952.05 C_5-C_7 level with unspecified spinal cord injury
- 952.06 C_5-C_7 level with complete lesion of spinal cord
- 952.07 C_5-C_7 level with anterior cord syndrome
- 952.08 C_5-C_7 level with central cord syndrome
- 952.09 C_5-C_7 level with other specified spinal cord injury
  - Incomplete spinal cord lesion at C_5-C_7 level:
    - NOS
    - with posterior cord syndrome

√5th 952.1 Dorsal [thoracic]
- 952.10 T_1-T_6 level with unspecified spinal cord injury
  - Spinal cord injury, thoracic region NOS
- 952.11 T_1-T_6 level with complete lesion of spinal cord
- 952.12 T_1-T_6 level with anterior cord syndrome
- 952.13 T_1-T_6 level with central cord syndrome
- 952.14 T_1-T_6 level with other specified spinal cord injury
  - Incomplete spinal cord lesion at T_1-T_6 level:
    - NOS
    - with posterior cord syndrome
- 952.15 T_7-T_{12} level with unspecified spinal cord injury
- 952.16 T_7-T_{12} level with complete lesion of spinal cord
- 952.17 T_7-T_{12} level with anterior cord syndrome
- 952.18 T_7-T_{12} level with central cord syndrome
- 952.19 T_7-T_{12} level with other specified spinal cord injury
  - Incomplete spinal cord lesion at T_7-T_{12} level:
    - NOS
    - with posterior cord syndrome

- 952.2 Lumbar
- 952.3 Sacral
- 952.4 Cauda equina
- 952.8 Multiple sites of spinal cord
- 952.9 Unspecified site of spinal cord

√4th 953 Injury to nerve roots and spinal plexus
- 953.0 Cervical root
- 953.1 Dorsal root
- 953.2 Lumbar root
- 953.3 Sacral root
- 953.4 Brachial plexus
- 953.5 Lumbosacral plexus
- 953.8 Multiple sites
- 953.9 Unspecified site

√4th 954 Injury to other nerve(s) of trunk, excluding shoulder and pelvic girdles
- 954.0 Cervical sympathetic
- 954.1 Other sympathetic
  - Celiac ganglion or plexus
  - Inferior mesenteric plexus
  - Splanchnic nerve(s)
  - Stellate ganglion
- 954.8 Other specified nerve(s) of trunk
- 954.9 Unspecified nerve of trunk

√4th 955 Injury to peripheral nerve(s) of shoulder girdle and upper limb
- 955.0 Axillary nerve
- 955.1 Median nerve
- 955.2 Ulnar nerve
- 955.3 Radial nerve
- 955.4 Musculocutaneous nerve
- 955.5 Cutaneous sensory nerve, upper limb
- 955.6 Digital nerve
- 955.7 Other specified nerve(s) of shoulder girdle and upper limb
- 955.8 Multiple nerves of shoulder girdle and upper limb
- 955.9 Unspecified nerve of shoulder girdle and upper limb

√4th 956 Injury to peripheral nerve(s) of pelvic girdle and lower limb
- 956.0 Sciatic nerve
- 956.1 Femoral nerve
- 956.2 Posterior tibial nerve
- 956.3 Peroneal nerve
- 956.4 Cutaneous sensory nerve, lower limb
- 956.5 Other specified nerve(s) of pelvic girdle and lower limb
- 956.8 Multiple nerves of pelvic girdle and lower limb
- 956.9 Unspecified nerve of pelvic girdle and lower limb

√4th 957 Injury to other and unspecified nerves
- 957.0 Superficial nerves of head and neck
- 957.1 Other specified nerve(s)
- 957.8 Multiple nerves in several parts
  - Multiple nerve injury NOS
- 957.9 Unspecified site
  - Nerve injury NOS

CERTAIN TRAUMATIC COMPLICATIONS AND UNSPECIFIED INJURIES (958-959)

√4th 958 Certain early complications of trauma
  - EXCLUDES: adult respiratory distress syndrome (518.5)
    - flail chest (807.4)
    - shock lung (518.5)
    - that occurring during or following medical procedures (996.0-999.9)
- 958.0 Air embolism
  - Pneumathemia
  - EXCLUDES: that complicating:
    - abortion (634-638 with .6, 639.6)
    - ectopic or molar pregnancy (639.6)
    - pregnancy, childbirth, or the puerperium (673.0)
  - DEF: Arterial obstruction due to introduction of air bubbles into the veins following surgery or trauma.
- 958.1 Fat embolism
  - EXCLUDES: that complicating:
    - abortion (634-638 with .6, 639.6)
    - pregnancy, childbirth, or the puerperium (673.8)
  - DEF: Arterial blockage due to the entrance of fat in circulatory system, after fracture of large bones or administration of corticosteroids.
- 958.2 Secondary and recurrent hemorrhage
- 958.3 Posttraumatic wound infection, not elsewhere classified
  - EXCLUDES: infected open wounds — code to complicated open wound of site
  - AHA: 4Q, '01, 53; S-O, '85, 10
- 958.4 Traumatic shock
  - Shock (immediate) (delayed) following injury
  - EXCLUDES: shock:
    - anaphylactic (995.0)
    - due to serum (999.4)
    - anesthetic (995.4)
    - electric (994.8)
    - following abortion (639.5)
    - lightning (994.0)
    - nontraumatic NOS (785.50)
    - obstetric (669.1)
    - postoperative (998.0)
  - DEF: Shock, immediate or delayed following injury.

INJURY AND POISONING

958.5 Traumatic anuria
Crush syndrome
Renal failure following crushing
EXCLUDES that due to a medical procedure (997.5)
DEF: Complete suppression of urinary secretion by kidneys due to trauma.

958.6 Volkmann's ischemic contracture
Posttraumatic muscle contracture
DEF: Muscle deterioration due to loss of blood supply from injury or tourniquet; causes muscle contraction and results in inability to extend the muscles fully.

958.7 Traumatic subcutaneous emphysema
EXCLUDES subcutaneous emphysema resulting from a procedure (998.81)

958.8 Other early complications of trauma
AHA: 2Q, '92, 13
DEF: Compartmental syndrome is abnormal pressure in confined anatomical space, as in swollen muscle restricted by fascia.

√5th 958.9 Traumatic compartment syndrome
EXCLUDES nontraumatic compartment syndrome (729.71-729.79)

- **958.90 Compartment syndrome, unspecified**
- **958.91 Traumatic compartment syndrome of upper extremity**
Traumatic compartment syndrome of shoulder, arm, forearm, wrist, hand, and fingers
- **958.92 Traumatic compartment syndrome of lower extremity**
Traumatic compartment syndrome of hip, buttock, thigh, leg, foot, and toes
- **958.93 Traumatic compartment syndrome of abdomen**
- **958.99 Traumatic compartment syndrome of other sites**

√4th 959 Injury, other and unspecified
INCLUDES injury NOS
EXCLUDES injury NOS of:
blood vessels (900.0-904.9)
eye (921.0-921.9)
internal organs (860.0-869.1)
intracranial sites (854.0-854.1)
nerves (950.0-951.9, 953.0-957.9)
spinal cord (952.0-952.9)

√5th 959.0 Head, face and neck

959.01 Head injury, unspecified
EXCLUDES concussion (850.1-850.9)
with head injury NOS (850.0-850.9)
head injury NOS with loss of consciousness (850.1-850.5)
specified injuries (850.0-854.1)
AHA: 4Q, '97, 46

959.09 Injury of face and neck
Cheek   Mouth
Ear   Nose
Eyebrow   Throat
Lip
AHA: 4Q, '97, 46

√5th 959.1 Trunk
EXCLUDES scapular region (959.2)
AHA: 4Q, '03, 78; 1Q, '99, 10

959.11 Other injury of chest wall
959.12 Other injury of abdomen
959.13 Fracture of corpus cavernosum penis ♂
959.14 Other injury of external genitals
959.19 Other injury of other sites of trunk
Injury of trunk NOS

959.2 Shoulder and upper arm
Axilla   Scapular region

959.3 Elbow, forearm, and wrist
AHA: 1Q, '97, 8

959.4 Hand, except finger

959.5 Finger
Fingernail   Thumb (nail)

959.6 Hip and thigh
Upper leg

959.7 Knee, leg, ankle, and foot

959.8 Other specified sites, including multiple
EXCLUDES multiple sites classifiable to the same four-digit category (959.0-959.7)

959.9 Unspecified site

POISONING BY DRUGS, MEDICINAL AND BIOLOGICAL SUBSTANCES (960-979)

INCLUDES overdose of these substances
wrong substance given or taken in error
EXCLUDES adverse effects ["hypersensitivity," "reaction," etc.] of correct substance properly administered. Such cases are to be classified according to the nature of the adverse effect, such as:
adverse effect NOS ▶(995.20)◀
allergic lymphadenitis (289.3)
aspirin gastritis (535.4)
blood disorders (280.0-289.9)
dermatitis:
contact (692.0-692.9)
due to ingestion (693.0-693.9)
nephropathy (583.9)
[The drug giving rise to the adverse effect may be identified by use of categories E930-E949.]
drug dependence (304.0-304.9)
drug reaction and poisoning affecting the newborn (760.0-779.9)
nondependent abuse of drugs (305.0-305.9)
pathological drug intoxication (292.2)
Use additional code to specify the effects of the poisoning
AHA: 2Q, '90, 11

√4th 960 Poisoning by antibiotics
EXCLUDES antibiotics:
ear, nose, and throat (976.6)
eye (976.5)
local (976.0)

960.0 Penicillins
Ampicillin   Cloxacillin
Carbenicillin   Penicillin G

960.1 Antifungal antibiotics
Amphotericin B   Nystatin
Griseofulvin   Trichomycin
EXCLUDES preparations intended for topical use (976.0-976.9)

960.2 Chloramphenicol group
Chloramphenicol Thiamphenicol

960.3 Erythromycin and other macrolides
Oleandomycin   Spiramycin

960.4 Tetracycline group
Doxycycline   Oxytetracycline
Minocycline

960.5 Cephalosporin group
Cephalexin   Cephaloridine
Cephaloglycin   Cephalothin

960.6 Antimycobacterial antibiotics
Cycloserine   Rifampin
Kanamycin   Streptomycin

INJURY AND POISONING

960.7 Antineoplastic antibiotics
Actinomycin such as: Actinomycin such as:
Bleomycin Daunorubicin
Cactinomycin Mitomycin
Dactinomycin

960.8 Other specified antibiotics
960.9 Unspecified antibiotic

✓4th **961 Poisoning by other anti-infectives**
EXCLUDES: anti-infectives:
ear, nose, and throat (976.6)
eye (976.5)
local (976.0)

961.0 Sulfonamides
Sulfadiazine Sulfamethoxazole
Sulfafurazole

961.1 Arsenical anti-infectives

961.2 Heavy metal anti-infectives
Compounds of: Compounds of:
antimony lead
bismuth mercury
EXCLUDES: mercurial diuretics (974.0)

961.3 Quinoline and hydroxyquinoline derivatives
Chiniofon Diiodohydroxyquin
EXCLUDES: antimalarial drugs (961.4)

961.4 Antimalarials and drugs acting on other blood protozoa
Chloroquine Proguanil [chloroguanide]
Cycloguanil Pyrimethamine
Primaquine Quinine

961.5 Other antiprotozoal drugs
Emetine

961.6 Anthelmintics
Hexylresorcinol Thiabendazole
Piperazine

961.7 Antiviral drugs
Methisazone
EXCLUDES: amantadine (966.4)
cytarabine (963.1)
idoxuridine (976.5)

961.8 Other antimycobacterial drugs
Ethambutol Para-aminosalicylic acid
Ethionamide derivatives
Isoniazid Sulfones

961.9 Other and unspecified anti-infectives
Flucytosine Nitrofuran derivatives

✓4th **962 Poisoning by hormones and synthetic substitutes**
EXCLUDES: oxytocic hormones (975.0)

962.0 Adrenal cortical steroids
Cortisone derivatives
Desoxycorticosterone derivatives
Fluorinated corticosteroids

962.1 Androgens and anabolic congeners
Methandriol Oxymetholone
Nandrolone Testosterone

962.2 Ovarian hormones and synthetic substitutes
Contraceptives, oral
Estrogens
Estrogens and progestogens, combined
Progestogens

962.3 Insulins and antidiabetic agents
Acetohexamide Insulin
Biguanide derivatives, Phenformin
oral Sulfonylurea derivatives,
Chlorpropamide oral
Glucagon Tolbutamide
AHA: M-A, '85, 8

962.4 Anterior pituitary hormones
Corticotropin Somatotropin [growth
Gonadotropin hormone]

962.5 Posterior pituitary hormones
Vasopressin
EXCLUDES: oxytocic hormones (975.0)

962.6 Parathyroid and parathyroid derivatives
962.7 Thyroid and thyroid derivatives
Dextrothyroxin Liothyronine
Levothyroxine sodium Thyroglobulin

962.8 Antithyroid agents
Iodides Thiourea
Thiouracil

962.9 Other and unspecified hormones and synthetic substitutes

✓4th **963 Poisoning by primarily systemic agents**

963.0 Antiallergic and antiemetic drugs
Antihistamines Diphenylpyraline
Chlorpheniramine Thonzylamine
Diphenhydramine Tripelennamine
EXCLUDES: phenothiazine-based tranquilizers (969.1)

963.1 Antineoplastic and immunosuppressive drugs
Azathioprine Cytarabine
Busulfan Fluorouracil
Chlorambucil Mercaptopurine
Cyclophosphamide thio-TEPA
EXCLUDES: antineoplastic antibiotics (960.7)

963.2 Acidifying agents
963.3 Alkalizing agents
963.4 Enzymes, not elsewhere classified
Penicillinase

963.5 Vitamins, not elsewhere classified
Vitamin A Vitamin D
EXCLUDES: nicotinic acid (972.2)
vitamin K (964.3)

963.8 Other specified systemic agents
Heavy metal antagonists

963.9 Unspecified systemic agent

✓4th **964 Poisoning by agents primarily affecting blood constituents**

964.0 Iron and its compounds
Ferric salts
Ferrous sulfate and other ferrous salts

964.1 Liver preparations and other antianemic agents
Folic acid

964.2 Anticoagulants
Coumarin Phenindione
Heparin Warfarin sodium
AHA: 1Q, '94, 22

964.3 Vitamin K [phytonadione]
964.4 Fibrinolysis-affecting drugs
Aminocaproic acid Streptokinase
Streptodornase Urokinase

964.5 Anticoagulant antagonists and other coagulants
Hexadimethrine Protamine sulfate

964.6 Gamma globulin
964.7 Natural blood and blood products
Blood plasma Packed red cells
Human fibrinogen Whole blood
EXCLUDES: transfusion reactions (999.4-999.8)

964.8 Other specified agents affecting blood constituents
Macromolecular blood substitutes
Plasma expanders

964.9 Unspecified agent affecting blood constituents

✓4th **965 Poisoning by analgesics, antipyretics, and antirheumatics**
EXCLUDES: drug dependence (304.0-304.9)
nondependent abuse (305.0-305.9)

✓5th **965.0 Opiates and related narcotics**
965.00 Opium (alkaloids), unspecified
965.01 Heroin
Diacetylmorphine
965.02 Methadone
965.09 Other
Codeine [methylmorphine]
Meperidine [pethidine]
Morphine

INJURY AND POISONING — Tabular List

965.1–970.9

965.1 Salicylates
- Acetylsalicylic acid [aspirin]
- Salicylic acid salts

AHA: N-D, '94, 15

965.4 Aromatic analgesics, not elsewhere classified
- Acetanilid
- Paracetamol [acetaminophen]
- Phenacetin [acetophenetidin]

965.5 Pyrazole derivatives
- Aminophenazone [aminopyrine]
- Phenylbutazone

√5th 965.6 Antirheumatics [antiphlogistics]
EXCLUDES salicylates (965.1)
steroids (962.0-962.9)

AHA: 4Q, '98, 50

965.61 Propionic acid derivatives
- Fenoprofen
- Flurbiprofen
- Ibuprofen
- Ketoprofen
- Naproxen
- Oxaprozin

AHA: 4Q, '98, 50

965.69 Other antirheumatics
- Gold salts
- Indomethacin

965.7 Other non-narcotic analgesics
- Pyrabital

965.8 Other specified analgesics and antipyretics
- Pentazocine

965.9 Unspecified analgesic and antipyretic

√4th 966 Poisoning by anticonvulsants and anti-Parkinsonism drugs

966.0 Oxazolidine derivatives
- Paramethadione
- Trimethadione

966.1 Hydantoin derivatives
- Phenytoin

966.2 Succinimides
- Ethosuximide
- Phensuximide

966.3 Other and unspecified anticonvulsants
- Primidone

EXCLUDES barbiturates (967.0)
sulfonamides (961.0)

966.4 Anti-Parkinsonism drugs
- Amantadine
- Ethopropazine [profenamine]
- Levodopa [L-dopa]

√4th 967 Poisoning by sedatives and hypnotics
EXCLUDES drug dependence (304.0-304.9)
nondependent abuse (305.0-305.9)

967.0 Barbiturates
- Amobarbital [amylobarbitone]
- Barbital [barbitone]
- Butabarbital [butabarbitone]
- Pentobarbital [pentobarbitone]
- Phenobarbital [phenobarbitone]
- Secobarbital [quinalbarbitone]

EXCLUDES thiobarbiturate anesthetics (968.3)

967.1 Chloral hydrate group
967.2 Paraldehyde
967.3 Bromine compounds
- Bromide
- Carbromal (derivatives)

967.4 Methaqualone compounds
967.5 Glutethimide group
967.6 Mixed sedatives, not elsewhere classified
967.8 Other sedatives and hypnotics
967.9 Unspecified sedative or hypnotic
- Sleeping:
  - drug
  - pill   } NOS
  - tablet

√4th 968 Poisoning by other central nervous system depressants and anesthetics
EXCLUDES drug dependence (304.0-304.9)
nondependent abuse (305.0-305.9)

968.0 Central nervous system muscle-tone depressants
- Chlorphenesin (carbamate)
- Mephenesin
- Methocarbamol

968.1 Halothane
968.2 Other gaseous anesthetics
- Ether
- Halogenated hydrocarbon derivatives, except halothane
- Nitrous oxide

968.3 Intravenous anesthetics
- Ketamine
- Methohexital [methohexitone]
- Thiobarbiturates, such as thiopental sodium

968.4 Other and unspecified general anesthetics
968.5 Surface [topical] and infiltration anesthetics
- Cocaine
- Lidocaine [lignocaine]
- Procaine
- Tetracaine

AHA: 1Q, '93, 25

968.6 Peripheral nerve- and plexus-blocking anesthetics
968.7 Spinal anesthetics
968.9 Other and unspecified local anesthetics

√4th 969 Poisoning by psychotropic agents
EXCLUDES drug dependence (304.0-304.9)
nondependent abuse (305.0-305.9)

969.0 Antidepressants
- Amitriptyline
- Imipramine
- Monoamine oxidase [MAO] inhibitors

969.1 Phenothiazine-based tranquilizers
- Chlorpromazine
- Fluphenazine
- Prochlorperazine
- Promazine

969.2 Butyrophenone-based tranquilizers
- Haloperidol
- Spiperone
- Trifluperidol

969.3 Other antipsychotics, neuroleptics, and major tranquilizers

969.4 Benzodiazepine-based tranquilizers
- Chlordiazepoxide
- Diazepam
- Flurazepam
- Lorazepam
- Medazepam
- Nitrazepam

969.5 Other tranquilizers
- Hydroxyzine
- Meprobamate

969.6 Psychodysleptics [hallucinogens]
- Cannabis (derivatives)
- Lysergide [LSD]
- Marihuana (derivatives)
- Mescaline
- Psilocin
- Psilocybin

969.7 Psychostimulants
- Amphetamine
- Caffeine

EXCLUDES central appetite depressants (977.0)

AHA: 2Q, '03, 11

969.8 Other specified psychotropic agents
969.9 Unspecified psychotropic agent

√4th 970 Poisoning by central nervous system stimulants

970.0 Analeptics
- Lobeline
- Nikethamide

970.1 Opiate antagonists
- Levallorphan
- Nalorphine
- Naloxone

970.8 Other specified central nervous system stimulants

AHA: 1Q, '05, 6

970.9 Unspecified central nervous system stimulant

Tabular List — INJURY AND POISONING — 971–977.2

✓4th 971 Poisoning by drugs primarily affecting the autonomic nervous system

- **971.0 Parasympathomimetics [cholinergics]**
  - Acetylcholine
  - Anticholinesterase: organophosphorus reversible
  - Pilocarpine
- **971.1 Parasympatholytics [anticholinergics and antimuscarinics] and spasmolytics**
  - Atropine
  - Homatropine
  - Hyoscine [scopolamine]
  - Quaternary ammonium derivatives
  - EXCLUDES: papaverine (972.5)
- **971.2 Sympathomimetics [adrenergics]**
  - Epinephrine [adrenalin]
  - Levarterenol [noradrenalin]
- **971.3 Sympatholytics [antiadrenergics]**
  - Phenoxybenzamine
  - Tolazolinehydrochloride
- **971.9 Unspecified drug primarily affecting autonomic nervous system**

✓4th 972 Poisoning by agents primarily affecting the cardiovascular system

- **972.0 Cardiac rhythm regulators**
  - Practolol
  - Procainamide
  - Propranolol
  - Quinidine
  - EXCLUDES: lidocaine (968.5)
- **972.1 Cardiotonic glycosides and drugs of similar action**
  - Digitalis glycosides
  - Digoxin
  - Strophanthins
- **972.2 Antilipemic and antiarteriosclerotic drugs**
  - Clofibrate
  - Nicotinic acid derivatives
- **972.3 Ganglion-blocking agents**
  - Pentamethonium bromide
- **972.4 Coronary vasodilators**
  - Dipyridamole
  - Nitrates [nitroglycerin]
  - Nitrites
- **972.5 Other vasodilators**
  - Cyclandelate
  - Diazoxide
  - Papaverine
  - EXCLUDES: nicotinic acid (972.2)
- **972.6 Other antihypertensive agents**
  - Clonidine
  - Guanethidine
  - Rauwolfia alkaloids
  - Reserpine
- **972.7 Antivaricose drugs, including sclerosing agents**
  - Sodium morrhuate
  - Zinc salts
- **972.8 Capillary-active drugs**
  - Adrenochrome derivatives
  - Metaraminol
- **972.9 Other and unspecified agents primarily affecting the cardiovascular system**

✓4th 973 Poisoning by agents primarily affecting the gastrointestinal system

- **973.0 Antacids and antigastric secretion drugs**
  - Aluminum hydroxide
  - Magnesium trisilicate
  - AHA: 1Q, '03, 19
- **973.1 Irritant cathartics**
  - Bisacodyl
  - Castor oil
  - Phenolphthalein
- **973.2 Emollient cathartics**
  - Dioctyl sulfosuccinates
- **973.3 Other cathartics, including intestinal atonia drugs**
  - Magnesium sulfate
- **973.4 Digestants**
  - Pancreatin
  - Papain
  - Pepsin
- **973.5 Antidiarrheal drugs**
  - Kaolin
  - Pectin
  - EXCLUDES: anti-infectives (960.0-961.9)
- **973.6 Emetics**
- **973.8 Other specified agents primarily affecting the gastrointestinal system**
- **973.9 Unspecified agent primarily affecting the gastrointestinal system**

✓4th 974 Poisoning by water, mineral, and uric acid metabolism drugs

- **974.0 Mercurial diuretics**
  - Chlormerodrin
  - Mercaptomerin
  - Mersalyl
- **974.1 Purine derivative diuretics**
  - Theobromine
  - Theophylline
  - EXCLUDES: aminophylline [theophylline ethylenediamine] (975.7)
  - caffeine (969.7)
- **974.2 Carbonic acid anhydrase inhibitors**
  - Acetazolamide
- **974.3 Saluretics**
  - Benzothiadiazides
  - Chlorothiazide group
- **974.4 Other diuretics**
  - Ethacrynic acid
  - Furosemide
- **974.5 Electrolytic, caloric, and water-balance agents**
- **974.6 Other mineral salts, not elsewhere classified**
- **974.7 Uric acid metabolism drugs**
  - Allopurinol
  - Colchicine
  - Probenecid

✓4th 975 Poisoning by agents primarily acting on the smooth and skeletal muscles and respiratory system

- **975.0 Oxytocic agents**
  - Ergot alkaloids
  - Oxytocin
  - Prostaglandins
- **975.1 Smooth muscle relaxants**
  - Adiphenine
  - Metaproterenol [orciprenaline]
  - EXCLUDES: papaverine (972.5)
- **975.2 Skeletal muscle relaxants**
- **975.3 Other and unspecified drugs acting on muscles**
- **975.4 Antitussives**
  - Dextromethorphan
  - Pipazethate
- **975.5 Expectorants**
  - Acetylcysteine
  - Guaifenesin
  - Terpin hydrate
- **975.6 Anti-common cold drugs**
- **975.7 Antiasthmatics**
  - Aminophylline [theophylline ethylenediamine]
- **975.8 Other and unspecified respiratory drugs**

✓4th 976 Poisoning by agents primarily affecting skin and mucous membrane, ophthalmological, otorhinolaryngological, and dental drugs

- **976.0 Local anti-infectives and anti-inflammatory drugs**
- **976.1 Antipruritics**
- **976.2 Local astringents and local detergents**
- **976.3 Emollients, demulcents, and protectants**
- **976.4 Keratolytics, keratoplastics, other hair treatment drugs and preparations**
- **976.5 Eye anti-infectives and other eye drugs**
  - Idoxuridine
- **976.6 Anti-infectives and other drugs and preparations for ear, nose, and throat**
- **976.7 Dental drugs topically applied**
  - EXCLUDES: anti-infectives (976.0)
  - local anesthetics (968.5)
- **976.8 Other agents primarily affecting skin and mucous membrane**
  - Spermicides [vaginal contraceptives]
- **976.9 Unspecified agent primarily affecting skin and mucous membrane**

✓4th 977 Poisoning by other and unspecified drugs and medicinal substances

- **977.0 Dietetics**
  - Central appetite depressants
- **977.1 Lipotropic drugs**
- **977.2 Antidotes and chelating agents, not elsewhere classified**

Additional Digit Required | Unspecified Code | Other Specified Code | Manifestation Code | ▶◀ Revised Text | ● New Code | ▲ Revised Code Title

2007 ICD•9•CM — Volume 1 — 289

INJURY AND POISONING

977.3 Alcohol deterrents
977.4 Pharmaceutical excipients
 Pharmaceutical adjuncts
977.8 Other specified drugs and medicinal substances
 Contrast media used for diagnostic x-ray procedures
 Diagnostic agents and kits
977.9 Unspecified drug or medicinal substance

√4th **978** Poisoning by bacterial vaccines
978.0 BCG
978.1 Typhoid and paratyphoid
978.2 Cholera
978.3 Plague
978.4 Tetanus
978.5 Diphtheria
978.6 Pertussis vaccine, including combinations with a pertussis component
978.8 Other and unspecified bacterial vaccines
978.9 Mixed bacterial vaccines, except combinations with a pertussis component

√4th **979** Poisoning by other vaccines and biological substances
 EXCLUDES gamma globulin (964.6)
979.0 Smallpox vaccine
979.1 Rabies vaccine
979.2 Typhus vaccine
979.3 Yellow fever vaccine
979.4 Measles vaccine
979.5 Poliomyelitis vaccine
979.6 Other and unspecified viral and rickettsial vaccines
 Mumps vaccine
979.7 Mixed viral-rickettsial and bacterial vaccines, except combinations with a pertussis component
 EXCLUDES combinations with a pertussis component (978.6)
979.9 Other and unspecified vaccines and biological substances

TOXIC EFFECTS OF SUBSTANCES CHIEFLY NONMEDICINAL AS TO SOURCE (980-989)

 EXCLUDES burns from chemical agents (ingested) (947.0-947.9)
 localized toxic effects indexed elsewhere (001.0-799.9)
 respiratory conditions due to external agents (506.0-508.9)
 Use additional code to specify the nature of the toxic effect

√4th **980** Toxic effect of alcohol
980.0 Ethyl alcohol
 Denatured alcohol Grain alcohol
 Ethanol
 Use additional code to identify any associated:
 acute alcohol intoxication (305.0)
 in alcoholism (303.0)
 drunkenness (simple) (305.0)
 pathological (291.4)
 AHA: 3Q, '96, 16
980.1 Methyl alcohol
 Methanol Wood alcohol
980.2 Isopropyl alcohol
 Dimethyl carbinol Rubbing alcohol
 Isopropanol
980.3 Fusel oil
 Alcohol: Alcohol:
  amyl   propyl
  butyl
980.8 Other specified alcohols
980.9 Unspecified alcohol

981 Toxic effect of petroleum products
 Benzine Petroleum:
 Gasoline   ether
 Kerosene   naphtha
 Paraffin wax   spirit

√4th **982** Toxic effect of solvents other than petroleum-based
982.0 Benzene and homologues
982.1 Carbon tetrachloride
982.2 Carbon disulfide
 Carbon bisulfide
982.3 Other chlorinated hydrocarbon solvents
 Tetrachloroethylene Trichloroethylene
 EXCLUDES chlorinated hydrocarbon preparations other than solvents (989.2)
982.4 Nitroglycol
982.8 Other nonpetroleum-based solvents
 Acetone

√4th **983** Toxic effect of corrosive aromatics, acids, and caustic alkalis
983.0 Corrosive aromatics
 Carbolic acid or phenol Cresol
983.1 Acids
 Acid: Acid:
  hydrochloric   sulfuric
  nitric
983.2 Caustic alkalis
 Lye Sodium hydroxide
 Potassium hydroxide
983.9 Caustic, unspecified

√4th **984** Toxic effect of lead and its compounds (including fumes)
 INCLUDES that from all sources except medicinal substances
984.0 Inorganic lead compounds
 Lead dioxide Lead salts
984.1 Organic lead compounds
 Lead acetate Tetraethyl lead
984.8 Other lead compounds
984.9 Unspecified lead compound

√4th **985** Toxic effect of other metals
 INCLUDES that from all sources except medicinal substances
985.0 Mercury and its compounds
 Minamata disease
985.1 Arsenic and its compounds
985.2 Manganese and its compounds
985.3 Beryllium and its compounds
985.4 Antimony and its compounds
985.5 Cadmium and its compounds
985.6 Chromium
985.8 Other specified metals
 Brass fumes Iron compounds
 Copper salts Nickel compounds
 AHA: 1Q, '88, 5
985.9 Unspecified metal

986 Toxic effect of carbon monoxide
 Carbon monoxide from any source

√4th **987** Toxic effect of other gases, fumes, or vapors
987.0 Liquefied petroleum gases
 Butane Propane
987.1 Other hydrocarbon gas
987.2 Nitrogen oxides
 Nitrogen dioxide Nitrous fumes
987.3 Sulfur dioxide
987.4 Freon
 Dichloromonofluoromethane
987.5 Lacrimogenic gas
 Bromobenzyl cyanide Ethyliodoacetate
 Chloroacetophenone

INJURY AND POISONING

987.6 Chlorine gas
987.7 Hydrocyanic acid gas
987.8 Other specified gases, fumes, or vapors
Phosgene   Polyester fumes
987.9 Unspecified gas, fume, or vapor
AHA: ▶3Q, '05, 10◀

✓4th 988 Toxic effect of noxious substances eaten as food
EXCLUDES: allergic reaction to food, such as:
gastroenteritis (558.3)
rash (692.5, 693.1)
food poisoning (bacterial) (005.0-005.9)
toxic effects of food contaminants, such as:
aflatoxin and other mycotoxin (989.7)
mercury (985.0)

988.0 Fish and shellfish
988.1 Mushrooms
988.2 Berries and other plants
988.8 Other specified noxious substances eaten as food
988.9 Unspecified noxious substance eaten as food

✓4th 989 Toxic effect of other substances, chiefly nonmedicinal as to source
989.0 Hydrocyanic acid and cyanides
Potassium cyanide   Sodium cyanide
EXCLUDES: gas and fumes (987.7)
989.1 Strychnine and salts
989.2 Chlorinated hydrocarbons
Aldrin   DDT
Chlordane   Dieldrin
EXCLUDES: chlorinated hydrocarbon solvents (982.0-982.3)
989.3 Organophosphate and carbamate
Carbaryl   Parathion
Dichlorvos   Phorate
Malathion   Phosdrin
989.4 Other pesticides, not elsewhere classified
Mixtures of insecticides
989.5 Venom
Bites of venomous snakes, lizards, and spiders
Tick paralysis
989.6 Soaps and detergents
989.7 Aflatoxin and other mycotoxin [food contaminants]
✓5th 989.8 Other substances, chiefly nonmedicinal as to source
AHA: 4Q, '95, 60

989.81 Asbestos
EXCLUDES: asbestosis (501)
exposure to asbestos (V15.84)
989.82 Latex
989.83 Silicone
EXCLUDES: silicone used in medical devices, implants and grafts (996.00-996.79)
989.84 Tobacco
989.89 Other
989.9 Unspecified substance, chiefly nonmedicinal as to source

OTHER AND UNSPECIFIED EFFECTS OF EXTERNAL CAUSES (990-995)

990 Effects of radiation, unspecified
Complication of: Radiation sickness
phototherapy
radiation therapy
EXCLUDES: specified adverse effects of radiation. Such conditions are to be classified according to the nature of the adverse effect, as:
burns (940.0-949.5)
dermatitis (692.7-692.8)
leukemia (204.0-208.9)
pneumonia (508.0)
sunburn (692.71, 692.76-692.77)
[The type of radiation giving rise to the adverse effect may be identified by use of the E codes.]

✓4th 991 Effects of reduced temperature
991.0 Frostbite of face
991.1 Frostbite of hand
991.2 Frostbite of foot
991.3 Frostbite of other and unspecified sites
991.4 Immersion foot
Trench foot
DEF: Paresthesia, edema, blotchy cyanosis of foot, the skin is soft (macerated), pale and wrinkled, and the sole is swollen with surface ridging and following sustained immersion in water.

991.5 Chilblains
Erythema pernio   Perniosis
DEF: Red, swollen, itchy skin; follows damp cold exposure; also associated with pruritus and a burning feeling, in hands, feet, ears, and face in children, legs and toes in women, and hands and fingers in men.

991.6 Hypothermia
Hypothermia (accidental)
EXCLUDES: hypothermia following anesthesia (995.89)
hypothermia not associated with low environmental temperature (780.99)
DEF: Reduced body temperature due to low environmental temperatures.

991.8 Other specified effects of reduced temperature
991.9 Unspecified effect of reduced temperature
Effects of freezing or excessive cold NOS

✓4th 992 Effects of heat and light
EXCLUDES: burns (940.0-949.5)
diseases of sweat glands due to heat (705.0-705.9)
malignant hyperpyrexia following anesthesia (995.86)
sunburn (692.71, 692.76-692.77)

992.0 Heat stroke and sunstroke
Heat apoplexy   Siriasis
Heat pyrexia   Thermoplegia
Ictus solaris
DEF: Headache, vertigo, cramps and elevated body temperature due to high environmental temperatures.

992.1 Heat syncope
Heat collapse
992.2 Heat cramps
992.3 Heat exhaustion, anhydrotic
Heat prostration due to water depletion
EXCLUDES: that associated with salt depletion (992.4)
992.4 Heat exhaustion due to salt depletion
Heat prostration due to salt (and water) depletion
992.5 Heat exhaustion, unspecified
Heat prostration NOS
992.6 Heat fatigue, transient

992.7–995.29 INJURY AND POISONING

992.7 Heat edema
DEF: Fluid retention due to high environmental temperatures.

992.8 Other specified heat effects

992.9 Unspecified

√4th **993** Effects of air pressure

993.0 Barotrauma, otitic
Aero-otitis media   Effects of high altitude on ears
DEF: Ringing ears, deafness, pain and vertigo due to air pressure changes.

993.1 Barotrauma, sinus
Aerosinusitis
Effects of high altitude on sinuses

993.2 Other and unspecified effects of high altitude
Alpine sickness   Hypobaropathy
Andes disease   Mountain sickness
Anoxia due to high altitude
AHA: 3Q, '88, 4

993.3 Caisson disease
Bends   Decompression sickness
Compressed-air disease   Divers' palsy or paralysis
DEF: Rapid reduction in air pressure while breathing compressed air; symptoms include skin lesions, joint pains, respiratory and neurological problems.

993.4 Effects of air pressure caused by explosion

993.8 Other specified effects of air pressure

993.9 Unspecified effect of air pressure

√4th **994** Effects of other external causes
EXCLUDES   certain adverse effects not elsewhere classified (995.0-995.8)

994.0 Effects of lightning
Shock from lightning   Struck by lightning NOS
EXCLUDES   burns (940.0-949.5)

994.1 Drowning and nonfatal submersion
Bathing cramp   Immersion
AHA: 3Q, '88, 4

994.2 Effects of hunger
Deprivation of food   Starvation

994.3 Effects of thirst
Deprivation of water

994.4 Exhaustion due to exposure

994.5 Exhaustion due to excessive exertion
Overexertion

994.6 Motion sickness
Air sickness   Travel sickness
Seasickness

994.7 Asphyxiation and strangulation
Suffocation (by):   Suffocation (by):
  bedclothes   plastic bag
  cave-in   pressure
  constriction   strangulation
  mechanical
EXCLUDES   asphyxia from:
  carbon monoxide (986)
  inhalation of food or foreign body (932-934.9)
  other gases, fumes, and vapors (987.0-987.9)

994.8 Electrocution and nonfatal effects of electric current
Shock from electric current
EXCLUDES   electric burns (940.0-949.5)

994.9 Other effects of external causes
Effects of:
  abnormal gravitational [G] forces or states
  weightlessness

Continuum of Illness Due to Infection
Bacteremia → Septicemia → Sepsis
Severe Sepsis with Septic Shock ← Severe Sepsis ←
↓
MODS (Multiple Organ Dysfunction Syndrome) → Death

√4th **995** Certain adverse effects not elsewhere classified
EXCLUDES   complications of surgical and medical care (996.0-999.9)

995.0 Other anaphylactic shock
Allergic shock   } NOS or due to adverse effect of
Anaphylactic   correct medicinal
  reaction   substance properly
Anaphylaxis   administered
Use additional E code to identify external cause, such as:
  adverse effects of correct medicinal substance properly administered [E930-E949]
EXCLUDES   anaphylactic reaction to serum (999.4)
    anaphylactic shock due to adverse food reaction (995.60-995.69)
AHA: 4Q, '93, 30
DEF: Immediate sensitivity response after exposure to specific antigen; results in life-threatening respiratory distress; usually followed by vascular collapse, shock, urticaria, angioedema and pruritus.

995.1 Angioneurotic edema
Giant urticaria
EXCLUDES   urticaria:
  due to serum (999.5)
  other specified (698.2, 708.0-708.9, 757.33)
DEF: Circulatory response of deep dermis, subcutaneous or submucosal tissues; causes localized edema and wheals.

▲ √5th **995.2** Other and unspecified adverse effect of drug, medicinal and biological substance
Adverse effect   } (due) to correct medicinal
Allergic reaction   substance properly
Hypersensitivity   administered
Idiosyncrasy
Drug: Drug:
  hypersensitivity NOS   reaction NOS
EXCLUDES   pathological drug intoxication (292.2)
AHA: 2Q, '97, 12; 3Q, '95, 13; 3Q, '92, 16

• **995.20** Unspecified adverse effect of unspecified drug, medicinal and biological substance
• **995.21** Arthus phenomenon
Arthus reaction
• **995.22** Unspecified adverse effect of anesthesia
• **995.23** Unspecified adverse effect of insulin
• **995.27** Other drug allergy
Drug allergy NOS
Drug hypersensitivity NOS
• **995.29** Unspecified adverse effect of other drug, medicinal and biological substance

INJURY AND POISONING

995.3 Allergy, unspecified
Allergic reaction NOS Idiosyncrasy NOS
Hypersensitivity NOS
EXCLUDES: allergic reaction NOS to correct
  medicinal substance properly
  administered ▶(995.27)◀
  ▶allergy to existing dental restorative
  materials (525.66)◀
  specific types of allergic reaction, such as:
  allergic diarrhea (558.3)
  dermatitis (691.0-693.9)
  hayfever (477.0-477.9)

995.4 Shock due to anesthesia
Shock due to anesthesia in which the correct substance was properly administered
EXCLUDES: complications of anesthesia in labor or delivery (668.0-668.9)
  overdose or wrong substance given (968.0-969.9)
  postoperative shock NOS (998.0)
  specified adverse effects of anesthesia classified elsewhere, such as:
  anoxic brain damage (348.1)
  hepatitis (070.0-070.9), etc.
  unspecified adverse effect of anesthesia ▶(995.22)◀

√5th 995.5 Child maltreatment syndrome
Use additional code(s), if applicable, to identify any associated injuries
Use additional E code to identify:
  nature of abuse (E960-E968)
  perpetrator (E967.0-E967.9)
AHA: 1Q, '98, 11

995.50 Child abuse, unspecified

995.51 Child emotional/psychological abuse
AHA: 4Q, '96, 38, 40

995.52 Child neglect (nutritional)
AHA: 4Q, '96, 38, 40

995.53 Child sexual abuse
AHA: 4Q, '96, 39, 40

995.54 Child physical abuse
Battered baby or child syndrome
EXCLUDES: shaken infant syndrome (995.55)
AHA: 3Q, '99, 14; 4Q, '96, 39, 40

995.55 Shaken infant syndrome
Use additional code(s) to identify any associated injuries
AHA: 4Q, '96, 40, 43

995.59 Other child abuse and neglect
Multiple forms of abuse

√5th 995.6 Anaphylactic shock due to adverse food reaction
Anaphylactic shock due to nonpoisonous foods
AHA: 4Q, '93, 30

995.60 Due to unspecified food
995.61 Due to peanuts
995.62 Due to crustaceans
995.63 Due to fruits and vegetables
995.64 Due to tree nuts and seeds
995.65 Due to fish
995.66 Due to food additives
995.67 Due to milk products
995.68 Due to eggs
995.69 Due to other specified food

995.7 Other adverse food reactions, not elsewhere classified
Use additional code to identify the type of reaction, such as:
  hives (708.0)
  wheezing (786.07)
EXCLUDES: anaphylactic shock due to adverse food reaction (995.60-995.69)
  asthma (493.0, 493.9)
  dermatitis due to food (693.1)
  in contact with the skin (692.5)
  gastroenteritis and colitis due to food (558.3)
  rhinitis due to food (477.1)

√5th 995.8 Other specified adverse effects, not elsewhere classified

995.80 Adult maltreatment, unspecified
Abused person NOS
Use additional code to identify:
  any associated injury
  perpetrator (E967.0-E967.9)
AHA: 4Q, '96, 41, 43

995.81 Adult physical abuse
Battered: Battered:
  person syndrome spouse
  NEC   woman
                man
Use additional code to identify:
  any association injury
  nature of abuse (E960-E968)
  perpetrator (E967.0-E967.9)
AHA: 4Q, '96, 42, 43

995.82 Adult emotional/psychological abuse
Use additional E code to identify perpetrator (E967.0-E967.9)

995.83 Adult sexual abuse
Use additional code to identify:
  any associated injury
  perpetrator (E967.0-E967.9)

995.84 Adult neglect (nutritional)
Use addition code to identify:
  intent of neglect (E904.0, E968.4)
  perpetrator (E967.0-E967.9)

995.85 Other adult abuse and neglect
Multiple forms of abuse and neglect
Use additional code to identify:
  any associated injury
  intent of neglect (E904.0, E968.4)
  nature of abuse (E960-E968)
  perpetrator (E967.0-E967.9)

995.86 Malignant hyperthermia
Malignant hyperpyrexia due to anesthesia
AHA: 4Q, '98, 51

995.89 Other
Hypothermia due to anesthesia
AHA: 2Q, '04, 18; 3Q, '03, 12

INJURY AND POISONING

995.9 Systemic inflammatory response syndrome (SIRS)
AHA: 2Q, '04, 16; 4Q, '02, 71

DEF: Clinical response to infection or trauma that can trigger an acute inflammatory reaction and progresses to coagulation, impaired fibrinolysis, and organ failure; manifested by two or more of the following symptoms: fever, tachycardia, tachypnea, leukocytosis or leukopenia.

995.90 Systemic inflammatory response syndrome, unspecified
SIRS NOS

995.91 Sepsis
▶Systemic inflammatory response syndrome due to infectious process without acute organ dysfunction◀
▶Code first underlying infection◀
EXCLUDES ▶ sepsis with acute organ dysfunction (995.92)
sepsis with multiple organ dysfunction (995.92)
severe sepsis (995.92)◀
AHA: 2Q, '04, 16; 4Q, '03, 79

995.92 Severe sepsis
▶Sepsis with acute organ dysfunction
Sepsis with multiple organ dysfunction (MOD)
Systemic inflammatory response syndrome due to infectious process with acute organ dysfunction
Code first underlying infection◀
Use additional code to specify ▶acute◀ organ dysfunction, such as:
acute renal failure (584.5-584.9)
acute respiratory failure (518.81)
critical illness myopathy (359.81)
critical illness polyneuropathy (357.82)
▶disseminated intravascular coagulopathy [DIC] (286.6)◀
encephalopathy (348.31)
hepatic failure (570)
septic shock (785.52)
AHA: 2Q, '05, 18-19; 1Q, '05, 7; 1Q, '05, 7; 2Q, '04, 16; 4Q, '03, 73, 79

995.93 Systemic inflammatory response syndrome due to noninfectious process without acute organ dysfunction
▶Code first underlying conditions, such as:
acute pancreatitis (577.0)
trauma◀
EXCLUDES ▶ systemic inflammatory response syndrome due to noninfectious process with acute organ dysfunction (995.94)◀

995.94 Systemic inflammatory response syndrome due to noninfectious process with acute organ dysfunction
▶Code first underlying conditions, such as:
acute pancreatitis (577.0)
trauma◀
Use additional code to specify ▶acute◀ organ dysfunction, such as:
acute renal failure (584.5-584.9)
acute respiratory failure (518.81)
critical illness myopathy (359.81)
critical illness polyneuropathy (357.82)
▶disseminated intravascular coagulopathy [DIC] syndrome (286.6)◀
encephalopathy (348.31)
hepatic failure (570)
EXCLUDES ▶ severe sepsis (995.92)◀
AHA: 4Q, '03, 79

COMPLICATIONS OF SURGICAL AND MEDICAL CARE, NOT ELSEWHERE CLASSIFIED (996-999)

EXCLUDES adverse effects of medicinal agents (001.0-799.9, 995.0-995.8)
burns from local applications and irradiation (940.0-949.5)
complications of:
conditions for which the procedure was performed
surgical procedures during abortion, labor, and delivery (630-676.9)
poisoning and toxic effects of drugs and chemicals (960.0-989.9)
postoperative conditions in which no complications are present, such as:
artificial opening status (V44.0-V44.9)
closure of external stoma (V55.0-V55.9)
fitting of prosthetic device (V52.0-V52.9)
specified complications classified elsewhere
anesthetic shock (995.4)
electrolyte imbalance (276.0-276.9)
postlaminectomy syndrome (722.80-722.83)
postmastectomy lymphedema syndrome (457.0)
postoperative psychosis (293.0-293.9)
any other condition classified elsewhere in the Alphabetic Index when described as due to a procedure

996 Complications peculiar to certain specified procedures
INCLUDES complications, not elsewhere classified, in the use of artificial substitutes [e.g., Dacron, metal, Silastic, Teflon] or natural sources [e.g., bone] involving:
anastomosis (internal)
graft (bypass) (patch)
implant
internal device:
catheter
electronic
fixation
prosthetic
reimplant
transplant
EXCLUDES accidental puncture or laceration during procedure (998.2)
complications of internal anastomosis of:
gastrointestinal tract (997.4)
urinary tract (997.5)
mechanical complication of respirator (V46.14)
other specified complications classified elsewhere, such as:
hemolytic anemia (283.1)
functional cardiac disturbances (429.4)
serum hepatitis (070.2-070.3)
AHA: 1Q, '94, 3

996.0 Mechanical complication of cardiac device, implant, and graft
Breakdown (mechanical)   Obstruction, mechanical
Displacement   Perforation
Leakage   Protrusion
AHA: 2Q, '93, 9

996.00 Unspecified device, implant, and graft
996.01 Due to cardiac pacemaker (electrode)
AHA: 2Q, '99, 11

996.02 Due to heart valve prosthesis
996.03 Due to coronary bypass graft
EXCLUDES atherosclerosis of graft (414.02, 414.03)
embolism [occlusion NOS] [thrombus] of graft (996.72)
AHA: 2Q, '95, 17; N-D, '86, 5

INJURY AND POISONING

996.04 Due to automatic implantable cardiac defibrillator
AHA: 2Q, '05, 3

996.09 Other
AHA: 2Q, '93, 9

996.1 Mechanical complication of other vascular device, implant, and graft
femoral-popliteal bypass graft
Mechanical complications involving:
  aortic (bifurcation) graft (replacement)
  arteriovenous:
    dialysis catheter
    fistula   } surgically created
    shunt
  balloon (counterpulsation) device, intra-aortic
  carotid artery bypass graft
  umbrella device, vena cava

EXCLUDES atherosclerosis of biological graft (440.30-440.32)
          embolism [occulsion NOS] [thrombus] of (biological) (synthetic) graft (996.74)
          peritoneal dialysis catheter (996.56)

AHA: 2Q, '05, 8; 1Q, '02, 13; 1Q, '95, 3

996.2 Mechanical complication of nervous system device, implant, and graft
Mechanical complications involving:
  dorsal column stimulator
  electrodes implanted in brain [brain "pacemaker"]
  peripheral nerve graft
  ventricular (communicating) shunt

AHA: 2Q, '99, 4; S-O, '87, 10

✓5th 996.3 Mechanical complication of genitourinary device, implant, and graft
AHA: 3Q, '01, 13; S-O, '85, 3

996.30 Unspecified device, implant, and graft

996.31 Due to urethral [indwelling] catheter

996.32 Due to intrauterine contraceptive device ♀

996.39 Other
Cystostomy catheter
Prosthetic reconstruction of vas deferens
Repair (graft) of ureter without mention of resection

EXCLUDES complications due to:
          external stoma of urinary tract (997.5)
          internal anastomosis of urinary tract (997.5)

✓5th 996.4 Mechanical complication of internal orthopedic device, implant, and graft
Mechanical complications involving:
  external (fixation) device utilizing internal screw(s), pin(s) or other methods of fixation
  grafts of bone, cartilage, muscle, or tendon
  internal (fixation) device such as nail, plate, rod, etc.
Use additional code to identify prosthetic joint with mechanical complication (V43.60-V43.69)

EXCLUDES complications of external orthopedic device, such as:
          pressure ulcer due to cast (707.00-707.09)

AHA: 4Q, '05, 91; 2Q, '99, 10; 2Q, '98, 19; 2Q, '96, 11; 3Q, '95, 16; N-D, '85, 11

996.40 Unspecified mechanical complication of internal orthopedic device, implant, and graft

996.41 Mechanical loosening of prosthetic joint
Aseptic loosening
AHA: 4Q, '05, 112

996.42 Dislocation of prosthetic joint
Instability of prosthetic joint
Subluxation of prosthetic joint

996.43 Prosthetic joint implant failure
Breakage (fracture) of prosthetic joint

996.44 Peri-prosthetic fracture around prosthetic joint
AHA: 4Q, '05, 93

996.45 Peri-prosthetic osteolysis
▶Use additional code to identify major osseous defect, if applicable (731.3)◀

996.46 Articular bearing surface wear of prosthetic joint

996.47 Other mechanical complication of prosthetic joint implant
Mechanical complication of prosthetic joint NOS

996.49 Other mechanical complication of other internal orthopedic device, implant, and graft

EXCLUDES mechanical complication of prosthetic joint implant (996.41-996.47)

✓5th 996.5 Mechanical complication of other specified prosthetic device, implant, and graft
Mechanical complications involving:
  prosthetic implant in: prosthetic implant in:
    bile duct   chin
    breast   orbit of eye
  nonabsorbable surgical material NOS
  other graft, implant, and internal device, not elsewhere classified

AHA: 1Q, '98, 11

996.51 Due to corneal graft

996.52 Due to graft of other tissue, not elsewhere classified
Skin graft failure or rejection

EXCLUDES failure of artificial skin graft (996.55)
          failure of decellularized allodermis (996.55)
          sloughing of temporary skin allografts or xenografts (pigskin)—omit code

AHA: 1Q, '96, 10

996.53 Due to ocular lens prosthesis

EXCLUDES contact lenses—code to condition

AHA: 1Q, '00, 9

996.54 Due to breast prosthesis
Breast capsule (prosthesis)
Mammary implant
AHA: 2Q, '98, 14; 3Q, '92, 4

996.55 Due to artificial skin graft and decellularized allodermis
Dislodgement   Non-adherence
Displacement   Poor incorporation
Failure   Shearing
AHA: 4Q, '98, 52

996.56 Due to peritoneal dialysis catheter

EXCLUDES mechanical complication of arteriovenous dialysis catheter (996.1)

AHA: 4Q, '98, 54

996.57 Due to insulin pump
AHA: 4Q, '03, 81-82

996.59 Due to other implant and internal device, not elsewhere classified
Nonabsorbable surgical material NOS
Prosthetic implant in:
  bile duct
  chin
  orbit of eye
AHA: 2Q, '99, 13; 3Q, '94, 7

INJURY AND POISONING — 996.6–996.99

996.6 ☑5th Infection and inflammatory reaction due to internal prosthetic device, implant, and graft

Infection (causing obstruction) } due to (presence of) any device, implant, and graft classifiable to 996.0-996.5
Inflammation

Use additional code to identify specified infections
AHA: 2Q, '89, 16; J-F, '87, 14

- **996.60** Due to unspecified device, implant, and graft
- **996.61** Due to cardiac device, implant, and graft
  - Cardiac pacemaker or defibrillator:
    - electrode(s), lead(s)
    - pulse generator
    - subcutaneous pocket
  - Coronary artery bypass graft
  - Heart valve prosthesis
- **996.62** Due to other vascular device, implant and graft
  - Arterial graft
  - Arteriovenous fistula or shunt
  - Infusion pump
  - Vascular catheter (arterial) (dialysis) (venous)

  AHA: 2Q, '04, 16; 1Q, '04, 5; 4Q, '03, 107, 111; 2Q, '03, 7; 2Q, '94, 13
- **996.63** Due to nervous system device, implant and graft
  - Electrodes implanted in brain
  - Peripheral nerve graft
  - Spinal canal catheter
  - Ventricular (communicating) shunt (catheter)
- **996.64** Due to indwelling urinary catheter
  - Use additional code to identify specified infections, such as:
    - Cystitis (595.0-595.9)
    - Sepsis (038.0-038.9)

  AHA: 3Q, '93, 6
- **996.65** Due to other genitourinary device, implant and graft
  - Intrauterine contraceptive device

  AHA: 1Q, '00, 15
- **996.66** Due to internal joint prosthesis
  - Use additional code to identify infected prosthetic joint (V43.60-V43.69)

  AHA: 4Q, '05, 91, 113; 2Q, '91, 18
- **996.67** Due to other internal orthopedic device implant and graft
  - Bone growth stimulator (electrode)
  - Internal fixation device (pin) (rod) (screw)
- **996.68** Due to peritoneal dialysis catheter
  - Exit-site infection or inflammation

  AHA: 4Q, '98, 54
- **996.69** Due to other internal prosthetic device, implant and graft
  - Breast prosthesis
  - Ocular lens prosthesis
  - Prosthetic orbital implant

  AHA: 4Q, '03, 108; 4Q, '98, 52

996.7 ☑5th Other complications of internal (biological) (synthetic) prosthetic device, implant, and graft

Complication NOS
occlusion NOS
Embolism
Fibrosis   } due to (presence of) any
Hemorrhage   device, implant, and
Pain   graft classifiable to
Stenosis   996.0-996.5
Thrombus

▶Use additional code to identify complication, such as:
  pain due to presence of device, implant or graft (338.18-338.19, 338.28-338.29)◀

EXCLUDES transplant rejection (996.8)

AHA: 4Q, '05, 94; 1Q, '89, 9; N-D, '86, 5

- **996.70** Due to unspecified device, implant, and graft
- **996.71** Due to heart valve prosthesis
- **996.72** Due to other cardiac device, implant, and graft
  - Cardiac pacemaker or defibrillator:
    - electrode(s), lead(s)
    - subcutaneous pocket
  - Coronary artery bypass (graft)

  EXCLUDES occlusion due to atherosclerosis (414.02-414.06)

  AHA: 3Q, '01, 20
- **996.73** Due to renal dialysis device, implant, and graft

  AHA: 2Q, '91, 18
- **996.74** Due to other vascular device, implant, and graft

  EXCLUDES occlusion of biological graft due to atherosclerosis (440.30-440.32)

  AHA: 1Q, '03, 16, 17
- **996.75** Due to nervous system device, implant, and graft
- **996.76** Due to genitourinary device, implant, and graft

  AHA: 1Q, '00, 15
- **996.77** Due to internal joint prosthesis

  AHA: 4Q, '05, 91
- **996.78** Due to other internal orthopedic device, implant, and graft

  AHA: 2Q, '03, 14
- **996.79** Due to other internal prosthetic device, implant, and graft

  AHA: 2Q, '04, 7; 1Q, '01, 8; 3Q, '95, 14; 3Q, '92, 4

996.8 ☑5th Complications of transplanted organ
  Transplant failure or rejection
  Use additional code to identify nature of complication, such as:
    Cytomegalovirus (CMV) infection (078.5)

  AHA: 3Q, '01, 12; 3Q, '93, 3, 4; 2Q, '93, 11; 1Q, '93, 24

- **996.80** Transplanted organ, unspecified
- **996.81** Kidney
  AHA: 3Q, '03, 16; 3Q, '98, 6, 7; 3Q, '94, 8; 2Q, '94, 9; 1Q, '93, 24
- **996.82** Liver
  AHA: 3Q, '03, 17; 3Q, '98, 3, 4
- **996.83** Heart
  AHA: 3Q, '03, 16; 4Q, '02, 53; 3Q, '98, 5
- **996.84** Lung
  AHA: 2Q, '03, 12; 3Q, '98, 5
- **996.85** Bone marrow
  Graft-versus-host disease (acute) (chronic)
  AHA: 4Q, '90, 4
- **996.86** Pancreas
- **996.87** Intestine
- **996.89** Other specified transplanted organ
  AHA: 3Q, '94, 5

996.9 ☑5th Complications of reattached extremity or body part
- **996.90** Unspecified extremity
- **996.91** Forearm
- **996.92** Hand
- **996.93** Finger(s)
- **996.94** Upper extremity, other and unspecified
- **996.95** Foot and toe(s)
- **996.96** Lower extremity, other and unspecified
- **996.99** Other specified body part

INJURY AND POISONING

✓4th 997 Complications affecting specified body systems, not elsewhere classified
Use additional code to identify complications
EXCLUDES the listed conditions when specified as:
  causing shock (998.0)
  complications of:
    anesthesia:
      adverse effect (001.0-799.9, 995.0-995.8)
      in labor or delivery (668.0-668.9)
      poisoning (968.0-969.9)
    implanted device or graft (996.0-996.9)
    obstetrical procedures (669.0-669.4)
    reattached extremity (996.90-996.96)
    transplanted organ (996.80-996.89)
AHA: 1Q, '94, 4; 1Q, '93, 26

✓5th 997.0 Nervous system complications
  997.00 Nervous system complication, unspecified
  997.01 Central nervous system complication
    Anoxic brain damage   Cerebral hypoxia
    EXCLUDES cerebrovascular hemorrhage or infarction (997.02)
  997.02 Iatrogenic cerebrovascular infarction or hemorrhage
    Postoperative stroke
    AHA: 2Q, '04, 8; 4Q, '95, 57
  997.09 Other nervous system complications

997.1 Cardiac complications
  Cardiac:
    arrest
    insufficiency   } during or resulting
  Cardiorespiratory failure   from a procedure
  Heart failure
  EXCLUDES the listed conditions as long-term effects of cardiac surgery or due to the presence of cardiac prosthetic device (429.4)
  AHA: 2Q, '02, 12

997.2 Peripheral vascular complications
  Phlebitis or thrombophlebitis during or resulting from a procedure
  EXCLUDES the listed conditions due to:
    implant or catheter device (996.62)
    infusion, perfusion, or transfusion (999.2)
    complications affecting blood vessels (997.71-997.79)
  AHA: 1Q, '03, 6; 3Q, '02, 24-26

997.3 Respiratory complications
  Mendelson's syndrome } resulting from a
  Pneumonia (aspiration)   procedure
  EXCLUDES iatrogenic [postoperative] pneumothorax (512.1)
    iatrogenic pulmonary embolism (415.11)
    Mendelson's syndrome in labor and delivery (668.0)
    specified complications classified elsewhere, such as:
      adult respiratory distress syndrome (518.5)
      pulmonary edema, postoperative (518.4)
      respiratory insufficiency, acute, postoperative (518.5)
      shock lung (518.5)
      tracheostomy complications (519.00-519.09)
    ▶transfusion related acute lung injury [TRALI] (518.7)◀
  AHA: 1Q, '97, 10; 2Q, '93, 3; 2Q, '93, 9; 4Q, '90, 25
  DEF: Mendelson's syndrome: acid pneumonitis due to aspiration of gastric acids, may occur after anesthesia or sedation.

997.4 Digestive system complications
  Complications of:
    intestinal (internal) anastomosis and bypass, not elsewhere classified, except that involving urinary tract
  Hepatic failure   }
  Hepatorenal syndrome   } specified as due to
  Intestinal obstruction NOS } a procedure
  EXCLUDES gastrostomy complications (536.40-536.49)
    specified gastrointestinal complications classified elsewhere, such as:
      blind loop syndrome (579.2)
      colostomy and enterostomy complications (569.60-569.69)
      gastrojejunal ulcer (534.0-534.9)
      infection of esophagostomy (530.86)
      infection of external stoma (569.61)
      mechanical complication of esophagostomy (530.87)
      pelvic peritoneal adhesions, female (614.6)
      peritoneal adhesions (568.0)
      peritoneal adhesions with obstruction (560.81)
      postcholecystectomy syndrome (576.0)
      postgastric surgery syndromes (564.2)
      vomiting following gastrointestinal surgery (564.3)
  AHA: 2Q, '01, 4-6; 3Q, '99, 4; 2Q, '99, 14; 3Q, '97, 7; 1Q, '97, 11; 2Q, '95, 7; 1Q, '93, 26; 3Q, '92, 15; 2Q, '89, 15; 1Q, '88, 14

997.5 Urinary complications
  Complications of:
    external stoma of urinary tract
    internal anastomosis and bypass of urinary tract, including that involving intestinal tract
  Oliguria or anuria
  Renal:
    failure (acute)   } specified as due to
    insufficiency (acute)   } procedure
  Tubular necrosis (acute)
  EXCLUDES specified complications classified elsewhere, such as:
    postoperative stricture of:
      ureter (593.3)
      urethra (598.2)
  AHA: 3Q, '03, 13; 3Q, '96, 10, 15; 4Q, '95, 73; 1Q, '92, 13; 2Q, '89, 16; M-A, '87, 10; S-O, '85, 3

✓5th 997.6 Amputation stump complication
  EXCLUDES admission for treatment for a current traumatic amputation — code to complicated traumatic amputation
    phantom limb (syndrome) (353.6)
  AHA: 4Q, '95, 82
  997.60 Unspecified complication
  997.61 Neuroma of amputation stump
    DEF: Hyperplasia generated nerve cell mass following amputation.
  997.62 Infection (chronic)
    Use additional code to identify organism
    AHA: 1Q, '05, 14; 4Q, '96, 46
  997.69 Other
    AHA: 1Q, '05, 15

✓5th 997.7 Vascular complications of other vessels
  EXCLUDES peripheral vascular complications (997.2)
  997.71 Vascular complications of mesenteric artery
    AHA: 4Q, '01, 53
  997.72 Vascular complications of renal artery
  997.79 Vascular complications of other vessels

INJURY AND POISONING

✓5th 997.9 Complications affecting other specified body systems, not elsewhere classified
EXCLUDES specified complications classified elsewhere, such as:
broad ligament laceration syndrome (620.6)
postartificial menopause syndrome (627.4)
postoperative stricture of vagina (623.2)

997.91 Hypertension
EXCLUDES essential hypertension (401.0-401.9)
AHA: 4Q, '95, 57

997.99 Other
Vitreous touch syndrome
AHA: 2Q, '94, 12; 1Q, '94, 17
DEF: Vitreous touch syndrome: vitreous protruding through pupil and attaches to corneal epithelium; causes aqueous fluid in vitreous body; marked by corneal edema, loss of lucidity; complication of cataract surgery.

✓4th 998 Other complications of procedures, not elsewhere classified
AHA: 1Q, '94, 4

998.0 Postoperative shock
Collapse NOS
Shock (endotoxic) (hypovolemic) (septic) } during or resulting from a surgical procedure

EXCLUDES shock:
anaphylactic due to serum (999.4)
anesthetic (995.4)
electric (994.8)
following abortion (639.5)
obstetric (669.1)
traumatic (958.4)

✓5th 998.1 Hemorrhage or hematoma or seroma complicating a procedure
EXCLUDES hemorrhage, hematoma, or seroma: complicating cesarean section or puerperal perineal wound (674.3)

998.11 Hemorrhage complicating a procedure
AHA: 3Q, '03, 13; 1Q, '03, 4; 4Q, '97, 52; 1Q, '97, 10

998.12 Hematoma complicating a procedure
AHA: 1Q, '03, 6; 3Q, '02, 24, 26

998.13 Seroma complicating a procedure
AHA: 4Q, '96, 46; 1Q, '93, 26; 2Q, '92, 15; S-O, '87, 8

998.2 Accidental puncture or laceration during a procedure
Accidental perforation by catheter or other instrument during a procedure on:
blood vessel
nerve
organ

EXCLUDES iatrogenic [postoperative] pneumothorax (512.1)
puncture or laceration caused by implanted device intentionally left in operation wound (996.0-996.5)
specified complications classified elsewhere, such as:
broad ligament laceration syndrome (620.6)
trauma from instruments during delivery (664.0-665.9)
AHA: 3Q, '02, 24, 26; 3Q, '94, 6; 3Q, '90, 17; 3Q, '90, 18

✓5th 998.3 Disruption of operation wound
Dehiscence
Rupture } of operation wound

EXCLUDES disruption of:
cesarean wound (674.1)
perineal wound, puerperal (674.2)
AHA: 4Q, '02, 73; 1Q, '93, 19

998.31 Disruption of internal operation wound
998.32 Disruption of external operation wound
Disruption of operation wound NOS
AHA: 1Q, '05, 11; 4Q, '03, 104, 106

998.4 Foreign body accidentally left during a procedure
Adhesions
Obstruction
Perforation } due to foreign body accidentally left in operative wound or body cavity during a procedure

EXCLUDES obstruction or perforation caused by implanted device intentionally left in body (996.0-996.5)
AHA: 1Q, '89, 9

✓5th 998.5 Postoperative infection
EXCLUDES ▶bleb associated endophthalmitis (379.63)◀
infection due to:
implanted device (996.60-996.69)
infusion, perfusion, or transfusion (999.3)
postoperative obstetrical wound infection (674.3)

998.51 Infected postoperative seroma
Use additional code to identify organism
AHA: 4Q, '96, 46

998.59 Other postoperative infection
Abscess:
intra-abdominal
stitch
subphrenic
wound
} postoperative

Use additional code to identify infection
AHA: 4Q, '04, 76; 4Q, '03, 104, 106-107; 3Q, '98, 3; 3Q, '95, 5; 2Q, '95, 7; 3Q, '94, 6; 1Q, '93, 19; J-F, '87, 14

998.6 Persistent postoperative fistula
AHA: J-F, '87, 14

998.7 Acute reaction to foreign substance accidentally left during a procedure
Peritonitis: aseptic
Peritonitis: chemical

✓5th 998.8 Other specified complications of procedures, not elsewhere classified
AHA: 4Q, '94, 46; 1Q, '89, 9

998.81 Emphysema (subcutaneous) (surgical) resulting from a procedure
998.82 Cataract fragments in eye following cataract surgery
998.83 Non-healing surgical wound
AHA: 4Q, '96, 47

998.89 Other specified complications
AHA: 3Q, '05, 16; 3Q, '99, 13; 2Q, '98, 16

998.9 Unspecified complication of procedure, not elsewhere classified
Postoperative complication NOS
EXCLUDES complication NOS of obstetrical, surgery or procedure (669.4)
AHA: 4Q, '93, 37

INJURY AND POISONING

✓4ᵗʰ 999 Complications of medical care, not elsewhere classified

INCLUDES: complications, not elsewhere classified, of:
- dialysis (hemodialysis) (peritoneal) (renal)
- extracorporeal circulation
- hyperalimentation therapy
- immunization
- infusion
- inhalation therapy
- injection
- inoculation
- perfusion
- transfusion
- vaccination
- ventilation therapy

EXCLUDES: specified complications classified elsewhere such as:
- complications of implanted device (996.0-996.9)
- contact dermatitis due to drugs (692.3)
- dementia dialysis (294.8)
  - transient (293.9)
- dialysis disequilibrium syndrome (276.0-276.9)
- poisoning and toxic effects of drugs and chemicals (960.0-989.9)
- postvaccinal encephalitis ▶(323.51)◀
- water and electrolyte imbalance (276.0-276.9)

999.0 Generalized vaccinia
DEF: Skin eruption, self-limiting; follows vaccination; due to transient viremia with virus localized in skin.

999.1 Air embolism
Air embolism to any site following infusion, perfusion, or transfusion

EXCLUDES: embolism specified as:
- complicating:
  - abortion (634-638 with .6, 639.6)
  - ectopic or molar pregnancy (639.6)
  - pregnancy, childbirth, or the puerperium (673.0)
- due to implanted device (996.7)
- traumatic (958.0)

999.2 Other vascular complications
Phlebitis } following infusion,
Thromboembolism } perfusion, or
Thrombophlebitis } transfusion

EXCLUDES: the listed conditions when specified as:
- due to implanted device (996.61-996.62, 996.72-996.74)
- postoperative NOS (997.2, 997.71-997.79)

AHA: 2Q, '97, 5

999.3 Other infection
Infection } following infusion, injection,
Sepsis } transfusion, or
Septicemia } vaccination

EXCLUDES: the listed conditions when specified as:
- due to implanted device (996.60-996.69)
- postoperative NOS (998.51-998.59)

AHA: 2Q, '01, 11, 12; 2Q, '97, 5; J-F, '87, 14

999.4 Anaphylactic shock due to serum
EXCLUDES: shock:
- allergic NOS (995.0)
- anaphylactic:
  - NOS (995.0)
  - due to drugs and chemicals (995.0)

DEF: Life-threatening hypersensitivity to foreign serum; causes respiratory distress, vascular collapse, and shock.

999.5 Other serum reaction
- Intoxication by serum
- Protein sickness
- Serum rash
- Serum sickness
- Urticaria due to serum

EXCLUDES: serum hepatitis (070.2-070.3)

DEF: Serum sickness: Hypersensitivity to foreign serum; causes fever, hives, swelling, and lymphadenopathy.

999.6 ABO incompatibility reaction
Incompatible blood transfusion
Reaction to blood group incompatibility in infusion or transfusion

999.7 Rh incompatibility reaction
Elevation of Rh titer
Reactions due to Rh factor in infusion or transfusion

999.8 Other transfusion reaction
Septic shock due to transfusion
Transfusion reaction NOS

EXCLUDES: postoperative shock (998.0)
▶transfusion related acute lung injury [TRALI] (518.7)◀

AHA: 3Q, '00, 9

999.9 Other and unspecified complications of medical care, not elsewhere classified
Complications, not elsewhere classified, of:
- electroshock }
- inhalation } therapy
- ultrasound }
- ventilation }

Unspecified misadventure of medical care

EXCLUDES: unspecified complication of:
- phototherapy (990)
- radiation therapy (990)

AHA: 1Q, '03, 19; 2Q, '97, 5

Tabular List — V CODES — V01–V04.89

SUPPLEMENTARY CLASSIFICATION OF FACTORS INFLUENCING HEALTH STATUS AND CONTACT WITH HEALTH SERVICES ►(V01-V86)◄

This classification is provided to deal with occasions when circumstances other than a disease or injury classifiable to categories 001-999 (the main part of ICD) are recorded as "diagnoses" or "problems." This can arise mainly in three ways:

a) When a person who is not currently sick encounters the health services for some specific purpose, such as to act as a donor of an organ or tissue, to receive prophylactic vaccination, or to discuss a problem which is in itself not a disease or injury. This will be a fairly rare occurrence among hospital inpatients, but will be relatively more common among hospital outpatients and patients of family practitioners, health clinics, etc.

b) When a person with a known disease or injury, whether it is current or resolving, encounters the health care system for a specific treatment of that disease or injury (e.g., dialysis for renal disease; chemotherapy for malignancy; cast change).

c) When some circumstance or problem is present which influences the person's health status but is not in itself a current illness or injury. Such factors may be elicited during population surveys, when the person may or may not be currently sick, or be recorded as an additional factor to be borne in mind when the person is receiving care for some current illness or injury classifiable to categories 001-999.

In the latter circumstances the V code should be used only as a supplementary code and should not be the one selected for use in primary, single cause tabulations. Examples of these circumstances are a personal history of certain diseases, or a person with an artificial heart valve in situ.

AHA: J-F, '87, 8

PERSONS WITH POTENTIAL HEALTH HAZARDS RELATED TO COMMUNICABLE DISEASES (V01-V06)

EXCLUDES *family history of infectious and parasitic diseases (V18.8)*
personal history of infectious and parasitic diseases (V12.0)

√4th **V01** Contact with or exposure to communicable diseases
- **V01.0** Cholera
  - Conditions classifiable to 001
- **V01.1** Tuberculosis
  - Conditions classifiable to 010-018
- **V01.2** Poliomyelitis
  - Conditions classifiable to 045
- **V01.3** Smallpox
  - Conditions classifiable to 050
- **V01.4** Rubella
  - Conditions classifiable to 056
- **V01.5** Rabies
  - Conditions classifiable to 071
- **V01.6** Venereal diseases
  - Conditions classifiable to 090-099
- √5th **V01.7** Other viral diseases
  - Conditions classifiable to 042-078 and V08, except as above
  - **AHA:** 2Q, '92, 11
  - **V01.71** Varicella
  - **V01.79** Other viral diseases
- √5th **V01.8** Other communicable diseases
  - Conditions classifiable to 001-136, except as above
  - **AHA:** J-A, '87, 24
  - **V01.81** Anthrax
    - **AHA:** 4Q, '02, 70, 78
  - **V01.82** Exposure to SARS-associated coronavirus
    - **AHA:** 4Q, '03, 46-47
  - **V01.83** Escherichia coli (E. coli)
  - **V01.84** Meningococcus
  - **V01.89** Other communicable diseases
- **V01.9** Unspecified communicable disease

√4th **V02** Carrier or suspected carrier of infectious diseases
AHA: 3Q, '95, 18; 3Q, '94, 4
- **V02.0** Cholera
- **V02.1** Typhoid
- **V02.2** Amebiasis
- **V02.3** Other gastrointestinal pathogens
- **V02.4** Diphtheria
- √5th **V02.5** Other specified bacterial diseases
  - **V02.51** Group B streptococcus
    - **AHA:** 1Q, '02, 14; 4Q, '98, 56
  - **V02.52** Other streptococcus
  - **V02.59** Other specified bacterial diseases
    - Meningococcal Staphylococcal
- √5th **V02.6** Viral hepatitis
  - Hepatitis Australian-antigen [HAA] [SH] carrier
  - Serum hepatitis carrier
  - **V02.60** Viral hepatitis carrier, unspecified
    - **AHA:** 4Q, '97, 47
  - **V02.61** Hepatitis B carrier
    - **AHA:** 4Q, '97, 47
  - **V02.62** Hepatitis C carrier
    - **AHA:** 4Q, '97, 47
  - **V02.69** Other viral hepatitis carrier
    - **AHA:** 4Q, '97, 47
- **V02.7** Gonorrhea
- **V02.8** Other venereal diseases
- **V02.9** Other specified infectious organism
  - **AHA:** 3Q, '95, 18; 1Q, '93, 22; J-A, '87, 24

√4th **V03** Need for prophylactic vaccination and inoculation against bacterial diseases
EXCLUDES *vaccination not carried out (V64.00-V64.09)*
vaccines against combinations of diseases (V06.0-V06.9)
- **V03.0** Cholera alone
- **V03.1** Typhoid-paratyphoid alone [TAB]
- **V03.2** Tuberculosis [BCG]
- **V03.3** Plague
- **V03.4** Tularemia
- **V03.5** Diphtheria alone
- **V03.6** Pertussis alone
- **V03.7** Tetanus toxoid alone
- √5th **V03.8** Other specified vaccinations against single bacterial diseases
  - **V03.81** Hemophilus influenza, type B [Hib]
  - **V03.82** Streptococcus pneumoniae [pneumococcus]
  - **V03.89** Other specified vaccination
    - **AHA:** 2Q, '00, 9
- **V03.9** Unspecified single bacterial disease

√4th **V04** Need for prophylactic vaccination and inoculation against certain viral diseases
EXCLUDES *vaccines against combinations of diseases (V06.0-V06.9)*
- **V04.0** Poliomyelitis
- **V04.1** Smallpox
- **V04.2** Measles alone
- **V04.3** Rubella alone
- **V04.4** Yellow fever
- **V04.5** Rabies
- **V04.6** Mumps alone
- **V04.7** Common cold
- √5th **V04.8** Other viral diseases
  - **AHA:** 4Q, '03, 83
  - **V04.81** Influenza
  - **V04.82** Respiratory syncytial virus (RSV)
  - **V04.89** Other viral diseases

√4th √5th Additional Digit Required   Unspecified Code   Other Specified Code   Manifestation Code   ►◄ Revised Text   ● New Code   ▲ Revised Code Title

2007 ICD•9•CM

V CODES — Tabular List

V05–V09.91

✓4th V05 Need for other prophylactic vaccination and inoculation against single diseases
- EXCLUDES: vaccines against combinations of diseases (V06.0-V06.9)
- **V05.0** Arthropod-borne viral encephalitis
- **V05.1** Other arthropod-borne viral diseases
- **V05.2** Leishmaniasis
- **V05.3** Viral hepatitis
- **V05.4** Varicella
  - Chickenpox
- **V05.8** Other specified disease
  - AHA: 1Q, '01, 4; 3Q, '91, 20
- **V05.9** Unspecified single disease

✓4th V06 Need for prophylactic vaccination and inoculation against combinations of diseases
- Note: Use additional single vaccination codes from categories V03-V05 to identify any vaccinations not included in a combination code.
- **V06.0** Cholera with typhoid-paratyphoid [cholera+TAB]
- **V06.1** Diphtheria-tetanus-pertussis, combined [DTP] [DTaP]
  - AHA: 4Q, '03, 83; 3Q, '98, 13
- **V06.2** Diphtheria-tetanus-pertussis with typhoid-paratyphoid [DTP+TAB]
- **V06.3** Diphtheria-tetanus-pertussis with poliomyelitis [DTP+polio]
- **V06.4** Measles-mumps-rubella [MMR]
- **V06.5** Tetanus-diphtheria [Td] [DT]
  - AHA: 4Q, '03, 83
- **V06.6** Streptococcus pneumoniae [pneumococcus] and influenza
- **V06.8** Other combinations
  - EXCLUDES: multiple single vaccination codes (V03.0-V05.9)
  - AHA: 1Q, '94, 19
- **V06.9** Unspecified combined vaccine

PERSONS WITH NEED FOR ISOLATION, OTHER POTENTIAL HEALTH HAZARDS AND PROPHYLACTIC MEASURES (V07-V09)

✓4th V07 Need for isolation and other prophylactic measures
- EXCLUDES: prophylactic organ removal (V50.41-V50.49)
- **V07.0** Isolation
  - Admission to protect the individual from his surroundings or for isolation of individual after contact with infectious diseases
- **V07.1** Desensitization to allergens
- **V07.2** Prophylactic immunotherapy
  - Administration of: antivenin, immune sera [gamma globulin]
  - Administration of: RhoGAM, tetanus antitoxin
- **✓5th V07.3** Other prophylactic chemotherapy
  - **V07.31** Prophylactic fluoride administration
  - **V07.39** Other prophylactic chemotherapy
    - EXCLUDES: maintenance chemotherapy following disease ▶(V58.11)◄
- **V07.4** Hormone replacement therapy (postmenopausal) ♀
- **V07.8** Other specified prophylactic measure
  - AHA: 1Q, '92, 11
- **V07.9** Unspecified prophylactic measure

V08 Asymptomatic human immunodeficiency virus [HIV] infection status
- HIV positive NOS
- Note: This code is ONLY to be used when NO HIV infection symptoms or conditions are present. If any HIV infection symptoms or conditions are present, see code 042.
- EXCLUDES:
  - AIDS (042)
  - human immunodeficiency virus [HIV] disease (042)
  - exposure to HIV (V01.79)
  - nonspecific serologic evidence of HIV (795.71)
  - symptomatic human immunodeficiency virus [HIV] infection (042)
- AHA: 2Q, '04, 11; 2Q, '99, 8; 3Q, '95, 18

✓4th V09 Infection with drug-resistant microorganisms
- Note: This category is intended for use as an additional code for infectious conditions classified elsewhere to indicate the presence of drug-resistance of the infectious organism.
- AHA: 3Q, '94, 4; 4Q, '93, 22
- **V09.0** Infection with microorganisms resistant to penicillins [SDx]
  - Methicillin-resistant staphylococcus aureus (MRSA)
  - AHA: 4Q, '03, 104, 106
- **V09.1** Infection with microorganisms resistant to cephalosporins and other B-lactam antibiotics [SDx]
- **V09.2** Infection with microorganisms resistant to macrolides [SDx]
- **V09.3** Infection with microorganisms resistant to tetracyclines [SDx]
- **V09.4** Infection with microorganisms resistant to aminoglycosides [SDx]
- **✓5th V09.5** Infection with microorganisms resistant to quinolones and fluoroquinolones
  - **V09.50** Without mention of resistance to multiple quinolones and fluoroquinoles [SDx]
  - **V09.51** With resistance to multiple quinolones and fluoroquinoles [SDx]
- **V09.6** Infection with microorganisms resistant to sulfonamides [SDx]
- **✓5th V09.7** Infection with microorganisms resistant to other specified antimycobacterial agents
  - EXCLUDES: Amikacin (V09.4), Kanamycin (V09.4), Streptomycin [SM] (V09.4)
  - **V09.70** Without mention of resistance to multiple antimycobacterial agents [SDx]
  - **V09.71** With resistance to multiple antimycobacterial agents [SDx]
- **✓5th V09.8** Infection with microorganisms resistant to other specified drugs
  - Vancomycin (glycopeptide) intermediate staphylococcus aureus (VISA/GISA)
  - Vancomycin (glycopeptide) resistant enterococcus (VRE)
  - Vancomycin (glycopeptide) resistant staphylococcus aureus (VRSA/GRSA)
  - **V09.80** Without mention of resistance to multiple drugs [SDx]
  - **V09.81** With resistance to multiple drugs [SDx]
- **✓5th V09.9** Infection with drug-resistant microorganisms, unspecified
  - Drug resistance, NOS
  - **V09.90** Without mention of multiple drug resistance [SDx]
  - **V09.91** With multiple drug resistance [SDx]
    - Multiple drug resistance NOS

V CODES

PERSONS WITH POTENTIAL HEALTH HAZARDS RELATED TO PERSONAL AND FAMILY HISTORY

EXCLUDES obstetric patients where the possibility that the fetus might be affected is the reason for observation or management during pregnancy (655.0-655.9)

AHA: J-F, '87, 1

V10 Personal history of malignant neoplasm
AHA: 4Q, '02, 80; 4Q, '98, 69; 1Q, '95, 4; 3Q, '92, 5; M-J, '85, 10; 2Q, '90, 9

- **V10.0 Gastrointestinal tract**
  History of conditions classifiable to 140-159
  - V10.00 Gastrointestinal tract, unspecified
  - V10.01 Tongue
  - V10.02 Other and unspecified oral cavity and pharynx
  - V10.03 Esophagus
  - V10.04 Stomach
  - V10.05 Large intestine
    AHA: 3Q, '99, 7; 1Q, '95, 4
  - V10.06 Rectum, rectosigmoid junction, and anus
  - V10.07 Liver
  - V10.09 Other
    AHA: 4Q, '03, 111

- **V10.1 Trachea, bronchus, and lung**
  History of conditions classifiable to 162
  - V10.11 Bronchus and lung
  - V10.12 Trachea

- **V10.2 Other respiratory and intrathoracic organs**
  History of conditions classifiable to 160, 161, 163-165
  - V10.20 Respiratory organ, unspecified
  - V10.21 Larynx
    AHA: 4Q, '03, 108, 110
  - V10.22 Nasal cavities, middle ear, and accessory sinuses
  - V10.29 Other

- **V10.3 Breast**
  History of conditions classifiable to 174 and 175
  AHA: 2Q, '03, 5; 4Q, '01, 66; 4Q, '98, 65; 4Q, '97, 50; 1Q, '91, 16; 1Q, '90, 21

- **V10.4 Genital organs**
  History of conditions classifiable to 179-187
  - V10.40 Female genital organ, unspecified ♀
  - V10.41 Cervix uteri ♀
  - V10.42 Other parts of uterus ♀
  - V10.43 Ovary ♀
  - V10.44 Other female genital organs ♀
  - V10.45 Male genital organ, unspecified ♂
  - V10.46 Prostate ♂
  - V10.47 Testis ♂
  - V10.48 Epididymis ♂
  - V10.49 Other male genital organs ♂

- **V10.5 Urinary organs**
  History of conditions classifiable to 188 and 189
  - V10.50 Urinary organ, unspecified
  - V10.51 Bladder
  - V10.52 Kidney
    EXCLUDES renal pelvis (V10.53)
    AHA: 2Q, '04, 4
  - V10.53 Renal pelvis
    AHA: 4Q, '01, 55
  - V10.59 Other

- **V10.6 Leukemia**
  Conditions classifiable to 204-208
  EXCLUDES leukemia in remission (204-208)
  AHA: 2Q, '92, 13; 4Q, '91, 26; 4Q, '90, 3
  - V10.60 Leukemia, unspecified
  - V10.61 Lymphoid leukemia
  - V10.62 Myeloid leukemia
  - V10.63 Monocytic leukemia
  - V10.69 Other

- **V10.7 Other lymphatic and hematopoietic neoplasms**
  Conditions classifiable to 200-203
  EXCLUDES listed conditions in 200-203 in remission
  AHA: M-J, '85, 18
  - V10.71 Lymphosarcoma and reticulosarcoma
  - V10.72 Hodgkin's disease
  - V10.79 Other

- **V10.8 Personal history of malignant neoplasm of other sites**
  History of conditions classifiable to 170-173, 190-195
  - V10.81 Bone
    AHA: 2Q, '03, 13
  - V10.82 Malignant melanoma of skin
  - V10.83 Other malignant neoplasm of skin
  - V10.84 Eye
  - V10.85 Brain
    AHA: 1Q, '01, 6
  - V10.86 Other parts of nervous system
    EXCLUDES peripheral sympathetic, and parasympathetic nerves (V10.89)
  - V10.87 Thyroid
  - V10.88 Other endocrine glands and related structures
  - V10.89 Other

- **V10.9 Unspecified personal history of malignant neoplasm**

V11 Personal history of mental disorder
- **V11.0 Schizophrenia**
  EXCLUDES that in remission (295.0-295.9 with fifth-digit 5)
- **V11.1 Affective disorders**
  Personal history of manic-depressive psychosis
  EXCLUDES that in remission (296.0-296.6 with fifth-digit 5, 6)
- **V11.2 Neurosis**
- **V11.3 Alcoholism**
- **V11.8 Other mental disorders**
- **V11.9 Unspecified mental disorder**

V12 Personal history of certain other diseases
AHA: 3Q, '92, 11

- **V12.0 Infectious and parasitic diseases**
  EXCLUDES personal history of infectious diseases specific to a body system
  - V12.00 Unspecified infectious and parasitic disease
  - V12.01 Tuberculosis
  - V12.02 Poliomyelitis
  - V12.03 Malaria
  - V12.09 Other

- **V12.1 Nutritional deficiency**

- **V12.2 Endocrine, metabolic, and immunity disorders**
  EXCLUDES history of allergy (V14.0-V14.9, V15.01-V15.09)

- **V12.3 Diseases of blood and blood-forming organs**

- **V12.4 Disorders of nervous system and sense organs**
  - V12.40 Unspecified disorder of nervous system and sense organs
  - V12.41 Benign neoplasm of the brain
    AHA: 4Q, '97, 48
  - V12.42 Infections of the central nervous system
    Encephalitis   Meningitis
    AHA: ►4Q, '05, 95◄
  - V12.49 Other disorders of nervous system and sense organs
    AHA: 4Q, '98, 59

V CODES — Tabular List
V12.5–V15.81

- ✓5th **V12.5 Diseases of circulatory system**
  - EXCLUDES: old myocardial infarction (412)
  - postmyocardial infarction syndrome (411.0)
  - AHA: 4Q, '95, 61
  - **V12.50** Unspecified circulatory disease
  - **V12.51** Venous thrombosis and embolism
    - Pulmonary embolism
    - AHA: 4Q, '03, 108; 1Q, '02, 15
  - **V12.52** Thrombophlebitis
  - **V12.59** Other
    - AHA: 4Q, '99, 4; 4Q, '98, 88; 4Q, '97, 37
- ✓5th **V12.6 Diseases of respiratory system**
  - EXCLUDES: tuberculosis (V12.01)
  - **V12.60** Unspecified disease of respiratory system
  - **V12.61** Pneumonia (recurrent)
    - AHA: ▶4Q, '05, 95◀
  - **V12.69** Other diseases of respiratory system
- ✓5th **V12.7 Diseases of digestive system**
  - AHA: 1Q, '95, 3; 2Q, '89, 16
  - **V12.70** Unspecified digestive disease
  - **V12.71** Peptic ulcer disease
  - **V12.72** Colonic polyps
    - AHA: 3Q, '02, 15
  - **V12.79** Other
- ✓4th **V13 Personal history of other diseases**
  - ✓5th **V13.0 Disorders of urinary system**
    - **V13.00** Unspecified urinary disorder
    - **V13.01** Urinary calculi
    - **V13.02** Urinary (tract) infection
      - AHA: ▶4Q, '05, 95◀
    - **V13.03** Nephrotic syndrome
      - AHA: ▶4Q, '05, 95◀
    - **V13.09** Other
  - **V13.1** Trophoblastic disease ♀
    - EXCLUDES: supervision during a current pregnancy (V23.1)
  - ✓5th **V13.2** Other genital system and obstetric disorders
    - EXCLUDES: supervision during a current pregnancy of a woman with poor obstetric history (V23.0-V23.9)
    - habitual aborter (646.3) without current pregnancy (629.9)
    - **V13.21** Personal history of pre-term labor ♀
      - EXCLUDES: current pregnancy with history of pre-term labor (V23.41)
      - AHA: 4Q, '02, 78
    - **V13.29** Other genital system and obstetric disorders ♀
  - **V13.3** Diseases of skin and subcutaneous tissue
  - **V13.4** Arthritis
  - **V13.5** Other musculoskeletal disorders
  - ✓5th **V13.6** Congenital malformations
    - AHA: 4Q, '98, 63
    - **V13.61** Hypospadias [SDx] ♂
    - **V13.69** Other congenital malformations
      - AHA: 1Q, '04, 16
  - **V13.7** Perinatal problems
    - EXCLUDES: low birth weight status (V21.30-V21.35)
  - **V13.8** Other specified diseases
  - **V13.9** Unspecified disease
- ✓4th **V14 Personal history of allergy to medicinal agents**
  - **V14.0** Penicillin [SDx]
  - **V14.1** Other antibiotic agent [SDx]
  - **V14.2** Sulfonamides [SDx]
  - **V14.3** Other anti-infective agent [SDx]
  - **V14.4** Anesthetic agent [SDx]
  - **V14.5** Narcotic agent [SDx]
  - **V14.6** Analgesic agent [SDx]
  - **V14.7** Serum or vaccine [SDx]
  - **V14.8** Other specified medicinal agents [SDx]
  - **V14.9** Unspecified medicinal agent [SDx]
- ✓4th **V15 Other personal history presenting hazards to health**
  - ✓5th **V15.0 Allergy, other than to medicinal agents**
    - EXCLUDES: allergy to food substance used as base for medicinal agent (V14.0-V14.9)
    - AHA: 4Q, '00, 42, 49
    - **V15.01** Allergy to peanuts [SDx]
    - **V15.02** Allergy to milk products [SDx]
      - EXCLUDES: lactose intolerance (271.3)
      - AHA: 1Q, '03, 12
    - **V15.03** Allergy to eggs [SDx]
    - **V15.04** Allergy to seafood [SDx]
      - Seafood (octopus) (squid) ink
      - Shellfish
    - **V15.05** Allergy to other foods [SDx]
      - Food additives   Nuts other than peanuts
    - **V15.06** Allergy to insects [SDx]
      - Bugs   Spiders
      - Insect bites and stings
    - **V15.07** Allergy to latex [SDx]
      - Latex sensitivity
    - **V15.08** Allergy to radiographic dye [SDx]
      - Contrast media used for diagnostic x-ray procedures
    - **V15.09** Other allergy, other than to medicinal agents [SDx]
  - **V15.1** Surgery to heart and great vessels [SDx]
    - EXCLUDES: replacement by transplant or other means (V42.1-V42.2, V43.2-V43.4)
    - AHA: 1Q, '04, 16
  - **V15.2** Surgery to other major organs [SDx]
    - EXCLUDES: replacement by transplant or other means (V42.0-V43.8)
  - **V15.3** Irradiation [SDx]
    - Previous exposure to therapeutic or other ionizing radiation
  - ✓5th **V15.4 Psychological trauma**
    - EXCLUDES: history of condition classifiable to 290-316 (V11.0-V11.9)
    - **V15.41** History of physical abuse [SDx]
      - Rape
      - AHA: 3Q, '99, 15
    - **V15.42** History of emotional abuse [SDx]
      - Neglect
      - AHA: 3Q, '99, 15
    - **V15.49** Other [SDx]
      - AHA: 3Q, '99, 15
  - **V15.5** Injury [SDx]
  - **V15.6** Poisoning [SDx]
  - **V15.7** Contraception
    - EXCLUDES: current contraceptive management (V25.0-V25.4)
    - presence of intrauterine contraceptive device as incidental finding (V45.5)
  - ✓5th **V15.8 Other specified personal history presenting hazards to health**
    - AHA: 4Q, '95, 62
    - **V15.81** Noncompliance with medical treatment [SDx]
      - AHA: 2Q, '03, 7; 2Q, '01, 11; 12, 13; 2Q '99, 17; 2Q, '97, 11; 1Q, '97, 12; 3Q, '96, 9

V CODES — V15.82–V21.33

- **V15.82** History of tobacco use [SDx]
  - EXCLUDES: tobacco dependence (305.1)
- **V15.84** Exposure to asbestos [SDx]
- **V15.85** Exposure to potentially hazardous body fluids [SDx]
- **V15.86** Exposure to lead [SDx]
- **V15.87** History of extracorporeal membrane oxygenation [ECMO] [SDx]
  - AHA: 4Q, '03, 84
- **V15.88** History of fall
  - At risk for falling
  - AHA: 4Q, '05, 95
- **V15.89** Other [SDx]
  - AHA: 1Q, '90, 21; N-D, '84, 12
- **V15.9** Unspecified personal history presenting hazards to health [SDx]

✓4th V16 Family history of malignant neoplasm
- **V16.0** Gastrointestinal tract
  - Family history of condition classifiable to 140-159
  - AHA: 1Q, '99, 4
- **V16.1** Trachea, bronchus, and lung
  - Family history of condition classifiable to 162
- **V16.2** Other respiratory and intrathoracic organs
  - Family history of condition classifiable to 160-161, 163-165
- **V16.3** Breast
  - Family history of condition classifiable to 174
  - AHA: 4Q, '04, 107; 2Q, '03, 4; 2Q, '00, 8; 1Q, '92, 11
- **✓5th V16.4** Genital organs
  - Family history of condition classifiable to 179-187
  - AHA: 4Q, '97, 48
  - **V16.40** Genital organ, unspecified
  - **V16.41** Ovary
  - **V16.42** Prostate
  - **V16.43** Testis
  - **V16.49** Other
- **✓5th V16.5** Urinary organs
  - Family history of condition classifiable to 189
  - **V16.51** Kidney
  - **V16.59** Other
- **V16.6** Leukemia
  - Family history of condition classifiable to 204-208
- **V16.7** Other lymphatic and hematopoietic neoplasms
  - Family history of condition classifiable to 200-203
- **V16.8** Other specified malignant neoplasm
  - Family history of other condition classifiable to 140-199
- **V16.9** Unspecified malignant neoplasm

✓4th V17 Family history of certain chronic disabling diseases
- **V17.0** Psychiatric condition
  - EXCLUDES: family history of mental retardation (V18.4)
- **V17.1** Stroke (cerebrovascular)
- **V17.2** Other neurological diseases
  - Epilepsy   Huntington's chorea
- **V17.3** Ischemic heart disease
- **V17.4** Other cardiovascular diseases
  - AHA: 1Q, '04, 6
- **V17.5** Asthma
- **V17.6** Other chronic respiratory conditions
- **V17.7** Arthritis
- **✓5th V17.8** Other musculoskeletal diseases
  - **V17.81** Osteoporosis
    - AHA: 4Q, '05, 95
  - **V17.89** Other musculoskeletal diseases

✓4th V18 Family history of certain other specific conditions
- **V18.0** Diabetes mellitus
  - AHA: 1Q, '04, 8
- **V18.1** Other endocrine and metabolic diseases
- **V18.2** Anemia
- **V18.3** Other blood disorders
- **V18.4** Mental retardation
- **✓5th V18.5** Digestive disorders
  - ● **V18.51** Colonic polyps
    - EXCLUDES: family history of malignant neoplasm of gastrointestinal tract (V16.0)
  - ● **V18.59** Other digestive disorders
- **✓5th V18.6** Kidney diseases
  - **V18.61** Polycystic kidney
  - **V18.69** Other kidney diseases
- **V18.7** Other genitourinary diseases
- **V18.8** Infectious and parasitic diseases
- **V18.9** Genetic disease carrier
  - AHA: 4Q, '05, 95

✓4th V19 Family history of other conditions
- **V19.0** Blindness or visual loss
- **V19.1** Other eye disorders
- **V19.2** Deafness or hearing loss
- **V19.3** Other ear disorders
- **V19.4** Skin conditions
- **V19.5** Congenital anomalies
- **V19.6** Allergic disorders
- **V19.7** Consanguinity
- **V19.8** Other condition

PERSONS ENCOUNTERING HEALTH SERVICES IN CIRCUMSTANCES RELATED TO REPRODUCTION AND DEVELOPMENT (V20-V29)

✓4th V20 Health supervision of infant or child
- **V20.0** Foundling [PDx] [P]
- **V20.1** Other healthy infant or child receiving care [PDx] [P]
  - Medical or nursing care supervision of healthy infant in cases of:
    - maternal illness, physical or psychiatric
    - socioeconomic adverse condition at home
    - too many children at home preventing or interfering with normal care
  - AHA: 1Q, '00, 25; 3Q, '89, 14
- **V20.2** Routine infant or child health check [PDx] [P]
  - Developmental testing of infant or child
  - Immunizations appropriate for age
  - ▶Initial and subsequent routine newborn check◀
  - Routine vision and hearing testing
  - Use additional code(s) to identify:
    - special screening examination(s) performed (V73.0-V82.9)
  - EXCLUDES: special screening for developmental handicaps (V79.3)
  - AHA: 1Q, '04, 15

✓4th V21 Constitutional states in development
- **V21.0** Period of rapid growth in childhood [SDx]
- **V21.1** Puberty [SDx]
- **V21.2** Other adolescence [SDx]
- **✓5th V21.3** Low birth weight status
  - EXCLUDES: history of perinatal problems (V13.7)
  - AHA: 4Q, '00, 51
  - **V21.30** Low birth weight status, unspecified [SDx]
  - **V21.31** Low birth weight status, less than 500 grams [SDx]
  - **V21.32** Low birth weight status, 500-999 grams [SDx]
  - **V21.33** Low birth weight status, 1000-1499 grams [SDx]

V CODES

V21.34–V25.9

- **V21.34** Low birth weight status, 1500-1999 grams [SDx]
- **V21.35** Low birth weight status, 2000-2500 grams [SDx]
- **V21.8** Other specified constitutional states in development [SDx]
- **V21.9** Unspecified constitutional state in development [SDx]

✓4th V22 Normal pregnancy
EXCLUDES pregnancy examination or test, pregnancy unconfirmed (V72.40)

- **V22.0** Supervision of normal first pregnancy [PDx] ♀
  AHA: 3Q, '99, 16
- **V22.1** Supervision of other normal pregnancy [PDx] ♀
  AHA: 3Q, '99, 16
- **V22.2** Pregnant state, incidental [SDx] ♀
  Pregnant state NOS

✓4th V23 Supervision of high-risk pregnancy
AHA: 1Q, 90, 10

- **V23.0** Pregnancy with history of infertility [M] ♀
- **V23.1** Pregnancy with history of trophoblastic disease [M] ♀
  Pregnancy with history of:
  hydatidiform mole
  vesicular mole
  EXCLUDES that without current pregnancy (V13.1)
- **V23.2** Pregnancy with history of abortion [M] ♀
  Pregnancy with history of conditions classifiable to 634-638
  EXCLUDES habitual aborter:
  care during pregnancy (646.3)
  that without current pregnancy (629.9)
- **V23.3** Grand multiparity [M] ♀
  EXCLUDES care in relation to labor and delivery (659.4)
  that without current pregnancy (V61.5)

✓5th V23.4 Pregnancy with other poor obstetric history
Pregnancy with history of other conditions classifiable to 630-676
- **V23.41** Pregnancy with history of pre-term labor [M] ♀
  AHA: 4Q, '02, 79
- **V23.49** Pregnancy with other poor obstetric history [M] ♀

- **V23.5** Pregnancy with other poor reproductive history [M] ♀
  Pregnancy with history of stillbirth or neonatal death
- **V23.7** Insufficient prenatal care [M] ♀
  History of little or no prenatal care

✓5th V23.8 Other high-risk pregnancy
AHA: 4Q, '98, 56, 63
- **V23.81** Elderly primigravida [M] ♀
  First pregnancy in a woman who will be 35 years of age or older at expected date of delivery
  EXCLUDES elderly primigravida complicating pregnancy (659.5)
- **V23.82** Elderly multigravida [M] ♀
  Second or more pregnancy in a woman who will be 35 years of age or older at expected date of delivery
  EXCLUDES elderly multigravida complicating pregnancy (659.6)
- **V23.83** Young primigravida [M] ♀
  First pregnancy in a female less than 16 years old at expected date of delivery
  EXCLUDES young primigravida complicating pregnancy (659.8)
- **V23.84** Young multigravida [M] ♀
  Second or more pregnancy in a female less than 16 years old at expected date of delivery
  EXCLUDES young multigravida complicating pregnancy (659.8)
- **V23.89** Other high-risk pregnancy [M] ♀

- **V23.9** Unspecified high-risk pregnancy [M] ♀

✓4th V24 Postpartum care and examination
- **V24.0** Immediately after delivery [PDx][M] ♀
  Care and observation in uncomplicated cases
- **V24.1** Lactating mother [PDx] ♀
  Supervision of lactation
- **V24.2** Routine postpartum follow-up [PDx] ♀

✓4th V25 Encounter for contraceptive management
AHA: 4Q, '92, 24

✓5th V25.0 General counseling and advice
- **V25.01** Prescription of oral contraceptives ♀
- **V25.02** Initiation of other contraceptive measures
  Fitting of diaphragm
  Prescription of foams, creams, or other agents
  AHA: 3Q, '97, 7
- **V25.03** Encounter for emergency contraceptive counseling and prescription
  Encounter for postcoital contraceptive counseling and prescription
  AHA: 4Q, '03, 84
- **V25.09** Other
  Family planning advice

- **V25.1** Insertion of intrauterine contraceptive device ♀
- **V25.2** Sterilization
  Admission for interruption of fallopian tubes or vas deferens
- **V25.3** Menstrual extraction ♀
  Menstrual regulation

✓5th V25.4 Surveillance of previously prescribed contraceptive methods
Checking, reinsertion, or removal of contraceptive device
Repeat prescription for contraceptive method
Routine examination in connection with contraceptive maintenance
EXCLUDES presence of intrauterine contraceptive device as incidental finding (V45.5)
- **V25.40** Contraceptive surveillance, unspecified
- **V25.41** Contraceptive pill ♀
- **V25.42** Intrauterine contraceptive device ♀
  Checking, reinsertion, or removal of intrauterine device
- **V25.43** Implantable subdermal contraceptive ♀
- **V25.49** Other contraceptive method
  AHA: 3Q, '97, 7

- **V25.5** Insertion of implantable subdermal contraceptive ♀
  AHA: 3Q, '92, 9
- **V25.8** Other specified contraceptive management
  Postvasectomy sperm count
  EXCLUDES sperm count following sterilization reversal (V26.22)
  sperm count for fertility testing (V26.21)
  AHA: 3Q, '96, 9
- **V25.9** Unspecified contraceptive management

Tabular List — V CODES — V26–V31

- √4th **V26 Procreative management**
  - **V26.0 Tuboplasty or vasoplasty after previous sterilization**
    - AHA: 2Q, '95, 10
  - **V26.1 Artificial insemination** ♀
  - √5th **V26.2 Investigation and testing**
    - EXCLUDES: postvasectomy sperm count (V25.8)
    - AHA: 4Q, '00, 56
    - **V26.21 Fertility testing**
      - Fallopian insufflation
      - Sperm count for fertility testing
      - EXCLUDES: genetic counseling and testing ▶(V26.31-V26.39)◀
    - **V26.22 Aftercare following sterilization reversal**
      - Fallopian insufflation following sterilization reversal
      - Sperm count following sterilization reversal
    - **V26.29 Other investigation and testing**
      - AHA: 2Q, '96, 9; N-D, '85, 15
  - √5th **V26.3 Genetic counseling and testing**
    - EXCLUDES: fertility testing (V26.21)
      ▶nonprocreative genetic screening (V82.71, V82.79)◀
    - AHA: 4Q, '05, 96
    - ▲ **V26.31 Testing of female for genetic disease carrier status** ♀
    - ▲ **V26.32 Other genetic testing of female** ♀
      - ▶Use additional code to identify habitual aborter (629.81, 646.3)◀
    - **V26.33 Genetic counseling**
    - ● **V26.34 Testing of male for genetic disease carrier status** ♂
    - ● **V26.35 Encounter for testing of male partner of habitual aborter** ♂
    - ● **V26.39 Other genetic testing of male** ♂
  - **V26.4 General counseling and advice**
  - √5th **V26.5 Sterilization status**
    - **V26.51 Tubal ligation status** SDx ♀
      - EXCLUDES: infertility not due to previous tubal ligation (628.0-628.9)
    - **V26.52 Vasectomy status** SDx ♂
  - **V26.8 Other specified procreative management**
  - **V26.9 Unspecified procreative management**

- √4th **V27 Outcome of delivery**
  - Note: This category is intended for the coding of the outcome of delivery on the mother's record.
  - AHA: 2Q, '91, 16
  - **V27.0 Single liveborn** M SDx
    - AHA: 4Q, '05, 81; 2Q, '03, 9; 2Q, '02, 10; 1Q, '01, 10; 3Q, '00, 5; 4Q, '98, 77; 4Q, '95, 59; 1Q, '92, 9
  - **V27.1 Single stillborn** M SDx ♀
  - **V27.2 Twins, both liveborn** M SDx ♀
  - **V27.3 Twins, one liveborn and one stillborn** M SDx ♀
  - **V27.4 Twins, both stillborn** M SDx ♀
  - **V27.5 Other multiple birth, all liveborn** M SDx ♀
  - **V27.6 Other multiple birth, some liveborn** M SDx ♀
  - **V27.7 Other multiple birth, all stillborn** M SDx ♀
  - **V27.9 Unspecified outcome of delivery** M SDx ♀
    - Single birth } outcome to infant unspecified
    - Multiple birth

- ▲ √4th **V28 Encounter for antenatal screening of mother**
  - EXCLUDES: abnormal findings on screening — code to findings
    routine prenatal care (V22.0-V23.9)
  - AHA: 1Q, '04, 11
  - **V28.0 Screening for chromosomal anomalies by amniocentesis** M ♀
  - **V28.1 Screening for raised alpha-fetoprotein levels in amniotic fluid** M ♀
  - **V28.2 Other screening based on amniocentesis** M ♀
  - **V28.3 Screening for malformation using ultrasonics** ♀
  - **V28.4 Screening for fetal growth retardation using ultrasonics** ♀
  - **V28.5 Screening for isoimmunization** ♀
  - **V28.6 Screening for Streptococcus B** M ♀
    - AHA: 4Q, '97, 46
  - **V28.8 Other specified antenatal screening** ♀
    - AHA: 3Q, '99, 16
  - **V28.9 Unspecified antenatal screening** ♀

- √4th **V29 Observation and evaluation of newborns and infants for suspected condition not found**
  - Note: This category is to be used for newborns, within the neonatal period, (the first 28 days of life) who are suspected of having an abnormal condition resulting from exposure from the mother or the birth process, but without signs or symptoms, and, which after examination and observation, is found not to exist.
  - AHA: 1Q, '00, 25; 4Q, '94, 47; 1Q, '94, 9; 4Q, '92, 21
  - [1] **V29.0 Observation for suspected infectious condition** N PDx
    - AHA: 1Q, '01, 10
  - [1] **V29.1 Observation for suspected neurological condition** N PDx
  - [1] **V29.2 Observation for suspected respiratory condition** N PDx
  - [1] **V29.3 Observation for suspected genetic or metabolic condition** N PDx
    - AHA: 2Q, '05, 21; 4Q, '98, 59, 68
  - [1] **V29.8 Observation for other specified suspected condition** N PDx
    - AHA: 2Q, '03, 15
  - [1] **V29.9 Observation for unspecified suspected condition** N PDx
    - AHA: 1Q, '02, 6

LIVEBORN INFANTS ACCORDING TO TYPE OF BIRTH (V30–V39)

Note: These categories are intended for the coding of liveborn infants who are consuming health care [e.g., crib or bassinet occupancy].

The following fourth-digit subdivisions are for use with categories V30–V39:
- √5th 0 Born in hospital N
- 1 Born before admission to hospital N
- 2 Born outside hospital and not hospitalized

The following two fifth-digits are for use with the fourth-digit .0, Born in hospital:
- 0 delivered without mention of cesarean delivery
- 1 delivered by cesarean delivery

AHA: 1Q, '01, 10

- √4th **V30 Single liveborn** PDx
  - AHA: 2Q, '03, 9; 4Q, '98, 46, 59; 1Q, '94, 9; For code V30.00: 1Q, '04, 8, 16; 4Q, '03, 68; For code V30.01: 4Q, '05, 88
- √4th **V31 Twin, mate liveborn** PDx
  - AHA: 3Q, '92, 10

[1] A code from the V30–V39 series may be sequenced before the V29 on the newborn medical record.

√4th √5th Additional Digit Required | Unspecified Code | Other Specified Code | Manifestation Code | ▶◀ Revised Text | ● New Code | ▲ Revised Code Title

V CODES — Tabular List

V32–V45.01

- ☑4th **V32** Twin, mate stillborn [PDx]
- ☑4th **V33** Twin, unspecified [PDx]
- ☑4th **V34** Other multiple, mates all liveborn [PDx]
- ☑4th **V35** Other multiple, mates all stillborn [PDx]
- ☑4th **V36** Other multiple, mates live- and stillborn [PDx]
- ☑4th **V37** Other multiple, unspecified [PDx]
- ☑4th **V39** Unspecified [PDx]

PERSONS WITH A CONDITION INFLUENCING THEIR HEALTH STATUS (V40-V49)

Note: These categories are intended for use when these conditions are recorded as "diagnoses" or "problems."

- ☑4th **V40** Mental and behavioral problems
  - **V40.0** Problems with learning
  - **V40.1** Problems with communication [including speech]
  - **V40.2** Other mental problems
  - **V40.3** Other behavioral problems
  - **V40.9** Unspecified mental or behavioral problem
- ☑4th **V41** Problems with special senses and other special functions
  - **V41.0** Problems with sight
  - **V41.1** Other eye problems
  - **V41.2** Problems with hearing
  - **V41.3** Other ear problems
  - **V41.4** Problems with voice production
  - **V41.5** Problems with smell and taste
  - **V41.6** Problems with swallowing and mastication
  - **V41.7** Problems with sexual function
    - EXCLUDES: marital problems (V61.10)
    - psychosexual disorders (302.0-302.9)
  - **V41.8** Other problems with special functions
  - **V41.9** Unspecified problem with special functions
- ☑4th **V42** Organ or tissue replaced by transplant
  - INCLUDES: homologous or heterologous (animal) (human) transplant organ status
  - AHA: 3Q, '98, 3, 4
  - **V42.0** Kidney [SDx]
    - AHA: 1Q, '03, 10; 3Q, '01, 12
  - **V42.1** Heart [SDx]
    - AHA: 3Q, '03, 16; 3Q, '01, 13
  - **V42.2** Heart valve [SDx]
  - **V42.3** Skin [SDx]
  - **V42.4** Bone [SDx]
  - **V42.5** Cornea [SDx]
  - **V42.6** Lung [SDx]
  - **V42.7** Liver [SDx]
  - ☑5th **V42.8** Other specified organ or tissue
    - AHA: 4Q, '98, 64; 4Q, '97, 49
    - **V42.81** Bone marrow [SDx]
    - **V42.82** Peripheral stem cells [SDx]
    - **V42.83** Pancreas [SDx]
      - AHA: 1Q, '03, 10; 2Q, '01, 16
    - **V42.84** Intestines [SDx]
      - AHA: 4Q, '00, 48, 50
    - **V42.89** Other [SDx]
  - **V42.9** Unspecified organ or tissue [SDx]
- ☑4th **V43** Organ or tissue replaced by other means
  - INCLUDES: organ or tissue assisted by other means
    replacement of organ by:
      artificial device
      mechanical device
      prosthesis
  - EXCLUDES: cardiac pacemaker in situ (V45.01)
    fitting and adjustment of prosthetic device (V52.0-V52.9)
    renal dialysis status (V45.1)
  - **V43.0** Eye globe [SDx]
  - **V43.1** Lens [SDx]
    - Pseudophakos
    - AHA: 4Q, '98, 65
  - ☑5th **V43.2** Heart
    - Fully implantable artificial heart
    - Heart assist device
    - AHA: 4Q, '03, 85
    - **V43.21** Heart assist device
    - **V43.22** Fully implantable artificial heart
  - **V43.3** Heart valve [SDx]
    - AHA: 3Q, '02, 13, 14
  - **V43.4** Blood vessel [SDx]
  - **V43.5** Bladder [SDx]
  - ☑5th **V43.6** Joint
    - AHA: ▶4Q, '05, 91◀
    - **V43.60** Unspecified joint [SDx]
    - **V43.61** Shoulder [SDx]
    - **V43.62** Elbow [SDx]
    - **V43.63** Wrist [SDx]
    - **V43.64** Hip [SDx]
      - AHA: ▶4Q, '05, 93, 112;◀ 2Q, '04, 15
    - **V43.65** Knee [SDx]
    - **V43.66** Ankle [SDx]
    - **V43.69** Other [SDx]
  - **V43.7** Limb [SDx]
  - ☑5th **V43.8** Other organ or tissue
    - **V43.81** Larynx [SDx]
      - AHA: 4Q, '95, 55
    - **V43.82** Breast [SDx]
      - AHA: 4Q, '95, 55
    - **V43.83** Artificial skin [SDx]
    - **V43.89** Other [SDx]
- ☑4th **V44** Artificial opening status
  - EXCLUDES: artificial openings requiring attention or management (V55.0-V55.9)
  - **V44.0** Tracheostomy [SDx]
    - AHA: 4Q, '03, 103, 107, 111; 1Q, '01, 6
  - **V44.1** Gastrostomy [SDx]
    - AHA: 4Q, '03, 103, 107-108, 110; 1Q, '01, 12; 3Q, '97, 12; 1Q, '93, 26
  - **V44.2** Ileostomy [SDx]
  - **V44.3** Colostomy [SDx]
    - AHA: 4Q, '03, 110
  - **V44.4** Other artificial opening of gastrointestinal tract [SDx]
  - ☑5th **V44.5** Cystostomy
    - **V44.50** Cystostomy, unspecified [SDx]
    - **V44.51** Cutaneous-vesicostomy [SDx]
    - **V44.52** Appendico-vesicostomy [SDx]
    - **V44.59** Other cystostomy [SDx]
  - **V44.6** Other artificial opening of urinary tract [SDx]
    - Nephrostomy   Urethrostomy
    - Ureterostomy
  - **V44.7** Artificial vagina [SDx]
  - **V44.8** Other artificial opening status [SDx]
  - **V44.9** Unspecified artificial opening status [SDx]
- ☑4th **V45** Other postprocedural states
  - EXCLUDES: aftercare management (V51-V58.9)
    malfunction or other complication — code to condition
  - AHA: 4Q, '03, 85
  - ☑5th **V45.0** Cardiac device in situ
    - EXCLUDES: artificial heart (V43.22)
      heart assist device (V43.21)
    - **V45.00** Unspecified cardiac device [SDx]
    - **V45.01** Cardiac pacemaker [SDx]

Tabular List — V CODES

V45.02 Automatic implantable cardiac defibrillator [SDx]
V45.09 Other specified cardiac device [SDx]
    Carotid sinus pacemaker in situ

V45.1 Renal dialysis status [SDx]
    Hemodialysis status
    Patient requiring intermittent renal dialysis
    Peritoneal dialysis status
    Presence of arterial-venous shunt (for dialysis)
    EXCLUDES *admission for dialysis treatment or session (V56.0)*
    AHA: 4Q, '05, 96; 1Q, '04, 22-23; 2Q, '03, 7; 2Q, '01, 12, 13

V45.2 Presence of cerebrospinal fluid drainage device [SDx]
    Cerebral ventricle (communicating) shunt, valve, or device in situ
    EXCLUDES *malfunction (996.2)*
    AHA: 4Q, '03, 106

V45.3 Intestinal bypass or anastomosis status [SDx]
    EXCLUDES ▶ *bariatric surgery status (V45.86)*
    gastric bypass status (V45.86)
    obesity surgery status (V45.86) ◀

V45.4 Arthrodesis status [SDx]
    AHA: N-D, '84, 18

V45.5 Presence of contraceptive device
    EXCLUDES *checking, reinsertion, or removal of device (V25.42)*
    complication from device (996.32)
    insertion of device (V25.1)

  V45.51 Intrauterine contraceptive device [SDx] ♀
  V45.52 Subdermal contraceptive implant [SDx]
  V45.59 Other [SDx]

V45.6 States following surgery of eye and adnexa
    Cataract extraction
    Filtering bleb   } state following eye surgery
    Surgical eyelid adhesion
    EXCLUDES *aphakia (379.31)*
    artificial eye globe (V43.0)
    AHA: 4Q, '98, 65; 4Q, '97, 49

  V45.61 Cataract extraction status [SDx]
    Use additional code for associated artificial lens status (V43.1)
  V45.69 Other states following surgery of eye and adnexa [SDx]
    AHA: 2Q, '01, 16; 1Q, '98, 10; 4Q, '97, 19

V45.7 Acquired absence of organ
    AHA: 4Q, '98, 65; 4Q, '97, 50

  V45.71 Acquired absence of breast
    AHA: 4Q, '01, 66; 4Q, '97, 50
  V45.72 Acquired absence of intestine (large) (small)
  V45.73 Acquired absence of kidney
  V45.74 Other parts of urinary tract
    Bladder
    AHA: 4Q, '00, 51
  V45.75 Stomach
    AHA: 4Q, '00, 51
  V45.76 Lung
    AHA: 4Q, '00, 51
  V45.77 Genital organs
    EXCLUDES *female genital mutilation status* ▶*(629.20-629.29)*◀
    AHA: 1Q, '03, 13, 14; 4Q, '00, 51
  V45.78 Eye
    AHA: 4Q, '00, 51
  V45.79 Other acquired absence of organ
    AHA: 4Q, '00, 51

V45.8 Other postprocedural status
  V45.81 Aortocoronary bypass status [SDx]
    AHA: 4Q, '03, 105; 3Q, '01, 15; 3Q, '97, 16
  V45.82 Percutaneous transluminal coronary angioplasty status [SDx]
  V45.83 Breast implant removal status [SDx]
    AHA: 4Q, '95, 55
  V45.84 Dental restoration status [SDx]
    Dental crowns status
    Dental fillings status
    AHA: 4Q, '01, 54
  V45.85 Insulin pump status [SDx]
  V45.86 Bariatric surgery status [SDx]
    Gastric banding status
    Gastric bypass status for obesity
    Obesity surgery status
    EXCLUDES *bariatric surgery status complicating pregnancy, childbirth or the puerperium (649.2)*
    intestinal bypass or anastomosis status (V45.3)
  V45.89 Other [SDx]
    Presence of neuropacemaker or other electronic device
    EXCLUDES *artificial heart valve in situ (V43.3)*
    vascular prosthesis in situ (V43.4)
    AHA: 1Q, '95, 11

V46 Other dependence on machines
  V46.0 Aspirator [SDx]
  V46.1 Respirator [Ventilator]
    Iron lung
    AHA: 4Q, '05, 96; 4Q, '03, 103; 1Q, '01, 12; J-F, '87, 7 3
    V46.11 Dependence on respirator, status [SDx]
    AHA: 4Q, '04, 100
    V46.12 Encounter for respirator dependence during power failure [PDx]
    AHA: 4Q, '04, 100
    V46.13 Encounter for weaning from respirator [ventilator] [PDx]
    V46.14 Mechanical complication of respirator [ventilator]
      Mechanical failure of respirator [ventilator]
  V46.2 Supplemental oxygen [SDx]
    Long-term oxygen therapy
    AHA: 4Q, '03, 108; 4Q, '02, 79
  V46.8 Other enabling machines [SDx]
    Hyperbaric chamber
    Possum [Patient-Operated-Selector-Mechanism]
    EXCLUDES *cardiac pacemaker (V45.0)*
    kidney dialysis machine (V45.1)
  V46.9 Unspecified machine dependence [SDx]

V47 Other problems with internal organs
  V47.0 Deficiencies of internal organs
  V47.1 Mechanical and motor problems with internal organs
  V47.2 Other cardiorespiratory problems
    Cardiovascular exercise intolerance with pain (with):
      at rest
      less than ordinary activity
      ordinary activity
  V47.3 Other digestive problems
  V47.4 Other urinary problems
  V47.5 Other genital problems
  V47.9 Unspecified

V CODES

V48 Problems with head, neck, and trunk
- **V48.0** Deficiencies of head
  - EXCLUDES: deficiencies of ears, eyelids, and nose (V48.8)
- **V48.1** Deficiencies of neck and trunk
- **V48.2** Mechanical and motor problems with head
- **V48.3** Mechanical and motor problems with neck and trunk
- **V48.4** Sensory problem with head
- **V48.5** Sensory problem with neck and trunk
- **V48.6** Disfigurements of head
- **V48.7** Disfigurements of neck and trunk
- **V48.8** Other problems with head, neck, and trunk
- **V48.9** Unspecified problem with head, neck, or trunk

V49 Other conditions influencing health status
- **V49.0** Deficiencies of limbs
- **V49.1** Mechanical problems with limbs
- **V49.2** Motor problems with limbs
- **V49.3** Sensory problems with limbs
- **V49.4** Disfigurements of limbs
- **V49.5** Other problems of limbs
- **V49.6** Upper limb amputation status
  - AHA: 4Q, '05, 94; 4Q, '98, 42; 4Q, '94, 39
  - **V49.60** Unspecified level
  - **V49.61** Thumb
  - **V49.62** Other finger(s)
    - AHA: 2Q, '05, 7
  - **V49.63** Hand
  - **V49.64** Wrist
    - Disarticulation of wrist
  - **V49.65** Below elbow
  - **V49.66** Above elbow
    - Disarticulation of elbow
  - **V49.67** Shoulder
    - Disarticulation of shoulder
- **V49.7** Lower limb amputation status
  - AHA: 4Q, '05, 94; 4Q, '98, 42; 4Q, '94, 39
  - **V49.70** Unspecified level
  - **V49.71** Great toe
  - **V49.72** Other toe(s)
  - **V49.73** Foot
  - **V49.74** Ankle
    - Disarticulation of ankle
  - **V49.75** Below knee
  - **V49.76** Above knee
    - Disarticulation of knee
    - AHA: 2Q, '05, 14
  - **V49.77** Hip
    - Disarticulation of hip
- **V49.8** Other specified conditions influencing health status
  - AHA: 4Q, '00, 51
  - **V49.81** Asymptomatic postmenopausal status (age-related) (natural) [A] ♀
    - EXCLUDES: menopausal and premenopausal disorders (627.0-627.9)
      postsurgical menopause (256.2)
      premature menopause (256.31)
      symptomatic menopause (627.0-627.9)
    - AHA: 4Q, '02, 79; 4Q, '00, 54
  - **V49.82** Dental sealant status [SDx]
    - AHA: 4Q, '01, 54
  - **V49.83** Awaiting organ transplant status [SDx]
  - **V49.84** Bed confinement status
    - AHA: 4Q, '05, 96
- **V49.89** Other specified conditions influencing health status
  - AHA: 4Q, '05, 94
- **V49.9** Unspecified

PERSONS ENCOUNTERING HEALTH SERVICES FOR SPECIFIC PROCEDURES AND AFTERCARE (V50-V59)

Note: Categories V51-V58 are intended for use to indicate a reason for care in patients who may have already been treated for some disease or injury not now present, or who are receiving care to consolidate the treatment, to deal with residual states, or to prevent recurrence.

EXCLUDES: follow-up examination for medical surveillance following treatment (V67.0-V67.9)

V50 Elective surgery for purposes other than remedying health states
- **V50.0** Hair transplant
- **V50.1** Other plastic surgery for unacceptable cosmetic appearance
  - Breast augmentation or reduction
  - Face-lift
  - EXCLUDES: plastic surgery following healed injury or operation (V51)
- **V50.2** Routine or ritual circumcision ♂
  - Circumcision in the absence of significant medical indication
- **V50.3** Ear piercing
- **V50.4** Prophylactic organ removal
  - EXCLUDES: organ donations (V59.0-V59.9)
    therapeutic organ removal — code to condition
  - AHA: 4Q, '94, 44
  - **V50.41** Breast
    - AHA: 4Q, '04, 107
  - **V50.42** Ovary ♀
  - **V50.49** Other
- **V50.8** Other
- **V50.9** Unspecified

V51 Aftercare involving the use of plastic surgery
Plastic surgery following healed injury or operation
- EXCLUDES: cosmetic plastic surgery (V50.1)
  plastic surgery as treatment for current injury — code to condition
  repair of scarred tissue — code to scar

V52 Fitting and adjustment of prosthetic device and implant
- INCLUDES: removal of device
- EXCLUDES: malfunction or complication of prosthetic device (996.0-996.7)
  status only, without need for care (V43.0-V43.8)
- AHA: 4Q, '05, 94; 4Q, '95, 55; 1Q, '90, 7
- **V52.0** Artificial arm (complete) (partial)
- **V52.1** Artificial leg (complete) (partial)
- **V52.2** Artificial eye
- **V52.3** Dental prosthetic device
- **V52.4** Breast prosthesis and implant ♀
  - EXCLUDES: admission for implant insertion (V50.1)
  - AHA: 4Q, '95, 80, 81
- **V52.8** Other specified prosthetic device
  - AHA: 2Q, '02, 12, 16
- **V52.9** Unspecified prosthetic device

V53 Fitting and adjustment of other device
- INCLUDES: removal of device
  replacement of device
- EXCLUDES: status only, without need for care (V45.0-V45.8)
- **V53.0** Devices related to nervous system and special senses
  - AHA: 4Q, '98, 66; 4Q, '97, 51
  - **V53.01** Fitting and adjustment of cerebral ventricular (communicating) shunt
    - AHA: 4Q, '97, 51

| Tabular List | V CODES | V53.02–V55.1 |

V53.02 Neuropacemaker (brain) (peripheral nerve) (spinal cord)

V53.09 Fitting and adjustment of other devices related to nervous system and special senses
  Auditory substitution device
  Visual substitution device
  AHA: 2Q, '99, 4

V53.1 Spectacles and contact lenses

V53.2 Hearing aid

√5th **V53.3** Cardiac device
  Reprogramming
  AHA: 3Q, '92, 3; 1Q, '90, 7; M-J, '87, 8 ; N-D, '84, 18

  V53.31 Cardiac pacemaker
    EXCLUDES mechanical complication of cardiac pacemaker (996.01)
    AHA: 1Q, '02, 3

  V53.32 Automatic implantable cardiac defibrillator
    AHA: 3Q, '05, 8

  V53.39 Other cardiac device

V53.4 Orthodontic devices

V53.5 Other intestinal appliance
  EXCLUDES colostomy (V55.3)
            ileostomy (V55.2)
            other artificial opening of digestive tract (V55.4)

V53.6 Urinary devices
  Urinary catheter
  EXCLUDES cystostomy (V55.5)
            nephrostomy (V55.6)
            ureterostomy (V55.6)
            urethrostomy (V55.6)

V53.7 Orthopedic devices
  Orthopedic: Orthopedic:
    brace   corset
    cast   shoes
  EXCLUDES other orthopedic aftercare (V54)

V53.8 Wheelchair

√5th **V53.9** Other and unspecified device
  AHA: 2Q, '03, 6

  V53.90 Unspecified device

  V53.91 Fitting and adjustment of insulin pump
    Insulin pump titration

  V53.99 Other device

√4th **V54** Other orthopedic aftercare
  EXCLUDES fitting and adjustment of orthopedic devices (V53.7)
            malfunction of internal orthopedic device (996.40-996.49)
            other complication of nonmechanical nature (996.60-996.79)
  AHA: 3Q, '95, 3

√5th **V54.0** Aftercare involving internal fixation device
  EXCLUDES malfunction of internal orthopedic device (996.40-996.49)
            other complication of nonmechanical nature (996.60-996.79)
            removal of external fixation device (V54.89)
  AHA: 4Q, '03, 87

  V54.01 Encounter for removal of internal fixation device

  V54.02 Encounter for lengthening/adjustment of growth rod

  V54.09 Other aftercare involving internal fixation device

√5th **V54.1** Aftercare for healing traumatic fracture
  EXCLUDES ▶aftercare for amputation stump (V54.89)◀
  AHA: 4Q, '02, 80

V54.10 Aftercare for healing traumatic fracture of arm, unspecified

V54.11 Aftercare for healing traumatic fracture of upper arm

V54.12 Aftercare for healing traumatic fracture of lower arm

V54.13 Aftercare for healing traumatic fracture of hip
  AHA: 4Q, '03, 103, 105; 2Q, '03, 16

V54.14 Aftercare for healing traumatic fracture of leg, unspecified

V54.15 Aftercare for healing traumatic fracture of upper leg
  EXCLUDES aftercare for healing traumatic fracture of hip (V54.13)

V54.16 Aftercare for healing traumatic fracture of lower leg

V54.17 Aftercare for healing traumatic fracture of vertebrae

V54.19 Aftercare for healing traumatic fracture of other bone
  AHA: 1Q, '05, 13; 4Q, '02, 80

√5th **V54.2** Aftercare for healing pathologic fracture
  AHA: 4Q, '02, 80

  V54.20 Aftercare for healing pathologic fracture of arm, unspecified

  V54.21 Aftercare for healing pathologic fracture of upper arm

  V54.22 Aftercare for healing pathologic fracture of lower arm

  V54.23 Aftercare for healing pathologic fracture of hip

  V54.24 Aftercare for healing pathologic fracture of leg, unspecified

  V54.25 Aftercare for healing pathologic fracture of upper leg
    EXCLUDES aftercare for healing pathologic fracture of hip (V54.23)

  V54.26 Aftercare for healing pathologic fracture of lower leg

  V54.27 Aftercare for healing pathologic fracture of vertebrae
    AHA: 4Q, '03, 108

  V54.29 Aftercare for healing pathologic fracture of other bone
    AHA: 4Q, '02, 80

√5th **V54.8** Other orthopedic aftercare
  AHA: 3Q, '01, 19; 4Q, '99, 5

  V54.81 Aftercare following joint replacement
    Use additional code to identify joint replacement site (V43.60-V43.69)
    AHA: 2Q, '04, 15; 4Q, '02, 80

  V54.89 Other orthopedic aftercare
    Aftercare for healing fracture NOS

V54.9 Unspecified orthopedic aftercare

√4th **V55** Attention to artificial openings
  INCLUDES adjustment or repositioning of catheter
            closure
            passage of sounds or bougies
            reforming
            removal or replacement of catheter
            toilet or cleansing
  EXCLUDES complications of external stoma (519.00-519.09, 569.60-569.69, 997.4, 997.5)
            status only, without need for care (V44.0-V44.9)

V55.0 Tracheostomy

V55.1 Gastrostomy
  AHA: 4Q, '99, 9; 3Q, '97, 7, 8; 1Q, '96, 14; 3Q, '95, 13

V55.2–V58.44 V CODES Tabular List

- **V55.2** Ileostomy
- **V55.3** Colostomy
  AHA: 2Q, '05, 4; 3Q, '97, 9
- **V55.4** Other artificial opening of digestive tract
  AHA: 2Q, '05, 14; 1Q, '03, 10
- **V55.5** Cystostomy
- **V55.6** Other artificial opening of urinary tract
  Nephrostomy   Urethrostomy
  Ureterostomy
- **V55.7** Artificial vagina
- **V55.8** Other specified artificial opening
- **V55.9** Unspecified artificial opening

√4th **V56 Encounter for dialysis and dialysis catheter care**
  Use additional code to identify the associated condition
  EXCLUDES: dialysis preparation — code to condition
  AHA: 4Q, '98, 66; 1Q, '93, 29

- **V56.0** Extracorporeal dialysis [PDx]
  Dialysis (renal) NOS
  EXCLUDES: dialysis status (V45.1)
  AHA: 4Q, '05, 79; 1Q, '04, 23; 4Q, '00, 40; 3Q, '98, 6; 2Q, '98, 20
- **V56.1** Fitting and adjustment of extracorporeal dialysis catheter
  Removal or replacement of catheter
  Toilet or cleansing
  Use additional code for any concurrent extracorporeal dialysis (V56.0)
  AHA: 2Q, '98, 20
- **V56.2** Fitting and adjustment of peritoneal dialysis catheter
  Use additional code for any concurrent peritoneal dialysis (V56.8)
  AHA: 4Q, '98, 55

√5th **V56.3** Encounter for adequacy testing for dialysis
  AHA: 4Q, '00, 55
  - **V56.31** Encounter for adequacy testing for hemodialysis
  - **V56.32** Encounter for adequacy testing for peritoneal dialysis
    Peritoneal equilibration test
- **V56.8** Other dialysis
  Peritoneal dialysis
  AHA: 4Q, '98, 55

√4th **V57 Care involving use of rehabilitation procedures**
  Use additional code to identify underlying condition
  AHA: 1Q, '02, 19; 3Q, '97, 12; 1Q, '90, 6; S-O, '86, 3

- **V57.0** Breathing exercises [PDx]
- **V57.1** Other physical therapy [PDx]
  Therapeutic and remedial exercises, except breathing
  AHA: 2Q, '04, 15; 4Q, '02, 56; 4Q, '99, 5

√5th **V57.2** Occupational therapy and vocational rehabilitation
  - **V57.21** Encounter for occupational therapy [PDx]
    AHA: 4Q, '99, 7
  - **V57.22** Encounter for vocational therapy [PDx]
- **V57.3** Speech therapy [PDx]
  AHA: 4Q, '97, 36
- **V57.4** Orthoptic training [PDx]

√5th **V57.8** Other specified rehabilitation procedure
  - **V57.81** Orthotic training [PDx]
    Gait training in the use of artificial limbs
  - **V57.89** Other [PDx]
    Multiple training or therapy
    AHA: 4Q, '03, 105-106, 108; 2Q, '03, 16; 1Q, '02, 16; 3Q, '01, 21; 3Q, '97, 11, 12; S-O, '86, 4
- **V57.9** Unspecified rehabilitation procedure [PDx]

√4th **V58 Encounter for other and unspecified procedures and aftercare**
  EXCLUDES: convalescence and palliative care (V66)
- **V58.0** Radiotherapy [PDx]
  Encounter or admission for radiotherapy
  EXCLUDES: encounter for radioactive implant — code to condition
    radioactive iodine therapy — code to condition
  AHA: 3Q, '92, 5; 2Q, '90, 7; J-F, '87, 13

√5th **V58.1** Encounter for antineoplastic chemotherapy and immunotherapy
  Encounter or admission for chemotherapy
  EXCLUDES: chemotherapy and immunotherapy for nonneoplastic conditions — code to condition
    prophylactic chemotherapy against disease which has never been present (V03.0-V07.9)
  AHA: 1Q, '04, 13; 2Q, '03, 16; 3Q, '93, 4; 2Q, '92, 6; 2Q, '91, 17; 2Q, '90, 7; S-O, '84, 5
  - **V58.11** Encounter for antineoplastic chemotherapy [PDx]
    AHA: 4Q, '05, 98
  - **V58.12** Encounter for antineoplastic immunotherapy [PDx]
    AHA: 4Q, '05, 98
- **V58.2** Blood transfusion, without reported diagnosis

▲ √5th **V58.3** Attention to dressings and sutures
  ▶Change or removal of wound packing◀
  EXCLUDES: ▶attention to drains (V58.49)
    planned postoperative wound closure (V58.41)◀
  AHA: 2Q, '05, 14
  • **V58.30** Encounter for change or removal of nonsurgical wound dressing
    Encounter for change or removal of wound dressing NOS
  • **V58.31** Encounter for change or removal of surgical wound dressing
  • **V58.32** Encounter for removal of sutures
    Encounter for removal of staples

√5th **V58.4** Other aftercare following surgery
  EXCLUDES: aftercare following sterilization reversal surgery (V26.22)
    attention to artificial openings (V55.0-V55.9)
    orthopedic aftercare (V54.0-V54.9)
  Note: Codes from this subcategory should be used in conjunction with other aftercare codes to fully identify the reason for the aftercare encounter
  AHA: 4Q, '99, 9; N-D, '87, 9
  - **V58.41** Encounter for planned postoperative wound closure
    EXCLUDES: disruption of operative wound (998.3)
      ▶encounter for dressings and suture aftercare (V58.30-V58.32)◀
    AHA: 4Q, '99, 15
  - **V58.42** Aftercare following surgery for neoplasm
    Conditions classifiable to 140-239
    AHA: 4Q, '02, 80
  - **V58.43** Aftercare following surgery for injury and trauma
    Conditions classifiable to 800-999
    EXCLUDES: aftercare for healing traumatic fracture (V54.10-V54.19)
    AHA: 4Q, '02, 80
  - **V58.44** Aftercare following organ transplant
    Use additional code to identify the organ transplanted (V42.0-V42.9)
    AHA: 4Q, '04, 101

V CODES

V58.49 Other specified aftercare following surgery
▶Change or removal of drains◀
AHA: 1Q, '96, 8, 9

V58.5 Orthodontics
EXCLUDES: fitting and adjustment of orthodontic device (V53.4)

✓5ᵗʰ V58.6 Long-term (current) drug use
EXCLUDES: drug abuse (305.00-305.93)
drug dependence (304.00-304.93)
hormone replacement therapy (postmenopausal) (V07.4)
AHA: 4Q, '03, 85; 4Q, '02, 84; 3Q, '02, 15; 4Q, '95, 61

V58.61 Long-term (current) use of anticoagulants [SDx]
EXCLUDES: long-term (current) use of aspirin (V58.66)
AHA: 3Q, '04, 7; 4Q, '03, 108; 3Q, '02, 13-16; 1Q, '02, 15, 16

V58.62 Long-term (current) use of antibiotics [SDx]
AHA: 4Q, '98, 59

V58.63 Long-term (current) use of antiplatelets/antithrombotics [SDx]
EXCLUDES: long-term (current) use of aspirin (V58.66)

V58.64 Long-term (current) use of non-steroidal anti-inflammatories (NSAID)
EXCLUDES: long-term (current) use of aspirin (V58.66)

V58.65 Long-term (current) use of steroids [SDx]

V58.66 Long-term (current) use of aspirin [SDx]
AHA: 4Q, '04, 102

V58.67 Long-term (current) use of insulin [SDx]
AHA: 4Q, '04, 55-56, 103

V58.69 Long-term (current) use of other medications [SDx]
High-risk medications
AHA: 2Q, '04, 10; 1Q, '03, 11; 2Q, '00, 8; 3Q, '99, 13; 2Q, '99, 17; 1Q, '97, 12; 2Q, '96, 7

✓5ᵗʰ V58.7 Aftercare following surgery to specified body systems, not elsewhere classified
Note: Codes from this subcategory should be used in conjunction with other aftercare codes to fully identify the reason for the aftercare encounter
EXCLUDES: aftercare following organ transplant (V58.44)
aftercare following surgery for neoplasm (V58.42)
AHA: 4Q, '03, 104; 4Q, '02, 80

V58.71 Aftercare following surgery of the sense organs, NEC
Conditions classifiable to 360-379, 380-389

V58.72 Aftercare following surgery of the nervous system, NEC
Conditions classifiable to 320-359
EXCLUDES: aftercare following surgery of the sense organs, NEC (V58.71)

V58.73 Aftercare following surgery of the circulatory system, NEC
Conditions classifiable to 390-459
AHA: 4Q, '03, 105

V58.74 Aftercare following surgery of the respiratory system, NEC
Conditions classifiable to 460-519

V58.75 Aftercare following surgery of the teeth, oral cavity and digestive system, NEC
Conditions classifiable to 520-579
AHA: 2Q, '05, 14

V58.76 Aftercare following surgery of the genitourinary system, NEC
Conditions classifiable to 580-629
EXCLUDES: aftercare following sterilization reversal (V26.22)
AHA: 1Q, '05, 11-12

V58.77 Aftercare following surgery of the skin and subcutaneous tissue, NEC
Conditions classifiable to 680-709

V58.78 Aftercare following surgery of the musculoskeletal system, NEC
Conditions classifiable to 710-739

✓5ᵗʰ V58.8 Other specified procedures and aftercare
AHA: 4Q, '94, 45; 2Q, '94, 8

V58.81 Fitting and adjustment of vascular catheter
Removal or replacement of catheter
Toilet or cleansing
EXCLUDES: complication of renal dialysis (996.73)
complication of vascular catheter (996.74)
dialysis preparation — code to condition
encounter for dialysis (V56.0-V56.8)
fitting and adjustment of dialysis catheter (V56.1)

V58.82 Fitting and adjustment of nonvascular catheter, NEC
Removal or replacement of catheter
Toilet or cleansing
EXCLUDES: fitting and adjustment of peritoneal dialysis catheter (V56.2)
fitting and adjustment of urinary catheter (V53.6)

V58.83 Encounter for therapeutic drug monitoring
Use additional code for any associated long-term (current) drug use (V58.61-V58.69)
EXCLUDES: blood-drug testing for medico-legal reasons (V70.4)
AHA: 2Q, '04, 10; 1Q, '04, 13; 4Q, '03, 85; 4Q, '02, 84; 3Q, '02, 13-16
DEF: Drug monitoring: Measurement of the level of a specific drug in the body or measurement of a specific function to assess effectiveness of a drug.

V58.89 Other specified aftercare
AHA: 4Q, '98, 59

V58.9 Unspecified aftercare

✓4ᵗʰ V59 Donors
EXCLUDES: examination of potential donor (V70.8)
self-donation of organ or tissue — code to condition
AHA: 4Q, '95, 62; 1Q, '90, 10; N-D, '84, 8

✓5ᵗʰ V59.0 Blood
V59.01 Whole blood [PDx]
V59.02 Stem cells [PDx]
V59.09 Other [PDx]

V59.1 Skin [PDx]
V59.2 Bone [PDx]
V59.3 Bone marrow [PDx]
V59.4 Kidney [PDx]
V59.5 Cornea [PDx]
V59.6 Liver [PDx]

✓5ᵗʰ V59.7 Egg (oocyte) (ovum)
AHA: 4Q, '05, 99

V59.70 Egg (oocyte) (ovum) donor, unspecified [PDx ♀]

V59.71 Egg (oocyte) (ovum) donor, under age 35, anonymous recipient [PDx ♀]
Egg donor, under age 35 NOS

V CODES — Tabular List

V59.72 Egg (oocyte) (ovum) donor, under age 35, designated recipient [PDx] ♀

V59.73 Egg (oocyte) (ovum) donor, age 35 and over, anonymous recipient [PDx] ♀
   Egg donor, age 35 and over NOS

V59.74 Egg (oocyte) (ovum) donor, age 35 and over, designated recipient [PDx] ♀

V59.8 Other specified organ or tissue
   AHA: 3Q, '02, 20

V59.9 Unspecified organ or tissue [PDx]

PERSONS ENCOUNTERING HEALTH SERVICES IN OTHER CIRCUMSTANCES (V60-V69)

✓4th **V60** Housing, household, and economic circumstances

   V60.0 Lack of housing [SDx]
      Hobos   Transients
      Social migrants Vagabonds
      Tramps

   V60.1 Inadequate housing [SDx]
      Lack of heating   Technical defects in home
      Restriction of space   preventing adequate care

   V60.2 Inadequate material resources [SDx]
      Economic problem   Poverty NOS

   V60.3 Person living alone [SDx]

   V60.4 No other household member able to render care [SDx]
      Person requiring care (has) (is):
         family member too handicapped, ill, or otherwise unsuited to render care
         partner temporarily away from home
         temporarily away from usual place of abode
      EXCLUDES holiday relief care (V60.5)

   V60.5 Holiday relief care [SDx]
      Provision of health care facilities to a person normally cared for at home, to enable relatives to take a vacation

   V60.6 Person living in residential institution [SDx]
      Boarding school resident

   V60.8 Other specified housing or economic circumstances [SDx]

   V60.9 Unspecified housing or economic circumstance [SDx]

✓4th **V61** Other family circumstances
   INCLUDES when these circumstances or fear of them, affecting the person directly involved or others, are mentioned as the reason, justified or not, for seeking or receiving medical advice or care
   AHA: 1Q, '90, 9

   V61.0 Family disruption
      Divorce   Estrangement

   ✓5th **V61.1** Counseling for marital and partner problems
      EXCLUDES problems related to:
         psychosexual disorders (302.0-302.9)
         sexual function (V41.7)

      V61.10 Counseling for marital and partner problems, unspecified
         Marital conflict
         Marital relationship problem
         Partner conflict
         Partner relationship problem

      V61.11 Counseling for victim of spousal and partner abuse
         EXCLUDES encounter for treatment of current injuries due to abuse (995.80-995.85)

      V61.12 Counseling for perpetrator of spousal and partner abuse

   ✓5th **V61.2** Parent-child problems

      V61.20 Counseling for parent-child problem, unspecified
         Concern about behavior of child
         Parent-child conflict
         Parent-child relationship problem

      V61.21 Counseling for victim of child abuse
         Child battering   Child neglect
         EXCLUDES current injuries due to abuse (995.50-995.59)

      V61.22 Counseling for perpetrator of parental child abuse
         EXCLUDES counseling for non-parental abuser (V62.83)

      V61.29 Other
         Problem concerning adopted or foster child
         AHA: 3Q, '99, 16

   V61.3 Problems with aged parents or in-laws

   ✓5th **V61.4** Health problems within family
      V61.41 Alcoholism in family
      V61.49 Other
         Care of   } sick or handicapped person
         Presence of } in family or household

   V61.5 Multiparity
   V61.6 Illegitimacy or illegitimate pregnancy Ⓜ♀
   V61.7 Other unwanted pregnancy Ⓜ♀
   V61.8 Other specified family circumstances
      Problems with family members NEC
      Sibling relationship problem

   V61.9 Unspecified family circumstance

✓4th **V62** Other psychosocial circumstances
   INCLUDES those circumstances or fear of them, affecting the person directly involved or others, mentioned as the reason, justified or not, for seeking or receiving medical advice or care
   EXCLUDES previous psychological trauma (V15.41-V15.49)

   V62.0 Unemployment [SDx]
      EXCLUDES circumstances when main problem is economic inadequacy or poverty (V60.2)

   V62.1 Adverse effects of work environment [SDx]

   V62.2 Other occupational circumstances or maladjustment [SDx]
      Career choice problem
      Dissatisfaction with employment
      Occupational problem

   V62.3 Educational circumstances
      Academic problem
      Dissatisfaction with school environment
      Educational handicap

   V62.4 Social maladjustment [SDx]
      Acculturation problem
      Cultural deprivation
      Political, religious, or sex discrimination
      Social:
         isolation
         persecution

   V62.5 Legal circumstances [SDx]
      Imprisonment   Litigation
      Legal investigation Prosecution

   V62.6 Refusal of treatment for reasons of religion or conscience [SDx]

   ✓5th **V62.8** Other psychological or physical stress, not elsewhere classified

      V62.81 Interpersonal problems, not elsewhere classified [SDx]
         Relational problem NOS

      V62.82 Bereavement, uncomplicated [SDx]
         EXCLUDES bereavement as adjustment reaction (309.0)

Ⓝ Newborn Age: 0   Ⓟ Pediatric Age: 0-17   Ⓜ Maternity Age: 12-55   Ⓐ Adult Age: 15-124

 Secondary Diagnosis   Primary Diagnosis

V CODES

V62.83 Counseling for perpetrator of physical/sexual abuse [SDx]
  EXCLUDES: *counseling for perpetrator of parental child abuse (V61.22)*
  counseling for perpetrator of spousal and partner abuse (V61.12)

V62.84 Suicidal ideation [SDx]
  EXCLUDES: *suicidal tendencies (300.9)*
  AHA: 4Q, '05, 96
  DEF: Thoughts of committing suicide; no actual attempt of suicide has been made.

V62.89 Other [SDx]
  Borderline intellectual functioning
  Life circumstance problems
  Phase of life problems
  Religious or spiritual problem

V62.9 Unspecified psychosocial circumstance [SDx]

✓4th V63 Unavailability of other medical facilities for care
AHA: 1Q, '91, 21

V63.0 Residence remote from hospital or other health care facility

V63.1 Medical services in home not available
  EXCLUDES: *no other household member able to render care (V60.4)*
  AHA: 4Q, '01, 67; 1Q, '01, 12

V63.2 Person awaiting admission to adequate facility elsewhere

V63.8 Other specified reasons for unavailability of medical facilities
  Person on waiting list undergoing social agency investigation

V63.9 Unspecified reason for unavailability of medical facilities

✓4th V64 Persons encountering health services for specific procedures, not carried out

✓5th V64.0 Vaccination not carried out
  AHA: 4Q, '05, 99

  V64.00 Vaccination not carried out, unspecified reason [SDx]
  V64.01 Vaccination not carried out because of acute illness [SDx]
  V64.02 Vaccination not carried out because of chronic illness or condition [SDx]
  V64.03 Vaccination not carried out because of immune compromised state [SDx]
  V64.04 Vaccination not carried out because of allergy to vaccine or component [SDx]
  V64.05 Vaccination not carried out because of caregiver refusal [SDx]
  V64.06 Vaccination not carried out because of patient refusal [SDx]
  V64.07 Vaccination not carried out for religious reasons [SDx]
  V64.08 Vaccination not carried out because patient had disease being vaccinated against [SDx]
  V64.09 Vaccination not carried out for other reason [SDx]

V64.1 Surgical or other procedure not carried out because of contraindication [SDx]

V64.2 Surgical or other procedure not carried out because of patient's decision [SDx]
  AHA: 2Q, '01, 8

V64.3 Procedure not carried out for other reasons [SDx]

✓5th V64.4 Closed surgical procedure converted to open procedure
  AHA: 4Q, '03, 87; 4Q, '98, 68; 4Q, '97, 52

  V64.41 Laparoscopic surgical procedure converted to open procedure [SDx]
  V64.42 Thoracoscopic surgical procedure converted to open procedure [SDx]
  V64.43 Arthroscopic surgical procedure converted to open procedure [SDx]

✓4th V65 Other persons seeking consultation

V65.0 Healthy person accompanying sick person
  Boarder

✓5th V65.1 Person consulting on behalf of another person
  Advice or treatment for nonattending third party
  EXCLUDES: *concern (normal) about sick person in family (V61.41-V61.49)*
  AHA: 4Q, '03, 84

  V65.11 Pediatric pre-birth visit for expectant mother [M] ♀
  V65.19 Other person consulting on behalf of another person

V65.2 Person feigning illness
  Malingerer   Peregrinating patient
  AHA: 3Q, '99, 20

V65.3 Dietary surveillance and counseling
  Dietary surveillance and counseling (in):
    NOS
    colitis
    diabetes mellitus
    food allergies or intolerance
    gastritis
    hypercholesterolemia
    hypoglycemia
    obesity
  ▶Use additional code to identify Body Mass Index (BMI), if known (V85.0-V85.54)◀
  AHA: 4Q, '05, 96

✓5th V65.4 Other counseling, not elsewhere classified
  Health: advice   Health: instruction
  Health: education
  EXCLUDES: *counseling (for):*
    contraception (V25.40-V25.49)
    genetic ▶(V26.31-V26.39)◀
    on behalf of third party (V65.11-V65.19)
    procreative management (V26.4)

  V65.40 Counseling NOS
  V65.41 Exercise counseling
  V65.42 Counseling on substance use and abuse
  V65.43 Counseling on injury prevention
  V65.44 Human immunodeficiency virus [HIV] counseling
  V65.45 Counseling on other sexually transmitted diseases
  V65.46 Encounter for insulin pump training
  V65.49 Other specified counseling
    AHA: 2Q, '00, 8

V65.5 Person with feared complaint in whom no diagnosis was made
  Feared condition not demonstrated
  Problem was normal state
  "Worried well"

V65.8 Other reasons for seeking consultation
  EXCLUDES: *specified symptoms*
  AHA: 3Q, '92, 4

V65.9 Unspecified reason for consultation

✓4th V66 Convalescence and palliative care

V66.0 Following surgery [PDx]
V66.1 Following radiotherapy [PDx]
V66.2 Following chemotherapy [PDx]

V CODES — Tabular List

V66.3 Following psychotherapy and other treatment for mental disorder [PDx]
V66.4 Following treatment of fracture [PDx]
V66.5 Following other treatment [PDx]
V66.6 Following combined treatment [PDx]
V66.7 Encounter for palliative care [SDx]
　　End-of-life care　　Terminal care
　　Hospice care
　　Code first underlying disease
　　AHA: 2Q, '05, 9; 4Q, '03, 107; 1Q, '98, 11; 4Q, '96, 47, 48
V66.9 Unspecified convalescence [PDx]
　　AHA: 4Q, '99, 8

✓4th **V67** Follow-up examination
　　INCLUDES　surveillance only following completed treatment
　　EXCLUDES　surveillance of contraception (V25.40-V25.49)
　　AHA: 2Q, '03, 5; 4Q, '94, 48

✓5th **V67.0** Following surgery
　　AHA: 4Q, '00, 56; 4Q, '98, 69; 4Q, '97, 50; 2Q, '95, 8; 1Q, '95, 4; 3Q, '92, 11
　　V67.00 Following surgery, unspecified
　　V67.01 Follow-up vaginal pap smear ♀
　　　Vaginal pap-smear, status-post hysterectomy for malignant condition
　　　Use additional code to identify:
　　　　acquired absence of uterus (V45.77)
　　　　personal history of malignant neoplasm (V10.40-V10.44)
　　　EXCLUDES　vaginal pap smear status-post hysterectomy for non-malignant condition (V76.47)
　　V67.09 Following other surgery
　　　EXCLUDES　sperm count following sterilization reversal (V26.22)
　　　　sperm count for fertility testing (V26.21)
　　AHA: 3Q, '03, 16; 3Q, '02, 15

V67.1 Following radiotherapy
V67.2 Following chemotherapy
　　Cancer chemotherapy follow-up
V67.3 Following psychotherapy and other treatment for mental disorder
V67.4 Following treatment of healed fracture
　　EXCLUDES　current (healing) fracture aftercare (V54.0-V54.9)
　　AHA: 1Q, '90, 7

✓5th **V67.5** Following other treatment
　　V67.51 Following completed treatment with high-risk medications, not elsewhere classified
　　　EXCLUDES　long-term (current) drug use (V58.61-V58.69)
　　AHA: 1Q, '99, 5, 6; 4Q, '95, 61; 1Q, '90, 18
　　V67.59 Other
V67.6 Following combined treatment
V67.9 Unspecified follow-up examination

✓4th **V68** Encounters for administrative purposes
V68.0 Issue of medical certificates [PDx]
　　Issue of medical certificate of:
　　　cause of death
　　　fitness
　　　incapacity
　　EXCLUDES　encounter for general medical examination (V70.0-V70.9)

V68.1 Issue of repeat prescriptions [PDx]
　　Issue of repeat prescription for:
　　　appliance
　　　glasses
　　　medications
　　EXCLUDES　repeat prescription for contraceptives (V25.41-V25.49)
V68.2 Request for expert evidence

✓5th **V68.8** Other specified administrative purpose
　　V68.81 Referral of patient without examination or treatment [PDx]
　　V68.89 Other [PDx]
V68.9 Unspecified administrative purpose [PDx]

✓4th **V69** Problems related to lifestyle
　　AHA: 4Q, '94, 48
V69.0 Lack of physical exercise
V69.1 Inappropriate diet and eating habits
　　EXCLUDES　anorexia nervosa (307.1)
　　　bulimia (783.6)
　　　malnutrition and other nutritional deficiencies (260-269.9)
　　　other and unspecified eating disorders (307.50-307.59)
V69.2 High-risk sexual behavior
V69.3 Gambling and betting
　　EXCLUDES　pathological gambling (312.31)
V69.4 Lack of adequate sleep
　　Sleep deprivation
　　EXCLUDES　insomnia (780.52)
V69.5 Behavioral insomnia of childhood [P]
　　AHA: 4Q, '05, 99
　　DEF: Behaviors on the part of the child or caregivers that cause negative compliance with a child's sleep schedule; results in lack of adequate sleep.
V69.8 Other problems related to lifestyle
　　Self-damaging behavior
V69.9 Problem related to lifestyle, unspecified

PERSONS WITHOUT REPORTED DIAGNOSIS ENCOUNTERED DURING EXAMINATION AND INVESTIGATION OF INDIVIDUALS AND POPULATIONS ▶(V70-V82)◀

　Note: Nonspecific abnormal findings disclosed at the time of these examinations are classifiable to categories 790-796.

✓4th **V70** General medical examination
　　Use additional code(s) to identify any special screening examination(s) performed (V73.0-V82.9)
V70.0 Routine general medical examination at a health care facility [PDx]
　　Health checkup
　　EXCLUDES　health checkup of infant or child (V20.2)
　　　pre-procedural general physical examination (V72.83)
V70.1 General psychiatric examination, requested by the authority [PDx]
V70.2 General psychiatric examination, other and unspecified [PDx]

 Newborn Age: 0　　 Pediatric Age: 0-17　　 Maternity Age: 12-55　　 Adult Age: 15-124

SDx Secondary Diagnosis　　PDx Primary Diagnosis

V CODES

V70.3 Other medical examination for administrative purposes [PDx]
General medical examination for:
- admission to old age home
- adoption
- camp
- driving license
- immigration and naturalization
- insurance certification
- marriage
- prison
- school admission
- sports competition

EXCLUDES attendance for issue of medical certificates (V68.0)
pre-employment screening (V70.5)

AHA: 1Q, '90, 6

V70.4 Examination for medicolegal reasons [PDx]
Blood-alcohol tests   Paternity testing
Blood-drug tests

EXCLUDES examination and observation following:
accidents (V71.3, V71.4)
assault (V71.6)
rape (V71.5)

V70.5 Health examination of defined subpopulations [PDx]
- Armed forces personnel
- Inhabitants of institutions
- Occupational health examinations
- Pre-employment screening
- Preschool children
- Prisoners
- Prostitutes
- Refugees
- School children
- Students

V70.6 Health examination in population surveys [PDx]
EXCLUDES special screening (V73.0-V82.9)

V70.7 Examination of participant in clinical trial
Examination of participant or control in clinical research
AHA: 4Q, '01, 55

V70.8 Other specified general medical examinations [PDx]
Examination of potential donor of organ or tissue

V70.9 Unspecified general medical examination [PDx]

√4th **V71 Observation and evaluation for suspected conditions not found**
INCLUDES This category is to be used when persons without a diagnosis are suspected of having an abnormal condition, without signs or symptoms, which requires study, but after examination and observation, is found not to exist. This category is also for use for administrative and legal observation status.
AHA: 4Q, '94, 47; 2Q, '90, 5; M-A, '87, 1

√5th **V71.0 Observation for suspected mental condition**
V71.01 Adult antisocial behavior [A] [PDx]
Dyssocial behavior or gang activity in adult without manifest psychiatric disorder

V71.02 Childhood or adolescent antisocial behavior [PDx]
Dyssocial behavior or gang activity in child or adolescent without manifest psychiatric disorder

V71.09 Other suspected mental condition [PDx]

V71.1 Observation for suspected malignant neoplasm [PDx]
V71.2 Observation for suspected tuberculosis [PDx]
V71.3 Observation following accident at work [PDx]
V71.4 Observation following other accident [PDx]
Examination of individual involved in motor vehicle traffic accident

V71.5 Observation following alleged rape or seduction [PDx]
Examination of victim or culprit

V71.6 Observation following other inflicted injury [PDx]
Examination of victim or culprit

V71.7 Observation for suspected cardiovascular disease [PDx]
AHA: 1Q, '04, 6; 3Q, '90, 10; S-O, '87, 10

√5th **V71.8 Observation and evaluation for other specified suspected conditions**
AHA: 4Q, '00, 54 ; 1Q, '90, 19

V71.81 Abuse and neglect [PDx]
EXCLUDES adult abuse and neglect (995.80-995.85)
child abuse and neglect (995.50-995.59)
AHA: 4Q, '00, 55

V71.82 Observation and evaluation for suspected exposure to anthrax [PDx]
AHA: 4Q, '02, 70, 85

V71.83 Observation and evaluation for suspected exposure to other biological agent [PDx]
AHA: 4Q, '03, 47

V71.89 Other specified suspected conditions [PDx]
AHA: 2Q, '03, 15

V71.9 Observation for unspecified suspected condition [PDx]
AHA: 1Q, '02, 6

√4th **V72 Special investigations and examinations**
INCLUDES routine examination of specific system
EXCLUDES general medical examination (V70.0-V70.4)
general screening examination of defined population groups (V70.5, V70.6, V70.7)
routine examination of infant or child (V20.2)
Use additional code(s) to identify any special screening examination(s) performed (V73.0-V82.9)

V72.0 Examination of eyes and vision [PDx]
AHA: 1Q, '04, 15

√5th **V72.1 Examination of ears and hearing**
AHA: 1Q, '04, 15

▶◀ **V72.11 Encounter for hearing examination following failed hearing screening** [PDx]
▶◀ **V72.19 Other examination of ears and hearing** [PDx]

V72.2 Dental examination [PDx]

√5th **V72.3 Gynecological examination**
EXCLUDES cervical Papanicolaou smear without general gynecological examination (V76.2)
routine examination in contraceptive management (V25.40-V25.49)

V72.31 Routine gynecological examination [PDx] ♀
General gynecological examination with or without Papanicolaou cervical smear
Pelvic examination (annual) (periodic)
Use additional code to identify routine vaginal Papanicolaou smear (V76.47)
AHA: 4Q, '05, 98

V72.32 Encounter for Papanicolaou cervical smear to confirm findings of recent normal smear following initial abnormal smear [PDx] ♀

√5th **V72.4 Pregnancy examination or test**
AHA: 4Q, '05, 98

V72.40 Pregnancy examination or test, pregnancy unconfirmed ♀
Possible pregnancy, not (yet) confirmed

V72.41 Pregnancy examination or test, negative result ♀

V72.42 Pregnancy examination or test, positive result [M] ♀

V CODES — Tabular List

V72.5 Radiological examination, not elsewhere classified
  Routine chest x-ray
  EXCLUDES: examination for suspected tuberculosis (V71.2)
  AHA: 1Q, '90, 19

V72.6 Laboratory examination
  EXCLUDES: that for suspected disorder (V71.0-V71.9)
  AHA: 1Q, '90, 22

V72.7 Diagnostic skin and sensitization tests [PDx]
  Allergy tests   Skin tests for hypersensitivity
  EXCLUDES: diagnostic skin tests for bacterial diseases (V74.0-V74.9)

√5th **V72.8** Other specified examinations
  V72.81 Pre-operative cardiovascular examination [PDx]
    Pre-procedural cardiovascular examination
  V72.82 Pre-operative respiratory examination [PDx]
    Pre-procedural respiratory examination
    AHA: 3Q, '96, 14
  V72.83 Other specified pre-operative examination [PDx]
    Other pre-procedural examination
    Pre-procedural general physical examination
    EXCLUDES: routine general medical examination (V70.0)
    AHA: 3Q, '96, 14
  V72.84 Pre-operative examination, unspecified [PDx]
    Pre-procedural examination, unspecified
  V72.85 Other specified examination [PDx]
    AHA: ▶4Q, '05, 9◀; 1Q, '04, 12
  V72.86 Encounter for blood typing

V72.9 Unspecified examination [PDx]

√4th **V73** Special screening examination for viral and chlamydial diseases
  AHA: 1Q, '04, 11
  V73.0 Poliomyelitis
  V73.1 Smallpox
  V73.2 Measles
  V73.3 Rubella
  V73.4 Yellow fever
  V73.5 Other arthropod-borne viral diseases
    Dengue fever   Viral encephalitis:
    Hemorrhagic fever   mosquito-borne
                tick-borne
  V73.6 Trachoma
  √5th **V73.8** Other specified viral and chlamydial diseases
    V73.88 Other specified chlamydial diseases
    V73.89 Other specified viral diseases
  √5th **V73.9** Unspecified viral and chlamydial disease
    V73.98 Unspecified chlamydial disease
    V73.99 Unspecified viral disease

√4th **V74** Special screening examination for bacterial and spirochetal diseases
  INCLUDES: diagnostic skin tests for these diseases
  AHA: 1Q, '04, 11
  V74.0 Cholera
  V74.1 Pulmonary tuberculosis
  V74.2 Leprosy [Hansen's disease]
  V74.3 Diphtheria
  V74.4 Bacterial conjunctivitis
  V74.5 Venereal disease
  V74.6 Yaws

V74.8 Other specified bacterial and spirochetal diseases
  Brucellosis   Tetanus
  Leptospirosis   Whooping cough
  Plague

V74.9 Unspecified bacterial and spirochetal disease

√4th **V75** Special screening examination for other infectious diseases
  AHA: 1Q, '04, 11
  V75.0 Rickettsial diseases
  V75.1 Malaria
  V75.2 Leishmaniasis
  V75.3 Trypanosomiasis
    Chagas' disease   Sleeping sickness
  V75.4 Mycotic infections
  V75.5 Schistosomiasis
  V75.6 Filariasis
  V75.7 Intestinal helminthiasis
  V75.8 Other specified parasitic infections
  V75.9 Unspecified infectious disease

√4th **V76** Special screening for malignant neoplasms
  AHA: 1Q, '04, 11
  V76.0 Respiratory organs
  √5th **V76.1** Breast
    AHA: 4Q, '98, 67
    V76.10 Breast screening, unspecified ♀
    V76.11 Screening mammogram for high-risk patient ♀
      AHA: 2Q, '03, 4
    V76.12 Other screening mammogram
      AHA: 2Q, '03, 3-4
    V76.19 Other screening breast examination
  V76.2 Cervix ♀
    Routine cervical Papanicolaou smear
    EXCLUDES: that as part of a general gynecological examination (V72.31)
  V76.3 Bladder
  √5th **V76.4** Other sites
    V76.41 Rectum
    V76.42 Oral cavity
    V76.43 Skin
    V76.44 Prostate ♂
    V76.45 Testis ♂
    V76.46 Ovary ♀
      AHA: 4Q, '00, 52
    V76.47 Vagina ♀
      Vaginal pap smear status-post hysterectomy for non-malignant condition
      Use additional code to identify acquired absence of uterus (V45.77)
      EXCLUDES: vaginal pap smear status-post hysterectomy for malignant condition (V67.01)
      AHA: 4Q, '00, 52
    V76.49 Other sites
      AHA: 1Q, '99, 4
  √5th **V76.5** Intestine
    AHA: 4Q, '00, 52
    V76.50 Intestine, unspecified
    V76.51 Colon
      EXCLUDES: rectum (V76.41)
      AHA: 4Q, '01, 56
    V76.52 Small intestine

 Newborn Age: 0   Pediatric Age: 0-17   Maternity Age: 12-55   [A] Adult Age: 15-124

318 — Volume 1 • February 2006   [SDx] Secondary Diagnosis   [PDx] Primary Diagnosis   2007 ICD•9•CM

V CODES

V76.8 Other neoplasm
AHA: 4Q, '00, 52

    V76.81 Nervous system
    V76.89 Other neoplasm

V76.9 Unspecified

V77 Special screening for endocrine, nutritional, metabolic, and immunity disorders
AHA: 1Q, '04, 11

  V77.0 Thyroid disorders
  V77.1 Diabetes mellitus
  V77.2 Malnutrition
  V77.3 Phenylketonuria [PKU]
  V77.4 Galactosemia
  V77.5 Gout
  V77.6 Cystic fibrosis
    Screening for mucoviscidosis
  V77.7 Other inborn errors of metabolism
  V77.8 Obesity
  V77.9 Other and unspecified endocrine, nutritional, metabolic, and immunity disorders
AHA: 4Q, '00, 53

    V77.91 Screening for lipoid disorders
      Screening cholesterol level
      Screening for hypercholesterolemia
      Screening for hyperlipidemia
    V77.99 Other and unspecified endocrine, nutritional, metabolic, and immunity disorders

V78 Special screening for disorders of blood and blood-forming organs
AHA: 1Q, '04, 11

  V78.0 Iron deficiency anemia
  V78.1 Other and unspecified deficiency anemia
  V78.2 Sickle cell disease or trait
  V78.3 Other hemoglobinopathies
  V78.8 Other disorders of blood and blood-forming organs
  V78.9 Unspecified disorder of blood and blood-forming organs

V79 Special screening for mental disorders and developmental handicaps
AHA: 1Q, '04, 11

  V79.0 Depression
  V79.1 Alcoholism
  V79.2 Mental retardation
  V79.3 Developmental handicaps in early childhood
  V79.8 Other specified mental disorders and developmental handicaps
  V79.9 Unspecified mental disorder and developmental handicap

V80 Special screening for neurological, eye, and ear diseases
AHA: 1Q, '04, 11

  V80.0 Neurological conditions
  V80.1 Glaucoma
  V80.2 Other eye conditions
    Screening for:
      cataract
      congenital anomaly of eye
      senile macular lesions
    EXCLUDES general vision examination (V72.0)
  V80.3 Ear diseases
    EXCLUDES general hearing examination (V72.1)

V81 Special screening for cardiovascular, respiratory, and genitourinary diseases
AHA: 1Q, '04, 11

  V81.0 Ischemic heart disease
  V81.1 Hypertension
  V81.2 Other and unspecified cardiovascular conditions
  V81.3 Chronic bronchitis and emphysema
  V81.4 Other and unspecified respiratory conditions
    EXCLUDES screening for:
      lung neoplasm (V76.0)
      pulmonary tuberculosis (V74.1)
  V81.5 Nephropathy
    Screening for asymptomatic bacteriuria
  V81.6 Other and unspecified genitourinary conditions

V82 Special screening for other conditions
AHA: 1Q, '04, 11

  V82.0 Skin conditions
  V82.1 Rheumatoid arthritis
  V82.2 Other rheumatic disorders
  V82.3 Congenital dislocation of hip
  V82.4 Maternal postnatal screening for chromosomal anomalies ♀
    EXCLUDES antenatal screening by amniocentesis (V28.0)
  V82.5 Chemical poisoning and other contamination
    Screening for:
      heavy metal poisoning
      ingestion of radioactive substance
      poisoning from contaminated water supply
      radiation exposure
  V82.6 Multiphasic screening
  V82.7 Genetic screening
    EXCLUDES genetic testing for procreative management (V26.31-V26.32)
    V82.71 Screening for genetic disease carrier status
    V82.79 Other genetic screening
  V82.8 Other specified conditions
AHA: 4Q, '00, 53

    V82.81 Osteoporosis
      Use additional code to identify:
        hormone replacement therapy (postmenopausal) status (V07.4)
        postmenopausal (age-related) (natural) status (V49.81)
AHA: 4Q, '00, 54

    V82.89 Other specified conditions
  V82.9 Unspecified condition

►GENETICS (V83-V84)◄

V83 Genetic carrier status
AHA: 4Q, '02, 79; 4Q, '01, 54

  V83.0 Hemophilia A carrier
    V83.01 Asymptomatic hemophilia A carrier
    V83.02 Symptomatic hemophilia A carrier
  V83.8 Other genetic carrier status
    V83.81 Cystic fibrosis gene carrier
    V83.89 Other genetic carrier status

V84 Genetic susceptibility to disease
INCLUDES confirmed abnormal gene
Use additional code, if applicable, for any associated family history of the disease (V16-V19)
AHA: 4Q, '04, 106

V CODES

V84.0 Genetic susceptibility to malignant neoplasm
Code first, if applicable, any current malignant neoplasms (140.0-195.8, 200.0-208.9, 230.0-234.9)
Use additional code, if applicable, for any personal history of malignant neoplasm (V10.0-V10.9)

- **V84.01** Genetic susceptibility to malignant neoplasm of breast [SDx]
  AHA: 4Q, '04, 107
- **V84.02** Genetic susceptibility to malignant neoplasm of ovary [SDx] ♀
- **V84.03** Genetic susceptibility to malignant neoplasm of prostate [SDx] ♂
- **V84.04** Genetic susceptibility to malignant neoplasm of endometrium [SDx] ♀
- **V84.09** Genetic susceptibility to other malignant neoplasm [SDx]

V84.8 Genetic susceptibility to other disease [SDx]

►BODY MASS INDEX (V85)◄

V85 Body Mass Index [BMI]
Kilograms per meters squared
Note: BMI adult codes are for use for persons over 20 years old
AHA: 4Q, '05, 97

- **V85.0** Body Mass Index less than 19, adult [SDx] [A]
- **V85.1** Body Mass Index between 19-24, adult [SDx] [A]
- **V85.2** Body Mass Index between 25-29, adult [SDx] [A]
  - V85.21 Body Mass Index 25.0-25.9, adult [SDx] [A]
  - V85.22 Body Mass Index 26.0-26.9, adult [SDx] [A]
  - V85.23 Body Mass Index 27.0-27.9, adult [SDx] [A]
  - V85.24 Body Mass Index 28.0-28.9, adult [SDx] [A]
  - V85.25 Body Mass Index 29.0-29.9, adult [SDx] [A]
- **V85.3** Body Mass Index between 30-39, adult
  - V85.30 Body Mass Index 30.0-30.9, adult [SDx] [A]
  - V85.31 Body Mass Index 31.0-31.9, adult [SDx] [A]
  - V85.32 Body Mass Index 32.0-32.9, adult [SDx] [A]
  - V85.33 Body Mass Index 33.0-33.9, adult [SDx] [A]
  - V85.34 Body Mass Index 34.0-34.9, adult [SDx] [A]
  - V85.35 Body Mass Index 35.0-35.9, adult [SDx] [A]
  - V85.36 Body Mass Index 36.0-36.9, adult [SDx] [A]
  - V85.37 Body Mass Index 37.0-37.9, adult [SDx] [A]
  - V85.38 Body Mass Index 38.0-38.9, adult [SDx] [A]
  - V85.39 Body Mass Index 39.0-39.9, adult [SDx] [A]
- **V85.4** Body Mass Index 40 and over, adult [SDx] [A]
- **V85.5** Body Mass Index, pediatric
  Note: BMI pediatric codes are for use for persons age 2-20 years old. These percentiles are based on the growth charts published by the Centers for Disease Control and Prevention (CDC)
  - V85.51 Body Mass Index, pediatric, less than 5th percentile for age [SDx] [P]
  - V85.52 Body Mass Index, pediatric, 5th percentile to less than 85th percentile for age [SDx] [P]
  - V85.53 Body Mass Index, pediatric, 85th percentile to less than 95th percentile for age [SDx] [P]
  - V85.54 Body Mass Index, pediatric, greater than or equal to 95th percentile for age [SDx] [P]

►ESTROGEN RECEPTOR STATUS (V86)◄

V86 Estrogen receptor status
Code first malignant neoplasm of breast (174.0-174.9, 175.0-175.9)

- **V86.0** Estrogen receptor positive status [ER+] [SDx]
- **V86.1** Estrogen receptor negative status [ER-] [SDx]

SUPPLEMENTARY CLASSIFICATION OF EXTERNAL CAUSES OF INJURY AND POISONING (E800-E999)

This section is provided to permit the classification of environmental events, circumstances, and conditions as the cause of injury, poisoning, and other adverse effects. Where a code from this section is applicable, it is intended that it shall be used in addition to a code from one of the main chapters of ICD-9-CM, indicating the nature of the condition. Certain other conditions which may be stated to be due to external causes are classified in Chapters 1 to 16 of ICD-9-CM. For these, the "E" code classification should be used as an additional code for more detailed analysis.

Machinery accidents [other than those connected with transport] are classifiable to category E919, in which the fourth-digit allows a broad classification of the type of machinery involved. If a more detailed classification of type of machinery is required, it is suggested that the "Classification of Industrial Accidents according to Agency," prepared by the International Labor Office, be used in addition. This is reproduced in Appendix D for optional use.

Categories for "late effects" of accidents and other external causes are to be found at E929, E959, E969, E977, E989, and E999.

DEFINITIONS AND EXAMPLES RELATED TO TRANSPORT ACCIDENTS

(a) A **transport accident** (E800-E848) is any accident involving a device designed primarily for, or being used at the time primarily for, conveying persons or goods from one place to another.

INCLUDES accidents involving:
- aircraft and spacecraft (E840-E845)
- watercraft (E830-E838)
- motor vehicle (E810-E825)
- railway (E800-E807)
- other road vehicles (E826-E829)

In classifying accidents which involve more than one kind of transport, the above order of precedence of transport accidents should be used.

Accidents involving agricultural and construction machines, such as tractors, cranes, and bulldozers, are regarded as transport accidents only when these vehicles are under their own power on a highway [otherwise the vehicles are regarded as machinery]. Vehicles which can travel on land or water, such as hovercraft and other amphibious vehicles, are regarded as watercraft when on the water, as motor vehicles when on the highway, and as off-road motor vehicles when on land, but off the highway.

EXCLUDES accidents:
- *in sports which involve the use of transport but where the transport vehicle itself was not involved in the accident*
- *involving vehicles which are part of industrial equipment used entirely on industrial premises*
- *occurring during transportation but unrelated to the hazards associated with the means of transportation [e.g., injuries received in a fight on board ship; transport vehicle involved in a cataclysm such as an earthquake]*
- *to persons engaged in the maintenance or repair of transport equipment or vehicle not in motion, unlesss injured by another vehicle in motion*

(b) A **railway accident** is a transport accident involving a railway train or other railway vehicle operated on rails, whether in motion or not.

EXCLUDES accidents:
- *in repair shops*
- *in roundhouse or on turntable*
- *on railway premises but not involving a train or other railway vehicle*

(c) A **railway train** or **railway vehicle** is any device with or without cars coupled to it, designed for traffic on a railway.

INCLUDES
- interurban:
  - electric car
  - streetcar

  (operated chiefly on its own right-of-way, not open to other traffic)
- railway train, any power [diesel] [electric] [steam]
- funicular
- monorail or two-rail
- subterranean or elevated
- other vehicle designed to run on a railway track

EXCLUDES *interurban electric cars [streetcars] specified to be operating on a right-of-way that forms part of the public street or highway [definition (n)]*

(d) A **railway** or **railroad** is a right-of-way designed for traffic on rails, which is used by carriages or wagons transporting passengers or freight, and by other rolling stock, and which is not open to other public vehicular traffic.

(e) A **motor vehicle accident** is a transport accident involving a motor vehicle. It is defined as a motor vehicle traffic accident or as a motor vehicle nontraffic accident according to whether the accident occurs on a public highway or elsewhere.

EXCLUDES
- *injury or damage due to cataclysm*
- *injury or damage while a motor vehicle, not under its own power, is being loaded on, or unloaded from, another conveyance*

(f) A **motor vehicle traffic accident** is any motor vehicle accident occurring on a public highway [i.e., originating, terminating, or involving a vehicle partially on the highway]. A motor vehicle accident is assumed to have occurred on the highway unless another place is specified, except in the case of accidents involving only off-road motor vehicles which are classified as nontraffic accidents unless the contrary is stated.

(g) A **motor vehicle nontraffic accident** is any motor vehicle accident which occurs entirely in any place other than a public highway.

(h) A **public highway [trafficway]** or **street** is the entire width between property lines [or other boundary lines] of every way or place, of which any part is open to the use of the public for purposes of vehicular traffic as a matter of right or custom. A **roadway** is that part of the public highway designed, improved, and ordinarily used, for vehicular travel.

INCLUDES approaches (public) to:
- docks
- public building
- station

EXCLUDES
- *driveway (private)*
- *parking lot*
- *ramp*
- *roads in:*
  - *airfield*
  - *farm*
  - *industrial premises*
  - *mine*
  - *private grounds*
  - *quarry*

E CODES

Tabular List

(i) A **motor vehicle** is any mechanically or electrically powered device, not operated on rails, upon which any person or property may be transported or drawn upon a highway. Any object such as a trailer, coaster, sled, or wagon being towed by a motor vehicle is considerd a part of the motor vehicle.

INCLUDES
- automobile [any type]
- bus
- construction machinery, farm and industrial machinery, steam roller, tractor, army tank, highway grader, or similar vehicle on wheels or treads, while in transport under own power
- fire engine (motorized)
- motorcycle
- motorized bicycle [moped] or scooter
- trolley bus not operating on rails
- truck
- van

EXCLUDES *devices used solely to move persons or materials within the confines of a building and its premises, such as:*
- *building elevator*
- *coal car in mine*
- *electric baggage or mail truck used solely within a railroad station*
- *electric truck used solely within an industrial plant*
- *moving overhead crane*

(j) A **motorcycle** is a two-wheeled motor vehicle having one or two riding saddles and sometimes having a third wheel for the support of a sidecar. The sidecar is considered part of the motorcycle.

INCLUDES motorized:
- bicycle [moped]
- scooter
- tricycle

(k) An **off-road motor vehicle** is a motor vehicle of special design, to enable it to negotiate rough or soft terrain or snow. Examples of special design are high construction, special wheels and tires, driven by treads, or support on a cushion of air.

INCLUDES
- all terrain vehicle [ATV]
- army tank
- hovercraft, on land or swamp
- snowmobile

(l) A **driver** of a motor vehicle is the occupant of the motor vehicle operating it or intending to operate it. A **motorcyclist** is the driver of a motorcycle. Other authorized occupants of a motor vehicle are **passengers**.

(m) An **other road vehicle** is any device, except a motor vehicle, in, on, or by which any person or property may be transported on a highway.

INCLUDES
- animal carrying a person or goods
- animal-drawn vehicles
- animal harnessed to conveyance
- bicycle [pedal cycle]
- streetcar
- tricycle (pedal)

EXCLUDES *pedestrian conveyance [definition (q)]*

(n) A **streetcar** is a device designed and used primarily for transporting persons within a municipality, running on rails, usually subject to normal traffic control signals, and operated principally on a right-of-way that forms part of the traffic way. A trailer being towed by a streetcar is considered a part of the streetcar.

INCLUDES
- interurban or intraurban electric or streetcar, when specified to be operating on a street or public highway
- tram (car)
- trolley (car)

(o) A **pedal cycle** is any road transport vehicle operated solely by pedals.

INCLUDES
- bicycle
- pedal cycle
- tricycle

EXCLUDES *motorized bicycle [definition (i)]*

(p) A **pedal cyclist** is any person riding on a pedal cycle or in a sidecar attached to such a vehicle.

(q) A **pedestrian conveyance** is any human powered device by which a pedestrian may move other than by walking or by which a walking person may move another pedestrian.

INCLUDES
- baby carriage
- coaster wagon
- ice skates
- perambulator
- pushcart
- pushchair
- roller skates
- scooter
- skateboard
- skis
- sled
- wheelchair

(r) A **pedestrian** is any person involved in an accident who was not at the time of the accident riding in or on a motor vehicle, railroad train, streetcar, animal-drawn or other vehicle, or on a bicycle or animal.

INCLUDES person:
- changing tire of vehicle
- in or operating a pedestrian conveyance
- making adjustment to motor of vehicle
- on foot

(s) A **watercraft** is any device for transporting passengers or goods on the water.

(t) A **small boat** is any watercraft propelled by paddle, oars, or small motor, with a passenger capacity of less than ten.

INCLUDES
- boat NOS
- canoe
- coble
- dinghy
- punt
- raft
- rowboat
- rowing shell
- scull
- skiff
- small motorboat

EXCLUDES
- *barge*
- *lifeboat (used after abandoning ship)*
- *raft (anchored) being used as a diving platform*
- *yacht*

(u) An **aircraft** is any device for transporting passengers or goods in the air.

INCLUDES
- airplane [any type]
- balloon
- bomber
- dirigible
- glider (hang)
- military aircraft
- parachute

(v) A **commercial transport aircraft** is any device for collective passenger or freight transportation by air, whether run on commercial lines for profit or by government authorities, with the exception of military craft.

Tabular List — E CODES

RAILWAY ACCIDENTS (E800-E807)

Note: For definitions of railway accident and related terms see definitions (a) to (d).

EXCLUDES accidents involving railway train and:
  aircraft (E840.0-E845.9)
  motor vehicle (E810.0-E825.9)
  watercraft (E830.0-E838.9)

The following fourth-digit subdivisions are for use with categories E800-E807 to identify the injured person:

.0 Railway employee
  Any person who by virtue of his employment in connection with a railway, whether by the railway company or not, is at increased risk of involvement in a railway accident, such as:
  catering staff of train
  driver
  guard
  porter
  postal staff on train
  railway fireman
  shunter
  sleeping car attendant

.1 Passenger on railway
  Any authorized person traveling on a train, except a railway employee.
  EXCLUDES intending passenger waiting at station (.8)
  unauthorized rider on railway vehicle (.8)

.2 Pedestrian
  See definition (r)

.3 Pedal cyclist
  See definition (p)

.8 Other specified person
  Intending passenger or bystander waiting at station
  Unauthorized rider on railway vehicle

.9 Unspecified person

✓4th E800 Railway accident involving collision with rolling stock
INCLUDES
  collision between railway trains or railway vehicles, any kind
  collision NOS on railway
  derailment with antecedent collision with rolling stock or NOS

✓4th E801 Railway accident involving collision with other object
INCLUDES collision of railway train with:
  buffers
  fallen tree on railway
  gates
  platform
  rock on railway
  streetcar
  other nonmotor vehicle
  other object

EXCLUDES collision with:
  aircraft (E840.0-E842.9)
  motor vehicle (E810.0-E810.9, E820.0-E822.9)

✓4th E802 Railway accident involving derailment without antecedent collision

✓4th E803 Railway accident involving explosion, fire, or burning
EXCLUDES explosion or fire, with antecedent derailment (E802.0-E802.9)
  explosion or fire, with mention of antecedent collision (E800.0-E801.9)

✓4th E804 Fall in, on, or from railway train
INCLUDES fall while alighting from or boarding railway train
EXCLUDES fall related to collision, derailment, or explosion of railway train (E800.0-E803.9)

✓4th E805 Hit by rolling stock
INCLUDES
  crushed
  injured
  killed   } by railway train or part
  knocked down
  run over

EXCLUDES pedestrian hit by object set in motion by railway train (E806.0-E806.9)

✓4th E806 Other specified railway accident
INCLUDES
  hit by object falling in railway train
  injured by door or window on railway train
  nonmotor road vehicle or pedestrian hit by object set in motion by railway train
  railway train hit by falling:
    earth NOS
    rock
    tree
    other object

EXCLUDES railway accident due to cataclysm (E908-E909)

✓4th E807 Railway accident of unspecified nature
INCLUDES
  found dead   } on railway right-of-way
  injured   NOS

  railway accident NOS

MOTOR VEHICLE TRAFFIC ACCIDENTS (E810-E819)

Note: For definitions of motor vehicle traffic accident, and related terms, see definitions (e) to (k).

EXCLUDES accidents involving motor vehicle and aircraft (E840.0-E845.9)

The following fourth-digit subdivisions are for use with categories E810-E819 to identify the injured person:

.0 Driver of motor vehicle other than motorcycle
  See definition (1)

.1 Passenger in motor vehicle other than motorcycle
  See definition (1)

.2 Motorcyclist
  See definition (1)

.3 Passenger on motorcycle
  See definition (1)

.4 Occupant of streetcar

.5 Rider of animal; occupant of animal-drawn vehicle

.6 Pedal cyclist
  See definition (p)

.7 Pedestrian
  See definition (r)

.8 Other specified person
  Occupant of vehicle other than above
  Person in railway train involved in accident
  Unauthorized rider of motor vehicle

.9 Unspecified person

✓4th E810 Motor vehicle traffic accident involving collision with train
EXCLUDES motor vehicle collision with object set in motion by railway train (E815.0-E815.9)
  railway train hit by object set in motion by motor vehicle (E818.0-E818.9)

✓4th E811 Motor vehicle traffic accident involving re-entrant collision with another motor vehicle
INCLUDES collision between motor vehicle which accidentally leaves the roadway then re-enters the same roadway, or the opposite roadway on a divided highway, and another motor vehicle

EXCLUDES collision on the same roadway when none of the motor vehicles involved have left and re-entered the highway (E812.0-E812.9)

E812 Other motor vehicle traffic accident involving collision with motor vehicle

INCLUDES: collision with another motor vehicle parked, stopped, stalled, disabled, or abandoned on the highway
motor vehicle collision NOS

EXCLUDES: collision with object set in motion by another motor vehicle (E815.0-E815.9)
re-entrant collision with another motor vehicle (E811.0-E811.9)

E813 Motor vehicle traffic accident involving collision with other vehicle

INCLUDES: collision between motor vehicle, any kind, and:
other road (nonmotor transport) vehicle, such as:
- animal carrying a person
- animal-drawn vehicle
- pedal cycle
- streetcar

EXCLUDES: collision with:
- object set in motion by nonmotor road vehicle (E815.0-E815.9)
- pedestrian (E814.0-E814.9)
nonmotor road vehicle hit by object set in motion by motor vehicle (E818.0-E818.9)

E814 Motor vehicle traffic accident involving collision with pedestrian

INCLUDES: collision between motor vehicle, any kind, and pedestrian
pedestrian dragged, hit, or run over by motor vehicle, any kind

EXCLUDES: pedestrian hit by object set in motion by motor vehicle (E818.0-E818.9)

E815 Other motor vehicle traffic accident involving collision on the highway

INCLUDES: collision (due to loss of control) (on highway) between motor vehicle, any kind, and:
- abutment (bridge) (overpass)
- animal (herded) (unattended)
- fallen stone, traffic sign, tree, utility pole
- guard rail or boundary fence
- interhighway divider
- landslide (not moving)
- object set in motion by railway train or road vehicle (motor) (nonmotor)
- object thrown in front of motor vehicle
- other object, fixed, movable, or moving
- safety island
- temporary traffic sign or marker
- wall of cut made for road

EXCLUDES: collision with:
- any object off the highway (resulting from loss of control) (E816.0-E816.9)
- any object which normally would have been off the highway and is not stated to have been on it (E816.0-E816.9)
- motor vehicle parked, stopped, stalled, disabled, or abandoned on highway (E812.0-E812.9)
moving landslide (E909)
motor vehicle hit by object:
- set in motion by railway train or road vehicle (motor) (nonmotor) (E818.0-E818.9)
- thrown into or on vehicle (E818.0-E818.9)

E816 Motor vehicle traffic accident due to loss of control, without collision on the highway

INCLUDES: motor vehicle:
- failing to make curve
- going out of control (due to):
  - blowout
  - burst tire
  - driver falling asleep
  - driver inattention
  - excessive speed
  - failure of mechanical part

and:
- colliding with object off the highway
- overturning
- stopping abruptly off the highway

EXCLUDES: collision on highway following loss of control (E810.0-E815.9)
loss of control of motor vehicle following collision on the highway (E810.0-E815.9)

E817 Noncollision motor vehicle traffic accident while boarding or alighting

INCLUDES:
- fall down stairs of motor bus
- fall from car in street
- injured by moving part of the vehicle
- trapped by door of motor bus

while boarding or alighting

E818 Other noncollision motor vehicle traffic accident

INCLUDES:
- accidental poisoning from exhaust gas generated by
- breakage of any part of
- explosion of any part of
- fall, jump, or being accidentally pushed from
- fire starting in
- hit by object thrown into or on
- injured by being thrown against some part of, or object in
- injury from moving part of
- object falling in or on
- object thrown on

motor vehicle while in motion

- collision of railway train or road vehicle except motor vehicle, with object set in motion by motor vehicle
- motor vehicle hit by object set in motion by railway train or road vehicle (motor) (nonmotor)
- pedestrian, railway train, or road vehicle (motor) (nonmotor) hit by object set in motion by motor vehicle

EXCLUDES: collision between motor vehicle and:
- object set in motion by railway train or road vehicle (motor) (nonmotor) (E815.0-E815.9)
- object thrown towards the motor vehicle (E815.0-E815.9)
person overcome by carbon monoxide generated by stationary motor vehicle off the roadway with motor running (E868.2)

E819 Motor vehicle traffic accident of unspecified nature

INCLUDES: motor vehicle traffic accident NOS
traffic accident NOS

---

§ Requires fourth-digit. See beginning of section E810-E819 for codes and definitions.

E CODES — E820–E824

MOTOR VEHICLE NONTRAFFIC ACCIDENTS (E820-E825)

Note: For definitions of motor vehicle nontraffic accident and related terms see definition (a) to (k).

INCLUDES
- accidents involving motor vehicles being used in recreational or sporting activities off the highway
- collision and noncollision motor vehicle accidents occurring entirely off the highway

EXCLUDES
- accidents involving motor vehicle and:
  - aircraft (E840.0-E845.9)
  - watercraft (E830.0-E838.9)
- accidents, not on the public highway, involving agricultural and construction machinery but not involving another motor vehicle (E919.0, E919.2, E919.7)

The following fourth-digit subdivisions are for use with categories E820-E825 to identify the injured person:

- **.0 Driver of motor vehicle other than motorcycle**
  - See definition (l)
- **.1 Passenger in motor vehicle other than motorcycle**
  - See definition (l)
- **.2 Motorcyclist**
  - See definition (l)
- **.3 Passenger on motorcycle**
  - See definition (l)
- **.4 Occupant of streetcar**
- **.5 Rider of animal; occupant of animal-drawn vehicle**
- **.6 Pedal cyclist**
  - See definition (p)
- **.7 Pedestrian**
  - See definition (r)
- **.8 Other specified person**
  - Occupant of vehicle other than above
  - Person on railway train involved in accident
  - Unauthorized rider of motor vehicle
- **.9 Unspecified person**

✓4th E820 Nontraffic accident involving motor-driven snow vehicle

INCLUDES
- breakage of part of / fall from / hit by / overturning of / run over or dragged by } motor-driven snow vehicle (not on public highway)
- collision of motor-driven snow vehicle with:
  - animal (being ridden) (-drawn vehicle)
  - another off-road motor vehicle
  - other motor vehicle, not on public highway
  - railway train
  - other object, fixed or movable
- injury caused by rough landing of motor-driven snow vehicle (after leaving ground on rough terrain)

EXCLUDES
- accident on the public highway involving motor driven snow vehicle (E810.0-E819.9)

✓4th E821 Nontraffic accident involving other off-road motor vehicle

INCLUDES
- breakage of part of / fall from / hit by / overturning of / run over or dragged by / thrown against some part of or object in } off-road motor vehicle, except snow vehicle (not on public highway)
- collision with:
  - animal (being ridden) (-drawn vehicle)
  - another off-road motor vehicle, except snow vehicle
  - other motor vehicle, not on public highway
  - other object, fixed or movable

EXCLUDES
- accident on public highway involving off-road motor vehicle (E810.0-E819.9)
- collision between motor driven snow vehicle and other off-road motor vehicle (E820.0-E820.9)
- hovercraft accident on water (E830.0-E838.9)

✓4th E822 Other motor vehicle nontraffic accident involving collision with moving object

INCLUDES
- collision, not on public highway, between motor vehicle, except off-road motor vehicle and:
  - animal
  - nonmotor vehicle
  - other motor vehicle, except off-road motor vehicle
  - pedestrian
  - railway train
  - other moving object

EXCLUDES
- collision with:
  - motor-driven snow vehicle (E820.0-E820.9)
  - other off-road motor vehicle (E821.0-E821.9)

✓4th E823 Other motor vehicle nontraffic accident involving collision with stationary object

INCLUDES
- collision, not on public highway, between motor vehicle, except off-road motor vehicle, and any object, fixed or movable, but not in motion

✓4th E824 Other motor vehicle nontraffic accident while boarding and alighting

INCLUDES
- fall / injury from moving part of motor vehicle / trapped by door of motor vehicle } while boarding or alighting from motor vehicle, except off-road motor vehicle, not on public highway

E825–E829 E CODES

§ ✓4ᵗʰ **E825 Other motor vehicle nontraffic accident of other and unspecified nature**

INCLUDES:
- accidental poisoning from carbon monoxide generated by
- breakage of any part of
- explosion of any part of
- fall, jump, or being accidentally pushed from
- fire starting in
- hit by object thrown into, towards, or on
- injured by being thrown against some part of, or object in
- injury from moving part of
- object falling in or on

} motor vehicle while in motion, not on public highway

motor vehicle nontraffic accident NOS

EXCLUDES:
- fall from or in stationary motor vehicle (E884.9, E885.9)
- overcome by carbon monoxide or exhaust gas generated by stationary motor vehicle off the roadway with motor running (E868.2)
- struck by falling object from or in stationary motor vehicle (E916)

OTHER ROAD VEHICLE ACCIDENTS (E826-E829)

Note: Other road vehicle accidents are transport accidents involving road vehicles other than motor vehicles. For definitions of other road vehicle and related terms see definitions (m) to (o).

INCLUDES: accidents involving other road vehicles being used in recreational or sporting activities

EXCLUDES: collision of other road vehicle [any] with:
- aircraft (E840.0-E845.9)
- motor vehicle (E813.0-E813.9, E820.0-E822.9)
- railway train (E801.0-E801.9)

The following fourth-digit subdivisions are for use with categories E826-E829 to identify the injured person.
- .0 Pedestrian
  - See definition (r)
- .1 Pedal cyclist
  - See definition (p)
- .2 Rider of animal
- .3 Occupant of animal-drawn vehicle
- .4 Occupant of streetcar
- .8 Other specified person
- .9 Unspecified person

✓4ᵗʰ **E826 Pedal cycle accident**
[0-9]

INCLUDES:
- breakage of any part of pedal cycle
- collision between pedal cycle and:
  - animal (being ridden) (herded) (unattended)
  - another pedal cycle
  - any pedestrian
  - nonmotor road vehicle
  - other object, fixed, movable, or moving, not set in motion by motor vehicle, railway train, or aircraft
- entanglement in wheel of pedal cycle
- fall from pedal cycle
- hit by object falling or thrown on the pedal cycle
- pedal cycle accident NOS
- pedal cycle overturned

✓4ᵗʰ **E827 Animal-drawn vehicle accident**
[0,2-4,8,9]

INCLUDES:
- breakage of any part of vehicle
- collision between animal-drawn vehicle and:
  - animal (being ridden) (herded) (unattended)
  - nonmotor road vehicle, except pedal cycle
  - pedestrian, pedestrian conveyance, or pedestrian vehicle
  - other object, fixed, movable, or moving, not set in motion by motor vehicle, railway train, or aircraft
- fall from
- knocked down by
- overturning of
- run over by
- thrown from

} animal-drawn vehicle

EXCLUDES: collision of animal-drawn vehicle with pedal cycle (E826.0-E826.9)

✓4ᵗʰ **E828 Accident involving animal being ridden**
[0,2,4,8,9]

INCLUDES:
- collision between animal being ridden and:
  - another animal
  - nonmotor road vehicle, except pedal cycle, and animal-drawn vehicle
  - pedestrian, pedestrian conveyance, or pedestrian vehicle
  - other object, fixed, movable, or moving, not set in motion by motor vehicle, railway train, or aircraft
- fall from
- knocked down by
- thrown from
- trampled by

} animal being ridden

- ridden animal stumbled and fell

EXCLUDES: collision of animal being ridden with:
- animal-drawn vehicle (E827.0-E827.9)
- pedal cycle (E826.0-E826.9)

✓4ᵗʰ **E829 Other road vehicle accidents**
[0,4,8,9]

INCLUDES:
- accident while
  - boarding or alighting from
- blow from object in
- breakage of any part of
- caught in door of-
- derailment of
- fall in, on, or from
- fire in

} streetcar nonmotor road vehicle not classifiable to E826-E828

- collision between streetcar or nonmotor road vehicle, except as in E826-E828, and:
  - animal (not being ridden)
  - another nonmotor road vehicle not classifiable to E826-E828
  - pedestrian
  - other object, fixed, movable, or moving, not set in motion by motor vehicle, railway train, or aircraft
- nonmotor road vehicle accident NOS
- streetcar accident NOS

EXCLUDES: collision with:
- animal being ridden (E828.0-E828.9)
- animal-drawn vehicle (E827.0-E827.9)
- pedal cycle (E826.0-E826.9)

---

§ Requires fourth-digit. Valid digits are in [brackets] under each code. See beginning of section E820-E825 for codes and definitions.

WATER TRANSPORT ACCIDENTS (E830-E838)

Note: For definitions of water transport accident and related terms see definitions (a), (s), and (t).

INCLUDES watercraft accidents in the course of recreational activities

EXCLUDES accidents involving both aircraft, including objects set in motion by aircraft, and watercraft (E840.0-E845.9)

The following fourth-digit subdivisions are for use with categories E830-E838 to identify the injured person:

.0 Occupant of small boat, unpowered
.1 Occupant of small boat, powered
   See definition (t)
   EXCLUDES water skier (.4)
.2 Occupant of other watercraft — crew
   Persons:
      engaged in operation of watercraft
      providing passenger services [cabin attendants, ship's physician, catering personnel]
      working on ship during voyage in other capacity [musician in band, operators of shops and beauty parlors]
.3 Occupant of other watercraft — other than crew
   Passenger
   Occupant of lifeboat, other than crew, after abandoning ship
.4 Water skier
.5 Swimmer
.6 Dockers, stevedores
   Longshoreman employed on the dock in loading and unloading ships
.8 Other specified person
   Immigration and custom officials on board ship
   Person:
      accompanying passenger or member of crew visiting boat
   Pilot (guiding ship into port)
.9 Unspecified person

√4th E830 Accident to watercraft causing submersion
INCLUDES submersion and drowning due to:
   boat overturning
   boat submerging
   falling or jumping from burning ship
   falling or jumping from crushed watercraft
   ship sinking
   other accident to watercraft

√4th E831 Accident to watercraft causing other injury
INCLUDES any injury, except submersion and drowning, as a result of an accident to watercraft
   burned while ship on fire
   crushed between ships in collision
   crushed by lifeboat after abandoning ship
   fall due to collision or other accident to watercraft
   hit by falling object due to accident to watercraft
   injured in watercraft accident involving collision
   struck by boat or part thereof after fall or jump from damaged boat

EXCLUDES burns from localized fire or explosion on board ship (E837.0-E837.9)

√4th E832 Other accidental submersion or drowning in water transport accident
INCLUDES submersion or drowning as a result of an accident other than accident to the watercraft, such as:
   fall:
      from gangplank
      from ship
   overboard
   thrown overboard by motion of ship
   washed overboard

EXCLUDES submersion or drowning of swimmer or diver who voluntarily jumps from boat not involved in an accident (E910.0-E910.9)

√4th E833 Fall on stairs or ladders in water transport
EXCLUDES fall due to accident to watercraft (E831.0-E831.9)

√4th E834 Other fall from one level to another in water transport
EXCLUDES fall due to accident to watercraft (E831.0-E831.9)

√4th E835 Other and unspecified fall in water transport
EXCLUDES fall due to accident to watercraft (E831.0-E831.9)

√4th E836 Machinery accident in water transport
INCLUDES injuries in water transport caused by:
   deck
   engine room
   galley   } machinery
   laundry
   loading

√4th E837 Explosion, fire, or burning in watercraft
INCLUDES explosion of boiler on steamship
   localized fire on ship

EXCLUDES burning ship (due to collision or explosion) resulting in:
   submersion or drowning (E830.0-E830.9)
   other injury (E831.0-E831.9)

√4th E838 Other and unspecified water transport accident
INCLUDES accidental poisoning by gases or fumes on ship
   atomic power plant malfunction in watercraft
   crushed between ship and stationary object [wharf]
   crushed between ships without accident to watercraft
   crushed by falling object on ship or while loading or unloading
   hit by boat while water skiing
   struck by boat or part thereof (after fall from boat)
   watercraft accident NOS

AIR AND SPACE TRANSPORT ACCIDENTS (E840-E845)

Note: For definition of aircraft and related terms see definitions (u) and (v).

The following fourth-digit subdivisions are for use with categories E840-E845 to identify the injured person. Valid fourth digits are in [brackets] under codes E842-E845.

.0 Occupant of spacecraft
.1 Occupant of military aircraft, any
    Crew in military aircraft [air force] [army] [national guard] [navy]
    Passenger (civilian) (military) in military aircraft [air force] [army] [national guard] [navy]
    Troops in military aircraft [air force] [army] [national guard] [navy]
    EXCLUDES *occupants of aircraft operated under jurisdiction of police departments (.5)*
        parachutist (.7)
.2 Crew of commercial aircraft (powered) in surface to surface transport
.3 Other occupant of commercial aircraft (powered) in surface to surface transport
    Flight personnel:
        not part of crew
        on familiarization flight
    Passenger on aircraft (powered) NOS
.4 Occupant of commercial aircraft (powered) in surface to air transport
    Occupant [crew] [passenger] of aircraft (powered) engaged in activities, such as:
        aerial spraying (crops) (fire retardants)
        air drops of emergency supplies
        air drops of parachutists, except from military craft
        crop dusting
        lowering of construction material [bridge or telephone pole]
        sky writing
.5 Occupant of other powered aircraft
    Occupant [crew][passenger] of aircraft [powered] engaged in activities, such as:
        aerobatic flying
        aircraft racing
        rescue operation
        storm surveillance
        traffic surveillance
    Occupant of private plane NOS
.6 Occupant of unpowered aircraft, except parachutist
    Occupant of aircraft classifiable to E842
.7 Parachutist (military) (other)
    Person making voluntary descent
    EXCLUDES *person making descent after accident to aircraft (.1-.6)*
.8 Ground crew, airline employee
    Persons employed at airfields (civil) (military) or launching pads, not occupants of aircraft
.9 Other person

√4th E840 Accident to powered aircraft at takeoff or landing

INCLUDES
- collision of aircraft with any object, fixed, movable, or moving — while taking off or landing
- crash — while taking off or landing
- explosion on aircraft — while taking off or landing
- fire on aircraft — while taking off or landing
- forced landing

√4th E841 Accident to powered aircraft, other and unspecified

INCLUDES
- aircraft accident NOS
- aircraft crash or wreck NOS
- any accident to powered aircraft while in transit or when not specified whether in transit, taking off, or landing
- collision of aircraft with another aircraft, bird, or any object, while in transit
- explosion on aircraft while in transit
- fire on aircraft while in transit

√4th E842 Accident to unpowered aircraft
[6-9]

INCLUDES any accident, except collision with powered aircraft, to:
- balloon
- glider
- hang glider
- kite carrying a person
- hit by object falling from unpowered aircraft

√4th E843 Fall in, on, or from aircraft
[0-9]

INCLUDES
- accident in boarding or alighting from aircraft, any kind
- fall in, on, or from aircraft [any kind], while in transit, taking off, or landing, except when as a result of an accident to aircraft

√4th E844 Other specified air transport accidents
[0-9]

INCLUDES
- hit by:
  - aircraft
  - object falling from aircraft
- injury by or from:
  - machinery on aircraft — without accident to aircraft
  - rotating propeller — without accident to aircraft
  - voluntary parachute descent — without accident to aircraft
- poisoning by carbon monoxide from aircraft while in transit — without accident to aircraft
- sucked into jet
- any accident involving other transport vehicle (motor) (nonmotor) due to being hit by object set in motion by aircraft (powered)

EXCLUDES
- *air sickness (E903)*
- *effects of:*
  - *high altitude (E902.0-E902.1)*
  - *pressure change (E902.0-E902.1)*
- *injury in parachute descent due to accident to aircraft (E840.0-E842-9)*

√4th E845 Accident involving spacecraft
[0,8,9]

INCLUDES launching pad accident

EXCLUDES *effects of weightlessness in spacecraft (E928.0)*

E CODES

VEHICLE ACCIDENTS NOT ELSEWHERE CLASSIFIABLE (E846-E848)

E846 Accidents involving powered vehicles used solely within the buildings and premises of industrial or commercial establishment

Accident to, on, or involving:
- battery powered airport passenger vehicle
- battery powered trucks (baggage) (mail)
- coal car in mine
- logging car
- self propelled truck, industrial
- station baggage truck (powered)
- tram, truck, or tub (powered) in mine or quarry

Collision with:
- pedestrian
- other vehicle or object within premises

Explosion of } powered vehicle, industrial
Fall from } or commercial
Overturning of
Struck by

EXCLUDES accidental poisoning by exhaust gas from vehicle not elsewhere classifiable (E868.2)
injury by crane, lift (fork), or elevator (E919.2)

E847 Accidents involving cable cars not running on rails

Accident to, on, or involving:
- cable car, not on rails
- ski chair-lift
- ski-lift with gondola
- téléférique

Breakage of cable
Caught or dragged by } cable car, not on rails
Fall or jump from
Object thrown from or in

E848 Accidents involving other vehicles, not elsewhere classifiable

Accident to, on, or involving:
- ice yacht
- land yacht
- nonmotor, nonroad vehicle NOS

✓4th E849 Place of occurrence

The following category is for use to denote the place where the injury or poisoning occurred.

E849.0 Home
- Apartment
- Boarding house
- Farm house
- Home premises
- House (residential)
- Noninstitutional place of residence
- Private: driveway
- Private: garage
- Private: garden
- Private: home
- Private: walk
- Swimming pool in private house or garden
- Yard of home

EXCLUDES home under construction but not yet occupied (E849.3)
institutional place of residence (E849.7)

E849.1 Farm
Farm:
- buildings
- land under cultivation

EXCLUDES farm house and home premises of farm (E849.0)

E849.2 Mine and quarry
- Gravel pit
- Sand pit
- Tunnel under construction

E849.3 Industrial place and premises
- Building under construction
- Dockyard
- Dry dock
- Factory
  - building
  - premises
- Garage (place of work)
- Industrial yard
- Loading platform (factory) (store)
- Plant, industrial
- Railway yard
- Shop (place of work)
- Warehouse
- Workhouse

E849.4 Place for recreation and sport
- Amusement park
- Baseball field
- Basketball court
- Beach resort
- Cricket ground
- Fives court
- Football field
- Golf course
- Gymnasium
- Hockey field
- Holiday camp
- Ice palace
- Lake resort
- Mountain resort
- Public park
- Racecourse
- Resort NOS
- Riding school
- Rifle range
- Seashore resort
- Skating rink
- Sports palace
- Stadium
- Swimming pool, public
- Tennis court
- Vacation resort
- Playground, including school playground

EXCLUDES that in private house or garden (E849.0)

E849.5 Street and highway

E849.6 Public building
Building (including adjacent grounds) used by the general public or by a particular group of the public, such as:
- airport
- bank
- café
- casino
- church
- cinema
- clubhouse
- courthouse
- dance hall
- garage building (for car storage)
- hotel
- market (grocery or other commodity)
- movie house
- music hall
- nightclub
- office
- office building
- opera house
- post office
- public hall
- radio broadcasting station
- restaurant
- school (state) (public) (private)
- shop, commercial
- station (bus) (railway)
- store
- theater

EXCLUDES home garage (E849.0)
industrial building or workplace (E849.3)

E849.7 Residential institution
- Children's home
- Dormitory
- Hospital
- Jail
- Old people's home
- Orphanage
- Prison
- Reform school

E849.8 Other specified places
- Beach NOS
- Canal
- Caravan site NOS
- Derelict house
- Desert
- Dock
- Forest
- Harbor
- Hill
- Lake NOS
- Mountain
- Parking lot
- Parking place
- Pond or pool (natural)
- Prairie
- Public place NOS
- Railway line
- Reservoir
- River
- Sea
- Seashore NOS
- Stream
- Swamp
- Trailer court
- Woods

E849.9 Unspecified place

ACCIDENTAL POISONING BY DRUGS, MEDICINAL SUBSTANCES, AND BIOLOGICALS (E850-E858)

INCLUDES: accidental overdose of drug, wrong drug given or taken in error, and drug taken inadvertently
accidents in the use of drugs and biologicals in medical and surgical procedures

EXCLUDES: administration with suicidal or homicidal intent or intent to harm, or in circumstances classifiable to E980-E989 (E950.0-E950.5, E962.0, E980.0-E980.5)
correct drug properly administered in therapeutic or prophylactic dosage, as the cause of adverse effect (E930.0-E949.9)

See Alphabetic Index for more complete list of specific drugs to be classified under the fourth-digit subdivisions. The American Hospital Formulary numbers can be used to classify new drugs listed by the American Hospital Formulary Service (AHFS). See Appendix C.

✓4th **E850 Accidental poisoning by analgesics, antipyretics, and antirheumatics**
- E850.0 Heroin
  - Diacetylmorphine
- E850.1 Methadone
- E850.2 Other opiates and related narcotics
  - Codeine [methylmorphine]
  - Meperidine [pethidine]
  - Morphine
  - Opium (alkaloids)
- E850.3 Salicylates
  - Acetylsalicylic acid [aspirin]
  - Amino derivatives of salicylic acid
  - Salicylic acid salts
- E850.4 Aromatic analgesics, not elsewhere classified
  - Acetanilid
  - Paracetamol [acetaminophen]
  - Phenacetin [acetophenetidin]
- E850.5 Pyrazole derivatives
  - Aminophenazone [amidopyrine]
  - Phenylbutazone
- E850.6 Antirheumatics [antiphlogistics]
  - Gold salts
  - Indomethacin
  - **EXCLUDES**: salicylates (E850.3)
    steroids (E858.0)
- E850.7 Other non-narcotic analgesics
  - Pyrabital
- E850.8 Other specified analgesics and antipyretics
  - Pentazocine
- E850.9 Unspecified analgesic or antipyretic

E851 Accidental poisoning by barbiturates
- Amobarbital [amylobarbitone]
- Barbital [barbitone]
- Butabarbital [butabarbitone]
- Pentobarbital [pentobarbitone]
- Phenobarbital [phenobarbitone]
- Secobarbital [quinalbarbitone]
- **EXCLUDES**: thiobarbiturates (E855.1)

✓4th **E852 Accidental poisoning by other sedatives and hypnotics**
- E852.0 Chloral hydrate group
- E852.1 Paraldehyde
- E852.2 Bromine compounds
  - Bromides
  - Carbromal (derivatives)
- E852.3 Methaqualone compounds
- E852.4 Glutethimide group
- E852.5 Mixed sedatives, not elsewhere classified
- E852.8 Other specified sedatives and hypnotics
- E852.9 Unspecified sedative or hypnotic
  - Sleeping:
    - drug
    - pill } NOS
    - tablet

✓4th **E853 Accidental poisoning by tranquilizers**
- E853.0 Phenothiazine-based tranquilizers
  - Chlorpromazine
  - Fluphenazine
  - Prochlorperazine
  - Promazine
- E853.1 Butyrophenone-based tranquilizers
  - Haloperidol
  - Spiperone
  - Trifluperidol
- E853.2 Benzodiazepine-based tranquilizers
  - Chlordiazepoxide
  - Diazepam
  - Flurazepam
  - Lorazepam
  - Medazepam
  - Nitrazepam
- E853.8 Other specified tranquilizers
  - Hydroxyzine
  - Meprobamate
- E853.9 Unspecified tranquilizer

✓4th **E854 Accidental poisoning by other psychotropic agents**
- E854.0 Antidepressants
  - Amitriptyline
  - Imipramine
  - Monoamine oxidase [MAO] inhibitors
- E854.1 Psychodysleptics [hallucinogens]
  - Cannabis derivatives
  - Lysergide [LSD]
  - Marihuana (derivatives)
  - Mescaline
  - Psilocin
  - Psilocybin
- E854.2 Psychostimulants
  - Amphetamine
  - Caffeine
  - **EXCLUDES**: central appetite depressants (E858.8)
- E854.3 Central nervous system stimulants
  - Analeptics
  - Opiate antagonists
- E854.8 Other psychotropic agents

✓4th **E855 Accidental poisoning by other drugs acting on central and autonomic nervous system**
- E855.0 Anticonvulsant and anti-Parkinsonism drugs
  - Amantadine
  - Hydantoin derivatives
  - Levodopa [L-dopa]
  - Oxazolidine derivatives [paramethadione] [trimethadione]
  - Succinimides
- E855.1 Other central nervous system depressants
  - Ether
  - Gaseous anesthetics
  - Halogenated hydrocarbon derivatives
  - Intravenous anesthetics
  - Thiobarbiturates, such as thiopental sodium
- E855.2 Local anesthetics
  - Cocaine
  - Lidocaine [lignocaine]
  - Procaine
  - Tetracaine
- E855.3 Parasympathomimetics [cholinergics]
  - Acetylcholine
  - Anticholinesterase:
    - organophosphorus
    - reversible
  - Pilocarpine
- E855.4 Parasympatholytics [anticholinergics and antimuscarinics] and spasmolytics
  - Atropine
  - Homatropine
  - Hyoscine [scopolamine]
  - Quaternary ammonium derivatives
- E855.5 Sympathomimetics [adrenergics]
  - Epinephrine [adrenalin]
  - Levarterenol [noradrenalin]
- E855.6 Sympatholytics [antiadrenergics]
  - Phenoxybenzamine
  - Tolazoline hydrochloride
- E855.8 Other specified drugs acting on central and autonomic nervous systems
- E855.9 Unspecified drug acting on central and autonomic nervous systems

E856 Accidental poisoning by antibiotics

E857 Accidental poisoning by other anti-infectives

✓4th **E858 Accidental poisoning by other drugs**
- E858.0 Hormones and synthetic substitutes
- E858.1 Primarily systemic agents
- E858.2 Agents primarily affecting blood constituents
- E858.3 Agents primarily affecting cardiovascular system
- E858.4 Agents primarily affecting gastrointestinal system

Tabular List — E CODES

E858.5–E865.9

- **E858.5** Water, mineral, and uric acid metabolism drugs
- **E858.6** Agents primarily acting on the smooth and skeletal muscles and respiratory system
- **E858.7** Agents primarily affecting skin and mucous membrane, ophthalmological, otorhinolaryngological, and dental drugs
- **E858.8** Other specified drugs
  - Central appetite depressants
- **E858.9** Unspecified drug

ACCIDENTAL POISONING BY OTHER SOLID AND LIQUID SUBSTANCES, GASES, AND VAPORS (E860-E869)

Note: Categories in this section are intended primarily to indicate the external cause of poisoning states classifiable to 980-989. They may also be used to indicate external causes of localized effects classifiable to 001-799.

✓4th E860 Accidental poisoning by alcohol, not elsewhere classified
- **E860.0** Alcoholic beverages
  - Alcohol in preparations intended for consumption
- **E860.1** Other and unspecified ethyl alcohol and its products
  - Denatured alcohol
  - Ethanol NOS
  - Grain alcohol NOS
  - Methylated spirit
- **E860.2** Methyl alcohol
  - Methanol
  - Wood alcohol
- **E860.3** Isopropyl alcohol
  - Dimethyl carbinol
  - Isopropanol
  - Rubbing alcohol subsitute
  - Secondary propyl alcohol
- **E860.4** Fusel oil
  - Alcohol: amyl
  - butyl
  - Alcohol: propyl
- **E860.8** Other specified alcohols
- **E860.9** Unspecified alcohol

✓4th E861 Accidental poisoning by cleansing and polishing agents, disinfectants, paints, and varnishes
- **E861.0** Synthetic detergents and shampoos
- **E861.1** Soap products
- **E861.2** Polishes
- **E861.3** Other cleansing and polishing agents
  - Scouring powders
- **E861.4** Disinfectants
  - Household and other disinfectants not ordinarily used on the person
  - **EXCLUDES** carbolic acid or phenol (E864.0)
- **E861.5** Lead paints
- **E861.6** Other paints and varnishes
  - Lacquers
  - Oil colors
  - Paints, other than lead
  - White washes
- **E861.9** Unspecified

✓4th E862 Accidental poisoning by petroleum products, other solvents and their vapors, not elsewhere classified
- **E862.0** Petroleum solvents
  - Petroleum: ether
  - benzine
  - Petroleum: naphtha
- **E862.1** Petroleum fuels and cleaners
  - Antiknock additives to petroleum fuels
  - Gas oils
  - Gasoline or petrol
  - Kerosene
  - **EXCLUDES** kerosene insecticides (E863.4)
- **E862.2** Lubricating oils
- **E862.3** Petroleum solids
  - Paraffin wax
- **E862.4** Other specified solvents
  - Benzene
- **E862.9** Unspecified solvent

✓4th E863 Accidental poisoning by agricultural and horticultural chemical and pharmaceutical preparations other than plant foods and fertilizers
EXCLUDES plant foods and fertilizers (E866.5)
- **E863.0** Insecticides of organochlorine compounds
  - Benzene hexachloride
  - Chlordane
  - DDT
  - Dieldrin
  - Endrine
  - Toxaphene
- **E863.1** Insecticides of organophosphorus compounds
  - Demeton
  - Diazinon
  - Dichlorvos
  - Malathion
  - Methyl parathion
  - Parathion
  - Phenylsulphthion
  - Phorate
  - Phosdrin
- **E863.2** Carbamates
  - Aldicarb
  - Carbaryl
  - Propoxur
- **E863.3** Mixtures of insecticides
- **E863.4** Other and unspecified insecticides
  - Kerosene insecticides
- **E863.5** Herbicides
  - 2, 4-Dichlorophenoxyacetic acid [2, 4-D]
  - 2, 4, 5-Trichlorophenoxyacetic acid [2, 4, 5-T]
  - Chlorates
  - Diquat
  - Mixtures of plant foods and fertilizers with herbicides
  - Paraquat
- **E863.6** Fungicides
  - Organic mercurials (used in seed dressing)
  - Pentachlorophenols
- **E863.7** Rodenticides
  - Fluoroacetates
  - Squill and derivatives
  - Thallium
  - Warfarin
  - Zinc phosphide
- **E863.8** Fumigants
  - Cyanides
  - Methyl bromide
  - Phosphine
- **E863.9** Other and unspecified

✓4th E864 Accidental poisoning by corrosives and caustics, not elsewhere classified
EXCLUDES those as components of disinfectants (E861.4)
- **E864.0** Corrosive aromatics
  - Carbolic acid or phenol
- **E864.1** Acids
  - Acid: hydrochloric
  - nitric
  - Acid: sulfuric
- **E864.2** Caustic alkalis
  - Lye
- **E864.3** Other specified corrosives and caustics
- **E864.4** Unspecified corrosives and caustics

✓4th E865 Accidental poisoning from poisonous foodstuffs and poisonous plants
INCLUDES any meat, fish, or shellfish
plants, berries, and fungi eaten as, or in mistake for, food, or by a child
EXCLUDES anaphylactic shock due to adverse food reaction (995.60-995.69)
food poisoning (bacterial) (005.0-005.9)
poisoning and toxic reactions to venomous plants (E905.6-E905.7)
- **E865.0** Meat
- **E865.1** Shellfish
- **E865.2** Other fish
- **E865.3** Berries and seeds
- **E865.4** Other specified plants
- **E865.5** Mushrooms and other fungi
- **E865.8** Other specified foods
- **E865.9** Unspecified foodstuff or poisonous plant

✓4th Fourth-digit Required ▶◀ Revised Text ● New Code ▲ Revised Code Title

2007 ICD•9•CM

E866–E872.5 — E CODES — Tabular List

✓4th E866 Accidental poisoning by other and unspecified solid and liquid substances

> EXCLUDES these substances as a component of:
> medicines (E850.0-E858.9)
> paints (E861.5-E861.6)
> pesticides (E863.0-E863.9)
> petroleum fuels (E862.1)

- E866.0 Lead and its compounds and fumes
- E866.1 Mercury and its compounds and fumes
- E866.2 Antimony and its compounds and fumes
- E866.3 Arsenic and its compounds and fumes
- E866.4 Other metals and their compounds and fumes
  - Beryllium (compounds)   Iron (compounds)
  - Brass fumes   Manganese (compounds)
  - Cadmium (compounds)   Nickel (compounds)
  - Copper salts   Thallium (compounds)
- E866.5 Plant foods and fertilizers
  > EXCLUDES mixtures with herbicides (E863.5)
- E866.6 Glues and adhesives
- E866.7 Cosmetics
- E866.8 Other specified solid or liquid substances
- E866.9 Unspecified solid or liquid substance

E867 Accidental poisoning by gas distributed by pipeline

Carbon monoxide from incomplete combustion of piped gas
Coal gas NOS
Liquefied petroleum gas distributed through pipes (pure or mixed with air)
Piped gas (natural) (manufactured)

✓4th E868 Accidental poisoning by other utility gas and other carbon monoxide

- E868.0 Liquefied petroleum gas distributed in mobile containers
  - Butane
  - Liquefied hydrocarbon gas NOS   } or carbon monoxide from incomplete combustion of these gases
  - Propane
- E868.1 Other and unspecified utility gas
  - Acetylene
  - Gas NOS used for lighting, heating, or cooking   } or carbon monoxide from incomplete combustion of these gases
  - Water gas
- E868.2 Motor vehicle exhaust gas
  - Exhaust gas from:
    - farm tractor, not in transit
    - gas engine
    - motor pump
    - motor vehicle, not in transit
    - any type of combustion engine not in watercraft
  > EXCLUDES poisoning by carbon monoxide from:
  > aircraft while in transit (E844.0-E844.9)
  > motor vehicle while in transit (E818.0-E818.9)
  > watercraft whether or not in transit (E838.0-E838.9)
- E868.3 Carbon monoxide from incomplete combustion of other domestic fuels
  - Carbon monoxide from incomplete combustion of:
    - coal
    - coke
    - kerosene   } in domestic stove or fireplace
    - wood
  > EXCLUDES carbon monoxide from smoke and fumes due to conflagration (E890.0-E893.9)
- E868.8 Carbon monoxide from other sources
  - Carbon monoxide from:
    - blast furnace gas
    - incomplete combustion of fuels in industrial use
    - kiln vapor
- E868.9 Unspecified carbon monoxide

✓4th E869 Accidental poisoning by other gases and vapors

> EXCLUDES effects of gases used as anesthetics (E855.1, E938.2)
> fumes from heavy metals (E866.0-E866.4)
> smoke and fumes due to conflagration or explosion (E890.0-E899)

- E869.0 Nitrogen oxides
- E869.1 Sulfur dioxide
- E869.2 Freon
- E869.3 Lacrimogenic gas [tear gas]
  - Bromobenzyl cyanide   Ethyliodoacetate
  - Chloroacetophenone
- E869.4 Second-hand tobacco smoke
- E869.8 Other specified gases and vapors
  - Chlorine   Hydrocyanic acid gas
- E869.9 Unspecified gases and vapors

MISADVENTURES TO PATIENTS DURING SURGICAL AND MEDICAL CARE (E870-E876)

> EXCLUDES accidental overdose of drug and wrong drug given in error (E850.0-E858.9)
> surgical and medical procedures as the cause of abnormal reaction by the patient, without mention of misadventure at the time of procedure (E878.0-E879.9)

✓4th E870 Accidental cut, puncture, perforation, or hemorrhage during medical care

- E870.0 Surgical operation
- E870.1 Infusion or transfusion
- E870.2 Kidney dialysis or other perfusion
- E870.3 Injection or vaccination
- E870.4 Endoscopic examination
- E870.5 Aspiration of fluid or tissue, puncture, and catheterization
  - Abdominal paracentesis   Lumbar puncture
  - Aspirating needle biopsy   Thoracentesis
  - Blood sampling
  > EXCLUDES heart catheterization (E870.6)
- E870.6 Heart catheterization
- E870.7 Administration of enema
- E870.8 Other specified medical care
- E870.9 Unspecified medical care

✓4th E871 Foreign object left in body during procedure

- E871.0 Surgical operation
- E871.1 Infusion or transfusion
- E871.2 Kidney dialysis or other perfusion
- E871.3 Injection or vaccination
- E871.4 Endoscopic examination
- E871.5 Aspiration of fluid or tissue, puncture, and catheterization
  - Abdominal paracentesis   Lumbar puncture
  - Aspiration needle biopsy Thoracentesis
  - Blood sampling
  > EXCLUDES heart catheterization (E871.6)
- E871.6 Heart catheterization
- E871.7 Removal of catheter or packing
- E871.8 Other specified procedures
- E871.9 Unspecified procedure

✓4th E872 Failure of sterile precautions during procedure

- E872.0 Surgical operation
- E872.1 Infusion or transfusion
- E872.2 Kidney dialysis and other perfusion
- E872.3 Injection or vaccination
- E872.4 Endoscopic examination
- E872.5 Aspiration of fluid or tissue, puncture, and catheterization
  - Abdominal paracentesis   Lumbar puncture
  - Aspiration needle biopsy   Thoracentesis
  - Blood sampling
  > EXCLUDES heart catheterization (E872.6)

| Tabular List | E CODES | E872.6–E879.9 |

E872.6 Heart catheterization
E872.8 Other specified procedures
E872.9 Unspecified procedure

✓4ᵗʰ **E873 Failure in dosage**
> **EXCLUDES** accidental overdose of drug, medicinal or biological substance (E850.0-E858.9)

E873.0 Excessive amount of blood or other fluid during transfusion or infusion
E873.1 Incorrect dilution of fluid during infusion
E873.2 Overdose of radiation in therapy
E873.3 Inadvertent exposure of patient to radiation during medical care
E873.4 Failure in dosage in electroshock or insulin-shock therapy
E873.5 Inappropriate [too hot or too cold] temperature in local application and packing
E873.6 Nonadministration of necessary drug or medicinal substance
E873.8 Other specified failure in dosage
E873.9 Unspecified failure in dosage

✓4ᵗʰ **E874 Mechanical failure of instrument or apparatus during procedure**
E874.0 Surgical operation
E874.1 Infusion and transfusion
    Air in system
E874.2 Kidney dialysis and other perfusion
E874.3 Endoscopic examination
E874.4 Aspiration of fluid or tissue, puncture, and catheterization
    Abdominal paracentesis Lumbar puncture
    Aspiration needle biopsy Thoracentesis
    Blood sampling
> **EXCLUDES** heart catheterization (E874.5)

E874.5 Heart catheterization
E874.8 Other specified procedures
E874.9 Unspecified procedure

✓4ᵗʰ **E875 Contaminated or infected blood, other fluid, drug, or biological substance**
> **INCLUDES** presence of:
> bacterial pyrogens
> endotoxin-producing bacteria
> serum hepatitis-producing agent

E875.0 Contaminated substance transfused or infused
E875.1 Contaminated substance injected or used for vaccination
E875.2 Contaminated drug or biological substance administered by other means
E875.8 Other
E875.9 Unspecified

✓4ᵗʰ **E876 Other and unspecified misadventures during medical care**
E876.0 Mismatched blood in transfusion
E876.1 Wrong fluid in infusion
E876.2 Failure in suture and ligature during surgical operation
E876.3 Endotracheal tube wrongly placed during anesthetic procedure
E876.4 Failure to introduce or to remove other tube or instrument
> **EXCLUDES** foreign object left in body during procedure (E871.0-E871.9)

E876.5 Performance of inappropriate operation
E876.8 Other specified misadventures during medical care
    Performance of inappropriate treatment NEC
E876.9 Unspecified misadventure during medical care

SURGICAL AND MEDICAL PROCEDURES AS THE CAUSE OF ABNORMAL REACTION OF PATIENT OR LATER COMPLICATION, WITHOUT MENTION OF MISADVENTURE AT THE TIME OF PROCEDURE (E878-E879)

> **INCLUDES** procedures as the cause of abnormal reaction, such as:
> displacement or malfunction of prosthetic device
> hepatorenal failure, postoperative
> malfunction of external stoma
> postoperative intestinal obstruction
> rejection of transplanted organ
>
> **EXCLUDES** anesthetic management properly carried out as the cause of adverse effect (E937.0-E938.9)
> infusion and transfusion, without mention of misadventure in the technique of procedure (E930.0-E949.9)

✓4ᵗʰ **E878 Surgical operation and other surgical procedures as the cause of abnormal reaction of patient, or of later complication, without mention of misadventure at the time of operation**
E878.0 Surgical operation with transplant of whole organ
    Transplantation of: Transplantation of:
      heart   liver
      kidney
E878.1 Surgical operation with implant of artificial internal device
    Cardiac pacemaker Heart valve prosthesis
    Electrodes implanted in brain Internal orthopedic device
E878.2 Surgical operation with anastomosis, bypass, or graft, with natural or artificial tissues used as implant
    Anastomosis: Graft of blood vessel,
      arteriovenous   tendon, or skin
      gastrojejunal
> **EXCLUDES** external stoma (E878.3)

E878.3 Surgical operation with formation of external stoma
    Colostomy Gastrostomy
    Cystostomy Ureterostomy
    Duodenostomy
E878.4 Other restorative surgery
E878.5 Amputation of limb(s)
E878.6 Removal of other organ (partial) (total)
E878.8 Other specified surgical operations and procedures
E878.9 Unspecified surgical operations and procedures

✓4ᵗʰ **E879 Other procedures, without mention of misadventure at the time of procedure, as the cause of abnormal reaction of patient, or of later complication**
E879.0 Cardiac catheterization
E879.1 Kidney dialysis
E879.2 Radiological procedure and radiotherapy
> **EXCLUDES** radio-opaque dyes for diagnostic x-ray procedures (E947.8)

E879.3 Shock therapy
    Electroshock therapy
    Insulin-shock therapy
E879.4 Aspiration of fluid
    Lumbar puncture
    Thoracentesis
E879.5 Insertion of gastric or duodenal sound
E879.6 Urinary catheterization
E879.7 Blood sampling
E879.8 Other specified procedures
    Blood transfusion
E879.9 Unspecified procedure

✓4ᵗʰ Fourth-digit Required   ▶◀ Revised Text   ● New Code   ▲ Revised Code Title

ACCIDENTAL FALLS (E880-E888)

EXCLUDES falls (in or from):
- burning building (E890.8, E891.8)
- into fire (E890.0-E899)
- into water (with submersion or drowning) (E910.0-E910.9)
- machinery (in operation) (E919.0-E919.9)
- on edged, pointed, or sharp object (E920.0-E920.9)
- transport vehicle (E800.0-E845.9)
- vehicle not elsewhere classifiable (E846-E848)

✓4th **E880 Fall on or from stairs or steps**
- E880.0 Escalator
- E880.1 Fall on or from sidewalk curb
  - **EXCLUDES** fall from moving sidewalk (E885.9)
- E880.9 Other stairs or steps

✓4th **E881 Fall on or from ladders or scaffolding**
- E881.0 Fall from ladder
- E881.1 Fall from scaffolding

E882 Fall from or out of building or other structure
Fall from:
- balcony
- bridge
- building
- flagpole
- tower
- turret
- viaduct
- wall
- window

Fall through roof

EXCLUDES
- collapse of a building or structure (E916)
- fall or jump from burning building (E890.8, E891.8)

✓4th **E883 Fall into hole or other opening in surface**
INCLUDES fall into:
- cavity
- dock
- hole
- pit
- quarry
- shaft
- swimming pool
- tank
- well

EXCLUDES
- fall into water NOS (E910.9)
- that resulting in drowning or submersion without mention of injury (E910.0-E910.9)

- E883.0 Accident from diving or jumping into water [swimming pool]
  Strike or hit:
  - against bottom when jumping or diving into water
  - wall or board of swimming pool
  - water surface

  EXCLUDES
  - diving with insufficient air supply (E913.2)
  - effects of air pressure from diving (E902.2)

- E883.1 Accidental fall into well
- E883.2 Accidental fall into storm drain or manhole
- E883.9 Fall into other hole or other opening in surface

✓4th **E884 Other fall from one level to another**
- E884.0 Fall from playground equipment
  - **EXCLUDES** recreational machinery (E919.8)
- E884.1 Fall from cliff
- E884.2 Fall from chair
- E884.3 Fall from wheelchair
- E884.4 Fall from bed
- E884.5 Fall from other furniture
- E884.6 Fall from commode
  - Toilet
- E884.9 Other fall from one level to another
  Fall from:
  - embankment
  - haystack
  - stationary vehicle
  - tree

✓4th **E885 Fall on same level from slipping, tripping, or stumbling**
- E885.0 Fall from (nonmotorized) scooter
- E885.1 Fall from roller skates
  - In-line skates
- E885.2 Fall from skateboard
- E885.3 Fall from skis
- E885.4 Fall from snowboard
- E885.9 Fall from other slipping, tripping, or stumbling
  - Fall on moving sidewalk

✓4th **E886 Fall on same level from collision, pushing, or shoving, by or with other person**
  - **EXCLUDES** crushed or pushed by a crowd or human stampede (E917.1, E917.6)
- E886.0 In sports
  - Tackles in sports
  - **EXCLUDES** kicked, stepped on, struck by object, in sports (E917.0, E917.5)
- E886.9 Other and unspecified
  - Fall from collision of pedestrian (conveyance) with another pedestrian (conveyance)

E887 Fracture, cause unspecified

✓4th **E888 Other and unspecified fall**
- Accidental fall NOS
- Fall on same level NOS
- E888.0 Fall resulting in striking against sharp object
  - Use additional external cause code to identify object (E920)
- E888.1 Fall resulting in striking against other object
- E888.8 Other fall
- E888.9 Unspecified fall
  - Fall NOS

ACCIDENTS CAUSED BY FIRE AND FLAMES (E890-E899)

INCLUDES
- asphyxia or poisoning due to conflagration or ignition
- burning by fire
- secondary fires resulting from explosion

EXCLUDES
- arson (E968.0)
- fire in or on:
  - machinery (in operation) (E919.0-E919.9)
  - transport vehicle other than stationary vehicle (E800.0-E845.9)
  - vehicle not elsewhere classifiable (E846-E848)

✓4th **E890 Conflagration in private dwelling**
INCLUDES conflagration in:
- apartment
- boarding house
- camping place
- caravan
- farmhouse
- house
- lodging house
- mobile home
- private garage
- rooming house
- tenement

conflagration originating from sources classifiable to E893-E898 in the above buildings

- E890.0 Explosion caused by conflagration
- E890.1 Fumes from combustion of polyvinylchloride [PVC] and similar material in conflagration
- E890.2 Other smoke and fumes from conflagration
  - Carbon monoxide
  - Fumes NOS
  - Smoke NOS
  } from conflagration in private building
- E890.3 Burning caused by conflagration
- E890.8 Other accident resulting from conflagration
  - Collapse of
  - Fall from
  - Hit by object falling from
  - Jump from
  } burning private building
- E890.9 Unspecified accident resulting from conflagration in private dwelling

---
✓4th Fourth-digit Required ▶◀ Revised Text ● New Code ▲ Revised Code Title

E CODES

☑4th E891 Conflagration in other and unspecified building or structure

Conflagration in:
- barn
- church
- convalescent and other residential home
- dormitory of educational institution
- factory
- farm outbuildings
- hospital
- hotel
- school
- store
- theater

Conflagration originating from sources classifiable to E893-E898, in the above buildings

E891.0 Explosion caused by conflagration

E891.1 Fumes from combustion of polyvinylchloride [PVC] and similar material in conflagration

E891.2 Other smoke and fumes from conflagration

Carbon monoxide / Fumes NOS / Smoke NOS } from conflagration in building or structure

E891.3 Burning caused by conflagration

E891.8 Other accident resulting from conflagration

Collapse of / Fall from / Hit by object falling from / Jump from } burning building or structure

E891.9 Unspecified accident resulting from conflagration of other and unspecified building or structure

E892 Conflagration not in building or structure

Fire (uncontrolled) (in) (of):
- forest
- grass
- hay
- lumber
- mine
- prairie
- transport vehicle [any], except while in transit
- tunnel

☑4th E893 Accident caused by ignition of clothing

> **EXCLUDES** ignition of clothing:
> from highly inflammable material (E894)
> with conflagration (E890.0-E892)

E893.0 From controlled fire in private dwelling

Ignition of clothing from:
normal fire (charcoal) (coal) (electric) (gas) (wood) in: brazier / fireplace / furnace / stove } in private dwelling (as listed in E890)

E893.1 From controlled fire in other building or structure

Ignition of clothing from:
normal fire (charcoal) (coal) (electric) (gas) (wood) in: brazier / fireplace / furnace / stove } in other building or structure (as listed in E81)

E893.2 From controlled fire not in building or structure

Ignition of clothing from:
- bonfire (controlled)
- brazier fire (controlled), not in building or structure
- trash fire (controlled)

> **EXCLUDES** conflagration not in building (E892)
> trash fire out of control (E892)

E893.8 From other specified sources

Ignition of clothing from:
- blowlamp
- blowtorch
- burning bedspread
- candle
- cigar
- cigarette
- lighter
- matches
- pipe
- welding torch

E893.9 Unspecified source

Ignition of clothing (from controlled fire NOS) (in building NOS) NOS

E894 Ignition of highly inflammable material

Ignition of:
- benzine
- gasoline
- fat
- kerosene
- paraffin
- petrol
} (with ignition of clothing)

> **EXCLUDES** ignition of highly inflammable material with:
> conflagration (E890.0-E892)
> explosion (E923.0-E923.9)

E895 Accident caused by controlled fire in private dwelling

Burning by (flame of) normal fire (charcoal) (coal) (electric) (gas) (wood) in: brazier / fireplace / furnace / stove } in private dwelling (as listed in E890)

> **EXCLUDES** burning by hot objects not producing fire or flames (E924.0-E924.9)
> ignition of clothing from these sources (E893.0)
> poisoning by carbon monoxide from incomplete combustion of fuel (E867-E868.9)
> that with conflagration (E890.0-E890.9)

E896 Accident caused by controlled fire in other and unspecified building or structure

Burning by (flame of) normal fire (charcoal) (coal) (electric) (gas) (wood) in: brazier / fireplace / furnace / stove } in other building or structure (as listed in E891)

> **EXCLUDES** burning by hot objects not producing fire or flames (E924.0-E924.9)
> ignition of clothing from these sources (E893.1)
> poisoning by carbon monoxide from incomplete combustion of fuel (E867-E868.9)
> that with conflagration (E891.0-E891.9)

E897 Accident caused by controlled fire not in building or structure

Burns from flame of:
- bonfire
- brazier fire, not in building or structure
- trash fire
} controlled

> **EXCLUDES** ignition of clothing from these sources (E893.2)
> trash fire out of control (E892)
> that with conflagration (E892)

☑4th E898 Accident caused by other specified fire and flames

> **EXCLUDES** conflagration (E890.0-E892)
> that with ignition of:
> clothing (E893.0-E893.9)
> highly inflammable material (E894)

E898.0 Burning bedclothes

Bed set on fire NOS

E898.1 Other

Burning by:
- blowlamp
- blowtorch
- candle
- cigar
- cigarette
- fire in room NOS
- lamp
- lighter
- matches
- pipe
- welding torch

E899 Accident caused by unspecified fire

Burning NOS

ACCIDENTS DUE TO NATURAL AND ENVIRONMENTAL FACTORS (E900-E909)

☑4th E900 Excessive heat

E900.0 Due to weather conditions

Excessive heat as the external cause of:
- ictus solaris
- siriasis
- sunstroke

E900.1 Of man-made origin
    Heat (in):
        boiler room
        drying room
        factory
        furnace room
    Heat (in):
        generated in transport vehicle
        kitchen

E900.9 Of unspecified origin

✓4th E901 Excessive cold

E901.0 Due to weather conditions
    Excessive cold as the cause of:
        chilblains NOS
        immersion foot

E901.1 Of man-made origin
    Contact with or inhalation of:
        dry ice
        liquid air
        liquid hydrogen
        liquid nitrogen
    Prolonged exposure in:
        deep freeze unit
        refrigerator

E901.8 Other specified origin

E901.9 Of unspecified origin

✓4th E902 High and low air pressure and changes in air pressure

E902.0 Residence or prolonged visit at high altitude
    Residence or prolonged visit at high altitude as the cause of:
        Acosta syndrome
        Alpine sickness
        altitude sickness
        Andes disease
        anoxia, hypoxia
        barotitis, barodontalgia, barosinusitis, otitic barotrauma
        hypobarism, hypobaropathy
        mountain sickness
        range disease

E902.1 In aircraft
    Sudden change in air pressure in aircraft during ascent or descent as the cause of:
        aeroneurosis
        aviators' disease

E902.2 Due to diving
    High air pressure from rapid descent in water
    Reduction in atmospheric pressure while surfacing from deep water diving
    as the cause of:
        caisson disease
        divers' disease
        divers' palsy or paralysis

E902.8 Due to other specified causes
    Reduction in atmospheric pressure while surfacing from underground

E902.9 Unspecified cause

E903 Travel and motion

✓4th E904 Hunger, thirst, exposure, and neglect

> **EXCLUDES** any condition resulting from homicidal intent (E968.0-E968.9)
> hunger, thirst, and exposure resulting from accidents connected with transport (E800.0-E848)

E904.0 Abandonment or neglect of infants and helpless persons
    Exposure to weather conditions } resulting from abandonment or neglect
    Hunger or thirst
    Desertion of newborn
    Inattention at or after birth
    Lack of care (helpless person) (infant)

> **EXCLUDES** criminal [purposeful] neglect (E968.4)

E904.1 Lack of food
    Lack of food as the cause of:
        inanition
        insufficient nourishment
        starvation

> **EXCLUDES** hunger resulting from abandonment or neglect (E904.0)

E904.2 Lack of water
    Lack of water as the cause of:
        dehydration
        inanition

> **EXCLUDES** dehydration due to acute fluid loss (276.51)

E904.3 Exposure (to weather conditions), not elsewhere classifiable
    Exposure NOS
    Humidity
    Struck by hailstones

> **EXCLUDES** struck by lightning (E907)

E904.9 Privation, unqualified
    Destitution

✓4th E905 Venomous animals and plants as the cause of poisoning and toxic reactions

> **INCLUDES** chemical released by animal
> insects
> release of venom through fangs, hairs, spines, tentacles, and other venom apparatus

> **EXCLUDES** eating of poisonous animals or plants (E865.0-E865.9)

E905.0 Venomous snakes and lizards
    Cobra
    Copperhead snake
    Coral snake
    Fer de lance
    Gila monster
    Krait
    Mamba
    Rattlesnake
    Sea snake
    Snake (venomous)
    Viper
    Water moccasin

> **EXCLUDES** bites of snakes and lizards known to be nonvenomous (E906.2)

E905.1 Venomous spiders
    Black widow spider
    Brown spider
    Tarantula (venomous)

E905.2 Scorpion

E905.3 Hornets, wasps, and bees
    Yellow jacket

E905.4 Centipede and venomous millipede (tropical)

E905.5 Other venomous arthropods
    Sting of:
        ant
        caterpillar

E905.6 Venomous marine animals and plants
    Puncture by sea urchin spine
    Sting of:
        coral
        jelly fish
        nematocysts
        sea anemone
        sea cucumber
        other marine animal or plant

> **EXCLUDES** bites and other injuries caused by nonvenomous marine animal (E906.2-E906.8)
> bite of sea snake (venomous) (E905.0)

E905.7 Poisoning and toxic reactions caused by other plants
    Injection of poisons or toxins into or through skin by plant thorns, spines, or other mechanisms

> **EXCLUDES** puncture wound NOS by plant thorns or spines (E920.8)

E905.8 Other specified

E905.9 Unspecified
    Sting NOS
    Venomous bite NOS

✓4th E906 Other injury caused by animals

> **EXCLUDES** poisoning and toxic reactions caused by venomous animals and insects (E905.0-E905.9)
> road vehicle accident involving animals (E827.0-E828.9)
> tripping or falling over an animal (E885.9)

Tabular List — E CODES

- **E906.0** Dog bite
- **E906.1** Rat bite
- **E906.2** Bite of nonvenomous snakes and lizards
- **E906.3** Bite of other animal except arthropod
  - Cats
  - Moray eel
  - Rodents, except rats
  - Shark
- **E906.4** Bite of nonvenomous arthropod
  - Insect bite NOS
- **E906.5** Bite by unspecified animal
  - Animal bite NOS
- **E906.8** Other specified injury caused by animal
  - Butted by animal
  - Fallen on by horse or other animal, not being ridden
  - Gored by animal
  - Implantation of quills of porcupine
  - Pecked by bird
  - Run over by animal, not being ridden
  - Stepped on by animal, not being ridden
  - **EXCLUDES** injury by animal being ridden (E828.0-E828.9)
- **E906.9** Unspecified injury caused by animal

E907 Lightning
- **EXCLUDES** injury from:
  - fall of tree or other object caused by lightning (E916)
  - fire caused by lightning (E890.0-E892)

✓4th E908 Cataclysmic storms, and floods resulting from storms
- **EXCLUDES** collapse of dam or man-made structure causing flood (E909.3)
- **E908.0** Hurricane
  - Storm surge
  - "Tidal wave" caused by storm action
  - Typhoon
- **E908.1** Tornado
  - Cyclone
  - Twisters
- **E908.2** Floods
  - Torrential rainfall
  - Flash flood
  - **EXCLUDES** collapse of dam or man-made structure causing flood (E909.3)
- **E908.3** Blizzard (snow) (ice)
- **E908.4** Dust storm
- **E908.8** Other cataclysmic storms
  - Cloudburst
- **E908.9** Unspecified cataclysmic storms, and floods resulting from storms
  - Storm NOS

✓4th E909 Cataclysmic earth surface movements and eruptions
- **E909.0** Earthquakes
- **E909.1** Volcanic eruptions
  - Burns from lava
  - Ash inhalation
- **E909.2** Avalanche, landslide, or mudslide
- **E909.3** Collapse of dam or man-made structure
- **E909.4** Tidalwave caused by earthquake
  - Tidalwave NOS
  - Tsunami
  - **EXCLUDES** tidalwave caused by tropical storm (E908.0)
- **E909.8** Other cataclysmic earth surface movements and eruptions
- **E909.9** Unspecified cataclysmic earth surface movements and eruptions

ACCIDENTS CAUSED BY SUBMERSION, SUFFOCATION, AND FOREIGN BODIES (E910-E915)

✓4th E910 Accidental drowning and submersion
- **INCLUDES**
  - immersion
  - swimmers' cramp
- **EXCLUDES**
  - diving accident (NOS) (resulting in injury except drowning) (E883.0)
  - diving with insufficient air supply (E913.2)
  - drowning and submersion due to:
    - cataclysm (E908-E909)
    - machinery accident (E919.0-E919.9)
    - transport accident (E800.0-E845.9)
  - effect of high and low air pressure (E902.2)
  - injury from striking against objects while in running water (E917.2)
- **E910.0** While water-skiing
  - Fall from water skis with submersion or drowning
  - **EXCLUDES** accident to water-skier involving a watercraft and resulting in submersion or other injury (E830.4, E831.4)
- **E910.1** While engaged in other sport or recreational activity with diving equipment
  - Scuba diving NOS
  - Skin diving NOS
  - Underwater spear fishing NOS
- **E910.2** While engaged in other sport or recreational activity without diving equipment
  - Fishing or hunting, except from boat or with diving equipment
  - Ice skating
  - Playing in water
  - Surfboarding
  - Swimming NOS
  - Voluntarily jumping from boat, not involved in accident, for swim NOS
  - Wading in water
  - **EXCLUDES** jumping into water to rescue another person (E910.3)
- **E910.3** While swimming or diving for purposes other than recreation or sport
  - Marine salvage
  - Pearl diving
  - Placement of fishing nets
  - Rescue (attempt) of another person
  - Underwater construction or repairs
  - (with diving equipment)
- **E910.4** In bathtub
- **E910.8** Other accidental drowning or submersion
  - Drowning in: quenching tank
  - Drowning in: swimming pool
- **E910.9** Unspecified accidental drowning or submersion
  - Accidental fall into water NOS
  - Drowning NOS

E911 Inhalation and ingestion of food causing obstruction of respiratory tract or suffocation
- Aspiration and inhalation of food [any] (into respiratory tract) NOS
- Asphyxia by
- Choked on
- Suffocation by
  - food [including bone, seed in food, regurgitated food]
- Compression of trachea
- Interruption of respiration
- Obstruction of respiration
  - by food lodged in esophagus
- Obstruction of pharynx by food (bolus)
- **EXCLUDES**
  - injury, except asphyxia and obstruction of respiratory passage, caused by food (E915)
  - obstruction of esophagus by food without mention of asphyxia or obstruction of respiratory passage (E915)

E912 Inhalation and ingestion of other object causing obstruction of respiratory tract or suffocation
Aspiration and inhalation of foreign body except food (into respiratory tract) NOS
Foreign object [bean] [marble] in nose
Obstruction of pharynx by foreign body
Compression
Interruption of respiration } by foreign body in esophagus
Obstruction of respiration

> **EXCLUDES** injury, except asphyxia and obstruction of respiratory passage, caused by foreign body (E915)
> obstruction of esophagus by foreign body without mention of asphyxia or obstruction in respiratory passage (E915)

✓4ᵗʰ E913 Accidental mechanical suffocation

> **EXCLUDES** mechanical suffocation from or by:
> accidental inhalation or ingestion of:
> food (E911)
> foreign object (E912)
> cataclysm (E908-E909)
> explosion (E921.0-E921.9, E923.0-E923.9)
> machinery accident (E919.0-E919.9)

E913.0 In bed or cradle
> **EXCLUDES** suffocation by plastic bag (E913.1)

E913.1 By plastic bag

E913.2 Due to lack of air (in closed place)
Accidentally closed up in refrigerator or other airtight enclosed space
Diving with insufficient air supply
> **EXCLUDES** suffocation by plastic bag (E913.1)

E913.3 By falling earth or other substance
Cave-in NOS
> **EXCLUDES** cave-in caused by cataclysmic earth surface movements and eruptions (E909)
> struck by cave-in without asphyxiation or suffocation (E916)

E913.8 Other specified means
Accidental hanging, except in bed or cradle

E913.9 Unspecified means
Asphyxia, mechanical NOS   Suffocation NOS
Strangulation NOS

E914 Foreign body accidentally entering eye and adnexa
> **EXCLUDES** corrosive liquid (E924.1)

E915 Foreign body accidentally entering other orifice
> **EXCLUDES** aspiration and inhalation of foreign body, any, (into respiratory tract) NOS (E911-E912)

OTHER ACCIDENTS (E916-E928)

E916 Struck accidentally by falling object
Collapse of building, except on fire
Falling:
  rock
  snowslide NOS
  stone
  tree
Object falling from:
  machine, not in operation
  stationary vehicle

Code first:
  collapse of building on fire (E890.0-E891.9)
  falling object in:
    cataclysm (E908-E909)
    machinery accidents (E919.0-E919.9)
    transport accidents (E800.0-E845.9)
    vehicle accidents not elsewhere classifiable (E846-E848)
  object set in motion by:
    explosion (E921.0-E921.9, E923.0-E923.9)
    firearm (E922.0-E922.9)
    projected object (E917.0-E917.9)

✓4ᵗʰ E917 Striking against or struck accidentally by objects or persons
> **INCLUDES** bumping into or against
> colliding with
> kicking against } object (moving) (projected) (stationary)
> stepping on   pedestrian conveyance
> struck by   person

> **EXCLUDES** fall from:
> collision with another person, except when caused by a crowd (E886.0-E886.9)
> stumbling over object (E885.9)
> fall resulting in striking against object (E888.0, E888.1)
> injury caused by:
> assault (E960.0-E960.1, E967.0-E967.9)
> cutting or piercing instrument (E920.0-E920.9)
> explosion (E921.0-E921.9, E923.0-E923.9)
> firearm (E922.0-E922.9)
> machinery (E919.0-E919.9)
> transport vehicle (E800.0-E845.9)
> vehicle not elsewhere classifiable (E846-E848)

E917.0 In sports without subsequent fall
Kicked or stepped on during game (football) (rugby)
Struck by hit or thrown ball
Struck by hockey stick or puck

E917.1 Caused by a crowd, by collective fear or panic without subsequent fall
Crushed
Pushed   } by crowd or human stampede
Stepped on

E917.2 In running water without subsequent fall
> **EXCLUDES** drowning or submersion (E910.0-E910.9)
> that in sports (E917.0, E917.5)

E917.3 Furniture without subsequent fall
> **EXCLUDES** fall from furniture (E884.2, E884.4-E884.5)

E917.4 Other stationary object without subsequent fall
Bath tub
Fence
Lamp-post

E917.5 Object in sports with subsequent fall
Knocked down while boxing

E917.6 Caused by a crowd, by collective fear or panic with subsequent fall

E917.7 Furniture with subsequent fall
> **EXCLUDES** fall from furniture (E884.2, E884.4-E884.5)

E917.8 Other stationary object with subsequent fall
Bath tub
Fence
Lamp-post

E917.9 Other striking against with or without subsequent fall

E918 Caught accidentally in or between objects
Caught, crushed, jammed, or pinched in or between moving or stationary objects, such as:
escalator
folding object
hand tools, appliances, or implements
sliding door and door frame
under packing crate
washing machine wringer

> **EXCLUDES** injury caused by:
> cutting or piercing instrument (E920.0-E920.9)
> machinery (E919.0-E919.9)
> transport vehicle (E800.0-E845.9)
> vehicle not elsewhere classifiable (E846-E848)
> struck accidentally by:
> falling object (E916)
> object (moving) (projected) (E917.0-E917.9)

✓4th E919 Accidents caused by machinery

INCLUDES: machinery (accident):
- burned by
- caught in (moving parts of)
- collapse of
- crushed by
- cut or pierced by
- drowning or submersion caused by
- explosion of, on, in
- fall from or into moving part of
- fire starting in or on
- mechanical suffocation caused by
- object falling from, on, in motion by
- overturning of
- pinned under
- run over by
- struck by
- thrown from

caught between machinery and other object
machinery accident NOS

EXCLUDES:
- accidents involving machinery, not in operation (E884.9, E916-E918)
- injury caused by:
  - electric current in connection with machinery (E925.0-E925.9)
  - escalator (E880.0, E918)
  - explosion of pressure vessel in connection with machinery (E921.0-E921.9)
  - moving sidewalk (E885.9)
  - powered hand tools, appliances, and implements (E916-E918, E920.0-E921.9, E923.0-E926.9)
  - transport vehicle accidents involving machinery (E800.0-E848)
  - poisoning by carbon monoxide generated by machine (E868.8)

E919.0 Agricultural machines
- Animal-powered agricultural machine
- Combine
- Derrick, hay
- Farm machinery NOS
- Farm tractor
- Harvester
- Hay mower or rake
- Reaper
- Thresher

EXCLUDES:
- that in transport under own power on the highway (E810.0-E819.9)
- that being towed by another vehicle on the highway (E810.0-E819.9, E827.0-E827.9, E829.0-E829.9)
- that involved in accident classifiable to E820-E829 (E820.0-E829.9)

E919.1 Mining and earth-drilling machinery
- Bore or drill (land) (seabed)
- Shaft hoist
- Shaft lift
- Under-cutter

EXCLUDES: coal car, tram, truck, and tub in mine (E846)

E919.2 Lifting machines and appliances
- Chain hoist
- Crane
- Derrick
- Elevator (building) (grain)
- Forklift truck
- Lift
- Pulley block
- Winch

except in agricultural or mining operations

EXCLUDES:
- that being towed by another vehicle on the highway (E810.0-E819.9, E827.0-E827.9, E829.0-829.9)
- that in transport under own power on the highway (E810.0-E819.9)
- that involved in accident classifiable to E820-E829 (E820.0-E829.9)

E919.3 Metalworking machines
- Abrasive wheel
- Forging machine
- Lathe
- Mechanical shears
- Metal:
  - drilling machine
  - milling machine
  - power press
  - rolling-mill
  - sawing machine

E919.4 Woodworking and forming machines
- Band saw
- Bench saw
- Circular saw
- Molding machine
- Overhead plane
- Powered saw
- Radial saw
- Sander

EXCLUDES: hand saw (E920.1)

E919.5 Prime movers, except electrical motors
- Gas turbine
- Internal combustion engine
- Steam engine
- Water driven turbine

EXCLUDES:
- that being towed by other vehicle on the highway (E810.0-E819.9, E827.0-E827.9, E829.0-E829.9)
- that in transport under own power on the highway (E810.0-E819.9)

E919.6 Transmission machinery
- Transmission:
  - belt
  - cable
  - chain
  - gear
  - pinion
  - pulley
  - shaft

E919.7 Earth moving, scraping, and other excavating machines
- Bulldozer
- Road scraper
- Steam shovel

EXCLUDES:
- that being towed by other vehicle on the highway (E810.0-E819.9, E827.0-E827.9, E829.0-E829.9)
- that in transport under own power on the highway (E810.0-E819.9)

E919.8 Other specified machinery
- Machines for manufacture of:
  - clothing
  - foodstuffs and beverages
  - paper
- Printing machine
- Recreational machinery
- Spinning, weaving, and textile machines

E919.9 Unspecified machinery

✓4th E920 Accidents caused by cutting and piercing instruments or objects

INCLUDES: accidental injury (by) object:
- edged
- pointed
- sharp

E920.0 Powered lawn mower

E920.1 Other powered hand tools
Any powered hand tool [compressed air] [electric] [explosive cartridge] [hydraulic power], such as:
- drill
- hand saw
- hedge clipper
- rivet gun
- snow blower
- staple gun

EXCLUDES:
- band saw (E919.4)
- bench saw (E919.4)

E920.2 Powered household appliances and implements
- Blender
- Electric:
  - beater or mixer
  - can opener
- Electric:
  - fan
  - knife
  - sewing machine
- Garbage disposal appliance

E920.3 Knives, swords, and daggers

E920.4 Other hand tools and implements
- Axe
- Can opener NOS
- Chisel
- Fork
- Hand saw
- Hoe
- Ice pick
- Needle (sewing)
- Paper cutter
- Pitchfork
- Rake
- Scissors
- Screwdriver
- Sewing machine, not powered
- Shovel

E920.5 Hypodermic needle
- Contaminated needle
- Needle stick

E920.8 Other specified cutting and piercing instruments or objects
- Arrow
- Broken glass
- Dart
- Edge of stiff paper
- Lathe turnings
- Nail
- Plant thorn
- Splinter
- Tin can lid

EXCLUDES animal spines or quills (E906.8)
flying glass due to explosion (E921.0-E923.9)

E920.9 Unspecified cutting and piercing instrument or object

✓4th E921 Accident caused by explosion of pressure vessel
INCLUDES accidental explosion of pressure vessels, whether or not part of machinery
EXCLUDES explosion of pressure vessel on transport vehicle (E800.0-E845.9)

E921.0 Boilers

E921.1 Gas cylinders
- Air tank
- Pressure gas tank

E921.8 Other specified pressure vessels
- Aerosol can
- Automobile tire
- Pressure cooker

E921.9 Unspecified pressure vessel

✓4th E922 Accident caused by firearm, and air gun missile

E922.0 Handgun
- Pistol
- Revolver

EXCLUDES Verey pistol (E922.8)

E922.1 Shotgun (automatic)
E922.2 Hunting rifle
E922.3 Military firearms
- Army rifle
- Machine gun

E922.4 Air gun
- BB gun
- Pellet gun

E922.5 Paintball gun
E922.8 Other specified firearm missile
- Verey pistol [flare]

E922.9 Unspecified firearm missile
- Gunshot wound NOS
- Shot NOS

✓4th E923 Accident caused by explosive material
INCLUDES flash burns and other injuries resulting from explosion of explosive material
ignition of highly explosive material with explosion

EXCLUDES explosion:
in or on machinery (E919.0-E919.9)
on any transport vehicle, except stationary motor vehicle (E800.0-E848)
with conflagration (E890.0, E891.0, E892)
secondary fires resulting from explosion (E890.0-E899)

E923.0 Fireworks

E923.1 Blasting materials
- Blasting cap
- Detonator
- Dynamite
- Explosive [any] used in blasting operations

E923.2 Explosive gases
- Acetylene
- Butane
- Coal gas
- Explosion in mine NOS
- Fire damp
- Gasoline fumes
- Methane
- Propane

E923.8 Other explosive materials
- Bomb
- Explosive missile
- Grenade
- Mine
- Shell
- Torpedo
- Explosion in munitions:
  - dump
  - factory

E923.9 Unspecified explosive material
- Explosion NOS

✓4th E924 Accident caused by hot substance or object, caustic or corrosive material, and steam
EXCLUDES burning NOS (E899)
chemical burn resulting from swallowing a corrosive substance (E860.0-E864.4)
fire caused by these substances and objects (E890.0-E894)
radiation burns (E926.0-E926.9)
therapeutic misadventures (E870.0-E876.9)

E924.0 Hot liquids and vapors, including steam
Burning or scalding by:
- boiling water
- hot or boiling liquids not primarily caustic or corrosive
- liquid metal
- steam
- other hot vapor

EXCLUDES hot (boiling) tap water (E924.2)

E924.1 Caustic and corrosive substances
Burning by:
- acid [any kind]
- ammonia
- caustic oven cleaner or other substance
- corrosive substance
- lye
- vitriol

E924.2 Hot (boiling) tap water

E924.8 Other
Burning by:
- heat from electric heating appliance
- hot object NOS
- light bulb
- steam pipe

E924.9 Unspecified

✓4th E925 Accident caused by electric current
INCLUDES electric current from exposed wire, faulty appliance, high voltage cable, live rail, or open electric socket as the cause of:
- burn
- cardiac fibrillation
- convulsion
- electric shock
- electrocution
- puncture wound
- respiratory paralysis

EXCLUDES burn by heat from electrical appliance (E924.8)
lightning (E907)

E925.0 Domestic wiring and appliances

E925.1 Electric power generating plants, distribution stations, transmission lines
- Broken power line

E925.2 Industrial wiring, appliances, and electrical machinery
- Conductors
- Control apparatus
- Electrical equipment and machinery
- Transformers

E925.8 Other electric current
Wiring and appliances in or on:
- farm [not farmhouse]
- outdoors
- public building
- residential institutions
- schools

E925.9 Unspecified electric current
Burns or other injury from electric current NOS
Electric shock NOS
Electrocution NOS

✓4th E926 Exposure to radiation
EXCLUDES abnormal reaction to or complication of treatment without mention of misadventure (E879.2)
atomic power plant malfunction in water transport (E838.0-E838.9)
misadventure to patient in surgical and medical procedures (E873.2-E873.3)
use of radiation in war operations (E996-E997.9)

E926.0 Radiofrequency radiation
Overexposure to: microwave radiation, radar radiation, radiofrequency radiation [any] from: high-powered radio and television transmitters, industrial radiofrequency induction heaters, radar installations

E926.1 Infrared heaters and lamps
Exposure to infrared radiation from heaters and lamps as the cause of:
blistering
burning
charring
inflammatory change

EXCLUDES physical contact with heater or lamp (E924.8)

E926.2 Visible and ultraviolet light sources
Arc lamps   Oxygas welding torch
Black light sources   Sun rays
Electrical welding arc   Tanning bed

EXCLUDES excessive heat from these sources (E900.1-E900.9)

E926.3 X-rays and other electromagnetic ionizing radiation
Gamma rays   X-rays (hard) (soft)

E926.4 Lasers

E926.5 Radioactive isotopes
Radiobiologicals   Radiopharmaceuticals

E926.8 Other specified radiation
Artificially accelerated beams of ionized particles generated by:
betatrons
synchrotrons

E926.9 Unspecified radiation
Radiation NOS

E927 Overexertion and strenuous movements
Excessive physical exercise   Strenuous movements in:
Overexertion (from):   recreational activities
  lifting   other activities
  pulling
  pushing

✓4th E928 Other and unspecified environmental and accidental causes

E928.0 Prolonged stay in weightless environment
Weightlessness in spacecraft (simulator)

E928.1 Exposure to noise
Noise (pollution)   Supersonic waves
Sound waves

E928.2 Vibration

E928.3 Human bite

E928.4 External constriction caused by hair

E928.5 External constriction caused by other object

E928.8 Other

E928.9 Unspecified accident
Accident NOS
Blow NOS
Casualty (not due to war)
Decapitation
} stated as accidentally inflicted

Knocked down
Killed
Injury [any part of body, or unspecified]
Mangled
Wound
} stated as accidentally inflicted, but not otherwise specified

EXCLUDES fracture, cause unspecified (E887)
injuries undetermined whether accidentally or purposely inflicted (E980.0-E989)

LATE EFFECTS OF ACCIDENTAL INJURY (E929)
Note: This category is to be used to indicate accidental injury as the cause of death or disability from late effects, which are themselves classifiable elsewhere. The "late effects" include conditions reported as such, or as sequelae which may occur at any time after the attempted suicide or self-inflicted injury.

✓4th E929 Late effects of accidental injury
EXCLUDES late effects of:
surgical and medical procedures (E870.0-E879.9)
therapeutic use of drugs and medicines (E930.0-E949.9)

E929.0 Late effects of motor vehicle accident
Late effects of accidents classifiable to E810-E825

E929.1 Late effects of other transport accident
Late effects of accidents classifiable to E800-E807, E826-E838, E840-E848

E929.2 Late effects of accidental poisoning
Late effects of accidents classifiable to E850-E858, E860-E869

E929.3 Late effects of accidental fall
Late effects of accidents classifiable to E880-E888

E929.4 Late effects of accident caused by fire
Late effects of accidents classifiable to E890-E899

E929.5 Late effects of accident due to natural and environmental factors
Late effects of accidents classifiable to E900-E909

E929.8 Late effects of other accidents
Late effects of accidents classifiable to E910-E928.8

E929.9 Late effects of unspecified accident
Late effects of accidents classifiable to E928.9

DRUGS, MEDICINAL AND BIOLOGICAL SUBSTANCES CAUSING ADVERSE EFFECTS IN THERAPEUTIC USE (E930-E949)

INCLUDES correct drug properly administered in therapeutic or prophylactic dosage, as the cause of any adverse effect including allergic or hypersensitivity reactions

EXCLUDES accidental overdose of drug and wrong drug given or taken in error (E850.0-E858.9)
accidents in the technique of administration of drug or biological substance, such as accidental puncture during injection, or contamination of drug (E870.0-E876.9)
administration with suicidal or homicidal intent or intent to harm, or in circumstances classifiable to E980-E989 (E950.0-E950.5, E962.0, E980.0-E980.5)

See Alphabetic Index for more complete list of specific drugs to be classified under the fourth-digit subdivisions. The American Hospital Formulary numbers can be used to classify new drugs listed by the American Hospital Formulary Service (AHFS). See Appendix C.

✓4th E930 Antibiotics
EXCLUDES that used as eye, ear, nose, and throat [ENT], and local anti-infectives (E946.0-E946.9)

- **E930.0 Penicillins**
  - Natural
  - Synthetic
  - Semisynthetic, such as:
    - ampicillin
  - Semisynthetic, such as:
    - cloxacillin
    - nafcillin
    - oxacillin
- **E930.1 Antifungal antibiotics**
  - Amphotericin B
  - Griseofulvin
  - Hachimycin [trichomycin]
  - Nystatin
- **E930.2 Chloramphenicol group**
  - Chloramphenicol
  - Thiamphenicol
- **E930.3 Erythromycin and other macrolides**
  - Oleandomycin
  - Spiramycin
- **E930.4 Tetracycline group**
  - Doxycycline
  - Minocycline
  - Oxytetracycline
- **E930.5 Cephalosporin group**
  - Cephalexin
  - Cephaloglycin
  - Cephaloridine
  - Cephalothin
- **E930.6 Antimycobacterial antibiotics**
  - Cycloserine
  - Kanamycin
  - Rifampin
  - Streptomycin
- **E930.7 Antineoplastic antibiotics**
  - Actinomycins, such as:
    - Bleomycin
    - Cactinomycin
    - Dactinomycin
  - Actinomycins, such as:
    - Daunorubicin
    - Mitomycin
  - *EXCLUDES* other antineoplastic drugs (E933.1)
- **E930.8 Other specified antibiotics**
- **E930.9 Unspecified antibiotic**

✓4ᵗʰ **E931 Other anti-infectives**
  - *EXCLUDES* ENT, and local anti-infectives (E946.0-E946.9)
- **E931.0 Sulfonamides**
  - Sulfadiazine
  - Sulfafurazole
  - Sulfamethoxazole
- **E931.1 Arsenical anti-infectives**
- **E931.2 Heavy metal anti-infectives**
  - Compounds of:
    - antimony
    - bismuth
  - Compounds of:
    - lead
    - mercury
  - *EXCLUDES* mercurial diuretics (E944.0)
- **E931.3 Quinoline and hydroxyquinoline derivatives**
  - Chiniofon
  - Diiodohydroxyquin
  - *EXCLUDES* antimalarial drugs (E931.4)
- **E931.4 Antimalarials and drugs acting on other blood protozoa**
  - Chloroquine phosphate
  - Cycloguanil
  - Primaquine
  - Proguanil [chloroguanide]
  - Pyrimethamine
  - Quinine (sulphate)
- **E931.5 Other antiprotozoal drugs**
  - Emetine
- **E931.6 Anthelmintics**
  - Hexylresorcinol
  - Male fern oleoresin
  - Piperazine
  - Thiabendazole
- **E931.7 Antiviral drugs**
  - Methisazone
  - *EXCLUDES* amantadine (E936.4)
    - cytarabine (E933.1)
    - idoxuridine (E946.5)
- **E931.8 Other antimycobacterial drugs**
  - Ethambutol
  - Ethionamide
  - Isoniazid
  - Para-aminosalicylic acid derivatives
  - Sulfones
- **E931.9 Other and unspecified anti-infectives**
  - Flucytosine
  - Nitrofuranderivatives

✓4ᵗʰ **E932 Hormones and synthetic substitutes**
- **E932.0 Adrenal cortical steroids**
  - Cortisone derivatives
  - Desoxycorticosterone derivatives
  - Fluorinated corticosteroid
- **E932.1 Androgens and anabolic congeners**
  - Nandrolone phenpropionate
  - Oxymetholone
  - Testosterone and preparations
- **E932.2 Ovarian hormones and synthetic substitutes**
  - Contraceptives, oral
  - Estrogens
  - Estrogens and progestogens combined
  - Progestogens
- **E932.3 Insulins and antidiabetic agents**
  - Acetohexamide
  - Biguanide derivatives, oral
  - Chlorpropamide
  - Glucagon
  - Insulin
  - Phenformin
  - Sulfonylurea derivatives, oral
  - Tolbutamide
  - *EXCLUDES* adverse effect of insulin administered for shock therapy (E879.3)
- **E932.4 Anterior pituitary hormones**
  - Corticotropin
  - Gonadotropin
  - Somatotropin [growth hormone]
- **E932.5 Posterior pituitary hormones**
  - Vasopressin
  - *EXCLUDES* oxytocic agents (E945.0)
- **E932.6 Parathyroid and parathyroid derivatives**
- **E932.7 Thyroid and thyroid derivatives**
  - Dextrothyroxine
  - Levothyroxine sodium
  - Liothyronine
  - Thyroglobulin
- **E932.8 Antithyroid agents**
  - Iodides
  - Thiouracil
  - Thiourea
- **E932.9 Other and unspecified hormones and synthetic substitutes**

✓4ᵗʰ **E933 Primarily systemic agents**
- **E933.0 Antiallergic and antiemetic drugs**
  - Antihistamines
  - Chlorpheniramine
  - Diphenhydramine
  - Diphenylpyraline
  - Thonzylamine
  - Tripelennamine
  - *EXCLUDES* phenothiazine-based tranquilizers (E939.1)
- **E933.1 Antineoplastic and immunosuppressive drugs**
  - Azathioprine
  - Busulfan
  - Chlorambucil
  - Cyclophosphamide
  - Cytarabine
  - Fluorouracil
  - Mechlorethamine hydrochloride
  - Mercaptopurine
  - Triethylenethiophosphoramide [thio-TEPA]
  - *EXCLUDES* antineoplastic antibiotics (E930.7)
- **E933.2 Acidifying agents**
- **E933.3 Alkalizing agents**
- **E933.4 Enzymes, not elsewhere classified**
  - Penicillinase
- **E933.5 Vitamins, not elsewhere classified**
  - Vitamin A
  - Vitamin D
  - *EXCLUDES* nicotinic acid (E942.2)
    - vitamin K (E934.3)
- **E933.8 Other systemic agents, not elsewhere classified**
  - Heavy metal antagonists
- **E933.9 Unspecified systemic agent**

✓4ᵗʰ **E934 Agents primarily affecting blood constituents**
- **E934.0 Iron and its compounds**
  - Ferric salts
  - Ferrous sulphate and other ferrous salts
- **E934.1 Liver preparations and other antianemic agents**
  - Folic acid
- **E934.2 Anticoagulants**
  - Coumarin
  - Heparin
  - Phenindione
  - Prothrombin synthesis inhibitor
  - Warfarin sodium
- **E934.3 Vitamin K [phytonadione]**
- **E934.4 Fibrinolysis-affecting drugs**
  - Aminocaproic acid
  - Streptodornase
  - Streptokinase
  - Urokinase

Tabular List — E CODES

E934.5 Anticoagulant antagonists and other coagulants
  Hexadimethrine bromide
  Protamine sulfate
E934.6 Gamma globulin
E934.7 Natural blood and blood products
  Blood plasma   Packed red cells
  Human fibrinogen Whole blood
E934.8 Other agents affecting blood constituents
  Macromolecular blood substitutes
E934.9 Unspecified agent affecting blood constituents

√4ᵗʰ **E935 Analgesics, antipyretics, and antirheumatics**
  E935.0 Heroin
    Diacetylmorphine
  E935.1 Methadone
  E935.2 Other opiates and related narcotics
    Codeine [methylmorphine]   Morphine
    Meperidine [pethidine]   Opium (alkaloids)
  E935.3 Salicylates
    Acetylsalicylic acid [aspirin]
    Amino derivatives of salicylic acid
    Salicylic acid salts
  E935.4 Aromatic analgesics, not elsewhere classified
    Acetanilid
    Paracetamol [acetaminophen]
    Phenacetin [acetophenetidin]
  E935.5 Pyrazole derivatives
    Aminophenazone [aminopyrine]
    Phenylbutazone
  E935.6 Antirheumatics [antiphlogistics]
    Gold salts   Indomethacin
    EXCLUDES salicylates (E935.3)
             steroids (E932.0)
  E935.7 Other non-narcotic analgesics
    Pyrabital
  E935.8 Other specified analgesics and antipyretics
    Pentazocine
  E935.9 Unspecified analgesic and antipyretic

√4ᵗʰ **E936 Anticonvulsants and anti-Parkinsonism drugs**
  E936.0 Oxazolidine derivatives
    Paramethadione
    Trimethadione
  E936.1 Hydantoin derivatives
    Phenytoin
  E936.2 Succinimides
    Ethosuximide
    Phensuximide
  E936.3 Other and unspecified anticonvulsants
    Beclamide
    Primidone
  E936.4 Anti-Parkinsonism drugs
    Amantadine
    Ethopropazine [profenamine]
    Levodopa [L-dopa]

√4ᵗʰ **E937 Sedatives and hypnotics**
  E937.0 Barbiturates
    Amobarbital [amylobarbitone]
    Barbital [barbitone]
    Butabarbital [butabarbitone]
    Pentobarbital [pentobarbitone]
    Phenobarbital [phenobarbitone]
    Secobarbital [quinalbarbitone]
    EXCLUDES thiobarbiturates (E938.3)
  E937.1 Chloral hydrate group
  E937.2 Paraldehyde
  E937.3 Bromine compounds
    Bromide
    Carbromal (derivatives)
  E937.4 Methaqualone compounds
  E937.5 Glutethimide group
  E937.6 Mixed sedatives, not elsewhere classified
  E937.8 Other sedatives and hypnotics
  E937.9 Unspecified
    Sleeping:
      drug ⎫
      pill ⎬ NOS
      tablet⎭

√4ᵗʰ **E938 Other central nervous system depressants and anesthetics**
  E938.0 Central nervous system muscle-tone depressants
    Chlorphenesin (carbamate)
    Mephenesin
    Methocarbamol
  E938.1 Halothane
  E938.2 Other gaseous anesthetics
    Ether
    Halogenated hydrocarbon derivatives, except halothane
    Nitrous oxide
  E938.3 Intravenous anesthetics
    Ketamine
    Methohexital [methohexitone]
    Thiobarbiturates, such as thiopental sodium
  E938.4 Other and unspecified general anesthetics
  E938.5 Surface and infiltration anesthetics
    Cocaine   Procaine
    Lidocaine [lignocaine] Tetracaine
  E938.6 Peripheral nerve- and plexus-blocking anesthetics
  E938.7 Spinal anesthetics
  E938.9 Other and unspecified local anesthetics

√4ᵗʰ **E939 Psychotropic agents**
  E939.0 Antidepressants
    Amitriptyline
    Imipramine
    Monoamine oxidase [MAO] inhibitors
  E939.1 Phenothiazine-based tranquilizers
    Chlorpromazine   Prochlorperazine
    Fluphenazine   Promazine
    Phenothiazine
  E939.2 Butyrophenone-based tranquilizers
    Haloperidol   Trifluperidol
    Spiperone
  E939.3 Other antipsychotics, neuroleptics, and major tranquilizers
  E939.4 Benzodiazepine-based tranquilizers
    Chlordiazepoxide   Lorazepam
    Diazepam   Medazepam
    Flurazepam   Nitrazepam
  E939.5 Other tranquilizers
    Hydroxyzine   Meprobamate
  E939.6 Psychodysleptics [hallucinogens]
    Cannabis (derivatives) Mescaline
    Lysergide [LSD]   Psilocin
    Marihuana (derivatives) Psilocybin
  E939.7 Psychostimulants
    Amphetamine   Caffeine
    EXCLUDES central appetite depressants (E947.0)
  E939.8 Other psychotropic agents
  E939.9 Unspecified psychotropic agent

√4ᵗʰ **E940 Central nervous system stimulants**
  E940.0 Analeptics
    Lobeline   Nikethamide
  E940.1 Opiate antagonists
    Levallorphan   Naloxone
    Nalorphine
  E940.8 Other specified central nervous system stimulants
  E940.9 Unspecified central nervous system stimulant

√4ᵗʰ **E941 Drugs primarily affecting the autonomic nervous system**
  E941.0 Parasympathomimetics [cholinergics]
    Acetylcholine
    Anticholinesterase:
      organophosphorus
      reversible
    Pilocarpine

E941.1 Parasympatholytics [anticholinergics and antimuscarinics] and spasmolytics
 Atropine Hyoscine [scopolamine]
 Homatropine Quaternary ammonium derivatives
 EXCLUDES papaverine (E942.5)

E941.2 Sympathomimetics [adrenergics]
 Epinephrine [adrenalin] Levarterenol [noradrenalin]

E941.3 Sympatholytics [antiadrenergics]
 Phenoxybenzamine
 Tolazolinehydrochloride

E941.9 Unspecified drug primarily affecting the autonomic nervous system

✓4th **E942 Agents primarily affecting the cardiovascular system**

E942.0 Cardiac rhythm regulators
 Practolol Propranolol
 Procainamide Quinidine

E942.1 Cardiotonic glycosides and drugs of similar action
 Digitalis glycosides Strophanthins
 Digoxin

E942.2 Antilipemic and antiarteriosclerotic drugs
 Cholestyramine Nicotinic acid derivatives
 Clofibrate Sitosterols
 EXCLUDES dextrothyroxine (E932.7)

E942.3 Ganglion-blocking agents
 Pentamethonium bromide

E942.4 Coronary vasodilators
 Dipyridamole Nitrites
 Nitrates [nitroglycerin] Prenylamine

E942.5 Other vasodilators
 Cyclandelate Hydralazine
 Diazoxide Papaverine

E942.6 Other antihypertensive agents
 Clonidine Rauwolfia alkaloids
 Guanethidine Reserpine

E942.7 Antivaricose drugs, including sclerosing agents
 Monoethanolamine Zinc salts

E942.8 Capillary-active drugs
 Adrenochrome derivatives
 Bioflavonoids
 Metaraminol

E942.9 Other and unspecified agents primarily affecting the cardiovascular system

✓4th **E943 Agents primarily affecting gastrointestinal system**

E943.0 Antacids and antigastric secretion drugs
 Aluminum hydroxide
 Magnesium trisilicate

E943.1 Irritant cathartics
 Bisacodyl Phenolphthalein
 Castor oil

E943.2 Emollient cathartics
 Sodium dioctyl sulfosuccinate

E943.3 Other cathartics, including intestinal atonia drugs
 Magnesium sulfate

E943.4 Digestants
 Pancreatin Pepsin
 Papain

E943.5 Antidiarrheal drugs
 Bismuth subcarbonate Pectin or Kaolin
 EXCLUDES anti-infectives (E930.0-E931.9)

E943.6 Emetics

E943.8 Other specified agents primarily affecting the gastrointestinal system

E943.9 Unspecified agent primarily affecting the gastrointestinal system

✓4th **E944 Water, mineral, and uric acid metabolism drugs**

E944.0 Mercurial diuretics
 Chlormerodrin Mercurophylline
 Mercaptomerin Mersalyl

E944.1 Purine derivative diuretics
 Theobromine Theophylline
 EXCLUDES aminophylline [theophylline ethylenediamine] (E945.7)

E944.2 Carbonic acid anhydrase inhibitors
 Acetazolamide

E944.3 Saluretics
 Benzothiadiazides Chlorothiazide group

E944.4 Other diuretics
 Ethacrynic acid Furosemide

E944.5 Electrolytic, caloric, and water-balance agents

E944.6 Other mineral salts, not elsewhere classified

E944.7 Uric acid metabolism drugs
 Cinchophen and congeners Phenoquin
 Colchicine Probenecid

✓4th **E945 Agents primarily acting on the smooth and skeletal muscles and respiratory system**

E945.0 Oxytocic agents
 Ergot alkaloids
 Prostaglandins

E945.1 Smooth muscle relaxants
 Adiphenine
 Metaproterenol [orciprenaline]
 EXCLUDES papaverine (E942.5)

E945.2 Skeletal muscle relaxants
 Alcuronium chloride
 Suxamethonium chloride

E945.3 Other and unspecified drugs acting on muscles

E945.4 Antitussives
 Dextromethorphan Pipazethate hydrochloride

E945.5 Expectorants
 Acetylcysteine Ipecacuanha
 Cocillana Terpin hydrate
 Guaifenesin [glyceryl guaiacolate]

E945.6 Anti-common cold drugs

E945.7 Antiasthmatics
 Aminophylline [theophylline ethylenediamine]

E945.8 Other and unspecified respiratory drugs

✓4th **E946 Agents primarily affecting skin and mucous membrane, ophthalmological, otorhinolaryngological, and dental drugs**

E946.0 Local anti-infectives and anti-inflammatory drugs

E946.1 Antipruritics

E946.2 Local astringents and local detergents

E946.3 Emollients, demulcents, and protectants

E946.4 Keratolytics, kerstoplastics, other hair treatment drugs and preparations

E946.5 Eye anti-infectives and other eye drugs
 Idoxuridine

E946.6 Anti-infectives and other drugs and preparations for ear, nose, and throat

E946.7 Dental drugs topically applied

E946.8 Other agents primarily affecting skin and mucous membrane
 Spermicides

E946.9 Unspecified agent primarily affecting skin and mucous membrane

✓4th **E947 Other and unspecified drugs and medicinal substances**

E947.0 Dietetics

E947.1 Lipotropic drugs

E947.2 Antidotes and chelating agents, not elsewhere classified

E947.3 Alcohol deterrents

E947.4 Pharmaceutical excipients

E947.8 Other drugs and medicinal substances
 Contrast media used for diagnostic x-ray procedures
 Diagnostic agents and kits

E947.9 Unspecified drug or medicinal substance

✓4th **E948 Bacterial vaccines**

E948.0 BCG vaccine

E948.1 Typhoid and paratyphoid
E948.2 Cholera
E948.3 Plague
E948.4 Tetanus
E948.5 Diphtheria
E948.6 Pertussis vaccine, including combinations with a pertussis component
E948.8 Other and unspecified bacterial vaccines
E948.9 Mixed bacterial vaccines, except combinations with a pertussis component

☑4th E949 Other vaccines and biological substances
EXCLUDES gamma globulin (E934.6)
E949.0 Smallpox vaccine
E949.1 Rabies vaccine
E949.2 Typhus vaccine
E949.3 Yellow fever vaccine
E949.4 Measles vaccine
E949.5 Poliomyelitis vaccine
E949.6 Other and unspecified viral and rickettsial vaccines
Mumps vaccine
E949.7 Mixed viral-rickettsial and bacterial vaccines, except combinations with a pertussis component
EXCLUDES combinations with a pertussis component (E948.6)
E949.9 Other and unspecified vaccines and biological substances

SUICIDE AND SELF-INFLICTED INJURY (E950-E959)
INCLUDES injuries in suicide and attempted suicide
self-inflicted injuries specified as intentional

☑4th E950 Suicide and self-inflicted poisoning by solid or liquid substances
E950.0 Analgesics, antipyretics, and antirheumatics
E950.1 Barbiturates
E950.2 Other sedatives and hypnotics
E950.3 Tranquilizers and other psychotropic agents
E950.4 Other specified drugs and medicinal substances
E950.5 Unspecified drug or medicinal substance
E950.6 Agricultural and horticultural chemical and pharmaceutical preparations other than plant foods and fertilizers
E950.7 Corrosive and caustic substances
Suicide and self-inflicted poisoning by substances classifiable to E864
E950.8 Arsenic and its compounds
E950.9 Other and unspecified solid and liquid substances

☑4th E951 Suicide and self-inflicted poisoning by gases in domestic use
E951.0 Gas distributed by pipeline
E951.1 Liquefied petroleum gas distributed in mobile containers
E951.8 Other utility gas

☑4th E952 Suicide and self-inflicted poisoning by other gases and vapors
E952.0 Motor vehicle exhaust gas
E952.1 Other carbon monoxide
E952.8 Other specified gases and vapors
E952.9 Unspecified gases and vapors

☑4th E953 Suicide and self-inflicted injury by hanging, strangulation, and suffocation
E953.0 Hanging
E953.1 Suffocation by plastic bag
E953.8 Other specified means
E953.9 Unspecified means

E954 Suicide and self-inflicted injury by submersion [drowning]

☑4th E955 Suicide and self-inflicted injury by firearms, air guns and explosives
E955.0 Handgun
E955.1 Shotgun
E955.2 Hunting rifle
E955.3 Military firearms
E955.4 Other and unspecified firearm
Gunshot NOS   Shot NOS
E955.5 Explosives
E955.6 Air gun
BB gun   Pellet gun
E955.7 Paintball gun
E955.9 Unspecified

E956 Suicide and self-inflicted injury by cutting and piercing instrument

☑4th E957 Suicide and self-inflicted injuries by jumping from high place
E957.0 Residential premises
E957.1 Other man-made structures
E957.2 Natural sites
E957.9 Unspecified

☑4th E958 Suicide and self-inflicted injury by other and unspecified means
E958.0 Jumping or lying before moving object
E958.1 Burns, fire
E958.2 Scald
E958.3 Extremes of cold
E958.4 Electrocution
E958.5 Crashing of motor vehicle
E958.6 Crashing of aircraft
E958.7 Caustic substances, except poisoning
EXCLUDES poisoning by caustic substance (E950.7)
E958.8 Other specified means
E958.9 Unspecified means

E959 Late effects of self-inflicted injury
Note: This category is to be used to indicate circumstances classifiable to E950-E958 as the cause of death or disability from late effects, which are themselves classifiable elsewhere. The "late effects" include conditions reported as such, or as sequelae which may occur at any time after the attempted suicide or self-inflicted injury.

HOMICIDE AND INJURY PURPOSELY INFLICTED BY OTHER PERSONS (E960-E969)
INCLUDES injuries inflicted by another person with intent to injure or kill, by any means
EXCLUDES injuries due to:
legal intervention (E970-E978)
operations of war (E990-E999)
terrorism (E979)

☑4th E960 Fight, brawl, rape
E960.0 Unarmed fight or brawl
Beatings NOS
Brawl or fight with hands, fists, feet
Injured or killed in fight NOS
EXCLUDES homicidal:
injury by weapons (E965.0-E966, E969)
strangulation (E963)
submersion (E964)
E960.1 Rape

E961 Assault by corrosive or caustic substance, except poisoning
Injury or death purposely caused by corrosive or caustic substance, such as:
acid [any]
corrosive substance
vitriol
EXCLUDES burns from hot liquid (E968.3)
chemical burns from swallowing a corrosive substance (E962.0-E962.9)

E CODES

✓4ᵗʰ **E962 Assault by poisoning**
  E962.0 Drugs and medicinal substances
    Homicidal poisoning by any drug or medicinal substance
  E962.1 Other solid and liquid substances
  E962.2 Other gases and vapors
  E962.9 Unspecified poisoning

E963 Assault by hanging and strangulation
  Homicidal (attempt):
    garrotting or ligature
    hanging
  Homicidal (attempt):
    strangulation
    suffocation

E964 Assault by submersion [drowning]

✓4ᵗʰ **E965 Assault by firearms and explosives**
  E965.0 Handgun
    Pistol   Revolver
  E965.1 Shotgun
  E965.2 Hunting rifle
  E965.3 Military firearms
  E965.4 Other and unspecified firearm
  E965.5 Antipersonnel bomb
  E965.6 Gasoline bomb
  E965.7 Letter bomb
  E965.8 Other specified explosive
    Bomb NOS (placed in):   Dynamite
      car
      house
  E965.9 Unspecified explosive

E966 Assault by cutting and piercing instrument
  Assassination (attempt), homicide (attempt) by any instrument classifiable under E920
  Homicidal:
    cut
    puncture   } any part of body
    stab
    Stabbed

✓4ᵗʰ **E967 Perpetrator of child and adult abuse**
  Note: Selection of the correct perpetrator code is based on the relationship between the perpetrator and the victim
  E967.0 By father, stepfather, or boyfriend
    Male partner of child's parent or guardian
  E967.1 By other specified person
  E967.2 By mother, stepmother, or girlfriend
    Female partner of child's parent or guardian
  E967.3 By spouse or partner
    Abuse of spouse or partner by ex-spouse or ex-partner
  E967.4 By child
  E967.5 By sibling
  E967.6 By grandparent
  E967.7 By other relative
  E967.8 By non-related caregiver
  E967.9 By unspecified person

✓4ᵗʰ **E968 Assault by other and unspecified means**
  E968.0 Fire
    Arson
    Homicidal burns NOS
    EXCLUDES burns from hot liquid (E968.3)
  E968.1 Pushing from a high place
  E968.2 Striking by blunt or thrown object
  E968.3 Hot liquid
    Homicidal burns by scalding
  E968.4 Criminal neglect
    Abandonment of child, infant, or other helpless person with intent to injure or kill
  E968.5 Transport vehicle
    Being struck by other vehicle or run down with intent to injure
    Pushed in front of, thrown from, or dragged by moving vehicle with intent to injure
  E968.6 Air gun
    BB gun
    Pellet gun
  E968.7 Human bite
  E968.8 Other specified means
  E968.9 Unspecified means
    Assassination (attempt) NOS
    Homicidal (attempt):
      injury NOS
      wound NOS
    Manslaughter (nonaccidental)
    Murder (attempt) NOS
    Violence, non-accidental

E969 Late effects of injury purposely inflicted by other person
  Note: This category is to be used to indicate circumstances classifiable to E960-E968 as the cause of death or disability from late effects, which are themselves classifiable elsewhere. The "late effects" include conditions reported as such, or as sequelae which may occur at any time after injury purposely inflicted by another person.

LEGAL INTERVENTION (E970-E978)

INCLUDES injuries inflicted by the police or other law-enforcing agents, including military on duty, in the course of arresting or attempting to arrest lawbreakers, suppressing disturbances, maintaining order, and other legal action
legal execution

EXCLUDES injuries caused by civil insurrections (E990.0-E999)

E970 Injury due to legal intervention by firearms
  Gunshot wound   Injury by:
  Injury by: rifle pellet or
    machine gun   rubber bullet
    revolver   shot NOS

E971 Injury due to legal intervention by explosives
  Injury by: Injury by:
    dynamite   grenade
    explosive shell   mortar bomb

E972 Injury due to legal intervention by gas
  Asphyxiation by gas   Poisoning by gas
  Injury by tear gas

E973 Injury due to legal intervention by blunt object
  Hit, struck by: Hit, struck by:
    baton (nightstick)   stave
    blunt object

E974 Injury due to legal intervention by cutting and piercing instrument
  Cut   Injured by bayonet
  Incised wound   Stab wound

E975 Injury due to legal intervention by other specified means
  Blow   Manhandling

E976 Injury due to legal intervention by unspecified means

E977 Late effects of injuries due to legal intervention
  Note: This category is to be used to indicate circumstances classifiable to E970-E976 as the cause of death or disability from late effects, which are themselves classifiable elsewhere. The "late effects" include conditions reported as such, or as sequelae, which may occur at any time after the injury due to legal intervention.

E978 Legal execution
  All executions performed at the behest of the judiciary or ruling authority [whether permanent or temporary] as:
    asphyxiation by gas
    beheading, decapitation (by guillotine)
    capital punishment
    electrocution
    hanging
    poisoning
    shooting
    other specified means

TERRORISM (E979)

☑4th **E979 Terrorism**
Injuries resulting from the unlawful use of force or violence against persons or property to intimidate or coerce a Government, the civilian population, or any segment thereof, in furtherance of political or social objective

E979.0 Terrorism involving explosion of marine weapons
Depth-charge
Marine mine
Mine NOS, at sea or in harbour
Sea-based artillery shell
Torpedo
Underwater blast

E979.1 Terrorism involving destruction of aircraft
Aircraft used as a weapon
Aircraft:
  burned
  exploded
  shot down
Crushed by falling aircraft

E979.2 Terrorism involving other explosions and fragments
Antipersonnel bomb (fragments)
Blast NOS
Explosion (of):
  artillery shell
  breech-block
  cannon block
  mortar bomb
  munitions being used in terrorism
  NOS
Fragments from:
  artillery shell
  bomb
  grenade
  guided missile
  land-mine
  rocket
  shell
  shrapnel
Mine NOS

E979.3 Terrorism involving fires, conflagration and hot substances
Burning building or structure:
  collapse of
  fall from
  hit by falling object in
  jump from
Conflagration NOS
Fire (causing):
  Asphyxia
  Burns
  NOS
  Other injury
Melting of fittings and furniture in burning
Petrol bomb
Smouldering building or structure

E979.4 Terrorism involving firearms
Bullet:
  carbine
  machine gun
  pistol
  rifle
  rubber (rifle)
Pellets (shotgun)

E979.5 Terrorism involving nuclear weapons
Blast effects
Exposure to ionizing radiation from nuclear weapon
Fireball effects
Heat from nuclear weapon
Other direct and secondary effects of nuclear weapons

E979.6 Terrorism involving biological weapons
Anthrax
Cholera
Smallpox

E979.7 Terrorism involving chemical weapons
Gases, fumes, chemicals
Hydrogen cyanide
Phosgene
Sarin

E979.8 Terrorism involving other means
Drowning and submersion
Lasers
Piercing or stabbing instruments
Terrorism NOS

E979.9 Terrorism, secondary effects
Note: This code is for use to identify conditions occurring subsequent to a terrorist attack not those that are due to the initial terrorist act
EXCLUDES late effect of terrorist attack (E999.1)

INJURY UNDETERMINED WHETHER ACCIDENTALLY OR PURPOSELY INFLICTED (E980-E989)

Note: Categories E980-E989 are for use when it is unspecified or it cannot be determined whether the injuries are accidental (unintentional), suicide (attempted), or assault.

☑4th **E980 Poisoning by solid or liquid substances, undetermined whether accidentally or purposely inflicted**
E980.0 Analgesics, antipyretics, and antirheumatics
E980.1 Barbiturates
E980.2 Other sedatives and hypnotics
E980.3 Tranquilizers and other psychotropic agents
E980.4 Other specified drugs and medicinal substances
E980.5 Unspecified drug or medicinal substance
E980.6 Corrosive and caustic substances
  Poisoning, undetermined whether accidental or purposeful, by substances classifiable to E864
E980.7 Agricultural and horticultural chemical and pharmaceutical preparations other than plant foods and fertilizers
E980.8 Arsenic and its compounds
E980.9 Other and unspecified solid and liquid substances

☑4th **E981 Poisoning by gases in domestic use, undetermined whether accidentally or purposely inflicted**
E981.0 Gas distributed by pipeline
E981.1 Liquefied petroleum gas distributed in mobile containers
E981.8 Other utility gas

☑4th **E982 Poisoning by other gases, undetermined whether accidentally or purposely inflicted**
E982.0 Motor vehicle exhaust gas
E982.1 Other carbon monoxide
E982.8 Other specified gases and vapors
E982.9 Unspecified gases and vapors

☑4th **E983 Hanging, strangulation, or suffocation, undetermined whether accidentally or purposely inflicted**
E983.0 Hanging
E983.1 Suffocation by plastic bag
E983.8 Other specified means
E983.9 Unspecified means

E984 Submersion [drowning], undetermined whether accidentally or purposely inflicted

☑4th **E985 Injury by firearms, air guns and explosives, undetermined whether accidentally or purposely inflicted**
E985.0 Handgun
E985.1 Shotgun
E985.2 Hunting rifle
E985.3 Military firearms
E985.4 Other and unspecified firearm
E985.5 Explosives
E985.6 Air gun
  BB gun   Pellet gun
E985.7 Paintball gun

E986 Injury by cutting and piercing instruments, undetermined whether accidentally or purposely inflicted

✓4ᵗʰ E987 Falling from high place, undetermined whether accidentally or purposely inflicted
- E987.0 Residential premises
- E987.1 Other man-made structures
- E987.2 Natural sites
- E987.9 Unspecified site

✓4ᵗʰ E988 Injury by other and unspecified means, undetermined whether accidentally or purposely inflicted
- E988.0 Jumping or lying before moving object
- E988.1 Burns, fire
- E988.2 Scald
- E988.3 Extremes of cold
- E988.4 Electrocution
- E988.5 Crashing of motor vehicle
- E988.6 Crashing of aircraft
- E988.7 Caustic substances, except poisoning
- E988.8 Other specified means
- E988.9 Unspecified means

E989 Late effects of injury, undetermined whether accidentally or purposely inflicted

> Note: This category is to be used to indicate circumstances classifiable to E980-E988 as the cause of death or disability from late effects, which are themselves classifiable elsewhere. The "late effects" include conditions reported as such, or as sequelae, which may occur at any time after injury, undetermined whether accidentally or purposely inflicted.

INJURY RESULTING FROM OPERATIONS OF WAR (E990-E999)

INCLUDES injuries to military personnel and civilians caused by war and civil insurrections and occurring during the time of war and insurrection

EXCLUDES accidents during training of military personnel manufacture of war material and transport, unless attributable to enemy action

✓4ᵗʰ E990 Injury due to war operations by fires and conflagrations

INCLUDES asphyxia, burns, or other injury originating from fire caused by a fire-producing device or indirectly by any conventional weapon

- E990.0 From gasoline bomb
- E990.9 From other and unspecified source

✓4ᵗʰ E991 Injury due to war operations by bullets and fragments
- E991.0 Rubber bullets (rifle)
- E991.1 Pellets (rifle)
- E991.2 Other bullets
    Bullet [any, except rubber bullets and pellets]
        carbine
        machine gun
        pistol
        rifle
        shotgun
- E991.3 Antipersonnel bomb (fragments)
- E991.9 Other and unspecified fragments
    Fragments from: Fragments from:
        artillery shell   land mine
        bombs, except   rockets
            anti-personnel   shell
        grenade   Shrapnel
        guided missile

E992 Injury due to war operations by explosion of marine weapons
    Depth charge   Sea-based artillery shell
    Marine mines   Torpedo
    Mine NOS, at sea or in harbor   Underwater blast

E993 Injury due to war operations by other explosion
    Accidental explosion of   Explosion of:
        munitions being used   artillery shell
        in war   breech block
    Accidental explosion of own   cannon block
        weapons   mortar bomb
    Air blast NOS   Injury by weapon burst
    Blast NOS
    Explosion NOS

E994 Injury due to war operations by destruction of aircraft
    Airplane: Airplane:
        burned   shot down
        exploded   Crushed by falling
                                airplane

E995 Injury due to war operations by other and unspecified forms of conventional warfare
    Battle wounds
    Bayonet injury
    Drowned in war operations

E996 Injury due to war operations by nuclear weapons
    Blast effects
    Exposure to ionizing radiation from nuclear weapons
    Fireball effects
    Heat
    Other direct and secondary effects of nuclear weapons

✓4ᵗʰ E997 Injury due to war operations by other forms of unconventional warfare
- E997.0 Lasers
- E997.1 Biological warfare
- E997.2 Gases, fumes, and chemicals
- E997.8 Other specified forms of unconventional warfare
- E997.9 Unspecified form of unconventional warfare

E998 Injury due to war operations but occurring after cessation of hostilities
    Injuries due to war operations but occurring after cessation of hostilities by any means classifiable under E990-E997
    Injuries by explosion of bombs or mines placed in the course of operations of war, if the explosion occurred after cessation of hostilities

✓4ᵗʰ E999 Late effect of injury due to war operations and terrorism

> Note: This category is to be used to indicate circumstances classifiable to E979, E990-E998 as the cause of death or disability from late effects, which are themselves classifiable elsewhere. The "late effects" include conditions reported as such, or as sequelae, which may occur at any time after the injury, resulting from operations of war or terrorism

- E999.0 Late effect of injury due to war operations
- E999.1 Late effect of injury due to terrorism

Official ICD-9-CM Government Appendixes

MORPHOLOGY OF NEOPLASMS

The World Health Organization has published an adaptation of the International Classification of Diseases for oncology (ICD-O). It contains a coded nomenclature for the morphology of neoplasms, which is reproduced here for those who wish to use it in conjunction with Chapter 2 of the International Classification of Diseases, 9th Revision, Clinical Modification.

The morphology code numbers consist of five digits; the first four identify the histological type of the neoplasm and the fifth indicates its behavior. The one-digit behavior code is as follows:

/0 Benign
/1 Uncertain whether benign or malignant
   Borderline malignancy
/2 Carcinoma in situ
   Intraepithelial
   Noninfiltrating
   Noninvasive
/3 Malignant, primary site
/6 Malignant, metastatic site
   Secondary site
/9 Malignant, uncertain whether primary or metastatic site

In the nomenclature below, the morphology code numbers include the behavior code appropriate to the histological type of neoplasm, but this behavior code should be changed if other reported information makes this necessary. For example, "chordoma (M9370/3)" is assumed to be malignant; the term "benign chordoma" should be coded M9370/0. Similarly, "superficial spreading adenocarcinoma (M8143/3)" described as "noninvasive" should be coded M8143/2 and "melanoma (M8720/3)" described as "secondary" should be coded M8720/6.

The following table shows the correspondence between the morphology code and the different sections of Chapter 2:

Morphology Code Histology/Behavior		ICD-9-CM Chapter 2	
Any	0	210-229	Benign neoplasms
M8000-M8004	1	239	Neoplasms of unspecified nature
M8010+	1	235-238	Neoplasms of uncertain behavior
Any	2	230-234	Carcinoma in situ
Any	3	140-195 200-208	Malignant neoplasms, stated or presumed to be primary
Any	6	196-198	Malignant neoplasms, stated or presumed to be secondary

The ICD-O behavior digit /9 is inapplicable in an ICD context, since all malignant neoplasms are presumed to be primary (/3) or secondary (/6) according to other information on the medical record.

Only the first-listed term of the full ICD-O morphology nomenclature appears against each code number in the list below. The ICD-9-CM Alphabetical Index (Volume 2), however, includes all the ICD-O synonyms as well as a number of other morphological names still likely to be encountered on medical records but omitted from ICD-O as outdated or otherwise undesirable.

A coding difficulty sometimes arises where a morphological diagnosis contains two qualifying adjectives that have different code numbers. An example is "transitional cell epidermoid carcinoma." "Transitional cell carcinoma NOS" is M8120/3 and "epidermoid carcinoma NOS" is M8070/3. In such circumstances, the higher number (M8120/3 in this example) should be used, as it is usually more specific.

CODED NOMENCLATURE FOR MORPHOLOGY OF NEOPLASMS

M800 Neoplasms NOS
M8000/0 Neoplasm, benign
M8000/1 Neoplasm, uncertain whether benign or malignant
M8000/3 Neoplasm, malignant
M8000/6 Neoplasm, metastatic
M8000/9 Neoplasm, malignant, uncertain whether primary or metastatic
M8001/0 Tumor cells, benign
M8001/1 Tumor cells, uncertain whether benign or malignant
M8001/3 Tumor cells, malignant
M8002/3 Malignant tumor, small cell type
M8003/3 Malignant tumor, giant cell type
M8004/3 Malignant tumor, fusiform cell type

M801-M804 Epithelial neoplasms NOS
M8010/0 Epithelial tumor, benign
M8010/2 Carcinoma in situ NOS
M8010/3 Carcinoma NOS
M8010/6 Carcinoma, metastatic NOS
M8010/9 Carcinomatosis
M8011/0 Epithelioma, benign
M8011/3 Epithelioma, malignant
M8012/3 Large cell carcinoma NOS
M8020/3 Carcinoma, undifferentiated type NOS
M8021/3 Carcinoma, anaplastic type NOS
M8022/3 Pleomorphic carcinoma
M8030/3 Giant cell and spindle cell carcinoma
M8031/3 Giant cell carcinoma
M8032/3 Spindle cell carcinoma
M8033/3 Pseudosarcomatous carcinoma
M8034/3 Polygonal cell carcinoma
M8035/3 Spheroidal cell carcinoma
M8040/1 Tumorlet
M8041/3 Small cell carcinoma NOS
M8042/3 Oat cell carcinoma
M8043/3 Small cell carcinoma, fusiform cell type

M805-M808 Papillary and squamous cell neoplasms
M8050/0 Papilloma NOS (except Papilloma of urinary bladder M8120/1)
M8050/2 Papillary carcinoma in situ
M8050/3 Papillary carcinoma NOS
M8051/0 Verrucous papilloma
M8051/3 Verrucous carcinoma NOS
M8052/0 Squamous cell papilloma
M8052/3 Papillary squamous cell carcinoma
M8053/0 Inverted papilloma
M8060/0 Papillomatosis NOS
M8070/2 Squamous cell carcinoma in situ NOS
M8070/3 Squamous cell carcinoma NOS
M8070/6 Squamous cell carcinoma, metastatic NOS
M8071/3 Squamous cell carcinoma, keratinizing type NOS
M8072/3 Squamous cell carcinoma, large cell, nonkeratinizing type
M8073/3 Squamous cell carcinoma, small cell, nonkeratinizing type
M8074/3 Squamous cell carcinoma, spindle cell type
M8075/3 Adenoid squamous cell carcinoma
M8076/2 Squamous cell carcinoma in situ with questionable stromal invasion
M8076/3 Squamous cell carcinoma, microinvasive
M8080/2 Queyrat's erythroplasia
M8081/2 Bowen's disease
M8082/3 Lymphoepithelial carcinoma

M809-M811 Basal cell neoplasms
M8090/1 Basal cell tumor
M8090/3 Basal cell carcinoma NOS
M8091/3 Multicentric basal cell carcinoma
M8092/3 Basal cell carcinoma, morphea type
M8093/3 Basal cell carcinoma, fibroepithelial type
M8094/3 Basosquamous carcinoma
M8095/3 Metatypical carcinoma
M8096/0 Intraepidermal epithelioma of Jadassohn
M8100/0 Trichoepithelioma
M8101/0 Trichofolliculoma
M8102/0 Tricholemmoma
M8110/0 Pilomatrixoma

M812-M813 Transitional cell papillomas and carcinomas
M8120/0 Transitional cell papilloma NOS
M8120/1 Urothelial papilloma
M8120/2 Transitional cell carcinoma in situ
M8120/3 Transitional cell carcinoma NOS
M8121/0 Schneiderian papilloma
M8121/1 Transitional cell papilloma, inverted type
M8121/3 Schneiderian carcinoma
M8122/3 Transitional cell carcinoma, spindle cell type
M8123/3 Basaloid carcinoma
M8124/3 Cloacogenic carcinoma
M8130/3 Papillary transitional cell carcinoma

M814-M838 Adenomas and adenocarcinomas
M8140/0 Adenoma NOS
M8140/1 Bronchial adenoma NOS
M8140/2 Adenocarcinoma in situ
M8140/3 Adenocarcinoma NOS
M8140/6 Adenocarcinoma, metastatic NOS
M8141/3 Scirrhous adenocarcinoma
M8142/3 Linitis plastica
M8143/3 Superficial spreading adenocarcinoma
M8144/3 Adenocarcinoma, intestinal type
M8145/3 Carcinoma, diffuse type
M8146/0 Monomorphic adenoma
M8147/3 Basal cell adenoma
M8150/0 Islet cell adenoma
M8150/3 Islet cell carcinoma
M8151/0 Insulinoma NOS
M8151/3 Insulinoma, malignant
M8152/0 Glucagonoma NOS
M8152/3 Glucagonoma, malignant
M8153/1 Gastrinoma NOS

APPENDIX A: MORPHOLOGY OF NEOPLASMS

Code	Description
M8153/3	Gastrinoma, malignant
M8154/3	Mixed islet cell and exocrine adenocarcinoma
M8160/0	Bile duct adenoma
M8160/3	Cholangiocarcinoma
M8161/0	Bile duct cystadenoma
M8161/3	Bile duct cystadenocarcinoma
M8170/0	Liver cell adenoma
M8170/3	Hepatocellular carcinoma NOS
M8180/0	Hepatocholangioma, benign
M8180/3	Combined hepatocellular carcinoma and cholangiocarcinoma
M8190/0	Trabecular adenoma
M8190/3	Trabecular adenocarcinoma
M8191/0	Embryonal adenoma
M8200/0	Eccrine dermal cylindroma
M8200/3	Adenoid cystic carcinoma
M8201/3	Cribriform carcinoma
M8210/0	Adenomatous polyp NOS
M8210/3	Adenocarcinoma in adenomatous polyp
M8211/0	Tubular adenoma NOS
M8211/3	Tubular adenocarcinoma
M8220/0	Adenomatous polyposis coli
M8220/3	Adenocarcinoma in adenomatous polyposis coli
M8221/0	Multiple adenomatous polyps
M8230/3	Solid carcinoma NOS
M8231/3	Carcinoma simplex
M8240/1	Carcinoid tumor NOS
M8240/3	Carcinoid tumor, malignant
M8241/1	Carcinoid tumor, argentaffin NOS
M8241/3	Carcinoid tumor, argentaffin, malignant
M8242/1	Carcinoid tumor, nonargentaffin NOS
M8242/3	Carcinoid tumor, nonargentaffin, malignant
M8243/3	Mucocarcinoid tumor, malignant
M8244/3	Composite carcinoid
M8250/1	Pulmonary adenomatosis
M8250/3	Bronchiolo-alveolar adenocarcinoma
M8251/0	Alveolar adenoma
M8251/3	Alveolar adenocarcinoma
M8260/0	Papillary adenoma NOS
M8260/3	Papillary adenocarcinoma NOS
M8261/1	Villous adenoma NOS
M8261/3	Adenocarcinoma in villous adenoma
M8262/3	Villous adenocarcinoma
M8263/0	Tubulovillous adenoma
M8270/0	Chromophobe adenoma
M8270/3	Chromophobe carcinoma
M8280/0	Acidophil adenoma
M8280/3	Acidophil carcinoma
M8281/0	Mixed acidophil-basophil adenoma
M8281/3	Mixed acidophil-basophil carcinoma
M8290/0	Oxyphilic adenoma
M8290/3	Oxyphilic adenocarcinoma
M8300/0	Basophil adenoma
M8300/3	Basophil carcinoma
M8310/0	Clear cell adenoma
M8310/3	Clear cell adenocarcinoma NOS
M8311/1	Hypernephroid tumor
M8312/3	Renal cell carcinoma
M8313/0	Clear cell adenofibroma
M8320/3	Granular cell carcinoma
M8321/0	Chief cell adenoma
M8322/0	Water-clear cell adenoma
M8322/3	Water-clear cell adenocarcinoma
M8323/0	Mixed cell adenoma
M8323/3	Mixed cell adenocarcinoma
M8324/0	Lipoadenoma
M8330/0	Follicular adenoma
M8330/3	Follicular adenocarcinoma NOS
M8331/3	Follicular adenocarcinoma, well differentiated type
M8332/3	Follicular adenocarcinoma, trabecular type
M8333/3	Microfollicular adenoma
M8334/0	Macrofollicular adenoma
M8340/3	Papillary and follicular adenocarcinoma
M8350/3	Nonencapsulated sclerosing carcinoma
M8360/1	Multiple endocrine adenomas
M8361/1	Juxtaglomerular tumor
M8370/0	Adrenal cortical adenoma NOS
M8370/3	Adrenal cortical carcinoma
M8371/0	Adrenal cortical adenoma, compact cell type
M8372/0	Adrenal cortical adenoma, heavily pigmented variant
M8373/0	Adrenal cortical adenoma, clear cell type
M8374/0	Adrenal cortical adenoma, glomerulosa cell type
M8375/0	Adrenal cortical adenoma, mixed cell type
M8380/0	Endometrioid adenoma NOS
M8380/1	Endometrioid adenoma, borderline malignancy
M8380/3	Endometrioid carcinoma
M8381/0	Endometrioid adenofibroma NOS
M8381/1	Endometrioid adenofibroma, borderline malignancy
M8381/3	Endometrioid adenofibroma, malignant
M839-M842	**Adnexal and skin appendage neoplasms**
M8390/0	Skin appendage adenoma
M8390/3	Skin appendage carcinoma
M8400/0	Sweat gland adenoma
M8400/1	Sweat gland tumor NOS
M8400/3	Sweat gland adenocarcinoma
M8401/0	Apocrine adenoma
M8401/3	Apocrine adenocarcinoma
M8402/0	Eccrine acrospiroma
M8403/0	Eccrine spiradenoma
M8404/0	Hidrocystoma
M8405/0	Papillary hydradenoma
M8406/0	Papillary syringadenoma
M8407/0	Syringoma NOS
M8410/0	Sebaceous adenoma
M8410/3	Sebaceous adenocarcinoma
M8420/0	Ceruminous adenoma
M8420/3	Ceruminous adenocarcinoma
M843	**Mucoepidermoid neoplasms**
M8430/1	Mucoepidermoid tumor
M8430/3	Mucoepidermoid carcinoma
M844-M849	**Cystic, mucinous, and serous neoplasms**
M8440/0	Cystadenoma NOS
M8440/3	Cystadenocarcinoma NOS
M8441/0	Serous cystadenoma NOS
M8441/1	Serous cystadenoma, borderline malignancy
M8441/3	Serous cystadenocarcinoma NOS
M8450/0	Papillary cystadenoma NOS
M8450/1	Papillary cystadenoma, borderline malignancy
M8450/3	Papillary cystadenocarcinoma NOS
M8460/0	Papillary serous cystadenoma NOS
M8460/1	Papillary serous cystadenoma, borderline malignancy
M8460/3	Papillary serous cystadenocarcinoma
M8461/0	Serous surface papilloma NOS
M8461/1	Serous surface papilloma, borderline malignancy
M8461/3	Serous surface papillary carcinoma
M8470/0	Mucinous cystadenoma NOS
M8470/1	Mucinous cystadenoma, borderline malignancy
M8470/3	Mucinous cystadenocarcinoma NOS
M8471/0	Papillary mucinous cystadenoma NOS
M8471/1	Papillary mucinous cystadenoma, borderline malignancy
M8471/3	Papillary mucinous cystadenocarcinoma
M8480/0	Mucinous adenoma
M8480/3	Mucinous adenocarcinoma
M8480/6	Pseudomyxoma peritonei
M8481/3	Mucin-producing adenocarcinoma
M8490/3	Signet ring cell carcinoma
M8490/6	Metastatic signet ring cell carcinoma
M850-M854	**Ductal, lobular, and medullary neoplasms**
M8500/2	Intraductal carcinoma, noninfiltrating NOS
M8500/3	Infiltrating duct carcinoma
M8501/2	Comedocarcinoma, noninfiltrating
M8501/3	Comedocarcinoma NOS
M8502/3	Juvenile carcinoma of the breast
M8503/0	Intraductal papilloma
M8503/2	Noninfiltrating intraductal papillary adenocarcinoma
M8504/0	Intracystic papillary adenoma
M8504/2	Noninfiltrating intracystic carcinoma
M8505/0	Intraductal papillomatosis NOS
M8506/0	Subareolar duct papillomatosis
M8510/3	Medullary carcinoma NOS
M8511/3	Medullary carcinoma with amyloid stroma
M8512/3	Medullary carcinoma with lymphoid stroma
M8520/2	Lobular carcinoma in situ
M8520/3	Lobular carcinoma NOS
M8521/3	Infiltrating ductular carcinoma
M8530/3	Inflammatory carcinoma
M8540/3	Paget's disease, mammary
M8541/3	Paget's disease and infiltrating duct carcinoma of breast
M8542/3	Paget's disease, extramammary (except Paget's disease of bone)
M855	**Acinar cell neoplasms**
M8550/0	Acinar cell adenoma
M8550/1	Acinar cell tumor
M8550/3	Acinar cell carcinoma
M856-M858	**Complex epithelial neoplasms**
M8560/3	Adenosquamous carcinoma
M8561/0	Adenolymphoma
M8570/3	Adenocarcinoma with squamous metaplasia
M8571/3	Adenocarcinoma with cartilaginous and osseous metaplasia
M8572/3	Adenocarcinoma with spindle cell metaplasia
M8573/3	Adenocarcinoma with apocrine metaplasia
M8580/0	Thymoma, benign
M8580/3	Thymoma, malignant
M859-M867	**Specialized gonadal neoplasms**
M8590/1	Sex cord-stromal tumor
M8600/0	Thecoma NOS
M8600/3	Theca cell carcinoma
M8610/0	Luteoma NOS
M8620/1	Granulosa cell tumor NOS
M8620/3	Granulosa cell tumor, malignant
M8621/1	Granulosa cell-theca cell tumor
M8630/0	Androblastoma, benign
M8630/1	Androblastoma NOS
M8630/3	Androblastoma, malignant
M8631/0	Sertoli-Leydig cell tumor
M8632/1	Gynandroblastoma
M8640/0	Tubular androblastoma NOS
M8640/3	Sertoli cell carcinoma
M8641/0	Tubular androblastoma with lipid storage

APPENDIX A: MORPHOLOGY OF NEOPLASMS

M8650/0	Leydig cell tumor, benign	M8813/0	Fascial fibroma	M8990/1	Mesenchymoma NOS
M8650/1	Leydig cell tumor NOS	M8813/3	Fascial fibrosarcoma	M8990/3	Mesenchymoma, malignant
M8650/3	Leydig cell tumor, malignant	M8814/3	Infantile fibrosarcoma	M8991/3	Embryonal sarcoma
M8660/0	Hilar cell tumor	M8820/0	Elastofibroma	**M900-M903**	**Fibroepithelial neoplasms**
M8670/0	Lipid cell tumor of ovary	M8821/1	Aggressive fibromatosis	M9000/0	Brenner tumor NOS
M8671/0	Adrenal rest tumor	M8822/1	Abdominal fibromatosis	M9000/1	Brenner tumor, borderline malignancy
M868-M871	**Paragangliomas and glomus tumors**	M8823/1	Desmoplastic fibroma	M9000/3	Brenner tumor, malignant
M8680/1	Paraganglioma NOS	M8830/0	Fibrous histiocytoma NOS	M9010/0	Fibroadenoma NOS
M8680/3	Paraganglioma, malignant	M8830/1	Atypical fibrous histiocytoma	M9011/0	Intracanalicular fibroadenoma NOS
M8681/1	Sympathetic paraganglioma	M8830/3	Fibrous histiocytoma, malignant	M9012/0	Pericanalicular fibroadenoma
M8682/1	Parasympathetic paraganglioma	M8831/0	Fibroxanthoma NOS	M9013/0	Adenofibroma NOS
M8690/1	Glomus jugulare tumor	M8831/1	Atypical fibroxanthoma	M9014/0	Serous adenofibroma
M8691/1	Aortic body tumor	M8831/3	Fibroxanthoma, malignant	M9015/0	Mucinous adenofibroma
M8692/1	Carotid body tumor	M8832/0	Dermatofibroma NOS	M9020/0	Cellular intracanalicular fibroadenoma
M8693/1	Extra-adrenal paraganglioma NOS	M8832/1	Dermatofibroma protuberans	M9020/1	Cystosarcoma phyllodes NOS
M8693/3	Extra-adrenal paraganglioma, malignant	M8832/3	Dermatofibrosarcoma NOS	M9020/3	Cystosarcoma phyllodes, malignant
M8700/0	Pheochromocytoma NOS	**M884**	**Myxomatous neoplasms**	M9030/0	Juvenile fibroadenoma
M8700/3	Pheochromocytoma, malignant	M8840/0	Myxoma NOS	**M904**	**Synovial neoplasms**
M8710/3	Glomangiosarcoma	M8840/3	Myxosarcoma	M9040/0	Synovioma, benign
M8711/0	Glomus tumor	**M885-M888**	**Lipomatous neoplasms**	M9040/3	Synovial sarcoma NOS
M8712/0	Glomangioma	M8850/0	Lipoma NOS	M9041/3	Synovial sarcoma, spindle cell type
M872-M879	**Nevi and melanomas**	M8850/3	Liposarcoma NOS	M9042/3	Synovial sarcoma, epithelioid cell type
M8720/0	Pigmented nevus NOS	M8851/0	Fibrolipoma		
M8720/3	Malignant melanoma NOS	M8851/3	Liposarcoma, well differentiated type	M9043/3	Synovial sarcoma, biphasic type
M8721/3	Nodular melanoma			M9044/3	Clear cell sarcoma of tendons and aponeuroses
M8722/0	Balloon cell nevus	M8852/0	Fibromyxolipoma		
M8722/3	Balloon cell melanoma	M8852/3	Myxoid liposarcoma	**M905**	**Mesothelial neoplasms**
M8723/0	Halo nevus	M8853/3	Round cell liposarcoma	M9050/0	Mesothelioma, benign
M8724/1	Fibrous papule of the nose	M8854/3	Pleomorphic liposarcoma	M9050/3	Mesothelioma, malignant
M8725/0	Neuronevus	M8855/3	Mixed type liposarcoma	M9051/0	Fibrous mesothelioma, benign
M8726/0	Magnocellular nevus	M8856/0	Intramuscular lipoma	M9051/3	Fibrous mesothelioma, malignant
M8730/0	Nonpigmented nevus	M8857/0	Spindle cell lipoma	M9052/0	Epithelioid mesothelioma, benign
M8730/3	Amelanotic melanoma	M8860/0	Angiomyolipoma	M9052/3	Epithelioid mesothelioma, malignant
M8740/0	Junctional nevus	M8860/3	Angiomyoliposarcoma		
M8740/3	Malignant melanoma in junctional nevus	M8861/0	Angiolipoma NOS	M9053/0	Mesothelioma, biphasic type, benign
		M8861/1	Angiolipoma, infiltrating		
M8741/2	Precancerous melanosis NOS	M8870/0	Myelolipoma	M9053/3	Mesothelioma, biphasic type, malignant
M8741/3	Malignant melanoma in precancerous melanosis	M8880/0	Hibernoma		
		M8881/0	Lipoblastomatosis	M9054/0	Adenomatoid tumor NOS
M8742/2	Hutchinson's melanotic freckle	**M889-M892**	**Myomatous neoplasms**	**M906-M909**	**Germ cell neoplasms**
M8742/3	Malignant melanoma in Hutchinson's melanotic freckle	M8890/0	Leiomyoma NOS	M9060/3	Dysgerminoma
		M8890/1	Intravascular leiomyomatosis	M9061/3	Seminoma NOS
M8743/3	Superficial spreading melanoma	M8890/3	Leiomyosarcoma NOS	M9062/3	Seminoma, anaplastic type
M8750/0	Intradermal nevus	M8891/1	Epithelioid leiomyoma	M9063/3	Spermatocytic seminoma
M8760/0	Compound nevus	M8891/3	Epithelioid leiomyosarcoma	M9064/3	Germinoma
M8761/1	Giant pigmented nevus	M8892/1	Cellular leiomyoma	M9070/3	Embryonal carcinoma NOS
M8761/3	Malignant melanoma in giant pigmented nevus	M8893/0	Bizarre leiomyoma	M9071/3	Endodermal sinus tumor
		M8894/0	Angiomyoma	M9072/3	Polyembryoma
M8770/0	Epithelioid and spindle cell nevus	M8894/3	Angiomyosarcoma	M9073/1	Gonadoblastoma
M8771/3	Epithelioid cell melanoma	M8895/0	Myoma	M9080/0	Teratoma, benign
M8772/3	Spindle cell melanoma NOS	M8895/3	Myosarcoma	M9080/1	Teratoma NOS
M8773/3	Spindle cell melanoma, type A	M8900/0	Rhabdomyoma NOS	M9080/3	Teratoma, malignant NOS
M8774/3	Spindle cell melanoma, type B	M8900/3	Rhabdomyosarcoma NOS	M9081/3	Teratocarcinoma
M8775/3	Mixed epithelioid and spindle cell melanoma	M8901/3	Pleomorphic rhabdomyosarcoma	M9082/3	Malignant teratoma, undifferentiated type
		M8902/3	Mixed type rhabdomyosarcoma		
M8780/0	Blue nevus NOS	M8903/0	Fetal rhabdomyoma	M9083/3	Malignant teratoma, intermediate type
M8780/3	Blue nevus, malignant	M8904/0	Adult rhabdomyoma		
M8790/0	Cellular blue nevus	M8910/3	Embryonal rhabdomyosarcoma	M9084/0	Dermoid cyst
M880	**Soft tissue tumors and sarcomas NOS**	M8920/3	Alveolar rhabdomyosarcoma	M9084/3	Dermoid cyst with malignant transformation
		M893-M899	**Complex mixed and stromal neoplasms**		
M8800/0	Soft tissue tumor, benign			M9090/0	Struma ovarii NOS
M8800/3	Sarcoma NOS	M8930/3	Endometrial stromal sarcoma	M9090/3	Struma ovarii, malignant
M8800/9	Sarcomatosis NOS	M8931/1	Endolymphatic stromal myosis	M9091/1	Strumal carcinoid
M8801/3	Spindle cell sarcoma	M8932/0	Adenomyoma	**M910**	**Trophoblastic neoplasms**
M8802/3	Giant cell sarcoma (except of bone M9250/3)	M8940/0	Pleomorphic adenoma	M9100/0	Hydatidiform mole NOS
		M8940/3	Mixed tumor, malignant NOS	M9100/1	Invasive hydatidiform mole
M8803/3	Small cell sarcoma	M8950/3	Mullerian mixed tumor	M9100/3	Choriocarcinoma
M8804/3	Epithelioid cell sarcoma	M8951/3	Mesodermal mixed tumor	M9101/3	Choriocarcinoma combined with teratoma
M881-M883	**Fibromatous neoplasms**	M8960/1	Mesoblastic nephroma		
M8810/0	Fibroma NOS	M8960/3	Nephroblastoma NOS	M9102/3	Malignant teratoma, trophoblastic
M8810/3	Fibrosarcoma NOS	M8961/3	Epithelial nephroblastoma	**M911**	**Mesonephromas**
M8811/0	Fibromyxoma	M8962/3	Mesenchymal nephroblastoma	M9110/0	Mesonephroma, benign
M8811/3	Fibromyxosarcoma	M8970/3	Hepatoblastoma	M9110/1	Mesonephric tumor
M8812/0	Periosteal fibroma	M8980/3	Carcinosarcoma NOS	M9110/3	Mesonephroma, malignant
M8812/3	Periosteal fibrosarcoma	M8981/3	Carcinosarcoma, embryonal type	M9111/1	Endosalpingioma
		M8982/0	Myoepithelioma		
		M8990/0	Mesenchymoma, benign		

APPENDIX A: MORPHOLOGY OF NEOPLASMS

M912-M916	**Blood vessel tumors**	M9301/0	Calcifying odontogenic cyst	M9530/3	Meningioma, malignant
M9120/0	Hemangioma NOS	M9310/0	Ameloblastoma NOS	M9531/0	Meningotheliomatous meningioma
M9120/3	Hemangiosarcoma	M9310/3	Ameloblastoma, malignant	M9532/0	Fibrous meningioma
M9121/0	Cavernous hemangioma	M9311/0	Odontoameloblastoma	M9533/0	Psammomatous meningioma
M9122/0	Venous hemangioma	M9312/0	Squamous odontogenic tumor	M9534/0	Angiomatous meningioma
M9123/0	Racemose hemangioma	M9320/0	Odontogenic myxoma	M9535/0	Hemangioblastic meningioma
M9124/3	Kupffer cell sarcoma	M9321/0	Odontogenic fibroma NOS	M9536/0	Hemangiopericytic meningioma
M9130/0	Hemangioendothelioma, benign	M9330/0	Ameloblastic fibroma	M9537/0	Transitional meningioma
M9130/1	Hemangioendothelioma NOS	M9330/3	Ameloblastic fibrosarcoma	M9538/1	Papillary meningioma
M9130/3	Hemangioendothelioma, malignant	M9340/0	Calcifying epithelial odontogenic tumor	M9539/3	Meningeal sarcomatosis
M9131/0	Capillary hemangioma			M954-M957	**Nerve sheath tumor**
M9132/0	Intramuscular hemangioma	M935-M937	**Miscellaneous tumors**	M9540/0	Neurofibroma NOS
M9140/3	Kaposi's sarcoma	M9350/1	Craniopharyngioma	M9540/1	Neurofibromatosis NOS
M9141/0	Angiokeratoma	M9360/1	Pinealoma	M9540/3	Neurofibrosarcoma
M9142/0	Verrucous keratotic hemangioma	M9361/1	Pineocytoma	M9541/0	Melanotic neurofibroma
M9150/0	Hemangiopericytoma, benign	M9362/3	Pineoblastoma	M9550/0	Plexiform neurofibroma
M9150/1	Hemangiopericytoma NOS	M9363/0	Melanotic neuroectodermal tumor	M9560/0	Neurilemmoma NOS
M9150/3	Hemangiopericytoma, malignant	M9370/3	Chordoma	M9560/1	Neurinomatosis
M9160/0	Angiofibroma NOS	M938-M948	**Gliomas**	M9560/3	Neurilemmoma, malignant
M9161/1	Hemangioblastoma	M9380/3	Glioma, malignant	M9570/0	Neuroma NOS
M917	**Lymphatic vessel tumors**	M9381/3	Gliomatosis cerebri	M958	**Granular cell tumors and alveolar soft part sarcoma**
M9170/0	Lymphangioma NOS	M9382/3	Mixed glioma		
M9170/3	Lymphangiosarcoma	M9383/1	Subependymal glioma	M9580/0	Granular cell tumor NOS
M9171/0	Capillary lymphangioma	M9384/1	Subependymal giant cell astrocytoma	M9580/3	Granular cell tumor, malignant
M9172/0	Cavernous lymphangioma			M9581/3	Alveolar soft part sarcoma
M9173/0	Cystic lymphangioma	M9390/0	Choroid plexus papilloma NOS	M959-M963	**Lymphomas, NOS or diffuse**
M9174/0	Lymphangiomyoma	M9390/3	Choroid plexus papilloma, malignant	M9590/0	Lymphomatous tumor, benign
M9174/1	Lymphangiomyomatosis			M9590/3	Malignant lymphoma NOS
M9175/0	Hemolymphangioma	M9391/3	Ependymoma NOS	M9591/3	Malignant lymphoma, non Hodgkin's type
M918-M920	**Osteomas and osteosarcomas**	M9392/3	Ependymoma, anaplastic type		
M9180/0	Osteoma NOS	M9393/1	Papillary ependymoma	M9600/3	Malignant lymphoma, undifferentiated cell type NOS
M9180/3	Osteosarcoma NOS	M9394/1	Myxopapillary ependymoma		
M9181/3	Chondroblastic osteosarcoma	M9400/3	Astrocytoma NOS	M9601/3	Malignant lymphoma, stem cell type
M9182/3	Fibroblastic osteosarcoma	M9401/3	Astrocytoma, anaplastic type	M9602/3	Malignant lymphoma, convoluted cell type NOS
M9183/3	Telangiectatic osteosarcoma	M9410/3	Protoplasmic astrocytoma		
M9184/3	Osteosarcoma in Paget's disease of bone	M9411/3	Gemistocytic astrocytoma	M9610/3	Lymphosarcoma NOS
		M9420/3	Fibrillary astrocytoma	M9611/3	Malignant lymphoma, lymphoplasmacytoid type
M9190/3	Juxtacortical osteosarcoma	M9421/3	Pilocytic astrocytoma		
M9191/0	Osteoid osteoma NOS	M9422/3	Spongioblastoma NOS	M9612/3	Malignant lymphoma, immunoblastic type
M9200/0	Osteoblastoma	M9423/3	Spongioblastoma polare		
M921-M924	**Chondromatous neoplasms**	M9430/3	Astroblastoma	M9613/3	Malignant lymphoma, mixed lymphocytic-histiocytic NOS
M9210/0	Osteochondroma	M9440/3	Glioblastoma NOS		
M9210/1	Osteochondromatosis NOS	M9441/3	Giant cell glioblastoma	M9614/3	Malignant lymphoma, centroblastic-centrocytic, diffuse
M9220/0	Chondroma NOS	M9442/3	Glioblastoma with sarcomatous component		
M9220/1	Chondromatosis NOS			M9615/3	Malignant lymphoma, follicular center cell NOS
M9220/3	Chondrosarcoma NOS	M9443/3	Primitive polar spongioblastoma		
M9221/0	Juxtacortical chondroma	M9450/3	Oligodendroglioma NOS	M9620/3	Malignant lymphoma, lymphocytic, well differentiated NOS
M9221/3	Juxtacortical chondrosarcoma	M9451/3	Oligodendroglioma, anaplastic type		
M9230/0	Chondroblastoma NOS	M9460/3	Oligodendroblastoma	M9621/3	Malignant lymphoma, lymphocytic, intermediate differentiation NOS
M9230/3	Chondroblastoma, malignant	M9470/3	Medulloblastoma NOS		
M9240/3	Mesenchymal chondrosarcoma	M9471/3	Desmoplastic medulloblastoma	M9622/3	Malignant lymphoma, centrocytic
M9241/0	Chondromyxoid fibroma	M9472/3	Medullomyoblastoma	M9623/3	Malignant lymphoma, follicular center cell, cleaved NOS
M925	**Giant cell tumors**	M9480/3	Cerebellar sarcoma NOS		
M9250/1	Giant cell tumor of bone NOS	M9481/3	Monstrocellular sarcoma	M9630/3	Malignant lymphoma, lymphocytic, poorly differentiated NOS
M9250/3	Giant cell tumor of bone, malignant	M949-M952	**Neuroepitheliomatous neoplasms**		
M9251/0	Giant cell tumor of soft parts NOS	M9490/0	Ganglioneuroma	M9631/3	Prolymphocytic lymphosarcoma
M9251/3	Malignant giant cell tumor of soft parts	M9490/3	Ganglioneuroblastoma	M9632/3	Malignant lymphoma, centroblastic type NOS
		M9491/0	Ganglioneuromatosis		
M926	**Miscellaneous bone tumors**	M9500/3	Neuroblastoma NOS	M9633/3	Malignant lymphoma, follicular center cell, noncleaved NOS
M9260/3	Ewing's sarcoma	M9501/3	Medulloepithelioma NOS		
M9261/3	Adamantinoma of long bones	M9502/3	Teratoid medulloepithelioma	M964	**Reticulosarcomas**
M9262/0	Ossifying fibroma	M9503/3	Neuroepithelioma NOS	M9640/3	Reticulosarcoma NOS
M927-M934	**Odontogenic tumors**	M9504/3	Spongioneuroblastoma	M9641/3	Reticulosarcoma, pleomorphic cell type
M9270/0	Odontogenic tumor, benign	M9505/1	Ganglioglioma		
M9270/1	Odontogenic tumor NOS	M9506/0	Neurocytoma	M9642/3	Reticulosarcoma, nodular
M9270/3	Odontogenic tumor, malignant	M9507/0	Pacinian tumor	M965-M966	**Hodgkin's disease**
M9271/0	Dentinoma	M9510/3	Retinoblastoma NOS	M9650/3	Hodgkin's disease NOS
M9272/0	Cementoma NOS	M9511/3	Retinoblastoma, differentiated type	M9651/3	Hodgkin's disease, lymphocytic predominance
M9273/0	Cementoblastoma, benign	M9512/3	Retinoblastoma, undifferentiated type		
M9274/0	Cementifying fibroma			M9652/3	Hodgkin's disease, mixed cellularity
M9275/0	Gigantiform cementoma	M9520/3	Olfactory neurogenic tumor		
M9280/0	Odontoma NOS	M9521/3	Esthesioneurocytoma	M9653/3	Hodgkin's disease, lymphocytic depletion NOS
M9281/0	Compound odontoma	M9522/3	Esthesioneuroblastoma		
M9282/0	Complex odontoma	M9523/3	Esthesioneuroepithelioma	M9654/3	Hodgkin's disease, lymphocytic depletion, diffuse fibrosis
M9290/0	Ameloblastic fibro-odontoma	M953	**Meningiomas**		
M9290/3	Ameloblastic odontosarcoma	M9530/0	Meningioma NOS	M9655/3	Hodgkin's disease, lymphocytic depletion, reticular type
M9300/0	Adenomatoid odontogenic tumor	M9530/1	Meningiomatosis NOS		

APPENDIX A: MORPHOLOGY OF NEOPLASMS

M9656/3	Hodgkin's disease, nodular sclerosis NOS
M9657/3	Hodgkin's disease, nodular sclerosis, cellular phase
M9660/3	Hodgkin's paragranuloma
M9661/3	Hodgkin's granuloma
M9662/3	Hodgkin's sarcoma

M969   **Lymphomas, nodular or follicular**
- M9690/3   Malignant lymphoma, nodular NOS
- M9691/3   Malignant lymphoma, mixed lymphocytic-histiocytic, nodular
- M9692/3   Malignant lymphoma, centroblastic-centrocytic, follicular
- M9693/3   Malignant lymphoma, lymphocytic, well differentiated, nodular
- M9694/3   Malignant lymphoma, lymphocytic, intermediate differentiation, nodular
- M9695/3   Malignant lymphoma, follicular center cell, cleaved, follicular
- M9696/3   Malignant lymphoma, lymphocytic, poorly differentiated, nodular
- M9697/3   Malignant lymphoma, centroblastic type, follicular
- M9698/3   Malignant lymphoma, follicular center cell, noncleaved, follicular

M970   **Mycosis fungoides**
- M9700/3   Mycosis fungoides
- M9701/3   Sezary's disease

M971-M972   **Miscellaneous reticuloendothelial neoplasms**
- M9710/3   Microglioma
- M9720/3   Malignant histiocytosis
- M9721/3   Histiocytic medullary reticulosis
- M9722/3   Letterer-Siwe's disease

M973   **Plasma cell tumors**
- M9730/3   Plasma cell myeloma
- M9731/0   Plasma cell tumor, benign
- M9731/1   Plasmacytoma NOS
- M9731/3   Plasma cell tumor, malignant

M974   **Mast cell tumors**
- M9740/1   Mastocytoma NOS
- M9740/3   Mast cell sarcoma
- M9741/3   Malignant mastocytosis

M975   **Burkitt's tumor**
- M9750/3   Burkitt's tumor

M980-M994   **Leukemias**

M980   **Leukemias NOS**
- M9800/3   Leukemia NOS
- M9801/3   Acute leukemia NOS
- M9802/3   Subacute leukemia NOS
- M9803/3   Chronic leukemia NOS
- M9804/3   Aleukemic leukemia NOS

M981   **Compound leukemias**
- M9810/3   Compound leukemia

M982   **Lymphoid leukemias**
- M9820/3   Lymphoid leukemia NOS
- M9821/3   Acute lymphoid leukemia
- M9822/3   Subacute lymphoid leukemia
- M9823/3   Chronic lymphoid leukemia
- M9824/3   Aleukemic lymphoid leukemia
- M9825/3   Prolymphocytic leukemia

M983   **Plasma cell leukemias**
- M9830/3   Plasma cell leukemia

M984   **Erythroleukemias**
- M9840/3   Erythroleukemia
- M9841/3   Acute erythremia
- M9842/3   Chronic erythremia

M985   **Lymphosarcoma cell leukemias**
- M9850/3   Lymphosarcoma cell leukemia

M986   **Myeloid leukemias**
- M9860/3   Myeloid leukemia NOS
- M9861/3   Acute myeloid leukemia
- M9862/3   Subacute myeloid leukemia
- M9863/3   Chronic myeloid leukemia
- M9864/3   Aleukemic myeloid leukemia
- M9865/3   Neutrophilic leukemia
- M9866/3   Acute promyelocytic leukemia

M987   **Basophilic leukemias**
- M9870/3   Basophilic leukemia

M988   **Eosinophilic leukemias**
- M9880/3   Eosinophilic leukemia

M989   **Monocytic leukemias**
- M9890/3   Monocytic leukemia NOS
- M9891/3   Acute monocytic leukemia
- M9892/3   Subacute monocytic leukemia
- M9893/3   Chronic monocytic leukemia
- M9894/3   Aleukemic monocytic leukemia

M990-M994   **Miscellaneous leukemias**
- M9900/3   Mast cell leukemia
- M9910/3   Megakaryocytic leukemia
- M9920/3   Megakaryocytic myelosis
- M9930/3   Myeloid sarcoma
- M9940/3   Hairy cell leukemia

M995-M997   **Miscellaneous myeloproliferative and lymphoproliferative disorders**
- M9950/1   Polycythemia vera
- M9951/1   Acute panmyelosis
- M9960/1   Chronic myeloproliferative disease
- M9961/1   Myelosclerosis with myeloid metaplasia
- M9962/1   Idiopathic thrombocythemia
- M9970/1   Chronic lymphoproliferative disease

Appendix B was officially deleted October 1, 2004

APPENDIX C: CLASSIFICATION OF DRUGS BY AHFS LIST

CLASSIFICATION OF DRUGS BY AMERICAN HOSPITAL FORMULARY SERVICE LIST NUMBER AND THEIR ICD-9-CM EQUIVALENTS

The coding of adverse effects of drugs is keyed to the continually revised Hospital Formulary of the American Hospital Formulary Service (AHFS) published under the direction of the American Society of Hospital Pharmacists.

The following section gives the ICD-9-CM diagnosis code for each AHFS list.

	AHFS* List	ICD-9-CM Diagnosis Code
4:00	ANTIHISTAMINE DRUGS	963.0
8:00	ANTI-INFECTIVE AGENTS	
8:04	Amebacides	961.5
	hydroxyquinoline derivatives	961.3
	arsenical anti-infectives	961.1
8:08	Anthelmintics	961.6
	quinoline derivatives	961.3
8:12.04	Antifungal Antibiotics	960.1
	nonantibiotics	961.9
8:12.06	Cephalosporins	960.5
8:12.08	Chloramphenicol	960.2
8:12.12	The Erythromycins	960.3
8:12.16	The Penicillins	960.0
8:12.20	The Streptomycins	960.6
8:12.24	The Tetracyclines	960.4
8:12.28	Other Antibiotics	960.8
	antimycobacterial antibiotics	960.6
	macrolides	960.3
8:16	Antituberculars	961.8
	antibiotics	960.6
8:18	Antivirals	961.7
8:20	Plasmodicides (antimalarials)	961.4
8:24	Sulfonamides	961.0
8:26	The Sulfones	961.8
8:28	Treponemicides	961.2
8:32	Trichomonacides	961.5
	hydroxyquinoline derivatives	961.3
	nitrofuran derivatives	961.9
8:36	Urinary Germicides	961.9
	quinoline derivatives	961.3
8:40	Other Anti-Infectives	961.9
10:00	ANTINEOPLASTIC AGENTS	963.1
	antibiotics	960.7
	progestogens	962.2
12:00	AUTONOMIC DRUGS	
12:04	Parasympathomimetic (Cholinergic) Agents	971.0
12:08	Parasympatholytic (Cholinergic Blocking) Agents	971.1
12:12	Sympathomimetic (Adrenergic) Agents	971.2
12:16	Sympatholytic (Adrenergic Blocking) Agents	971.3
12:20	Skeletal Muscle Relaxants	975.2
	central nervous system muscle-tone depressants	968.0
16:00	BLOOD DERIVATIVES	964.7
20:00	BLOOD FORMATION AND COAGULATION	
20:04	Antianemia Drugs	964.1
20:04.04	Iron Preparations	964.0
20:04.08	Liver and Stomach Preparations	964.1
20:12.04	Anticoagulants	964.2
20:12.08	Antiheparin Agents	964.5
20:12.12	Coagulants	964.5
20:12.16	Hemostatics	964.5
	capillary-active drugs	972.8
	fibrinolysis-affecting agents	964.4
	natural products	964.7
24:00	CARDIOVASCULAR DRUGS	
24:04	Cardiac Drugs	972.9
	cardiotonic agents	972.1
	rhythm regulators	972.0
24:06	Antilipemic Agents	972.2
	thyroid derivatives	962.7
24:08	Hypotensive Agents	972.6
	adrenergic blocking agents	971.3
	ganglion-blocking agents	972.3
	vasodilators	972.5
24:12	Vasodilating Agents	972.5
	coronary	972.4
	nicotinic acid derivatives	972.2
24:16	Sclerosing Agents	972.7
28:00	CENTRAL NERVOUS SYSTEM DRUGS	
28:04	General Anesthetics	968.4
	gaseous anesthetics	968.2
	halothane	968.1
	intravenous anesthetics	968.3
28:08	Analgesics and Antipyretics	965.9
	antirheumatics	965.61-965.69
	aromatic analgesics	965.4
	non-narcotics NEC	965.7
	opium alkaloids	965.00
	heroin	965.01
	methadone	965.02
	specified type NEC	965.09
	pyrazole derivatives	965.5
	salicylates	965.1
	specified type NEC	965.8
28:10	Narcotic Antagonists	970.1
28:12	Anticonvulsants	966.3
	barbiturates	967.0
	benzodiazepine-based tranquilizers	969.4
	bromides	967.3
	hydantoin derivatives	966.1
	oxazolidine derivative	966.0
	succinimides	966.2
28:16.04	Antidepressants	969.0
28:16.08	Tranquilizers	969.5
	benzodiazepine-based	969.4
	butyrophenone-based	969.2
	major NEC	969.3
	phenothiazine-based	969.1
28:16.12	Other Psychotherapeutic Agents	969.8
28:20	Respiratory and Cerebral Stimulants	970.9
	analeptics	970.0
	anorexigenic agents	977.0
	psychostimulants	969.7
	specified type NEC	970.8
28:24	Sedatives and Hypnotics	967.9
	barbiturates	967.0
	benzodiazepine-based tranquilizers	969.4
	chloral hydrate group	967.1
	glutethamide group	967.5
	intravenous anesthetics	968.3
	methaqualone	967.4
	paraldehyde	967.2
	phenothiazine-based tranquilizers	969.1
	specified type NEC	967.8
	thiobarbiturates	968.3
	tranquilizer NEC	969.5
36:00	DIAGNOSTIC AGENTS	977.8
40:00	ELECTROLYTE, CALORIC, AND WATER BALANCE AGENTS NEC	974.5
40:04	Acidifying Agents	963.2
40:08	Alkalinizing Agents	963.3
40:10	Ammonia Detoxicants	974.5
40:12	Replacement Solutions NEC	974.5
	plasma volume expanders	964.8
40:16	Sodium-Removing Resins	974.5
40:18	Potassium-Removing Resins	974.5
40:20	Caloric Agents	974.5
40:24	Salt and Sugar Substitutes	974.5
40:28	Diuretics NEC	974.4
	carbonic acid anhydrase inhibitors	974.2
	mercurials	974.0
	purine derivatives	974.1
	saluretics	974.3
40:36	Irrigating Solutions	974.5
40:40	Uricosuric Agents	974.7
44:00	ENZYMES NEC	963.4
	fibrinolysis-affecting agents	964.4
	gastric agents	973.4

APPENDIX C: CLASSIFICATION OF DRUGS BY AHFS LIST

AHFS* List		ICD-9-CM Diagnosis Code
48:00	EXPECTORANTS AND COUGH PREPARATIONS	
	antihistamine agents	963.0
	antitussives	975.4
	codeine derivatives	965.09
	expectorants	975.5
	narcotic agents NEC	965.09
52:00	EYE, EAR, NOSE, AND THROAT PREPARATIONS	
52:04	Anti-Infectives	
	ENT	976.6
	ophthalmic	976.5
52:04.04	Antibiotics	
	ENT	976.6
	ophthalmic	976.5
52:04.06	Antivirals	
	ENT	976.6
	ophthalmic	976.5
52:04.08	Sulfonamides	
	ENT	976.6
	ophthalmic	976.5
52:04.12	Miscellaneous Anti-Infectives	
	ENT	976.6
	ophthalmic	976.5
52:08	Anti-Inflammatory Agents	
	ENT	976.6
	ophthalmic	976.5
52:10	Carbonic Anhydrase Inhibitors	974.2
52:12	Contact Lens Solutions	976.5
52:16	Local Anesthetics	968.5
52:20	Miotics	971.0
52:24	Mydriatics	
	adrenergics	971.2
	anticholinergics	971.1
	antimuscarinics	971.1
	parasympatholytics	971.1
	spasmolytics	971.1
	sympathomimetics	971.2
52:28	Mouth Washes and Gargles	976.6
52:32	Vasoconstrictors	971.2
52:36	Unclassified Agents	
	ENT	976.6
	ophthalmic	976.5
56:00	GASTROINTESTINAL DRUGS	
56:04	Antacids and Absorbents	973.0
56:08	Anti-Diarrhea Agents	973.5
56:10	Antiflatulents	973.8
56:12	Cathartics NEC	973.3
	emollients	973.2
	irritants	973.1
56:16	Digestants	973.4
56:20	Emetics and Antiemetics	
	antiemetics	963.0
	emetics	973.6
56:24	Lipotropic Agents	977.1
60:00	GOLD COMPOUNDS	965.69
64:00	HEAVY METAL ANTAGONISTS	963.8
68:00	HORMONES AND SYNTHETIC SUBSTITUTES	
68:04	Adrenals	962.0
68:08	Androgens	962.1
68:12	Contraceptives	962.2
68:16	Estrogens	962.2
68:18	Gonadotropins	962.4
68:20	Insulins and Antidiabetic Agents	962.3
68:20.08	Insulins	962.3
68:24	Parathyroid	962.6
68:28	Pituitary	
	anterior	962.4
	posterior	962.5
68:32	Progestogens	962.2
68:34	Other Corpus Luteum Hormones	962.2
68:36	Thyroid and Antithyroid	
	antithyroid	962.8
	thyroid	962.7

AHFS* List		ICD-9-CM Diagnosis Code
72:00	LOCAL ANESTHETICS NEC	968.9
	topical (surface) agents	968.5
	infiltrating agents (intradermal) (subcutaneous) (submucosal)	968.5
	nerve blocking agents (peripheral) (plexus) (regional)	968.6
	spinal	968.7
76:00	OXYTOCICS	975.0
78:00	RADIOACTIVE AGENTS	990
80:00	SERUMS, TOXOIDS, AND VACCINES	
80:04	Serums	979.9
	immune globulin (gamma) (human)	964.6
80:08	Toxoids NEC	978.8
	diphtheria	978.5
	and tetanus	978.9
	with pertussis component	978.6
	tetanus	978.4
	and diphtheria	978.9
	with pertussis component	978.6
80:12	Vaccines NEC	979.9
	bacterial NEC	978.8
	with	
	other bacterial component	978.9
	pertussis component	978.6
	viral and rickettsial component	979.7
	rickettsial NEC	979.6
	with	
	bacterial component	979.7
	pertussis component	978.6
	viral component	979.7
	viral NEC	979.6
	with	
	bacterial component	979.7
	pertussis component	978.6
	rickettsial component	979.7
84:00	SKIN AND MUCOUS MEMBRANE PREPARATIONS	
84:04	Anti-Infectives	976.0
84:04.04	Antibiotics	976.0
84:04.08	Fungicides	976.0
84:04.12	Scabicides and Pediculicides	976.0
84:04.16	Miscellaneous Local Anti-Infectives	976.0
84:06	Anti-Inflammatory Agents	976.0
84:08	Antipruritics and Local Anesthetics	
	antipruritics	976.1
	local anesthetics	968.5
84:12	Astringents	976.2
84:16	Cell Stimulants and Proliferants	976.8
84:20	Detergents	976.2
84:24	Emollients, Demulcents, and Protectants	976.3
84:28	Keratolytic Agents	976.4
84:32	Keratoplastic Agents	976.4
84:36	Miscellaneous Agents	976.8
86:00	SPASMOLYTIC AGENTS	975.1
	antiasthmatics	975.7
	papaverine	972.5
	theophyllin	974.1
88:00	VITAMINS	
88:04	Vitamin A	963.5
88:08	Vitamin B Complex	963.5
	hematopoietic vitamin	964.1
	nicotinic acid derivatives	972.2
88:12	Vitamin C	963.5
88:16	Vitamin D	963.5
88:20	Vitamin E	963.5
88:24	Vitamin K Activity	964.3
88:28	Multivitamin Preparations	963.5
92:00	UNCLASSIFIED THERAPEUTIC AGENTS	977.8

* American Hospital Formulary Service

APPENDIX D: INDUSTRIAL ACCIDENTS ACCORDING TO AGENCY

CLASSIFICATION OF INDUSTRIAL ACCIDENTS ACCORDING TO AGENCY
Annex B to the Resolution concerning Statistics of Employment Injuries adopted by the Tenth International Conference of Labor Statisticians on 12 October 1962

1 MACHINES

11	**Prime-Movers, except Electrical Motors**
111	*Steam engines*
112	*Internal combustion engines*
119	*Others*
12	**Transmission Machinery**
121	*Transmission shafts*
122	*Transmission belts, cables, pulleys, pinions, chains, gears*
129	*Others*
13	**Metalworking Machines**
131	*Power presses*
132	*Lathes*
133	*Milling machines*
134	*Abrasive wheels*
135	*Mechanical shears*
136	*Forging machines*
137	*Rolling-mills*
139	*Others*
14	**Wood and Assimilated Machines**
141	*Circular saws*
142	*Other saws*
143	*Molding machines*
144	*Overhand planes*
149	*Others*
15	**Agricultural Machines**
151	*Reapers (including combine reapers)*
152	*Threshers*
159	*Others*
16	**Mining Machinery**
161	*Under-cutters*
169	*Others*
19	**Other Machines Not Elsewhere Classified**
191	*Earth-moving machines, excavating and scraping machines, except means of transport*
192	*Spinning, weaving and other textile machines*
193	*Machines for the manufacture of foodstuffs and beverages*
194	*Machines for the manufacture of paper*
195	*Printing machines*
199	*Others*

2 MEANS OF TRANSPORT AND LIFTING EQUIPMENT

21	**Lifting Machines and Appliances**
211	*Cranes*
212	*Lifts and elevators*
213	*Winches*
214	*Pulley blocks*
219	*Others*
22	**Means of Rail Transport**
221	*Inter-urban railways*
222	*Rail transport in mines, tunnels, quarries, industrial establishments, docks, etc.*
229	*Others*
23	**Other Wheeled Means of Transport, Excluding Rail Transport**
231	*Tractors*
232	*Lorries*
233	*Trucks*
234	*Motor vehicles, not elsewhere classified*
235	*Animal-drawn vehicles*
236	*Hand-drawn vehicles*
239	*Others*
24	**Means of Air Transport**
25	**Means of Water Transport**
251	*Motorized means of water transport*
252	*Non-motorized means of water transport*
26	**Other Means of Transport**
261	*Cable-cars*
262	*Mechanical conveyors, except cable-cars*
269	*Others*

3 OTHER EQUIPMENT

31	**Pressure Vessels**
311	*Boilers*
312	*Pressurized containers*
313	*Pressurized piping and accessories*
314	*Gas cylinders*
315	*Caissons, diving equipment*
319	*Others*
32	**Furnaces, Ovens, Kilns**
321	*Blast furnaces*
322	*Refining furnaces*
323	*Other furnaces*
324	*Kilns*
325	*Ovens*
33	**Refrigerating Plants**
34	**Electrical Installations, Including Electric Motors, but Excluding Electric Hand Tools**
341	*Rotating machines*
342	*Conductors*
343	*Transformers*
344	*Control apparatus*
349	*Others*
35	**Electric Hand Tools**
36	**Tools, Implements, and Appliances, Except Electric Hand Tools**
361	*Power-driven hand tools, except electric hand tools*
362	*Hand tools, not power-driven*
369	*Others*
37	**Ladders, Mobile Ramps**
38	**Scaffolding**
39	**Other Equipment, Not Elsewhere Classified**

4 MATERIALS, SUBSTANCES AND RADIATIONS

41	**Explosives**
42	**Dusts, Gases, Liquids and Chemicals, Excluding Explosives**
421	*Dusts*
422	*Gases, vapors, fumes*
423	*Liquids, not elsewhere classified*
424	*Chemicals, not elsewhere classified*
43	**Flying Fragments**
44	**Radiations**
441	*Ionizing radiations*
449	*Others*
49	**Other Materials and Substances Not Elsewhere Classified**

5 WORKING ENVIRONMENT

51	**Outdoor**
511	*Weather*
512	*Traffic and working surfaces*
513	*Water*
519	*Others*
52	**Indoor**
521	*Floors*
522	*Confined quarters*
523	*Stairs*
524	*Other traffic and working surfaces*
525	*Floor openings and wall openings*
526	*Environmental factors (lighting, ventilation, temperature, noise, etc.)*
529	*Others*
53	**Underground**
531	*Roofs and faces of mine roads and tunnels, etc.*
532	*Floors of mine roads and tunnels, etc.*
533	*Working-faces of mines, tunnels, etc.*
534	*Mine shafts*
535	*Fire*
536	*Water*
539	*Others*

6 OTHER AGENCIES, NOT ELSEWHERE CLASSIFIED

61	**Animals**
611	*Live animals*
612	*Animal products*
69	**Other Agencies, Not Elsewhere Classified**

7 AGENCIES NOT CLASSIFIED FOR LACK OF SUFFICIENT DATA

APPENDIX E: LIST OF THREE-DIGIT CATEGORIES

LIST OF THREE-DIGIT CATEGORIES

1. INFECTIOUS AND PARASITIC DISEASES

Intestinal infectious diseases (001-009)
- 001 Cholera
- 002 Typhoid and paratyphoid fevers
- 003 Other salmonella infections
- 004 Shigellosis
- 005 Other food poisoning (bacterial)
- 006 Amebiasis
- 007 Other protozoal intestinal diseases
- 008 Intestinal infections due to other organisms
- 009 Ill-defined intestinal infections

Tuberculosis (010-018)
- 010 Primary tuberculous infection
- 011 Pulmonary tuberculosis
- 012 Other respiratory tuberculosis
- 013 Tuberculosis of meninges and central nervous system
- 014 Tuberculosis of intestines, peritoneum, and mesenteric glands
- 015 Tuberculosis of bones and joints
- 016 Tuberculosis of genitourinary system
- 017 Tuberculosis of other organs
- 018 Miliary tuberculosis

Zoonotic bacterial diseases (020-027)
- 020 Plague
- 021 Tularemia
- 022 Anthrax
- 023 Brucellosis
- 024 Glanders
- 025 Melioidosis
- 026 Rat-bite fever
- 027 Other zoonotic bacterial diseases

Other bacterial diseases (030-042)
- 030 Leprosy
- 031 Diseases due to other mycobacteria
- 032 Diphtheria
- 033 Whooping cough
- 034 Streptococcal sore throat and scarlatina
- 035 Erysipelas
- 036 Meningococcal infection
- 037 Tetanus
- 038 Septicemia
- 039 Actinomycotic infections
- 040 Other bacterial diseases
- 041 Bacterial infection in conditions classified elsewhere and of unspecified site

Human immunodeficiency virus (042)
- 042 Human immunodeficiency virus [HIV] disease

Poliomyelitis and other non-arthropod-borne viral diseases of central nervous system (045-049)
- 045 Acute poliomyelitis
- 046 Slow virus infection of central nervous system
- 047 Meningitis due to enterovirus
- 048 Other enterovirus diseases of central nervous system
- 049 Other non-arthropod-borne viral diseases of central nervous system

Viral diseases accompanied by exanthem (050-057)
- 050 Smallpox
- 051 Cowpox and paravaccinia
- 052 Chickenpox
- 053 Herpes zoster
- 054 Herpes simplex
- 055 Measles
- 056 Rubella
- 057 Other viral exanthemata

Arthropod-borne viral diseases (060-066)
- 060 Yellow fever
- 061 Dengue
- 062 Mosquito-borne viral encephalitis
- 063 Tick-borne viral encephalitis
- 064 Viral encephalitis transmitted by other and unspecified arthropods
- 065 Arthropod-borne hemorrhagic fever
- 066 Other arthropod-borne viral diseases

Other diseases due to viruses and Chlamydiae (070-079)
- 070 Viral hepatitis
- 071 Rabies
- 072 Mumps
- 073 Ornithosis
- 074 Specific diseases due to Coxsackievirus
- 075 Infectious mononucleosis
- 076 Trachoma
- 077 Other diseases of conjunctiva due to viruses and Chlamydiae
- 078 Other diseases due to viruses and Chlamydiae
- 079 Viral infection in conditions classified elsewhere and of unspecified site

Rickettsioses and other arthropod-borne diseases (080-088)
- 080 Louse-borne [epidemic] typhus
- 081 Other typhus
- 082 Tick-borne rickettsioses
- 083 Other rickettsioses
- 084 Malaria
- 085 Leishmaniasis
- 086 Trypanosomiasis
- 087 Relapsing fever
- 088 Other arthropod-borne diseases

Syphilis and other venereal diseases (090-099)
- 090 Congenital syphilis
- 091 Early syphilis, symptomatic
- 092 Early syphilis, latent
- 093 Cardiovascular syphilis
- 094 Neurosyphilis
- 095 Other forms of late syphilis, with symptoms
- 096 Late syphilis, latent
- 097 Other and unspecified syphilis
- 098 Gonococcal infections
- 099 Other venereal diseases

Other spirochetal diseases (100-104)
- 100 Leptospirosis
- 101 Vincent's angina
- 102 Yaws
- 103 Pinta
- 104 Other spirochetal infection

Mycoses (110-118)
- 110 Dermatophytosis
- 111 Dermatomycosis, other and unspecified
- 112 Candidiasis
- 114 Coccidioidomycosis
- 115 Histoplasmosis
- 116 Blastomycotic infection
- 117 Other mycoses
- 118 Opportunistic mycoses

Helminthiases (120-129)
- 120 Schistosomiasis [bilharziasis]
- 121 Other trematode infections
- 122 Echinococcosis
- 123 Other cestode infection
- 124 Trichinosis
- 125 Filarial infection and dracontiasis
- 126 Ancylostomiasis and necatoriasis
- 127 Other intestinal helminthiases
- 128 Other and unspecified helminthiases
- 129 Intestinal parasitism, unspecified

Other infectious and parasitic diseases (130-136)
- 130 Toxoplasmosis
- 131 Trichomoniasis
- 132 Pediculosis and phthirus infestation
- 133 Acariasis
- 134 Other infestation
- 135 Sarcoidosis
- 136 Other and unspecified infectious and parasitic diseases

Late effects of infectious and parasitic diseases (137-139)
- 137 Late effects of tuberculosis
- 138 Late effects of acute poliomyelitis
- 139 Late effects of other infectious and parasitic diseases

2. NEOPLASMS

Malignant neoplasm of lip, oral cavity, and pharynx (140-149)
- 140 Malignant neoplasm of lip
- 141 Malignant neoplasm of tongue
- 142 Malignant neoplasm of major salivary glands
- 143 Malignant neoplasm of gum
- 144 Malignant neoplasm of floor of mouth
- 145 Malignant neoplasm of other and unspecified parts of mouth
- 146 Malignant neoplasm of oropharynx
- 147 Malignant neoplasm of nasopharynx
- 148 Malignant neoplasm of hypopharynx
- 149 Malignant neoplasm of other and ill-defined sites within the lip, oral cavity, and pharynx

Malignant neoplasm of digestive organs and peritoneum (150-159)
- 150 Malignant neoplasm of esophagus
- 151 Malignant neoplasm of stomach
- 152 Malignant neoplasm of small intestine, including duodenum
- 153 Malignant neoplasm of colon
- 154 Malignant neoplasm of rectum, rectosigmoid junction, and anus
- 155 Malignant neoplasm of liver and intrahepatic bile ducts
- 156 Malignant neoplasm of gallbladder and extrahepatic bile ducts
- 157 Malignant neoplasm of pancreas
- 158 Malignant neoplasm of retroperitoneum and peritoneum
- 159 Malignant neoplasm of other and ill-defined sites within the digestive organs and peritoneum

Malignant neoplasm of respiratory and intrathoracic organs (160-165)
- 160 Malignant neoplasm of nasal cavities, middle ear, and accessory sinuses
- 161 Malignant neoplasm of larynx
- 162 Malignant neoplasm of trachea, bronchus, and lung
- 163 Malignant neoplasm of pleura
- 164 Malignant neoplasm of thymus, heart, and mediastinum
- 165 Malignant neoplasm of other and ill-defined sites within the respiratory system and intrathoracic organs

Malignant neoplasm of bone, connective tissue, skin, and breast (170-176)
- 170 Malignant neoplasm of bone and articular cartilage
- 171 Malignant neoplasm of connective and other soft tissue
- 172 Malignant melanoma of skin
- 173 Other malignant neoplasm of skin
- 174 Malignant neoplasm of female breast
- 175 Malignant neoplasm of male breast
- 176 Kaposi's sarcoma

Malignant neoplasm of genitourinary organs (179-189)
- 179 Malignant neoplasm of uterus, part unspecified
- 180 Malignant neoplasm of cervix uteri
- 181 Malignant neoplasm of placenta
- 182 Malignant neoplasm of body of uterus
- 183 Malignant neoplasm of ovary and other uterine adnexa
- 184 Malignant neoplasm of other and unspecified female genital organs
- 185 Malignant neoplasm of prostate

APPENDIX E: LIST OF THREE-DIGIT CATEGORIES

186 Malignant neoplasm of testis
187 Malignant neoplasm of penis and other male genital organs
188 Malignant neoplasm of bladder
189 Malignant neoplasm of kidney and other unspecified urinary organs

Malignant neoplasm of other and unspecified sites (190-199)
190 Malignant neoplasm of eye
191 Malignant neoplasm of brain
192 Malignant neoplasm of other and unspecified parts of nervous system
193 Malignant neoplasm of thyroid gland
194 Malignant neoplasm of other endocrine glands and related structures
195 Malignant neoplasm of other and ill-defined sites
196 Secondary and unspecified malignant neoplasm of lymph nodes
197 Secondary malignant neoplasm of respiratory and digestive systems
198 Secondary malignant neoplasm of other specified sites
199 Malignant neoplasm without specification of site

Malignant neoplasm of lymphatic and hematopoietic tissue (200-208)
200 Lymphosarcoma and reticulosarcoma
201 Hodgkin's disease
202 Other malignant neoplasm of lymphoid and histiocytic tissue
203 Multiple myeloma and immunoproliferative neoplasms
204 Lymphoid leukemia
205 Myeloid leukemia
206 Monocytic leukemia
207 Other specified leukemia
208 Leukemia of unspecified cell type

Benign neoplasms (210-229)
210 Benign neoplasm of lip, oral cavity, and pharynx
211 Benign neoplasm of other parts of digestive system
212 Benign neoplasm of respiratory and intrathoracic organs
213 Benign neoplasm of bone and articular cartilage
214 Lipoma
215 Other benign neoplasm of connective and other soft tissue
216 Benign neoplasm of skin
217 Benign neoplasm of breast
218 Uterine leiomyoma
219 Other benign neoplasm of uterus
220 Benign neoplasm of ovary
221 Benign neoplasm of other female genital organs
222 Benign neoplasm of male genital organs
223 Benign neoplasm of kidney and other urinary organs
224 Benign neoplasm of eye
225 Benign neoplasm of brain and other parts of nervous system
226 Benign neoplasm of thyroid gland
227 Benign neoplasm of other endocrine glands and related structures
228 Hemangioma and lymphangioma, any site
229 Benign neoplasm of other and unspecified sites

Carcinoma in situ (230-234)
230 Carcinoma in situ of digestive organs
231 Carcinoma in situ of respiratory system
232 Carcinoma in situ of skin
233 Carcinoma in situ of breast and genitourinary system
234 Carcinoma in situ of other and unspecified sites

Neoplasms of uncertain behavior (235-238)
235 Neoplasm of uncertain behavior of digestive and respiratory systems
236 Neoplasm of uncertain behavior of genitourinary organs
237 Neoplasm of uncertain behavior of endocrine glands and nervous system
238 Neoplasm of uncertain behavior of other and unspecified sites and tissues

Neoplasms of unspecified nature (239)
239 Neoplasm of unspecified nature

3. ENDOCRINE, NUTRITIONAL AND METABOLIC DISEASES, AND IMMUNITY DISORDERS

Disorders of thyroid gland (240-246)
240 Simple and unspecified goiter
241 Nontoxic nodular goiter
242 Thyrotoxicosis with or without goiter
243 Congenital hypothyroidism
244 Acquired hypothyroidism
245 Thyroiditis
246 Other disorders of thyroid

Diseases of other endocrine glands (250-259)
250 Diabetes mellitus
251 Other disorders of pancreatic internal secretion
252 Disorders of parathyroid gland
253 Disorders of the pituitary gland and its hypothalamic control
254 Diseases of thymus gland
255 Disorders of adrenal glands
256 Ovarian dysfunction
257 Testicular dysfunction
258 Polyglandular dysfunction and related disorders
259 Other endocrine disorders

Nutritional deficiencies (260-269)
260 Kwashiorkor
261 Nutritional marasmus
262 Other severe protein-calorie malnutrition
263 Other and unspecified protein-calorie malnutrition
264 Vitamin A deficiency
265 Thiamine and niacin deficiency states
266 Deficiency of B-complex components
267 Ascorbic acid deficiency
268 Vitamin D deficiency
269 Other nutritional deficiencies

Other metabolic disorders and immunity disorders (270-279)
270 Disorders of amino-acid transport and metabolism
271 Disorders of carbohydrate transport and metabolism
272 Disorders of lipoid metabolism
273 Disorders of plasma protein metabolism
274 Gout
275 Disorders of mineral metabolism
276 Disorders of fluid, electrolyte, and acid-base balance
277 Other and unspecified disorders of metabolism
278 Overweight, obesity and other hyperalimentation
279 Disorders involving the immune mechanism

4. DISEASES OF BLOOD AND BLOOD-FORMING ORGANS (280-289)
280 Iron deficiency anemias
281 Other deficiency anemias
282 Hereditary hemolytic anemias
283 Acquired hemolytic anemias
284 Aplastic anemia
285 Other and unspecified anemias
286 Coagulation defects
287 Purpura and other hemorrhagic conditions
288 Diseases of white blood cells
289 Other diseases of blood and blood-forming organs

5. MENTAL DISORDERS

Organic psychotic conditions (290-294)
290 Senile and presenile organic psychotic conditions
291 Alcoholic psychoses
292 Drug psychoses
293 Transient organic psychotic conditions
294 Other organic psychotic conditions (chronic)

Other psychoses (295-299)
295 Schizophrenic psychoses
296 Affective psychoses
297 Paranoid states
298 Other nonorganic psychoses
299 Psychoses with origin specific to childhood

Neurotic disorders, personality disorders, and other nonpsychotic mental disorders (300-316)
300 Neurotic disorders
301 Personality disorders
302 Sexual deviations and disorders
303 Alcohol dependence syndrome
304 Drug dependence
305 Nondependent abuse of drugs
306 Physiological malfunction arising from mental factors
307 Special symptoms or syndromes, not elsewhere classified
308 Acute reaction to stress
309 Adjustment reaction
310 Specific nonpsychotic mental disorders following organic brain damage
311 Depressive disorder, not elsewhere classified
312 Disturbance of conduct, not elsewhere classified
313 Disturbance of emotions specific to childhood and adolescence
314 Hyperkinetic syndrome of childhood
315 Specific delays in development
316 Psychic factors associated with diseases classified elsewhere

Mental retardation (317-319)
317 Mild mental retardation
318 Other specified mental retardation
319 Unspecified mental retardation

6. DISEASES OF THE NERVOUS SYSTEM AND SENSE ORGANS

Inflammatory diseases of the central nervous system (320-326)
320 Bacterial meningitis
321 Meningitis due to other organisms
322 Meningitis of unspecified cause
323 Encephalitis, myelitis, and encephalomyelitis
324 Intracranial and intraspinal abscess
325 Phlebitis and thrombophlebitis of intracranial venous sinuses
326 Late effects of intracranial abscess or pyogenic infection

Organic Sleep Disorders (327)
327 Organic sleep disorders

Hereditary and degenerative diseases of the central nervous system (330-337)
330 Cerebral degenerations usually manifest in childhood
331 Other cerebral degenerations
332 Parkinson's disease
333 Other extrapyramidal diseases and abnormal movement disorders
334 Spinocerebellar disease
335 Anterior horn cell disease
336 Other diseases of spinal cord
337 Disorders of the autonomic nervous system

Pain (338)
338 Pain, not elsewhere classified

APPENDIX E: LIST OF THREE-DIGIT CATEGORIES

Other disorders of the central nervous system (340-349)
340 Multiple sclerosis
341 Other demyelinating diseases of central nervous system
342 Hemiplegia and hemiparesis
343 Infantile cerebral palsy
344 Other paralytic syndromes
345 Epilepsy and recurrent seizures
346 Migraine
347 Cataplexy and narcolepsy
348 Other conditions of brain
349 Other and unspecified disorders of the nervous system

Disorders of the peripheral nervous system (350-359)
350 Trigeminal nerve disorders
351 Facial nerve disorders
352 Disorders of other cranial nerves
353 Nerve root and plexus disorders
354 Mononeuritis of upper limb and mononeuritis multiplex
355 Mononeuritis of lower limb
356 Hereditary and idiopathic peripheral neuropathy
357 Inflammatory and toxic neuropathy
358 Myoneural disorders
359 Muscular dystrophies and other myopathies

Disorders of the eye and adnexa (360-379)
360 Disorders of the globe
361 Retinal detachments and defects
362 Other retinal disorders
363 Chorioretinal inflammations and scars and other disorders of choroid
364 Disorders of iris and ciliary body
365 Glaucoma
366 Cataract
367 Disorders of refraction and accommodation
368 Visual disturbances
369 Blindness and low vision
370 Keratitis
371 Corneal opacity and other disorders of cornea
372 Disorders of conjunctiva
373 Inflammation of eyelids
374 Other disorders of eyelids
375 Disorders of lacrimal system
376 Disorders of the orbit
377 Disorders of optic nerve and visual pathways
378 Strabismus and other disorders of binocular eye movements
379 Other disorders of eye

Diseases of the ear and mastoid process (380-389)
380 Disorders of external ear
381 Nonsuppurative otitis media and Eustachian tube disorders
382 Suppurative and unspecified otitis media
383 Mastoiditis and related conditions
384 Other disorders of tympanic membrane
385 Other disorders of middle ear and mastoid
386 Vertiginous syndromes and other disorders of vestibular system
387 Otosclerosis
388 Other disorders of ear
389 Hearing loss

7. DISEASES OF THE CIRCULATORY SYSTEM

Acute rheumatic fever (390-392)
390 Rheumatic fever without mention of heart involvement
391 Rheumatic fever with heart involvement
392 Rheumatic chorea

Chronic rheumatic heart disease (393-398)
393 Chronic rheumatic pericarditis
394 Diseases of mitral valve
395 Diseases of aortic valve
396 Diseases of mitral and aortic valves
397 Diseases of other endocardial structures
398 Other rheumatic heart disease

Hypertensive disease (401-405)
401 Essential hypertension
402 Hypertensive heart disease
403 Hypertensive kidney disease
404 Hypertensive heart and kidney disease
405 Secondary hypertension

Ischemic heart disease (410-414)
410 Acute myocardial infarction
411 Other acute and subacute form of ischemic heart disease
412 Old myocardial infarction
413 Angina pectoris
414 Other forms of chronic ischemic heart disease

Diseases of pulmonary circulation (415-417)
415 Acute pulmonary heart disease
416 Chronic pulmonary heart disease
417 Other diseases of pulmonary circulation

Other forms of heart disease (420-429)
420 Acute pericarditis
421 Acute and subacute endocarditis
422 Acute myocarditis
423 Other diseases of pericardium
424 Other diseases of endocardium
425 Cardiomyopathy
426 Conduction disorders
427 Cardiac dysrhythmias
428 Heart failure
429 Ill-defined descriptions and complications of heart disease

Cerebrovascular disease (430-438)
430 Subarachnoid hemorrhage
431 Intracerebral hemorrhage
432 Other and unspecified intracranial hemorrhage
433 Occlusion and stenosis of precerebral arteries
434 Occlusion of cerebral arteries
435 Transient cerebral ischemia
436 Acute but ill-defined cerebrovascular disease
437 Other and ill-defined cerebrovascular disease
438 Late effects of cerebrovascular disease

Diseases of arteries, arterioles, and capillaries (440-448)
440 Atherosclerosis
441 Aortic aneurysm and dissection
442 Other aneurysm
443 Other peripheral vascular disease
444 Arterial embolism and thrombosis
445 Atheroembolism
446 Polyarteritis nodosa and allied conditions
447 Other disorders of arteries and arterioles
448 Diseases of capillaries

Diseases of veins and lymphatics, and other diseases of circulatory system (451-459)
451 Phlebitis and thrombophlebitis
452 Portal vein thrombosis
453 Other venous embolism and thrombosis
454 Varicose veins of lower extremities
455 Hemorrhoids
456 Varicose veins of other sites
457 Noninfective disorders of lymphatic channels
458 Hypotension
459 Other disorders of circulatory system

8. DISEASES OF THE RESPIRATORY SYSTEM

Acute respiratory infections (460-466)
460 Acute nasopharyngitis [common cold]
461 Acute sinusitis
462 Acute pharyngitis
463 Acute tonsillitis
464 Acute laryngitis and tracheitis
465 Acute upper respiratory infections of multiple or unspecified sites
466 Acute bronchitis and bronchiolitis

Other diseases of upper respiratory tract (470-478)
470 Deviated nasal septum
471 Nasal polyps
472 Chronic pharyngitis and nasopharyngitis
473 Chronic sinusitis
474 Chronic disease of tonsils and adenoids
475 Peritonsillar abscess
476 Chronic laryngitis and laryngotracheitis
477 Allergic rhinitis
478 Other diseases of upper respiratory tract

Pneumonia and influenza (480-487)
480 Viral pneumonia
481 Pneumococcal pneumonia [Streptococcus pneumoniae pneumonia]
482 Other bacterial pneumonia
483 Pneumonia due to other specified organism
484 Pneumonia in infectious diseases classified elsewhere
485 Bronchopneumonia, organism unspecified
486 Pneumonia, organism unspecified
487 Influenza

Chronic obstructive pulmonary disease and allied conditions (490-496)
490 Bronchitis, not specified as acute or chronic
491 Chronic bronchitis
492 Emphysema
493 Asthma
494 Bronchiectasis
495 Extrinsic allergic alveolitis
496 Chronic airways obstruction, not elsewhere classified

Pneumoconioses and other lung diseases due to external agents (500-508)
500 Coal workers' pneumoconiosis
501 Asbestosis
502 Pneumoconiosis due to other silica or silicates
503 Pneumoconiosis due to other inorganic dust
504 Pneumopathy due to inhalation of other dust
505 Pneumoconiosis, unspecified
506 Respiratory conditions due to chemical fumes and vapors
507 Pneumonitis due to solids and liquids
508 Respiratory conditions due to other and unspecified external agents

Other diseases of respiratory system (510-519)
510 Empyema
511 Pleurisy
512 Pneumothorax
513 Abscess of lung and mediastinum
514 Pulmonary congestion and hypostasis
515 Postinflammatory pulmonary fibrosis
516 Other alveolar and parietoalveolar pneumopathy
517 Lung involvement in conditions classified elsewhere
518 Other diseases of lung
519 Other diseases of respiratory system

9. DISEASES OF THE DIGESTIVE SYSTEM

Diseases of oral cavity, salivary glands, and jaws (520-529)
520 Disorders of tooth development and eruption
521 Diseases of hard tissues of teeth
522 Diseases of pulp and periapical tissues
523 Gingival and periodontal diseases
524 Dentofacial anomalies, including malocclusion
525 Other diseases and conditions of the teeth and supporting structures
526 Diseases of the jaws
527 Diseases of the salivary glands

APPENDIX E: LIST OF THREE-DIGIT CATEGORIES

528 Diseases of the oral soft tissues, excluding lesions specific for gingiva and tongue
529 Diseases and other conditions of the tongue

Diseases of esophagus, stomach, and duodenum (530-538)
530 Diseases of esophagus
531 Gastric ulcer
532 Duodenal ulcer
533 Peptic ulcer, site unspecified
534 Gastrojejunal ulcer
535 Gastritis and duodenitis
536 Disorders of function of stomach
537 Other disorders of stomach and duodenum
538 Gastrointestinal mucositis (ulcerative)

Appendicitis (540-543)
540 Acute appendicitis
541 Appendicitis, unqualified
542 Other appendicitis
543 Other diseases of appendix

Hernia of abdominal cavity (550-553)
550 Inguinal hernia
551 Other hernia of abdominal cavity, with gangrene
552 Other hernia of abdominal cavity, with obstruction, but without mention of gangrene
553 Other hernia of abdominal cavity without mention of obstruction or gangrene

Noninfective enteritis and colitis (555-558)
555 Regional enteritis
556 Ulcerative colitis
557 Vascular insufficiency of intestine
558 Other noninfective gastroenteritis and colitis

Other diseases of intestines and peritoneum (560-569)
560 Intestinal obstruction without mention of hernia
562 Diverticula of intestine
564 Functional digestive disorders, not elsewhere classified
565 Anal fissure and fistula
566 Abscess of anal and rectal regions
567 Peritonitis and retroperitoneal infections
568 Other disorders of peritoneum
569 Other disorders of intestine

Other diseases of digestive system (570-579)
570 Acute and subacute necrosis of liver
571 Chronic liver disease and cirrhosis
572 Liver abscess and sequelae of chronic liver disease
573 Other disorders of liver
574 Cholelithiasis
575 Other disorders of gallbladder
576 Other disorders of biliary tract
577 Diseases of pancreas
578 Gastrointestinal hemorrhage
579 Intestinal malabsorption

10. DISEASES OF THE GENITOURINARY SYSTEM

Nephritis, nephrotic syndrome, and nephrosis (580-589)
580 Acute glomerulonephritis
581 Nephrotic syndrome
582 Chronic glomerulonephritis
583 Nephritis and nephropathy, not specified as acute or chronic
584 Acute renal failure
585 Chronic kidney disease (CKD)
586 Renal failure, unspecified
587 Renal sclerosis, unspecified
588 Disorders resulting from impaired renal function
589 Small kidney of unknown cause

Other diseases of urinary system (590-599)
590 Infections of kidney
591 Hydronephrosis
592 Calculus of kidney and ureter
593 Other disorders of kidney and ureter
594 Calculus of lower urinary tract
595 Cystitis
596 Other disorders of bladder
597 Urethritis, not sexually transmitted, and urethral syndrome
598 Urethral stricture
599 Other disorders of urethra and urinary tract

Diseases of male genital organs (600-608)
600 Hyperplasia of prostate
601 Inflammatory diseases of prostate
602 Other disorders of prostate
603 Hydrocele
604 Orchitis and epididymitis
605 Redundant prepuce and phimosis
606 Infertility, male
607 Disorders of penis
608 Other disorders of male genital organs

Disorders of breast (610-611)
610 Benign mammary dysplasias
611 Other disorders of breast

Inflammatory disease of female pelvic organs (614-616)
614 Inflammatory disease of ovary, fallopian tube, pelvic cellular tissue, and peritoneum
615 Inflammatory diseases of uterus, except cervix
616 Inflammatory disease of cervix, vagina, and vulva

Other disorders of female genital tract (617-629)
617 Endometriosis
618 Genital prolapse
619 Fistula involving female genital tract
620 Noninflammatory disorders of ovary, fallopian tube, and broad ligament
621 Disorders of uterus, not elsewhere classified
622 Noninflammatory disorders of cervix
623 Noninflammatory disorders of vagina
624 Noninflammatory disorders of vulva and perineum
625 Pain and other symptoms associated with female genital organs
626 Disorders of menstruation and other abnormal bleeding from female genital tract
627 Menopausal and postmenopausal disorders
628 Infertility, female
629 Other disorders of female genital organs

11. COMPLICATIONS OF PREGNANCY, CHILDBIRTH AND THE PUERPERIUM

Ectopic and molar pregnancy and other pregnancy with abortive outcome (630-639)
630 Hydatidiform mole
631 Other abnormal product of conception
632 Missed abortion
633 Ectopic pregnancy
634 Spontaneous abortion
635 Legally induced abortion
636 Illegally induced abortion
637 Unspecified abortion
638 Failed attempted abortion
639 Complications following abortion and ectopic and molar pregnancies

Complications mainly related to pregnancy (640-649)
640 Hemorrhage in early pregnancy
641 Antepartum hemorrhage, abruptio placentae, and placenta previa
642 Hypertension complicating pregnancy, childbirth, and the puerperium
643 Excessive vomiting in pregnancy
644 Early or threatened labor
645 Prolonged pregnancy
646 Other complications of pregnancy, not elsewhere classified
647 Infective and parasitic conditions in the mother classifiable elsewhere but complicating pregnancy, childbirth, and the puerperium
648 Other current conditions in the mother classifiable elsewhere but complicating pregnancy, childbirth, and the puerperium
649 Other conditions or status of the mother complicating pregnancy, childbirth, or puerperium

Normal delivery, and other indications for care in pregnancy, labor, and delivery (650-659)
650 Normal delivery
651 Multiple gestation
652 Malposition and malpresentation of fetus
653 Disproportion
654 Abnormality of organs and soft tissues of pelvis
655 Known or suspected fetal abnormality affecting management of mother
656 Other fetal and placental problems affecting management of mother
657 Polyhydramnios
658 Other problems associated with amniotic cavity and membranes
659 Other indications for care or intervention related to labor and delivery and not elsewhere classified

Complications occurring mainly in the course of labor and delivery (660-669)
660 Obstructed labor
661 Abnormality of forces of labor
662 Long labor
663 Umbilical cord complications
664 Trauma to perineum and vulva during delivery
665 Other obstetrical trauma
666 Postpartum hemorrhage
667 Retained placenta or membranes, without hemorrhage
668 Complications of the administration of anesthetic or other sedation in labor and delivery
669 Other complications of labor and delivery, not elsewhere classified

Complications of the puerperium (670-677)
670 Major puerperal infection
671 Venous complications in pregnancy and the puerperium
672 Pyrexia of unknown origin during the puerperium
673 Obstetrical pulmonary embolism
674 Other and unspecified complications of the puerperium, not elsewhere classified
675 Infections of the breast and nipple associated with childbirth
676 Other disorders of the breast associated with childbirth, and disorders of lactation
677 Late effect of complication of pregnancy, childbirth, and the puerperium

12. DISEASES OF THE SKIN AND SUBCUTANEOUS TISSUE

Infections of skin and subcutaneous tissue (680-686)
680 Carbuncle and furuncle
681 Cellulitis and abscess of finger and toe
682 Other cellulitis and abscess
683 Acute lymphadenitis
684 Impetigo
685 Pilonidal cyst
686 Other local infections of skin and subcutaneous tissue

Other inflammatory conditions of skin and subcutaneous tissue (690-698)
690 Erythematosquamous dermatosis
691 Atopic dermatitis and related conditions
692 Contact dermatitis and other eczema
693 Dermatitis due to substances taken internally
694 Bullous dermatoses
695 Erythematous conditions
696 Psoriasis and similar disorders

APPENDIX E: LIST OF THREE-DIGIT CATEGORIES

697 Lichen
698 Pruritus and related conditions

Other diseases of skin and subcutaneous tissue (700-709)
700 Corns and callosities
701 Other hypertrophic and atrophic conditions of skin
702 Other dermatoses
703 Diseases of nail
704 Diseases of hair and hair follicles
705 Disorders of sweat glands
706 Diseases of sebaceous glands
707 Chronic ulcer of skin
708 Urticaria
709 Other disorders of skin and subcutaneous tissue

13. DISEASES OF THE MUSCULOSKELETAL SYSTEM AND CONNECTIVE TISSUE

Arthropathies and related disorders (710-719)
710 Diffuse diseases of connective tissue
711 Arthropathy associated with infections
712 Crystal arthropathies
713 Arthropathy associated with other disorders classified elsewhere
714 Rheumatoid arthritis and other inflammatory polyarthropathies
715 Osteoarthrosis and allied disorders
716 Other and unspecified arthropathies
717 Internal derangement of knee
718 Other derangement of joint
719 Other and unspecified disorder of joint

Dorsopathies (720-724)
720 Ankylosing spondylitis and other inflammatory spondylopathies
721 Spondylosis and allied disorders
722 Intervertebral disc disorders
723 Other disorders of cervical region
724 Other and unspecified disorders of back

Rheumatism, excluding the back (725-729)
725 Polymyalgia rheumatica
726 Peripheral enthesopathies and allied syndromes
727 Other disorders of synovium, tendon, and bursa
728 Disorders of muscle, ligament, and fascia
729 Other disorders of soft tissues

Osteopathies, chondropathies, and acquired musculoskeletal deformities (730-739)
730 Osteomyelitis, periostitis, and other infections involving bone
731 Osteitis deformans and osteopathies associated with other disorders classified elsewhere
732 Osteochondropathies
733 Other disorders of bone and cartilage
734 Flat foot
735 Acquired deformities of toe
736 Other acquired deformities of limbs
737 Curvature of spine
738 Other acquired deformity
739 Nonallopathic lesions, not elsewhere classified

14. CONGENITAL ANOMALIES

740 Anencephalus and similar anomalies
741 Spina bifida
742 Other congenital anomalies of nervous system
743 Congenital anomalies of eye
744 Congenital anomalies of ear, face, and neck
745 Bulbus cordis anomalies and anomalies of cardiac septal closure
746 Other congenital anomalies of heart
747 Other congenital anomalies of circulatory system
748 Congenital anomalies of respiratory system
749 Cleft palate and cleft lip
750 Other congenital anomalies of upper alimentary tract
751 Other congenital anomalies of digestive system
752 Congenital anomalies of genital organs
753 Congenital anomalies of urinary system
754 Certain congenital musculoskeletal deformities
755 Other congenital anomalies of limbs
756 Other congenital musculoskeletal anomalies
757 Congenital anomalies of the integument
758 Chromosomal anomalies
759 Other and unspecified congenital anomalies

15. CERTAIN CONDITIONS ORIGINATING IN THE PERINATAL PERIOD

Maternal causes of perinatal morbidity and mortality (760-763)
760 Fetus or newborn affected by maternal conditions which may be unrelated to present pregnancy
761 Fetus or newborn affected by maternal complications of pregnancy
762 Fetus or newborn affected by complications of placenta, cord, and membranes
763 Fetus or newborn affected by other complications of labor and delivery

Other conditions originating in the perinatal period (764-779)
764 Slow fetal growth and fetal malnutrition
765 Disorders relating to short gestation and unspecified low birthweight
766 Disorders relating to long gestation and high birthweight
767 Birth trauma
768 Intrauterine hypoxia and birth asphyxia
769 Respiratory distress syndrome
770 Other respiratory conditions of fetus and newborn
771 Infections specific to the perinatal period
772 Fetal and neonatal hemorrhage
773 Hemolytic disease of fetus or newborn, due to isoimmunization
774 Other perinatal jaundice
775 Endocrine and metabolic disturbances specific to the fetus and newborn
776 Hematological disorders of fetus and newborn
777 Perinatal disorders of digestive system
778 Conditions involving the integument and temperature regulation of fetus and newborn
779 Other and ill-defined conditions originating in the perinatal period

16. SYMPTOMS, SIGNS, AND ILL-DEFINED CONDITIONS

Symptoms (780-789)
780 General symptoms
781 Symptoms involving nervous and musculoskeletal systems
782 Symptoms involving skin and other integumentary tissue
783 Symptoms concerning nutrition, metabolism, and development
784 Symptoms involving head and neck
785 Symptoms involving cardiovascular system
786 Symptoms involving respiratory system and other chest symptoms
787 Symptoms involving digestive system
788 Symptoms involving urinary system
789 Other symptoms involving abdomen and pelvis

Nonspecific abnormal findings (790-796)
790 Nonspecific findings on examination of blood
791 Nonspecific findings on examination of urine
792 Nonspecific abnormal findings in other body substances
793 Nonspecific abnormal findings on radiological and other examination of body structure
794 Nonspecific abnormal results of function studies
795 Nonspecific abnormal histological and immunological findings
796 Other nonspecific abnormal findings

Ill-defined and unknown causes of morbidity and mortality (797-799)
797 Senility without mention of psychosis
798 Sudden death, cause unknown
799 Other ill-defined and unknown causes of morbidity and mortality

17. INJURY AND POISONING

Fracture of skull (800-804)
800 Fracture of vault of skull
801 Fracture of base of skull
802 Fracture of face bones
803 Other and unqualified skull fractures
804 Multiple fractures involving skull or face with other bones

Fracture of spine and trunk (805-809)
805 Fracture of vertebral column without mention of spinal cord lesion
806 Fracture of vertebral column with spinal cord lesion
807 Fracture of rib(s), sternum, larynx, and trachea
808 Fracture of pelvis
809 Ill-defined fractures of bones of trunk

Fracture of upper limb (810-819)
810 Fracture of clavicle
811 Fracture of scapula
812 Fracture of humerus
813 Fracture of radius and ulna
814 Fracture of carpal bone(s)
815 Fracture of metacarpal bone(s)
816 Fracture of one or more phalanges of hand
817 Multiple fractures of hand bones
818 Ill-defined fractures of upper limb
819 Multiple fractures involving both upper limbs, and upper limb with rib(s) and sternum

Fracture of lower limb (820-829)
820 Fracture of neck of femur
821 Fracture of other and unspecified parts of femur
822 Fracture of patella
823 Fracture of tibia and fibula
824 Fracture of ankle
825 Fracture of one or more tarsal and metatarsal bones
826 Fracture of one or more phalanges of foot
827 Other, multiple, and ill-defined fractures of lower limb
828 Multiple fractures involving both lower limbs, lower with upper limb, and lower limb(s) with rib(s) and sternum
829 Fracture of unspecified bones

Dislocation (830-839)
830 Dislocation of jaw
831 Dislocation of shoulder
832 Dislocation of elbow
833 Dislocation of wrist
834 Dislocation of finger
835 Dislocation of hip
836 Dislocation of knee
837 Dislocation of ankle
838 Dislocation of foot
839 Other, multiple, and ill-defined dislocations

Sprains and strains of joints and adjacent muscles (840-848)
840 Sprains and strains of shoulder and upper arm
841 Sprains and strains of elbow and forearm
842 Sprains and strains of wrist and hand
843 Sprains and strains of hip and thigh

APPENDIX E: LIST OF THREE-DIGIT CATEGORIES

844 Sprains and strains of knee and leg
845 Sprains and strains of ankle and foot
846 Sprains and strains of sacroiliac region
847 Sprains and strains of other and unspecified parts of back
848 Other and ill-defined sprains and strains

Intracranial injury, excluding those with skull fracture (850-854)
850 Concussion
851 Cerebral laceration and contusion
852 Subarachnoid, subdural, and extradural hemorrhage, following injury
853 Other and unspecified intracranial hemorrhage following injury
854 Intracranial injury of other and unspecified nature

Internal injury of chest, abdomen, and pelvis (860-869)
860 Traumatic pneumothorax and hemothorax
861 Injury to heart and lung
862 Injury to other and unspecified intrathoracic organs
863 Injury to gastrointestinal tract
864 Injury to liver
865 Injury to spleen
866 Injury to kidney
867 Injury to pelvic organs
868 Injury to other intra-abdominal organs
869 Internal injury to unspecified or ill-defined organs

Open wound of head, neck, and trunk (870-879)
870 Open wound of ocular adnexa
871 Open wound of eyeball
872 Open wound of ear
873 Other open wound of head
874 Open wound of neck
875 Open wound of chest (wall)
876 Open wound of back
877 Open wound of buttock
878 Open wound of genital organs (external), including traumatic amputation
879 Open wound of other and unspecified sites, except limbs

Open wound of upper limb (880-887)
880 Open wound of shoulder and upper arm
881 Open wound of elbow, forearm, and wrist
882 Open wound of hand except finger(s) alone
883 Open wound of finger(s)
884 Multiple and unspecified open wound of upper limb
885 Traumatic amputation of thumb (complete) (partial)
886 Traumatic amputation of other finger(s) (complete) (partial)
887 Traumatic amputation of arm and hand (complete) (partial)

Open wound of lower limb (890-897)
890 Open wound of hip and thigh
891 Open wound of knee, leg [except thigh], and ankle
892 Open wound of foot except toe(s) alone
893 Open wound of toe(s)
894 Multiple and unspecified open wound of lower limb
895 Traumatic amputation of toe(s) (complete) (partial)
896 Traumatic amputation of foot (complete) (partial)
897 Traumatic amputation of leg(s) (complete) (partial)

Injury to blood vessels (900-904)
900 Injury to blood vessels of head and neck
901 Injury to blood vessels of thorax
902 Injury to blood vessels of abdomen and pelvis
903 Injury to blood vessels of upper extremity
904 Injury to blood vessels of lower extremity and unspecified sites

Late effects of injuries, poisonings, toxic effects, and other external causes (905-909)
905 Late effects of musculoskeletal and connective tissue injuries
906 Late effects of injuries to skin and subcutaneous tissues
907 Late effects of injuries to the nervous system
908 Late effects of other and unspecified injuries
909 Late effects of other and unspecified external causes

Superficial injury (910-919)
910 Superficial injury of face, neck, and scalp except eye
911 Superficial injury of trunk
912 Superficial injury of shoulder and upper arm
913 Superficial injury of elbow, forearm, and wrist
914 Superficial injury of hand(s) except finger(s) alone
915 Superficial injury of finger(s)
916 Superficial injury of hip, thigh, leg, and ankle
917 Superficial injury of foot and toe(s)
918 Superficial injury of eye and adnexa
919 Superficial injury of other, multiple, and unspecified sites

Contusion with intact skin surface (920-924)
920 Contusion of face, scalp, and neck except eye(s)
921 Contusion of eye and adnexa
922 Contusion of trunk
923 Contusion of upper limb
924 Contusion of lower limb and of other and unspecified sites

Crushing injury (925-929)
925 Crushing injury of face, scalp, and neck
926 Crushing injury of trunk
927 Crushing injury of upper limb
928 Crushing injury of lower limb
929 Crushing injury of multiple and unspecified sites

Effects of foreign body entering through orifice (930-939)
930 Foreign body on external eye
931 Foreign body in ear
932 Foreign body in nose
933 Foreign body in pharynx and larynx
934 Foreign body in trachea, bronchus, and lung
935 Foreign body in mouth, esophagus, and stomach
936 Foreign body in intestine and colon
937 Foreign body in anus and rectum
938 Foreign body in digestive system, unspecified
939 Foreign body in genitourinary tract

Burns (940-949)
940 Burn confined to eye and adnexa
941 Burn of face, head, and neck
942 Burn of trunk
943 Burn of upper limb, except wrist and hand
944 Burn of wrist(s) and hand(s)
945 Burn of lower limb(s)
946 Burns of multiple specified sites
947 Burn of internal organs
948 Burns classified according to extent of body surface involved
949 Burn, unspecified

Injury to nerves and spinal cord (950-957)
950 Injury to optic nerve and pathways
951 Injury to other cranial nerve(s)
952 Spinal cord injury without evidence of spinal bone injury
953 Injury to nerve roots and spinal plexus
954 Injury to other nerve(s) of trunk excluding shoulder and pelvic girdles
955 Injury to peripheral nerve(s) of shoulder girdle and upper limb
956 Injury to peripheral nerve(s) of pelvic girdle and lower limb
957 Injury to other and unspecified nerves

Certain traumatic complications and unspecified injuries (958-959)
958 Certain early complications of trauma
959 Injury, other and unspecified

Poisoning by drugs, medicinals and biological substances (960-979)
960 Poisoning by antibiotics
961 Poisoning by other anti-infectives
962 Poisoning by hormones and synthetic substitutes
963 Poisoning by primarily systemic agents
964 Poisoning by agents primarily affecting blood constituents
965 Poisoning by analgesics, antipyretics, and antirheumatics
966 Poisoning by anticonvulsants and anti-Parkinsonism drugs
967 Poisoning by sedatives and hypnotics
968 Poisoning by other central nervous system depressants and anesthetics
969 Poisoning by psychotropic agents
970 Poisoning by central nervous system stimulants
971 Poisoning by drugs primarily affecting the autonomic nervous system
972 Poisoning by agents primarily affecting the cardiovascular system
973 Poisoning by agents primarily affecting the gastrointestinal system
974 Poisoning by water, mineral, and uric acid metabolism drugs
975 Poisoning by agents primarily acting on the smooth and skeletal muscles and respiratory system
976 Poisoning by agents primarily affecting skin and mucous membrane, ophthalmological, otorhinolaryngological, and dental drugs
977 Poisoning by other and unspecified drugs and medicinals
978 Poisoning by bacterial vaccines
979 Poisoning by other vaccines and biological substances

Toxic effects of substances chiefly nonmedicinal as to source (980-989)
980 Toxic effect of alcohol
981 Toxic effect of petroleum products
982 Toxic effect of solvents other than petroleum-based
983 Toxic effect of corrosive aromatics, acids, and caustic alkalis
984 Toxic effect of lead and its compounds (including fumes)
985 Toxic effect of other metals
986 Toxic effect of carbon monoxide
987 Toxic effect of other gases, fumes, or vapors
988 Toxic effect of noxious substances eaten as food
989 Toxic effect of other substances, chiefly nonmedicinal as to source

Other and unspecified effects of external causes (990-995)
990 Effects of radiation, unspecified
991 Effects of reduced temperature
992 Effects of heat and light
993 Effects of air pressure
994 Effects of other external causes
995 Certain adverse effects, not elsewhere classified

Complications of surgical and medical care, not elsewhere classified (996-999)
996 Complications peculiar to certain specified procedures
997 Complications affecting specified body systems, not elsewhere classified
998 Other complications of procedures, not elsewhere classified

APPENDIX E: LIST OF THREE-DIGIT CATEGORIES

999 Complications of medical care, not elsewhere classified

SUPPLEMENTARY CLASSIFICATION OF FACTORS INFLUENCING HEALTH STATUS AND CONTACT WITH HEALTH SERVICES

Persons with potential health hazards related to communicable diseases (V01-V09)
- V01 Contact with or exposure to communicable diseases
- V02 Carrier or suspected carrier of infectious diseases
- V03 Need for prophylactic vaccination and inoculation against bacterial diseases
- V04 Need for prophylactic vaccination and inoculation against certain viral diseases
- V05 Need for other prophylactic vaccination and inoculation against single diseases
- V06 Need for prophylactic vaccination and inoculation against combinations of diseases
- V07 Need for isolation and other prophylactic measures
- V08 Asymptomatic human immunodeficiency virus [HIV] infection status
- V09 Infection with drug-resistant microorganisms

Persons with potential health hazards related to personal and family history (V10-V19)
- V10 Personal history of malignant neoplasm
- V11 Personal history of mental disorder
- V12 Personal history of certain other diseases
- V13 Personal history of other diseases
- V14 Personal history of allergy to medicinal agents
- V15 Other personal history presenting hazards to health
- V16 Family history of malignant neoplasm
- V17 Family history of certain chronic disabling diseases
- V18 Family history of certain other specific conditions
- V19 Family history of other conditions

Persons encountering health services in circumstances related to reproduction and development (V20-V29)
- V20 Health supervision of infant or child
- V21 Constitutional states in development
- V22 Normal pregnancy
- V23 Supervision of high-risk pregnancy
- V24 Postpartum care and examination
- V25 Encounter for contraceptive management
- V26 Procreative management
- V27 Outcome of delivery
- V28 Antenatal screening
- V29 Observation and evaluation of newborns and infants for suspected condition not found

Liveborn infants according to type of birth (V30-V39)
- V30 Single liveborn
- V31 Twin, mate liveborn
- V32 Twin, mate stillborn
- V33 Twin, unspecified
- V34 Other multiple, mates all liveborn
- V35 Other multiple, mates all stillborn
- V36 Other multiple, mates live- and stillborn
- V37 Other multiple, unspecified
- V39 Unspecified

Persons with a condition influencing their health status (V40-V49)
- V40 Mental and behavioral problems
- V41 Problems with special senses and other special functions
- V42 Organ or tissue replaced by transplant
- V43 Organ or tissue replaced by other means
- V44 Artificial opening status
- V45 Other postprocedural states
- V46 Other dependence on machines
- V47 Other problems with internal organs
- V48 Problems with head, neck, and trunk
- V49 Problems with limbs and other problems

Persons encountering health services for specific procedures and aftercare (V50-V59)
- V50 Elective surgery for purposes other than remedying health states
- V51 Aftercare involving the use of plastic surgery
- V52 Fitting and adjustment of prosthetic device
- V53 Fitting and adjustment of other device
- V54 Other orthopedic aftercare
- V55 Attention to artificial openings
- V56 Encounter for dialysis and dialysis catheter care
- V57 Care involving use of rehabilitation procedures
- V58 Encounter for other and unspecified procedures and aftercare
- V59 Donors

Persons encountering health services in other circumstances (V60-V69)
- V60 Housing, household, and economic circumstances
- V61 Other family circumstances
- V62 Other psychosocial circumstances
- V63 Unavailability of other medical facilities for care
- V64 Persons encountering health services for specific procedures, not carried out
- V65 Other persons seeking consultation
- V66 Convalescence and palliative care
- V67 Follow-up examination
- V68 Encounters for administrative purposes
- V69 Problems related to lifestyle

Persons without reported diagnosis encountered during examination and investigation of individuals and populations (V70-V82)
- V70 General medical examination
- V71 Observation and evaluation for suspected conditions not found
- V72 Special investigations and examinations
- V73 Special screening examination for viral and chlamydial diseases
- V74 Special screening examination for bacterial and spirochetal diseases
- V75 Special screening examination for other infectious diseases
- V76 Special screening for malignant neoplasms
- V77 Special screening for endocrine, nutritional, metabolic, and immunity disorders
- V78 Special screening for disorders of blood and blood-forming organs
- V79 Special screening for mental disorders and developmental handicaps
- V80 Special screening for neurological, eye, and ear diseases
- V81 Special screening for cardiovascular, respiratory, and genitourinary diseases
- V82 Special screening for other conditions

Genetics (V83-V84)
- V83 Genetic carrier status
- V84 Genetic susceptibility to disease

Body mass index (V85)
- V85 Body Mass Index

Estrogen receptor status (V86)
- V86 Estrogen receptor status

SUPPLEMENTARY CLASSIFICATION OF EXTERNAL CAUSES OF INJURY AND POISONING

Railway accidents (E800-E807)
- E800 Railway accident involving collision with rolling stock
- E801 Railway accident involving collision with other object
- E802 Railway accident involving derailment without antecedent collision
- E803 Railway accident involving explosion, fire, or burning
- E804 Fall in, on, or from railway train
- E805 Hit by rolling stock
- E806 Other specified railway accident
- E807 Railway accident of unspecified nature

Motor vehicle traffic accidents (E810-E819)
- E810 Motor vehicle traffic accident involving collision with train
- E811 Motor vehicle traffic accident involving re-entrant collision with another motor vehicle
- E812 Other motor vehicle traffic accident involving collision with another motor vehicle
- E813 Motor vehicle traffic accident involving collision with other vehicle
- E814 Motor vehicle traffic accident involving collision with pedestrian
- E815 Other motor vehicle traffic accident involving collision on the highway
- E816 Motor vehicle traffic accident due to loss of control, without collision on the highway
- E817 Noncollision motor vehicle traffic accident while boarding or alighting
- E818 Other noncollision motor vehicle traffic accident
- E819 Motor vehicle traffic accident of unspecified nature

Motor vehicle nontraffic accidents (E820-E825)
- E820 Nontraffic accident involving motor-driven snow vehicle
- E821 Nontraffic accident involving other off-road motor vehicle
- E822 Other motor vehicle nontraffic accident involving collision with moving object
- E823 Other motor vehicle nontraffic accident involving collision with stationary object
- E824 Other motor vehicle nontraffic accident while boarding and alighting
- E825 Other motor vehicle nontraffic accident of other and unspecified nature

Other road vehicle accidents (E826-E829)
- E826 Pedal cycle accident
- E827 Animal-drawn vehicle accident
- E828 Accident involving animal being ridden
- E829 Other road vehicle accidents

Water transport accidents (E830-E838)
- E830 Accident to watercraft causing submersion
- E831 Accident to watercraft causing other injury
- E832 Other accidental submersion or drowning in water transport accident
- E833 Fall on stairs or ladders in water transport
- E834 Other fall from one level to another in water transport
- E835 Other and unspecified fall in water transport
- E836 Machinery accident in water transport
- E837 Explosion, fire, or burning in watercraft
- E838 Other and unspecified water transport accident

Air and space transport accidents (E840-E845)
- E840 Accident to powered aircraft at takeoff or landing
- E841 Accident to powered aircraft, other and unspecified
- E842 Accident to unpowered aircraft
- E843 Fall in, on, or from aircraft
- E844 Other specified air transport accidents
- E845 Accident involving spacecraft

Vehicle accidents, not elsewhere classifiable (E846-E849)
- E846 Accidents involving powered vehicles used solely within the buildings and premises of an industrial or commercial establishment
- E847 Accidents involving cable cars not running on rails
- E848 Accidents involving other vehicles, not elsewhere classifiable
- E849 Place of occurrence

APPENDIX E: LIST OF THREE-DIGIT CATEGORIES

Accidental poisoning by drugs, medicinal substances, and biologicals (E850-E858)
E850 Accidental poisoning by analgesics, antipyretics, and antirheumatics
E851 Accidental poisoning by barbiturates
E852 Accidental poisoning by other sedatives and hypnotics
E853 Accidental poisoning by tranquilizers
E854 Accidental poisoning by other psychotropic agents
E855 Accidental poisoning by other drugs acting on central and autonomic nervous systems
E856 Accidental poisoning by antibiotics
E857 Accidental poisoning by anti-infectives
E858 Accidental poisoning by other drugs

Accidental poisoning by other solid and liquid substances, gases, and vapors (E860-E869)
E860 Accidental poisoning by alcohol, not elsewhere classified
E861 Accidental poisoning by cleansing and polishing agents, disinfectants, paints, and varnishes
E862 Accidental poisoning by petroleum products, other solvents and their vapors, not elsewhere classified
E863 Accidental poisoning by agricultural and horticultural chemical and pharmaceutical preparations other than plant foods and fertilizers
E864 Accidental poisoning by corrosives and caustics, not elsewhere classified
E865 Accidental poisoning from poisonous foodstuffs and poisonous plants
E866 Accidental poisoning by other and unspecified solid and liquid substances
E867 Accidental poisoning by gas distributed by pipeline
E868 Accidental poisoning by other utility gas and other carbon monoxide
E869 Accidental poisoning by other gases and vapors

Misadventures to patients during surgical and medical care (E870-E876)
E870 Accidental cut, puncture, perforation, or hemorrhage during medical care
E871 Foreign object left in body during procedure
E872 Failure of sterile precautions during procedure
E873 Failure in dosage
E874 Mechanical failure of instrument or apparatus during procedure
E875 Contaminated or infected blood, other fluid, drug, or biological substance
E876 Other and unspecified misadventures during medical care

Surgical and medical procedures as the cause of abnormal reaction of patient or later complication, without mention of misadventure at the time of procedure (E878-E879)
E878 Surgical operation and other surgical procedures as the cause of abnormal reaction of patient, or of later complication, without mention of misadventure at the time of operation
E879 Other procedures, without mention of misadventure at the time of procedure, as the cause of abnormal reaction of patient, or of later complication

Accidental falls (E880-E888)
E880 Fall on or from stairs or steps
E881 Fall on or from ladders or scaffolding
E882 Fall from or out of building or other structure
E883 Fall into hole or other opening in surface
E884 Other fall from one level to another
E885 Fall on same level from slipping, tripping, or stumbling
E886 Fall on same level from collision, pushing or shoving, by or with other person
E887 Fracture, cause unspecified
E888 Other and unspecified fall

Accidents caused by fire and flames (E890-E899)
E890 Conflagration in private dwelling
E891 Conflagration in other and unspecified building or structure
E892 Conflagration not in building or structure
E893 Accident caused by ignition of clothing
E894 Ignition of highly inflammable material
E895 Accident caused by controlled fire in private dwelling
E896 Accident caused by controlled fire in other and unspecified building or structure
E897 Accident caused by controlled fire not in building or structure
E898 Accident caused by other specified fire and flames
E899 Accident caused by unspecified fire

Accidents due to natural and environmental factors (E900-E909)
E900 Excessive heat
E901 Excessive cold
E902 High and low air pressure and changes in air pressure
E903 Travel and motion
E904 Hunger, thirst, exposure, and neglect
E905 Venomous animals and plants as the cause of poisoning and toxic reactions
E906 Other injury caused by animals
E907 Lightning
E908 Cataclysmic storms, and floods resulting from storms
E909 Cataclysmic earth surface movements and eruptions

Accidents caused by submersion, suffocation, and foreign bodies (E910-E915)
E910 Accidental drowning and submersion
E911 Inhalation and ingestion of food causing obstruction of respiratory tract or suffocation
E912 Inhalation and ingestion of other object causing obstruction of respiratory tract or suffocation
E913 Accidental mechanical suffocation
E914 Foreign body accidentally entering eye and adnexa
E915 Foreign body accidentally entering other orifice

Other accidents (E916-E928)
E916 Struck accidentally by falling object
E917 Striking against or struck accidentally by objects or persons
E918 Caught accidentally in or between objects
E919 Accidents caused by machinery
E920 Accidents caused by cutting and piercing instruments or objects
E921 Accident caused by explosion of pressure vessel
E922 Accident caused by firearm missile
E923 Accident caused by explosive material
E924 Accident caused by hot substance or object, caustic or corrosive material, and steam
E925 Accident caused by electric current
E926 Exposure to radiation
E927 Overexertion and strenuous movements
E928 Other and unspecified environmental and accidental causes

Late effects of accidental injury (E929)
E929 Late effects of accidental injury

Drugs, medicinal and biological substances causing adverse effects in therapeutic use (E930-E949)
E930 Antibiotics
E931 Other anti-infectives
E932 Hormones and synthetic substitutes
E933 Primarily systemic agents
E934 Agents primarily affecting blood constituents
E935 Analgesics, antipyretics, and antirheumatics
E936 Anticonvulsants and anti-Parkinsonism drugs
E937 Sedatives and hypnotics
E938 Other central nervous system depressants and anesthetics
E939 Psychotropic agents
E940 Central nervous system stimulants
E941 Drugs primarily affecting the autonomic nervous system
E942 Agents primarily affecting the cardiovascular system
E943 Agents primarily affecting gastrointestinal system
E944 Water, mineral, and uric acid metabolism drugs
E945 Agents primarily acting on the smooth and skeletal muscles and respiratory system
E946 Agents primarily affecting skin and mucous membrane, ophthalmological, otorhinolaryngological, and dental drugs
E947 Other and unspecified drugs and medicinal substances
E948 Bacterial vaccines
E949 Other vaccines and biological substances

Suicide and self-inflicted injury (E950-E959)
E950 Suicide and self-inflicted poisoning by solid or liquid substances
E951 Suicide and self-inflicted poisoning by gases in domestic use
E952 Suicide and self-inflicted poisoning by other gases and vapors
E953 Suicide and self-inflicted injury by hanging, strangulation, and suffocation
E954 Suicide and self-inflicted injury by submersion [drowning]
E955 Suicide and self-inflicted injury by firearms and explosives
E956 Suicide and self-inflicted injury by cutting and piercing instruments
E957 Suicide and self-inflicted injuries by jumping from high place
E958 Suicide and self-inflicted injury by other and unspecified means
E959 Late effects of self-inflicted injury

Homicide and injury purposely inflicted by other persons (E960-E969)
E960 Fight, brawl, and rape
E961 Assault by corrosive or caustic substance, except poisoning
E962 Assault by poisoning
E963 Assault by hanging and strangulation
E964 Assault by submersion [drowning]
E965 Assault by firearms and explosives
E966 Assault by cutting and piercing instrument
E967 Child and adult battering and other maltreatment
E968 Assault by other and unspecified means
E969 Late effects of injury purposely inflicted by other person

Legal intervention (E970-E978)
E970 Injury due to legal intervention by firearms
E971 Injury due to legal intervention by explosives
E972 Injury due to legal intervention by gas
E973 Injury due to legal intervention by blunt object
E974 Injury due to legal intervention by cutting and piercing instruments
E975 Injury due to legal intervention by other specified means
E976 Injury due to legal intervention by unspecified means
E977 Late effects of injuries due to legal intervention
E978 Legal execution

APPENDIX E: LIST OF THREE-DIGIT CATEGORIES

Terrorism (E979)
E979 Terrorism

Injury undetermined whether accidentally or purposely inflicted (E980-E989)
E980 Poisoning by solid or liquid substances, undetermined whether accidentally or purposely inflicted
E981 Poisoning by gases in domestic use, undetermined whether accidentally or purposely inflicted
E982 Poisoning by other gases, undetermined whether accidentally or purposely inflicted
E983 Hanging, strangulation, or suffocation, undetermined whether accidentally or purposely inflicted
E984 Submersion [drowning], undetermined whether accidentally or purposely inflicted
E985 Injury by firearms and explosives, undetermined whether accidentally or purposely inflicted
E986 Injury by cutting and piercing instruments, undetermined whether accidentally or purposely inflicted
E987 Falling from high place, undetermined whether accidentally or purposely inflicted
E988 Injury by other and unspecified means, undetermined whether accidentally or purposely inflicted
E989 Late effects of injury, undetermined whether accidentally or purposely inflicted

Injury resulting from operations of war (E990-E999)
E990 Injury due to war operations by fires and conflagrations
E991 Injury due to war operations by bullets and fragments
E992 Injury due to war operations by explosion of marine weapons
E993 Injury due to war operations by other explosion
E994 Injury due to war operations by destruction of aircraft
E995 Injury due to war operations by other and unspecified forms of conventional warfare
E996 Injury due to war operations by nuclear weapons
E997 Injury due to war operations by other forms of unconventional warfare
E998 Injury due to war operations but occurring after cessation of hostilities
E999 Late effects of injury due to war operations

Valid Three-digit ICD-9-CM Codes

Three-digit ICD-9-CM codes are used to identify a condition or disease only when a fourth or fifth digit is not available. The following are the only ICD-9-CM codes that are valid without further specificity.

024	Glanders
025	Melioidosis
035	Erysipelas
037	Tetanus
042	Human immunodeficiency virus (HIV) disease
048	Other enterovirus diseases of central nervous system
061	Dengue
064	Viral encephalitis transmitted by other and unspecified arthropods
071	Rabies
075	Infectious mononucleosis
080	Louse-borne [epidemic] typhus
096	Late syphilis, latent
101	Vincent's angina
118	Opportunistic mycoses
124	Trichinosis
129	Intestinal parasitism, unspecified
135	Sarcoidosis
138	Late effects of acute poliomyelitis
179	Malignant neoplasm of uterus, part unspecified
181	Malignant neoplasm of placenta
185	Malignant neoplasm of prostate
193	Malignant neoplasm of thyroid glands
217	Benign neoplasm of breast
220	Benign neoplasm of ovary
226	Benign neoplasm of thyroid glands
243	Congenital hypothyroidism
260	Kwashiorkor
261	Nutritional marasmus
262	Other severe, protein-calorie malnutrition
267	Ascorbic acid deficiency
311	Depressive disorder, not elsewhere classified
316	Psychic factors associated with diseases classified elsewhere
317	Mild mental retardation
319	Unspecified mental retardation
325	Phlebitis and thrombophlebitis of intracranial venous sinuses
326	Late effects of intracranial abscess or pyogenic infection
340	Multiple sclerosis
390	Rheumatic fever without mention of heart involvement
393	Chronic rheumatic pericarditis
412	Old myocardial infarction
430	Subarachnoid hemorrhage
431	Intracerebral hemorrhage
436	Acute, but ill-defined, cerebrovascular disease
452	Portal vein thrombosis
460	Acute nasopharyngitis [common cold]
462	Acute pharyngitis
463	Acute tonsillitis
470	Deviated nasal septum
475	Peritonsillar abscess
481	Pneumococcal pneumonia (streptococcus pneumoniae pneumonia)
485	Bronchopneumonia, organism unspecified
486	Pneumonia, organism unspecified
490	Bronchitis, not specified as acute or chronic
496	Chronic airway obstruction, not elsewhere classified
500	Coal workers' pneumoconiosis
501	Asbestosis
502	Pneumoconiosis due to other silica or silicates
503	Pneumoconiosis due to other inorganic dust
504	Pneumonopathy due to inhalation of other dust
505	Pneumoconiosis, unspecified
514	Pulmonary congestion and hypostasis
515	Postinflammatory pulmonary fibrosis
538	Gastrointestinal mucositis (ulcerative)
541	Appendicitis, unqualified
542	Other appendicitis
566	Abscess of anal and rectal regions
570	Acute and subacute necrosis of liver
586	Renal failure, unspecified
587	Renal sclerosis, unspecified
591	Hydronephrosis
605	Redundant prepuce and phimosis
630	Hydatidiform mole
631	Other abnormal product of conception
632	Missed abortion
650	Normal delivery
677	Late effect of complication of pregnancy, childbirth, and the puerperium
683	Acute lymphadenitis
684	Impetigo
700	Corns and callosities
725	Polymyalgia rheumatica
734	Flat foot
769	Respiratory distress syndrome
797	Senility without mention of psychosis
920	Contusion of face, scalp, and neck except eye(s)
931	Foreign body in ear
932	Foreign body in nose
936	Foreign body in intestine and colon
937	Foreign body in anus and rectum
938	Foreign body in digestive system, unspecified
981	Toxic effect of petroleum products
986	Toxic effect of carbon monoxide
990	Effects of radiation, unspecified
V08	Asymptomatic human immunodeficiency virus [HIV] infection status
V51	Aftercare involving the use of plastic surgery

Resources

Abortion	Spontaneous Abortion (accidental) (early) (late) (miscarriage) (recurrent)				Spontaneous Abortion (accidental) (early) (late) (miscarriage) (recurrent)			
	Incomplete (part of the products of conception are retained)	Complete (all of the products of conception are expelled)	Complication following abortion (separate epidosde of care)	Unspecified	Incomplete (part of the products of conception are retained)	Complete (all of the products of conception are expelled)	Unspecified	Complication following abortion (separate epidosde of care)
Without complication	634.91	634.92	634.90		635.91	635.92	635.90	
With complication of:								
Afibrinogenemia						635.12	635.10	639.1
Atrophy, acute yellow	634.71	634.72	634.70	639.8	635.71	635.72	635.70	639.8
Cardiac arrest	634.71	634.72	634.70	639.8	635.71	635.72	635.70	639.8
Cardiac failure	634.71	634.72	634.70	639.8	635.71	635.72	635.70	639.8
Cerebral anoxia	634.71	634.72	634.70	639.8	635.71	635.72	635.70	639.8
Circulatory collapse	634.51	634.52	634.50	639.5	635.51	635.52	635.50	639.5
Defibrination syndrome	634.11	634.12	634.10	639.1	635.11	635.12	635.10	639.1
Electrolyte imbalance	634.41	634.42	634.40	639.4	635.41	635.42	635.40	639.4
Embolism (any type)	634.61	634.62	634.60	639.6	635.61	635.62	635.60	639.6
Endometritis	634.01	634.02	634.00	639.0	635.01	635.02	635.00	639.0
Genital tract infection	634.01	634.02	634.00	639.0	635.01	635.02	635.00	639.0
Hemorrhage, delayed or excessive	634.11	634.12	634.10	639.1	635.11	635.12	635.10	639.1
Intravascular hemolysis	634.11	634.12	634.10	639.1	635.11	635.12	635.10	639.1
Laceration of:								
bladder	634.21	634.22	634.20	639.2	635.21	635.22	635.20	639.2
bowel	634.21	634.22	634.20	639.2	635.21	635.22	635.20	639.2
broad ligament	634.21	634.22	634.20	639.2	635.21	635.22	635.20	639.2
cervix	634.21	634.22	634.20	639.2	635.21	635.22	635.20	639.2
periurethral tissue	634.21	634.22	634.20	639.2	635.21	635.22	635.20	639.2
uterus	634.21	634.22	634.20	639.2	635.21	635.22	635.20	639.2
vagina	634.21	634.22	634.20	639.2	635.21	635.22	635.20	639.2
Metabolic disorder	634.41	634.42	634.40	639.4	635.41	635.42	635.40	639.4
Necrosis of liver	634.71	634.72	634.70	639.8	635.71	635.72	635.70	639.8
Oliguria	634.31	634.32	634.30	639.3	635.31	635.32	635.30	639.3
Other specified complication	634.71	634.72	634.70	639.8	635.71	635.72	635.70	639.8
Parametritis	634.01	634.02	634.00	639.0	635.01	635.02	635.00	639.0
Pelvic infection	634.01	634.02	634.00	639.0	635.01	635.02	635.00	639.0
Pelvic peritonitis	634.01	634.02	634.00	639.0	635.01	635.02	635.00	639.0
Perforation — see Abortion, by type, laceration								
Renal failure (acute)	634.31	634.32	634.30	639.3	635.31	635.32	635.30	639.3
Renal shutdown	634.31	634.32	634.30	639.3	635.31	635.32	635.30	639.3
Renal tubular necrosis	634.31	634.32	634.30	639.3	635.31	635.32	635.30	639.3
Salpingitis	634.01	634.02	634.00	639.0	635.01	635.02	635.00	639.0
Salpingo-oophoritis	634.01	634.02	634.00	639.0	635.01	635.02	635.00	639.0
Sepsis NOS	634.01	634.02	634.00	639.0	635.01	635.02	635.00	639.0
Septicemia NOS	634.01	634.02	634.00	639.0	635.01	635.02	635.00	639.0
Shock (postoperative)(septic)	634.51	634.52	634.50	639.5	635.51	635.52	635.50	639.5
Tear — see Abortion, by type, laceration								
Unspecified complications	634.81	634.82	634.80	639.9	635.81	635.82	635.80	639.9
Uremia	634.31	634.32	634.30	639.3	635.31	635.32	635.30	639.3
Urinary tract infection	634.71	634.72	634.70	639.8	635.71	635.72	635.70	639.8
UTI (urinary tract infection)	634.71	634.72	634.70	639.8	635.71	635.72	635.70	639.8

Abortion	Illegally Induced Abortion (criminal) (homicidal) (self-induced)				Unspecified Abortion — Retained product of conception following abortion, not classifiable elsewhere or not otherwise specified			
	Incomplete (part of the products of conception are retained)	Complete (all of the products of conception are expelled)	Unspecified	Complication following abortion (separate epidosde of care)	Incomplete (part of the products of conception are retained)	Complete (all of the products of conception are expelled)	Unspecified	Complication following abortion (separate epidosde of care)
Without complication	636.91	636.92	636.90		637.91	637.92	637.90	
With complication of:								
Afibrinogenemia	636.11	636.12	636.10	639.1	637.11	637.12	637.10	639.1
Atrophy, acute yellow	636.71	636.72	636.70	639.8	637.71	637.72	637.70	639.8
Cardiac arrest	636.71	636.72	636.70	639.8	637.71	637.72	637.70	639.8
Cardiac failure	636.71	636.72	636.70	639.8	637.71	637.72	637.70	639.8
Cerebral anoxia	636.71	636.72	636.70	639.8	637.71	637.72	637.70	639.8
Circulatory collapse	636.51	636.52	636.50	639.5	637.51	637.52	637.50	639.5
Defibrination syndrome	636.11	636.12	636.10	639.1	637.11	637.12	637.10	639.1
Electrolyte imbalance	636.41	636.42	636.40	639.4	637.41	637.42	637.40	639.4
Embolism (any type)	636.61	636.62	636.60	639.6	637.61	637.62	637.60	639.6
Endometritis	636.01	636.02	636.00	639.0	637.01	637.02	637.00	639.0
Genital tract infection	636.01	636.02	636.00	639.0	637.01	637.02	637.00	639.0
Hemorrhage, delayed or excessive	636.11	636.12	636.10	639.1	637.11	637.12	637.10	639.1
Intravascular hemolysis	636.11	636.12	636.10	639.1	637.11	637.12	637.10	639.1
Laceration of:								
bladder	636.21	636.22	636.20	639.2	637.21	637.22	637.20	639.2
bowel	636.21	636.22	636.20	639.2	637.21	637.22	637.20	639.2
broad ligament	636.21	636.22	636.20	639.2	637.21	637.22	637.20	639.2
cervix	636.21	636.22	636.20	639.2	637.21	637.22	637.20	639.2
periurethral tissue	636.21	636.22	636.20	639.2	637.21	637.22	637.20	639.2
uterus	636.21	636.22	636.20	639.2	637.21	637.22	637.20	639.2
vagina	636.21	636.22	636.20	639.2	637.21	637.22	637.20	639.2
Metabolic disorder	636.41	636.42	636.40	639.4	637.41	637.42	637.40	639.4

Resources

Abortion Table

Abortion	Illegally Induced Abortion (criminal) (homicidal) (self-induced)				Unspecified Abortion — Retained products of conception following abortion, not classifiable elsewhere or not otherwise specified			
	Incomplete (part of the products of conception are retained)	Complete (all of the products of conception are expelled)	Unspecified	Complication following abortion (separate epidosde of care)	Incomplete (part of the products of conception are retained)	Complete (all of the products of conception are expelled)	Unspecified	Complication following abortion (separate epidosde of care)
Necrosis of liver	636.71	636.72	636.70	639.8	637.71	637.72	637.70	639.8
Oliguria	636.31	636.32	636.30	639.3	637.31	637.32	637.30	639.3
Other specified complication	636.71	636.72	636.70	639.8	637.71	637.72	637.70	639.8
Parametritis	636.01	636.02	636.00	639.0	637.01	637.02	637.00	639.0
Pelvic infection	636.01	636.02	636.00	639.0	637.01	637.02	637.00	639.0
Pelvic peritonitis	636.01	636.02	636.00	639.0	637.01	637.02	637.00	639.0
Perforation — see Abortion, by type, laceration								
Renal failure (acute)	636.31	636.32	636.30	639.3	637.31	637.32	637.30	639.3
Renal shutdown	636.31	636.32	636.30	639.3	637.31	637.32	637.30	639.3
Renal tubular necrosis	636.31	636.32	636.30	639.3	637.31	637.32	637.30	639.3
Salpingitis	636.01	636.02	636.00	639.0	637.01	637.02	637.00	639.0
Salpingo-oophoritis	636.01	636.02	636.00	639.0	637.01	637.02	637.00	639.0
Sepsis NOS	636.01	636.02	636.00	639.0	637.01	637.02	637.00	639.0
Septicemia NOS	636.01	636.02	636.00	639.0	637.01	637.02	637.00	639.0
Shock (postoperative) (septic)	636.51	636.52	636.50	639.5	637.51	637.52	637.50	639.5
Specified complication NEC	636.71	636.72	636.70	639.8				
Tear — see Abortion, by type, laceration								
Unspecified complications	636.81	636.82	636.80	639.9	637.81	637.82	637.80	639.9
Uremia	636.31	636.32	636.30	639.3	637.31	637.32	637.30	639.3
Urinary tract infection	636.71	636.72	636.70	639.8	637.71	637.72	637.70	639.8
UTI (urinary tract infection)	636.71	636.72	636.70	639.8	637.71	637.72	637.70	639.8

Abortion	Failed Attempted Abortion / Hydatidiform Mole / Missed Abortion / Other Abnormal Product of Conception			
	Failed Attempted Abortion	Hydatidiform Mole	Missed Abortion (all products of conception retained)	Other abnormal product of conception (blighted ovum, fleshy mole, stone mole, carneous mole, mole NOS)
Without complication	638.9	630	632	631
With complication of:				
Afibrinogenemia	638.1	639.1	639.1	639.1
Atrophy, acute yellow	638.7	639.8	639.8	639.8
Cardiac arrest	638.7	639.8	639.8	639.8
Cardiac failure	638.7	639.8	639.8	639.8
Cerebral anoxia	638.7	639.8	639.8	639.8
Circulatory collapse	638.5	639.5	639.5	639.5
Defibrination syndrome	638.1	639.1	639.1	639.1
Electrolyte imbalance	638.4	639.4	639.4	639.4
Embolism (any type)	638.6	639.6	639.6	639.6
Endometritis	638.0	639.0	639.0	639.0
Genital tract infection	638.0	639.0	639.0	639.0
Hemorrhage, delayed or excessive	638.1	639.1	639.1	639.1
Intravascular hemolysis	638.1	639.1	639.1	639.1
Laceration of:				
bladder	638.2	639.2	639.2	639.2
bowel	638.2	639.2	639.2	639.2
broad ligament	638.2	639.2	639.2	639.2
cervix	638.2	639.2	639.2	639.2
periurethral tissue	638.2	639.2	639.2	639.2
uterus	638.2	639.2	639.2	639.2
vagina	638.2	639.2	639.2	639.2
Metabolic disorder	638.4	639.4	639.4	639.4
Necrosis of liver	638.7	639.8	639.8	639.8
Oliguria	638.3	639.3	639.3	639.3
Other specified complications	638.7	639.8	639.8	639.8
Parametritis	638.0	639.0	639.0	639.0
Pelvic infection	638.0	639.0	639.0	639.0
Pelvic peritonitis	638.0	639.0	639.0	639.0
Perforation — see Abortion, by type, laceration				
Renal failure (acute)	638.3	639.3	639.3	639.3
Renal shutdown	638.3	639.3	639.3	639.3
Renal tubular necrosis	638.3	639.3	639.3	639.3
Salpingitis	638.0	639.0	639.0	639.0
Salpingo-oophoritis	638.0	639.0	639.0	639.0
Sepsis NOS	638.0	639.0	639.0	639.0
Septicemia NOS	638.0	639.0	639.0	639.0
Shock (postoperative) (septic)	638.5	639.5	639.5	639.5
Tear — see Abortion, by type, laceration				
Unspecified complications	638.8	639.9	639.9	639.9
Urinary tract infection	638.7	639.8	639.8	639.8
UTI (urinary tract infection)	638.7	639.8	639.8	639.8

Resources

Burn (acid) (cathode ray) (caustic) (chemical) (electric heating appliance) (electricicity) (fire) (flame) (hot liquid or object) (irradiation) (lime) (radiation) (steam) (thermal) (x-ray)	Unspecified Degree	First Degree [erythema]	Second Degree [blisters, epidermal loss]	Third Degree NOS [full-thickness skin loss]	Deep Third Degree [without mention of loss of body part]	Deep Third Degree [with loss of a body part]
Abdomen, abdominal (wall) (muscle)	942.03	942.13	942.23	942.33	942.43	942.53
with trunk	942.09	942.19	942.29	942.39	942.49	942.59
Ankle	945.03	945.13	945.23	945.33	945.43	945.53
with lower limb	945.09	945.19	945.29	945.39	945.49	945.59
Anus	942.09	942.19	942.29	942.39	942.49	942.59
Arm(s)	943.00	943.10	943.20	943.30	943.40	943.50
lower	943.01	943.11	943.21	943.31	943.41	943.51
multiple sites, except hand(s) or wrist(s)	943.09	943.19	943.29	943.39	943.49	943.59
upper	943.03	943.13	943.23	943.33	943.43	943.53
Auditory canal (external)	941.01	941.11	941.21	941.31	941.41	941.51
with face or head	941.09	941.19	941.29	941.39	941.49	941.59
Auricle (ear)	941.01	941.11	941.21	941.31	941.41	941.51
with face or head	941.09	941.19	941.29	941.39	941.49	941.59
Axilla	943.04	943.14	943.24	943.34	943.44	943.54
with upper limb, except hand(s) or wrist(s)	943.09	943.19	943.29	943.39	943.49	943.59
Back	942.04	942.14	942.24	942.34	942.44	942.54
with trunk	942.09	942.19	942.29	942.39	942.49	942.59
Biceps						
brachii	943.03	943.13	943.23	943.33	943.43	943.53
femoris	945.06	945.16	945.26	945.36	945.46	945.56
Breast(s)	942.01	942.11	942.21	942.31	942.41	942.51
with trunk	942.09	942.19	942.29	942.39	942.49	942.59
Brow	941.07	941.17	941.27	941.37	941.47	941.57
Buttock(s)	942.04	942.14	942.24	942.34	942.44	942.54
Cheek (cutaneous)	941.07	941.17	941.27	941.37	941.47	941.57
with face or head	941.09	941.19	941.29	941.39	941.49	941.59
Chest wall (anterior)	942.02	942.12	942.22	942.32	942.42	942.52
with trunk	942.09	942.19	942.29	942.39	942.49	942.59
Chin	941.04	941.14	941.24	941.34	941.44	941.54
with face or head	941.09	941.19	941.29	941.39	941.49	941.59
Clitoris	942.05	942.15	942.25	942.35	942.45	942.55
Ear (drum) (external)	941.01	941.11	941.21	941.31	941.41	941.51
with face or head	941.09	941.19	941.29	941.39	941.49	941.59
Elbow	943.02	943.12	943.22	943.32	943.42	943.52
with hand(s) and wrist(s)	946.0	946.1	946.2	946.3	946.4	946.5
with upper limb, except hand(s) or wrist(s)	943.09	943.19	943.29	943.39	943.49	943.59
Entire body	946.0	946.1	946.2	946.3	946.4	946.5
Epididymis	942.05	942.15	942.25	942.35	942.45	942.55
Epigastric region	942.03	942.13	942.23	942.33	942.43	942.53
Extremity						
arm	943.00	943.10	943.20	943.30	943.40	943.50
lower	943.01	943.11	943.21	943.31	943.41	943.51
multiple sites	943.09	943.19	943.29	943.39	943.49	943.59
upper	943.03	943.13	943.23	943.33	943.43	943.53
leg	945.00	945.10	945.20	945.30	945.40	945.50
lower	945.04	945.14	945.24	945.34	945.44	945.54
multiple sites	945.09	945.19	945.29	945.39	945.49	945.59
upper	945.06	945.16	945.26	945.36	945.46	945.56
Eye(s), only — see Eye, eyeball, burn						
with						
face, head or neck	941.02	941.12	941.22	941.32	941.42	941.52
other sites	946.0	946.1	946.2	946.3	946.4	946.5
Face	941.00	941.10	941.20	941.30	941.40	941.50
multiple sites	941.09	941.19	941.29	941.39	941.49	941.59
with eye(s)	941.02	941.12	941.22	941.32	941.42	941.52
Finger (nail) (subungual)	944.01	944.11	944.21	944.31	944.41	944.41
with						
hand(s)	944.08	944.18	944.28	944.38	944.48	944.58
other sites	946.0	946.1	946.2	946.3	946.4	946.5
thumb	944.04	944.14	944.24	944.34	944.44	944.54
multiple digits	944.03	944.13	944.23	944.33	944.43	944.53
with thumb	944.04	944.14	944.24	944.34	944.44	944.54
Foot	945.02	945.12	945.22	945.32	945.42	945.52
with lower limb	945.09	945.19	945.29	945.39	945.49	945.59
Forearm(s)	943.01	943.11	943.21	943.31	943.41	943.51
with upper limb, except hand(s) or wrist(s)	943.09	943.19	943.29	943.39	943.49	943.59
Forehead	941.07	941.17	941.27	941.37	941.47	941.57
with face or head	941.09	941.19	941.29	941.39	941.49	941.59
Genitourinary organ(s)						
external	942.05	942.15	942.25	942.35	942.45	942.55
internal—see specific organ or site, burn						
Groin	942.03	942.13	942.23	942.33	942.43	942.53
Hand(s) (and wrist)	944.00	944.10	944.20	944.30	944.40	944.50
back (doral surface)	944.06	944.16	944.26	944.36	944.46	944.56
multiple sites	944.08	944.18	944.28	944.38	944.48	944.58
Head (and face)	941.00	941.10	941.20	941.30	941.40	941.50
multiple sites	941.09	941.19	941.29	941.39	941.49	941.59
Heel	945.02	945.12	945.22	945.32	945.42	945.52
Hip	942.09	942.19	942.29	942.39	942.49	942.59
Internal organ(s) — see specific organ or site, burn						
Knee	945.05	945.15	945.25	945.35	945.45	945.55
with lower limb	945.09	945.19	945.29	945.39	945.49	945.59
Labium (majus) (minus)	942.05	942.15	942.25	942.35	942.45	942.55

Resources

Complications Table

Burn (acid) (cathode ray) (caustic) (chemical) (electric heating appliance) (electricity) (fire) (flame) (hot liquid or object) (irradiation) (lime) (radiation) (steam) (thermal) (x-ray)	Unspecified Degree	First Degree [erythema]	Second Degree [blisters, epidermal loss]	Third Degree NOS [full-thickness skin loss]	Deep Third Degree [without mention of loss of body part]	Deep Third Degree [with loss of a body part]
Leg	945.00	945.10	945.20	945.30	945.40	945.50
lower	945.04	945.14	945.24	945.34	945.44	945.54
multiple sites	945.09	945.19	945.29	945.39	945.49	945.59
upper	945.06	945.16	945.26	945.36	945.46	945.56
Lip(s)	941.03	941.13	941.23	941.33	941.43	941.53
with face or head	941.09	941.19	941.29	941.39	941.49	941.59
Lumbar region	942.04	942.14	942.24	942.34	942.44	942.54
Malar region	941.07	941.17	941.27	941.37	941.47	941.57
Mastoid region	941.06	941.16	941.26	941.36	941.46	941.56
Membrane, tympanic	941.01	941.11	941.21	941.31	941.41	941.51
Multiple, specified sites, classifiable to more than one category in 940–945	946.0	946.1	946.2	946.3	946.4	946.5
Nasal (septum)	941.05	941.15	941.25	941.35	941.45	941.55
Neck	941.08	941.18	941.28	941.38	941.48	941.58
with face or head	941.09	941.19	941.29	941.39	941.49	941.59
Nose	941.05	941.15	941.25	941.35	941.45	941.55
with face or head	941.09	941.19	941.29	941.39	941.49	941.59
Palm(s)	944.05	944.15	944.25	944.35	944.45	944.55
with hand(s) or wrist(s)	944.08	944.18	944.28	944.38	944.48	944.58
Penis	942.05	942.15	942.25	942.35	942.45	942.55
Perineum	942.05	942.15	942.25	942.35	942.45	942.55
Pubic region	942.05	942.15	942.25	942.35	942.45	942.55
Sacral region	942.04	942.14	942.24	942.34	942.44	942.54
Scalp	941.06	941.16	941.26	941.36	941.46	941.56
with face or head	941.09	941.19	941.29	941.39	941.49	941.59
Scapular region	943.06	943.16	943.26	943.36	943.46	943.56
with upper limb, except hand(s) or wrist(s)	943.09	943.19	943.29	943.39	943.49	943.59
Scrotum	942.05	942.15	942.25	942.35	942.45	942.55
Shoulder(s)	943.05	943.15	943.25	943.35	943.45	943.55
with						
hand(s) and wrist(s)	946.0	946.1	946.2	946.3	946.4	946.5
upper limb, except hand(s) or wrist(s)	943.09	943.19	943.29	943.39	943.49	943.59
Skin, unspecified site	949.0	949.1	949.2	949.3	949.4	949.5
Skull	941.00	941.10	941.20	941.30	941.40	941.50
Submental region	941.04	941.14	941.24	941.34	941.44	941.54
Supraclavicular fossa	941.08	941.18	941.28	941.38	941.48	941.58
Temple	941.06	941.16	941.26	941.36	941.46	941.56
Testicle	942.05	942.15	942.25	942.35	942.45	942.55
Thigh	945.06	945.16	945.26	945.36	945.46	945.56
with lower limb	945.09	945.19	945.29	945.39	945.49	945.59
Thumb(s) (nail)	944.02	944.12	944.22	944.32	944.42	944.52
with finger(s)	944.04	944.14	944.24	944.34	944.44	944.54
with hand(s) or wrist(s)	944.08	944.18	944.28	944.38	944.48	944.58
Toe (nail)	945.01	945.11	945.21	945.31	945.41	945.51
with lower limb	945.09	945.19	945.29	945.39	945.49	945.59
Trunk	942.00	942.10	942.20	942.30	942.40	942.50
multiple sites	942.09	942.19	942.29	942.39	942.49	942.59
specified site, NEC	942.09	942.19	942.29	942.39	942.49	942.59
Tunica vaginalis	942.05	942.15	942.25	942.35	942.45	942.55
Unspecified site	949.0	949.1	949.2	949.3	949.4	949.5
Vulva	942.05	942.15	942.25	942.35	942.45	942.55
Wrist(s)	944.07	944.17	944.27	944.37	944.47	944.57
with hand(s)	944.08	944.18	944.28	944.38	944.48	944.58

Complications due to (presence of)	Mechanical	Infection/inflammatory reaction	Other
Aortocoronary bypass graft	996.03	996.61	996.72
Arteriovenous			
fistula	996.1	996.62	996.74
shunt		996.62	996.74
Artificial heart		996.61	
Artificial skin graft	996.55	996.69	996.79
Bile duct	996.59	996.69	996.79
Blood vessel graft		996.62	996.74
Bone growth stimulator	996.40	996.67	996.78
Bone marrow transplant	996.85	996.85	996.85
Breast implant	996.54	996.69	996.79
Bypass graft			
aortocoronary	996.03	996.61	996.72
blood vessel		996.62	996.74
carotid artery		996.62	996.74
coronary artery	996.03	996.61	996.72
femoral-popliteal		996.62	996.74
Cardiac			
defibrillator	996.04	996.61	996.72
pulse generator	996.04	996.61	
subcutaneous pocket		996.61	996.72
pacemaker		996.61	996.72
pulse generator		996.61	
subcutaneous pocket		996.61	996.72
valve prosthesis	996.02	996.61	996.71
Carotid artery bypass graft		996.62	996.74

Resources

Complications Table

Complications due to (presence of)	Mechanical	Infection/inflammatory reaction	Other
Catheter			
cystostomy	996.39	996.65	996.76
dialysis		996.62	996.73
peritoneal	996.56	996.68	996.73
spinal	996.2	996.63	996.75
urinary, indwelling	996.31	996.64	996.76
vascular		996.62	996.74
Chin implant	996.59	996.69	996.79
Contraceptive device (intrauterine)	996.32	996.65	996.76
Corneal graft	996.51	996.69	996.79
Coronary artery bypass graft	996.03	996.61	996.72
Decellularized alodermis	996.55	996.69	996.79
Dialysis catheter		996.62	996.73
peritoneal	996.56	996.68	996.73
Dorsal column stimulator	996.2	996.63	996.75
Electrodes			
brain	996.2	996.63	996.75
heart	996.01	996.61	996.72
Esophagostomy	530.87	530.86	
External fixator device	996.40	996.67	996.78
Genitourinary device	996.39	996.65	996.76
unspecified	996.30	996.65	996.70
Graft			
artificial skin	996.52	996.69	996.79
blood vessel		996.62	996.74
bone	996.40	996.67	996.78
cartilage	996.40	996.67	996.78
carotid artery		996.62	996.74
corneal	996.51	996.69	996.79
coronary artery	996.03	996.61	996.72
femoral-popliteal		996.62	996.74
muscle	996.40	996.67	996.78
peripheral nerve	996.2	996.62	996.75
skin	996.52	996.69	996.79
tendon	996.40	996.67	996.78
ureter	996.39	996.65	996.76
Heart assist device		996.61	
Heart transplant	996.83	996.83	996.83
Infusion pump		996.62	996.74
Insulin pump	996.57	996.69	
Internal fixator device			
nail	996.40	996.67	996.78
plate	996.40	996.67	996.78
rod	996.40	996.67	996.78
screw	996.40	996.67	996.78
Intraaortic balloon		996.62	996.74
Joint prosthesis, internal	996.40	996.66	996.77
Articular bearing surface wear	996.46		
Aseptic loosening	996.41		
Breakage (fracture) of prosthetic joint	996.43		
Dislocation of prosthetic joint, 996.42	996.42		
Failure of prosthetic joint implant	996.43		
Instability of prosthetic joint	996.42		
Loosening of prosthetic joint	996.41		
Peri-prosthetic fracture	996.44		
Peri-prosthetic osteolysis	996.45		
Subluxation of prosthetic joint	996.42		
Liver transplant	996.82	996.82	996.82
Lung transplant	996.84	996.84	996.84
Mammary implant	996.54	996.69	996.79
Nervous system device	996.2	996.63	996.75
Nonabsorbable surgical material NOS	996.59	996.69	996.79
Other vascular device		996.62	996.70
Pancreas transplant	996.86	996.86	996.86
Prosthetic implant			
bile duct	996.59	996.69	996.79
breast	996.54	996.69	996.79
chin	996.59	996.69	996.79
ocular lens	996.53	996.69	996.79
orbit of eye	996.59	996.69	996.79
vas deferens	996.39	996.65	996.76
Shunt			
arteriovenous		996.62	996.74
ventricular	996.2	996.63	996.75
Transplanted organ			
bone marrow	996.85	996.85	996.85
heart	996.83	996.83	996.83
liver	996.82	996.82	996.82
lung	996.84	996.84	996.84
other specified organ	996.89	996.89	996.89
pancreas	996.86	996.86	996.86
unspecified organ	996.80	996.80	996.80
Umbrella device, vena cava		996.62	996.74
Unspecified cardiac device		996.60	996.70
Vascular catheter		996.62	996.74
Ventricular shunt	996.2	996.63	996.75

Resources

Diabetes Table

Diabetes (brittle) (congenital) (familial) (mellitus) (severe) (slight)	TYPE I		TYPE II or unspecified type The codes found in these columns are for use even if the patient requires insulin.		Additional Code Required	
	Controlled or not stated as uncontrolled	Uncontrolled	Controlled or not stated as uncontrolled	Uncontrolled	Other metabolic disorders or conditions	List these codes after the diabetes code
Without complication or manifestation	250.01	250.03	250.00	250.02		
With complication or manifestation						
coma (ketoacidosis)	250.31	250.33	250.30	250.32		
hyperosmolar (nonketotic)	250.21	250.23	250.20	250.22		
complication NOS	250.91	250.93	250.90	250.92		
specified NEC	250.81	250.83	250.80	250.82		
gangrene	250.71	250.73	250.70	250.72		785.4
hyperosmolarity	250.21	250.23	250.20	250.22		
ketosis, ketoacidosis	250.11	250.13	250.10	250.12		
osteomyelitis	250.81	250.83	250.80	250.82		731.8
specified manifestations NEC	250.81	250.83	250.80	250.82		
Abnormal glucose NOS						
NOS					790.29	
non-fasting					790.29	
fasting					790.21	
tolerance test					790.22	
Abnormal glucose tolerance test (GTT), elevated glucose tolerance test					790.22	
Acetonemia	250.11	250.13	250.10	250.12		
Acidosis	250.11	250.13	250.10	250.12		
Amyotrophy	250.61	250.63	250.60	250.62		358.1
Angiopathia, angiopathy (peripheral)	250.71	250.73	250.70	250.72		443.81
retinalis (juvenilis)	250.51	250.53	250.50	250.52		362.01
Arthritis, arthropathy	250.61	250.63	250.60	250.62		713.5
Charcôt's	250.61	250.63	250.60	250.62		713.5
neuropathic (Charcôt's)	250.61	250.63	250.60	250.62		713.5
Asymptomatic elevated (abnormal glucose)					790.29	
Ataxia, ataxy, ataxic, locomotor (progressive)	250.61	250.63	250.60	250.62		337.1
Autonomic neuropathy (peripheral)	250.61	250.63	250.60	250.62		337.1
Bone change	250.81	250.83	250.80	250.82		731.8
Bronze, bronzed					275.0	
Cataract diabetic	250.51	250.53	250.50	250.52		366.41
senile (non diabetic)	250.01	250.03	250.00	250.02		366.17
snowflake	250.51	250.53	250.50	250.52		366.41
Charcôt's joint (disease)	250.61	250.63	250.60	250.62		713.5
Chemical					790.29	
Coma (with ketoacidosis)	250.31	250.33	250.30	250.32		
hyperglycemic	250.31	250.33	250.30	250.32		
hyperosmolar (nonketotic)	250.21	250.23	250.20	250.22		
hypoglycemic	250.31	250.33	250.30	250.32		
nondiabetic					251.0	
insulin	250.31	250.33	250.30	250.32		
nondiabetic					251.0	
Kussmaul's	250.31	250.33	250.30	250.32		
prediabetic	250.21	250.23	250.20	250.22		
Complication NOS	250.91	250.93	250.90	250.92		
specified NEC	250.81	250.83	250.80	250.82		
Dermopathy	250.81	250.83	250.80	250.82		709.8
Dietary supervision					V65.3	
Ebstein's disease	250.41	250.43	250.40	250.42		581.81
Edema (macula) (retina)	250.51	250.53	250.50	250.52		362.01
Family History					V18.0	
Gangrene	250.71	250.73	250.70	250.72		785.4
Gastroparalysis/Gastroparesis	250.61	250.63	250.60	250.62		536.3
Gestational diabetes						
antepartum					648.83	
delivered w/o antepartum condition					648.81	
postpartum					648.84	
unspecified. episode. of care					648.80	
with antepartum condition					648.82	
with long term (current) insulin use						V58.67
Glaucoma	250.51	250.53	250.50	250.52		365.44
Glomerulohyalinosis — diabetic syndrome	250.41	250.43	250.40	250.42		581.81
Glomerulonephritis, chronic	250.41	250.43	250.40	250.42		583.81
with nephrotic syndrome	250.41	250.43	250.40	250.42		581.81
Glomerulosclerosis (intercapillary)	250.41	250.43	250.40	250.42		581.81
Glucose Intolerance					790.22	
Glycogenosis, secondary	250.81	250.83	250.80	250.82		259.8
Hemochromatosis					275.0	
Hirschfeld's disease	250.01	250.01	250.00	250.02		
Hyperglycemia						
with coma	250.31	250.33	250.30	250.32		
diabetic	250.11	250.13	250.10	250.12		
neonatal (transient)					775.1	
nondiabetic					790.6	
postpancreatectomy					251.3	
Hyperosmolar coma	250.21	250.23	250.20	250.22		

Resources

Diabetes (brittle) (congenital) (familial) (mellitus) (severe) (slight)	TYPE I		TYPE II or unspecified type The codes found in these columns are for use even if the patient requires insulin.			Additional Code Required
	Controlled or not stated as uncontrolled	Uncontrolled	Controlled or not stated as uncontrolled	Uncontrolled	Other metabolic disorders or conditions	List these codes after the diabetes code
Hyperosmolarity	250.21	250.23	250.20	250.22		
Hypertension nephrosis syndrome	250.41	250.43	250.40	250.42		581.81
Hypoglycemia (diabetic) without coma	250.81	250.83	250.80	250.82		
with coma	250.31	250.33	250.30	250.32		
neonatal, transient					775.0	
nondiabetic						
with coma					251.0	
without coma					251.1	
NOS (spontaneous)					251.2	
Hypoglycemic shock	250.81	250.83	250.80	250.82		
Hypoinsulinemia, postsurgical					251.3	
Impaired fasting glucose					790.21	
Impotence	250.61	250.63	250.60	250.62		607.84
Insipidus					253.5	
nephrogenic					588.1	
pituitary					253.5	
vasopressin-resistant					588.1	
Insulin, long term (current) use						V58.67
Insulin overdose	250.x1	250.x3	250.x0	250.x2	962.3	
Insulin underdoes (code to diabetes only)						
Intercapillary glomerulosclerosis	250.41	250.43	250.40	250.42		581.81
Iridis rubeosis/Iritis	250.51	250.53	250.50	250.53		364.42
Ketosis, ketoacidosis	250.11	250.13	250.10	250.12		
Kimmelstiel (-Wilson) disease or syndrome	250.41	250.43	250.40	250.42		581.81
Kussmaul's coma	250.31	250.33	250.30	250.32		
Lancereaux's (diabetes mellitus with marked emaciation)	250.81	250.83	250.80	250.82		261
Latent (chemical)					790.29	
Lipoidosis	250.81	250.83	250.80	250.82		272.7
Macular edema	250.51	250.53	250.50	250.52		362.01
Microangiopathy (peripheral)	250.71	250.73	250.70	250.72		443.81
Mononeuropathy, mononeuritis, unspecified site	250.61	250.63	250.60	250.62		355.9
lower limb, unspecified	250.61	250.63	250.60	250.62		355.8
upper limb, unspecified	250.61	250.63	250.60	250.62		354.9
Myasthenic syndrome, myasthenia	250.61	250.63	250.60	250.62		358.1
Myelopathy	250.61	250.63	250.60	250.62		336.3
Necrobiosis lipoidica	250.81	250.83	250.80	250.82		709.3
Neonatal, transient hyperglycemia					775.1	
hypoglycemia					775.0	
Nephritis, chronic	250.41	250.43	250.40	250.42		583.81
with nephrotic syndrome	250.41	250.43	250.40	250.42		581.81
Nephropathy	250.41	250.43	250.40	250.42		583.81
Nephrosis (Ebsteins) (syndrome)	250.41	250.43	250.40	250.42		581.81
Neuralgia	250.61	250.63	250.60	250.62		357.2
Neuritis	250.61	250.63	250.60	250.62		357.2
Neurogenic arthropathy	250.61	250.63	250.60	250.62		713.5
Neuropathic arthritis	250.61	250.63	250.60	250.62	713.5	
Neuropathy	250.61	250.63	250.60	250.62		357.2
peripheral	250.61	250.63	250.60	250.62		337.1
Neurophthisis	250.61	250.63	250.60	250.62		357.2
Nonclinical					790.29	
Ophthalmoplegia	250.51	250.53	250.50	250.52		378.86
Osteomyelitis	250.81	250.83	250.80	250.82		731.8
Peripheral angiopathy	250.71	250.73	250.70	250.72		443.81
Peripheral autonomic neuropathy	250.61	250.63	250.60	250.62		337.1
Peripheral vascular disease (occlusive)	250.71	250.73	250.70	250.72		443.81
Pre-diabetes NOS					790.29	
Phosphate					275.3	
Polyneuropathy, polyneuritis	250.61	250.63	250.60	250.62		357.2
Postpancreatectomy					251.3	
Postsurgical (hypoinsulinemia)					251.3	
Prediabetes					790.29	
Pseudotabes	250.61	250.63	250.60	250.62		337.1
Renal disease, chronic	250.41	250.43	250.40	250.42		585.9
End Stage	250.41	250.43	250.40	250.42		585.6
Stage I	250.41	250.43	250.40	250.42		585.1
Stage II	250.41	250.43	250.40	250.42		585.2
Stage III	250.41	250.43	250.40	250.42		585.3
Stage IV	250.41	250.43	250.40	250.42		585.4
Stage V	250.41	250.43	250.40	250.42		585.5
Renal glycosuria (true)					271.4	
Retinal						
edema	250.51	250.53	250.50	250.52		362.07
hemorrhage	250.51	250.53	250.50	250.52		362.01
Retinitis	250.51	250.53	250.50	250.52		362.01
Retinopathy	250.51	250.53	250.50	250.52		362.01
background (simple)	250.51	250.53	250.50	250.52		362.01
nonproliferative, NOS	250.51	250.53	250.50	250.52		362.03
nonproliferative, mild	250.51	250.53	250.50	250.52		362.04
nonproliferative, moderate	250.51	250.53	250.50	250.52		362.05
nonproliferative, severe	250.51	250.53	250.50	250.52		362.06
proliferative	250.51	250.53	250.50	250.52		362.02
Rubeosis iridis	250.51	250.53	250.50	250.52		364.42

Diabetes (brittle) (congenital) (familial) (mellitus) (severe) (slight)

	TYPE I		TYPE II or unspecified type The codes found in these columns are for use even if the patient requires insulin.		Other metabolic disorders or conditions	Additional Code Required — List these codes after the diabetes code
	Controlled or not stated as uncontrolled	Uncontrolled	Controlled or not stated as uncontrolled	Uncontrolled		
Secondary						
postsurgical					251.3	
steroid induced					251.8	E932.0
Skin						
dermopathy	250.81	250.83	250.80	250.82		709.8
necrobiosis lipoidica diabeticorum	250.81	250.83	250.80	250.82		709.3
Screening					V77.1	
Steroid induced						
correct substance properly administered					251.8	E932.0
overdose or wrong substance given or taken					962.0	
Stress					790.29	
Subclinical					790.29	
Subliminal					790.29	
Syndrome						
diabetes-dwarfism-obesity (juvenile)					258.1	
diabetes mellitus in newborn infant					775.1	
diabetes-nephrosis	250.41	250.43	250.40	250.42		581.81
diabetic amyotrophy	250.61	250.63	250.60	250.62		358.1
Hanot-Chauffard (-Troisier) (bronze diabetes)					275.0	
nephrotic	250.41	250.43	250.40	250.42		581.81
Oppenheim-Urbach (necrobiosis lipoidica diabeticorum)	250.81	250.83	250.80	250.82		709.3
Pierre Mauriac's (diabetes-dwarfism-obesity)					258.1	
renal glomerulohyalinosis-diabetic	250.41	250.43	250.40	250.42		581.81
Troisier-Hanot-Chauffard (bronze diabetes)					275.0	
Urbach-Oppenheim (necrobiosis lipoidica diabeticorum)	250.81	250.83	250.80	250.82		709.3
Ulcer (skin), unspecified site	250.81	250.83	250.80	250.82		707.9
lower extremity, unspecified	250.81	250.83	250.80	250.82		707.19
lower extremity, ankle	250.81	250.83	250.80	250.82		707.13
lower extremity, calf	250.81	250.83	250.80	250.82		707.12
lower extremity, heel and midfoot	250.81	250.83	250.80	250.82		707.14
lower extremity, thigh	250.81	250.83	250.80	250.82		707.11
lower extremity, toes	250.81	250.83	250.80	250.82		707.15
specified site NEC	250.81	250.83	250.80	250.82		707.8
unspecified complication	250.91	250.93	250.90	250.92		
Willis' disease	250.01	250.03	250.00	250.02		
Xanthoma diabeticorum, xanthomatosis	250.81	250.83	250.80	250.82		272.2

Hernia Table

Site of Hernia	Without Obstruction	With Obstruction	Gangrene (with or without obstruction)
Abdomen (wall)	553.20	552.20	551.20
recurrent	553.21	552.21	551.21
Abdominal, specified site NEC	553.8	552.8	551.8
Appendix	553.8	552.8	551.8
Bilateral — *see* Hernia, by site			
Bladder (sphincter)			
congenital (female) (male)	756.71		
female			
lateral	618.02		
midline	618.01		
male		596.8	
Brain (acquired) (stem)	348.4		
congenital	742.0		
Broad ligament	553.8		
Bubonocele — *see* Hernia, inguinal			
Cecocele — *see also* Hernia, by site	553.9	552.9	551.9
Cerebral (acquired)	348.4		
congenital (endaural)	742.0		
Ciliary body (acquired)	364.8		
traumatic	871.1		
Colic	553.9		
Colon	553.9	552.9	551.9
Colostomy	569.69		
Cooper's	553.8	552.8	551.8
Crural — *see* Hernia, femoral			
Diaphragm(atic)	553.3	552.3	551.3
congenital (gross defect)	756.6		
traumatic	862.0		
with open wound	862.1		
Direct — *see* Hernia, inguinal			
Disc, intervertebral — *see* Displacement, intervertebral disc			
Diverticulum (intestine)	553.9	552.9	551.9
Double — *see* Hernia, inguinal			
Duodenojejunal	553.8	552.8	551.8
Encysted — *see* Hernia, inguinal			
En glissade — *see* Hernia, inguinal			
Enterocele — *see also* Hernia, by site	553.9	552.9	551.9
Enterostomy	569.69		

Resources

Site of Hernia	Without Obstruction	With Obstruction	Gangrene (with or without obstruction)
Epigastric	553.29	552.29	551.29
recurrent	553.21	552.21	551.21
Epigastrocele	553.29	552.29	551.29
recurrent	553.21	552.21	551.21
Epiplocele	553.9	552.9	551.9
Epiplosarcomphalocele	553.1	552.1	551.1
Esophageal (hiatal)	553.3	552.3	551.3
congenital	750.6		
Eventration (chest to colon)	553.3	552.3	551.3
congenital (gross defect)	756.6		
External — *see* Hernia, inguinal			
Fallopian tube	620.4		
Fascia	728.89		
Fat (pad)	729.30		
eye, eyelid	374.34		
knee		729.31	
orbit		374.34	
retro-orbital	374.34		
retropatellar	729.31		
specified site NEC	729.39		
Female			
complete	618.3		
cystocele			
lateral	618.02		
midline	618.01		
with prolapse	618.4		
incomplete	618.2		
fallopian tube	620.4		
ovary, oviduct	620.4		
rectovaginal	618.6		
uterus	621.8		
vaginal	618.6		
vesical			
congenital	756.71		
lateral	618.02		
midline	618.01		
Femoral (unilateral)	553.00	552.00	551.00
bilateral	553.02	552.02	551.02
recurrent	553.03	552.03	551.03
recurrent (unilateral)	553.01	552.01	551.01
Foramen			
Bochdale (acquired)	553.3	552.3	551.3
congenital	756.6		
magnum	348.4		
Morgagni (an) (acquired)	553.3	552.3	551.3
congenital	756.6		
Furnicular (umbilical)	553.1	552.1	551.1
spermatic cord—*see* Hernia, inguinal			
Gastric mucosa	537.89		
Gastrointestinal tract	553.9	552.9	551.9
Gluteal — *see* Hernia, femoral			
Gruber's	553.8	552.8	551.8
Hesselbach's	553.8	552.8	551.8
Hiatal (esophageal) (sliding)	553.3	552.3	551.3
Holthouse's — *see* Hernia, inguinal			
Incarcerated — *see* Hernia, by site, with obstruction			
Incisional	553.21	552.21	551.21
lumbar	553.8	552.8	551.8
Indirect — *see* Hernia, inguinal			
Infantile — *see* Hernia, inguinal			
Infrapatellar fat pad	729.31		
Inguinal (unilateral) (direct) (double) ((encysted) (external) (furnicular) (indirect) (infantile) (internal) (interstial) (oblique) (scrotal) (sliding)	550.90	550.10	550.00
bilateral	550.92	550.12	550.02
recurrent	550.93	550.13	550.03
recurrent (unilateral)	550.91	550.11	550.01
Internal	553.8	552.8	551.8
Interstitial	553.9	552.9	551.9
Intervertebral cartilage — *see* Displacement, intervertebral disc			
Intestine(al)	553.9	552.9	551.9
Intra-abdominal	553.9	552.9	551.9
Intraparietal	553.9	552.9	551.9
Iris (acquired)	364.8		
traumatic	871.1		
Irreducible — *see* Hernia, by site, with obstruction			
Ischiatic	553.8	552.8	551.8
Lens (acquired)	379.32		
traumatic	871.1		
Linea alba	553.29	552.29	551.29
recurrent	553.21	552.21	551.21
Linea semilunaris	553.29	552.29	551.29
Littre's	553.9	552.9	551.9
Lumbar	553.8	552.8	551.8
intervertebral disc	722.10		

Hernia Table

Site of Hernia	Without Obstruction	With Obstruction	Gangrene (with or without obstruction)
Lung (acquired)	518.89		
congenital	748.69		
Male			
chylocele	608.84		
cystocele	596.8		
scrotal — *see* Hernia, inguinal			
spermatocele	608.1		
congenital	752.8		
testis	550.90	550.10	550.00
bilateral	550.92	550.12	550.02
recurrent	550.93	550.13	550.03
recurrent (unilateral)	550.91	550.11	550.01
vesical	596.8		
congenital	756.71		
Mediastinum	519.3		
Merocele — *see* Hernia, femoral			
Mesenteric (internal)	553.8	552.8	551.8
Mesocolon	553.8	552.8	551.8
Muscle (sheath)	728.89		
Nucleus polpous — *see* Displacement, intervertebral disc			
Oblique — *see* Hernia, inguinal			
Obstructive — *see* Hernia, by site with obstruction			
Orbturator	553.8	552.8	551.8
Omental	553.8	552.8	551.8
Omentocele	553.8	552.8	551.8
Orbital fat pad	374.34		
Ovary, oviduct	620.4		
Paracolostomy	569.69		
Paraduodenal	553.8	552.8	551.8
Paraesophageal	553.8	552.8	551.8
congenital	750.6		
Parahiatal	553.8	552.8	551.8
Paraumbilical	553.1	552.1	551.1
Parietal	553.9	552.9	551.9
Perineal	553.8	552.8	551.8
Peritoneal sac, lesser	553.8	552.8	551.8
Petit's	553.8	552.8	551.8
intervertebral disc	722.10		
Popliteal fat pad	729.31		
Postoperative	553.21	552.21	551.21
Prevesical	596.8		
Properitoneal	553.8	552.8	551.8
Pudendal	553.8	552.8	551.8
Rectovaginal	618.6		
Retroperitoneal	553.8	552.8	551.8
Richter's	553.9	552.9	551.9
Rieux's, Reix's	553.8	552.8	551.8
Saint's, triad — *see* Hernia, Diaphragm			
Sarcopiplocele	553.9	552.9	551.9
Sarcoepiplomphalocele	553.9	552.9	551.9
Sciatic	553.8	552.8	551.8
Scrotum, scrotal — *see* Hernia, inguinal			
Sliding			
hiatal	553.3	552.3	551.3
congenital	750.6		
inguinal — *see* Hernia, inguinal			
Spermatocele	608.1		
congenital	752.8		
Spigelian	553.29	552.29	551.29
Spinal — *see* Spina Bifida			
Strangulated — *see* Hernia, by site, wth obstruction			
Supraumbilicus	553.29	552.29	551.29
recurrent	553.21	552.21	551.21
Tendon	727.9		
Testis (nontraumatic)	550.90	550.10	550.00
bilateral	550.92	550.12	550.02
recurrent	550.93	550.13	550.03
recurrent (unilateral)	550.91	550.11	550.01
Thoracic stomach	553.8	552.8	551.8
Treitz's	553.8	552.8	551.8
Triad, Saint's — *see* Hernia, diaphragm			
Umbilical, umbilicus	553.1	552.1	551.1
Unspecified site NEC	553.9	552.9	551.9
Ureter	593.89	593.4	
Uterus	621.8		
Vaginal	618.6		
Velpeau's — *see* Hernia, femoral			
Ventral	553.20	552.20	551.20
incisional	553.21	552.21	551.21
recurrent	553.21	552.21	551.21
Vertebral cartilage — *see* Displacement, intervertebral disc			
Vesical			
congenital (female) (male)	756.71		
female			
lateral	618.02		
midline	618.01		
male		596.8	

Resources

Site of Hernia	Without Obstruction	With Obstruction	Gangrene (with or without obstruction)
Vitreous (acquired)	379.21		
traumatic	871.1		

Ectopic Pregnancy

	Abdominal pregnancy (Intraperitoneal pregnancy)	Tubal pregnancy (Fallopian pregnancy, rupture of fallopian tube due to pregnancy, tubal abortion)	Ovarian pregnancy	Other ectopic pregnancy (Includes the following pregnancy(s): cervical, cornual mural mesometric intraligamentou)	Unspecified ectopic pregnancy
Without complication					
with intrauterine pregnancy	633.01	633.11	633.21	633.81	633.91
without intrauterine pregnancy	633.00	633.10	633.20	633.80	633.90
With complication of:					
Afibrinogenemia	639.1	639.1	639.1	639.1	639.1
Atrophy, acute yellow	639.8	639.8	639.8	639.8	639.8
Cardiac arrest	639.8	639.8	639.8	639.8	639.8
Cardiac failure	639.8	639.8	639.8	639.8	639.8
Cerebral anoxia	639.8	639.8	639.8	639.8	639.8
Circulatory collapse	639.5	639.5	639.5	639.5	639.5
Defibrination syndrome	639.1	639.1	639.1	639.1	639.1
Electrolyte imbalance	639.4	639.4	639.4	639.4	639.4
Embolism (any type)	639.6	639.6	639.6	639.6	639.6
Endometritis	639.0	639.0	639.0	639.0	639.0
Genital tract infection	639.0	639.0	639.0	639.0	639.0
Hemorrhage, delayed or excessive	639.1	639.1	639.1	639.1	639.1
Intravascular hemolysis	639.1	639.1	639.1	639.1	639.1
Laceration of:					
bladder	639.2	639.2	639.2	639.2	639.2
bowel	639.2	639.2	639.2	639.2	639.2
broad ligament	639.2	639.2	639.2	639.2	639.2
cervix	639.2	639.2	639.2	639.2	639.2
periurethral tissue	639.2	639.2	639.2	639.2	639.2
uterus	639.2	639.2	639.2	639.2	639.2
vagina	639.2	639.2	639.2	639.2	639.4
Metabolic disorder	639.4	639.4	639.4	639.4	639.8
Necrosis of liver	639.8	639.8	639.8	639.8	639.3
Oliguria	639.3	639.3	639.3	639.3	639.8
Other specified complication	639.8	639.8	639.8	639.8	639.0
Parametritis	639.0	639.0	639.0	639.0	639.0
Pelvic infection	639.0	639.0	639.0	639.0	639.0
Pelvic peritonitis	639.0	639.0	639.0	639.0	
Perforation — *see* Abortion, by type, laceration:					
Renal failure (acute)	639.3	639.3	639.3	639.3	639.3
Renal shutdown	639.3	639.3	639.3	639.3	639.3
Renal tubular necrosis	639.3	639.3	639.3	639.3	639.0
Salpingitis	639.0	639.0	639.0	639.0	639.0
Salpingo-oophoritis	639.0	639.0	639.0	639.0	639.0
Sepsis NOS	639.0	639.0	639.0	639.0	639.5
Septicemia NOS	639.0	639.0	639.0	639.0	
Shock (postoperative)(septic)	639.5	639.5	639.5	639.5	
Tear — *see* Abortion, by type, laceration:					
Unspecified complications	639.9	639.9	639.9	639.9	639.9
Urinary tract infection	639.8	639.8	639.8	639.8	639.8
UTI	639.8	639.8	639.8	639.8	639.8

Normal Pregnancy

Pregnancy/Delivery, current (Normal) (Single) (Uterine) (without Sickness)	Code	Special Notes
Examination (pregnancy test)		
negative results	V72.41	
positive results	V72.42	
unconfirmed	V72.40	
Normal delivery	650	This code is always a primary diagnosis.
Normal pregnancy		
with other condition not affecting the pregnancy	V22.2	V22.2 should be used in place of any other pregnancy codes and listed second on the claim form. The condition, which does not affect the pregnancy, must be listed first.
first pregnancy	V22.0	Codes V22.0 and V22.1 should never be used in conjunction with any codes from cataegories 640-648 and 651-676.
second or other normal pregnancy	V22.1	Meaning 2nd, 3rd, 4th etc. pregnancy
Postpartum care and examination		
immediately after delivery	V24.0	Normal uncomplicated cases
lactating mother	V24.1	Supervision of lactating mother
routine postpartum follow-up	V24.2	Care within 6 weeks after delivery
Previous (not effecting current pregnancy)		These codes may be used in conjunction with chapter 11 codes. A thorough review of any pertinent excludes notes (found in the tabular list) is necessary to be certain that these V codes are being used properly.
abortion	V23.2	
difficult delivery	V23.49	
forceps delivery	V23.49	
hemorrhage, antepartum or postpartum	V23.49	
hydatidiform mole	V23.1	
infertility	V23.0	
malignancy NEC	V23.89	
neonatal death	V23.5	
nonobstetrical conditions	V23.89	
premature delivery	V23.41	

2007 ICD•9•CM

Resources

Normal Pregnancy

Pregnancy/Delivery, current (Normal) (Single) (Uterine) (without Sickness)	Code	Special Notes
Previous (not effecting current pregnancy) — *continued*		
pre-term labor	V23.41	
specified NEC	V23.89	
stillbirth	V23.5	
trophoblastic disease	V23.1	
unspecified condition	V23.9	
vesicular mole	V23.1	
Screening, prenatal (for)		If the abnormal finding is known—code the screening and the findings as additional codes
by		
amniocentesis		
chromosomal anomalies	V28.0	N/A
raised alpha-fetoprotein levels (amniotic fluid)	V28.1	N/A
specified, NEC	V28.2	N/A
ultrasound		
fetal growth retardation	V28.4	N/A
malformation	V28.3	N/A
isoimmunization	V28.5	N/A
other specified screening	V28.8	N/A
Streptococcus B	V28.6	N/A
unspecified, screening	V28.9	N/A
Supervision (of) (for)		These codes may be used in conjunction with chapter 11 codes. A thorough review of any pertinent excludes notes (found in the tabular list) is necessary to be certain that these V codes are being used properly.
high-risk	V23.9	
insufficient prenatal care	V23.7	
specified problem NEC	V23.89	
multigravida		Second or more pregnancy
elderly	V23.82	35 years of age or older at expected date of delivery
young	V23.84	Younger than 16 years of age at expected date of delivery
multiparity	V23.3	
normal NEC	V22.1	
first pregnancy	V22.0	
poor		
obstetric history	V23.49	
reproductive history	V23.5	
primigravida		First pregnancy
elderly	V23.81	35 years of age or older at expected date of delivery
young	V23.83	Younger than 16 years of age at expected date of delivery
Unwanted NEC	V61.7	

Antepartum Pregnancy Condition or Complication; affecting management of mother	Antepartum condition or complication	Delivered, with or without mention of antepartum condition	Unspecified episode of care	Assign additional code to describe the...	Affecting fetus (coded on the newborn chart only)
Ablatio placentae	641.23	641.21	641.20	N/A	762.1
Abnormal NEC	646.93	646.91	646.90	condition	761.9
amnion	658.93	658.91	658.90	N/A	762.9
cervix	654.63	654.61	654.60	N/A	763.89
causing obstructed labor	660.23	660.21	660.20	cause	763.1
chorion	658.93	658.91	658.90	N/A	762.9
cord (umbilical)	663.93	663.91	663.90	N/A	762.6
fetal chromosomes (suspected)	655.13	655.11	655.10	N/A	758.89
fetal					
heart rate	659.73	659.71	659.70	N/A	763.83
before onset of labor	659.73	659.71	659.70	N/A	763.81
during labor	659.73	659.71	659.70	N/A	763.82
heart rhythm	659.73	659.71	659.70	N/A	763.8
before onset of labor	659.73	659.71	659.70	N/A	763.81
during labor	659.73	659.71	659.70	N/A	763.82
fetus, fetal (suspected) NEC	655.93	655.91	655.90	N/A	779.9
acid-base balance	656.83	656.81	656.80	N/A	768.4
causing disproportion	653.73	653.71	653.70	N/A	763.1
causing obstructed labor	660.13	660.11	660.10	cause	763.1
specified NEC	655.83	655.81	655.80	N/A	779.8
findings, nonspecific (a code from 640-648 should be used first when the management of the mother is affected by the abnormal findings)	796.5	N/A	N/A	N/A	
glucose tolerance test	648.83	648.81	648.80	condition	775.0
labor (forces of) NEC	661.93	661.91	661.90	condition	763.7
pelvic organs or tissues NEC	654.93	654.91	654.90	N/A	763.89
causing obstructed labor	660.23	660.21	660.20	cause	763.1
pelvis (bony)	653.03	653.01	653.00	N/A	763.1
causing obstructed labor	660.13	660.11	660.10	cause	763.1
perineum or vulva	654.83	654.81	654.80	N/A	763.89
causing obstructed labor	660.23	660.21	660.20	cause	763.1
placenta, placental (vessel)	656.73	656.71	656.70	N/A	762.2
with hemorrhage	641.83	641.81	641.80	N/A	762.1
position					
cervix	654.43	654.41	654.40	N/A	763.89
causing obstructed labor	660.23	660.21	660.20	cause	763.1
fetus	652.93	652.91	652.90	N/A	763.1
causing obstructed labor	660.03	660.01	660.00	cause	763.1

Resources

Antepartum Pregnancy Condition or Complication; affecting management of mother	Antepartum condition or complication	Delivered, with or without mention of antepartum condition	Unspecified episode of care	Assign additional code to describe the...	Affecting fetus (coded on the newborn chart only)
Abnormal NEC – *continued*					
placenta (low implantation) (previa)	641.03	641.01	641.00	N/A	762.0
with hemorrhage	641.13	641.11	641.10	N/A	762.1
uterus	654.43	654.41	654.40	N/A	763.89
causing obstructed labor	660.23	660.21	660.20	cause	763.1
product(s) of conception NEC	631	N/A	N/A	N/A	
quality of milk	676.83	676.81	676.80	N/A	
shape of uterus	654.43	654.41	654.40	N/A	763.89
causing obstructed labor	660.23	660.21	660.20	cause	763.1
size of fetus	653.53	653.51	653.50	N/A	763.1
causing obstructed labor	660.13	660.11	660.10	cause	763.1
umbilical cord NEC	663.83	663.81	663.80	N/A	762.6
uterus (congenital)	654.03	654.01	654.00	N/A	763.89
causing obstructed labor	660.23	660.21	660.20	cause	763.1
vagina	654.73	654.71	654.70	N/A	763.89
causing obstructed labor	660.23	660.21	660.20	cause	763.1
vulva (acquired) (congenital)	654.83	654.81	654.80	N/A	763.89
causing obstructed labor	660.23	660.21	660.20	cause	763.1
weight gain	646.13	646.11	646.10	condition	761.8
with					
hypertension (mild) (pre-eclamptic)	642.43	642.41	642.40	N/A	760.0
convulsions	642.63	642.61	642.60	N/A	760.0
pre-existing hypertension	642.73	642.71	642.70	N/A	760.0
severe hypertension	642.53	642.51	642.50	N/A	760.0
Aborter, habitual or recurrent	646.33	646.31	646.30	condition	761.8
Abruption of placenta	641.23	641.21	641.20	N/A	762.1
Abscess					
areola (acute) (chronic)	675.13	675.11	675.10	N/A	
Bartholin's gland	646.63	646.61	646.60	condition	760.8
bladder	646.63	646.61	646.60	condition	760.1
breast (acute) (chronic)	675.13	675.11	675.10	N/A	
kidney	646.63	646.61	646.60	condition	760.1
labium (majus) (minus)	646.63	646.61	646.60	condition	760.8
milk		675.13	675.11	675.10	N/A
nipple	675.03	675.01	675.00	N/A	
subareolar	675.13	675.11	675.10	N/A	
urethra	646.63	646.61	646.60	condition	760.1
vulva	646.63	646.61	646.60	condition	760.8
Absorption (of) (through placenta)					
suspected damage to fetus					760.70
chemical	655.53	655.51	655.50	N/A	760.70
drug	655.53	655.51	655.50	N/A	760.70
Acidosis (fetal) (intrauterine)	656.83	656.81	656.80	N/A	768.4
Addiction					
alcoholic	648.43	648.41	648.40	condition	760.71
suspected fetal damage	655.43	655.41	655.40	N/A	760.71
Adhesion(s), adhesive					
amnion to fetus	658.83	658.81	658.80	N/A	762.8
uterus to abdominal wall	654.43	654.41	654.40	N/A	763.89
causing obstructed labor	660.23	660.21	660.20	cause	763.1
Advanced maternal age (multigravida)	659.63	659.61	659.60	N/A	761.8
primigravida	659.53	659.51	659.50	N/A	761.8
Aerocele	673.03	673.01	673.00	N/A	
AFP (screening for raised levels in amniotic fluid)	V28.1	N/A	N/A	N/A	
Agalactia	676.43	676.41	676.40	N/A	
Air embolism	673.03	673.01	673.00	N/A	
Age					
elderly (35 years of age or older at expected date of delivery)					
multigravida (second or more pregnancy)	659.63	659.61	659.60	N/A	
primigravida (first pregnancy)	659.53	659.51	659.50	N/A	
young (less than 16 years old at expected date of delivery)	659.83	659.81	659.80		
Albuminuria (gravidarum)	646.23	646.21	646.20	condition	760.1
with hypertension (and edema)					760.1
mild	642.43	642.41	642.40	N/A	760.0
severe	642.53	642.51	642.50	N/A	760.0
gestational	646.23	646.21	646.20	condition	760.1
pre-eclamptic (mild)	642.23	642.21	642.20	N/A	760.0
severe	642.53	642.51	642.50	N/A	760.0
Alcohol, alcoholic					
addiction (maternal)	648.43	648.41	648.40	condition	760.71
with suspected fetal damage	655.43	655.41	655.40	N/A	760.71
Alphafetoprotein (screening for raised levels in amniotic fluid)	V28.1	N/A	N/A	N/A	
Amnion (nodosum)	658.83	658.81	658.80	N/A	762.9
Amnionitis	658.43	658.41	658.40	N/A	762.7
Amniotic fluid embolism	673.13	673.11	673.10	N/A	
Amputation of cervix	654.63	654.61	654.60	N/A	763.89
causing obstructed labor	660.23	660.21	660.20	cause	763.1
Android pelvis					
with disproportion (fetopelvic)	653.33	653.31	653.30	N/A	763.1
causing obstructed labor	660.13	660.11	660.10	cause	763.1

2007 ICD•9•CM

Resources

Antepartum Pregnancy Table

Antepartum Pregnancy Condition or Complication; affecting management of mother	Antepartum condition or complication	Delivered, with or without mention of antepartum condition	Unspecified episode of care	Assign additional code to describe the...	Affecting fetus (coded on the newborn chart only)
Anemia	648.23	648.21	648.20	condition	760.8
aplastic	648.23	648.21	648.20	condition	760.8
iron (Fe) deficiency	648.23	648.21	648.20	condition	760.8
macrocytic	648.23	648.21	648.20	condition	760.8
megaloblastic	648.23	648.21	648.20	condition	760.8
pernicious	648.23	648.21	648.20	condition	760.8
postpartum	648.23	648.21	648.20	condition	
Anencephalus, anencephaly (fetal)	655.03	655.01	655.00	N/A	
Anesthesia, anesthetic					
complications NEC	668.83	668.81	668.80	condition	
cardiac	668.13	668.11	668.10	condition	763.5
central nervous system	668.23	668.21	668.20	condition	763.5
pulmonary	668.03	668.01	668.00	condition	763.5
death (from) during delivery	668.93	668.91	668.90	condition	761.6
Anomaly, anomalous (congenital)					
cardiovascular system	648.53	648.51	648.50	condition	
cervix	654.63	654.61	654.60	N/A	763.89
causing obstructed labor	660.23	660.21	660.20	cause	763.1
pelvis (bony)	653.03	653.01	653.00	N/A	763.1
causing obstructed labor	660.13	660.11	660.10	cause	763.1
uterus	654.03	654.01	654.00	N/A	763.89
causing obstructed labor	660.23	660.21	660.20	cause	763.1
Anoxia cerebral					
complicating delivery (cesarean) (instrumental)	669.43	669.41	669.40	N/A	
due to obstetric anesthesia or sedation	668.23	668.21	668.20	complication	
Anteversion					
uterus, uterine (cervix)	654.43	654.41	654.40	N/A	763.89
causing obstructed labor	660.23	660.21	660.20	cause	763.1
Anthropoid pelvis					
with disproportion (fetopelvic)	653.23	653.21	653.20	N/A	763.1
causing obstructed labor	660.13	660.11	660.10	cause	763.1
Antibodies (incompatibility)					
ABO	656.23	656.21	656.20	N/A	773.2
anti-C	656.13	656.11	656.10	N/A	773.0
anti-D, cord blood	656.13	656.11	656.10	N/A	773.0
anti-E	656.13	656.11	656.10	N/A	773.0
blood group (ABO)	656.23	656.21	656.20	N/A	773.1
Rh (blood group) (factor)	656.13	656.11	656.10	N/A	773.0
Apoplexia, apoplexy, apoplectic					
placenta	641.23	641.21	641.20	N/A	762.1
uteroplacental	641.23	641.21	641.20	N/A	762.1
Arrest, arrested					
active phase of labor	661.13	661.11	661.10	N/A	763.7
any plane in pelvis complicating delivery	660.13	660.11	660.10	cause	763.1
cardiac					
anesthesia, complicating	668.13	668.11	668.10	N/A	
delivery (cesarean) (instrumental)	669.43	669.41	669.40	N/A	
deep transverse	660.33	660.31	660.30	cause	763.1
development or growth of fetus	656.53	656.51	656.50	N/A	764.90
transverse (deep)	660.33	660.31	660.30	cause	763.1
Ascites					
fetal, causing fetopelvic disproportion	653.73	653.71	653.70	N/A	763.1
causing obstructed labor	660.13	660.11	660.10	cause	763.1
Aspiration					
acid-pulmonary (syndrome)	668.03	668.01	668.00	complication	
pneumonitis	668.03	668.01	668.00	complication	
Assimilation, pelvis					
with disproportion	653.23	653.21	653.20	N/A	763.1
causing obstructed labor	660.13	660.11	660.10	cause	763.1
Asymmetry					
pelvis with disproportion	653.03	653.01	653.00	N/A	763.1
causing obstructed labor	660.13	660.11	660.10	cause	763.1
Atresia, atretic					
cervix	654.63	654.61	654.60	N/A	763.89
causing obstructed labor	660.23	660.21	660.20	cause	763.1
Atrophy, atrophic					
breast	676.33	676.31	676.30		
liver (acute) (subacute) (yellow)	646.73	646.71	646.70	complication	
Avulsion (traumatic)					
symphyseal cartilage (inner)	N/A	665.61	665.60	N/A	
Bacilluria, asymptomatic	646.53	646.51	646.50	complication	
Bacteremia					
during labor	659.33	659.31	659.30	N/A	
during pregnancy	647.83	647.81	647.80	condition	
Bacteriuria, asymptomatic	646.53	646.51	646.50	complication	
Band(s), amniotic	658.83	658.81	658.80	N/A	760.1
Bandl's ring (contraction)	661.43	661.41	661.40	N/A	762.8
Bariatric surgery	649.23	649.21	649.20	N/A	763.7
Bicornis or Bicornuate uterus	654.03	654.01	654.00	N/A	763.89
causing obstructed labor	660.23	660.21	660.20	cause	763.1
Bleeding	641.93	641.91	641.90	N/A	
accidental	641.23	641.21	641.20	N/A	
before 22 completed weeks gestation NEC	640.93	640.91	640.90	N/A	762.1
cerebrovascular	674.03	674.01	674.00	N/A	
due to					

2007 ICD•9•CM

Resources

Antepartum Pregnancy Condition or Complication; affecting management of mother	Antepartum condition or complication	Delivered, with or without mention of antepartum condition	Unspecified episode of care	Assign additional code to describe the...	Affecting fetus (coded on the newborn chart only)
Bleeding — continued					
afibrinogenemia or other coagulation defect	641.33	641.31	641.30	N/A	762.1
fibroids	641.83	641.81	641.80	N/A	762.1
marginal sinus (rupture)	641.23	641.21	641.20	N/A	762.1
premature separation, placenta	641.23	641.21	641.20	N/A	
trauma	641.83	641.81	641.80	N/A	
early (before 22 completed weeks gestation)	640.93	640.91	640.90	N/A	
threatened abortion	640.03	640.01	640.00	N/A	
unavoidable	641.13	641.11	641.10	N/A	
Bone disorders	648.73	648.71	648.70	condition	
Borderline pelvis	653.13	653.11	653.10	N/A	763.1
with obstruction during labor	660.13	660.11	660.10	cause	763.1
Braxton Hicks contractions	644.13	N/A	644.10	N/A	
Breech presentation (buttocks) (complete) (frank)	652.23	652.21	652.20	N/A	761.7
with successful version	652.13	652.11	652.10	N/A	763.1
before labor	652.23	652.21	652.20	N/A	761.7
during labor	652.23	652.21	652.20	N/A	763.0
Brow presentation					
complicating delivery	652.43	652.41	652.40		763.1
Bruise					
umbilical cord	663.63	663.61	663.60	N/A	762.6
Caked breast	676.23	676.21	676.20	N/A	
Cardiomyopathy	674.53	674.51	674.50		
Cardiovascular disease	648.63	648.61	648.60	condition	
congenital	648.53	648.51	648.50	condition	
Cellulitis, breast	675.13	675.11	675.10	N/A	
Cephalopelvic disproportion NOS	653.43	653.41	653.40	N/A	763.1
with obstruction during labor	660.13	660.11	660.10	cause	763.1
Cerebrovascular disorders	674.03	674.01	674.00	condition	
Cervicitis	646.63	646.61	646.60	condition	760.8
Cervix					
adhesions	654.63	654.61	654.60	N/A	
anaplasia	654.63	654.61	654.60	N/A	
atypism	654.63	654.61	654.60	N/A	
bands	654.63	654.61	654.60	N/A	
with obstruction during labor	660.23	660.21	660.20	cause	763.1
cervicitis	654.63	654.61	654.60	N/A	
cicatrix	654.63	654.61	654.60	N/A	
cyst		654.63	654.61	654.60	N/A
dysplasia	654.63	654.61	654.60	N/A	
ectropion	654.63	654.61	654.60	N/A	
endocervicitis	654.63	654.61	654.60	N/A	
erosion	654.63	654.61	654.60	N/A	
hypertrophic elongation	654.63	654.61	654.60	N/A	
incompetence	654.53	654.51	654.50	N/A	761.0
leukoplakia	654.63	654.61	654.60	N/A	
Nabothian (gland) cyst or follicle	654.63	654.61	654.60	N/A	
old laceration	654.63	654.61	654.60	N/A	
polyp		654.63	654.61	654.60	N/A
stricture and stenosis	654.63	654.61	654.60	N/A	
ulcer		654.63	654.61	654.60	N/A
Cesarean delivery, section NEC	N/A	669.71	669.70	N/A	763.4
post mortem	N/A	669.71	669.70	N/A	761.6
previous	654.23	654.21	654.20	N/A	
causing obstructed labor	660.23	660.21	660.20	cause	763.1
Chiari-Frommel syndrome	676.63	676.61	676.60	N/A	
Chloasma (gravidarum)	646.83	646.81	646.80	condition	
Chorioamnionitis	658.43	658.41	658.40	N/A	762.7
Cicatrix					
cervix	654.63	654.61	654.60	N/A	
causing obstructed labor	660.23	660.21	660.20	cause	763.1
vagina	654.73	654.71	654.70	N/A	
causing obstructed labor	660.23	660.21	660.20	cause	763.1
Coagulation defects	649.33	649.31	649.30	286.0-286.9	
Collapse (during or after labor and delivery)					
circulatory (peripheral)	669.13	669.11	669.10	N/A	779.8
lung		668.03	668.01	668.00	N/A
vascular (peripheral)	669.13	669.11	669.10	N/A	
Colporrhexis	N/A	665.41	665.40	N/A	
Complications NEC	646.93	646.91	646.90	condition	761.9
delivery	669.93	669.91	669.90	N/A	
procedure (instrumental) (manual) (surgical)	669.43	669.41	669.40	N/A	
specified type NEC	669.83	669.81	669.80	N/A	
umbilical cord	663.93	663.91	663.90	N/A	762.6
specified type NEC	663.83	663.81	663.80	N/A	762.6
labor and delivery	669.93	669.91	669.90	N/A	
anesthesia (sedation)	668.93	668.91	668.90	N/A	763.5
cardiac	668.13	668.11	668.10	N/A	
central nervous system	668.23	668.21	668.20	N/A	
pulmonary	668.03	668.01	668.00	N/A	
specified type NEC	668.83	668.81	668.80	N/A	
specified condition NEC	669.83	669.81	669.80	N/A	
intrauterine contraceptive device (IUD)	655.83	655.81	655.80	N/A	

2007 ICD•9•CM

Antepartum Pregnancy Table

Antepartum Pregnancy Condition or Complication; affecting management of mother	Antepartum condition or complication	Delivered, with or without mention of antepartum condition	Unspecified episode of care	Assign additional code to describe the...	Affecting fetus (coded on the newborn chart only)
Compound presentation					
complicating delivery	652.83	652.81	652.80	N/A	763.1
causing obstructed labor	660.03	660.01	660.00	cause	763.1
Compression, umbilical cord					
complicating delivery	663.23	663.21	663.20	N/A	762.5
cord around neck	663.13	663.11	663.10	N/A	762.5
cord prolapsed	663.03	663.01	663.00	N/A	762.4
Conjoined twins, causing disproportion (fetopelvic)	653.73	653.71	653.70	N/A	763.1
with obstruction during labor	660.13	660.11	660.10	cause	763.1
Constriction					
ring (uterus)	661.43	661.41	661.40	N/A	763.7
Contractions					
before 37 weeks	644.03	N/A	644.00	N/A	
Braxton Hicks	644.13	N/A	644.10	N/A	
Hicks'	644.13	N/A	644.10	N/A	
hourglass uterus	661.43	661.41	661.40	N/A	763.7
pelvis, complicating delivery	653.13	653.11	653.10	N/A	763.1
causing obstructed labor	660.13	660.11	660.10	cause	763.1
generally contracted	653.13	653.11	653.10	N/A	763.1
causing obstructed labor	660.13	660.11	660.10	cause	763.1
inlet	653.23	653.21	653.20	N/A	763.1
causing obstructed labor	660.13	660.11	660.10	cause	763.1
midpelvic	653.83	653.81	653.80	N/A	763.1
causing obstructed labor	660.13	660.11	660.10	cause	763.1
midplane	653.83	653.81	653.80	N/A	763.1
causing obstructed labor	660.13	660.11	660.10	cause	763.1
outlet	653.33	653.31	653.30	N/A	763.1
causing obstructed labor	660.13	660.11	660.10	cause	763.1
ring (Bandl's)	661.43	661.41	661.40	N/A	763.7
uterus					
abnormal	661.93	661.91	661.90	N/A	763.7
clonic, hourglass or tetanic	661.43	661.41	661.40	N/A	763.7
dyscoordinate	661.43	661.41	661.40	N/A	763.7
hourglass	661.43	661.41	661.40	N/A	763.7
incoordinate	661.43	661.41	661.40	N/A	763.7
inefficient or poor	661.23	661.21	661.20	N/A	763.7
irregular	661.23	661.21	661.20	N/A	763.7
tetanic	661.43	661.41	661.40	N/A	763.7
Convulsions (eclamptic) (uremic)	642.63	642.61	642.60	N/A	760.0
with pre-existing hypertension	642.73	642.71	642.70	N/A	760.0
Cord, complicating delivery				N/A	
around neck (tightly) (with compression)	663.13	663.11	663.10	N/A	762.5
without compression	663.33	663.31	663.30	N/A	762.6
prolapse, complicating delivery	663.03	663.01	663.00	N/A	762.4
Cornual — see Ectopic pregnancy					
CPD	653.43	653.41	653.40	N/A	761.4
causing obstructed labor	653.43	653.41	653.40	N/A	763.1
Cracked nipple	676.13	676.11	676.10	N/A	
Cretin, pelvis (with disproportion) (fetopelvic)	653.13	653.11	653.10	N/A	763.1
causing obstructed labor	660.13	660.11	660.10	cause	763.1
Cross birth (of fetus) complicating delivery	652.33	652.31	652.30	N/A	763.1
with successful version	652.13	652.11	652.10	N/A	763.1
causing obstructed labor	660.03	660.01	660.00	cause	763.1
Cyst					
amnion, amniotic	658.83	658.81	658.80	N/A	763.89
chorion	658.83	658.81	658.80	N/A	763.89
ovary	654.43	654.41	654.40	N/A	763.89
causing obstructed labor	660.23	660.21	660.20	cause	763.1
pelvic	654.43	654.41	654.40	N/A	763.89
causing obstructed labor	660.23	660.21	660.20	cause	763.1
Cystitis	646.63	646.61	646.60	condition	760.1
Cystocele	654.43	654.41	654.40	N/A	763.89
causing obstructed labor	660.23	660.21	660.20	cause	763.1
Damage					
coccyx, complicating delivery	N/A	665.61	665.60	N/A	763.89
pelvic (during delivery)					
joint or ligament	N/A	665.61	665.60	N/A	763.89
organ		N/A	665.51	665.50	N/A
Dates vs uterine size discrepancy	646.83	646.81	646.80		
Dead, fetus					
retained in utero (after 22 completed weeks' gestation)	656.43	656.41	656.40	N/A	779.9
before 22 weeks — see Abortion, missed					
syndrome	641.33	641.31	641.30		779.9
Death					
fetal NEC	646.93	646.91	646.90	condition	779.9
early before 22 weeks gestation — see Abortion, missed					
near term	656.43	656.41	656.40	N/A	779.9
maternal, NEC	646.93	646.91	646.90	condition	761.6
during delivery	668.93	668.91	668.90	N/A	
sudden, during delivery	669.93	669.91	669.90	N/A	761.6
under anesthesia NEC	668.93	668.91	668.90	N/A	761.6
Deciduitis	646.63	646.61	646.60	N/A	760.8
Decreased fetal movements	655.73	655.71	655.70	N/A	

Resources

Antepartum Pregnancy Condition or Complication; affecting management of mother	Antepartum condition or complication	Delivered, with or without mention of antepartum condition	Unspecified episode of care	Assign additional code to describe the...	Affecting fetus (coded on the newborn chart only)
Defect, defective					
coagulation (factor)	641.33	641.31	641.30	N/A	762.1
causing hemorrhage of pregnancy or delivery	641.33	641.31	641.30	N/A	762.1
Deficiency, deficient					
coagulation (factor)	641.33	641.31	641.30	N/A	762.1
causing hemorrhage of pregnancy or delivery	641.33	641.31	641.30	N/A	762.1
Deformity					
fetal					
with fetopelvic disproportion	653.73	653.71	653.70	N/A	763.1
causing obstructed labor	660.13	660.11	660.10	N/A	763.1
known or suspected	655.93	655.91	655.90	N/A	763.89
pelvic, pelvis					
with disproportion (fetopelvic)	653.03	653.01	653.00	N/A	763.1
causing obstructed labor	660.13	660.11	660.10	cause	763.1
soft part, organs or tissues NEC	654.93	654.91	654.90	cause	763.89
causing obstructed labor	660.23	660.21	660.20	cause	763.1
Delay, delayed					
any plane in pelvis, complicating delivery	660.13	660.11	660.10	cause	763.1
birth or delivery NEC	662.13	662.11	662.10	N/A	763.89
second twin, triplet, or multiple mate	662.33	662.31	662.30	N/A	763.89
Dependence, maternal					
alcohol, with suspected fetal damage	655.43	655.41	655.40	N/A	779.5
drug	648.33	648.31	648.30	condition	779.5
suspected damage to fetus	655.53	655.51	655.50	N/A	779.5
Depression	648.43	648.41	648.40	condition	
Dermatitis, gestationis	646.83	646.81	646.80	condition	
Detachment					
cervix, annular	N/A	665.31	665.30	N/A	763.89
Development					
incomplete (fetus or newborn)	656.53	656.51	656.50	N/A	763.89
Diabetes					
condition present before pregnancy	648.03	648.01	648.00	condition	775.0
gestational (chemical) (latent)	648.83	648.81	648.80	condition	775.0
with long term (current) insulin use				V58.67	775.0
Diastasis, recti (abdomen) complicating delivery	665.83	665.81	665.80	N/A	763.89
Difficult delivery NEC	669.93	669.91	669.90	N/A	763.89
Dilatation					
bladder (sphincter)	654.43	654.41	654.40	N/A	763.89
causing obstructed labor	660.23	660.21	660.20	cause	763.1
cervix, complicating delivery	654.63	654.61	654.60	N/A	763.89
incomplete, poor, slow	661.03	661.01	661.00	N/A	763.7
Discrepancy-uterine size to dates	646.83	646.81	646.80	N/A	
Disease, diseased NEC	646.93	646.91	646.90	condition	
breast NEC	676.33	676.31	676.30	N/A	
cerebrovascular, NEC	674.03	674.01	674.00	N/A	
Frommel's	676.63	676.61	676.60	N/A	
heart	656.73	656.71	656.70	N/A	762.2
placenta	656.73	656.71	656.70	N/A	762.2
renal NEC	646.23	646.21	646.20	condition	760.1
Valsuani's (progressive pernicious anemia, puerperal)	648.23	648.21	648.20	condition	
venereal NEC	647.23	647.21	647.20	condition	
virus NEC	647.63	647.61	647.60	condition	
with fetal damage	655.33	655.31	655.30	N/A	763.89
Disorders					
breast	676.33	676.31	676.30	N/A	
genital tract or organ	646.63	646.61	646.60	condition	760.8
lactation	676.93	676.91	676.90	N/A	
liver	646.73	646.71	646.70	condition	760.8
mental	648.43	648.41	648.40	condition	
metabolism NEC (in labor and delivery)	669.03	669.01	669.00	N/A	763.89
Displacement, uterus NEC	654.43	654.41	654.40	N/A	763.89
causing obstructed labor	660.23	660.21	660.20	cause	763.1
Disproportion	653.93	653.91	653.90		763.1
caused by					
conjoined twins	653.73	653.71	653.70	N/A	763.1
contraction, pelvis (general)	653.13	653.11	653.10	N/A	763.1
inlet	653.23	653.21	653.20	N/A	763.1
midpelvic	653.83	653.81	653.80	N/A	763.1
midplane	653.83	653.81	653.80	N/A	763.1
outlet	653.33	653.31	653.30	N/A	763.1
fetal NEC	653.53	653.51	653.50	N/A	763.1
ascites	653.73	653.71	653.70	N/A	763.1
hydrocephalus	653.63	653.61	653.60	N/A	763.1
hydrops	653.73	653.71	653.70	N/A	763.1
meningomyelocele	653.73	653.71	653.70	N/A	763.1
sacral teratoma	653.73	653.71	653.70	N/A	763.1
tumor	653.73	653.71	653.70	N/A	763.1
hydrocephalic fetus	653.63	653.61	653.60	N/A	763.1
pelvis, pelvic, abnormality (bony) NEC	653.03	653.01	653.00	N/A	763.1
unusually large fetus	653.53	653.51	653.50	N/A	763.1
causing obstructed labor	660.13	660.11	660.10	cause	763.1
cephalopelvic, normally formed fetus	653.43	653.41	653.40	N/A	763.1
fetopelvic, normally formed fetus	653.43	653.41	653.40	N/A	763.1
causing obstructed labor	660.13	660.11	660.10	cause	763.1

2007 ICD·9·CM

Antepartum Pregnancy Table

Antepartum Pregnancy Condition or Complication; affecting management of mother	Antepartum condition or complication	Delivered, with or without mention of antepartum condition	Unspecified episode of care	Assign additional code to describe the...	Affecting fetus (coded on the newborn chart only)
Disproportion — *continued*					
pelvis, pelvic (bony) NEC	653.13	653.11	653.10	N/A	763.1
causing obstructed labor	660.13	660.11	660.10	cause	763.1
specified type NEC	653.83	653.81	653.80	N/A	763.1
Distortion					
lumbar spine				N/A	
with disproportion (fetopelvic)	653.03	653.01	653.00	N/A	763.1
causing obstructed labor	660.13	660.11	660.10	cause	763.1
maternal	669.03	669.01	669.00	N/A	
Distress (fetal)	656.83	656.81	656.80	N/A	763.89
Double uterus	654.03	654.01	654.00	N/A	763.89
causing obstructed labor	660.23	660.21	660.20	cause	763.1
Dropsy, amnion	657.03	657.01	657.00	N/A	761.3
Drug dependence	648.33	648.31	648.30	condition	
Dyscrasia, blood					
with antepartum hemorrhage	641.33	641.31	641.30	N/A	762.1
Dysfunction					
thyroid	648.13	648.11	648.10	condition	
uterus, complicating delivery	661.93	661.91	661.90	N/A	763.7
hypertonic	661.43	661.41	661.40	N/A	763.7
hypotonic, primary	661.03	661.01	661.00	N/A	763.7
secondary	661.13	661.11	661.10	N/A	763.7
Dysplasia of cervix	654.63	654.61	654.60	N/A	763.89
causing obstructed labor	660.23	660.21	660.20	cause	763.1
Dystocia	660.93	660.91	660.90	cause	763.1
cervical	661.03	661.01	661.00	N/A	763.7
contraction ring	661.43	661.41	661.40	N/A	763.7
fetal	660.93	660.91	660.90	cause	763.1
abnormal size	653.53	653.51	653.50	N/A	763.1
causing obstructed labor	660.13	660.11	660.10	cause	763.1
deformity	653.73	653.71	653.70	N/A	763.1
causing obstructed labor	660.13	660.11	660.10	cause	763.1
maternal	660.93	660.91	660.90	N/A	763.1
positional	660.03	660.01	660.00	cause	763.1
shoulder (girdle)	660.43	660.41	660.40	cause	763.1
uterine NEC	661.43	661.41	661.40	N/A	763.7
Early onset of delivery (spontaneous)	N/A	644.21	644.20	N/A	
Preterm neonate birthweight					
Extreme immaturity (code also weeks of gestation, codes 765.20-765.29)					
unspecified (weight)					765.00
< 500 gms					765.01
500-749 gms					765.02
750-999 gms					765.03
1,000-1,249 gms					765.04
1,250-1,499 gms					765.05
1,500-1,749 gms					765.06
1,750-1,999 gms					765.07
2,000-2,499 gms					765.08
≥ 2,500 gms					765.09
Other preterm (code also weeks of gestation, codes 765.20-765.29)					
unspecified (weight)					765.10
< 500 gms					765.11
500-749 gms					765.12
750-999 gms					765.13
1,000-1,249 gms					765.14
1,250-1,499 gms					765.15
1,500-1,749 gms					765.16
1,750-1,999 gms					765.17
2,000-2,499 gms					765.18
≥ 2,500 gms					765.19
Preterm neonate weeks of gestation (code in addition to birthweight, subcategory codes 765.0 and 765.1)					
unspecified weeks of gestation					765.20
< 24 completed weeks of gestation					765.21
24 completed weeks of gestation					765.22
25-26 completed weeks of gestation					765.23
27-28 completed weeks of gestation					765.24
29-30 completed weeks of gestation					765.25
31-32 completed weeks of gestation					765.26
33-34 completed weeks of gestation					765.27
35-36 completed weeks of gestation					765.28
≥ 37 completed weeks of gestation					765.29
Eclampsia, eclamptic (coma) (convulsions) (delirium)	642.63	642.61	642.60	N/A	760.0
with pre-existing hypertension	642.73	642.71	642.70	N/A	760.0
Edema	646.13	646.11	646.10	condition	
with hypertension — *see* Pregnancy, toxemia					
Effect, adverse					
anesthetic (in labor and delivery) NEC	668.93	668.91	668.90	N/A	763.5
radiation (suspected damage to fetus)	655.63	655.61	655.60	N/A	condition
Effusion, amniotic fluid	658.13	658.11	658.10	N/A	761.1
delayed delivery following	658.23	658.21	658.20	N/A	761.1

Resources

Antepartum Pregnancy Condition or Complication; affecting management of mother	Antepartum condition or complication	Delivered, with or without mention of antepartum condition	Unspecified episode of care	Assign additional code to describe the...	Affecting fetus (coded on the newborn chart only)
Electrolyte imbalance with hyperemesis gravidarum (before 22 completed weeks' gestation)	643.13	643.11	643.10	N/A	761.8
Embolism					
air (pulmonary)	673.03	673.01	673.00	N/A	
amniotic fluid	673.13	673.11	673.10	N/A	
blood clot	673.23	673.21	673.20	N/A	
brain		674.03	674.01	674.00	N/A
cerebral	674.03	674.01	674.00	N/A	
fat (cerebral) (pulmonary) (systemic)	673.83	673.81	673.80	N/A	
intracranial (venous sinus) (nonpyogenic)	671.53	671.51	671.50	N/A	
pulmonary NEC	673.23	673.21	673.20	N/A	
pyemic	673.33	673.31	673.30	N/A	
septic	673.33	673.31	673.30	N/A	
Emesis (gravidarum) — see Pregnancy, vomiting					
Endometritis	646.63	646.61	646.60	condition	760.8
decidual	646.63	646.61	646.60	condition	760.8
Engorgement, breast	676.23	676.21	676.20	N/A	
Entanglement, umbilical cord(s)	663.33	663.31	663.30	N/A	762.5
with compression	663.23	663.21	663.20	N/A	762.5
around neck with compression	663.13	663.11	663.10	N/A	762.5
twins in monoamniotic sac	663.23	663.21	663.20	N/A	762.5
Epilepsy	649.43	649.41	649.40	345.00-345.91	
Excessive					
large (fetus)	656.63	656.61	656.60	N/A	766.0
with obstructed labor	660.13	660.11	660.10	cause	763.1
causing disproportion	653.53	653.51	653.50	N/A	763.1
causing obstructed labor	660.13	660.11	660.10	cause	763.1
milk secretion	676.63	676.61	676.60	N/A	
weight gain	646.13	646.11	646.10	condition	
Exhaustion (complicating delivery)	669.83	669.81	669.80	N/A	763.89
Extraction					
breech NEC	N/A	669.61	669.60	N/A	763.0
manual NEC	669.83	669.81	669.80	N/A	763.89
Face presentation	652.43	652.41	652.40	N/A	763.1
causing obstructed labor	660.03	660.01	660.00	cause	763.1
Failure, failed					
cervical dilation in labor	661.03	661.01	661.00	N/A	763.7
descent of head (at term)	652.53	652.51	652.50	N/A	763.1
in labor	660.03	660.01	660.00	cause	763.1
engagement of head NEC	652.53	652.51	652.50	N/A	763.1
in labor	660.03	660.01	660.00	cause	763.1
fetal head to enter pelvic brim	652.53	652.51	652.50	N/A	763.1
in labor	660.03	660.01	660.00	cause	763.1
forceps NEC	660.73	660.71	660.70	cause	763.1
heart, complicating					
delivery (cesarean) (instrumental)	669.43	669.41	669.40	N/A	
obstetric anesthesia or sedation	668.13	668.11	668.10	N/A	
induction (of labor)	659.13	659.11	659.10	N/A	763.89
by oxytocic drugs (Pitocin)	659.13	659.11	659.10	N/A	763.89
instrumental	659.03	659.01	659.00	N/A	763.89
mechanical	659.03	659.01	659.00	N/A	763.89
medical	659.13	659.11	659.10	N/A	763.89
surgical	659.03	659.01	659.00	N/A	763.89
lactation	676.43	676.41	676.40	N/A	
to progress	661.23	661.21	661.20	N/A	763.89
trial of labor NOS	660.63	660.61	660.60	cause	763.1
vacuum extraction delivery NOS	660.73	660.71	660.70	cause	763.1
ventouse NOS	660.73	660.71	660.70	cause	763.1
False labor (pains)	644.13	N/A	644.10	N/A	
Fatigue	646.83	646.81	646.80	condition	
Fatty metamorphosis of liver	646.73	646.71	646.70	condition	760.8
Female genital mutilation	649.93	648.91	648.90	629.20-629	
Fetal					
acidosis	656.33	656.31	656.30	N/A	763.89
bradycardia	659.73	659.71	659.70	N/A	763.83
before onset of labor	659.73	659.71	659.70	N/A	763.81
during labor	659.73	659.71	659.70	N/A	763.82
decreased movements	655.73	655.71	655.70	N/A	763.89
demise (near term)	656.43	656.41	656.40	N/A	cause
early (before 22 weeks completed gestation)	632	N/A	N/A	N/A	761.8
deformity	653.73	653.71	653.70	N/A	763.1
causing obstructed labor	660.13	660.11	660.10	cause	763.1
distress	656.83	656.81	656.80	N/A	
heart rate, abnormal	659.73	659.71	659.70	N/A	763.83
before onset of labor	659.73	659.71	659.70	N/A	763.81
during labor	659.73	659.71	659.70	N/A	763.82
heart rhythm, abnormal	659.73	659.71	659.70	N/A	763.83
before onset of labor	659.73	659.71	659.70	N/A	763.81
during labor	659.73	659.71	659.70	N/A	763.82
movements, decreased	655.73	655.71	655.70	N/A	
Fetomaternal hemorrhage	656.03	656.01	656.00	N/A	772.0
Fibrinolysis	641.33	641.31	641.30	N/A	762.1
Fibroid tumor(s)	654.13	654.11	654.10	N/A	763.89
causing obstructed labor	660.23	660.21	660.20	cause	763.1
Fibromyoma (uterus)	654.13	654.11	654.10	N/A	763.89
causing obstructed labor	660.23	660.21	660.20	cause	763.1

Antepartum Pregnancy Table

Antepartum Pregnancy Condition or Complication; affecting management of mother	Antepartum condition or complication	Delivered, with or without mention of antepartum condition	Unspecified episode of care	Assign additional code to describe the...	Affecting fetus (coded on the newborn chart only)
Fibrosis, fibrotic					
amnion	658.83	658.81	658.80	N/A	
chorion	658.83	658.81	658.80	N/A	
perineum	654.83	654.81	654.80	N/A	763.8
causing obstructed labor	660.23	660.21	660.20	cause	763.1
Fissure, nipple	676.13	676.11	676.10	N/A	
Fistula					
breast	675.13	675.11	675.10	N/A	
mammary gland	675.13	675.11	675.10	N/A	
Flat, pelvis					
with disproportion (fetopelvic)	653.23	653.21	653.20	N/A	763.1
causing obstructed labor	660.13	660.11	660.10	cause	763.1
Footling presentation	652.83	652.81	652.80	N/A	
with successful version	652.13	652.11	652.10	N/A	
Forced birth or delivery NEC	N/A	669.81	669.80	N/A	763.89
Forceps delivery NEC	N/A	669.51	669.50	N/A	763.2
Fractured coccyx complicating delivery	N/A	665.61	665.60	N/A	
Frommel's disease	676.63	676.61	676.60	N/A	
Frommel-Chiari syndrome	676.63	676.61	676.60	N/A	
Funnel pelvis with disproportion (fetopelvic)	653.33	653.31	653.30	N/A	763.1
causing obstructed labor	660.13	660.11	660.10	cause	763.1
Fusion, hymeno-urethral					
causing obstructed labor	660.13	660.11	660.10	cause	763.1
Galactocele (breast)	676.83	676.81	676.80	N/A	
Galactorrhea	676.63	676.61	676.60	N/A	
Genital (female) mutilation	648.93	648.91	648.90	629.20-629.29	
Goiter	648.13	648.11	648.10	condition	
Gonococcal infection	647.13	647.11	647.10	condition	760.2
Gonorrhea	647.13	647.11	647.10	condition	760.2
Grand multiparity, affecting labor and delivery	659.43	659.41	659.40	N/A	
Growth fetal (poor)	656.53	656.51	656.50	N/A	764.90
Heart (fetal)					
abnormal					
rate		659.73	659.71	659.70	N/A
before onset of labor	659.73	659.71	659.70	N/A	763.81
during labor	659.73	659.71	659.70	N/A	763.82
rhythm	659.73	659.71	659.70	N/A	763.83
before onset of labor	659.73	659.71	659.70	N/A	763.81
during labor	659.73	659.71	659.70	N/A	763.82
HELLP (Hemolysis, Elevated Liver function and Low Platelets)	642.53	642.51	642.50	N/A	
Hematoma					
amnion	658.83	658.81	658.80	N/A	
broad ligament	N/A	665.71	665.70	N/A	
complicating delivery (perineum) (vulva)	N/A	664.51	664.50	N/A	
pelvic					
vagina	N/A	N/A	665.71	665.70	N/A
pelvis, complicating delivery	N/A	665.71	665.70	N/A	
perineal wound complicating delivery	N/A	664.51	664.50	N/A	
umbilical cord	663.63	663.61	663.60	N/A	762.6
vagina	N/A	665.71	665.70	N/A	
vulva, complicating delivery	N/A	664.51	664.50	N/A	767.8
Hemolysis, intravascular	641.33	641.31	641.30	N/A	762.1
Hemolysis, elevated liver function, low platelets syndrome (HELLP)	642.53	642.51	642.50	N/A	
Hemorrhage					
accidental	641.23	641.21	641.20	N/A	762.1
before 22 completed weeks gestation NEC	640.93	640.91	640.90	N/A	
brain		674.03	674.01	674.00	N/A
cerebrovascular	674.03	674.01	674.00	N/A	
complicating delivery	641.93	641.91	641.90	N/A	762.1
associated with					
afibrinogenemia	641.33	641.31	641.30	N/A	763.89
coagulation defect	641.33	641.31	641.30	N/A	763.89
hyperfibrinolysis	641.33	641.31	641.30	N/A	763.89
hypofibrinogenemia	641.33	641.31	641.30	N/A	763.89
concealed	641.93	641.91	641.90	N/A	762.1
due to					
afibrinogenemia or other coagulation defect	641.33	641.31	641.30	condition	763.89
fibroids	641.83	641.81	641.80	N/A	763.89
low-lying placenta	641.13	641.11	641.10	N/A	762.0
marginal sinus (rupture)	641.23	641.21	641.20	N/A	762.1
placenta previa	641.13	641.11	641.10	N/A	762.0
premature separation, placenta	641.23	641.21	641.20	N/A	762.1
trauma	641.83	641.81	641.80	N/A	763.89
umbilicus, umbilical cord	663.83	663.81	663.80	N/A	772.0
due to					
afibrinogenemia or other coagulation defect	641.33	641.31	641.30	condition	762.1
fibroids	641.83	641.81	641.80	N/A	762.1
low-lying placenta	641.13	641.11	641.10	N/A	762.1
marginal sinus					
(rupture)	641.23	641.21	641.20	N/A	762.1
placenta previa	641.13	641.11	641.10	N/A	762.0
premature separation, placenta	641.23	641.21	641.20	N/A	762.1
trauma	641.83	641.81	641.80	N/A	763.89

Resources

Antepartum Pregnancy Condition or Complication; affecting management of mother	Antepartum condition or complication	Delivered, with or without mention of antepartum condition	Unspecified episode of care	Assign additional code to describe the...	Affecting fetus (coded on the newborn chart only)
Hemorrhage – *continued*					
umbilicus, umbilical cord	663.83	663.81	663.80	N/A	772.0
early (before 22 completed weeks gestation)	640.93	640.91	640.90	N/A	762.1
fetomaternal	656.03	656.01	656.00	N/A	772.0
funis (complicating delivery)	663.83	663.81	663.80	N/A	772.0
intracranial	674.03	674.01	674.00	N/A	
marginal sinus	641.23	641.21	641.20	N/A	762.1
placenta NEC	641.93	641.91	641.90	N/A	762.1
from surgical or instrumental damage	641.83	641.81	641.80	N/A	762.1
previa	641.13	641.11	641.10	N/A	762.0
retroplacental	641.23	641.21	641.20	N/A	762.1
subarachnoid	674.03	674.01	674.00	N/A	
subdural	674.03	674.01	674.00	N/A	
threatened abortion	640.03	640.01	640.00	N/A	
umbilicus, umbilical cord (complicating delivery)	663.83	663.81	663.80	N/A	772.0
unavoidable	641.13	641.11	641.10	N/A	762.0
vasa previa	663.53	663.51	663.50	N/A	772.0
Hemorrhoids	671.83	671.81	671.80	N/A	
Hepatitis	646.73	646.71	646.70	condition	
viral	647.63	647.61	647.60	647.60	condition
Herniation of uterus	654.43	654.41	654.40	N/A	
causing obstructed labor	660.23	660.21	660.20	cause	763.1
Herpes, herpetic	647.63	647.61	647.60	condition	
gestationis	646.83	646.81	646.80	condition	
High head at term	652.43	652.41	652.40	N/A	763.1
HIV	647.63	647.61	647.60	647.60	042
asymptomatic	647.63	647.61	647.60	V08	
Hourglass uterus	661.43	661.41	661.40	N/A	763.7
Hydatidiform mole	630	N/A	N/A	N/A	
previous pregnancy, affecting management of current pregnancy	V23.1	V23.1	V23.1	N/A	
Hydramnios	657.03	657.01	657.00	N/A	761.3
Hydroa gestationis	646.83	646.81	646.80	condition	
Hydrocephalic fetus	655.03	655.01	655.00	N/A	763.1
causing disproportion	653.63	653.61	653.60	N/A	763.1
with obstructed labor	660.13	660.11	660.10	cause	763.1
Hydrops amnii	657.03	657.01	657.00	N/A	
Hydrorrhea	658.13	658.11	658.10	N/A	
Hyperemesis					
before 22 completed weeks of gestation	643.03	643.01	643.00	N/A	761.8
with					
carbohydrate depletion	643.13	643.11	643.10	N/A	761.8
dehydration	643.13	643.11	643.10	N/A	761.8
electrolyte imbalance	643.13	643.11	643.10	N/A	761.8
metabolic disturbance	643.13	643.11	643.10	N/A	761.8
mild	643.03	643.01	643.00	N/A	761.8
severe with metabolic disturbance	643.13	643.11	643.10	N/A	761.8
late (starting 23rd week of gestation)	643.23	643.21	643.20	N/A	761.8
Hypersecretion of milk	676.63	676.61	676.60	N/A	
Hypertension	642.93	642.91	642.90	N/A	760.0
with					
albuminuria (and edema) (mild)	642.43	642.41	642.40	N/A	760.0
severe	642.53	642.51	642.50	N/A	760.0
edema (mild)	642.43	642.41	642.40	N/A	760.0
severe	642.53	642.51	642.50	N/A	760.0
heart disease	642.23	642.21	642.20	N/A	760.0
and renal disease	642.23	642.21	642.20	N/A	760.0
pre-eclampsia or eclampsia	642.73	642.71	642.70	N/A	760.0
renal disease	642.23	642.21	642.20	N/A	760.0
and heart disease	642.23	642.21	642.20	N/A	760.0
benign	642.03	642.01	642.00	N/A	760.0
chronic	642.03	642.01	642.00	N/A	760.0
pre-existing	642.03	642.01	642.00	N/A	760.0
chronic	642.03	642.01	642.00	N/A	760.0
essential	642.03	642.01	642.00	N/A	760.0
with pre-eclampsia or eclampsia	642.73	642.71	642.70	N/A	
gestational	642.33	642.31	642.30	N/A	
malignant	642.23	642.21	642.20	N/A	760.0
chronic	642.23	642.21	642.20	N/A	760.0
with pre-eclampsia or eclampsia	642.73	642.71	642.70	N/A	
pre-existing	642.23	642.21	642.20	N/A	
pre-existing	642.03	642.01	642.00	N/A	760.0
secondary to renal disease	642.13	642.11	642.10	N/A	760.0
with pre-eclampsia or eclampsia	642.73	642.71	642.70	N/A	
transient	642.33	642.31	642.30	N/A	

Resources

Antepartum Pregnancy Table

Antepartum Pregnancy Condition or Complication; affecting management of mother	Antepartum condition or complication	Delivered, with or without mention of antepartum condition	Unspecified episode of care	Assign additional code to describe the...	Affecting fetus (coded on the newborn chart only)
Hypertensive					
heart and renal disease	642.23	642.21	642.20	N/A	760.0
heart disease	642.23	642.21	642.20	N/A	760.0
renal disease	642.23	642.21	642.20	N/A	760.0
Hyperthyroidism	648.13	648.11	648.10	condition	
Hypertonicity	648.13	648.11	648.10	condition	763.7
Hypertrophy					
breast	676.33	676.31	676.30	N/A	
Hypotension (following labor and delivery)	669.23	669.21	669.20	N/A	
Hypothyroidism	648.13	648.11	648.10	condition	
Hysteralgia	646.83	646.81	646.80	condition	
Icterus gravis	646.73	646.71	646.70	condition	760.8
Illegitimate	V61.6	V61.6	V61.6	N/A	
Imbalance					
electrolyte with hyperemesis gravidarum (before 22 completed weeks' gestation)	643.13	643.11	643.10	N/A	
Immunization					
ABO	656.23	656.21	656.20	N/A	773.1
Rh factor	656.13	656.11	656.10	N/A	773.0
Immunodeficiency to Rh factor	656.13	656.11	656.10	N/A	773.0
Impacted shoulder	660.43	660.41	660.40	cause	763.1
Inadequate development of fetus	656.53	656.51	656.50	N/A	764.90
Incarceration, uterus	654.33	654.31	654.30	N/A	763.1
causing obstructed labor	660.23	660.21	660.20	cause	763.1
Incompatibility, blood groups (ABO)					
ABO	656.23	656.21	656.20	N/A	773.1
Blood (group) (Duffy) (E) (K(ell)) (Kidd) (Lewis) (M) (N) (P) (S) NEC	656.23	656.21	656.20	N/A	773.2
Rh(esus) (blood group) (factor)	656.13	656.11	656.10	N/A	773.0
Incompetent cervix (os)	654.53	654.51	654.50	N/A	761.0
causing obstructed labor	660.23	660.21	660.20	cause	763.1
Incoordinate uterus (action) (contractions)	661.43	661.41	661.40	N/A	763.7
In double uterus	654.03	654.01	654.00	N/A	
causing obstructed labor	660.23	660.21	660.20	cause	763.1
Induced					
failed by method of					
drugs					
mechanical		659.13	659.11	659.10	N/A
successful — assign code to indicate the reason for the induction	659.03	659.01	659.00	N/A	763.89
Indurated breast	676.33	676.31	676.30	N/A	
Inertia, uterus NEC					
primary	661.03	661.01	661.00	N/A	763.7
secondary	661.13	661.11	661.10	N/A	763.7
Infantile					
genitalia, genitals	654.43	654.41	654.40	N/A	763.89
causing obstructed labor	660.23	660.21	660.20	cause	763.1
pelvis	653.13	653.11	653.10	N/A	763.1
causing obstructed labor	660.13	660.11	660.10	cause	763.1
Infarct, infarction					
amnion	658.83	658.81	658.80	N/A	
brain (stem)	674.03	674.01	674.00	N/A	
chorion	658.83	658.81	658.80	N/A	
lung — see Pregnancy, embolism					
placenta	656.73	656.71	656.70	N/A	762.2
Infection	647.93	647.91	647.90	condition	760.2
amniotic fluid	658.43	658.41	658.40	condition	762.7
bladder	646.63	646.61	646.60	condition	
breast (mammary gland)	675.23	675.21	675.20	N/A	
with nipple	675.93	675.91	675.90	N/A	
specified type NEC	675.83	675.81	675.80	N/A	
nonpurulent	675.23	675.21	675.20	N/A	
purulent	675.13	675.11	675.10	N/A	
chorionic plate	658.83	658.81	658.80	N/A	
genital organs	646.63	646.61	646.60	condition	760.8
minor or localized	646.63	646.61	646.60	condition	760.8
intrauterine, complicating delivery	646.63	646.61	646.60	condition	
kidney	646.63	646.61	646.60	condition	760.1
nipple	675.03	675.01	675.00	N/A	
with breast	675.93	675.91	675.90	N/A	
specified type NEC	675.83	675.81	675.80	N/A	
perineal wound minor	646.63	646.61	646.60	condition	760.1
urinary (tract)	646.63	646.61	646.60	condition	760.1
asymptomatic	646.53	646.51	646.50	condition	760.1
UTI	646.63	646.61	646.60	condition	760.1
asymptomatic	646.53	646.51	646.50	condition	760.1
Infective and parasitic diseases NEC	647.83	647.81	647.80	complication	
Infestation	647.93	647.91	647.90	condition	760.8
Inflammation					
areola	675.03	675.01	675.00	N/A	
bladder	646.63	646.61	646.60	condition	760.8
breast (mammary gland)	675.23	675.21	675.20	N/A	
fetal membranes (acute)	658.43	658.41	658.40	N/A	762.7
genital organ	646.63	646.61	646.60	condition	760.8
urinary tract NEC	646.63	646.61	646.60	condition	760.8

Resources

Antepartum Pregnancy Condition or Complication; affecting management of mother	Antepartum condition or complication	Delivered, with or without mention of antepartum condition	Unspecified episode of care	Assign additional code to describe the...	Affecting fetus (coded on the newborn chart only)
Inhalation of stomach contents or secretions in labor and delivery	668.03	668.01	668.00	N/A	
Injury	648.93	648.91	648.90	condition	
birth canal NEC	665.93	665.91	665.90	N/A	763.89
coccyx, complicating delivery	N/A	665.61	665.60	N/A	
genital organs, obstetrical					
trauma NEC	665.93	665.91	665.90	N/A	763.89
instrumental, obstetrical NEC	665.93	665.91	665.90	N/A	763.89
bladder	N/A	665.51	665.50	N/A	763.89
cervix	N/A	665.31	665.30	N/A	763.89
high vaginal	N/A	665.41	665.40	N/A	763.89
perineal NEC	N/A	664.91	664.90	N/A	763.89
urethra	N/A	665.51	665.50	N/A	763.89
uterus	N/A	665.51	665.50	N/A	763.89
obstetrical NEC	665.93	665.91	665.90	N/A	763.89
pelvic, complicating delivery					
floor	N/A	664.11	664.10	N/A	763.89
joint or ligament	N/A	665.61	665.60	N/A	763.89
organs	N/A	665.51	665.50	N/A	763.89
periurethral tissue, complicating delivery	N/A	665.51	665.50	N/A	763.89
symphysis pubis, complicating delivery	N/A	665.61	665.60	N/A	763.89
Insertion of umbilical cord, lateral or velamentous	663.53	663.51	663.50	N/A	762.6
Insufficient					
prenatal care	V23.7	N/A	N/A	N/A	
weight gain	646.83	646.81	646.80	condition	
Interstitial — *see also* Ectopic pregnancy table	633.8	N/A	N/A	N/A	761.4
Intraligamentous — *see also* Ectopic pregnancy	633.8	N/A	N/A	N/A	761.4
Intramural — *see also* Ectopic pregnancy	633.8	N/A	N/A	N/A	761.4
Intraperitoneal — *see also* Ectopic pregnancy	633.0	N/A	N/A	N/A	761.4
Intoxication					
chemical via placenta or breast milk, suspected	655.53	655.51	655.50	N/A	760.70
drug					
obstetric anesthetic or sedation	668.93	668.91	668.90	N/A	763.5
via placenta or breast milk, suspected	655.53	655.51	655.50	N/A	760.70
septic					
during labor	659.33	659.31	659.30	N/A	
Intrauterine fetal death					
early (before 22 completed weeks of gestation)	632	N/A	N/A	N/A	
near term NEC	656.43	656.41	656.40	N/A	
Isoimmunization (ABO)	656.23	656.21	656.20	N/A	
Rh(esus)	656.13	656.11	656.10	N/A	
Isthmian (with rupture) — *see also* Ectopic Pregnancy	633.1	N/A	N/A	N/A	761.4
Inversion					
nipple	676.33	676.31	676.30		
Ischemia, cerebral	674.03	674.01	674.00	N/A	
Joint disorders	648.73	648.71	648.70	condition	
Knot, umbilical cord (true)	663.23	663.21	663.20	N/A	762.5
Labor					
abnormal NEC	661.93	661.91	661.90	N/A	763.7
arrested active phase	661.13	661.11	661.10	N/A	763.7
desultory	661.23	661.21	661.20	N/A	763.7
dyscoordinate	661.43	661.41	661.40	N/A	763.7
early onset (22-36 weeks gestation)	N/A3	644.21	644.20	N/A	763.7
failed					763.7
induction	659.13	659.11	659.10	N/A	763.89
mechanical	659.03	659.01	659.00	N/A	763.89
medical (drug)	659.13	659.11	659.10	N/A	763.89
surgical	659.03	659.01	659.00	N/A	763.89
trial (vaginal delivery)	660.63	660.61	660.60	cause	763.1
false		644.13	N/A	644.10	N/A
hypertonic	661.43	661.41	661.40	N/A	763.7
hypotonic, primary	661.03	661.01	661.00	N/A	763.7
secondary	661.13	661.11	661.10	N/A	763.7
incoordinate	661.43	661.41	661.40	N/A	763.7
irregular	661.23	661.21	661.20	N/A	763.7
long	662.13	662.11	662.10	N/A	763.89
first stage	662.03	662.01	662.00	N/A	763.89
second stage	662.23	662.21	662.20	N/A	763.89
missed (at or near term)	656.43	656.41	656.40	N/A	
obstructed NEC	660.93	660.91	660.90	cause	763.1
specified cause NEC	660.83	660.81	660.80	cause	763.1
pains, spurious	644.13	N/A	644.10	N/A	
precipitate	661.33	661.31	661.30	N/A	763.6
premature	N/A3	644.21	644.20	N/A	
threatened	644.03	N/A	644.00	N/A	
prolonged or protracted	662.13	662.11	662.10	N/A	763.89
first stage	662.03	662.01	662.00	N/A	763.89
second stage	662.23	662.21	662.20	N/A	763.89
threatened NEC	644.13	N/A	644.10	N/A	
undelivered	644.13	N/A	644.10	N/A	
Laceration (obstetrical trauma)					
anus (complicating delivery)	N/A	664.21	664.20	N/A	
with laceration of anal or rectal mucosa	N/A	664.31	664.30	N/A	
bladder	N/A	665.51	665.50	N/A	

Antepartum Pregnancy Table

Antepartum Pregnancy Condition or Complication; affecting management of mother	Antepartum condition or complication	Delivered, with or without mention of antepartum condition	Unspecified episode of care	Assign additional code to describe the...	Affecting fetus (coded on the newborn chart only)
Laceration (obstetrical trauma) — *continued*					
bowel		N/A	665.51	665.50	N/A
broad ligament	N/A	665.61	665.60	N/A	
central, complicating delivery	N/A	664.41	664.40	N/A	
cervix (uteri)	N/A	665.31	665.30	N/A	
fourchette, complicating delivery	N/A	664.01	664.00	N/A	
labia, complicating delivery	N/A	664.01	664.00	N/A	
pelvic (complicating delivery)					
floor (muscles)	N/A	664.11	664.10	N/A	
organ NEC (obstetrical trauma)	N/A	665.51	665.50	N/A	763.89
perineum, complicating delivery	N/A	664.41	664.40	N/A	
first degree	N/A	664.01	664.00	N/A	
second degree	N/A	664.11	664.10	N/A	
third degree	N/A	664.21	664.20	N/A	
fourth degree	N/A	664.31	664.30	N/A	
involving					
anal sphincter	N/A	664.21	664.20	N/A	
fourchette	N/A	664.01	664.00	N/A	
hymen	N/A	664.01	664.00	N/A	
labia		N/A	664.01	664.00	N/A
pelvic floor	N/A	664.11	664.10	N/A	
perineal muscles	N/A	664.11	664.10	N/A	
rectovaginal with septum	N/A	664.21	664.20	N/A	
with anal mucosa	N/A	664.31	664.30	N/A	
skin		N/A	664.01	664.00	N/A
sphincter (anal)	N/A	664.21	664.20	N/A	
with anal mucosa	N/A	664.31	664.30	N/A	
vagina	N/A	664.01	664.00	N/A	
vaginal muscles	N/A	664.11	664.10	N/A	
vulva		N/A	664.01	664.00	N/A
peritoneum (obstetrical trauma)	N/A	665.51	665.50	N/A	
periurethral tissue (obstetrical trauma)	N/A	665.51	665.50	N/A	
rectovaginal septum	N/A	665.41	665.40	N/A	
with perineum	N/A	664.21	664.20	N/A	
involving anal or rectal mucosa	N/A	664.31	664.30	N/A	
urethra (obstetrical trauma)	N/A	665.51	665.50	N/A	
uterus (obstetrical trauma NEC)	N/A	665.11	665.10	N/A	
vagina (complicating delivery)	N/A	665.41	665.40	N/A	
with perineal involvement	N/A	664.01	664.00	N/A	
first degree	N/A	664.01	664.00	N/A	
second degree	N/A	664.11	664.10	N/A	
third degree	N/A	664.21	664.20	N/A	
fourth degree	N/A	664.31	664.30	N/A	
high	N/A	664.41	664.40	N/A	
muscles	N/A	664.11	664.10	N/A	
sulcus	N/A	665.41	665.40	N/A	
wall	N/A	665.41	665.40	N/A	
vulva (complicating delivery)	N/A	664.01	664.00	N/A	
Lactation, lactating (breast)					
defective	676.43	676.41	676.40	N/A	
disorder	676.93	676.91	676.90	N/A	
specified type NEC	676.83	676.81	676.80	N/A	
examination and/or care of mother	V24.1	V24.1	V24.1	N/A	
excessive	676.63	676.61	676.60	N/A	
failed		676.43	676.41	676.40	N/A
mastitis NEC	675.23	675.21	675.20	N/A	
suppressed	676.53	676.51	676.50	N/A	
Large					
fetus causing disproportion	653.53	653.51	653.50	N/A	763.1
with obstructed labor	660.13	660.11	660.10	cause	763.1
for-dates (fetus)	656.63	656.61	656.60	N/A	766.1
exceptionally (weight of 4500 grams or more)	656.63	656.61	656.60	N/A	766.0
Late effect(s) (of)					
childbirth complication(s)	677	677	677	condition	
complication(s) of					
childbirth	677	677	677	condition	
delivery	677	677	677	condition	
postpartum	677	677	677	condition	
pregnancy	677	677	677	condition	
puerperium	677	677	677	condition	
Lateroversion, uterus	654.43	654.41	654.40	N/A	763.89
causing obstructed labor	660.23	660.21	660.20	cause	763.1
Leakage					
amniotic fluid	658.13	658.11	658.10	N/A	761.1
with delayed delivery	658.23	658.21	658.20	N/A	761.1
blood (microscopic), fetal, into maternal circulation	656.03	656.01	656.00	N/A	
Lesion, vascular of umbilical cord	663.63	663.61	663.60	N/A	762.6
Light-for-dates	656.53	656.51	656.50	N/A	764.00
with signs of fetal malnutrition	656.53	656.51	656.50	N/A	764.10
Listeriosis, suspected fetal damage	655.43	655.41	655.40	N/A	771.2
Lithopedion	656.83	656.81	656.80	N/A	
Locked twins	660.53	660.51	660.50	cause	763.1
Lymphadenitis, breast	675.23	675.21	675.20	N/A	
breast	675.23	675.21	675.20	N/A	
Malaria	647.43	647.41	647.40	condition	

Resources

Antepartum Pregnancy Condition or Complication; affecting management of mother	Antepartum condition or complication	Delivered, with or without mention of antepartum condition	Unspecified episode of care	Assign additional code to describe the...	Affecting fetus (coded on the newborn chart only)
Male type pelvis with disproportion (fetopelvic)	653.23	653.21	653.20	N/A	763.1
causing obstructed labor	660.13	660.11	660.10	cause	763.1
Malformation					
pelvic organs or tissues	654.93	654.91	654.90	N/A	763.89
causing obstructed labor	660.23	660.21	660.20	cause	763.1
placenta	656.73	656.71	656.70	N/A	
umbilical cord (complicating delivery)	663.93	663.91	663.90	N/A	762.6
uterus (congenital)	654.03	654.01	654.00	N/A	
causing obstructed labor	660.23	660.21	660.20	cause	763.1
Malnutrition	648.93	648.91	648.90	condition	
Fetal malnutrition					
Without mention of "light-for dates"					
unspecified (weight)					764.20
< 500 gms					764.21
500-749 gms					764.22
750-999 gms					764.23
1,000-1,249 gms					764.24
1,250-1,499 gms					764.25
1,500-1,749 gms					764.26
1,750-1,999 gms					764.27
2,000-2,499 gms					764.28
≥ 2,500 gms					764.29
With mention of "light-for dates" unspecified (weight)					764.10
< 500 gms					764.11
500-749 gms					764.12
750-999 gms					764.13
1,000-1,249 gms					764.14
1,250-1,499 gms					764.15
1,500-1,749 gms					764.16
1,750-1,999 gms					764.17
2,000-2,499 gms					764.18
≥ 2,500 gms					764.19
Malposition					
fetal NEC	652.93	652.91	652.90	N/A	763.1
with successful version	652.13	652.11	652.10	N/A	763.1
before labor	652.93	652.91	652.90	N/A	763.1
in multiple gestation	652.63	652.61	652.60	N/A	763.1
with locking	660.53	660.51	660.50	cause	763.1
causing obstructed labor	660.03	660.01	660.00	cause	763.1
pelvic organs or tissues	654.43	654.41	654.40	N/A	763.89
causing obstructed labor	660.23	660.21	660.20	cause	763.1
specified type NEC	652.83	652.81	652.80	N/A	763.1
causing obstructed labor	660.03	660.01	660.00	cause	763.1
uterus or cervix	654.43	654.41	654.40	N/A	763.89
causing obstructed labor	660.23	660.21	660.20	cause	763.1
Malpresentation					
fetal	652.93	652.91	652.90	N/A	763.1
with successful version	652.13	652.11	652.10	N/A	763.1
in multiple gestation	652.63	652.61	652.60	N/A	763.1
specified type NEC	652.83	652.81	652.80	N/A	763.1
causing obstructed labor	660.03	660.01	660.00	cause	763.1
uterus or cervix	654.43	654.41	654.40	N/A	
causing obstructed labor	660.03	660.01	660.00	cause	763.1
Mammillitis, puerperal	675.23	675.21	675.20	N/A	
Mammitis, puerperal	675.23	675.21	675.20	N/A	
Marginal sinus hemorrhage or rupture	641.23	641.21	641.20	N/A	762.1
Mastitis					
lactational	675.23	675.21	675.20	N/A	
puerperal, (interstitial) (nonpurulent) (parenchymatous)	675.23	675.21	675.20	N/A	
purulent	675.13	675.11	675.10	N/A	
stagnation	675.23	675.21	675.20	N/A	
puerperalis	675.23	675.21	675.20	N/A	
retromammary	675.13	675.11	675.10	N/A	
submammary	675.13	675.11	675.10	N/A	
Maternal obesity syndrome	646.13	646.11	646.10	condition	
Meconium in liquor (staining)	656.83	656.81	656.80	N/A	
Membranitis, fetal	658.43	658.41	658.40	N/A	762.7
Mendelson's syndrome	668.03	668.01	668.00	N/A	
Menstruation during pregnancy	640.83	640.81	640.80	N/A	
Mental disorders	648.43	648.41	648.40	condition	
Mentum presentation	652.43	652.41	652.40	N/A	763.1
causing obstructed labor	660.03	660.01	660.00	cause	763.1
Metaplasia squamous cell amnion	658.83	658.81	658.80	N/A	763.89
Milk					
excess secretion	676.63	676.61	676.60	N/A	
Milk leg (deep vessels)	671.33	671.31	671.30	N/A	
Missed					
delivery (at or near term)	656.43	656.41	656.40	N/A	763.89
labor (at or near term)	656.43	656.41	656.40	N/A	763.89
Morning sickness	643.03	643.01	643.00	N/A	
Multiparity (grand)	659.43	659.41	659.40	N/A	763.8

Resources

Antepartum Pregnancy Table

Antepartum Pregnancy Condition or Complication; affecting management of mother	Antepartum condition or complication	Delivered, with or without mention of antepartum condition	Unspecified episode of care	Assign additional code to describe the...	Affecting fetus (coded on the newborn chart only)
Myelomeningocele fetal, causing fetopelvic disproportion	653.73	653.71	653.70	N/A	763.1
causing obstructed labor	660.13	660.11	660.10	cause	763.1
Myoma uterus (cervix) (corpus)	654.13	654.11	654.10	N/A	763.89
causing obstructed labor	660.23	660.21	660.20	cause	763.1
Nägele's pelvis with disproportion (fetopelvic)	653.03	653.01	653.00	N/A	763.1
causing obstructed labor	660.13	660.11	660.10	cause	763.1
Necrosis					
genital organ or tract	646.63	646.61	646.60	condition	760.8
kidney, cortical (acute)	646.23	646.21	646.20	condition	760.1
tubular	646.23	646.21	646.20	condition	760.1
liver	646.73	646.71	646.70	condition	760.8
placenta	656.73	656.71	656.70	N/A	762.2
renal, cortical	646.23	646.21	646.20	condition	760.1
Nephritis, nephrosis	646.23	646.21	646.20	condition	760.1
with hypertension	642.13	642.11	642.10	N/A	760.0
Nephropathy NEC	646.23	646.21	646.20	condition	
Neuritis (peripheral)	646.43	646.41	646.40	condition	
Nonengagement of head NEC	652.53	652.51	652.50	N/A	763.1
in labor	660.03	660.01	660.00	cause	763.1
Noxious substances transmitted through placenta or breast milk, suspected, unspecified	655.53	655.51	655.50	N/A	760.70
Nuchal hitch (arm)	652.83	652.81	652.80	N/A	763.1
causing obstructed labor	660.03	660.01	660.00	cause	763.1
Nutritional deficiency	648.93	648.91	648.90	condition	
Obesity					
excessive weight gain during pregnancy	646.13	646.11	646.10	complication	
morbid	649.13	649.11	649.10	278.01, V85.39-V85.4	
Oblique lie or presentation	652.33	652.31	652.30	N/A	763.1
with successful version	652.13	652.11	652.10	N/A	763.1
causing obstructed labor	660.03	660.01	660.00	cause	763.1
Obstetrical trauma NEC (complicating delivery)	665.93	665.91	665.90	N/A	763.89
Obstruction, obstructed, obstructive					
labor	660.93	660.91	660.90	cause	763.1
borderline pelvis	660.13	660.11	660.10	cause	763.1
by					
bony pelvis	660.13	660.11	660.10	cause	763.1
deep transverse arrest	660.33	660.31	660.30	cause	763.1
impacted shoulder	660.43	660.41	660.40	cause	763.1
locked twins	660.53	660.51	660.50	cause	763.1
malposition (fetus)	660.03	660.01	660.00	cause	763.1
head during labor	660.33	660.31	660.30	cause	763.1
persistent occipitoposterior position	660.33	660.31	660.30	cause	763.1
soft tissue, pelvic	660.23	660.21	660.20	cause	763.1
Occlusion, precerebral artery NEC	674.03	674.01	674.00	condition	
Oligohydramnios NEC	658.03	658.01	658.00	N/A	761.2
due to premature rupture of membranes	658.13	658.11	658.10	N/A	761.2
Oliguria	646.23	646.21	646.20	condition	
with hypertension — see Pregnancy, toxemia					
Oophoritis	646.63	646.61	646.60	condition	
Oversize fetus (weight of 4500 grams or more)	656.63	656.61	656.60	N/A	766.0
causing disproportion	653.53	653.51	653.50	N/A	763.1
with obstructed labor	660.13	660.11	660.10	cause	763.1
Pain(s)	646.83	646.81	646.80	condition	
false labor	644.13	N/A	644.10	N/A	
Papyraceous fetus	646.03	646.01	646.00	condition	779.8
Paralysis, bladder	N/A	665.51	665.50	N/A	
Patent cervix	654.53	654.51	654.50	N/A	761.0
causing obstructed labor	660.23	660.21	660.20	cause	763.1
Pendulous	654.43	654.41	654.40	N/A	763.89
causing obstructed labor	660.23	660.21	660.20	cause	763.1
complication of delivery	N/A	665.11	665.10	N/A	763.89
Perforation					
bladder	N/A	665.51	665.50	N/A	
bowel	N/A	665.51	665.50	N/A	
broad ligament	N/A	665.61	665.60	N/A	
cervix	N/A	665.31	665.30	N/A	
instrumental (complicating delivery)	665.93	665.91	665.90	N/A	
pelvic (floor)	N/A	664.11	664.10	N/A	
organ	N/A	665.51	665.50	N/A	763.89
urethral	N/A	665.51	665.50	N/A	763.89
uterus	N/A	665.51	665.50	N/A	763.89
Persistence					
hymen (tag)	654.83	654.81	654.80	N/A	
causing obstructed labor	660.23	660.21	660.20	cause	763.1
occiput (anterior or posterior)	660.33	660.31	660.30	cause	763.1
Phlebitis	671.93	671.91	671.90	N/A	760.3
deep	671.33	671.31	671.30	N/A	760.3
intracranial	671.53	671.51	671.50	N/A	
lower extremities	671.23	671.21	671.20	N/A	760.3
specified site NEC	671.53	671.51	671.50	N/A	
superficial	671.23	671.21	671.20	N/A	760.3
Phlegmasia	671.33	671.31	671.30	N/A	760.3
PID	646.63	646.61	646.60	condition	

Resources

Antepartum Pregnancy Condition or Complication; affecting management of mother	Antepartum condition or complication	Delivered, with or without mention of antepartum condition	Unspecified episode of care	Assign additional code to describe the...	Affecting fetus (coded on the newborn chart only)
Pithecoid pelvis (fetopelvic)	653.23	653.21	653.20	N/A	763.1
obstructed labor	660.13	660.11	660.10	cause	763.1
Placenta, placental					
abnormal	656.73	656.71	656.70	N/A	762.2
with hemorrhage	641.83	641.81	641.80	N/A	762.1
abruptio or ablatio	641.23	641.21	641.20	N/A	762.1
absorption (suspected) of					
chemical	655.53	655.51	655.50	N/A	760.79
drug (NEC)	655.53	655.51	655.50	N/A	760.79
accessory lobe	656.73	656.71	656.70	N/A	762.2
with hemorrhage	641.83	641.81	641.80	N/A	762.1
apoplexy	641.23	641.21	641.20	N/A	762.1
battledore	656.73	656.71	656.70	N/A	762.2
with hemorrhage	641.83	641.81	641.80	N/A	762.1
bilobate	656.73	656.71	656.70	N/A	762.2
with hemorrhage	641.83	641.81	641.80	N/A	762.1
bipartita	656.73	656.71	656.70	N/A	762.2
with hemorrhage	641.83	641.81	641.80	N/A	762.1
centralis	641.03	641.01	641.00	N/A	762.0
with hemorrhage	641.13	641.11	641.10	N/A	762.1
circumvallata	656.73	656.71	656.70	N/A	762.2
with hemorrhage	641.83	641.81	641.80	N/A	762.1
cyst (amniotic)	656.73	656.71	656.70	N/A	762.2
with hemorrhage	641.83	641.81	641.80	N/A	762.1
deficiency	656.53	656.51	656.50	N/A	762.2
degeneration	656.53	656.51	656.50	N/A	762.2
detachment	641.23	641.21	641.20	N/A	762.1
dimidiata	656.73	656.71	656.70	N/A	762.2
with hemorrhage	641.83	641.81	641.80	N/A	762.1
disease	656.73	656.71	656.70	N/A	762.2
with hemorrhage	641.83	641.81	641.80	N/A	762.1
duplex	656.73	656.71	656.70	N/A	762.2
with hemorrhage	641.83	641.81	641.80	N/A	762.1
dysfunction	656.53	656.51	656.50	N/A	762.2
fenestrata	656.73	656.71	656.70	N/A	762.2
with hemorrhage	641.83	641.81	641.80	N/A	762.1
fibrosis	656.73	656.71	656.70	N/A	762.2
with hemorrhage	641.83	641.81	641.80	N/A	762.1
hematoma	656.73	656.71	656.70	N/A	762.2
with hemorrhage	641.83	641.81	641.80	N/A	762.1
hemorrhage	641.23	641.21	641.20	N/A	762.1
hormone disturbance	656.73	656.71	656.70	N/A	762.2
with hemorrhage	641.83	641.81	641.80	N/A	762.1
hyperplasia	656.73	656.71	656.70	N/A	762.2
with hemorrhage	641.83	641.81	641.80	N/A	762.1
infarct	656.73	656.71	656.70	N/A	762.2
with hemorrhage	641.83	641.81	641.80	N/A	762.1
insertion, vicious	641.03	641.01	641.00	N/A	762.0
with hemorrhage	641.13	641.11	641.10	N/A	762.1
insufficiency	656.53	656.51	656.50	N/A	762.2
lateral	641.03	641.01	641.00	N/A	762.0
with hemorrhage	641.13	641.11	641.10	N/A	762.1
low implantation	641.03	641.01	641.00	N/A	762.0
with hemorrhage	641.13	641.11	641.10	N/A	762.1
low lying	641.03	641.01	641.00	N/A	762.0
with hemorrhage	641.13	641.11	641.10	N/A	762.1
malformation	656.73	656.71	656.70	N/A	762.2
with hemorrhage	641.83	641.81	641.80	N/A	762.1
malposition	641.03	641.01	641.00	N/A	762.2
with hemorrhage	641.13	641.11	641.10	N/A	762.1
marginalis, marginata	641.03	641.01	641.00	N/A	762.0
with hemorrhage	641.13	641.11	641.10	N/A	762.1
marginal sinus (hemorrhage)	641.23	641.21	641.20	N/A	762.1
membranacea	656.73	656.71	656.70	N/A	762.2
with hemorrhage	641.83	641.81	641.80	N/A	762.1
multiload	656.73	656.71	656.70	N/A	762.2
with hemorrhage	641.83	641.81	641.80	N/A	762.1
necrosis	656.73	656.71	656.70	N/A	762.2
with hemorrhage	641.83	641.81	641.80	N/A	762.1
previa	641.03	641.01	641.00	N/A	762.0
with hemorrhage	641.13	641.11	641.10	N/A	762.1
separation (premature) (undelivered)	641.23	641.21	641.20	N/A	762.1
septuplex	656.73	656.71	656.70	N/A	762.2
with hemorrhage	641.83	641.81	641.80	N/A	762.1
small	656.53	656.51	656.50	N/A	762.2
softening	656.73	656.71	656.70	N/A	762.2
with hemorrhage	641.83	641.81	641.80	N/A	762.1
spuria	656.73	656.71	656.70	N/A	762.2
with hemorrhage	641.83	641.81	641.80	N/A	762.1
succenturiata	656.73	656.71	656.70	N/A	762.2
with hemorrhage	641.83	641.81	641.80	N/A	762.1
syphilitic	647.03	647.01	647.00	condition	760.2
manifest syphilis in the infant or fetus	647.03	647.01	647.00	condition	090.0
transfusion syndromes (fetus)	N/A	N/A	N/A	N/A	762.3

Resources

Antepartum Pregnancy Table

Antepartum Pregnancy Condition or Complication; affecting management of mother	Antepartum condition or complication	Delivered, with or without mention of antepartum condition	Unspecified episode of care	Assign additional code to describe the...	Affecting fetus (coded on the newborn chart only)
Placenta, placental – *continued*					
transmission of chemical substance (suspected, affecting pregnancy)	655.53	655.51	655.50	N/A	760.70
trilobate	656.73	656.71	656.70	N/A	762.2
with hemorrhage	641.83	641.81	641.80	N/A	762.1
triplex	656.73	656.71	656.70	N/A	762.2
with hemorrhage	641.83	641.81	641.80	N/A	762.1
varicose vessel	656.73	656.71	656.70	N/A	762.2
with hemorrhage	641.83	641.81	641.80	N/A	762.1
vicious insertion	641.03	641.01	641.00	N/A	
with hemorrhage	641.13	641.11	641.10	N/A	762.0
Placentitis	658.43	658.41	658.40	N/A	762.7
Platypelloid pelvis (disproportion)	653.23	653.21	653.20	N/A	763.1
obstructed labor	660.13	660.11	660.10	cause	763.1
Pneumonitis					
aspiration	668.03	668.01	668.00	condition	770.18
postanesthetic	668.03	668.01	668.00	condition	
postoperative	668.03	668.01	668.00	N/A	
Polygalactia	676.63	676.61	676.60	N/A	
Polyhydramnios	657.03	657.01	657.00	N/A	761.3
Polyp					
cervix	654.63	654.61	654.60	N/A	763.89
obstructed labor	660.23	660.21	660.20	cause	763.1
uterus	654.13	654.11	654.10	N/A	763.89
obstructed labor	660.23	660.21	660.20	cause	763.1
Poor					
contractions labor	661.23	661.21	661.20	N/A	763.7
fetal growth, affecting management	656.53	656.51	656.50	N/A	
Fetal growth retardation					
unspecified (weight)					764.90
< 500 gms					764.91
500-749 gms					764.92
750-999 gms					764.93
1,000-1,249 gms					764.94
1,250-1,499 gms					764.95
1,500-1,749 gms					764.96
1,750-1,999 gms					764.97
2,000-2,499 gms					764.98
≥ 2,500 gms					764.99
obstetrical history	V23.4	N/A	N/A	N/A	
Position – *see also* Presentation, fetal	652.93	652.91	652.90	N/A	763.1
causing obstructed labor	660.03	660.01	660.00	cause	763.1
Post-term (over 40 to 42 completed weeks)	645.13	645.11	645.10	N/A	766.21
Prediabetes	648.83	648.81	648.80	condition	
Prolonged (over 42 completed weeks)	645.23	645.21	645.20	N/A	766.22
Pre-eclampsia (mild)	642.43	642.41	642.40	N/A	760.0
with convulsions	642.63	642.61	642.60	N/A	760.0
severe	642.53	642.51	642.50	N/A	760.0
superimposed on pre-existing hypertensive disease	642.73	642.71	642.70	N/A	760.0
Pre-existing condition (prior to pregnancy) affecting current pregnancy					
abnormal glucose tolerance	648.83	648.81	648.80	condition	
anemia	648.23	648.21	648.20	condition	
bone and joint (lower limb)	648.73	648.71	648.70	condition	
cardiovascular	648.63	648.61	648.60	condition	
congenital	648.53	648.51	648.50	condition	
cerebrovascular	674.03	674.01	674.00	N/A	
diabetic	648.03	648.01	648.00	condition	
drug dependence	648.33	648.31	648.30	condition	
genital organ or tract	646.63	646.61	646.60	condition	
gonorrheal	647.13	647.11	647.10	condition	
hypertensive	642.23	642.21	642.20	N/A	
renal		642.13	642.11	642.10	N/A
infectious	647.93	647.91	647.90	condition	
specified type NEC	647.83	647.81	647.80	condition	
liver		646.73	646.71	646.70	condition
malarial	647.43	647.41	647.40	condition	
nutritional deficiency	648.93	648.91	648.90	condition	
parasitic NEC	647.83	647.81	647.80	condition	
renal		646.23	646.21	646.20	condition
hypertensive	642.13	642.11	642.10	N/A	
rubella	647.53	647.51	647.50	condition	
specified condition NEC	648.93	648.91	648.90	condition	
syphilitic	647.03	647.01	647.00	condition	
thyroid	648.13	648.11	648.10	condition	
tuberculous	647.33	647.31	647.30	condition	
urinary	646.63	646.61	646.60	condition	
venereal	647.23	647.21	647.20	condition	
viral NEC	647.63	647.61	647.60	condition	
Premature					
labor		N/A	644.21	644.20	N/A
threatened	644.03	N/A	644.00	N/A	
rupture of membranes or amnion	658.13	658.11	658.10	N/A	761.1
with delayed delivery	658.23	658.21	658.20	N/A	

Resources

Antepartum Pregnancy Condition or Complication; affecting management of mother	Antepartum condition or complication	Delivered, with or without mention of antepartum condition	Unspecified episode of care	Assign additional code to describe the...	Affecting fetus (coded on the newborn chart only)
Presentation, fetal					
abnormal	652.93	652.91	652.90	N/A	763.1
with successful version	652.13	652.11	652.10	N/A	761.7
causing obstructed labor	660.03	660.01	660.00	cause	763.1
in multiple gestation (one or more)	652.63	652.61	652.60	N/A	763.1
causing obstructed labor	660.03	660.01	660.00	cause	763.1
specified NEC	652.83	652.81	652.80	N/A	763.1
causing obstructed labor	660.03	660.01	660.00	cause	763.1
arm	652.73	652.71	652.70	N/A	763.1
causing obstructed labor	660.03	660.01	660.00	cause	763.1
breech	652.23	652.21	652.20	N/A	761.7
with successful version	652.13	652.11	652.10	N/A	761.7
causing obstructed labor	660.03	660.01	660.00	cause	763.0
brow	652.43	652.41	652.40	N/A	763.1
causing obstructed labor	660.03	660.01	660.00	cause	763.1
cord	663.03	663.01	663.00	N/A	762.5
extended head	652.43	652.41	652.40	N/A	763.1
causing obstructed labor	660.03	660.01	660.00	cause	763.1
face	652.43	652.41	652.40	N/A	763.1
causing obstructed labor	660.03	660.01	660.00	cause	763.1
to pubes	652.83	652.81	652.80	N/A	763.1
causing obstructed labor	660.33	660.31	660.30	cause	763.1
hand, leg, or foot NEC	652.83	652.81	652.80	N/A	763.1
causing obstructed labor	660.03	660.01	660.00	cause	763.1
mentum	652.43	652.41	652.40	N/A	763.1
causing obstructed labor	660.03	660.01	660.00	cause	763.1
multiple gestation (one fetus or more)	652.63	652.61	652.60	N/A	763.1
causing obstructed labor	660.03	660.01	660.00	cause	763.1
oblique	652.33	652.31	652.30	N/A	763.1
with successful version	652.13	652.11	652.10	N/A	763.1
causing obstructed labor	660.03	660.01	660.00	cause	763.1
shoulder	652.83	652.81	652.80	N/A	763.1
causing obstructed labor	660.03	660.01	660.00	cause	763.1
transverse	652.33	652.31	652.30	N/A	763.1
with successful version	652.13	652.11	652.10	N/A	763.1
causing obstructed labor	660.03	660.01	660.00	cause	763.1
umbilical cord	663.03	663.01	663.00	N/A	
unstable	652.03	652.01	652.00	N/A	763.1
causing obstructed labor	660.03	660.01	660.00	cause	763.1
Previous					
abortion	V23.2	N/A	N/A	N/A	
infertility	V23.0	N/A	N/A	N/A	
nonobstetric condition	V23.89	N/A	N/A	N/A	
poor obstetrical history	V23.49		N/A	N/A	N/A
premature delivery	V23.41		N/A	N/A	N/A
trophoblastic disease	V23.1	N/A	N/A	N/A	
Primigravida, elderly	659.53	659.51	659.50	N/A	763.89
Primipara, old	659.53	659.51	659.50	N/A	763.89
Problem (with)					
fetus NOS	656.93	656.91	656.90	N/A	779.9
specified type NEC	656.83	656.81	656.80	N/A	779.8
placenta NOS	656.93	656.91	656.90	N/A	762.2
specified type NEC	656.83	656.81	656.80	N/A	762.2
Prolapse, prolapsed					
arm or hand, complicating delivery	652.73	652.71	652.70	N/A	763.1
causing obstructed labor	660.03	660.01	660.00	cause	763.1
cervix, anterior lip (obstructing labor)	660.23	660.21	660.20	cause	763.1
fetal extremity, complicating delivery	652.83	652.81	652.80	N/A	763.1
causing obstructed labor	660.03	660.01	660.00	cause	763.1
leg, complicating delivery	652.83	652.81	652.80	N/A	763.1
causing obstructed labor	660.03	660.01	660.00	cause	763.1
umbilical cord, complicating delivery	663.03	663.01	663.00	N/A	762.4
uterus	654.43	654.41	654.40	N/A	763.1
causing obstructed labor	660.23	660.21	660.20	cause	763.1
Prolonged					
labor		662.13	662.11	662.10	N/A
first stage	662.03	662.01	662.00	N/A	763.89
second stage	662.23	662.21	662.20	N/A	763.89
pregnancy over 40 completed weeks to 42 completed weeks	645.13	645.11	645.10	N/A	766.21
pregnancy over 42 completed weeks	645.23	645.21	645.20	N/A	766.22
rupture of membranes (24 hours or more prior to onset of labor)	658.23	658.21	658.20	N/A	761.8
uterine contractions in labor	661.43	661.41	661.40	N/A	763.7
PROM	658.13	658.11	658.10	N/A	761.1
with delayed delivery	658.23	658.21	658.20	N/A	761.8
Prominence, ischial spine or sacral promontory					
with disproportion (fetopelvic)	653.33	653.31	653.30	N/A	763.1
causing obstructed labor	660.13	660.11	660.10	cause	763.1
Proteinuria (gestational)	646.23	646.21	646.20	condition	
with toxemia (mild) (pre-eclamptic)	642.43	642.41	642.40	N/A	760.0
convulsions	642.63	642.61	642.60	N/A	760.0
pre-existing hypertension	642.73	642.71	642.70	N/A	760.0
severe	642.53	642.51	642.50	N/A	760.0
Pruritus, pruritic	646.83	646.81	646.80	condition	

Resources

Antepartum Pregnancy Table

Antepartum Pregnancy Condition or Complication; affecting management of mother	Antepartum condition or complication	Delivered, with or without mention of antepartum condition	Unspecified episode of care	Assign additional code to describe the...	Affecting fetus (coded on the newborn chart only)
Psychosis or psychoneurosis	648.43	648.41	648.40	condition	
Ptyalism	646.83	646.81	646.80	condition	
Pyelitis	646.63	646.61	646.60	condition	760.1
Pyrexia (of unknown origin) (PUO), during labor	659.23	659.21	659.20	N/A	
Quadruplet NEC	651.23	651.21	651.20	N/A	761.5
with fetal loss and retention of one or more fetus(es)	651.53	651.51	651.50	N/A	
reduction, multiple gestation (elective)	651.73	651.71	651.70	N/A	
Quintuplet NEC	651.83	651.81	651.80	N/A	761.5
with fetal loss and retention of one or more fetus(es)	651.63	651.61	651.60	N/A	
reduction, multiple gestation (elective)	651.73	651.71	651.70	N/A	
Rachitic with disproportion (fetopelvic)	653.23	653.21	653.20	N/A	763.1
causing obstructed labor	660.13	660.11	660.10	cause	763.1
Rapid second stage (delivery)	661.33	661.31	661.30	N/A	763.6
Reaction obstetric anesthetic or analgesic NEC	668.93	668.91	668.90	N/A	763.5
Rectocele	654.43	654.41	654.40	N/A	763.1
causing obstructed labor	660.23	660.21	660.20	cause	763.1
Reduction, multiple gestation (elective)	651.73	651.71	651.70	N/A	
Renal					
disease or failure NEC	646.23	646.21	646.20	condition	
with secondary hypertension	642.13	642.11	642.10	N/A	
hypertensive	642.23	642.21	642.20	N/A	
Repair of pelvic floor, previous	654.43	654.41	654.40	N/A	763.89
causing obstructed labor	660.23	660.21	660.20	cause	763.1
Retardation fetal growth (intrauterine)	656.53	656.51	656.50	N/A	764.90
Retention, retained					
dead					
fetus (after 22 completed weeks gestation)	656.43	656.41	656.40	N/A	cause
early fetal death (before 22 completed weeks gestation)	632	N/A	N/A	N/A	
ovum		631	N/A	N/A	N/A
Retinitis	646.83	646.81	646.80	condition	
Retraction					
nipple	676.03	676.01	676.00	N/A	
ring, uterus (Bandl's) (pathological)	661.43	661.41	661.40	N/A	763.7
Retroversion, uterus	654.33	654.31	654.30	N/A	763.89
causing obstructed labor	660.23	660.21	660.20	cause	763.1
Rh immunization, incompatibility, or sensitization	656.13	656.11	656.10	N/A	773.0
Rigid, rigidity					
cervix	654.63	654.61	654.60	N/A	763.89
causing obstructed labor	660.23	660.21	660.20	cause	763.1
pelvic floor	654.43	654.41	654.40	N/A	763.89
causing obstructed labor	660.23	660.21	660.20	cause	763.1
perineum or vulva	654.83	654.81	654.80	N/A	763.89
causing obstructed labor	660.23	660.21	660.20	cause	763.1
vagina	654.73	654.71	654.70	N/A	763.89
causing obstructed labor	660.23	660.21	660.20	cause	763.1
Ring(s), complicating delivery					
Bandl's	661.43	661.41	661.40	N/A	763.7
contraction	661.43	661.41	661.40	N/A	763.7
retraction, uterus, pathological	661.43	661.41	661.40	N/A	763.7
Robert's pelvis with disproportion (fetopelvic)	653.03	653.01	653.00	N/A	763.1
causing obstructed labor	660.13	660.11	660.10	cause	763.1
Rubella (German measles)	647.53	647.51	647.50	condition	760.2
with suspected fetal damage	655.33	655.31	655.30	N/A	771.0
Rupture					
abdominal viscera (obstetrical trauma)	N/A	665.51	665.50	N/A	
amnion (premature)	658.13	658.11	658.10	N/A	763.89
with delayed delivery	658.23	658.21	658.20	N/A	763.89
bladder (sphincter), obstetrical trauma	N/A	665.51	665.50	N/A	
cervix (uteri), obstetrical trauma	N/A	665.31	665.30	N/A	
marginal sinus (hemorrhage)	641.23	641.21	641.20	N/A	762.1
membranes (premature)	658.13	658.11	658.10	N/A	761.1
with delayed delivery	658.23	658.21	658.20	N/A	761.1
artificial with delayed delivery following	658.33	658.31	658.30	N/A	761.1
pelvic floor, complicating delivery	N/A	664.11	664.10	N/A	
perineum during delivery	N/A	664.41	664.40	N/A	
umbilical cord	663.83	663.81	663.80	N/A	772.0
urethra (obstetrical trauma)	N/A	665.51	665.50	N/A	
uterus					
before onset of labor	665.03	665.01	665.00	N/A	763.89
during labor	N/A	665.11	665.10	N/A	763.89
vulva, complicating delivery	N/A	664.01	664.00	N/A	
Sacculation, complicating delivery	654.43	654.41	654.40	N/A	763.1
causing obstructed labor	660.23	660.21	660.20	cause	763.1
Salivation (excessive)	646.83	646.81	646.80	condition	
Salpingitis	646.63	646.61	646.60	condition	760.8
Salpingo-oophoritis	646.63	646.61	646.60	condition	760.8
Scar, scarring					
cervix	654.63	654.61	654.60	N/A	763.89
causing obstructed labor	660.23	660.21	660.20	cause	763.1
uterus NEC	654.93	654.91	654.90	N/A	763.89
from previous cesarean delivery	654.23	654.21	654.20	N/A	763.89
causing obstructed labor	660.23	660.21	660.20	cause	763.1
Scoliotic pelvis with disproportion (fetopelvic)	653.03	653.01	653.00	N/A	763.1
causing obstructed labor	660.13	660.11	660.10	cause	763.1

Resources

Antepartum Pregnancy Condition or Complication; affecting management of mother	Antepartum condition or complication	Delivered, with or without mention of antepartum condition	Unspecified episode of care	Assign additional code to describe the...	Affecting fetus (coded on the newborn chart only)
Screening, prenatal (for)					
If the abnormal finding is known — code the findings					
by					
amniocentesis					
chromosomal anomalies	V28.0	N/A	N/A		
raised alpha-fetoprotein levels (amniotic fluid)	V28.1	N/A	N/A		
specified, NEC	V28.2	N/A	N/A		
ultrasound					
fetal growth retardation	V28.4	N/A	N/A		
malformation	V28.3	N/A	N/A		
isoimmunization	V28.5	N/A	N/A		
other specified screening	V28.8	N/A	N/A		
Streptococcus B	V28.6	N/A	N/A		
unspecified, screening	V28.9	N/A	N/A		
Separation (obstetrical trauma)					
pubic bone	N/A	665.61	665.60	N/A	
symphysis pubis	N/A	665.61	665.60	N/A	
Sepsis, complicating labor	659.33	659.31	659.30	N/A	
Septicemia	647.83	647.81	647.80	condition	
Septum, vagina	654.73	654.71	654.70	N/A	763.89
causing obstructed labor	660.23	660.21	660.20	cause	763.1
Sextuplet NEC	651.83	651.81	651.80	N/A	761.5
with fetal loss and retention of one or more fetus(es)	651.63	651.61	651.60	N/A	
reduction, multiple gestation (elective)	651.73	651.71	651.70	N/A	
Shirodkar suture	654.53	654.51	654.50	N/A	
causing obstructed labor	660.23	660.21	660.20	cause	763.1
Shock					
complicating labor and delivery	669.13	669.11	669.10	N/A	
following labor and delivery	669.13	669.11	669.10	N/A	
Short, shortening, shortness of umbilical cord	663.43	663.41	663.40	N/A	762.6
Sinus, marginal, rupture or bleeding	641.23	641.21	641.20	N/A	762.1
Slow fetal growth	656.53	656.51	656.50	N/A	764.90
Small					
for-dates fetus	656.53	656.51	656.50	N/A	764.00
pelvis					
with disproportion (fetopelvic)	653.13	653.11	653.10	N/A	763.1
causing obstructed labor	660.13	660.11	660.10	cause	763.1
Spasms					
cervix, complicating delivery	661.43	661.41	661.40	N/A	763.7
uterus	646.83	646.81	646.80	condition	
complicating delivery	661.43	661.41	661.40	N/A	763.7
complicating labor	661.43	661.41	661.40	N/A	763.7
Specified condition NEC	646.83	646.81	646.80	condition	
Spina bifida (aperta), suspected fetal	655.03	655.01	655.00	N/A	
Spondylolisthesis with disproportion (fetopelvic)	653.33	653.31	653.30	N/A	763.1
causing obstructed labor	660.13	660.11	660.10	cause	763.1
Spondylolysis with disproportion (fetopelvic)	653.33	653.31	653.30	N/A	763.1
causing obstructed labor	660.13	660.11	660.10	cause	763.1
Spondylosis with disproportion (fetopelvic)	653.33	653.31	653.30	N/A	763.1
causing obstructed labor	660.13	660.11	660.10	cause	763.1
Spotting					
antepartum hemorrhage	641.93	641.91	641.90	N/A	
spotting	649.53	649.51	649.50		
Spurious labor pains	644.13	N/A	644.10	N/A	
Stenosis (cicatricial)					
cervix, cervical (canal)	654.63	654.61	654.60	N/A	763.89
causing obstructed labor	660.23	660.21	660.20	cause	763.1
vagina	654.73	654.71	654.70	N/A	763.89
causing obstructed labor	660.23	660.21	660.20	cause	763.1
Stricture, cervix (canal)	654.63	654.61	654.60	N/A	763.89
causing obstructed labor	660.23	660.21	660.20	cause	763.1
Sudden death					
during childbirth	669.93	669.91	669.90	N/A	
Supervision (of) (for)					
high-risk	V23.9	N/A	N/A	N/A	
insufficient prenatal care	V23.7	N/A	N/A	N/A	
specified problem NEC	V23.89	N/A	N/A	N/A	
multiparity	V23.3	N/A	N/A	N/A	
normal NEC	V22.1	N/A	N/A	N/A	
first pregnancy	V22.0	N/A	N/A	N/A	
poor		N/A	N/A	N/A	
obstetric history	V23.49		N/A	N/A	N/A
reproductive history	V23.5	N/A	N/A	N/A	
Suppression of lactation	676.53	676.51	676.50	N/A	
Suppurative, breast, mammary gland	675.13	675.11	675.10	N/A	

Resources

Antepartum Pregnancy Table

Antepartum Pregnancy Condition or Complication; affecting management of mother	Antepartum condition or complication	Delivered, with or without mention of antepartum condition	Unspecified episode of care	Assign additional code to describe the...	Affecting fetus (coded on the newborn chart only)
Surgery, previous					
cervix	654.63	654.61	654.60	N/A	763.89
causing obstructed labor	660.23	660.21	660.20	cause	763.1
pelvic soft tissues NEC	654.93	654.91	654.90	N/A	763.89
causing obstructed labor	660.23	660.21	660.20	cause N/A	763.1
perineum or vulva	654.83	654.81	654.80	N/A	
uterus NEC	654.93	654.91	654.90	N/A	763.89
causing obstructed labor	660.23	660.21	660.20	cause	763.1
from previous cesarean delivery	654.23	654.21	654.20	N/A	
causing obstructed labor	660.23	660.21	660.20	cause	763.1
vagina	654.73	654.71	654.70	N/A	
causing obstructed labor	660.23	660.21	660.20	cause	763.1
Suspended uterus	654.43	654.41	654.40	N/A	763.89
causing obstructed labor	660.23	660.21	660.20	cause	763.1
Suture, Shirodkar (with or without cervical incompetence)	654.53	654.51	654.50	N/A	
causing obstructed labor	660.23	660.21	660.20	cause	763.1
Syncope complicating delivery	669.23	669.21	669.20	N/A	
Syndrome					
acid pulmonary aspiration (Mendelson's)	668.03	668.01	668.00	N/A	
Chiari-Frommel	676.63	676.61	676.60	N/A	
dead fetus	641.33	641.31	641.30	N/A	
dystocia, dystrophia	654.93	654.91	654.90	N/A	
causing obstructed labor	660.23	660.21	660.20	cause	763.1
Frommel-Chiari	676.63	676.61	676.60	N/A	
H.E.L.L.P (Hemolysis, Elevated Liver function and Low Platelets)	642.53	642.51	642.50	N/A	
hypotension, maternal	669.23	669.21	669.20	N/A	
maternal hypotension	669.23	669.21	669.20	N/A	
Mendelson's (during labor) (obstetric)	668.03	668.01	668.00	N/A	
vanishing twin	651.33	N/A	N/A	N/A	
Syphilis	647.03	647.01	647.00	condition	760.2
Tear, torn					
anus, anal (sphincter), complicating delivery	N/A	664.21	664.20	N/A	763.89
with mucosa	N/A	664.31	664.30	N/A	763.89
bladder, obstetrical trauma	N/A	665.51	665.50	N/A	763.89
bowel, obstetrical trauma	N/A	665.51	665.50	N/A	763.89
broad ligament, obstetrical trauma	N/A	665.51	665.50	N/A	763.89
cervix, obstetrical trauma	N/A	665.31	665.30	N/A	763.89
pelvic					
floor, complicating delivery	N/A	664.11	664.10	N/A	763.89
organ NEC, obstetrical trauma	N/A	665.51	665.50	N/A	763.89
perineum, obstetrical trauma	N/A	665.51	665.50	N/A	763.89
periurethral, obstetrical trauma	N/A	665.51	665.50	N/A	763.89
umbilical cord, complicating delivery	663.83	663.81	663.80	N/A	772.0
urethra, obstetrical trauma	N/A	665.51	665.50	N/A	
vulva, complicating delivery	N/A	664.01	664.00	N/A	763.89
Teratoma, fetal sacral, causing fetopelvic disproportion	653.73	653.71	653.70	N/A	763.1
causing obstructed labor	660.23	660.21	660.20	cause	763.1
Thelitis	675.03	675.01	675.00	N/A	
Threatened				N/A	
abortion or miscarriage	640.03	640.01	640.00	N/A	762.1
labor	644.13	N/A	644.10	N/A	761.8
before 22 completed weeks gestation	640.03	640.01	640.00	N/A	762.1
premature delivery	N/A	644.21	644.20	N/A	761.8
premature labor	644.03	N/A	644.00	N/A	761.8
Thrombophlebitis	671.23	671.21	671.20	N/A	760.3
cerebral (sinus) (vein), nonpyogenic	671.53	671.51	671.50	N/A	760.3
deep	671.33	671.31	671.30	N/A	760.3
intracranial venous sinus, nonpyogenic	671.53	671.51	671.50	N/A	760.3
specified site NEC	671.53	671.51	671.50	N/A	760.3
superficial	671.23	671.21	671.20	N/A	760.3
deep	671.33	671.31	671.30	N/A	760.3
Thrombosis	671.93	671.91	671.90	N/A	
brain (artery) (stem)	674.03	674.01	674.00	N/A	
intracranial, venous sinus (nonpyogenic origin)	671.53	671.51	671.50	N/A	
deep	671.33	671.31	671.30	N/A	760.3
spinal cord	671.53	671.51	671.50	N/A	
superficial	671.23	671.21	671.20	N/A	
umbilical cord (vessels)	663.63	663.61	663.60	N/A	762.6
venous (superficial)	671.23	671.21	671.20	N/A	
deep	671.33	671.31	671.30	N/A	760.3
Thyroid dysfunction	648.13	648.11	648.10	condition	
Thyroiditis	648.13	648.11	648.10	condition	
Thyrotoxicosis	648.13	648.11	648.10	condition	
Tipping pelvis with disproportion (fetopelvic)	653.03	653.01	653.00	N/A	763.1
causing obstructed labor	660.13	660.11	660.10	cause	763.1
Tobacco use disorder	649.03	649.01	649.00		
Torsion of uterus	654.43	654.41	654.40	N/A	
causing obstructed labor	660.23	660.21	660.20	cause	763.1
Toxemia (mild) (pre-eclamptic)	642.43	642.41	642.40	N/A	760.0
with					760.0
convulsions	642.63	642.61	642.60	N/A	760.0
pre-existing hypertension	642.73	642.71	642.70	N/A	760.0

Resources

Antepartum Pregnancy Condition or Complication; affecting management of mother	Antepartum condition or complication	Delivered, with or without mention of antepartum condition	Unspecified episode of care	Assign additional code to describe the...	Affecting fetus (coded on the newborn chart only)
Toxemia (mild) (pre-eclamptic)	642.43	642.41	642.40	N/A	760.0
eclamptic	642.63	642.61	642.60	N/A	760.0
with pre-existing hypertension	642.73	642.71	642.70	N/A	760.0
severe	642.53	642.51	642.50	N/A	760.0
Transmission of chemical substances through the placenta, suspected	655.53	655.51	655.50	N/A	760.70
Transverse					
arrest (deep), in labor	660.33	660.31	660.30	cause	763.1
lie or presentation	652.33	652.31	652.30	N/A	761.7
with successful version	652.13	652.11	652.10		763.1
causing obstructed labor	660.03	660.01	660.00	cause	763.1
Trauma	648.93	648.91	648.90	condition	
causing hemorrhage	641.83	641.81	641.80	N/A	760.5
during delivery NEC	665.93	665.91	665.90	N/A	760.5
obstetrical	665.93	665.91	665.90	N/A	760.5
previous pregnancy (major), affecting management of current pregnancy, childbirth or puerperium	V23.89	V23.89	V23.89	N/A	
Triplet NEC	651.13	651.11	651.10	N/A	761.5
with fetal loss and retention of one or more fetus(es)	651.43	651.41	651.40	N/A	761.5
reduction, multiple gestation (elective)	651.73	651.71	651.70	N/A	
Trophoblastic disease	630	N/A	N/A	N/A	
previous pregnancy, affecting management of current pregnancy	V23.1	V23.1	V23.1	N/A	
Tubal (with rupture)	633.1	N/A	N/A	N/A	761.4
Tuberculosis	647.33	647.31	647.30	condition	760.2
Tumor					
cervix	654.63	654.61	654.60	N/A	763.89
causing obstructed labor	660.23	660.21	660.20	cause	763.1
fetal, causing disproportion	653.73	653.71	653.70	N/A	763.1
causing obstructed labor	660.13	660.11	660.10	cause	763.1
ovary	654.43	654.41	654.40	N/A	763.89
causing obstructed labor	660.23	660.21	660.20	cause	763.1
pelvic	654.93	654.91	654.90	N/A	763.89
causing obstructed labor	660.23	660.21	660.20	cause	763.1
pelvic organs or tissue NEC	654.43	654.41	654.40	N/A	763.89
causing obstructed labor	660.23	660.21	660.20	cause	763.1
uterus	654.13	654.11	654.10	N/A	763.89
causing obstructed labor	660.23	660.21	660.20	cause	763.1
vagina	654.73	654.71	654.70	N/A	763.89
causing obstructed labor	660.23	660.21	660.20	cause	763.1
vulva	654.83	654.81	654.80	N/A	763.89
causing obstructed labor	660.23	660.21	660.20	cause	763.1
Twin NEC	651.03	651.01	651.00	N/A	761.5
with fetal loss and retention of one or more fetus(es)	651.33	651.31	651.30	N/A	761.5
reduction, multiple gestation (elective)	651.73	651.71	651.70	N/A	
Unstable lie	652.03	652.01	652.00	N/A	761.7
causing obstructed labor	660.03	660.01	660.00	cause	763.1
Unwanted NEC	V61.7	N/A	N/A	N/A	
Uremia (renal disease or failure) NEC	646.23	646.21	646.20	condition	760.1
with secondary hypertension	642.13	642.11	642.10	N/A	760.0
hypertensive	642.23	642.21	642.20	N/A	760.0
Urethritis	646.63	646.61	646.60	condition	760.1
Uterine size date discrepancy	649.63	649.61	649.60		
UTI	646.63	646.61	646.60	condition	760.1
Vaginitis or vulvitis	646.63	646.61	646.60	condition	760.8
Valsuani's disease	648.23	648.21	648.20	condition	
Vanishing twin	651.33	N/A	N/A	N/A	
Varicose					
placental vessels	656.73	656.71	656.70	N/A	
veins (legs)	671.03	671.01	671.00	N/A	
perineum	671.13	671.11	671.10	N/A	
vulva	671.13	671.11	671.10	N/A	
Varicosity, labia or vulva	671.13	671.11	671.10	N/A	
Varix (lower extremity)	671.03	671.01	671.00	N/A	
perineum	671.13	671.11	671.10	N/A	
Vulva	671.13	671.11	671.10		
Vasa previa	663.53	663.51	663.50	N/A	762.6
hemorrhage	663.53	663.51	663.50	N/A	772.0
Venereal disease NEC	647.23	647.21	647.20	disease	
Ventouse delivery NEC	N/A	669.51	669.50	N/A	763.3
Version					
before labor	652.13	652.11	652.10	N/A	761.7
causing obstructed labor	660.03	660.01	660.00	cause	763.1
cephalic (correcting previous malposition)	652.13	652.11	652.10	N/A	763.1
causing obstructed labor	660.03	660.01	660.00	cause	763.1
Viral disease NEC	647.63	647.61	647.60	disease	
Vomiting	643.93	643.91	643.90	N/A	761.8
due to					
organic disease or other cause	643.83	643.81	643.80	N/A	761.8
specific cause NEC	643.83	643.81	643.80	N/A	761.8
early (mild) (before 22 completed weeks gestation)	643.03	643.01	643.00	N/A	761.8
with					761.8
carbohydrate depletion	643.13	643.11	643.10	N/A	761.8

Resources

Antepartum Pregnancy Condition or Complication; affecting management of mother	Antepartum condition or complication	Delivered, with or without mention of antepartum condition	Unspecified episode of care	Assign additional code to describe the...	Affecting fetus (coded on the newborn chart only)
Vomiting – *continued*					761.8
dehydration	643.13	643.11	643.10	N/A	761.8
electrolyte imbalance	643.13	643.11	643.10	N/A	761.8
late (after 22 completed weeks gestation)	643.23	643.21	643.20	N/A	761.8
severe (with metabolic disturbance)	643.13	643.11	643.10	N/A	761.8
Vulvitis	646.63	646.61	646.60	condition	760.8
Weight gain	646.13	646.11	646.10	condition	
insufficient	646.83	646.81	646.80	condition	
Young maternal age	659.83	659.81	659.80	N/A	

Postpartum Pregnancy Condition or Complication; affecting management of mother	Postpartum condition or complication	Delivered with mention of postpartum complication	Unspecified episode of care	Assign additional code to describe the...	Affecting newborn (coded on the newborn chart only)
Abnormal NEC					
cervix	654.64	654.62	654.60	N/A	763.89
glucose tolerance test	648.84	648.82	648.80	condition	775.0
pelvic organs or tissues NEC	654.94	654.92	654.90	N/A	763.89
perineum or vulva	654.84	654.82	654.80	N/A	763.89
position					
cervix	654.44	654.42	654.40	N/A	763.89
uterus	654.44	654.42	654.40	N/A	763.89
quality of milk	676.84	676.82	676.80	N/A	
shape of uterus	654.44	654.42	654.40	N/A	763.89
uterus (congenital)	654.04	654.02	654.00	N/A	763.89
vagina	654.74	654.72	654.70	N/A	763.89
vulva (acquired) (congenital)	654.84	654.82	654.80	N/A	763.89
weight gain	646.14	646.12	646.10	condition	761.8
with hypertension (mild) (pre-eclamptic)	642.44	642.42	642.40	N/A	760.0
with					
convulsions	642.64	642.62	642.60	N/A	760.0
pre-existing hypertension	642.74	642.72	642.70	N/A	760.0
with severe hypertension	642.54	642.52	642.50	N/A	760.0
Abscess					
areola (acute) (chronic)	675.14	675.12	675.10	N/A	
Bartholin's gland	646.64	646.62	646.60	condition	760.8
bladder	646.64	646.62	646.60	condition	760.1
breast (acute) (chronic)	675.14	675.12	675.10		
cervix (uteri)	670.04	670.02	670.00	N/A	
fallopian tube	670.04	670.02	670.00		
genital organ or tract NEC (postpartum)	670.04	670.02	670.00		
kidney	646.64	646.62	646.60	condition	760.1
labium (majus) (minus)	646.64	646.62	646.60	condition	760.8
mesosalpinx	670.04	670.02	670.00	N/A	
milk	675.14	675.12	675.10	N/A	
nabothian	646.64	646.62	646.60	condition	
nipple	675.04	675.02	675.00	N/A	
ovary	670.04	670.02	670.00	N/A	
oviduct	670.04	670.02	670.00	N/A	
para-uterine	670.04	670.02	670.00	N/A	
pelvic	670.04	670.02	670.00	N/A	
perimetric	670.04	670.02	670.00	N/A	
peritoneum, peritoneal (perforated) (ruptured) postpartum	670.04	670.02	670.00	N/A	
periuterine	670.04	670.02	670.00	N/A	
retro-uterine	670.04	670.02	670.00	N/A	
subareolar postpartum	675.14	675.12	675.10	N/A	
suprapelvic	670.04	670.02	670.00	N/A	
tubal (ruptured)	670.04	670.02	670.00	N/A	
tubo-ovarian	670.04	670.02	670.00	N/A	
urethra	646.64	646.62	646.60	condition	760.1
urinary tract NEC	646.64	646.62	646.60	condition	
uterine, uterus	670.04	670.02	670.00	N/A	
vagina (wall)	646.64	646.62	646.60	condition	
vaginorectal	646.64	646.62	646.60	condition	
vulva	646.64	646.62	646.60	condition	760.8
vulvovaginal gland	646.64	646.62	646.60	condition	
Accreta placenta	667.04	667.02	667.00	N/A	
with hemorrhage	666.04	666.02	666.00	N/A	
Accident	674.94	674.92	674.90	N/A	
Addiction					
alcoholic	648.44	648.42	648.40	condition	760.71
Adherent placenta	667.04	667.02	667.00	N/A	
with hemorrhage	666.04	666.02	666.00	N/A	
Adhesion(s), adhesive					
cervicovaginal (postpartum)	674.84	674.82	674.80	N/A	
uterus to abdominal wall	654.44	654.42	654.40	N/A	763.89
Adnexitis	670.04	670.02	670.00	N/A	
Aerocele	673.04	673.02	673.00	N/A	
Afibrinogenemia (postpartum)	666.34	666.32	666.30	N/A	
AFP (screening for raised levels in amniotic fluid)	V28.1	N/A	N/A	N/A	
Agalactia	676.44	676.42	676.40	N/A	
Air embolism	673.04	673.02	673.00	N/A	

Resources

Postpartum Pregnancy Condition or Complication; affecting management of mother	Postpartum condition or complication	Delivered with mention of postpartum complication	Unspecified episode of care	Assign additional code to describe the...	Affecting newborn (coded on the newborn chart only)
Albuminuria (gravidarum)	646.24	646.22	646.20	condition	760.1
with hypertension (and edema)					760.1
mild	642.44	642.42	642.40	N/A	760.0
severe	642.54	642.52	642.50	N/A	760.0
gestational	646.24	646.22	646.20	condition	760.1
pre-eclamptic (mild)	642.24	642.22	642.20	N/A	760.0
severe	642.54	642.52	642.50	N/A	760.0
Alcohol, alcoholic					
addiction (maternal)	648.44	648.42	648.40	condition	760.71
Alphafetoprotein (screening for raised levels in amniotic fluid)	V28.1	N/A	N/A	N/A	
Amniotic fluid embolism	673.14	673.12	673.10	N/A	
Amputation of cervix	654.64	654.62	654.60	N/A	763.8
Anemia	648.24	648.22	648.20	condition	760.8
aplastic	648.24	648.22	648.20	condition	760.8
iron (Fe) deficiency	648.24	648.22	648.20	condition	760.8
macrocytic	648.24	648.22	648.20	condition	760.8
megaloblastic	648.24	648.22	648.20	condition	760.8
pernicious	648.24	648.22	648.20	condition	760.8
postpartum	648.24	648.22	648.20	condition	
Anesthesia, anesthetic					
complications NEC	668.84	668.82	668.80	condition	763.5
cardiac	668.14	668.12	668.10	condition	763.5
central nervous system	668.24	668.22	668.20	condition	763.5
pulmonary	668.04	668.02	668.00	condition	763.5
death (from) during delivery	668.94	668.92	668.90	condition	761.6
Anomaly, anomalous (congenital)					
cardiovascular system	648.54	648.52	648.50	condition	
cervix	654.64	654.62	654.60	N/A	763.89
uterus	654.04	654.02	654.00	N/A	763.89
Anoxia cerebral					
complicating delivery (cesarean) (instrumental)	669.44	669.42	669.40	N/A	
due to obstetric anesthesia or sedation	668.24	668.22	668.20	complication	
Anteversion					
uterus, uterine (cervix)	654.44	654.42	654.40	N/A	763.89
Anuria, postpartum	669.34	669.32	669.30	N/A	
Apoplexy	674.04	674.02	674.00	N/A	
Arrest, arrested					
cardiac					
anesthesia, complicating delivery (cesarean)	668.14	668.12	668.10	N/A	
(instrumental)	669.44	669.42	669.40	N/A	
Aspiration					
acid-pulmonary (syndrome)	668.04	668.02	668.00	complication	
pneumonitis	668.04	668.02	668.00	complication	
Atresia, atretic					
cervix	654.64	654.62	654.60	N/A	763.89
Atrophy, atrophic					
breast, postpartum	676.34	676.32	676.30		
postpartum	674.84	674.82	674.80	N/A	
Atonia, atony, atonic	666.14	666.12	666.10		
Avulsion (traumatic)					
symphyseal cartilage (inner)	665.64	N/A	665.60	N/A	
Bacilluria, asymptomatic	646.54	646.52	646.50	complication	760.1
Bacteremia	647.84	647.82	647.80	condition	
Bacteriuria, asymptomatic	646.54	646.52	646.50	complication	760.1
Bariatric surgery	649.24	649.22	649.20	N/A	
Bicornis or Bicornuate uterus	654.04	654.02	654.00	N/A	763.89
Bleeding				N/A	
atonic, following delivery	666.14	666.12	666.10	N/A	
cerebrovascular	674.04	674.02	674.00	N/A	
due to					
subinvolution, postpartum	666.24	666.22	666.20	N/A	
Blood, dyscrasia (postpartum)	666.34	666.32	666.30	N/A	
Bone disorders	648.74	648.72	648.70	condition	
Breakdown, perineum	674.24	674.22	674.20	N/A	
Breastfeeding difficulties	676.84	676.82	676.80		
Caked breast (postpartum)	676.24	676.22	676.20	N/A	
Cardiomyopathy	674.54	674.52	674.50	N/A	
Cardiovascular disease	648.64	648.62	648.60	condition	
congenital	648.54	648.52	648.50	condition	
Cellulitis (postpartum)					
breast	675.14	675.12	675.10	N/A	
pelvis		670.04	670.02	670.00	N/A
Cerebrovascular disorders	674.04	674.02	674.00	condition	
Cervicitis	646.64	646.62	646.60	condition	760.8
Cervix					
adhesions	654.64	654.62	654.60	N/A	
anaplasia	654.64	654.62	654.60	N/A	
atypism	654.64	654.62	654.60	N/A	
bands	654.64	654.62	654.60	N/A	
cervicitis	654.64	654.62	654.60	N/A	
cicatrix	654.64	654.62	654.60	N/A	
cyst		654.64	654.62	654.60	N/A
dysplasia	654.64	654.62	654.60	N/A	
ectropion	654.64	654.62	654.60	N/A	

Postpartum Pregnancy Table

Postpartum Pregnancy Condition or Complication; affecting management of mother	Postpartum condition or complication	Delivered with mention of postpartum complication	Unspecified episode of care	Assign additional code to describe the...	Affecting newborn (coded on the newborn chart only)
Cervix — *contiued*					
endocervicitis	654.64	654.62	654.60	N/A	
erosion	654.64	654.62	654.60	N/A	
hypertrophic elongation	654.64	654.62	654.60	N/A	
incompetence	654.54	654.52	654.50	N/A	761.0
leukoplakia	654.64	654.62	654.60	N/A	
Nabothian (gland) cyst or follicle	654.64	654.62	654.60	N/A	
old laceration	654.64	654.62	654.60	N/A	
polyp		654.64	654.62	654.60	N/A
stricture and stenosis	654.64	654.62	654.60	N/A	
ulcer		654.64	654.62	654.60	N/A
Chiari-Frommel syndrome	676.64	676.62	676.60	N/A	
Childbed fever	670.04	670.02	670.00	N/A	
Chloasma (gravidarum)	646.84	646.82	646.80	condition	
Cicatrix					
cervix	654.64	654.62	654.60	N/A	
vagina	654.74	654.72	654.70	N/A	
Circulating anticoagulants	666.34	666.32	666.30	N/A	
Coagulation defects	649.34	649.32	649.30	286.0-286.9	
Collapse (during or after labor and delivery)					
circulatory (peripheral)	669.14	669.12	669.10	N/A	779.8
lung		668.04	668.02	668.00	N/A
vascular (peripheral)	669.14	669.12	669.10	N/A	
Colporrhexis	665.44	N/A	665.40	N/A	
Complications NEC					
cesarean section wound	674.34	674.32	674.30	N/A	
delivery	669.94	669.92	669.90	N/A	
procedure (instrumental) (manual) (surgical)	669.44	669.42	669.40	N/A	
specified type NEC	669.84	669.82	669.80	N/A	
labor and delivery	669.94	669.92	669.90	N/A	
anesthesia (sedation)	668.94	668.92	668.90	N/A	763.5
cardiac	668.14	668.12	668.10	N/A	
central nervous system	668.24	668.22	668.20	N/A	
pulmonary	668.04	668.02	668.00	N/A	
specified type NEC	668.84	668.82	668.80	N/A	
specified condition NEC	669.84	669.82	669.80	N/A	
perineal repair	674.34	674.32	674.30	N/A	
disruption	674.24	674.22	674.20	N/A	
postpartum NEC	674.94	674.92	674.90	N/A	
surgical wound	674.34	674.32	674.30	N/A	
Convulsions (eclamptic) (uremic)	642.64	642.62	642.60	N/A	760.0
with pre-existing hypertension	642.74	642.72	642.70	N/A	760.0
Cracked nipple (postpartum)	676.14	676.12	676.10	N/A	
Cyst					
ovary	654.44	654.42	654.40	N/A	763.89
pelvic	654.44	654.42	654.40	N/A	763.89
Cystitis	646.64	646.62	646.60	condition	760.1
Cystocele	654.44	654.42	654.40	N/A	763.89
Damage					
coccyx, complicating delivery	665.64	N/A	665.60	N/A	763.89
pelvic (during delivery)					
joint or ligament	665.64	N/A	665.60	N/A	763.89
organ	665.54	N/A	665.50	N/A	763.89
Death, maternal, NEC					
during delivery	668.94	668.92	668.90	N/A	761.6
postpartum (cause not stated) (sudden)	674.94	674.92	674.90	N/A	
sudden, during delivery	669.94	669.92	669.90	N/A	761.6
under anesthesia NEC	668.94	668.92	668.90	N/A	761.6
Deciduitis	646.64	646.62	646.60	N/A	760.8
postpartum	670.04	670.02	670.00	N/A	
Defect, defective coagulation (factor)					
postpartum	666.34	666.32	666.30	N/A	
Deficiency, deficient coagulation (factor)					
postpartum	666.34	666.32	666.30	N/A	
Deformity					
pelvic, pelvis					
soft part, organs or tissues NEC	654.94	654.92	654.90	cause	763.89
Dehiscence (postpartum)					
cesarean wound	674.14	674.12	674.10	N/A	
episiotomy	674.24	674.22	674.20	N/A	
perineal wound	674.24	674.22	674.20	N/A	
uterine wound	674.14	674.12	674.10	N/A	
Dependence, maternal					
drug	648.34	648.32	648.30	condition	779.5
Depression, postpartum	648.44	648.42	648.40	condition	
Dermatitis, gestationis	646.84	646.82	646.80	condition	
Detachment					
cervix, annular	665.34	N/A	665.30	N/A	763.89
Diabetes					
with long term (current) insulin use				V58.67	775.0
condition present before pregnancy	648.04	648.02	648.00	condition	775.0
gestational (chemical) (latent)	648.84	648.82	648.80	condition	775.0
Diastasis, recti (abdomen) complicating delivery	665.84	665.82	665.80	N/A	763.89
Difficult delivery NEC	669.94	669.92	669.90	N/A	763.89

Resources

Postpartum Pregnancy Condition or Complication; affecting management of mother	Postpartum condition or complication	Delivered with mention of postpartum complication	Unspecified episode of care	Assign additional code to describe the...	Affecting newborn (coded on the newborn chart only)
Difficulty with breast feeding	676.84	676.82	676.80		
Dilatation					
bladder (sphincter)	654.44	654.42	654.40	N/A	763.89
Disease, NEC (postpartum)	674.94	674.92	674.90	N/A	
breast NEC	676.34	676.32	676.30	N/A	
cerebrovascular, NEC	674.04	674.02	674.00	N/A	
Frommel's	676.64	676.62	676.60	N/A	
heart	648.64	648.62	648.60	condition	760.8
postpartum	674.84	674.82	674.80	N/A	
renal NEC	646.24	646.22	646.20	condition	760.1
Valsuani's (progressive pernicious anemia, puerperal)	648.24	648.22	648.20	condition	
venereal NEC	647.24	647.22	647.20	condition	
virus NEC	647.64	647.62	647.60	condition	
Disorders					
breast, postpartum	676.34	676.32	676.30	N/A	
genital tract or organ	646.64	646.62	646.60	condition	760.8
lactation	676.94	676.92	676.90	N/A	
mental	648.44	648.42	648.40	condition	
metabolism NEC (in labor and delivery)	669.04	669.02	669.00	N/A	763.8
specified type NEC	676.84	676.82	676.80	N/A	
Displacement, uterus NEC	654.44	654.42	654.40	N/A	763.8
Disruption, wound					
cesarean operation	674.14	674.12	674.10	N/A	
episiotomy	674.24	674.22	674.20	N/A	
perineal (obstetric)	674.24	674.22	674.20	N/A	
uterine	674.14	674.12	674.10	N/A	
Distortion					
maternal	669.04	669.02	669.00	N/A	
Double uterus	654.04	654.02	654.00	N/A	763.89
Drug dependence	648.34	648.32	648.30	condition	
Dyscrasia, blood					
postpartum	666.34	666.32	666.30	N/A	
Dysfunction					
thyroid	648.14	648.12	648.10	condition	
Dysplasia of cervix	654.64	654.62	654.60	N/A	763.89
Eclampsia, eclamptic	642.64	642.62	642.60	N/A	760.0
with pre-existing hypertension	642.74	642.72	642.70	N/A	760.0
Edema	646.14	646.12	646.10	condition	
with hypertension — *see* Pregnancy, toxemia					
cervix (postpartum)	674.84	674.82	674.80	N/A	
Effect, adverse					
anesthetic (in labor and delivery) NEC	668.94	668.92	668.90	N/A	763.5
Embolism					
air (pulmonary)	673.04	673.02	673.00	N/A	
amniotic fluid	673.14	673.12	673.10	N/A	
blood clot	673.24	673.22	673.20	N/A	
brain (postpartum)	674.04	674.02	674.00	N/A	
cerebral (postpartum)	674.04	674.02	674.00	N/A	
fat (cerebral) (pulmonary) (systemic)	673.84	673.82	673.80	N/A	
heart	674.84	674.82	674.80	N/A	
intracranial (venous sinus) (nonpyogenic)	671.54	671.52	671.50	N/A	
pulmonary NEC	673.24	673.22	673.20	N/A	
pyemic	673.34	673.32	673.30	N/A	
septic	673.34	673.32	673.30	N/A	
specified NEC	674.84	674.82	674.80	N/A	
spinal cord	671.54	671.52	671.50	N/A	
Emesis (gravidarum) — *see* Pregnancy, vomiting					
Endometritis	646.64	646.62	646.60	condition	760.8
decidual	646.64	646.62	646.60	condition	760.8
postpartum	670.04	670.02	670.00	N/A	
Engorgement, breast (postpartum)	676.24	676.22	676.20	N/A	
Epilepsy	649.44	649.42	649.40	345.00-345.91	
Erysipelas (postpartum, childbirth)	670.04	670.02	670.00	N/A	
Eversion, uterus					
complicating delivery	665.24	665.22	665.20	N/A	763.89
postpartum	674.84	674.82	674.80	N/A	
Excessive					
milk secretion	676.64	676.62	676.60	N/A	
weight gain	646.14	646.12	646.10	condition	
Exhaustion (complicating delivery)	669.84	669.82	669.80	N/A	763.89
Extraction					
manual NEC	669.84	669.82	669.80	N/A	763.89
Extroversion, uterus (complicating delivery)	665.24	665.22	665.20	N/A	763.89
Failure, failed					
heart, complicating					
delivery (cesarean) (instrumental)	669.44	669.42	669.40	N/A	
obstetric anesthesia or sedation	668.14	668.12	668.10	N/A	
lactation	676.44	676.42	676.40	N/A	
renal following labor and delivery (acute)	669.34	669.32	669.30	N/A	
Fatigue	646.84	646.82	646.80	condition	
Febris puerperalis	672.04	672.02	672.00	N/A	
Female genital mutilation	648.94	648.92	648.90	629.20-629.29	

Resources

Postpartum Pregnancy Table

Postpartum Pregnancy Condition or Complication; affecting management of mother	Postpartum condition or complication	Delivered with mention of postpartum complication	Unspecified episode of care	Assign additional code to describe the...	Affecting newborn (coded on the newborn chart only)
Fever	672.04	672.02	672.00	N/A	
childbed	670.04	670.02	670.00	N/A	
milk	672.04	672.02	672.00	N/A	
sepsis	670.04	670.02	670.00	N/A	
Fibrinolysis postpartum	666.34	666.32	666.30	N/A	
Fibroid tumor(s)	654.14	654.12	654.10	N/A	763.89
Fibromyoma (uterus)	654.14	654.12	654.10	N/A	763.89
Fibrosis, fibrotic					
perineum	654.84	654.82	654.80	N/A	763.89
Fissure, nipple (postpartum)	676.14	676.12	676.10	N/A	
Fistula (postpartum)					
breast, mammary gland	675.14	675.12	675.10	N/A	
nipple	675.04	675.02	675.00	N/A	
Forced birth or delivery NEC	669.84	669.82	669.80	N/A	763.89
Fractured coccyx complicating delivery	665.64	N/A	665.60	N/A	
Frommel's disease	676.64	676.62	676.60	N/A	
Frommel-Chiari syndrome	676.64	676.62	676.60	N/A	
Galactocele (breast), postpartum	676.84	676.82	676.80	N/A	
Galactorrhea	676.64	676.62	676.60	N/A	
Gangrene					
gas (bacillus) postpartum, childbirth	670.04	670.02	670.00	N/A	
Genital (female) mutilation	648.94	648.92	648.90	629.20-629.29	
Goiter	648.14	648.12	648.10	condition	
Gonococcal infection	647.14	647.12	647.10	condition	760.2
Gonorrhea	647.14	647.12	647.10	condition	760.2
HELLP	642.54	642.52	642.50	N/A	
Hematoma					
broad ligament	665.74	665.72	665.70	N/A	
cesarean section wound	674.34	674.32	674.30	N/A	
complicating delivery (perineum) (vulva)	664.54	N/A	664.50	N/A	
pelvic	665.74	665.72	665.70	N/A	
vagina	665.74	665.72	665.70	N/A	
episiotomy	674.34	674.32	674.30	N/A	
obstetrical surgical wound	674.34	674.32	674.30	N/A	
pelvis, complicating delivery	665.74	665.72	665.70	N/A	
perineal wound	674.34	674.32	674.30	N/A	
complicating delivery	664.54	N/A	664.50	N/A	
vagina	665.74	665.72	665.70	N/A	
vulva, complicating delivery	664.54	N/A	664.50	N/A	767.8
Hematosalpinx, infectional	670.04	670.02	670.00	N/A	
Hemiplegia, cerebral	674.04	674.02	674.00	N/A	
Hemolysis, liver dysfunction, low platelets syndrome	642.54	642.52	642.50		
Hemorrhage					
brain (postpartum, childbirth)	674.04	674.02	674.00	N/A	
bulbar	674.04	674.02	674.00	N/A	
cerebrovascular	674.04	674.02	674.00	N/A	
cesarean section wound	674.34	674.32	674.30	N/A	
retained					
placenta	666.04	666.02	666.00	N/A	
secundines	666.24	666.22	666.20	N/A	
delayed, postpartum	666.24	666.22	666.20	N/A	
due to					
episiotomy	674.34	674.32	674.30	N/A	
extradural	674.04	674.02	674.00	N/A	
internal capsule	674.04	674.02	674.00	N/A	
intracranial, postpartum, childbirth	674.04	674.02	674.00	N/A	
intrapontine	674.04	674.02	674.00	N/A	
obstetrical surgical wound	674.34	674.32	674.30	N/A	
perineal wound	674.34	674.32	674.30	N/A	
postpartum (atonic) (following delivery of placenta)	666.14	666.12	666.10	N/A	
pontine	674.04	674.02	674.00	N/A	
subarachnoid	674.04	674.02	674.00	N/A	
subcortical	674.04	674.02	674.00	N/A	
subdural	674.04	674.02	674.00	N/A	
delayed or secondary (after 24 hours)	666.24	666.22	666.20	N/A	
retained placenta	666.04	666.02	666.00	N/A	
third stage	666.04	666.02	666.00	N/A	
subarachnoid, postpartum, childbirth	674.04	674.02	674.00	N/A	
subdural, postpartum, childbirth	674.04	674.02	674.00	N/A	
third stage	666.04	666.02	666.00	N/A	
uterine, delayed	666.24	666.22	666.20	N/A	
ventricular	674.04	674.02	674.00	N/A	
Hemorrhoids	671.84	671.82	671.80	N/A	
Hepatitis, viral	647.64	647.62	647.60	condition	
Hepatorenal syndrome	674.84	674.82	674.80	N/A	
Herniation of uterus	654.44	654.42	654.40	N/A	
Herpes, herpetic	647.64	647.62	647.60	condition	
gestationis	646.84	646.82	646.80	condition	
Hydroa gestationis	646.84	646.82	646.80	condition	
Hypersecretion of milk	676.64	676.62	676.60	N/A	

Resources

Postpartum Pregnancy Condition or Complication; affecting management of mother	Postpartum condition or complication	Delivered with mention of postpartum complication	Unspecified episode of care	Assign additional code to describe the...	Affecting newborn (coded on the newborn chart only)
Hypertension	642.94	642.92	642.90	N/A	760.0
with					
albuminuria (and edema) (mild)	642.44	642.42	642.40	N/A	760.0
severe	642.54	642.52	642.50	N/A	760.0
edema (mild)	642.44	642.42	642.40	N/A	760.0
severe	642.54	642.52	642.50	N/A	760.0
heart disease	642.24	642.22	642.20	N/A	760.0
and renal disease	642.24	642.22	642.20	N/A	760.0
pre-eclampsia or eclampsia	642.74	642.72	642.70	N/A	760.0
renal disease	642.24	642.22	642.20	N/A	760.0
and heart disease	642.24	642.22	642.20	N/A	760.0
benign	642.04	642.02	642.00	N/A	760.0
chronic	642.04	642.02	642.00	N/A	760.0
pre-existing	642.04	642.02	642.00	N/A	760.0
chronic	642.04	642.02	642.00	N/A	760.0
essential	642.04	642.02	642.00	N/A	
with pre-eclampsia or eclampsia	642.74	642.72	642.70	N/A	760.0
gestational	642.34	642.32	642.30	N/A	
malignant	642.24	642.22	642.20	N/A	760.0
chronic	642.24	642.22	642.20	N/A	760.0
with pre-eclampsia or eclampsia	642.74	642.72	642.70	N/A	760.0
pre-existing	642.24	642.22	642.20	N/A	760.0
pre-existing	642.04	642.02	642.00	N/A	
secondary to renal disease	642.14	642.12	642.10	N/A	760.0
with pre-eclampsia or eclampsia	642.74	642.72	642.70	N/A	760.0
transient	642.34	642.32	642.30	N/A	
Hypertensive					
heart and renal disease	642.24	642.22	642.20	N/A	760.0
heart disease	642.24	642.22	642.20	N/A	760.0
renal disease	642.24	642.22	642.20	N/A	760.0
Hyperthyroidism	648.14	648.12	648.10	condition	
Hypotonic uterus	666.14	666.12	666.10		
Hypertonicity	648.14	648.12	648.10	condition	763.7
Hypertrophy					
breast (postpartum)	676.34	676.32	676.30	N/A	
uterus (postpartum)	674.84	674.82	674.80	N/A	
Hypotension (following labor and delivery)	669.24	669.22	669.20	N/A	
Hypothyroidism	648.14	648.12	648.10	condition	
Hysteralgia	646.84	646.82	646.80	condition	
Incarceration, uterus	654.34	654.32	654.30	N/A	763.1
Incompetent cervix (os)	654.54	654.52	654.50	N/A	761.0
Increased anticoagulants (postpartum)	666.34	666.32	666.30	N/A	
In double uterus	654.04	654.02	654.00	N/A	763.89
Indurated breast (postpartum)	676.34	676.32	676.30	N/A	
Inertia of uterus	666.14	666.12	666.10		
Infantile					
genitalia, genitals	654.44	654.42	654.40	N/A	763.89
Infarct, infarction					
brain (stem), postpartum, childbirth	674.04	674.02	674.00	N/A	
Infection	647.94	647.92	647.90	condition	760.2
Bartholin's gland	646.64	646.62	646.60	condition	
bladder	646.64	646.62	646.60	condition	
breast (mammary gland), postpartum	675.24	675.22	675.20	N/A	
with nipple	675.94	675.92	675.90	N/A	
specified type NEC	675.84	675.82	675.80	N/A	
nonpurulent	675.24	675.22	675.20	N/A	
purulent	675.14	675.12	675.10	N/A	
cervix (uteri)	646.64	646.62	646.60	condition	
cesarean section wound	674.34	674.32	674.30	N/A	
endocervix	646.64	646.62	646.60	condition	
episiotomy	674.34	674.32	674.30	N/A	
fallopian tube	670.04	670.02	670.00	N/A	
generalized	670.04	670.02	670.00	N/A	
genital organs	646.64	646.62	646.60	condition	760.8
postpartum, childbirth	670.04	670.02	670.00	N/A	760.8
major	670.04	670.02	670.00	N/A	760.8
minor or localized	646.64	646.62	646.60	condition	760.8
intrauterine, complicating delivery	646.64	646.62	646.60	condition	
kidney	646.64	646.62	646.60	condition	760.1
nipple	675.04	675.02	675.00	N/A	
with breast	675.94	675.92	675.90	N/A	
specified type NEC	675.84	675.82	675.80	N/A	
ovary	670.04	670.02	670.00	N/A	
pelvic	670.04	670.02	670.00	N/A	
perineal wound (obstetrical)	674.34	674.32	674.30	N/A	
postpartum (major)	670.04	670.02	670.00	N/A	
minor	646.64	646.62	646.60	condition	
renal	646.64	646.62	646.60	condition	
tubo-ovarian	670.04	670.02	670.00	N/A	
urinary (tract)	646.64	646.62	646.60	condition	760.1
asymptomatic	646.54	646.52	646.50	condition	760.1
UTI	646.64	646.62	646.60	condition	760.1
asymptomatic	646.54	646.52	646.50	condition	760.1
vagina	646.64	646.62	646.60	condition	
Infective and parasitic diseases NEC	647.84	647.82	647.80	complication	

Resources

Postpartum Pregnancy Table

Postpartum Pregnancy Condition or Complication; affecting management of mother	Postpartum condition or complication	Delivered with mention of postpartum complication	Unspecified episode of care	Assign additional code to describe the...	Affecting newborn (coded on the newborn chart only)
Infestation	647.94	647.92	647.90	condition	760.8
Inflammation					
areola, postpartum	675.04	675.02	675.00	N/A	
Bartholin's gland	646.64	646.62	646.60	condition	
bladder	646.64	646.62	646.60	condition	760.8
breast (mammary gland), postpartum	675.24	675.22	675.20	N/A	
breast	675.24	675.22	675.20	N/A	
cervix (uteri)	646.64	646.62	646.60	condition	
fallopian tube	670.04	670.02	670.00	N/A	
genital organ	646.64	646.62	646.60	condition	760.8
urinary tract NEC	646.64	646.62	646.60	condition	760.8
Inhalation of stomach contents or secretions in labor and delivery	668.04	668.02	668.00	N/A	
Injury	648.94	648.92	648.90	condition	
birth canal NEC	665.94	665.92	665.90	N/A	763.89
coccyx, complicating delivery	665.64	N/A	665.60	N/A	
genital organs, obstetrical trauma NEC	665.94	665.92	665.90	N/A	763.89
instrumental, obstetrical NEC	665.94	665.92	665.90	N/A	763.89
bladder	665.54	N/A	665.50	N/A	763.89
cervix	665.34	N/A	665.30	N/A	763.89
high vaginal	665.44	N/A	665.40	N/A	763.89
perineal NEC	664.94	N/A	664.90	N/A	763.89
urethra	665.54	N/A	665.50	N/A	763.89
uterus	665.54	N/A	665.50	N/A	763.89
obstetrical NEC	665.94	665.92	665.90	N/A	763.89
pelvic, complicating delivery					
floor	664.14	N/A	664.10	N/A	763.89
joint or ligament	665.64	N/A	665.60	N/A	763.89
organs	665.54	N/A	665.50	N/A	763.89
periurethral tissue, complicating delivery	665.54	N/A	665.50	N/A	763.89
symphysis pubis, complicating delivery	665.64	N/A	665.60	N/A	763.89
Insufficient					
prenatal care	V23.7	N/A	N/A	N/A	
weight gain	646.84	646.82	646.80	condition	
Newborn "light-for-dates" without mention of fetal malnutrition					
unspecified (weight)					764.00
< 500 gms					764.01
500-749 gms					764.02
750-999 gms					764.03
1,000-1,249 gms					764.04
1,250-1,499 gms					764.05
1,500-1,749 gms					764.06
1,750-1,999 gms					764.07
2,000-2,499 gms					764.08
≥ 2,500 gms					764.09
Intoxication					
drug					
obstetric anesthetic or sedation	668.94	668.92	668.90	N/A	763.5
septic, postpartum, childbirth	670.04	670.02	670.00	N/A	
Inversion					
nipple, postpartum	676.34	676.32	676.30		
uterus, complicating delivery	665.24	665.22	665.20		763.89
Ischemia, cerebral (postpartum, childbirth)	674.04	674.02	674.00	N/A	
Joint disorders	648.74	648.72	648.70	condition	
Laceration (obstetrical trauma)					
anus	664.24	N/A	664.20	N/A	
with laceration of anal or rectal mucosa	664.34	N/A	664.30	N/A	
bladder	665.54	N/A	665.50	N/A	
bowel	665.54	N/A	665.50	N/A	
broad ligament	665.64	N/A	665.60	N/A	
central	664.44	N/A	664.40	N/A	
cervix (uteri)	665.34	N/A	665.30	N/A	
fourchette	664.04	N/A	664.00	N/A	
labia	664.04	N/A	664.00	N/A	
pelvic					
floor (muscles)	664.14	N/A	664.10	N/A	
organ NEC	665.54	N/A	665.50	N/A	
perineum	664.44	N/A	664.40	N/A	
first degree	664.04	N/A	664.00	N/A	
second degree	664.14	N/A	664.10	N/A	
third degree	664.24	N/A	664.20	N/A	
fourth degree	664.34	N/A	664.30	N/A	
central	664.44	N/A	664.40	N/A	
involving					
anal sphincter	664.24	N/A	664.20	N/A	
fourchette	664.04	N/A	664.00	N/A	
hymen	664.04	N/A	664.00	N/A	
labia	664.04	N/A	664.00	N/A	
pelvic floor	664.14	N/A	664.10	N/A	
perineal muscles	664.14	N/A	664.10	N/A	
rectovaginal with septum	664.24	N/A	664.20	N/A	
with anal mucosa	664.34	N/A	664.30	N/A	
skin	664.04	N/A	664.00	N/A	
sphincter (anal)	664.24	N/A	664.20	N/A	
with anal mucosa	664.34	N/A	664.30	N/A	

Resources

Postpartum Pregnancy Condition or Complication; affecting management of mother	Postpartum condition or complication	Delivered with mention of postpartum complication	Unspecified episode of care	Assign additional code to describe the...	Affecting newborn (coded on the newborn chart only)
Laceration (obstetrical trauma) — continued					
vagina	664.04	N/A	664.00	N/A	
vaginal muscles	664.14	N/A	664.10	N/A	
vulva	664.04	N/A	664.00	N/A	
secondary	674.24	674.22	674.20	N/A	
peritoneum (obstetrical trauma)	665.54	N/A	665.50	N/A	
periurethral tissue (obstetrical trauma)	665.54	N/A	665.50	N/A	
rectovaginal septum	665.44	N/A	665.40	N/A	
with perineum	664.24	N/A	664.20	N/A	
involving anal or rectal mucosa	664.34	N/A	664.30	N/A	
urethra (obstetrical trauma)	665.54	N/A	665.50	N/A	
vagina (complicating delivery)	665.44	N/A	665.40	N/A	
with perineal involvement	664.04	N/A	664.00	N/A	
first degree	664.04	N/A	664.00	N/A	
second degree	664.14	N/A	664.10	N/A	
third degree	664.24	N/A	664.20	N/A	
fourth degree	664.34	N/A	664.30	N/A	
high	664.44	N/A	664.40	N/A	
muscles	664.14	N/A	664.10	N/A	
sulcus	665.44	N/A	665.40	N/A	
wall	665.44	N/A	665.40	N/A	
vulva (complicating delivery)	664.04	N/A	664.00	N/A	
Lactation, lactating (breast) (postpartum)					
defective	676.44	676.42	676.40	N/A	
disorder	676.94	676.92	676.90	N/A	
specified type NEC	676.84	676.82	676.80	N/A	
examination and/or care of mother	V24.1	V24.1	V24.1	N/A	
excessive	676.64	676.62	676.60	N/A	
failed	676.44	676.42	676.40	N/A	
mastitis NEC	675.24	675.22	675.20	N/A	
suppressed	676.54	676.52	676.50	N/A	
Late effect(s) (of)					
childbirth complication(s)	677	677	677	condition	
complication(s) of					
childbirth	677	677	677	condition	
delivery	677	677	677	condition	
postpartum	677	677	677	condition	
pregnancy	677	677	677	condition	
puerperium	677	677	677	condition	
Lateroversion, uterus	654.44	654.42	654.40	N/A	763.89
Lymphadenitis, breast postpartum	675.24	675.22	675.20	N/A	
Lymphangitis (postpartum)	670.04	670.02	670.00	N/A	
breast	675.24	675.22	675.20	N/A	
Malaria	647.44	647.42	647.40	condition	
Malformation					
pelvic organs or tissues	654.94	654.92	654.90	N/A	763.89
uterus (congenital)	654.04	654.02	654.00	N/A	
Malnutrition	648.94	648.92	648.90	condition	
Malposition					
pelvic organs or tissues	654.44	654.42	654.40	N/A	763.89
uterus or cervix	654.44	654.42	654.40	N/A	763.89
Malpresentation					
uterus or cervix	654.44	654.42	654.40	N/A	
Mammillitis, puerperal, postpartum	675.24	675.22	675.20	N/A	
Mammitis, puerperal, postpartum	675.24	675.22	675.20	N/A	
Mastitis					
lactational	675.24	675.22	675.20	N/A	
puerperal, postpartum, (interstitial) (nonpurulent) (parenchymatous)	675.24	675.22	675.20	N/A	
purulent	675.14	675.12	675.10	N/A	
stagnation	675.24	675.22	675.20	N/A	
puerperalis	675.24	675.22	675.20	N/A	
retromammary (puerperal, postpartum)	675.14	675.12	675.10	N/A	
submammary (puerperal, postpartum)	675.14	675.12	675.10	N/A	
Maternal obesity syndrome	646.14	646.12	646.10	condition	
Membrane, retained (complicating delivery) (with hemorrhage)	666.24	666.22	666.20	N/A	
without hemorrhage	667.14	667.12	667.10	N/A	
Mendelson's syndrome	668.04	668.02	668.00	N/A	
Mental disorders	648.44	648.42	648.40	condition	
Metritis (puerperal, postpartum, childbirth)	670.04	670.02	670.00	N/A	
Metroperitonitis	670.04	670.02	670.00	N/A	
Metrorrhagia	666.24	666.22	666.20	N/A	
Metrorrhagia, postpartum	666.24	666.22	666.20	N/A	
Metrosalpingitis	670.04	670.02	670.00	N/A	
Metrovaginitis	670.04	670.02	670.00	N/A	
Milk					
excess secretion	676.64	676.62	676.60	N/A	
fever	672.04	672.02	672.00	N/A	
retention	672.04	672.02	672.00	N/A	
Milk leg (deep vessels)	671.44	671.42	671.40	N/A	
Monoplegia, cerebral	674.04	674.02	674.00	N/A	
Myocardiopathy (postpartum)	674.84	674.82	674.80	N/A	
Myoma uterus (cervix) (corpus)	654.14	654.12	654.10	N/A	763.89
Myxedema (postpartum)	674.84	674.82	674.80	N/A	

Resources

Postpartum Pregnancy Table

Postpartum Pregnancy Condition or Complication; affecting management of mother	Postpartum condition or complication	Delivered with mention of postpartum complication	Unspecified episode of care	Assign additional code to describe the...	Affecting newborn (coded on the newborn chart only)
Necrosis					
genital organ or tract	646.64	646.62	646.60	condition	760.8
kidney, cortical (acute)	646.24	646.22	646.20	condition	760.1
following labor and delivery	669.34	669.32	669.30	N/A	
liver, puerperal, postpartum	674.84	674.82	674.80	N/A	
ovary	670.04	670.02	670.00	N/A	
renal, cortical	646.24	646.22	646.20	condition	760.1
tubular	646.24	646.22	646.20	condition	760.1
following labor and delivery	669.34	669.32	669.30	N/A	
Nephritis, nephrosis	646.24	646.22	646.20	condition	760.1
with hypertension	642.14	642.12	642.10	N/A	760.0
Nephropathy NEC	646.24	646.22	646.20	condition	
Neuritis (peripheral)	646.44	646.42	646.40	condition	
puerperal, postpartum	646.44	646.42	646.40	condition	
Nutritional deficiency	648.94	648.92	648.90	condition	
Obesity					
excessive weight gain during pregnancy	646.14	646.12	646.10	complication	
morbid	649.14	649.12	649.10	278.01, V85.39-V85.4	
Obstetrical trauma NEC (complicating delivery)	665.94	665.92	665.90	N/A	763.89
Occlusion, precerebral artery NEC (puerperal, postpartum, childbirth)	674.04	674.02	674.00	condition	
Oliguria	646.24	646.22	646.20	condition	
with hypertension — *see* Pregnancy, toxemia					
following labor and delivery (postpartum)	669.34	669.32	669.30	N/A	
Oophoritis	646.64	646.62	646.60	condition	
Pain(s),	646.84	646.82	646.80	condition	
Paralysis, bladder	665.54	N/A	665.50	N/A	
Paralytic stroke	674.04	674.02	674.00	N/A	
Parametritis	670.04	670.02	670.00	N/A	
Paravaginitis	646.64	646.62	646.60	condition	
Patent cervix	654.54	654.52	654.50	N/A	761.0
Pelvic inflammatory disease	646.64	646.62	646.60	condition	
Pelviperitonitis	670.04	670.02	670.00	N/A	
Pendulous abdomen	654.44	654.42	654.40	N/A	763.89
Perforation					
bladder	665.54	N/A	665.50	N/A	
bowel	665.54	N/A	665.50	N/A	
broad ligament	665.64	N/A	665.60	N/A	
cervix	665.34	N/A	665.30	N/A	
instrumental (complicating delivery)	665.94	665.92	665.90	N/A	
pelvic (floor)	664.14	N/A	664.10	N/A	
organ	665.54	N/A	665.50	N/A	763.89
urethral	665.54	N/A	665.50	N/A	763.89
uterus	665.54	N/A	665.50	N/A	763.89
Perimetritis	670.04	670.02	670.00	N/A	
Perimetrosalpingitis	670.04	670.02	670.00	N/A	
Perinephritis	646.64	646.62	646.60	condition	
Perioophoritis	670.04	670.02	670.00	N/A	
Perisalpingitis	670.04	670.02	670.00	N/A	
Peritoneal infection	670.04	670.02	670.00	N/A	
Peritonitis	670.04	670.02	670.00	N/A	
Perivaginitis	646.64	646.62	646.60	condition	
Persistence					
hymen (tag)	654.84	654.82	654.80	N/A	
Phlebitis	671.94	671.92	671.90	N/A	760.3
deep, postpartum	671.44	671.42	671.40	N/A	
intracranial	671.54	671.52	671.50	N/A	
lower extremities	671.24	671.22	671.20	N/A	760.3
specified site NEC	671.54	671.52	671.50	N/A	
superficial	671.24	671.22	671.20	N/A	760.3
Phlegmasia alba dolens	671.44	671.42	671.40	N/A	
PID	646.64	646.62	646.60	condition	
Placenta, placental					
accreta	667.04	667.02	667.00	N/A	
with hemorrhage	666.04	666.02	666.00	N/A	
adherent	667.04	667.02	667.00	N/A	
with hemorrhage	666.04	666.02	666.00	N/A	
increta	667.04	667.02	667.00	N/A	
with hemorrhage	666.04	666.02	666.00	N/A	
percreta	667.04	667.02	667.00	N/A	
with hemorrhage	666.04	666.02	666.00	N/A	
polyp	674.44	674.42	674.40	N/A	
retention (without hemorrhage)	667.04	667.02	667.00	N/A	
fragments (delayed hemorrhage)	666.24	666.22	666.20	N/A	
without hemorrhage	667.14	667.12	667.10	N/A	
hemorrhage	666.04	666.02	666.00	N/A	
postpartum	666.24	666.22	666.20	N/A	
syphilitic	647.04	647.02	647.00	condition	760.2
manifest syphilis in the infant or fetus	647.04	647.02	647.00	condition	090.0
trapped	667.04	667.02	667.00	N/A	
with hemorrhage	666.04	666.02	666.00	N/A	
Pneumonitis					
aspiration	668.04	668.02	668.00	condition	770.18
postanesthetic	668.04	668.02	668.00	condition	
postoperative	668.04	668.02	668.00	N/A	

Resources

Postpartum Pregnancy Condition or Complication; affecting management of mother	Postpartum condition or complication	Delivered with mention of postpartum complication	Unspecified episode of care	Assign additional code to describe the...	Affecting newborn (coded on the newborn chart only)
Polygalactia	676.64	676.62	676.60	N/A	
Polyp					
cervix	654.64	654.62	654.60	N/A	763.89
placenta	674.44	674.42	674.40	N/A	
uterus	654.14	654.12	654.10	N/A	763.89
Pyelocystitis	646.64	646.62	646.60	condition	
Pyelohydronephrosis	646.64	646.62	646.60	condition	
Pyelonephritis	646.64	646.62	646.60	condition	
Pyelonephrosis	646.64	646.62	646.60	condition	
Pyemia	670.04	670.02	670.00	N/A	
Pyocystitis	646.64	646.62	646.60	condition	
Pyohemia	670.04	670.02	670.00	N/A	
Pyometra	670.04	670.02	670.00	N/A	
Pyonephritis	646.64	646.62	646.60	condition	
Pyonephrosis	646.64	646.62	646.60	condition	
Pyo-oophoritis	670.04	670.02	670.00	N/A	
Pyosalpingitis	670.04	670.02	670.00	N/A	
Pyosalpinx	670.04	670.02	670.00	N/A	
Prediabetes	648.84	648.82	648.80	condition	
Pre-eclampsia (mild)	642.44	642.42	642.40	N/A	760.0
with convulsions	642.64	642.62	642.60	N/A	760.0
severe	642.54	642.52	642.50	N/A	760.0
superimposed on pre-existing hypertensive disease	642.74	642.72	642.70	N/A	760.0
Pre-existing condition (prior to pregnancy) affecting current pregnancy					
abnormal glucose tolerance	648.84	648.82	648.80	condition	
anemia	648.24	648.22	648.20	condition	
bone and joint (lower limb)	648.74	648.72	648.70	condition	
cardiovascular	648.64	648.62	648.60	condition	
congenital	648.54	648.52	648.50	condition	
cerebrovascular	674.04	674.02	674.00	N/A	
diabetic	648.04	648.02	648.00	condition	
drug dependence	648.34	648.32	648.30	condition	
genital organ or tract	646.64	646.62	646.60	condition	
gonorrheal	647.14	647.12	647.10	condition	
hypertensive	642.24	642.22	642.20	N/A	
renal	642.14	642.12	642.10	N/A	
infectious	647.94	647.92	647.90	condition	
specified type NEC	647.84	647.82	647.80	condition	
malarial	647.44	647.42	647.40	condition	
nutritional deficiency	648.94	648.92	648.90	condition	
parasitic NEC	647.84	647.82	647.80	condition	
renal	646.24	646.22	646.20	condition	
hypertensive	642.14	642.12	642.10	N/A	
rubella	647.54	647.52	647.50	condition	
specified condition NEC	648.94	648.92	648.90	condition	
syphilitic	647.04	647.02	647.00	condition	
thyroid	648.14	648.12	648.10	condition	
tuberculous	647.34	647.32	647.30	condition	
urinary	646.64	646.62	646.60	condition	
venereal	647.24	647.22	647.20	condition	
viral NEC	647.64	647.62	647.60	condition	
Proteinuria (gestational)	646.24	646.22	646.20	condition	
with toxemia (mild) (pre-eclamptic)	642.44	642.42	642.40	N/A	760.0
with convulsion	642.64	642.62	642.60	N/A	760.0
with pre-existing hypertension	642.74	642.72	642.70	N/A	760.0
severe	642.54	642.52	642.50	N/A	760.0
Pruritus, pruritic	646.84	646.82	646.80	condition	
Psychosis or psychoneurosis	648.44	648.42	648.40	condition	
Ptyalism	646.84	646.82	646.80	condition	
Pyelitis	646.64	646.62	646.60	condition	760.1
Pyrexia (of unknown origin) (PUO)					
postpartum	672.04	672.02	672.00	N/A	
Reaction obstetric anesthetic or analgesic NEC	668.94	668.92	668.90	N/A	763.5
Rectocele	654.44	654.42	654.40	N/A	763.1
Renal					
disease or failure NEC	646.24	646.22	646.20	condition	
with secondary hypertension	642.14	642.12	642.10	N/A	
hypertensive	642.24	642.22	642.20	N/A	
shutdown following labor and delivery	669.34	669.32	669.30	N/A	
Repair of pelvic floor, previous	654.44	654.42	654.40	N/A	763.89
Retention, retained					
decidua (following delivery) (fragments)	667.14	667.12	667.10	N/A	
with hemorrhage	666.24	666.22	666.20	N/A	
membranes (following delivery)	667.14	667.12	667.10	N/A	
with hemorrhage	666.24	666.22	666.20	N/A	
milk (postpartum)	676.24	676.22	676.20	N/A	
placenta (total) (without hemorrhage)	667.04	667.02	667.00	N/A	
with hemorrhage	666.04	666.02	666.00	N/A	
portions or fragments	667.14	667.12	667.10	N/A	
with hemorrhage	666.24	666.22	666.20	N/A	
secundines (following delivery)	667.14	667.12	667.10	N/A	
with hemorrhage	666.24	666.22	666.20	N/A	
complicating puerperium (delayed hemorrhage)	666.24	666.22	666.20	N/A	
Retinitis	646.84	646.82	646.80	condition	

Postpartum Pregnancy Table

Postpartum Pregnancy Condition or Complication; affecting management of mother	Postpartum condition or complication	Delivered with mention of postpartum complication	Unspecified episode of care	Assign additional code to describe the...	Affecting newborn (coded on the newborn chart only)
Retraction					
nipple (postpartum)	676.04	676.02	676.00	N/A	
Retroversion, uterus	654.34	654.32	654.30	N/A	763.89
Rigid, rigidity					
cervix	654.64	654.62	654.60	N/A	763.89
pelvic floor	654.44	654.42	654.40	N/A	763.89
perineum or vulva	654.84	654.82	654.80	N/A	763.89
vagina	654.74	654.72	654.70	N/A	763.89
Rubella (German measles)	647.54	647.52	647.50	condition	760.2
Rupture					
abdominal viscera	665.54	N/A	665.50	N/A	
bladder (sphincter)	665.54	N/A	665.50	N/A	
cervix (uteri	665.34	N/A	665.30	N/A	
pelvic floor	664.14	N/A	664.10	N/A	
perineum	664.44	N/A	664.40	N/A	
urethra	665.54	N/A	665.50	N/A	
vulva	664.04	N/A	664.00	N/A	
Sacculation	654.44	654.42	654.40	N/A	763.1
Salivation (excessive)	646.84	646.82	646.80	condition	
Salpingitis	646.64	646.62	646.60	condition	760.8
postpartum	670.04	670.02	670.00	N/A	
Salpingo-oophoritis	646.64	646.62	646.60	condition	760.8
postpartum	670.04	670.02	670.00	N/A	
Scar, scarring					
cervix	654.64	654.62	654.60	N/A	763.89
uterus NEC	654.94	654.92	654.90	N/A	763.89
Separation (obstetrical trauma)					
pubic bone	665.64	N/A	665.60	N/A	
symphysis pubis	665.64	N/A	665.60	N/A	
Sepsis, postpartum	670.04	670.02	670.00	N/A	
Septicemia	647.84	647.82	647.80	condition	771.81
postpartum	670.04	670.02	670.00	N/A	
Septum, vagina	654.74	654.72	654.70	N/A	763.89
Shirodkar suture	654.54	654.52	654.50	N/A	
Shock					
complicating labor and delivery	669.14	669.12	669.10	N/A	
following labor and delivery	669.14	669.12	669.10	N/A	
Spasms					
uterus	646.84	646.82	646.80	condition	
Specified condition NEC	646.84	646.82	646.80	condition	
Stenosis (cicatricial)					
cervix, cervical (canal)	654.64	654.62	654.60	N/A	763.89
vagina	654.74	654.72	654.70	N/A	763.89
Stricture, cervix (canal)	654.64	654.62	654.60	N/A	763.89
Subinvolution of uterus (postpartum)	674.84	674.82	674.80	N/A	
Sudden death					
during childbirth	669.94	669.92	669.90	N/A	
postpartum	674.94	674.92	674.90	N/A	
Suppression of lactation	676.54	676.52	676.50	N/A	
Suppuration, suppurative of breast or mammary gland (postpartum)	675.14	675.12	675.10	N/A	
Surgery, previous					
cervix	654.64	654.62	654.60	N/A	763.89
pelvic soft tissues NEC	654.94	654.92	654.90	N/A	763.89
perineum or vulva	654.84	654.82	654.80	N/A	
uterus NEC	654.94	654.92	654.90	N/A	763.89
vagina	654.74	654.72	654.70	N/A	
Suspended uterus	654.44	654.42	654.40	N/A	763.89
Suture, Shirodkar (with or without cervical incompetence)	654.54	654.52	654.50	N/A	
Syncope complicating delivery	669.24	669.22	669.20	N/A	
Syndrome					
acid pulmonary aspiration (Mendelson's)	668.04	668.02	668.00	N/A	
Chiari-Frommel	676.64	676.62	676.60	N/A	
dystocia, dystrophia	654.94	654.92	654.90	N/A	
Frommel-Chiari	676.64	676.62	676.60	N/A	
H.E.L.L.P (Hemolysis, Elevated Liver function and Low Platelets)	642.54	642.52	642.50	N/A	
hepatorenal following delivery	674.84	674.82	674.80	N/A	
hypotension, maternal	669.24	669.22	669.20	N/A	
maternal hypotension	669.24	669.22	669.20	N/A	
Mendelson's (during labor) (obstetric)	668.04	668.02	668.00	N/A	
Syphilis	647.04	647.02	647.00	condition	760.2
Tear, torn					
anus, anal (sphincter),	664.24	N/A	664.20	N/A	763.89
with mucosa	664.34	N/A	664.30	N/A	763.89
bladder	665.54	N/A	665.50	N/A	763.89
bowel	665.54	N/A	665.50	N/A	763.89
broad ligament	665.54	N/A	665.50	N/A	763.89
cervix	665.34	N/A	665.30	N/A	763.89
pelvic					
floor	664.14	N/A	664.10	N/A	763.89
organ NEC	665.54	N/A	665.50	N/A	763.89
perineum	665.54	N/A	665.50	N/A	763.89
periurethral	665.54	N/A	665.50	N/A	763.89

Resources

Postpartum Pregnancy Condition or Complication; affecting management of mother	Postpartum condition or complication	Delivered with mention of postpartum complication	Unspecified episode of care	Assign additional code to describe the...	Affecting newborn (coded on the newborn chart only)
Tear, torn — *continued*					
urethra	665.54	N/A	665.50	N/A	
vulva	664.04	N/A	664.00	N/A	
Tetanus, tetanic (puerperal, postpartum, childbirth)	670.04	670.02	670.00	N/A	763.89
Thelitis (puerperal, postpartum)	675.04	675.02	675.00	N/A	
Thrombocytopenia (postpartum)	666.34	666.32	666.30	N/A	
Thrombophlebitis	671.24	671.22	671.20	N/A	
cerebral (sinus) (vein), nonpyogenic	671.54	671.52	671.50	N/A	760.3
intracranial venous sinus, nonpyogenic	671.54	671.52	671.50	N/A	760.3
pelvic, postpartum	671.44	671.42	671.40	N/A	760.3
specified site NEC	671.54	671.52	671.50	N/A	760.3
superficial	671.24	671.22	671.20	N/A	760.3
Thrombosis	671.94	671.92	671.90	N/A	
brain (artery) (stem)	674.04	674.02	674.00	N/A	
intracranial, venous sinus (nonpyogenic origin)	671.54	671.52	671.50	N/A	
pelvic	671.44	671.42	671.40	N/A	
postpartum	671.94	671.92	671.90	N/A	
brain (artery) (stem)	674.04	674.02	674.00	N/A	
venous	671.54	671.52	671.50	N/A	760.3
cardiac	674.84	674.82	674.80	N/A	
cerebral (artery)	674.04	674.02	674.00	N/A	
venous	671.54	671.52	671.50	N/A	760.3
deep (vein)	671.44	671.42	671.40	N/A	
intracranial sinus (nonpyogenic) (venous)	671.54	671.52	671.50	N/A	760.3
pulmonary (artery)	673.24	673.22	673.20	N/A	
specified site NEC	671.54	671.52	671.50	N/A	
superficial	671.24	671.22	671.20	N/A	
spinal cord	671.54	671.52	671.50	N/A	
superficial	671.24	671.22	671.20	N/A	
venous (superficial)	671.24	671.22	671.20	N/A	
Thyroid dysfunction	648.14	648.12	648.10	condition	
Thyroiditis	648.14	648.12	648.10	condition	
Thyrotoxicosis	648.14	648.12	648.10	condition	
Tobacco use disorder	649.04	649.02	649.00		
Torsion of uterus					
Toxemia (mild) (pre-eclamptic)	654.44	654.42	654.40	N/A	
	642.44	642.42	642.40	N/A	760.0
with					760.0
convulsions	642.64	642.62	642.60	N/A	760.0
pre-existing hypertension	642.74	642.72	642.70	N/A	760.0
eclamptic	642.64	642.62	642.60	N/A	760.0
with pre-existing hypertension	642.74	642.72	642.70	N/A	760.0
severe	642.54	642.52	642.50	N/A	760.0
Trapped placenta (without hemorrhage)	666.04	666.02	666.00	N/A	
with hemorrhage	667.04	667.02	667.00	N/A	
Trauma	648.94	648.92	648.90	condition	
during delivery NEC	665.94	665.92	665.90	N/A	760.5
obstetrical	665.94	665.92	665.90	N/A	760.5
previous pregnancy (major), affecting childbirth or postpartum management	V23.89	V23.89	V23.89	N/A	
Tuberculosis	647.34	647.32	647.30	condition	760.2
Tumor					
cervix	654.64	654.62	654.60	N/A	763.89
ovary	654.44	654.42	654.40	N/A	763.89
pelvic	654.94	654.92	654.90	N/A	763.89
pelvic organs or tissue NEC	654.44	654.42	654.40	N/A	763.89
uterus	654.14	654.12	654.10	N/A	763.89
vagina	654.74	654.72	654.70	N/A	763.89
vulva	654.84	654.82	654.80	N/A	763.89
Uremia (renal disease or failure) NEC	646.24	646.22	646.20	condition	760.1
with secondary hypertension	642.14	642.12	642.10	N/A	760.0
complicating labor and delivery	669.34	669.32	669.30	N/A	
hypertensive	642.24	642.22	642.20	N/A	760.0
Urethritis	646.64	646.62	646.60	condition	760.1
Urinary Tract Infection	646.64	646.62	646.60	condition	760.1
Uterine size date discrepancy	649.64	649.62	649.60		
UTI	646.64	646.62	646.60	condition	760.1
Vaginitis or vulvitis	646.64	646.62	646.60	condition	760.8
Valsuani's disease (progressive pernicious anemia, puerperal)	648.24	648.22	648.20	condition	
Varicose					
veins (legs)	671.04	671.02	671.00	N/A	
perineum	671.14	671.12	671.10	N/A	
vulva	671.14	671.12	671.10	N/A	
Varicosity, labia or vulva	671.14	671.12	671.10	N/A	
Varix (lower extremity)	671.04	671.02	671.00	N/A	
perineum	671.14	671.12	671.10	N/A	
vulva	671.14	671.12	671.10	N/A	
Venereal disease NEC	647.24	647.22	647.20	disease	
Viral disease NEC	647.64	647.62	647.60	disease	
Vulvitis	646.64	646.62	646.60	condition	760.8
Weight gain	646.14	646.12	646.10	condition	
insufficient	646.84	646.82	646.80	condition	
White leg, postpartum, childbirth	671.44	671.42	671.40	N/A	

2007 ICD•9•CM